MW00345025

Enzinger and Weiss's

SOFT TISSUE TUMORS

SIXTH EDITION

Enzinger and Weiss's

SOFT TISSUE TUMORS

SIXTH EDITION

John R. Goldblum, MD, FCAP, FASCP, FACG
Chairman, Department of Anatomic Pathology, Cleveland Clinic
Professor of Pathology, Cleveland Clinic Lerner College of Medicine
Cleveland, Ohio

Andrew L. Folpe, MD
Professor of Laboratory Medicine and Pathology
Director, Bone and Soft Tissue Pathology Fellowship
College of Medicine
Mayo Clinic
Rochester, Minnesota

Sharon W. Weiss, MD
Professor of Pathology and Laboratory Medicine
Associate Dean for Faculty Affairs
Emory University School of Medicine and Hospital
Atlanta, Georgia

ELSEVIER
SAUNDERS

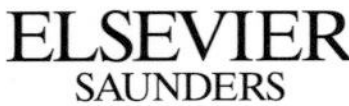

1600 John F. Kennedy Blvd.
Ste 1800
Philadelphia, PA 19103-2899

ENZINGER AND WEISS'S SOFT TISSUE TUMORS, ED. 6 ISBN: 978-0-323-08834-3

Notices

Knowledge and best practice in this field are constantly changing. As new research and experience broaden our understanding, changes in research methods, professional practices, or medical treatment may become necessary.

Practitioners and researchers must always rely on their own experience and knowledge in evaluating and using any information, methods, compounds, or experiments described herein. In using such information or methods they should be mindful of their own safety and the safety of others, including parties for whom they have a professional responsibility.

With respect to any drug or pharmaceutical products identified, readers are advised to check the most current information provided (i) on procedures featured or (ii) by the manufacturer of each product to be administered, to verify the recommended dose or formula, the method and duration of administration, and contraindications. It is the responsibility of practitioners, relying on their own experience and knowledge of their patients, to make diagnoses, to determine dosages and the best treatment for each individual patient, and to take all appropriate safety precautions.

To the fullest extent of the law, neither the Publisher nor the authors, contributors, or editors, assume any liability for any injury and/or damage to persons or property as a matter of products liability, negligence or otherwise, or from any use or operation of any methods, products, instructions, or ideas contained in the material herein.

Library of Congress Cataloging-in-Publication Data

Goldblum, John R.
Enzinger and Weiss's soft tissue tumors / John R. Goldblum, Andrew L. Folpe, Sharon W. Weiss.—6th ed.
p. ; cm.
Soft tissue tumors
Sharon W. Weiss's name appears first on prev. ed.
Includes bibliographical references and index.
ISBN 978-0-323-08834-3 (hardcover : alk. paper)
I. Folpe, Andrew L. II. Weiss, Sharon W. III. Enzinger, Franz M. Soft tissue tumors. IV. Weiss, Sharon W. Enzinger and Weiss's soft tissue tumors. V. Title. VI. Title: Soft tissue tumors.
[DNLM: 1. Soft Tissue Neoplasms. WD 375]
RC280.S66
616.99′4—dc23

2013010770

Executive Content Strategist: William R. Schmitt
Managing Editor: Kathryn DeFrancesco
Publishing Services Manager: Patricia Tannian
Project Manager: Amanda Mincher
Design Direction: Steven Stave

Printed in China

Last digit is the print number: 9 8 7 6 5 4 3 2 1

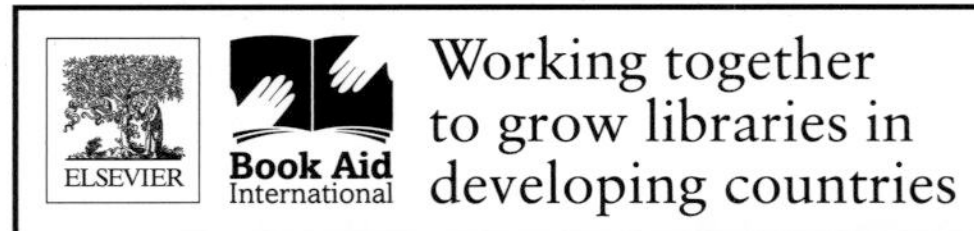

I would like to dedicate this book to my lovely wife Asmita, who has been my dearest companion for 33 years; to my four amazing children, Andrew, Ryan, Janavi, and Raedan; to my dear mother, Bette Jean, and my late father, Raymond; and to the rest of the Goldblum and Shirali families, whom I cherish.

—John R. Goldblum, MD, FCAP, FASCP, FACG

I would like to thank my wife, Ana, our children, Leah, Elizabeth, and Benjamin, my father, Herbert, and late mother, Susan, and all of our families for their support in this and all my other endeavors.

—Andrew L. Folpe, MD

To Bernie and Francine, who have brought sublime happiness and purpose to my life.

—Sharon W. Weiss, MD

Contributors

Fadi W. Abdul-Karim, MD
Department of Anatomic Pathology, Cleveland Clinic
Vice-Chair of Education, Robert J. Tomsich Pathology and Laboratory Medicine Institute
Professor of Pathology
Cleveland Clinic Lerner College of Medicine
Cleveland, Ohio

Hassana Barazi, MD
Musculoskeletal Radiology Fellow
Department of Diagnostic Radiology, Cleveland Clinic
Cleveland, Ohio

Paola Dal Cin, PhD
Associate Professor of Pathology
Cytogenetics Laboratory
Brigham and Women's Hospital
Boston, Massachusetts

Jonathan A. Fletcher, MD
Associate Professor of Pathology
Brigham and Women's Hospital
Boston, Massachusetts

Kim R. Geisinger, MD
Piedmont Pathology Associates
Hickory, North Carolina
Adjunct Professor
Department of Pathology and Laboratory Medicine
University of North Carolina at Chapel Hill
School of Medicine
Chapel Hill, North Carolina

Allen M. Gown, MD
Medical Director and Chief Pathologist
PhenoPath Laboratories
Seattle, Washington

Hakan Ilaslan, MD
Assistant Professor of Radiology
Department of Diagnostic Radiology, Cleveland Clinic
Assistant Professor of Radiology, Cleveland Clinic Lerner College of Medicine
Cleveland, Ohio

Marc Ladanyi, MD
William J. Ruane Chair
Molecular Oncology
Department of Diagnostic Molecular Pathology
Memorial Sloan-Kettering Cancer Center
New York, New York

Peter W.T. Pisters, MD, FACS
Professor of Surgery
Medical Director, Regional Care Centers
University of Texas
M.D. Anderson Cancer Center
Houston, Texas

Brian P. Rubin, MD, PhD
Professor, Department of Anatomic Pathology, Cleveland Clinic
Professor of Pathology, Cleveland Clinic Lerner College of Medicine
Cleveland, Ohio

Murali Sundaram, MD
Professor of Radiology
Department of Diagnostic Radiology, Cleveland Clinic
Professor of Radiology, Cleveland Clinic Lerner College of Medicine
Cleveland, Ohio

Preface to the Sixth Edition

Just over a hundred years ago, in 1910 to be exact, two events changed the landscape of American medicine. Dr. Abraham Flexner published his now famous report, The Flexner Report, which revolutionized American medical education and forever integrated science and the practice of clinical medicine into our medical curricula. And, coincidentally, that same year, as if to reinforce the interdependence of basic science and clinical medicine, Peyton Rous discovered a transmissible, sarcoma-producing virus in chickens (Rous sarcoma virus). Although initially not well accepted, this finding ultimately ignited interest in sarcomas as a specific form of cancer. In the several decades following that seminal event, work on sarcomas focused on defining and classifying these tumors; however, the last three decades have witnessed an explosive growth in understanding genetic alterations of these tumors. More recently, elucidation of the downstream consequences of the genetic alterations has spawned optimism for the identification of druggable targets. It has been six years since the fifth edition of *Enzinger and Weiss's Soft Tissue Tumors*, and although this may seem like a short interval between editions, the preceding advances suggest an exponential growth of new information worthy of dissemination. The editors and contributors of this edition, therefore, have extensively revised areas related to the molecular genetic alterations of soft tissue tumors, incorporated myriad recently described entities, reorganized chapters so that they are consistent with new views, and provided recent behavioral data that inform clinical decision-making. Our challenge and commitment have been to incorporate these recent advances into a framework that remains useful for the daily practice of pathology and related specialties. It is our hope that we have achieved this balance.

As we look forward to the release of the sixth edition of our textbook, we are also reminded that on the eve of the last edition we lost Dr. Franz Enzinger, whose name has forever become a part of this book's title. His contributions to soft tissue pathology were manifold, and his diagnostic virtuosity legendary. The exquisite detail and nuances embodied in his descriptions of epithelioid sarcoma and clear cell sarcoma, to name just two, are unmatched even today. Viewed in a larger context, his work offers more than an introduction to new entities; it underscores the importance of laying a sturdy foundation—based on accurate, consistent, and reproducible pathologic observations—on which subsequent scientific and clinical work can build and progress. For that lesson alone we owe him an enormous debt of gratitude.

We have many individuals to thank for assisting with the completion of this textbook. We would like to thank our superb group of co-authors, who have crafted outstanding and up-to-date chapters, and our superlative assistants, Ms. Kathleen Ranney and Ms. Susan Raven, who have yet again worked tirelessly on the manuscript. Many thanks to our dedicated young faculty, Drs. Alison Cheah, Darya Buehler, and Konstantinos Linos, for their excellent proofreading skills, and to Dr. Rish Pai for his technical support. Our most sincere thanks to each of you.

Sharon W. Weiss
John R. Goldblum
Andrew L. Folpe

Preface to the First Edition

Since the publication of the *AFIP Fascicle on Soft Tissue Tumors* by A.P. Stout in 1957 and the revised edition by A.P. Stout and R. Lattes in 1967, there have been numerous advances and changes both in the diagnosis and treatment of soft tissue tumors. This book combines traditional views, which have stood the test of time, and newer concepts and observations accrued over the past 20 years. Because a precise diagnosis is essential for planning of treatment and assessment of prognosis, emphasis has been placed throughout the book on clear and concise descriptions and differential diagnoses of the tumors discussed. Each chapter has been freely illustrated, and comprehensive references have been added with emphasis on recent publications.

The WHO Classification of Soft Tissue Tumors provided the basis for the classification in this book. However, since its publication in 1969 several modifications have become necessary. Fibrohistiocytic and extraskeletal cartilaginous and osseous tumors have been included as separate groups, and a number of changes have been made, especially in the classification of fibrous, vascular, and neural tumors. The role of histochemistry, electron microscopy, and immunohistochemistry has been noted when applicable. Relatively less emphasis, however, has been placed on the specifics of therapy because of the rapidly changing nature of this discipline. It is our hope that this blending of old and new will make this book valuable not only as a reference book for those specifically interested in soft tissue tumors but also as a diagnostic aid for the practicing general pathologist.

In many areas the contents of this book reflect our personal experience derived from approximately 5000 cases reviewed annually in the Department of Soft Tissue Pathology of the Armed Forces Institute of Pathology. The large number of cases has afforded us a unique opportunity for which we are extremely grateful.

We also wish to express our appreciation and gratitude to the many contributing pathologists who not only shared their interesting and problematic cases with us but also provided additional teaching material in the form of photographs, roentgenograms, and electron micrographs. We also owe thanks to our professional colleagues for their advice and support in this endeavor, to the photographic staff of the Institute, especially Mr. C. Edwards and Mr. B. Allen, for their skill and assistance in preparing the photographs, and to Mrs. P. Diaz and Mrs. J. Kozlay for typing the manuscript. We are also greatly indebted to our publishers for their cooperation and help throughout the production of this book. We are particularly indebted to our families for their patience and tolerance.

Franz M. Enzinger
Sharon W. Weiss

Contents

General Considerations

CHAPTER CONTENTS

Soft tissue can be defined as nonepithelial extraskeletal tissue of the body exclusive of the reticuloendothelial system, glia, and supporting tissue of various parenchymal organs. It is represented by the voluntary muscles, fat, and fibrous tissue, along with the vessels serving these tissues. By convention, it also includes the peripheral nervous system because tumors arising from nerves present as soft tissue masses and pose similar problems in differential diagnosis and therapy. Embryologically, soft tissue is derived principally from mesoderm, with some contribution from neuroectoderm.

Soft tissue tumors are a highly heterogeneous group of tumors that are classified by the line of differentiation, according to the adult tissue they resemble. Lipomas and liposarcomas, for example, are tumors that recapitulate to a varying degree normal fatty tissue; and hemangiomas and angiosarcomas contain cells resembling vascular endothelium. Within the various categories, soft tissue tumors are usually divided into benign and malignant forms.

Benign tumors, which more closely resemble normal tissue, have a limited capacity for autonomous growth. They exhibit little tendency to invade locally and are attended by a low rate of local recurrence following conservative therapy.

Malignant tumors, or *sarcomas*, in contrast, are locally aggressive and are capable of invasive or destructive growth, recurrence, and distant metastasis. Radical surgery is required to ensure the total removal of these tumors. Unfortunately, the term *sarcoma* does not indicate the likelihood or rapidity of metastasis. Some sarcomas, such as dermatofibrosarcoma protuberans, rarely metastasize, whereas others do so with alacrity. For these reasons, it is important to qualify the term *sarcoma* with a statement concerning the degree of differentiation or the histologic grade. "Well differentiated" and "poorly differentiated" are qualitative, and therefore subjective, terms used to indicate the relative maturity of the tumor with respect to normal adult tissue. Histologic grade is a means of quantitating the degree of differentiation by applying a set of histologic criteria. Usually, well-differentiated sarcomas are low-grade lesions, whereas poorly differentiated sarcomas are high-grade neoplasms. Tumors of intermediate or borderline malignancy are characterized by frequent recurrence but rarely metastasis.

INCIDENCE OF SOFT TISSUE TUMORS

The incidence of soft tissue tumors, especially the frequency of benign tumors relative to malignant ones, is nearly impossible to determine accurately. Benign soft tissue tumors outnumber malignant tumors by a wide margin. The fact that many benign tumors, such as lipomas and hemangiomas, do not undergo biopsy makes direct application of data from most hospital series invalid for the general population.

Malignant soft tissue tumors, on the other hand, ultimately come to medical attention. Soft tissue sarcomas, compared with carcinomas and other neoplasms, are relatively rare and constitute fewer than 1.5% of all cancers with an annual incidence of about 6 per 100,000 persons.[1] However, according to an analysis of the Surveillance, Epidemiology and End Results (SEER) database, the incidence changes with age[1]; for children younger than 10 years of age, the annual incidence was 0.9/100,000 children but rose to 18.2/100,000 adults over the age of 70 years. The most dramatic increases occurred at 30 and 70 years of age (Table 1-1).

There seems to be an upward trend in the incidence of soft tissue sarcomas, but it is not clear whether this represents a true increase or reflects better diagnostic capabilities and greater interest in this type of tumor. Data from the SEER database showed a marked increase in the age-adjusted incidence of soft tissue sarcomas between 1981 and 1987.[2] However, when patients with Kaposi sarcoma were eliminated from this analysis, the rates remained relatively unchanged throughout that time period. Judging from the available data, the incidence and distribution of soft tissue sarcomas seem to be similar in different regions of the world. Soft tissue sarcomas may occur anywhere in the body, but most arise from the large muscles of the extremities, the chest wall, the mediastinum, and the retroperitoneum. They occur at any age and, like carcinomas, are more common in older patients.

Soft tissue sarcomas occur more commonly in males, but gender and age-related incidences vary among the histologic types: for instance, embryonal rhabdomyosarcoma occurs almost exclusively in young individuals, whereas undifferentiated pleomorphic sarcoma is predominantly a tumor of old age and is rare in children younger than 10 years. There is also no proven racial variation.

PATHOGENESIS OF SOFT TISSUE TUMORS

As with other malignant neoplasms, the pathogenesis of most soft tissue tumors is still unknown. Recognized causes include various physical and chemical factors, exposure to ionizing

TABLE 1-1 Characteristics of Select Soft Tissue Sarcomas from the Surveillance Epidemiology and End Results Database (SEER)

SARCOMA TYPE	NUMBER OF CASES	MEDIAN AGE OF DIAGNOSIS	PERCENTAGE OF PATIENTS ≤19 YEARS (%)
Fibroblastic/ myofibroblastic tumors	3,037	54	9.4
Fibrohistiocytic tumors	14,599	57	3.7
Rhabdomyosarcomas	2,831	15	58.9
Malignant peripheral nerve sheath tumor	2,186	46	9.9
Ewing family of tumors	589	24	39.6
Liposarcomas	7,419	60	1.2
Leiomyosarcomas	13,135	59	0.9
Synovial sarcomas	1,859	35	17.6
Vascular tumors (not Kaposi)	2,742	65	2.1
Chondroosseous soft tissue tumors	680	55	3.8
Alveolar soft part sarcomas	164	25	28.7

Data from SEER database from 1973-2006. Modified from: Ferrari A, Sultan I, Huang TT, et al. Soft tissue sarcoma across the age spectrum: a population-based study from the surveillance epidemiology and end results database. Pediatr Blood Cancer 2011;57(6):943–9.

radiation, and inherited or acquired immunologic defects. An evaluation of the exact cause is often difficult because of the long latent period between the time of exposure and the development of sarcoma, as well as the possible effect of multiple environmental and hereditary factors during the induction period. The origin of sarcomas from benign soft tissue tumors is exceedingly rare, except for malignant peripheral nerve sheath tumors arising in neurofibromas, which are nearly always in patients with the manifestations of type 1 neurofibromatosis (von Recklinghausen disease).

Environmental Factors

Trauma is frequently implicated in the development of sarcomas. Many of these reports are anecdotal, however, and the integrity of the injured part was not clearly established before the injury. Consequently, trauma often seems to be an event that merely calls attention to the underlying neoplasm. Occasionally, there is reasonable evidence to suggest a causal relation. Rare soft tissue sarcomas have been reported as arising in scar tissue following surgical procedures or thermal or acid burns, at fracture sites, and in the vicinity of plastic or metal implants, usually after a latent period of several years.[3] Kirkpatrick et al. studied the histologic features in capsules surrounding the implantation site of a variety of biomaterials.[4] Interestingly, these authors noted a spectrum of change from focal proliferative lesions through preneoplastic proliferations to incipient sarcomas and suggested a model of multistage tumorigenesis akin to the adenoma-carcinoma sequence.

Environmental carcinogens have been related to the development of sarcomas, but their role is largely unexplored, and only a few substances have been identified as playing a role in the induction of sarcomas in humans. A variety of animal models now exist to induce sarcomas, allowing a better understanding of their pathogenesis.

Phenoxyacetic acid herbicides, chlorophenols, and their contaminants such as 2,3,7,8-tetrachlorodibenzo-para-dioxin (dioxin) have been linked to sarcomagenesis.[5-9] A series of case-control studies from Sweden from 1979 to 1990 reported an up to sixfold increased risk of soft tissue sarcoma associated with exposure to phenoxyacetic acids or chlorophenols in individuals exposed to these herbicides in agricultural or forestry work.[10-12] Similar reports of an increased risk of sarcoma associated with these herbicides were reported from Italy,[13] Great Britain,[14] and New Zealand.[15] Although a study by Leiss and Savitz linked the use of phenoxyacetic acid lawn pesticides with soft tissue sarcomas in children,[16] several other studies with more detailed exposure histories did not confirm this association.[17] These inconsistencies may be due in part to the predominant phenoxyacetic herbicide used in different locations. In the United States, 2,4-dichlorophenoxyacetic acid is the primary phenoxyacetic herbicide used, whereas in Sweden the main herbicides contain 2,4,5-trichlorophenoxyacetic acid and 2-methyl-4-chlorophenoxyacetic acid, both of which are more likely contaminated with dioxin.[18,19] High levels of dioxin exposure due to accidental environmental contamination near Seveso, Italy, from an explosion at a chemical factory was followed by a threefold increased risk of soft tissue sarcomas reported among individuals living near this factory.[13,20] Similarly, Collins et al. found a significantly higher risk of soft tissue sarcomas in trichlorophenol workers in Midland, Michigan, who were exposed to 2,3,7,8-tetrachlorodibenzo-para-dioxin.[9] In addition, the possibility of an increased incidence of sarcomas was claimed for some of the two million soldiers stationed in Vietnam between 1965 and 1970 who were exposed to Agent Orange, a defoliant that contained dioxin as a contaminant.[21,22] However, in several case-control and proportional mortality studies, no excess risk of soft tissue sarcoma was reported among those Vietnam veterans who were directly involved with the spraying of Agent Orange.[18]

Vinyl chloride exposure is clearly associated with the development of hepatic angiosarcoma.[23,24] There are also rare reports of extrahepatic angiosarcoma associated with this agent.[25]

Radiation exposure has been related to the development of sarcomas, but considering the frequency of radiotherapy, radiation-induced soft tissue sarcomas are quite uncommon. The incidence of postradiation sarcoma is difficult to estimate, but reports generally range from 0.03% to 0.80%.[26,27] Much of the data regarding the incidence of postradiation sarcomas are derived from large cohorts of breast cancer patients treated with postoperative radiation therapy.[28,29] To qualify as a postradiation sarcoma, there must be documentation that the sarcoma developed in the irradiated field, a histologic confirmation of the diagnosis, a period of latency of at least 3 years between irradiation and the appearance of a tumor, and documentation that the region bearing the tumor was normal before the administration of the radiation.[30] Nearly all postradiation sarcomas occur in adults, and women develop these tumors more frequently, an observation that reflects the common use of radiation for the treatment of breast and gynecologic malignancies.

Postradiation sarcomas do not display the wide range of appearances associated with sporadic non–radiation-induced tumors. The most common postradiation soft tissue sarcoma is undifferentiated pleomorphic sarcoma, which accounts for nearly 70% of cases. Unfortunately, most postradiation sarcomas are high-grade lesions and are detected at a relatively higher stage than their sporadic counterparts. Therefore, the survival rate associated with these lesions is quite poor.

The prognosis of postradiation sarcomas is most closely related to the anatomic site, which, in turn, probably reflects resectability. Patients with radiation-induced sarcomas of the extremities have the best survival (approximately 30% at 5 years), whereas those with lesions arising in the vertebral column, pelvis, and shoulder girdle generally have survival rates of less than 5% at 5 years.[28,31,32]

The total dose of radiation seems to influence the incidence of postradiation sarcoma; most are reported to occur at doses of 5000 cGy or more.[33] Mutations of the *p53* gene have been implicated in the pathogenesis of these tumors.[34] Extravasated Thorotrast (thorium dioxide), although no longer used for diagnostic or therapeutic purposes, has induced soft tissue sarcomas, particularly angiosarcomas, at the site of injection.[35,36]

Oncogenic Viruses

The role of oncogenic viruses in the evolution of soft tissue sarcomas is still poorly understood, although there is strong evidence that the human herpesvirus 8 (HHV8) is the causative agent of Kaposi sarcoma.[37,38] In addition, there is a large body of literature supporting the role of the Epstein-Barr virus in the pathogenesis of smooth muscle tumors in patients with immunodeficiency syndromes or following therapeutic immunosuppression in the transplant setting.[39] Aside from these settings, there is no conclusive evidence that human-transmissible viral agents constitute a major risk factor in the development of soft tissue sarcomas.

Immunologic Factors

As mentioned previously, immunodeficiency and therapeutic immunosuppression are also associated with the development of soft tissue sarcomas, particularly smooth muscle tumors and Kaposi sarcoma. In addition, acquired regional immunodeficiency, or loss of regional immune surveillance, may play a central role in the development of the relatively rare angiosarcomas that arise in the setting of chronic lymphedema,[40] secondary to radical mastectomy (Stewart-Treves syndrome)[41] or congenital or infectious conditions.[41,42]

Genetic Factors

A number of genetic diseases are associated with the development of soft tissue tumors, and the list will undoubtedly lengthen as we begin to understand the molecular underpinnings of mesenchymal neoplasia. Neurofibromatosis type 1, neurofibromatosis type 2, and familial adenomatous polyposis (FAP)/Gardner syndrome are classic examples of genetic diseases associated with soft tissue tumors. Familial cancer syndromes associated with soft tissue sarcomas are more fully described in Chapter 4.

CLASSIFICATION OF SOFT TISSUE TUMORS

The development of a useful, comprehensive histologic classification of soft tissue tumors has been a relatively slow process. Earlier classifications have been largely descriptive and based more on the nuclear configuration than the type of tumor cells. Terms such as *round cell sarcoma* and *spindle cell sarcoma* may be diagnostically convenient but should be discouraged because they convey little information as to the nature and potential behavior of a given tumor. Moreover, purely descriptive classifications do not clearly distinguish between tumors and tumor-like reactive processes. More recent classifications have been based principally on the line of differentiation of the tumor, that is, the type of tissue formed by the tumor rather than the type of tissue from which the tumor theoretically arose.

Over the past four decades, there have been several attempts to devise a useful, comprehensive classification of soft tissue tumors. The classification used herein is very similar but not identical to the revised 2013 World Health Organization (WHO) classification, a collective effort by pathologists throughout the world.

Each of the histologic categories is divided into a benign group and a malignant group. In addition, for several tumor categories, some tumors are classified as being of intermediate (borderline or low malignant potential) malignancy, implying a high rate of local recurrence and a small risk of metastasis. Most tumors retain the same pattern of differentiation in the primary and recurrent lesions, but, occasionally, they change their pattern of differentiation or may even differentiate along several cellular lines.

Undifferentiated pleomorphic sarcoma (formerly known as *malignant fibrous histiocytoma*) and liposarcoma are the most common soft tissue sarcomas of adults; together they account for 35% to 45% of all sarcomas. Rhabdomyosarcoma, neuroblastoma, and the Ewing family of tumors are the most frequent soft tissue sarcomas of childhood.

GRADING AND STAGING SOFT TISSUE SARCOMAS

With a few notable exceptions, histologic typing does not provide sufficient information for predicting the clinical course of a sarcoma and, therefore, must be accompanied by grading and staging information. *Grading* assesses the degree of malignancy of a sarcoma and is based on an evaluation of several histologic parameters (described in the following two sections), whereas *staging* provides shorthand information regarding the extent of the disease at a designated time, usually the time of initial diagnosis. Many variables affect the outcome of a sarcoma. Their relative importance may vary with time and with the sarcoma subtype. Grading and staging systems of necessity simplify these variables and emphasize the most important ones that seem to have the most universal applicability for all sarcomas. An extensive discussion related to grading systems and issues was provided by Deyrup and Weiss.[45]

Grading Systems

Grading of soft tissue sarcomas was first proposed in 1939 by Broders, who used a combination of mitotic activity, giant-cell tumors, and fibrous stroma in assigning a grade to fibrosarcomas.[46] Broders also acknowledged the importance of cellular differentiation in grading. He suggested that fibrosarcomas could be divided into several subtypes (fibrous, fibrocellular, and cellular), and that those that were highly cellular should be considered grade 4 regardless of the level of mitotic activity. These principles persist in grading systems today, namely that certain parameters (e.g., mitotic activity) should be evaluated in sarcomas, that some histologic subtypes *a priori* dictate a grade, and that the level of differentiation must be factored into the assignment of a grade. Over the ensuing decades following that publication, numerous studies reaffirmed the importance of grading and emphasized the primacy of necrosis and mitotic activity in assessing a grade.[47–50] Some studies have further proposed the use of Ki-67 immunoreactivity or MIB-1 score/index to accurately assess mitotic activity.[51–54]

The first large-scale effort to grade and stage sarcomas occurred in 1977 when Russell et al., using a database of 1000 cases and the tumor node metastasis (TNM) staging system showed that incorporating a grade into the staging system achieved predictions of outcome.[55] Most important, in the absence of metastatic disease, grade essentially defined the clinical stage. This study is most often cited as providing the first reliable grading system in the United States, yet, paradoxically, it did not provide objective criteria for grading. Rather, the grade was determined by a panel of experts based on their years of experience. The real contribution that the paper provided to grading was the implied concept that certain histologic types of sarcomas were inherently low grade and others were high grade, a premise of many grading systems.

Following that seminal publication, many grading systems were published internationally,[49,56-60] including one from the National Cancer Institute (NCI) (Table 1-2). Although differing in emphasis, most relied on mitotic activity and necrosis in deriving a grade, and some proposed that sarcoma-specific parameters should be used. The number of grades varies among the staging systems, ranging from two to four. Three-grade systems seem best suited for predicting patterns for survival and a likely response to therapy (Fig. 1-1). Four-grade systems usually show little difference between the two lowermost grades; two-grade systems, which distinguish between only low-grade and high-grade sarcomas, are more readily related to the type of surgical therapy but make it difficult to deal with sarcomas that lie between these two extremes.

The French system published by Trojani et al. in 1984 was developed by the French Federation of Cancer Centers Sarcoma Group (FNCLCC), based on an analysis of 155 adult patients with soft tissue sarcomas.[61] On the basis of a multivariate analysis of histologic features, a combination of cellular differentiation, mitotic rate, and tumor necrosis was determined to be the most useful parameters for sarcoma grading. This system assigns a score to each parameter and adds the scores together for a combined grade (Table 1-3). This study concluded that histologic grade was the single most important factor for predicting survival rates; tumor depth (superficial versus deep) was another important prognostic parameter. The reproducibility of this system was tested by 15 pathologists; an agreement was reached in 81% of the cases for tumor necrosis, 74% for tumor differentiation, 73% for mitotic rate, and 75% for overall tumor grade, although the agreement as to histologic type was 61% only.

Although the French system relies on a balanced evaluation of parameters (differentiation score, mitoses, necrosis), its principal weakness lies in the assignment of the differentiation score. The *differentiation score* is defined as the extent to which a tumor resembles adult mesenchymal tissue (score 1), the extent to which the histologic type is known (score 2), or the observation that the tumor is undifferentiated (score 3). Although a listing of the differentiation scores for the common tumors has been reported (Table 1-4), the rationale for some of these scores is not clear. It must also be remembered that this system has been derived from resected specimens unmodified by treatment, a situation that is not analogous to our current practices, which are heavily weighted toward grading on biopsies or on resection specimens following preoperative radiation or chemotherapy.

Despite these issues, the French system appears to be the most widely used grading system for sarcomas throughout the world. In a study of soft tissue pathologists from 30 countries, more preferred the French system (37.3%) over the NCI (24%), Broders' criteria (12%), Markhede's system (1.3%), and other (15.3%)[62] systems, probably because it is more precisely defined and, therefore, reproducible. It also performs superiorly to the NCI system in a large dataset comparison. The two systems were compared by Guillou et al. in adult patients with nonmetastatic soft tissue sarcomas.[63] By a univariate analysis, both systems were of prognostic value for predicting metastasis and overall survival. By a multivariate analysis, a tumor size of 10 cm or more, a deep location, and a high tumor grade, regardless of the system used, were found to be independent prognostic factors for predicting metastases. Interestingly, there were grade discrepancies using these two

TABLE 1-2 Assigned Histologic Grade According to Histologic Type in the NCI System

HISTOLOGIC TYPE	GRADE 1	GRADE 2	GRADE 3
Well-differentiated liposarcoma	+		
Myxoid liposarcoma	+		
Round cell liposarcoma		+	+
Pleomorphic liposarcoma			+
Fibrosarcoma		+	+
MFH, pleomorphic type*		+	+
MFH, inflammatory type*		+	+
MFH, myxoid type*		+	
MFH, pleomorphic type*		+	
DFSP	+		
Leiomyosarcoma	+	+	+
Malignant solitary fibrous tumor	+	+	+
Rhabdomyosarcoma (all types)			+
Chondrosarcoma	+	+	+
Myxoid chondrosarcoma	+	+	
Mesenchymal chondrosarcoma			+
Osteosarcoma			+
Extraskeletal Ewing sarcoma			+
Synovial sarcoma			+
Epithelioid sarcoma		+	+
Clear cell sarcoma		+	+
Superficial MPNST		+	
Epithelioid MPNST		+	+
Malignant triton tumor			+
Angiosarcoma		+	+
Alveolar soft part sarcoma			+
Kaposi sarcoma		+	+

Modified from Costa J, Wesley RA, Glatstein E, et al. The grading of soft tissue sarcomas: results of a clinicopathologic correlation in a series of 163 cases. Cancer 1984;53(3):530.

DFSP, dermatofibrosarcoma protuberans; MFH, malignant fibrous histiocytoma; MPNST, malignant peripheral nerve sheath tumor; NCI, National Cancer Institute.
*MFH is now referred to as undifferentiated pleomorphic sarcoma.

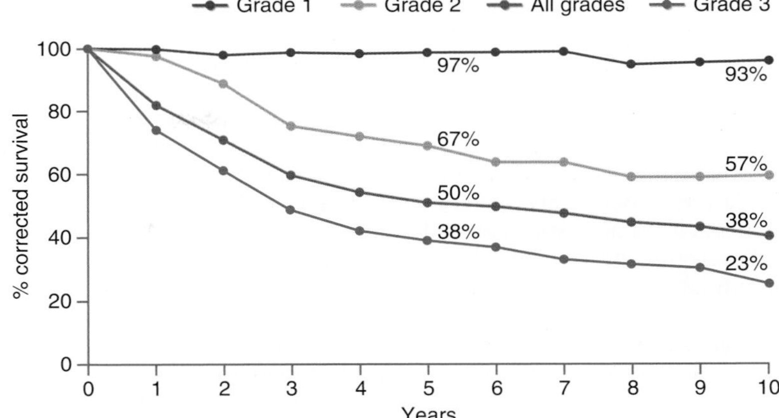

FIGURE 1-1. Grading system for soft tissue sarcomas based on three grades of malignancy. *(From Myhre Jensen O, Kaae S, Madsen EH, et al. Histopathological grading in soft-tissue tumours: relation to survival in 261 surgically treated patients. Acta Pathol Microbiol Immunol Scand 1983;91A:145.)*

TABLE 1-3 Definitions of Grading Parameters for the FNCLCC System

PARAMETER	CRITERION
Tumor Differentiation	
Score 1	Sarcoma closely resembling normal adult mesenchymal tissue (e.g., well-differentiated liposarcoma)
Score 2	Sarcomas for which histologic typing is certain (e.g., myxoid liposarcoma)
Score 3	Embryonal and undifferentiated sarcomas; sarcoma of uncertain type
Mitosis Count	
Score 1	0-9/10 HPF
Score 2	10-19/10 HPF
Score 3	≥20/10 HPF
Tumor Necrosis (Microscopic)	
Score 0	No necrosis
Score 1	≤50% tumor necrosis
Score 2	>50% tumor necrosis
Histologic Grade	
Grade 1	Total score 2, 3
Grade 2	Total score 4, 5
Grade 3	Total score 6, 7, 8

Modified from Coindre JM, Trojani M, Contesso G, et al. Reproducibility of a histopathologic grading system for adult soft tissue sarcomas. Cancer 1986;58(2):306.

FNCLCC, Fédération Nationale de Centres de Lutte Contre le Cancer; HPF, high-power field.

grading systems in 34.6% of the cases. The use of the FNCLCC system resulted in an increased number of grade 3 tumors, a reduced number of grade 2 tumors, and a better correlation with overall and metastasis-free survival when compared with the results from using the NCI system.

Limitations of Grading

Despite the widespread use of some form of grading system in the diagnosis and management of sarcomas, there is agreement among experts that no grading system performs well on every type of sarcoma. There are several reasons for this. In

TABLE 1-4 Tumor Differentiation Score According to Histologic Type in the Updated Version of the FNCLCC System

HISTOLOGIC TYPE	TUMOR DIFFERENTIATION SCORE
Well-differentiated liposarcoma	1
Myxoid liposarcoma	2
Round cell liposarcoma	3
Pleomorphic liposarcoma	3
Dedifferentiated liposarcoma	3
Fibrosarcoma	2
Myxofibrosarcoma	2
MFH*, pleomorphic type (patternless pleomorphic sarcoma)	3
Giant-cell and inflammatory MFH* (pleomorphic sarcoma, NOS, with giant cells or inflammatory cells)	3
Well-differentiated leiomyosarcoma	1
Conventional leiomyosarcoma	2
Poorly differentiated/ pleomorphic/epithelioid leiomyosarcoma	3
Biphasic/monophasic synovial sarcoma	3
Poorly differentiated synovial sarcoma	3
Pleomorphic rhabdomyosarcoma	3
Mesenchymal chondrosarcoma	3
Extraskeletal osteosarcoma	3
Ewing sarcoma/PNET**	3
Malignant rhabdoid tumor	3
Undifferentiated (spindle cell and pleomorphic) sarcoma	3

Rubin BP, et al. Protocol for the Examination of Specimens From Patients With Tumors of Soft Tissue. College of American Pathologists, June 2012. Modified from Guillou L, et al.[63]

Grading of malignant peripheral nerve sheath tumor, embryonal and alveolar rhabdomyosarcoma, angiosarcoma, extraskeletal myxoid chondrosarcoma, alveolar soft part sarcoma, clear cell sarcoma, and epithelioid sarcoma is not recommended.

*MFH is now referred to as undifferentiated pleomorphic sarcoma.

**PNET, primitive neuroectodermal tumor.

the most obvious situation, there are sarcomas in which the histologic subtype essentially defines behavior and, therefore, grade becomes redundant. This is best illustrated by a well-differentiated liposarcoma (atypical lipomatous neoplasm), an inherently low-grade, nonmetastasizing lesion, and the majority of round cell sarcomas (e.g., alveolar rhabdomyosarcoma), which are inherently high grade.

Also problematic are the rare sarcomas that are considered difficult, if not impossible, to grade. Epithelioid sarcoma, clear cell sarcoma, and alveolar soft part sarcoma are the most commonly cited examples of ungradable sarcomas, yet it is difficult to find a cogent explanation for this long-standing bias in the literature. It is possible that our grading systems fail to capture the correct histologic information in grading these rare sarcomas or, perhaps, when compared to other sarcomas, nonhistologic factors are far more influential in determining outcome than histologic factors. What is clear, however, is that there is a substantial risk of distant metastasis in the long term, whereas in the short term (5 years) where the interval for which traditional grading systems are most accurate, the risk may be low. Therefore, the assignment of grade to these tumors does not guarantee biologic equivalency to other sarcomas of comparable grade.

In a number of sarcomas, clinical features play a larger role in determining a prognosis. Cutaneous angiosarcomas are usually ungraded because multifocality and size are more predictive of outcome; paradoxically, angiosarcomas of deep soft tissue are probably amenable to grading. The difficulty of grading synovial sarcomas by histologic features has been noted in many studies, leading Bergh et al. to stratify synovial sarcoma into low- and high-risk groups using a combination of age, size, and presence or absence of poorly differentiated areas.[64] Myxoid chondrosarcoma, long considered a low-grade lesion histologically, has late metastasis in approximately 40% of cases. By stratifying lesions by age, distal versus proximal location, and grade, Meis-Kindblom et al. were able to predict an outcome.[65]

Leiomyosarcomas present another interesting paradigm. Various studies present conflicting views as to the predictive power of grading leiomyosarcomas, and there is some evidence that, as a group, myogenic tumors have a worse prognosis when matched for other variables.[66-68] The reasons for this are not clear. However, a study documenting the vascular origin of most somatic leiomyosarcomas speculated that early hematogenous dissemination may account in part for this aggressive behavior, and the authors proposed a risk model, taking into account the age, grade, and whether a tumor had been "disrupted" by prior surgical intervention.[69] Even among sarcomas that have traditionally been graded, we have begun to recognize the limitations of grading. For example, malignant peripheral nerve sheath tumors have customarily been graded, but the FNCLCC has indicated that an assigned grade does not predict metastasis.

Strictly speaking, these models are not grading systems because they incorporate histologic, clinical, and demographic variables. Nonetheless, their use gives some indication that we may gradually move in the direction of sarcoma-specific analyses, which may be used in conjunction with or, in some cases, instead of grade. The advantage of such an approach is that it allows the most appropriate criteria to be used for each sarcoma type to theoretically improve the ability to prognosticate. The disadvantage of this approach is that it presupposes an inordinate amount of clinical information for each sarcoma type, a challenge considering the rarity of some subtypes of these tumors. Moreover, the more specific these systems become, the more complicated they also become.

Another means of integrating clinical and pathologic data in a manner that accounts for sarcoma subtypes is the use of nomograms. This method collates multiple clinical and histologic parameters in a given patient and compares the data against a large population of patients with similar parameters whose outcome is known. A nomogram for a 12-year sarcoma-specific mortality has been devised by the Memorial Sloan–Kettering Cancer Center.[70,71] Ultimately, nomograms could incorporate new molecular information with a prognostic import.

Despite the limitations noted previously, grading remains one of the most powerful and inexpensive ways of assessing the prognosis in a sarcoma and is currently regarded as a major independent predictor of metastasis in the major histologic types of adult soft tissue sarcomas.[72] Consequently, a grade should be provided by the pathologist, whenever possible. Putative grade ranges for various sarcomas are shown in Figure 1-2. It should not be considered a substitute for an accurate histologic diagnosis, however. Grading, like diagnosing soft tissue sarcomas, requires representative, well-fixed, well-stained histologic material that should be obtained before neoadjuvant therapy because this process alters many of the features necessary for accurate grading. Thick or heavily stained sections are misleading because they may suggest less cellular differentiation than is actually present. Selection of the tissue sample and the length of fixation may also influence the degree of necrosis and the mitotic index. Necrosis may be prominent in tumors of which a biopsy has been previously performed or that have been irradiated or embolized and, therefore, cannot be accurately assessed in these situations. Grading is usually based on the least differentiated area of a tumor, unless it comprises a very minor component of the overall tumor.

Staging Systems

Several staging systems have been developed for soft tissue sarcomas in an attempt to predict a prognosis and to evaluate therapy by stratifying similar tumors according to prognostic factors such as the histologic grade, tumor size, compartmentalization of the tumor, and the presence or absence of metastasis. The two major staging systems used at present for adult soft tissue sarcomas were developed by The American Joint Committee on Cancer (AJCC)[55,73-75] and the Musculoskeletal Tumor Society.[76-78] Each of these systems has advantages and disadvantages, as described in the following sections.

AJCC Staging System

The original AJCC staging system was based on data obtained from a retrospective study of 702 sarcomas collected from 13 institutions. The study included only tumors that were diagnosed during the 15-year period of 1954 to 1969, were histologically confirmed, had adequate follow-up information, and underwent primary treatment in the institution that contributed the specimen. Because the sample was too small to gain sufficient data on all well-defined soft tissue sarcomas,

Histologic type	Histologic grade		
	I	II	III
Fibrosarcoma		—	—
Infantile fibrosarcoma	—	—	
Dermatofibrosarcoma protuberans	—		
Malignant fibrous histiocytoma	—	—	—
Liposarcoma	—	—	—
Well-differentiated liposarcoma	—		
Myxoid liposarcoma	—		
Round cell liposarcoma	—	—	—
Pleomorphic liposarcoma		—	—
Leiomyosarcoma	—	—	—
Rhabdomyosarcoma			—
Angiosarcoma	—	—	—
Malignant hemangiopericytoma	—	—	—
Synovial sarcoma	—	—	—
Malignant mesothelioma		—	—
Malignant PNST	—	—	—
Neuroblastoma			—
Ganglioneuroblastoma			—
Extraskeletal chondrosarcoma	—	—	—
Myxoid chondrosarcoma	—	—	—
Mesenchymal chondrosarcoma			—
Extraskeletal osteosarcoma		—	—
Malignant granular cell tumor		—	—
Alveolar soft part sarcoma		—	—
Epithelioid sarcoma		—	—
Clear cell sarcoma		—	—
Extraskeletal Ewing sarcoma/PNET			—

FIGURE 1-2. Soft tissue sarcomas. Estimated range of degree of malignancy based on histologic type and grade. Grade within the overall range depends on specific histologic features such as cellularity, cellular pleomorphism, mitotic activity, amount of stroma, infiltrative or expansive growth, and necrosis.

the staging system was limited to the eight most common types.[55,79] This system is based on the TNM staging system used for staging carcinomas, with the addition of histologic grade as a prognostic variable. The AJCC system published in 1992 was based on the size of the primary tumor (T), the involvement of lymph nodes (N), the presence of metastasis (M), and the type and grade of sarcoma (G).[80] In 1997, several important modifications were made to the AJCC staging system.[73] Tumor depth was subsequently incorporated into this staging system. In addition, grades 1 and 2 were grouped as low grade and grades 3 and 4 as high grade, whereas in a three-tiered grading system, grade 1 is considered low grade and grades 2 and 3 are high grade. In 2010, the AJCC published the seventh edition of its staging manual, updating the staging system for soft tissue sarcomas, as shown in Table 1-5.[75]

Musculoskeletal Tumor Society Staging System

The Enneking system, designed for sarcomas of soft tissue and bone, distinguishes two anatomic settings: T1, intracompartmental tumors confined within the boundaries of well-defined anatomic structures, such as a functional muscle group, joint, and subcutis; and T2, extracompartmental neoplasms that arise within or involve secondarily extrafascial spaces or planes that have no natural anatomic barriers to extension. There are two grades (G1 and G2) and three stages. In this system, two grades are favored because they can be better related to the two surgical procedures (wide and radical excisions) and because of the reported lack of any difference in the metastatic rate between intermediate- and high-grade tumors.[76,81] This staging system is summarized in Tables 1-6 and 1-7.

Advantages and Disadvantages of Staging Systems

These two principal staging systems serve as a valuable guide to therapy and provide useful prognostic information. Although the AJCC system is applicable to soft tissue sarcomas at any site, the development of this system was based on studies that included lesions from a variety of anatomic locations, including the extremities, retroperitoneum, and head and neck. It is difficult to compare data from patients with tumors at these sites, given the differences in the ability to eradicate tumors surgically in these anatomic locations.[82,83] The AJCC system also uses 5 cm as an important dimension for determining a prognosis, although the designation is somewhat arbitrary because size is a continuous variable. The Musculoskeletal Tumor Society system, with its emphasis on compartmentalization, is most popular with surgeons and is best tailored for lesions in the extremities. It does not include the type, size, or depth of the tumor as separate parameters; and its two-tiered grading system may be too narrow for the wide biologic range of soft tissue sarcomas. Because of the need for adequately defining compartmentalization, the system does not lend itself to retrospective staging. Furthermore, this system was devised before the routine use of

TABLE 1-5 Definitions and Staging System of the American Joint Committee on Cancer, 7th Edition

Primary Tumor (T)

TX	Primary tumor cannot be assessed
T0	No evidence of primary tumor
T1	Tumor 5 cm or less in greatest dimension*
T1a	Superficial tumor
T1b	Deep tumor
T2	Tumor more than 5 cm in greatest dimension*
T2a	Superficial tumor
T2b	Deep tumor

*Note: Superficial tumor is located exclusively above the superficial fascia without invasion of the fascia; deep tumor is located either exclusively beneath the superficial fascia, superficial to the fascia with invasion of or through the fascia, or both superficial yet beneath the fascia.

Regional Lymph Nodes (N)

NX	Regional lymph nodes cannot be assessed
N0	No regional lymph node metastasis
N1*	Regional lymph node metastasis

*Note: Presence of positive nodes (N1) in M0 tumors is considered Stage III.

Distant Metastasis (M)

M0	No distant metastasis
M1	Distant metastasis

	PRIMARY TUMOR	REGIONAL LYMPH NODES	DISTANT METASTASIS	GRADE
Stage IA	T1a	N0	M0	G1, GX
	T1b	N0	M0	G1, GX
Stage IB	T2a	N0	M0	G1, GX
	T2b	N0	M0	G1, GX
Stage IIA	T1a	N0	M0	G2, G3
	T1b	N0	M0	G2, G3
Stage IIB	T2a	N0	M0	G2
	T2b	N0	M0	G2
Stage III	T2a, T2b	N0	M0	G3
	Any T	N1	M0	Any G
Stage IV	Any T	Any N	M1	Any G

Histopathologic Grade (FNCLCC System Preferred)

GX	Grade cannot be assessed
G1	Grade 1
G2	Grade 2
G3	Grade 3

From AJCC Cancer Staging Handbook, 7th edition. Springer, New York, 2010.

TABLE 1-6 Definitions of Anatomic Extent in the Musculoskeletal Tumor Society Staging System

INTRACOMPARTMENTAL (T1)		EXTRACOMPARTMENTAL (T2)
Intra-articular	→	Soft tissue extension
Superficial to deep fascia	→	Deep fascial extension
Paraosseous	→	Intraosseous or extrafascial extension
Intrafascial compartment	→	Extrafascial compartment

Modified from Enneking WF, Spanier SS, Goodman MA. A system for the surgical staging of musculoskeletal sarcoma. Clin Orthop 1980; 153:106; and Peabody TD, Gibbs CP, Simon MA. Evaluation and staging of musculoskeletal neoplasms. J Bone Joint Surg [Am] 1998;80(8):1204.

TABLE 1-7 Musculoskeletal Tumor Society Staging System

STAGE	GRADE	SITE	METASTASIS
IA	G1	T1	M0
IB	G1	T2	M0
IIA	G2	T1	M0
IIB	G2	T2	M0
III	G1 or G2	T1 or T2	M1

Modified from Enneking WF, Spanier SS, Goodman MA. A system for the surgical staging of musculoskeletal sarcoma. Clin Orthop 1980; 153:106; and Peabody TD, Gibbs CP, Simon MA. Evaluation and staging of musculoskeletal neoplasms. J Bone Joint Surg [Am] 1998;80(8):1204.

advanced imaging techniques such as magnetic resonance imaging and before the widespread use of adjuvant therapy.[84] Obviously, staging soft tissue sarcomas requires a multidisciplinary approach with close cooperation among the clinician, oncologist, and pathologist. In view of the relative rarity of these tumors, staging and grading are ideally carried out in large medical centers with special interest and experience in the diagnosis and management of soft tissue sarcomas. Moreover, prospective rather than retrospective studies are necessary to test the value of the various staging systems.

References

1. Ferrari A, Sultan I, Huang TT, et al. Soft tissue sarcoma across the age spectrum: A population-based study from the surveillance epidemiology and end results database. Pediatr Blood Cancer 2011;57(6):943–9.
2. Ross JA, Severson RK, Davis S, et al. Trends in the incidence of soft tissue sarcomas in the United States from 1973 through 1987. Cancer 1993;72(2):486–90.
3. Piscitelli D, Ruggeri E, Fiore MG, et al. Undifferentiated high-grade pleomorphic sarcoma in a blind eye with a silicone prosthesis implant: a clinico-pathologic study. Orbit 2011;30(4):192–4.
4. Kirkpatrick CJ, Alves A, Köhler H, et al. Biomaterial-induced sarcoma: A novel model to study preneoplastic change. Am J Pathol 2000;156(4):1455–67.
5. Zambon P, Ricci P, Bovo E, et al. Sarcoma risk and dioxin emissions from incinerators and industrial plants: a population-based case-control study (Italy). Environ Health 2007;6:19.
6. Fingerhut MA, Halperin WE, Marlow DA, et al. Cancer mortality in workers exposed to 2,3,7,8-tetrachlorodibenzo-p-dioxin. N Engl J Med 1991;324(4):212–8.
7. Kogevinas M, Becher H, Benn T, et al. Cancer mortality in workers exposed to phenoxy herbicides, chlorophenols, and dioxins. An expanded and updated international cohort study. Am J Epidemiol 1997;145(12):1061–75.
8. Tessari R, Canova C, Canal F, et al. [Environmental pollution from dioxins and soft tissue sarcomas in the population of Venice and Mestre: an example of the use of current electronic information sources]. Epidemiol Prev 2006;30(3):191–8.
9. Collins JJ, Bodner K, Aylward LL, et al. Mortality rates among workers exposed to dioxins in the manufacture of pentachlorophenol. J Occup Environ Med 2009;51(10):1212–9.
10. Eriksson M, Hardell L, Adami HO. Exposure to dioxins as a risk factor for soft tissue sarcoma: a population-based case-control study. J Natl Cancer Inst 1990;82(6):486–90.
11. Hardell L, Eriksson M. The association between cancer mortality and dioxin exposure: a comment on the hazard of repetition of epidemiological misinterpretation. Am J Ind Med 1991;19(4):547–9.
12. Hardell L, Eriksson M, Axelson O. Agent Orange in war medicine: an aftermath myth. Int J Health Serv 1998;28(4):715–24.
13. Bertazzi PA, Consonni D, Bachetti S, et al. Health effects of dioxin exposure: a 20-year mortality study. Am J Epidemiol 2001;153(11):1031–44.
14. Balarajan R, Acheson ED. Soft tissue sarcomas in agriculture and forestry workers. J Epidemiol Community Health 1984;38(2):113–6.
15. Smith AH, Patterson DG Jr, Warner ML, et al. Serum 2,3,7,8-tetrachlorodibenzo-p-dioxin levels of New Zealand pesticide applicators and their implication for cancer hypotheses. J Natl Cancer Inst 1992;84(2):104–8.
16. Leiss JK, Savitz DA. Home pesticide use and childhood cancer: a case-control study. Am J Public Health 1995;85(2):249–52.
17. Pahwa P, McDuffie HH, Dosman JA, et al. Hodgkin lymphoma, multiple myeloma, soft tissue sarcomas, insect repellents, and phenoxyherbicides. J Occup Environ Med 2006;48(3):264–74.
18. Zahm SH, Fraumeni JF Jr. The epidemiology of soft tissue sarcoma. Semin Oncol 1997;24(5):504–14.
19. Zahm SH, Ward MH. Pesticides and childhood cancer. Environ Health Perspect 1998;106(Suppl. 3):893–908.
20. Bertazzi PA, Zocchetti C, Guercilena S, et al. Dioxin exposure and cancer risk: a 15-year mortality study after the "Seveso accident." Epidemiology 1997;8(6):646–52.
21. Clapp RW, Cupples LA, Colton T, et al. Cancer surveillance of veterans in Massachusetts, USA, 1982–1988. Int J Epidemiol 1991;20(1):7–12.
22. Kramárová E, Kogevinas M, Anh CT, et al. Exposure to Agent Orange and occurrence of soft-tissue sarcomas or non-Hodgkin lymphomas: an ongoing study in Vietnam. Environ Health Perspect 1998;106(Suppl. 2):671–8.
23. Sahmel J, Unice K, Scott P, et al. The use of multizone models to estimate an airborne chemical contaminant generation and decay profile: occupational exposures of hairdressers to vinyl chloride in hairspray during the 1960s and 1970s. Risk Anal 2009;29(12):1699–725.
24. Sherman M. Vinyl chloride and the liver. J Hepatol 2009;51(6):1074–81.
25. Rhomberg W. Exposure to polymeric materials in vascular soft-tissue sarcomas. Int Arch Occup Environ Health 1998;71(5):343–7.
26. Mark RJ, Poen JC, Tran LM, et al. Angiosarcoma. A report of 67 patients and a review of the literature. Cancer 1996;77(11):2400–6.
27. Inoue YZ, Frassica FJ, Sim FH, et al. Clinicopathologic features and treatment of postirradiation sarcoma of bone and soft tissue. J Surg Oncol 2000;75(1):42–50.
28. Billings SD, McKenney JK, Folpe AL, et al. Cutaneous angiosarcoma following breast-conserving surgery and radiation: an analysis of 27 cases. Am J Surg Pathol 2004;28(6):781–8.
29. Weaver J, Billings SD. Postradiation cutaneous vascular tumors of the breast: a review. Semin Diagn Pathol 2009;26(3):141–9.
30. Arlen M, Higinbotham NL, Huvos AG, et al. Radiation-induced sarcoma of bone. Cancer 1971;28(5):1087–99.
31. Fang Z, Matsumoto S, Ae K, et al. Postradiation soft tissue sarcoma: a multi-institutional analysis of 14 cases in Japan. J Orthop Sci 2004;9(3):242–6.
32. Patel SG, See AC, Williamson PA, et al. Radiation induced sarcoma of the head and neck. Head Neck 1999;21(4):346–54.
33. Yap J, Chuba PJ, Thomas R, et al. Sarcoma as a second malignancy after treatment for breast cancer. Int J Radiat Oncol Biol Phys 2002;52(5):1231–7.
34. Nakanishi H, Tomita Y, Myoui A, et al. Mutation of the p53 gene in postradiation sarcoma. Lab Invest 1998;78(6):727–33.
35. Balamurali G, du Plessis DG, Wengoy M, et al. Thorotrast-induced primary cerebral angiosarcoma: case report. Neurosurgery 2009;65(1):E210–211; discussion E211.
36. Lipshutz GS, Brennan TV, Warren RS. Thorotrast-induced liver neoplasia: a collective review. J Am Coll Surg 2002;195(5):713–8.
37. Chang Y, Cesarman E, Pessin MS, et al. Identification of herpesvirus-like DNA sequences in AIDS-associated Kaposi's sarcoma. Science 1994;266(5192):1865–9.
38. Mesri EA, Cesarman E, Boshoff C. Kaposi's sarcoma and its associated herpesvirus. Nat Rev Cancer 2010;10(10):707–19.
39. Deyrup AT, Lee VK, Hill CE, et al. Epstein-Barr virus-associated smooth muscle tumors are distinctive mesenchymal tumors reflecting multiple infection events: a clinicopathologic and molecular analysis of 29 tumors from 19 patients. Am J Surg Pathol 2006;30(1):75–82.
40. Shon W, Ida CM, Boland-Froemming JM, et al. Cutaneous angiosarcoma arising in massive localized lymphedema of the morbidly obese: a report of five cases and review of the literature. J Cutan Pathol 2011;38(7):560–4.
41. Dawlatly SL, Dramis A, Sumathi VP, et al. Stewart-treves syndrome and the use of positron emission tomographic scanning. Ann Vasc Surg 2011;25(5):699.e1–3.
42. Roy P, Clark MA, Thomas JM. Stewart-Treves syndrome–treatment and outcome in six patients from a single centre. Eur J Surg Oncol 2004;30(9):982–6.
43. Fletcher CDM. The evolving classification of soft tissue tumours: an update based on the new WHO classification. Histopathology 2006;48(1):3–12.
44. Fletcher C, Bridges J, Hogendoorn P, et al. WHO classification of tumours of soft issue and bone. Lyon: IARC; 2013.
45. Deyrup AT, Weiss SW. Grading of soft tissue sarcomas: the challenge of providing precise information in an imprecise world. Histopathology 2006;48(1):42–50.
46. Broders A, Hargrave R, Meyerding H. Pathological features of soft tissue fibrosarcoma: with special reference to the grading of its malignancy. Surg Gynecol Obstet 1939;(69):267.
47. Coindre JM, Terrier P, Bui NB, et al. Prognostic factors in adult patients with locally controlled soft tissue sarcoma. A study of 546 patients from the French Federation of Cancer Centers Sarcoma Group. J Clin Oncol 1996;14(3):869–77.
48. Coindre JM, Trojani M, Contesso G, et al. Reproducibility of a histopathologic grading system for adult soft tissue sarcoma. Cancer 1986;58(2):306–9.
49. Costa J, Wesley RA, Glatstein E, et al. The grading of soft tissue sarcomas. Results of a clinicohistopathologic correlation in a series of 163 cases. Cancer 1984;53(3):530–41.
50. Parham DM, Webber BL, Jenkins JJ 3rd, et al. Nonrhabdomyosarcomatous soft tissue sarcomas of childhood: formulation of a simplified system for grading. Mod Pathol 1995;8(7):705–10.
51. Jensen V, Høyer M, Sørensen FB, et al. MIB-1 expression and iododeoxyuridine labelling in soft tissue sarcomas: an immunohistochemical study including correlations with p53, bcl-2 and histological characteristics. Histopathology 1996;28(5):437–44.
52. Jensen V, Sørensen FB, Bentzen SM, et al. Proliferative activity (MIB-1 index) is an independent prognostic parameter in patients with high-grade soft tissue sarcomas of subtypes other than malignant fibrous

histiocytomas: a retrospective immunohistological study including 216 soft tissue sarcomas. Histopathology 1998;32(6):536–46.
53. Hasegawa T. Histological grading and MIB-1 labeling index of soft-tissue sarcomas. Pathol Int 2007;57(3):121–5.
54. Hasegawa T, Yamamoto S, Yokoyama R, et al. Prognostic significance of grading and staging systems using MIB-1 score in adult patients with soft tissue sarcoma of the extremities and trunk. Cancer 2002;95(4):843–51.
55. Russell WO, Cohen J, Enzinger F, et al. A clinical and pathological staging system for soft tissue sarcomas. Cancer 1977;40(4):1562–70.
56. Jensen OM, Høgh J, Ostgaard SE, et al. Histopathological grading of soft tissue tumours. Prognostic significance in a prospective study of 278 consecutive cases. J Pathol 1991;163(1):19–24.
57. Hashimoto H, Daimaru Y, Takeshita S, et al. Prognostic significance of histologic parameters of soft tissue sarcomas. Cancer 1992;70(12):2816–22.
58. van Unnik JA, Coindre JM, Contesso C, et al. Grading of soft tissue sarcomas: experience of the EORTC Soft Tissue and Bone Sarcoma Group. Eur J Cancer 1993;29A(15):2089–93.
59. Gustafson P. Soft tissue sarcoma. Epidemiology and prognosis in 508 patients. Acta Orthop Scand Suppl 1994;259:1–31.
60. Markhede G, Angervall L, Stener B. A multivariate analysis of the prognosis after surgical treatment of malignant soft-tissue tumors. Cancer 1982;49(8):1721–33.
61. Trojani M, Contesso G, Coindre JM, et al. Soft-tissue sarcomas of adults; study of pathological prognostic variables and definition of a histopathological grading system. Int J Cancer 1984;33(1):37–42.
62. Golouh R, Bracko M. What is the current practice in soft tissue sarcoma grading? Radiol Oncol 2001;35(1):47.
63. Guillou L, Coindre JM, Bonichon F, et al. Comparative study of the National Cancer Institute and French Federation of Cancer Centers Sarcoma Group grading systems in a population of 410 adult patients with soft tissue sarcoma. J Clin Oncol 1997;15(1):350–62.
64. Bergh P, Meis-Kindblom JM, Gherlinzoni F, et al. Synovial sarcoma: identification of low and high risk groups. Cancer 1999;85(12):2596–607.
65. Meis-Kindblom JM, Bergh P, Gunterberg B, et al. Extraskeletal myxoid chondrosarcoma: a reappraisal of its morphologic spectrum and prognostic factors based on 117 cases. Am J Surg Pathol 1999;23(6):636–50.
66. Deyrup AT, Haydon RC, Huo D, et al. Myoid differentiation and prognosis in adult pleomorphic sarcomas of the extremity: an analysis of 92 cases. Cancer 2003;98(4):805–13.
67. Fletcher CD, Gustafson P, Rydholm A, et al. Clinicopathologic re-evaluation of 100 malignant fibrous histiocytomas: prognostic relevance of subclassification. J Clin Oncol 2001;19(12):3045–50.
68. Koea JB, Leung D, Lewis JJ, et al. Histopathologic type: an independent prognostic factor in primary soft tissue sarcoma of the extremity? Ann Surg Oncol 2003;10(4):432–40.
69. Farshid G, Pradhan M, Goldblum J, et al. Leiomyosarcoma of somatic soft tissues: a tumor of vascular origin with multivariate analysis of outcome in 42 cases. Am J Surg Pathol 2002;26(1):14–24.
70. Eilber FC, Kattan MW. Sarcoma nomogram: validation and a model to evaluate impact of therapy. J Am Coll Surg 2007;205(Suppl. 4):S90–95.
71. Kattan MW, Heller G, Brennan MF. A competing-risks nomogram for sarcoma-specific death following local recurrence. Stat Med 2003;22(22):3515–25.
72. Coindre JM, Terrier P, Guillou L, et al. Predictive value of grade for metastasis development in the main histologic types of adult soft tissue sarcomas: a study of 1240 patients from the French Federation of Cancer Centers Sarcoma Group. Cancer 2001;91(10):1914–26.
73. Fleming ID, Cooper J, Henson D. AJCC Cancer Staging Manual. 5th ed. Philadelphia: Lippincott-Raven; 1997.
74. Greene F, Page D, Fleming I. AJCC Cancer Staging Manual. 6th ed. New York: Springer; 2002.
75. Edge S, Byrd D, Compton C, et al. AJCC Cancer Staging Manual. 7th ed. New York: Springer; 2010.
76. Enneking WF, Spanier SS, Goodman MA. A system for the surgical staging of musculoskeletal sarcoma. Clin Orthop Relat Res 1980;(153):106–20.
77. Enneking WF, Spanier SS, Goodman MA. A system for the surgical staging of musculoskeletal sarcoma. 1980. Clin Orthop Relat Res 2003;(415):4–18.
78. Saddegh MK, Lindholm J, Lundberg A, et al. Staging of soft-tissue sarcomas. Prognostic analysis of clinical and pathological features. J Bone Joint Surg Br 1992;74(4):495–500.
79. Russell W, Cohen J, Cutler S, et al. Staging system for soft tissue sarcoma. In: Task Force on Soft Tissue Sarcoma. American Joint Committee for Cancer Staging and End Results Reporting. Chicago: American College of Surgeons; 1980.
80. Beahrs O, Henson D, Hutter R, et al. Manual for Staging of Cancer. 3rd ed. Philadelphia: Lippincott; 1992.
81. Enneking WF, Spanier SS, Malawer MM. The effect of the Anatomic setting on the results of surgical procedures for soft parts sarcoma of the thigh. Cancer 1981;47(5):1005–22.
82. Kotilingam D, Lev DC, Lazar AJF, et al. Staging soft tissue sarcoma: evolution and change. CA Cancer J Clin 2006;56(5):282–91; quiz 314–315.
83. Lahat G, Tuvin D, Wei C, et al. New perspectives for staging and prognosis in soft tissue sarcoma. Ann Surg Oncol 2008;15(10):2739–48.
84. Peabody TD, Gibbs CP Jr, Simon MA. Evaluation and staging of musculoskeletal neoplasms. J Bone Joint Surg Am 1998;80(8):1204–18.

Clinical Evaluation and Treatment of Soft Tissue Tumors

PETER W.T. PISTERS

CHAPTER CONTENTS

INTRODUCTION

Although soft tissue sarcomas (STS) are a heterogeneous group of neoplasms, their clinical evaluation and treatment follow common principles. This chapter will focus on the clinical evaluation, determinants of prognosis and outcome, and treatment of patients with STS.

The frequency and anatomic distribution of 7563 consecutive patients with STS, referred to the University of Texas MD Anderson Cancer Center, are outlined in Figure 2-1. The data illustrate that the extremity is the most common anatomic site, accounting for approximately one-half of all cases. Other important anatomic sites include the retroperitoneum, head and neck, and body wall. The site-specific distribution of histologic subtypes is outlined in Figure 2-1. Of note, the distribution of histologic subtypes is very dependent on the anatomic site; for example, in the extremity, undifferentiated pleomorphic sarcoma (so-called malignant fibrous histiocytoma), liposarcoma, and synovial sarcoma are common. In contrast, in the retroperitoneum, synovial sarcoma and undifferentiated pleomorphic sarcoma are relatively uncommon, and other histologic subtypes, particularly leiomyosarcoma and liposarcoma, predominate. The reasons for this regional variation in histologic subtype are not understood.

CLINICAL EVALUATION

Clinical Presentation and Assessment

Most patients with suspected soft tissue neoplasms present with a painless mass, although pain is reported in one-third of cases.[1] A delay in diagnosis is common; the most common

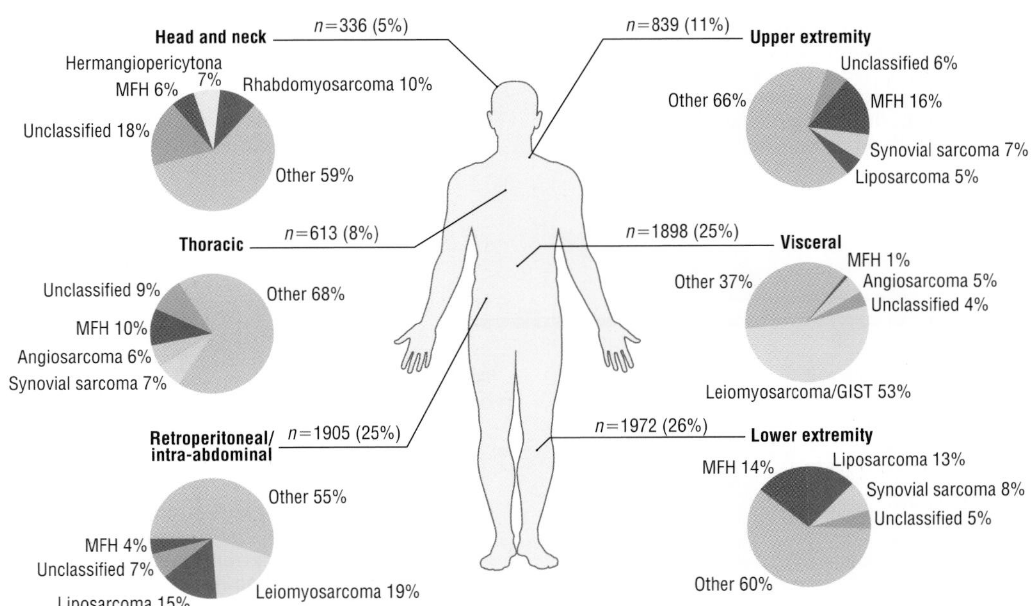

FIGURE 2-1. Anatomic distribution and site-specific histologic subtypes of 7563 consecutive STS seen at the University of Texas MD Anderson Cancer Center. *(From MDACC Sarcoma Database, June 1996 to June 2006.)*

misdiagnoses include posttraumatic or spontaneous hematoma and lipoma. A late diagnosis of patients with retroperitoneal sarcomas is very common because of the large size of the retroperitoneal space, generally slow growth rate, and the tendency of sarcomas to gradually displace rather than to invade and compromise adjacent viscera. Therefore, retroperitoneal sarcomas can reach a considerable size before the diagnosis (Fig. 2-2).

The physical examination should include an assessment of tumor size, relative mobility, and fixation. Patients with extremity soft tissue tumors should be evaluated for tumor-related neuropathy. An examination of regional lymph node basins should also be performed with the understanding that nodal metastases are relatively uncommon, occurring in less than 15% of patients with extremity STS.[2]

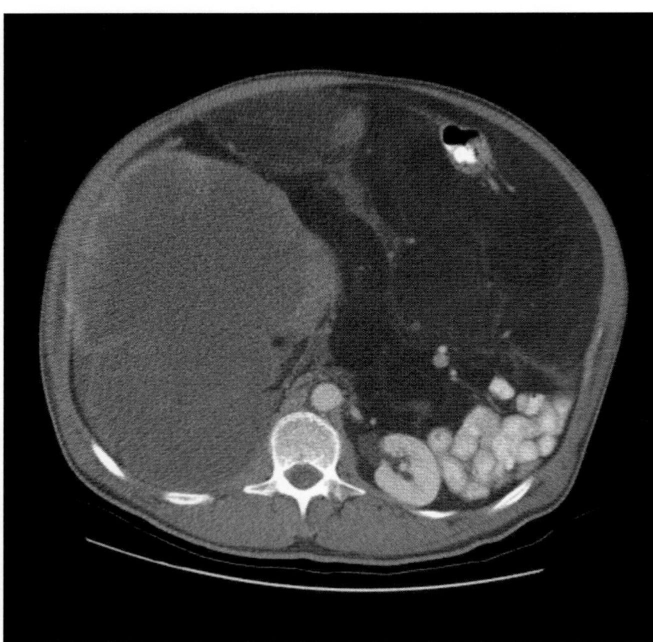

FIGURE 2-2. Contrast-enhanced CT scan of a 52-year-old patient with retroperitoneal dedifferentiated liposarcoma. The CT findings illustrate features of both well-differentiated and dedifferentiated forms of liposarcoma that frequently coexist. The dedifferentiated component is the more solid-appearing, low-density mass situated in the right retroperitoneum, whereas the well-differentiated component has similar density to the subcutaneous (normal) fat and fills the retroperitoneum, displacing the contrast-filled small bowel to the anatomic left side and posterior.

Pretreatment Evaluation

The pretreatment evaluation of the patient with a suspected soft tissue malignancy includes a biopsy diagnosis and radiologic staging to establish the extent of the disease. Practical algorithms for the evaluation of patients with extremity and retroperitoneal soft tissue masses are outlined in Figures 2-3 and 2-4.

Biopsy

A pretreatment biopsy of the primary tumor is essential for most patients presenting with soft tissue masses. In general, any soft tissue mass that is enlarging or is larger than 5 cm should be considered for a biopsy. The preferred biopsy method is generally the least invasive technique that allows for a definitive histologic assessment, including an assessment of grade. Grade is particularly important to clinicians because it impacts treatment planning and treatment options.

A percutaneous core-needle biopsy (CNB) provides satisfactory diagnostic tissue for the diagnosis of most soft tissue neoplasms. A CNB can be performed "blindly" in the clinic by clinicians without real-time radiologic control. However, many centers have moved to an image-guided CNB performed by interventional radiologists. Image-guided approaches allow for a biopsy from the areas of the tumor felt to be most likely to harbor a viable tumor (i.e., avoiding centrally necrotic areas). The use of real-time imaging also minimizes the risks for biopsy-related vascular or adjacent organ injury. In many centers, image-guided biopsy also allows for real-time pathology quality control by having a pathologist immediately available in the biopsy suite to evaluate the quality of tissue retrieved and its probable suitability for a definitive diagnosis. Studies comparing a CNB to the traditional open surgical biopsy have demonstrated the safety, reliability, and cost-effectiveness of this approach.[3-5] Additional issues related to a pathologic interpretation of the CNB are discussed in Chapter 5.

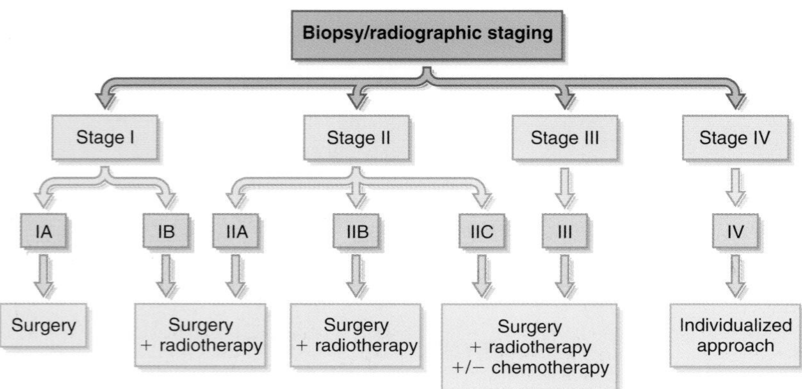

FIGURE 2-3. Pretreatment evaluation and staging algorithm for assessment of the patient presenting with an extremity soft tissue mass. AJCC, American Joint Committee on Cancer. *(From Pisters PW. Combined modality treatment of extremity soft tissue sarcomas. Ann Surg Oncol 1998;5(5):464–72.)*

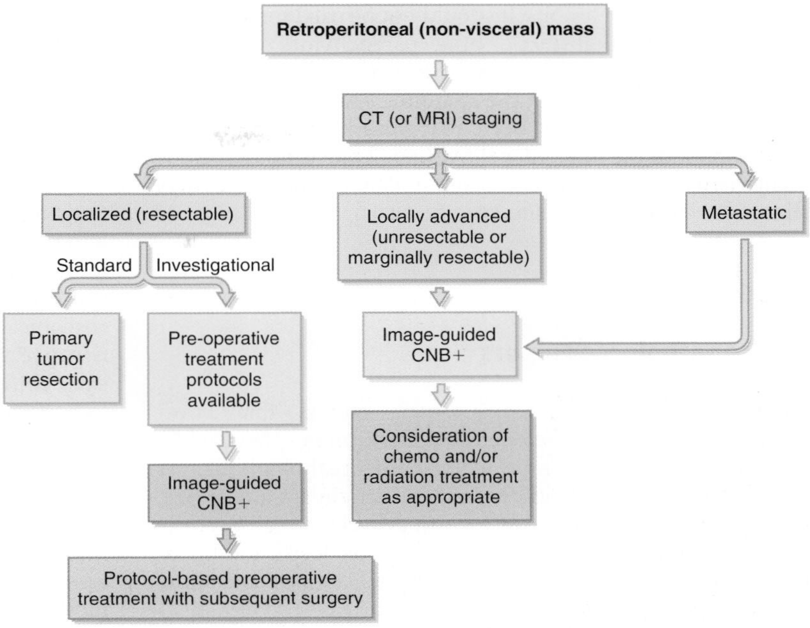

FIGURE 2-4. Pretreatment evaluation, staging, and treatment algorithm for assessment of the patient presenting with a retroperitoneal (nonvisceral) mass. Patients should undergo pretreatment cross-sectional imaging by CT or MRI. Localized, radiologically resectable masses that are believed to be neoplastic can be treated by diagnostic and therapeutic primary tumor resection. In clinical settings, where preoperative treatment protocols are available, pretreatment image-guided CNB should be used to establish the diagnosis of sarcoma for protocol eligibility. Patients with locally advanced (radiologically unresectable) or metastatic disease should undergo CNB for diagnosis followed by consideration of nonsurgical treatments. In general, CNB is sufficient for diagnosis, and surgery performed exclusively for diagnostic purposes (e.g., laparotomy for incisional biopsy) should be avoided whenever possible. CNB, core-needle biopsy.

Tumor recurrence in the needle track after a percutaneous CNB is extremely rare. Indeed, there are only case reports in the literature. However, these rare cases have led some physicians to advocate tattooing the biopsy site for subsequent excision.[6]

We have generally taken a practical approach to this issue and perform an en-bloc resection of the needle track and percutaneous entry point when feasible but not if a resection of the biopsy track requires a second incision or substantial modification of the surgical plan. The rare risks for needle track recurrence do not justify the added morbidity risk imposed by major alterations in the surgical plan.

An incisional biopsy is occasionally required to establish a definitive diagnosis for some soft tissue neoplasms. It has the advantage over a CNB of providing more tissue for a pathologic analysis and often additional tissue for tumor banking purposes. However, the morbidity of an incisional biopsy can be considerable and includes the risks for anesthesia, bleeding, and wound healing problems. Given these risks and the greater financial costs of an incisional biopsy, the incisional biopsy is generally a secondary technique that may best be reserved for cases where a definitive diagnosis cannot be established by a CNB.

An excisional biopsy may be appropriate for some patients who present with small superficial neoplasms located on the extremity or superficial body wall where the morbidity from this procedure is minimal. Although an incisional biopsy may allow for a single diagnostic and therapeutic procedure in some clinical settings, its main disadvantage is that the malignant potential of the neoplasm is unknown at the time of the biopsy, and informed decisions on surgical margins are not possible. This leaves the operating surgeon with the choice of narrow or nonexistent surgical margins with generally lower risks for wound and functional morbidity or deliberately wide margins with generally greater risks for wound and functional morbidity. The oncologic appropriateness of the surgical margin cannot be assessed preoperatively and is difficult to assess with precision intraoperatively. This disadvantage makes an excisional biopsy appropriate for only a small subset of patients who have small, superficial neoplasms and for whom a re-excision is feasible if the final diagnosis indicates a malignant lesion with compromised margins.

A percutaneous fine-needle aspiration (FNA) biopsy can also be used for cytologic assessment of some soft tissue neoplasms.[7,8] Accurate FNA diagnosis requires the availability of an expert cytopathologist experienced in the diagnosis of STS by cytology. From a practical standpoint, most centers (even academic centers) will not have a cytopathologist with sufficient experience to allow for the use of FNA for routine diagnosis and classification of primary soft tissue neoplasms. Given the frequent difficulty in histopathologic diagnosis and classification of STS, the major utility of FNA cytology in most centers is for the diagnosis of patients with suspected recurrent sarcoma. In such settings, there is already an established pathologic diagnosis such that only confirmation of a recurrence with similar features is required.

Staging

The relative rarity of STS, the anatomic heterogeneity of these lesions, and the presence of more than 50 recognized histologic subtypes of variable grades have made it difficult to establish a functional system that can accurately stage all forms of this disease. The staging system (seventh edition) of the American Joint Committee on Cancer (AJCC) and the Union for International Cancer Control (UICC) (formerly named International Union Against Cancer) is the most widely used staging system for STS and is presented in Chapter 1.[9] The system is designed to optimally stage extremity tumors but is also applicable to the torso, head and neck, and retroperitoneal lesions; it should not be used for sarcomas of the gastrointestinal tract or other parenchymal organs.

A major limitation of the present staging system is that it does not take into account the anatomic site of STS. The anatomic site, however, has been recognized as an important determinant of the outcome.[10,11] Although site is not a specific component of any present staging system, outcome data should be reported on a site-specific basis.

PROGNOSTIC FACTORS

Clinicopathologic Factors

Understanding the clinicopathologic factors that affect outcome is essential in formulating a treatment plan for the patient with STS. The three major clinicopathologic factors that establish the risk profile for a given patient are tumor size, anatomic depth relative to the investing fascia of the extremity or body wall musculature (superficial versus deep), and histologic grade.[12-14] Indeed, these factors are all components of the AJCC staging system for STS.

In addition to the foregoing factors, the anatomic site, histologic subtype, and margin status are also significant, but this information is not captured by the current staging system. Moreover, unlike other solid tumors, factors that predict local recurrence are different from those that predict distant metastasis and tumor-related death (Table 2-1).[12] In other words, patients with a constellation of adverse prognostic factors for local recurrence are not necessarily at increased risk for distant metastasis or tumor-related, death, and vice versa. Therefore, clinicians and pathologists should be careful about using the terminology *high-risk disease* without qualification of which end point (local recurrence or overall survival) for which the patient is believed to be at increased risk.

TABLE 2-1 Multivariate Analysis of Prognostic Factors in Patients with Extremity STS

END POINT	ADVERSE PROGNOSTIC FACTOR	RELATIVE RISK (%)
Local recurrence	Fibrosarcoma	2.5
	Local recurrence at presentation	2.0
	Microscopically positive margin	1.8
	Malignant peripheral nerve sheath tumor	1.8
	Age >50 years	1.6
Distant recurrence	High grade	4.3
	Deep location	2.5
	Size 5.0-9.9 cm	1.9
	Leiomyosarcoma	1.7
	Nonliposarcoma histology	1.6
	Local recurrence at presentation	1.5
	Size ≥10.0 cm	1.5
Disease-specific survival	High grade	4.0
	Deep location	2.8
	Size ≥10.0 cm	2.1
	Malignant peripheral nerve sheath tumor	1.9
	Leiomyosarcoma	1.9
	Microscopically positive margin	1.7
	Lower extremity site	1.6
	Local recurrence at presentation	1.5

From Pisters PW, Leung DH, Woodruff J, et al. Analysis of prognostic factors in 1041 patients with localized soft tissue sarcomas of the extremities. J Clin Oncol 1996;14(5):1679–89.

Adverse prognostic factors identified are independent by Cox regression analysis.

Classification and Prognostic Significance of Surgical Margins

Surgeons should use the UICC resection (designated by the letter *R*) classification system for integration of the operative findings and the final microscopic surgical margins. Under this classification system, an R0 resection is defined as a macroscopically complete sarcoma resection with microscopically negative surgical margins; an R1 resection is a macroscopically complete sarcoma resection with microscopically positive surgical margins, and an R2 resection is a macroscopically incomplete (i.e., with gross residual disease) and microscopically positive surgical margins.

All therapeutic surgical procedures should be described in medical records using the R classification. To do so, surgeons must await the final pathology report, including margin assessment and then integrate the observed operative findings, including the presence or absence of a residual gross tumor with the final assessment of microscopic surgical margins. The operative report, discharge summary, and related medical records should describe the procedure using the R classification. As an example, a surgical procedure that involved a wide local resection of a left anterior thigh soft tissue leiomyosarcoma with satisfactory gross tumor margins, no operatively defined residual gross tumor, and negative microscopic surgical margins would be described as "R0 resection of left anterior thigh leiomyosarcoma."

The type of microscopically positive surgical margins also appears important. For example, an R1 resection for a low-grade liposarcoma or an R1 after preoperative radiation treatment in which a microscopically positive margin is anticipated (and accepted) in order to preserve critical structures has a relatively low risk (<10%) for local recurrence.[15]

In contrast, patients undergoing "unplanned" excision followed by a re-excision with positive margins (i.e., R1 re-resection) or patients with unanticipated positive margins after primary resection are at increased risk for local recurrence, with rates approaching 30%. Therefore, the specific clinical setting needs to be considered when interpreting the relative risk for local recurrence after an R1 resection.

Nomograms for Assessment of Individual Patient Prognosis

Kattan et al. from the Memorial Sloan–Kettering Cancer Center (MSKCC) have used a database of over 2000 prospectively followed adult patients with STS to predict the probability of sarcoma-specific death by 12 years.[10]

The results have been used to construct and internally validate a nomogram to predict sarcoma-specific death (Fig. 2-5). This nomogram matches a patient's prognostic score against those of previously treated patients with comparable tumor and patient factors to estimate individual patient risk for sarcoma-related death. The MSKCC nomogram has been externally validated[16,17] and is considered to be an extremely valuable tool for individual patient counseling and determination of the frequency for individual

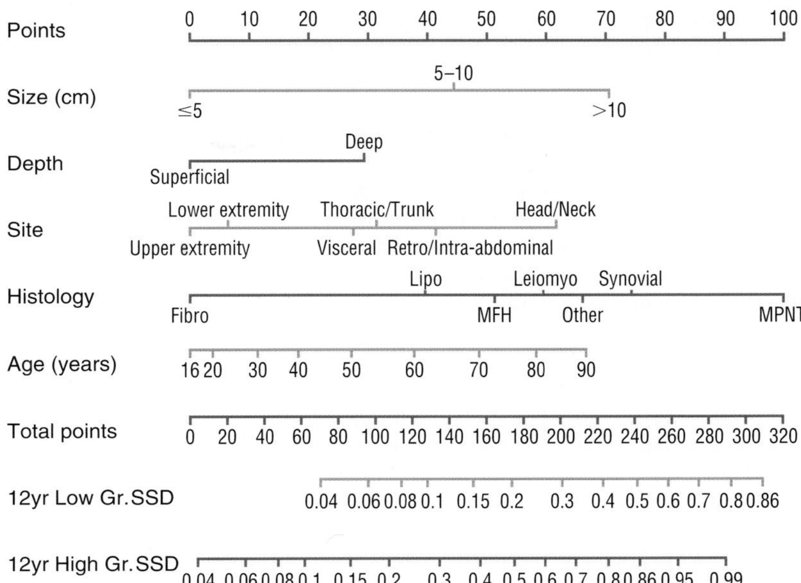

Instructions for physician: Locate the patient's tumor size on the size axis. Draw a line straight upwards to the points axis to determine how many points towards sarcoma-specific death the patient receives for his tumor size. Repeat this process for the other axis, each time drawing straight upward to the points axis. Sum the points achieved for each predictor and locate this sum on the Total Points axis. Draw a line straight down to either the Low Grade or High Grade axis to find the patient's probability of dying from sarcoma within 12 years assuming he or she does not die of another cause first.

Instruction to patient: "If we had 100 patients exactly like you, we would expect between <predicted percentage from nomogram −8%> and <predicted percentage + 8%> to die of sarcoma within 12 years if they did not die of another cause first, and death from sarcoma after 12 years is still possible."

FIGURE 2-5. Postoperative nomogram for 12-year sarcoma-specific deaths, in 2163 patients treated at the MSKCC. Fibro, fibrosarcoma; GR, grade; Lipo, liposarcoma; Leiomyo, leiomyosarcoma; MFH, malignant fibrous histiocytoma; MPNT, malignant peripheral-nerve sheath tumor; SSD, sarcoma-specific death. *(From Kattan MW, Leung DH, Brennan MF. Postoperative nomogram for 12-year sarcoma-specific death. J Clin Oncol 2002;20(3):791–6.)*

patient follow-up. The nomogram is available online at www.nomograms.org.

TREATMENT OF LOCALIZED PRIMARY EXTREMITY SARCOMAS

Surgery

Surgical resection remains the cornerstone of therapy for localized primary STS. The following discussion focuses on STS in the limbs, the most common anatomic site of origin, but the principles of treatment are generally applicable for patients with sarcomas at other anatomic sites.

Historically, amputation was the primary treatment for patients with extremity STS. However, there has been a marked decline in the rate of amputation as the primary therapy for extremity STS. With the widespread application of multimodality treatment strategies, the vast majority of patients with localized STS of the extremities undergo limb-sparing treatment, and less than 10% of patients presently undergo amputation.[18,19]

Satisfactory local resection involves resection of the primary tumor with a margin of normal tissue around the lesion. Dissection along the tumor pseudocapsule (enucleation or "shelling out") is associated with local recurrence rates ranging between 33% and 63%.[20-22]

In contrast, wide local excision with a margin of normal tissue around the lesion is associated with lower local recurrence rates in the range of 10% to 31%, as demonstrated in the surgery-alone control arms of randomized trials evaluating postoperative radiotherapy (RT) and in single-institution reports.[23-25]

The issue of what constitutes an acceptable gross surgical margin is complex, and there are limited prospective data specifically addressing surgical margins in STS surgery. Circumferential margin assessment in sarcomas is imprecise owing to the complex anatomy of each tumor and the tendency of soft tissue around the tumor to collapse and adopt its inherent shape when not under the continuous tension that is applied to the tissues as part of modern soft tissue surgery. This can result in significant discordance between the intraoperative perception and the pathologic evaluation of the gross surgical margin.

Unlike resections for cutaneous melanoma in which gross surgical margins can be measured with a ruler at the time of surgery, a gross margin assessment for STS cannot be measured so precisely. In addition, it is likely that not all soft tissues provide an equivalent barrier to tumor extension. For example, it is believed that a smaller gross margin that includes a fascial barrier is, in general, a more secure margin than a comparable gross margin that does not include fascia. For many of these reasons, a margin assessment for sarcomas by both surgeons and pathologists will continue to have an unavoidable degree of imprecision that probably exceeds the inherent imprecision in the assessment of gross margins of other solid tumors.

Combined Modality Limb-Sparing Treatment

Currently, approximately 90% of patients with localized extremity sarcomas undergo limb-sparing treatment.[18,26]

The use of limb-sparing multimodality treatment approaches for extremity sarcoma was based on an important phase III trial from the U.S. National Cancer Institute (NCI) in which patients with extremity sarcomas amenable to limb-sparing surgery were randomly assigned to receive amputation or limb-sparing surgery with postoperative RT.[27,28]

Both arms of this trial included postoperative chemotherapy with doxorubicin, cyclophosphamide, and methotrexate. With more than 9 years of follow-up information, this study established that for patients for whom limb-sparing surgery is an option, limb-sparing surgery combined with postoperative RT and chemotherapy yielded disease-related survival rates comparable to those for amputation and simultaneously preserved a functional extremity.[27,28]

This trial established limb-sparing treatment as the standard treatment for patients with localized extremity STS. Amputation is used in only clinical settings in which local tumor anatomy precludes limb-sparing approaches, most commonly as a result of tumor involvement of functionally significant neurovascular structures.

Today, a discussion of limb-preserving approaches must be linked to a discussion of the role of adjuvant therapies, most commonly radiation treatment. Several randomized, controlled trials have addressed issues surrounding the use of adjuvant therapy and collectively have established important milestones in the evolution of the local management of STS.

Yang et al. randomized 91 patients with high-grade extremity lesions following limb-sparing surgery to receive adjuvant chemotherapy alone or concurrent chemotherapy and RT.[24]

An additional 50 patients with low-grade tumors were to receive adjuvant RT or no further treatment following limb-sparing surgery. The local control rate for those who received RT was 99% compared to 70% in the non-RT group (p <0.0001).[24]

The results were similar for high- and low-grade tumors (Table 2-2).

Adjuvant radiation using brachytherapy (BRT) was also evaluated at the MSKCC in a randomized trial of 126 cases treated between 1982 and 1987 (see Table 2-2).[23]

Patients with localized extremity and superficial trunk sarcomas undergoing surgery were randomly assigned to be treated by surgery alone or by a combination of surgery and BRT. BRT was administered postoperatively through an iridium-192 implant that delivered 42 to 45 Gy over 4 to 6 days. At 5 years, the local control rate for high-grade tumors was 91% with BRT compared to 70% in surgery-alone controls (p <0.04). Of note, no improvement in local control with BRT was evident for patients with low-grade tumors. The local control rate was 74% with surgery alone and 64% with BRT. The full explanation for grade-specific differences in local control with BRT remains unresolved, although one suggestion implicates the relatively long cell cycle of low-grade tumors; low-grade tumor cells may not enter the radiosensitive phases of the cell cycle during the relatively short BRT time.[23]

Taken together, the NCI and MSKCC randomized trials have provided the evidence to support surgery plus radiation as the standard approach for most patients with operable extremity and superficial trunk sarcomas. At this time, there are no controlled trials evaluating the use of radiation treatment for patients with sarcomas in non-extremity sites. However, most multidisciplinary groups have extrapolated from the foregoing data and have assumed that radiation improves local control for patients with non-extremity sarcomas as well.

Treatment by Surgery Alone—without Radiotherapy

Radiation provides the unquestioned clinical benefit of decreasing local recurrence for the majority of patients with STS. However, the known secondary adverse effects of radiation, which include edema, fibrosis, and radiation-induced second malignancies, have also prompted clinicians to try to identify a subset of patients who could be treated by surgery alone without compromising local disease control. Careful patient selection for unimodality treatment by surgery alone is essential. Important criteria include an R0 resection in clinical settings in which the anatomic site clearly allows for adequate surgical margins. The importance of anatomic site in considering treatment by surgery alone is illustrated by the hypothetical cases of two patients with 4-cm, high-grade sarcomas: one in the anterior thigh and the second case with an identically sized tumor located in the wrist. Clearly, the first patient could undergo satisfactory treatment by surgery alone because the surgical margins can and should be satisfactory. However, this is not the case for the second patient because

TABLE 2-2 Phase III Trials of Adjuvant Radiotherapy for Localized Extremity and Trunk Sarcoma Stratified by Grade

HISTOLOGIC GRADE	FIRST AUTHOR/ INSTITUTION	TREATMENT GROUP	RADIATION DOSE, GY	NO. OF PATIENTS	NO. OF LOCAL FAILURES (%)	LRFS (%)	OS (%)
High grade	Pisters/MSKCC[23]	Surgery + BRT	42-45	56	5 (9)	89	27
		Surgery	–	63	19 (30)	66	67
	Yang[24]	Surgery + XRT	45 + 18 (boost)	47	0 (0)	100	75
		Surgery	–	44	9 (20)	78	74
Low grade	Pisters[23]	Surgery + BRT	42-45	22	8 (36)	73	96
		Surgery	–	23	6 (26)	73	95
	Yang[24]	Surgery + BRT	45 + 18 (boost)	26	1 (4)	96	NR
		Surgery	–	24	8 (33)	63	NR

MSKCC, Memorial Sloan-Kettering Cancer Center; BRT, brachytherapy; LRFS, local recurrence-free survival; OS, overall survival; NCI, National Cancer Institute; XRT, external-beam radiotherapy; NR, not reported.

the wrist or other anatomically similar site is not amenable to wide margins without amputation and sacrifice of neurovascular structures. Table 2-2 summarizes recent reports of patients treated by surgery alone and demonstrates that very acceptable local control rates of 10% or less can be achieved in carefully selected patients treated by surgery alone.

Amputation

Although sparingly used, amputation is still the appropriate treatment for a subset of patients who present with locally advanced primary tumors. The criteria for patient selection for amputation include:

- Radiologically defined major vascular, bony, or nerve involvement such that a "limb sparing" primary tumor resection will result in critical loss of function or tissue viability
- Localized nonmetastatic disease (Amputation is usually not considered for patients with established metastatic disease.)

For patients without limb-sparing surgical options, amputation offers excellent local tumor control and the prospect of prompt rehabilitation; therefore, there remains a small but well-defined role for amputation in the management of patients with extremity STS.

Management of Regional Lymph Nodes

There is no role for routine regional lymph node dissection in most patients with localized STS given the low (2% to 3%) incidence of lymph node metastasis in adults with sarcomas.[2,29] However, patients with angiosarcoma, embryonal/alveolar rhabdomyosarcoma, clear cell sarcoma, and epithelioid sarcoma are at increased risk for lymph node metastasis and should be carefully examined for lymphadenopathy. These patients should be considered for a sentinel lymph node biopsy as part of a definitive surgical treatment. A therapeutic lymph node dissection should be considered for patients with pathologically proven lymph node involvement who do not have radiologically defined metastatic disease. A therapeutic lymph node dissection may result in survival rates as high as 34%.[2]

The prognosis of patients with pathologically positive metastatic disease to lymph nodes has been generally regarded as similar to patients with visceral metastatic disease. However, a recent series of patients with isolated lymph node metastasis treated intensively with combined modality treatment showed somewhat better outcomes, approaching those of patients with localized, high-risk (stage III) disease. This report and the relative rarity of nodal involvement in patients with STS raise questions as to whether nodal involvement should be reconsidered in the future editions of the AJCC staging system.[30,31]

Radiotherapy

Rationale for Combining Radiotherapy with Surgery

The use of RT in combination with surgery for STS is supported by two phase III clinical trials (see Table 2-2)[23,24] and is based on two premises: microscopic foci or residual disease can be destroyed by RT, and less radical surgery can be performed when surgery and RT are combined. Although the traditional belief was that STS is resistant to RT, radiosensitivity assays performed on sarcoma cell lines grown in vitro have confirmed that the radiosensitivity of sarcomas is similar to that of other malignancies; this confirmation supports the first premise.[32,33]

The second premise stresses the philosophy of preservation of form (including cosmesis where possible) and function as a goal for many patients with extremity, truncal, breast, and head and neck sarcomas.[34-36]

Similar principles govern the frequent use of RT for sarcomas at anatomically challenging sites, such as the retroperitoneum, head and neck, or paravertebral regions.

Sequencing of Radiotherapy and Surgery

The optimal sequencing of surgery and radiation is a subject of considerable controversy and debate. Advantages of preoperative radiation include a generally lower radiation dose (50 Gy) and small field size with reduced risks for long-term treatment sequelae, including edema and fibrosis. These advantages occur at the cost of increased risk for surgical wound complications resulting from radiation-related impairment in wound healing. Advantages of postoperative radiation treatment include the ability to treat pathologically diagnosed and staged patients with known margin status. However, postoperative radiation is usually administered to a higher dose (65 Gy) and is associated with greater risks for treatment-related, long-term complications, including edema and fibrosis. Therefore, treatment-sequencing involves complicated trade-off issues that need to be individualized and carefully discussed with the patient.

The NCI of Canada/Canadian Sarcoma Group SR2 clinical trial (Fig. 2-6) is the only prospective, randomized comparison of preoperative versus postoperative RT.[37]

Patients were randomly assigned to be treated by surgery with either preoperative or postoperative radiation (with a radiation boost dose for patients with microscopically positive surgical margins). The primary end point of the trial was major wound complications. The SR2 trial demonstrated that wound complications were twice as common with preoperative RT as with postoperative RT (35% versus 17%, respectively), although the increased risk was almost exclusively confined to patients with sarcomas of the lower extremity. Of interest, a recent report from the University of Texas MD Anderson Cancer Center, using the same criteria for classifying wound complications as were used in the Canadian NCI trial, found almost identical results.[38]

The SR2 trial also provided important data on long-term, treatment-related complications. Patients randomized to postoperative radiation had significantly greater rates of generally irreversible fibrosis and edema.[39]

This observation is potentially important because patients with significant fibrosis, joint stiffness, or limb edema had significantly lower-limb function scores at these later time points.[39]

The analysis of late-treatment effects demonstrated that the radiation field size was associated with greater degrees of fibrosis and joint stiffness and also may be related to edema.[40]

The SR2 trial was neither designed nor statistically powered to compare traditional oncologic end points such as local control and overall survival (these were secondary end points in the trial). The 5-year results for preoperative versus postoperative, respectively, include: local control, 93% versus 92%;

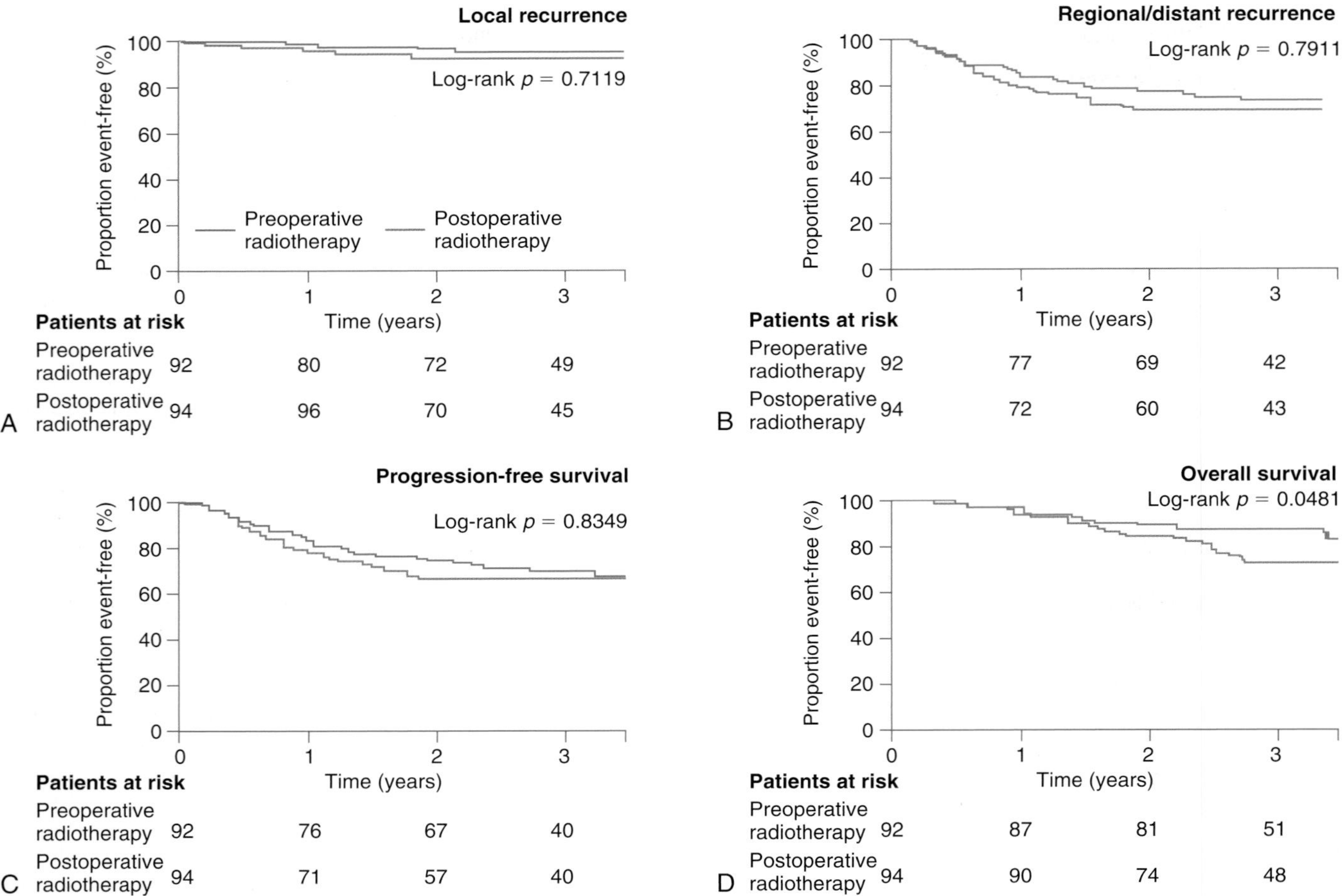

FIGURE 2-6. A-D, Kaplan–Meier plots for probability of local recurrence, metastasis (local and regional recurrence), progression-free survival, and overall survival in the Canadian Sarcoma Group randomized trial of the National Cancer Institute of Canada Clinical Trials Group comparing preoperative and postoperative radiotherapy. *(Reproduced with permission of The Lancet Ltd. from O'Sullivan B, Davis AM, Turcotte R, et al. Preoperative versus postoperative radiotherapy in soft-tissue sarcoma of the limbs: a randomised trial. Lancet 2002;359(9325):2235–41.)*

metastatic-relapse free, 67% versus 69%; recurrence-free survival, 58% versus 59%; overall survival, 73% versus 67% ($p = 0.48$); cause-specific survival, 78% versus 73% ($p = 0.64$).[41]

Cox modeling showed only resection margins as significant for local control. Tumor size and grade were the only significant factors for metastatic relapse, overall survival, and cause-specific survival. Grade was the only consistent predictor of recurrence-free survival.[41]

For the present, decisions about preoperative versus postoperative RT should be individualized, taking into account tumor location, tumor size, RT field size, comorbidities, and risks. In general, preoperative RT provides some advantages over postoperative RT but exposes the patient to significantly increased risks of serious (generally reversible) postoperative wound complications. A summary of the relative indications that can be used to select patients for preoperative RT is provided in Table 2-3.

Radiation Treatment Techniques

External beam radiation treatment (EBRT) and BRT are used for patients with STS. There are no prospective trials that directly compare EBRT and BRT, but each of these techniques has been compared with surgery alone.[23,24]

EBRT is the most commonly used radiation treatment technique for patients with STS. EBRT is widely available and can be administered by all radiation oncologists. It is also effective for patients with both high- and low-grade sarcomas. Treatment is usually administered on an outpatient basis in daily fractions of 1.8 to 2.0 Gy (Monday to Friday) to total doses of 50 Gy (preop dose; 5-week duration) or 60 to 66 Gy (postop dose; 6½ weeks).

In contrast, BRT for STS is available in only specific centers where there are trained radiation oncologists and appropriate radiation isotope storage and handling facilities, but BRT does offer several advantages. Because of the shorter treatment time (4 to 6 days) compared to EBRT, it is usually administered on an inpatient basis during the same hospital stay and is more easily integrated into treatment protocols that include systemic chemotherapy. Because irradiated tissue volume is less, BRT may confer long-term functional advantages. BRT also costs $1200 per patient, which is less than the cost of EBRT.[42]

One specific limitation of BRT is that it should be used for patients with only high-grade sarcomas (as well as R0 cases) because the only randomized trial that evaluated this technique demonstrated that BRT does not appear effective for

TABLE 2-3 Relative Indications for Preoperative RT, Despite Concerns Related to Wound Complications

TREATMENT CONTEXT/SARCOMA SITE	ISSUES OF CONCERN	COMMENTS
Head and neck Paranasal sinus	Proximity to optic apparatus (eye, orbit, chiasma)	Major visual functional deficit can be minimized
Skull base	Proximity to spinal cord, brainstem	Other "lesser" morbidities (dental, xerostomia) may also be less due to reduced doses and volumes
Cheek and face		
Split-thickness skin graft reconstruction (especially lower limb)	Skin graft breakdown and consequent infection	Many months to years of recreational and/or vocational disability may occur during healing (rare)
Retroperitoneum	Proximity to bowel, liver, kidney	Critical organs may be displaced by tumor or not fixed or adherent as is likely in postoperative setting
	Large-volume GTV or CTV occupying coelomic cavities	Entire tumor treated before possible contamination of cavity
Some small bowel lesions	Proximity to critical anatomy, especially intestine with side wall adherence	Contamination of abdominal cavity renders postoperative RT unsuitable
Thoracic wall/pleura	Proximity to lung or cardiac structures	Lung may be displaced by chest wall or pleural tumor and can be avoided with preoperative RT, or permits GTV to be treated before operative contamination
Abdominal trunk walls, pelvic side wall	Proximity to kidney, bowel, liver, ovaries	Avoid CT encroachment on vulnerable anatomy GTV adjacent to dose-limiting critical anatomy
Thoracic inlet/upper chest	Proximity to brachial plexus	Dose limitation of critical anatomy lends itself to preoperative wall low neck RT. Additional volume considerations
Medial thigh (young male)	Proximity to testes	Permanent infertility may be avoided
Central limb tumor	Proximity to other compartments	Permits partial circumferential sparing, which would not be feasible in postoperative setting

From O'Sullivan B, Wylie J, Catton C, et al. The local management of soft tissue sarcoma. Semin Radiat Oncol 1999;9(4):328–48

CTV, clinical target volume; GTV, gross tumor volume; RT, radiotherapy.

patients with low-grade sarcomas (see Table 2-2),[24,43-44] and retrospective data suggest that BRT may not provide optimal local control for R1 cases.[45]

BRT may also have an advantage in the following situations in which normal-tissue tolerance to conventional external beam radiation has been compromised: (1) a postoperative boost in patients who have received preoperative RT or (2) radiation for local recurrence in a previously irradiated field.[46-49]

Intensity modulated radiation treatment is a radiation delivery technique that allows external beams designed with variable intensity to be delivered across their profiles, in contrast to the uniform flat profile used in traditional external beam RT. These variable-intensity beams are not only shaped according to the needs of the target but also take into account the dose provided by the others. This allows the beams to closely conform to the target while avoiding other structures. It may be particularly valuable for tumors of complex shape, such as sarcomas, and has recently been used to treat large intra-abdominal targets, including retroperitoneal sarcomas.[50] Clinical results are anticipated from studies of these improvements in RT planning and delivery.

Chemotherapy

Chemotherapy is the mainstay of therapy for patients with metastatic (stage IV) STS. The use of chemotherapy in the adjuvant setting has been controversial but is gaining increased acceptance when used selectively.

Chemotherapy Following Primary Surgical Resection

Although local or locoregional recurrence is a problem for a small subset of patients following primary therapy, the major risk to life in sarcoma patients is uncontrolled microscopic or macroscopic systemic disease. Increasingly, major sarcoma centers are taking a histology-specific approach to selecting patients for consideration of adjuvant treatment.

Adjuvant chemotherapy is an appropriate standard of care for the Ewing family of tumors and for rhabdomyosarcoma.[51-53] However, for more common STSs such as leiomyosarcoma, liposarcoma, and high-grade undifferentiated pleomorphic sarcoma, the benefit for chemotherapy, if there is one, is small.[54] Because adjuvant therapy is used by many practitioners for more common diseases where the benefit is a relatively small one, such as stage I breast cancer and stage II colon cancer, this small potential benefit is an issue that needs to be discussed on an individual basis with patients. Certainly, the lack of available effective agents for metastatic sarcoma has impeded progress in this area, but the utility of imatinib in a gastrointestinal stromal tumor gives hope that new agents will contribute to the ultimate goal of any type of systemic therapy, specifically to increase the cure rate of new patients.

There have been over a dozen studies of anthracycline-based adjuvant chemotherapy for STS, which date back nearly as long as the initial development of doxorubicin.[55,56] These will not be reviewed here because anthracycline/ifosfamide-based therapy constitutes a better standard of care in patients offered adjuvant chemotherapy, and only one of the studies completed by 1992 had used ifosfamide. The best summary of

TABLE 2-4 Hazard Ratios for Individual Patient Data Meta-Analysis in 1568 Adults from 14 Trials of Doxorubicin-Based Chemotherapy for STS

HAZARD RATIO	OUTCOME	95% CONFIDENCE Intervals	P value
Local RFI	0.73	0.56-0.94	0.016
Distant RFI	0.70	0.57-0.85	0.0003
Overall recurrence-free survival	0.75	0.64-0.87	0.0001
Overall survival	0.89	0.76-1.03	0.12

From Verweij J and Seynaeve C. The reason for confining the use of adjuvant chemotherapy in soft tissue sarcoma to the investigational setting. Semin Radiat Oncol 1999;9(4):352–9.

RFI, recurrent-free survival.
Data from the Sarcoma Data Base Meta-Analysis Collaboration.

anthracycline-containing adjuvant-based chemotherapy for extremity sarcomas to date was the 1997 meta-analysis of 14 studies encompassing sarcomas of all anatomic sites.[57] In this study, 23 potential studies were considered, and 14 ultimately selected, constituting 1568 patients with STS of extremity and non-extremity sites with a median follow-up of 9.4 years. Pathology review was not centralized. The results of the meta-analysis, including the actuarial outcome probabilities and the hazard ratios, are summarized in Table 2-4. Disease-free survival at 10 years was improved with chemotherapy from 45% to a highly statistically significant 55%, as was seen in several of the individual studies comprising this population. Furthermore, local disease-free survival was also improved at 10 years with chemotherapy, from 75% to 81% ($p = 0.016$). Most important, overall survival also improved from 50% to 54% at 10 years, but was a favorable trend only, and not statistically significant ($p = 0.12$). The largest difference in overall survival was found in a post-hoc analysis of the 886 patients examined with extremity sarcomas. Overall survival was shown to improve by 7% in the group receiving chemotherapy ($p = 0.029$).

Many important interpretation issues have been summarized in a commentary on this meta-analysis. As pointed out by Verweij and Seynaeve,[58] these data have to be interpreted with caution because of the following: (1) the subset analysis was unplanned, (2) 18% of patients did not have histology available for review, (3) ineligibility rates were high, and (4) 6% of the patients from the largest contributing study to this meta-analysis did not have sarcoma after a repeat pathology review. Although the meta-analysis cannot replace a well-designed, randomized study, it reinforces many of the findings from smaller studies that local and distant recurrence-free survival is definitely improved, but the same may not be true for overall survival.

Adjuvant and Neoadjuvant Studies Since the 1997 Meta-Analysis

The relevance of these older data to more modern practice may be limited because of improved imaging, widespread acceptance of limb-sparing surgery, introduction of ifosfamide, more sophisticated pathological diagnosis, and better supportive care such as that offered by hematopoietic growth factors. Therefore, the post-meta-analysis modern (i.e., modern chemotherapy drugs, dosing, and schedule) randomized trials may be the best group of studies to examine the question of the utility of adjuvant chemotherapy.

The largest modern-generation randomized trial was performed by the Italian Sarcoma Study Group in patients with primary or recurrent resected STS of the extremity or limb girdle treated or not treated with radiation.[59] One hundred and four patients with localized high-risk disease were randomized to receive no chemotherapy or to receive ifosfamide (1800 mg/m^2/day for 5 consecutive days with mesna) and epirubicin (60 mg/m^2 on 2 consecutive days), with filgrastim support. Interim analysis in 1996 led to an early conclusion of the trial when the study reached its primary end point of improved disease-free survival. Unfortunately, had this study commenced after the meta-analysis, it might have been constructed with a primary end point of overall survival. At a median follow-up of 36 months, overall survival in the chemotherapy arm was 72% compared to 55% for the control arm ($p = 0.002$). However, with longer-term follow-up, the overall survival difference is now no longer statistically significant on an intention-to-treat analysis.[59] This study was the strongest argument in the literature for the use of adjuvant chemotherapy. Nonetheless, interpretation of the study is made more difficult with the observation of equivalent distant and local recurrence rates at 4 years. There are also subtle imbalances in the distribution of patients on the control and treatment arms of the study, which are difficult to evaluate given the heterogeneous nature of STS histology.

The data from this well-executed Italian study must also be taken into consideration with other data from two smaller studies. To examine the possible benefit of increased dose intensity in an adjuvant setting, an Austrian group studied 59 patients receiving no chemotherapy or doxorubicin 50 mg/m^2/cycle, dacarbazine 800 mg/m^2/cycle, and ifosfamide 6 g/m^2/cycle every 2 weeks with mesna and filgrastim support following surgical resection of the primary sarcoma. Overall survival and relapse-free survival did not differ significantly between the treatment arms at a mean follow-up of 41 months.[60] There were trends to improved recurrence-free survival, but the study was underpowered to detect a small difference in overall survival or disease-free survival. A randomized, phase II neoadjuvant study of doxorubicin 50 mg/m^2 and ifosfamide 5 g/m^2 by the European Organization for Research and Treatment of Cancer (EORTC) and Canadian NCI also failed to show a survival advantage for the use of chemotherapy (estimated 5-year overall survival 64% for the control arm, 65% for the treatment arm).[61] Neoadjuvant chemotherapy is discussed in greater detail in the following section. Finally, the EORTC has completed accrual in December 2003, to an adjuvant trial (Study 62931) for high-grade STS for all sites, using doxorubicin 75 mg/m^2 and ifosfamide 5000 mg/m^2 with filgrastim. Analysis will not be feasible until there has been sufficient follow-up.

Preoperative (Neoadjuvant) Chemotherapy

Preoperative chemotherapy has theoretical advantages over postoperative treatment. First, preoperative chemotherapy provides an in vivo test of chemotherapy sensitivity. Patients whose tumors show objective evidence of response are presumed to be the subset that may benefit most from further postoperative systemic treatment. In contrast, it is assumed that the population of non-responding patients will derive minimal or no benefit from further chemotherapy and can, therefore, be spared its toxicity. However, there are alternative ways to consider the subsets of patients identified by preoperative chemotherapy, that is, the "responders" and the "non-responders." It is conceivable that patients who have tumors that respond well to preoperative chemotherapy simply have biologically less aggressive tumors that are destined to do well regardless of whether they receive chemotherapy (i.e., that response to chemotherapy simply selects biologically favorable tumors). Using this perspective, one might also conclude that patients who have tumors that appear resistant to chemotherapy have biologically more aggressive tumors not apparently impacted by conventional chemotherapy. This subset of patients is a group that could potentially benefit the most from the discovery of more effective systemic treatments.

A second potential advantage of preoperative chemotherapy is that it treats occult microscopic metastatic disease as soon as possible after the cancer diagnosis. This may theoretically prevent the development of chemotherapy resistance by isolated clones of metastatic cells or prevent the postoperative growth of microscopic metastases, but, given the nature of the growth of sarcomas, at most one or two doublings of the tumor would be affected, far fewer than the greater than 35 typically required in the development of a tumor larger than 1 cm.

A third potential advantage of preoperative chemotherapy treatment is that chemotherapy-induced cytoreduction may permit a less radical and consequently less morbid surgical resection than would have been required initially. In patients with large STS of the extremities, a chemotherapy-associated response may reduce the morbidity of limb-sparing surgical procedures and even allow patients who might otherwise have required an amputation to undergo limb-sparing surgery.

Investigators from the University of Texas MD Anderson Cancer Center reported long-term results with doxorubicin-based preoperative chemotherapy for AJCC stages IIC and III (formerly AJCC stage IIIB) extremity STS.[62] In a series of 76 patients treated with doxorubicin-based preoperative chemotherapy, radiologic response rates were as follows: complete response, 9%; partial response, 19%; minor response, 13%; stable disease, 30%; and disease progression, 30%. The overall objective major response rate (complete plus partial responses) was 27%. At a median follow-up of 85 months, 5-year actuarial rates of local recurrence-free survival, distant metastasis-free survival, disease-free survival, and overall survival were 83%, 52%, 46%, and 59%, respectively. The event-free outcomes reported from the University of Texas MD Anderson Cancer Center are similar to those observed with chemotherapy in the phase III postoperative chemotherapy trials. Furthermore, a comparison of responding patients (complete and partial responses) and non-responding patients did not reveal any significant differences in event-free outcome.

In a prospective study from MSKCC, 29 patients with AJCC (fourth edition) stage IIIB STS larger than 10 cm were treated with two cycles of a doxorubicin-based regimen before local therapy.[63] Subjective changes in the degree of primary tumor firmness and in imaging characteristics of the tumor (intratumoral necrosis and hemorrhage) were observed in many patients but were not quantifiable. Only one patient met the standard criteria for a partial response. Survival results in this population of high-risk patients were similar to those in historic controls treated with postoperative doxorubicin or patients treated with local therapy alone. The reasons for the apparent discrepancy in response rates between the reports from the University of Texas MD Anderson Cancer Center and MSKCC remain unclear. Possible explanations include that the population treated at MSKCC appears to be a higher-risk population, with all patients having high-grade lesions larger than 10 cm, as is discussed in the next section in studies examining retrospective data from both institutions. Moreover, the patients treated at MSKCC received a lower doxorubicin dose (60 mg/m^2) for fewer cycles (two). This may be important, given the known dose-response relationship with doxorubicin.[64]

Recently, ifosfamide-containing combinations have been used in the preoperative setting. Selected patients treated with aggressive ifosfamide-based regimens have had major responses, and preliminary results suggest that response rates may be higher than in historic controls treated with non-ifosfamide-containing regimens.[65] However, as noted previously, the randomized phase II neoadjuvant study of doxorubicin and ifosfamide chemotherapy showed no benefit for the treatment arm, although the study was not specifically designed to determine a survival advantage.[61]

Recent Analyses of Multicenter Data Regarding Adjuvant Therapy for STS

It is well recognized that different sarcoma subtypes have different chemosensitivity patterns. For example, malignant peripheral nerve sheath tumors are typically less sensitive to doxorubicin, and leiomyosarcomas are less sensitive to ifosfamide than other forms of sarcoma. Synovial sarcoma and myxoid/round cell liposarcoma appear to be more sensitive to chemotherapy in the metastatic setting than other subtypes of sarcoma and may well be two subtypes that respond to both anthracyclines and ifosfamide.[66] This argues that adjuvant chemotherapy should be examined on a subtype-specific basis. Combined non-randomized data from the University of California, Los Angeles and MSKCC showed that adjuvant chemotherapy may, indeed, be useful for synovial sarcomas and myxoid/round cell liposarcoma, and argued for the use of chemotherapy in the neoadjuvant setting for all types of STS based on MSKCC and Dana-Farber institutional databases.[67-69] Interestingly, data of all patients treated or not treated with chemotherapy from the University of Texas MD Anderson Cancer Center and MSKCC indicated in the adjuvant or neoadjuvant setting that there was no statistical difference in overall survival in the group of patients who received chemotherapy versus those who did not.[70] However, these data are inherently biased in that it is likely that younger, healthier patients with larger, high-grade tumors were those selected to receive chemotherapy. Even though there was no statistically significant difference in the group of patients who received chemotherapy and those who did not, there is still some shift toward patients with larger sarcomas and liposarcomas receiving chemotherapy, thereby possibly creating selection bias that allowed a group of patients with an inherently poorer outcome to do as well as those with a better outcome.

In summary, for AJCC stage III STS, if there is a benefit to chemotherapy in the adjuvant setting, it appears to be a small one. Therefore, dialogue with patients must include careful comparison of the small potential benefit and well-defined risks of systemic therapy. Above all, treatment must be individualized to the clinical setting. Younger patients with chemosensitive subtypes (e.g., myxoid/round cell liposarcoma, synovial sarcoma) may benefit most in this highly heterogeneous patient population.

TREATMENT OF LOCALLY ADVANCED DISEASE

Hyperthermic Isolated Limb Perfusion

Hyperthermic isolated limb perfusion (HILP), an investigational technique in the United States (although recently approved by regulatory agencies in other parts of the world), has received considerable attention in the treatment of locally advanced, unresectable sarcomas of nonosseous tissues. HILP has been evaluated in two settings: (1) attempted limb preservation in cases of locally advanced extremity lesions surgically amenable to amputation only and (2) functional extremity preservation for the short-term in cases of locally advanced extremity lesions and synchronous pulmonary metastases (stage IV disease).

A multicenter phase II trial has evaluated a series of 55 patients with radiologically unresectable extremity STS using HILP with high-dose tumor necrosis factor-α, interferon-α, and melphalan.[71] A major tumor response was seen in 87% of patients: complete responses in 20 (36%) and partial responses in 28 (51%). Limb salvage was achieved in 84% of patients. Regional toxicity was limited, and systemic toxicity was minimal to moderate. There were no treatment-related deaths. This approach is being further evaluated in ongoing trials in Europe.

Radiation Alone

Apart from patients with some very radiosensitive subtypes of sarcomas, most patients who undergo RT as the sole treatment modality for sarcoma have been deemed to have locally advanced unresectable disease. RT alone is a rare treatment choice that should be done only at centers skilled in the management of sarcomas; medically fit patients with grossly unresectable but nonmetastatic disease should always be referred to a specialty center for multidisciplinary management, which may combine surgery, RT, and sometimes chemotherapy. For example, proximal inguinal or axillary tumors that encircle major vascular structures in the proximal arm may be resected along with the involved vasculature and the vessels reconstructed. Adjuvant RT is also generally used. Rarely, a patient with truly inoperable locally advanced disease may require RT alone, with either photon or particle (proton, neutron, or pion) beams.[72-76] No formal clinical trials have been performed to compare these strategies to each other, and they are generally administered in an adverse clinical setting. Local control has been reported in 40% to 70% of such cases treated with neutrons; treatment with photons produces local control in approximately 30% of cases.[73,74]

MANAGEMENT OF LOCAL RECURRENCE

If an isolated local recurrence is identified, the treatment goals are the same as for patients with primary tumors, namely, optimal local control while maintaining as much function, and cosmesis as possible.[48] Early identification of local relapse may improve the chance of successful salvage therapy, and, like newly diagnosed patients, these patients are probably best managed in specialized multidisciplinary sarcoma centers. An approach to the evaluation and management of locally recurrent STS is summarized in Figure 2-7. The initial evaluation must include a full review of previous therapy because this will have a bearing on the therapeutic options available. Therefore, all prior surgery and pathology reports should be

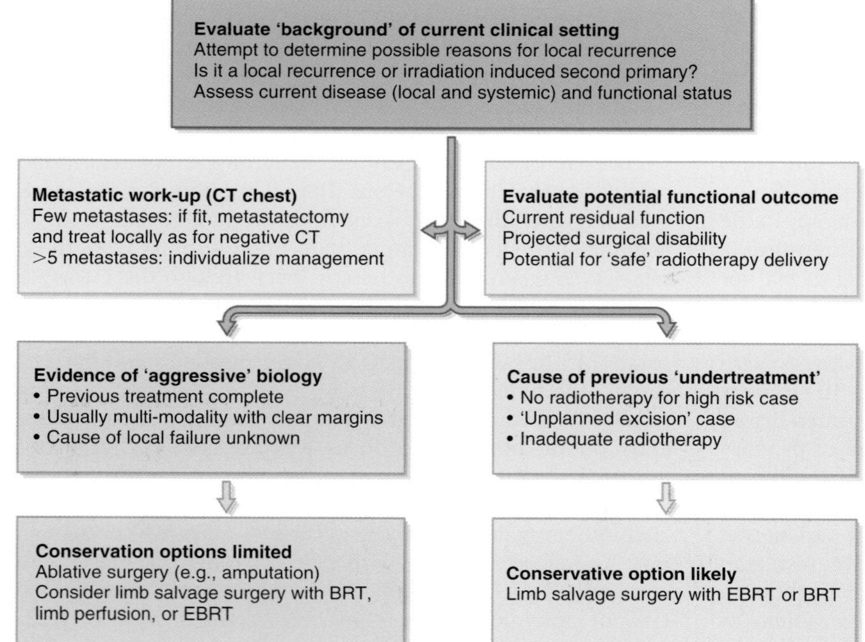

FIGURE 2-7. Schema for approaching the patient with local recurrence of soft-tissue sarcoma. The schema is oriented toward extremity lesions but is equally applicable to other anatomic sites (e.g., head and neck and retroperitoneum). BRT, brachytherapy; EBRT, external-beam radiotherapy. *(From Catton CN, Swallow CJ, O'Sullivan B. Approaches to local salvage of soft tissue sarcoma after primary site failure. Semin Radiat Oncol 1999 Oct;9(4):378–88.)*

examined, as should reports on previous chemotherapy and previous RT, especially volume treated, dose, and energy of radiation.

Several distinct clinical settings are evident under the rubric of locally recurrent disease: (1) cases in which prior treatment did not include RT; (2) cases treated with RT in the past; (3) cases in which distant metastases are also present; and (4) cases in which it is difficult to distinguish between recurrence and secondary tumors induced by RT. Although the therapeutic options available are more limited in recurrent disease and the challenge posed by these cases are that much more formidable, a proportion of these patients can be cured. Clinical experience is needed to determine which therapeutic options are appropriate in a given case of recurrent disease.

KEY POINTS

- Core-needle biopsy is the preferred biopsy method for most patients with suspected sarcoma.
- Pretreatment staging should include an MRI (or CT) of the primary tumor site, chest X-ray, and chest CT (for patients with high-grade sarcomas).
- Surgery and preoperative or postoperative EBRT is the primary local treatment for most patients with localized disease. In many clinical settings, preoperative radiation should be considered because of the lower dose, smaller treatment volume, and lower risks for post-treatment edema and fibrosis.
- The role for routine administration of adjuvant chemotherapy treatment remains unclear.
- Patients with metastatic disease should be considered for chemotherapy treatment with carefully selected cases considered for metastasectomy.

References

1. Lawrence W Jr, Donegan WL, Natarajan N, et al. Adult soft tissue sarcomas. A pattern of care survey of the American College of Surgeons. Ann Surg 1987;205(4):349–59.
2. Fong Y, Coit DG, Woodruff JM, et al. Lymph node metastasis from soft tissue sarcoma in adults. Analysis of data from a prospective database of 1772 sarcoma patients. Ann Surg 1993;217(1):72–7.
3. Ball AB, Fisher C, Pittam M, et al. Diagnosis of soft tissue tumours by Tru-Cut biopsy. Br J Surg 1990;77(7):756–58.
4. Skrzynski MC, Biermann JS, Montag A, et al. Diagnostic accuracy and charge-savings of outpatient core needle biopsy compared with open biopsy of musculoskeletal tumors. J Bone Joint Surg Am 1996;78(5):644–49.
5. Heslin MJ, Lewis JJ, Woodruff JM, et al. Core needle biopsy for diagnosis of extremity soft tissue sarcoma. Ann Surg Oncol 1997;4(5):425–31.
6. Schwartz HS, Spengler DM. Needle tract recurrences after closed biopsy for sarcoma: three cases and review of the literature. Ann Surg Oncol 1997;4(3):228–36.
7. Akerman M. Fine-needle aspiration cytology of soft tissue sarcoma: benefits and limitations. Sarcoma 1998;2(3-4):155–61.
8. Kissin MW, Fisher C, Webb AJ, et al. Value of fine needle aspiration cytology in the diagnosis of soft tissue tumours: a preliminary study on the excised specimen. Br J Surg 1987;74(6):479–80.
9. Edge S, Byrd D, Compton C, et al. American Joint Committee on Cancer (AJCC) Staging Manual. 7th ed. New York: Springer; 2010.
10. Kattan MW, Leung DH, Brennan MF. Postoperative nomogram for 12-year sarcoma-specific death. J Clin Oncol 2002;20(3):791–96.
11. Stojadinovic A, Yeh A, Brennan MF. Completely resected recurrent soft tissue sarcoma: primary anatomic site governs outcomes. J Am Coll Surg 2002;194(4):436–47.
12. Pisters PW, Leung DH, Woodruff J, et al. Analysis of prognostic factors in 1,041 patients with localized soft tissue sarcomas of the extremities. J Clin Oncol 1996;14(5):1679–89.
13. Coindre JM, Terrier P, Bui NB, et al. Prognostic factors in adult patients with locally controlled soft tissue sarcoma. A study of 546 patients from the French Federation of Cancer Centers Sarcoma Group. J Clin Oncol 1996;14(3):869–77.
14. Gaynor JJ, Tan CC, Casper ES, et al. Refinement of clinicopathologic staging for localized soft tissue sarcoma of the extremity: a study of 423 adults. J Clin Oncol 1992;10(8):1317–29.
15. Gerrand CH, Wunder JS, Kandel RA, et al. Classification of positive margins after resection of soft-tissue sarcoma of the limb predicts the risk of local recurrence. J Bone Joint Surg Br 2001;83(8):1149–55.
16. Eilber FC, Brennan MF, Eilber FR, et al. Validation of the postoperative nomogram for 12-year sarcoma-specific mortality. Cancer 2004;101(10):2270–75.
17. Mariani L, Miceli R, Kattan MW, et al. Validation and adaptation of a nomogram for predicting the survival of patients with extremity soft tissue sarcoma using a three-grade system. Cancer 2005;103(2):402–08.
18. Williard WC, Collin C, Casper ES, et al. The changing role of amputation for soft tissue sarcoma of the extremity in adults. Surg Gynecol Obstet 1992;175(5):389–96.
19. Williard WC, Collin C, Casper ES, et al. Comparison of amputation with limb-sparing operations for adult soft tissue sarcoma of the extremity. Ann Surg 1992;215(3):269–75.
20. Bowden L, Booher RJ. The principles and technique of resection of soft parts for sarcoma. Surgery 1958;44(6):963–77.
21. Cantin J, McNeer GP, Chu FC, et al. The problem of local recurrence after treatment of soft tissue sarcoma. Ann Surg 1968;168(1):47–53.
22. Gerner RE, Moore GE, Pickren JW. Soft tissue sarcomas. Ann Surg 1975;181(6):803–8.
23. Pisters PW, Harrison LB, Leung DH, et al. Long-term results of a prospective randomized trial of adjuvant brachytherapy in soft tissue sarcoma. J Clin Oncol 1996;14(3):859–68.
24. Yang JC, Chang AE, Baker AR, et al. Randomized prospective study of the benefit of adjuvant radiation therapy in the treatment of soft tissue sarcomas of the extremity. J Clin Oncol 1998;16(1):197–203.
25. Karakousis CP, Proimakis C, Walsh DL. Primary soft tissue sarcoma of the extremities in adults. Br J Surg 1995;82(9):1208–12.
26. Brennan MF, Casper ES, Harrison LB, et al. The role of multimodality therapy in soft-tissue sarcoma. Ann Surg 1991;214(3):328–36.
27. Yang JC, Rosenberg SA. Surgery for adult patients with soft tissue sarcomas. Semin Oncol 1989;16(4):289–96.
28. Rosenberg SA, Tepper J, Glatstein E, et al. The treatment of soft-tissue sarcomas of the extremities: prospective randomized evaluations of (1) limb-sparing surgery plus radiation therapy compared with amputation and (2) the role of adjuvant chemotherapy. Ann Surg 1982;196(3):305–15.
29. Weingrad DN, Rosenberg SA. Early lymphatic spread of osteogenic and soft-tissue sarcomas. Surgery 1978;84(2):231–40.
30. Behranwala KA, A'Hern R, Omar AM, et al. Prognosis of lymph node metastasis in soft tissue sarcoma. Ann Surg Oncol 2004;11(7):714–19.
31. Riad S, Griffin AM, Liberman B, et al. Lymph node metastasis in soft tissue sarcoma in an extremity. Clin Orthop Relat Res 2004;426:129–34.
32. Ruka W, Taghian A, Gioioso D, et al. Comparison between the in vitro intrinsic radiation sensitivity of human soft tissue sarcoma and breast cancer cell lines. J Surg Oncol 1996;61(4):290–94.
33. Weichselbaum RR, Beckett MA, Simon MA, et al. In vitro radiobiological parameters of human sarcoma cell lines. Int J Radiat Oncol Biol Phys 1988;15(4):937–42.
34. O'Sullivan B, Wylie J, Catton C, et al. The local management of soft tissue sarcoma. Semin Radiat Oncol 1999;9(4):328–48.
35. Le Vay J, O'Sullivan B, Catton C, et al. An assessment of prognostic factors in soft-tissue sarcoma of the head and neck. Arch Otolaryngol Head Neck Surg 1994;120(9):981–86.
36. McGowan TS, Cummings BJ, O'Sullivan B, et al. An analysis of 78 breast sarcoma patients without distant metastases at presentation. Int J Radiat Oncol Biol Phys 2000;46(2):383–90.
37. O'Sullivan B, Davis AM, Turcotte R, et al. Preoperative versus postoperative radiotherapy in soft-tissue sarcoma of the limbs: a randomised trial. Lancet 2002;359(9325):2235–41.
38. Tseng JF, Ballo MT, Langstein HN, et al. The effect of preoperative radiotherapy and reconstructive surgery on wound complications after resection of extremity soft-tissue sarcomas. Ann Surg Oncol 2006;13(9):1209–15.

39. Davis AM, O'Sullivan B, Turcotte R, et al. Late radiation morbidity following randomization to preoperative versus postoperative radiotherapy in extremity soft tissue sarcoma. Radiother Oncol 2005;75(1):48–53.
40. O'Sullivan B, Davis AM. A randomized phase III trial of preoperative compared to postoperative radiotherapy in extremity soft tissue sarcoma. Proc Astro 2001;51(3):151.
41. O'Sullivan B, Davis AM, Turcotte R. Five-year results of a randomized phase III trial of pre-operative vs post-operative radiotherapy in extremity soft tissue sarcoma. Proc Am Soc Clin Oncol 2004;23:815.
42. Janjan NA, Yasko AW, Reece GP, et al. Comparison of charges related to radiotherapy for soft-tissue sarcomas treated by preoperative external-beam irradiation versus interstitial implantation. Ann Surg Oncol 1994;1(5):415–22.
43. Suit HD, Mankin HJ, Wood WC, et al. Treatment of the patient with stage M0 soft tissue sarcoma. J Clin Oncol 1988;6(5):854–62.
44. Pisters PW, Harrison LB, Woodruff JM, et al. A prospective randomized trial of adjuvant brachytherapy in the management of low-grade soft tissue sarcomas of the extremity and superficial trunk. J Clin Oncol 1994;12(6):1150–55.
45. Alektiar KM, Velasco J, Zelefsky MJ, et al. Adjuvant radiotherapy for margin-positive high-grade soft tissue sarcoma of the extremity. Int J Radiat Oncol Biol Phys 2000;48(4):1051–58.
46. Catton C, Swallow CJ, O'Sullivan B. A pilot study of external beam radiotherapy and pulsed dose rate brachytherapy for resectable retroperitoneal sarcomas. Radiother Oncol 1998;47(Suppl. 1):Ss30.
47. Catton CN, Davis AM, Bell RS. Soft tissue sarcoma of the extremity. Limb salvage after failure of combined conservative therapy. Radiother Oncol 1996:41(3):209.
48. Catton CN, Swallow CJ, O'Sullivan B. Approaches to local salvage of soft tissue sarcoma after primary site failure. Semin Radiat Oncol 1999;9(4):378–88.
49. Pearlstone DB, Janjan NA, Feig BW, et al. Re-resection with brachytherapy for locally recurrent soft tissue sarcoma arising in a previously radiated field. Cancer J Sci Am 1999;5(1):26–33.
50. Hong L, Alektiar K, Chui C, et al. IMRT of large fields: whole-abdomen irradiation. Int J Radiat Oncol Biol Phys 2002;54(1):278–89.
51. Souhami RL, Craft AW, Van der Eijken JW, et al. Randomised trial of two regimens of chemotherapy in operable osteosarcoma: a study of the European Osteosarcoma Intergroup. Lancet 1997;350(9082):911–17.
52. Grier HE, Krailo MD, Tarbell NJ, et al. Addition of ifosfamide and etoposide to standard chemotherapy for Ewing's sarcoma and primitive neuroectodermal tumor of bone. N Engl J Med 2003;348(8):694–701.
53. Crist WM, Anderson JR, Meza JL, et al. Intergroup rhabdomyosarcoma study-IV: results for patients with nonmetastatic disease. J Clin Oncol 2001;19(12):3091–102.
54. Bramwell VH. Adjuvant chemotherapy for adult soft tissue sarcoma: is there a standard of care? J Clin Oncol 2001;19(5):1235–37.
55. Wang JJ, Cortes E, Sinks LF, et al. Therapeutic effect and toxicity of adriamycin in patients with neoplastic disease. Cancer 1971;28(4):837–43.
56. Benjamin RS, Wiernik PH, Bachur NR. Adriamycin chemotherapy–efficacy, safety, and pharmacologic basis of an intermittent single high-dosage schedule. Cancer 1974;33(1):19–27.
57. Sarcoma Meta-analysis Collaboration. Adjuvant chemotherapy for localised resectable soft-tissue sarcoma of adults: meta-analysis of individual data. Lancet 1997;350:1647.
58. Verweij J, Seynaeve C. The reason for confining the use of adjuvant chemotherapy in soft tissue sarcoma to the investigational setting. Semin Radiat Oncol 1999;9(4):352–9.
59. Frustaci S, De Paoli A, Bidoli E, et al. Ifosfamide in the adjuvant therapy of soft tissue sarcomas. Oncology 2003;65(Suppl. 2):80–4.
60. Brodowicz T, Schwameis E, Widder J, et al. Intensified adjuvant IFADIC chemotherapy for adult soft tissue sarcoma: a prospective randomized feasibility trial. Sarcoma 2000;4(4):151–60.
61. Gortzak E, Azzarelli A, Buesa J, et al. A randomised phase II study on neo-adjuvant chemotherapy for 'high-risk' adult soft-tissue sarcoma. Eur J Cancer 2001;37(9):1096–103.
62. Pisters PW, Patel SR, Varma DG, et al. Preoperative chemotherapy for stage IIIB extremity soft tissue sarcoma: long-term results from a single institution. J Clin Oncol 1997;15(12):3481–87.
63. Casper ES, Gaynor JJ, Harrison LB, et al. Preoperative and postoperative adjuvant combination chemotherapy for adults with high grade soft tissue sarcoma. Cancer 1994;73(6):1644–51.
64. O'Bryan RM, Baker LH, Gottlieb JE, et al. Dose response evaluation of adriamycin in human neoplasia. Cancer 1977;39(5):1940–48.
65. Patel SR, Vadhan-Raj S, Papadopolous N, et al. High-dose ifosfamide in bone and soft tissue sarcomas: results of phase II and pilot studies–dose-response and schedule dependence. J Clin Oncol 1997;15(6):2378–84.
66. Rosen G, Forscher C, Lowenbraun S, et al. Synovial sarcoma. Uniform response of metastases to high dose ifosfamide. Cancer 1994;73(10):2506–11.
67. Eilber FC, Eilber FR, Eckardt J. Impact of ifosfamide-based chemotherapy on survival in patients with primary extremity synovial sarcoma. J Clin Oncol 2004;22(4):9017.
68. Eilber FC, Eilber FR, Eckardt J, et al. The impact of chemotherapy on the survival of patients with high-grade primary extremity liposarcoma. Ann Surg 2004;240(4):686–95.
69. Grobmyer SR, Maki RG, Demetri GD, et al. Neo-adjuvant chemotherapy for primary high-grade extremity soft tissue sarcoma. Ann Oncol 2004;15(11):1667–72.
70. Cormier JN, Huang X, Xing Y, et al. Cohort analysis of patients with localized, high-risk, extremity soft tissue sarcoma treated at two cancer centers: chemotherapy-associated outcomes. J Clin Oncol 2004;22(22):4567–74.
71. Eggermont AM, Schraffordt Koops H, Liénard D, et al. Isolated limb perfusion with high-dose tumor necrosis factor-alpha in combination with interferon-gamma and melphalan for nonresectable extremity soft tissue sarcomas: a multicenter trial. J Clin Oncol 1996;14(10):2653–65.
72. Isacsson U, Hagberg H, Johansson KA, et al. Potential advantages of protons over conventional radiation beams for paraspinal tumours. Radiother Oncol 1997;45(1):63–70.
73. Pickering DG, Stewart JS, Rampling R, et al. Fast neutron therapy for soft tissue sarcoma. Int J Radiat Oncol Biol Phys 1987;13(10):1489–95.
74. Tepper JE, Suit HD. Radiation therapy alone for sarcoma of soft tissue. Cancer 1985;56(3):475–79.
75. Slater JD, McNeese MD, Peters LJ. Radiation therapy for unresectable soft tissue sarcomas. Int J Radiat Oncol Biol Phys 1986;12(10):1729–34.
76. Greiner RH, Blattmann HJ, Thum P, et al. Dynamic pion irradiation of unresectable soft tissue sarcomas. Int J Radiat Oncol Biol Phys 1989;17(5):1077–83.

Radiologic Evaluation of Soft Tissue Tumors

Hakan Ilaslan, Hassana Barazi, and Murali Sundaram

CHAPTER CONTENTS

INTRODUCTION

Over the past few decades, remarkable advancements have been seen in the use of imaging for diagnosing, staging, and following up cases of soft tissue neoplasms. In this chapter, radiologic evaluation of soft tissue tumors will be covered, touching on the modalities of radiography, ultrasound, computed tomography (CT)-positron emission tomography (PET), and magnetic resonance imaging (MRI). Recent advances in technology will be reviewed with an emphasis on the importance of an MRI for the most comprehensive evaluation of soft tissue tumors. Finally, the value of image-guided percutaneous biopsy in the diagnosis of soft tissue tumors will be covered briefly.

IMAGING MODALITIES

Radiography

Radiographs, although often invaluable in the diagnosis of bony lesions, have limited utility in the evaluation of soft tissue neoplasms. Radiographs can be helpful in determining whether there is any bony involvement, and fatty tumors may present as areas of lucency on a radiograph. Additionally, radiographs of vascular tumors may show phleboliths, often the key to diagnosing this condition. The greatest value of radiography lies in its ability to detect the presence of matrix mineralization. The pattern of mineralization can be an important indication as to the nature of a lesion; therefore, appropriate characterization of mineralization on radiography may allow for a quick and accurate diagnosis. Characterization of mineralization may be difficult or misleading with an MRI alone, so plain films should always be interpreted alongside an MRI in the evaluation of soft tissue tumors.

Ultrasonography

In recent years, ultrasonography has gained popularity for the evaluation of soft tissue neoplasms, particularly in Europe and Asia, where ultrasonography is the preferred modality for the initial evaluation of palpable soft tissue masses. The advantages of ultrasound include its wide availability; low-cost, real-time imaging capabilities; and lack of ionizing radiation. In the United States, ultrasound is the diagnostic imaging modality of choice for pediatric patients. In small and superficial lesions, ultrasonography is particularly useful for differentiating between cystic and solid masses. Ultrasound can also be used to detect mineralization before it can be seen on radiographs or CT scans. Ultrasonography is the most sensitive modality for detecting the zone phenomenon in myositis ossificans, which presents as a thin, round zone of increased echogenicity corresponding to the area of calcification. The drawback to ultrasonography lies in its operator-dependent nature and its inability to definitively characterize lesions. Many lesions demonstrate a nonspecific appearance on ultrasound, although several studies have shown that lesions greater than 5 cm that have infiltrative margins are almost certainly malignant in nature.[1] In the United States, ultrasound is not routinely used for oncologic staging; instead, it is mainly used to confirm the presence of a suspected soft tissue lesion and to clarify its character.

Computed Tomography

There has been rapid growth in recent years in the use of CT as an adjunct to an MRI for the evaluation of soft tissue neoplasms. The advent of multidetector CT permits multiplanar reformatted thin slice imaging and 3D rendering of images. Faster examination times with CT than with an MRI lead to improved patient tolerance and decreased patient motion artifact. Additionally, CT has a high accuracy rate in the detection of calcifications and ossification that may be missed on an MRI or may be too subtle to detect on radiographs. CT is also helpful in evaluating the relationship between a soft tissue neoplasm and the adjacent bony cortex or marrow. Diagnostic CT angiography has replaced conventional angiography in the evaluation of vascular structures, in most cases, as a result of the less invasive nature of the procedure. A disadvantage of CT is its exposure of patients to ionizing radiation. In addition, CT has a much lower soft tissue contrast resolution than an MRI, which may make fine detail (e.g., a tumor's relationship to neurovascular involvement) difficult to ascertain.

Positron Emission Tomography–Computed Tomography

Although anatomically based imaging modalities are considered the standard of care for the diagnosis of soft tissue neoplasms, functional imaging (PET-CT) is beginning to play a larger role as an adjuvant option. With PET-CT, a radiotracer is administered, generally fluorine-18 fluorodeoxyglucose ([^{18}F] FDG), which is an analogue of glucose that is more avidly trapped in malignant cells than in noncancerous cells. Standardized uptake value (SUV) is often used to characterize lesions on PET-CT; the higher number of SUV indicates increased metabolic activity. Many conditions, such as insufficiency fractures, infectious or inflammatory conditions, postoperative changes, and heterotopic ossification, may have positive PET-CT simulating an aggressive process.[2] The primary benefit of PET-CT is that it allows for whole-body functional evaluation, which makes PET-CT ideal for staging malignant soft tissue tumors. PET-CT is also helpful in assessing response to therapy and monitoring for residual or recurrent soft tissue masses after treatment. In general, effective therapy leads to decreased tumor vascularity and metabolic activity, which results in less uptake of [^{18}F] FDG in the remaining soft tissues, indicating that treatment was successful. PET-CT is a relatively safe imaging modality, with only minor incidences of allergic reactions reported.

Magnetic Resonance Imaging

An MRI is indispensable in the evaluation of soft tissue tumors and has become the modality of choice for orthopedic oncologic imaging. An MRI allows for delineation of anatomic involvement, definition of fascial planes, evaluation of bony involvement, and demonstration of a lesion's relationship to nearby neurovascular bundles. An MRI also offers improved soft tissue contrast when compared to CT. Although, in many instances, an MRI cannot provide a histologic diagnosis, it can provide a reasonable differential based on signal characteristics, morphology, multiplicity, and location of the lesion when this information is considered in combination with the relevant clinical history. Because there are considerable similarities between the appearances of benign and malignant soft tissue tumors on an MRI, a lesion should not be classified as benign unless it can be definitively characterized and named based on specific MRI criteria. When a soft tissue mass cannot be definitively named, based on MRI characteristics, location of the mass, and patient age, it must be classified as an indeterminate mass and clinically managed as a malignancy until proven otherwise.

An MRI is also useful for surgical planning and follow-up. In the case of a sarcoma, an MRI can demonstrate the delineation of the tumor margins, which allows the surgical team to decide on the appropriate surgical approach. It should be noted, however, that there is some overlap between the appearances of tumor recurrence, edema, hemorrhage, and postoperative inflammatory change, which may complicate the interpretation of follow-up images.

One major drawback to an MRI is its unreliability in the detection of calcifications and ossifications. In such situations, radiography and CT are more useful and may, at times, provide clinicians with the diagnosis.

Many pulse sequences are used to evaluate soft tissue tumors on MRI. Standard spin echo T1- and T2-weighted images are the most common pulse sequences used in two or more orthogonal planes (one of which must be axial). In recent years, many institutions have begun using faster imaging techniques, most commonly the fast spin echo method, to produce higher resolution T2-weighted images with reduced examination time and decreased artifact from patient motion. Fat suppression is another important tool in the MRI evaluation of soft tissue tumors. Fat suppression can be used to characterize fat-containing tumors, improve the dynamic range for soft tissue contrast display, and enable more accurate discrimination of signal differences between different tissues on T1- and T2-weighted sequences. A short inversion time inversion recovery (STIR) sequence can be used to suppress signal from fat. STIR sequences also eliminate chemical shift artifact at fat-water interfaces, which can lead to improved lesion-background contrast. When fat suppression is used, a nonsuppressed T1-weighted sequence should also be acquired, which helps identify intralesional fat versus hemorrhage and subtle marrow signal changes in the adjacent bones.

The appearance of soft tissue tumors on an MRI is fairly consistent. On T1-weighted sequences, most soft tissue tumors demonstrate signal intensity similar to that of muscle; on T2-weighted sequences, most soft tissue tumors demonstrate signal intensity higher than that of muscle. There are cases in which a tumor demonstrates signal characteristics specific to that lesion. In these cases, the signal characteristics of the lesion are a direct reflection of the histologic makeup of the mass. This is most often the case in benign lesions but may also occur in a few malignant soft tissue tumors.

Gadolinium-diethylenetriamine pentaacetic acid (Gd-DTPA) enhancement is not believed to be particularly useful in the evaluation of most soft tissue tumors, and so it is not routinely used. There are some cases (e.g., vascular and neural lesions) for which the addition of contrast may provide additional diagnostic information. Gd-DTPA is used in special circumstances only (e.g., distinguishing a cyst from a necrotic or myxoid mass).

One area of soft tissue tumor imaging that often poses a conundrum for the interpreting radiologist is the benign-appearing mass. This type of lesion, interpreted as appearing benign (i.e., a small, superficial, homogeneous, well-defined lesion without evidence of infiltration), may be inappropriately treated with a resection. Pathologic examination may later demonstrate that the lesion is a sarcoma; by then, the time for optimal surgical management may have passed. It has been reported that more than 30% of soft tissue sarcomas may be superficial in location or small in size (i.e., less than 5 cm).[1] Therefore, all soft tissue masses that cannot be definitively characterized by the MRI are classified as *Indeterminate*.

IMAGING FEATURES OF COMMON BENIGN SOFT TISSUE TUMORS

Lipomas, Lipoma Variants, and Atypical Lipomatous Tumors/Well-Differentiated Liposarcomas

Lipomatous tumors are very common in clinical practice. Lipoma variants are defined as fatty tumors with variable amounts of fibrous tissue, chondroid, or bone matrix. The terms *atypical lipomatous tumor* (*ALT*) and *well-differentiated liposarcoma* (*WDL*) are synonyms, with the former term preferred in both superficial and deep locations in the extremities, and the latter term reserved for tumors involving the retroperitoneum and inguinal regions. Dedifferentiation of ALT/WDL is more frequently encountered in deep lesions of the trunk and is rare in extremity lesions. Various authors have suggested that entrapped muscle fibers are a feature of ALT/WDL,[3] and increased patient age and lesion size (greater than 20 cm) have been associated with ALT/WDL compared to lipomas.[3]

MRI findings for lipomatous masses are usually sufficiently characteristic to suggest this diagnosis; however, the distinction among lipoma, lipoma variants, and ALT/WDL is less clear because there is overlap in the MRI features of these lesions. On an MRI, a typical lipoma will demonstrate homogeneous fat signal intensity on all pulse sequences, an appearance similar to that of subcutaneous fat, and complete saturation of signal on fat-suppressed sequences (Figure 3-1). A subtle capsule or pseudocapsule is frequently seen on MR images of superficial lipomas, as are thin septations. Deeper tumors are more likely to have ill-defined and infiltrating margins (Figure 3-2).

Certain MRI features of ALT/WDL may help differentiate these lesions from typical lipomas, such as thickened septa, nodularity, and hyperintensity on fluid-sensitive MRI sequences.[3] Some of these findings are also associated with traumatized benign lipomas with fat necrosis and lipoma variants with nonfatty components (Figure 3-3). The various amounts of fibrous tissue, chondroid, and bone matrix in lipoma variants produce heterogeneity on MR images. Hibernoma is a lipoma variant in which brown fat predominates; brown fat typically demonstrates a slightly different signal intensity than subcutaneous fat on all sequences, resulting in a unique MRI appearance (Figure 3-4).

Benign Neurogenic Tumors

Solitary benign peripheral neurogenic tumors comprise two major groups: schwannoma (neurilemoma) and neurofibroma. Schwannomas are slightly less common than neurofibromas, and together these lesions constitute about 10% of all benign soft tissue tumors.[4] Unlike many other soft tissue tumors, neurogenic tumors may have specific imaging and clinical features, which may be helpful in the diagnosis.

Schwannoma is a slow-growing tumor arising from the outer sheath of a peripheral nerve. The tumor is typically eccentric to the nerve fibers, which may be diagnosed prospectively, especially if proximal and distal nerve fibers are visualized on the MRI (Figure 3-5). It may be difficult to recognize the associated nerve fiber when tumors arise from small nerve branches. The flexor surfaces of the extremities (particularly the ulnar and peroneal nerves), mediastinum, retroperitoneum, head, and neck are the most common

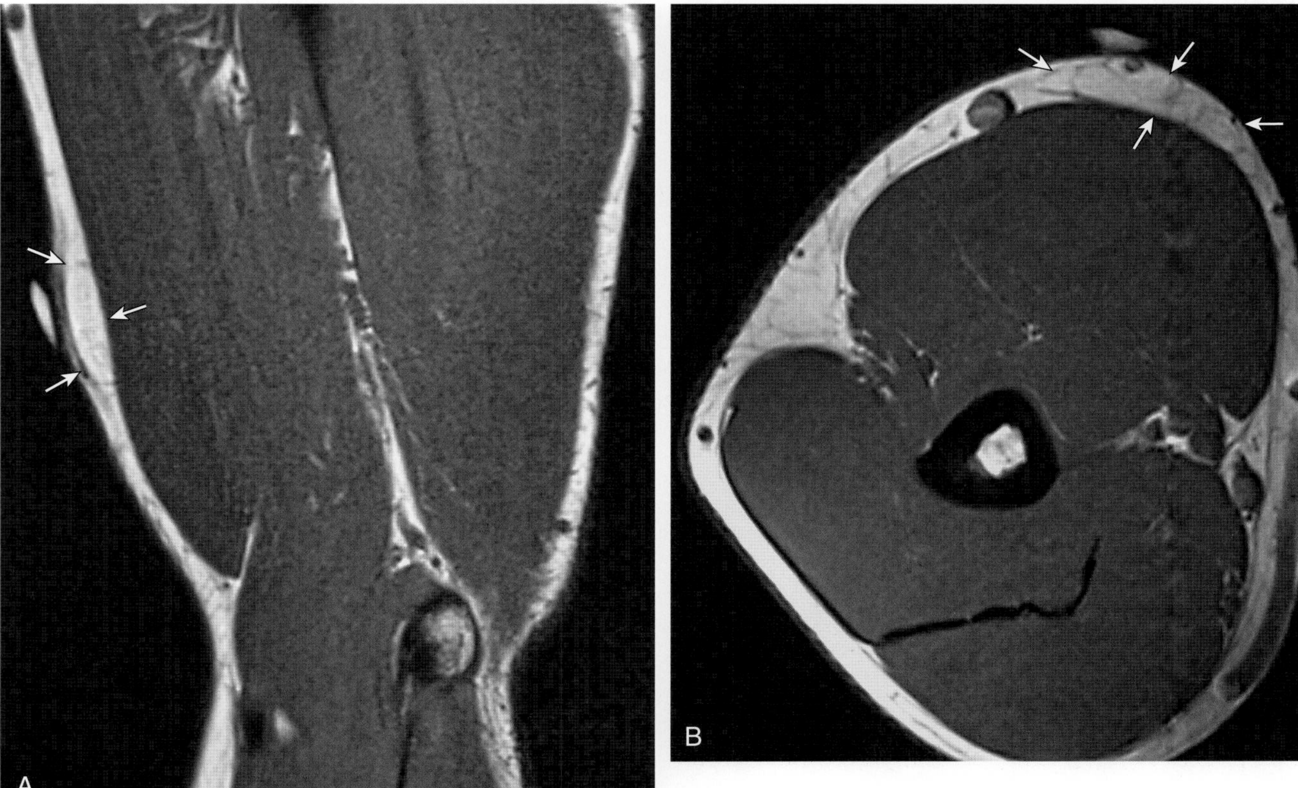

FIGURE 3-1. Sagittal (A) and axial (B) T1-weighted images showing a small subcutaneous mass with signal intensity identical with adjacent subcutaneous fat surrounded by a thin capsule (arrows) consistent with a lipoma. Complete saturation of fat signal on the fat saturated T2-weighted axial images (C). *Continued*

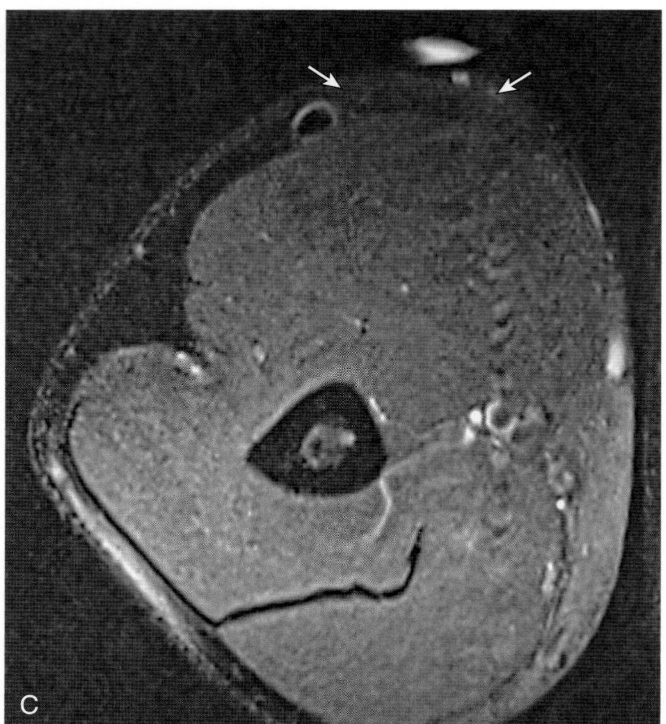

FIGURE 3-1, cont'd

sites. Long-standing and large lesions, known as giant ancient schwannomas, may have cystic changes, calcification, hemorrhage, and fibrosis that may be mistaken for more aggressive tumors on imaging.[5]

Localized or solitary neurofibromas are also slow-growing lesions with a centrally entering and exiting nerve, which gives a fusiform shape to the tumor. Unlike schwannomas, neurofibromas often lack a capsule, and the tumor tissue cannot be separated from normal nerve fibers on imaging and at surgery. Neurofibromas are usually seen in the second and third decades of life.[4]

Schwannomas and neurofibromas share many imaging features on an MRI. Both present as well-defined, often elongated masses that rarely exceed 5 cm in diameter.[4] Paraspinal lesions typically have a dumbbell shape, which may enlarge the surrounding neural foramen through pressure erosion over a long period of time. Continuity with a nerve, the most helpful diagnostic MRI feature, is usually evident on images of lesions arising from larger nerves. Differentiation of schwannomas and neurofibromas based on the position of the tumor relative to the nerve (eccentric versus central) is often difficult, especially when smaller nerves are involved. Intramuscular neurogenic tumors may be surrounded by a thin rim of fat; this creates the split-fat sign on T1-weighted MR images, especially along the long axis of the extremity as a result of slow growth over an extended period of time (Figure 3-6). Most

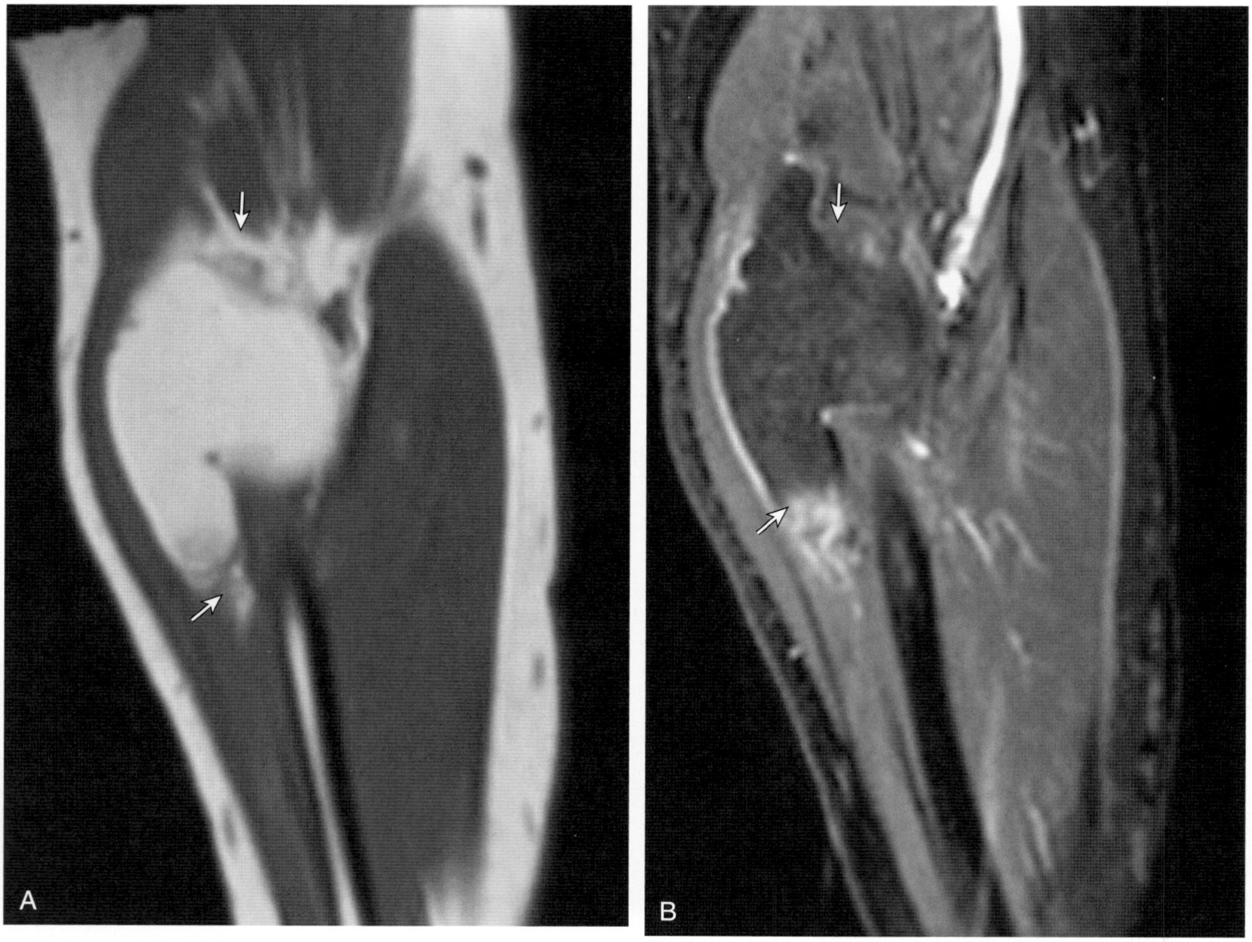

FIGURE 3-2. T1-weighted coronal images of the left forearm (A) shows a deep seated lipoma with poorly defined margins (arrows). Postcontrast T1-weighted fat saturated images in coronal plane shows mild septal enhancement and poorly defined margins (B).

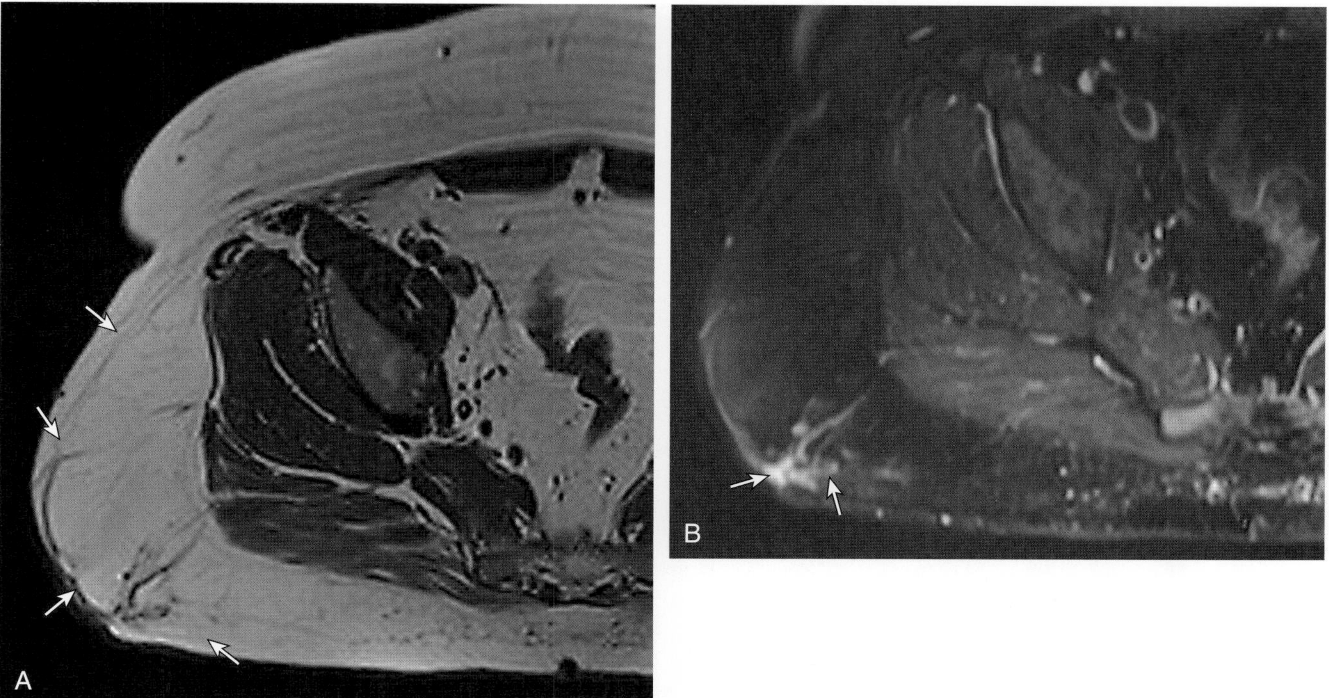

FIGURE 3-3. Axial T1-weighted image of the pelvis (A) shows a large fatty mass with ill-defined margins (arrows). Linear areas of nonfatty tissue (arrows) shows hyperintense signal on fat-suppressed T2-weighted axial images (B) corresponding to fat necrosis on histologic examination.

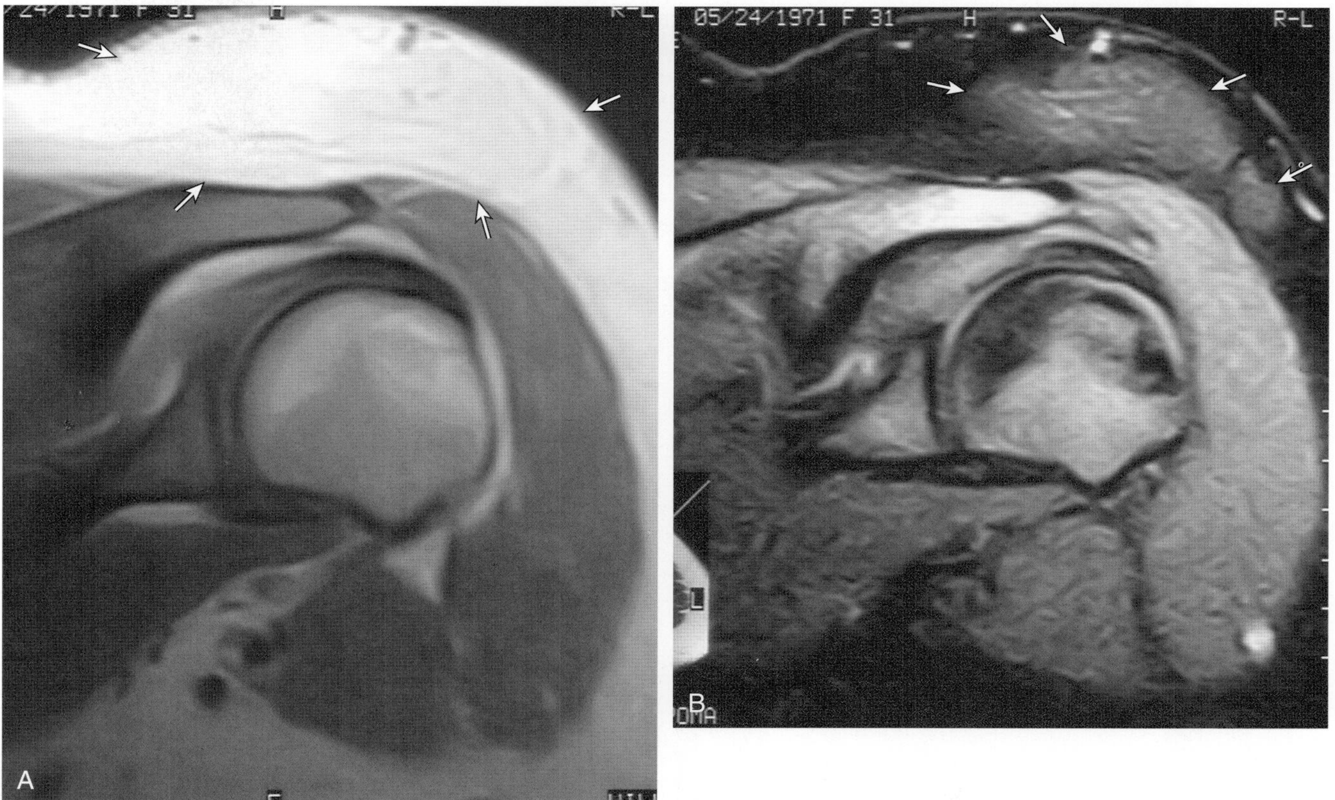

FIGURE 3-4. Coronal T1-weighted images of the left shoulder (A) shows a subcutaneous mass with signal intensity similar to that of adjacent subcutaneous tissues and ill-defined margins (arrows). Fat-suppressed T2-weighted coronal images shows incomplete saturation of signal within this mass, not typical of simple lipoma (B). Excisional biopsy revealed a hibernoma.

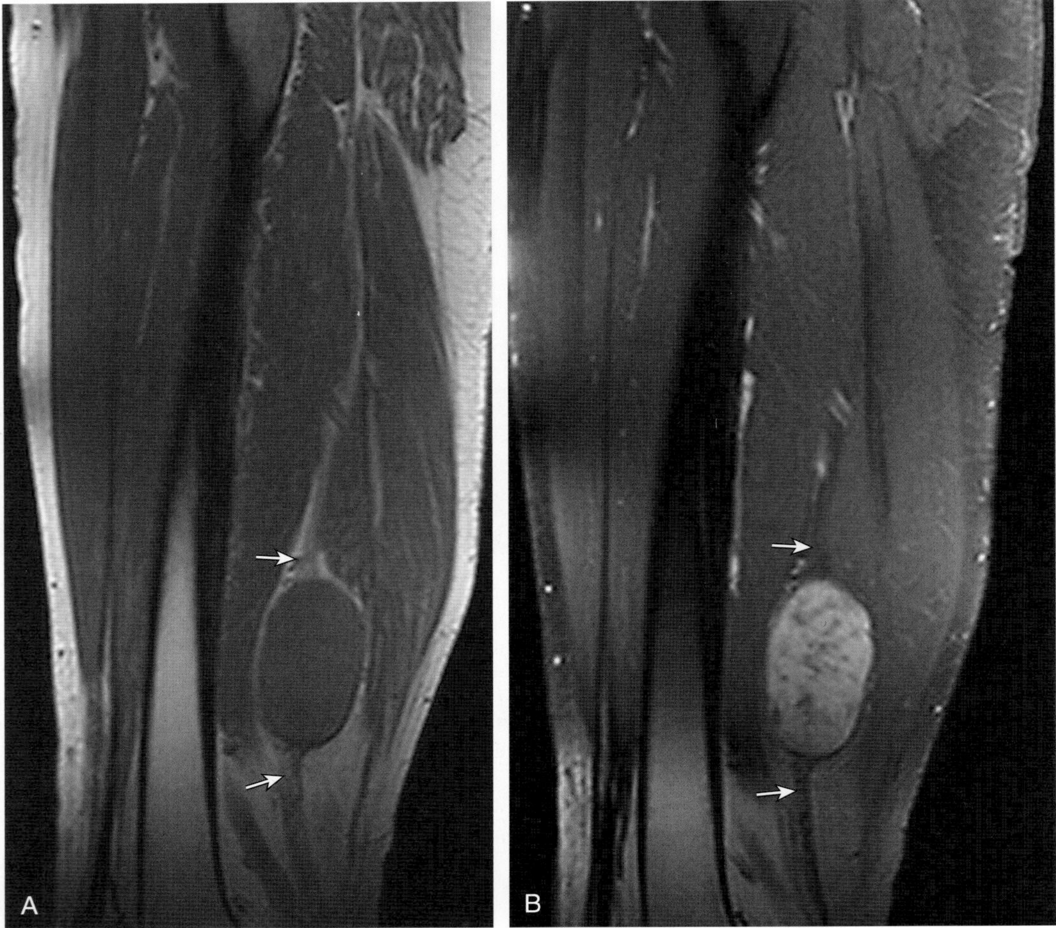

FIGURE 3-5. Sagittal T1-weighted (A) and sagittal T2-weighted fat suppressed (B) images of left thigh show an intermuscular ovoid mass associated with the sciatic nerve. Nerve fibers are visualized proximal and distal to the mass (arrows).

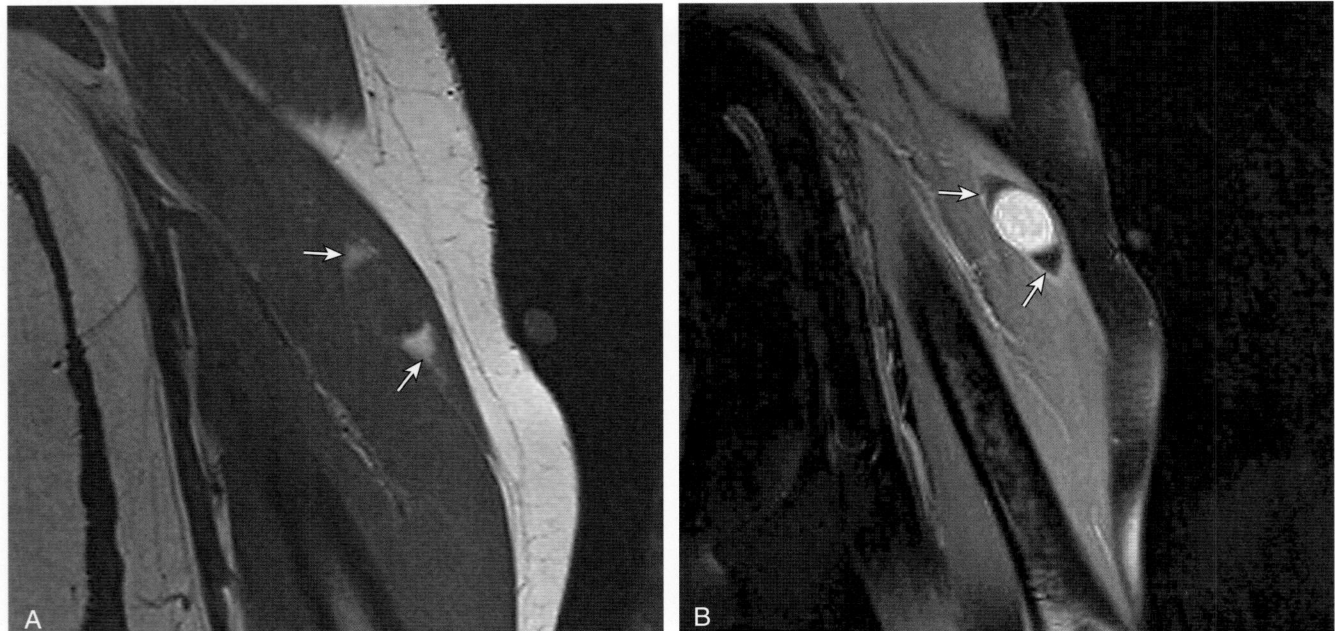

FIGURE 3-6. Coronal T1-weighted (A) and T2-weighted (B) images of the left arm show an ovoid mass with proximal and distal curved linear areas of fat signal intensity consistent with split fat sign, typical of a schwannoma. Postcontrast T1-weighted fat suppressed image (C) shows heterogeneous enhancement pattern (arrow heads).

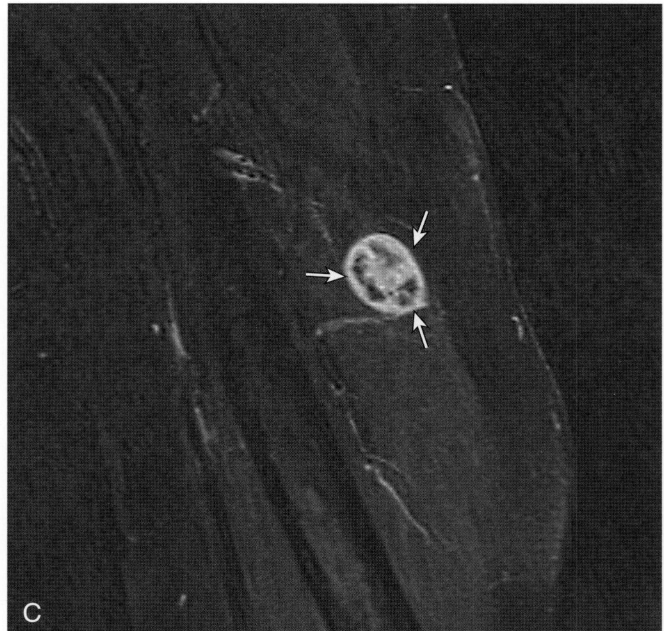

FIGURE 3-6, cont'd

benign neurogenic tumors are isointense or slightly hyperintense to muscle on T1-weighted images and are markedly hyperintense to fat with a variable degree of heterogeneity on T2-weighted images. On fluid-sensitive sequences, these tumors may exhibit high signal intensity in the periphery and low-to-intermediate signal intensity centrally. This appearance is likely caused by myxoid material peripherally and fibrous tissue centrally, so-called *target sign*.[4] Although the target sign was initially thought to be pathognomonic of neurofibromas, it has also been observed in schwannomas and even in malignant peripheral nerve sheath tumors (MPNSTs). Multiple small ring-like structures (*fascicular sign*) within the neurogenic tumors may be visualized on an MRI, representing the fascicular bundles.[4]

On contrast-enhanced images, small neurogenic tumors often show intense and relatively homogeneous enhancement, whereas large lesions may demonstrate predominantly peripheral, central, or heterogeneous nodular enhancement. Atrophy of innervated muscles distal to the tumor is another imaging finding that is suggestive of neurogenic tumors.

Neurofibromas are typically associated with neurofibromatosis type 1 (NF1). Neurofibromas can occur in anywhere in the body, including skin, subcutaneous tissues, and viscera. There are three types of neurofibromas: localized, diffuse, and plexiform.

All three types of neurofibromas may be associated with NF1. Localized neurofibroma is the most common type seen with NF1. Although less common, plexiform neurofibromas are essentially pathognomonic of NF1 (Figure 3-7). Plexiform neurofibromas usually develop during childhood and adolescence and can precede the appearance of cutaneous neurofibromas. Because of their large size, these lesions commonly extend beyond the epineurium into the surrounding tissue. Plexiform neurofibromas may be associated with massive and disfiguring enlargement of an extremity called *elephantiasis neuromatosa*, which may be associated with bony hypertrophy. Growth of neurofibromas is usually slow,

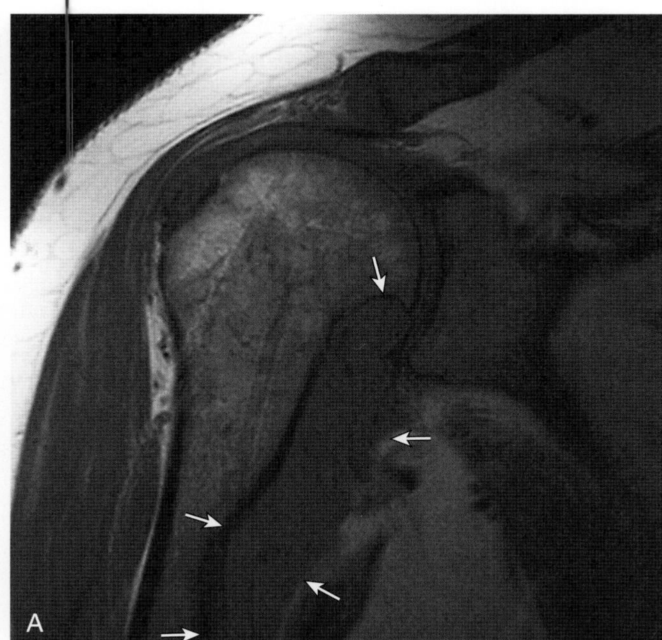

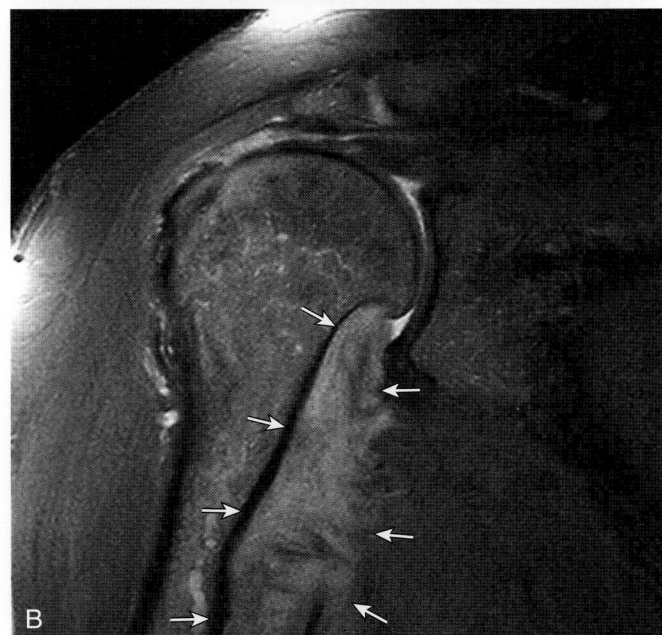

FIGURE 3-7. T1-weighted coronal image (A) of the right shoulder shows a tubular large lesion with ill-defined margins extending along the proximal humerus medially (arrows) with smooth erosion of the humeral cortex. Moderately diffuse enhancement of this mass (arrows) on postcontrast T1-weighted fat saturated images (B).

although faster growth can be seen during pregnancy, puberty, or malignant transformation.[6]

Benign Vascular Lesions

Several classification systems have been proposed for vascular anomalies. In 1996, the International Society for the Study of Vascular Anomalies adopted and expanded two leading classification systems.[7] Two categories of vascular anomalies are considered: vascular tumors (with infantile hemangioma being the most common) and vascular malformations (VMs). Benign VMs and tumors comprise a wide, heterogeneous spectrum of lesions that sometimes create diagnostic and therapeutic challenges for clinicians. VMs are the outcome of defects in vascular formation during embryonic development. These lesions do not proliferate, although the dilated blood vessels within these lesions may gradually enlarge as the child grows. VMs are subcategorized according to the type of their flow as low-flow (capillary, venous, lymphatic) lesions, high-flow lesions (arterial malformations, such as arteriovenous malformations [AVMs] or arteriovenous fistulas [AVFs]) or combined low-flow/high-flow lesions.

Low-Flow Vascular Malformations

Venous malformations are the most common peripheral VM.[8] Venous malformations are usually septated lesions and mistakenly often called a *hemangioma* by radiologists. Extremities are the most common location where they account for almost two-thirds of VMs.[8] Venous malformations are present at birth, but symptoms usually appear in late childhood or early adulthood. These lesions show intermediate to hypointense signal intensity on T1-weighted images and increased signal intensity on T2-weighted and STIR images. Internal fluid-fluid levels are rare, likely caused by hemorrhage. In cases of thrombosis or hemorrhage, heterogeneous signal intensity can be observed on T1-weighted images (Figure 3-8). Presence of phleboliths often confirms the diagnosis. Phleboliths are difficult to recognize on an MRI, where they appear as small, low-signal-intensity foci on all pulse sequences and easily seen on radiographs (Figure 3-9). Venous malformations commonly have fat interspersed between blood vessels. When fat becomes the dominant part of the mass, it may be confused with a lipoma variant.

Lymphatic malformations are the second most common type of VM.[9] They are usually located in the neck and rarely in the extremities.[8]

Lymphatic malformations consist of lymph-filled cysts lined with endothelium, resulting from sequestered lymphatic sacs that fail to communicate with peripheral draining channels. Lymphatic malformations present as microcystic (composed of multiple cysts smaller than 2 mm in a background of solid matrix) or macrocystic (larger cysts of variable sizes) types.[8]

On an MRI, lymphatic malformations are usually seen as lobulated, septated solid-appearing masses with intermediate to decreased signal intensity on T1-weighted images and increased signal intensity on T2-weighted and STIR images (Figs. 3-10 and 3-11). Internal fluid-fluid levels are common. Lymphatic malformations tend to be infiltrative and involve multiple tissue planes, giving an aggressive imaging appearance.

Contrast-enhanced MRI is very helpful in the diagnosis of lymphatic malformations. There is usually no significant enhancement of microcystic type, whereas macrocystic type may have a peripheral and septal enhancement with no enhancement in the center. Central enhancement may be seen in some cases of microcystic type, which is typically caused by septal enhancement of the small cysts or enhancement of the venous component in mixed malformations.[8]

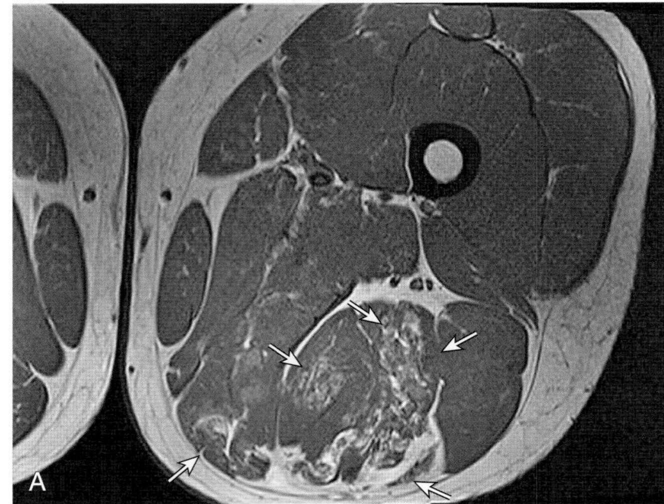

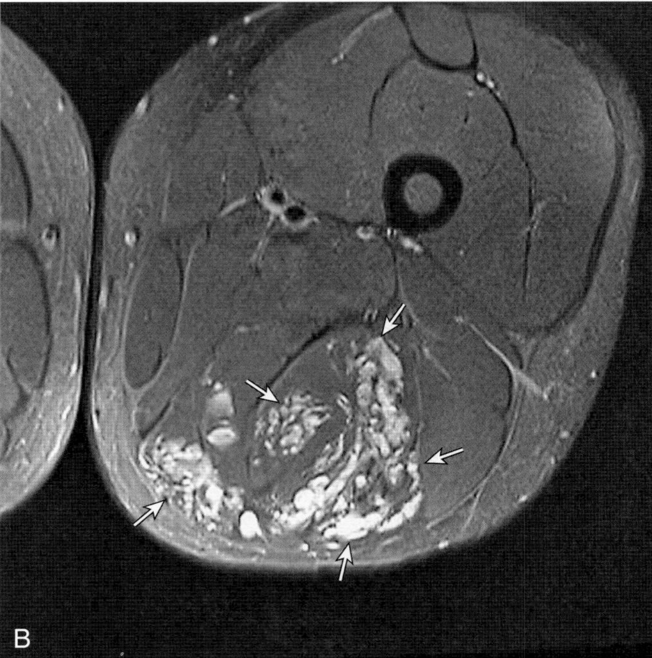

FIGURE 3-8. Axial T1-weighted (A) and T2-weighted (B) images of the left thigh show an ill-defined mass-like region composed of tubular structures consistent with blood vessels (arrows). Note fat-like signal intermixed between these blood vessels.

Capillary malformations are areas of congenital ectasia of thin-walled, small-caliber vessels of the skin and in 0.3% of children at birth and demonstrate cutaneous red discoloration.[9] They predominantly involve the head-neck region[10] and typically are confined to the dermis or mucous membranes, although they may also be a sign of more complex underlying anomalies, such as Sturge-Weber, Klippel-Trenaunay, and Parkes Weber syndromes.[10] The diagnosis of capillary malformation is usually made clinically without a need for imaging, unless an underlying syndrome is suspected. MR imaging findings of capillary malformations are subtle and nonspecific, such as thickening of overlying skin or subcutaneous tissues if no deeper involvement is present.

Capillary-venous malformations are low-flow malformations formed from dysplastic capillary vessels and enlarged postcapillary vascular spaces.

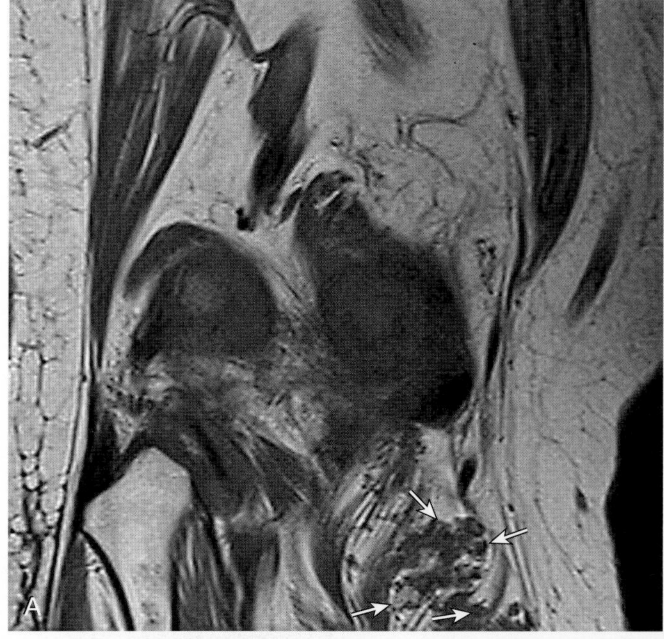

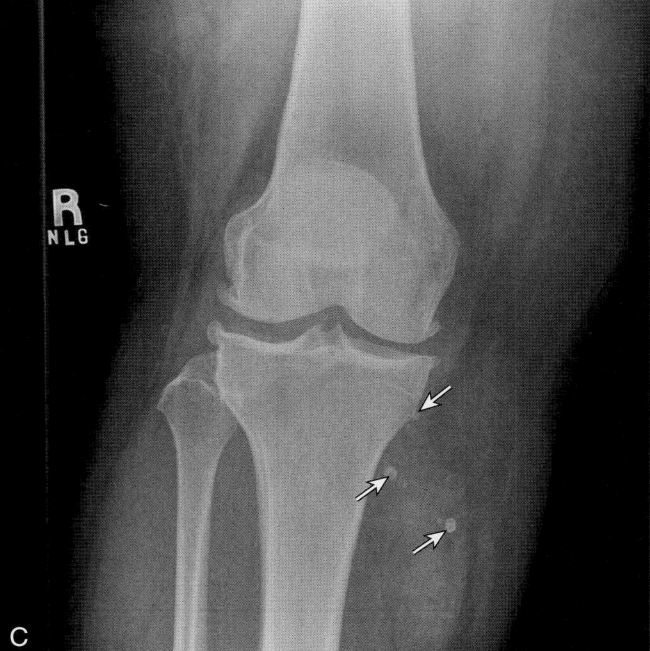

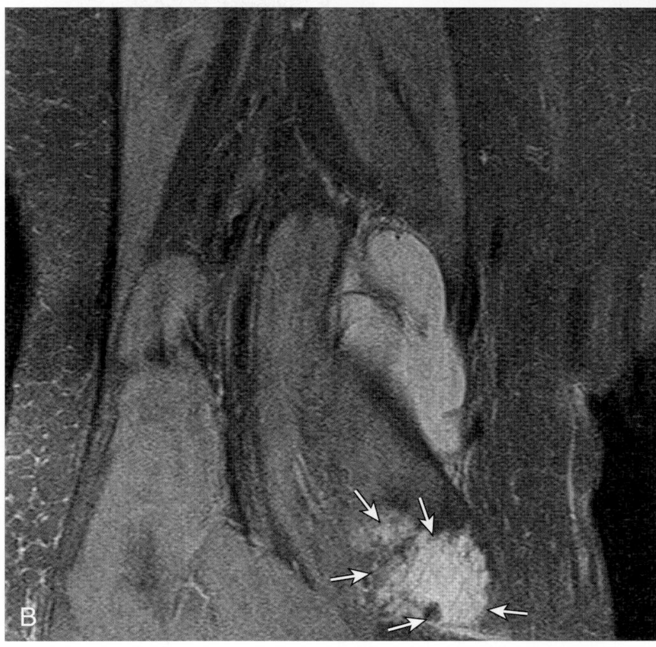

FIGURE 3-9. Coronal T1-weighted (A) and coronal T2-weighted (B) images of the right knee show prominent blood vessels intermixed with fat (arrows) typical of a venous malformation. Subtle hypointense signal on MRI (arrows) correspond to calcified phleboliths easily visible on the knee radiograph (C).

Imaging findings are nonspecific and similar to those of venous malformations. MR imaging can be helpful because capillary-venous malformations typically show early homogeneous enhancement when a dynamic contrast-enhanced study is obtained.[8]

High-Flow Vascular Malformations

High-flow malformations are less common, representing approximately 10% of VMs in the extremities.[11]

AVMs are complex anomalies that consist of feeding arteries, draining veins, and a nidus composed of multiple dysplastic vascular channels that connect the arteries and veins. AVFs are much simpler, formed by a single vascular communication between an artery and a vein.

Although present at birth, AVMs do not usually become evident until childhood or adulthood. Like other VMs, they generally increase proportionally in size as the child grows. The growth of AVMs may be increased because of hormonal changes during puberty or pregnancy or as a result of trauma, thrombosis, or infection.

MRI findings of AVMs include high-flow serpentine and enlarged feeding arteries and draining veins, which appear as large flow voids with absence of an encapsulated mass (Figure 3-12). Areas of high signal intensity on T1-weighted images may represent areas of hemorrhage, intravascular thrombosis, or flow-related enhancement if contrast

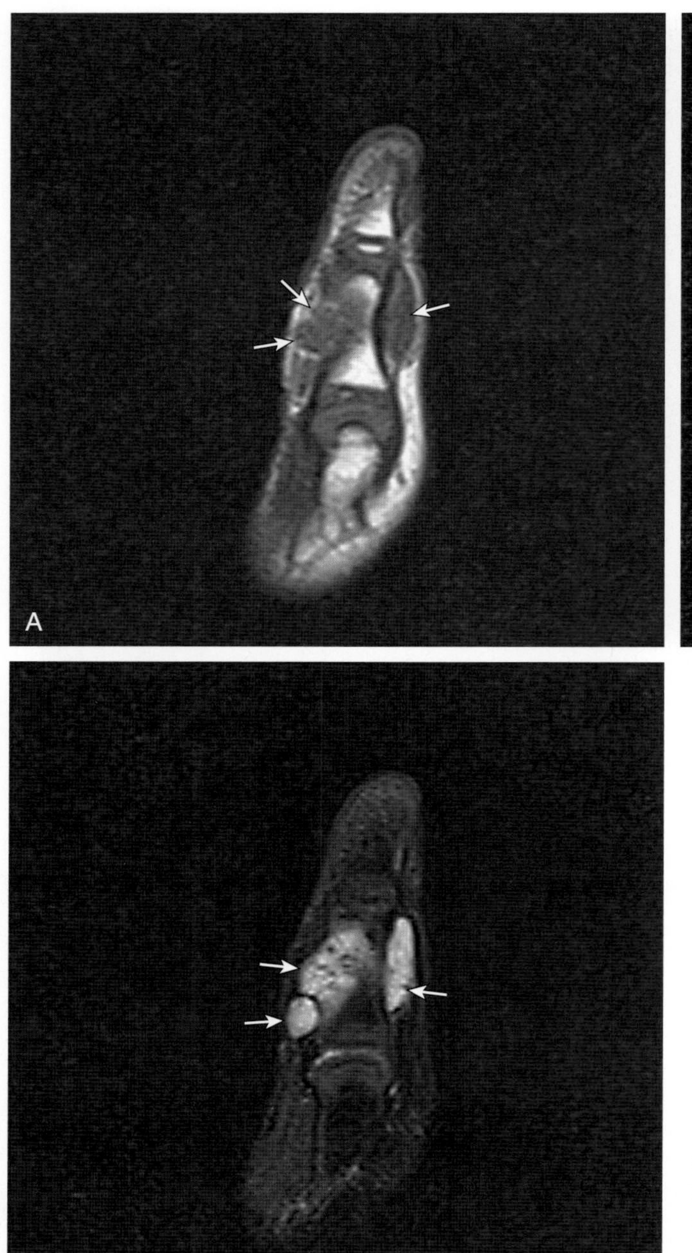

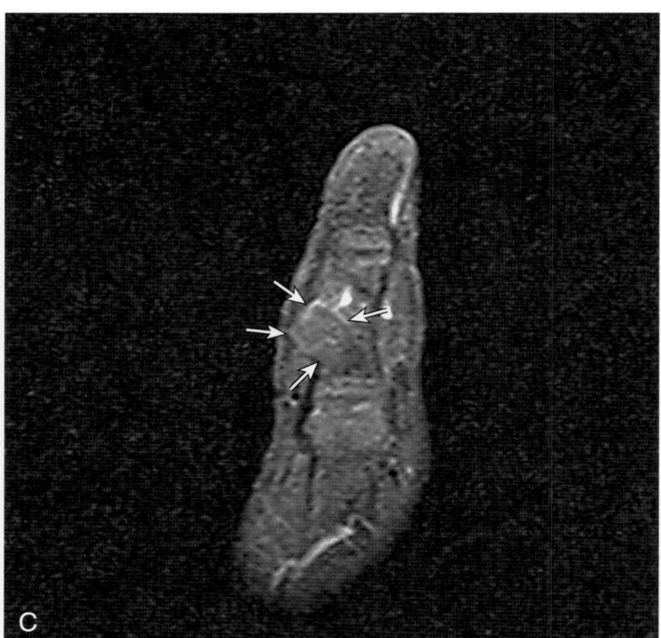

FIGURE 3-10. Sagittal T1-weighted (A) and fat-suppressed T2-weighted (B) MR images of the left thumb in a 4-year-old male show lobulated multiseptated mass wrapping around the proximal phalanx. Postcontrast T1-weighted fat saturated images (C) show minimal peripheral enhancement (arrows) and no central enhancement typical of a lymphatic malformation.

was given.[12] Contrast-enhanced studies (CT or MR angiogram) are useful in demonstrating the feeding arteries and draining veins.

Congenital AVFs usually occur in the head and neck. The more common acquired AVFs are typically a consequence of a traumatic or iatrogenic injury. MR imaging shows the arterial and venous components with large signal voids without a well-defined mass. Arterial enhancement of a vein is usually diagnostic of this entity. Chronic secondary AVFs may result in the enlargement of proximal supplying arteries and distal draining veins simulating the appearance of AVMs. When a soft tissue mass arising from blood vessels is found and an acquired vascular lesion is suspected, other possibilities should be considered in the differential diagnosis, such as pseudoaneurysms that can occur in the setting of trauma (e.g., femoral vessel injury from iatrogenic catheterization). In these cases, it is important to make the diagnosis prospectively and to avoid biopsy.

Hemangiomas

The term *hemangioma* is used to define a heterogeneous group of benign endothelial neoplasms that include common hemangioma of infancy or infantile hemangioma and congenital hemangioma.[12]

Infantile hemangioma is the most common vascular tumor of infancy,[12] with a prevalence of about 2% to 3% in children, although a higher prevalence (10%) is noted among premature infants of very low birth weight.[12] The most common location

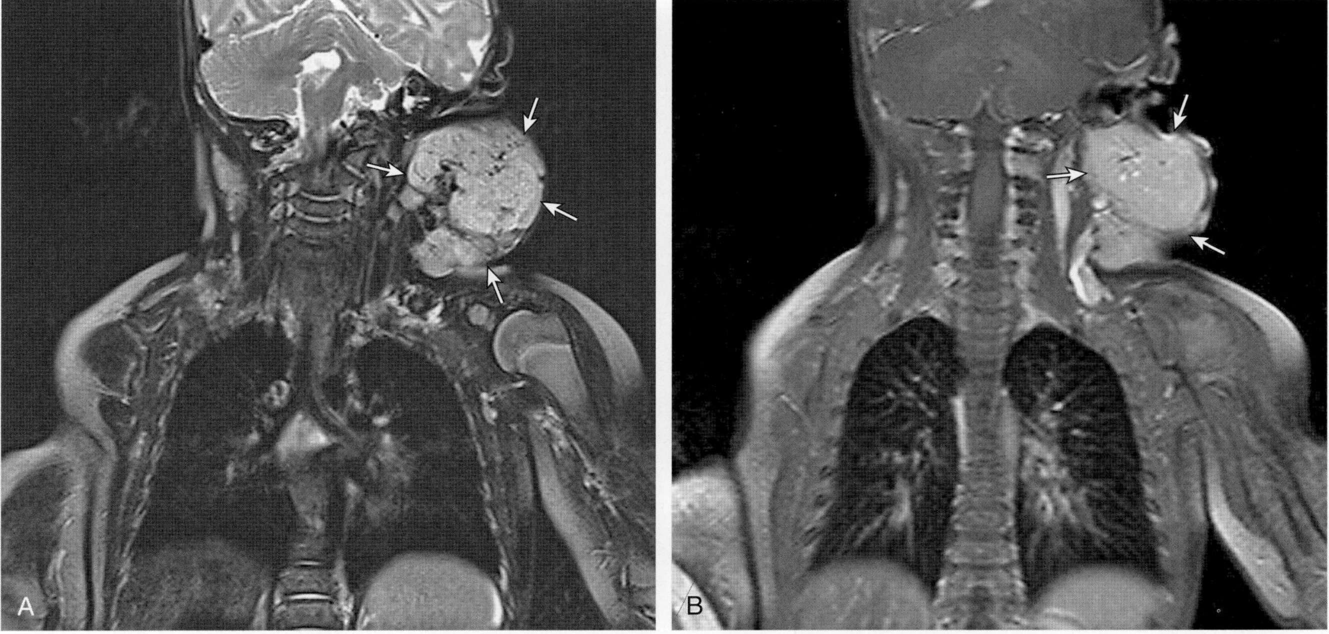

FIGURE 3-11. Coronal T2-weighted (A) and coronal T1-weighted fat saturated postcontrast (B) MR images of an 18-month-old girl show a large mass in the left side of the neck with heterogeneous signal and diffuse enhancement (arrows).

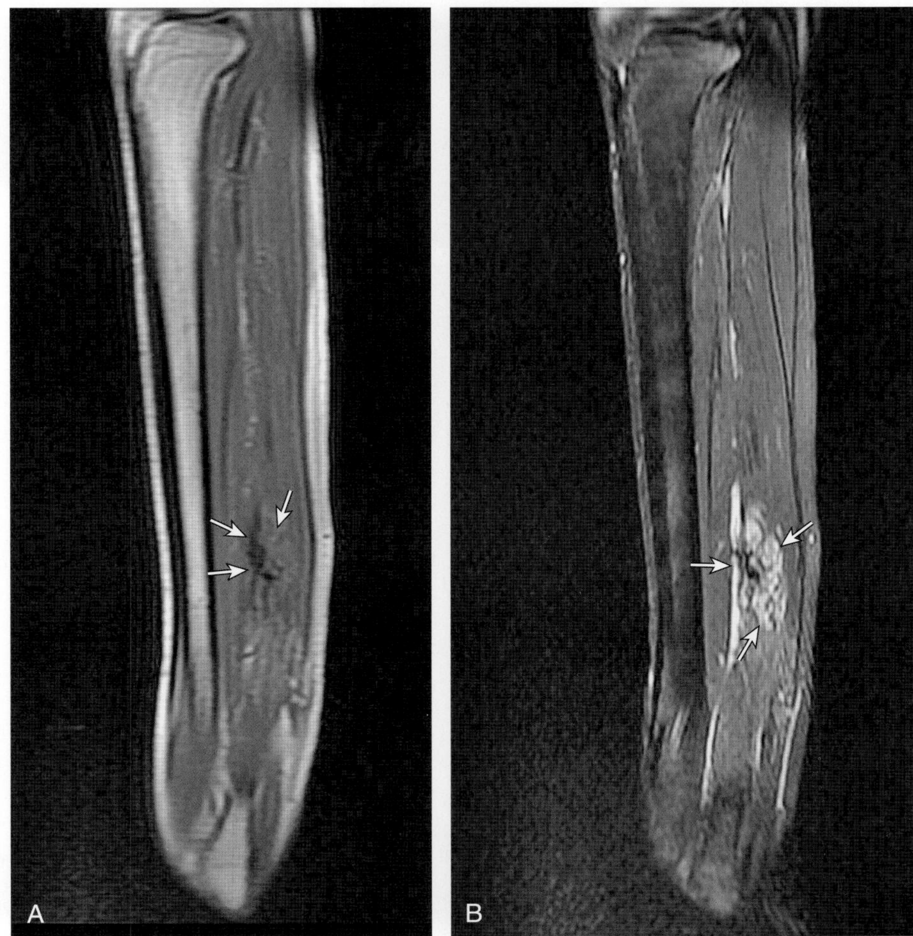

FIGURE 3-12. Sagittal T1-weighted (A) and T2-weighted fat-suppressed (B) images show a vascular malformation with flow voids, suggestive of an AVM.

is the head and neck (60%), followed by the trunk (25%) and extremities (15%).[12]

Infantile hemangiomas are normally not seen at birth but manifest during the first few weeks as rapidly growing subcutaneous lesions that resemble the surface of a strawberry. Diagnosis is made with visual inspection without a need for imaging. The diagnosis is made clinically, in most cases. MR imaging may be obtained in deep lesions with no skin manifestations, or guiding therapy, and follow-up after treatment.

MR imaging features of infantile hemangiomas are variable, depending on the biologic phase. In the proliferating phase, they typically appear as well-defined lobulated masses with high-arterial type flow and enhancement without arteriovenous shunting (Figure 3-13). After a proliferating phase

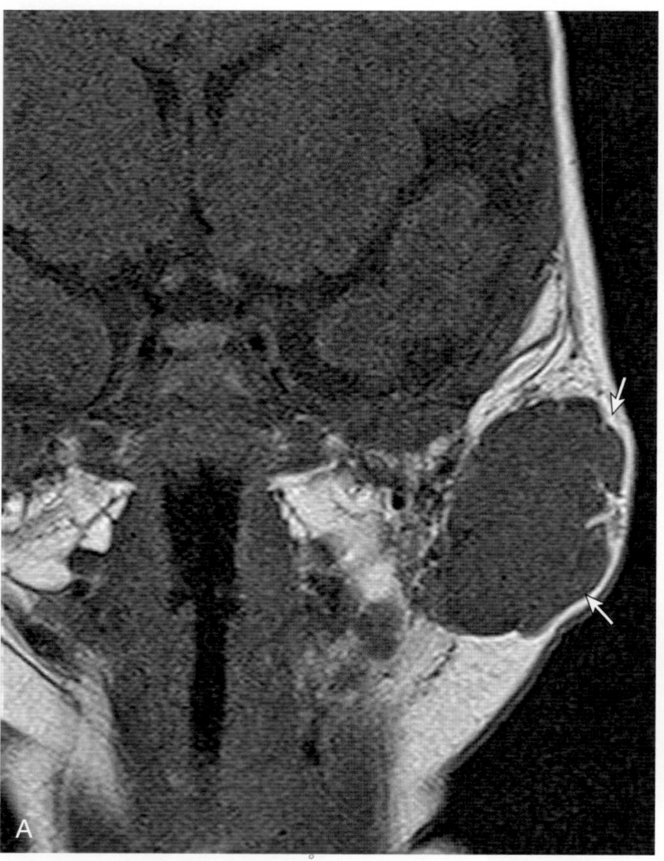

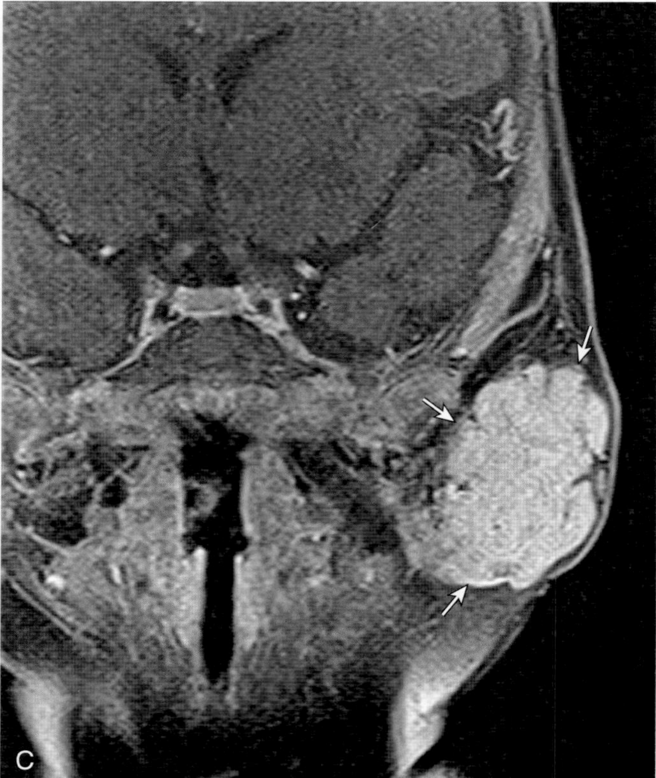

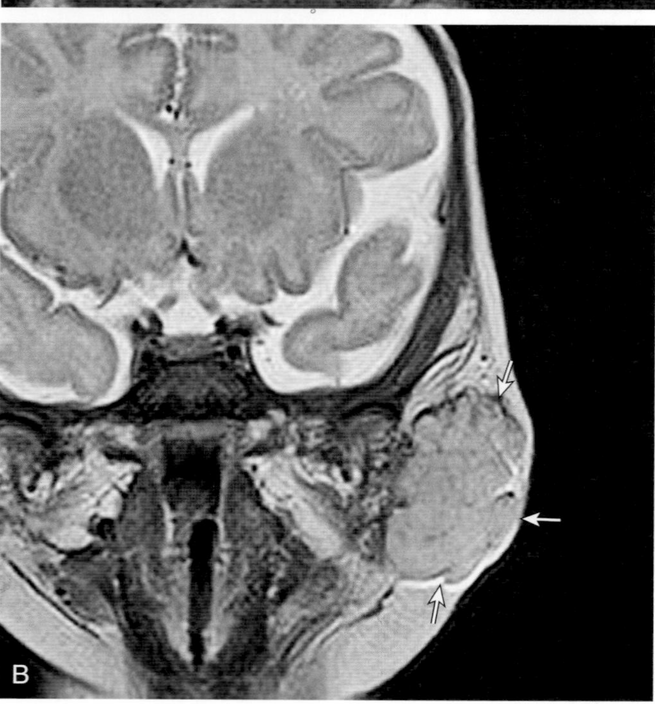

FIGURE 3-13. Coronal T1-weighted (A) and coronal T2-weighted (B) MR images of a 6-month-old boy show a left-sided solid mass (arrows). Diffuse contrast enhancement was observed on coronal T1-weighted fat saturated image (C).

in infancy, a slow but constant regression (involuting phase) can be seen, with the process usually being completed by 7 to 10 years of age.[12] During the involuting phase, MRI appearances are more variable with increasing amounts of fat replacing the lesion and less enhancement in postcontrast studies.[12]

Congenital Hemangioma

Congenital hemangioma is fully grown and clinically evident at birth, although much less common than infantile hemangioma.[8] There are two subtypes of this lesion: rapidly involuting congenital hemangiomas (completely regressed during the first 2 years of life) and noninvoluting congenital hemangiomas (growth proportional to that of the child without regression).[12]

MRI findings are similar to those of infantile hemangioma. Findings such as aneurysms, intravascular thrombus formation, and arteriovenous shunting differ from infantile hemangioma.

Desmoid Tumors

Desmoid tumors (also known as *fibromatosis* or *aggressive fibromatosis*) are rare monoclonal fibroblastic proliferations of musculoaponeurotic structures. Despite their benign nature, these tumors can damage nearby structures through compression and infiltration. Most cases of desmoid tumors are sporadic, and 9% to 18% are associated with familial adenomatous polyposis.[13] Desmoid tumors are locally aggressive and tend to recur, even after complete resection, in nearby tissues.

On T1-weighted MR images, desmoid tumors typically show a hypointense or isointense signal relative to skeletal muscle. On fluid-sensitive sequences, the typical signal intensity is low, although high signal is seen in more cellular lesions (Figure 3-14). Contrast enhancement is variable, with absent or mild enhancement seen in most lesions and intense enhancement seen in more cellular lesions. When the lesions are small, they may be difficult to visualize because they have a signal intensity similar to that of the surrounding muscle; this is especially true for small intramuscular or intermuscular lesions (Figure 3-15). Desmoid tumors appear infiltrative without a well-defined capsule or pseudocapsule (see Figure 3-14).

Myxomas

A myxoma of the soft tissue is a benign neoplasm arising from fibroblasts that produce an excessive amount of

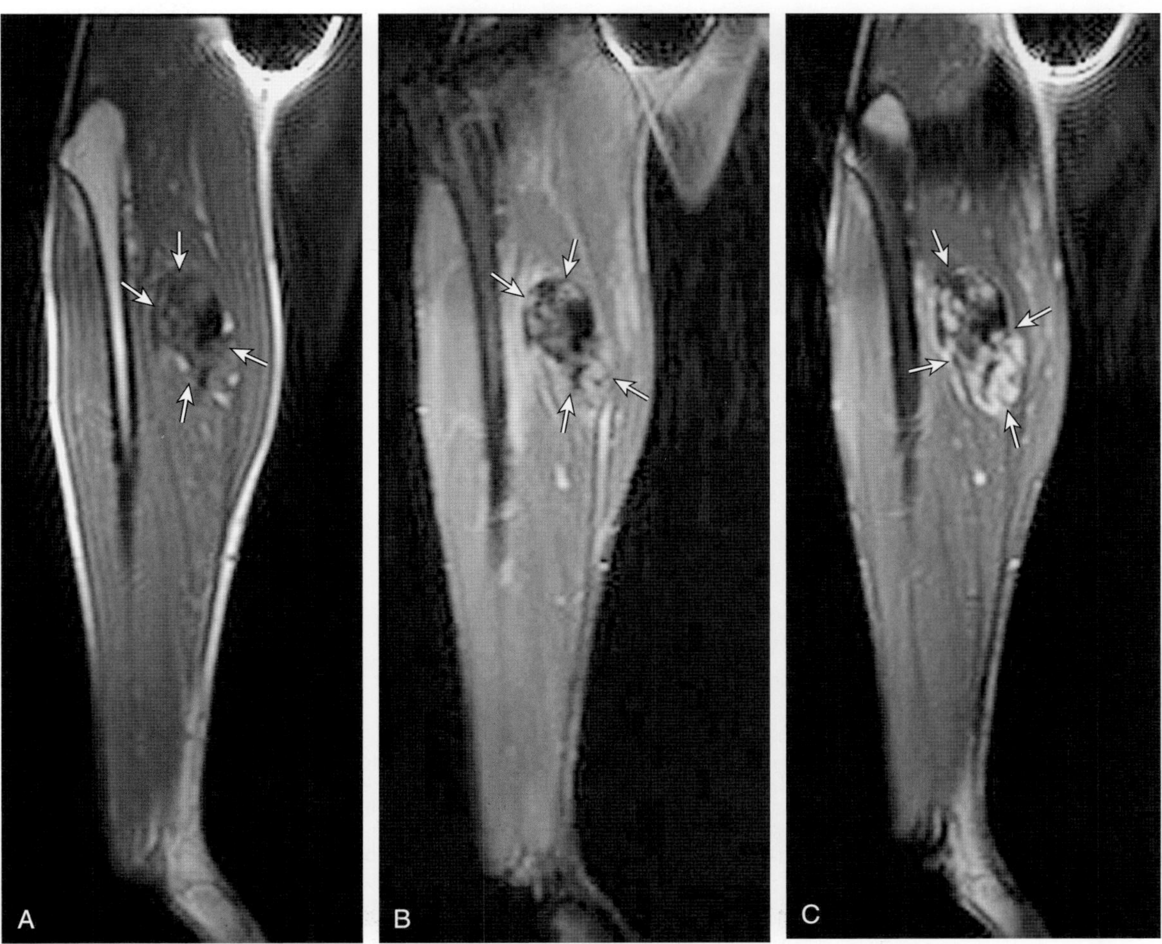

FIGURE 3-14. Coronal T1-weighted (A) and T2-weighted (B) images show a soft tissue mass in the posterior compartment with predominantly low signal on both pulse sequences (arrowheads). Postcontrast T1-weighted fat saturated image (C) shows heterogeneous enhancement of this mass. Note poorly defined infiltrative appearing margins on all pulse sequences.

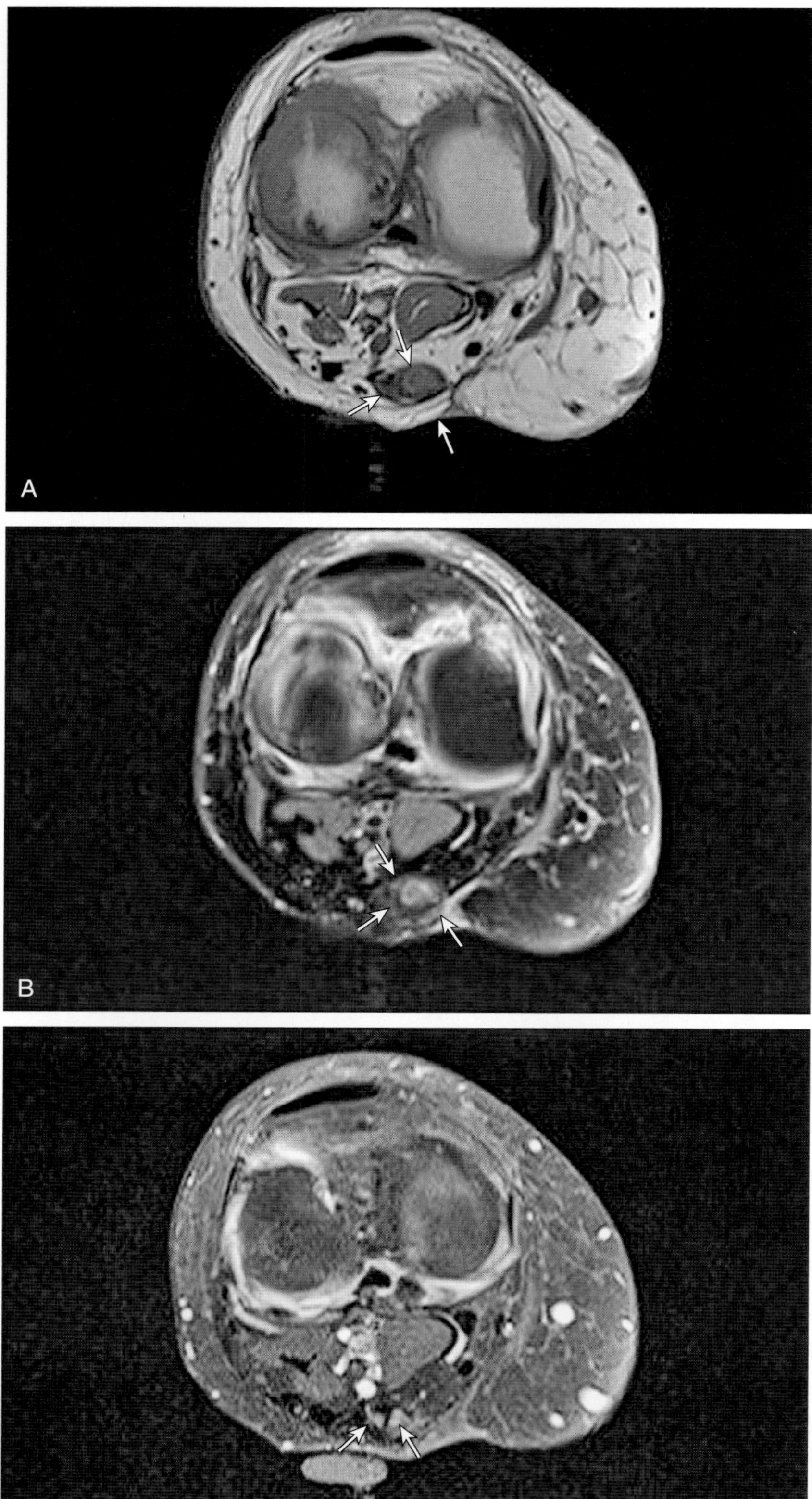

FIGURE 3-15. Soft tissue mass in the popliteal fossa with signal intensity similar to adjacent muscles on T1-weighted (A) and T2-weighted (B) images (arrows). No significant enhancement was observed in postcontrast images (C).

mucopolysaccharide. Myxomas may occasionally be associated with fibrous dysplasia of bone (Mazabraud syndrome).[14]

The intrinsic CT and MRI characteristics of soft tissue myxomas are similar to those of a cyst because myxomas demonstrate high mucin content, a large amount of water, and a low amount of collagen. The large amount of water in myxomas accounts for the hypoechoic appearance of these tumors on ultrasound, low attenuation at CT similar to simple fluid density, low signal intensity on T1-weighted MR images relative to skeletal muscle, and markedly high signal intensity on T2-weighted MR images (Figure 3-16). Intramuscular ganglia are rare, except in periarticular locations or rotator cuff muscles, where they may occur because of delaminating partial tears of rotator cuff tendons. An isolated cystic-appearing intramuscular lesion should raise suspicion, and contrast should be administered to these patients before imaging. Contrast-enhanced MRI more accurately reflects the solid, though hypocellular, nature of myxomas by showing the internal enhancement of these tumors (see Figure 3-16). However, the amount of enhancement can be variable and subtle, so a careful inspection of all images is required. Imaging findings for myxomas and low-grade myxoid sarcomas may overlap; therefore, a differential diagnosis, based on imaging studies, should include both entities.

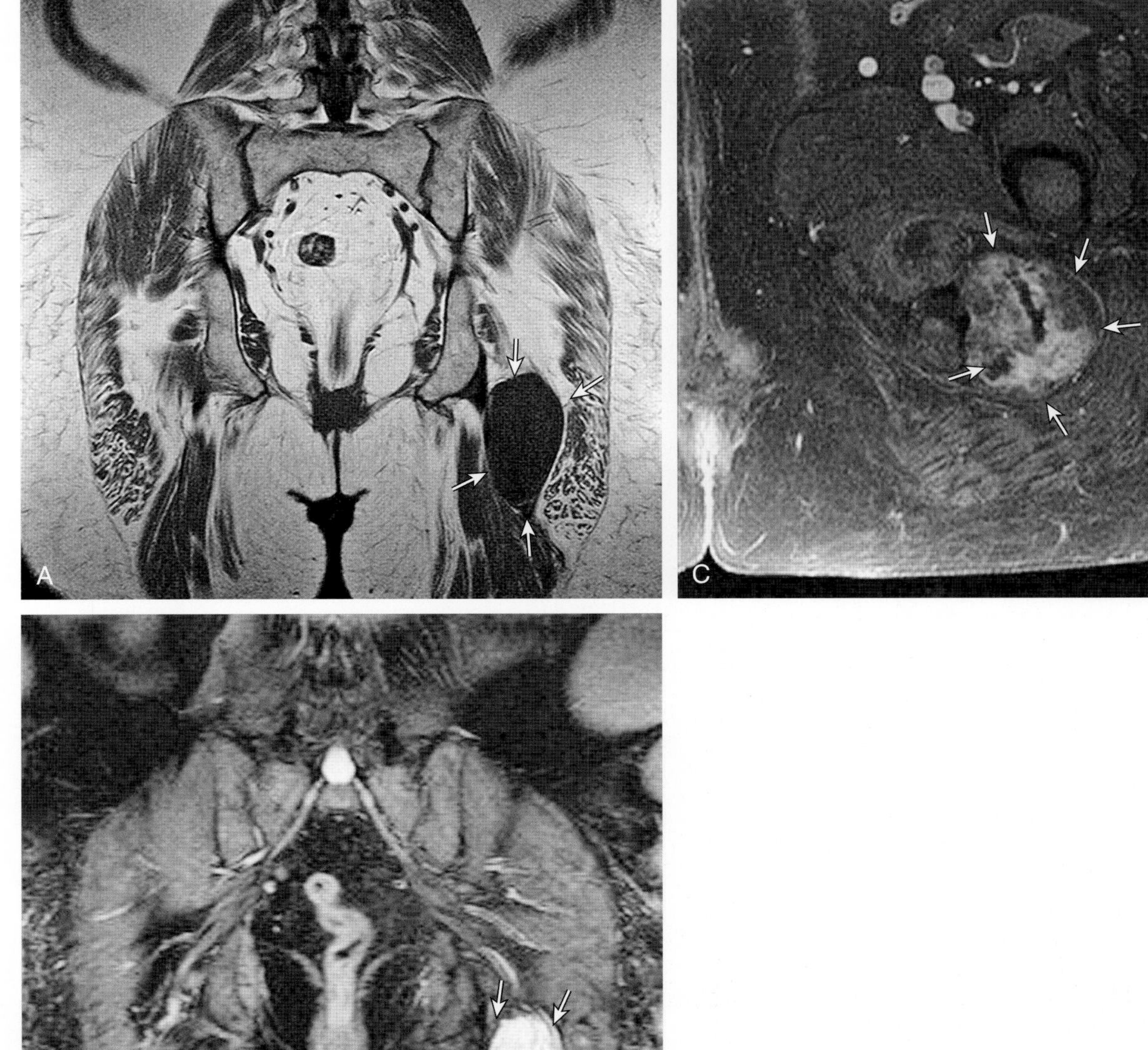

FIGURE 3-16. Coronal T1-weighted (A) and T2-weighted (B) images of the left hip show a large soft tissue mass with hypointense T1- and hyperintense T2-weighted signal intensities (arrows). Postcontrast T1-weighted fat saturated coronal image (C) shows subtle intralesional enhancement (arrowheads) excluding a cyst.

UNCOMMON BENIGN SOFT TISSUE TUMORS

Desmoplastic Fibroblastomas

A desmoplastic fibroblastoma (collagenous fibroma) is a rare benign tumor that is characterized by fibroblastic cells that are sparsely distributed in a collagenous and fibromyxoid background. The growth of this tumor is generally indolent, and most tumors are small, subcutaneous lesions, although larger tumors up to 23 cm have been reported.[15] They tend to behave in a nonaggressive manner, and several studies have reported no recurrences even after marginal excision. These lesions have been found in the arm, shoulder, posterior neck, upper back, abdominal wall, and around the hip joint.[15] Patients usually present with a firm, mobile, painless, slow-growing mass located in the subcutaneous tissues or deeper in the skeletal muscle. Fascia and muscle involvement are frequently seen.

On an MRI, a desmoplastic fibroblastoma has a low signal on both T1-weighted and T2-weighted pulse sequences because of the large amounts of collagen and low cellularity (Figure 3-17). Differential diagnosis for this tumor typically includes desmoid tumor (fibromatosis), which has a similar MRI appearance but is seen usually in younger patients.

Leiomyomas

A leiomyoma is a benign smooth muscle neoplasm that frequently involves the uterus. On an MRI, uterine leiomyomas

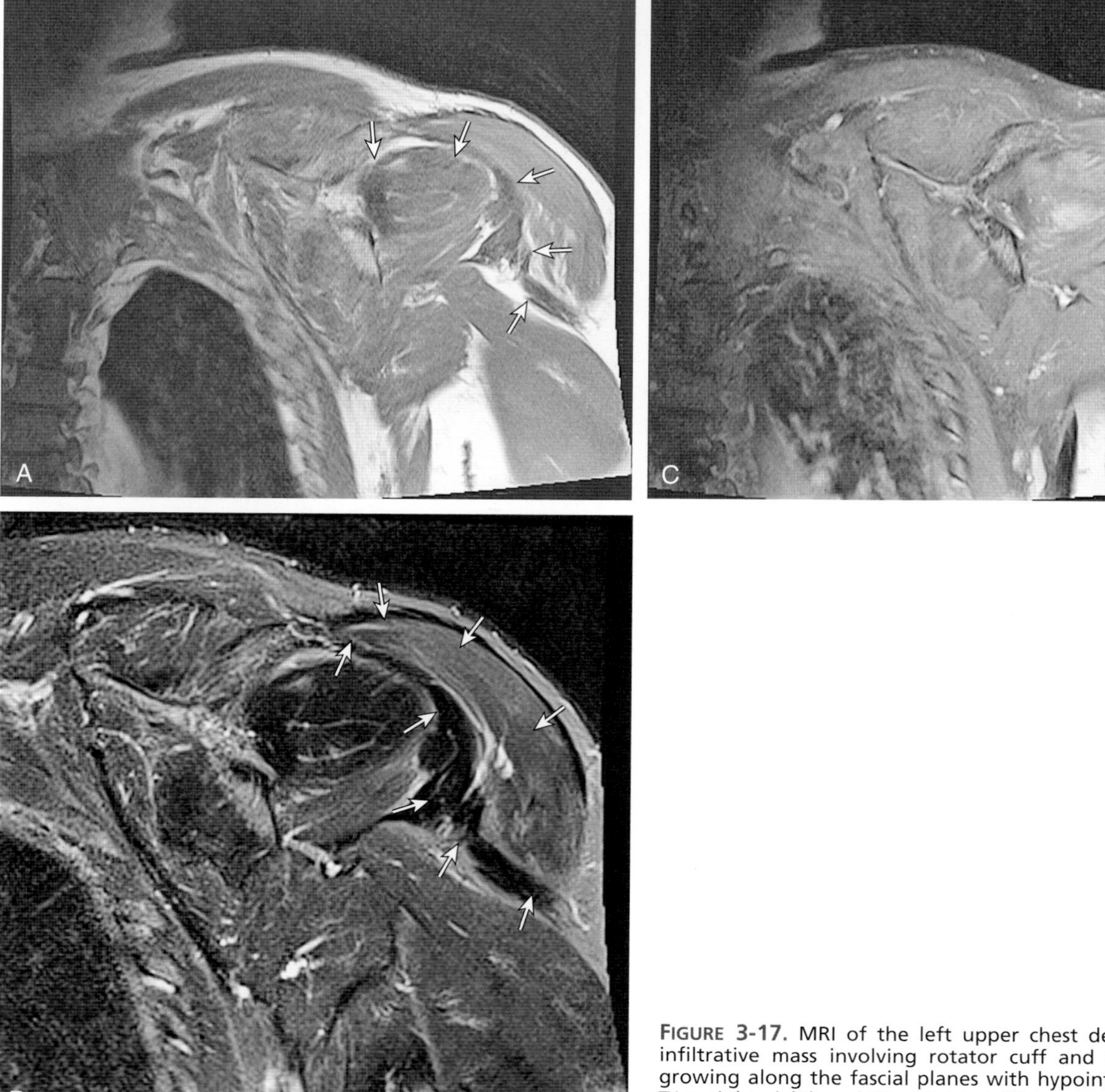

FIGURE 3-17. MRI of the left upper chest demonstrates a large, infiltrative mass involving rotator cuff and deltoid musculature growing along the fascial planes with hypointense signal on both T1-weighted (A) and T2-weighted (B) images (arrows). No significant enhancement was observed on postcontrast images (C).

typically demonstrate low signal intensity relative to that of the myometrium on T2-weighted images and intermediate signal intensity on T1-weighted images (Figure 3-18).[16] Other sites of involvement may include the ovaries, urinary bladder, lung, and gastrointestinal tract.

The skin and subcutaneous soft tissues may also be involved as a result of small vessel involvement, as is the case with vascular leiomyomas. Leiomyomas may also involve larger vessels arising from the smooth muscle of the vessel wall. When in the soft tissues, leiomyomas are usually small and cutaneous or subcutaneous in location. Rarely, leiomyomas may be encountered in the deep soft tissues, which tend to be larger than their superficial counterparts.[16] Soft tissue leiomyomas can be subdivided into three distinct groups. The most common form, the cutaneous leiomyoma, arises from the erector pili muscles of the skin and the deep dermis of the scrotum, labia major, and nipple. The cutaneous leiomyomas are quite small and often present as clustered papules measuring approximately several millimeters each. These lesions are considered dermatologic lesions and are rarely evaluated by imaging.[17]

The second group is called *angioleiomyomas* (angiomyomas or vascular leiomyomas), which are subcutaneous lesions composed of a conglomeration of thick-walled vessels associated with smooth muscle tissue. These lesions are typically small (less than 2 cm) and located in the extremities, with the lower extremity most frequently involved.[17]

The third group, leiomyomas of the deep soft tissues, may be located in the deep soft tissues of the extremities or the retroperitoneum. The retroperitoneal variety is more commonly found in females, likely reflecting an origin from hormonally sensitive smooth muscle similar to uterine lesions.[16]

MRI findings for extremity leiomyomas are nonspecific, with an isointense or hypointense T1-weighted signal relative to skeletal muscle and heterogeneously increased T2-weighted signal with a variable enhancement pattern. Areas of fibrosis and calcification have been reported in deep soft tissue lesions.[17]

Glomus Tumors

The glomus body is a highly specialized arteriovenous anastomosis responsible for thermoregulation. The normal glomus body is located in the stratum reticulare throughout the body but is more concentrated in the subungual region of the digits and the deep dermis of the palm, wrist, forearm, and foot. Glomus tumors are small, usually benign neoplasms closely resembling the normal glomus body, and represent up to 5% of soft tissue tumors of the hand.[18] Multiple glomus tumors are present in only 2% to 3% of cases.[18]

Radiographs in patients with glomus tumors often appear normal, although smooth pressure erosion of the cortex may

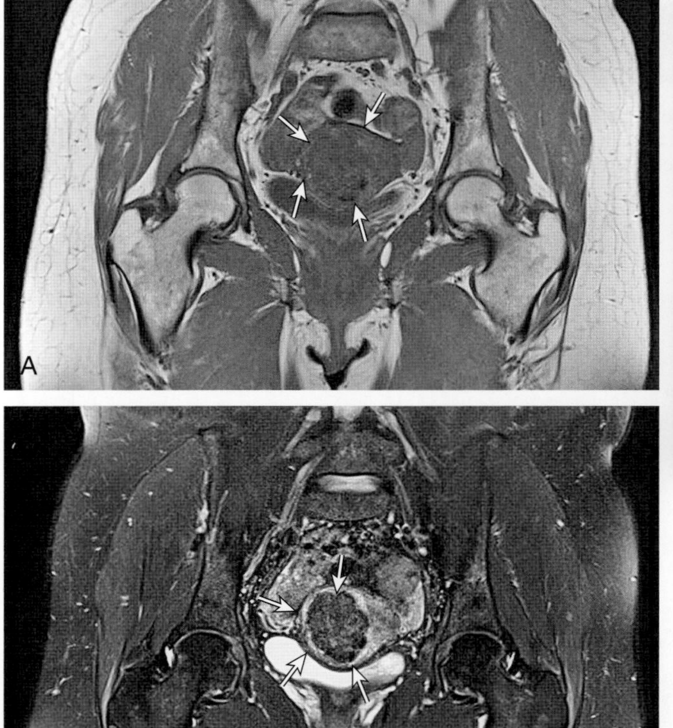

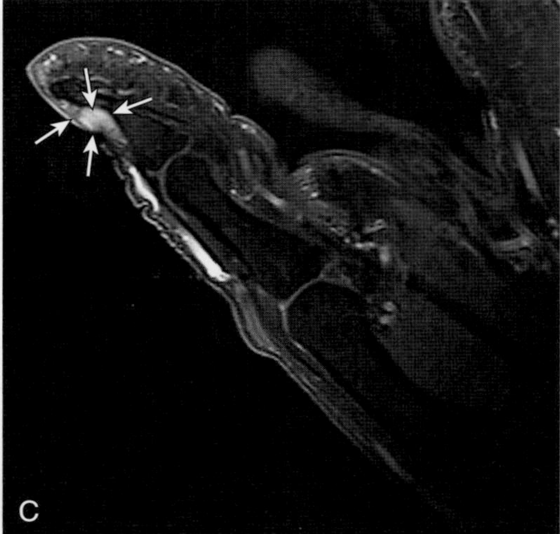

FIGURE 3-18. A 32-year-old female with uterine fibroids. Coronal T1- (A) and T2-weighted (B, C) images show an enlarged uterus with hypointense masses consistent with fibroids (arrows).

be seen. On an MRI, a typical glomus tumor shows nonspecific low T1-weighted and increased T2-weighted signal with avid contrast enhancement because of the highly vascular nature of the tumor (Figure 3-19). When the tumor is located in the nail bed and has intense contrast enhancement, a glomus tumor can usually be diagnosed if the patient presents with an appropriate history. Multiple glomus tumors should be considered in the differential diagnosis when multiple avidly enhancing intramuscular or subcutaneous nodules are seen on Gd-enhanced images (Figure 3-20), especially when sensitivity to temperature or pressure is elucidated in the patient's history.

Fibromas of Tendon Sheath

Tendon sheath fibroma is a rare, slow-growing benign lesion seen in adults between the ages of 20 and 50 years.[19] It is

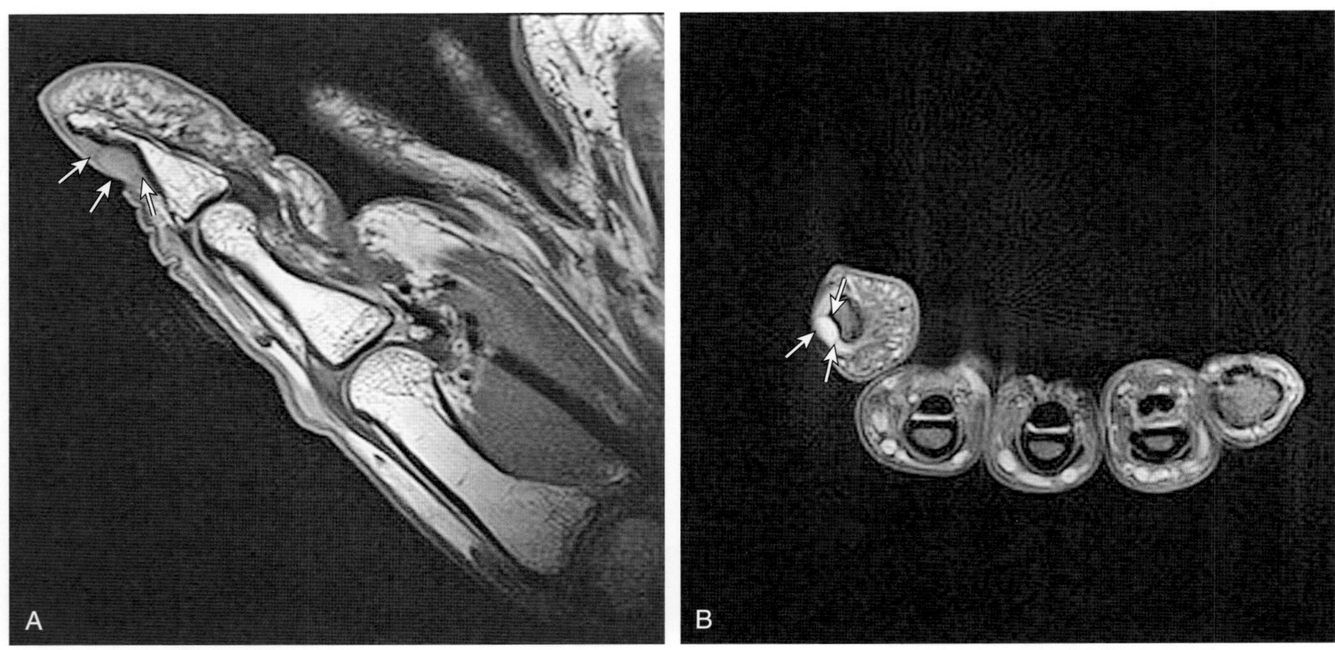

FIGURE 3-19. Small soft tissue mass in the thumb nail bed with subtle erosion of the underlying cortex. This mass demonstrates slightly hyperintense signal compared to muscle on T1-weighted images (A) and markedly hyperintense signal on T2-weighted fat suppressed images (B). There is avid contrast enhancement in postcontrast images typical of hypervascular glomus tumors.

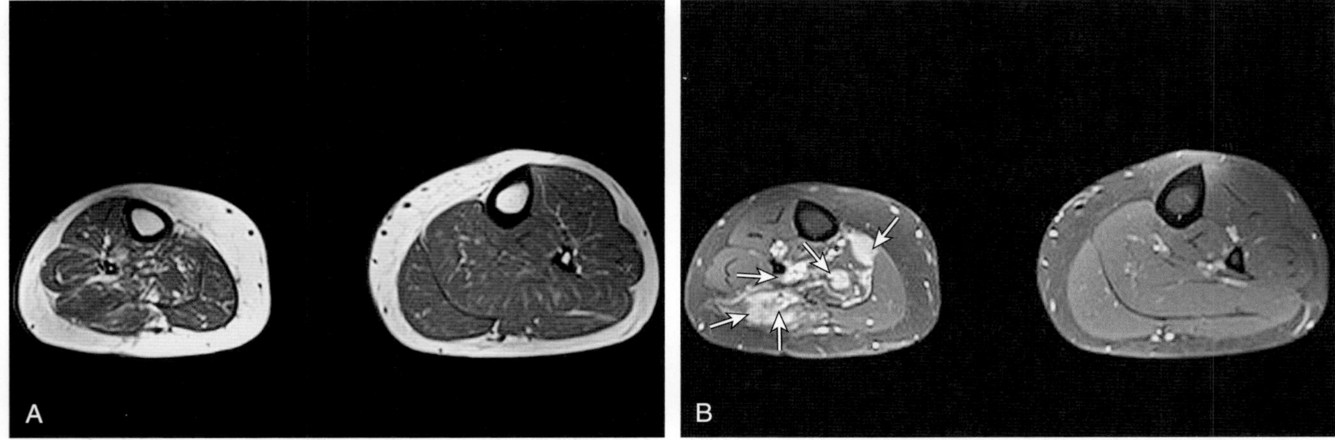

FIGURE 3-20. (A, B) Axial T1-weighted precontrast image shows small intramuscular masses with signal intensity similar to adjacent skeletal muscle. T1-weighted fat saturated axial image shows avid enhancement of these lesions typical of hypervascular glomus tumors (arrows).

difficult prospectively to diagnose fibroma of the tendon sheath because the lesion shares imaging features with giant cell tumor of the tendon sheath. In addition to their common site of origin adjacent to a tendon or tendon sheath, these two lesions are similar in size, location, and MR imaging features.

Most of these lesions are located in the extremities, particularly the fingers, hands, and wrists (82%).[20] These lesions usually present as painless soft tissue masses. In the past, tendon sheath fibroma has been considered a reactive lesion. Recent studies showed a chromosome 2;11 translocation abnormality associated with this condition, suggestive of a true neoplastic etiology.[21]

On an MRI, this lesion is typically seen within tendon sheath abutting the tendon. The lesion typically has a signal intensity that is isointense or hypointense to skeletal muscle on T1- and T2-weighted images, likely because of the large quantities of collagen within the tumor. These imaging features overlap with those of a giant cell tumor of the tendon sheath. In these cases, gradient-echo MR sequences can be used to differentiate between these entities. A giant cell tumor of the tendon sheath may show a blooming artifact (i.e., foci of very low signal intensity within the lesion from chronic hemorrhage), a feature that is not associated with a fibroma of the tendon sheath.

Areas of increased T2-weighted signal intensity may be seen in lesions with increased cellularity or myxoid change. The contrast-enhancement pattern in these tumors is variable, ranging from no appreciable enhancement to marked enhancement.

Myofibromas

Infantile myofibromas and myofibromatosis (multicentric) are the most common fibrous tumors during infancy. The majority of these tumors occur in children under the age of 2 years (88%).[22] The solitary form is more frequently seen in boys involving the head, neck, and trunk. The multicentric form may be present in the soft tissues, bones, and viscera (25% to 35%).[22]

MR imaging characteristics of these lesions are nonspecific and include low signal intensity on T1-weighted images and a variable appearance on T2-weighted images (Figure 3-21). These tumors may show a target sign after the administration of intravenous Gd, likely because of central necrosis.

Granular Cell Tumors

Granular cell tumors are rare tumors showing schwannian differentiation, most commonly occurring in the tongue, breast, skin, and subcutaneous tissues.[23] Most of the tumors are benign, with less than 50 malignant lesions reported.[24] Benign granular cell tumors are usually less than 4 cm in size, round or oval in shape, and superficial in location.[24] On an MRI, these tumors typically have an isointense or hyperintense signal compared to skeletal muscle on T1-weighted sequences and hyperintense peripheral signal, as well as a hypointense central signal intensity on T2-weighted sequences, with variable enhancement in postcontrast images (Figure 3-22).[24]

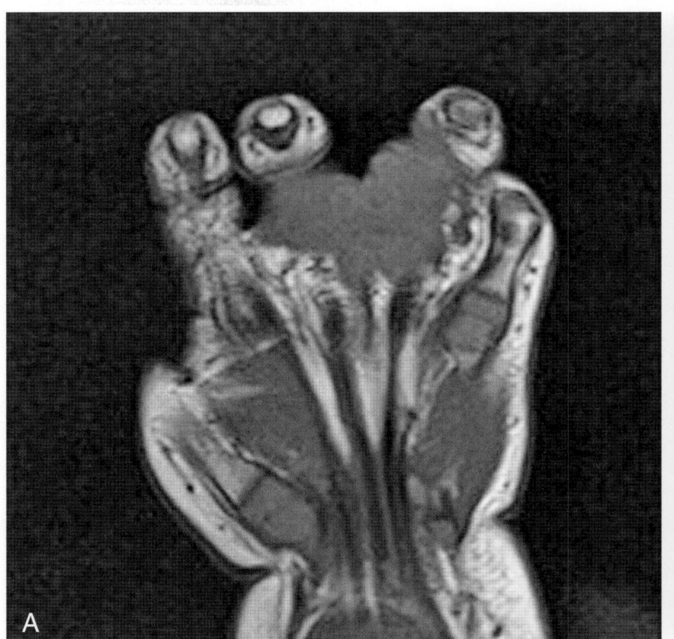

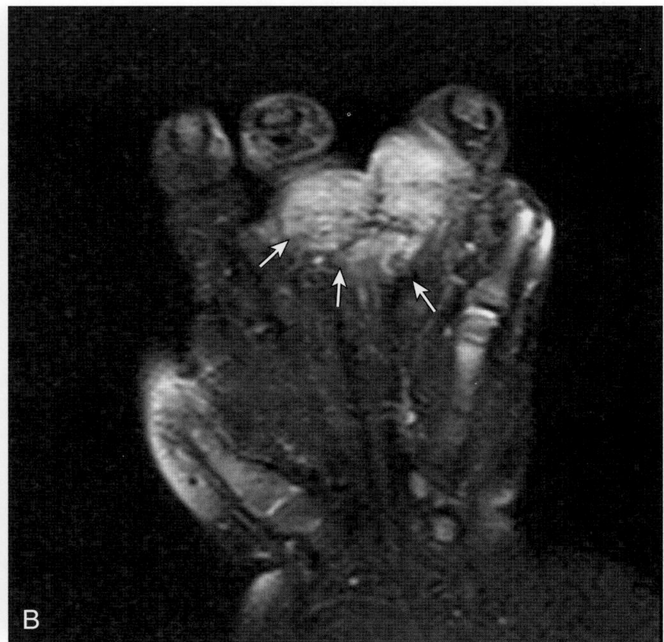

FIGURE 3-21. Coronal MRI of the right hand demonstrates an aggressive, infiltrative lesion involving the third and fourth digits (arrows) with hypointense signal on T1-weighted (A) and hyperintense signal on T2-weighted (B) images with evident contrast enhancement (C).

Continued

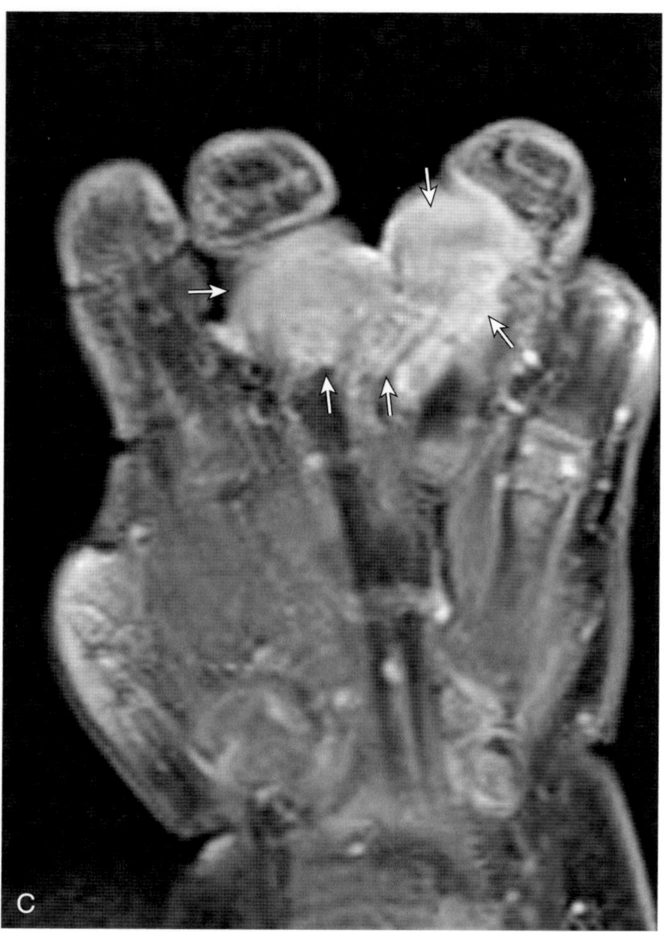

FIGURE 3-21, cont'd

Soft tissue chondromas or osteochondromas are rare benign tumors. They are most commonly seen in the Hoffa fat pad where a typical intracapsular soft tissue chondroma may present as a small round mass on MR imaging (Figure 3-23). These lesions are intermediate or low signal intensity on T1-weighted images relative to skeletal muscle and a variable heterogeneous signal on T2-weighted images.[25] Foci of signal void represent calcifications that may be visualized on radiographs. Prospective diagnoses of these entities are often difficult in other locations where they may appear as an aggressive lesion (Figure 3-24).

Soft Tissue Sarcomas

Soft tissue sarcomas usually present as a painless lump and are often larger than 5 cm at the time of diagnosis. The extremities, especially the thigh, are the most common sites for these tumors, followed by the head, neck, and trunk; however, these tumors can occur anywhere in the body. Men are slightly more likely than women to have soft tissue sarcomas.

On an MRI, a soft tissue sarcoma will typically appear as a soft tissue mass adjacent to the long bones in the extremities. A capsule or pseudocapsule with well-defined margins is usually present (Figure 3-25). The lesion typically displays intermediate T1-weighted signal intensity relative to skeletal muscle and heterogeneous high T2-weighted signal intensity; however, relatively low signal intensity may be seen in lesions with increased fibrous content such as fibrosarcomas. In myxoid sarcomas (e.g., myxofibrosarcomas), the T1-weighted signal tends to be lower because of a high

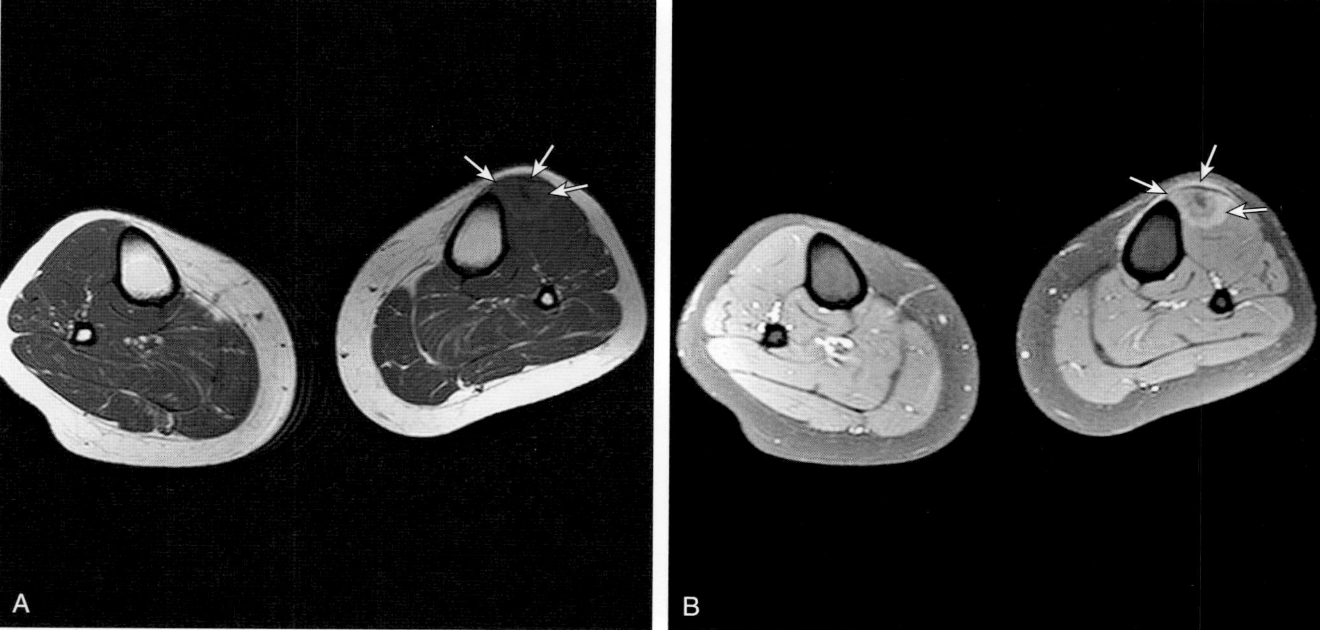

FIGURE 3-22. Axial MR images through left proximal leg show a soft tissue mass in the anterior compartment and abutting tibial cortex (arrows). There is a hyperintense rim of the lesion on T1-weighted images with subtle hypointensity centrally (A). There is more prominent hyperintensity of the rim with central hypointensity on T2-weighted images (B).

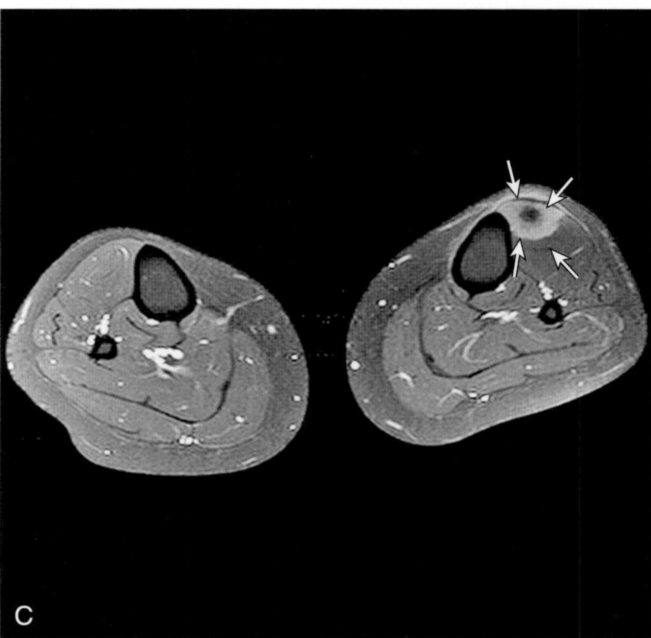

FIGURE 3-22, cont'd. There is thick peripheral enhancement in the postcontrast images (C).

volume of water, with a markedly increased T2-weighted signal (Figure 3-26). Cystic areas and hemorrhage are commonly seen, features that may simulate the appearance of a hematoma (Figure 3-27). Enhancement of solid components with a Gd contrast agent is typically seen. A lack of enhancement, typically in the center of the tumor, correlates with an area of necrosis and could be an important imaging feature for tumors with large areas of necrotic tissue and hemorrhage (see Figure 3-27). Bone involvement is uncommon, although direct invasion may be seen, especially in advanced cases.

Malignant fibrous histiocytoma (MFH) was previously thought to be the most common soft tissue sarcoma in adults. However, the morphologic pattern seen with pleomorphic MFH is actually shared by a variety of poorly differentiated malignant neoplasms. For these reasons, the World Health Organization (also known as WHO) suggested new terminology for the various subtypes of MFH in 2002. The term *undifferentiated pleomorphic sarcoma* that replaced MFH is now used for the small group of pleomorphic sarcomas that do not show a definable line of differentiation, which constitutes approximately 5% of adult soft tissue sarcomas.[26]

Dermatofibrosarcoma protuberans (DFSP) is an uncommon mesenchymal tumor of borderline (intermediate) malignancy that is typically seen in middle-aged adults. Unlike most soft tissue sarcomas, DFSP presents as a slow-growing subcutaneous mass or nodule.[27] The trunk and proximal extremities are most frequently involved.[27] The tumor originates in the dermis and extends gradually into the deeper tissues, although muscle and bone involvement is uncommon. The overlying skin may be discolored (reddish-blue or purple), which may simulate benign lesions, such as a VM or hemangioma. On an MRI, DFSP presents as a superficial soft tissue mass generally

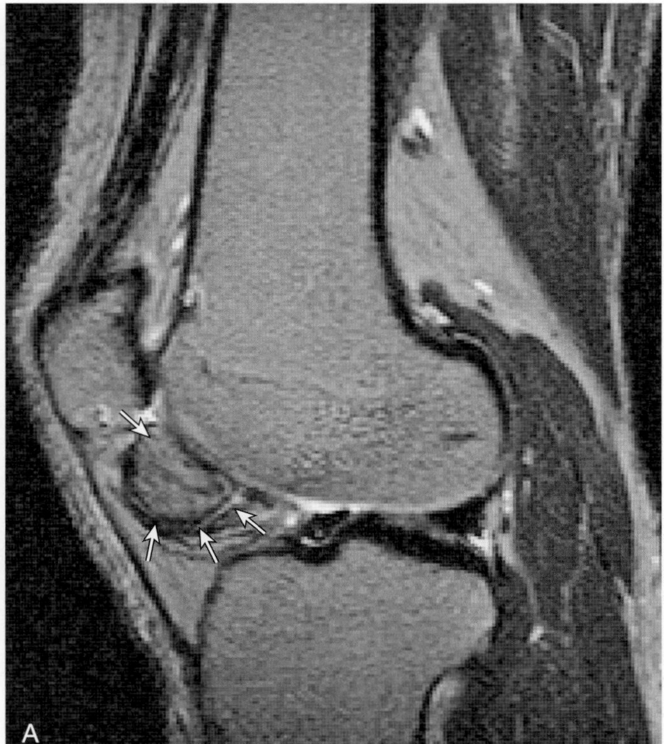

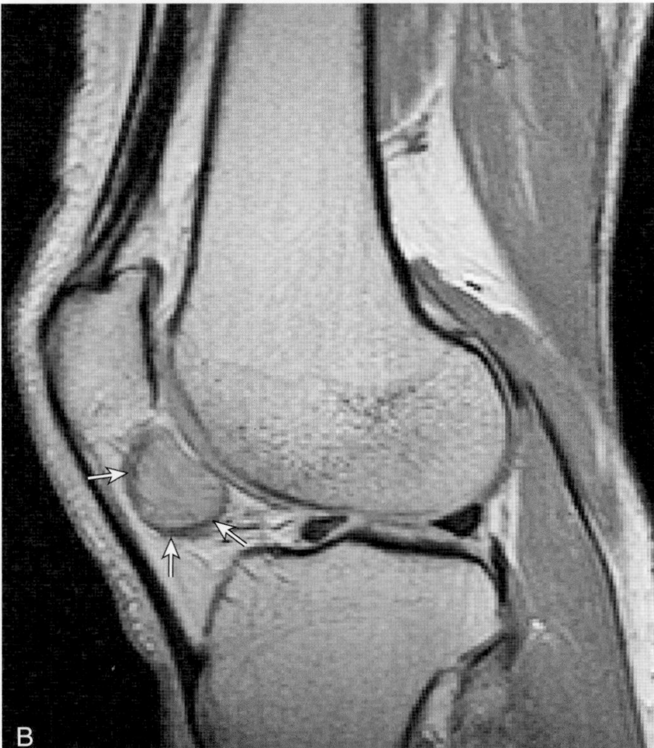

FIGURE 3-23. Sagittal T2-weighted (A) and proton density-weighted (B) images of the right knee demonstrate a well-defined synovial-based mass (arrows) in the Hoffa fat pad with hypointense foci, suggestive of calcification.

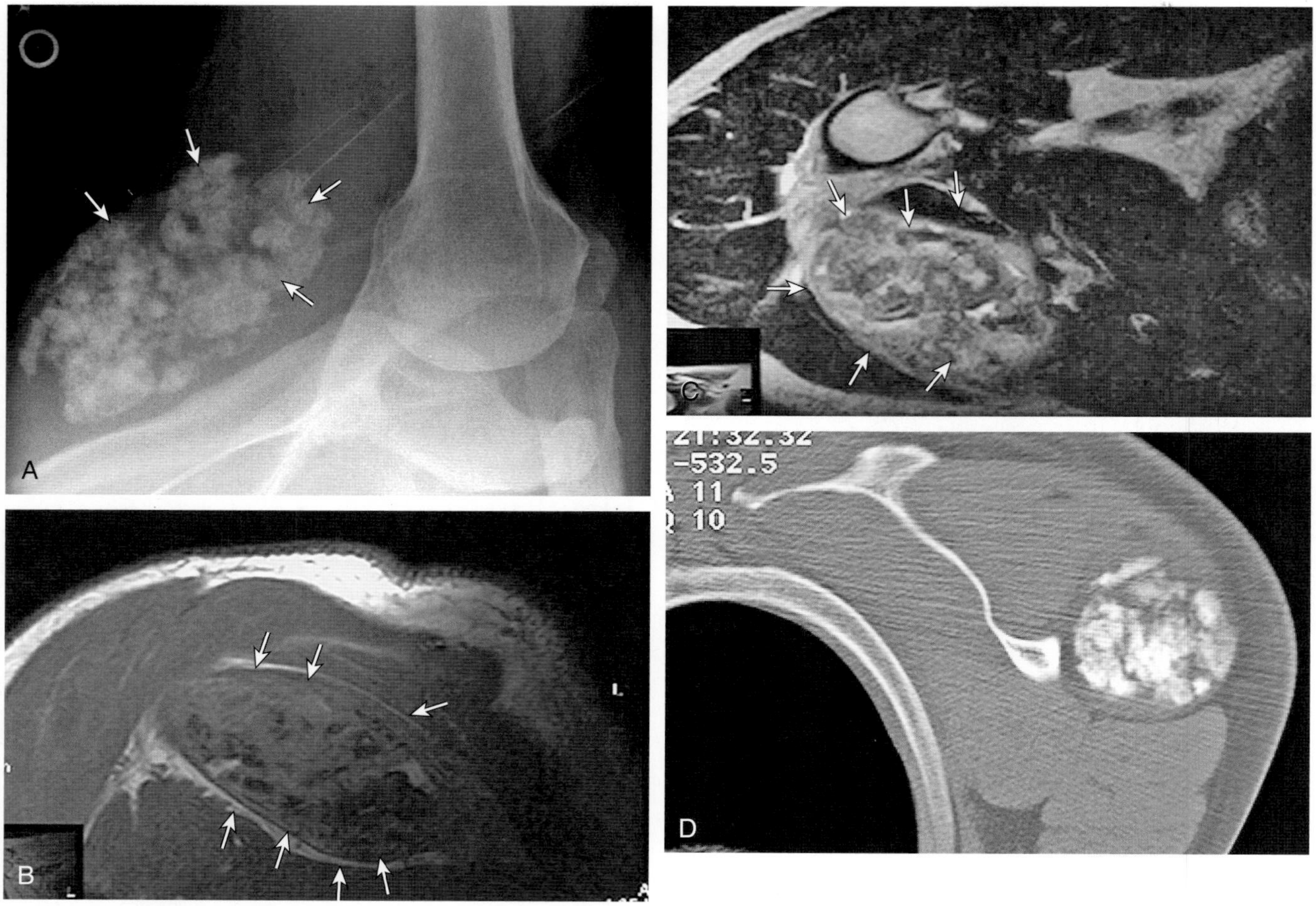

FIGURE 3-24. Axillary radiograph of the right shoulder shows a heavily mineralized mass (A). Intramuscular location is noted on the T1-weighted coronal (B) and T2-weighted axial (C) images (arrows). CT images confirm the mineralized mass, which has the appearance of chondroid matrix (D).

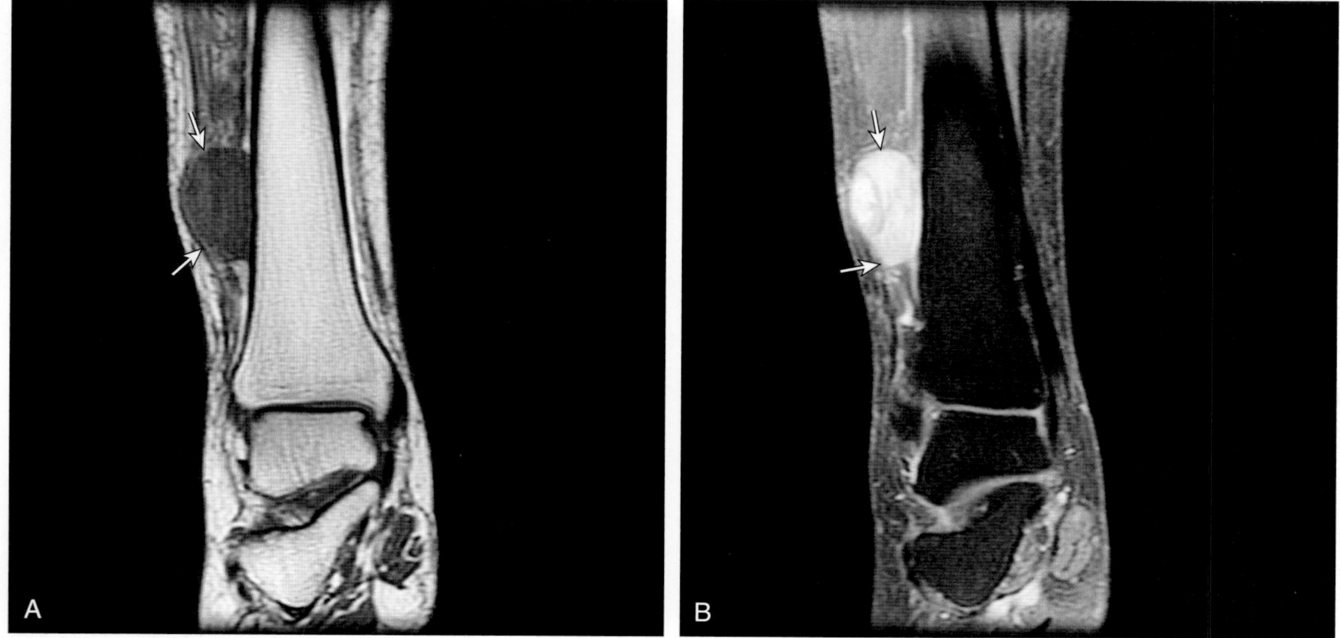

FIGURE 3-25. Myxofibrosarcoma in a 69-year-old female. Coronal T1-weighted image (A) and T2-weighted nonfat suppressed image (C) of the right leg show a deep soft tissue mass abutting the tibial cortex with well-defined margins (arrows). Note diffuse contrast enhancement (B).

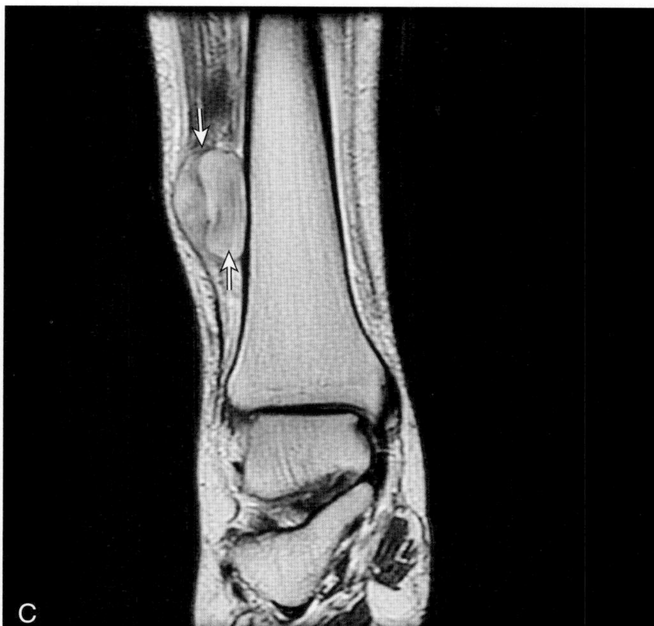

FIGURE 3-25, cont'd

confined to the skin and subcutaneous tissues (Figure 3-28). The mass is usually isointense or hypointense to muscle on T1-weighted images and is hyperintense on T2-weighted images. In the postcontrast images, uniform or patchy enhancement may be seen. Appropriate use of imaging sequences and MRI coils help in precise demonstrations of these tumors, especially when they involve web spaces of hand and feet where artifacts may confound the appearance of the neoplasm.

Myxoid liposarcoma spans a spectrum from typical low-grade lesions to fully malignant, high-grade tumors (round cell liposarcoma). It is the second most common type of liposarcoma, representing up to 50% of all liposarcomas.[28] Extremity myxoid liposarcomas are most commonly intermuscular (70% to 80% of cases); intramuscular and subcutaneous lesions are less common.[28] On an MRI, these lesions are typically well defined. Low signal intensity on T1-weighted images and markedly high signal on T2-weighted images reflect the high water content of the lesions, typical of myxoid neoplasms (Figure 3-29). Most myxoid liposarcomas show scattered small fatty foci, often appearing as thin septa or small nodules (see Figure 3-29). The differential diagnosis for a myxoid-appearing soft tissue lesion on an MRI includes myxoid liposarcoma, myxofibrosarcoma, myxoid chondrosarcoma, and myxoma.

Large areas (greater than 25%) of enhancing nonfatty tissue on MR images of fatty masses should be considered dedifferentiated liposarcoma until proven otherwise (Figure 3-30). In some cases, the low grade portion of the dedifferentiated sarcoma may not be apparent on imaging, and the entire tumor appears high grade.

Synovial sarcoma is a relatively common soft tissue malignancy that typically occurs in younger patients ages 15 to 35 years without sex predilection. Synovial sarcomas account for approximately 5% to 10% of soft tissue sarcomas. Most tumors occur in the extremities (60% to 70% in the lower extremities),[29] with the popliteal fossa being the most common location. A periarticular location is typical for synovial sarcoma, with most tumors occurring within 5 cm of a joint; an intra-articular location is rare.[29] Adjacent bone involvement, such as cortical remodeling, periosteal reactions, or invasion, is seen in 70% of cases.[30] Intratumoral calcification, often stippled, is present in 25% to 30% of cases.[31]

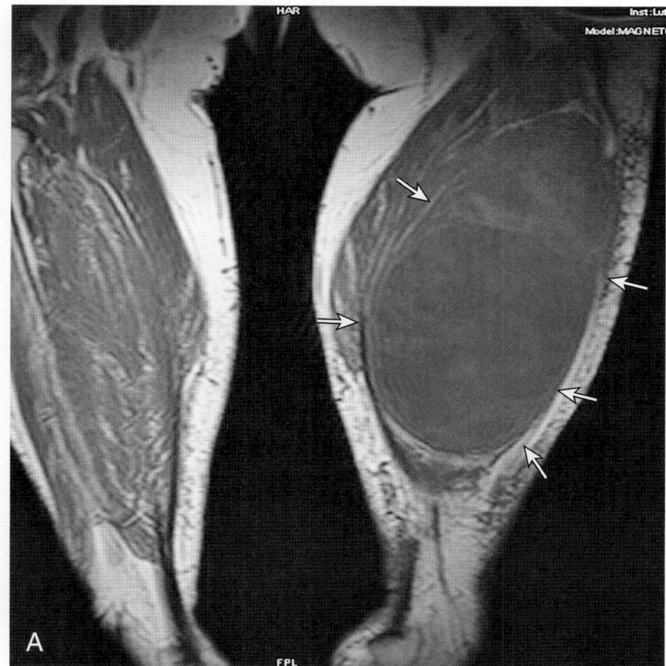

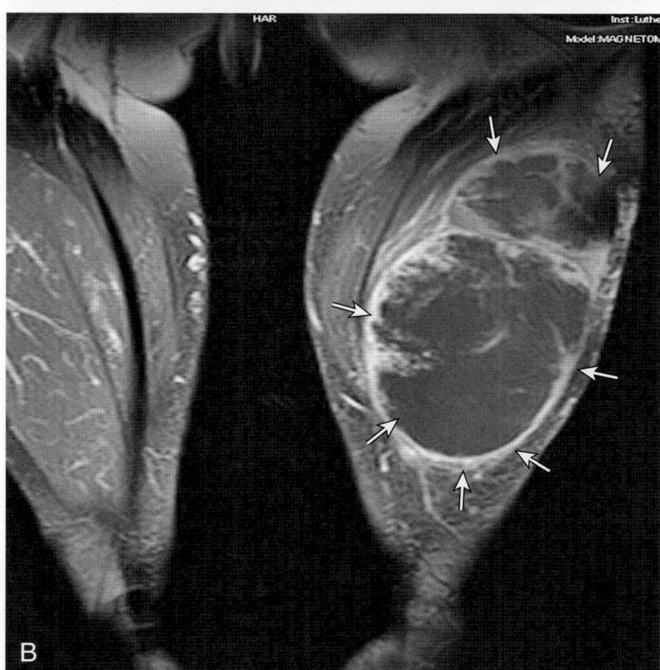

FIGURE 3-26. Coronal MR images of the left leg show a large soft tissue mass in the calf with well-demarcated margins. There is predominantly hypointense signal on T1-weighted (A) and enhancement particularly in the periphery of the tumor on T1-weighted fat-saturated postcontrast image (B).

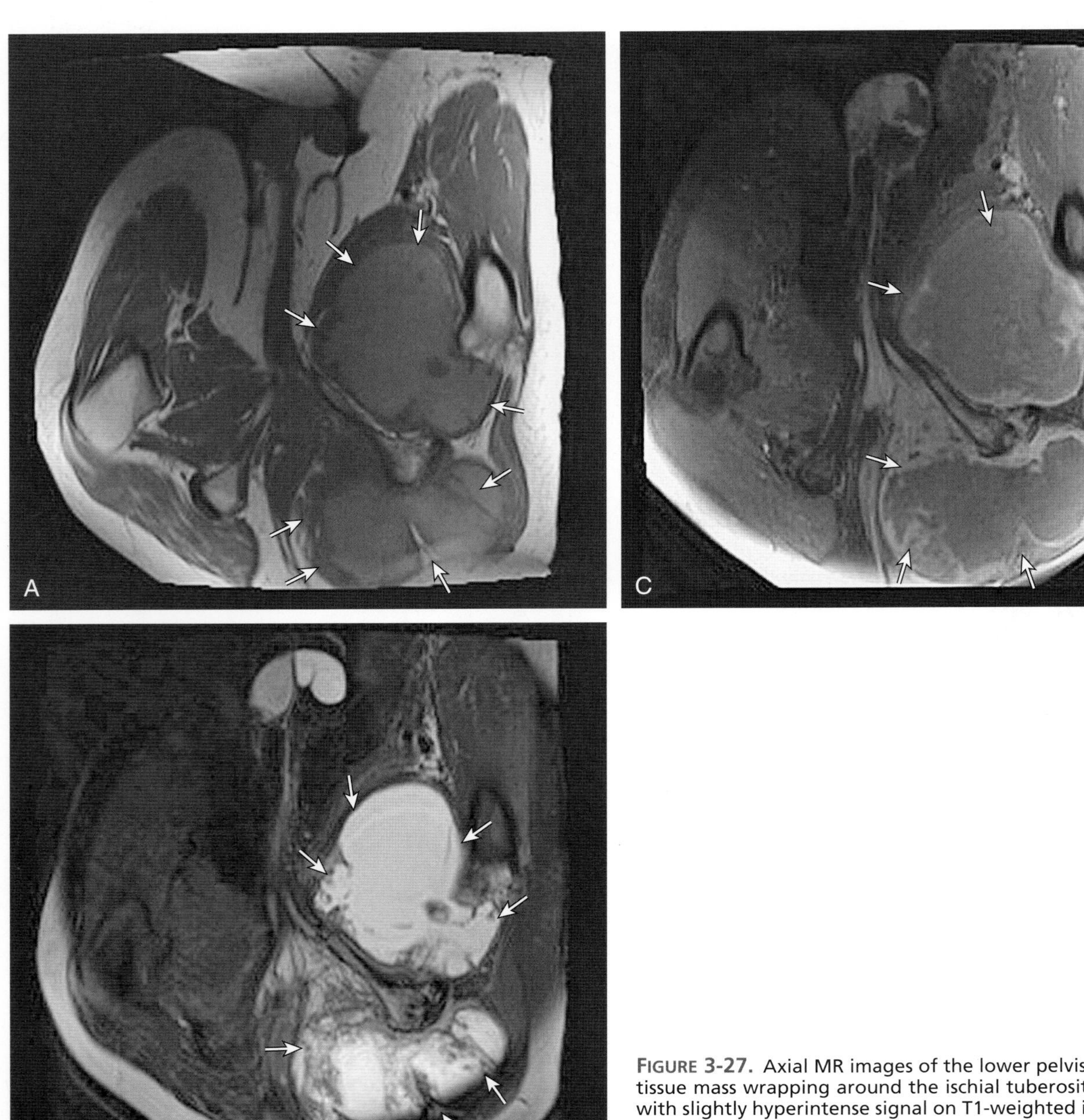

FIGURE 3-27. Axial MR images of the lower pelvis show a large soft tissue mass wrapping around the ischial tuberosity and pubic bone with slightly hyperintense signal on T1-weighted images (A). Hyperintense signal with areas of hypointense signal is noted on T2-weighted images (B). Postcontrast T1-weighted fat saturated images show a predominantly peripheral enhancement, suggestive of central necrosis (C) (arrows).

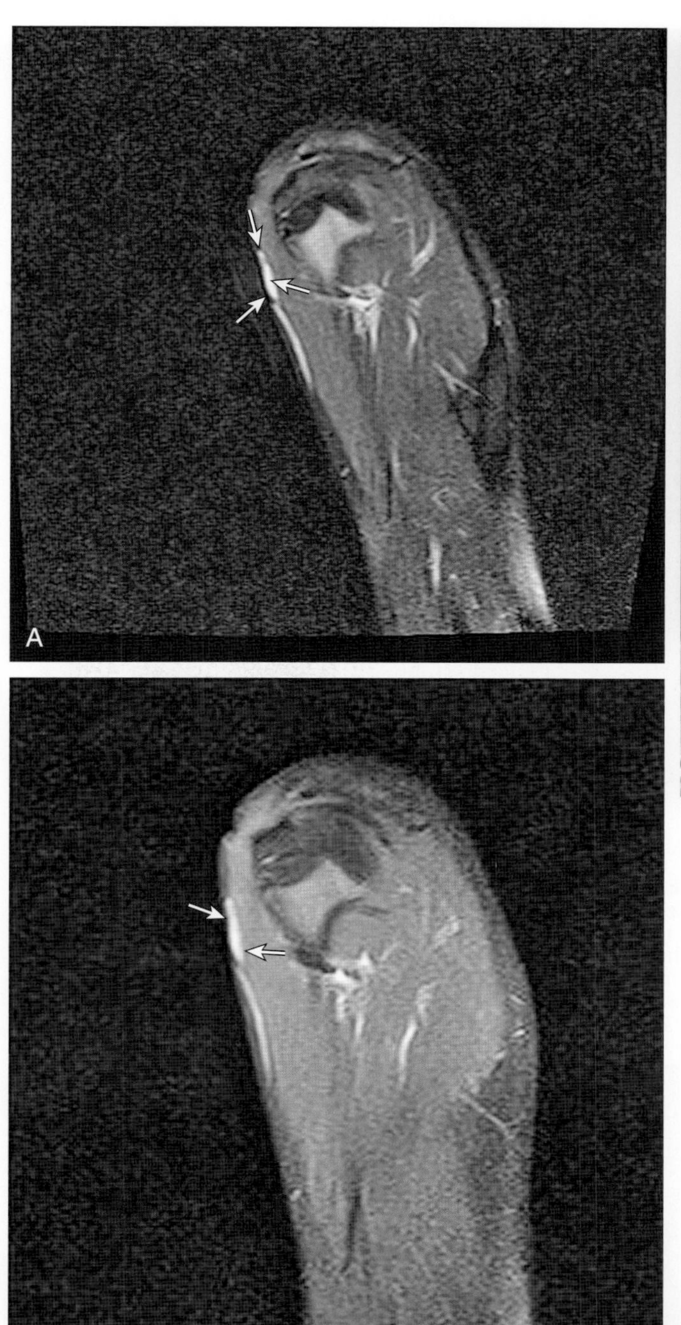

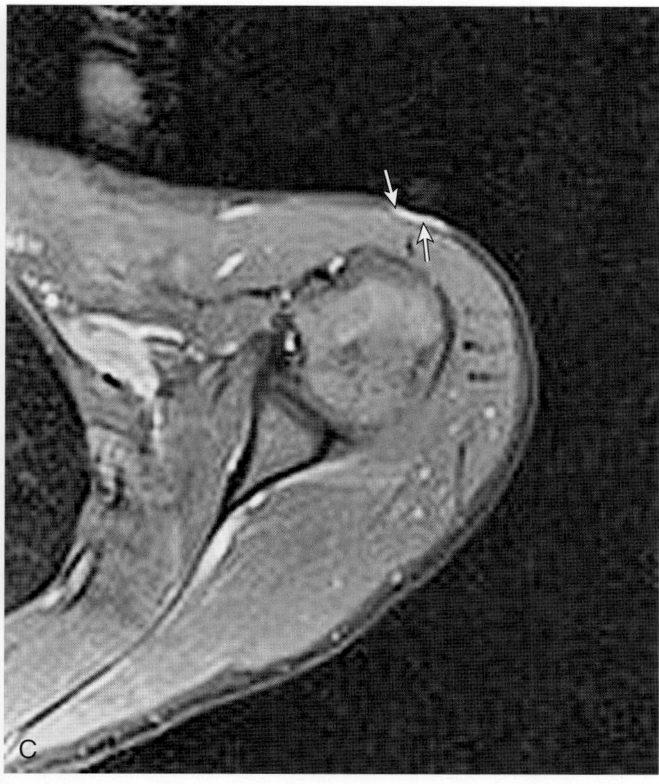

FIGURE 3-28. A 19-year-old female with dermatofibrosarcoma protuberans. Sagittal T2-weighted image (A) of the right arm shows a subtle subcutaneous hyperintense signal mass (arrows). Postcontrast T1-weighted fat-saturated sagittal (B) and axial plane (C) images show diffuse enhancement of this mass.

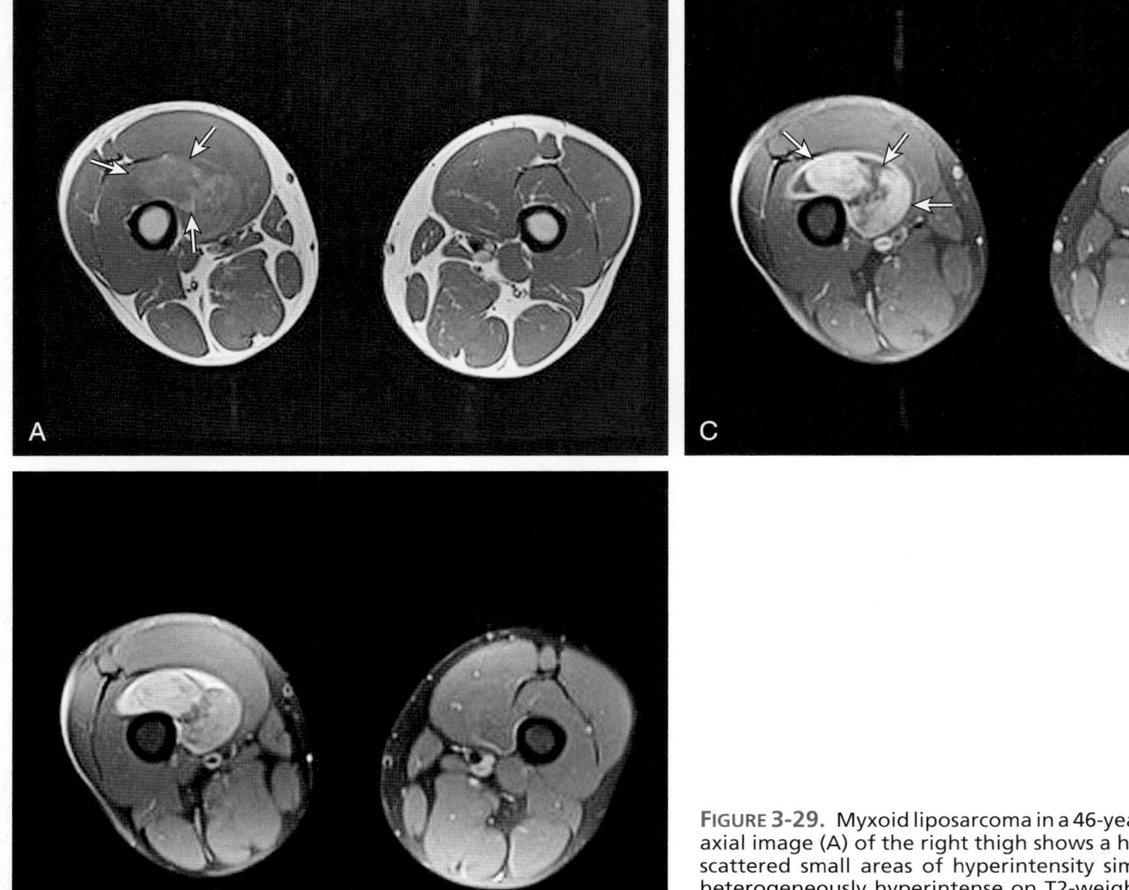

FIGURE 3-29. Myxoid liposarcoma in a 46-year-old male. T1-weighted axial image (A) of the right thigh shows a heterogeneous mass with scattered small areas of hyperintensity similar to fat. This mass is heterogeneously hyperintense on T2-weighted image (B). Postcontrast T1-weighted fat saturated image (C) shows fairly diffuse enhancement with small foci of nonenhancing areas centrally and laterally.

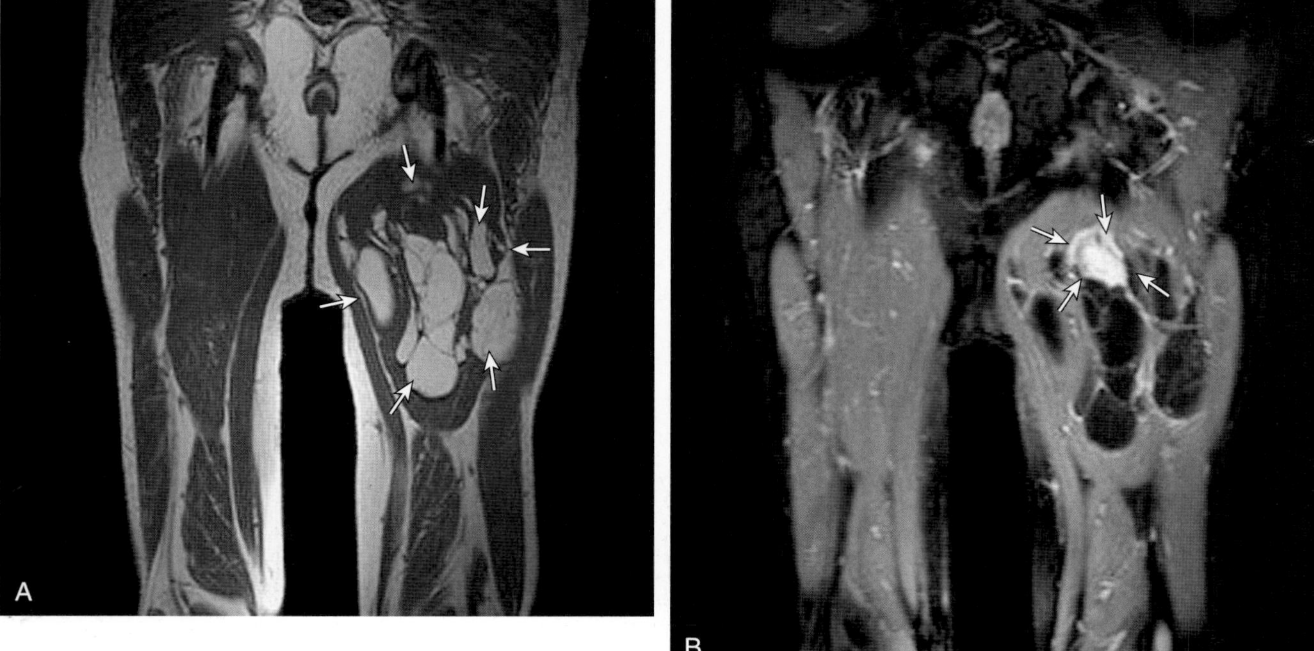

FIGURE 3-30. A 79-year-old male with dedifferentiated liposarcoma. Coronal T1-weighted images (A) of the left show a large, predominantly fatty mass (arrows) with lobulated contours and thick septations. Prominent focus of nonfatty nodule proximally, which appears hyperintense on STIR images (arrows) (B).

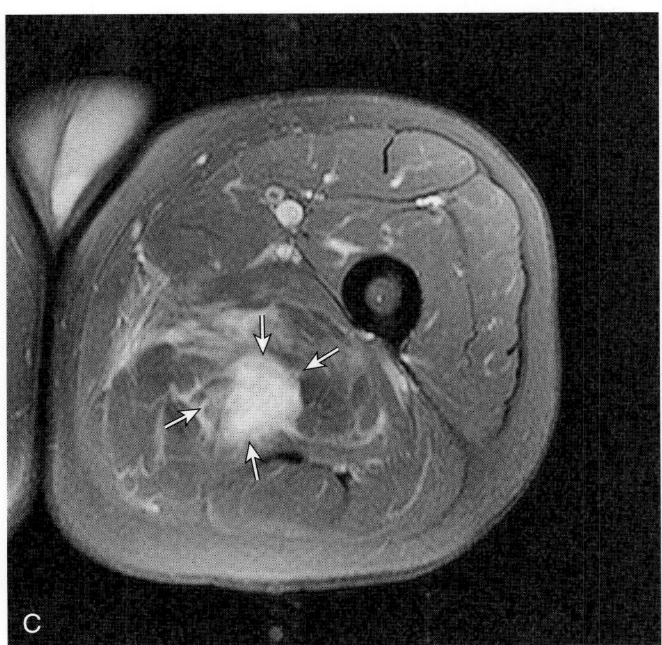

FIGURE 3-30, cont'd. On axial T1-weighted fat saturated image (C), there is diffuse enhancement of this nodular dedifferentiated component (arrows).

An MRI may demonstrate a heterogeneous mass with areas that are hyperintense, isointense, or hypointense to fat on T2-weighted imaging (Figure 3-31). This nonspecific triple sign is seen in 30% to 50% of cases and represents the mixture of hemorrhage, necrosis, and solid components in the tumor.[31] Smaller lesions may have a homogeneously high signal on T2-weighted images and simulate a cyst or a ganglion, especially near a joint. On T1-weighted images, a slightly increased signal should raise the suspicion for a solid neoplasm, and contrast should be administered to confirm this suspicion. Enhancement is variable in these tumors, with nonenhancing necrotic areas present, especially in the larger tumors.

MPNSTs account for 5% to 10% of soft tissue sarcomas and usually affect patients ages 20 to 50 years, with a slight female predilection.[32,33] MPNST is associated with NF1 in 25% to 70% of cases.[33] A sudden increase in the size of a previously known lesion in a patient with NF1 should always raise suspicion for MPNST. MPNST usually affects medium to large deep-seated nerves, with the sciatic nerve, brachial plexus, and sacral plexus most commonly involved. Distinguishing MPNST from benign peripheral nerve sheath tumor (BPNST) can be challenging because the lesions can appear very similar on imaging studies (Figure 3-32). Worrisome findings on an MRI include marked progression of tumor size on a follow-up study, cortical destruction, and marrow invasion of adjacent

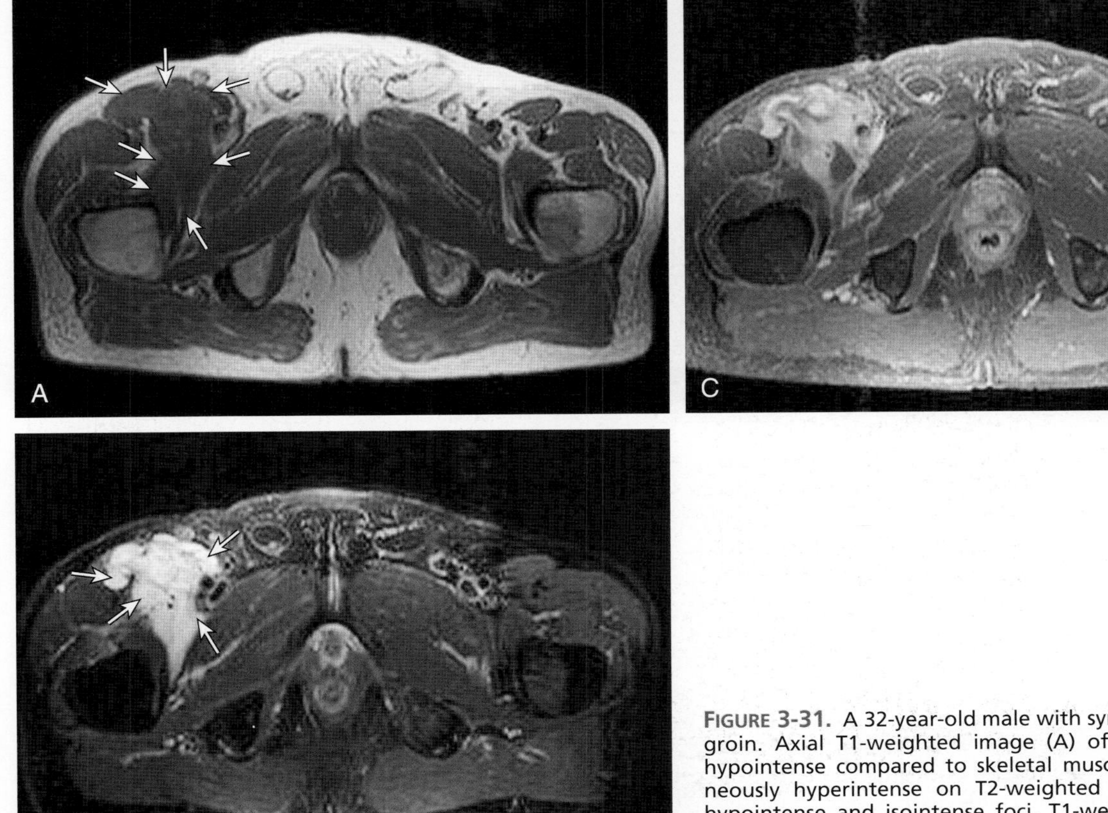

FIGURE 3-31. A 32-year-old male with synovial sarcoma of the right groin. Axial T1-weighted image (A) of the pelvis shows a mass hypointense compared to skeletal muscle. This mass is heterogeneously hyperintense on T2-weighted image (B) with areas of hypointense and isointense foci. T1-weighted fat-saturated post-contrast image (C) shows fairly diffuse contrast enhancement with a small nonenhancing focus in the midportion of the tumor.

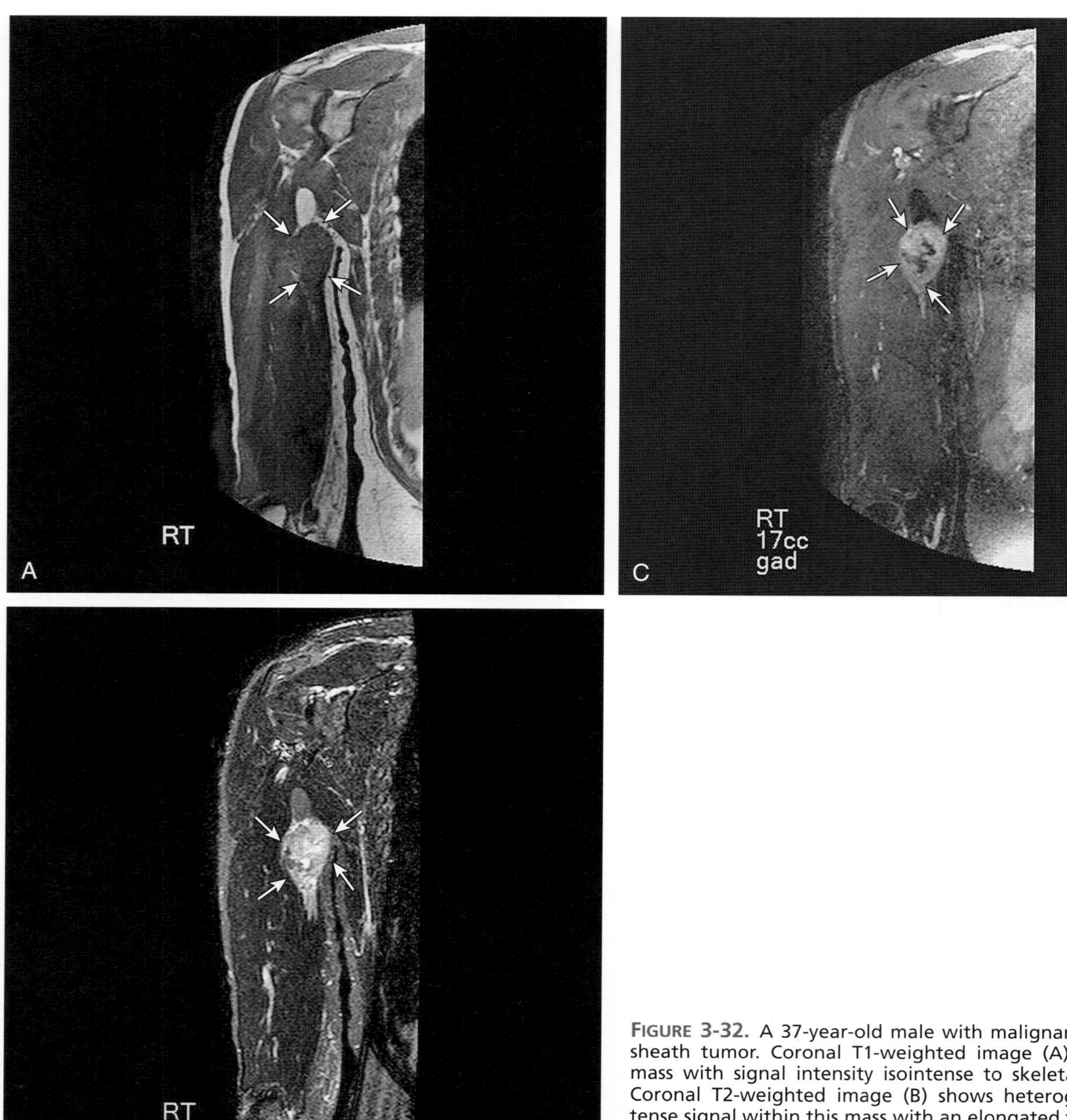

FIGURE 3-32. A 37-year-old male with malignant peripheral nerve sheath tumor. Coronal T1-weighted image (A) shows a fusiform mass with signal intensity isointense to skeletal muscle (arrows). Coronal T2-weighted image (B) shows heterogeneously hyperintense signal within this mass with an elongated tail distally, suggestive of neurogenic etiology. Postcontrast T1-weighted fat-saturated and shows thick nodular enhancement of the periphery with lack of central enhancement, suggestive of necrosis (C).

bones. Fludeoxyglucose F18 and 11C-methionine PET scans can differentiate between MPNST and BPNST, based on differences in SUV (Figure 3-33). PET-CT is used in complex cases to differentiate between these two entities. PET-MRI may also prove to be useful when imaging patients with NF1.

UNCOMMON MALIGNANT SOFT TISSUE TUMORS

In the absence of bone involvement, it is uncommon to see metastases and myeloma of muscles and other soft tissues. Clinically or radiologically detectable extraosseous masses occur in approximately 5% of patients with multiple myeloma,[34] and the incidence of extraosseous disease has increased in recent decades.[34] This increased incidence may be the result of prolonged survival of patients and improved imaging methods such as PET-CT and whole-body MRI. It is important to differentiate solitary plasmacytoma from multiple myeloma because the two entities have significantly different prognoses and require different treatments: solitary plasmacytoma represents focal malignant clonal plasma cell proliferation without bone marrow involvement and may arise from soft tissues. The imaging features of extraosseous myeloma are nonspecific and can mimic other malignancies. In patients with known multiple myeloma, newly developed focal soft tissue masses should be considered highly suspicious for myelomatous involvement, particularly after stem cell transplantation.

Solitary soft tissue metastasis without a known primary malignancy is a rare occurrence, with an incidence of approximately 0.8%.[35] Lung cancer is the most common underlying primary tumor.[35] Soft tissues, especially skeletal muscles, are infrequently involved in metastatic disease (Figure 3-34). The imaging features of soft tissue metastases are nonspecific and may simulate a sarcoma, therefore requiring biopsy confirmation. Unsuspected soft tissue metastases have become more frequent in recent years (especially in patients with advanced disease), likely because of the widespread use of whole-body imaging modalities.

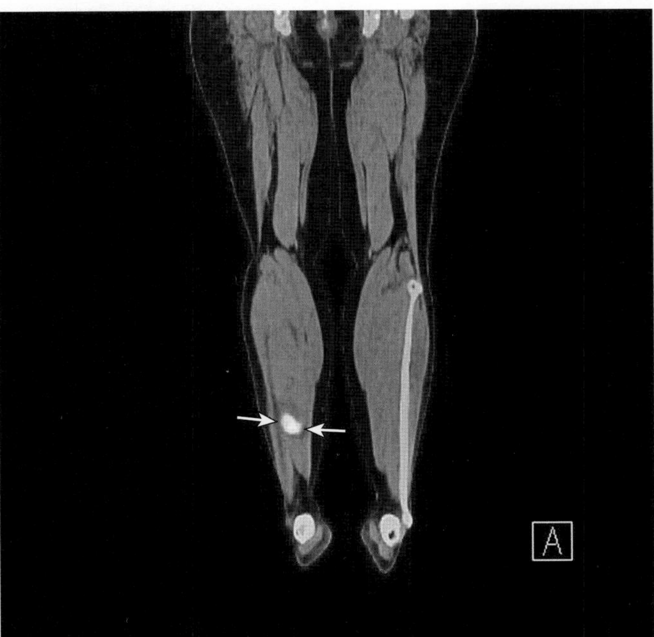

FIGURE 3-33. A 37-year-old male with malignant peripheral nerve sheath tumor. Coronal image shows a metabolically active lesion in the right calf with an SUV of 8.5, typical of an aggressive neoplasm.

Lymphoma of skeletal muscle is rare, representing 1.5% of cases of non-Hodgkin lymphoma and 0.3% of cases of Hodgkin lymphoma.[36] Most lymphoma cases involving skeletal muscle are caused by extension of lymphomatous deposits in adjacent lymph nodes and bone as a manifestation of systemic disease. Extranodal primary lymphoma of skeletal muscle is the least common form of the disease. Lymphoma can involve any muscle in the body, but the most common sites are the thigh, trunk, upper extremity, and leg.[36]

On an MRI, long segmental involvement is typically seen, with orientation of the tumor along muscle fascicles.[36] Muscle enlargement is typical, and associated subcutaneous stranding with or without cutaneous involvement is frequently seen (Figure 3-35). Multicompartmental involvement is also common.[36] MRI signal characteristics are nonspecific, with T1-weighted images typically showing low signal intensity compared to muscle and T2-weighted images showing variable signal intensity. The enhancement pattern, although variable, is often diffuse.

Clear cell sarcoma (malignant melanoma of soft parts) is a rare, slow growing soft tissue sarcoma showing melanocytic differentiation, with a predilection for the foot. De Beuckeleer et al.[37] reported slightly increased signal intensity on T1-weighted images compared with muscle in the majority of their cases, presumably a result of melanin content of the tumor. This finding is rarely seen in other soft tissue tumors and should raise suspicion for clear cell sarcoma or melanoma metastases (Figure 3-36). The appearance of this tumor is variable on T2-weighted images and often hyperintense, a nonspecific finding. Moderate-to-avid enhancement is seen with contrast.[37]

Epithelioid sarcoma is a rare, high-grade malignancy with a known propensity for local recurrence, although rare epithelioid sarcoma represents the most common primary soft tissue sarcoma of the hand[38] and typically involves aponeuroses and surrounding structures. An MRI is often helpful to detect tumor involvement of deeper tissues and its tendency to creep

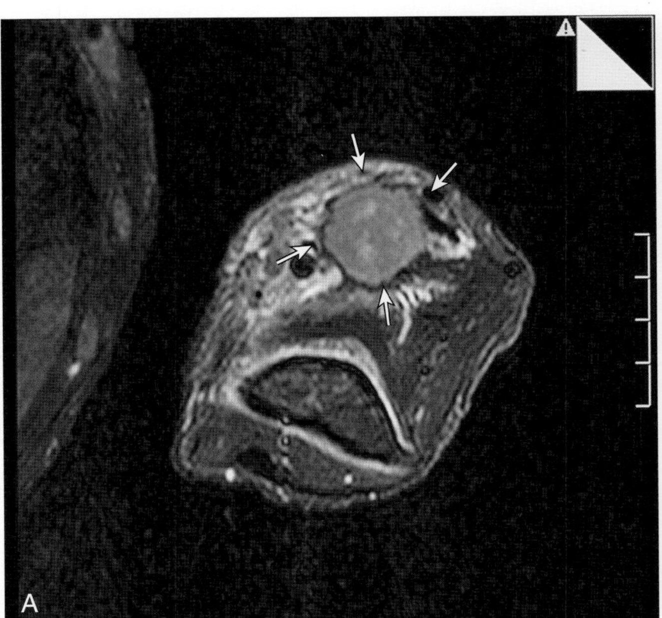

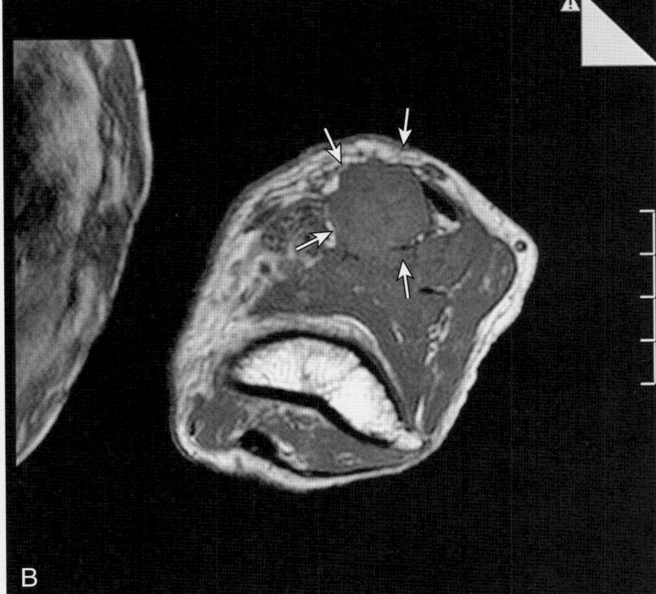

FIGURE 3-34. A 57-year-old male with adenocarcinoma of the lung. (A, B) Axial T1- and T2-weighted images show a mass in distal arm with a surrounding edema-like signal (arrows).

Continued

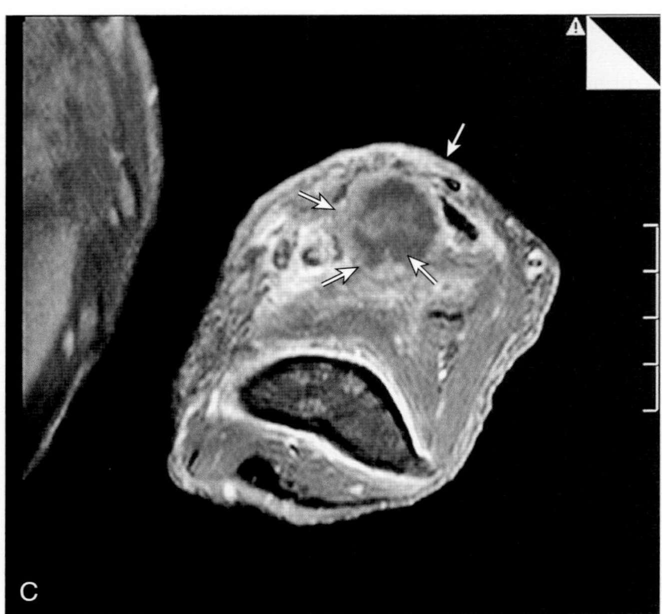

FIGURE 3-34, cont'd. (C) Axial T1-weighted fat-saturated post-contrast image shows mild intratumoral and peritumoral enhancement.

along tendon sheaths and metastasize to lymph nodes. MRI signal characteristics are nonspecific, with hypointense T1-weighted and hyperintense T2-weighted signal and avid contrast enhancement. Location and intimacy to tendons are often the clue to diagnosis (Figure 3-37).

Primitive neuroectodermal tumors (PNET) are rare in the extremities. PNET is a very aggressive neoplasm with a peak age of incidence in adolescence and young adulthood.[39] The most common locations of peripheral PNETs have been the thoracic region, the retroperitoneum, paravertebral region, the head and neck region, and the intra-abdominal and pelvic soft tissues and extremities.[39] The MR imaging features are nonspecific, similar to those of other aggressive soft tissue sarcomas and small blue cell neoplasms with nonspecific hypointense T1-weighted and heterogeneous on T2-weighted sequences with hyperintense T2-weighted signal intensity (Figure 3-38). Enhancement pattern is variable, often confounded by the degree of necrosis.

COMMON TUMOR-LIKE CONDITIONS

Elastofibromas

An elastofibroma is a degenerative or reactive fibrous lesion that is generally thought to be the result of long-standing mechanical irritation. Elastofibroma dorsi is typically found in the infrascapular regions, deep to the serratus anterior and latissimus dorsi musculature in elderly patients. Autopsy studies have demonstrated the presence of subscapular elastofibromas in 11.2% of men and 24.4% of women older than 55 years.[40] Elastofibromas are bilateral in approximately 25% of cases.[40] Extrascapular sites are uncommon, typically involving pressure points such as over the greater trochanter and the olecranon at the elbow.[41] On CT, a poorly defined soft tissue mass in the infrascapular or subscapular region with attenuation similar to that of the adjacent skeletal muscle confirms

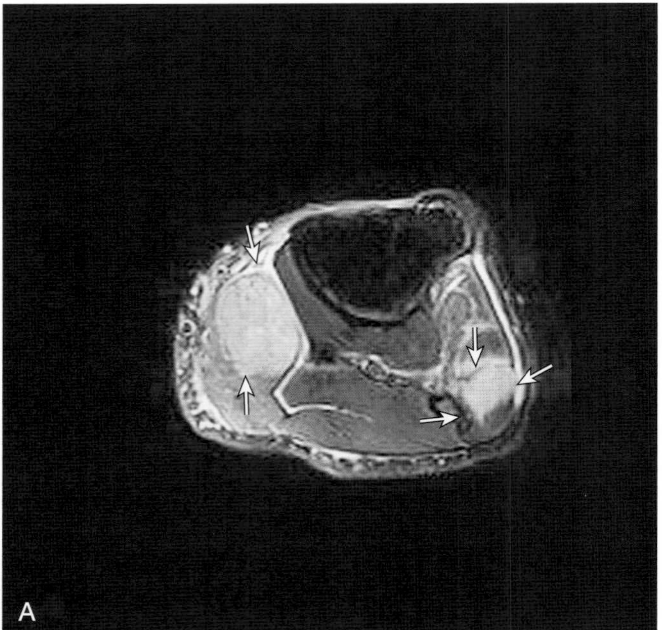

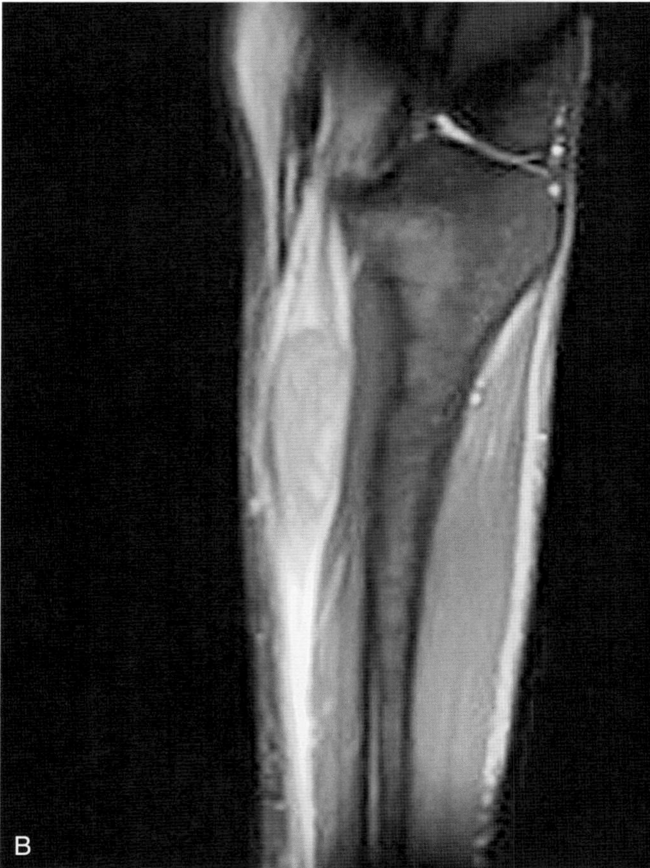

FIGURE 3-35. A 23-year-old male with left leg muscular lymphoma. Axial T2-weighted image (A) of the proximal calf shows two soft tissue masses medially and laterally (arrows). Coronal T2-weighted image (B) shows the larger medial soft tissue mass extending along the muscle fibers.

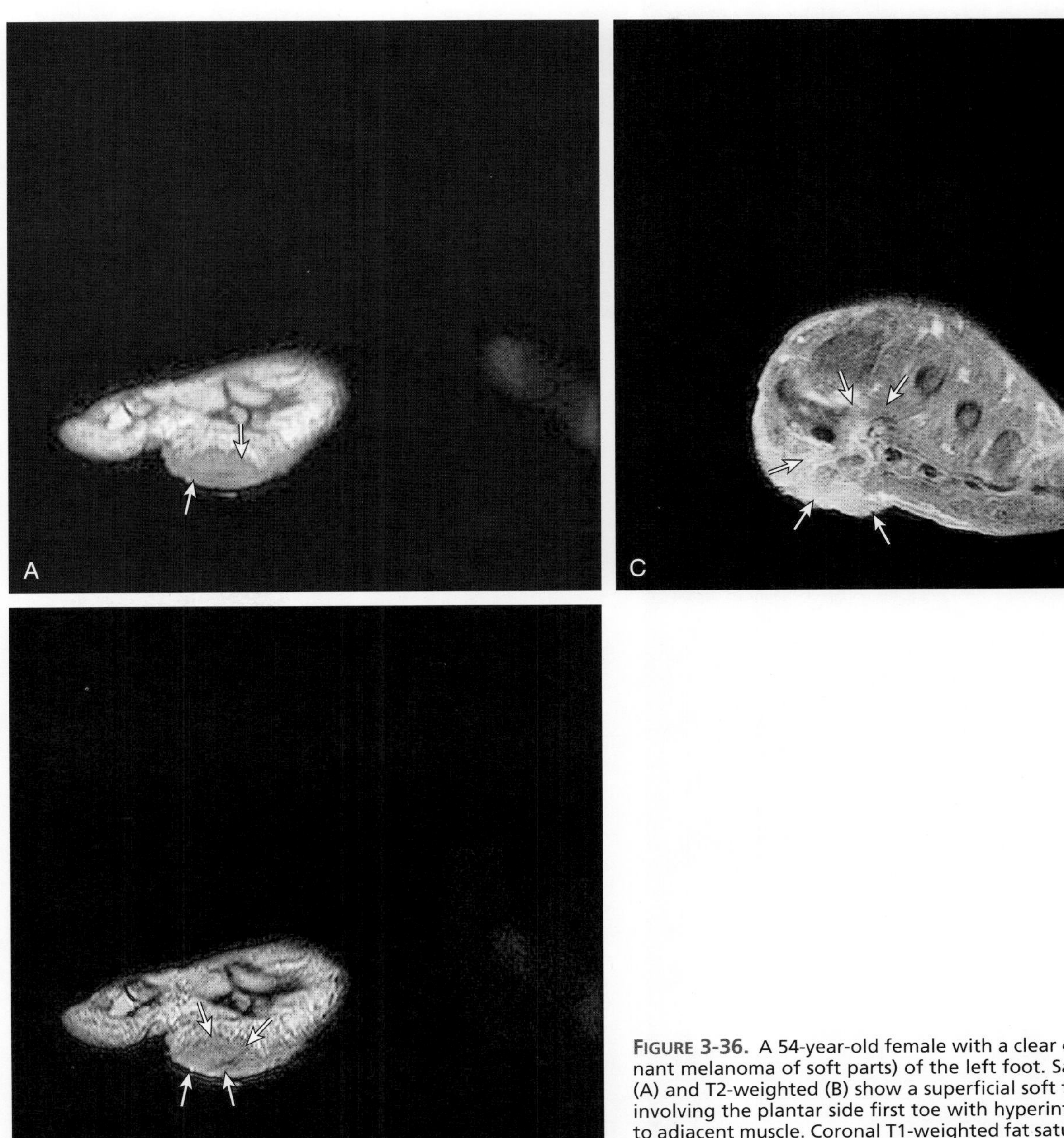

FIGURE 3-36. A 54-year-old female with a clear cell sarcoma (malignant melanoma of soft parts) of the left foot. Sagittal T1-weighted (A) and T2-weighted (B) show a superficial soft tissue mass (arrows) involving the plantar side first toe with hyperintense intense signal to adjacent muscle. Coronal T1-weighted fat saturated image shows diffuse enhancement of this mass extending to the underlying metatarsal (arrows) (C).

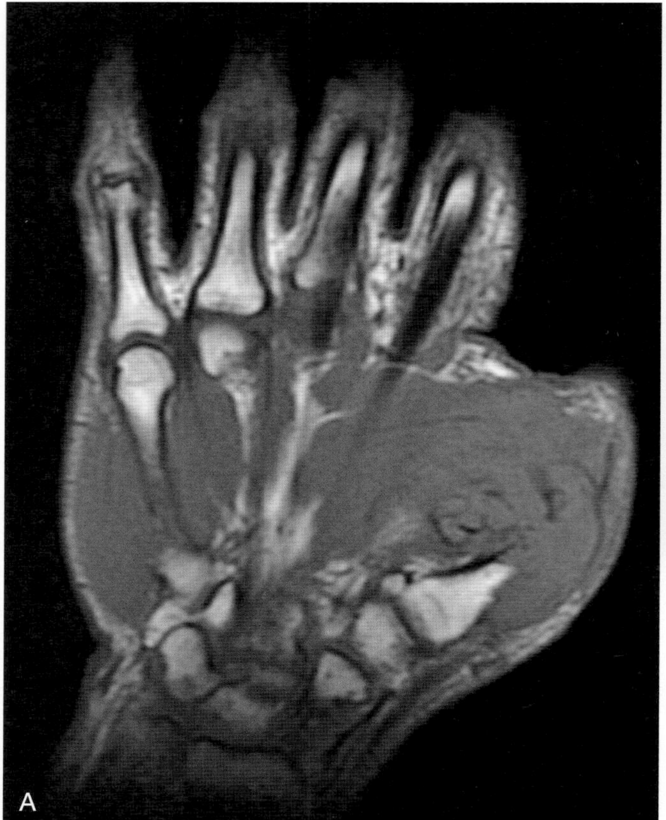

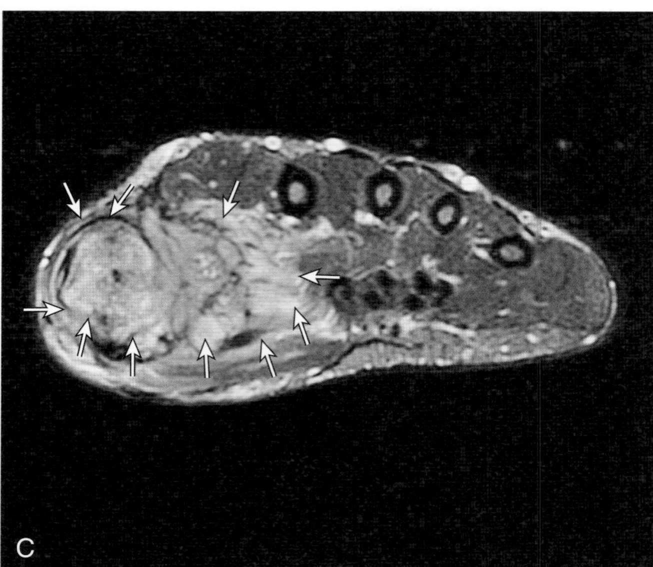

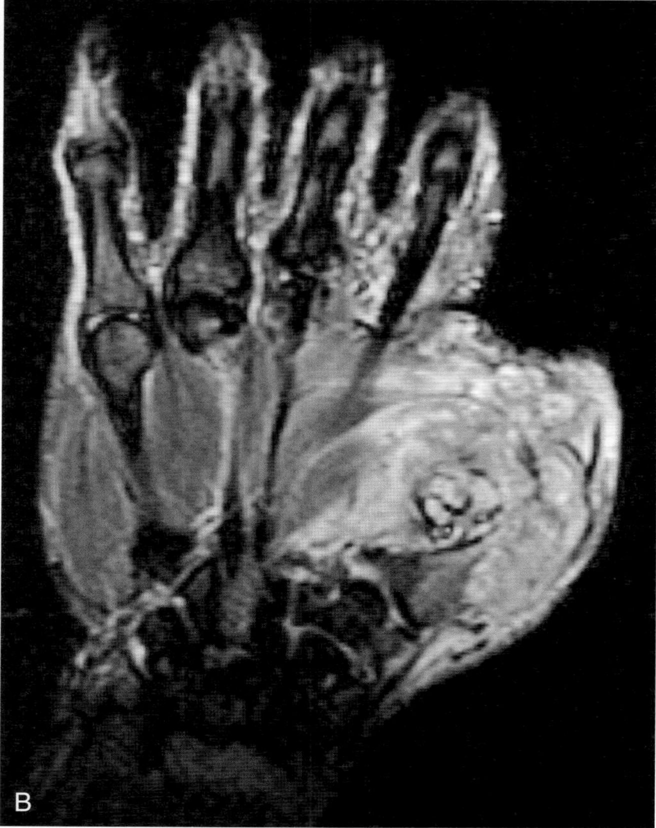

FIGURE 3-37. A 43-year-old male with an epithelioid sarcoma of the right hand. Coronal T1-weighted image (A) shows a large soft tissue mass centered around the distal two-thirds of the first metacarpal with isointense signal to adjacent muscle. T2-weighted coronal (B) and axial (C) images show heterogeneously increased T2 signal and destruction of first metacarpal and the phalanges.

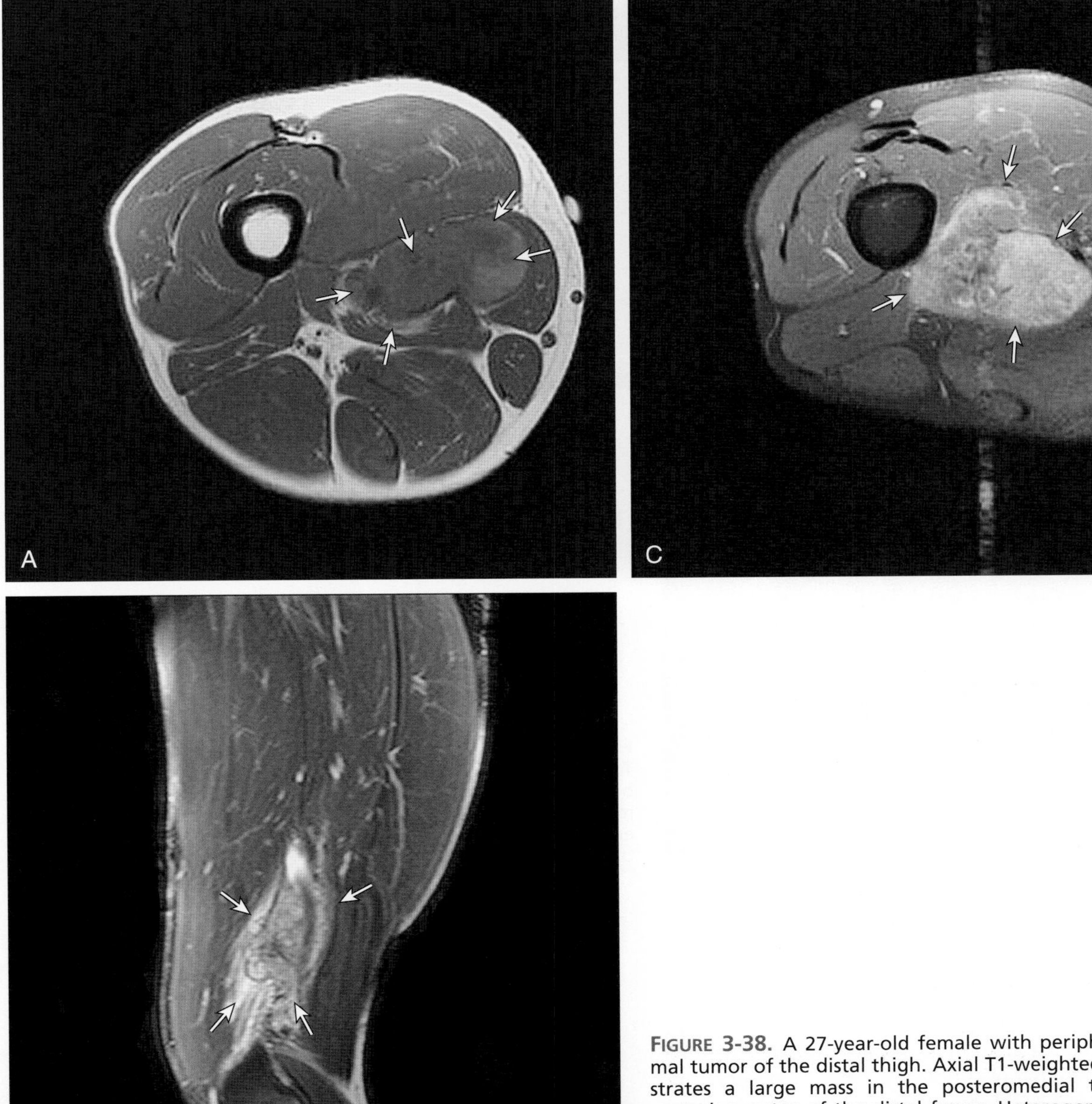

FIGURE 3-38. A 27-year-old female with peripheral neuroectodermal tumor of the distal thigh. Axial T1-weighted image (A) demonstrates a large mass in the posteromedial thigh abutting the posterior cortex of the distal femur. Heterogeneously hypointense signal is noted in the T2-weighted sagittal image (arrows) (B). There is avid contrast enhancement in the postcontrast T1-weighted axial image (C).

the diagnosis of elastofibroma, especially if internal striations or scattered areas of fat attenuation are seen. On MR images, elastofibromas are typically well-defined lesions with a capsule (Figure 3-39). The tumors display heterogeneous signal intensity similar to that of skeletal muscle and frequently demonstrate intermixed linear or curvilinear streaks of fat signal intensity. Contrast enhancement is typically heterogeneous on an MRI. Given a characteristic lesion location in the chest wall of a middle-aged or elderly patient deep to the scapula and typical MRI signal characteristics, a prospective MRI diagnosis of elastofibroma often can be made with a high degree of confidence.

Hematomas

A hematoma usually presents as a superficial soft tissue mass after trauma with typical overlying skin discoloration. These cases are generally managed clinically and without imaging. When there is a deep hematoma, especially in the absence of significant trauma, imaging is frequently performed to rule out a sarcoma. If a history of trauma is not present, one should search for a history of anticoagulation treatment, especially in elderly patients.

The MRI is the modality of choice for assessing deep hematomas, whereas the ultrasound is useful in evaluating

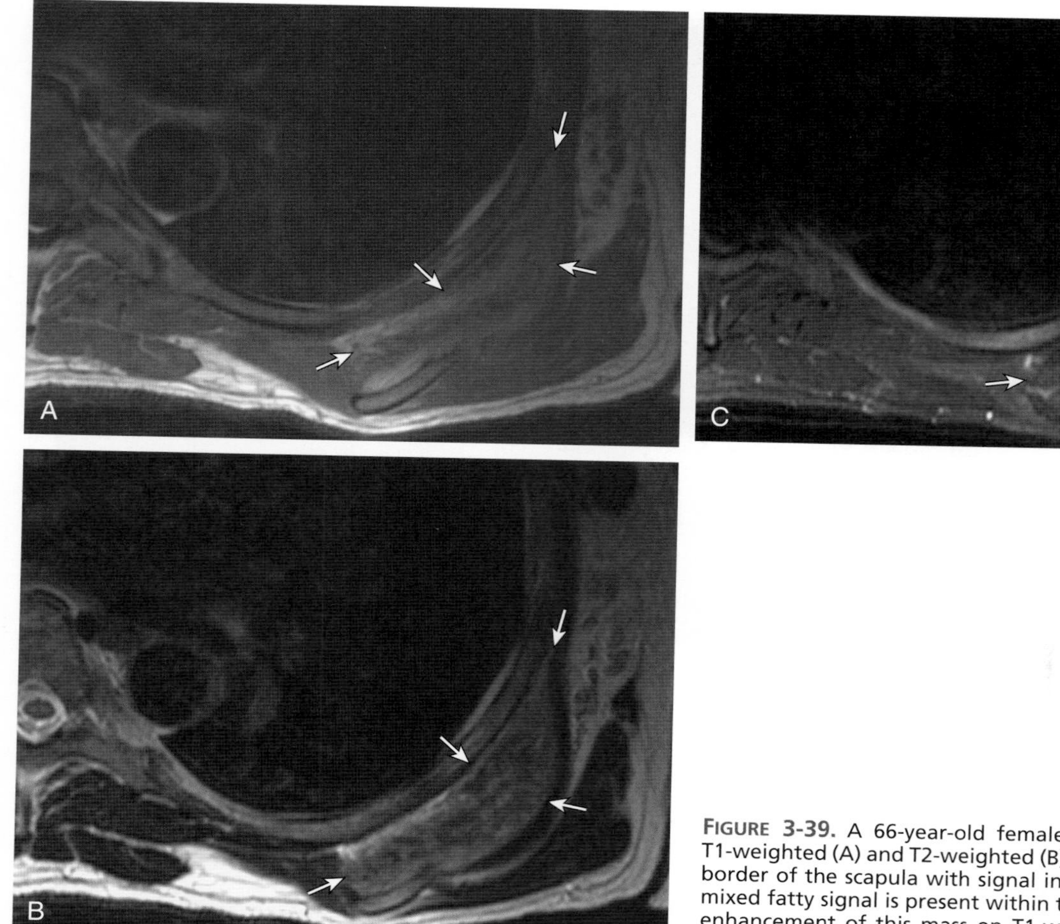

FIGURE 3-39. A 66-year-old female with an elastofibroma. Axial T1-weighted (A) and T2-weighted (B) images show a mass to inferior border of the scapula with signal intensity similar to muscle. Intermixed fatty signal is present within this mass (arrows). There is mild enhancement of this mass on T1-weighted fat-saturated postcontrast image (C).

superficial locations. On an MRI, hematomas display a variable appearance on T1-weighted images, showing slight hyperintensity relative to skeletal muscle in the acute phase and marked hyperintense areas in the subacute phase. Hypointense signal similar to that of simple fluid may be observed in chronic hematomas. T2-weighted images of hematomas are frequently heterogeneously hyperintense. Surrounding edema and fluid-like signal is typically seen extending between the muscle and fascial planes, especially in the acute and subacute stages, with no definable capsule or pseudocapsule. Because of the similarities between MRI features of hematomas and hemorrhagic sarcomas, contrast enhancement is usually required to differentiate between these entities. With a hematoma, contrast enhancement should be confined to the periphery (Figure 3-40); any internal enhancement should raise suspicion for a sarcoma. In patients with contrast allergy or renal insufficiency, clinical or imaging follow-up may be used in place of imaging with contrast enhancement. Most hematomas subside within several weeks, although some may persist and require further imaging. Chronic expanding hematoma is a rare persistent hematoma manifesting as an enlarging space-occupying mass simulating a neoplasm.[42] The etiology of such gradually enlarging hematomas is still unclear. The irritant effects of blood and its breakdown products, causing repeated bleeding from capillaries in the granulation tissue, have been speculated to be the cause of these conditions.[43]

Pigmented Villonodular Synovitis

Pigmented villonodular synovitis (PVNS) is a type of synovial proliferative lesion of the joint, bursa, or tendon sheath. The term *PVNS* is used when diffuse intra-articular involvement is present. The term *giant cell tumor of the tendon sheath* is preferred when the extra-articular form of the same disease process occurs, typically involving the tendon sheath. Imaging plays an important role in the localization of the disease process. PVNS is usually a monoarticular process of the large joints, affecting the knee in 80% of cases and also known to affect the hip, ankle, shoulder, and elbow joints.[44,45] Progressive pain, swelling, decreased range of motion, and history of recurrent bloody joint effusions are the most common clinical findings.

The MRI is the preferred modality for diagnosing PVNS because of its very specific imaging features, which help distinguish PVNS from other synovial processes. On an MRI, synovial-based masses with low signal intensity on T1- and T2-weighted pulse sequences are seen (Figure 3-41). Magnetic susceptibility artifact (blooming) within the affected

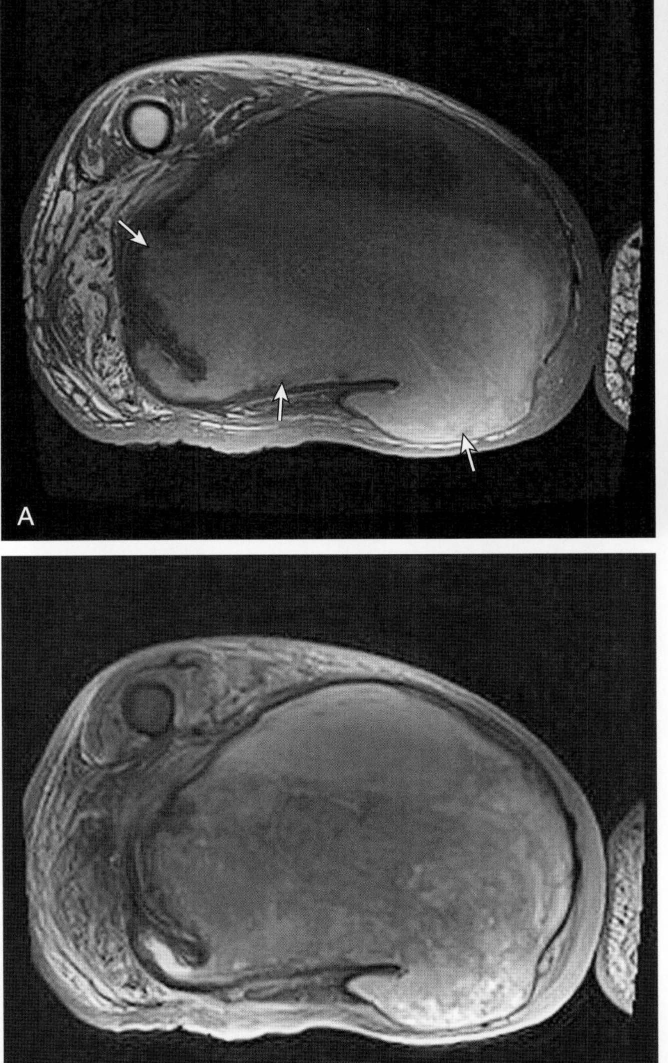

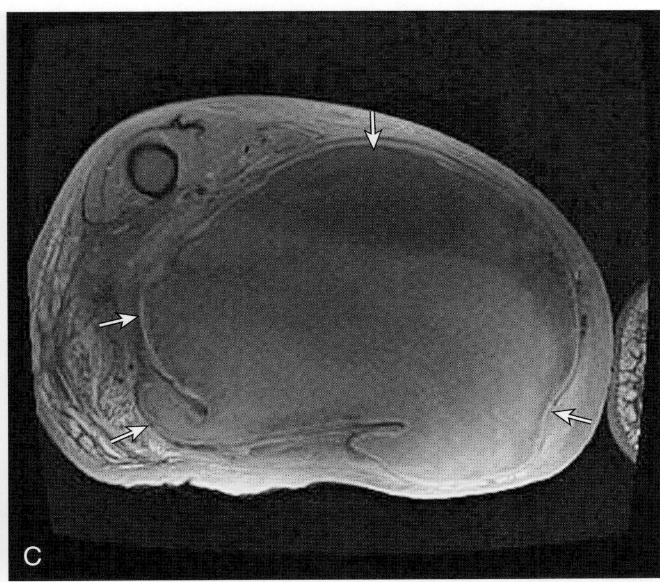

FIGURE 3-40. A 62-year-old female with a large thigh hematoma. Axial T1-weighted image (A) shows a large mass-like collection in the medial thigh with areas of hyperintense signal, suggestive of subacute blood products (arrows). On T2-weighted axial image (B), there is a hypointense rim that is also suggestive of blood products. On the postcontrast T1-weighted fat-saturated image (C), there is minimal peripheral enhancement, typical of a hematoma.

joint space on gradient recalled echo sequences is characteristic as a result of the presence of hemosiderin in the lesion (see Figure 3-41).[44,45] Areas of variable signal intensity, with foci of brighter T1 and T2 signals that indicate relatively low concentrations of hemosiderin, perhaps represent more recent hemorrhage. Although the degree of contrast enhancement in PVNS can vary, moderate to marked enhancement of the synovium is common because of the hypervascular nature of the disease.[44,45] A radiologic differential usually includes synovial chondromatosis, which tends to have multiple mineralized intra-articular bodies that are readily identifiable on radiographs. Other differential diagnostic considerations include nodular synovitis, gouty tophus, amyloid, and hemophilic arthropathy. Gout and amyloid are systemic illnesses with multiple sites of involvement. Osseous changes seen in hemophilia are not a feature of PVNS.[44]

Synovial Chondromatosis

Synovial chondromatosis is a proliferative and metaplastic condition of the synovium of the joints and bursa. An initial phase consisting of metaplastic cartilaginous masses within the synovium is followed by a transitional phase consisting of cartilaginous nodules detached from the involved synovium and forming free bodies. In the final, inactive phase, synovial proliferation is resolved but loose bodies remain, which may be a sequela of osteoarthritis; this is sometimes referred to as *secondary synovial chondromatosis*. Cartilaginous nodules typically become calcified or ossified, which is sometimes referred to as *synovial osteochondromatosis*. The term *synovial chondromatosis* is preferred, given the absence of calcification in 5% to 30% of cases.[46]

An MRI appearance of this condition is variable and depends on the relative preponderance of synovial

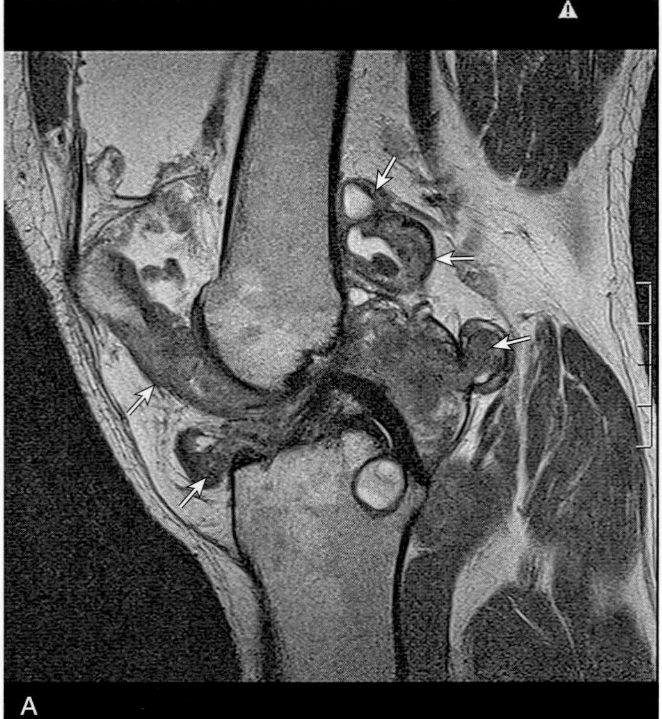

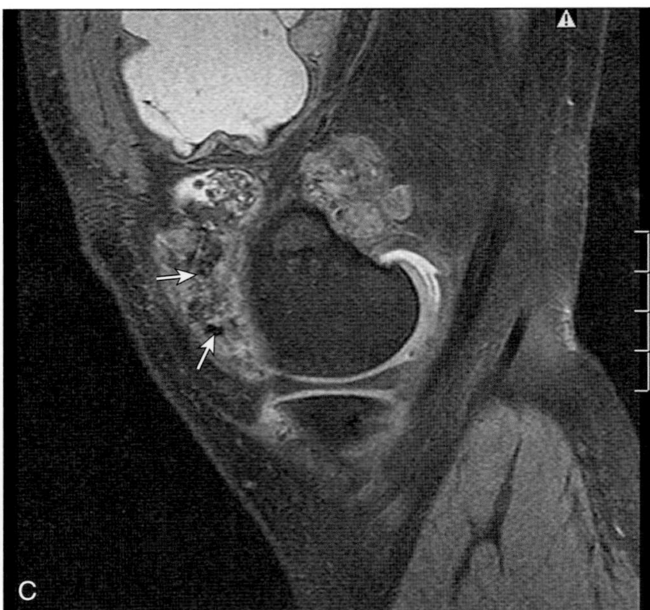

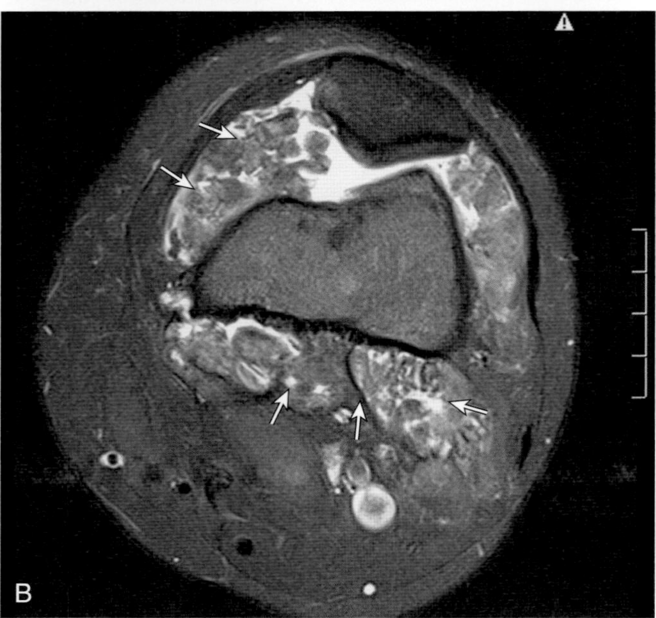

FIGURE 3-41. A 27-year-old male with pigmented villonodular synovitis of the left knee. Sagittal (A) and axial (B) T2-weighted image shows intra-articular synovial-based mass is predominantly hypointense signal intensity (arrows). Gradient echo sequence sagittal plane image shows susceptibility artifacts (arrows) from hemosiderin deposition within this mass is quite typical of pigmented villonodular synovitis (C).

proliferation and loose body formation, as well as the extent of calcification or ossification. There is an overlap between synovial chondromatosis and PVNS on an MRI, with both conditions displaying synovial-based masses. Synovial masses with lobulated borders and with or without associated intra-articular loose bodies are the most common MRI finding for synovial chondromatosis.[46] Noncalcified synovial masses typically show high signal intensity on T2-weighted images, reflecting hyaline cartilage content (Figure 3-42). Foci of signal void as a result of mineralization within synovial masses are common, but low signal intensity is only occasionally seen on T2-weighted images. Calcified loose bodies appear as foci of signal void, whereas ossified loose bodies show signal intensity characteristics of marrow fat centrally, surrounded by cortical bone peripherally.

Ganglia, Synovial Cysts, and Bursitis

Ganglia and synovial cysts have identical imaging features on an MRI, so some do not attempt to differentiate between these two entities. Both entities are periarticular in location and are commonly seen on the hands and feet. Synovial cysts represent true herniation of the synovial membrane through the joint capsule. Communication with the nearby joint through a narrow neck may be demonstrated on an MRI confirming the diagnosis of a synovial cyst. On MR images, both lesions typically appear as round or ovoid masses that are uniloculated or multiloculated, with smooth or slightly lobulated surfaces (Figure 3-43). These masses are in close proximity to a joint or tendon. Although McEvedy[47] found attachment of the ganglia to the joint capsule in an overwhelming majority of 150 cases examined at surgery, at arthrography and MRI, ganglia are not always seen to communicate with the adjacent joint. Signal characteristics of ganglia and synovial cysts are similar to those of simple

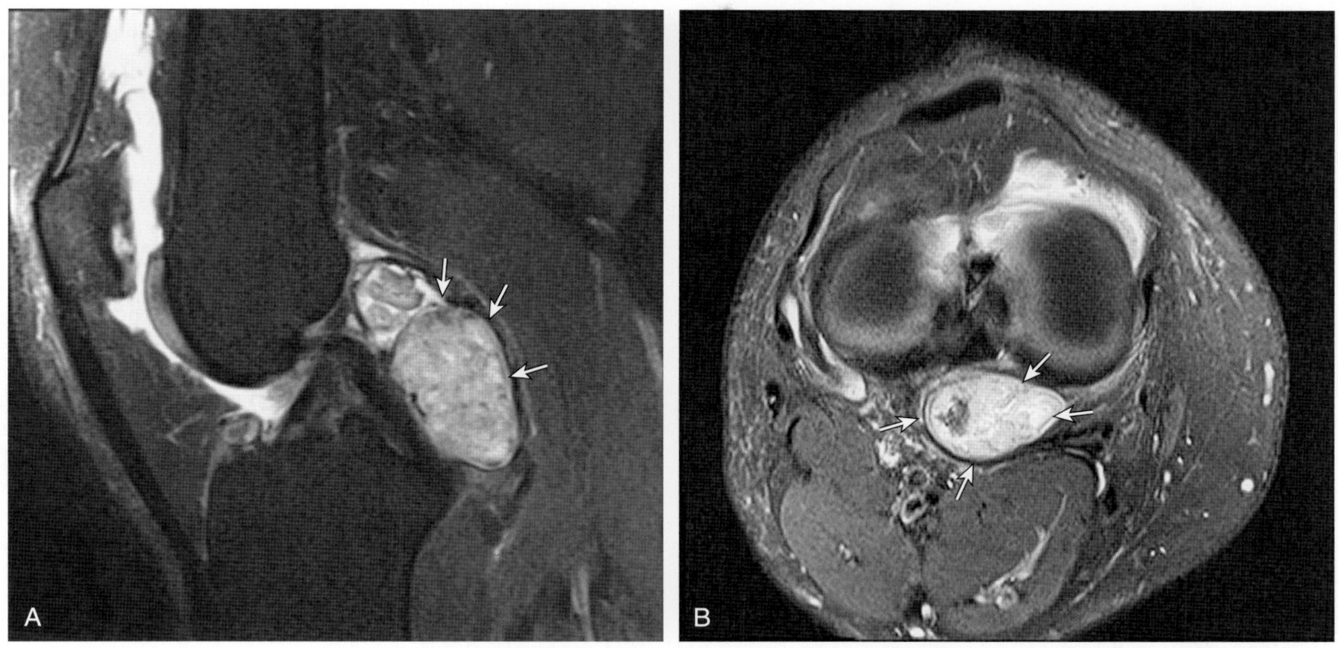

FIGURE 3-42. A 36-year-old male with synovial chondromatosis of the right knee. Sagittal (A) and axial T2-weighted (B) images show synovial bodies especially around the posterior aspect of the joint (arrows). Hyperintense T2 signal within the synovial bodies is typical of noncalcified synovial chondromatosis.

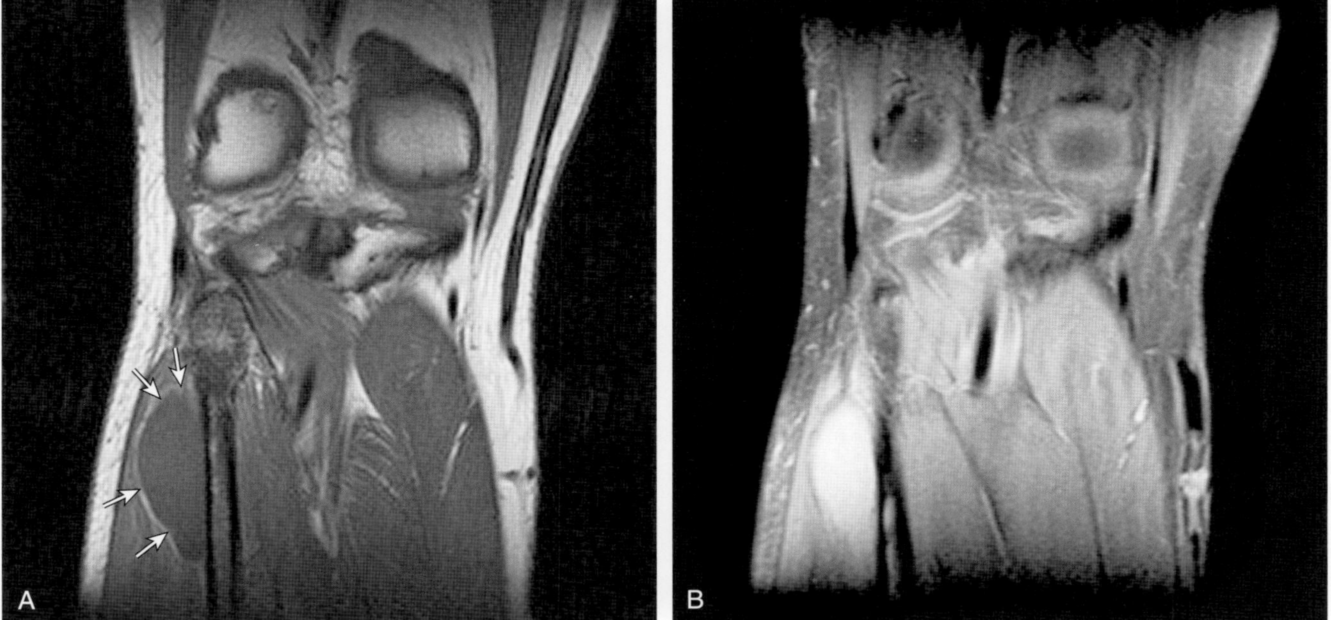

FIGURE 3-43. A 52-year-old male with a proximal tibiofibular joint ganglion. Coronal T1-weighted (A) and T2-weighted (B) images show a collection associated with the tibiofibular joint extending into adjacent soft tissues (arrows). Minimal peripheral enhancement of this collection is noted in the postcontrast T1-weighted fat-saturated coronal image (C).

Continued

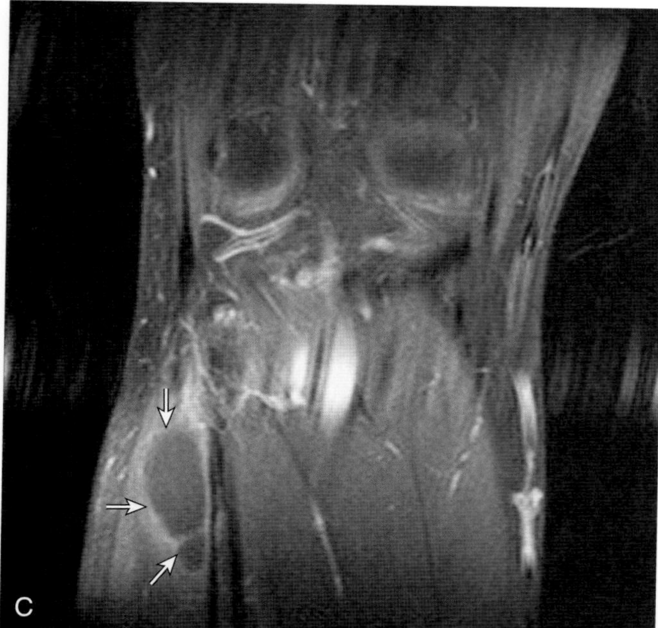

FIGURE 3-43, cont'd

fluid: hypointense to skeletal muscle on T1-weighted images and markedly hyperintense on fluid sensitive T2-weighted or STIR images. A slightly hyperintense signal can sometimes be seen on T1-weighted images; this may be the result of intralesional hemorrhage or accumulation of mucoid material (Figure 3-44). These cases require further imaging with contrast to rule out a solid neoplasm such as synovial sarcoma. Contrast enhancement in ganglia and synovial cysts is strictly peripheral, with no intralesional enhancement expected. If there is a delay in the MR imaging after contrast injection, secretion of contrast into the joint fluid and cyst would possibly confuse the radiologist. Because synovial cysts and ganglia do not occur away from periarticular locations, an intramuscular cystic-appearing mass without communication with a nearby joint should be examined as a possible neoplasm, typically a myxoid tumor. Rotator cuff musculature is an exception to this because delaminating partial thickness tears can form intramuscular ganglia (Figure 3-45). In addition, cystic structures with imaging features identical to those of synovial cysts and ganglia may be seen in the setting of meniscal and labral tears around the acetabular or glenoid labrum.

Bursal collections (bursitis) also usually occur near joints. Precise knowledge of anatomy allows localization of fluid collection in these locations, confirming the diagnosis of bursitis. Some bursa may communicate with nearby joints, such as popliteal cysts (Figure 3-46). Bursal collections may have associated tendon pathology in certain locations (i.e., subacromial-subdeltoid bursa and rotator cuff or retrocalcaneal bursa and Achilles tendon). Sebaceous cysts are often complex and easily recognized in the subcutaneous location abutting the dermis.

Postoperative Collections

Postoperative fluid collections within the surgical bed are frequently encountered on follow-up MRI examinations. These collections could represent hematomas, especially in the early postoperative period. Lymphocele and seroma are the most common fluid collections to occur after the immediate postoperative period. Both lymphocele and seroma demonstrate imaging features similar to those of simple fluid and almost identical to those of synovial cysts and ganglia, with low T1-weighted and increased T2-weighted signals (Figure 3-47). These collections may appear complex, in some cases, perhaps as a result of hemorrhage. These cases may require imaging with contrast, especially in the setting of prior tumor resection to exclude solid elements. Minimal peripheral enhancement is typically seen on postcontrast images. In general, these collections remain stable or become smaller over a long-term follow-up.

Abscesses

Soft tissue abscesses can often be diagnosed clinically without the need for imaging. For cases in which deep extension or osteomyelitis is suspected, the MRI is the modality of choice. On MRI, an abscess may simulate a necrotic sarcoma, particularly on postcontrast images that show nodular peripheral enhancement (Figure 3-48). On T1-weighted images, abscesses tend to be slightly hyperintense to skeletal muscle, with heterogeneous hyperintensity on fluid-sensitive T2-weighted and STIR sequences. There are typically inflammatory changes surrounding the abscesses on MRI, which is an unusual finding in the setting of a sarcoma (see Figure 3-48).

Heterotopic Ossification

Heterotopic ossification (myositis ossificans) is a localized, self-limiting, reparative lesion of the soft tissues. Some prefer the term *heterotopic ossification* over myositis ossificans because these lesions can arise outside of the muscles. The cause of heterotopic ossification is soft tissue injury, in most cases, secondary to an obvious trauma. In the remaining cases, minor repetitive trauma, ischemia, and inflammation are thought to be the causative agents. The lesion may develop anywhere in the body but occurs most frequently in those areas more likely to be exposed to trauma, especially the anterior compartments of the thigh and arm. Patients may be asymptomatic or may present with pain, swelling, and, occasionally, elevated inflammatory markers. In bedridden patients, heterotopic ossification may appear at pressure points in the pelvis and surrounding hip joints.

The imaging appearance of heterotopic ossification on imaging studies varies, depending on the stage of the lesion.[48] Heterotopic ossification evolves from nonspecific soft tissue mass to a dense rim of peripheral ossification and, eventually, an ossified mass. In the first few weeks after the lesion appears, calcification is rarely seen on radiographs. Calcification can become apparent from 3 to 8 weeks after onset of the lesion, starting peripherally and progressing centrally in a typical zonal pattern (Figure 3-49). The MR appearance of heterotopic ossification also varies as the lesion evolves. Early lesions appear as poorly defined masses on an MRI, isointense on T1-weighted images and heterogeneously hyperintense on T2-weighted images with diffuse surrounding soft tissue

Text continued on p. 67

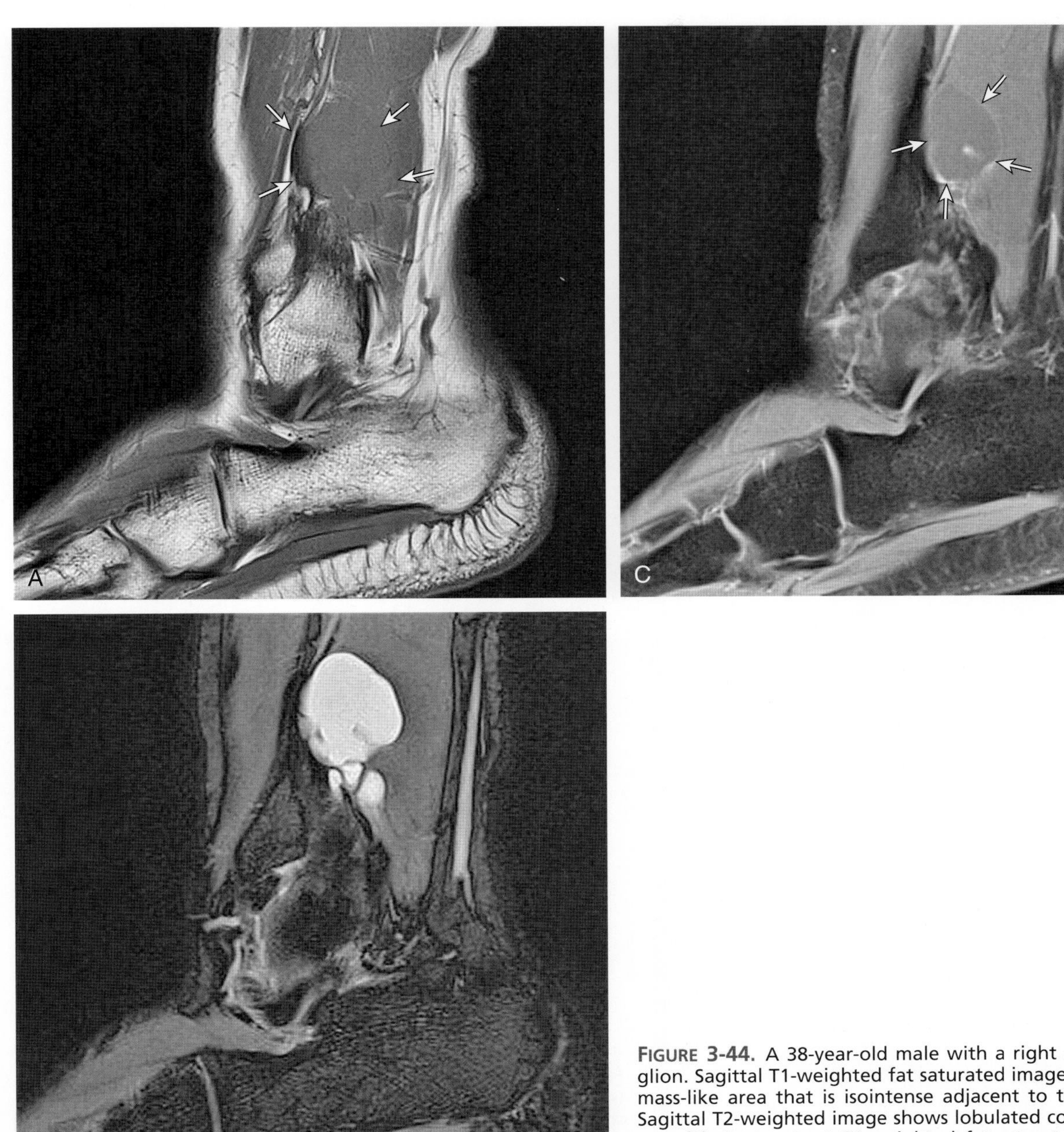

FIGURE 3-44. A 38-year-old male with a right ankle complex ganglion. Sagittal T1-weighted fat saturated image (A) demonstrates a mass-like area that is isointense adjacent to the muscle (arrows). Sagittal T2-weighted image shows lobulated contours of this structure (B). Postcontrast T1-weighted fat-saturated image (C) shows minimal peripheral enhancement of this mass, typical of a ganglion or synovial cyst (arrows).

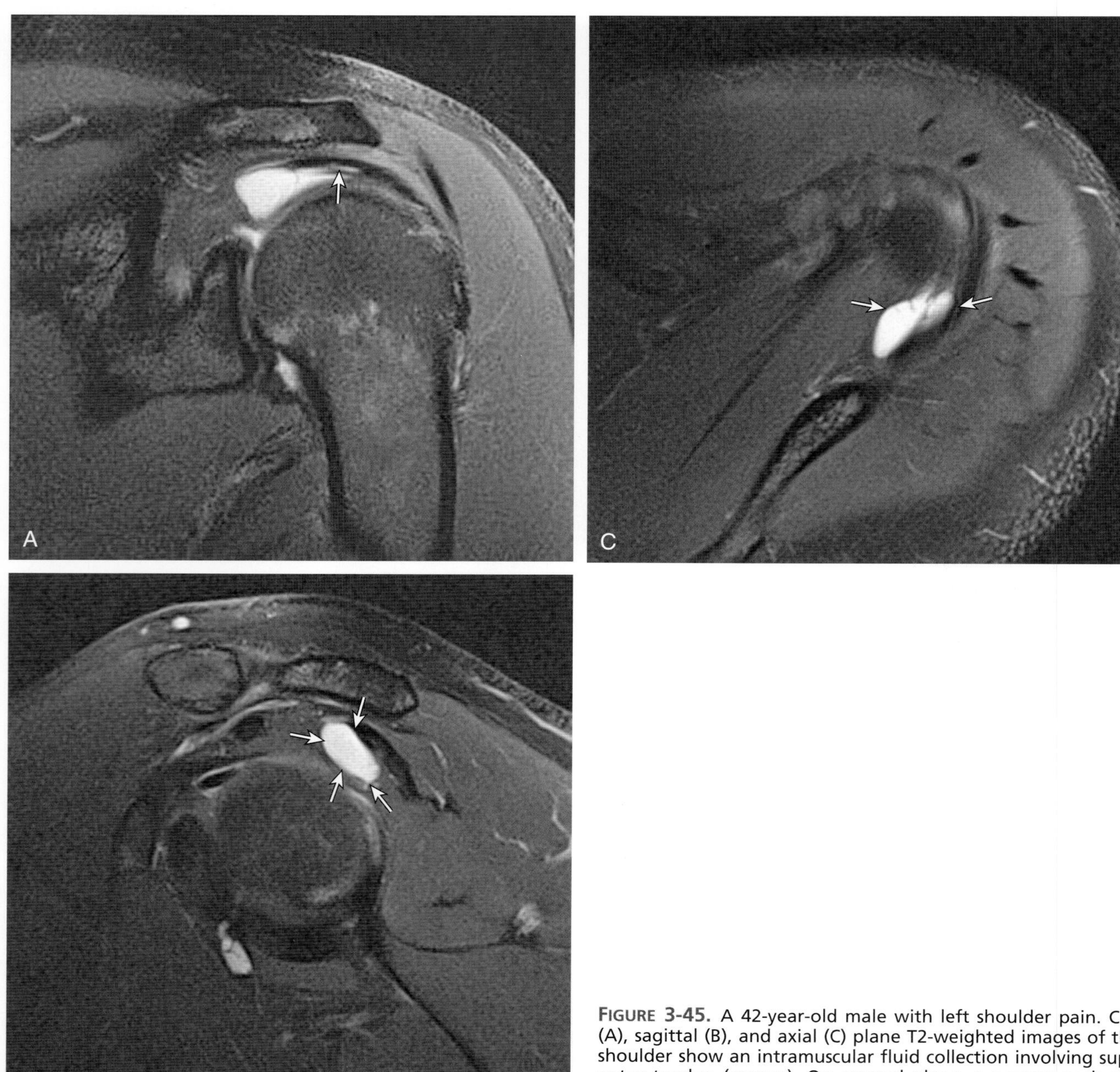

FIGURE 3-45. A 42-year-old male with left shoulder pain. Coronal (A), sagittal (B), and axial (C) plane T2-weighted images of the left shoulder show an intramuscular fluid collection involving supraspinatus tendon (arrows). On coronal plane, a narrow neck of fluid extending into the tendon surface (arrowhead) is noted consistent with partial tear.

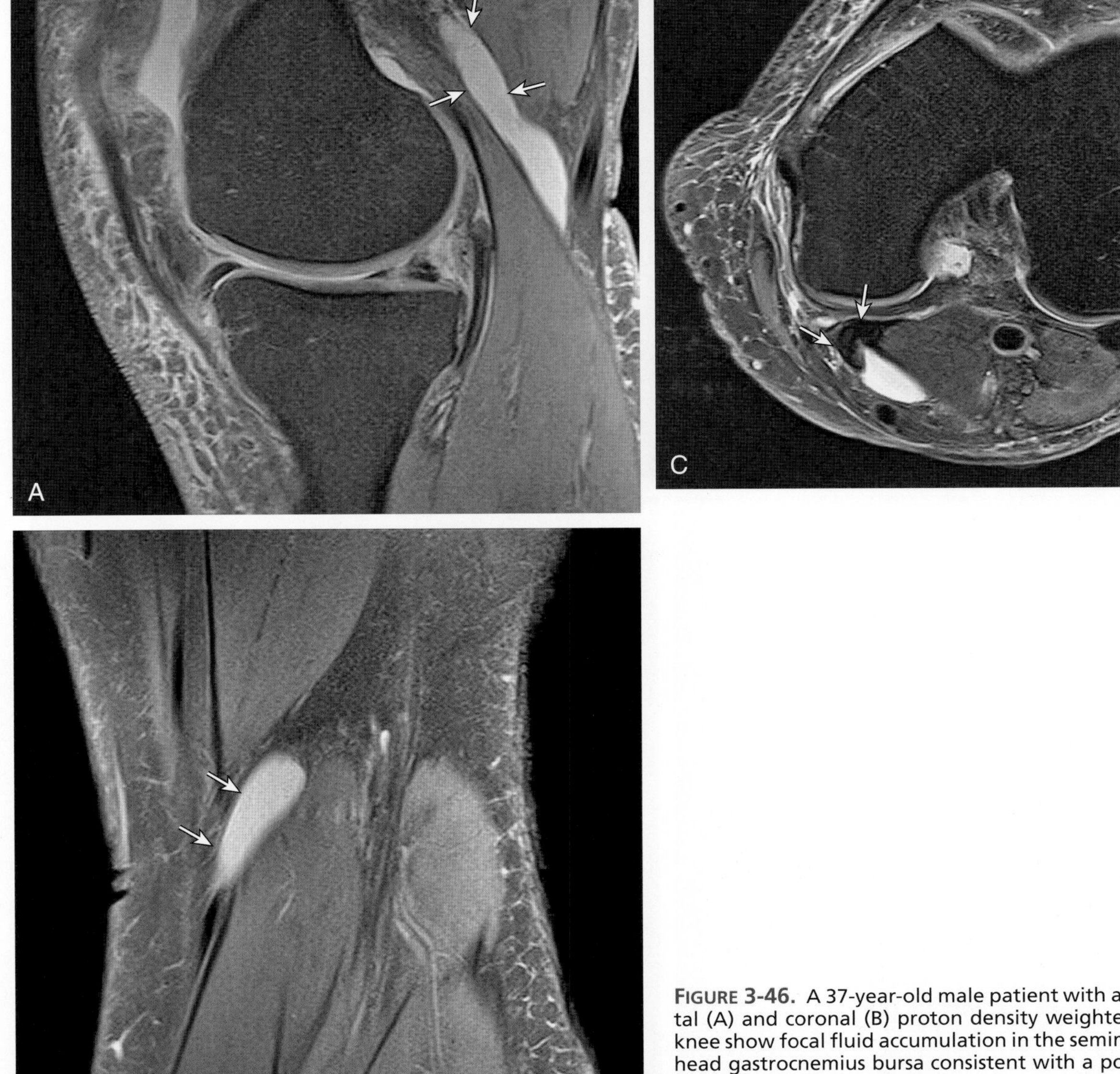

FIGURE 3-46. A 37-year-old male patient with a popliteal cyst. Sagittal (A) and coronal (B) proton density weighted images of the left knee show focal fluid accumulation in the semimembranosus-medial head gastrocnemius bursa consistent with a popliteal cyst (arrows). On axial T2-weighted images (C), semimembranosus and medial head gastrocnemius tendons are noted anterior to the popliteal cyst (arrows).

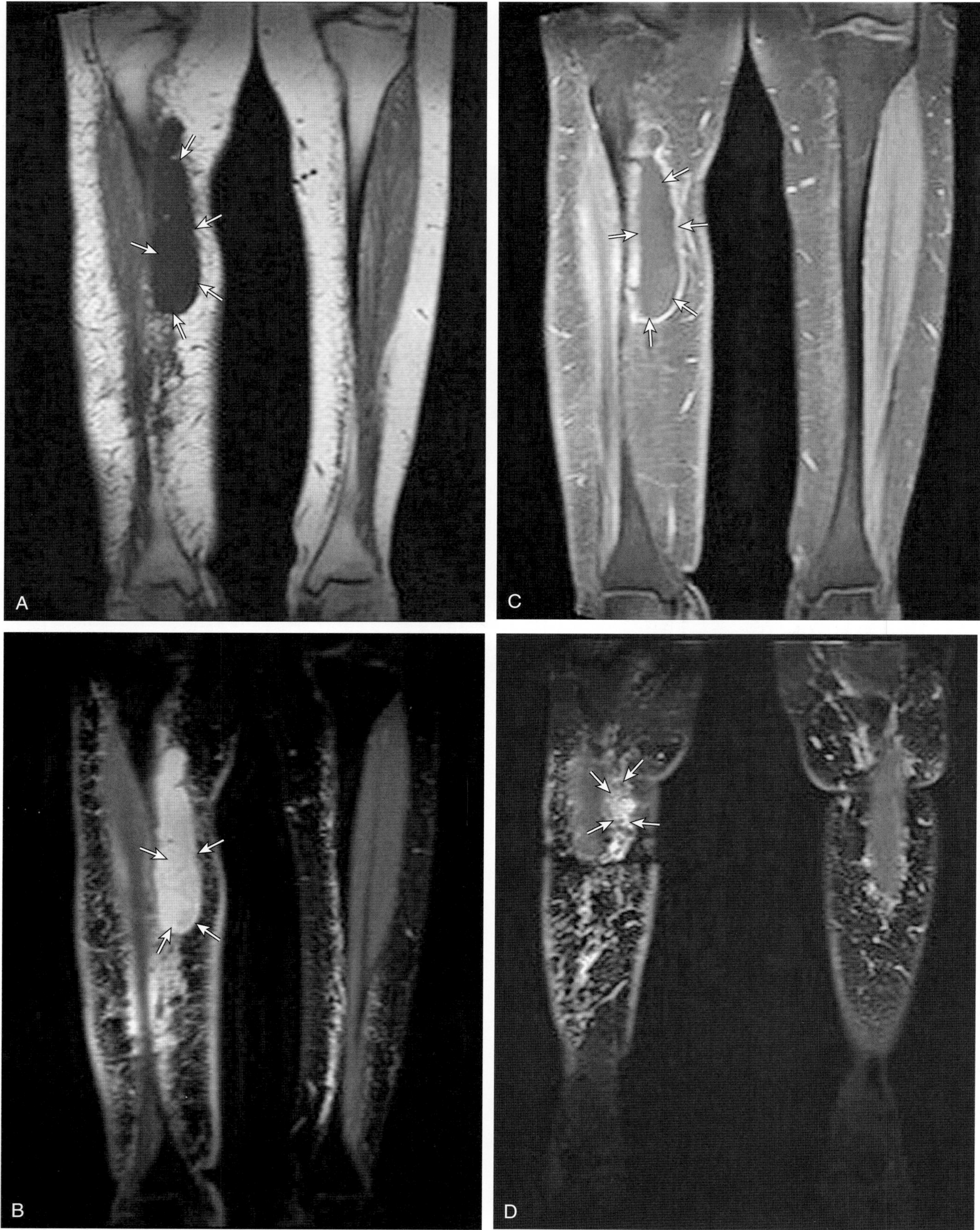

FIGURE 3-47. A 67-year-old female status post right tibial sarcoma resection. Six-month follow-up of the surgery shows a postoperative collection representing seroma or lymphocele hypointense on coronal T1-weighted image (A) and hyperintense on coronal STIR image (B) similar to simple fluid. Mild peripheral enhancement is noted in the postcontrast T1-weighted fat suppressed images (C). Two-year follow-up MRI shows marked decrease in the size of this mass on coronal STIR (D) and axial T2-weighted (E) images.

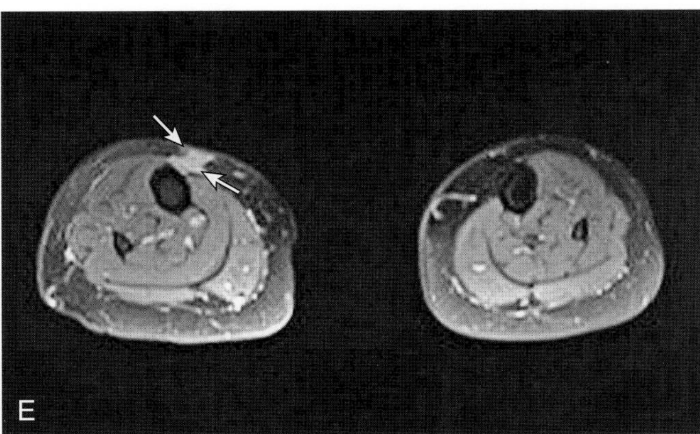

FIGURE 3-47, cont'd

edema.[48] As peripheral calcification develops, peripheral low signal intensity may be seen on the MRI.[48] Immature or non-calcified heterotopic ossification may appear because a complex fluid collection with diffuse enhancement can be mistaken for soft-tissue infection such as an abscess or phlegmon (Figure 3-50). Zonal pattern of mineralization is difficult to recognize on an MRI and best appreciated on radiographs or CT images.

Accessory or Hypertrophied Muscles

A large number of supernumerary and accessory musculature have been described in the anatomic, surgical, and radiology literature. In the majority of cases, accessory muscles are asymptomatic and represent incidental findings on imaging,[49] although they have been implicated as a potential source of clinical symptoms (Figure 3-51). These symptoms may be related to a palpable swelling or may be the result of mass effect on neurovascular structures, typically in fibro-osseous tunnels such as flexor digitorum accessorius longus-tarsal tunnel syndrome (see Figure 3-51), anconeus epitrochlearis muscle-cubital tunnel syndrome, or accessory flexor digitorum superficialis indicis muscle-carpal tunnel syndrome.[49] For cases in which an obvious cause for such symptoms is not evident, recognition and careful evaluation of accessory muscles may aid in a diagnosis.

UNCOMMON TUMOR-LIKE CONDITIONS

Decubital Ischemic Fasciitis (Atypical Decubital Fibroplasia or Ischemic Fasciitis)

Decubital ischemic fasciitis is a reactive, non-neoplastic lesion found in the deep subcutaneous tissue at pressure points or over bony prominences.[50] These lesions are typically encountered in patients who are debilitated, confined to the bed, or wheelchair-bound. Because this lesion simulates soft tissue sarcoma both clinically and histologically, it is important to be familiar with the MRI features of decubital ischemic fasciitis so that sarcoma is not mistakenly diagnosed.

Decubital ischemic fasciitis is found to demonstrate non-specific isointense signal intensity relative to muscle on T1-weighted sequences and heterogeneously hyperintense

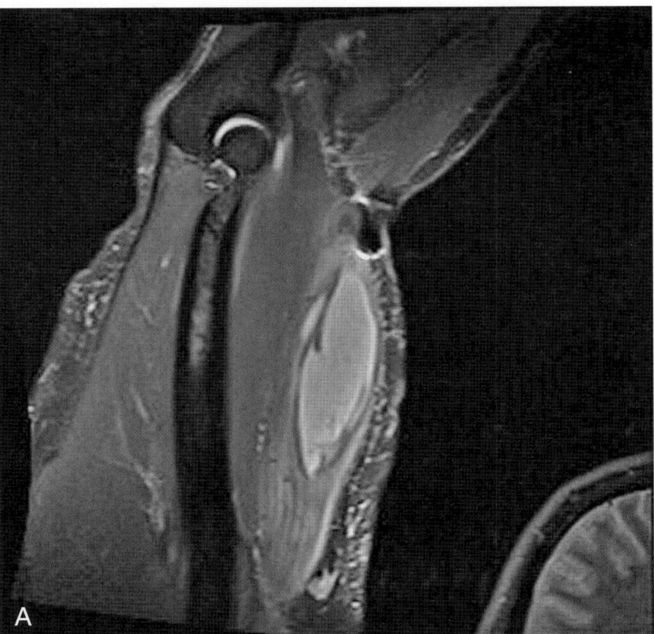

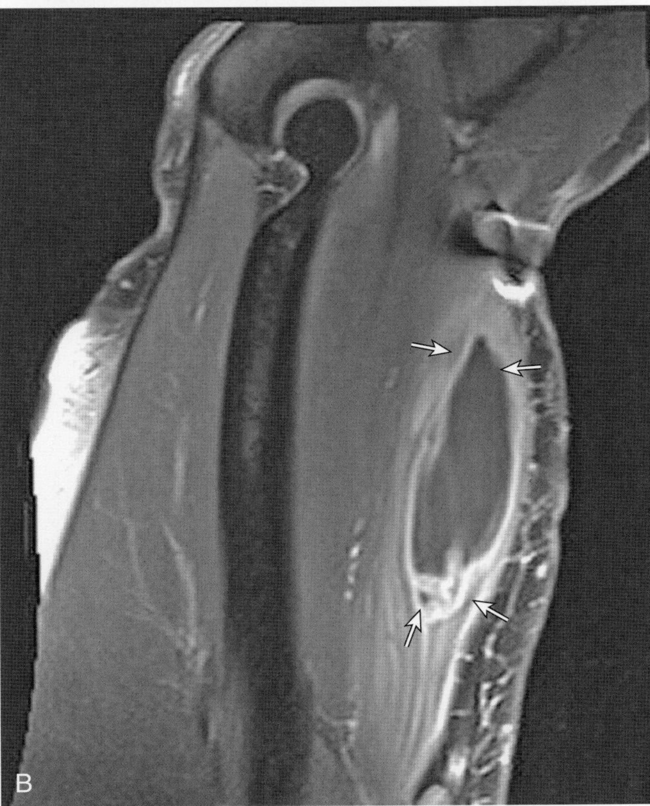

FIGURE 3-48. A 27-year-old male with right arm abscess. T2-weighted sagittal image (A) of the right arm shows a large intramuscular collection with surrounding reactive edema. Nodular enhancement is noted in the periphery of the collection on T1-weighted fat saturated postcontrast image (arrows) (B), typical of an abscess.

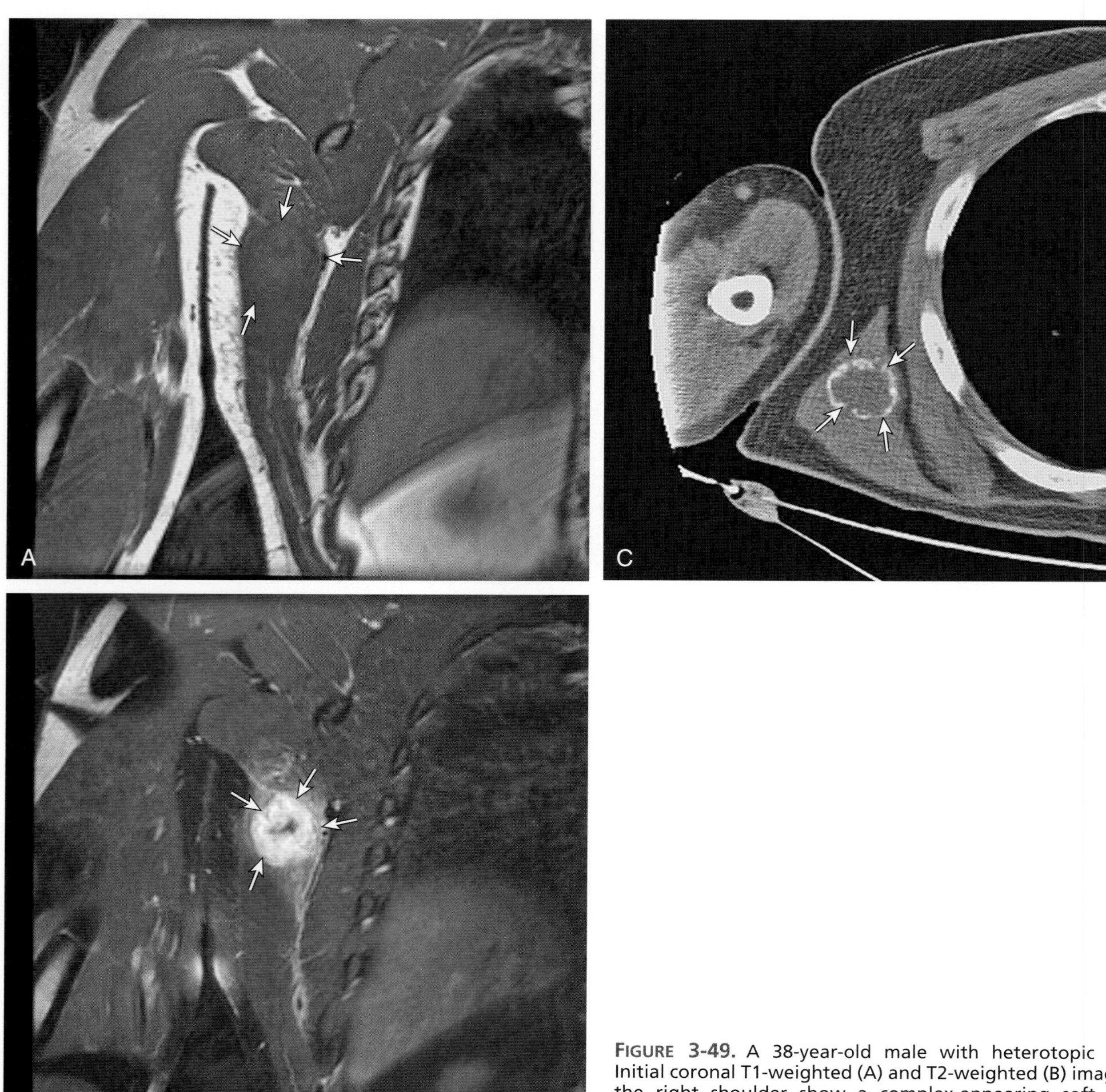

FIGURE 3-49. A 38-year-old male with heterotopic ossification. Initial coronal T1-weighted (A) and T2-weighted (B) images through the right shoulder show a complex-appearing soft tissue mass with increased T2 signal intensity and surrounding muscle edema (arrows). Follow-up CT (C) after 2 weeks shows zonal pattern of heterotopic ossification (arrows).

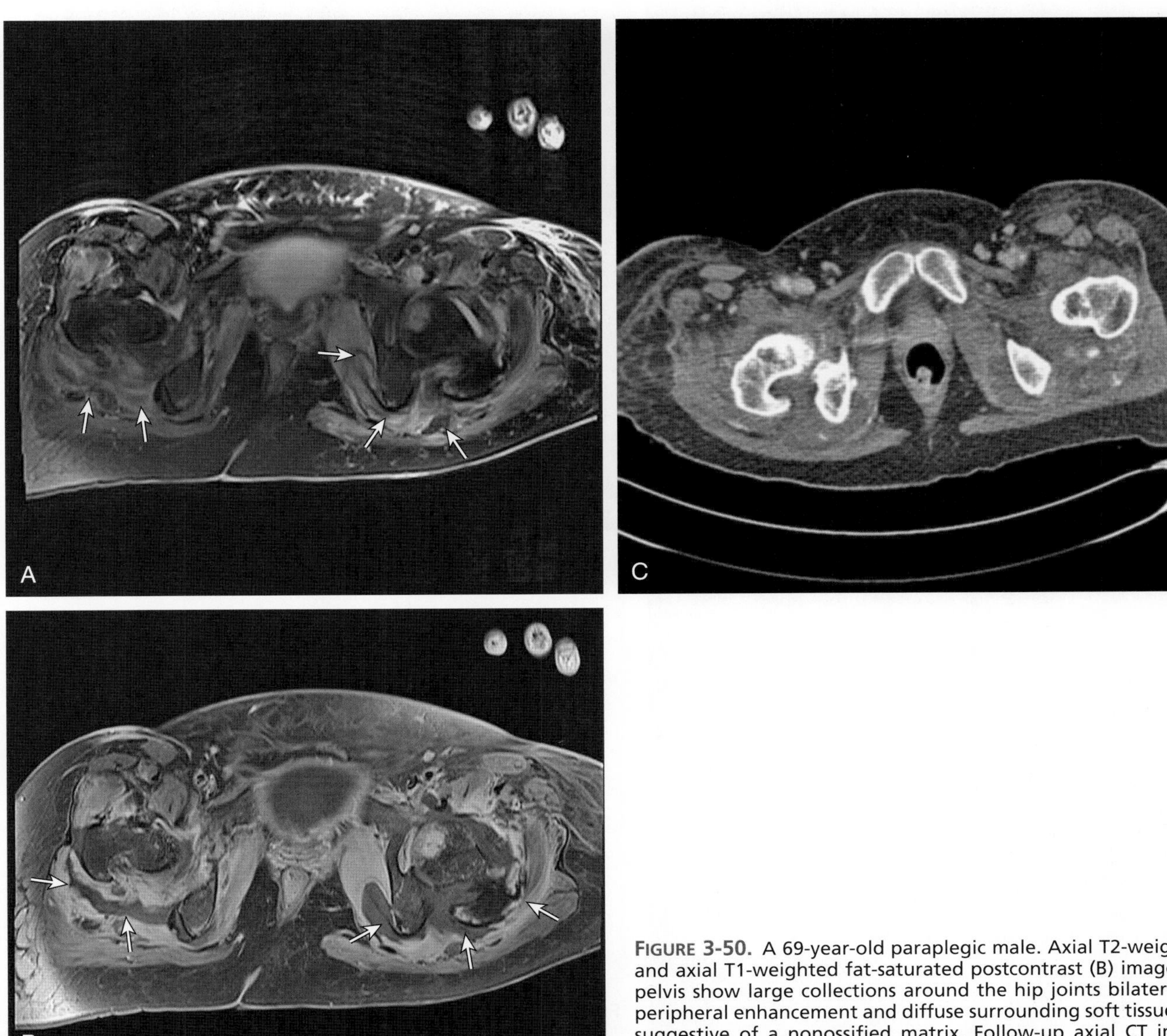

FIGURE 3-50. A 69-year-old paraplegic male. Axial T2-weighted (A) and axial T1-weighted fat-saturated postcontrast (B) images of the pelvis show large collections around the hip joints bilaterally with peripheral enhancement and diffuse surrounding soft tissue edema, suggestive of a nonossified matrix. Follow-up axial CT image (C) shows foci of heterotopic ossification (arrows).

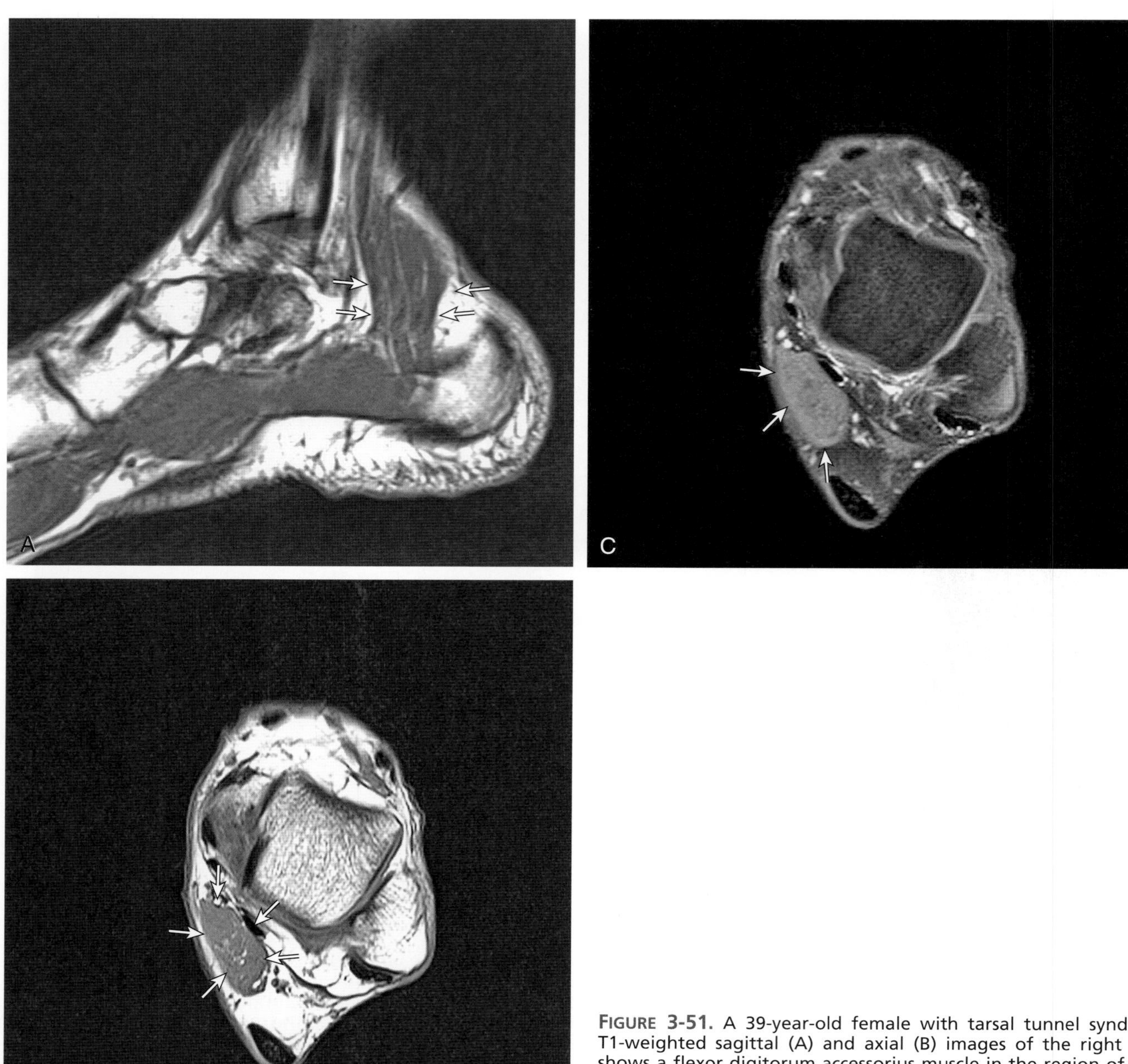

FIGURE 3-51. A 39-year-old female with tarsal tunnel syndrome. T1-weighted sagittal (A) and axial (B) images of the right ankle shows a flexor digitorum accessorius muscle in the region of tarsal tunnel. Anterior displacement neurovascular bundle is noted as a result of mass effect of this accessory muscle on proton-density-weighted axial images (C).

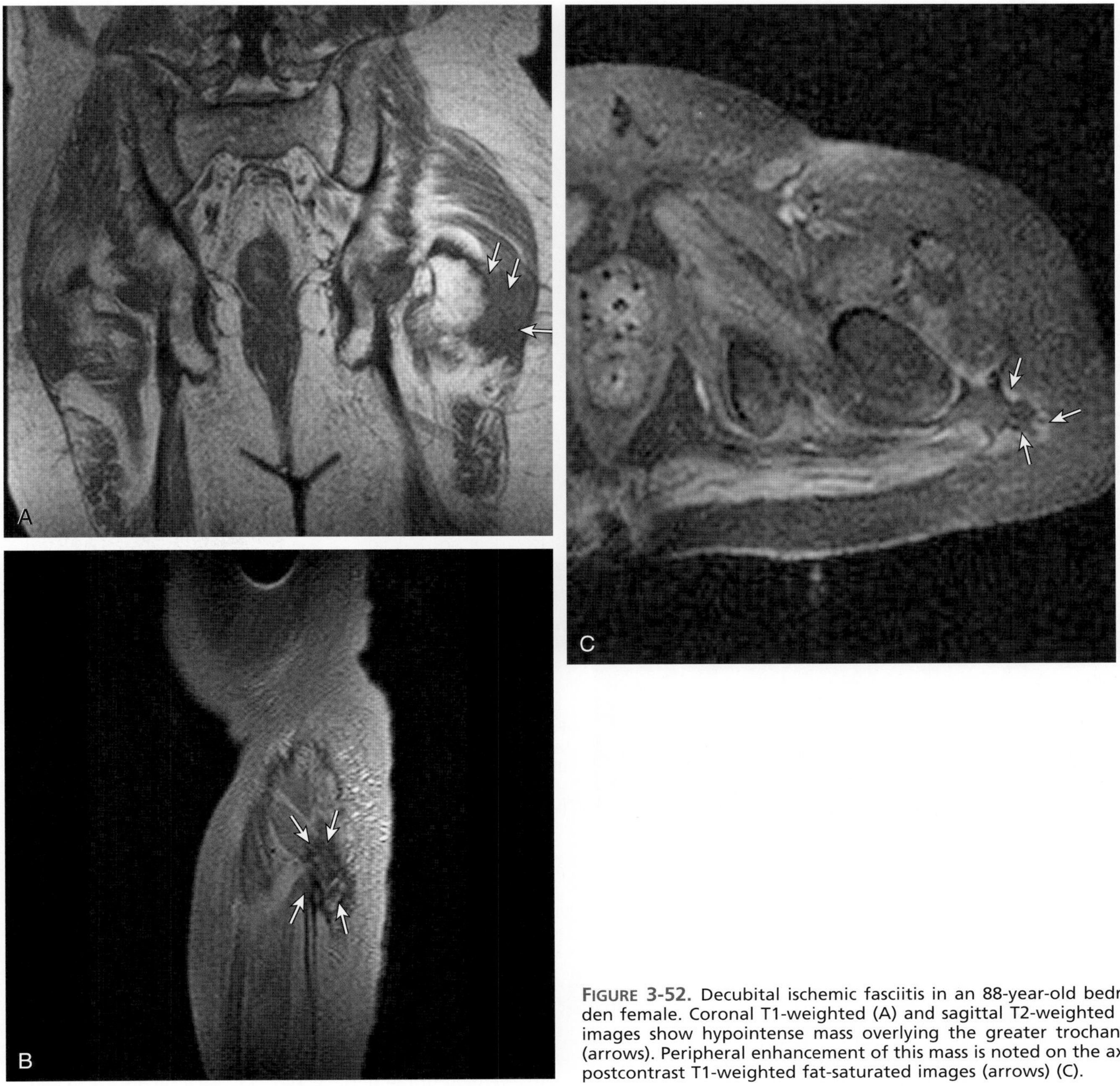

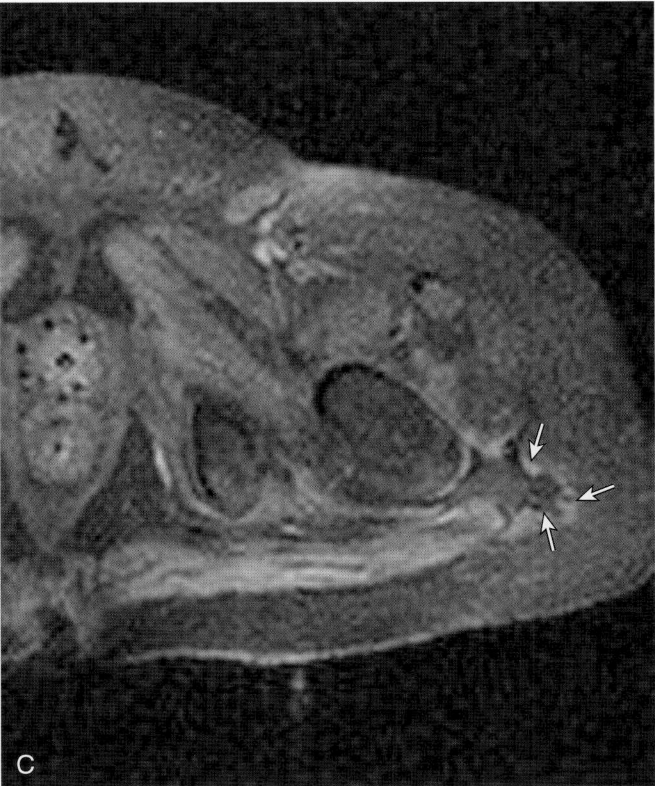

FIGURE 3-52. Decubital ischemic fasciitis in an 88-year-old bedridden female. Coronal T1-weighted (A) and sagittal T2-weighted (B) images show hypointense mass overlying the greater trochanter (arrows). Peripheral enhancement of this mass is noted on the axial postcontrast T1-weighted fat-saturated images (arrows) (C).

signal intensity on T2-weighted images. Intense peripheral enhancement is typically seen with a nonenhancing region in the center, indicating necrotic foci (Figure 3-52). The most distinctive feature of these lesions is their location over pressure points. Lesions most commonly occur over the greater trochanter (see Figure 3-52). These lesions may also be found in the shoulder, sacral area, posterior chest wall, and vulvovagina.[50]

Nodular Fasciitis

Nodular fasciitis is a benign proliferation of fibroblasts and myofibroblasts.[51] These lesions may be mistaken for a sarcomatous lesion because of its rapid growth, nonspecific imaging appearance, and histology. Patients typically present with a rapidly growing and painful soft tissue mass. Most cases arise from the upper extremities, particularly the volar aspect of the forearm.[51] Other sites of involvement include the trunk, head and neck, and lower extremities. Most of these lesions are small (usually smaller than 2 cm).[52] There are three subtypes of nodular fasciitis: subcutaneous, intramuscular, and fascial lesions.[52,53] Typical cases of nodular fasciitis are a subcutaneous small mass with well-defined margins abutting fascia (Figure 3-53). Intramuscular lesions may mimic soft tissue malignancies on imaging because of their larger size, deeper location, and less-defined borders.[53]

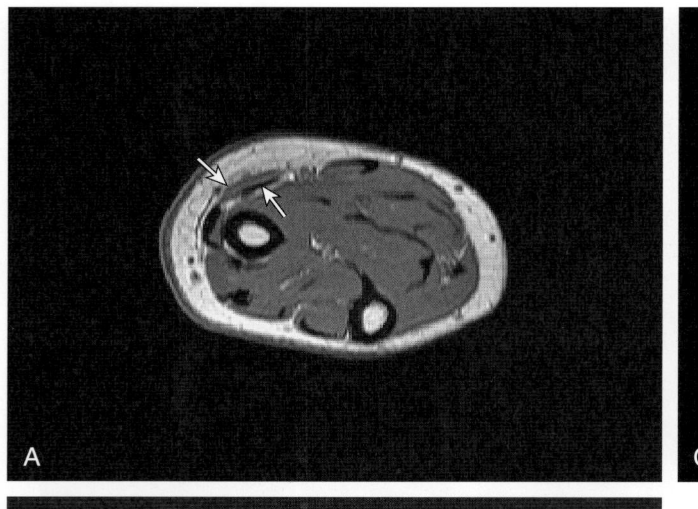

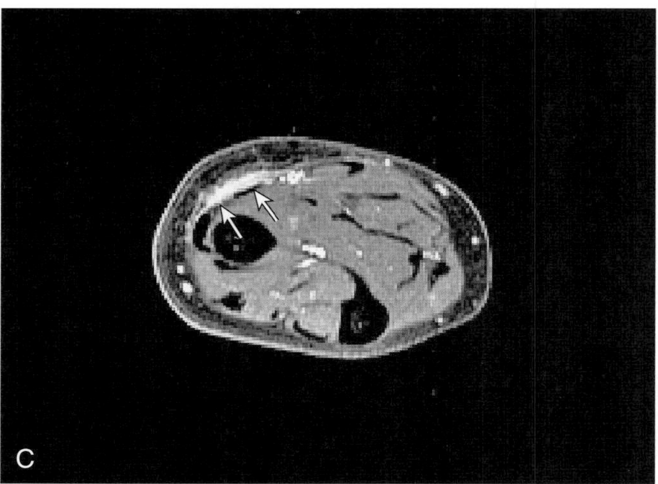

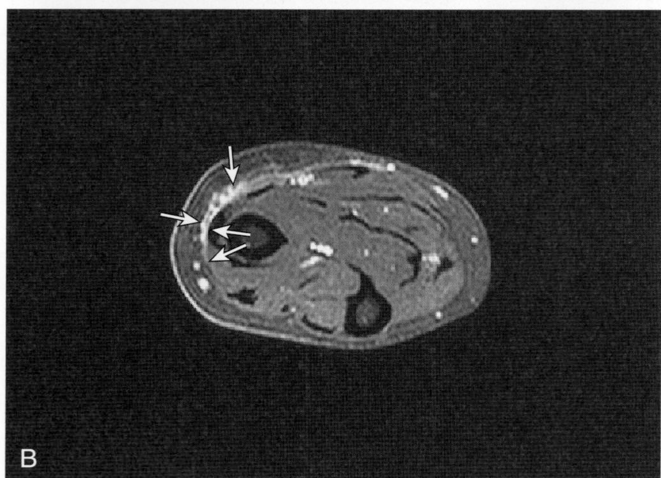

FIGURE 3-53. Nodular fasciitis in a 39-year-old female. Axial T1-weighted (A) and T2-weighted (C) images show small mass with ill-defined margins on the ulnar side of the distal forearm abutting the fascia (arrows). Mild-to-moderate enhancement is noted in the postcontrast T1-weighted fat-saturated image (arrows) (B).

The histologic diversity of nodular fasciitis is reflected on a variable imaging appearance of these lesions on an MRI. The signal in hypercellular lesions appears nearly isointense relative to muscle on T1-weighted images and hyperintense on T2-weighted images.[52] Highly collagenous lesions display a hypointense signal on all MRI sequences. Contrast enhancement is typically diffuse but may be peripheral, in some cases.[53]

Lipomatosis of Nerves

Lipomatosis of the nerve, formerly known as *fibrolipomatous hamartoma*, is the abnormal growth of fibrofatty tissue between nerve fibers.[54] Histologic changes in the nerves with this condition are identical to those seen in cases of macrodystrophia lipomatosa. Although lipomatosis of the nerve is typically first noted in early childhood, patients may not seek treatment until they reach adulthood. Median nerve and its digital branches are the most frequently involved, followed by the ulnar nerve,[50] although it can affect any nerve, including cranial nerves and the brachial plexus. These patients usually present with a gradually enlarging mass with or without associated motor or sensory deficits. Women are more likely to have associated macrodactyly.[54]

Fatty tissue between nerve fascicles resulting in fusiform enlargement of the nerve is typically seen on an MRI (Figure 3-54). The amount of fat varies and can be barely detectable, in some cases, which may make diagnosing this condition difficult. If typical MRI findings are present, biopsy or surgical excision of the involved nerve is not indicated because this can result in a neurologic deficit. Decompression may be helpful in tight spaces such as the median nerve in the carpal tunnel.

Subcutaneous Granuloma Annulare

Granuloma annulare is an uncommon benign dermatosis that can present as localized, generalized, perforating, or subcutaneous lesions.[55] Subcutaneous granuloma annulare most often manifests as a painless, nonmobile, subcutaneous mass with no associated overlying cutaneous abnormality at any time

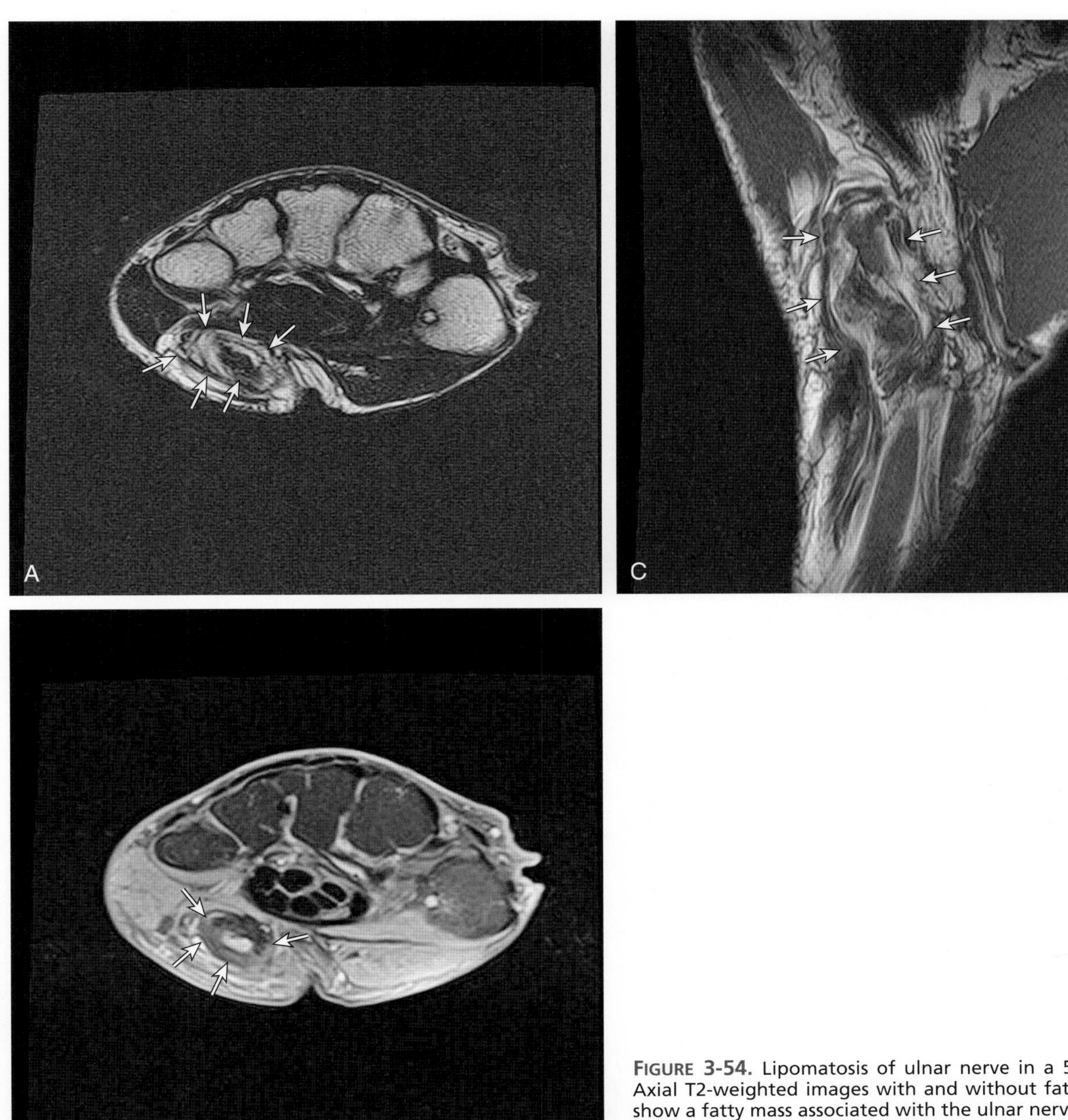

FIGURE 3-54. Lipomatosis of ulnar nerve in a 54-year-old female. Axial T2-weighted images with and without fat suppression (A, B) show a fatty mass associated with the ulnar nerve (arrows). Coronal T1-weighted images demonstrate the extent of the mass (arrows) (C). Note low-signal strands in this mass, representing fibrous elements.

from infancy to young adulthood.[55] The mass may rapidly enlarge over the course of a few weeks. Subcutaneous granuloma annulare generally occurs in the lower extremities (typically in a pretibial location) and is often a solitary lesion. Lesions have also been reported to occur in the upper extremities, buttocks, and face or scalp.[55] Local or distal recurrence may be seen in 19% to 75% of cases.[55,56] The lesion will spontaneously regress, even if it is recurrent.[55,56]

MRI features of this condition are nonspecific, with lesions isointense or hypointense to muscle on T1-weighted images and with heterogeneous but predominantly high signal intensity on T2-weighted or STIR sequences (Figure 3-55). Contrast enhancement may be diffuse or heterogeneous.[55,56] Ill-defined and infiltrative-appearing margins of the lesions could be attributed to inflammatory nature and increased vascularity (see Figure 3-55).

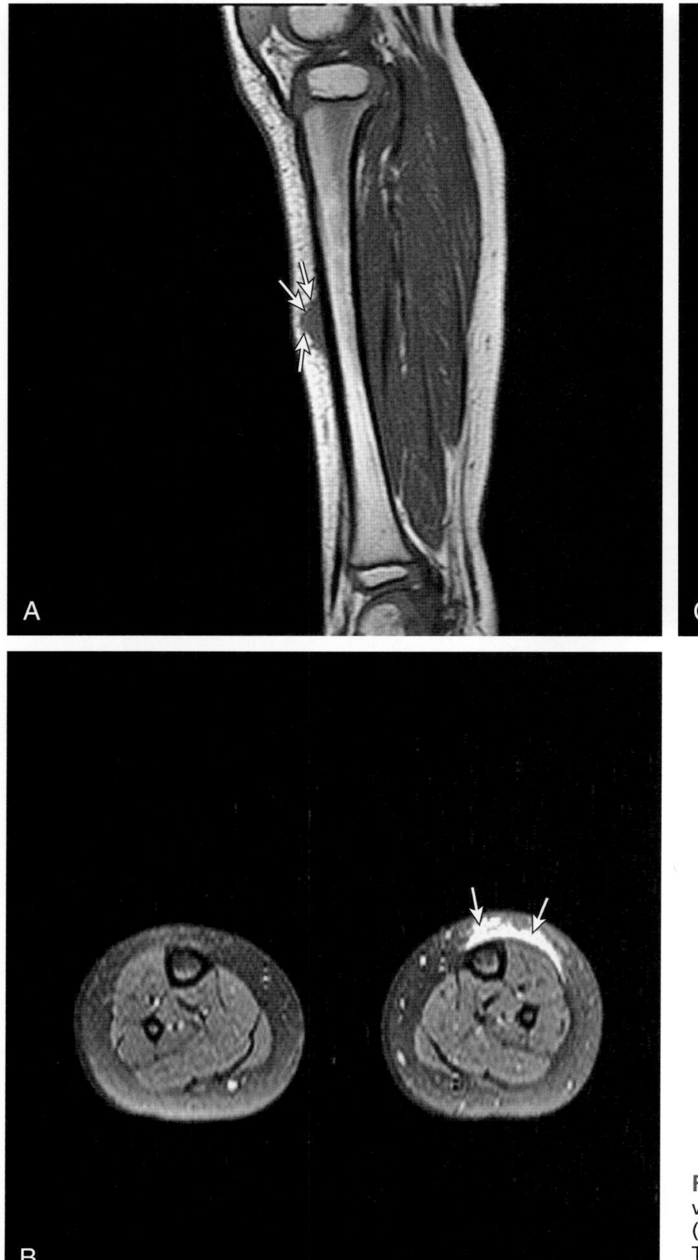

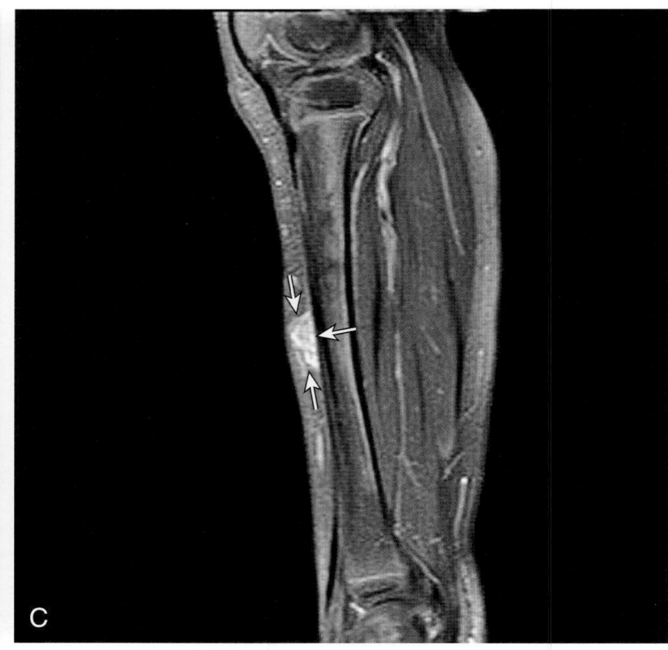

FIGURE 3-55. A 4-year-old female with granuloma annulare. (A) T1-weighted sagittal image of the left leg shows a pretibial mass (arrows) with hyperintense signal and ill-defined margins. (B) Axial T2-weighted image shows hyperintense signal. (C) Postcontrast images show diffuse enhancement of this mass (arrows).

References

1. Fisher C. Soft tissue sarcomas: diagnosis, classification and prognostic factors. Br J Plast Surg 1996;49:27–33.
2. Costelloe CM, Murphy WA Jr, Chasen BA. Musculoskeletal pitfalls in 18F-FDG PET/CT: pictorial review. AJR Am J Roentgenol 2009;193: S26–30; doi:10.2214/AJR.09.7178.
3. Hosono M, Kobayashi H, Fujimoto R, et al. Septum-like structures in lipoma and liposarcoma: MR imaging and pathologic correlation. Skeletal Radiol 1997;26:150–4.
4. Kransdorf MJ, Murphey MD. Neurogenic tumors. Imaging of soft tissue tumors. Philadelphia, Pa: Saunders; 1997. p. 235–73.
5. Isobe K, Shimizu T, Akahane T, et al. Imaging of ancient Schwannoma. AJR Am J Roentgenol 2004;183(2):331–6.
6. Murphey MD, Smith WS, Smith SE, et al. Imaging of musculoskeletal neurogenic tumors: radiologic-pathologic correlation. Radiographics 1999; 19:1253–80.
7. Enjolras O. Classification and management of the various superficial vascular anomalies. J Dermatol 1997;24(11):701–10.
8. Flors L, Leiva-Salinas C, Maged IM, et al. MR imaging of soft-tissue vascular malformations: diagnosis, classification, and therapy follow-up. Radiographics 2011;31(5):1321–40.
9. Marler JJ, Mulliken JB. Current management of hemangiomas and vascular malformations. Clin Plast Surg 2005;32(1):99–116.
10. Ernemann U, Kramer U, Miller S, et al. Current concepts in the classification, diagnosis and treatment of vascular anomalies. Eur J Radiol 2010; 75(1):2–11.
11. Dobson MJ, Hartley RW, Ashleigh R, et al. MR angiography and MR imaging of symptomatic vascular malformations. Clin Radiol 1997;52(8): 595–602.
12. Navarro OM, Laffan EE, Ngan BY. Pediatric soft-tissue tumors and pseudotumors: MR imaging features with pathologic correlation. I. Imaging approach, pseudotumors, vascular lesions, and adipocytic tumors. Radiographics 2009;29(3):887–906.

13. Azizi L, Balu M, Belkacem A, et al. MRI features of mesenteric desmoid tumors in familial adenomatous polyposis. AJR Am J Roentgenol 2005; 184:1128–35.
14. Iwasko N, Steinbach L, Disler D, et al. Imaging findings in Mazabraud's syndrome: seven new cases. Skeletal Radiol 2002;31(2):81–7.
15. Merriman DJ, Deavers MT, Czerniak BA, et al. Massive desmoplastic fibroblastoma with scapular invasion. Orthopedics 2010;33(8).
16. Hwang JW, Ahn JM, Kang HS, et al. Vascular leiomyoma of an extremity: MR imaging-pathology correlation. AJR Am J Roentgenol 1998;171: 981–5.
17. Kransdorf MJ, Murphey MD. Imaging of soft tissue tumors. Philadelphia, Pa: Saunders; 2006. p. 298–300.
18. Dalrymple NC, Hayes J, Bessinger VJ, et al. MRI of multiple glomus tumors of the finger. Skeletal Radiol 1997;26:664–6.
19. Chung EB, Enzinger FM. Fibroma of tendon sheath. Cancer 1979; 44:1945–54.
20. Fox M, Kransdorf MJ, Bancroft LW, et al. MR imaging of fibroma of the tendon sheath. AJR Am J Roentgenol 2003;180:1449–53.
21. Dal Cin P, Sciot R, De Smet L, et al. Translocation 2;11 in a fibroma of tendon sheath. Histopathology 1998;32(5):433–5.
22. Wiswell TE, Davis J, Cunningham BE, et al. Infantile myofibromatosis: the most common fibrous tumor of infancy. J Pediatr Surg 1988;23: 315–18.
23. Enginger FM, Weiss S. Granular cell tumor. In: Soft tissue tumors. 4th ed. St Louis, Mo: CV Mosby; 2004. p. 1178–87.
24. Blacksin MF, White LM, Hameed M, et al. Granular cell tumor of the extremity: magnetic resonance imaging characteristics with pathologic correlation. Skeletal Radiol 2005;34(10):625–31.
25. Stacy GS, Heck RK, Peabody TD, et al. Neoplastic and tumorlike lesions detected on MR imaging of the knee in patients with suspected internal derangement: part 2, articular and juxtaarticular entities. AJR Am J Roentgenol 2002;178(3):595–9.
26. Matushansky I, Charytonowicz E, Mills J, et al. MFH classification: differentiating undifferentiated pleomorphic sarcoma in the 21st century. Expert Rev Anticancer Ther 2009;9(8):1135–44.
27. Torreggiani WC, Al-Ismail K, Munk PL, et al. Dermatofibrosarcoma protuberans: MR imaging features. AJR Am J Roentgenol 2002;178(4): 989–93.
28. Murphey MD, Arcara LK, Fanburg-Smith J. Imaging of musculoskeletal liposarcoma with radiologic-pathologic correlation. Radiographics 2005;25(5):1371–95.
29. Chotel F, Unnithan A, Chandrasekar CR, et al. Variability in the presentation of synovial sarcoma in children: a plea for greater awareness. J Bone Joint Surg Br 2008;90:1090–6.
30. Kransdorf MJ, Meis JM. Extraskeletal osseous and cartilaginous tumors of the extremities. Radiographics 1993;13(4):853–84.
31. Sánchez Reyes JM, Alcaraz Mexia M, Quiñones Tapia D, et al. Extensively calcified synovial sarcoma. Skeletal Radiol 1997;26(11):671–3.
32. Kransdorf MJ. Malignant soft-tissue tumors in large referral population: distribution of diagnoses by age, sex, location. AJR Am J Roentgenol 1995;164:129–34.
33. Enzinger FM, Weiss SW. Malignant tumors of the peripheral nerves. In: Soft tissue tumors. 3rd ed. St Louis, Mo: Mosby; 1995. p. 889–928.
34. Damaj G, Mohty M, Vey N, et al. Features of extramedullary and extraosseous multiple myeloma: a report of 19 patients from a single center. Eur J Haematol 2004;73:402–6.
35. Glockner J, Sundaram M, White L. Incidence of solitary soft-tissue metastases revealed by MR imaging. AJR Am J Roentgenol 2002;179(6): 1644.
36. Chun CW, Jee WH, Park HJ, et al. MRI features of skeletal muscle lymphoma. AJR Am J Roentgenol 2010;195(6):1355–60.
37. De Beuckeleer LH, De Schepper AM, Vandevenne JE, et al. MR imaging of clear cell sarcoma (malignant melanoma of the soft parts): a multicenter correlative MRI-pathology study of 21 cases and literature review. Skeletal Radiol 2000;29(4):187–95.
38. Spillane AJ, Thomas JM, Fisher C. Epithelioid sarcoma: the clinicopathological complexities of this rare soft tissue sarcoma. Ann Surg Oncol 2000;7(3):218–25.
39. Schmidt D. Malignant peripheral neuroectodermal tumor. Curr Top Pathol 1995;89:297–312.
40. Jarvi OH, Lansimies PH. Subclinical elastofibromas in the scapular region at autopsy series. Acta Pathol Microbiol Scand 1975;83:87–108.
41. Nagamine N, Nohara Y, Ito E. Elastofibroma in Okinawa: a clinicopathologic study of 170 cases. Cancer 1982;50:1794–805.
42. Aoki T, Nakata H, Watanabe H, et al. The radiological findings in chronic expanding hematoma. Skeletal Radiol 1999;28:396–401.
43. Reid JD, Kommareddi S, Lankerani M, et al. Chronic expanding hematomas: a clinicopathologic entity. JAMA 1980;244:2441–2.
44. Dorwart RH, Genant HK, Johnston WH, et al. Pigmented villonodular synovitis of synovial joints: clinical, pathologic, and radiologic features. AJR Am J Roentgenol 1984;143:877–85.
45. Llauger J, Palmer J, Roson N, et al. Pigmented villonodular synovitis and giant cell tumors of the tendon sheath: radiologic and pathologic features. AJR Am J Roentgenol 1999;172:1087–91.
46. Murphey MD, Vidal JA, Fanburg-Smith JC, et al. Imaging of synovial chondromatosis with radiologic-pathologic correlation. Radiographics 2007;27(5):1465–88.
47. McEvedy BV. Simple ganglia. Br J Surg 1962;49:585–94.
48. Ledermann HP, Schweitzer ME, Morrison WB. Pelvic heterotopic ossification: MR imaging characteristics. Radiology 2002;222(1):189–95.
49. Sookur PA, Naraghi AM, Bleakney RR, et al. Accessory muscles: anatomy, symptoms, and radiologic evaluation. Radiographics 2008;28(2): 481–99.
50. Ilaslan H, Joyce M, Bauer T, et al. Decubital ischemic fasciitis: clinical, pathologic, and MRI features of pseudosarcoma. Am J Roentgenol 2006;187:1338–41.
51. Dinauer PA, Brixey CJ, Moncur JT, et al. Pathologic and MR imaging features of benign fibrous soft-tissue tumors in adults. Radiographics 2007;27(1):173–87.
52. Wang XL, DeSchepper AM, Vanhoenacker F, et al. Nodular fasciitis: correlation of MRI findings and histopathology. Skeletal Radiol 2002;31(3): 155–61.
53. Leung LY, Shu SJ, Chan AC, et al. Nodular fasciitis: MRI appearance and literature review. Skeletal Radiol 2002;31:9–13.
54. Toms AP, Anastakis D, Bleakney RR, et al. Lipofibromatous hamartoma of the upper extremity: a review of the radiologic findings for 15 patients. AJR Am J Roentgenol 2006;186(3):805–11.
55. Chung S, Frush DP, Prose NS, et al. Subcutaneous granuloma annulare: MR imaging features in six children and literature review. Radiology 1999;210(3):845–9.
56. Kransdorf MJ, Murphey MD, Temple HT. Subcutaneous granuloma annulare: radiologic appearance. Skeletal Radiol 1998;27:266–70.

Cytogenetic and Molecular Genetic Pathology of Soft Tissue Tumors

MARC LADANYI, JONATHAN A. FLETCHER, and PAOLA DAL CIN

CHAPTER CONTENTS

INTRODUCTION

Historically, much of the knowledge of the genetic pathology of sarcomas was based on conventional karyotypic analysis, and, for many years, the molecular consequences of the cytogenetic alterations remained largely obscure. Chromosomal translocations, deletions, and amplifications provided novel diagnostic markers, even if their biology was not understood. Beginning in the early 1990s, as more and more of the genetic underpinnings were identified, namely the gene fusions resulting from the translocations, the tumor suppressor genes subject to deletion, and the oncogenes undergoing amplification, a more integrated understanding of the molecular genetic pathology of mesenchymal neoplasms began to emerge. This process of discovery was accelerated with the application of microarray-based approaches and, more recently, with the development of massively parallel, next-generation sequencing technologies, which is covered later. Broad themes have become apparent at several levels, and these have been useful in organizing thoughts in this area. *At the cytogenetic level*, contrasting sarcomas with complex karyotypes and those with simple karyotypes have led to novel insights. *At the biologic level*, oncogenic mechanisms have fallen into two broad categories: transcriptional deregulation and deregulated signaling. *At the practical level*, the rapid translation of tumor-type-specific genetic alterations into molecular diagnostic markers stands in sharp contrast to the slow clinical adoption of less specific progression-related genetic alterations as prognostic markers. In this chapter, a survey of the major cytogenetic and molecular genetic alterations in soft tissue tumors is provided, focusing on those that are relevant to pathologic diagnosis and the development of more rational classification schemes, to clinical management and therapy selection, and to the understanding of the fundamental biology of these neoplasms.

GENERAL CONCEPTS IN CANCER GENETICS

In a landmark 2000 review, Hanahan and Weinberg[1] distilled the pathobiology of cancer into six key features or hallmarks: self-sufficiency in growth signals, insensitivity to growth-inhibitory signals, evasion of programmed cell death (apoptosis), limitless replicative potential, sustained angiogenesis, and tissue invasion and metastasis. More recently, additional cancer hallmarks have been proposed,[2] including genomic instability, reprogramming of energy metabolism, evasion of immune destruction, and the enabling stromal features that make up the tumor microenvironment, such as inflammation. The acquisition of the tumor cell-inherent hallmark features involves an essentially darwinian process of random mutation followed by natural selection, the selection in this context being for increasingly autonomous proliferation. The pathways by which different cancers acquire their hallmark capabilities clearly vary in terms of the specific genes involved, and this variability may also apply within a single tumor, resulting in intratumoral heterogeneity for some but not all genetic alterations. Whereas this hallmark model also applies to sarcomas, the widely held notion of multistep carcinogenesis arising from the study of epithelial neoplasia, which encompasses a progression from preneoplastic lesions to invasive cancer, does not translate well to sarcomas, especially the so-called translocation sarcomas. In translocation sarcomas, no preneoplastic phase has been recognized, and, in many cases, the translocation is the only identifiable genetic alteration, suggesting that the translocation may, by itself, provide several of the hallmarks of cancer. Furthermore, assuming that differences between sarcoma types are as great, if not greater than differences between epithelial cancers arising from different organs, the likelihood of cell type specificity of oncogenic mechanisms takes on a special importance.

The genetic alterations that allow a clone of cells to acquire the hallmark properties of cancer affect three broad types of cancer genes: oncogenes, tumor suppressor genes, and caretaker genes.[3,4] These designations refer to how these genes contribute to cancer development and do not constitute specific gene families in terms of similarity of sequence or function. Oncogenes are cancer genes that typically achieve their oncogenic effect through increased or deregulated activity of one of the two copies of the gene in question.[3] This activation can occur by a mutation that alters the sequence of the protein in such a way that its function is aberrantly enhanced, by an increase in the number of gene copies (gene amplification), by a translocation that brings its expression under the control of the regulatory sequences (promoter) of another gene, or by a combination of all of these. Examples relevant to mesenchymal tumors include *KIT* and *PDGFRA*, both activated by mutations; *MYCN* and *MDM2*, both activated by gene amplification; and *PLAG1* and *HMGA1*, activated by translocation-mediated promoter juxtaposition (see later text). In addition, translocations that fuse the coding sequences of two genes to generate chimeric proteins are generally considered a special variety of oncogenes, known as fusion oncogenes, of which there are numerous examples in sarcomas.

Tumor suppressor genes, in contrast, typically exert their oncogenic effects through a loss of both functional gene copies.[3] This can be caused by one or more of the following mechanisms: mutations that result in a truncated or inactive protein, mutations that result in a dominant negative protein that interferes with the function of the normal protein produced by the remaining unmutated gene copy, large deletions affecting the gene, replacement of the remaining unmutated copy of the gene by the inactive copy (loss of heterozygosity by mitotic recombination), reduced expression caused by hypermethylation of the regulatory sequences of the gene, or interruption of the gene by a nonrecurrent translocation. Key examples in sarcomas include the generic tumor suppressors *TP53 (p53)*, *RB1*, and *CDKN2A*, as well as more sarcoma-selective suppressors, such as *NF1* and *SMARCB1* (*INI1*). Classical tumor suppressor genes act through complete or near-complete loss of function of the protein in question within the cancer cell. However, for some nonclassic tumor suppressors, haploinsufficiency, that is, a loss of one copy resulting in 50% decreased protein function in the cell, may be pathogenetically significant,[5] but the extent of this type of mechanism in sarcomas requires further study.

The third major class of cancer genes are the caretaker genes.[3] These genes contribute to oncogenesis through a loss of function mechanism but differ from conventional tumor suppressor genes in that this does not directly cause a malignant phenotype but enables cancer cells to acquire other hallmark properties of cancer.[2] The loss of function of caretaker genes increases the likelihood that oncogene activation or conventional tumor suppressor inactivation will occur. Caretaker genes are involved in the maintenance of genomic and chromosomal integrity and, therefore, have also been referred to as *genomic stability genes*. This class of cancer genes seems to have a more limited role in sarcomas than in lymphomas, leukemias, and carcinomas. Examples relevant to mesenchymal tumors include the occurrence of soft tissue sarcomas in Werner syndrome.[6]

In terms of functional classes, the vast majority of cancer genes belong to one of three groups: protein kinases, transcription factors, and DNA maintenance and repair proteins. Whereas the last group corresponds to the caretaker genes, the various protein kinases and transcription factors can function as either oncogenes or tumor suppressor genes. Another class of cancer genes that has more recently gained prominence is involved in cancer cellular metabolism, such as the isocitrate dehydrogenase genes *IDH1* and *IDH2*,[7-9] and the succinate dehydrogenase (SDH) subunit genes,[10] to mention two examples relevant to sarcomas.

GENERAL PRINCIPLES OF TRANSLOCATIONS

The importance of specific, recurrent chromosomal translocations to the biology and diagnosis of sarcomas warrants a more detailed discussion of this special class of genetic alterations. Biologically, these gene fusions operate either by overexpression of the encoded protein, by promoter substitution, or by the formation of aberrant chimeric proteins. In the latter, the coding regions of two genes become fused and the new fusion gene encodes an abnormal, oncogenic protein with a novel combination of functional domains.

Chromosomal translocations constitute the majority of specific genetic alterations associated with sarcomas. As a whole, fusion gene-related sarcomas may account for approximately a third of all sarcomas. These chromosomal translocations produce highly specific gene fusions. The specificity of these gene fusions and their prevalence in selected sarcomas have become a defining feature of many of these entities.[11,12] Two key concepts in translocation sarcomas are (1) they contain their fusion gene from their earliest presentation and do not show a benign or premalignant phase, and (2) the fusion gene is present in all tumor cells and is expressed throughout the clinical course. One of the key concepts relating to the structure of these translocations is that the genomic (DNA-level) breaks almost always occur within introns (not within exons) and that the exon sequences flanking the chimeric intron are then joined by transcription and splicing to form a chimeric mRNA (Fig. 4-1). Because introns can be quite large and the genomic breaks can occur almost anywhere within them, it explains why tumor genomic DNA rarely provides a usable starting point for detecting such translocations by polymerase chain reaction (PCR). In contrast, the consistent joining of the flanking exons by transcript splicing makes mRNA an extremely convenient target for PCR-based molecular diagnosis by reverse-transcriptase (RT) PCR (see Fig. 4-1) or, as demonstrated more recently, for whole transcriptome sequencing as a pan-genomic diagnostic or discovery approach (see later text).

Most of the major *cytogenetically* described translocations in sarcomas by now have been cloned. Table 4-1 lists the major specific recurrent translocations reported in soft tissue neoplasms. Until a translocation is reported in more than one case of a given tumor, it is by definition nonrecurrent. For many of the translocations in Table 4-1, rare nonrecurrent variants have also been reported. These unique fusions have been reported in several sarcoma types, and some are presented in the following individual sarcoma sections.

In sarcomas that have been extensively karyotyped, it is likely that only rare variant gene fusions remain to be identified. However, novel fusions continue to be discovered in sarcomas with only limited cytogenetic data, or if the fusions are generated by translocations or intrachromosomal rearrangements that are difficult to detect in Giemsa-stained chromosomal preparations, or because the translocations occur in a

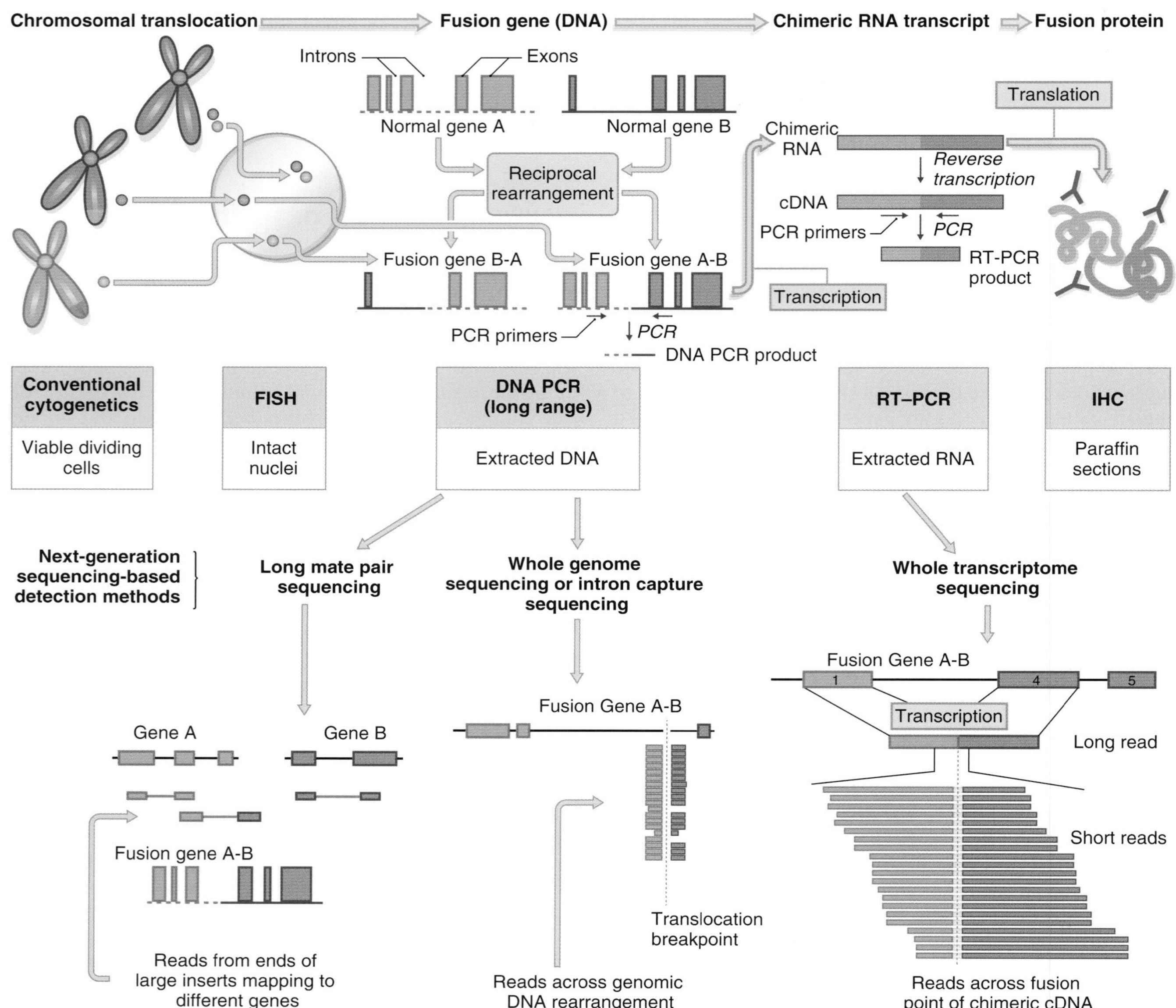

FIGURE 4-1. General principles of sarcoma translocation detection. The different approaches to the detection of a reciprocal translocation are schematized, ranging from conventional cytogenetics to the demonstration of the resulting fusion protein, along with the material needed for each assay. A break-apart FISH assay design is shown. Note that long-range DNA PCR and IHC detection are possible in only a minority of sarcoma translocations. IHC approaches usually use antibodies to one or both components of the fusion protein but are rarely specific for the fusion point. In the bottom half of the figure, the next-generation sequencing strategies for gene fusion detection are shown. These include (left) analyzing rearrangements by long mate pair sequencing, where the ends of large genomic fragments are sequenced in tandem, (middle) sequencing across the genomic junction of rearrangements by whole genome sequencing or sequencing of target introns following hybrid capture, and (right) sequencing across the cDNA junction by long read or short read transcriptome sequencing.

TABLE 4-1 Recurrent Chromosomal Translocations in Benign and Malignant Soft Tissue Tumors

SOFT TISSUE TUMOR	TRANSLOCATION	GENE FUSION	APPROXIMATE PREVALENCE
Alveolar rhabdomyosarcoma	t(2;13)(q35;q14)	*PAX3-FOXO1*	75%
	t(1;13)(p36;q14)	*PAX7-FOXO1*	20%
	Other t with 2q35	*PAX3*	5%
Alveolar soft part sarcoma	t(X;17)(p11.2;q25)	*ASPSCR1-TFE3*	>95%
Angiofibroma	t(5;8)(p15;q13)	*AHRR-NCOA2*	NA
Angiomatoid fibrous histiocytoma	t(2;22)(q34;q12)	*EWSR1-CREB1*	72%
	t(12;22)(q13;q12)	*EWSR1-ATF1*	21%
	t(12;16)(q13;p11)	*FUS-ATF1*	7%
Clear cell sarcoma	t(12;22)(q13;q12)	*EWSR1-ATF1*	90% soft tissue 10% GI tract
	t(2;22)(q34;q12)	*EWSR1-CREB1*	90% GI tract 10% soft tissue
Dermatofibrosarcoma protuberans/ giant cell fibroblastoma	+ring/marker chromosome from t(17;22)(q22;q13)	*COL1A1-PDGFB*	>90%

TABLE 4-1 Recurrent Chromosomal Translocations in Benign and Malignant Soft Tissue Tumors—cont'd

SOFT TISSUE TUMOR	TRANSLOCATION	GENE FUSION	APPROXIMATE PREVALENCE
Desmoplastic fibroblastoma	t(2;11)(q31;q12)	Unknown	NA
Desmoplastic small round cell tumor	t(11;22)(p13;q12)	*EWSR1-WT1*	>95%
Epithelioid sarcoma-like hemangioendothelioma	t(7;9)(q22;q13)	Unknown	NA
Epithelioid hemangioendothelioma	t(1;3)(p36.3;q25)	*WWTR1-CAMTA1*	85%
	t(X;11)(p11.2;q22.1)	*TFE3-YAP1*	NA
Ewing sarcoma	t(11;22)(q24;q12)	*EWSR1-FLI1*	90%
	t(21;22)(q22;q12)	*EWSR1-ERG*	5%
	Other t with 22q12	*EWSR1* fusion with various ETS partners: *ETV1* (7p22), *FEV* (2q36), *ETV4* (17q21)	<1%
	t(16;21)(p11;q22)	*FUS-ERG*	<1%
Ewing sarcoma-like	t(20;22)(q13;q12)	*EWSR1-NFATC2*	NA
	t(4;19)(q35;q13)	*CIC-DUX4*	NA
	t(10;19)(q26.3;q13)	*CIC-DUX4*	NA
	inv(X)(p11.4p11.22)	*BCOR-CCNB3*	NA
Extraskeletal myxoid chondrosarcoma	t(9;22)(q22;q12)	*EWSR1-NR4A3*	75%
	t(9;17)(q22:q11)	*TAF15-NR4A3*	15%
	t(9;15)(q22;q21)	*TCF12-NR4A3*	<1%
	t(3;9)(q12;q22)	*TFG-NR4A3*	<1%
Infantile fibrosarcoma	t(12;15)(p13;q25)	*ETV6-NTRK3*	>95%
Inflammatory myofibroblastic tumor	t with 2p23	*ALK* fusion with: *TPM4* (19p13.1), *TPM3* (1q21), *CLTC* (17q23), *RANBP2* (2q13), *ATIC* (2q35), *SEC31A* (4q21), *CARS* (11p15)	75%
Lipoblastoma	t with 8q12	*PLAG1* fusions	80%
Lipoma, ordinary	t with 12q14.3	*HMGA2* fusions	30%
	t with 6p21	*HMGA1 fusions*	10%
Lipoma, chondroid	t(11;16)(q13;p13)	*C11orf95-MKL2*	NA
Low-grade fibromyxoid sarcoma	t(7;16)(q33;p11)	*FUS-CREB3L2*	>95%
	t(11;16)(p11;p11)	*FUS-CREB3L1*	<5%
Mesenchymal chondrosarcoma	del(8)(q13.3q21.1)	*HEY1-NCOA2*	>90%
Myoepithelioma, soft tissue	t(19;22)(q13;q12)	*EWSR1-ZNF444*	NA
	t(1;22)(q23;q12)	*EWSR1-PBX1*	NA
	t(6;22)(p21;q12)	*EWSR1-POU5F1*	NA
	t with 16p11	*FUS*	NA
Myxoid/round cell liposarcoma	t(12;16)(q13;p11)	*FUS-DDIT3*	>90%
	t(12;22)(q13;q12)	*EWSR1-DDIT3*	<10%
Myxoinflammatory fibroblastic sarcoma/hemosiderotic fibrolipomatous tumor	der(10)t(1;10)(p22;q24)	*TGFBR3-MGEA5*	NA
Nodular fasciitis	t(17;22)(p13;q13.1)	*MYH9-USP6*	90%
Ossifying fibromyxoid tumor	t with 6p21	*PHF1* fusions	40%-50%
Pericytoma	t(7;12)(7p22;q13)	*ACTB-GLI1*	NA
Sclerosing epithelioid fibrosarcoma	t(7;16)(q33;p11.2)	*FUS-CREB3L2*	NA
	t(11;16)(p13;p11.2)	*FUS-CREB3L1*	NA
Solitary fibrous tumor	inv(12)(q13q13)	*NAB2-STAT6*	>95%
Spindle cell rhabdomyosarcoma	t with 8q13	*NCOA2* fusion with: *SRF*(6p21),*TEAD1*(11p15)	NA
Synovial sarcoma	t(X;18)(p11.2;q11.2)	*SS18-SSX1*	65%
		SS18-SSX2	35%
		SS18-SSX4	<1%
Tenosynovial giant cell tumor	t(1;2)(p13;q37)	*CSF1-COL6A3*	NA
	other t with 1p13	*CSF1*	NA

NA = not available due to insufficient data to estimate prevalence.
Note: *HMGA1* rearrangements and *TGFBR3–MGEA5* usually do not result in fusion transcripts (see text for details).

setting of highly complex karyotypes. As discussed later, the pathobiology of the oncogenic fusion proteins involves, in almost all instances, either transcriptional deregulation (most) or aberrant signaling (some).

The perennial question of how and why translocations arise has been extensively discussed.[13] Comparing genes involved in translocations to control genes, striking differences emerge in overall gene size, average intron length, and length of the longest intron, all three of which are significantly greater in genes involved in translocations.[14] However, so-called recombinogenic DNA sequence elements are not more frequent in translocated genes. This is notable because these DNA sequences had been previously proposed as explanations for the development of translocations. Overall, these data support the concept that the intronic breaks that lead to specific recurrent chromosomal translocations in cancer are largely random events (i.e., the risk of breaks is simply proportional to intron length) that become fixed through natural selection if they provide a growth advantage to the cell. Cellular factors that predispose to translocations include cellular stresses causing DNA damage followed by incorrect repair, the increased availability of the genes for rearrangement that is created by the open, less protected chromatin conformation associated with gene transcription or replication, and the unexpected proximity of some translocation partner genes caused by the three-dimensional arrangement of chromosomes in the nucleus.[13] In rare cases, sarcoma translocations appear etiologically related to radiotherapy-induced DNA damage, as mainly reported in synovial sarcoma.[15-17]

Although the above discussion applies to recurrent reciprocal translocations, one should keep in mind that nonreciprocal or unbalanced translocations, even if recurrent, usually have different oncogenic consequences (exception: alveolar soft part sarcoma [see later text]), essentially representing a mechanism for gains or losses of genetic material. A notable recurrent unbalanced translocation in several sarcomas is the der(16)t(1;16),[18-20] but the gene or genes whose gain or loss drives selection for this translocation remain unknown.

DIAGNOSTIC METHODS

Chromosome, Fluorescence In Situ Hybridization, and Gene Nomenclature

According to standard chromosome nomenclature, chromosome regions are subdivided into bands and, at higher resolution, subbands. For example, the designation *12q13* indicates chromosome 12, the long arm (q), region 1, band 3. On the ideogram, chromosome bands are numbered in an ascending fashion from centromere to telomere on each arm of the chromosome. Note that a limited number of bands is defined in each region, so that, on a given chromosome arm, band 13 may be followed by band 21, for example.

Because of the increase in the amount and variety of data on chromosome aberrations associated with neoplasia and the development and implementation of fluorescence in situ hybridization (FISH), a revised terminology was needed for describing acquired aberrations.[21,22] A fairly sophisticated set of rules governs the description of chromosomal abnormalities. The convention is to first specify the total number of chromosomes followed by the sex chromosomes (e.g., the normal male karyotype is given as 46,XY). The autosomes are indicated when only an aberration or variant is present. In the description of a karyotype with chromosomal abnormalities, sex chromosome aberrations are given first, followed by abnormalities of the autosomes listed in numeric order irrespective of the type of aberration. Aberrations are considered in two categories: numeric or structural. Numeric changes include either gain (+) or loss (−) of chromosomes (e.g., +7 indicates an extra copy of chromosome 7, or trisomy 7). The chromosome(s) involved in a structural change is specified in parentheses, directly following the symbol identifying the type of rearrangement, for example, a translocation between chromosomes 12 and 16 as t(12;16). In all structural changes, the location of any given chromosome break is specified by the chromosome band in which that break has occurred; for example, t(12;16)(q13;p11) describes a balanced translocation between the q13 band of chromosome 12 and the p11 band of chromosome 16. It is important to note that the chromosomes involved in a translocation are listed in numeric order, and, therefore, this nomenclature does not specify the order of the genes involved in the oncogenic fusion product. For example, in the classic t(11;22) of Ewing sarcoma (ES), chromosome 22 contributes the *EWSR1* (*EWS*) gene, which is the 5' end (first part) of the fusion oncogene. The most frequent structural changes in sarcomas include translocation (t), in which chromatin is exchanged between two or between more chromosomes; deletion (del), in which there is a net loss of chromatin; (add), in which there is additional material whose origin is uncertain by conventional G-banding; and derivative chromosome (der), in which one or more rearrangements within a single chromosome occur. For instance, a derivative chromosome may be the result of a reciprocal translocation that is followed by loss of one of the two rearranged chromosomes (also known as *unbalanced translocation*).

In the past two decades, FISH analysis and related molecular cytogenetic techniques have been very effectively used to identify chromosomal regions, to reveal cryptic abnormalities, to describe complex chromosomal rearrangements, and to detect chromosomal rearrangements in interphase nuclei, including those in paraffin-embedded, formalin-fixed tissues. The complementary use of conventional cytogenetic analysis and FISH has provided a remarkably powerful tool for cancer cytogenetics. Therefore, the current nomenclature, International System for Human Cytogenetic Nomenclature (known as *ISCN*), also incorporates FISH data.[21] A type of probe commonly used in sarcomas is referred to as a *break-apart probe*. A break-apart probe set consists of a pair of probes that flank a gene locus of interest, labeled in two different fluorochromes, and is especially useful for detecting chromosomal rearrangements of genes, such as *EWSR1*, for which the translocation partners are variable.

Information of interest in interphase/nuclear in situ hybridization (nuc ish) includes the number of signals and their position relative to each other. For instance, a break-apart probe (e.g., *EWSR1*) is made of two DNA probes (*5'EWSR1* and *3'EWSR1*) from the same locus (22q12) that are labeled with different fluorophores to give, on normal chromosomes 22, either a single-color signal (e.g., yellow) or overlapping red and green signals, depending on the level of chromosome/DNA contraction in the individual interphase cells. When a chromosomal rearrangement, such as a translocation, causes a separation of the paired probes, two signals of different colors (e.g., orange and green) are seen, typically separated by at least the width of two signal diameters. Therefore, abnormal cells will be described as nuc ish (*EWSR1*x2)(*5'EWSR1* sep *3'EWSR1* x1), meaning two *EWSR1* signals, one of which has separation (sep) of the 5' and 3' probe components caused by a gene rearrangement. An abbreviated list of symbols used to designate chromosomal abnormalities as well as abbreviations used in describing results obtained by in situ hybridization in cancer cytogenetics are given in Table 4-2.

Note that the nomenclature used to describe human genes in the chapter is the official name as assigned by the Human Gene Nomenclature Committee (see http://www.genenames.org/). However, if another name was more commonly used in the past, it is indicated in brackets the first time the gene is mentioned in the text, such as *DDIT3* (*CHOP*), the former being the HUGO name and the latter an older name. Human genes and transcripts are written in uppercase italics,

TABLE 4-2 Partial List of Symbols and Abbreviated Terms Used in Cancer Cytogenetics

SYMBOL	DEFINITION
Chromosome Abnormalities	
add	Additional material of unknown origin
cen	Centromere
cp	Composite karyotype
cth	Chromothripsis
del	Deletion
der	Derivative chromosome
dic	Dicentric chromosome
dmin	Double minute chromosome
dup	Duplication
hsr	Homogeneously staining region
i	Isochromosome
inc	Incomplete karyotype
ins	Insertion
inv	Inversion
mar	Marker chromosome
minus (−)	Loss
p	Short arm of a chromosome
plus (+)	Gain
q	Long arm of a chromosome
r	Ring chromosome
t	Translocation
In Situ Hybridization (ISH)	
amp	Amplified signal
con	Connected signals (signals are adjacent)
dim	Diminished signal intensity
FISH	Fluorescence in situ hybridization
double plus (++)	Duplication on a specific chromosome
ish	In situ hybridization on metaphases
minus (-)	Absent from a specific chromosome
multiplication sign (x)	Precedes the number of signal seen
nuc ish	Nuclear or interphase in situ hybridization
period (.)	Separates cytogenetics observation from results of ISH
plus (+)	Present on a specific chromosome
semicolon (;)	Separates probes on different derivative chromosomes
sep	Separated signals (signals are separated)
wcp	Whole chromosome paint

Data from Shaffer LG, McGowan-Jordan J, Schmid M. ISCN 2013: An international system for human cytogenetic nomenclature (2013). Recommendations of the international standing committee on human cytogenetic nomenclature. Basel: Karger; 2013.

whereas the corresponding proteins are uppercase but not italicized.

Methodologic Considerations

The application of long-term collagenase treatment for tissue disaggregation,[23] starting in the mid-1980s, greatly accelerated work in solid tumor cytogenetics. During the years in which these cytogenetic methodologies were being developed, adapted, and further refined for solid tumors, many differences arose among laboratories. However, today the protocols are more similar than dissimilar, despite that there is a need to adapt them to the specific needs and conditions of each laboratory. There are several technical pitfalls that can affect cytogenetic analyses of clinical tumor samples:

1. Unpredictable growth of the neoplastic cells in tissue culture
2. Overgrowth of neoplastic cells by reactive non-neoplastic cells
3. Contamination of tumor cultures by bacteria or fungi
4. Predominance of nonviable tumor (necrotic sample)

A successful cytogenetic analysis is based on a successful culture. The procedure for solid tumors begins in the operating room when the tumor is removed. The tissue sample sent for cytogenetics must be sterile, representative, and viable (i.e., not in a fixative solution). Optimally, the tumor biopsy is divided by the pathologist into sections to be used for pathologic diagnosis, cytogenetics (culture), and molecular analyses (snap-frozen). At least 80% of all soft tissue tumors can be cultured successfully if the specimens are carefully selected by the pathologist to minimize necrotic and non-neoplastic components.

Solid tumor samples generally must be disaggregated by mechanical (mincing) and enzymatic (collagenase) methods before the cells are placed in a tissue culture. To shorten the time in culture and avoid overgrowth of fibroblastic stroma, disaggregated cells are grown in chamber slides, which have the advantage of requiring only a small number of cells, and metaphases can be both harvested and stained using in situ techniques. Cell attachment, proliferation, and mitotic rate are monitored by daily examination of each culture through an inverted microscope. Selection of an appropriate point at which to harvest the cultures, as well as optimization of exposure to a mitotic spindle inhibitor that inhibits cell division at metaphase (e.g., colchicine) are also determined by daily monitoring.

Most mesenchymal tumors can be karyotyped within 7 days after culture initiation, and metaphases are best harvested after 1 to 3 days in culture, despite that the yield of metaphases may be low at this point. This is because growth of some neoplastic populations slows after 1 to 2 days in culture or are overgrown by fibroblasts or other non-neoplastic elements. Therefore, metaphase harvesting at multiple time points improves the likelihood of a successful analysis. Overgrowth by non-neoplastic cells is the most common explanation for a normal diploid karyotype obtained from malignant soft tissue tumor specimens.

The availability of fresh tumor, the differential diagnosis, and the need for rapid diagnostic cytogenetic results are factors in determining the order of performing molecular cytogenetic or molecular techniques (i.e., FISH and RT-PCR) or conventional cytogenetic analysis.

Molecular Cytogenetics

The greater resolution afforded by molecular cytogenetics bridges the gap between classic cytogenetics and molecular genetics. Molecular cytogenetic techniques provide a critical role in both the diagnostic (e.g., detection of submicroscopic chromosomal aberrations) and research arenas (e.g., localization and mapping of chromosomal breakpoints and candidate disease genes).[24] FISH analysis is well suited to identify submicroscopic changes and define cryptic, and often complex, chromosomal rearrangements. Moreover, FISH extends the application of diagnostic cytogenetics to all stages of the cell cycle because dividing cells are no longer a prerequisite. As a result, with carefully designed probes, certain chromosomal rearrangements (such as translocations) can be detected in nondividing (interphase) nuclei without the need for cell culture. Therefore, interphase cytogenetics using FISH provides cytogenetic information on specimens that are difficult or impossible to culture (e.g., fine-needle aspirates, paraffin-embedded fixed tissues). FISH differs from conventional cytogenetics, however, in that effective application and interpretation of FISH rely upon an a priori knowledge of the targeted aberration and appropriate rational probe design. Validated FISH assays are assessed for reproducibility, specificity, and sensitivity, all of which must be established within each laboratory for every diagnostic probe. Such validation must also include testing of appropriate and relevant tissue samples.

A variety of different types of probes is used to detect chromosome abnormalities; however, the most frequently used probes in soft tissue neoplasms are alpha-satellite DNA probes (for pericentromeric repeat sequences specific for each chromosome) and unique locus-specific (or gene-specific) DNA sequences. Alpha-satellite probes to pericentromeric repeats allow the detection of monosomies, trisomies, and other aneuploidies. These probes are also often used as a control for ploidy status when, for instance, using a gene locus-specific probe to determine amplification. However, the ability to detect numeric abnormalities in a small neoplastic subpopulation within a specimen (e.g., to assess minimal residual disease) is often hampered by hybridization inefficiencies, false background signals, and incomplete probe penetration in intact nuclei.

FISH probes that identify unique, locus-specific DNA sequences are typically genomic clones corresponding to hundreds of kilobases of target genome containing, or located strategically adjacent to, a gene of interest. In most clinic cytogenetics laboratories, the detection of chromosome abnormalities is limited to probes that are commercially available, although some laboratories may develop home-brew probes for special studies or new sarcoma translocation genes. In sarcomas, the most frequently used method to detect a chromosome translocation is to use DNA probes from one of the two loci involved. This type of probe design is referred to as a *break-apart probe* as described previously (Fig. 4-2A). Another variation on FISH assays based on break-apart probes, frequently used in hematologic disorders, is the selection of two pairs of DNA probes that span respectively both rearranged loci. A commonly used dual-fusion cocktail involves probes that span the *IGH@* and *BCL2* loci, respectively, so that the

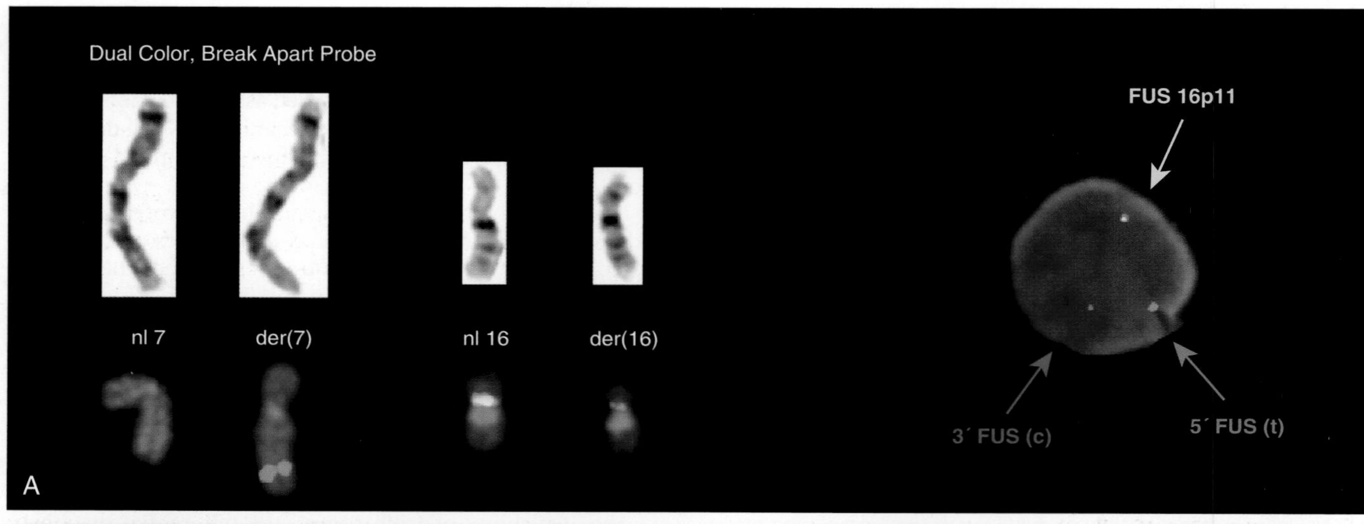

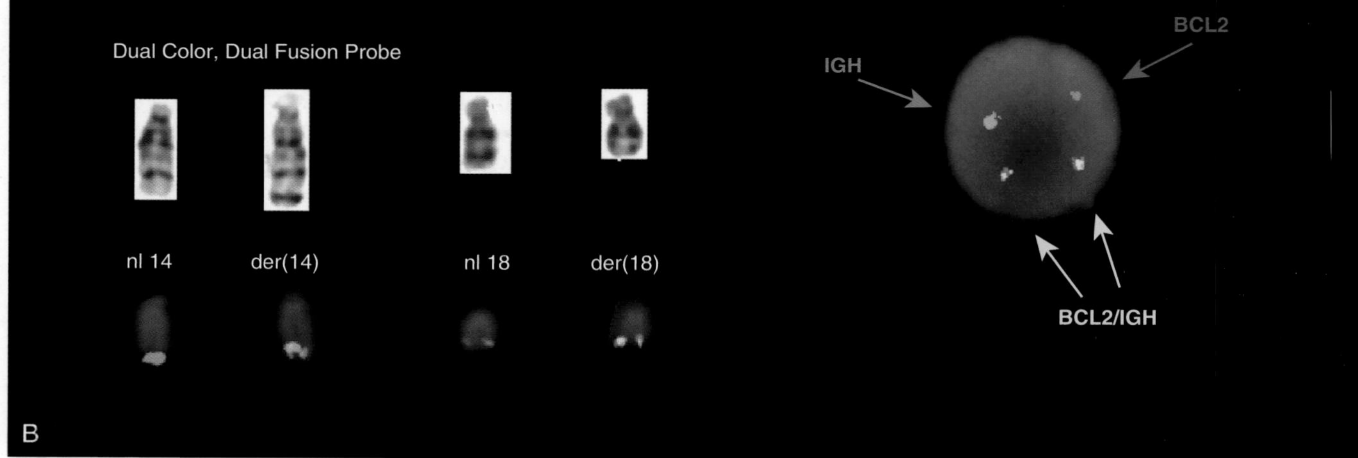

FIGURE 4-2. Two types of FISH assay designs for translocation detection (see text for details). nl, normal; c, centromeric; der, derivative chromosome; t, telomeric.

hybridization pattern in a cell with a t(14;18)(q32;q21) shows not one but two yellow fusion signals, that is, *IGH-BCL2* fusion on the der(14) and *BCL2-IGH* fusion on the der(18), improving the specificity of the assay (Fig. 4-2B). Finally, FISH using differentially labeled probes allows simultaneous detection of multiple regions, which is particularly valuable when analyzing multiple abnormalities within a single cell.

As with any technique, it is necessary to understand the limitations of FISH; in certain instances, molecular analysis may be of greater sensitivity and utility.

In terms of sensitivity, break-apart probes are optimal for the detection of rearrangements consistently involving a single chromosomal region (e.g., *EWSR1*) in concert with several different chromosomal partners; however, by the same token, this design cannot identify the translocation partner and, therefore, will not distinguish between specific rearrangements, other than to confirm involvement of the common locus. In contrast, dual-fusion probes distinguish between different chromosomal partners in rearrangements but require a separate assay for each combination, for example, detection of *EWSR1* rearrangement in a t(11;22) or a t(21;22).

Chromogenic in situ hybridization (CISH) is an alternative method in which the DNA probe is detected using a simple immunohistochemistry (IHC)-like peroxidase reaction. CISH is emerging as a practical, cost-effective, and valid alternative to FISH in testing for certain gene alterations.[25,26] CISH has some advantages over FISH: with CISH, a bright field microscope is sufficient for scoring results; the methodology is less cumbersome and more economical; and the signal intensity is not light-sensitive and, therefore, the signal does not fade over time. Because CISH signals can be correlated with histopathology, better evaluation of heterogeneous samples can be accomplished. On the other hand, with CISH, the number of colors that can be distinguished by light microscopy is limited, and, for this reason, most CISH applications have been directed toward the detection of numeric alterations (e.g., aneuploidy, amplification).

Interphase FISH/CISH can be performed using nuclei from touch or smear preparations, body fluid cell suspensions, or fresh tissue samples following enzymatic disaggregation, as well as from histologic sections of archival, formalin-fixed, paraffin-embedded tissue. With the latter, the thickness of tissue sections can affect hybridization quality and results of interpretation. Specifically, the use of standard thickness histologic sections (4 or 5 µm) in FISH/CISH assays can cause missed signals whenever sections cut through nuclei; analysis of many more cells is consequently necessary. This is a concern for the analysis of deletions or translocations but is less problematic for the detection of amplifications. In contrast, the use of 50-µ-thick sections followed by enzymatic isolation of intact nuclei allows the evaluation of intact nuclei and, therefore, circumvents the problems associated with sectioned nuclei, although nuclear morphology and FISH signal quality often suffer in nuclei isolated from thick sections.[27]

Multicolor FISH methods, for example, spectral karyotyping, multicolor FISH, combined binary ratio (COBRA)-FISH in which entire chromosomes are distinguished by different fluorescent labeling, can readily reveal complex interchromosomal rearrangements in a single hybridization experiment.[28] Their successful application depends upon the availability of a sufficient number of cells that can be evaluated in metaphase. However, such techniques are not suitable for detecting intrachromosomal rearrangements. Comparative genomic hybridization (CGH), as originally developed, involved labeling tumor DNA as a complex FISH probe and hybridizing it to normal metaphase chromosomes along with a reference DNA labeled with a different fluorophore to define regions of gains or losses across all chromosomal regions.[29] Therefore, this technique does not require viable or dividing tumor cells. Because this is a method in which bulk tumor DNA is extracted, normal DNA from admixed non-neoplastic cells can cause CGH to underestimate low-level copy number changes such as hemizygous loss or low amplification. However, conventional CGH was made obsolete by the advent of array CGH, in which the tumor DNA is hybridized instead to high-density arrays of probes covering the entire genome.[30] Array CGH provides a much higher resolution genome-wide definition of genetic gains and losses. However, conventional and array-based CGH do not detect balanced chromosome translocations, a hallmark of many soft tissue tumors. Array-based CGH data in sarcomas are further discussed in later text.

Reverse-Transcriptase-Polymerase Chain Reaction

The second major diagnostic method for sarcoma translocations is RT-PCR. RT-PCR assays detect the specific fusion RNA transcribed from the fusion gene by using forward and reverse primers bracketing the fusion point in the RNA. To be used in the PCR reaction, the RNA has to be converted into a complementary DNA (cDNA) using the enzyme RT. It should be noted that PCR using genomic DNA is usually not practical for the detection of most fusion genes because the genomic breakpoints are often scattered in large introns and only at the RNA level is there a highly consistent molecular structure. Therefore, RT-PCR is the standard molecular approach for the detection of translocation-associated gene fusions. It is especially powerful because the splicing of the transcripts encoded by fusion genes typically results in very consistent fusion points that can be tightly bracketed by appropriate primers to generate relatively small RT-PCR products (e.g., 100 to 300 bp).

However, RT-PCR, as an RNA-based assay, is susceptible to failure because of poor RNA quality. As a PCR-based assay, it is also susceptible to false-positives because of PCR cross-contamination. It is critical to include two types of contamination controls: controls lacking only the template RNA (to detect contamination of the PCR reagents) and controls lacking only the RT (to detect contamination of the patient RNA sample). Biologically, specific gene fusions are tumor-specific and appear necessary in the pathogenesis of specific cancers and, therefore, make excellent tumor markers. However, in practice, it is important to remember that technical limitations or errors in the detection of these translocations can lead to false-positives or false-negatives.

Although RT-PCR is more sensitive and provides more detailed fusion information than FISH, it is less adaptable to paraffin material, and frozen tissue is generally preferred. Another important consideration for RT-PCR assays is that they require extensive knowledge of the specific exons involved by the gene fusions and of the variability in exon composition of some fusions. Real-time RT-PCR, which uses highly sensitive fluorescent detection of PCR products as they are generated (in real time), has also been applied to the detection of sarcoma fusion transcripts in archival pathology material,[31,32] with the added benefit of reducing cross-contamination risks by the closed tube detection of product and the avoidance of nested PCR.

RT-PCR and FISH are complementary methods for detecting sarcoma translocations. The use of one or the other as the first-line approach often reflects differences in local expertise. Studies comparing both techniques in the sarcoma setting often conclude that optimal diagnostic accuracy can be achieved when both are available.[33-36] The College of American Pathologists offers regular proficiency testing for sarcoma translocation detection by FISH and RT-PCR.

The practical need for molecular testing in modern sarcoma diagnosis has been objectively evaluated in various clinical settings such as, for instance, in the diagnosis of synovial sarcomas and Ewing sarcoma (ES).[31,37,38] Based on these studies, after standard IHC panels are used, molecular confirmation of translocation status is more useful in diagnosing synovial sarcomas (useful in approximately 50%) than ES (useful in approximately 10% to 15%). Some of the most common settings or indications for molecular diagnostic translocation testing in sarcomas include (1) the differential diagnosis of undifferentiated small round cell sarcomas, Ewing/peripheral neuroectodermal tumor (PNET) versus desmoplastic small round cell tumor (DSRCT) versus poorly differentiated synovial sarcoma versus neuroblastoma; (2) the confirmation of alveolar subtype in rhabdomyosarcoma (as a prognostic factor); (3) the distinction of monophasic synovial sarcoma from other spindle cell sarcomas; and (4) the confirmation of typical sarcomas in an unusual demographic setting or with unusual histologic/immunocytochemical features.

New Hybridization-Based Methods for Fusion Transcript Detection

With the ever-increasing number of gene fusions identified in sarcomas, the need for more efficient, multiplexed methods for their detection is becoming more pressing. The NanoString nCounter system is a fluorescence-based platform to detect individual mRNA molecules without PCR amplification in a quantitative and highly multiplexed fashion.[39] It has been applied to gene fusion detection, including in sarcomas.[40] Other hybridization-based methods include custom oligonucleotide arrays,[41] the quantitative Nuclease Protection Assay,[42] and the antibody detection of translocations assay.[43] Beyond these multiplexed assays lie approaches based on next-generation sequencing that holds the promise of detecting any gene fusion in a given sarcoma tumor sample.

Applications of Next-Generation Sequencing to Gene Fusion Discovery or Diagnosis

Recently, massively parallel (next generation) sequencing approaches have been applied to the detection of known and novel gene rearrangements in sarcomas. Among the first successes of this approach in sarcoma translocation discovery is the *BCOR-CCNB3* gene fusion identified through whole transcriptome sequencing analysis of small blue round cell tumors lacking an *EWSR1-ETS* (E-twenty-six) family translocation,[44] the *WWTR1-CAMTA1* gene fusion generated by the t(1;3)(p36;q25) chromosomal translocation of epithelioid hemangioendothelioma,[45] and the highly recurrent *NAB2-STAT6* fusion in solitary fibrous tumor.[46,47] As shown in Figure 4-1, the different next-generation sequencing strategies for gene fusion detection include (1) obtaining sequencing reads across the genomic junction by whole genome sequencing or sequencing of target introns following hybrid capture, (2) obtaining sequencing reads across the cDNA junction by whole transcriptome sequencing, or (3) analyzing structural rearrangements in mate pair sequencing, where the ends of large genomic fragments are sequenced in tandem.[48] The translation of these new approaches based on next-generation sequencing into routine diagnostic assays for sarcoma fusions is moving quickly,[49,50] but there remain significant hurdles to their routine implementation for diagnosis, principally the requirement for relatively large amounts of high quality nucleic acids.

Immunohistochemical Markers of Genetic Alterations

Many translocations can be converted into immunohistochemistry (IHC) assays based on the phenomenon of discordance in the expression levels of the amino- and carboxy-terminal ends of the product of gene B in tumors with A-B gene fusions, the markedly aberrant expression of the carboxy-terminal encoded by gene B in the context of these fusion proteins, or their expression in aberrant cell types or aberrant cellular compartments. This has been used as a basis for the IHC detection of oncogenic fusion proteins.[51] In sarcomas, this approach has been applied to the detection of the EWSR1-WT1 protein (Fig. 4-3A),[52,53] ASPSCR1-TFE3 protein (Fig. 4-3B),[54] EWSR1-FLI1 protein,[55] EWSR1-ERG protein,[56] and ALK fusion proteins, among others.[57,58] Another strategy for converting molecular translocation detection into an IHC assay is provided by the rare gene fusions where a 5' exon of gene B that is not normally translated becomes translated in the context of the fusion protein and, therefore, represents a novel peptide sequence that can be used to generate a fusion protein-specific antibody. This approach was elegantly demonstrated for FUS-DDIT3 and EWS-DDIT3 detection in myxoid liposarcomas,[59] but the antibody did not become widely available.

Although recurrent translocations are by far the most widely used markers, certain other genetic alterations are so closely associated with specific sarcomas that they can also form the basis for confirmatory IHC assays. This is the case with *KIT* (and *PDGFRA*) mutations in gastrointestinal stromal tumors (GISTs).[60,61] However, KIT immunoreactivity in GIST is related to tumor cell lineage more than to the underlying mutation. Coamplification of *MDM2* and *CDK4* in well-differentiated and dedifferentiated liposarcomas caused by 12q amplification has emerged as a potentially useful marker in certain settings,[62,63] and this has been translated into an IHC assay.[64,65] Mutations involving the WNT pathway (in *APC* or in the beta-catenin gene) are characteristic of (but not specific for) aggressive desmoid-type fibromatosis (see later text). These mutations result in nuclear beta-catenin accumulation readily detected by IHC.[66,67] IHC analysis can be used to confirm the pathognomonic loss of SMARCB1 (INI1) in malignant rhabdoid tumors and epithelioid sarcomas, and it

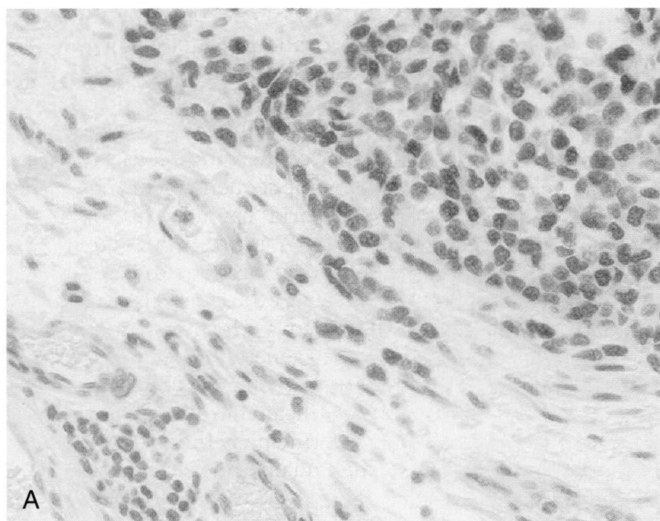

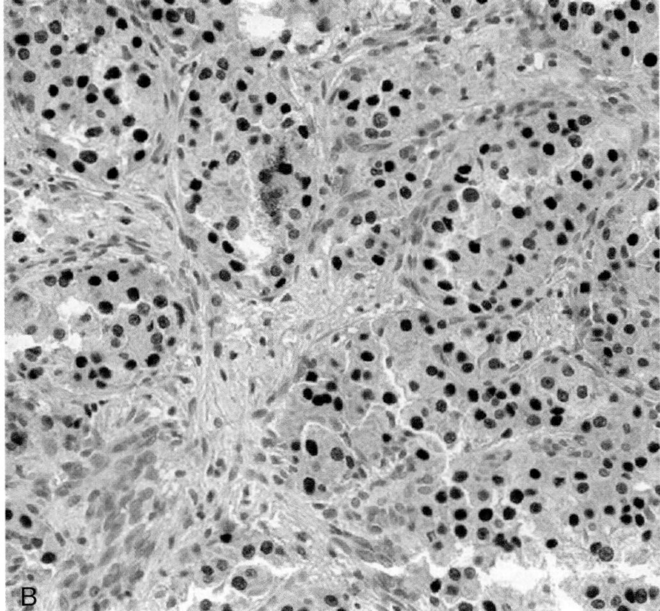

FIGURE 4-3. Two examples of IHC detection of translocation fusion proteins. (A) The detection of the EWSR1-WT1 protein using antibody to the WT1 carboxy-terminal. (B) The detection of the ASPSCR1-TFE3 protein using antibody to a portion of TFE3 included in the fusion protein.

appears fairly specific for these entities among sarcomas,[68,69] with rare exceptions.[70,71]

MAJOR PATHOGENETIC CLASSES OF SARCOMAS

For the discussion of genetic alterations in specific soft tissue tumors, tumors are grouped into broad categories that integrate their cytogenetic features and their presumed oncogenic mechanisms. These generally parallel each other insofar as sarcomas driven by transcriptional or signaling deregulation harbor specific translocations or point mutations and show relatively simple karyotypes with few changes. This is in contrast to sarcomas with highly complex karyotypes that are generally considered to have a different biology. The contrasting features of sarcomas with specific translocations (translocation sarcomas) and those with complex karyotypes (Table 4-3) have become a widely used approach for discussing their biology.[12,72] However, these groupings should be considered a conceptual framework that highlights the key shared features of different sarcomas, rather than an actual classification. For instance, the outcome of ES[73] and myxoid liposarcomas[74,75] is dramatically worsened by p53/p14ARF pathway alterations; in contrast, most sarcomas lacking specific translocations show more frequent p53 alterations,[76,77] but these typically seem to have a more modest clinic impact.[78] Another striking contrast emerges in telomere maintenance mechanisms, of which two main types have been described in human tumors: telomerase activation and the alternative lengthening of telomeres (ALT) mechanism. A predominance of telomerase activation in the absence of ALT appears to characterize sarcomas with specific chromosomal translocations, whereas a high prevalence of ALT is seen in sarcomas with nonspecific complex karyotypes.[79-81] The recent discovery that the ALT phenotype is associated with, and is possibly a result of, mutations in the alpha-thalassemia X-linked mental retardation protein/death domain associated protein (also referred to as ATRX/DAXX) chromatin remodeling complex is of great interest, but soft tissue sarcomas have yet to be screened systematically for these mutations.[82,83]

TABLE 4-3 Some Contrasting Aspects of Sarcomas with Specific Translocations and Sarcomas with Complex Karyotypes

	SARCOMAS WITH SPECIFIC TRANSLOCATIONS	SARCOMAS WITH OTHER GENETIC ALTERATIONS
Karyotypes	Usually simple	Usually complex
Translocations	Reciprocal and specific, producing fusion genes	Nonreciprocal and nonspecific, causing gene copy number changes
Telomere maintenance mechanisms	Telomerase expression common, ALT mechanism rare	ALT mechanism more common than telomerase
P53 pathway alterations	Relatively rare, but strong prognostic impact	More frequent, but limited or no prognostic impact
Incidence in bilateral retinoblastoma and Li-Fraumeni syndrome	Rare, if ever	Common
Similarity of gene expression profiles within each sarcoma type	Strong	Weak

ALT, alternative lengthening of telomeres.

SARCOMAS WITH CHIMERIC TRANSCRIPTION FACTORS

The fusion genes produced by most sarcoma translocations encode chimeric transcription factors that cause transcriptional deregulation. Transcription factors have a modular structure consisting, at a minimum, of a transcription regulatory domain and a DNA-binding domain. Transcription regulatory domains, because they do not show strong sequence conservation, are typically defined by functional assays and can either stimulate or repress gene transcription. DNA-binding domains show strong sequence conservation that allows them to be grouped into families. One general rule of sarcomas with chimeric transcription factors is that all translocation variants associated with a specific sarcoma involve genes from the same transcription factor family as defined by the type of DNA-binding domain. Translocations that lead to the production of novel chimeric transcription factors generally either fuse two transcription factor genes or fuse one transcription factor gene with another gene encoding a domain that can function as a transcriptional activation domain. The modular structure of transcription factors allows their domains to be reshuffled by these translocations, leading to new combinations of domains with aberrant properties.

Several features endow chimeric transcription factors with aberrant functional properties. Relative to the native translocation partners, there may be acquisition of new protein interactions (with coactivators, corepressors, chromatin binding proteins), acquisition of new target gene specificities (even if the primary structure of DNA-binding domain is not altered by the gene fusion), and deregulation of expression relative to normal expression levels, cell type, developmental stage, or cell cycle timing. Transcription factors, as master regulators of the expression of multiple downstream target genes, are themselves under tight control by other transcription factors that determine their expression by binding to the promoter region, located in the vicinity of their first exon. Within the context of fusion of genes A and B, the expression of the A-B fusion gene as a whole is largely driven by the promoter region of gene A, and this defines one aberrant aspect of chimeric transcription factors.

In broad terms, chimeric transcription factors are thought to deregulate the expression of specific repertoires of target genes, possibly orchestrating multiple oncogenic hits. The identities of the specific target genes deregulated by each type of chimeric transcription factor are being gradually elucidated, but a discussion of these studies is beyond the scope of this chapter. In general, the significance of individual target genes remains unclear, and few, if any, have clear diagnostic implications, at present. The key role of these chimeric transcription factors in sarcoma pathogenesis is supported by the in vitro growth requirement of these factors on their respective sarcoma cell lines and by the impact that relatively minor variations in their structure (e.g., cytogenetic or molecular breakpoints) have on tumor phenotype, the most striking example being seen in synovial sarcoma (see later text).

The specificity of chromosomal translocations in sarcomas is remarkable. The specificity of sarcoma gene fusions for certain tumor types may reflect a dynamic relationship with the cellular environment.[84] In this model, the gene fusion is oncogenic in a specific susceptible cell type at a particular developmental stage, and, in turn, the gene fusion may then modify the phenotype of the susceptible cell. The need to target a very specific mesenchymal cell type may account for the difficulty of transgenic mouse models for this class of sarcomas.[85-87] Aberrant transcription factors may be tolerated and transforming in only a very specific cell type. It has also become apparent that chimeric transcription factors may have a strong effect on cell lineage markers, in effect, redirecting differentiation (reprogramming). Therefore, the phenotype of the precursor cells may be difficult to infer from the phenotype of the translocation sarcoma, and, moreover, the precursor cells for a given type of translocation sarcoma may not be exactly identical from case to case. It has been found that introduction of the *EWSR1-FLI1* gene into neuroblastoma cells or embryonal rhabdomyosarcoma (ERMS) cells can shift their differentiation program to that of ES/PNET.[88,89] Likewise, *FUS-DDIT3* can induce fibrosarcoma cells to display features of liposarcoma. This also raises the possibility that the precursor cells for different sarcomas may be similar. For instance, the introduction of *EWSR1-FLI1* or *FUS-DDIT3* into primary mesenchymal progenitor cells leads to the formation of tumors with features of ES/PNET or liposarcoma, respectively.[90,91] Indeed, a recent study of ES cell lines suggests that they originate from mesenchymal stem cells.[92]

The following sections describe the genetic alterations in the major sarcomas driven by the transcriptional deregulation mediated by translocation-derived chimeric transcription factors. The major recurrent translocations are listed in Table 4-1. Partial karyotypes of 16 major translocations in sarcomas are shown in Fig. 4-4.

Ewing Sarcoma/Peripheral Neuroectodermal Tumor

At the molecular level, ES/PNET is characterized by chromosomal translocations that fuse *EWSR1 (EWS)*, located at 22q12, and a gene of the ETS family of transcription factors defined by the presence of an ETS DNA-binding domain. In 90% to 95% of cases, the gene fusion is *EWSR1-FLI1*, encoding a chimeric protein containing the N-terminal portion of EWSR1 and the C-terminal portion of FLI1, including the ETS DNA-binding domain. An *EWSR1-ERG* fusion, where the *ERG* gene from 21q22 substitutes for *FLI1*, is found in 5% to 10% of cases.[93,94] Very rare cases of ES/PNET show fusions of *EWSR1* to other *ETS* family genes, such as *ETV1*, *ETV4 (E1AF)*, and *FEV*,[95,96] or the *FUS-ERG* fusion.[97] These gene fusions are presumed to be the initiating oncogenic event in ES/PNET and appear to play a critical role in the proliferation and tumorigenesis of ES/PNET cells. The EWSR1 amino-terminal domain can function as a strong transactivation domain, and its promoter is strongly and broadly activated, leading to relatively unrestricted high-level expression of the resulting fusion genes. In contrast, expression of native FLI1 is tightly regulated and lineage-restricted. Details of the biology of native EWSR1 and FLI1, as well as the functional aspects of EWSR1-FLI1, are reviewed in detail elsewhere.[98]

EWSR1-FLI1 is structurally heterogeneous, with up to 18 possible types of in-frame *EWSR1-FLI1* chimeric transcripts, most of which have been observed in vivo.[93,96] The two main types, fusion of *EWSR1* exon 7 to *FLI1* exon 6 (type 1) and fusion of *EWSR1* exon 7 to *FLI1* exon 5 (type 2), account for about 85% to 90% of *EWSR1-FLI1* fusions. In spite of this heterogeneity, each EWSR1-FLI1 fusion protein invariably contains the amino-terminal domain of EWSR1 (exons 1 to 7) and the intact DNA-binding domain of FLI1 (exon 9). Historically, the survival of patients whose tumor contains the type

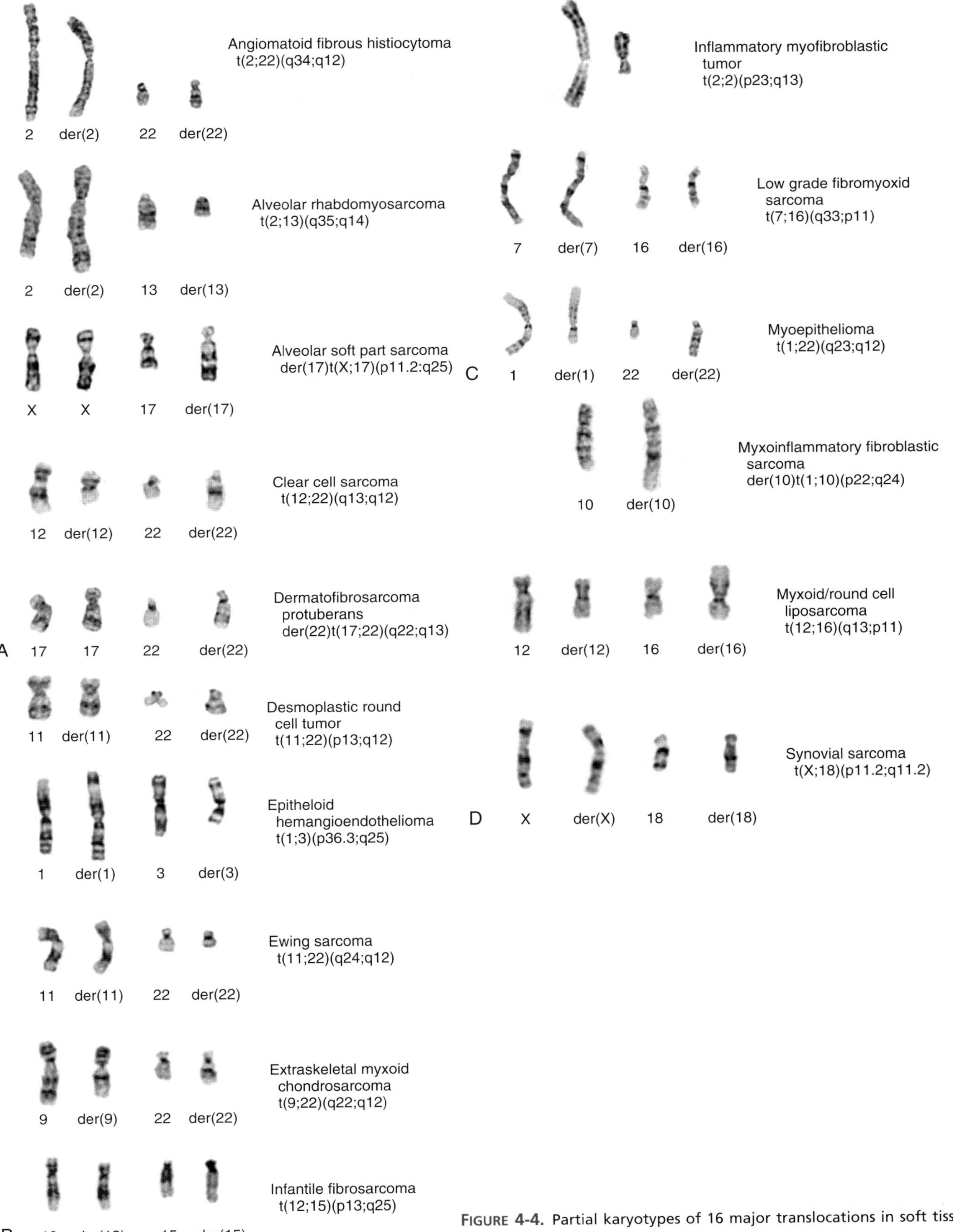

FIGURE 4-4. Partial karyotypes of 16 major translocations in soft tissue sarcomas.

1 *EWSR1-FLI1* fusion appeared statistically better than those with other *EWSR1-FLI1* fusion types,[99,100] but these survival differences are no longer apparent with current treatment protocols.[101,102]

The variant *EWSR1-ERG* fusion has been found to be associated with clinical phenotypes indistinguishable from *EWSR1-FLI1*-positive ES/PNET.[103] The more immediate practical significance of *EWSR1-FLI1* structural variability is that not all forms of the *EWSR1-FLI1* fusion transcript may be detected in clinical material with a single RT-PCR primer pair, leading to a risk of false-negative results. Therefore, several RT-PCR assays with different primer pairs are typically needed to reliably exclude the presence of a *EWSR1-FLI1* fusion. The same concern applies to *EWSR1-ERG* detection but to a lesser extent. When using FISH for *EWSR1* rearrangement as a diagnostic method, it is important to recall that *EWSR1* is a promiscuous gene that is rearranged with other partner genes in a variety of other mesenchymal tumors,[104] as well as in certain skin adnexal and salivary gland carcinomas.[105,106] Therefore, a positive result of FISH for *EWSR1* rearrangement must always be interpreted in the context of the histologic and immunophenotypic findings.

ES/PNET are also heterogeneous for the occurrence of genetic alterations involving certain critical regulators of cell-cycle progression and apoptosis, in particular p16/p14ARF (encoded by *CDKN2A*) and p53 (encoded by *TP53*). Alterations in p53 or p16/p14ARF are found in about 25% of ES/PNET and define a subset with highly aggressive behavior and poor chemoresponse.[73]

In recent years, rare undifferentiated small round cell sarcomas with fusions of *EWSR1* to non-ETS family transcription factor genes such as *SP3, PATZ1, SMARCA5, POU5F1, NFATC2,* have been reported, often as single cases, as reviewed elsewhere.[96] Their nosologic relationship to classic ES/PNET is unclear. For instance, it has been proposed that the EWSR1–NFATC2 fusion protein, although it does not contain an ETS DNA-binding domain, may activate a subset of ETS targets known to be deregulated by EWSR1-FLI1, through interactions with other transcriptional proteins.[107] In addition to these rare undifferentiated small round cell sarcomas with fusions of *EWSR1* to non-ETS family transcription factor genes, there are accumulating data supporting two other groups of ES-like tumors defined by highly recurrent fusions involving neither *EWSR1* nor ETS family transcription factor genes. These two emerging entities, which together appear to account for the majority of *EWSR1*-fusion negative ES-like tumors, are discussed in following sections.

Undifferentiated Small Round Cell Sarcomas with *CIC-DUX4*

Cases of soft tissue sarcoma diagnosed as Ewing-like sarcoma, cytogenetically characterized by t(4;19)(q35;q13), contain a *CIC-DUX4* fusion joining the *CIC* high mobility group box transcription factor gene to the double homeodomain gene *DUX4*.[108] More recently, a variant translocation has been described that involves another copy of *DUX4* present in the subtelomeric region of chromosome 10, t(10;19)(q26.3;q13).[109] These aggressive sarcomas typically arise in children and young adults, with a preference for males, and show variable CD99 immunoreactivity.[109,110]

Undifferentiated Small Round Cell Sarcomas with *BCOR-CCNB3*

Another new entity that appears to account for many *EWSR1*-fusion negative ES-like tumors is a bone and soft tissue sarcoma of children and young adults defined by a *BCOR-CCNB3* gene fusion.[44] This fusion results from a paracentric inversion on the short arm (p) of the X-chromosome between *BCOR* (exon 5) at Xp11.4 and *CCNB3* (exon 5) on Xp11.2. By IHC, these tumors are variably immunoreactive for CD99 but are consistently positive for CCNB3.[44]

Alveolar Rhabdomyosarcoma

Alveolar rhabdomyosarcoma (ARMS) is associated with recurrent translocations fusing genes from the *PAX* family of transcription factors to *FOXO1* (*FKHR*). Approximately 60% to 70% of histologically diagnosed ARMS involve a t(2;13)(q35;q14) leading to *PAX3-FOXO1* gene fusion, and 10% to 20% have a t(1;13)(p36;q14) representing the variant *PAX7- FOXO1* gene fusion.[111] However, approximately 20% of histologic ARMS fail to exhibit any of these translocations.[112,113] These cases represent a genetically heterogeneous subgroup, with some that have variant translocations involving related members of the *PAX* and/or *FOXO1* gene families (e.g., *PAX3–NCOA1, PAX3–NCOA2, PAX3–FOXO4*) and some that truly lack rearrangements or have other types of genetic abnormalities.[114,115]

Morphologic evaluation alone is sometimes insufficient to make a sharp distinction between ARMS and some ERMS because some ARMS lack alveolar architecture, and ERMS can be cellular and poorly differentiated.[116] Because this distinction is clinically critical in assigning patients to high-risk regimens, evaluation for evidence of *FOXO1* fusion is one of the most requested sarcoma translocation assays. Furthermore, recent detailed molecular and clinical analyses have confirmed that genuinely fusion-negative ARMS are more like ERMS than like fusion-positive ARMS,[117,118] underscoring the importance of routinely performing fusion confirmation in all morphologically diagnosed ARMS cases.[119] Among fusion-positive ARMS, *PAX3- FOXO1*-positive ARMS appear to be more aggressive tumors than those containing *PAX7-FOXO1*.[113,120-122] *PAX3-FOXO1* and *PAX7-FOXO1*-expressing ARMS appear morphologically identical.

The PAX3-FOXO1 DNA-binding domain, contributed by the *PAX3* gene, consists of the paired box domain and an adjacent homeodomain. Interestingly, both PAX3 and PAX7 have well-studied roles in normal embryonic muscle development, representing a rare instance in which the physiologic role of one of the translocation partners in a sarcoma gene fusion can be linked to the phenotype of the associated sarcoma. Additional details on the biology of *PAX3-FOXO1* fusions in ARMS can be found in recent reviews.[123]

An interesting distinctive feature of ARMS with the *PAX7-FOXO1* fusion is that the fusion gene is often duplicated or amplified.[124,125] Fusion-positive ARMS cases also show various other chromosomal gains and losses, some of which may function as secondary, cooperating genetic alterations.[126,127]

Spindle Cell Rhabdomyosarcoma

Pediatric cases of spindle cell rhabdomyosarcoma, a specific subtype of ERMS, contain fusions of the *NCOA2* gene at 8q13, with *SRF* and *TEAD1* being reported as fusion partners.[128] Notably, *NCOA2* is also involved in fusions with *PAX3* in rare cases of ARMS.[115] Adult spindle cell rhabdomyosarcoma does not appear to contain *NCOA2* rearrangements. This probably reflects the fact that lesions reported as spindle cell rhabdomyosarcoma in adults are not analogous to the pediatric lesions and more likely are examples of embryonal or another form of rhabdomyosarcoma with a prominent degree of spindling.

Desmoplastic Small Round Cell Tumor

DSRCT contains the characteristic *EWSR1-WT1* gene fusion in essentially all cases.[52,129] In the EWSR1-WT1 chimeric protein, the RNA-binding domain of EWSR1 is replaced by a truncated but functional portion of the WT1 DNA-binding domain (three of four zinc fingers). This truncated WT1 DNA-binding domain is associated with altered binding affinity and specificity, resulting in only limited overlap between WT1 and EWSR1-WT1 transcriptional targets. At model promoters, the encoded chimeric EWSR1-WT1 protein functions as a strong transactivator. Additional details on the biology of EWSR1-WT1 can be found elsewhere.[130] Occasional *EWSR1-WT1* fusion structure variants have been reported.[131] Demonstration of the *EWSR1-WT1* fusion has been useful in establishing the diagnosis of DSRCT in extra-abdominal locations and other atypical settings.

Clear Cell Sarcoma

At least 90% of clear cell sarcomas (CCSs) are characterized cytogenetically by a recurrent chromosomal translocation, t(12;22), resulting in fusion of the *EWSR1* gene with the *ATF1* gene (activating transcription factor-1) on 12q13.[132-136] In the resulting chimeric protein, the C-terminal of EWSR1 is replaced by a functional basic DNA binding and leucine zipper dimerization (bZIP) DNA-binding domain of ATF1. ATF1 is a member of a subgroup of bZIP transcription factors that includes the cAMP-response-element-binding protein (CREB1). There is molecular heterogeneity among *EWSR1-ATF1* transcripts. Most cases show an in-frame transcript resulting from the fusion of *EWSR1* exon 8 to *ATF1* exon 4 (type 1). Some cases have a different *EWSR1-ATF1* fusion structure in which the junction is between *EWSR1* exon 7 and *ATF1* exon 5 or between *EWSR1* exon 10 and *ATF1* exon 5.[133,134] In addition, some cases express two different fusion transcripts derived from the same fusion gene.[32,135]

A recurring theme in sarcoma translocations is that closely related gene family members can substitute for each other as translocation partners. Therefore, *EWSR1-CREB1* is a variant fusion present in about 10% of CCS of soft tissue, generated by a t(2;22)(q34;q12).[137] Because this novel fusion was initially found in three CCS cases that arose in the gastrointestinal tract, it was suggested that this variant fusion may be preferentially associated with a gastrointestinal location. However, nongastrointestinal CCSs can also harbor the *EWSR1-CREB1* fusion.[135,136] One notable feature of gastrointestinal tract CCSs with either *EWSR1–ATF1* or *EWSR1–CREB1* is that they lack melanocytic markers, in contrast to soft tissue CCSs.

Whereas most CCS share a melanocytic gene expression signature with melanomas,[138] the two are also clearly genetically distinct. CCS typically lack the *BRAF* mutations commonly seen in melanomas,[139] whereas melanomas never contain the *EWSR1-ATF1* fusion.[32,140-142]

When detecting fusions for diagnostic confirmation, it is important to recall that the spectrum of tumors with *EWSR1-ATF1* and *EWSR1-CREB1* fusions has further expanded to include angiomatoid fibrous histiocytoma,[143] hyalinizing clear cell carcinoma of the salivary gland,[106] and primary pulmonary myxoid sarcoma,[144] as reviewed elsewhere.[145]

Angiomatoid Fibrous Histiocytoma

Molecular and cytogenetic studies of angiomatoid fibrous hystiocytoma (AFH) have revealed three related translocations: a t(12;16)(q13;p11) associated with *FUS-ATF1* fusion, a t(12;22)(q13;q12) associated with *EWSR1–ATFI* gene fusion, and a t(2;22)(q34;q12) associated with *EWSR1–CREB1* gene fusion.[143,146,147] The *EWSR1* rearrangement is the most frequent genetic event in AFH, and the *EWSR1–CREB1* is the most common fusion.[143,148,149] These EWSR1 fusion proteins include the bZIP domain of CREB1 or ATF1 mediating DNA binding and dimerization. CREB1 and ATF1 are highly related members of the cAMP response element-binding (CREB) family of transcription factors. Indeed, their sequence similarity is such that it can be difficult to design PCR primers entirely specific for one or the other. As described previously, these fusions have also been found in hyalinizing clear cell carcinoma of the salivary gland and primary pulmonary myxoid sarcoma.[145]

Myxoid Liposarcoma

The karyotypic hallmark of myxoid liposarcoma, including cases with round cell components, is the t(12;16)(q13;p11) present in approximately 95% of cases. The translocation leads to the fusion of the *DDIT3(CHOP)* and *FUS(TLS)* genes at 12q13 and 16p11, respectively. The resulting fusion gene encodes a FUS-DDIT3 chimeric protein.[150,151] The remaining 5% of cases harbor a variant translocation, t(12;22)(q13;q12), in which *DDIT3* fuses instead with *EWSR1*.[152] *FUS-DDIT3* fusion transcripts occur as different recurrent structural variants based on the presence or absence of *FUS* exons 6 to 8 in the fusion product.[75,153,154]

Molecular detection of *FUS-DDIT3* or *EWSR1-DDIT3* has been used to confirm the monoclonal origin of multifocal myxoid liposarcoma/round cell liposarcoma.[155,156] These two related fusions are highly specific for myxoid liposarcoma and are not found in morphologic mimics such as the predominantly myxoid well-differentiated liposarcomas of the retroperitoneum and myxofibrosarcomas.[157] *TP53* alterations and activating *PIK3CA* mutations are sometimes observed, and they are both associated with a more aggressive clinical course.[74,75,158,159]

Extraskeletal Myxoid Chondrosarcoma

Approximately 75% of extraskeletal myxoid chondrosarcoma contain a characteristic t(9;22)(q22;q12) in which the *EWSR1* gene is fused to a gene located at 9q22 encoding an orphan nuclear receptor transcription factor belonging to the steroid /thyroid receptor gene superfamily, *NR4A3* (formerly *CHN* or *TEC* or *NOR1*) which contains a zinc finger DNA-binding domain.[160-163] In another 15% to 20% of extraskeletal myxoid chondrosarcoma, a gene at 17q11 highly related to *EWSR1*, *TAF15* (formerly *RBP56* or *TAF2N* or $hTAF_{II}68$), fuses with *NR4A3*.[163-166] In addition, two additional rare variant fusions involving *NR4A3* have been reported, *TCF12-NR4A3* and *TFG-NR4A3*, resulting from t(9;15)(q22;q21) and t(3;9)(q12;q22), respectively.[167,168]

EWSR1-NR4A3 rearrangements show considerable variability in terms of exon composition, with fusions joining *EWSR1* exon 12 to *NR4A3* exon 3 (type 1 fusion) in approximately two-thirds of cases and *EWSR1* exon 7 to *NR4A3* exon 2 (type 2 fusion) in another 20%.[163] The remaining 12% of *EWSR1-NR4A3* cases have other exon combinations.

The application of *EWSR1-NR4A3* detection has helped further define extraskeletal myxoid chondrosarcoma as an entity distinct from skeletal myxoid chondrosarcomas[169,170] and myoepithelial carcinoma of soft tissue[171] which uniformly lacks this gene fusion. FISH using *EWSR1* and *NR4A3* break-apart probes can be used to confirm the diagnosis of extraskeletal myxoid chondrosarcoma, helping distinguish it from other myxoid sarcomas.[172,173]

Mesenchymal Chondrosarcoma

Approximately 10% to 20% of mesenchymal chondrosarcomas are extraskeletal. A highly recurrent *HEY1-NCOA2* fusion was recently detected in this distinctive bone and soft tissue tumor by a genome-wide screen of exon-level expression data.[174] The *HEY1-NCOA2* fusion includes the HEY1 bHLH DNA binding/dimerization domain. As these two chromosome 8 genes are only ~10 Mb apart, the cytogenetic basis for this fusion may be a cryptic interstitial deletion between 8q13.3 and 8q21.1.[174] So far, this fusion appears to be present in all cases with adequate material,[174,175] with the exception of a single case that showed a t(1;5)(q42;q32) generating a novel *IRF2BP2-CDX1* fusion.[176] More work is needed to define the extent of genetic heterogeneity in mesenchymal chondrosarcoma.

Synovial Sarcoma

Synovial sarcoma is characterized by the t(X;18)(p11.2;q11.2), which juxtaposes the *SS18* (*SYT*) gene on chromosome 18 to either the *SSX1* or the *SSX2* gene, both located at Xp11.2.[177-179] A rare but recurrent variant, which appears cytogenetically identical, is a *SS18-SSX4* fusion.[180] Also, there is another variant, *SS18L1-SSX1*, so far described in a single case only.[181] The term *SS18-SSX* is sometimes used to refer collectively to *SS18-SSX1* and *SS18-SSX2* (and *SS18-SSX4*). Although the SS18-SSX1 and SS18-SSX2 fusion proteins differ at 13 amino acid positions only,[182] the type of fusion is strongly correlated with epithelial differentiation (i.e., biphasic histology) in synovial sarcoma, being observed in 35% to 50% of synovial sarcoma with *SS18-SSX1* fusion but less than 10% of synovial sarcoma with *SS18-SSX2*. Therefore, cases with *SS18-SSX1* are approximately five times more likely to show glandular epithelial differentiation.[183,184] Also, synovial sarcoma arising in women is twice as likely to contain the *SS18-SSX2* fusion type compared to those in men.[183,185,186] There is also a moderate association of *SS18-SSX1* fusion type with earlier distant recurrence and poorer metastasis-free survival in some studies[183,187,188] but not others.[185,186] The SS18-SSX chimeric transcriptional protein differs from most sarcoma translocation fusion proteins in that neither SS18 nor the SSX proteins contain DNA-binding domains. Instead, they appear to be transcriptional regulators whose effects on gene expression are mediated primarily through protein–protein interactions.[189,190]

The only secondary mutations described with any frequency in synovial sarcoma have been in genes encoding Wnt signaling pathway components. Mutations in several genes in this regulatory network have been reported in synovial sarcoma, specifically in the E-cadherin gene (13%), *APC* (8%), the beta-catenin gene *CTNNB1* (8%), as well as in *PTEN* (8%).[158,191-195] *SS18-SSX* translocation detection is frequently requested to help distinguish monophasic synovial sarcoma from other spindle cell sarcomas, such as fibrosarcoma or malignant peripheral nerve sheath tumor (MPNSTs). These assays have also helped establish the diagnosis of synovial sarcoma in many organ sites, most notably in the kidney.[196]

Alveolar Soft Part Sarcoma

Alveolar soft part sarcoma (ASPS) is unusual in that its canonical translocation is usually unbalanced, specifically as a der(17)t(X;17)(p11;q25). The der(17)t(X;17) has sometimes been described as an add(17)(q25) when the quality of the banding did not allow for positive identification of the additional material as the short arm of X. This translocation causes the fusion of the *TFE3* transcription factor gene (from Xp11.2) with a novel gene at 17q25, designated *ASPSCR1* (or *ASPL*).[197] The TFE3 transcription factor contains a basic helix-loop-helix DNA-binding domain and bZIP domain. The *ASPSCR1*-TFE3 fusion replaces the amino-terminal portion of TFE3 with ASPSCR1 sequences, while retaining the TFE3 DNA-binding region, activation domain, and nuclear localization signal. The *ASPSCR1*-TFE3 fusion protein localizes to the nucleus and can function as an aberrant transcription factor.[198] Although the presence of the *ASPSCR1-TFE3* fusion is highly specific and sensitive for *ASPSCR1* among sarcomas,[197,199,200] the same gene fusion is also found in a small but unique subset of renal adenocarcinomas.[201] Two forms of the *ASPSCR1-TFE3* fusion transcript are known and differ in the inclusion of an additional *TFE3* exon in the less common fusion structure, designated type 2.[197] As mentioned previously, IHC for overexpression of the TFE3 C-terminal portion has been applied to the diagnostic detection of this fusion.[54,199,200,202]

Low-Grade Fibromyxoid Sarcoma

Low-grade fibromyxoid sarcoma contains a recurrent t(7;16)(q33;p11) that represents the formation of an *FUS-CREB3L2* fusion gene.[203] Rarely, evidence of this fusion has been found in ring chromosomes derived from chromosomes 7 and 16.[204] The detection of this fusion by FISH, RT-PCR, or DNA PCR has emerged as a useful confirmatory marker for this sometimes problematic diagnosis.[205-207] CREB3L2 contains a basic DNA binding and bZIP motif. It belongs to the CREB transcription factor family but is not closely related to ATF1 or CREB1. A peculiar feature of this gene fusion is that the molecular structure of the *FUS-CREB3L2* fusion transcript varies from case to case because no simple recurrent exon-to-exon junctions are observed.[208] The t(7;16)/*FUS–CREB3L2* fusion is also present in hyalinizing spindle cell tumors with giant rosettes (a variant of low-grade fibromyxoid sarcoma) and sclerosing epithelioid fibrosarcoma.[209,210] Variant translocations, including a t(11;16)(p11;p11) leading to a *FUS-CREB3L1* fusion [208,210] and a variant *EWSR1-CREB3L1* fusion,[211] have been reported in a small minority of cases.

Epithelioid Hemangioendothelioma

A recurrent t(1;3)(p36.3;q25) resulting in a *WWTR1-CAMTA1* fusion is found in most cases of epithelioid hemangioendothelioma but not in epithelioid hemangioma or other epithelioid vascular neoplasms, for example, hemangioendothelioma, epithelioid angiosarcoma, or epithelioid sarcoma–like hemangioendothelioma.[45,212]

This fusion protein contains the amino terminus of WWTR1 and the carboxy terminus of CAMTA1 under the transcriptional control of the *WWTR1* promoter. So far, at least four molecular variants have been described: *WWTR1* exon 4-*CAMTA1* exon 8, *WWTR1* exon 4-*CAMTA1* exon 9, *WWTR1* exon 2-*CAMTA1* exon 9, and *WWTR1* exon 3-*CAMTA1* exon 9. The diversity of these variants has been used to address the question of whether multifocal epithelioid hemangioendothelioma represents an unusual pattern of metastasis or multiple separate primary tumors. Molecular evidence supports the former.[213] More recently, a small subset of epithelioid hemangioendothelioma has been found to harbor *TFE3* fusions instead of the *WWTR1-CAMTA1* fusion.[214]

Myoepithelioma of Soft Tissue

Myoepithelial tumors represent a family of lesions with variable terminology that can differ based on anatomic location. They typically occur in children or young adults, in the deep soft tissues of the extremities, or more superficially, in the head and neck. Approximately 50% show *EWSR1* (22q12) rearrangement.[215] A t(6;22)(p21;q12) involving the *EWSR1* and *POU5F1* genes was identified in a subset of deep seated tumors of extremities, in children, or young adults with distinct clear cell morphology.[216] A t(1;22)(q23;q12) involving *EWSR1* and *PBX1* genes was identified in a different subset of tumors with a deceptively bland, fibromatosis-like appearance.[216,217] A third rare t(19;22)(q13;q12) involving *EWSR1* and *ZNF444* genes has also been reported.[216,218] Over half of the *EWSR1* fusion positive tumors are histologically malignant, whereas myoepithelial tumors lacking an *EWSR1* fusion are typically benign.[216] Recently, a case of soft tissue myoepithelioma with an *EWSR1-ATF1* fusion was reported.[219] In another small subset of benign myoepitheliomas of the skin and soft tissues, *PLAG1* rearrangements have been detected by FISH, supporting a common pathogenesis with their salivary gland counterparts.[220] It should also be noted that the *EWSR1–POU5F1* fusion has been reported in cutaneous hidradenoma, mucoepidermoid carcinoma of salivary gland, and in undifferentiated sarcomas of bone or soft tissue.[105,221,222]

Solitary Fibrous Tumor

Virtually all solitary fibrous tumors contain a fusion oncogene, *NAB2-STAT6*, which has not been encountered in other soft tissue tumors and, therefore, appears to be diagnostically specific.[42,46] *NAB2* and *STAT6* are adjacent genes in chromosome band 12q13, and the pathognomonic *NAB2-STAT6* fusion results from a highly localized inversion event that is undetectable by standard G-banding karyotyping assays. Therefore, although the cytogenetic literature includes reports of various nonrecurrent chromosome aberrations in solitary fibrous tumor, the *NAB2-STAT6* fusion was recognized only when next-generation sequencing methods were applied.[42,46] The NAB2 protein functions normally as a repressor of transcription factors EGR1 and EGR2, but, in the context of the NAB2-STAT6 fusion, to which STAT6 contributes a transcriptional activation domain, NAB2 functions as an EGR activator, leading to upregulation of EGR-dependent genes such as *IGF2* and *FGFR1*. *NAB2* itself is an EGR-dependent gene, and, therefore, the *NAB2-STAT6* oncogene positively regulates its own expression. Notably, *NAB2-STAT6* appears to be ubiquitous in solitary fibrous tumor; therefore, other genetic mechanisms presumably account for the biologic and clinic variation within solitary fibrous tumors, including the clinically aggressive behavior seen in approximately 10% of cases.

Myopericytoma with a t(7;12)

This is a rare but novel class of pericytic spindle cell tumors arising in soft tissue or bone with a t(7;12)(p22;q13) that generates a fusion of *ACTB* and *GLI1 (GLI)*, leading to dysregulated *GLI1* expression.[223,224]

Myxoinflammatory Fibroblastic Sarcoma/ Hemosiderotic Fibrolipomatous Tumor

A characteristic but typically unbalanced translocation, der(10)t(1;10)(p22;q24), has been observed in two related tumors, myxoinflammatory fibroblastic sarcoma and hemosiderotic fibrolipomatous tumor (also referred to as *early pleomorphic hyalinizing angiectatic tumor*). This translocation is unusual because it consistently involves the *TGFBR3* gene at 1p22 and the *MGEA5* gene at 10q24, but, because these two genes are transcribed in opposite directions, no chimeric fusion transcript is detectable.[225,226] Because of the unbalanced nature of the translocation, the 5' portions of *TGFBR3* and *MGEA5* are lost and the der(10) chromosome contains the residual 3' portions of the two genes. The rearrangement is proposed to cause transcriptional upregulation of the nearby *FGF8* gene.[225] Additional chromosome aberrations involving chromosome 3 (e.g., ring or marker chromosomes), with amplification of 3p11.1–12.1, have been also observed.[225,226]

Ossifying Fibromyxoid Tumor

The *PHF1* gene at 6p21, previously shown to be involved in fusion gene formation in some endometrial stromal tumors,[227] is also recurrently rearranged in ossifying fibromyxoid tumor,[228] a rare soft tissue and bone tumor displaying multilineage differentiation.[229] The fusion partner *EP400* has been identified in at least one case.[228]

SARCOMAS WITH GENETIC DEREGULATION OF KINASE SIGNALING

A second group of sarcomas is characterized by recurrent genetic alterations that directly result in a deregulation of kinase signaling pathways. Three types of such alterations have been observed: (1) translocations forming chimeric protein tyrosine kinases, (2) translocations encoding a chimeric autocrine growth factor, and (3) activating mutations in specific kinases. The fusion of the catalytic domain of a protein tyrosine kinase with a ubiquitously expressed protein providing a dimerization domain produces a chimeric tyrosine kinase that is constitutively activated in a ligand-independent fashion. This type of mechanism is involved in the pathogenesis of inflammatory myofibroblastic tumor as a result of *ALK* rearrangements (*TPM3-ALK*, etc.) and congenital fibrosarcoma as a result of the *ETV6-NTRK3* fusion.

A less common mechanism implicated in sarcomas with chromosomal translocations is the formation of a chimeric autocrine growth factor, exemplified by the *COL1A1-PDGFB* fusion in dermatofibrosarcoma protuberans[230] and the *COL6A3– CSF1* fusion identified in giant cell tumor of tendon sheath.[231] Finally, GIST is one example of a sarcoma with activating intragenic mutations in specific kinases, including *KIT*, *PDGFRA* and, rarely, *BRAF*. These different types of kinase-dependent sarcomas are discussed in the following sections. Notably, although fusion kinase oncogenes were once thought to be diagnostically specific, it is increasingly evident that the same fusion tyrosine kinase oncogene can have a transforming role in a variety of contexts. These observations suggest that oncogenic transformation in distinct cell types may be mediated by the activation of the same tyrosine kinase signaling pathway, independent of lineage constraints and without affecting differentiation programs. *ETV6-NTRK3* and *ALK* fusion oncogenes are cases in point, with transforming roles in mesenchymal, hematologic, and epithelial contexts. The *NTRK3* fusions are found in congenital fibrosarcoma,[232] acute myelogenous leukemia,[233] and secretory breast carcinoma,[234] whereas *ALK* fusions are found in inflammatory myofibroblastic tumor,[235,236] anaplastic large cell lymphoma,[237,238] and lung adenocarcinoma.[239]

Inflammatory Myofibroblastic Tumor

The inflammatory myofibroblastic tumor affects mainly children and young adults and is composed of varying proportions of myofibroblasts, plasma cells, and lymphocytes. Genetic studies have shown chromosomal abnormalities of 2p23 and rearrangement of the *ALK* gene.[240] Molecular studies have identified *ALK* fusions involving the genes for tropomyosins 3 and 4 (*TPM3* and *TPM4*),[235] the clathrin heavy chain (*CLTC*),[236] the cysteinyl-tRNA synthetase (*CARS*),[241] and the Ran-binding protein 2 (*RANBP2*),[242] and this list continues to grow.[58] Inflammatory myofibroblastic tumors with the *RANBP2-ALK* fusion have ALK IHC staining in a nuclear membrane pattern, have an aggressive clinical course,[243] and can benefit from ALK inhibitor therapy.[244] The common characteristic shared by these *ALK* fusion partners is the presence of an amino-terminal oligomerization motif, which, once fused to a truncated tyrosine kinase (in this case, ALK), leads to activation of the kinase catalytic domain in a constitutive fashion.[245] ALK IHC studies show upregulated ALK protein expression in about 60% of cases, although the percentage is lower in adult cases.[246] IHC using newer, more sensitive ALK antibodies may identify additional positive cases [58] but it is also possible that other related kinase fusions may be present in *ALK*-fusion negative inflammatory myofibroblastic tumors. ALK positivity is not entirely specific for inflammatory myofibroblastic tumor and can be observed in some other mesenchymal neoplasms.[247]

Infantile Fibrosarcoma

Infantile fibrosarcoma generally presents at birth or within the first two years of life and is associated with a much better prognosis than adult fibrosarcoma. Cytogenetically, it shows a recurrent t(12;15)(p13;q25), resulting in the *ETV6-NTRK3* fusion.[232,248] The *ETV6-NTRK3* rearrangement is demonstrated convincingly by FISH methods, whereas the t(12;15) is often cryptic when assessed by conventional cytogenetic banding studies. Trisomies for chromosomes 8, 11, 17, and 20 are nearly as characteristic as the *ETV6-NTRK3* and appear to be acquired as secondary events after the *ETV6-NTRK3*.[249,250] NTRK3 is a transmembrane surface receptor for neurotrophin-3 and is primarily expressed in the central nervous system, where it is involved in growth and survival of neuronal cells.[251] ETV6 is a member of ETS transcription factor family, and the *ETV6* gene is frequently targeted by chromosomal translocations in human cancer, especially in leukemias.[251] In leukemia translocations, ETV6 either contributes its ETS-type DNA domain or its dimerization domain. In congenital fibrosarcoma, the oligomerization domain of ETV6 is fused to the kinase domain of NTRK3, mediating ligand-independent dimerization and resultant kinase activation. The *ETV6-NTRK3* fusion is absent in adult-type fibrosarcoma or in other pediatric cellular fibroblastic lesions such as infantile fibromatosis and myofibromatosis and, therefore, can be used as a molecular diagnostic test for congenital fibrosarcoma. However, *ETV6-NTRK3* is not specific for congenital fibrosarcoma but is found also in the cellular and mixed variants of congenital mesoblastic nephroma,[232,250] which is a renal tumor resembling congenital fibrosarcoma. It is also found in secretory breast carcinoma, mammary analogue secretory carcinoma of salivary glands, and a minor subset of acute myeloid leukemias.[234,252,253]

Dermatofibrosarcoma Protuberans/Giant Cell Fibroblastoma

The recurrent t(17;22)(q21;q13) resulting in *COL1A1-PDGFB* fusion has been reported as a consistent finding in both dermatofibrosarcoma protuberans (DFSP) and giant cell fibroblastoma (GCF) supporting the concept of a common pathogenetic entity.[230,254] Adult DFSP typically have three or so copies of the *COL1A-PDGFB* fusion gene that are repeated tandemly in supernumerary ring chromosomes.[255] GCF and pediatric DFSP more often have a single copy of the *COL1A-PDGFB* fusion gene, seen as a conventional translocation chromosome, rather than the ring chromosome. Studies of GCF and composite GCF-DFSP cases have shown the presence of a single translocation t(17;22), and the resultant *COL1A1-PDGFB* fusion, in the GCF component, with acquisition of additional copies of the fusion oncogene being associated with progression to DFSP.[256] The t(17;22)fuses the strongly expressed collagen 1 alpha 1 (*COL1A1*) gene on chromosome 17 to the second exon of the platelet-derived growth factor-B (*PDGFB*) gene on chromosome 22. This distinctive translocation mechanism results in transcriptional upregulation of the *PDGFB* gene. The posttranslational processed form of the fusion protein gives rise to a fully functional and mature PDGFB protein, which induces activation of its receptor, PDGFRB, through autocrine or paracrine mechanisms.[257] Clinical studies have shown a high response rate to imatinib therapy in both locally advanced and metastatic DFSP.[258-261] As imatinib blocks PDGFRB signaling, these results support the concept that DFSP cells are dependent on aberrant activation of PDGFRB for cellular proliferation and survival.

Tenosynovial Giant Cell Tumor

Localized and diffuse tenosynovial giant cell tumor (TGCT) is composed of a mixture of giant cells, mononuclear cells, and inflammatory cells and has also been referred to as pigmented villonodular synovitis. The neoplastic nature of TGCT, long controversial, was resolved by the identification of a recurrent t(1;2)(p13;q37), resulting in a *CSF1–COL6A3* fusion, in a substantial number of both localized and diffuse tumors.[231] This translocation results in overexpression of CSF1, which is detected in a minority of the intratumoral cells. However, the majority of cells express CSF1R, as detected by in situ hybridization. Therefore, only a minority of cells in TGCT seem to be neoplastic, whereas the remaining cells are apparently non-neoplastic and are recruited by the local overexpression of CSF1. This phenomenon, described as a tumor-landscaping effect, indicates that aberrant CSF1 expression in the neoplastic cells leads to abnormal accumulation of CSF1R-positive non-neoplastic cells.[231] These findings reconcile the distinctive histologic features of TGCT with the underlying biology, in which CSF1 mediates proliferation, differentiation, and activation of macrophages and their precursors. In these tumors, the cells expressing CSF1 also express CD68, but lack CD163, suggesting that the CSF1-expressing neoplastic cells may be derived from synovial lining cells.[231] Synovial lining cells in reactive synovitis express CSF1, providing additional support for this hypothesis. Approximately 60% of TGCT contain the *CSF1–COL6A3* fusion leading to CSF1 overexpression. Most of the remaining cases show high CSF1 without evidence of rearrangement.[262] The biologic evidence of a central role for CSF1 in the pathogenesis of TGCT is further supported by clinical experience, in which pigmented villonodular synovitis responded therapeutically to imatinib, which is also active as a CSF1R-inhibitor.[263]

Gastrointestinal Stromal Tumors

Constitutive activation of either the KIT or PDGFRA receptor tyrosine kinases by oncogenic mutations plays a central pathogenetic role in the GIST.[264,265] The *KIT* gene maps to 4q12, in the vicinity of the genes encoding for *PDGFRA* and *KDR* receptor tyrosine kinases. KIT belongs to the class III of receptor tyrosine kinases, together with CSF1R (colony stimulating factor 1 receptor), PDGFRB and PDGFRA, based on their sequence homology and similar conformational structure. The KIT receptor plays a critical role in the normal development and function of the interstitial cells of Cajal (ICC),[266-268] as well as in hematopoiesis, gametogenesis and melanogenesis during embryonic development and in the postnatal organism. Activating *KIT* mutations have also been implicated in the pathogenesis of several other human tumors, including seminomas,[269] mastocytosis,[270] acute myelogenous leukemias,[271] and a subset of melanomas.[272]

In GIST, the initiating (primary) *KIT* mutations can involve either the extracellular or the cytoplasmic domains of the receptor. Most of these mutations (70% to 75%) involve the cytoplasmic juxtamembrane domain in a hotspot region encoded by the 5' end of exon 11, codons 550-560.[273,274] By analogy with other receptor tyrosine kinases, the juxtamembrane domain may function as a negative regulator of the KIT kinase, and disruption of the conformational integrity of this domain may impair its negative regulatory function. Therefore, the oncogenic potential of juxtamembrane domain mutations is attributed to the loss of this inhibitory function. The types of mutations occurring in this hotspot are quite heterogeneous and include in-frame deletions of variable sizes, point mutations, or deletions accompanied by substitutions. A second, less common, hotspot in the juxtamembrane domain is located at the 3' end of exon 11; these mutations are often internal tandem duplications (ITDs).[273,275] The subtype of exon 11 mutation appears to have clinicopathologic relevance in GIST. Exon 11 deletions (compared to exon 11 substitution mutations) seem to be found in GISTs with more aggressive behavior.[276] Specifically, deletions affecting codons 557 and 558 predict a poor prognosis.[277,278] In contrast, GIST patients harboring the previously mentioned ITDs at the 3' end of exon 11 follow a more indolent clinical course, and their tumors are typically gastric.[273,275]

KIT exon 9 primary mutations occur in 10% to 15% of patients and define a distinct subset of GISTs that are often located in the small bowel and show more aggressive behavior.[273,279] In contrast to the more common *KIT* mutations in exons 9 and 11, mutations have been rarely described in the kinase domain (exon 13 and 17).[280,281]

Approximately one-third of GISTs lacking *KIT* mutations harbor a mutation in *PDGFRA,* within exons 12, 14, or 18.[265,282-284] *PDGFRA*-mutated GISTs show a preference for gastric location, epithelioid morphology, variable or absent KIT expression by IHC, and a more indolent clinical behavior.[265,284,285] In about 10% of patients, no detectable mutation is identified in either *KIT* or *PDGFRA*. These *KIT/PDGFRA*-wildtype GISTs can have mutations in one of the *SDH* genes, or in *NF1*, *KRAS*, or *BRAF*.[286-288] In particular, GISTs that occur in pediatric or neurofibromatosis type I patients almost never show mutations in *KIT* and *PDGFRA*.[289-291] The *SDH* gene mutations are inactivating and are associated with loss of SDH protein expression.

These SDH-deficient GISTs arise in the stomach and are typically diagnosed in young adults but can also be found in older individuals.[286] In some patients, the SDH mutations are germline, causing the Carney-Stratakis syndrome of GIST and paraganglioma.[292]

Although the pathologic diagnosis of GIST can be rendered on morphologic grounds in the majority of cases, as supported by KIT (CD117) immunoreactivity, in approximately 4% of cases, the KIT IHC is negative.[293] When compared to KIT-positive GISTs, these KIT-negative cases are more likely to have epithelioid morphology, contain *PDGFRA* mutations, and arise outside of the gastrointestinal tract. Because some GISTs that are negative for KIT by IHC, nonetheless, contain imatinib-sensitive *KIT* or *PDGFRA* mutations, these patients should not be denied imatinib therapy based on the negative IHC result alone.

Most activating mutations in *KIT* or *PDGFRA* in GISTs are sporadic and somatically acquired in the tumor cells. However, various kindreds have been reported to carry a germline mutation in either *KIT* or *PDGFRA*.[294-296] Affected individuals in these kindreds develop GISTs that are usually multiple, smaller, and occur in a background of ICC hyperplasia, both adjacent to and remote from the neoplastic lesions. The consistent ICC hyperplasia suggests that constitutive activation of KIT (or PDGFRA), through oncogenic mutation, is directly responsible for a polyclonal expansion of this subset of cells. Whereas *KIT* mutation appears to be sufficient for the expansion of the myenteric plexus, additional somatic genetic alterations are presumably required to generate the neoplastic proliferations recognized as GIST. In addition, a significant number of familial GIST patients have cutaneous hyperpigmentation and, in rare cases, abnormalities of mast cells, such as urticaria pigmentosa or systemic mast cell disease. The observation that *KIT* activating mutations may be inherited suggested that it might be possible to develop murine models harboring a germline gain of function mutation, as an experimental tool for the study of KIT oncogenic signaling mechanisms. Indeed, two such models have been created.[297,298]

Cytogenetically, GISTs show rather simple karyotypes with common losses of chromosomes 14 and 22, as early genetic events, independent of the tumor site, clinical outcome, or *KIT* genotype.[299,300] Additional chromosomal changes occur preferentially in high risk and recurrent GIST, including loss of 9p and 1p, among others. GISTs have a very distinctive gene expression profile that distinguishes them as a group from other soft tissue sarcomas.[301,302] When comparing different pathologic or molecular subsets of GISTs, there is some heterogeneity in gene expression patterns that can be correlated with tumor location and *KIT* genotype.[303,304]

Imatinib mesylate (Gleevec, Novartis Pharmaceuticals, Basel, Switzerland) is a selective tyrosine kinase inhibitor whose targets include KIT, PDGFRA, and ABL1. Imatinib treatment achieves a partial response or stable disease in about 80% of patients with metastatic GIST.[305] GISTs with *KIT* exon 11 mutations are potently inhibited by imatinib, whereas those with *KIT* exon 9 mutations are less responsive.[282,306,307] Although imatinib achieves a partial response or stable disease in the majority of GIST patients, complete and lasting responses are rare. Most patients who initially benefit from imatinib treatment eventually develop a drug resistance. The most common mechanism of acquired resistance is through a second *KIT* mutation, usually located in the kinase domain.[308] The secondary mutations are generally located in the KIT ATP-binding pocket, encoded by exons 13 and 14, or in the KIT activation loop, encoded by exon 17. The ATP-binding pocket mutations create steric and charge alterations that interfere with imatinib binding, but are potentially inhibited by sunitinib,[309,310] a smaller compound than imatinib. The activation loop mutations, by contrast, are cross-resistant to sunitinib[309,310] but appear to be at least partially inhibited by other KIT kinase inhibitors, such as regorafenib.

SARCOMAS WITH COMPLEX KARYOTYPES

The majority of malignant soft tissue tumors are not associated with specific chromosomal translocations or simple point mutations. In these sarcomas, many complex cytogenetic aberrations leading to numerous genomic gains and losses have been described. Soft tissue sarcomas with complex unbalanced karyotypes lacking specific translocations include pleomorphic and dedifferentiated liposarcomas, angiosarcoma, leiomyosarcoma, adult fibrosarcoma, and undifferentiated pleomorphic sarcoma (malignant fibrous histiocytoma). Common cytogenetic findings in these sarcomas are listed in Table 4-4.

How do these sarcomas accumulate these complex karyotypic changes? The process is not simply age-related because some sarcomas in this group are pediatric (e.g., osteosarcoma). Several possible pathways to karyotypic complexity have been suggested, some by mouse models, and some by cancer genomics studies. Two mouse models have been

TABLE 4-4 Common Chromosome Changes in Benign and Malignant Soft Tissue Tumors (Other Than Recurrent Translocations)

SOFT TISSUE TUMOR	CYTOGENETIC FINDING	MOLECULAR EVENT
Atypical lipomatous tumor, well differentiated liposarcoma, and dedifferentiated liposarcoma	Ring/long marker	*MDM2, HMGA2, CDK4* amplification
Embryonal rhabdomyosarcoma	Loss 11p15.5 +2,+8,+11,+12,+13,+20	*IGF2, H19, CDKN1C*
Desmoid type fibromatosis	Trisomy 8 and 20 Deletion of 5q	 *APC* loss CTNNB1 (β-catenin) mutation
Epithelioid sarcoma, proximal type	t/del (22)(q11.2)	*SMARCB1* loss
Gastrointestinal stromal tumor	Monosomy/partial loss 14 and 22 Deletion of 1p Deletion of 9p	 *CDKN2A/B* loss
Perineurioma	Deletion 22q	*NF2* loss
Rhabdoid tumor (extrarenal)	t/del (22)(q11.2)	*SMARCB1* loss
Spindle cell/ pleomorphic lipoma	Deletion 13q or 16q	Unknown
Schwannoma	Deletion of 22q	*NF2* loss

proposed, both in the setting of abrogation of p53 checkpoint function. In the first, progressive telomere erosion results in associations between heterologous telomeres leading to chromosomal fusion-bridge-breakage cycles and nonreciprocal translocations, as observed in some human sarcomas.[311,312] The unbalanced karyotype is then stabilized by the reactivation of telomerase or by the mechanism of ALT, also described in human sarcomas.[313] In a second murine model of karyotypic complexity, impaired joining of nonhomologous ends promotes chromosomal translocations, amplifications, and deletions, as a result of an increase in unrepaired double-strand breaks. This mechanism has led to formation of soft tissue sarcomas in mice of the same histologic types as human sarcomas lacking specific translocations.[314] More recently, next-generation sequencing studies have identified a novel genomic phenomenon, termed chromothripsis, in which dozens to hundreds of genomic rearrangements occur in a single catastrophic cellular event, generating a characteristic alternation between two copy number states in one or more chromosome arms.[315,316] It appears that chromothripsis may be more frequent in complex karyotype sarcomas than in most other cancers, but more data are needed to confirm this.[315,317]

Inactivation of the p53 pathway appears to be a key differentiating factor between sarcomas with simple genetic alterations and those with karyotypic complexity (see Table 4-3). Among sarcomas with complex unbalanced karyotypes, p53 pathway alterations are generally more prevalent[76] but often have a weaker prognostic value than in translocation sarcomas and require large numbers of patients to show statistically significant differences.[78,318] This suggests that, in sarcomas with nonspecific genetic alterations, p53 pathway inactivation may be a common early event required to overcome checkpoints triggered by senescence, telomere erosion, or double-strand breaks in the progression of these sarcomas. Its more widespread role in this class of sarcomas may account for its limited ability to define distinct clinical subsets in these tumors.

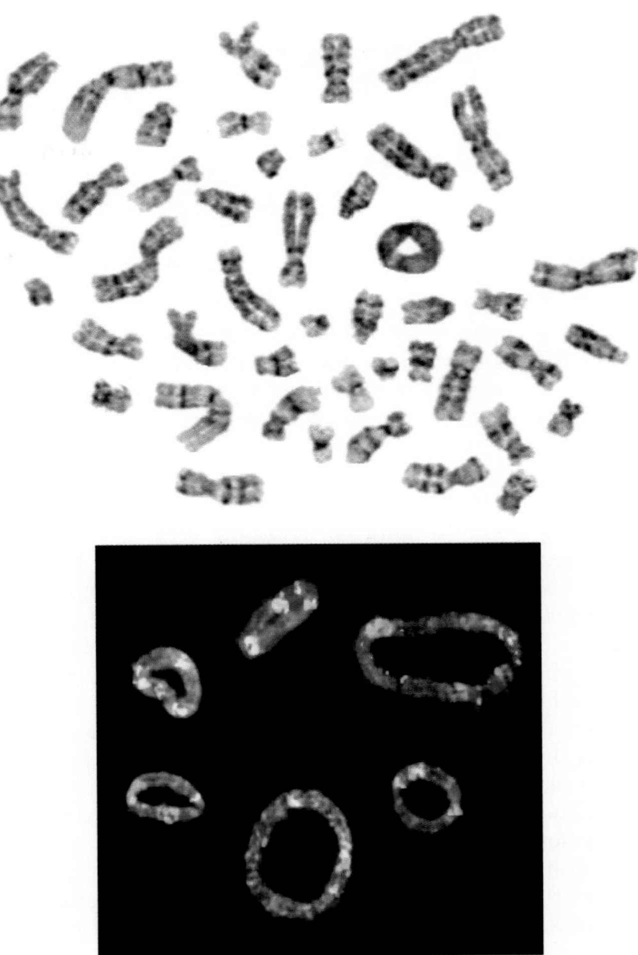

FIGURE 4-5. Ring and giant marker chromosomes in atypical lipoma (AL)/well-differentiated liposarcoma (WDLPS). Top panel shows Giemsa-stained metaphase chromosomes. Bottom panel shows ring chromosomes analyzed by spectral karyotyping (COBRA-FISH).

High-Grade Pleomorphic Sarcomas

High-grade pleomorphic sarcomas, including many tumors formerly called malignant fibrous histiocytoma, generally have complex and nondistinctive karyotypes[319,320] and may represent the most undifferentiated state of other sarcomas, such as leiomyosarcomas[321] or liposarcomas. High-grade pleomorphic sarcomas representing end-stage dedifferentiated liposarcomas can be suspected based on the characteristic rings or giant markers derived from chromosome 12q, in addition to complex aberrations, and occurrence in the retroperitoneum (see later text).[322]

Atypical Lipomatous Neoplasm (Well-Differentiated Liposarcoma) and Dedifferentiated Liposarcoma

Virtually all cases of atypical lipomatous neoplasm (ALN) and its deep counterpart (well-differentiated liposarcoma) share the same cytogenetic abnormality, which is supernumerary (extra) ring and/or giant marker chromosome(s) (Fig. 4-5). These ring and/or giant marker chromosomes generally represent the sole chromosome abnormality in ALN and coexist with a few other numeric/structural abnormalities and nonrandom telomeric association. The tumor cells contain either a ring or a giant marker chromosome that can vary in size among the tumor cells in a given case because they are unstable during cell division. At the molecular level, these ring or marker chromosomes are composed predominantly of amplicons involving the q13-q15 region of chromosome 12. Similar rings and giant marker chromosomes are also seen in dedifferentiated liposarcoma, although a more complex karyotype is frequently observed. Recent next-generation sequencing studies have provided a detailed picture of the structure of these highly characteristic amplicons.[323] This 12q region overlaps with the 12q14-15 region that is rearranged in a large number of lipomas and that contains numerous putative and established oncogenes. These include *MDM2, CDK4, HMGA2, GLI1*, and *DDIT3*, among others.[158,324] Functionally, the potential roles of *MDM2, CDK4*, and *HMGA2* have been examined most extensively.[158,325] However, the structure of these amplicons is complex, and other genes may well also be significant, such as *YEATS4*[158] and *FRS2*.[326] Amplification of the *JUN* gene at 1p32 and of the *MAP3K5* gene at 6q22 have been linked to impaired adipocytic differentiation in dedifferentiated liposarcomas,[327,328] and other copy number losses at 11q23-24 and 19q13 have been linked to genomic complexity and poor prognosis, respectively.[329] FISH for *MDM2* amplification is a highly sensitive ancillary test for the distinction of ALT from lipoma.[330]

Leiomyosarcoma

Marked aneuploidy with complex chromosomal rearrangements is the karyotypic feature of the majority of soft tissue leiomyosarcomas, as well as those arising in the uterus. No specific or recurrent change has been found in these tumors; however, some common gains or losses of genetic material have been detected by cytogenetic and CGH studies. Among nonsoft tissue leiomyosarcomas (mainly those of gastrointestinal and uterine origin), chromosome breaks at 1q21 are more frequent than those involving 1p13 or 10q22. Whereas losses involving 1q and 3p are more frequent among soft tissue leiomyosarcomas, losses of chromosomes 14, 15, and 22q are more frequent in nonsoft tissue leiomyosarcomas. These observations suggest that some aberrations may be more related to the site of origin than to the morphologic features of the tumors.[331] For instance, in leiomyosarcomas arising in the retroperitoneum, there is characteristically amplification of *MYOCD*, a gene at 17p11 encoding a transcriptional cofactor involved in smooth muscle development and differentiation.[332] It has also been noted that genomic copy number changes in poorly differentiated leiomyosarcomas overlap with those of many undifferentiated pleomorphic sarcomas, suggesting that many of the latter represent undifferentiated leiomyosarcomas.[333-335]

The patterns of oncogene and tumor suppressor mutations in leiomyoma and leiomyosarcoma differ, with leiomyomas (particularly those of uterine origin) featuring *HMGA2* and *HMGA1* rearrangements, whereas leiomyosarcomas often have *CDKN2A*, *PTEN*, and *TP53* inactivating mutations. However, *MED12* oncogenic mutations may be an exception. They are found frequently in both leiomyoma and leiomyosarcomas of uterine origin but infrequently in extrauterine ones.[336-339]

Embryonal Rhabdomyosarcoma

This subset of rhabdomyosarcoma harbors no characteristic translocations and instead typically shows multiple numeric chromosomal abnormalities. Two of the most frequent changes are gains of chromosomes 8 (most frequent), as well as of 2, 13, and 20, and loss of heterozygosity at 11p15 occurring through diverse mechanisms. The loss of heterozygosity at 11p15 may target the imprinted genes *IGF2*, *H19*, and *CDKN1C*.[340] Approximately 25% of ERMS contain activating mutations in kinase signaling genes, including *RAS* family genes, *PTPN11*, *BRAF*, *FGFR4*, and *PIK3CA*.[341-343] The RAS pathway is also activated by *NF1* deletions in another 15% of cases.[344] Activating *CTNNB1* mutations are present in 3% of ERMS.[341] There is an increased incidence of ERMS in syndromes with germline RAS/MAPK pathway mutations, including Noonan syndrome (OMIM: 163950), cardiofaciocutaneous syndrome (OMIM: 115150), and Costello syndrome (OMIM: 218040).[345] Along with *RAS* genes, *PTPN11* and *BRAF* are two of the most frequently mutated genes in this group of syndromes, with the germline mutations overlapping only partly with recurrent somatic mutations in these genes. ERMS is also seen in the familial pleuropulmonary blastoma-predisposition syndrome or DICER1 syndrome (OMIM: 601200) caused by germline mutations in *DICER1*, an endoribonuclease with a central role in microRNA biogenesis.[346] The syndrome includes ERMS, characteristically of uterine cervical origin.[347,348] Inactivating somatic mutations in *DICER1* are also rarely found in sporadic ERMS.[349]

PEComas

The family of tumors grouped under the term *PEComa* includes neoplasms with perivascular epithelioid cell phenotypes such as renal angiomyolipoma, lymphangioleiomyomatosis, and other visceral and soft tissue PEComas. PEComas are seen in the context of the tuberous sclerosis complex disorder caused by germline mutations in either *TSC1* (OMIM: 191100) or *TSC2* (OMIM:613254).[350,351] Sporadic PEComas often show complex karyotypes with loss of *TSC2*.[352] This has important implications for targeted therapy because *TSC2* loss leads to activation of the MTOR signaling pathway in PEComas [353] and, therefore, renders them sensitive to MTOR inhibitors.[354,355] A smaller subset of PEComas, approximately 10%, harbors *TFE3* fusions,[356] including *PSF-TFE3*,[357] but does not show *TSC2* loss.[358]

Neuroblastoma

Neuroblastoma, although not specifically within the scope of this edition, is included here because it enters into the differential diagnosis of small round blue cell tumors of childhood such as ES and others, and some of its genetic alterations, such as those involving *MYCN* and *ALK*, may be of confirmatory help. Neuroblastoma is a genetically heterogeneous tumor with a remarkably variable clinical behavior.[359] One of the key genetic alterations in neuroblastoma is *MYCN* amplification, presenting cytogenetically as double minute chromosomes (dmin) or homogeneously staining regions (HSR). Although it is a strong negative *prognostic* marker, *MYCN* amplification is a moderately specific, relatively insensitive *diagnostic* marker for neuroblastoma. It is present in only about 22% of neuroblastomas, including about 30% of advanced-stage tumors. It has also been found occasionally in other sarcomas, especially in ARMS, where it may also have a prognostic impact.[360] Another major genetic alteration that appears to be even more specific for neuroblastoma is somatic mutation of the *ALK* receptor tyrosine kinase gene,[361-363] present in about 6% to 10% of cases.[341,364,365]

CHROMOSOME CHANGES IN BENIGN MESENCHYMAL TUMORS

Many benign soft tissue tumors harbor specific genetic alterations that are quite distinct from those seen in sarcomas. This observation yet again highlights how seldom mesenchymal tumors progress from a preneoplastic to a benign and, ultimately, to a malignant lesion, compared to epithelial cancers. Table 4-4 lists the major cytogenetic findings in benign soft tissue tumors. Recurrent translocations in benign soft tissue tumors are included in Table 4-1.

Lipomas, the most common mesenchymal lesions studied cytogenetically, contain a recurrent t(3;12)(q28;q14). Clonal chromosomal abnormalities have been found in approximately 70% of these tumors, and the most frequently involved region is 12q13-q15. Although the t(3;12)(q28;q14) is found most often, virtually all chromosomes have been reported as partners in rearrangements involving 12q13-q15. Involvement of the same 12q region has been described in several other benign tumors, including uterine leiomyoma, endometrial polyps, pulmonary chondroid hamartoma, fibroadenoma, aggressive angiomyxoma, adenoma of the salivary glands, and soft tissue chondroma.

HMGA2 (formerly *HMGIC*), which maps to 12q14.4, encodes a member of the high-mobility group A, small, nonhistone, chromatin-associated proteins, HMGA2. It is consistently rearranged in all of the mesenchymal tumors described previously.[366,367] Although the 12q break appears homogeneous at the cytogenetic level, molecular studies have determined that the precise breakpoints are fairly heterogeneous. A variety of *HMGA2* rearrangements, some with an associated novel fusion transcript, have been demonstrated in these mesenchymal tumors. Most 12q rearrangements involve the large (140 kb) third intron of *HMGA2* and delete the 3' portion of the gene, which encodes the protein-binding domains.

The partner genes in the majority of *HMGA2* fusion transcripts are uncharacterized, novel DNA sequences. Most chimeric transcripts result in the addition of only a few amino acids (i.e., 1–10) to *HMGA2* exon 3. Consequently, one mechanistic possibility is that truncation of HMGA2 protein, rather than fusion to ectopic sequences, is the primary pathogenetic event. A few *HMGA2* fusion transcripts have been further characterized in lipoma, including *HMGA2-LPP*, *HMGA2-LHFP*, *HMGA2-CXCR7 (CMKOR1)*, *HMGA2-NFIB*, and *HMGA2-EBF1*.[368] Some specific *HMGA2* fusion genes (e.g., *HMGA2-LPP*, *HMGA2-NFIB*) have been found in different benign tumors, suggesting that they can transform a variety of cell types or that they occur in a pluripotent cell type.

In contrast to intragenic breaks, some benign tumors with 12q13-15 rearrangements show *HMGA2* breakpoints that fall outside of the coding region, suggesting that disruption of regulatory sequences may lead to abnormal *HMGA2* expression. This has been demonstrated in uterine leiomyoma with t(12;14)(q14.4;q24),[369] and in aggressive angiomyxoma with a t(11;12)(q23;q14.4).[370] Another proposed pathogenetic mechanism is that the rearrangements cause loss of the 3' untranslated portion of *HMGA2* that contains a binding site for the repressive let-7 miRNA, thereby resulting in higher expression of HMGA2,[371] but not all data in soft tissue tumors are consistent with that model.[372,373]

A second group of lipomas are characterized by 6p21 rearrangement, to which another member of the HMG family, *HMGA1* (*HMGIY*), maps. The majority of *HMGA1* breakpoints are located downstream of the coding region. It has been suggested that the dysregulation of *HMGA1* expression is mediated by replacement of negative regulatory sequences by enhancers from different translocation partners.[374] *HMGA1* rearrangements are also common in other benign tumors, including endometrial polyps and pulmonary chondroid hamartoma. In contrast to HMGA2 fusion products, few chimeric HMGA1 proteins have been characterized.[375] The different cytogenetic subgroups among lipomas have recently been surveyed.[376]

Furthermore, other benign adipose tissue tumors also show specific chromosomal rearrangements. The characteristic cytogenetic abnormality in *lipoblastoma*, for example, involves 8q12, the location of *PLAG1*. Two different fusion genes have been reported: *HAS1-PLAG1* and *COL1A2-PLAG1*.[377] The molecular consequence of these fusions is an activation of *PLAG1* transcription caused by promoter substitution, as has been described in pleomorphic adenoma of the salivary gland with a t(3;8)(p21;q12). Among soft tissue tumors, the presence of a *PLAG1* rearrangement in about 80% of lipoblastomas serves as a specific marker for this tumor.[378]

Several other benign soft tissue tumors are defined by recurrent gene fusions. *Hibernoma* is characterized by involvement of 11q13, affecting not only the derivative chromosome 11, but also the apparently normal homologue. Heterozygous and homozygous deletions have been detected that are not limited to the 11q13.1 region surrounding *MEN1* but extend to 11q13.5.[379] These deletions cause concomitant loss of the tumor suppressor genes, *MEN1* and *AIP*.[380] The recurrent t(11;16)(q13;p12-13) seen in *chondroid lipoma* results in a *c11orf95-MKL2* fusion gene.[381] *Soft tissue angiofibroma* is a recently defined benign tumor that is characterized by bland fibroblastic proliferation and a complex vascular network and harbors the recurrent translocation, t(5;8)(p15;q13), leading to the formation of a *AHRR-NCOA2* fusion gene.[382-384] In the predicted fusion protein, the two activation domains of NCOA2 replace the repressor domain of AHRR.[382] *Nodular fasciitis* is a clonal proliferation containing a fusion of the *MYH9* promoter region to the entire coding region of *USP6*, accounting for the overexpression of USP6 in this neoplasm.[385] The *USP6* and *MYH9* genes are located on the terminal white GTG-banded region of 17p13 and 22q13.1, respectively, explaining why t(17;22)(p13;q12) had been undetectable by conventional cytogenetic analysis.

GENETICS OF FAMILIAL SARCOMAS AND THEIR SPORADIC COUNTERPARTS

Numerous familial sarcoma syndromes have been described.[386] The genetic basis of many of these has been elucidated. Some are associated with a broad spectrum of soft tissue sarcomas. For example, Li-Fraumeni syndrome is associated with germline *P53* mutation, in most cases, and bone and soft tissue sarcomas are one of the classic syndromic tumors in this syndrome, along with breast carcinoma, brain cancers, and adrenocortical carcinoma.[348,387,388] Indeed, sarcomas account for approximately 25% of cancers in Li-Fraumeni syndrome, and the vast majority are diagnosed before age 50.[348] The reported histologies of the soft tissue sarcomas have been rhabdomyosarcoma (usually embryonal), undifferentiated pleomorphic sarcoma, fibrosarcoma, and leiomyosarcoma.[348] Significant genotype-phenotype correlations and age-dependent variations in sarcoma types are observed in individuals with

TABLE 4-5 Germline Genetic Syndromes with Soft Tissue Tumors as a Common or Rare Manifestation

DISORDER (OMIM NUMBER)[1]	INHERITANCE	LOCUS[2]	GENE	SOFT TISSUE TUMOR[3]
Bannayan-Riley-Ruvalcaba syndrome (153480)	AD	10q23	*PTEN*	Lipomas, hemangiomas
Beckwith-Wiedemann syndrome (130650)	Sporadic/AD	11p15	multiple	Embryonal rhabdomyosarcomas, myxomas, fibromas, hamartomas
Blue rubber bleb nevus syndrome (112200)	AD	unknown	unknown	Cavernous hemangiomas
Carney complex,[4] type I (160980)	AD	17q24	*PRKAR1A*	Myxoma, melanotic schwannoma
Carney complex,[4] type II (605244)	AD	2p16	unknown	Myxoma, melanotic schwannoma
Costello syndrome (218040)	Sporadic	11p15	*HRAS*	Rhabdomyosarcomas, neuroblastomas
Cowden syndrome (158350)	AD	10q23	*PTEN*	Cutaneous sclerotic fibromas
Familial adenomatous polyposis (175100), familial infiltrative fibromatosis (135290)	AD	5q21	*APC*	Desmoid tumors
Familial GIST syndrome (606764)	AD	4q12	*KIT*	GISTs
		4q12	*PDGFRA*	
Familial glomus tumor (138000)	AD	1p22	*GLMN*	Glomus tumors
Familial paragangliomas and GIST (606864)	AD	11q23	*SDHD*	Paragangliomas, GIST
		1q21	*SDHC*	
		1p36	*SDHB*	
		5p15	*SDHA*	
Fumarate hydratase deficiency (150800)	AD	1q42	*FH*	Leiomyomas (skin, uterus)
Juvenile hyaline fibromatosis/Infantile systemic hyalinosis (228600)	AR	4q21	*ANTXR2*	Hyaline fibromatosis
Li-Fraumeni syndrome (151623)	AD	17p13	*TP53*	Rhabdomyosarcomas, other sarcomas
		22q11	*CHEK2*	
Lipomas, familial multiple (151900)	AD	12q14.3	*HMGA2*	Lipomas
Maffucci syndrome (166000)	Somatic mosaic	2q33.3	*IDH1*	Hemangiomas, angiosarcomas
	Sporadic	15q26	*IDH2*	
		3p22	*PTH1R*	
Nevoid basal cell carcinoma syndrome (Gorlin) (109400)	AD	9q31	*PTCH1*	Fetal rhabdomyomas, embryonal rhabdomyosarcomas, leiomyomas, leiomyosarcomas
Neurofibromatosis type 1 (162200)	AD	17q11	*NF1*	Neurofibromas, malignant peripheral nerve sheath tumors, paragangliomas, GIST
Neurofibromatosis type 2 (101000)	AD	22q12	*NF2*	Schwannomas
Nijmegen breakage syndrome (251260)	AR	8q21	*NBN*	Perianal rhabdomyosarcomas
Proteus syndrome (176920)	Sporadic	14q32	AKT1	Lipomas
		10q23	PTEN	
Retinoblastoma (180200)	AD	13q14	*RB1*	Rhabdomyosarcomas, leiomyosarcomas
Rhabdoid predisposition syndrome 1 (601607)	AD	22q11	*SMARCB1*	Malignant rhabdoid tumors
Rhabdoid predisposition syndrome 2 (613325)	AD	19p13	*SMARCA4*	
Rubinstein-Taybi syndrome (180849)	AD	16p13	*CREBBP*	Rhabdomyosarcomas, neuroblastomas
Tuberous sclerosis, type 1 (191100)	AD	9q34	*TSC1*	Lymphangioleiomyomatosis, cutaneous angiofibroma, subungual fibromas
Tuberous sclerosis, type 2 (613254)	AD	16p13	*TSC2*	As above + PEComas
Venous malformations with glomus cells (138000)	AD	1p21-22	unknown	Glomus tumors
Von Hippel-Lindau (193300)	AD	3p25	*VHL*	Ocular hemangioblastomas
Werner syndrome (277700)	AR	8p12	*WRN*	Undifferentiated pleomorphic sarcoma, leiomyosarcomas, fibrosarcomas

1. Online Mendelian Inheritance in Man database (www.ncbi.nlm.nih.gov/entrez/query.fcgi?db=OMIM)
2. AD, autosomal dominant; AR, autosomal recessive; sporadic indicates that syndrome occurs as a new germline mutation with little or no data on transmission.
3. For syndromes not primarily associated with sarcomas, data on types of sarcomas should be considered tentative because of the lack of histopathologic detail of many reports.
4. Not to be confused with Carney triad (gastric stromal sarcoma, paraganglioma, pulmonary chondroma), which is not familial.

germline TP53 mutations: missense mutations in exons encoding the DNA-binding domain of TP53 are associated with sarcoma development in childhood or adolescence, typically rhabdomyosarcoma or osteosarcoma, whereas truncating mutations and missense mutations outside of the DNA-binding domain are associated with leiomyosarcoma, typically in young adults.[348] It should be noted that patients with sarcoma but without a significant personal or family history are unlikely to harbor germline *TP53* mutations.[389,390] However, recent data suggest that certain germline DNA sequence polymorphisms that affect p53 pathway function may be associated with early-onset sporadic sarcomas from the complex karyotype group.[76,391] For instance, other familial sarcoma syndromes are associated with very specific sarcomas, and the understanding of their genetic predisposition also illuminates understanding of their sporadic counterparts. Familial GIST, tuberous sclerosis, DICER1 syndrome, and germline RAS/MAPK pathway syndromes have been described previously. Several notable syndromes are briefly discussed later. Other notable genetic syndromes associated with sarcomas, either as a primary or a rare manifestation, are listed in Table 4-5.

Neurofibromatosis Type 1 and Malignant Peripheral Nerve Sheath Tumor

Neurofibromatosis type 1 (NF1) (OMIM: 162200) is caused by germline inactivating mutations in the *NF1* gene and is defined by a variety of tumors, with neurofibroma and MPNST being most relevant to this section. In neurofibromas arising in NF1 patients, a double-hit model for *NF1* involving inactivation of the remaining functional copy of the *NF1* gene is well established.[392] This scenario has also been supported by mouse models of the NF1 syndrome.[393] In sporadic neurofibromas, acquired genetic alterations inactivating both copies of *NF1* have been documented.[394,395] MPNST is also associated with bi-allelic inactivation of *NF1*,[396] but its development additionally requires additional mutations in *CDKN2A* or *P53*, both in familial and sporadic cases,[396-399] as well as in animal models.[393]

Familial Adenomatous Polyposis and Desmoids

Familial adenomatous polyposis (FAP) is caused by mutations in the adenomatous polyposis coli (*APC*) gene. Some cases are associated with extracolonic tumors (Gardner syndrome) (OMIM: 175100), most notably deep (desmoid-type) fibromatoses, and this is correlated with the location of the mutation in the *APC* gene, specifically with mutations that result in truncation of the protein after codon 1444.[400,401] Notably, deep fibromatoses may be the first diagnostic clue to FAP,[402] or they may, in rare cases, be associated with mild colonic disease only.[403] The APC protein is involved in the regulation of beta-catenin signaling. In the absence of functional APC, beta-catenin moves to the nucleus. This forms the basis for the nuclear immunolocalization for beta-catenin, a pattern helpful in the diagnosis of familial and sporadic desmoid-type fibromatoses.[66,404] In contrast to FAP-associated desmoids, most sporadic desmoids show activating mutations in the beta-catenin gene (*CTNNB1*) instead of inactivation of APC.[405] Desmoids with beta-catenin 45F mutations may have an increased risk of recurrence.[67]

Sarcomas in Hereditary Nonpolyposis Colorectal Cancer

Although sarcomas are not formally part of the hereditary nonpolyposis colorectal cancer (HNPCC) syndrome (OMIM: 276300), several types of sarcomas have been recurrently reported in individuals with HNPCC, including liposarcoma, leiomyosarcomas, and rhabdomyosarcoma.[406-409] Microsatellite instability caused by loss of mismatch repair proteins has also been reported in sporadic sarcomas.[410]

Familial Rhabdoid Predisposition Syndrome and Malignant Extrarenal Rhabdoid Tumors

Inactivation of the *SMARCB1* (*INI1*) tumor suppressor gene, which resides on the long arm of chromosome 22, is the molecular hallmark of extrarenal (and renal) rhabdoid tumors.[411,412] Among sarcomas, *SMARCB1* loss is seen in all cases of extrarenal rhabdoid tumors and has also been reported in a subset of epithelioid sarcomas.[413,414] Other cancers with discrete rhabdoid components do not show *SMARCB1* loss, even in areas of rhabdoid morphology.[415] The *SMARCB1* gene encodes a protein involved in chromatin remodeling that is thought to regulate the access of certain transcription factors to their target genes. Its inactivation is thought to promote neoplasia by altering gene expression secondary to its effect upon chromatin structure.[411] The inactivation occurs by loss of both copies or an inactivating mutation in one copy with loss of the other copy (through monosomy or mitotic recombination with loss of heterozygosity).[416,417] *SMARCB1* loss may require FISH and/or molecular techniques for detection, but IHC for loss of nuclear staining is emerging as an attractive alternative.[68] In familial rhabdoid predisposition syndrome type 1 (OMIM: 609322), affected family members carry one copy of *SMARCB1* with an inactivating mutation and then lose the remaining functional copy, leading to rhabdoid tumor development, both renal and extrarenal.[418]

CONTRIBUTIONS OF PAN-GENOMIC STUDIES TO SARCOMA DIAGNOSIS AND CLASSIFICATION

Since the late 1990s, high-density microarrays have been used to measure, in a comprehensive manner (profile), gene expression patterns (when tumor RNA is tested) or gene copy number changes (when tumor genomic DNA is tested). More recently, next-generation sequencing is increasingly replacing microarrays in these applications and also allows screening for mutations and rearrangements. Regardless of the specific technical platform, pan-genomic studies have proven very useful in addressing a wide variety of questions in sarcoma biology.[158,419-421] Here, discussion is limited to their application as a source of diagnostic markers for sarcoma diagnosis and their role in clarifying sarcoma classification. It is likely that, in the coming decade, next-generation sequencing will make further major contributions to the diagnosis and classification of sarcomas, just as translocation analysis and microarray-based gene expression profiling have provided in the past.

A general observation of pan-genomic expression profiling studies of sarcomas is that translocation-associated sarcomas are robustly clustered by expression profiling using cDNA microarrays, whereas so-called complex karyotype sarcomas tend to be less tightly clustered. This is perhaps not unexpected because, first, the aberrant transcriptional proteins encoded by most translocation-derived fusion genes act primarily through changes in gene expression. Second, genomic copy number changes are associated with changes in the expression of the corresponding genes. Therefore, complex karyotype sarcomas that often show different gains and losses from case to case are also likely to show more variability in gene expression patterns, leading to less robust unsupervised clustering of the expression profiles. Of course, this by itself does not mean that complex karyotype sarcomas are less discrete entities than translocation-associated sarcomas but may merely indicate that unsupervised clustering of expression data may not be the best approach to delineating them. Indeed, this tumor group may be more fruitfully studied by profiling of gene copy number changes using array-based CGH. For instance, a number of studies have used profiling of gene copy number changes to propose relationships of subsets of tumors designated as undifferentiated pleomorphic sarcoma (malignant fibrous histiocytoma) to leiomyosarcomas or liposarcomas.[422,423] Ultimately, integrated profiling of gene expression and genomic copy number changes may be the most efficient approach to understanding the biology and genetic heterogeneity of complex karyotype sarcomas.[158] Recently, a prognostic gene expression signature enriched in genes involved in mitosis and chromosome dynamics, designated complexity index in sarcomas (CINSARC), was derived and shown to be a robust independent predictor of clinical outcome in sarcomas.[424]

Although pan-genomic expression profiling still has no direct clinical application in sarcoma diagnosis, some of the data and insights that these studies have provided have had a practical impact because they have identified differentially expressed genes that have been translated into new sarcoma-specific IHC markers. For instance, TLE1, a nuclear protein that functions as a transcriptional repressor of Wnt/beta-catenin signaling, is one of the most consistent synovial sarcoma-associated genes in multiple expression microarray studies, and its application as a robust IHC marker for this sarcoma has recently been demonstrated.[425] Likewise, several studies have used microarrays to identify genes differentially expressed between ARMS and ERMS.[114,118,426] The gene encoding transcription factor AP2-beta (*TFAP2B*) has consistently stood out for its ARMS-associated expression, and transcription factor AP2-beta has now been validated as a useful marker for its distinction from ERMS.[427] Other new IHC markers emerging from profiling studies include ApoD as a novel marker for DFSP, among others.[428] Another important example of a useful diagnostic marker discovered through gene expression profiling is DOG1 (Discovered On GIST-1),[429] which has emerged as a sensitive and fairly specific marker for GIST, including GIST cases with *PDGFRA* mutation that can show poor immunoreactivity for KIT.[430-433]

Acknowledgments

The FISH image in Figure 4-5 was provided by David Gisselsson. An apology is extended to those colleagues whose papers could not be cited because of space considerations.

References

1. Hanahan D, Weinberg RA. The hallmarks of cancer. Cell 2000;100(1):57–70.
2. Hanahan D, Weinberg RA. Hallmarks of cancer: the next generation. Cell 2011;144(5):646–74.
3. Vogelstein B, Kinzler KW. Cancer genes and the pathways they control. Nat Med 2004;10(8):789–99.
4. Stratton MR, Campbell PJ, Futreal PA. The cancer genome. Nature 2009;458(7239):719–24.
5. Berger AH, Pandolfi PP. Haplo-insufficiency: a driving force in cancer. J Pathol 2011;223(2):137–46.
6. Goto M, Miller RW, Ishikawa Y, et al. Excess of rare cancers in Werner syndrome (adult progeria). Cancer Epidemiol Biomarkers Prev 1996;5(4):239–46.
7. Pansuriya TC, van ER, d'Adamo P, et al. Somatic mosaic IDH1 and IDH2 mutations are associated with enchondroma and spindle cell hemangioma in Ollier disease and Maffucci syndrome. Nat Genet 2011;43(12):1256–61.
8. Amary MF, Bacsi K, Maggiani F, et al. IDH1 and IDH2 mutations are frequent events in central chondrosarcoma and central and periosteal chondromas but not in other mesenchymal tumours. J Pathol 2011;224(3):334–43.
9. Amary MF, Damato S, Halai D, et al. Ollier disease and Maffucci syndrome are caused by somatic mosaic mutations of IDH1 and IDH2. Nat Genet 2011;43(12):1262–5.
10. Gill AJ. Succinate dehydrogenase (SDH) and mitochondrial driven neoplasia. Pathology 2012;44(4):285–92.
11. Mertens F, Antonescu CR, Hohenberger P, et al. Translocation-related sarcomas. Semin Oncol 2009;36(4):312–23.
12. Taylor BS, Barretina J, Maki RG, et al. Advances in sarcoma genomics and new therapeutic targets. Nat Rev Cancer 2011;11(8):541–57.
13. Mani RS, Chinnaiyan AM. Triggers for genomic rearrangements: insights into genomic, cellular and environmental influences. Nat Rev Genet 2010;11(12):819–29.
14. Novo FJ, Vizmanos JL. Chromosome translocations in cancer: computational evidence for the random generation of double-strand breaks. Trends Genet 2006;22(4):193–6.
15. van de Rijn M, Barr FG, Xiong QB, et al. Radiation-associated synovial sarcoma. Hum Pathol 1997;28(11):1325–8.
16. Egger JF, Coindre JM, Benhattar J, et al. Radiation-associated synovial sarcoma: clinicopathologic and molecular analysis of two cases. Mod Pathol 2002;15(9):998–1004.
17. Deraedt K, Debiec-Rychter M, Sciot R. Radiation-associated synovial sarcoma of the lung following radiotherapy for pulmonary metastasis of Wilms' tumour. Histopathology 2006;48(4):473–5.
18. Mrozek K, Bloomfield CD. Der(16)t(1;16) is a secondary chromosome aberration in at least eighteen different types of human cancer. Genes Chromosomes Cancer 1998;23(1):78–80.
19. Velagaleti GV, Miettinen M, Gatalica Z. Malignant peripheral nerve sheath tumor with rhabdomyoblastic differentiation (malignant triton tumor) with balanced t(7;9)(q11.2;p24) and unbalanced translocation der(16)t(1;16)(q23;q13). Cancer Genet Cytogenet 2004;149(1):23–7.
20. Kapels KM, Nishio J, Zhou M, et al. Embryonal rhabdomyosarcoma with a der(16)t(1;16) translocation. Cancer Genet Cytogenet 2007;174(1):68–73.
21. ISCN (2009). An international system for human cytogenetic nomenclature. Basel: Karger; 2009.
22. Brothman AR, Persons DL, Shaffer LG. Nomenclature evolution: changes in the ISCN from the 2005 to the 2009 edition. Cytogenet Genome Res 2009;127(1):1–4.
23. Limon J, Dal CP, Sandberg AA. Application of long-term collagenase disaggregation for the cytogenetic analysis of human solid tumors. Cancer Genet Cytogenet 1986;23(4):305–13.
24. Ried T. Cytogenetics–in color and digitized. N Engl J Med 2004;350(16):1597–600.
25. Summersgill B, Clark J, Shipley J. Fluorescence and chromogenic in situ hybridization to detect genetic aberrations in formalin-fixed paraffin embedded material, including tissue microarrays. Nat Protoc 2008;3(2):220–34.
26. Kumagai A, Motoi T, Tsuji K, et al. Detection of SYT and EWS gene rearrangements by dual-color break-apart CISH in liquid-based cytology samples of synovial sarcoma and Ewing sarcoma/primitive neuroectodermal tumor. Am J Clin Pathol 2010;134(2):323–31.
27. Kuchinka BD, Kalousek DK, Lomax BL, et al. Interphase cytogenetic analysis of single cell suspensions prepared from previously formalin-fixed and paraffin-embedded tissues. Mod Pathol 1995;8(2):183–6.
28. Speicher MR, Carter NP. The new cytogenetics: blurring the boundaries with molecular biology. Nat Rev Genet 2005;6(10):782–92.
29. Kallioniemi A, Kallioniemi OP, Sudar D, et al. Comparative genomic hybridization for molecular cytogenetic analysis of solid tumors. Science 1992;258(5083):818–21.
30. Pinkel D, Albertson DG. Comparative genomic hybridization. Annu Rev Genomics Hum Genet 2005;6:331–54.
31. Coindre JM, Pelmus M, Hostein I, et al. Should molecular testing be required for diagnosing synovial sarcoma? A prospective study of 204 cases. Cancer 2003;98(12):2700–7.
32. Coindre JM, Hostein I, Terrier P, et al. Diagnosis of clear cell sarcoma by real-time reverse transcriptase-polymerase chain reaction analysis of paraffin embedded tissues: clinicopathologic and molecular analysis of 44 patients from the French sarcoma group. Cancer 2006;107(5):1055–64.
33. Friedrichs N, Kriegl L, Poremba C, et al. Pitfalls in the detection of t(11;22) translocation by fluorescence in situ hybridization and RT-PCR. A single-blinded study. Diag Mol Pathol 2006;15(2):83–9.
34. Qian X, Jin L, Shearer BM, et al. Molecular diagnosis of Ewing's sarcoma/primitive neuroectodermal tumor in formalin-fixed paraffin-embedded tissues by RT-PCR and fluorescence in situ hybridization. Diagn Mol Pathol 2005;14(1):23–8.
35. Bridge RS, Rajaram V, Dehner LP, et al. Molecular diagnosis of Ewing sarcoma/primitive neuroectodermal tumor in routinely processed tissue: a comparison of two FISH strategies and RT-PCR in malignant round cell tumors. Mod Pathol 2006;19(1):1–8.

36. Nishio J, Althof PA, Bailey JM, et al. Use of a novel FISH assay on paraffin-embedded tissues as an adjunct to diagnosis of alveolar rhabdomyosarcoma. Lab Invest 2006;86(6):547–56.
37. Gamberi G, Cocchi S, Benini S, et al. Molecular diagnosis in Ewing family tumors: the Rizzoli experience–222 consecutive cases in four years. J Mol Diagn 2011;13(3):313–24.
38. Folpe AL, Goldblum JR, Rubin BP, et al. Morphologic and immunophenotypic diversity in Ewing family tumors: a study of 66 genetically confirmed cases. Am J Surg Pathol 2005;29(8):1025–33.
39. Geiss GK, Bumgarner RE, Birditt B, et al. Direct multiplexed measurement of gene expression with color-coded probe pairs. Nat Biotechnol 2008;26(3):317–25.
40. Luina-Contreras A, Jackson S, Ladanyi M. Highly multiplexed detection of translocation fusion transcripts without amplification using the NanoString platform. Mod Pathol 2010;23s1:426A.
41. Skotheim RI, Thomassen GO, Eken M, et al. A universal assay for detection of oncogenic fusion transcripts by oligo microarray analysis. Mol Cancer 2009;19(8):5. doi: 10.1186/1476-4598-8-5.:5–8.
42. Rimsza LM, Wright G, Schwartz M, et al. Accurate classification of diffuse large B-cell lymphoma into germinal center and activated B-cell subtypes using a nuclease protection assay on formalin-fixed, paraffin-embedded tissues. Clin Cancer Res 2011;17(11):3727–32.
43. Luo W, Milash B, Dalley B, et al. Antibody detection of translocations in Ewing sarcoma. EMBO Mol Med 2012;4(6):453–61.
44. Pierron G, Tirode F, Lucchesi C, et al. A new subtype of bone sarcoma defined by BCOR-CCNB3 gene fusion. Nat Genet 2012;44(4): 461–6.
45. Tanas MR, Sboner A, Oliveira AM, et al. Identification of a disease-defining gene fusion in epithelioid hemangioendothelioma. Sci Transl Med 2011;3(98):98ra82.
46. Robinson DR, Wu YM, Kalyana-Sundaram S, et al. Identification of recurrent NAB2-STAT6 gene fusions in solitary fibrous tumor by integrative sequencing. Nat Genet 2013;45(2):180–5.
47. Chmielecki J, Crago AM, Rosenberg M, et al. Whole-exome sequencing identifies a recurrent NAB2-STAT6 fusion in solitary fibrous tumors. Nat Genet 2013;45(2):131–2.
48. Meyerson M, Gabriel S, Getz G. Advances in understanding cancer genomes through second-generation sequencing. Nat Rev Genet 2010; 11(10):685–96.
49. Chmielecki J, Peifer M, Jia P, et al. Targeted next-generation sequencing of DNA regions proximal to a conserved GXGXXG signaling motif enables systematic discovery of tyrosine kinase fusions in cancer. Nucleic Acids Res 2010;38(20):6985–96.
50. Lipson D, Capelletti M, Yelensky R, et al. Identification of new ALK and RET gene fusions from colorectal and lung cancer biopsies. Nat Med 2012;18:382–4.
51. Falini B, Mason DY. Proteins encoded by genes involved in chromosomal alterations in lymphoma and leukemia: clinical value of their detection by immunocytochemistry. Blood 2002;99(2):409–26.
52. Gerald WL, Ladanyi M, de Alava E, et al. Clinical, pathologic, and molecular spectrum of tumors associated with t(11;22)(p13;q12): desmoplastic small round-cell tumor and its variants. J Clin Oncol 1998; 16(9):3028–36.
53. Barnoud R, Sabourin JC, Pasquier D, et al. Immunohistochemical expression of WT1 by desmoplastic small round cell tumor: a comparative study with other small round cell tumors. Am J Surg Pathol 2000; 24(6):830–6.
54. Argani P, Lal P, Hutchinson B, et al. Aberrant nuclear immunoreactivity for TFE3 in neoplasms with *TFE3* gene fusions. A sensitive and specific immunohistochemical assay. Am J Surg Pathol 2003;23: 750–61.
55. Folpe AL, Hill CE, Parham DM, et al. Immunohistochemical detection of FLI-1 protein expression: a study of 132 round cell tumors with emphasis on CD99-positive mimics of Ewing's sarcoma/primitive neuroectodermal tumor. Am J Surg Pathol 2000;24(12):1657–62.
56. Wang WL, Patel NR, Caragea M, et al. Expression of ERG, an Ets family transcription factor, identifies ERG-rearranged Ewing sarcoma. Mod Pathol 2012;25(10):1378–83.
57. Li XQ, Hisaoka M, Shi DR, et al. Expression of anaplastic lymphoma kinase in soft tissue tumors: an immunohistochemical and molecular study of 249 cases. Hum Pathol 2004;35(6):711–21.
58. Takeuchi K, Soda M, Togashi Y, et al. Pulmonary inflammatory myofibroblastic tumor expressing a novel fusion, PPFIBP1-ALK: reappraisal of anti-ALK immunohistochemistry as a tool for novel ALK fusion identification. Clin Cancer Res 2011;17(10):3341–8.
59. Oikawa K, Ishida T, Imamura T, et al. Generation of the novel monoclonal antibody against TLS/EWS-CHOP chimeric oncoproteins that is applicable to one of the most sensitive assays for myxoid and round cell liposarcomas. Am J Surg Pathol 2006;30(3):351–6.
60. Antonescu CR. Targeted therapy of cancer: new roles for pathologists in identifying GISTs and other sarcomas. Mod Pathol 2008;21(Suppl 2):S31–6. doi: 10.1038/modpathol.2008;9:S31–6.
61. Corless CL, Fletcher JA, Heinrich MC. Biology of gastrointestinal stromal tumors. J Clin Oncol 2004;22(18):3813–25.
62. Dei Tos AP, Doglioni C, Piccinin S, et al. Coordinated expression and amplification of the MDM2, CDK4, and HMGI-C genes in atypical lipomatous tumours. J Pathol 2000;190(5):531–6.
63. Weaver J, Downs-Kelly E, Goldblum JR, et al. Fluorescence in situ hybridization for MDM2 gene amplification as a diagnostic tool in lipomatous neoplasms. Mod Pathol 2008;21(8):943–9.
64. Binh MB, Sastre-Garau X, Guillou L, et al. MDM2 and CDK4 immunostainings are useful adjuncts in diagnosing well-differentiated and dedifferentiated liposarcoma subtypes: a comparative analysis of 559 soft tissue neoplasms with genetic data. Am J Surg Pathol 2005;29(10): 1340–7.
65. Weaver J, Rao P, Goldblum JR, et al. Can MDM2 analytical tests performed on core needle biopsy be relied upon to diagnose well-differentiated liposarcoma? Mod Pathol 2010;23(10):1301–6.
66. Bhattacharya B, Dilworth HP, Iacobuzio-Donahue C, et al. Nuclear beta-catenin expression distinguishes deep fibromatosis from other benign and malignant fibroblastic and myofibroblastic lesions. Am J Surg Pathol 2005;29(5):653–9.
67. Lazar AJ, Tuvin D, Hajibashi S, et al. Specific mutations in the beta-catenin gene (CTNNB1) correlate with local recurrence in sporadic desmoid tumors. Am J Pathol 2008;173(5):1518–27.
68. Hoot AC, Russo P, Judkins AR, et al. Immunohistochemical analysis of hSNF5/INI1 distinguishes renal and extra-renal malignant rhabdoid tumors from other pediatric soft tissue tumors. Am J Surg Pathol 2004;28(11):1485–91.
69. Hollmann TJ, Hornick JL. INI1-deficient tumors: diagnostic features and molecular genetics. Am J Surg Pathol 2011;35(10):e47–63.
70. Kreiger PA, Judkins AR, Russo PA, et al. Loss of INI1 expression defines a unique subset of pediatric undifferentiated soft tissue sarcomas. Mod Pathol 2009;22(1):142–50.
71. Arnold MA, Arnold CA, Li G, et al. A unique pattern of INI1 immunohistochemistry distinguishes synovial sarcoma from its histologic mimics. Hum Pathol 2013;44(5):881–7.
72. Mertens F, Panagopoulos I, Mandahl N. Genomic characteristics of soft tissue sarcomas. Virchows Archiv 2010;456(2):129–39.
73. Huang HY, Illei PB, Zhao Z, et al. Ewing sarcomas with p53 mutations or p16/p14ARF homozygous deletions: a highly aggressive subset associated with poor chemoresponse. J Clin Oncol 2005;23:548–58.
74. Oda Y, Yamamoto H, Takahira T, et al. Frequent alteration of p16(INK4a)/ p14(ARF) and p53 pathways in the round cell component of myxoid/ round cell liposarcoma: p53 gene alterations and reduced p14(ARF) expression both correlate with poor prognosis. J Pathol 2005;207(4): 410–21.
75. Antonescu CR, Tschernyavsky SJ, Decuseara R, et al. Prognostic impact of P53 status, TLS-CHOP fusion transcript structure, and histological grade in myxoid liposarcoma: a molecular and clinicopathologic study of 82 cases. Clin Cancer Res 2001;7(12):3977–87.
76. Ito M, Barys L, O'Reilly T, et al. Comprehensive mapping of p53 pathway alterations reveals an apparent role for both SNP309 and MDM2 amplification in sarcomagenesis. Clin Cancer Res 2011;17(3):416–26.
77. Perot G, Chibon F, Montero A, et al. Constant p53 pathway inactivation in a large series of soft tissue sarcomas with complex genetics. Am J Pathol 2010;177(4):2080–90.
78. Wurl P, Taubert H, Meye A, et al. Prognostic value of immunohistochemistry for p53 in primary soft-tissue sarcomas: a multivariate analysis of five antibodies. J Cancer Res Clin Oncol 1997;123(9):502–8.
79. Ulaner GA, Hoffman AR, Otero J, et al. Divergent patterns of telomere maintenance mechanisms among human sarcomas: sharply contrasting prevalence of the alternative lengthening of telomeres mechanism in Ewing's sarcomas and osteosarcomas. Genes Chromosomes Cancer 2004;41:155–62.
80. Montgomery E, Argani P, Hicks JL, et al. Telomere lengths of translocation-associated and nontranslocation-associated sarcomas differ dramatically. Am J Pathol 2004;164(5):1523–9.
81. Henson JD, Hannay JA, McCarthy SW, et al. A robust assay for alternative lengthening of telomeres in tumors shows the significance of

alternative lengthening of telomeres in sarcomas and astrocytomas. Clin Cancer Res 2005;11(1):217–25.
82. Heaphy CM, de Wilde RF, Jiao Y, et al. Altered telomeres in tumors with ATRX and DAXX mutations. Science 2011;333(6041):425.
83. Lovejoy CA, Li W, Reisenweber S, et al. Loss of ATRX, genome instability, and an altered DNA damage response are hallmarks of the alternative lengthening of telomeres pathway. PLoS Genet 2012;8(7): e1002772.
84. Barr FG. Translocations, cancer and the puzzle of specificity. Nat Genet 1998;19(2):121–4.
85. Keller C, Arenkiel BR, Coffin CM, et al. Alveolar rhabdomyosarcomas in conditional Pax3:Fkhr mice: cooperativity of Ink4a/ARF and Trp53 loss of function. Genes Dev 2004;18(21):2614–26.
86. Nishijo K, Chen QR, Zhang L, et al. Credentialing a preclinical mouse model of alveolar rhabdomyosarcoma. Cancer Res 2009;69(7): 2902–11.
87. Charytonowicz E, Terry M, Coakley K, et al. PPARgamma agonists enhance ET-743-induced adipogenic differentiation in a transgenic mouse model of myxoid round cell liposarcoma. J Clin Invest 2012; 122(3):886–98.
88. Rorie CJ, Thomas VD, Chen P, et al. The Ews/Fli-1 fusion gene switches the differentiation program of neuroblastomas to Ewing sarcoma/ peripheral primitive neuroectodermal tumors. Cancer Res 2004;64(4): 1266–77.
89. Hu-Lieskovan S, Zhang J, Wu L, et al. EWS-FLI1 fusion protein up-regulates critical genes in neural crest development and is responsible for the observed phenotype of Ewing's family of tumors. Cancer Res 2005;65(11):4633–44.
90. Riggi N, Cironi L, Provero P, et al. Expression of the FUS-CHOP fusion protein in primary mesenchymal progenitor cells gives rise to a model of myxoid liposarcoma. Cancer Res 2006;66(14):7016–23.
91. Riggi N, Cironi L, Provero P, et al. Development of Ewing's sarcoma from primary bone marrow-derived mesenchymal progenitor cells. Cancer Res 2005;65(24):11459–68.
92. Tirode F, Laud-Duval K, Prieur A, et al. Mesenchymal stem cell features of Ewing tumors. Cancer Cell 2007;11(5):421–9.
93. Zucman J, Melot T, Desmaze C, et al. Combinatorial generation of variable fusion proteins in the Ewing family of tumours. EMBO J 1993; 12:4481–7.
94. Sorensen PH, Lessnick SL, Lopez-Terrada D, et al. A second Ewing's sarcoma translocation, t(21;22), fuses the EWS gene to another ets-family transcription factor, ERG. Nature Genet 1994;6:146–51.
95. Wang L, Bhargava R, Zheng T, et al. Undifferentiated small round cell sarcomas with rare EWS gene fusions. Identification of a novel EWS-SP3 fusion and of additional cases with the EWS-ETV1 and EWS-FEV fusions. J Mol Diagn 2007;9:498–509.
96. Sankar S, Lessnick SL. Promiscuous partnerships in Ewing's sarcoma. Cancer Genet 2011;204(7):351–65.
97. Shing DC, McMullan DJ, Roberts P, et al. FUS/ERG gene fusions in Ewing's tumors. Cancer Res 2003;63(15):4568–76.
98. Lessnick SL, Ladanyi M. Molecular pathogenesis of Ewing sarcoma: new therapeutic and transcriptional targets. Annu Rev Pathol 2012;7: 145–59.
99. Zoubek A, Dockhorn-Dworniczak B, Delattre O, et al. Does expression of different EWS chimeric transcripts define clinically distinct risk groups of Ewing tumor patients? J Clin Oncol 1996;14(4):1245–51.
100. de Alava E, Kawai A, Healey JH, et al. EWS-FLI1 fusion transcript structure is an independent determinant of prognosis in Ewing's sarcoma. J Clin Oncol 1998;16:1248–55.
101. Le Deley MC, Delattre O, Schaefer KL, et al. Impact of EWS-ETS fusion type on disease progression in Ewing's sarcoma/peripheral primitive neuroectodermal tumor: prospective results from the cooperative Euro-E.W.I.N.G. 99 trial. J Clin Oncol 2010;28(12):1982–8.
102. van Doorninck JA, Ji L, Schaub B, et al. Current treatment protocols have eliminated the prognostic advantage of type 1 fusions in Ewing sarcoma: a report from the Children's Oncology Group. J Clin Oncol 2010; 28(12):1989–94.
103. Ginsberg JP, de Alava E, Ladanyi M, et al. EWS-FLI1 and EWS-ERG gene fusions are associated with similar clinical phenotypes in Ewing's sarcoma. J Clin Oncol 1999;17:1809–14.
104. Romeo S, Dei Tos AP. Soft tissue tumors associated with EWSR1 translocation. Virchows Arch 2010;456(2):219–34.
105. Moller E, Stenman G, Mandahl N, et al. POU5F1, encoding a key regulator of stem cell pluripotency, is fused to EWSR1 in hidradenoma of the skin and mucoepidermoid carcinoma of the salivary glands. J Pathol 2008;215(1):78–86.
106. Antonescu CR, Katabi N, Zhang L, et al. EWSR1-ATF1 fusion is a novel and consistent finding in hyalinizing clear-cell carcinoma of salivary gland. Genes Chromosomes Cancer 2011;50(7):559–70.
107. Szuhai K, IJszenga M, de Jong D, et al. The NFATc2 gene is involved in a novel cloned translocation in a Ewing sarcoma variant that couples its function in immunology to oncology. Clin Cancer Res 2009;15(7): 2259–68.
108. Kawamura-Saito M, Yamazaki Y, Kaneko K, et al. Fusion between CIC and DUX4 up-regulates PEA3 family genes in Ewing-like sarcomas with t(4;19)(q35;q13) translocation. Hum Mol Genet 2006;15: 2125–37.
109. Italiano A, Sung YS, Zhang L, et al. High prevalence of CIC fusion with double-homeobox (DUX4) transcription factors in EWSR1-negative undifferentiated small blue round cell sarcomas. Genes Chromosomes Cancer 2012;51(3):207–18.
110. Graham C, Chilton-MacNeill S, Zielenska M, et al. The CIC-DUX4 fusion transcript is present in a subgroup of pediatric primitive round cell sarcomas. Hum Pathol 2012;43(2):180–9.
111. Davis RJ, D'Cruz CM, Lovell MA, et al. Fusion of PAX7 to FKHR by the variant t(1;13)(p36;q14) translocation in alveolar rhabdomyosarcoma. Cancer Res 1994;54:2869–72.
112. Barr FG, Qualman SJ, Macris MH, et al. Genetic heterogeneity in the alveolar rhabdomyosarcoma subset without typical gene fusions. Cancer Res 2002;62(16):4704–10.
113. Sorensen PH, Lynch JC, Qualman SJ, et al. PAX3-FKHR and PAX7-FKHR gene fusions are prognostic indicators in alveolar rhabdomyosarcoma: a report from the children's oncology group. J Clin Oncol 2002; 20(11):2672–9.
114. Wachtel M, Dettling M, Koscielniak E, et al. Gene expression signatures identify rhabdomyosarcoma subtypes and detect a novel t(2;2)(q35;p23) translocation fusing PAX3 to NCOA1. Cancer Res 2004;64(16): 5539–45.
115. Sumegi J, Streblow R, Frayer RW, et al. Recurrent t(2;2) and t(2;8) translocations in rhabdomyosarcoma without the canonical PAX-FOXO1 fuse PAX3 to members of the nuclear receptor transcriptional coactivator family. Genes Chromosomes Cancer 2010;49(3): 224–36.
116. Parham DM, Qualman SJ, Teot L, et al. Correlation between histology and PAX/FKHR fusion status in alveolar rhabdomyosarcoma: a report from the Children's Oncology Group. Am J Surg Pathol 2007;31(6): 895–901.
117. Williamson D, Missiaglia E, de Reynies A, et al. Fusion gene-negative alveolar rhabdomyosarcoma is clinically and molecularly indistinguishable from embryonal rhabdomyosarcoma. J Clin Oncol 2010;28(13): 2151–8.
118. Davicioni E, Anderson MJ, Finckenstein FG, et al. Molecular classification of rhabdomyosarcoma–genotypic and phenotypic determinants of diagnosis: a report from the Children's Oncology Group. Am J Pathol 2009;174(2):550–64.
119. Wexler LH, Ladanyi M. Diagnosing alveolar rhabdomyosarcoma: morphology must be coupled with fusion confirmation. J Clin Oncol 2010;28(13):2126–8.
120. Kelly KM, Womer RB, Sorensen PH, et al. Common and variant gene fusions predict distinct clinical phenotypes in rhabdomyosarcoma. J Clin Oncol 1997;15:1831–6.
121. Anderson J, Gordon T, McManus A, et al. Detection of the PAX3-FKHR fusion gene in paediatric rhabdomyosarcoma: a reproducible predictor of outcome? Br J Cancer 2001;85(6):831–5.
122. Missiaglia E, Williamson D, Chisholm J, et al. PAX3/FOXO1 fusion gene status is the key prognostic molecular marker in rhabdomyosarcoma and significantly improves current risk stratification. J Clin Oncol 2012;30(14):1670–7.
123. Mercado GE, Barr FG. Fusions involving PAX and FOX genes in the molecular pathogenesis of alveolar rhabdomyosarcoma: recent advances. Curr Mol Med 2007;7(1):47–61.
124. Barr FG, Nauta LE, Davis RJ, et al. In vivo amplification of the PAX3-FKHR and PAX7-FKHR fusion genes in alveolar rhabdomyosarcoma. Hum Mol Genet 1996;5(1):15–21.
125. Weber-Hall S, McManus A, Anderson J, et al. Novel formation and amplification of the PAX7-FKHR fusion gene in a case of alveolar rhabdomyosarcoma. Genes Chromosomes Cancer 1996;17(1): 7–13.
126. Bridge JA, Liu J, Qualman SJ, et al. Genomic gains and losses are similar in genetic and histologic subsets of rhabdomyosarcoma, whereas amplification predominates in embryonal with anaplasia and alveolar subtypes. Genes Chromosomes Cancer 2002;33(3):310–21.

127. Reichek JL, Duan F, Smith LM, et al. Genomic and clinical analysis of amplification of the 13q31 chromosomal region in alveolar rhabdomyosarcoma: a report from the Children's Oncology Group. Clin Cancer Res 2011;17(6):1463–73.
128. Mosquera JM, Sboner A, Zhang L, et al. Recurrent NCOA2 gene rearrangements in congenital/infantile spindle cell rhabdomyosarcoma. Genes Chromosomes Cancer 2013;52(6):538–50.
129. Ladanyi M, Gerald W. Fusion of the EWS and WT1 genes in the desmoplastic small round cell tumor. Cancer Res 1994;54(11): 2837–40.
130. Gerald WL, Haber DA. The EWS-WT1 gene fusion in desmoplastic small round cell tumor. Semin Cancer Biol 2005;15(3):197–205.
131. Antonescu CR, Gerald WL, Magid MS, et al. Molecular variants of the EWS-WT1 gene fusion in desmoplastic small round cell tumor. Diagn Mol Pathol 1998;7:24–8.
132. Zucman J, Delattre O, Desmaze C, et al. EWS and ATF-1 gene fusion induced by t(12;22) translocation in malignant melanoma of soft parts. Nature Genet 1993;4:341–5.
133. Antonescu CR, Tschernyavsky SJ, Woodruff JM, et al. Molecular diagnosis of clear cell sarcoma: detection of EWS-ATF1 and MITF-M transcripts and histopathological and ultrastructural analysis of 12 cases. J Mol Diagn 2002;4(1):44–52.
134. Panagopoulos I, Mertens F, biec-Rychter M, et al. Molecular genetic characterization of the EWS/ATF1 fusion gene in clear cell sarcoma of tendons and aponeuroses. Int J Cancer 2002;99(4):560–7.
135. Wang WL, Mayordomo E, Zhang W, et al. Detection and characterization of EWSR1/ATF1 and EWSR1/CREB1 chimeric transcripts in clear cell sarcoma (melanoma of soft parts). Mod Pathol 2009;22(9):1201–9.
136. Hisaoka M, Ishida T, Kuo TT, et al. Clear cell sarcoma of soft tissue: a clinicopathologic, immunohistochemical, and molecular analysis of 33 cases. Am J Surg Pathol 2008;32(3):452–60.
137. Antonescu CR, Nafa K, Segal NH, et al. *EWS-CREB1*: a recurrent variant fusion in clear cell sarcoma. Association with gastrointestinal location and absence of melanocytic differentiation. Clin Cancer Res 2006;12(18): 5356–62.
138. Segal NH, Pavlidis P, Noble WS, et al. Classification of clear-cell sarcoma as a subtype of melanoma by genomic profiling. J Clin Oncol 2003;21(9): 1775–81.
139. Panagopoulos I, Mertens F, Isaksson M, et al. Absence of mutations of the BRAF gene in malignant melanoma of soft parts (clear cell sarcoma of tendons and aponeuroses). Cancer Genet Cytogenet 2005;156(1): 74–6.
140. Langezaal SM, Graadt van Roggen JF, Cleton-Jansen AM, et al. Malignant melanoma is genetically distinct from clear cell sarcoma of tendons and aponeurosis (malignant melanoma of soft parts). Br J Cancer 2001;84(4):535–8.
141. Patel RM, Downs-Kelly E, Weiss SW, et al. Dual-color, break-apart fluorescence in situ hybridization for EWS gene rearrangement distinguishes clear cell sarcoma of soft tissue from malignant melanoma. Mod Pathol 2005;18(12):1585–90.
142. Yang L, Chen Y, Cui T, et al. Identification of biomarkers to distinguish clear cell sarcoma from malignant melanoma. Hum Pathol 2012;43(9): 1463–70.
143. Antonescu CR, Dal CP, Nafa K, et al. EWSR1-CREB1 is the predominant gene fusion in angiomatoid fibrous histiocytoma. Genes Chromosomes Cancer 2007;46(12):1051–60.
144. Thway K, Nicholson AG, Lawson K, et al. Primary pulmonary myxoid sarcoma with EWSR1-CREB1 fusion: a new tumor entity. Am J Surg Pathol 2011;35(11):1722–32.
145. Thway K, Fisher C. Tumors with EWSR1-CREB1 and EWSR1-ATF1 fusions: the current status. Am J Surg Pathol 2012;36(7):e1–11.
146. Raddaoui E, Donner LR, Panagopoulos I. Fusion of the FUS and ATF1 genes in a large, deep-seated angiomatoid fibrous histiocytoma. Diagn Mol Pathol 2002;11(3):157–62.
147. Hallor KH, Mertens F, Jin Y, et al. Fusion of the EWSR1 and ATF1 genes without expression of the MITF-M transcript in angiomatoid fibrous histiocytoma. Genes Chromosomes Cancer 2005;44(1):97–102.
148. Rossi S, Szuhai K, IJszenga M, et al. EWSR1-CREB1 and EWSR1-ATF1 fusion genes in angiomatoid fibrous histiocytoma. Clin Cancer Res 2007;13(24):7322–8.
149. Tanas MR, Rubin BP, Montgomery EA, et al. Utility of FISH in the diagnosis of angiomatoid fibrous histiocytoma: a series of 18 cases. Mod Pathol 2010;23(1):93–7.
150. Crozat A, Aman P, Mandahl N, et al. Fusion of CHOP to a novel RNA-binding protein in human myxoid liposarcoma. Nature 1993;363: 640–4.
151. Rabbitts TH, Forster A, Larson R, et al. Fusion of the dominant negative transcription regulator CHOP with a novel gene FUS by translocation t(12;16) in malignant liposarcoma. Nature Genet 1993;4: 175–80.
152. Panagopoulos I, Hoglund M, Mertens F, et al. Fusion of the EWS and CHOP genes in myxoid liposarcoma. Oncogene 1996;12:489–94.
153. Panagopoulos I, Mandahl N, Ron D, et al. Characterization of the CHOP breakpoints and fusion transcripts in myxoid liposarcomas with the 12;16 translocation. Cancer Res 1994;54:6500–3.
154. Knight JC, Renwick PJ, Dal Cin P, et al. Translocation t(12;16)(q13;p11) in myxoid liposarcoma and round cell liposarcoma: molecular and cytogenetic analysis. Cancer Res 1995;55:24–7.
155. Antonescu CR, Elahi A, Healey JH, et al. Monoclonality of multifocal myxoid liposarcoma. Confirmation by analysis of TLS-CHOP or EWS-CHOP rearrangements. Clin Cancer Res 2000;6:2788–93.
156. de VR, de JD, Nederlof P, et al. Multifocal myxoid liposarcoma–metastasis or second primary tumor?: a molecular biological analysis. J Mol Diagn 2010;12(2):238–43.
157. Antonescu CR, Elahi A, Humphrey M, et al. Specificity of *TLS-CHOP* rearrangement for classic myxoid/round cell liposarcoma. Absence in predominantly myxoid well-differentiated liposarcomas. J Mol Diagn 2000;2:132–8.
158. Barretina J, Taylor BS, Banerji S, et al. Subtype-specific genomic alterations define new targets for soft-tissue sarcoma therapy. Nat Genet 2010;42(8):715–21.
159. Demicco EG, Torres KE, Ghadimi MP, et al. Involvement of the PI3K/Akt pathway in myxoid/round cell liposarcoma. Mod Pathol 2012;25(2):212–21.
160. Labelle Y, Zucman J, Stenman G, et al. Oncogenic conversion of a novel orphan nuclear receptor by chromosome translocation. Hum Mol Genet 1995;4:2219–26.
161. Clark J, Benjamin H, Gill S, et al. Fusion of EWS gene to CHN, a member of the steroid/thyroid receptor gene superfamily, in a human myxoid chondrosarcoma. Oncogene 1996;12(2):229–35.
162. Brody RI, Ueda T, Hamelin A, et al. Molecular analysis of the fusion of EWS to an orphan nuclear receptor gene in extraskeletal myxoid chondrosarcoma. Am J Pathol 1997;150(3):1049–58.
163. Panagopoulos I, Mertens F, Isaksson M, et al. Molecular genetic characterization of the EWS/CHN and RBP56/CHN fusion genes in extraskeletal myxoid chondrosarcoma. Genes Chromosomes Cancer 2002;35(4): 340–52.
164. Attwooll C, Tariq M, Harris M, et al. Identification of a novel fusion gene involving *hTAF$_{II}$68* and *CHN* from a t(9;17)(q22;q11.2) translocation in an extraskeletal myxoid chondrosarcoma. Oncogene 1999;18: 7599–601.
165. Panagopoulos I, Mencinger M, Dietrich CU, et al. Fusion of the *RBP56* and *CHN* genes in extraskeletal myxoid chondrosarcomas with translocation t(9;17)(q22;q11). Oncogene 1999;18:7594–8.
166. Sjogren H, Meis-Kindblom J, Kindblom LG, et al. Fusion of the *EWS*-related gene *TAF2N* to *TEC* in extraskeletal myxoid chondrosarcoma. Cancer Res 1999;59:5064–7.
167. Hisaoka M, Ishida T, Imamura T, et al. TFG is a novel fusion partner of NOR1 in extraskeletal myxoid chondrosarcoma. Genes Chromosomes Cancer 2004;40(4):325–8.
168. Sjogren H, Wedell B, Meis-Kindblom JM, et al. Fusion of the NH2-terminal domain of the basic helix-loop-helix protein TCF12 to TEC in extraskeletal myxoid chondrosarcoma with translocation t(9;15) (q22;q21). Cancer Res 2000;60(24):6832–5.
169. Antonescu CR, Argani P, Erlandson RA, et al. Skeletal and extraskeletal myxoid chondrosarcoma. A comparative clinicopathologic, ultrastructural and molecular study. Cancer 1998;83:1504–21.
170. Okamoto S, Hisaoka M, Ishida T, et al. Extraskeletal myxoid chondrosarcoma: a clinicopathologic, immunohistochemical, and molecular analysis of 18 cases. Hum Pathol 2001;32(10):1116–24.
171. Flucke U, Tops BB, Verdijk MA, et al. NR4A3 rearrangement reliably distinguishes between the clinicopathologically overlapping entities myoepithelial carcinoma of soft tissue and cellular extraskeletal myxoid chondrosarcoma. Virchows Arch 2012;460(6):621–8.
172. Wang WL, Mayordomo E, Czerniak BA, et al. Fluorescence in situ hybridization is a useful ancillary diagnostic tool for extraskeletal myxoid chondrosarcoma. Mod Pathol 2008;21(11):1303–10.
173. Noguchi H, Mitsuhashi T, Seki K, et al. Fluorescence in situ hybridization analysis of extraskeletal myxoid chondrosarcomas using EWSR1 and NR4A3 probes. Hum Pathol 2010;41(3):336–42.
174. Wang L, Motoi T, Khanin R, et al. Identification of a novel, recurrent HEY1-NCOA2 fusion in mesenchymal chondrosarcoma based on a

genome-wide screen of exon-level expression data. Genes Chromosomes Cancer 2012;51(2):127–39.
175. Nakayama R, Miura Y, Ogino J, et al. Detection of HEY1-NCOA2 fusion by fluorescence in-situ hybridization in formalin-fixed paraffin-embedded tissues as a possible diagnostic tool for mesenchymal chondrosarcoma. Pathol Int 2012;62(12):823–6.
176. Nyquist KB, Panagopoulos I, Thorsen J, et al. Whole-transcriptome sequencing identifies novel IRF2BP2-CDX1 fusion gene brought about by translocation t(1;5)(q42;q32) in mesenchymal chondrosarcoma. PLoS One 2012;7(11):e49705.
177. Clark J, Rocques PJ, Crew AJ, et al. Identification of novel genes, SYT and SSX, involved in t(X; 18)(p11.2;q11.2) translocation found in human synovial sarcoma. Nature Genet 1994;7:502–8.
178. Crew AJ, Clark J, Fisher C, et al. Fusion of SYT to two genes, SSX1 and SSX2, encoding proteins with homology to the Kruppel-associated box in human synovial sarcoma. EMBO J 1995;14:2333–40.
179. De Leeuw B, Balemans M, Olde Weghuis D, et al. Identification of two alternative fusion genes, SYT-SSX1 and SYT-SSX2, in t(X;18)(p11.2;q11.2)-positive synovial sarcomas. Hum Mol Genet 1995;4: 1097–9.
180. Skytting B, Nilsson G, Brodin B, et al. A novel fusion gene, SYT-SSX4, in synovial sarcoma. J Natl Cancer Inst 1999;91(11): 974–5.
181. Storlazzi CT, Mertens F, Mandahl N, et al. A novel fusion gene, SS18L1/SSX1, in synovial sarcoma. Genes Chromosomes Cancer 2003;37(2): 195–200.
182. Ladanyi M. Fusions of the *SYT* and *SSX* Genes in synovial sarcoma. Oncogene 2001;20:5755–62.
183. Ladanyi M, Antonescu CR, Leung DH, et al. Impact of *SYT-SSX* fusion type on the clinical behavior of synovial sarcoma. A multi-institutional retrospective study of 243 patients. Cancer Res 2002;62: 135–40.
184. Antonescu CR, Kawai A, Leung DH, et al. Strong association of *SYT-SSX* fusion type and morphologic epithelial differentiation in synovial sarcoma. Diagn Mol Pathol 2000;9:1–8.
185. Guillou L, Benhattar J, Bonichon F, et al. Histologic grade, but not SYT-SSX fusion type, is an important prognostic factor in patients with synovial sarcoma: a multicenter, retrospective analysis. J Clin Oncol 2004;22(20):4040–50.
186. Takenaka S, Ueda T, Naka N, et al. Prognostic implication of SYT-SSX fusion type in synovial sarcoma: a multi-institutional retrospective analysis in Japan. Oncol Rep 2008;19(2):467–76.
187. Canter RJ, Qin LX, Maki RG, et al. A synovial sarcoma-specific preoperative nomogram supports a survival benefit to ifosfamide-based chemotherapy and improves risk stratification for patients. Clin Cancer Res 2008;14(24):8191–7.
188. Sun Y, Sun B, Wang J, et al. Prognostic implication of SYT-SSX fusion type and clinicopathological parameters for tumor-related death, recurrence, and metastasis in synovial sarcoma. Cancer Sci 2009;100(6): 1018–25.
189. Garcia CB, Shaffer CM, Eid JE. Genome-wide recruitment to polycomb-modified chromatin and activity regulation of the synovial sarcoma oncogene SYT-SSX2. BMC Genomics 2012;13:189.
190. Su L, Sampaio AV, Jones KB, et al. Deconstruction of the SS18-SSX fusion oncoprotein complex: insights into disease etiology and therapeutics. Cancer Cell 2012;21(3):333–47.
191. Saito T, Oda Y, Sakamoto A, et al. Prognostic value of the preserved expression of the E-cadherin and catenin families of adhesion molecules and of beta-catenin mutations in synovial sarcoma. J Pathol 2000;192: 342–50.
192. Saito T, Oda Y, Sugimachi K, et al. E-cadherin gene mutations frequently occur in synovial sarcoma as a determinant of histological features. Am J Pathol 2001;159(6):2117–24.
193. Saito T, Oda Y, Sakamoto A, et al. APC mutations in synovial sarcoma. J Pathol 2002;196(4):445–9.
194. Saito T, Oda Y, Kawaguchi K, et al. PTEN and other tumor suppressor gene mutations as secondary genetic alterations in synovial sarcoma. Oncol Rep 2004;11(5):1011–15.
195. Subramaniam MM, Calabuig-Farinas S, Pellin A, et al. Mutational analysis of E-cadherin, beta-catenin and APC genes in synovial sarcomas. Histopathology 2010;57(3):482–6.
196. Argani P, Faria PA, Epstein JI, et al. Primary renal synovial sarcoma: molecular and morphologic delineation of an entity previously included among embryonal sarcomas of the kidney. Am J Surg Pathol 2000; 24(8):1087–96.
197. Ladanyi M, Lui MY, Antonescu CR, et al. The der(17)t(X;17)(p11;q25) of human alveolar soft part sarcoma fuses the *TFE3* transcription factor gene to *ASPL*, a novel gene at 17q25. Oncogene 2001;20(1):48–57.
198. Kobos R, Nagai M, Tsuda M, et al. Combining integrated genomics and functional genomics to dissect the biology of a cancer-associated, aberrant transcription factor, the ASPSCR1-TFE3 fusion oncoprotein. J Pathol 2013;229(5):743–54.
199. Williams A, Bartle G, Sumathi VP, et al. Detection of ASPL/TFE3 fusion transcripts and the TFE3 antigen in formalin-fixed, paraffin-embedded tissue in a series of 18 cases of alveolar soft part sarcoma: useful diagnostic tools in cases with unusual histological features. Virchows Arch 2011;458(3):291–300.
200. Tsuji K, Ishikawa Y, Imamura T. Technique for differentiating alveolar soft part sarcoma from other tumors in paraffin-embedded tissue: comparison of immunohistochemistry for TFE3 and CD147 and of reverse transcription polymerase chain reaction for ASPSCR1-TFE3 fusion transcript. Hum Pathol 2012;43(3):356–63.
201. Argani P, Antonescu CR, Illei PB, et al. Primary renal neoplasms with the ASPL-TFE3 gene fusion of alveolar soft part sarcoma: a distinctive tumor entity previously included among renal cell carcinomas of children and adolescents. Am J Pathol 2001;159(1):179–92.
202. Amin MB, Patel RM, Oliveira P, et al. Alveolar soft-part sarcoma of the urinary bladder with urethral recurrence: a unique case with emphasis on differential diagnoses and diagnostic utility of an immunohistochemical panel including TFE3. Am J Surg Pathol 2006;30(10):1322–5.
203. Storlazzi CT, Mertens F, Nascimento A, et al. Fusion of the FUS and BBF2H7 genes in low grade fibromyxoid sarcoma. Hum Mol Genet 2003;12(18):2349–58.
204. Bartuma H, Moller E, Collin A, et al. Fusion of the FUS and CREB3L2 genes in a supernumerary ring chromosome in low-grade fibromyxoid sarcoma. Cancer Genet Cytogenet 2010;199(2):143–6.
205. Panagopoulos I, Storlazzi CT, Fletcher CD, et al. The chimeric FUS/CREB3l2 gene is specific for low-grade fibromyxoid sarcoma. Genes Chromosomes Cancer 2004;40(3):218–28.
206. Matsuyama A, Hisaoka M, Shimajiri S, et al. DNA-based polymerase chain reaction for detecting FUS-CREB3L2 in low-grade fibromyxoid sarcoma using formalin-fixed, paraffin-embedded tissue specimens. Diagn Mol Pathol 2008;17(4):237–40.
207. Patel RM, Downs-Kelly E, Dandekar MN, et al. FUS (16p11) gene rearrangement as detected by fluorescence in-situ hybridization in cutaneous low-grade fibromyxoid sarcoma: a potential diagnostic tool. Am J Dermatopathol 2011;33(2):140–3.
208. Mertens F, Fletcher CD, Antonescu CR, et al. Clinicopathologic and molecular genetic characterization of low-grade fibromyxoid sarcoma, and cloning of a novel FUS/CREB3L1 fusion gene. Lab Invest 2005; 85(3):408–15.
209. Reid R, de Silva MV, Paterson L, et al. Low-grade fibromyxoid sarcoma and hyalinizing spindle cell tumor with giant rosettes share a common t(7;16)(q34;p11) translocation. Am J Surg Pathol 2003;27(9):1229–36.
210. Guillou L, Benhattar J, Gengler C, et al. Translocation-positive low-grade fibromyxoid sarcoma: clinicopathologic and molecular analysis of a series expanding the morphologic spectrum and suggesting potential relationship to sclerosing epithelioid fibrosarcoma: a study from the French Sarcoma Group. Am J Surg Pathol 2007;31(9):1387–402.
211. Doyle LA, Wang WL, Dal Cin P, et al. MUC4 is a sensitive and extremely useful marker for sclerosing epithelioid fibrosarcoma: association with FUS gene rearrangement. Am J Surg Pathol 2012;36(10): 1444–51.
212. Errani C, Zhang L, Sung YS, et al. A novel WWTR1-CAMTA1 gene fusion is a consistent abnormality in epithelioid hemangioendothelioma of different anatomic sites. Genes Chromosomes Cancer 2011;50(8): 644–53.
213. Errani C, Sung YS, Zhang L, et al. Monoclonality of multifocal epithelioid hemangioendothelioma of the liver by analysis of WWTR1-CAMTA1 breakpoints. Cancer Genet 2012;205(1-2):12–17.
214. Antonescu CR, Le Loarer F, Zhang L, et al. A novel subset of epithelioid hemangioendothelioma of soft tissue and bone occurring in yound adult show a TFE3 rearrangement, mainly as the result of a t(X;11)(p11.2;q22.1) associated with TFE3-YAPI fusion. Genes Chromosomes Cancer 2013;52(8):775–84.
215. Flucke U, Palmedo G, Blankenhorn N, et al. EWSR1 gene rearrangement occurs in a subset of cutaneous myoepithelial tumors: a study of 18 cases. Mod Pathol 2011;24(11):1444–50.
216. Antonescu CR, Zhang L, Chang NE, et al. EWSR1-POU5F1 fusion in soft tissue myoepithelial tumors. A molecular analysis of sixty-six cases,

including soft tissue, bone, and visceral lesions, showing common involvement of the EWSR1 gene. Genes Chromosomes Cancer 2010;49(12):1114–24.
217. Brandal P, Panagopoulos I, Bjerkehagen B, et al. Detection of a t(1;22)(q23;q12) translocation leading to an EWSR1-PBX1 fusion gene in a myoepithelioma. Genes Chromosomes Cancer 2008;47(7):558–64.
218. Brandal P, Panagopoulos I, Bjerkehagen B, et al. t(19;22)(q13;q12) Translocation leading to the novel fusion gene EWSR1-ZNF444 in soft tissue myoepithelial carcinoma. Genes Chromosomes Cancer 2009; 48(12):1051–6.
219. Flucke U, Mentzel T, Verdijk MA, et al. EWSR1-ATF1 chimeric transcript in a myoepithelial tumor of soft tissue: a case report. Hum Pathol 2012;43(5):764–8.
220. Bahrami A, Dalton JD, Krane JF, et al. A subset of cutaneous and soft tissue mixed tumors are genetically linked to their salivary gland counterpart. Genes Chromosomes Cancer 2012;51(2):140–8.
221. Yamaguchi S, Yamazaki Y, Ishikawa Y, et al. EWSR1 is fused to POU5F1 in a bone tumor with translocation t(6;22)(p21;q12). Genes Chromosomes Cancer 2005;43(2):217–22.
222. Deng FM, Galvan K, de la Roza G, et al. Molecular characterization of an EWSR1-POU5F1 fusion associated with a t(6;22) in an undifferentiated soft tissue sarcoma. Cancer Genet 2011;204(8):423–9.
223. Dahlen A, Fletcher CD, Mertens F, et al. Activation of the GLI oncogene through fusion with the beta-actin gene (ACTB) in a group of distinctive pericytic neoplasms: pericytoma with t(7;12). Am J Pathol 2004;164(5): 1645–53.
224. Bridge JA, Sanders K, Huang D, et al. Pericytoma with t(7;12) and ACTB-GLI1 fusion arising in bone. Hum Pathol 2012;43(9):1524–9.
225. Hallor KH, Sciot R, Staaf J, et al. Two genetic pathways, t(1;10) and amplification of 3p11-12, in myxoinflammatory fibroblastic sarcoma, haemosiderotic fibrolipomatous tumour, and morphologically similar lesions. J Pathol 2009;217(5):716–27.
226. Antonescu CR, Zhang L, Nielsen GP, et al. Consistent t(1;10) with rearrangements of TGFBR3 and MGEA5 in both myxoinflammatory fibroblastic sarcoma and hemosiderotic fibrolipomatous tumor. Genes Chromosomes Cancer 2011;50(10):757–64.
227. Chiang S, Ali R, Melnyk N, et al. Frequency of known gene rearrangements in endometrial stromal tumors. Am J Surg Pathol 2011;35(9): 1364–72.
228. Gebre-Medhin S, Nord KH, Moller E, et al. Recurrent rearrangement of the PHF1 gene in ossifying fibromyxoid tumors. Am J Pathol 2012;181(3):1069–77.
229. Graham RP, Dry S, Li X, et al. Ossifying fibromyxoid tumor of soft parts: a clinicopathologic, proteomic, and genomic study. Am J Surg Pathol 2011;35(11):1615–25.
230. Simon MP, Pedeutour F, Sirvent N, et al. Deregulation of the platelet-derived growth factor B-chain gene via fusion with collagen gene COL1A1 in dermatofibrosarcoma protuberans and giant-cell fibroblastoma. Nat Genet 1997;15(1):95–8.
231. West RB, Rubin BP, Miller MA, et al. A landscape effect in tenosynovial giant-cell tumor from activation of CSF1 expression by a translocation in a minority of tumor cells. Proc Natl Acad Sci U S A 2006;103(3): 690–5.
232. Knezevich SR, McFadden DE, Tao W, et al. A novel ETV6-NTRK3 gene fusion in congenital fibrosarcoma. Nat Genet 1998;18(2):184–7.
233. Kralik JM, Kranewitter W, Boesmueller H, et al. Characterization of a newly identified ETV6-NTRK3 fusion transcript in acute myeloid leukemia. Diagn Pathol 2011;6:19. doi: 10.1186/1746-1596-6-19.): 19–26.
234. Tognon C, Knezevich SR, Huntsman D, et al. Expression of the ETV6-NTRK3 gene fusion as a primary event in human secretory breast carcinoma. Cancer Cell 2002;2(5):367–76.
235. Lawrence B, Perez-Atayde A, Hibbard MK, et al. *TPM3-ALK* and *TPM4-ALK* oncogenes in inflammatory myofibroblastic tumors. Am J Pathol 2000;157(2):377–84.
236. Bridge JA, Kanamori M, Ma Z, et al. Fusion of the *ALK* gene to the clathrin heavy chain gene, *CLTC*, in inflammatory myofibroblastic tumor. Am J Pathol 2001;159(2):411–15.
237. Lamant L, Dastugue N, Pulford K, et al. A new fusion gene TPM3-ALK in anaplastic large cell lymphoma created by a (1;2)(q25;p23) translocation. Blood 1999;93(9):3088–95.
238. Touriol C, Greenland C, Lamant L, et al. Further demonstration of the diversity of chromosomal changes involving 2p23 in ALK-positive lymphoma: 2 cases expressing ALK kinase fused to CLTCL (clathrin chain polypeptide-like). Blood 2000;95(10):3204–7.
239. Soda M, Choi YL, Enomoto M, et al. Identification of the transforming EML4-ALK fusion gene in non-small-cell lung cancer. Nature 2007; 448(7153):561–6.
240. Griffin CA, Hawkins AL, Dvorak C, et al. Recurrent involvement of 2p23 in inflammatory myofibroblastic tumors. Cancer Res 1999;59(12): 2776–80.
241. Cools J, Wlodarska I, Somers R, et al. Identification of novel fusion partners of ALK, the anaplastic lymphoma kinase, in anaplastic large-cell lymphoma and inflammatory myofibroblastic tumor. Genes Chromosomes Cancer 2002;34(4):354–62.
242. Ma Z, Hill DA, Collins MH, et al. Fusion of ALK to the Ran-binding protein 2 (RANBP2) gene in inflammatory myofibroblastic tumor. Genes Chromosomes Cancer 2003;37(1):98–105.
243. Marino-Enriquez A, Wang WL, Roy A, et al. Epithelioid inflammatory myofibroblastic sarcoma: an aggressive intra-abdominal variant of inflammatory myofibroblastic tumor with nuclear membrane or perinuclear ALK. Am J Surg Pathol 2011;35(1):135–44.
244. Butrynski JE, D'Adamo DR, Hornick JL, et al. Crizotinib in ALK-rearranged inflammatory myofibroblastic tumor. N Engl J Med 2010; 363(18):1727–33.
245. Schlessinger J. Cell signaling by receptor tyrosine kinases. Cell 2002; 103(2):211–25.
246. Cook JR, Dehner LP, Collins MH, et al. Anaplastic lymphoma kinase (ALK) expression in the inflammatory myofibroblastic tumor: a comparative immunohistochemical study. Am J Surg Pathol 2001;25(11): 1364–71.
247. Cessna M. Expression of ALK1 and p80 in inflammatory myofibroblastic tumor and its mesenchymal mimics: a study of 135 cases. Modern Pathol 2002;15(9):931–8.
248. Bourgeois JM, Knezevich SR, Mathers JA, et al. Molecular detection of the ETV6-NTRK3 gene fusion differentiates congenital fibrosarcoma from other childhood spindle cell tumors. Am J Surg Pathol 2000; 24(7):937–46.
249. Schofield DE, Fletcher JA, Grier HE, et al. Fibrosarcoma in infants and children. Application of new techniques. Am J Surg Pathol 1994; 18(1):14–24.
250. Rubin BP, Chen CJ, Morgan TW, et al. Congenital mesoblastic nephroma t(12;15) is associated with *ETV6-NTRK3* gene fusion. Cytogenetic and molecular relationship to congenital (infantile) fibrosarcoma. Am J Pathol 1998;153:1451–8.
251. Lannon CL, Sorensen PH. ETV6-NTRK3: a chimeric protein tyrosine kinase with transformation activity in multiple cell lineages. Semin Cancer Biol 2005;15(3):215–23.
252. Eguchi M, Eguchi-Ishimae M, Tojo A, et al. Fusion of *ETV6* to neurotrophin-3 receptor *TRKC* in acute myeloid leukemia with t(12;15)(p13;q25). Blood 1999;93(4):1355–63.
253. Skalova A, Vanecek T, Sima R, et al. Mammary analogue secretory carcinoma of salivary glands, containing the ETV6-NTRK3 fusion gene: a hitherto undescribed salivary gland tumor entity. Am J Surg Pathol 2010;34(5):599–608.
254. Wang J, Hisaoka M, Shimajiri S, et al. Detection of COL1A1-PDGFB fusion transcripts in dermatofibrosarcoma protuberans by reverse transcription-polymerase chain reaction using archival formalin-fixed, paraffin-embedded tissues. Diagn Mol Pathol 1999;8(3):113–19.
255. Naeem R, Lux ML, Huang SF, et al. Ring chromosomes in dermatofibrosarcoma protuberans are composed of interspersed sequences from chromosomes 17 and 22. Am J Pathol 1995;147(6):1553–8.
256. Macarenco RS, Zamolyi R, Franco MF, et al. Genomic gains of COL1A1-PDFGB occur in the histologic evolution of giant cell fibroblastoma into dermatofibrosarcoma protuberans. Genes Chromosomes Cancer 2008; 47(3):260–5.
257. Sjoblom T, Shimizu A, O'Brien KP, et al. Growth inhibition of dermatofibrosarcoma protuberans tumors by the platelet-derived growth factor receptor antagonist STI571 through induction of apoptosis. Cancer Res 2001;61(15):5778–83.
258. Maki RG, Awan RA, Dixon RH, et al. Differential sensitivity to imatinib of 2 patients with metastatic sarcoma arising from dermatofibrosarcoma protuberans. Int J Cancer 2002;100(6):623–6.
259. Sirvent N, Maire G, Pedeutour F. Genetics of dermatofibrosarcoma protuberans family of tumors: from ring chromosomes to tyrosine kinase inhibitor treatment. Genes Chromosomes Cancer 2003;37(1):1–19.
260. McArthur GA, Demetri GD, Van Oosterom A, et al. Molecular and clinical analysis of locally advanced dermatofibrosarcoma protuberans treated with imatinib: Imatinib Target Exploration Consortium Study B2225. J Clin Oncol 2005;23(4):866–73.

261. Rutkowski P, Van GM, Rankin CJ, et al. Imatinib mesylate in advanced dermatofibrosarcoma protuberans: pooled analysis of two phase II clinical trials. J Clin Oncol 2010;28(10):1772–9.
262. Cupp JS, Miller MA, Montgomery KD, et al. Translocation and expression of CSF1 in pigmented villonodular synovitis, tenosynovial giant cell tumor, rheumatoid arthritis and other reactive synovitides. Am J Surg Pathol 2007;31(6):970–6.
263. Cassier PA, Gelderblom H, Stacchiotti S, et al. Efficacy of imatinib mesylate for the treatment of locally advanced and/or metastatic tenosynovial giant cell tumor/pigmented villonodular synovitis. Cancer 2012;118(6):1649–55.
264. Hirota S, Isozaki K, Moriyama Y, et al. Gain-of-function mutations of c-kit in human gastrointestinal stromal tumors. Science 1998;279(5350): 577–80.
265. Heinrich MC, Corless CL, Duensing A, et al. PDGFRA activating mutations in gastrointestinal stromal tumors. Science 2003;299(5607): 708–10.
266. Huizinga JD, Thuneberg L, Kluppel M, et al. W/kit gene required for interstitial cells of Cajal and for intestinal pacemaker activity. Nature 1995;373(6512):347–9.
267. Maeda H, Yamagata A, Nishikawa S, et al. Requirement of c-kit for development of intestinal pacemaker system. Development 1992;116(2): 369–75.
268. Torihashi S, Ward SM, Nishikawa S, et al. c-kit-dependent development of interstitial cells and electrical activity in the murine gastrointestinal tract. Cell Tissue Res 1995;280(1):97–111.
269. Tian Q, Frierson HF Jr, Krystal GW, et al. Activating c-kit gene mutations in human germ cell tumors. Am J Pathol 1999;154(6): 1643–7.
270. Nagata H, Worobec AS, Oh CK, et al. Identification of a point mutation in the catalytic domain of the protooncogene c-kit in peripheral blood mononuclear cells of patients who have mastocytosis with an associated hematologic disorder. Proceedings of the National Academy of Sciences of the United States of America 1995;92(23):10560–4.
271. Gari M, Goodeve A, Wilson G, et al. c-kit proto-oncogene exon 8 in-frame deletion plus insertion mutations in acute myeloid leukaemia. Br J Haematol 1999;105(4):894–900.
272. Willmore-Payne C, Holden JA, Tripp S, et al. Human malignant melanoma: detection of BRAF- and c-kit-activating mutations by high-resolution amplicon melting analysis. Hum Pathol 2005;36(5):486–93.
273. Antonescu CR, Sommer G, Sarran L, et al. Association of KIT exon 9 mutations with nongastric primary site and aggressive behavior: KIT mutation analysis and clinical correlates of 120 gastrointestinal stromal tumors. Clin Cancer Res 2003;9(9):3329–37.
274. Rubin BP, Singer S, Tsao C. KIT activation is a ubiquitous feature of gastrointestinal stromal tumors. Cancer Res 2001;61(22):8118–21.
275. Lasota J, Dansonka-Mieszkowska A, Stachura T, et al. Gastrointestinal stromal tumors with internal tandem duplications in 3' end of KIT juxtamembrane domain occur predominantly in stomach and generally seem to have a favorable course. Mod Pathol 2003;16(12):1257–64.
276. Andersson J, Bumming P, Meis-Kindblom JM, et al. Gastrointestinal stromal tumors with KIT exon 11 deletions are associated with poor prognosis. Gastroenterology 2006;130(6):1573–81.
277. Martin J, Poveda A, Llombart-Bosch A, et al. Deletions affecting codons 557-558 of the c-KIT gene indicate a poor prognosis in patients with completely resected gastrointestinal stromal tumors: a study by the Spanish Group for Sarcoma Research (GEIS). J Clin Oncol 2005; 23(25):6190–8.
278. Wardelmann E, Losen I, Hans V, et al. Deletion of Trp-557 and Lys-558 in the juxtamembrane domain of the c-kit protooncogene is associated with metastatic behavior of gastrointestinal stromal tumors. Int J Cancer 2003;106(6):887–95.
279. Lasota J, Kopczynski J, Sarlomo-Rikala M. KIT 1530ins6 mutation defines a subset of predominantly malignant gastrointestinal stromal tumors of intestinal origin. Hum Pathol 2003;34(12):1306–12.
280. Lasota J, Wozniak A, Sarlomo-Rikala M. Mutations in exons 9 and 13 of KIT gene are rare events in gastrointestinal stromal tumors. A study of 200 cases. Am J Pathol 2000;157(4):1091–5.
281. Lux ML, Rubin BP, Biase TL, et al. KIT extracellular and kinase domain mutations in gastrointestinal stromal tumors. Am J Pathol 2000; 156(3):791–5.
282. Heinrich MC, Corless CL, Demetri GD, et al. Kinase mutations and imatinib response in patients with metastatic gastrointestinal stromal tumor. J Clin Oncol 2003;21(23):4342–9.
283. Hirota S, Ohashi A, Nishida T, et al. Gain-of-function mutations of platelet-derived growth factor receptor alpha gene in gastrointestinal stromal tumors. Gastroenterology 2003;125(3):660–7.
284. Lasota J, nsonka-Mieszkowska A, Sobin LH, et al. A great majority of GISTs with PDGFRA mutations represent gastric tumors of low or no malignant potential. Lab Invest 2004;84(7):874–83.
285. Wardelmann E, Hrychyk A, Merkelbach-Bruse S, et al. Association of platelet-derived growth factor receptor alpha mutations with gastric primary site and epithelioid or mixed cell morphology in gastrointestinal stromal tumors. J Mol Diagn 2004;6(3):197–204.
286. Janeway KA, Kim SY, Lodish M, et al. Defects in succinate dehydrogenase in gastrointestinal stromal tumors lacking KIT and PDGFRA mutations. Proc Natl Acad Sci U S A 2011;108(1):314–18.
287. Agaram NP, Wong GC, Guo T, et al. Novel V600E BRAF mutations in imatinib-naive and imatinib-resistant gastrointestinal stromal tumors. Genes Chromosomes Cancer 2008;47(10):853–9.
288. Miranda C, Nucifora M, Molinari F, et al. KRAS and BRAF mutations predict primary resistance to imatinib in gastrointestinal stromal tumors. Clin Cancer Res 2012;18(6):1769–76.
289. Miettinen M, Lasota J, Sobin LH. Gastrointestinal stromal tumors of the stomach in children and young adults: a clinicopathologic, immunohistochemical, and molecular genetic study of 44 cases with long-term follow-up and review of the literature. Am J Surg Pathol 2005;29(10): 1373–81.
290. Miettinen M, Makhlouf H, Sobin LH, et al. Gastrointestinal stromal tumors of the jejunum and ileum: a clinicopathologic, immunohistochemical, and molecular genetic study of 906 cases before imatinib with long-term follow-up. Am J Surg Pathol 2006;30(4): 477–89.
291. Prakash S, Sarran L, Socci N, et al. Gastrointestinal stromal tumors in children and young adults: a clinicopathologic, molecular, and genomic study of 15 cases and review of the literature. J Pediatr Hematol Oncol 2005;27(4):179–87.
292. Pasini B, McWhinney SR, Bei T, et al. Clinical and molecular genetics of patients with the Carney-Stratakis syndrome and germline mutations of the genes coding for the succinate dehydrogenase subunits SDHB, SDHC, and SDHD. Eur J Hum Genet 2008;16(1):79–88.
293. Medeiros F, Corless CL, Duensing A, et al. KIT-negative gastrointestinal stromal tumors: proof of concept and therapeutic implications. Am J Surg Pathol 2004;28(7):889–94.
294. Nishida T, Hirota S, Taniguchi M, et al. Familial gastrointestinal stromal tumours with germline mutation of the KIT gene. Nat Genet 1998; 19(4):323–4.
295. Robson ME, Glogowski E, Sommer G, et al. Pleomorphic characteristics of a germ-line KIT mutation in a large kindred with gastrointestinal stromal tumors, hyperpigmentation, and dysphagia. Clin Cancer Res 2004;10(4):1250–4.
296. Isozaki K, Terris B, Belghiti J, et al. Germline-activating mutation in the kinase domain of KIT gene in familial gastrointestinal stromal tumors. Am J Pathol 2000;157(5):1581–5.
297. Sommer G, Agosti V, Ehlers I, et al. Gastrointestinal stromal tumors in a mouse model by targeted mutation of the Kit receptor tyrosine kinase. Proc Natl Acad Sci U S A 2003;100(11):6706–11.
298. Rubin BP, Antonescu CR, Scott-Browne JP, et al. A knock-in mouse model of gastrointestinal stromal tumor harboring kit K641E. Cancer Res 2005;65(15):6631–9.
299. Breiner JA, Meis-Kindblom J, Kindblom LG, et al. Loss of 14q and 22q in gastrointestinal stromal tumors (pacemaker cell tumors). Cancer Genet Cytogenet 2000;120(2):111–16.
300. el-Rifai W, Sarlomo-Rikala M, Miettinen M, et al. DNA copy number losses in chromosome 14: an early change in gastrointestinal stromal tumors. Cancer Res 1996;56(14):3230–3.
301. Allander SV, Nupponen NN, Ringner M, et al. Gastrointestinal stromal tumors with KIT mutations exhibit a remarkably homogeneous gene expression profile. Cancer Res 2001;61(24):8624–8.
302. Segal NH, Pavlidis P, Antonescu CR, et al. Classification and subtype prediction of adult soft tissue sarcoma by functional genomics. Am J Pathol 2003;163(2):691–700.
303. Antonescu CR, Viale A, Sarran L, et al. Gene expression in gastrointestinal stromal tumors is distinguished by KIT genotype and anatomic site. Clin Cancer Res 2004;10(10):3282–90.
304. Subramanian S, West RB, Corless CL, et al. Gastrointestinal stromal tumors (GISTs) with KIT and PDGFRA mutations have distinct gene expression profiles. Oncogene 2004;23(47):7780–90.
305. Demetri GD, von Mehren M, Blanke CD. Efficacy and safety of imatinib mesylate in advanced gastrointestinal stromal tumors. N Engl J Med 2002;347(7):472–80.
306. Debiec-Rychter M, Dumez H, Judson I. Use of c-KIT/PDGFRA mutational analysis to predict the clinical response to imatinib in patients with advanced gastrointestinal stromal tumours entered on phase I and

II studies of the EORTC Soft Tissue and Bone Sarcoma Group. Eur J Cancer 2004;40(5):689–95.
307. Yeh CN, Chen TW, Lee HL, et al. Kinase mutations and imatinib mesylate response for 64 Taiwanese with advanced GIST: preliminary experience from Chang Gung Memorial Hospital. Ann Surg Oncol 2007;14(3):1123–8.
308. Antonescu CR, Besmer P, Guo T, et al. Acquired resistance to imatinib in gastrointestinal stromal tumor occurs through secondary gene mutation. Clin Cancer Res 2005;11(11):4182–90.
309. Heinrich MC, Maki RG, Corless CL, et al. Primary and secondary kinase genotypes correlate with the biological and clinical activity of sunitinib in imatinib-resistant gastrointestinal stromal tumor. J Clin Oncol 2008;26(33):5352–9.
310. Gajiwala KS, Wu JC, Christensen J, et al. KIT kinase mutants show unique mechanisms of drug resistance to imatinib and sunitinib in gastrointestinal stromal tumor patients. Proc Natl Acad Sci U S A 2009;106(5):1542–7.
311. Gisselsson D, Pettersson L, Hoglund M, et al. Chromosomal breakage-fusion-bridge events cause genetic intratumor heterogeneity. Proc Natl Acad Sci U S A 2000;97(10):5357–62.
312. Gisselsson D, Jonson T, Petersen A, et al. Telomere dysfunction triggers extensive DNA fragmentation and evolution of complex chromosome abnormalities in human malignant tumors. Proc Natl Acad Sci U S A 2001;98(22):12683–8.
313. Scheel C, Schaefer KL, Jauch A, et al. Alternative lengthening of telomeres is associated with chromosomal instability in osteosarcomas. Oncogene 2001;20(29):3835–44.
314. Sharpless NE, Ferguson DO, O'Hagan RC, et al. Impaired nonhomologous end-joining provokes soft tissue sarcomas harboring chromosomal translocations, amplifications, and deletions. Mol Cell 2001;8(6): 1187–96.
315. Stephens PJ, Greenman CD, Fu B, et al. Massive genomic rearrangement acquired in a single catastrophic event during cancer development. Cell 2011;144(1):27–40.
316. Forment JV, Kaidi A, Jackson SP. Chromothripsis and cancer: causes and consequences of chromosome shattering. Nat Rev Cancer 2012;12(10): 663–70.
317. Molenaar JJ, Koster J, Zwijnenburg DA, et al. Sequencing of neuroblastoma identifies chromothripsis and defects in neuritogenesis genes. Nature 2012;483(7391):589–93.
318. Drobnjak M, Latres E, Pollack D, et al. Prognostic implications of p53 nuclear overexpression and high proliferation index of Ki-67 in adult soft-tissue sarcomas. J Natl Cancer Inst 1994;86(7): 549–54.
319. Mertens F, Fletcher CD, Dal Cin P, et al. Cytogenetic analysis of 46 pleomorphic soft tissue sarcomas and correlation with morphologic and clinical features: a report of the CHAMP Study Group. Chromosomes and MorPhology. Genes Chromosomes Cancer 1998;22(1): 16–25.
320. Fletcher CD, Dal Cin P, de Wever I, et al. Correlation between clinicopathological features and karyotype in spindle cell sarcomas. A report of 130 cases from the CHAMP study group. Am J Pathol 1999;154(6): 1841–7.
321. Carneiro A, Francis P, Bendahl PO, et al. Indistinguishable genomic profiles and shared prognostic markers in undifferentiated pleomorphic sarcoma and leiomyosarcoma: different sides of a single coin? Lab Invest 2009;89(6):668–75.
322. Coindre JM, Mariani O, Chibon F, et al. Most malignant fibrous histiocytomas developed in the retroperitoneum are dedifferentiated liposarcomas: a review of 25 cases initially diagnosed as malignant fibrous histiocytoma. Mod Pathol 2003;16(3):256–62.
323. Taylor BS, Decarolis PL, Angeles CV, et al. Frequent alterations and epigenetic silencing of differentiation pathway genes in structurally rearranged liposarcomas. Cancer Discov 2011;1(7):587–97.
324. Italiano A, Bianchini L, Keslair F, et al. HMGA2 is the partner of MDM2 in well-differentiated and dedifferentiated liposarcomas whereas CDK4 belongs to a distinct inconsistent amplicon. Int J Cancer 2008;122(10): 2233–41.
325. Italiano A, Bianchini L, Gjernes E, et al. Clinical and biological significance of CDK4 amplification in well-differentiated and dedifferentiated liposarcomas. Clin Cancer Res 2009;15(18):5696–703.
326. Zhang K, Chu K, Wu X, et al. Amplification of FRS2 and activation of FGFR/FRS2 signaling pathway in high-grade liposarcoma. Cancer Res 2013;73(4):1298–307.
327. Mariani O, Brennetot C, Coindre JM, et al. JUN oncogene amplification and overexpression block adipocytic differentiation in highly aggressive sarcomas. Cancer Cell 2007;11(4):361–74.
328. Chibon F, Mariani O, Derre J, et al. ASK1 (MAP3K5) as a potential therapeutic target in malignant fibrous histiocytomas with 12q14-q15 and 6q23 amplifications. Genes Chromosomes Cancer 2004;40(1): 32–7.
329. Crago AM, Socci ND, Decarolis P, et al. Copy number losses define subgroups of dedifferentiated liposarcoma with poor prognosis and genomic instability. Clin Cancer Res 2012;18(5):1334–40.
330. Kashima T, Halai D, Ye H, et al. Sensitivity of MDM2 amplification and unexpected multiple faint alphoid 12 (alpha 12 satellite sequences) signals in atypical lipomatous tumor. Mod Pathol 2012;25(10):1384–96.
331. Mandahl N, Fletcher CD, Dal Cin P, et al. Comparative cytogenetic study of spindle cell and pleomorphic leiomyosarcomas of soft tissues: a report from the CHAMP Study Group. Cancer Genet Cytogenet 2000;116(1):66–73.
332. Perot G, Derre J, Coindre JM, et al. Strong smooth muscle differentiation is dependent on myocardin gene amplification in most human retroperitoneal leiomyosarcomas. Cancer Res 2009;69(6):2269–78.
333. Derre J, Lagace R, Nicolas A, et al. Leiomyosarcomas and most malignant fibrous histiocytomas share very similar comparative genomic hybridization imbalances: an analysis of a series of 27 leiomyosarcomas. Lab Invest 2001;81(2):211–15.
334. Larramendy ML, Gentile M, Soloneski S, et al. Does comparative genomic hybridization reveal distinct differences in DNA copy number sequence patterns between leiomyosarcoma and malignant fibrous histiocytoma? Cancer Genet Cytogenet 2008;187(1):1–11.
335. Gibault L, Perot G, Chibon F, et al. New insights in sarcoma oncogenesis: a comprehensive analysis of a large series of 160 soft tissue sarcomas with complex genomics. J Pathol 2011;223(1):64–71.
336. Makinen N, Mehine M, Tolvanen J, et al. MED12, the mediator complex subunit 12 gene, is mutated at high frequency in uterine leiomyomas. Science 2011;334(6053):252–5.
337. Ravegnini G, Marino-Enriquez A, Slater J, et al. MED12 mutations in leiomyosarcoma and extrauterine leiomyoma. Mod Pathol 2013;26(5): 743–9.
338. Perot G, Croce S, Ribeiro A, et al. MED12 alterations in both human benign and malignant uterine soft tissue tumors. PLoS One 2012;7(6): e40015.
339. Matsubara A, Sekine S, Yoshida M, et al. Prevalence of MED12 mutations in uterine and extrauterine smooth muscle tumours. Histopathology 2013;62(4):657–61.
340. Xia SJ, Pressey JG, Barr FG. Molecular pathogenesis of rhabdomyosarcoma. Cancer Biol Ther 2002;1(2):97–104.
341. Shukla N, Ameur N, Yilmaz I, et al. Oncogene mutation profiling of pediatric solid tumors reveals significant subsets of embryonal rhabdomyosarcoma and neuroblastoma with mutated genes in growth signaling pathways. Clin Cancer Res 2012;18(3):748–57.
342. Martinelli S, McDowell HP, Vigne SD, et al. RAS signaling dysregulation in human embryonal rhabdomyosarcoma. Genes Chromosomes Cancer 2009;48(11):975–82.
343. Taylor JG, Cheuk AT, Tsang PS, et al. Identification of FGFR4-activating mutations in human rhabdomyosarcomas that promote metastasis in xenotransplanted models. J Clin Invest 2009;119(11):3395–407.
344. Paulson V, Chandler G, Rakheja D, et al. High-resolution array CGH identifies common mechanisms that drive embryonal rhabdomyosarcoma pathogenesis. Genes Chromosomes Cancer 2011;50(6): 397–408.
345. Kratz CP, Rapisuwon S, Reed H, et al. Cancer in Noonan, Costello, cardiofaciocutaneous and LEOPARD syndromes. Am J Med Genet C Semin Med Genet 2011;157(2):83–9.
346. Hill DA, Ivanovich J, Priest JR, et al. DICER1 mutations in familial pleuropulmonary blastoma. Science 2009;325(5943):965.
347. Foulkes WD, Bahubeshi A, Hamel N, et al. Extending the phenotypes associated with DICER1 mutations. Hum Mutat 2011;32(12):1381–4.
348. Ognjanovic S, Olivier M, Bergemann TL, et al. Sarcomas in TP53 germline mutation carriers: a review of the IARC TP53 database. Cancer 2012;118(5):1387–96.
349. Doros L, Yang J, Dehner L, et al. DICER1 mutations in embryonal rhabdomyosarcomas from children with and without familial PPB-tumor predisposition syndrome. Pediatr Blood Cancer 2012;59(3): 558–60.
350. Curatolo P, Bombardieri R, Jozwiak S. Tuberous sclerosis. Lancet 2008;372(9639):657–68.
351. Martignoni G, Pea M, Reghellin D, et al. Molecular pathology of lymphangioleiomyomatosis and other perivascular epithelioid cell tumors. Arch Pathol Lab Med 2010;134(1):33–40.
352. Pan CC, Chung MY, Ng KF, et al. Constant allelic alteration on chromosome 16p (TSC2 gene) in perivascular epithelioid cell tumour (PEComa):

genetic evidence for the relationship of PEComa with angiomyolipoma. J Pathol 2008;214(3):387–93.
353. Kenerson H, Folpe AL, Takayama TK, et al. Activation of the mTOR pathway in sporadic angiomyolipomas and other perivascular epithelioid cell neoplasms. Hum Pathol 2007;38(9):1361–71.
354. Wagner AJ, Malinowska-Kolodziej I, Morgan JA, et al. Clinical activity of mTOR inhibition with sirolimus in malignant perivascular epithelioid cell tumors: targeting the pathogenic activation of mTORC1 in tumors. J Clin Oncol 2010;28(5):835–40.
355. Dickson MA, Schwartz GK, Antonescu CR, et al. Extrarenal perivascular epithelioid cell tumors (PEComas) respond to mTOR inhibition: clinical and molecular correlates. Int J Cancer 2013;132(7):1711–17.
356. Argani P, Aulmann S, Illei PB, et al. A distinctive subset of PEComas harbors TFE3 gene fusions. Am J Surg Pathol 2010;34(10):1395–406.
357. Tanaka M, Kato K, Gomi K, et al. Perivascular epithelioid cell tumor with SFPQ/PSF-TFE3 gene fusion in a patient with advanced neuroblastoma. Am J Surg Pathol 2009;33(9):1416–20.
358. Malinowska I, Kwiatkowski DJ, Weiss S, et al. Perivascular epithelioid cell tumors (PEComas) harboring TFE3 gene rearrangements lack the TSC2 alterations characteristic of conventional PEComas: further evidence for a biological distinction. Am J Surg Pathol 2012;36(5):783–4.
359. Maris JM. Recent advances in neuroblastoma. N Engl J Med 2010; 362(23):2202–11.
360. Williamson D, Lu YJ, Gordon T, et al. Relationship between MYCN copy number and expression in rhabdomyosarcomas and correlation with adverse prognosis in the alveolar subtype. J Clin Oncol 2005;23(4): 880–8.
361. Janoueix-Lerosey I, Lequin D, Brugieres L, et al. Somatic and germline activating mutations of the ALK kinase receptor in neuroblastoma. Nature 2008;455(7215):967–70.
362. Chen Y, Takita J, Choi YL, et al. Oncogenic mutations of ALK kinase in neuroblastoma. Nature 2008;455(7215):971–4.
363. George RE, Sanda T, Hanna M, et al. Activating mutations in ALK provide a therapeutic target in neuroblastoma. Nature 2008;455(7215):975–8.
364. De BS, De PK, Kumps C, et al. Meta-analysis of neuroblastomas reveals a skewed ALK mutation spectrum in tumors with MYCN amplification. Clin Cancer Res 2010;16(17):4353–62.
365. Pugh TJ, Morozova O, Attiyeh EF, et al. The genetic landscape of high-risk neuroblastoma. Nat Genet 2013;45(3):279–84.
366. Hess JL. Chromosomal translocations in benign tumors: the HMGI proteins. Am J Clin Pathol 1998;109(3):251–61.
367. Tallini G, Dal Cin P. HMGI(Y) and HMGI-C dysregulation: a common occurrence in human tumors. Adv Anat Pathol 1999;6(5):237–46.
368. Nilsson M, Mertens F, Hoglund M, et al. Truncation and fusion of HMGA2 in lipomas with rearrangements of 5q32–>q33 and 12q14–>q15. Cytogenet Genome Res 2006;112(1-2):60–6.
369. Quade BJ, Weremowicz S, Neskey DM, et al. Fusion transcripts involving HMGA2 are not a common molecular mechanism in uterine leiomyomata with rearrangements in 12q15. Cancer Res 2003;63(6): 1351–8.
370. Micci F, Panagopoulos I, Bjerkehagen B, et al. Deregulation of HMGA2 in an aggressive angiomyxoma with t(11;12)(q23;q15). Virchows Arch 2006;448(6):838–42.
371. Mayr C, Hemann MT, Bartel DP. Disrupting the pairing between let-7 and Hmga2 enhances oncogenic transformation. Science 2007; 315(5818):1576–9.
372. Wang X, Hulshizer RL, Erickson-Johnson MR, et al. Identification of novel HMGA2 fusion sequences in lipoma: evidence that deletion of let-7 miRNA consensus binding site 1 in the HMGA2 3' UTR is not critical for HMGA2 transcriptional upregulation. Genes Chromosomes Cancer 2009;48(8):673–8.
373. Bianchini L, Saada E, Gjernes E, et al. Let-7 microRNA and HMGA2 levels of expression are not inversely linked in adipocytic tumors: analysis of 56 lipomas and liposarcomas with molecular cytogenetic data. Genes Chromosomes Cancer 2011;50(6):442–55.
374. Kazmierczak B, Dal CP, Wanschura S, et al. HMGIY is the target of 6p21.3 rearrangements in various benign mesenchymal tumors. Genes Chromosomes Cancer 1998;23(4):279–85.
375. Xiao S, Lux ML, Reeves R, et al. HMGI(Y) activation by chromosome 6p21 rearrangements in multilineage mesenchymal cells from pulmonary hamartoma. Am J Pathol 1997;150(3):901–10.
376. Bartuma H, Hallor KH, Panagopoulos I, et al. Assessment of the clinical and molecular impact of different cytogenetic subgroups in a series of 272 lipomas with abnormal karyotype. Genes Chromosomes Cancer 2007;46(6):594–606.
377. Hibbard MK, Kozakewich HP, Dal CP, et al. PLAG1 fusion oncogenes in lipoblastoma. Cancer Res 2000;60(17):4869–72.
378. Bartuma H, Domanski HA, Von Steyern FV, et al. Cytogenetic and molecular cytogenetic findings in lipoblastoma. Cancer Genet Cytogenet 2008;183(1):60–3.
379. Maire G, Forus A, Foa C, et al. 11q13 alterations in two cases of hibernoma: large heterozygous deletions and rearrangement breakpoints near GARP in 11q13.5. Genes Chromosomes Cancer 2003;37(4): 389–95.
380. Nord KH, Magnusson L, Isaksson M, et al. Concomitant deletions of tumor suppressor genes MEN1 and AIP are essential for the pathogenesis of the brown fat tumor hibernoma. Proc Natl Acad Sci U S A 2010;107(49):21122–7.
381. Huang D, Sumegi J, Dal CP, et al. C11orf95-MKL2 is the resulting fusion oncogene of t(11;16)(q13;p13) in chondroid lipoma. Genes Chromosomes Cancer 2010;49(9):810–18.
382. Jin Y, Moller E, Nord KH, et al. Fusion of the AHRR and NCOA2 genes through a recurrent translocation t(5;8)(p15;q13) in soft tissue angiofibroma results in upregulation of aryl hydrocarbon receptor target genes. Genes Chromosomes Cancer 2012;51(5):510–20.
383. Edgar MA, Lauer SR, Bridge JA, et al. Soft tissue angiofibroma: report of 2 cases of a recently described tumor. Hum Pathol 2013;44(3): 438–41.
384. Marino-Enriquez A, Fletcher CD. Angiofibroma of soft tissue: clinicopathologic characterization of a distinctive benign fibrovascular neoplasm in a series of 37 cases. Am J Surg Pathol 2012;36(4):500–8.
385. Erickson-Johnson MR, Chou MM, Evers BR, et al. Nodular fasciitis: a novel model of transient neoplasia induced by MYH9-USP6 gene fusion. Lab Invest 2011;91(10):1427–33.
386. Lynch HT, Deters CA, Hogg D, et al. Familial sarcoma: challenging pedigrees. Cancer 2003;98(9):1947–57.
387. Kleihues P, Schauble B, zur HA, et al. Tumors associated with p53 germline mutations: a synopsis of 91 families. Am J Pathol 1997;150(1): 1–13.
388. Olivier M, Goldgar DE, Sodha N, et al. Li-Fraumeni and related syndromes: correlation between tumor type, family structure, and TP53 genotype. Cancer Res 2003;63(20):6643–50.
389. Toguchida J, Yamaguchi T, Dayton SH, et al. Prevalence and spectrum of germline mutations of the p53 gene among patients with sarcoma. New Engl J Med 1992;326(20):1301–8.
390. Hwang SJ, Lozano G, Amos CI, et al. Germline p53 mutations in a cohort with childhood sarcoma: sex differences in cancer risk. Am J Hum Genet 2003;72(4):975–83.
391. Bond GL, Hirshfield KM, Kirchhoff T, et al. MDM2 SNP309 accelerates tumor formation in a gender-specific and hormone-dependent manner. Cancer Res 2006;66(10):5104–10.
392. Serra E, Puig S, Otero D, et al. Confirmation of a double-hit model for the NF1 gene in benign neurofibromas. Am J Hum Genet 1997;61(3): 512–19.
393. Cichowski K, Shih TS, Schmitt E, et al. Mouse models of tumor development in neurofibromatosis type 1. Science 1999;286(5447): 2172–6.
394. Storlazzi CT, Von Steyern FV, Domanski HA, et al. Biallelic somatic inactivation of the NF1 gene through chromosomal translocations in a sporadic neurofibroma. Int J Cancer 2005;117(6):1055–7.
395. De RT, Maertens O, Chmara M, et al. Somatic loss of wild type NF1 allele in neurofibromas: Comparison of NF1 microdeletion and non-microdeletion patients. Genes Chromosomes Cancer 2006;45(10): 893–904.
396. Birindelli S, Perrone F, Oggionni M, et al. Rb and TP53 pathway alterations in sporadic and NF1-related malignant peripheral nerve sheath tumors. Lab Invest 2001;81(6):833–44.
397. Legius E, Dierick H, Wu R, et al. TP53 mutations are frequent in malignant NF1 tumors. Genes Chromosomes Cancer 1994;10(4): 250–5.
398. Kourea HP, Orlow I, Scheithauer BW, et al. Deletions of the INK4A gene occur in malignant peripheral nerve sheath tumors but not in neurofibromas. Am J Pathol 1999;155(6):1855–60.
399. Perrone F, Tabano S, Colombo F, et al. p15INK4b, p14ARF, and p16INK4a inactivation in sporadic and neurofibromatosis type 1-related malignant peripheral nerve sheath tumors. Clin Cancer Res 2003;9(11): 4132–8.
400. Caspari R, Olschwang S, Friedl W, et al. Familial adenomatous polyposis: desmoid tumours and lack of ophthalmic lesions (CHRPE) associated with APC mutations beyond codon 1444. Hum Mol Genet 1995;4(3): 337–40.

401. Bertario L, Russo A, Sala P, et al. Genotype and phenotype factors as determinants of desmoid tumors in patients with familial adenomatous polyposis. Int J Cancer 2001;95(2):102–7.
402. Clark SK, Pack K, Pritchard J, et al. Familial adenomatous polyposis presenting with childhood desmoids. Lancet 1997;349(9050):471–2.
403. Scott RJ, Froggatt NJ, Trembath RC, et al. Familial infiltrative fibromatosis (desmoid tumours) (MIM135290) caused by a recurrent 3' APC gene mutation. Hum Mol Genet 1996;5(12):1921–4.
404. Ng TL, Gown AM, Barry TS, et al. Nuclear beta-catenin in mesenchymal tumors. Mod Pathol 2005;18(1):68–74.
405. Tejpar S, Nollet F, Li C, et al. Predominance of beta-catenin mutations and beta-catenin dysregulation in sporadic aggressive fibromatosis (desmoid tumor). Oncogene 1999;18(47):6615–20.
406. den Bakker MA, Seynaeve C, Kliffen M, et al. Microsatellite instability in a pleomorphic rhabdomyosarcoma in a patient with hereditary non-polyposis colorectal cancer. Histopathology 2003;43(3):297–9.
407. Nilbert M, Therkildsen C, Nissen A, et al. Sarcomas associated with hereditary nonpolyposis colorectal cancer: broad anatomical and morphological spectrum. Fam Cancer 2009;8(3):209–13.
408. Kratz CP, Holter S, Etzler J, et al. Rhabdomyosarcoma in patients with constitutional mismatch-repair-deficiency syndrome. J Med Genet 2009;46(6):418–20.
409. Urso E, Agostini M, Pucciarelli S, et al. Soft tissue sarcoma and the hereditary non-polyposis colorectal cancer (HNPCC) syndrome: formulation of an hypothesis. Mol Biol Rep 2012;39(10):9307–10.
410. Kawaguchi K, Oda Y, Takahira T, et al. Microsatellite instability and hMLH1 and hMSH2 expression analysis in soft tissue sarcomas. Oncol Rep 2005;13(2):241–6.
411. Versteege I, Sevenet N, Lange J, et al. Truncating mutations of hSNF5/INI1 in aggressive paediatric cancer. Nature 1998;394(6689):203–6.
412. Biegel JA, Zhou JY, Rorke LB, et al. Germ-Line and Acquired Mutations of *INI1* in Atypical Teratoid and Rhabdoid Tumors. Cancer Res 1999;59(1):74–9.
413. Sevenet N, Lellouch-Tubiana A, Schofield D, et al. Spectrum of hSNF5/INI1 somatic mutations in human cancer and genotype-phenotype correlations. Hum Mol Genet 1999;8(13):2359–68.
414. Modena P, Lualdi E, Facchinetti F, et al. SMARCB1/INI1 tumor suppressor gene is frequently inactivated in epithelioid sarcomas. Cancer Res 2005;65(10):4012–19.
415. Fuller CE, Pfeifer J, Humphrey P, et al. Chromosome 22q dosage in composite extrarenal rhabdoid tumors: clonal evolution or a phenotypic mimic? Hum Pathol 2001;32(10):1102–8.
416. Rousseau-Merck MF, Versteege I, Legrand I, et al. hSNF5/INI1 inactivation is mainly associated with homozygous deletions and mitotic recombinations in rhabdoid tumors. Cancer Res 1999;59(13):3152–6.
417. Biegel JA, Tan L, Zhang F, et al. Alterations of the hSNF5/INI1 gene in central nervous system atypical teratoid/rhabdoid tumors and renal and extrarenal rhabdoid tumors. Clin Cancer Res 2002;8(11):3461–7.
418. Sevenet N, Sheridan E, Amram D, et al. Constitutional mutations of the *hSNF5/INI1* gene predispose to a variety of cancers. Am J Hum Genet 1999;65(5):1342–8.
419. Khan J, Wei J, Ringner M, et al. Classification and diagnostic prediction of cancers using gene expression profiling and artificial neural networks. Nat Med 2001;7(6):673–9.
420. Baird K, Davis S, Antonescu CR, et al. Gene expression profiling of human sarcomas: insights into sarcoma biology. Cancer Res 2005;65(20):9226–35.
421. Nielsen TO, West RB. Translating gene expression into clinical care: sarcomas as a paradigm. J Clin Oncol 2010;28(10):1796–805.
422. Coindre JM, Hostein I, Maire G, et al. Inflammatory malignant fibrous histiocytomas and dedifferentiated liposarcomas: histological review, genomic profile, and MDM2 and CDK4 status favour a single entity. J Pathol 2004;203(3):822–30.
423. Idbaih A, Coindre JM, Derre J, et al. Myxoid malignant fibrous histiocytoma and pleomorphic liposarcoma share very similar genomic imbalances. Lab Invest 2005;85(2):176–81.
424. Chibon F, Lagarde P, Salas S, et al. Validated prediction of clinical outcome in sarcomas and multiple types of cancer on the basis of a gene expression signature related to genome complexity. Nat Med 2010;16(7):781–7.
425. Terry J, Saito T, Subramanian S, et al. TLE1 as a diagnostic immunohistochemical marker for synovial sarcoma emerging from gene expression profiling studies. Am J Surg Pathol 2007;31(2):240–6.
426. Laé M, Ahn EH, Mercado GE, et al. Global gene expression profiling of PAX-FKHR fusion-positive alveolar and PAX-FKHR fusion-negative embryonal rhabdomyosarcomas. J Pathol 2007;212(2):143–51.
427. Wachtel M, Runge T, Leuschner I, et al. Subtype and prognostic classification of rhabdomyosarcoma by immunohistochemistry. J Clin Oncol 2006;24(5):816–22.
428. West RB, Harvell J, Linn SC, et al. Apo D in soft tissue tumors: a novel marker for dermatofibrosarcoma protuberans. Am J Surg Pathol 2004;28(8):1063–9.
429. West RB, Corless CL, Chen X, et al. The novel marker, DOG1, is expressed ubiquitously in gastrointestinal stromal tumors irrespective of KIT or PDGFRA mutation status. Am J Pathol 2004;165(1):107–13.
430. Espinosa I, Lee CH, Kim MK, et al. A novel monoclonal antibody against DOG1 is a sensitive and specific marker for gastrointestinal stromal tumors. Am J Surg Pathol 2008;32(2):210–18.
431. Liegl B, Hornick JL, Corless CL, et al. Monoclonal antibody DOG1.1 shows higher sensitivity than KIT in the diagnosis of gastrointestinal stromal tumors, including unusual subtypes. Am J Surg Pathol 2009;33(3):437–46.
432. Miettinen M, Wang ZF, Lasota J. DOG1 antibody in the differential diagnosis of gastrointestinal stromal tumors: a study of 1840 cases. Am J Surg Pathol 2009;33(9):1401–8.
433. Novelli M, Rossi S, Rodriguez-Justo M, et al. DOG1 and CD117 are the antibodies of choice in the diagnosis of gastrointestinal stromal tumours. Histopathology 2010;57(2):259–70.

Fine-Needle Aspiration Biopsy of Soft Tissue Tumors

Kim R. Geisinger and *Fadi W. Abdul-Karim*

CHAPTER CONTENTS

INTRODUCTION

A fine-needle aspiration biopsy (FNAB) is an established tool in the diagnostic armamentarium of many clinical practices. The initial diagnosis of mass lesions in superficial (e.g., breast and thyroid) and deep (e.g., lung and pancreas) body sites is often readily assessed by FNAB. FNAB remains underutilized in the evaluation of primary soft tissue tumors, however, and, for some, is still controversial.[1-14]

ADVANTAGES AND DISADVANTAGES OF FINE-NEEDLE ASPIRATION

Several important challenges are inherent in the evaluation of soft tissue neoplasms. Many lesions, especially sarcomas, are rare so most practicing pathologists do not encounter these neoplasms on a routine basis and may not be familiar with their morphologic, clinical, and radiographic features. Soft tissue lesions also possess overlapping histopathologic and cytomorphologic attributes that are further compounded by the morphologic heterogeneity that may be present within some of these proliferations. For these reasons, some have advocated that the diagnosis and treatment of many soft tissue lesions, especially sarcomas, should generally occur within large, centralized medical facilities.[1-3,14]

FNAB of soft tissue masses possesses a number of distinct advantages.[1,2,11,14] Compared to other techniques, FNAB is a rapid outpatient procedure that permits on-site evaluation of specimen adequacy and may provide an immediate diagnosis. This allows the orthopedic surgeon to discuss potential additional diagnostic procedures and therapeutic options during the initial visit. The aspiration procedure is well tolerated, and local anesthesia is usually unnecessary. A major advantage of FNAB is that much greater sampling is possible. By altering the direction of the needle during a single puncture, multiple portions of the mass may be aspirated as compared to a core needle biopsy (CNB). If necessary, multiple separate FNAB punctures may be performed during a single patient visit. Cellular material may be obtained during the same biopsy setting for electron microscopy, cytogenetics, molecular biologic analysis, and cell blocks. Cell blocks are preferable to direct smears for immunocytochemical studies; these blocks provide excellent substrates for most ancillary investigations, including most molecular and genetic assays.

FNAB also has a very low rate of significant clinical complications. Rarely, patients may suffer bleeding or develop edema and tenderness at the biopsy site. The procedure does not disrupt tissue planes or contaminate the subsequent surgical site. If not diagnostic, FNAB can be followed by another biopsy procedure. No instance of needle tracking of sarcomatous tumor cells by a fine needle has been documented. According to Fleshman et al., some surgeons are therefore comfortable in not resecting the skin through which the aspiration needle traversed; this should reduce complications related to surgical closing and healing of the skin.[15] Finally, compared to all other biopsy techniques, FNAB is relatively inexpensive and viewed as very cost-effective.

FNAB possesses several distinct disadvantages, some of which are relatively specific to soft tissue lesions.[1-3,14] FNAB results in relatively small samples of a tumor. Inherent in the aspiration technique is a dispersion of individual cells and loss of recognizable diagnostic tissue patterns. These limitations inevitably hinder the cytopathologist's ability to distinguish specific histologic type and subtype of tumors. There may be even more difficulty in distinguishing among benign cellular lesions and low-grade sarcomas. Accurate grading of many sarcomas may not be possible when using current histopathologic classification schemes. In densely collagenized or sclerotic masses or highly vascular lesions, FNAB may provide only a sparse smear cellularity, making a benign versus malignant distinction impossible.

Although the exact role for FNAB in the clinical evaluation of soft tissue masses remains controversial, most published data and expert experiences strongly support its utility in accurately distinguishing between benign and malignant soft tissue tumors. Cytomorphologically, the most important feature in this decision process is the overall cellularity of the smears. Sarcomas usually yield moderately to highly cellular specimens, whereas benign mesenchymal lesions usually are more sparsely cellular. It is crucial to recognize, however, that there is overlap in this cellularity parameter. For example, aspirates of nodular fasciitis may yield numerous atypical-appearing spindle-shaped cells; the atypia is related to large open nuclei with prominent nucleoli, and not to well-developed hyperchromasia. Conversely, certain neoplasms, for example, low-grade fibromyxoid sarcoma and richly collagenized malignancies, may not provide numerous neoplastic elements. This can be further complicated by poor sampling of the mass and extensive necrosis within the tumor. The classic cytologic attributes of malignancy also support the diagnosis of sarcoma. It is important to find diffuse and uniform hyperchromasia among essentially all of the aspirated tumor cells. The presence of moderate to marked pleomorphism, although certainly not specific, also leads to a diagnosis of malignancy. Irregularly contoured and variably thickened nuclear membranes are features of sarcoma. A word of caution concerning nucleoli is warranted in that they may be prominent in benign proliferations (e.g., granulation tissue and pseudosarcomatous proliferations) and inconspicuous in some malignancies (e.g., myxoid sarcomas). The levels of reported diagnostic specificity and sensitivity are approximately 95% in establishing a diagnosis of sarcoma.[1,14] FNAB can also readily differentiate sarcomas from other malignancies that have spread to the soft tissues.

The diagnosis of a soft tissue tumor by aspiration biopsy necessitates the intimate cooperation of orthopedic surgeons, radiologists, and pathologists to optimize the integration of all clinically relevant information.[1,14] Whenever possible, an on-site evaluation by the pathologist is preferred because this expedites the opportunity for the pathologist to examine the patient, to review imaging studies, and to discuss the lesion with the surgeon. This also permits a timely assessment of specimen adequacy and possibly the rendering of an immediate interpretation.

Another important reason for on-site evaluation is that it allows the pathologist to suggest further triage of the sample. Therefore, additional needle punctures may be performed to obtain cellular material for cell blocks that may provide additional architectural data and a substrate for immunocytochemistry, cytogenetics, and a variety of molecular biologic assays.[16-22]

Generally, one can accurately subclassify soft tissue neoplasms on the basis of FNAB into clinically relevant categories that permit the initiation of therapy in many patients.[1,2,4,5,14,23,24] Soft tissue sarcomas in aspiration smears are classified into six general categories on the basis of the predominant appearance of the specimen: myxoid, spindle cell, pleomorphic, polygonal cell, round cell, and miscellaneous.[1] The following sections will expand upon this classification scheme. In general, these categories correlate relatively well with the grade of the malignancy.

Histologic grade is one of the most significant and perhaps the most crucial single factor in predicting a patient's prognosis.[15,25] Within certain limitations, many soft tissue sarcomas can be accurately graded in smears in a clinically relevant manner.[1,11-15,26-29] However, not all authorities subscribe to this approach, and some have discouraged this practice because of the limitations of FNAB.[25] The inability to assess mitotic figure counts, variability in cellularity from field to field, and the extent of tumor necrosis is prohibitive of accurate grading. The cytologist can state only that necrotic debris is absent or present in scant or large amounts. On the other hand, histologic subtype or degree of differentiation is somewhat different. In FNAB, a specific cell type can be identified in a large proportion of sarcomas.

Although many may not treat solely on the FNAB diagnosis, in some centers therapy is dictated by the FNAB interpretation. If tumors are considered low grade, surgery usually is the next step. However, if high grade, then preoperative radiation or chemotherapy may be administered to reduce or better define the extent of surgery. Pleomorphic and round cell sarcomas are almost always high grade. Pure myxoid sarcomas are low grade. Polygonal cell and especially the spindle cell categories pose the greatest difficulties.[26-28]

Some authorities have provided data on the complementary nature of FNAB and the CNB in the outpatient setting for the primary diagnosis of soft tissue neoplasms.[1,2] More recently, several groups have compared these two diagnostic modalities in this exact clinical scenario. Yang and Damron evaluated 50 consecutive patients.[30] These authors averaged six core needle passes per patient (this number is considered high), followed by FNAB. The first procedure was performed by the surgeon, whereas the pathologist performed the aspiration. The authors concluded that CNB has a higher level of diagnostic accuracy in determining the nature of the neoplasm, establishing a histologic type and grade, and a specific diagnosis. Domanski et al. evaluated 130 consecutive patients in which both biopsy procedures were performed by the pathologist.[31] These authors concluded that the two techniques were complementary. It should be pointed out that both of these series included osseous and soft tissue lesions. Although more data can generally be acquired by CNB, the complementary nature is related to the many advantages of FNAB.

MYXOID SARCOMAS

The myxoid sarcomas include myxoid liposarcoma, myxofibrosarcoma, low-grade fibromyxoid sarcoma, and extraskeletal myxoid chondrosarcoma. At low power, the most apparent feature of the smears is the voluminous extracellular matrix material (Fig. 5-1).[1,2,32-43] Often, the matrix fragments are irregularly shaped and moderately sized, with or without embedded tumor cells. Alternatively, the matrix may present as a thin film on the slide. With the Romanowsky stains, the matrix appears as homogeneous, fibrillar to structureless reddish purple material (Fig. 5-2). The matrix is typically metachromatic, especially in extraskeletal chondrosarcomas. With the Papanicolaou stain, the matrix is cyanophilic and often appears as a relatively watery pale-green substance (see Fig. 5-1). The edges of the fragments may be sharply defined or blend irregularly with the background as delicate spicules that extend from the fragment. In the smear, the sarcoma cells are present in moderate to high numbers as individually dispersed elements and in small aggregates, both embedded within the matrix and scattered in the background. Typically, the malignant cells are relatively small and have spindled, rounded, or stellate contours. Their precise shape is more apparent when they are unencumbered by the matrix. Most of the tumor cells are small to moderately sized, often with densely hyperchromatic solitary nuclei. Nucleoli are generally small and inconspicuous, or inapparent. A few multinucleated tumor giant cells may also be randomly distributed in the

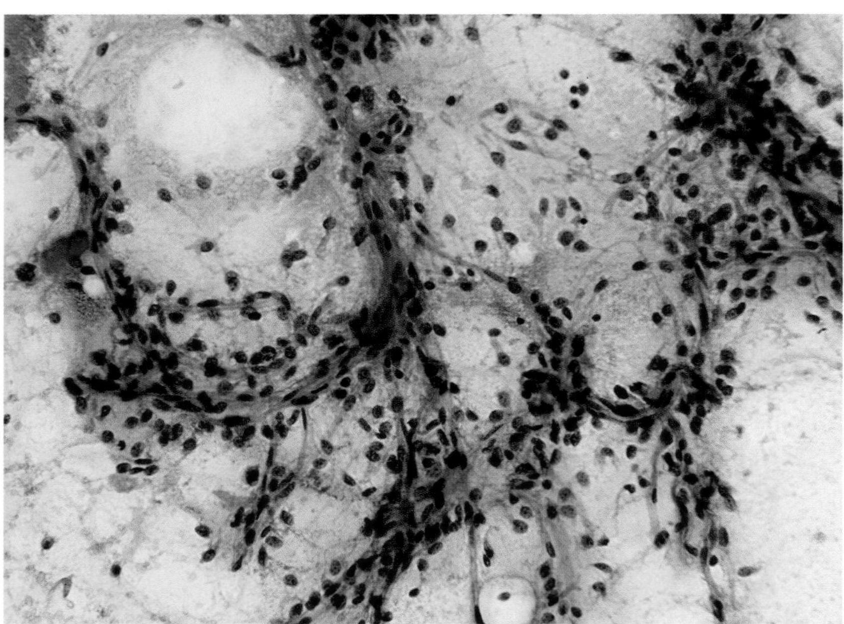

FIGURE 5-1. Myxoid liposarcoma. A moderate number of small neoplastic cells with solitary hyperchromatic nuclei and spindled, round, and stellate contours are embedded within abundant cyanophilic matrix. A few tumor cells contain cytoplasmic lipid. (Papanicolaou stain, ×400.)

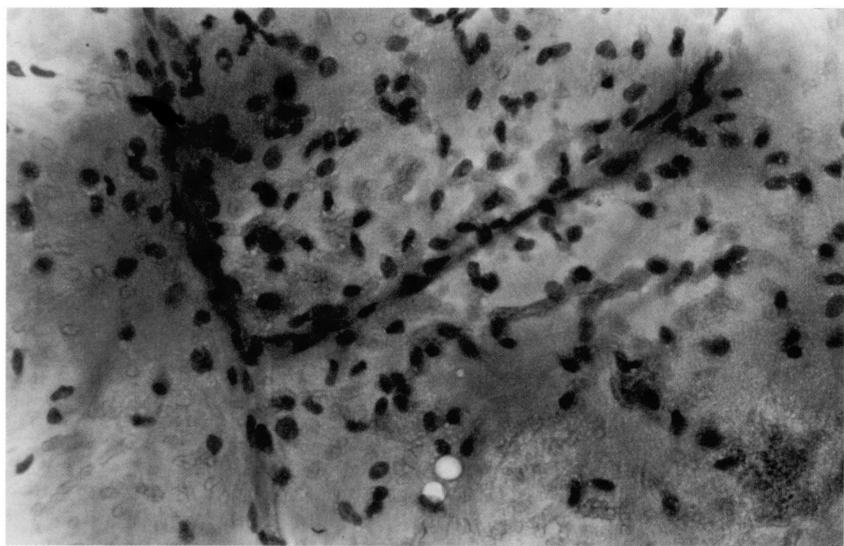

FIGURE 5-2. Myxoid liposarcoma. The small malignant cells are characterized by solitary darkly stained nuclei and high nuclear-to-cytoplasmic ratios. They appear to be fairly evenly scattered within the metachromatic matrix, which also contains a branched capillary. Two neoplastic cells have lipid vacuoles. (Diff-Quik stain, ×400.)

smears, primarily with myxoid malignant fibrous histiocytoma/myxofibrosarcomas (Fig. 5-3).

In aspirates from myxoid liposarcomas, the only cells of diagnostic value are lipoblasts.[1,2,31-34] Lipoblasts, however, may be sparse and require a careful search. They are characterized by rounded contours and scant-to-moderate cytoplasm occupied by one or more sharply defined lipid vacuoles. The latter may be uniform in size or vary in diameter but characteristically displace the nucleus eccentrically and indent or scallop its borders. Another highly distinctive feature of myxoid liposarcoma is the presence of branched delicate capillaries in the matrix material (see Figs. 5-1 and 5-2). Larger round tumor cells with high nuclear-to-cytoplasmic ratios and occasional lipid vacuoles are seen in smears of poorly differentiated myxoid liposarcoma (round cell liposarcoma) (Fig. 5-4). The finding of a low-grade component with malignant round cells in the same smear is a helpful clue to the correct classification. In smears, lipoblastoma may be indistinguishable from myxoid liposarcoma (this malignant entity does not manifest much in the way of adipocyte differentiation) or much more likely, well-differentiated liposarcoma; therefore, it is essential that patient age is integrated into the diagnosis.[35,41]

The most distinguishing feature of smears of myxoid malignant fibrous histiocytoma/myxofibrosarcoma is the presence of moderate numbers of scattered bizarre tumor giant cells, generally multinucleated, with voluminous cytoplasm; these cells have indistinct edges that appear to blend into the smear background (see Fig. 5-3).[1,32,33,36,39] Typically, the nuclei within a given cell vary in both size and outline.

The distinctive attribute of extraskeletal myxoid chondrosarcomas is the arrangement of the small-round tumor cells in linear chains or cords (Fig. 5-5). Elsewhere, cells are isolated

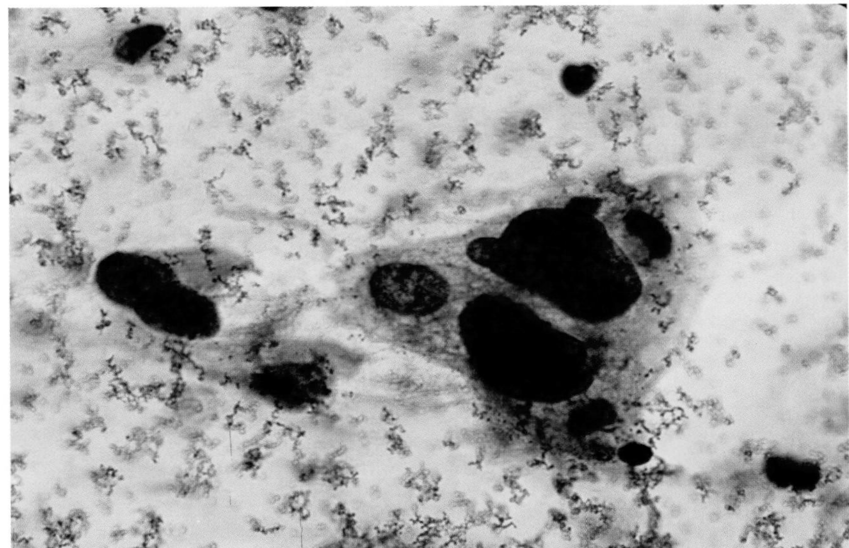

FIGURE 5-3. Myxoid malignant fibrous histiocytoma/myxofibrosarcoma. Nuclear hyperchromasia and pleomorphism of size and shape are obvious and include giant cells. Their wispy cytoplasm varies in quantity and blends into the smear background. Such giant cells are not expected in these numbers in other myxoid sarcomas. (Papanicolaou stain, ×400.)

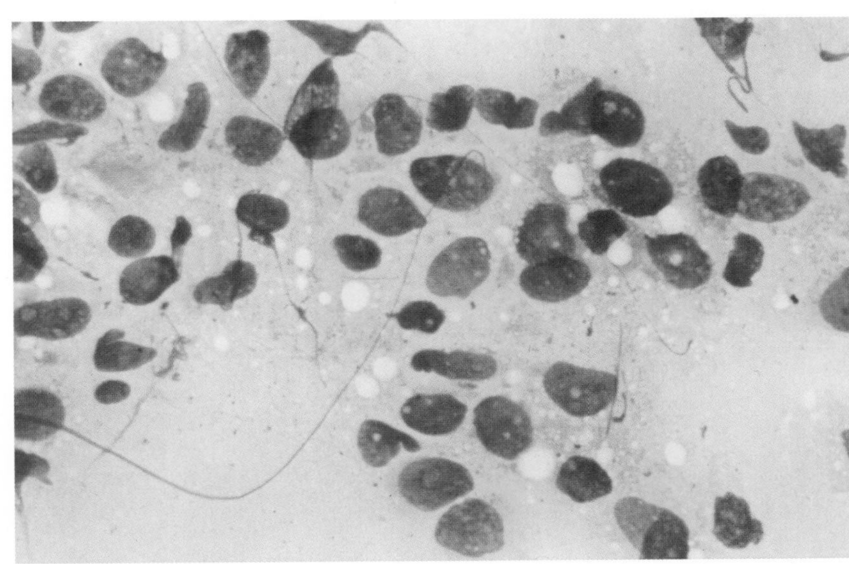

FIGURE 5-4. Round cell liposarcoma. The poorly differentiated variant of myxoid liposarcoma is composed of relatively small uniform malignant cells with round, large nuclei, scanty cytoplasm, and occasionally prominent nucleoli. Cytoplasmic lipid vacuoles may be seen within some of the cells. (Diff-Quik stain, ×400.)

or in nonspecific aggregates. In some instances, the avascular matrix manifests extreme metachromasia and a dense appearance,[32,33,37] features that contrast with the myxoid matrix of benign myxoid neoplasms.

Colin et al. reported that generally the cytomorphology of myxofibrosarcomas (and therefore on low-grade myxoid malignant fibrous histiocytoma) overlaps with that of other myxoid sarcomas, creating difficulty in rendering a specific diagnosis.[36] This includes the presence in the matrix of curvilinear blood vessels, which resemble the vasculature of myxoid liposarcoma, as seen in their illustrations. However, the tumor cells tend to be more spindled than is typical of other sarcomas in this category.

The differential diagnosis of myxoid sarcomas includes benign myxoid soft tissue tumors, most commonly ganglion cysts and intramuscular and juxta-articular myxomas.[32,33,40] These masses may yield viscous aspiration fluid, which is difficult to smear.[40] The smears are usually dominated by granular myxoid material in which paucicellular elements are embedded that resemble histiocytes. Although mitotic figures are sparse in aspirates of myxoid sarcomas, they are not present in samples of benign entities.

SPINDLE CELL SARCOMAS

This category includes fibrosarcoma, leiomyosarcoma, synovial sarcoma, malignant peripheral nerve sheath tumors, Kaposi sarcoma, low-grade fibromyxoid sarcoma, gastrointestinal stromal tumors, and some angiosarcomas.[1,2,7,8,18,22,26,27,36,38,44-61] This group poses the greatest diagnostic difficulties and has the greatest potential for false-negative diagnoses because of the difficulty in distinguishing benign proliferations from low-grade sarcomas. Conversely, a variety of benign spindle cell

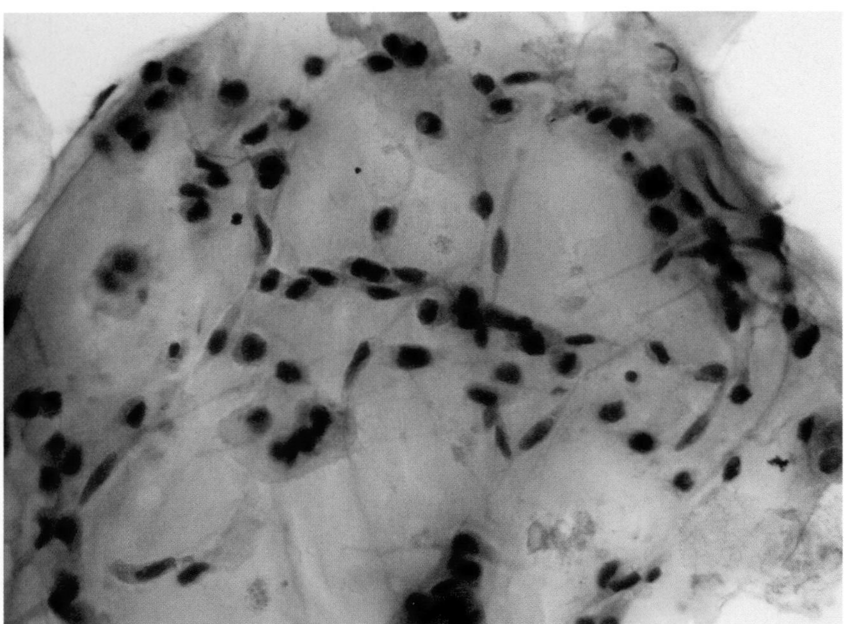

FIGURE 5-5. Extraskeletal myxoid chondrosarcoma. Each small round to spindled malignant cell has a single hyperchromatic nucleus without obvious nucleoli and high nuclear-to-cytoplasmic ratios. Many are arranged in linear chains within the homogeneous matrix material. (Diff-Quik stain, ×400.)

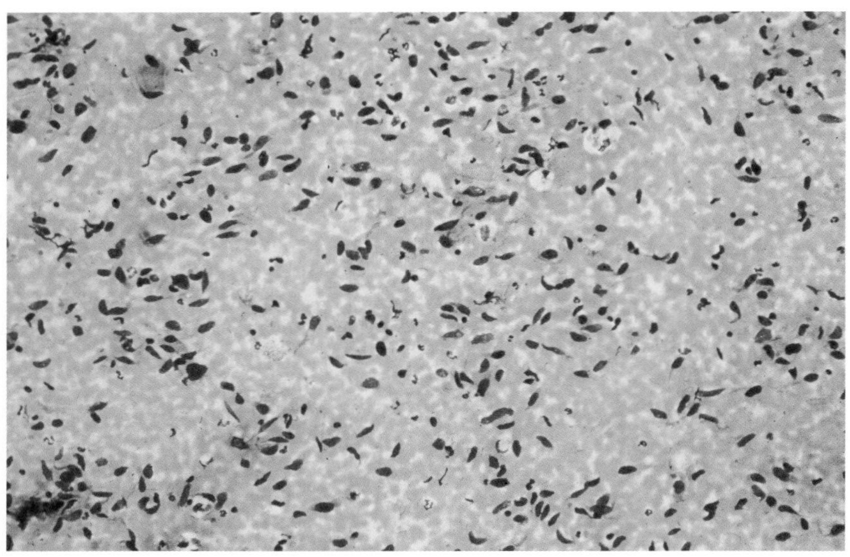

FIGURE 5-6. Malignant peripheral nerve sheath tumor. This extremely cellular aspirate is dominated by mildly pleomorphic and dissociated spindle-shaped malignant cells. There is almost no evidence of intercellular cohesion. The nuclear-to-cytoplasmic ratios appear high, although some possess elongated cytoplasmic tails. The spindle-shaped nuclei vary from smooth to buckled to wavy. (Diff-Quik stain, ×40.)

proliferations, for example, the fibromatoses and the pseudosarcomatous lesions,[55-58] may yield false-positive interpretations. The two major attributes that allow an aspirate to be designated as a sarcoma are moderate to high smear cellularity with some loss of cohesion and uniformly hyperchromatic nuclei. Based purely on the cytomorphology, it may be difficult or impossible to distinguish among the various spindle cell sarcomas and to grade them accurately. Neither nuclear configurations nor cytoplasmic features are of consistent value in distinguishing among these neoplasms, especially the high-grade tumors.

In general, aspiration biopsies yield moderately to highly cellular smears (Fig. 5-6).[1,2] The major feature is a predominance of cells with elongated or spindled nuclei, paralleling the shape of the cell (Figs. 5-7, 5-8, and 5-9). The degree of intercellular cohesion may vary markedly from patient to patient and among the various spindle cell sarcomas. Some specimens are dominated by individually dispersed tumor cells and small, loose aggregates, whereas in others, large tissue fragments predominate. The latter situation is most characteristic of leiomyosarcomas.[1,54] The edges of the neoplastic fragments are rendered indistinct by the detachment of cells from its surface. The neoplastic cells are usually mononuclear and monotonous. Their chromatin is finely to coarsely granular and may be either evenly or irregularly distributed. Generally, nucleoli are neither large nor prominent; if they are, the morphologist needs to consider nodular fasciitis and related proliferations.[55,56] The volume of cytoplasm varies from

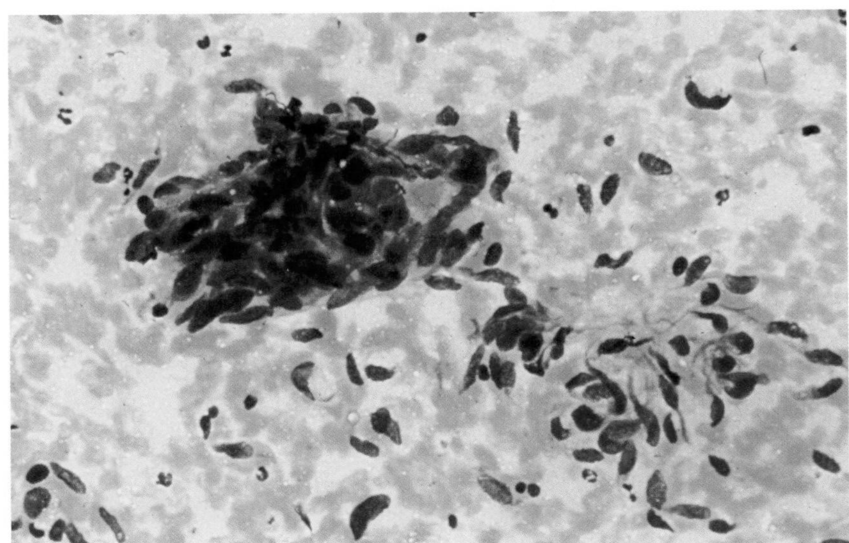

FIGURE 5-7. Synovial sarcoma. This highly cellular aspirate smear contains individual tumor cells, loose clusters, and a three-dimensional cohesive tumor fragment. The malignant cells are uniform, each possessing a single elongated nucleus and very high nuclear-to-cytoplasmic ratios. Nuclear contours vary from plump and ovoid to very elongated to comma-shaped. (Diff-Quik stain, ×250.)

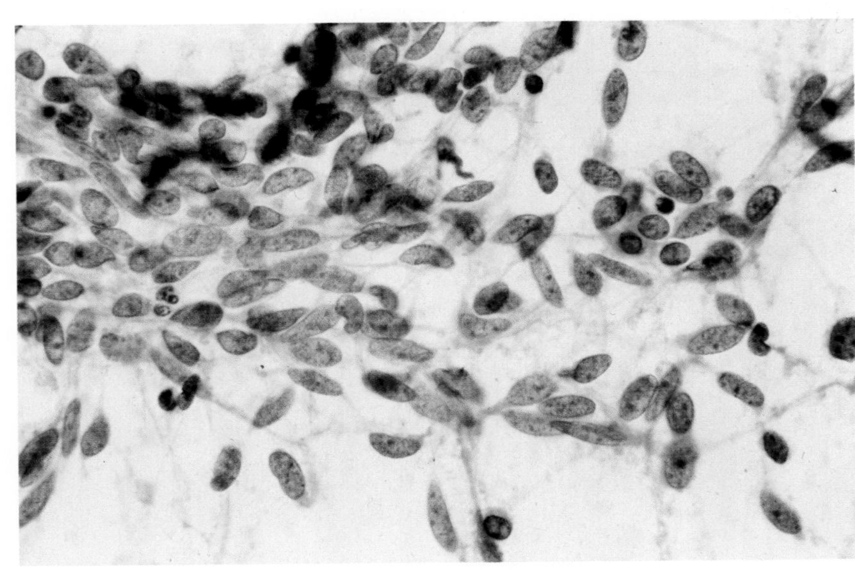

FIGURE 5-8. Malignant peripheral nerve sheath tumor. This cellular aspirate contains a loose aggregate of malignant cells. The edges of the aggregate appear irregular, resulting from individual cells falling away from its surface. Each cell has a solitary elongated nucleus with finely granulated, evenly distributed hyperchromatic chromatin and occasional minute nucleoli. No evidence of specific differentiation is seen. (Papanicolaou stain, ×400.)

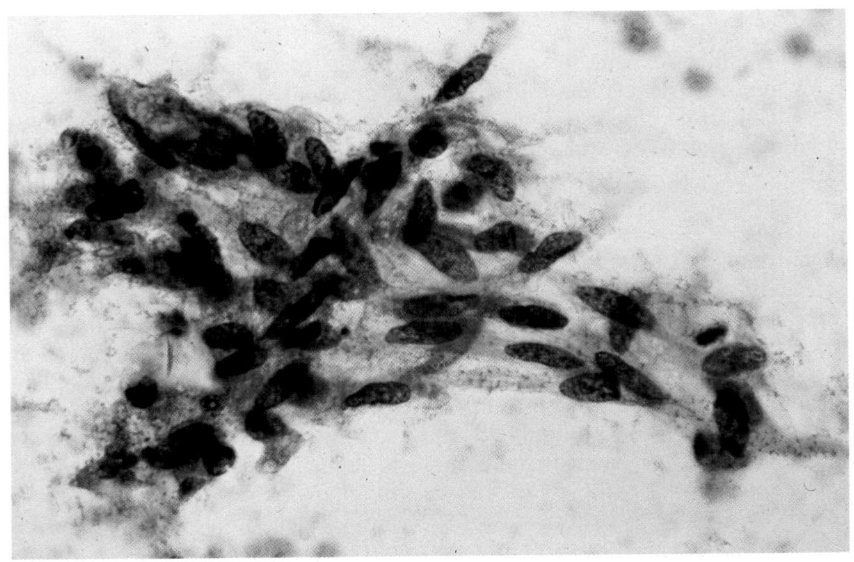

FIGURE 5-9. Leiomyosarcoma. The sarcomatous nuclei are large and hyperchromatic. Although the cells possess obvious dense cytoplasm, the cells are crowded because of high nuclear-to-cytoplasmic ratios. (Papanicolaou stain, ×400.)

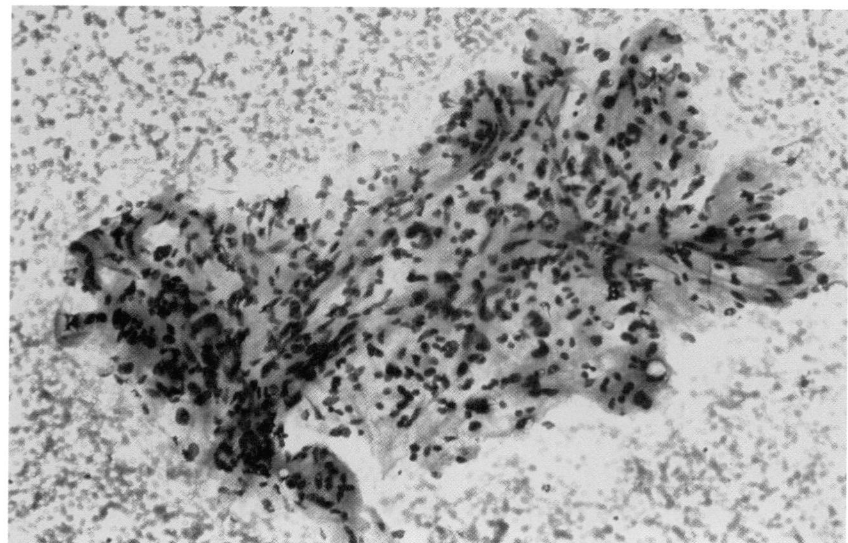

FIGURE 5-10. Schwannoma. This smear is characterized by a large cohesive fragment of tumor. Moderate numbers of neoplastic cells are situated within an abundant matrix. The pink-staining material represents both cytoplasm and collagen. Note the complete absence of individually dispersed tumor cells. (Diff-Quik stain, ×100.)

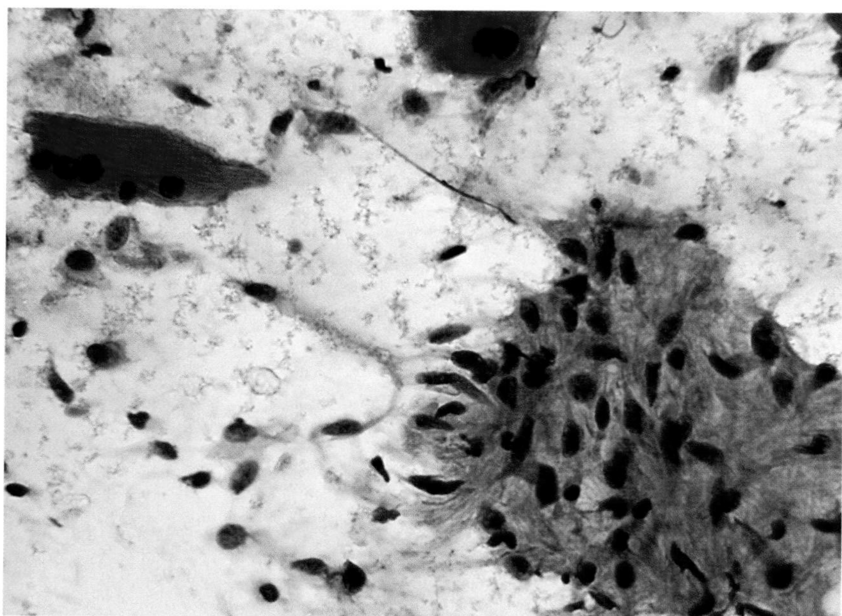

FIGURE 5-11. Nodular fasciitis. The classic loosely textured tissue-culture appearance is evident. Haphazardly arranged myofibroblasts are present within a pale fibrillated myxoid matrix. Other lesional cells with long tails of delicate cytoplasm are freely dispersed. Most nuclei are euchromatic, and some manifest distinct nucleoli. Fragments of muscle fibers are also present. (Papanicolaou stain, ×100.)

scant to moderate, and, in some neoplasms, the tumor cells have long, tapering cytoplasmic tails. The application of ancillary diagnostic procedures, such as immunocytochemistry, cytogenetics, and molecular assays of aspirated cellular material, may assist in arriving at a specific diagnosis.

The most commonly aspirated benign spindle cell soft tissue lesions are nerve sheath neoplasms and nodular fasciitis. In most benign nerve sheath tumors, the cellularity of the smear is low to moderate.[62] The vast majority of the aspirated cells are consistently present in cohesive tissue fragments with irregular contours and consisting of interlacing fascicles (Fig. 5-10). Most neoplastic cells have a solitary elongated nucleus with sharply pointed tips. Some of the nuclei may have a wavy outline. Although uncommon, hyperchromasia may be noted focally. Intranuclear vacuoles are present with some frequency. The cytoplasm of the tumor cells is generally inapparent and blends imperceptibly with the surrounding collagen in the fragments. Mitotic figures are not evident. One must be wary of two variants, namely, ancient and cellular schwannomas.[63,64] A clinical clue to the diagnosis of a nerve sheath tumor is that aspiration incites pain that radiates along the involved nerve.

In conjunction with the appropriate clinical presentation, the cytomorphology of aspirates of nodular fasciitis is often quite distinctive.[1,2,55,56] The smears are moderately to highly cellular and composed of singly dispersed cells, loose aggregates, and tissue fragments, all set in either a collagenous or myxoid material, or dispersed free in the smear. Within the fragments, the cells are loosely and haphazardly arranged, similar to the pattern of tissue cultures (Fig. 5-11). Although cellular shapes are variable, most are spindled with moderate volumes of faintly basophilic cytoplasm and one or two cytoplasmic tails. Most possess a solitary nucleus that is round with delicate, distinct membranes, vesicular chromatin, and distinct nucleoli that may be large and irregular in shape. This is referred to as nuclear-nucleolar dyssynchrony in that the huge nucleoli may suggest malignancy, but the thin, smooth

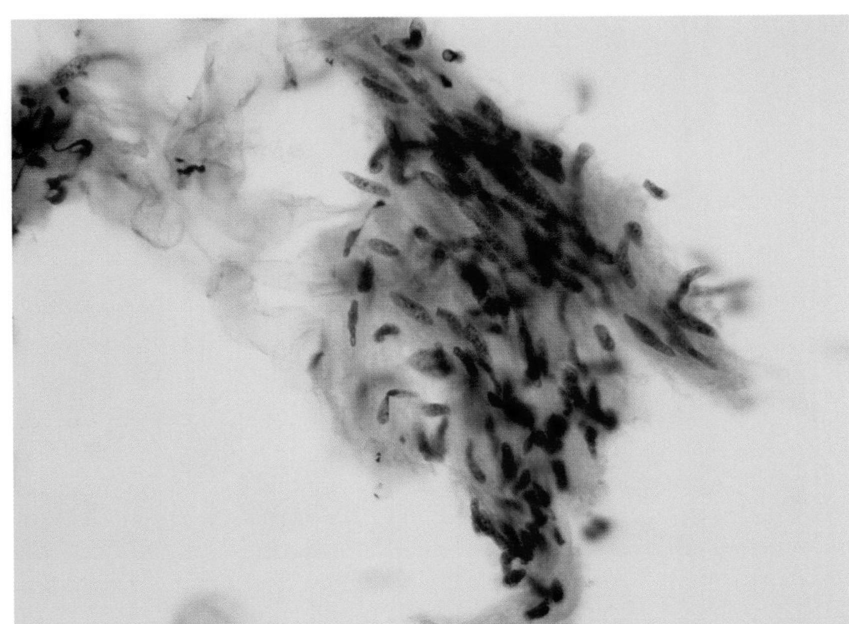

FIGURE 5-12. Fibromatosis. Set within a cohesive collagenous fragment are fibroblasts with solitary elongated nuclei with smooth delicate membranes, fine chromatin, and no obvious nucleoli. Note the parallel arrangement of many of the cells and their nuclei. (Papanicolaou stain, ×200.)

membranes and fine pale chromatin are in keeping with a benign process. Larger cells with more polygonal contours, resembling ganglion cells, may be present but are more numerous in proliferative myositis and fasciitis. Mitotic figures may also be present, at times numerous, but do not possess atypical morphologies. The cytologic picture is completed by the presence of inflammatory cells. A frequent clinical benefit of aspiration biopsy in these pseudosarcomatous lesions is that they spontaneously resolve within a number of weeks following the needle puncture.

FNAB of the fibromatoses notoriously may lead to false-negative (insufficient) specimens or false-positive diagnoses of sarcoma. The smears are variably cellular but tend to be less so than in sarcomas (Fig. 5-12).[1,2,57,58] Presumably, this is related to the abundant collagen within the lesion. These cells are present both singly and in small, loose aggregates. Proliferating fibroblasts have solitary, uniform, elongated nuclei with delicate membranes, even fine chromatin, and inconspicuous nucleoli. One may find bipolar, tapering, long cytoplasmic tails. The lesional cells may be individually dispersed or present in collagen-rich tissue fragments; in the latter, they may be arranged in a fascicular pattern. Mitotic figures are not expected. In some specimens, massive cells with multiple nuclei may be present as a minority component; these are derived from degenerated skeletal muscle. If not correctly recognized as such, they could lead to a false-positive diagnosis, but with experience with such elements, they are readily recognized for what they are (some may persist with cytoplasmic striations).

PLEOMORPHIC SARCOMAS

The vast majority of the neoplasms in this category are undifferentiated pleomorphic sarcomas (previously termed malignant fibrous histiocytomas) and pleomorphic liposarcomas.[1,2,15,39,65-68] However, many other sarcomas may occasionally enter the differential diagnosis. For example, bizarre giant cells may be a component of high-grade leiomyosarcomas.[54] In aspirate smears, pleomorphic sarcomas are almost always readily recognized as malignant and often as sarcomatous at low magnification. The direct smears are extremely cellular with little tendency for the malignant cells to aggregate.[1,2] An admixture of small, round cells with high nuclear-to-cytoplasmic ratios, large spindled or polygonal cells with scant to moderate volumes of cytoplasm, and numerous bizarre tumor giant cells may be observed within a single field (Figs. 5-13 and 5-14). The giant cells contain hyperchromatic, multilobated nuclei, often with huge nucleoli, and typically have moderate to abundant cytoplasm with cell borders that blend imperceptibly into the background. The latter frequently contains necrotic debris. In general, based solely on morphology, it is impossible to distinguish among the different pleomorphic sarcomas on smears. However, this limitation generally does not hinder subsequent clinical management of most patients, as emphasized by Fleshman.[15]

The most common entities in the differential diagnosis are pleomorphic carcinomas of diverse sites. Notable examples are giant cell or sarcomatoid carcinomas of the lung, kidney, thyroid, and pancreas. On the basis of cytomorphology alone, some of these aspirates may be completely indistinguishable from those of sarcomas. In addition to clinical history, the smears should be carefully searched for the presence of residual epithelial differentiation in the form of cohesive aggregates (including glands and papillae) of carcinoma cells with polygonal to columnar contours. Other malignancies that may fall into this morphologic pattern include melanoma, sarcomatoid mesothelioma, and anaplastic large-cell lymphoma. A few benign entities also need to be considered, including pleomorphic lipoma, ancient schwannoma, and proliferative fasciitis/myositis (Fig. 5-15).[55,56,63,69] In most instances, when the clinical data are integrated with the aspiration cytomorphology, the correct interpretation can be rendered. Although less likely to be overdiagnosed as sarcoma,

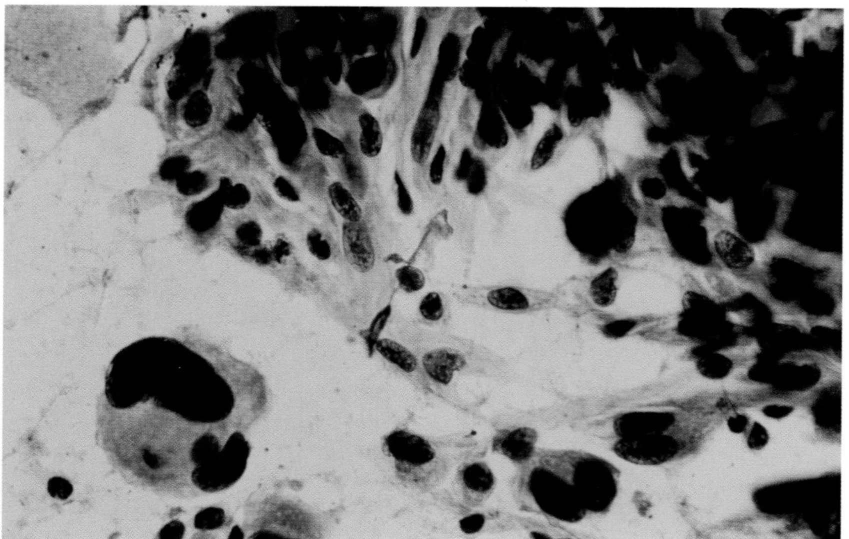

FIGURE 5-13. Undifferentiated pleomorphic sarcoma. Marked variability in the sizes and appearances of the malignant cells is apparent. Some tumor cells are relatively small with solitary hyperchromatic nuclei and inapparent cytoplasm. Others are larger with more polygonal or spindled shapes. Also present are several multinucleated tumor giant cells that have two or more extremely darkly stained nuclei and moderate-to-voluminous cytoplasm. Note that in several of the tumor giant cells, the nuclei form a characteristic acute angle with each other. (Papanicolaou stain, ×400.)

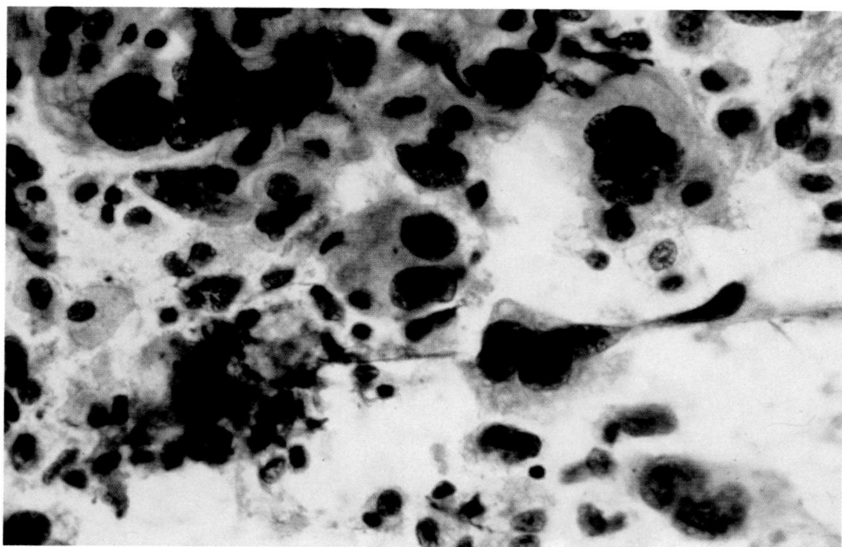

FIGURE 5-14. Undifferentiated pleomorphic sarcoma. Striking hyperchromasia and pleomorphism characterize the neoplastic nuclei and cells. Multinucleated tumor giant cells, some with bizarre appearances, are evident in association with malignant cells having a more histiocytoid appearance. (Papanicolaou stain, ×400.)

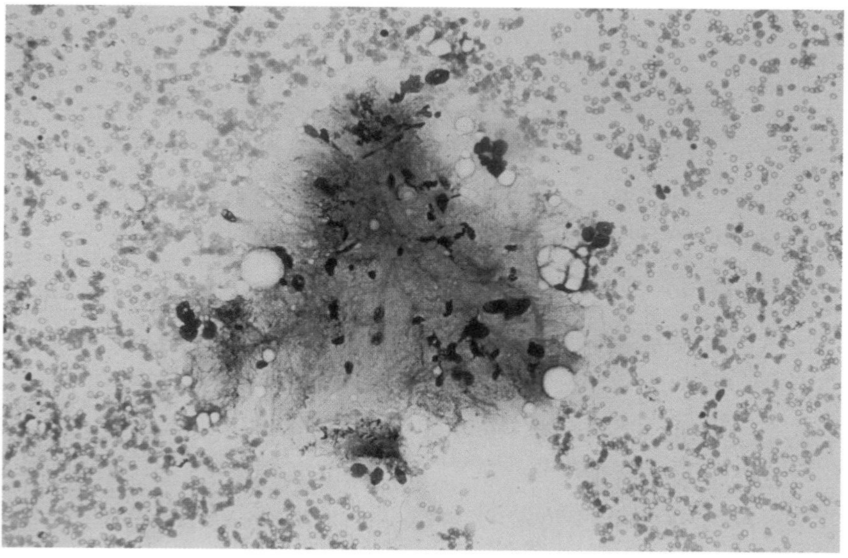

FIGURE 5-15. Pleomorphic lipoma. Scant cellularity characterizes this aspirate. Although most of the cells are small with solitary nuclei and apparently high nuclear-to-cytoplasmic ratios, others are larger. They vary from spindled to multinucleated tumor giant cells. A few neoplastic cells have prominent cytoplasmic lipid vacuoles. (Diff-Quik stain, ×40.)

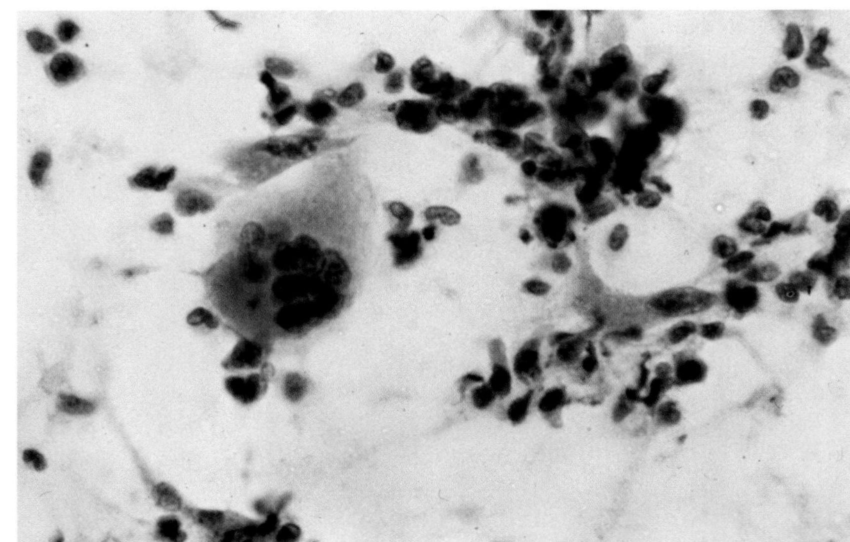

FIGURE 5-16. Giant cell tumor of tendon sheath. In contrast to the pleomorphic sarcomas, the nuclei within the giant cells are much smaller and more homogeneous. They have fine, even chromatin and small but distinct nucleoli. These giant cells have much more abundant cytoplasm and therefore lower nuclear-to-cytoplasmic ratios. In the proper clinical setting, this should never be confused with a pleomorphic sarcoma. (Papanicolaou stain, ×100.)

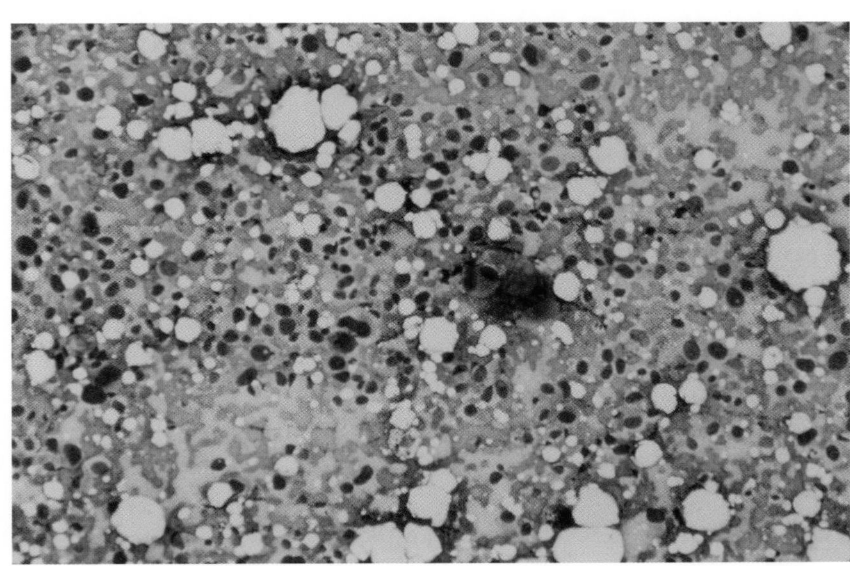

FIGURE 5-17. Clear cell sarcoma. Both high cellularity and a lack of cohesion characterize this aspirate. Most cells have large single nuclei with prominent nucleoli. A few larger and multinucleated neoplastic cells are also evident. (Diff-Quik stain, ×40.)

giant cell tumors of tendon sheath also need to be considered (Fig. 5-16).[1,70,71]

POLYGONAL CELL SARCOMAS

The least frequent of the FNAB categories of sarcomas is the polygonal or epithelial-like group. This includes epithelioid sarcoma, clear cell sarcoma, alveolar soft part sarcoma, malignant granular cell tumors, and the predominantly epithelioid types of other sarcomas (e.g., gastrointestinal stromal tumor and angiosarcoma).[1,2,45,46,72-79] Although smear cellularity is variable, it is usually moderate to high, often with a largely dissociative pattern. The smears contain numerous individually dispersed malignant cells and small, generally flat aggregates (Figs. 5-17 and 5-18). The tumor cells have round or polygonal shapes, well-defined cellular borders, and at least a moderate volume of cytoplasm (Fig. 5-19). Typically, they possess a solitary, often eccentrically positioned, round nucleus with a thick, distinct membrane, vesicular chromatin, and one or more large nucleoli. A small proportion of the neoplastic cells may be binucleated or even multinucleated. Alternatively, some cells have a spindled contour. In addition to subtle cytologic clues, an accurate clinical history and a judicious use of immunocytochemistry will allow distinction among these neoplasms.

Lemos et al. claim that a preoperative diagnosis of epithelioid sarcoma may be generated when the appropriate morphology and immunohistochemistry occurs in the proper clinical setting.[77] Features emphasized by them included a mixture of polygonal and spindled tumor cells with clearly malignant nuclei and voluminous dense cytoplasm mixed with an eosinophilic fibrillar material. In contrast to many mesenchymal lesions, the cells possessed well-defined borders.

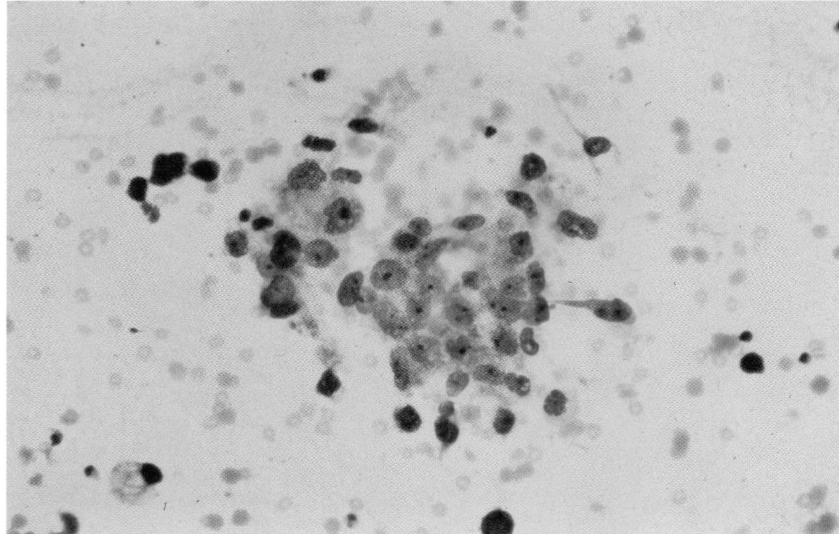

FIGURE 5-18. Epithelioid sarcoma. This cohesive aggregate has a distinct epithelioid appearance with the maintenance of cohesion, polygonal cell contours, and peripherally situated round nuclei. Nucleoli are also strikingly prominent. (Diff-Quik stain, ×250.)

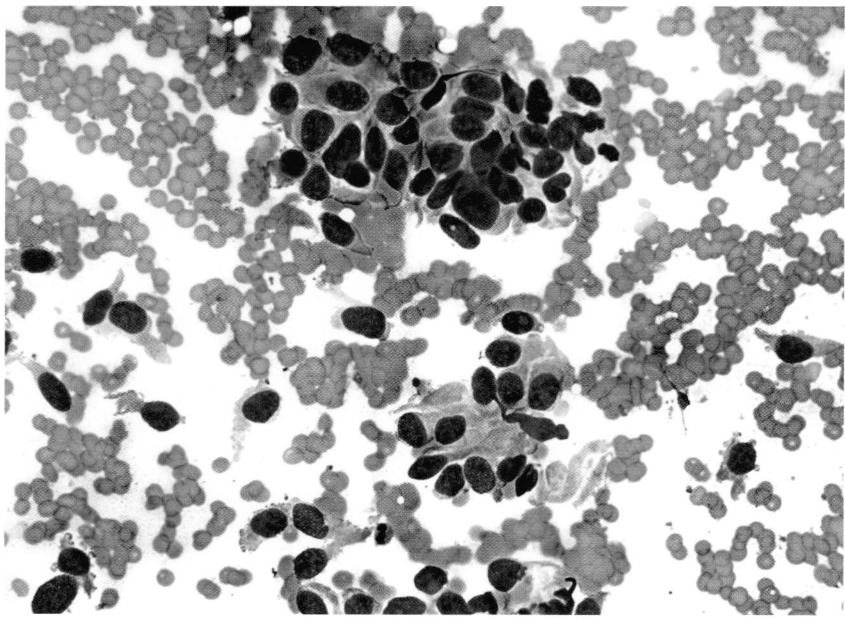

FIGURE 5-19. Epithelioid angiosarcoma. Polygonally contoured tumor cells with large nuclei, often with very prominent nucleoli, have high nuclear-to-cytoplasmic ratios. A minority of the neoplastic elements has blunt spindled shapes. This is not morphologically diagnostic for angiosarcoma. (Diff-Quik stain, ×200.)

The helpful immunoprofile was the coexpression of epithelial markers (keratin and epithelial membrane antigen), vimentin and CD34.

Although the characteristic cytoplasmic crystals of alveolar soft part sarcoma are recognized in only a minority of aspirates and there is overlap in morphology with other entities, some authors have been able to render specific diagnoses of this entity on aspiration specimens, again within the context of the proper clinical scenario and the results of ancillary testing. Features typical of the neoplasm include very large polygonal cells with abundant granular to vacuolated cytoplasm, numerous stripped nuclei, macronucleoli, cytoplasmic syncytia housing several neoplastic nuclei, and a background of granular material and/or obvious blood. Although Agarwal et al. found alveolar structures with some frequency in their specimens; Wakely et al. did not.[74,75]

In clear cell sarcoma, the cytoplasm may present as optically clear or pale staining.[72] Useful diagnostic attributes include nuclear pseudoinclusions and cytoplasmic melanin pigment.

It may be impossible in cytologic samples to distinguish between benign and malignant granular cell tumors because the latter may manifest little or no morphologic evidence of a potential for aggressive behavior. The same is true for histologic specimens, especially small samples such as core biopsies. In many of the rare granular cell tumors that prove to be sarcomatous, the nuclei have essentially the same appearance as their benign counterparts.

The differential diagnosis is rather limited. It includes carcinoma or melanoma metastatic to soft tissue. In smears, a greater degree of intercellular cohesion, large cytoplasmic vacuoles, and three-dimensional aggregates favor

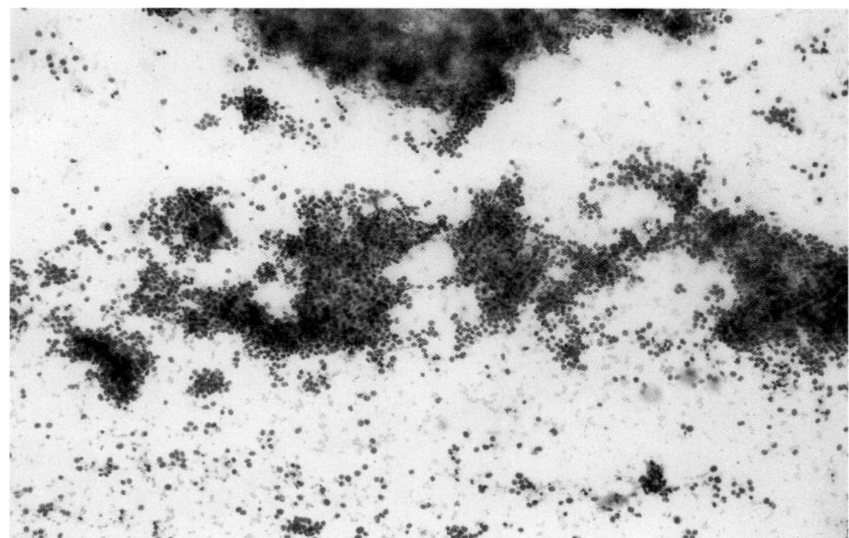

FIGURE 5-20. Alveolar rhabdomyosarcoma. High smear cellularity is apparent, with many of the tumor cells present in loosely cohesive fragments. This almost suggests a pseudoalveolar arrangement. In addition, individually dispersed neoplastic cells are evident. Even at this very low magnification, the striking uniformity of the cells is evident. Each cell possesses a solitary round nucleus that is surrounded by only a scanty rim of cytoplasm. (Diff-Quik stain, ×20.)

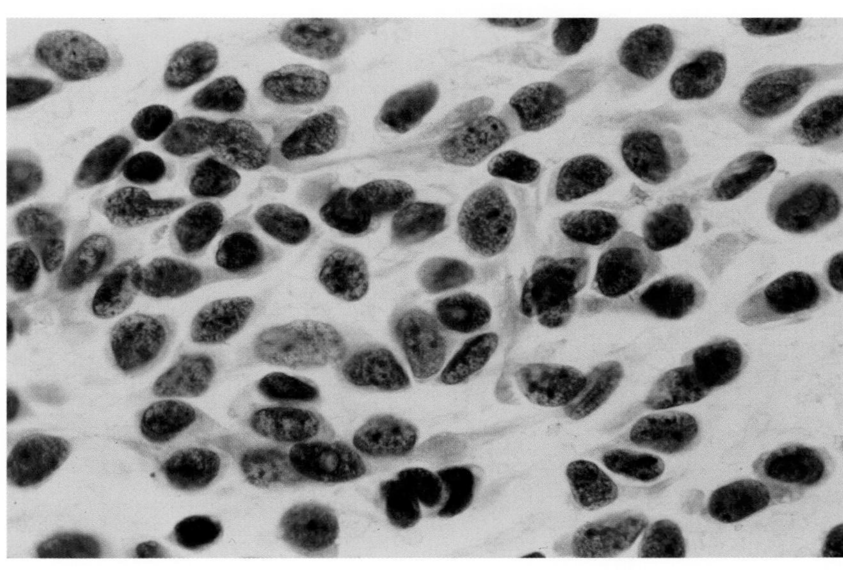

FIGURE 5-21. Embryonal rhabdomyosarcoma. Smear cellularity is high, and cohesion is poorly preserved. The neoplastic cells are quite homogeneous in appearance. Each has a single ovoid nucleus with fine, even, hyperchromatic chromatin and minute nucleoli. Most cells possess scant cytoplasm in which the nucleus appears to be eccentrically positioned. A few tumor cells have long tapering cytoplasmic tails. (Hematoxylin and eosin, ×400.)

metastatic carcinoma. As always, an accurate clinical history is paramount.

ROUND CELL SARCOMAS

Round cell sarcomas predominate in the pediatric population and young adults, and include rhabdomyosarcoma, the Ewing family of tumors (EFT), and intra-abdominal desmoplastic small round cell tumor (DSRCT).[1,2,21,80-88] Aspiration biopsies of these neoplasms typically yield highly cellular smears (although DSRCT may be less so) composed of relatively small, homogeneous malignant cells (Figs. 5-20 to 5-24). The tumor cells have solitary hyperchromatic nuclei with a high nuclear-to-cytoplasmic ratio. In embryonal rhabdomyosarcoma, however, a portion may have abundant cytoplasm and multiple nuclei (see Fig. 5-22). Tumor cells with cytoplasmic tails may be seen in any of these neoplasms. Although nucleoli are usually inconspicuous in EFT and DSRCT (see Fig. 5-23), they are more apt to be well developed in rhabdomyosarcoma. Within a given specimen, uniformity of the cells is expected in the former two neoplasms, whereas pleomorphism is quite variable in the last. This is the category in which ancillary diagnostic tests, performed on aspirated cellular material, are most helpful in determining an exact tumor type.

The major differential diagnosis is extranodal, primary non-Hodgkin B-cell lymphoma.[89] These tumors almost never demonstrate any evidence of true intercellular cohesion. The cells tend to be homogeneous with round to irregular nuclear membranes, variably prominent nucleoli, and scant cytoplasm. Lymphoglandular bodies are numerous in the background.

MISCELLANEOUS SARCOMAS

A neoplasm that does not fit into any of the previous categories is well-differentiated liposarcoma (atypical lipomatous neoplasm).[1,2,65,67,68] The aspiration cytomorphology of this neoplasm has only rarely been detailed. At best, smears are

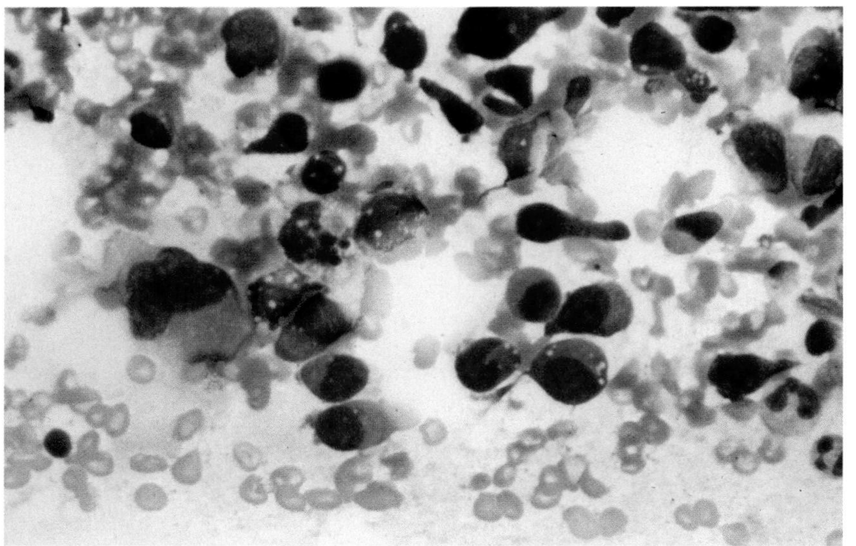

FIGURE 5-22. Embryonal rhabdomyosarcoma. A spectrum of cellular appearances is apparent. Most of the cells have solitary small round nuclei and rather high nuclear-to-cytoplasmic ratios. A tadpole cell is evident in the center of the field. Also note the presence of a large multinucleated tumor giant cell and the absence of intercellular cohesion. (Diff-Quik stain, ×400.)

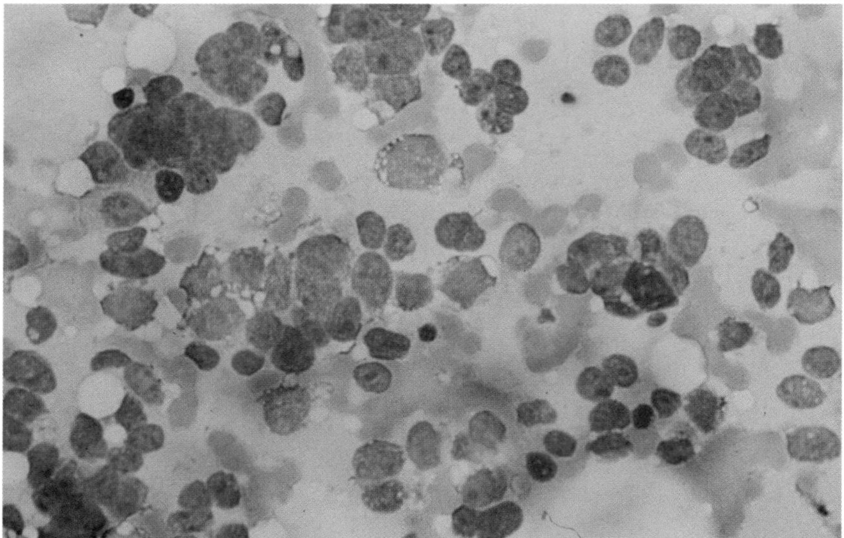

FIGURE 5-23. Primitive neuroectodermal tumor. Each malignant cell has a single round nucleus with very finely reticulated and evenly dispersed chromatin. For the most part, nucleoli are inconspicuous. In many cells, cytoplasm is barely visible, whereas others have small-to-large glycogen vacuoles. The presence of cohesion and the lack of lymphoglandular bodies help distinguish this from lymphoma. (Diff-Quik stain, ×400.)

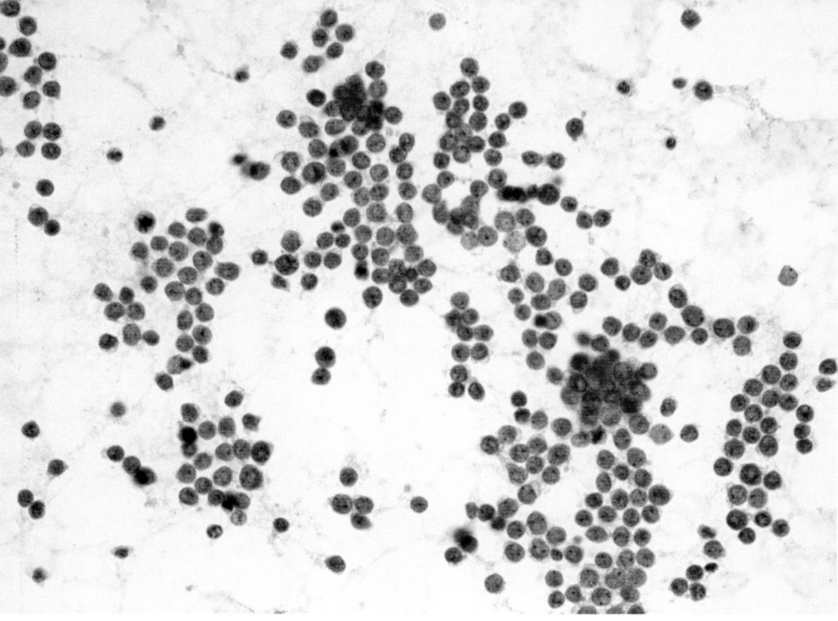

FIGURE 5-24. EFT. Numerous homogeneous neoplastic cells have perfectly round small nuclei, fine even dark chromatin, inconspicuous nucleoli, and exceedingly high nuclear-to-cytoplasmic ratios. Note the lack of lymphoglandular bodies. (Papanicolaou stain, ×40.)

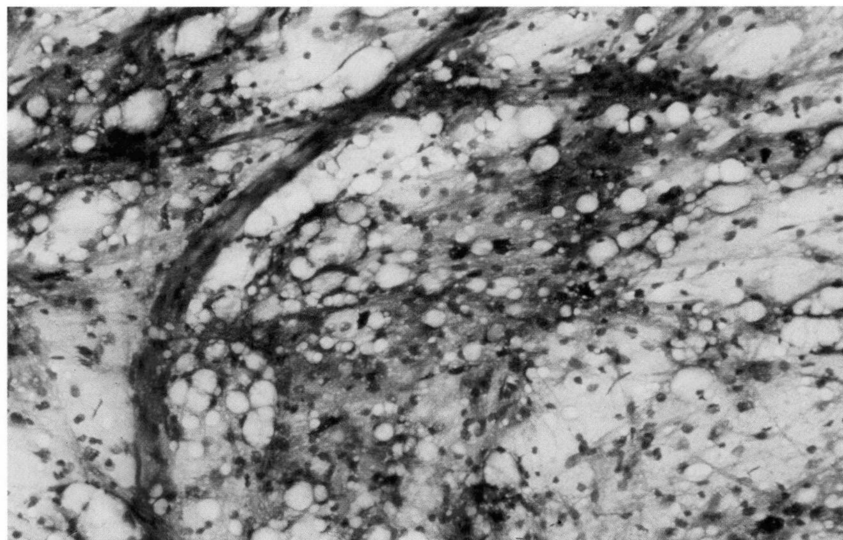

FIGURE 5-25. Well-differentiated liposarcoma. Unremarkable-appearing adipocytes are embedded within fibrous connective tissue. In addition, however, scattered cells have much larger nuclei. Some of these also appear to have cytoplasmic lipid vacuoles. In the proper clinical setting, this is diagnostic of liposarcoma. Vascularity is prominent. (Diff-Quik stain, ×100.)

moderately cellular, and the sample may be mistaken for benign adipose tissue because it is composed mostly of fragments of mature-appearing fat cells (Fig. 5-25). The diagnosis of liposarcoma requires the finding of unequivocal lipoblasts with cytoplasmic lipid vacuoles that compress and distort the nucleus. The distinction from lipoblastomatosis is not possible, based solely on the smear findings; here, patient age is critical. As a generalization, it is not preferable to perform only aspiration biopsies of tumors of adipose tissue because, often, one may not be capable of separating a lipoma from a well-differentiated liposarcoma.

Other neoplasms that may fall into this category are gastrointestinal stromal tumor and angiosarcoma.[45,46,50] Paralleling their histologic appearances, these neoplasms may show a spectrum of cell contours, ranging from almost completely spindled to pure epithelioid cells. Many will contain a combination of the two cell types, as well as transitional forms.

ACCURACY OF FINE-NEEDLE ASPIRATION

Only a few series with large numbers of patients have addressed the diagnostic accuracy of FNAB of soft tissue neoplasms.[1,3-5,9,12-14,90] There is a lack of standardization among these reports. Some studies have included patients with both benign and malignant neoplasms, whereas others have addressed only sarcomas or benign entities. Some series are dedicated to the primary diagnosis of a mass, whereas others include patients with recurrent or metastatic sarcomas. Several investigations have included aspiration biopsies of soft tissue and bone lesions, and it is not always clear as to how these statistical data are subdivided. Some authors have provided only the number of patients or specimens, whereas others have reported the levels of diagnostic sensitivity and specificity, rates of false-negative and false-positive diagnoses, or both.

Khalbuss et al. have published the largest series with 841 soft tissue lesions sampled, but their series also included 273 bone aspirates; much of their data is intertwined between the two tissue types.[90] They reported a sensitivity and specificity of 96% and 98%, respectively. However, as with some other publications, obvious limitations must be recognized: most malignancies were metastatic carcinomas, and sarcomas accounted for only 20% of the cancers. Further, of the sarcomas, a primary diagnosis had been rendered before the aspirate in 45%, so that many of these were recurrences or metastases.

Akerman and Willen evaluated 517 patients with an aspirate for a primary diagnosis of a soft tissue neoplasm; of these, 315 were benign and 202 were sarcomas.[14] This is the largest published series with this specific focus. The authors were able to distinguish benign from malignant in 94% of the patients. Their errors were equally divided between false-negative and false-positive diagnoses (14 each). As is the experience for many individuals, their area of greatest difficulty was spindle-cell neoplasms, followed by lipomatous tumors.

Brosjö et al. evaluated 342 patients with a relatively equal distribution between benign and malignant soft tissue tumors.[4] The cytologic diagnosis was conclusive in 300 patients (88%). There was a 5% false-negative rate among the 153 benign cytologic diagnoses, and a 2% false-positive rate among the 147 malignant interpretations. Therefore, a correct diagnosis was rendered in 97% of this population.

Oland et al. reported their experience with 196 patients who underwent FNAB of a soft tissue mass.[80] Patients who had a benign cytologic diagnosis (tumor or inflammation) were followed clinically. Sixteen were diagnosed with metastatic carcinoma without subsequent surgery. A total of 48 patients underwent histologic examination of their masses following the aspiration biopsy, and all 25 cytologic diagnoses of frank sarcoma were confirmed; therefore, there were no false-positive interpretations. Of the 17 benign soft tissue tumors diagnosed by cytology, 1 was a false-negative interpretation.

Jakowski et al. examined aspiration biopsies of palpable masses of a specific location, namely, the distal extremities; this included soft tissue and bony lesions.[43] Their specificity and sensitivity for malignancy were 96% and 100%, respectively.

Liu et al. examined a series of 89 aspirates that included samples from 20 benign and 69 malignant masses, including 11 metastatic melanomas.[9] Each aspirate was independently evaluated by four pathologists who differed in their years of experience. Each evaluated these specimens in two settings:

without and then later with the appropriate clinical history. In each of these two scenarios, each pathologist provided a precise cytopathologic diagnosis and classified the smears into one of four categories: benign, probably benign, probably malignant, and malignant. The data were then analyzed to create receiver operator characteristics curves. Without the benefit of clinical history, the proportion of correct diagnoses ranged from 0.19 to 0.44. With the addition of clinical history, the proportion of accurate interpretations was improved to a range of 0.48 to 0.66. The proportion of correct diagnoses improved for all four pathologists. Difficulty was especially noted for benign spindle cell neoplasms.[80]

GRADING AND FINE-NEEDLE ASPIRATION

As soon as a lesion is determined to be a sarcoma, the ability to grade it accurately is important. Despite the relative prognostic value of grade, little attention has been paid to this topic. One of the most detailed studies was by Palmer et al.[28] Their three-tiered cytologic grading scheme was an expansion of the one used by Weir et al.[26] Palmer used several criteria, including cellularity (and related nuclear overlap), variability in nuclear sizes, nuclear membrane irregularities, chromatin patterns, and nucleolar prominence.[28] When their grades were collapsed into a two-level system (1 versus 2 + 3), correlation with the histologic grade occurred in 90% of specimens. Most of their noncorrelations resulted in undergrading in aspirates, especially with myxoid tumors. As stated earlier, many find the spindle cell category to be the most problematic. Jones et al. graded a series of 107 sarcomas, which included bone neoplasms; although they did not specify the exact origin of their specimens, it would appear that at least one-third were osseous in type.[29] The authors found a tendency among observers to undergrade in aspiration smears compared to the histologic grade (only 72% had corresponding histology for comparison). These authors found only the degree of nuclear atypia in smears to correlate with histologic grade. To reemphasize, histologic grading of sarcomas relies in part on the mitotic figure count and the degree of necrosis; such cannot be determined accurately in smears.

CONCLUSIONS

FNAB of soft tissue neoplasms has important limitations. Samples may be limited in cellularity to the point of being insufficient for a diagnosis, because soft tissue neoplasms have several attributes that may lead to poor cellularity on the smear. There are certain neoplasms in which a benign versus malignant designation cannot be made with certainty from FNAB. In addition, it may be impossible to predict the grade on the basis of the smear preparation; this is most commonly encountered with the spindle cell neoplasms. Based purely on cytomorphology, the exact cell type of many soft tissue neoplasms cannot be stated accurately; this is more likely with adult rather than childhood tumors. However, many of these problems are obviated by the use of ancillary diagnostic procedures on aspirated cellular material.

Still, FNAB of soft tissue neoplasms possesses a number of advantages that overall outweigh the disadvantages. Aspiration biopsy is easily performed in the outpatient setting and, compared to other diagnostic procedures, is relatively inexpensive. Aspiration biopsy provides a rapid, relatively nontraumatic procedure for sampling both superficial and deep-seated mass lesions. Soft tissue neoplasms can be recognized and accurately designated as benign or malignant in many instances. Multiple samples can also be obtained during a single clinical visit, thereby increasing the likelihood of specimen adequacy, including tissue for ancillary tests. Grading of sarcomas in aspiration smears needs more investigative work. However, it does appear that in many patients, morphologic grading by cytology is valid, using some criteria different from those used in histopathology.

Obtaining both an aspiration and a CNB from the same mass may frequently prove more helpful because the two procedures yield diagnostically complementary specimens. The core may well be a better substrate for ancillary procedures. Doing both during the same patient visit adds little time and cost but may expedite appropriate care for many individuals.

References

1. Geisinger KR, Stanley MW, Raab SS, et al. Soft tissue and bone. In: Modern Cytopathology. Philadelphia: Churchill Livingstone: Elsevier; 2004. p. 813.
2. Nicolas MM, Nayar R, Abdul-Karim F. Soft tissue. In: Sidawy MK, Ali SZ, editors. Fine needle aspiration cytology. Churchill Livingstone: Elsevier; 2007.
3. Akerman M, Rydholm A, Persson BM. Aspiration cytology of soft tissue tumors: the 10-year experience of an orthopedic oncology center. Acta Orthop Scand 1985;56:407.
4. Brosjö O, Bauer HCF, Kreisbergers A, et al. Fine needle aspiration biopsy of soft tissue tumors. Acta Orthop Scand 1994;65(Suppl. 256):108.
5. Costa MJ, Campman SC, Davis RL, et al. Fine-needle aspiration cytology of sarcoma: retrospective review of diagnostic utility and specificity. Diagn Cytopathol 1996;15:23.
6. Layfield LJ, Liu K, Dodge RK. Logistic regression analysis of small round cell neoplasms: a cytologic study. Diagn Cytopathol 1999;20:271.
7. Liu K, Dodge RK, Dodd LG, et al. Logistic regression analysis of low grade spindle cell lesions. A cytologic study. Acta Cytol 1999;43:143.
8. Liu K, Dodge RK, Layfield LJ. Logistic regression analysis of high grade spindle cell neoplasms. A fine needle aspiration cytologic study. Acta Cytol 1999;43:593.
9. Liu K, Layfield LJ, Coogan AC, et al. Diagnostic accuracy in fine-needle aspiration of soft tissue and bone lesions. Influence of clinical history and experience. Am J Clin Pathol 1999;111:632.
10. Willén H, Akerman M, Carlén B. Fine needle aspiration (FNA) in the diagnosis of soft tissue tumours: a review of 22 years experience. Cytopathology 1995;6:236.
11. Wakely PE Jr, Kineisl JS. Soft tissue aspiration cytopathology. Cancer Cytopathol 2000;90(5):292.
12. Nagira K, Yamamoto T, Akisue T, et al. Reliability of fine-needle aspiration biopsy in the initial diagnosis of soft-tissue lesions. Diagn Cytopathol 2002;27(6):354.
13. Dey P, Mallik MK, Gupta SK, et al. Role of fine needle aspiration cytology in the diagnosis of soft tissue tumours and tumour-like lesions. Cytopathology 2004;15:32.
14. Akerman M, Willen H. Critical review of the role of fine needle aspiration in soft tissue tumors. Pathol Case Rev 1998;3:111.
15. Fleshman R, Mayerson J, Wakely PG Jr. Fine needle aspiration biopsy of high-grade sarcoma: a report of 107 cases. Cancer Cytopathol 2007;111:491.
16. Rekhi B, Bhatnagar D, Bhatnagar A, et al. Cytomorphological study of soft tissue neoplasms: role of fluorescent immunocytochemistry in diagnosis. Cytopathology 2005;16:219.
17. Kilpatrick SE, Bergman S, Pettenati MJ, et al. The usefulness of cytogenetic analysis in fine needle aspirates for the histologic subtyping of sarcomas. Modern Pathol 2006;19:815.
18. Geisinger KR, Silverman JF, Cappellari JO, et al. Fine-needle aspiration cytology of malignant hemangiopericytomas with ultrastructural and flow cytometric analyses. Arch Pathol Lab Med 1990;114:705.

19. Akhtar M, Ashraf AM, Sabbah R, et al. Small round cell tumor with divergent differentiation: cytologic, histologic and ultrastructural findings. Diagn Cytopathol 1994;11:159.
20. Alkan S, Eltoum IA, Tabbara S, et al. Usefulness of molecular detection of human herpesvirus-8 in the diagnosis of Kaposi sarcoma by fine-needle aspiration. Am J Clin Pathol 1999;111:91.
21. Sanati S, Lu DW, Schmidt E, et al. Cytologic diagnosis of Ewing sarcoma/peripheral neuroectodermal tumor with paired prospective molecular genetic analysis. Cancer Cytopathol 2007;111:192.
22. Akerman M, Ryd W, Skytting B. Fine-needle aspiration of synovial sarcoma: criteria for diagnosis: retrospective reexamination of 37 cases, including ancillary diagnostics. A Scandinavian Sarcoma Group study. Diagn Cytopathol 2003;28:232.
23. Kilpatrick SE, Ward WG, Cappellari JO, et al. Fine-needle aspiration biopsy of soft tissue sarcomas: a cytomorphologic analysis with emphasis on histologic subtyping, grading and therapeutic significance. Am J Clin Pathol 1999;112:179.
24. Kilpatrick SE, Cappellari JO, Bos GD, et al. Is fine needle aspiration biopsy a practical alternative to open biopsy for the primary diagnosis of sarcoma? Experience with 140 patients. Am J Clin Pathol 2001;115(1):59.
25. Guillou L, Coindre J-M. How should we grade soft tissue sarcomas and what are the limitations? Pathol Case Rev 1998;3:105.
26. Weir MM, Rosenberg AE, Bell DA. Grading of spindle cell sarcomas in fine-needle aspiration biopsy specimens. Am J Clin Pathol 1999;112:784.
27. Mathur S, Kapila K, Verma K. Accuracy of cytologic grading of spindle-cell sarcomas. Diagn Cytopathol 2003;29:79.
28. Palmer HE, Mukunyadzi P, Culbreth W, et al. Subgrouping and grading of soft-tissue sarcomas by fine-needle aspiration cytology: a histopathologic correlation study. Diagn Cytopathol 2001;24:307.
29. Jones C, Leu K, Hirschowitz S, et al. Concordance of histopathologic and cytologic grading in musculoskeletal sarcomas: can grades obtained from analysis of the fine-needle aspirates serve as the basis for therapeutic decisions? Cancer Cytopathol 2002;96:83.
30. Yang YJ, Damron TA. Comparison of needle core biopsy and fine needle aspiration for diagnostic accuracy in musculoskeletal lesions. Arch Pathol Lab Med 2004;128:759.
31. Domanski HA, Akerman M, Carlen B, et al. Core-needle biopsy performed by the cytopathologist: a technique to complement fine-needle aspiration of soft tissue and bone lesions. Cancer Cytopathol 2005;105:229.
32. Gonzalez-Campora R, Otal-Salaverri C, Helvia-Vazquez A, et al. Fine needle aspiration in myxoid tumors of the soft tissues. Acta Cytol 1990;34:179.
33. Wakely PE Jr, Geisinger KR, Cappellari JO, et al. Fine-needle aspiration cytopathology of soft tissue: chondromyxoid and myxoid lesions. Diagn Cytopathol 1995;12:101.
34. Szadowska A, Lasota J. Fine needle aspiration cytology of myxoid liposarcoma: a study of 18 tumors. Cytopathology 1993;4:99.
35. Kloboves-Prevodnik VV, Us-Krasovec M, Gale N, et al. Cytologic features of lipoblastoma: a report of three cases. Diagn Cytopathol 2005;33:195.
36. Colin P, Legacè R, Cailland J-M, et al. Fine-needle aspiration in myxofibrosarcoma: experience of Institut Curie. Diagn Cytopathol 2010;38:343.
37. Jakowski JD, Wakely PE Jr. Cytopathology of extraskeletal myxoid chondrosarcoma: a report of 8 cases. Cancer Cytopathol 2007;111:298.
38. Dawamneh MF, Amra NK, Amr SS. Low grade fibromyxoid sarcoma: a report of a case with fine needle aspiration cytology and histologic correlation. Acta Cytol 2006;50:208.
39. Klijanienko J, Cailland J-M, Lagace R, et al. Comparative fine-needle aspiration and pathologic study of malignant fibrous histiocytoma: cytodiagnosis of 95 tumors in 71 patients. Diagn Cytopathol 2003;29:320.
40. Wakely PE Jr, Bos GD, Mayerson I. The cytopathology of soft tissue myxomas: ganglia, juxta-articular myxoid lesions, and intramuscular myxoma. Am J Clin Pathol 2005;123:858.
41. Lopez-Ferver P, Jimenez-Heffernan JA, Yebenes L, et al. Fine-needle aspiration cytology of lipoblastoma: a report of two cases. Diagn Cytopathol 2005;32:32.
42. Damanski HA. Fine-needle aspiration cytology of soft tissue lesions: diagnostic challenges. Diagn Cytopathol 2009;35:368.
43. Jakowski JD, Meyerson J, Wakely PE Jr. Fine-needle aspiration biopsy of the distal extremities: a study of 141 cases. Am J Clin Pathol 2010; 133:224.
44. Powers CN, Berardo MD, Frable WJ. Fine needle aspiration biopsy: pitfalls in the diagnosis of spindle-cell lesions. Diagn Cytopathol 1994; 10:232.
45. Boucher LD, Swanson PE, Stanley MW, et al. Fine-needle aspiration of angiosarcoma. Acta Cytol 1998;42:1289.
46. Klijanienko J, Calliwad JM, Lagace R, et al. Cytohistologic correlations in angiosarcoma, including classic and epithelioid variants: Institut Curie's experience. Diag Cytopathol 2003;29:140.
47. Barbazza R, Chiarelli S, Quintarelli GF, et al. Role of fine-needle aspiration cytology in the preoperative evolution of smooth muscle tumors. Diagn Cytopathol 1997;16:326.
48. Gupta K, Dey P, Vasahist R. Fine-needle aspiration cytology of malignant peripheral nerve sheath tumors. Diagn Cytopathol 2004;31(1):1.
49. Klijanienko J, Cailland J-M, Lagacé R, et al. Cytohistologic correlations of 24 malignant peripheral nerve sheath tumor (MPNST) in 17 patients: the Institut Curie experience. Diagn Cytopathol 2002;27:103.
50. Elliott DD, Fanning CV, Caraway NP. The utility of fine-needle aspiration in the diagnosis of gastrointestinal stromal tumors. Cancer Cytopathol 2006;108(1):49.
51. Hales M, Bottles K, Miller T, et al. Diagnosis of Kaposi's sarcoma by fine-needle aspiration biopsy. Am J Clin Pathol 1987;88:20.
52. Viguer JM, Jiménez-Heffernan JA, Vicandi B, et al. Cytologic features of synovial sarcoma with emphasis on the monophasic fibrous variant: a morphologic and immunocytochemical analysis of bcl-2 protein expression. Cancer Cytopathol 1998;84:50.
53. Klijanienko J, Cailland J-M, Lagacé R, et al. Cytohistologic correlations in 56 synovial sarcomas in 36 patients: the Institut Curie experience. Diagn Cytopathol 2002;27:96.
54. Domonski HA, Akerman M, Rissler P, et al. Fine-needle aspiration of soft tissue leiomyosarcoma: an analysis of the most common cytologic findings and the value of ancillary techniques. Diagn Cytopathol 2006; 34:597.
55. Wong NL, Di F. Pseudosarcomatous fasciitis and myositis. Diagnosis by fine-needle aspiration cytology. Am J Clin Pathol 2009;132:857.
56. Kong CS, Cha I. Nodular fasciitis. Diagnosis by fine needle aspiration biopsy. Acta Cytol 2004;48:473.
57. Dalèn BPM, Meis-Kindblom JM, Sumathi VP, et al. Fine-needle aspiration cytology and core biopsy of the preoperative diagnosis of desmoid tumors. Aeta Orthopaedica 2006;77:926.
58. Owens C, Sharma R, Ali SZ. Deep fibromatosis (desmoid tumor): cytopathologic characteristics, clinicoradiologic features, and immunohistochemical findings on fine-needle aspiration. Cancer Cytopathol 2007; 111:166.
59. Lindberg GM, Maitra A, Gokaslan ST, et al. Low grade fibromyxoid sarcoma: fine-needle aspiration cytology with histologic, cytogenetic, immunohistochemical, and ultrastructural correlation. Cancer Cytopathol 1999;87:75.
60. Ewing CA, Zakowski MF, Lin O. Monophasic synovial sarcoma: a cytologic spectrum. Diagn Cytopathol 2004;30(1):19.
61. Domanski HA. FNA diagnosis of dermatofibroma protuberans. Diagn Cytopathol 2005;32:299.
62. Resnick JM, Fanning CV, Caraway NP, et al. Percutaneous needle biopsy diagnosis of benign neurogenic neoplasms. Diagn Cytopathol 1997;16:17.
63. Dodd LG, Marom EM, Dash RC, et al. Fine-needle aspiration cytology of "ancient" schwannoma. Diagn Cytopathol 1999;20:307.
64. Henke AC, Salomão DR, Hughes JH. Cellular schwannoma mimics a sarcoma: an example of a potential pitfall in aspiration cytodiagnosis. Diagn Cytopathol 1999;30:312.
65. Walaas L, Kindblom LG. Lipomatous tumors: a correlative cytologic and histologic study of 27 tumors examined by fine needle aspiration cytology. Hum Pathol 1985;16:6.
66. Walaas L, Angervall L, Hagmar B, et al. A correlative cytologic and histologic study of malignant fibrous histiocytoma: an analysis of 40 cases examined by fine needle aspiration cytology. Diagn Cytopathol 1986;2:46.
67. Nemanqani D, Mourad WA. Cytomorphologic features of fine-needle aspiration of liposarcoma. Diagn Cytopathol 1999;20:67.
68. Einarsdottir H, Skoog L, Soderlund V, et al. Accuracy of cytology for diagnosis of lipomatous tumors: comparison with magnetic resonance and computed tomography findings in 175 cases. Acta Radiol 2004; 45(8):840.
69. Yang M, Raza AS, Greaves TS, et al. Fine-needle aspiration of a pleomorphic lipoma of the head and neck: a case report. Diagn Cytopathol 2005;32:110.
70. Iyer VK, Kapila K, Verma K. Fine-needle aspiration cytology of giant cell tumor of tendon sheath. Diagn Cytopathol 2003;29(2):105.
71. Gupta K, Dey P, Goldsmith R, et al. Comparison of cytologic features of giant-cell tumor and giant-cell tumor of tendon sheath. Diagn Cytopathol 2004;30:14.

72. Creager AJ, Pitman MB, Geisinger KR. Cytologic features of clear cell sarcoma (malignant melanoma) of soft parts. A study of fine-needle aspirates and exfoliative specimens. Am J Clin Pathol 2002;117:217.
73. Lin O, Olgac S, Zakowski M. Cytological features of epithelioid mesenchymal neoplasms: a study of 21 cases. Diagn Cytopathol 2005;32:5.
74. Wakely PE Jr, McDermott JE, Ali SZ. Cytopathology of alveolar soft part sarcoma: a report of 10 cases. Cancer Cytopathol 2009;117:500.
75. Agarwal S, Gupta R, Iyer VK, et al. Cytopathological diagnosis of alveolar soft part sarcoma, a rare soft tissue neoplasm. Cytopathology 2011; 22:318.
76. Pohar-Marinsek Z, Zidar A. Epithelioid sarcoma in FNAB smears. Diagn Cytopathol 1994;11:367.
77. Lemos MM, Chaves P, Mendanca ME. Is preoperative cytologic diagnosis of epithelioid sarcoma possible? Diagn Cytopathol 2008;36:780.
78. Geisinger KR, Kawamoto EH, Marshall RB, et al. Aspiration and exfoliative cytology, including ultrastructure, of a malignant granular cell tumor. Acta Cytol 1985;29:593.
79. Dong Q, McKee G, Pitman M, et al. Epithelioid variant of gastrointestinal stromal tumor: diagnosis of fine-needle aspiration. Diagn Cytopathol 2003;29(2):55.
80. Oland J, Rosen A, Reif R, et al. Cytodiagnosis of soft tissue tumors. J Surg Oncol 1986;37:168.
81. Pettinato G, Swanson PE, Insabato L, et al. Undifferentiated small round-cell tumors of childhood: the immunocytochemical demonstration of myogenic differentiation in fine needle aspirates. Diagn Cytopathol 1989;5:194.
82. Seidal T, Mark J, Hagmar B, et al. Alveolar rhabdomyosarcoma: a cytometric and correlated cytological and histological study. Acta Pathol Microbiol Scand (A) 1982;90:345.
83. Seidal T, Walaas L, Kindblom LG, et al. Cytology of embryonal rhabdomyosarcoma: a cytologic, light microscopic, electron microscopic, and immunohistochemical study of seven cases. Diagn Cytopathol 1988;4:292.
84. Akhtar M, Ali MA, Bakry M, et al. Fine needle aspiration biopsy of childhood rhabdomyosarcoma: cytologic, histologic, and ultrastructural correlations. Diagn Cytopathol 1992;8:465.
85. Almeida M, Stastny JF, Wakely PE Jr, et al. Fine-needle aspiration biopsy of childhood rhabdomyosarcoma: reevaluation of the cytologic criteria for diagnosis. Diagn Cytopathol 1994;11:231.
86. Carraway NP, Fanning CV, Amato RJ, et al. Fine-needle aspiration of intra-abdominal desmoplastic small round cell tumor. Diagn Cytopathol 1993;9:465.
87. Logrono R, Kurtycz DF, Sproat IA, et al. Diagnosis of recurrent desmoplastic small round cell tumor by fine needle aspiration. A case report. Acta Cytol 1997;41:1402.
88. Klijanienko J, Couturier J, Bourdeaut F, et al. Fine-needle aspiration as a diagnostic technique in 50 cases of primary Ewing sarcoma/peripheral neuroectodermal tumor. Institut Curie's experience. Diagn Cytopathol 2012;40:19.
89. Meda BA, Buss DH, Woodruff RD, et al. Diagnosis and subclassification of primary and recurrent lymphoma. The usefulness and limitations of combined fine-needle aspiration cytomorphology and flow cytometry. Am J Clin Pathol 2000;113:688.
90. Khalbuss WE, Teot LA, Monaco SE. Diagnostic accuracy and limitations of fine-needle aspiration cytology of bone and soft tissue lesions: a review of 1114 cases with cytological-histological correlation. Cancer Cytopathol 2010;118:24.

Approach to the Diagnosis of Soft Tissue Tumors

CHAPTER CONTENTS

CLINICAL INFORMATION

The diagnosis of a soft tissue lesion requires a modicum of clinical information and adequate, well-processed tissue. At a minimum, the pathologist should be apprised of the age of the patient, the location of the tumor, and its growth characteristics. In some cases, the results of imaging studies, particularly magnetic resonance imaging, enhance one's understanding of the clinical extent of the lesion and its relationship to normal structures (see Chapter 3).

Although age rarely, if ever, suggests a particular diagnosis, it is important to know whether the patient is a child. In general, there is little overlap between soft tissue tumors occurring in children and those in adults. Therefore, this critical piece of information essentially presents the pathologist with two groups of tumors from which a differential diagnosis can be constructed. For example, undifferentiated pleomorphic sarcoma (malignant fibrous histiocytoma) is essentially unheard of during childhood, so one should consider other diagnoses for a pleomorphic tumor in a child. On the other hand, neuroblastoma rarely occurs after childhood, and such diagnoses should always be made cautiously in adults.

Location, too, provides ancillary help in the differential diagnosis. Sarcomas, for the most part, develop as deeply located masses and infrequently present as superficial lesions. Exceptions do occur, however, and include lesions such as dermatofibrosarcoma protuberans, epithelioid sarcoma, Kaposi sarcoma, and angiosarcoma (Box 6-1). It is also useful to recall that when carcinomas or melanomas metastasize to soft tissue, they do so usually as small, superficial nodules rather than as large, deeply situated masses. The most common carcinomas that present as soft tissue metastases are pulmonary and renal carcinomas, the former usually appearing as a subcutaneous mass on the chest wall and the latter as a soft tissue mass in nearly any location.

Unfortunately, there is a great deal of overlap in the presentation of benign and malignant soft tissue masses, so this information may be least helpful to the pathologist. Most soft tissue sarcomas of the extremities are detected by the patient as a slowly growing mass that has been present for about 6 months at the time of diagnosis. The duration of benign lesions may be similar, although such lesions are generally described as static or slowly growing. An exception to the foregoing observation is the rapid development of some cases of nodular fasciitis. These superficial, reactive lesions may develop rapidly over a period of 1 to 3 weeks, and we have even encountered some that evolved in a few days, a pattern of growth that seldom, if ever, is encountered with a sarcoma. Therefore, an astute general surgeon can sometimes suggest the diagnosis of fasciitis for a rapidly evolving superficial lesion of the extremity.

BIOPSY DIAGNOSIS

In the past, the choice of biopsy technique for soft tissue masses was dictated by the size and location of the lesion (see Chapter 2). An incisional biopsy was considered the gold standard for large, deeply situated masses and provided ample material for diagnosis and ancillary studies. Its principal disadvantages included spillage of tumor into adjacent compartments as a result of poor hemostasis or faulty biopsy placement, complications of wound infection, and the usual requirement for hospitalization of the patient. Excisional biopsy, although more expedient and providing the entire lesion for examination, was performed on only small, superficial lesions amenable to complete resection. The current reliance on minimally invasive techniques to procure tissue has significantly changed the biopsy paradigm in the direction of the use of a core needle biopsy. The incidence of core needle biopsies increased from less than 10% to nearly 80% during the early 1990s[1] and is performed in our hospitals on essentially all deep soft tissue masses. Consequently, the amount of material available to type and grade sarcomas has decreased, and this trend is likely to continue unabated because of the emphasis on less costly outpatient care. Therefore, it is important to be aware of the limitations and pitfalls of core needle biopsy and to keep in mind a few basic principles.[2]

First, the pathologist should be aware of the expectation of the clinician. In some instances, the goal of a core needle biopsy may be simply to establish that a soft tissue mass is a mesenchymal neoplasm as opposed to a lymphoma or metastatic lesion, a distinction that can usually be made in the majority of cases with the use of adjuvant immunohistochemistry.

BOX 6-1 Superficial Soft Tissue Sarcomas

Dermatofibrosarcoma protuberans
Epithelioid sarcoma
Angiomatoid fibrous histiocytoma
Plexiform fibrohistiocytic tumor
Myxoid undifferentiated pleomorphic sarcoma (myxoid malignant fibrous histiocytoma, high-grade myxofibrosarcoma)
Angiosarcoma
Kaposi sarcoma
Atypical fibroxanthoma

If definitive surgery will be performed following the needle biopsy, then the most important priority is to determine whether the lesion is a sarcoma. If, however, the intention is to provide preoperative (neoadjuvant) radiotherapy or chemotherapy, every attempt should be made not only to make the diagnosis of sarcoma but also to classify and grade the lesion. However, it is not always possible to reliably grade a sarcoma on the basis of a core needle biopsy. In particular, it is difficult to discriminate a grade 2 from a grade 3 lesion. Pathologists may find that the best assessment that they can give is the designation *low grade* or *high grade,* recognizing that high grade will encompass both grades 2 and 3 lesions. Information is inevitably lost when collapsing a three-tiered system into a two-tiered one; however, a two-tiered system still performs reasonably well and is consistent with therapeutic considerations.[3]

In grading core needle biopsies, one can usually accept the presence of high-grade areas in several needle cores as diagnostic of a high-grade sarcoma because of the improbability that additional material will result in downgrading the lesion. At the same time, one should also be unwilling to accept a lesion as low grade if the number of core biopsies is small, if the lesion has not been adequately sampled, or if imaging studies suggest features of a high-grade sarcoma (i.e., necrosis). Core needle biopsies containing necrosis usually imply a high-grade sarcoma, again because of the improbability that limited material captures a solitary or limited focus of necrosis. However, pathologists must be certain that necrosis is of the coagulative and not the hyaline type and is not reflective of prior therapy or surgical intervention. The corollary to the latter portion of this statement is that as soon as radiation or chemotherapy has been administered, grading becomes unreliable because of alterations in nuclear features, mitotic activity, cellularity, and interstitial hyalinization. Therapy also induces necrosis, although it is not possible to discriminate spontaneous from therapy-induced necrosis. Most important, interpreting core needle biopsies implies a close dialogue with clinicians to resolve any inconsistencies between clinical and pathologic diagnoses.

FROZEN SECTION DIAGNOSIS

In the past, frozen section examinations were performed commonly with the expectation that definitive surgery would be accomplished during the same intraoperative procedure, but this trend has changed. Frozen sections are now obtained primarily to assure the surgeon that she or he has obtained representative, viable tissue that is adequate for a permanent section diagnosis or to evaluate margins. The former may be accomplished by freezing a portion of the biopsy material or sometimes, as in the case of a needle biopsy, by performing a touch preparation. The presence of malignant cells in a nonnecrotic background on a touch preparation usually ensures that the specimen is adequate. A background of reactive or necrotic cells suggests that a biopsy has been performed on the pseudocapsule or that the specimen is largely necrotic, requiring additional material depending on the clinical impression.

EVALUATION OF RESECTION SPECIMENS

Because there is a preference to perform limb-sparing surgery for sarcomas of all types, if possible, the number of major amputation specimens received in the surgical pathology laboratory has decreased markedly. Most extremity sarcomas are removed with a wide local excision usually combined with preoperative or postoperative radiotherapy. Ideally, such specimens are received fresh and unfixed so that tissue for ancillary studies can be obtained. As with many other surgical specimens, the margins should be marked with permanent ink and blotted dry before the dissection of the specimen. After the incision, the gross characteristics of the tumor should be noted. If malignancy is suspected, a careful assessment of the tumor as to its surroundings is mandatory. This includes the location of the lesion (e.g., subcutis, muscle), its size, its relation to vital structures (e.g., bone, neurovascular bundle), and the relative amount of necrosis, if it can be judged grossly. Size is important for providing an accurate T descriptor for the surgeon if the lesion is a sarcoma. Lesions less than 5 cm are classified as *T1,* whereas those larger than 5 cm are classified as *T2.* An assessment of the degree of necrosis is important for untreated sarcomas because this parameter is used in some grading systems. The extent of necrosis in lesions treated with preoperative irradiation or chemotherapy is also important because it helps the clinician assess the efficacy of therapy, although it does not carry the same implication as necrosis in an untreated lesion. Often, the gross appearance of the tumor is deceptive. Sarcomas may appear well circumscribed, and benign tumors occasionally infiltrate. Use of the term *encapsulation* can be misleading and invite inadequate excision by shelling out, or enucleating, the tumor. In reality, sarcomas lack a true capsule and, instead, are surrounded by a compressed zone of normal tissue, known as a *pseudocapsule.*

There are no rigid guidelines for sampling soft tissue tumors; to some extent, sampling is dictated by the specific case. In the case of a known benign lesion, a few representative sections suffice (or the entire lesion if it is small). With a sarcoma, the questions to be answered are different. For example, it may be less important to submit numerous sections for a high-grade sarcoma than for a low-grade lesion in which the sampling is being driven by the need to rule out the presence of high-grade areas. We have generally obtained one section for each centimeter of tumor diameter, with no more than about 10 sections if the lesion appeared more or less uniform. Representative sections of the margins or sections designed to show impingement of vital structures are also obtained. We select blocks for margins judiciously, depending on the gross appearance of the lesion. Lesions several centimeters away from a margin seldom have positive margins microscopically, so extensive margin sampling in these situations is less critical than with excisions containing grossly close margins. One exception is epithelioid sarcoma, a lesion that may be grossly deceptive in its clinical extent. Digital images can be useful for providing visual data as to the orientation of the specimen and sampling sites.

Most specimens are handled adequately as described previously. In diagnostically challenging cases, it is useful to have frozen tissue in reserve if ancillary studies are required. Even though the ability to perform molecular tests on formalin-fixed material has diminished the need to have fresh tissue on every case, freezing tissue is an excellent practice, particularly because frozen tissue is often a requirement for patient entry into national protocols (e.g., childhood rhabdomyosarcoma). Approximately 1 cm^3 is sufficient, although less is acceptable from small biopsy specimens. The tissue should be cut into small 0.2 cm^3 fragments, stored at −70.0 C, and shipped on dry ice, if necessary.[4]

MICROSCOPIC EXAMINATION

The first and most important step in reaching a correct diagnosis is careful scrutiny of conventionally stained sections at low-power magnification. Useful microscopic features that can be identified at this point include the size and depth of the lesion, its relation to overlying skin and underlying fascia, and the nature of the borders (e.g., pushing, infiltrative).

The most important decision to be made initially is whether the lesion is reactive or neoplastic. Reactive lesions occur in either superficial or deep soft tissue but tend to be more frequent in the former location (Box 6-2). A number of histologic features are suggestive of a reactive process. First, many reactive lesions display a zonation. For example, in the case of fascial forms of nodular fasciitis and ischemic fasciitis, there is a cuff of proliferating fibroblasts that surround a central hypocellular zone of fibrinoid change. Myositis ossificans, too, displays zonation manifested by centrifugal maturation of fibroblastic to osteoblastic mesenchyme. Cells comprising reactive lesions often have the appearance of tissue culture fibroblasts with large vesicular nuclei, prominent nucleoli, and striking cytoplasmic basophilia, reflecting the presence of abundant, rough endoplasmic reticulum. Although mitotic figures may be numerous, important negative observations include the absence of atypical mitotic figures or nuclear atypia, as one would expect in a sarcoma.

When satisfied that a reactive lesion can be excluded, the pathologist proceeds with analysis of the neoplasm. At low power, the architectural pattern, appearance of the cells, and characteristics of the stroma should be noted. These characteristics lend themselves to the development of a number of differential diagnostic categories.

1. *Fasciculated spindle cell tumors*. These lesions comprise a large group of tumors (e.g., fibrosarcoma and synovial sarcoma) characterized by spindled cells arranged in long fascicles (Box 6-3). Cellular schwannoma and fibromatosis must be distinguished from the others because they are nonmetastasizing tumors. Unlike the others, fibromatosis is typically a lesion of low cellularity and nuclear grade. Cellular schwannoma, unlike the others, is characterized by diffuse, intense S100 protein immunoreactivity.
2. *Myxoid lesions* (Box 6-4). Although nearly any soft tissue tumor may appear myxoid from time to time, a number of

BOX 6-2 Reactive Lesions Simulating a Sarcoma

Nodular fasciitis
Intravascular and cranial fasciitis
Ischemic fasciitis (atypical decubital fibroplasia)
Proliferative fasciitis and myositis
Intravascular papillary endothelial hyperplasia
Myositis and panniculitis ossificans
Fibrodysplasia ossificans progressiva
Fibro-osseous pseudotumor of the digits
Localized massive lymphedema

BOX 6-3 Fasciculated Spindle Cell Tumors

Fibromatosis (desmoid tumor)
Cellular schwannoma
Fibrosarcoma
Leiomyosarcoma
Spindle cell rhabdomyosarcoma
Synovial sarcoma
Malignant peripheral nerve sheath tumor
Low-grade fibromyxoid sarcoma

BOX 6-4 Myxoid Soft Tissue Lesions

Myxoma, cutaneous, intramuscular*
Aggressive angiomyxoma*
Myxoid neurofibroma
Neurothekeoma, myxoid
Nerve sheath myxoma
Myxoid chondroma
Myxoid lipoma (including myxoid spindle cell lipoma)
Lipoblastoma
Low-grade fibromyxoid sarcoma (partially myxoid)
Ossifying fibromyxoid tumor of soft parts
Myxoid liposarcoma*
Extraskeletal myxoid chondrosarcoma*
Myxoid dermatofibrosarcoma protuberans
Myxoid undifferentiated pleomorphic sarcoma (myxoid malignant fibrous histiocytoma, high-grade myxofibrosarcoma)*
Botryoid embryonal rhabdomyosarcoma
Myxoid leiomyosarcoma (rare)

*Most consistently myxoid.

BOX 6-5 Epithelioid Soft Tissue Tumors

Alveolar soft part sarcoma
Epithelioid sarcoma
Epithelioid angiosarcoma
Epithelioid hemangioendothelioma
Epithelioid hemangioma
Extragastrointestinal stromal tumor
Epithelioid variant of malignant peripheral nerve sheath tumor
Epithelioid schwannoma
Malignant rhabdoid tumor
Sclerosing epithelioid fibrosarcoma
Synovial sarcoma (biphasic and predominantly monophasic epithelial)

BOX 6-6 Round Cell Soft Tissue Tumors

Alveolar rhabdomyosarcoma
Desmoplastic small-round-cell tumor of childhood
Embryonal rhabdomyosarcoma
Extraskeletal Ewing sarcoma/primitive neuroectodermal tumor (ES/PNET)
Round cell liposarcoma
Cellular forms of extraskeletal myxoid chondrosarcoma
Mesenchymal chondrosarcoma
Small-cell osteosarcoma
Malignant hemangiopericytoma/solitary fibrous tumor
Glomus tumor
Tenosynovial giant cell tumor

lesions display myxoid features consistently. In adults, the differential diagnosis of myxoid tumors includes myxoma, myxoid undifferentiated pleomorphic sarcoma (myxoid malignant fibrous histiocytoma, high-grade myxofibrosarcoma), myxoid liposarcoma, and extraskeletal myxoid chondrosarcoma. Analysis of the vascular pattern, degree of nuclear atypia, and occasionally the staining characteristics of the matrix aid in this distinction. For example, an intricate vasculature is a feature of both myxoid liposarcoma and myxoid undifferentiated pleomorphic sarcoma, but it is not a feature of extraskeletal myxoid chondrosarcoma or myxoma.

3. *Epithelioid tumors* (Box 6-5). For the differential diagnosis of epithelioid tumors, it is important to rule out metastatic carcinoma, melanoma, and even large-cell lymphomas before assuming that one is dealing with an epithelioid soft tissue tumor. Immunohistochemistry plays a decidedly pivotal role in this regard (discussed in greater detail in Chapter 7).
4. *Round cell tumors* (Box 6-6). Like epithelioid lesions, the differential diagnosis of round cell lesions can be broad; it presupposes excluding non-soft tissue lesions that may mimic a round cell sarcoma (e.g., lymphoma, carcinoma) and is greatly facilitated by the use of immunohistochemistry. One should also bear in mind that the round cell tumor is not synonymous with round cell sarcoma because benign lesions (e.g., glomus tumor, giant cell-poor forms of tenosynovial giant cell tumor) also enter the differential diagnosis. In general, the age of the patient helps narrow the possibilities. In children, these lesions include neuroblastoma, rhabdomyosarcoma, Ewing sarcoma/primitive neuroectodermal tumor (ES/PNET), and the rare desmoplastic small-round-cell tumor. Most of these diagnoses would not be considered in adults.
5. *Pleomorphic tumors* (Box 6-7). The differential diagnosis of pleomorphic sarcomas relies heavily on tumor sampling to identify areas of specific differentiation, sometimes in conjunction with immunohistochemistry. Undifferentiated pleomorphic sarcoma (malignant fibrous histiocytoma) is the most common pleomorphic sarcoma, but it should not be diagnosed in unusual situations, such as parenchymal organs, unless carcinoma, melanoma, and lymphoma have been excluded.

BOX 6-7 Pleomorphic Sarcomas

Undifferentiated pleomorphic sarcoma (malignant fibrous histiocytoma)
Pleomorphic liposarcoma
Dedifferentiated liposarcoma
Pleomorphic rhabdomyosarcoma
Pleomorphic malignant peripheral nerve sheath tumor
Pleomorphic leiomyosarcoma
Atypical fibroxanthoma

BOX 6-8 Hemorrhagic Lesions of Soft Tissue

Organizing hemorrhage/hematoma
Aneurysmal fibrous histiocytoma
Angiomatoid fibrous histiocytoma
Angiosarcoma
High-grade sarcomas of various types (occasional)

6. *Hemorrhagic and vascular lesions* (Box 6-8). Although sarcomas are generally highly vascularized, the number of soft tissue lesions that present as a hemorrhagic mass is limited and, interestingly, includes many nonvascular (i.e., nonendothelial) tumors. Conversely, some vascular tumors, such as intramuscular hemangiomas, do not have a hemorrhagic appearance. When evaluating vascular lesions, a good starting point is to ascertain whether the lesion is

BOX 6-9 Intravascular Tumors and Pseudotumors

Organizing thrombi and papillary endothelial hyperplasia
Intravascular fasciitis
Spindle cell hemangioma
Epithelioid hemangioendothelioma
Epithelioid hemangioma
Intimal sarcoma

BOX 6-10 Melanocytic Tumors of Soft Tissue

Clear cell sarcoma
Cellular blue nevus
Paraganglioma-like dermal melanocytic tumor
Perivascular epithelioid cell tumor (PEComa)
Pigmented neurofibroma
Melanotic schwannoma
Pigmented neuroectodermal tumor of infancy
Pigmented dermatofibrosarcoma protuberans (Bednar tumor)

TABLE 6-1 Evaluation of Vascular Lesions

PARAMETER	BENIGN VASCULAR LESION	ANGIOSARCOMA
Age	All	Adults
Anatomic site	All	Typically superficial soft tissues
Predisposing factors		Lymphedema, radiation
Intravascular vs. extravascular	Either	Virtually always extravascular
Lobular growth	Often, particularly capillary hemangioma	No
Circumscription	Variable	No
Thick-walled vessels	Yes, particularly intramuscular hemangioma, angiomatosis	No

predominantly intravascular or extravascular (Box 6-9).[5] Intravascular lesions are nearly always benign and include primarily organizing thrombus/hematoma followed by the occasional angiocentric vascular tumor (Table 6-1; see Box 6-9). Extravascular lesions may be benign or malignant; features that favor benignancy include sharp circumscription, lobular arrangement of vessels, and the presence of both large (thick-walled) and small vessels. Angiosarcomas, on the other hand, have irregular margins, lack a lobular arrangement of vessels, and are composed of naked endothelial cells that dissect randomly through tissue planes. They usually occur in adults in the superficial soft tissues.

7. *Melanocytic tumors*. Soft tissue tumors showing melanocytic differentiation are rare but important to distinguish from primary or metastatic malignant melanoma (Box 6-10).

Important information can be gleaned at low power about the growth pattern, degree of cellularity, and amount and type of matrix formation. Growth patterns vary, ranging from a fascicular, herringbone, or storiform (cartwheel, spiral nebula) pattern in fibroblastic, myofibroblastic, and fibrohistiocytic tumors to plexiform or endocrinoid patterns, palisading, and rosettes in various benign and malignant neural tumors. Biphasic cellular patterns with epithelial and spindle cell areas are characteristic of synovial sarcoma. Although not all growth patterns permit a definitive diagnosis, they are of great help in narrowing the various differential diagnostic possibilities. Table 6-2 lists some of the most common architectural patterns and the tumors in which they are found.

TABLE 6-2 Correlation of Growth Pattern and Tumor Type

GROWTH PATTERN	TUMOR TYPE
Alveolar	Alveolar soft part sarcoma; alveolar rhabdomyosarcoma
Acinar	Synovial sarcoma
Biphasic	Synovial sarcoma
Cording	Epithelioid hemangioendothelioma; myxoid chondrosarcoma; malignant peripheral nerve sheath tumor, epithelioid type; round cell liposarcoma (rare)
Fascicular	Fibromatosis (desmoid tumor); cellular schwannoma; fibrosarcoma; malignant peripheral nerve sheath tumor; synovial sarcoma, leiomyosarcoma
Endocrinoid (Zellballen)	Paraganglioma; alveolar soft part sarcoma
Lobular, nodular, nest-like	Lipoblastoma; liposarcoma; epithelioid sarcoma; clear cell sarcoma; fibrous hamartoma of infancy
Palisading	Schwannoma; malignant peripheral nerve sheath tumor; leiomyosarcoma; extragastrointestinal stromal tumor; synovial sarcoma (rare)
Plexiform	Neurofibroma; schwannoma; plexiform fibrohistiocytic tumor
Plexiform capillary	Myxoid liposarcoma; myxofibrosarcoma
Pericytoma	Hemangiopericytoma/solitary fibrous tumor; synovial sarcoma; mesenchymal chondrosarcoma; malignant peripheral nerve sheath tumor; myofibromatosis; liposarcoma (rare)
Rosettes, pseudorosettes	Neuroblastoma; primitive neuroectodermal tumor; schwannoma and low-grade fibromyxoid sarcoma (collagen rosettes)
Storiform (cartwheel)	Dermatofibrosarcoma protuberans; fibrous histiocytoma; undifferentiated pleomorphic sarcoma (malignant fibrous histiocytoma); neurofibroma; perineurioma

Abundant myxoid material is produced by a variety of benign and malignant soft tissue tumors, ranging from myxoma and myxoid neurofibroma to myxoid liposarcoma and myxoid chondrosarcoma, but is found consistently in a few only (see Box 6-4). In the past, histochemical analysis was commonly used to characterize the matrix and, therefore, narrow the differential diagnosis; newer techniques have rendered these studies archaic.

A prominent myxoid matrix is usually an indication of a relatively slow-growing tumor, and it has been shown that the

TABLE 6-3 Calcification, Chondroid, and Osseous Metaplasia in Soft Tissue Tumors

LESION	CALCIFICATION	CHONDROID	OSTEOID
Calcifying aponeurotic fibroma	+	+	–
Fibrodysplasia ossificans progressiva	+	+	+
Giant cell tumor of soft parts	+	–	+
Hemangioma	+	–	+
Lipoma	+	+	+
Leiomyoma	+	–	–
Pleomorphic undifferentiated sarcoma (malignant fibrous histiocytoma)	–	–	+
Melanocytic schwannoma	+ Psammoma bodies	–	–
Mesenchymal chondrosarcoma	–	+	+
Myofibromatosis	+	–	–
Myositis ossificans	–	+	+
Myxoid liposarcoma	–	+	–
Malignant mesenchymoma	–	+	+
Malignant peripheral nerve sheath tumor	–	+	–
Myxoid chondrosarcoma	–	+	–
Ossifying fibromyxoid tumor	–	+	+
Osteosarcoma	+	+	+
Panniculitis ossificans	–	–	+
Synovial sarcoma	+	+	+
Tumoral calcinosis	+	–	–

+, present (variable); –, usually absent.

degree of myxoid change in some malignant tumors is inversely related to the metastatic rate (e.g., myxoid undifferentiated pleomorphic sarcoma, myxoid liposarcoma). Abundant collagen formation is found more often in slowly growing tumors than in rapidly growing ones. However, this finding is not always significant because it may be a feature of some highly malignant sarcomas, such as synovial sarcoma, undifferentiated pleomorphic sarcoma, and postirradiation sarcomas. Deposits of calcium, osteoid, and chondroid are encountered in a limited number of soft tissue tumors summarized in Table 6-3.

The degree and type of cellular differentiation is best evaluated at medium or high power. Lipoblasts, for example, are characterized by the presence of sharply defined intracellular droplets of lipid and one or more centrally or peripherally placed round or scalloped nuclei. Round and spindle-shaped rhabdomyoblasts can usually be identified in conventionally stained hematoxylin-eosin sections by their deeply eosinophilic cytoplasm with whorls of eosinophilic fibrillary material near the nucleus and cytoplasmic cross-striations. When interpreting these cells, however, caution is indicated because occasionally entrapped normal or atrophic fat or muscle tissue may closely resemble lipoblasts or rhabdomyoblasts, respectively. Differentiated smooth muscle cells are characterized by

BOX 6-11 Benign Soft Tissue Tumors with Nuclear Atypia

Pleomorphic fibroma of the skin
Fibrous histiocytoma with bizarre cells
Pleomorphic lipoma
Schwannoma, ancient
Symplastic glomus tumor
Neurofibroma

their elongated shape, eosinophilic longitudinal fibrils, and long, slender (cigar-shaped) nuclei, often with terminal juxtanuclear vacuoles. Other spindle cells, such as neoplastic fibroblasts, myofibroblasts, and Schwann cells, are more difficult to evaluate cytologically. One relies more heavily on histologic context and immunohistochemistry. Cellular inclusions are rare in soft tissue tumors. They are represented principally by the intracellular periodic acid-Schiff-positive crystalline material in alveolar soft part sarcoma and the actin-rich eosinophilic inclusions in digital fibromatosis.

Mitotic figures are best evaluated at high power and their significance evaluated contextually. Atypical mitotic figures are rare in benign soft tissue tumors and usually indicate malignancy. Mitotic counts are useful for assessing malignancy in smooth muscle tumors, but they are of no importance in the diagnosis of nodular fasciitis, localized, and diffuse giant cell tumors or undifferentiated sarcoma, where the diagnosis is based on a constellation of other findings. Although nuclear atypia is more often associated with malignancy, it may occur as a degenerative feature in benign lesions (Box 6-11).

IMMUNOHISTOCHEMISTRY

Although not needed in every case, immunohistochemistry has assumed an increasingly important role in diagnosis. Although previously used principally to determine line of differentiation, immunostains are now often used as surrogate markers to identify specific molecular alterations (e.g., murine double minute 2 [MDM2] amplification in well-differentiated liposarcoma). Not only is it important to know the specificity of the antibody, but also one must be aware of the artifacts that can occur in these preparations, such as nonspecific staining of the edge of the tissue section (edge artifact) or within a necrotic zone, diffusion or uptake of antigen into adjacent tissues or cells (e.g., myoglobin), and the cross-reactivity of some antibodies.

To use immunostains in the most effective and cost-efficient way, having an algorithmic approach in mind and using the reagents in panels (see Chapter 7) is recommended. For example, a panel of antibodies to differentiate carcinomas, melanomas, sarcomas, and lymphomas from one another would be selected before a series of B- and T-cell markers. Immunohistochemistry is an important, if not obligate, part of the workup of certain soft tissue lesions, such as round cell sarcomas, epithelioid tumors, and pleomorphic tumors, particularly in the skin.

TABLE 6-4 FISH Testing in Soft Tissue Tumors, Common Usages

DIAGNOSTIC PROBLEM	DIFFERENTIAL DIAGNOSIS	FISH RESULT
Round cell sarcomas[8-10]	Ewing sarcoma	+*EWSR1* rearrangement
	Desmoplastic small-round-cell sarcoma	+*EWSR1* rearrangement
	Alveolar rhabdomyosarcoma	+*FOXO1* gene rearrangement
	Embryonal rhabdomyosarcoma	No FISH test
	Cellular myxoid chondrosarcoma (uncommon)[20]	+*EWSR1* rearrangement (two-thirds)
	Predominantly round cell liposarcoma	+*FUS* rearrangement or +*EWSR1* rearrangement (occasional)
	Round cell synovial sarcoma (uncommon)	+*SYT* rearrangement
Angiomatoid fibrous histiocytoma with round cell or pleomorphic features[11,12]		+*EWSR1* rearrangement or +*FUS* rearrangement (uncommon)
Melanocytic tumors[13]	Clear cell sarcoma (and variants)	+*EWSR1* rearrangement
	Cellular blue nevus	–*EWSR1* rearrangement
	Malignant melanoma	–*EWSR1* rearrangement
Myxoid tumors[14-16]	Myxoma	No FISH test
	Myxoid liposarcoma	+*FUS* rearrangement
	Myxoid liposarcoma	+*EWSR1* rearrangement (uncommon)
	Myxoid chondrosarcoma	+*EWSR1* rearrangement
	Low-grade fibromyxoid sarcoma[14]	+*FUS* rearrangement
	Myxoid undifferentiated pleomorphic sarcoma (myxofibrosarcoma)	No FISH test
Spindle cell sarcoma with fascicular growth pattern	Fibrosarcoma, not other specified	No FISH test
	Leiomyosarcoma	No FISH test
	Synovial sarcoma[21-23]	+*SYT* rearrangement
	Low-grade fibromyxoid sarcoma	+*FUS* rearrangement (some)
	Malignant peripheral nerve sheath tumor	No FISH test
Distinguish large, deep, or recurrent lipomas from well-differentiated liposarcomas[17,18]	Intramuscular and retroperitoneal lipoma	–*MDM2* amplification
	Well-differentiated liposarcoma	+*MDM2* amplification
Pleomorphic sarcomas	Undifferentiated pleomorphic sarcoma	+*MDM2* amplification strongly favors dedifferentiated liposarcoma
	Leiomyosarcoma	
	Dedifferentiated liposarcoma	
	Pleomorphic liposarcoma	
Vascular tumors[19]	Atypical vascular lesion with architectural complexity or other unusual features	–*MYC* amplification
	Postirradiation/lymphedema-associated angiosarcoma	+*MYC* amplification
DFSP with problematic features		
Myxoid DFSP	Cutaneous myxoma	+PDGF beta rearrangement in DFSP; others negative
	Myxoid liposarcoma	
Fibrosarcomatous DFSP	Superficial fibrosarcoma not arising in DFSP	
DFSP resembling fibrous histiocytoma	Cellular fibrous histiocytoma	
Inflammatory myofibroblastic tumor	Other spindle cell lesions with inflammation	+*ALK* rearrangement

DFSP, dermatofibrosarcoma protuberans.

MOLECULAR TESTS

Molecular studies have assumed an increasingly important role in the diagnosis of soft tissue neoplasms. It is estimated that about 10% of all referred soft tissue consultations benefit from molecular studies.[6] In fact, specific molecular alterations have become definitional for some sarcomas. The commonly used methods include conventional cytogenetics, reverse transcriptase-polymerase chain reaction (RT-PCR), and fluorescence in situ hybridization (FISH). The methods, advantages, and disadvantages of each are discussed in Chapter 4. Conventional cytogenetics, which requires fresh tissue, is used to evaluate the entire karyotype, whereas FISH and RT-PCR are used to identify specific translocations/amplifications associated with a given tumor type(s).[6,7] The latter two methods are considered complementary; the choice of one over the other will, to a large extent, be dictated by the expertise of the laboratory. In some laboratories, the methods are used sequentially, depending on the initial results. For example, a fusion-negative Ewing sarcoma by RT-PCR might be reexamined by FISH using a 22q12 break-apart probe to more inclusively detect variant translocations. Because FISH offers the advantage that, with a relatively few number of commercial probes, all of the common differential diagnostic problems can be addressed (Table 6-4),[8-23] it has become our front-line molecular test. In the experiences of the Cleveland Clinic, the situations in which FISH is highly desirable include evaluation of[6]: round cell sarcomas, spindle cell tumors, adipocytic tumors,[17,24] myxoid tumors, and melanocytic tumors.[6,11]

DIAGNOSTIC NOMENCLATURE

Even with complete sampling and ancillary studies, it may not be possible to accurately classify all sarcomas. In our consultation practices, approximately 10% of all sarcomas cannot be classified. Nonetheless, it is often possible for the pathologist to provide the clinician with sufficient information so that therapy can proceed unencumbered. For example, when evaluating moderately differentiated spindle-cell sarcomas, one cannot always distinguish a malignant

TABLE 6-5 Managerial Disease Categories

CLINICAL STATUS	BEHAVIOR	USUAL THERAPY	EXAMPLES
Benign	Local excision usually curative; rare recurrence but not destructive; no metastasis	Local excision	Histologically benign tumors and pseudotumors
Borderline or intermediate	Local recurrence common and often destructive; metastases vary from none to few	Extended local to wide excision, depending on circumstances	Fibromatosis (nonmetastasizing); dermatofibrosarcoma protuberans (rare metastasis)
Malignant	Local recurrence common; metastasis common; systemic disease sometimes present at onset	Wide excision; possible adjuvant therapy	Undifferentiated pleomorphic sarcoma

Modified from Kempson RL, Hendrickson MR. In: Weiss SW, Brooks JSJ, editors. An approach to the diagnosis of soft tissue tumors. In: Soft tissue tumors. Baltimore: Williams & Wilkins; 1996, with permission.

peripheral nerve sheath tumor from a fibrosarcoma. Yet this distinction is not critical if the pathologist can assure the clinician that the lesion is malignant and can provide a histologic grade. Likewise, it is not worthwhile to labor exhaustively over classifying a pleomorphic sarcoma when the therapy does not differ. In these ambiguous diagnostic situations, there is no substitute for a constructive dialogue among the surgeon, pathologist, and oncologist to define the therapeutically relevant pathologic information. This has led to a managerial classification of soft tissue lesions (Table 6-5).[25] Such a system emphasizes the expected behavior rather than the histologic type. When the pathologist cannot be certain of the exact diagnosis, a managerial system can bridge the gap. For example, a low-grade myxoid sarcoma that does not seem to fall clearly into a specific diagnostic category could be labeled *low-grade myxoid sarcoma* with a comment that local recurrence rather than metastasis would be the expected behavior. The diagnosis *myxoid tumor with locally recurring potential* expresses the same information.

STANDARDIZED REPORTING OF SOFT TISSUE SARCOMAS

In 2004, the American College of Surgeons Commission on Cancer mandated the use of checklists to ensure completeness of cancer reports as part of its Cancer Program Standards for approved cancer programs. Subsequently, the College of American Pathologists, in conjunction with a panel of expert soft tissue pathologists, proposed a standardized method of reporting both biopsy and resection specimens for sarcomas (Fig. 6-1).[4] This checklist may be modified or formatted to conform to institutional policies and preferences, as long as the essential information is retained. The three most important pieces of information that the pathologist provides in a surgical pathology report, apart from the diagnosis of sarcoma, are the grade, size, and depth of the lesion; each is an independent prognostic variable that figures prominently in the clinical stage (see Chapter 1).[26] Anatomic site does not directly enter into the staging of sarcomas. Nevertheless, site does affect outcome and should be recorded. Neurovascular and bone invasion, previously considered determinants of stage, are no longer used.

Grading system. The choice of a grading system is largely one of institutional, regional, or national preference, because all reported grading systems can be correlated with outcome (see Chapter 1).[27,28] The report should make clear the number of tiers in the grading system; for example, it is important to know whether a lesion is grade 2 of a four-tiered system or a three-tiered system. Alternatively, some prefer the simple labels *low grade* or *high grade,* particularly when dealing with a core needle biopsy (see previous text).

Tumor. The maximum dimensions of a tumor are given in metric units and in three dimensions, if possible.

Location and depth. These tumor parameters are addressed by indicating whether it is superficial (above the fascia), deep (below the fascia or in muscle), or in a body cavity. For purposes of staging, deep lesions are defined as those in muscle, a body cavity, or the head and neck.

Margins. Sarcomas excised with a less than 1.5- to 2.0-cm margin are prone to local recurrence[29] unless they are bordered by unbreached fascia or periosteum.[30] For this reason, all positive margins (ink on the tumor) should be reported as well as the distance from those that are judged to be close (<2.0 cm). Positive margins imply a greater chance for distant metastasis with high-risk extremity sarcomas.[31]

Necrosis. Because necrosis is an integral part of some grading systems, it is useful to indicate whether necrosis is absent, microscopically present, or macroscopically present. If macroscopically present, one should provide some estimate of the amount. It should be kept in mind, however, that grading systems that rely on assessment of necrosis imply examination of surgical specimens that have not been altered by preoperative irradiation or chemotherapy. As soon as therapy is given, it is difficult to know to what extent that necrosis is spontaneous versus therapy-induced. Nonetheless, if preoperative irradiation or chemotherapy has been undertaken, clinicians usually expect a statement as to the amount of viable tumor.

Ancillary studies. A report should indicate what tissue has been archived for future use (tissue bank) or referred to other laboratories for additional tests or consultation.

Optional information. There are several other features on which pathologists may comment, including the mitotic rate, vascular invasion, nature of the margin (e.g., circumscribed, infiltrating), presence of an inflammatory infiltrate, and a preexisting benign lesion (e.g., sarcoma arising in a neurofibroma). None translates directly into patient management, and, therefore, they are considered optional in the report. Although the mitotic rate need not be reported, it is assessed as part of the grading of a sarcoma.

CHECKLIST FOR STANDARD REPORTING OF SARCOMA RESECTION SPECIMENS

Procedure

___ Intralesional resection
___ Marginal resection
___ Wide resection
___ Radical resection
___ Other (specify)
___ Not specified

Tumor Site

Specify, if known ___
___ Not specified

Tumor Size

Greatest dimension ___ cm
Additional dimensions ___ cm X ___ cm
___ Indeterminate

Macroscopic Extent of Tumor

___ Superficial
  ___ Dermal
    ___ Subcutaneous/suprafascial
___ Deep
  ___ Fascial
  ___ Subfascial
  ___ Intramuscular
  ___ Mediastinal
  ___ Intraabdominal
  ___ Retroperitoneal
  ___ Head/Neck
  ___ Other
  ___ Indeterminate

Histologic Type

Specify: ___
Indeterminate/unclassified ___

Mitotic Rate (optional)

Specify: ___/10 HPF
(most proliferative area)

Necrosis

___ Not present
___ Present (Extent ___%)

Histologic Grade (Specify grading system e.g. FNCLCC)

___ Grade 1
___ Grade 2
___ Grade 3
___ Ungraded sarcoma
___ Cannot be assessed

Margins

___ Cannot be assessed
___ Negative
  Distance from closest margin ___ cm
  Specify margin
  Specify other close margins (<2 cm)
___ Positive
  Specify margins

Lymph-Vascular Invasion (optional)

___ Not present
___ Present
___ Indeterminate

Pathologic Stage (pTNM) TNM descriptors

___ m (multiple)
___ r (recurrent)
___ y (post treatment)

1. Primary Tumors (pT)

___ PTX: Primary tumor cannot be assessed
___ pT0: No tumor present
___ pT1a: Tumor 5 cm or less; superficial tumor
___ pT1b: Tumor 5 cm or less; deep tumor
___ pT2a: Tumor greater than 5 cm; superficial tumor
___ pT2b: Tumor greater than 5 cm; deep tumor

2. Regional lymph nodes

___ pNX: Regional nodes cannot be assessed
___ pN0: No regional lymph node metastases
___ pN1: Regional lymph nodes metastases
  Specify: Number examined ___
  Number positive ___

3. Distant Metastasis (pM)

___ Not applicable
___ pM1 Distant metastasis
  Specify site, if known ___

Additional pathologic findings: Specify

Ancillary studies

1. Immunohistochemistry
  ___ Not performed
  ___ Performed, specify
2. Cytogenetics
  ___ Not performed
  ___ Performed, specify
3. Molecular Pathology
  ___ Not performed
  ___ Performed, specify

Preresection treatment (select all that apply)

___ No therapy
___ Chemotherapy performed
___ Radiation therapy performed
___ Therapy performed, type not specified
___ Unknown

Treatment Effect

___ Not identified
___ Present
  Specify amount of viable tumor ___%
___ Cannot be determined

CHECKLIST FOR STANDARD REPORTING OF SOFT TISSUE BIOPSY

Procedure

___ Core needle biopsy
___ Incisional biopsy
___ Excisional biopsy
___ Other (specify)
___ Not specified

Tumor Site

Specify, if known ___
___ Not specified

Tumor Size

Greatest dimension ___ cm
Additional dimensions ___ cm X ___ cm
___ Cannot be determined

Macroscopic Extent of Tumor (select all that apply)

___ Superficial
  ___ Dermal
    ___ Subcutaneous
___ Deep
  ___ Fascial
  ___ Subfascial
  ___ Intramuscular
  ___ Mediastinal
  ___ Intra-abdominal
  ___ Retroperitoneal
  ___ Head and Neck
  ___ Other
  ___ Cannot be determined

Histologic Type

Specify: ___
___ Cannot be determined

Mitotic Rate: (optional)

Necrosis

___ Not identified
___ Present (Extent ___%)
___ Cannot be determined

Histologic grade

___ Grade 1
___ Grade 2
___ Grade 3

or

___ Low grade
___ High grade

or

___ Ungradable
___ Cannot be determined

Margins (for excisional biopsy only)

___ Cannot be assessed
___ Margins negative for sarcoma
  Distance of sarcoma from closest margin ___ cm (specify)
___ Margins positive for sarcoma (specify)

Ancillary studies: Immunohistochemistry, cytogenetics, molecular pathology (specify)

Pre-biopsy treatment

___ No therapy
___ Chemotherapy
___ Radiation
___ Therapy, not otherwise specified
___ Unknown

Treatment Effect:

___ Not identified
___ Present
  Specify % viable tumor ___%
___ Indeterminate

FIGURE 6-1. Checklists for standard reporting of sarcoma resection specimens and soft tissue biopsy. *Modified from Rubin BP, Cooper K, Fletcher CD, et al. Protocol for the examination of specimens from patients with tumors of soft tissue. Arch Pathol Lab Med 2010;134(4):e31–9.*

References

1. Heslin MJ, Lewis JJ, Woodruff JM. Core needle biopsy for diagnosis of extremity soft tissue sarcoma. Ann Surg Oncol 1997;44:425–31.
2. Deyrup AT, Weiss SW. Grading of soft tissue sarcomas: the challenge of providing precise information in an imprecise world. Histopathology 2006;48(1):42–50.
3. Kandel RA, Bell RS, Wunder JS, et al. Comparison between a 2- and 3-grade system in predicting metastatic-free survival in extremity soft-tissue sarcoma. J Surg Oncol 1999;72(2):77–82.
4. Rubin BP, Cooper K, Fletcher CD, et al. Protocol for the examination of specimens from patients with tumors of soft tissue. Arch Pathol Lab Med 2010;134(4):e31–39.
5. Weiss SW. The Vincent McGovern memorial lecture. Vascular tumors: a deductive approach to diagnosis. Surg Pathol 1989;2:185.
6. Tanas MR, Rubin BP, Tubbs RR, et al. Utilization of fluorescence in situ hybridization in the diagnosis of 230 mesenchymal neoplasms: an institutional experience. Arch Pathol Lab Med 2010;134(12):1797–803.
7. Tanas MR, Goldblum JR. Fluorescence in situ hybridization in the diagnosis of soft tissue neoplasms: a review. Adv Anat Pathol 2009;16(6): 383–91.
8. Machado I, Noguera R, Pellin A, et al. Molecular diagnosis of Ewing sarcoma family of tumors: a comparative analysis of 560 cases with FISH and RT-PCR. Diagn Mol Pathol 2009;18(4):189–99.
9. Terrier-Lacombe MJ, Guillou L, Chibon F, et al. Superficial primitive Ewing's sarcoma: a clinicopathologic and molecular cytogenetic analysis of 14 cases. Mod Pathol 2009;22(1):87–94.
10. Downs-Kelly E, Goldblum JR, Patel RM, et al. The utility of FOXO1 fluorescence in situ hybridization (FISH) in formalin-fixed paraffin-embedded specimens in the diagnosis of alveolar rhabdomyosarcoma. Diagn Mol Pathol 2009;18(3):138–43.
11. Tanas MR, Rubin BP, Montgomery EA, et al. Utility of FISH in the diagnosis of angiomatoid fibrous histiocytoma: a series of 18 cases. Mod Pathol 2010;23(1):93–7.
12. Antonescu CR, Dal Cin P, Nafa K, et al. EWSR1-CREB1 is the predominant gene fusion in angiomatoid fibrous histiocytoma. Genes Chromosomes Cancer 2007;46(12):1051–60.
13. Song JS, Choi J, Kim JH, et al. Diagnostic utility of EWS break-apart fluorescence in situ hybridization in distinguishing between non-cutaneous melanoma and clear cell sarcoma. Pathol Int 2010;60(9):608–13.
14. Patel R, Downs-Kelly E, Dandehar MN, et al. FUS (16q11) gene rearrangment as detected by fluorescence-in-situ hybridization in cutaneous low-grade fibromyxoid sarcoma: a potential diagnostic tool. Am J Dermatopathol 2011;33(2):140–3.
15. Sugita S, Seki K, Yokozawa K, et al. Analysis of CHOP rearrangement in pleomorphic liposarcomas using fluorescence in situ hybridization. Cancer Sci 2009;100(1):82–7.
16. Downs-Kelly E, Goldblum JR, Patel RM, et al. The utility of fluorescence in situ hybridization (FISH) in the diagnosis of myxoid soft tissue neoplasms. Am J Surg Pathol 2008;32(1):8–13.
17. Zhang H, Erickson-Johnson M, Wang X, et al. Molecular testing for lipomatous tumors: critical analysis and test recommendations based on the analysis of 405 extremity-based tumors. Am J Surg Pathol 2010;34(9):1304–11.
18. Weaver J, Rao P, Goldblum JR, et al. Can MDM2 analytical tests performed on core needle biopsy be relied upon to diagnose well-differentiated liposarcoma? Mod Pathol 2010;23(10):1301–6.
19. Fernandez A, Sun Y, Tubbs RR, et al. FISH for MYC amplification and anti-MYC immunohistochemistry: useful diagnostic tools in the assessment of secondary angiosarcoma and atypical vascular proliferations. J Cutan Pathol 2012;39:234–42.
20. Noguchi H, Mitsuhashi T, Seki K, et al. Fluorescence in situ hybridization analysis of extraskeletal myxoid chondrosarcomas using EWSR1 and NR4A3 probes. Hum Pathol 2010;41(3):336–42.
21. Sun B, Sun Y, Wang J, et al. The diagnostic value of SYT-SSX detected by reverse transcriptase-polymerase chain reaction (RT-PCR) and fluorescence in situ hybridization (FISH) for synovial sarcoma: a review and prospective study of 255 cases. Cancer Sci 2008;99(7):1355–61.
22. Ten Heuvel SE, Hoekstra HJ, Suurmeijer AJH. Diagnostic accuracy of FISH and RT-PCR in 50 routinely processed synovial sarcomas. Appl Immunohistochem Mol Morphol 2008;16(3):246–50.
23. Amary MF, Berisha F, Bernardi F del C, et al. Detection of SS18-SSX fusion transcripts in formalin-fixed paraffin-embedded neoplasms: analysis of conventional RT-PCR, qRT-PCR and dual color FISH as diagnostic tools for synovial sarcoma. Mod Pathol 2007;20(4):482–96.
24. Macarenco RS, Erickson-Johnson M, Wang X, et al. Retroperitoneal lipomatous tumors without cytologic atypia: are they lipomas? A clinicopathologic and molecular study of 19 cases. Am J Surg Pathol 2009; 33(10):1470–6.
25. Kempson RL, Hendrickson MR. In: Weiss SW, Brooks JSJ, editors. An approach to the diagnosis of soft tissue tumors, In: Soft tissue tumors. Williams & Wilkins: Baltimore; 1996.
26. AJCC cancer staging handbook, 7th ed. 2010. p. 291–8.
27. Coindre JM, Terrier P, Bui NB, et al. Prognostic factors in adult patients with locally controlled soft tissue sarcoma. A study of 546 patients from the French Federation of Cancer Centers Sarcoma Group. J Clin Oncol 1996;14(3):869–77.
28. Guillou L, Coindre JM, Bonichon F, et al. Comparative study of the National Cancer Institute and French Federation of Cancer Centers Sarcoma Group grading systems in a population of 410 adult patients with soft tissue sarcoma. J Clin Oncol 1997;15(1):350–62.
29. Pisters PW, Leung DH, Woodruff J, et al. Analysis of prognostic factors in 1,041 patients with localized soft tissue sarcomas of the extremities. J Clin Oncol 1996;14(5):1679–89.
30. Rydholm A, Rööser B. Surgical margins for soft-tissue sarcoma. J Bone Joint Surg Am 1987;69(7):1074–8.
31. Heslin MJ, Woodruff J, Brennan MF. Prognostic significance of a positive microscopic margin in high-risk extremity soft tissue sarcoma: implications for management. J Clin Oncol 1996;14(2):473–8.

Immunohistochemistry for Analysis of Soft Tissue Tumors

ANDREW L. FOLPE and ALLEN M. GOWN

CHAPTER CONTENTS

Immunohistochemistry is the use of antibody-based reagents for localization of specific epitopes in tissue sections. Over the past two decades, immunohistochemistry has become a powerful tool to assist the surgical pathologist in many clinically critical settings. It is important to recognize that immunohistochemistry has two components, each with its own strengths and weaknesses. These components may be thought of as the hardware (i.e., antibodies, detection systems) and the software (i.e., analytic processes). No matter how selective the antibodies or how powerful the detection system, the method fails if the analytic tools are inadequate. This chapter focuses on the antibody component of the hardware and some of the analytic processes in which immunohistochemistry assists in the diagnosis of soft tissue neoplasms.

It cannot be overemphasized that immunohistochemistry is an adjunctive diagnostic technique to traditional morphologic methods in soft tissue pathology, as in any other area of surgical pathology. It is critical to recognize that the diagnosis of many soft tissue tumors does not require immunohistochemistry (e.g., osteocartilaginous tumors), and that there are no markers or combinations of markers that will reliably distinguish benign from malignant tumors (e.g., the distinction of nodular fasciitis from leiomyosarcoma). Furthermore, reliable specific markers do not yet exist for certain mesenchymal cell types and their tumors, and there is a subset of soft tissue tumors that are better defined by their molecular rather than their immunophenotypic profile, and techniques other than immunohistochemistry, such as cytogenetic or molecular genetic studies, may prove more valuable in this setting. Last, it is important to acknowledge that a subset of soft tissue tumors defies classification, even with exhaustive immunohistochemistry or genetic study.

The expression of certain antigens, or clusters of antigens, is characteristic of some tumors. Although there are thousands of monoclonal and polyclonal antibodies available to assist in tumor diagnosis, only a small subset has proved to be of practical value in the diagnosis of soft tissue neoplasms. Tables 7-1 and 7-2 present an overview of the markers discussed in the following sections. The question marks highlight the gaps in the understanding of the cellular biology of many soft tissue tumors.

INTERMEDIATE FILAMENTS

The intermediate filaments comprise the major component of the cytoskeleton and consist of five major subgroups (vimentin, cytokeratins, desmin, neurofilaments, glial fibrillary acidic protein [GFAP]) and a small number of minor subgroups (e.g., nestin, peripherin).[1-3] Ultrastructurally, the intermediate filaments appear as wavy unbranched filaments that often occupy a perinuclear location in the cell. The original belief that intermediate filament expression was restricted to specific cell types (e.g., cytokeratins in carcinomas, vimentin in sarcomas) is now being recognized as an oversimplification. The following sections on intermediate filaments concentrate not only on the normal pattern of expression of these proteins but also on the situations in which intermediate filaments show anomalous expression.

Vimentin

Vimentin, a 57-kDa intermediate filament protein, is expressed in all mesenchymal cells. Vimentin is ubiquitously expressed in all cells during early embryogenesis and is gradually replaced in many cells by type-specific intermediate filaments.[1,4] In some mesenchymal tissues, vimentin is typically co-expressed along with the cell type-specific intermediate filaments (e.g., desmin and vimentin co-expression in muscle cells, vimentin and GFAP in some Schwann cells). Vimentin is expressed in virtually all mesenchymal tumors and is therefore of minimal value in identifying particular tumors. Given the frequent co-expression of vimentin along with cytokeratin

TABLE 7-1 Common Immunohistochemical Markers

ANTIBODIES TO:	EXPRESSED BY:
Cytokeratins	Carcinomas, epithelioid sarcoma, synovial sarcoma, some angiosarcomas and leiomyosarcomas, mesothelioma, rhabdoid tumor
Vimentin	Sarcomas, melanoma, lymphoma, some carcinomas
Desmin	Benign and malignant smooth and skeletal muscle tumors
Glial fibrillary acidic protein	Gliomas, some schwannomas
Neurofilaments	Neural and neuroblastic tumors
Smooth and skeletal muscle actins (HHF35)	Benign and malignant smooth and skeletal muscle tumors, myofibroblastic tumors and pseudotumors
Smooth muscle actin (1A4)	Benign and malignant smooth muscle tumors, myofibroblastic tumors and pseudotumors
Myogenic nuclear regulatory proteins (myogenin, MyoD1)	Rhabdomyosarcoma
S-100 protein	Melanoma, benign and malignant peripheral nerve sheath tumors, cartilaginous tumors, normal adipose tissue, Langerhans cells, many others
Epithelial membrane antigen	Carcinomas, epithelioid sarcoma, synovial sarcoma, perineurioma, meningioma, anaplastic large cell lymphoma
CD31	Benign and malignant vascular tumors
von Willebrand factor (factor VIII-related protein)	Benign and malignant vascular tumors
CD34	Benign and malignant vascular tumors, solitary fibrous tumor, epithelioid sarcoma, dermatofibrosarcoma protuberans, GIST
CD99 (MIC2 gene product)	Ewing family of tumors, some rhabdomyosarcomas, some synovial sarcomas, lymphoblastic lymphoma, mesenchymal chondrosarcoma, small cell osteosarcoma, many others
CD45 (leukocyte common antigen)	Non-Hodgkin lymphoma
CD30 (Ki-1)	Anaplastic large cell lymphoma, embryonal carcinoma
CD68	Macrophages, fibrohistiocytic tumors, granular cell tumors, various sarcomas, melanomas, carcinomas
Melanosome-specific antigens (HMB-45 defined gp100, Melan-A, tyrosinase, microphthalmia transcription factor)	Melanoma, PEComa, clear cell sarcoma, melanotic schwannoma
MDM2/CDK4	Atypical lipomatous tumor and dedifferentiated liposarcoma
Claudin-1	Perineurioma, synovial sarcoma, epithelioid sarcoma, some Ewing family of tumors
Glut-1	Perineurioma, infantile hemangioma
SMARCB1 (INI1)	Expression lost in extrarenal rhabdoid tumor, epithelioid sarcoma, some epithelioid malignant peripheral nerve sheath tumor, and extraskeletal myxoid chondrosarcomas
Protein kinase C-θ and DOG1	GIST
Bcl-2	Synovial sarcoma, solitary fibrous tumor, other spindle cell tumors

TABLE 7-2 Specific Tumor Types, Normal Counterparts, and Useful Markers

TUMOR TYPE	NORMAL CELL COUNTERPART	USEFUL MARKER(S)
Angiosarcoma	Endothelium	CD31, CD34, FLI-1, ERG, von Willebrand factor, claudin-5, type IV collagen
Leiomyosarcoma	Smooth muscle	Muscle (smooth) actins, desmin, caldesmon, myosin heavy chain, type IV collagen
Rhabdomyosarcoma	Skeletal muscle	MyoD1, myogenin; muscle (sarcomeric) actins; desmin
Ewing family of tumors	—	CD99 (p30/32-MIC2), FLI-1, NKX2.2
Synovial sarcoma	—	Cytokeratin, EMA, TLE1
Epithelioid sarcoma	—	Cytokeratin, CD34, SMARCB1 (INI1) loss
Malignant peripheral nerve sheath tumor	Nerve sheath (e.g., Schwann cell, perineurial cell)	S-100, CD57, NGF receptor, EMA, claudin-1, Glut-1, SOX10
Liposarcoma	Adipocyte	S-100 protein, MDM2, CDK4
Chondrosarcoma	Chondrocyte	S-100 protein
Osteogenic sarcoma	Osteocyte	Osteocalcin
Kaposi sarcoma	Endothelium	CD31, CD34, VEGFR3, podoplanin, LANA
Myofibroblastic lesions (e.g., nodular fasciitis)	Myofibroblast	Smooth muscle actins
Gastrointestinal stromal tumor	Interstitial cells of Cajal	CD117 (c-kit), CD34, protein kinase C-θ, DOG1
Solitary fibrous tumor	—	CD34, Bcl-2
Glomus tumors	Glomus cell	Smooth muscle actins, type IV collagen
Angiomatoid (malignant) fibrous histiocytoma	—	Desmin, EMA, CD68
Alveolar soft part sarcoma	—	TFE3
Perivascular epithelioid cell neoplasms (PEComas)	—	Smooth muscle actins, melanocytic markers

in carcinomas, vimentin expression is also of little value in the immunohistochemical distinction of carcinomas from sarcomas.[5-9] Vimentin immunoreactivity has been touted as a good marker of tissue preservation. However, vimentin expression, similar to that of all of the intermediate filaments, is rather hardy and may remain present in tissues in which all other immunoreactivity has been lost.[10] The absence of vimentin expression may occasionally be a clue to the diagnosis of rare vimentin-negative mesenchymal tumors, such as alveolar soft part sarcoma (ASPS) and perivascular epithelioid cell neoplasms.[11,12] In general, there is no value in performing vimentin immunostains on any spindle cell neoplasm.

Cytokeratins

Cytokeratins, the most complex members of the intermediate filament protein family, are a collection of more than 20 proteins. The cytokeratins may be grouped by their molecular

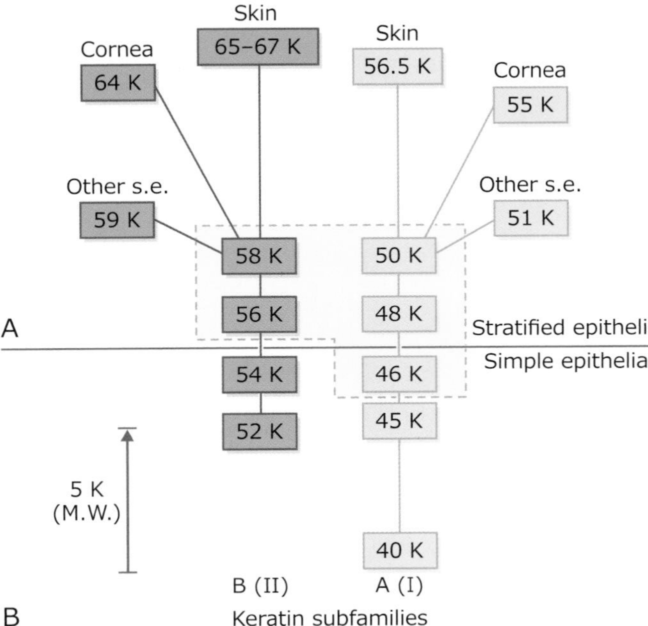

FIGURE 7-1. Subcategorization of acidic (A) and basic (B) cytokeratin subgroups within various tissues. *(Modified from Cooper D, Schermer A, Sun TT. Classification of human epithelium and their neoplasms using monoclonal antibodies to keratins: strategies, applications, and limitations. Lab Invest 1985; 52:243, with permission.)*

weights (40 to 67 kDa) into acidic and basic subfamilies or by their usual pattern of expression in simple or complex epithelium (Fig. 7-1). In practice, the cytokeratins are most commonly thought of in terms of low-molecular-weight cytokeratins (generally cytokeratins 8, 18, and 19) and high-molecular-weight cytokeratins (generally cytokeratins 1, 5, 10, and 14). Cytokeratins are highly sensitive markers for identifying carcinomas and are generally used as markers distinguishing epithelial from nonepithelial tumors (i.e., lymphomas, sarcomas, melanomas) (Fig. 7-2). Over the past decade, it has become abundantly clear that cytokeratin expression is not restricted to carcinomas.

Sarcomas with True Epithelial Differentiation: Epithelioid Sarcoma and Synovial Sarcoma

Among the sarcomas, there are two patterns of cytokeratin expression. A small subset of sarcomas displays true epithelial differentiation as defined by usual expression of cytokeratin and other epithelial proteins such as the desmoplakins and occludin (e.g., synovial sarcomas and epithelioid sarcomas).[13,14] Additionally, there is a larger group of tumors that occasionally display anomalous cytokeratin expression (i.e., cytokeratin expression by cells and tumors without true epithelial differentiation). Synovial sarcomas and epithelioid sarcomas are the best, if not the only, examples of sarcomas manifesting true epithelial differentiation (Fig. 7-3). Expression of both low- and high-molecular-weight cytokeratin isoforms is seen in both synovial sarcoma and epithelioid sarcoma, confirming the presence of true epithelial differentiation.[15,16] Antibodies to specific cytokeratins, such as cytokeratins 7 and 19 for synovial sarcoma and cytokeratins 5 and 6 in epithelioid sarcoma, may also be diagnostically useful in selected cases.[16-18]

Anomalous Cytokeratin Expression

Anomalous cytokeratin expression is typically characterized by immunostaining (even under optimal technical conditions) in only a subset of the target cell population. In those cells, cytokeratin is present in only a portion of the cytoplasm, often yielding a perinuclear or dot-like pattern of immunostaining. However, this dot-like pattern is not always an indication of anomalous cytokeratin because it is typically seen in some neuroendocrine carcinomas, including small cell carcinomas and Merkel cell tumors, and in extrarenal rhabdoid tumors (Fig. 7-4).[19-21] In addition, it is rare to find cytokeratins other than those corresponding to the Moll catalog 8 and 18 (corresponding to positivity with antibodies CAM5.2 or 35βH11) in tumors manifesting anomalous cytokeratin expression.[13]

Contrary to some earlier suggestions, anomalous cytokeratin expression is not a universal feature of sarcomas. It is, instead, a feature of a limited subset of nonepithelial tumors, particularly smooth muscle tumors, melanomas, and endothelial cell tumors; as such, it may serve as a clue to the diagnosis of these tumors. Interestingly, the normal cell counterparts of some of these tumors (i.e., smooth muscle cells and endothelial cells) have been found to express cytokeratins in nonmammalian species[22] and are frequently cytokeratin-positive in routinely processed sections, particularly with newer, more sensitive antibodies, such as the OSCAR wide spectrum cytokeratin antibody.

Smooth Muscle Cells and Smooth Muscle Tumors

Frozen sections of the smooth muscle cell-rich myometrium of the uterus (along with myocardial cells) were first reported to react with various anticytokeratin antibodies. Brown et al.[23] and Norton et al.[24] verified these findings using slightly different techniques, although Norton et al. failed to find corroborative biochemical evidence of cytokeratin expression by these smooth muscle cells. Biochemical documentation of true anomalous cytokeratin expression of cytokeratins 8 and 18 was first presented by Gown et al.,[25] in which immunostaining was corroborated by Western blots; it was further documented by two-color immunofluorescence studies of myometrial smooth muscle cells grown in vitro. Subsequent studies have shown that at least 30% of leiomyosarcomas manifest cytokeratin.[26-28]

Melanomas

Despite that many studies completed during the mid-1980s concluded that melanomas were vimentin-positive, cytokeratin-negative tumors,[29,30] Zarbo et al.[30] first confirmed the cytokeratin positivity of many melanomas and demonstrated the positive immunostaining as a function of tissue preparation and fixation (with 21% of cases positive in frozen sections but far fewer in formalin-fixed, paraffin-embedded sections). Zarbo et al.[30] also performed one- and two-dimensional gel electrophoresis with immunoblotting, confirming that cytokeratin 8 was expressed by the tumor cell population. Anomalous cytokeratin expression is generally a feature of metastatic, but not primary, melanomas.[31]

Angiosarcomas

Early reports suggested that vascular tumors manifesting epithelioid histologic features (e.g., epithelioid hemangioendothelioma and epithelioid angiosarcoma) express cytokeratin in

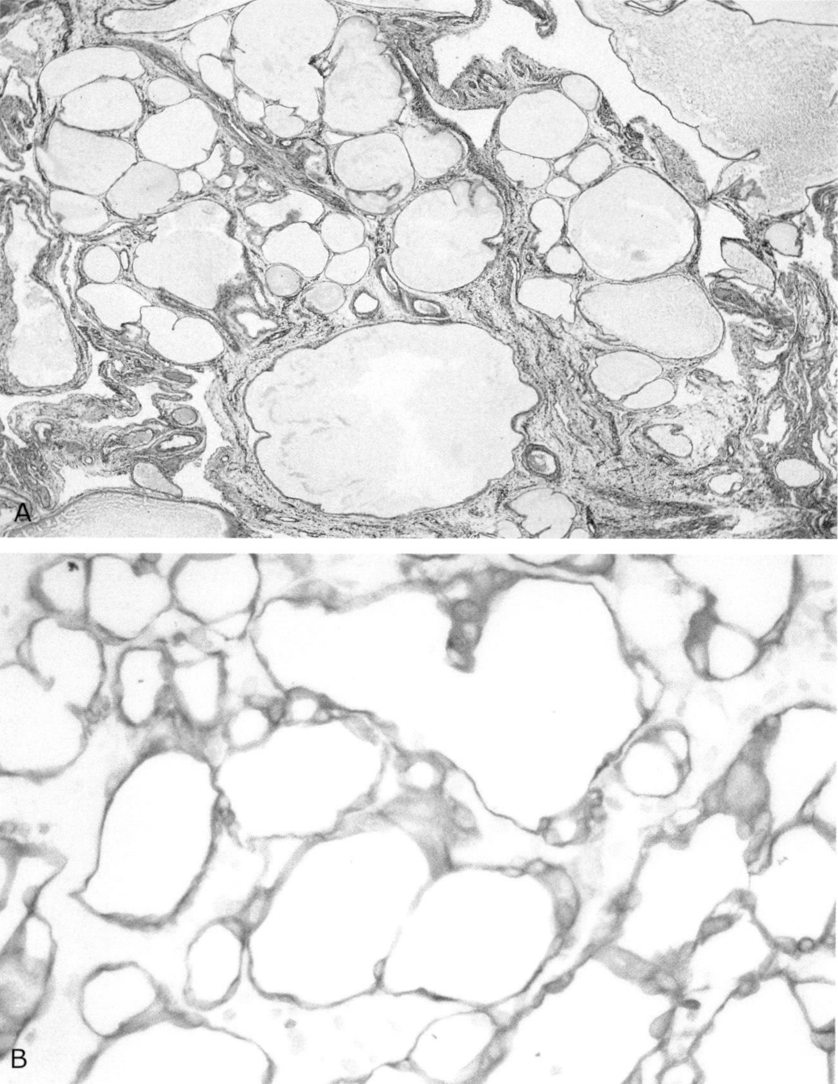

FIGURE 7-2. Cystic mesothelioma (A) immunostained for cytokeratin (B). Demonstration of strong cytokeratin expression is useful for distinguishing this entity from cystic lymphangioma.

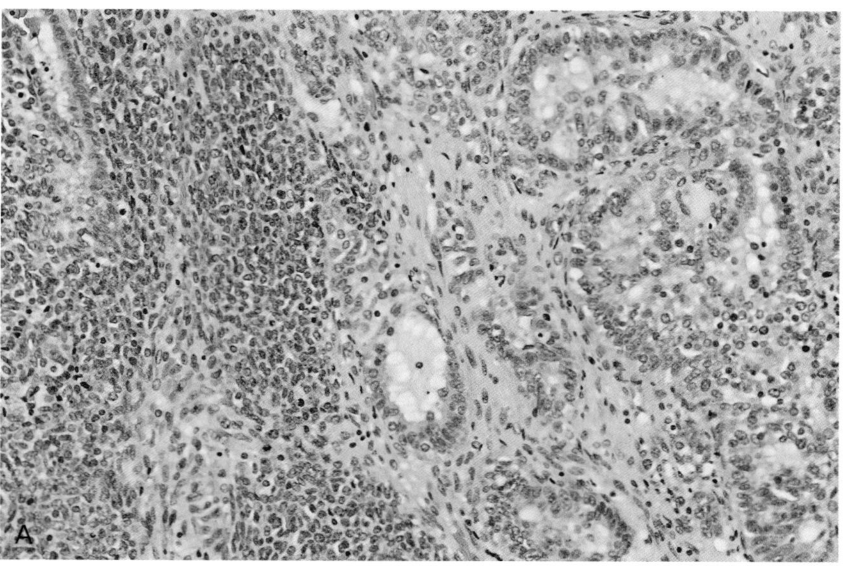

FIGURE 7-3. Biphasic synovial sarcoma with an evolving poorly differentiated cell population (A).

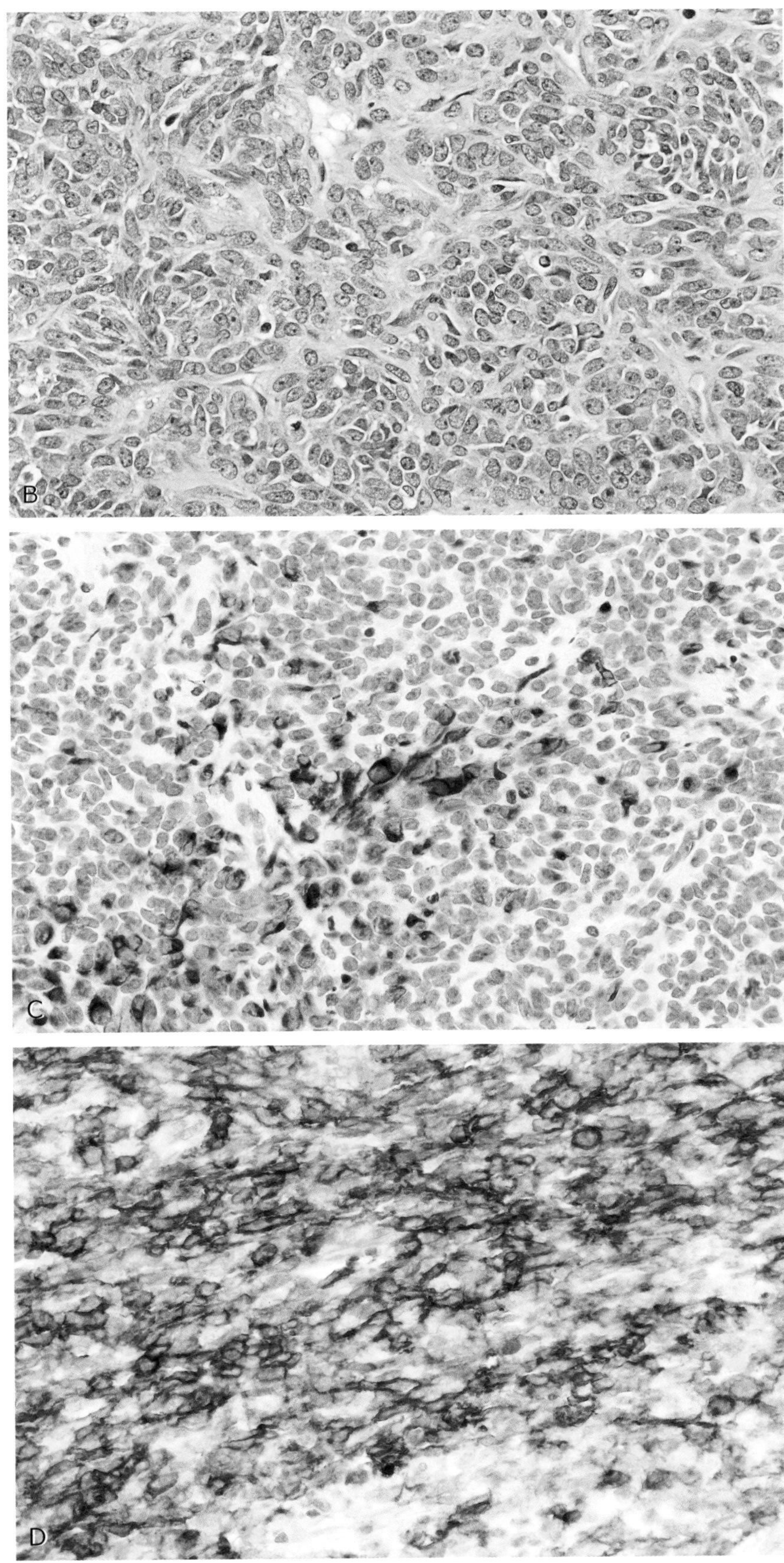

FIGURE 7-3, cont'd. Poorly differentiated synovial sarcoma (B) demonstrating focal expression of high-molecular-weight cytokeratins. (C) Expression of cytokeratin in synovial sarcomas may be focal, and some express only high-molecular-weight isoforms. Many poorly differentiated synovial sarcomas also express CD99 (D), and it is important not to mistake them for EFT.

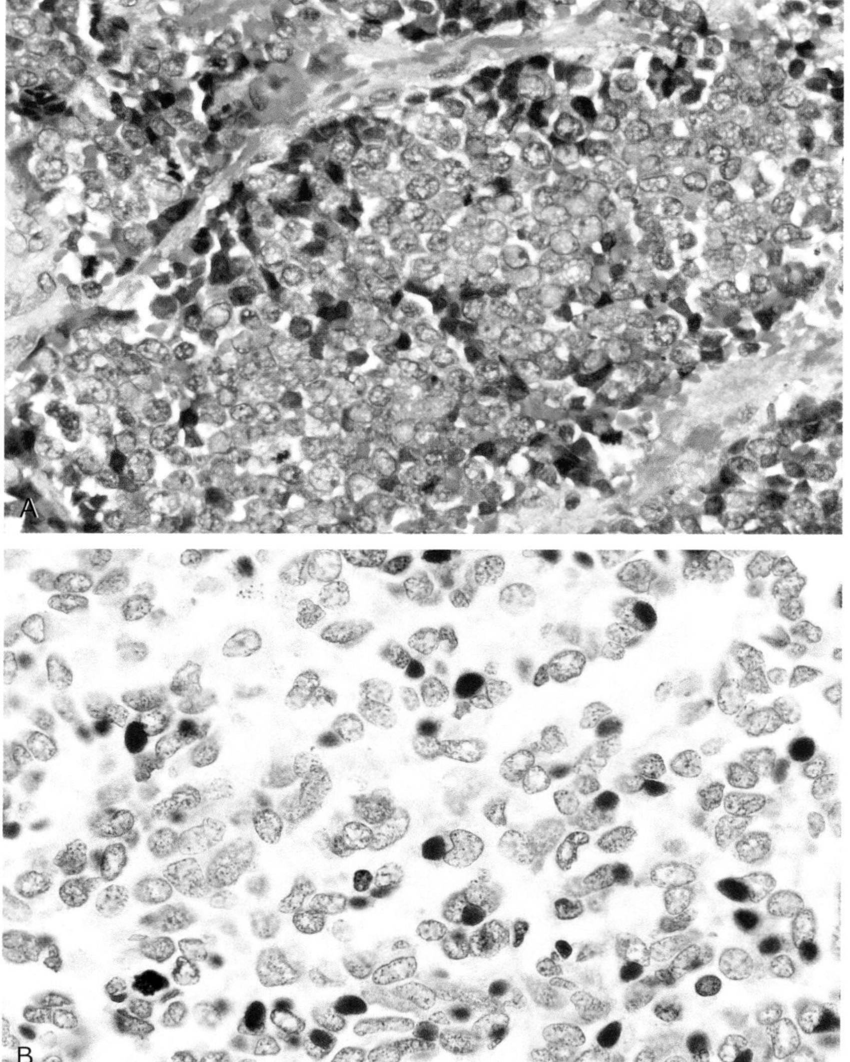

FIGURE 7-4. Merkel cell carcinoma (A) demonstrating characteristic expression of cytokeratin in a dot-like pattern (B). Dot-like expression of cytokeratin and other intermediate filaments is not specific for neuroendocrine carcinomas and may be seen in any small, blue round cell tumor. Dot-like expression may also be a clue to anomalous intermediate filament expression.

most cases (Fig. 7-5).[32-36] The largest published series of angiosarcomas of deep soft tissue has documented cytokeratin expression in about one-third of cases.[37]

Small Blue Round Cell Tumors

A surprising number of tumors in the category of small, blue round cell tumors of childhood typically co-express cytokeratin in a pattern much like that of anomalous cytokeratin expression. These tumors include Ewing family of tumors (EFT),[38-41] rhabdomyosarcoma (RMS),[42,43] Wilms tumor,[44,45] and desmoplastic small round cell tumor (DSRCT) of childhood.[46,47] Expression of low-molecular-weight cytokeratin isoforms may be seen in nearly 25% of EFT, usually confined to less than 20% of the neoplastic cells[38,39,41]; expression of high-molecular-weight cytokeratins is far less common and is restricted to the rare adamantinoma-like variant of EFT (Fig. 7-6).[41]

Cytokeratin Expression in Other Sarcomas

The literature is replete with reports of cytokeratin expression in other sarcomas, including undifferentiated pleomorphic sarcoma (also known as malignant fibrous histiocytoma),[48-51] chondrosarcoma,[52,53] osteosarcoma,[54,55] and malignant peripheral nerve sheath tumors.[18,56] Nonetheless, cytokeratin expression in these tumors is exceedingly rare.

It is important to remember that immunoreactivity and true antigen expression are not necessarily synonymous.[57] Several factors can theoretically account for positive cytokeratin immunostaining in tumors without true cytokeratin expression. This includes the use of antibodies at inappropriately high concentrations,[58,59] potentially altered specificities following the use of heat-induced epitope retrieval techniques (antigen retrieval),[58,59] and the cross-reactivity of anticytokeratin antibodies with other proteins, such as GFAP in gliomas and some schwannomas.[60,61] It is also important to distinguish reactive cytokeratin-positive cells, such as submesothelial fibroblasts, from the neoplastic cell population (Fig. 7-7). By using an approach to immunohistochemistry that includes use of a panel of antibodies, the pathologist can generally avoid misinterpretation that might result from a misbehavior of one antibody.

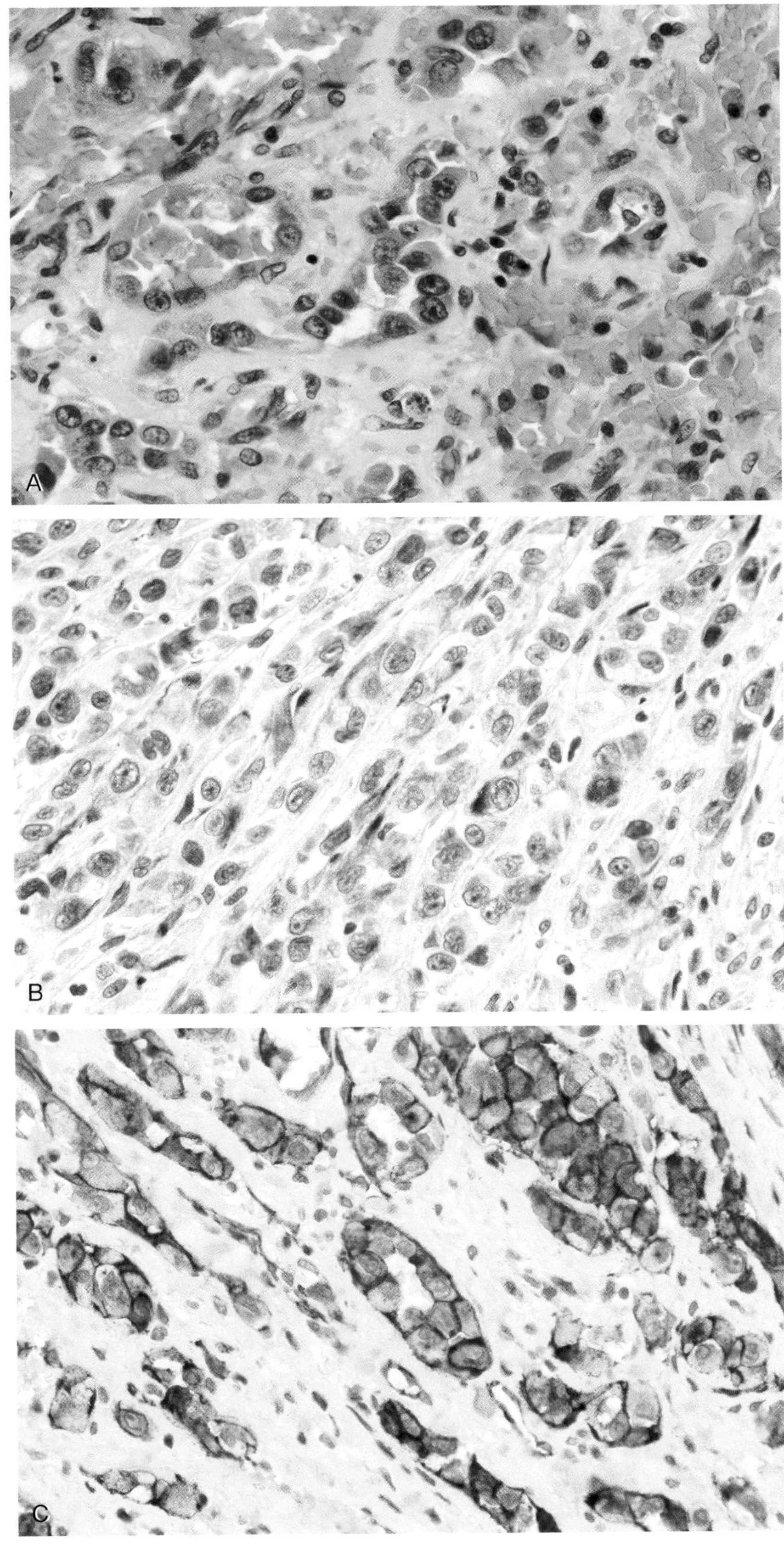

FIGURE 7-5. Epithelioid angiosarcoma (A) with strong expression of low-molecular-weight cytokeratin (B). Vascular tumors, particularly epithelioid ones, commonly express low-molecular-weight cytokeratins and may be mistaken for carcinoma. Expression of CD31 (C), a highly specific marker of endothelium, serves to distinguish keratin-positive angiosarcoma from carcinoma or epithelioid sarcoma.

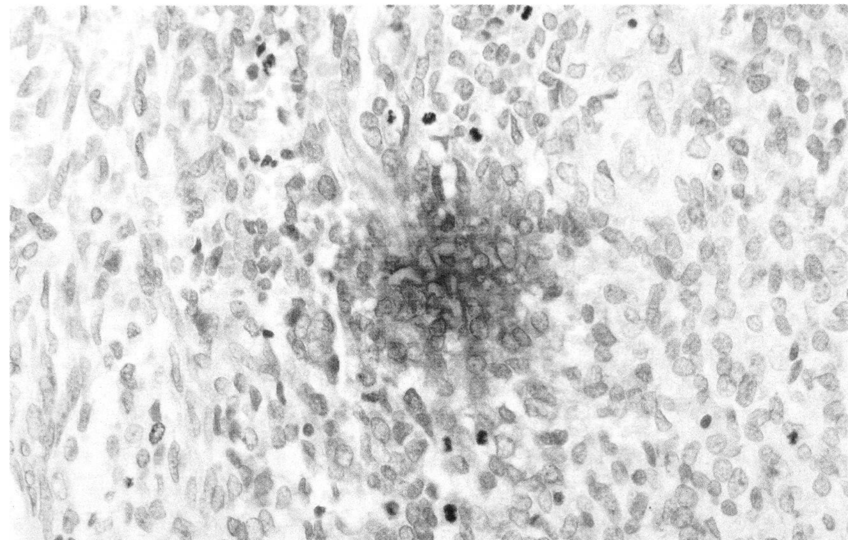

FIGURE 7-6. Overlay of dandruff on a slide, creating apparent focal cytokeratin expression.

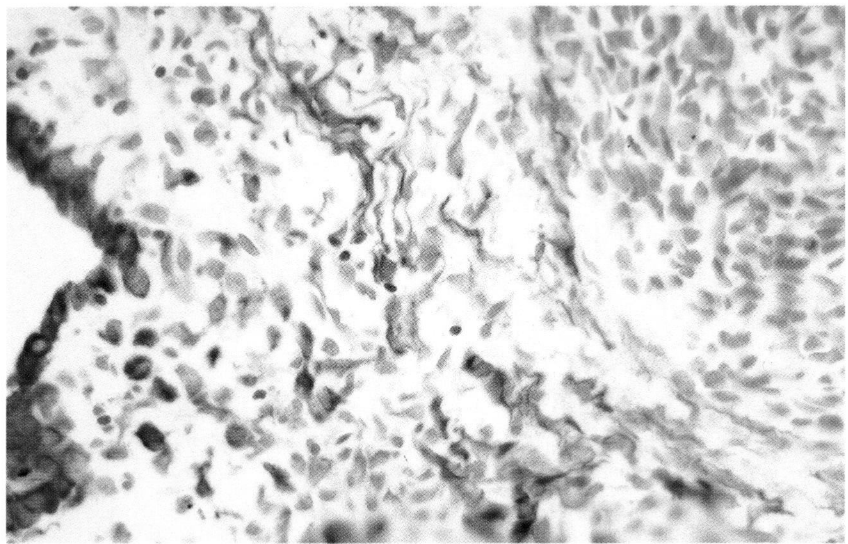

FIGURE 7-7. Low-molecular-weight cytokeratin expression in mesothelium (top) and in spindled submesothelial fibroblasts (middle). Expression of cytokeratin in these reactive submesothelial fibroblasts should be distinguished from cytokeratin expression in the adjacent infiltrating sarcoma (bottom).

EPITHELIAL MEMBRANE ANTIGEN

Epithelial membrane antigen (EMA) is an incompletely characterized antigen that is present in a group of carbohydrate-rich, protein-poor, high-molecular-weight molecules present on the surface of many normal types of epithelium, including those in the pancreas, stomach, intestine, salivary gland, respiratory tract, urinary tract, and breast.[62,63] Among normal mesenchymal cells, EMA expression is limited to perineurial cells[64-67] and meningeal cells.[67,68] There are a limited number of uses for EMA in sarcoma diagnosis. EMA expression is a more sensitive, but less specific, marker of poorly differentiated synovial sarcomas (PDSS); it may be helpful in cases with only focal (or absent) cytokeratin expression.[15] Perineuriomas and malignant peripheral nerve sheath tumors with perineurial differentiation are characterized by a sometimes subtle expression of EMA along cell processes as well as by claudin-1, GLUT-1, and type IV collagen expression (Fig. 7-8).[69-73] Ectopic meningiomas, like their meningeal counterparts, are characterized by EMA and vimentin expression in the absence of cytokeratin expression.[67,68] Patchy expression of EMA (along with desmin and CD68) is seen in roughly 50% of angiomatoid fibrous histiocytomas.[74] EMA expression has been documented in a significant subset of genetically confirmed low-grade fibromyxoid sarcomas, a potentially serious pitfall, given the morphologic similarities between these tumors and perineuriomas.[75] Patchy EMA immunoreactivity may be seen in a fairly broad range of mesenchymal tumors, emphasizing the need to use antibodies to EMA as part of a panel of immunostains.

MARKERS OF MUSCLE DIFFERENTIATION

There are three types of muscle differentiation. The first is skeletal muscle differentiation, as recapitulated in rhabdomyoma and RMS. The second is true smooth muscle differentiation, reflected in leiomyoma and leiomyosarcoma. The third is partial smooth muscle differentiation, as seen in the

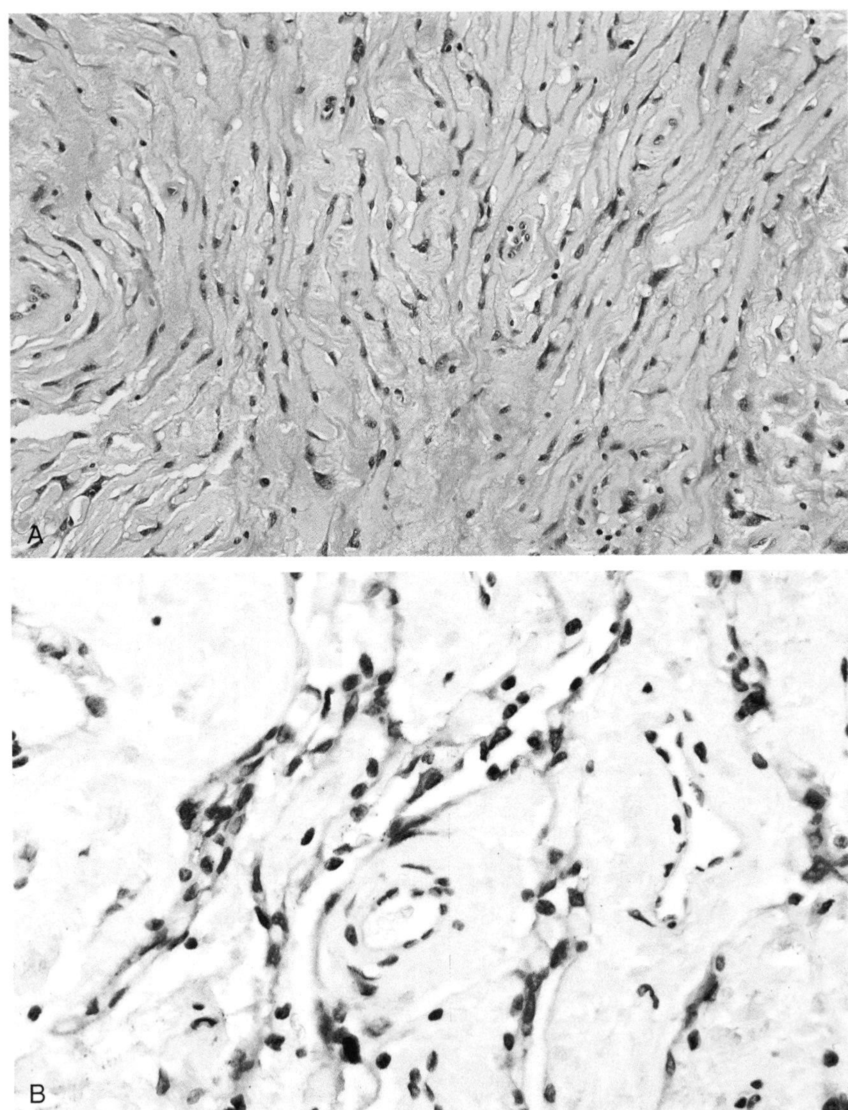

FIGURE 7-8. Malignant perineurioma (A) expressing epithelial membrane antigen (B).

myofibroblasts that constitute a significant population of cells in healing wounds and the stromal reaction to tumors. There is also a subset of soft tissue tumors (e.g., nodular fasciitis and myofibroblastoma), the phenotype of which bears a great resemblance to myofibroblasts rather than to true smooth muscle cells. The principal markers of muscle differentiation are the intermediate filament desmin, the various actin isoforms, and the myogenic regulatory proteins.

Desmin

Desmin is the intermediate filament protein associated with both smooth and skeletal muscle differentiation; it is rarely expressed by myofibroblasts and their corresponding tumors. In skeletal muscle, desmin is localized to the Z-zone between the myofibrils, where it presumably serves as binding material for the contractile apparatus.[76] In smooth muscle, it is associated with cytoplasmic dense bodies and subplasmalemmal dense plaques. Desmin may also be expressed by nonmuscle cells, including the fibroblastic reticulum cell of the lymph node,[77,78] the submesothelial fibroblast,[79] and endometrial stromal cells.[80] It is among the earliest muscle structural genes expressed in the myotome of embryos and has been regarded by some as the best single marker for the diagnosis of poorly differentiated RMS.[81,82] Although the early literature on desmin questioned its sensitivity in formalin-fixed, deparaffinized tissue sections,[83-85] more recent studies have borne out its excellent sensitivity. With the use of heat-induced epitope retrieval techniques and modern antibodies such as D33, desmin is the most sensitive marker of skeletal and smooth muscle differentiation in terms of both the fraction of tumors so identified and the fraction of tumor cells in given tumors that are positive. Desmin expression is present in nearly 100% of RMS of all subtypes, including very poorly differentiated ones (Fig. 7-9).[71,85-92]

Desmin expression is apparently not as specific for muscle tumors as was originally thought, as it has also been described in EFT,[41,93] DSRCT,[46,47,94] neuroblastoma,[95] mesothelial cells and tumors,[96] the blastemal component of Wilms tumor,[97]

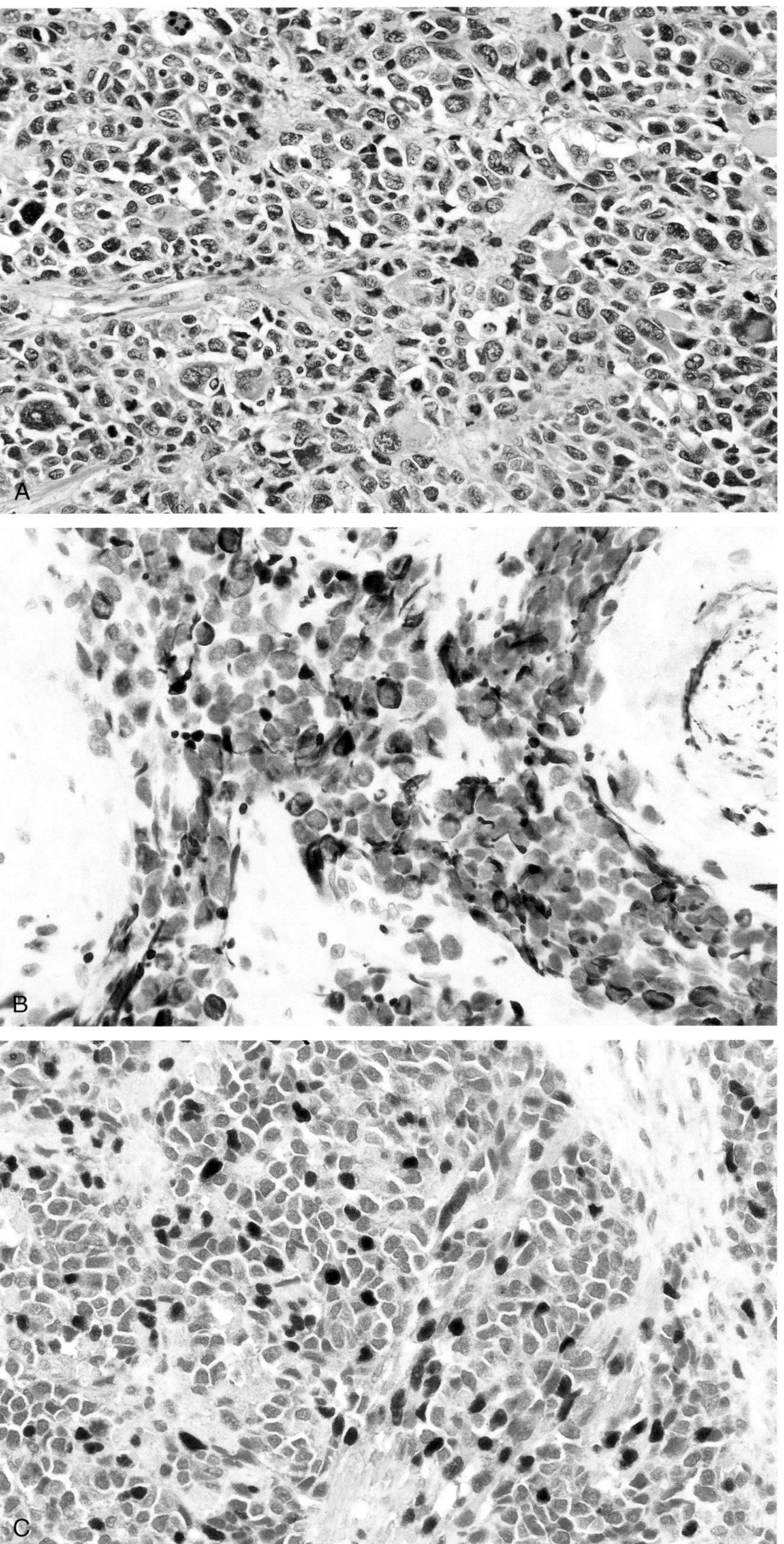

FIGURE 7-9. Alveolar rhabdomyosarcoma (A) demonstrating intense expression of desmin (B). Although desmin is a highly sensitive marker of myogenous sarcomas, it may also be expressed in a variety of nonmyogenous tumors. The most specific markers of rhabdomyosarcoma are antibodies to myogenic nuclear regulatory proteins, such as MyoD1 or myogenin (C). Only a nuclear pattern of expression of these proteins should be accepted.

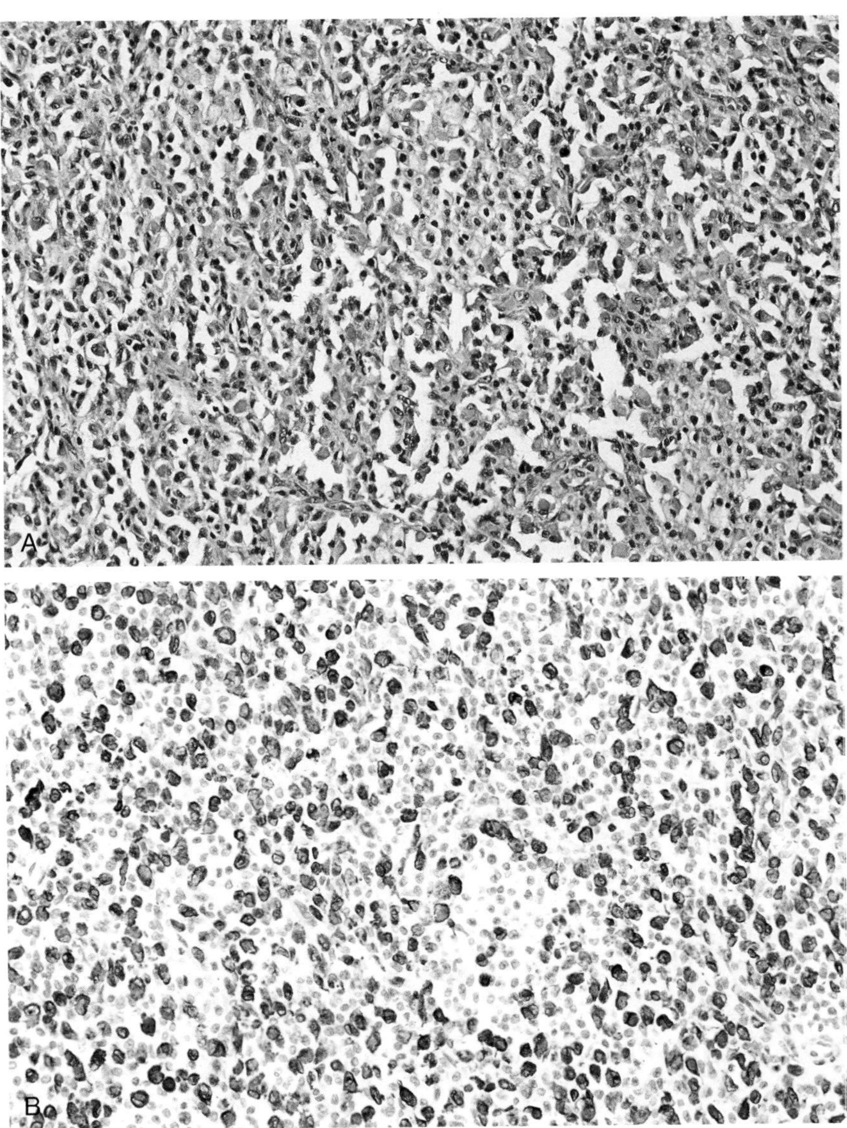

FIGURE 7-10. Diffuse-type tenosynovial giant cell tumor with a prominent population of large eosinophilic cells (A). These eosinophilic cells may show intense positivity with antibodies to desmin (B) and may result in an erroneous diagnosis of rhabdomyosarcoma. Such desmin-positive cells are present in approximately 40% of tenosynovial giant cell tumors.

giant cell tumors of the tendon sheath,[98] and ossifying fibromyxoid tumors of soft parts;[99] in none of these contexts is there thought to be true muscle differentiation (Fig. 7-10). Expression of desmin along with EMA and CD68, in the absence of other muscle markers, is highly characteristic of angiomatoid fibrous histiocytomas (Fig. 7-11).[74,100] Occasional desmin-positive melanomas and schwannomas have also been seen. Definitive identification of tumors manifesting skeletal muscle differentiation, therefore, may require the additional use of antibodies to myogenic transcription factors such as myogenin and myoD1 (see the following sections).

Actin

Actin, a ubiquitous protein, is expressed by all cell types; high concentrations of actins and unique isoforms, however, help make actin a marker of muscle differentiation. In general, actins can be grouped into muscle and nonmuscle isoforms, which differ by only a few amino acids in a protein with a molecular weight of 43,000. It has, nevertheless, been possible to generate antibodies specific to muscle actins versus nonmuscle actins and to specific actin isotypes with respect to the various muscle types (e.g., smooth muscle versus skeletal muscle).[9,101-103] Although an early body of literature speaks to the specificity of anti-actin polyclonal antibodies for muscle cells, in most of these studies, it is a quantitative rather than a qualitative phenomenon: that is, muscle cells have far more actin than many other cells, and demonstration of positivity is determined on this basis alone. Whereas there are monoclonal antibodies that can identify all actin isoforms (i.e., the C4 clone[101]), given the sensitive immunohistochemical techniques available, this antibody cannot be used to distinguish muscle from nonmuscle actins. The antibody HHF35, which has been widely used to identify muscle cells and tumors, displays specificity for all muscle (versus nonmuscle) actins.[104] Antibody 1A4 is a monoclonal antibody that specifically identifies smooth muscle actin isoforms; therefore, it can distinguish smooth from skeletal muscle cells and tumors.[102] Smooth muscle actin isoforms are also expressed by myofibroblasts,

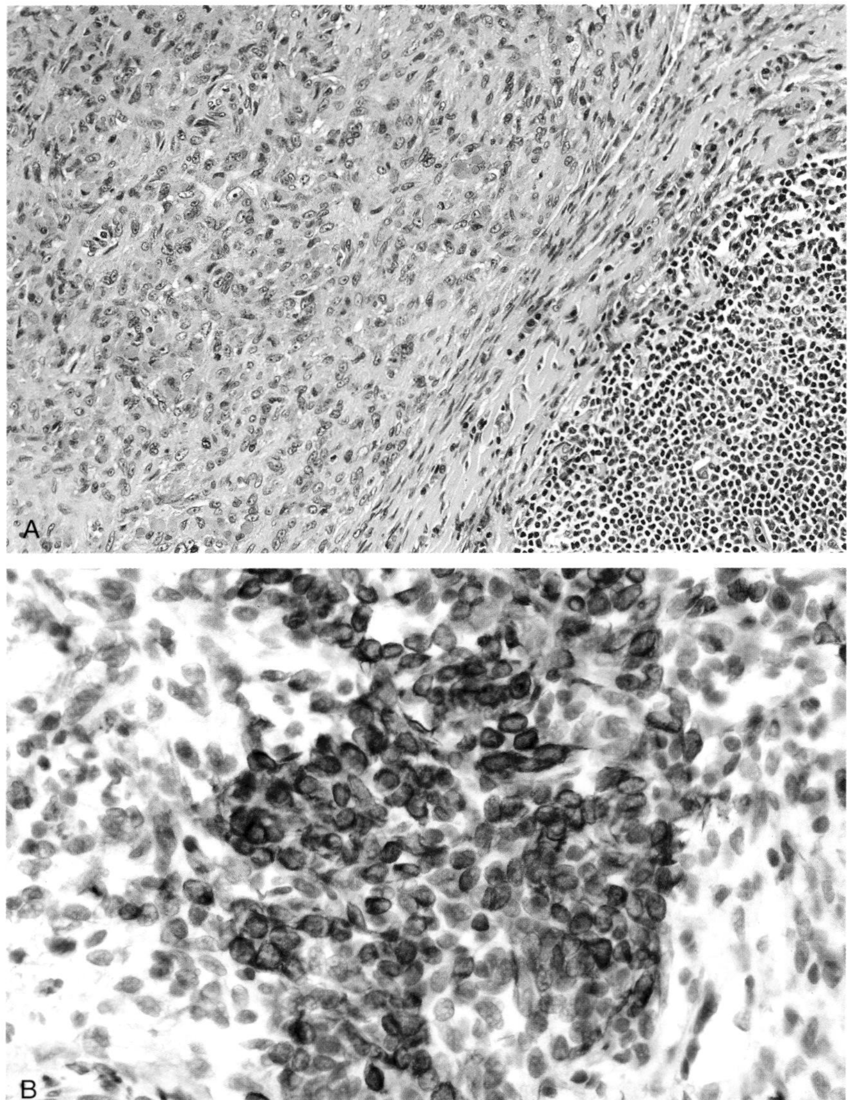

FIGURE 7-11. Angiomatoid fibrous histiocytoma (A) with strong expression of desmin (B). These tumors characteristically co-express desmin, EMA, and CD68 but are negative for all other muscle-related markers.

and the characteristic pattern of actin expression in these cells may help distinguish them from true smooth muscle cells. In general, myofibroblasts show expression of smooth muscle actin only at the periphery of their cytoplasm (tram-track pattern); this is in contrast to the uniform cytoplasmic expression in smooth muscle (Fig. 7-12). On occasion, this tram-track pattern is a clue that one is dealing with a myofibroblastic process (e.g., fasciitis) rather than a leiomyosarcoma. Antibody asr-1 is monoclonal and specifically identifies sarcomeric actins (skeletal, cardiac); it identifies RMS but not leiomyosarcoma.[105] One should be aware that some RMS, particularly the paratesticular spindle cell type, can express low levels of smooth muscle actins.[89]

Myogenic Transcription Factors

Myogenic regulatory proteins (i.e., transcription factors of the MyoD [myogenic determination] family) play a critical role in the commitment and differentiation of mesenchymal progenitor cells to the myogenic lineage and subsequent maintenance of the skeletal muscle phenotype. MyoD1 and myogenin are members of the basic helix-loop-helix family of DNA binding myogenic nuclear regulatory proteins; the other members include Myf5 and MRF4.[106,107] These genes encode transcription factors, whose introduction into non-muscle cells in culture can initiate muscle-specific gene expression and muscle differentiation.[107] In addition, such regulatory factors are expressed much earlier in the normal skeletal muscle differentiation program than structural proteins such as desmin, actin, and myosin; indeed, expression of these myogenic regulatory proteins leads to activation of the latter.[108,109] Antibodies to both MyoD1 and myogenin, but not the other myogenic nuclear regulatory proteins, have been studied in terms of diagnosing RMS. Both MyoD1 and myogenin are expressed in more than 90% of RMS of all subtypes.[86-88,110-117] Antibodies to both MyoD1 and myogenin show excellent specificity (see Fig. 7-9). There is only a single report of nuclear immunoreactivity for MyoD1 in formalin-fixed, paraffin-embedded sections in a pleomorphic

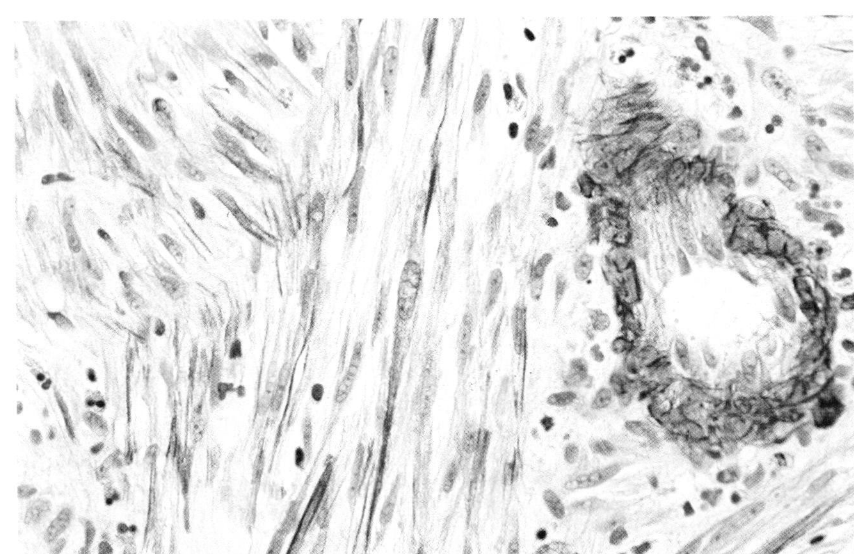

FIGURE 7-12. Immunostain for smooth muscle actin demonstrating the characteristic tram-track pattern of expression in myofibroblasts (left). This is in contrast to the uniform intracellular staining seen in true smooth muscle (right).

liposarcoma.[114,117,118] Four ASPS have been demonstrated to express MyoD1 by immunohistochemistry on frozen sections and by Western blot.[119] There have been no reports of myogenin immunoreactivity in nonrhabdomyosarcomas. Cytoplasmic immunoreactivity for MyoD1 has been reported in a small number of nonrhabdomyosarcomas, including EFT, Wilms tumor, and undifferentiated sarcoma.[120] Only nuclear immunoreactivity for MyoD1 should be taken as evidence of skeletal muscle differentiation because the epitope recognized by the most commonly used antibody to MyoD1, 5.8A, includes amino acid sequences with close homology to the class 1 major histocompatibility antigen and transcription factors E2A and ITF-1,[110] suggesting that cytoplasmic immunoreactivity may represent a cross-reaction rather than true MyoD1 expression.

As noted previously, both MyoD1 and myogenin are expressed by greater than 95% of embryonal and alveolar rhabdomyosarcomas (ARMS), including the well-differentiated spindle cell variant of embryonal rhabdomyosarcoma (ERMS) and the solid variant of ARMS.[86-88,110-118] In general, ARMS express very high levels of myogenin and comparatively less MyoD1, whereas ERMS show the opposite pattern, or equal levels of expression.[115] The recently described sclerosing variant of RMS typically shows very strong expression of MyoD1, but only very focal myogenin expression.[86,87,116,121] Pleomorphic RMS are less frequently MyoD1 or myogenin positive, with a recent large series documenting expression in only 53% and 56% of cases, respectively[88]; in addition, pleomorphic RMS may show only a small percentage of positive tumor cells.

Although the available evidence appears to strongly support the view that MyoD1 and myogenin expression are highly specific for rhabdomyoblastic differentiation, it is important to realize that their expression does not obligate a diagnosis of RMS. Expression of MyoD1 and/or myogenin may be seen in a variety of rare tumors with rhabdomyoblastic differentiation, including Wilms tumors with myogenous differentiation, neuroendocrine carcinoma (including Merkel cell carcinoma) with rhabdomyoblastic differentiation,[122] malignant glial tumors with myoblastic differentiation, malignant peripheral nerve sheath tumors with rhabdomyoblastic differentiation (malignant Triton tumor), and teratomas with rhabdomyoblastic differentiation.[118] It is also important not to mistake myogenin and MyoD1 expression in degenerating and regenerating skeletal muscle for tumor cell expression, particularly in the setting of diffuse skeletal muscle infiltration by a nonmyogenous small, blue round cell tumor, such as lymphoma.

Myoglobin and Other Less Commonly Used Markers

Antibodies to myoglobin, an oxygen-binding heme protein found in skeletal and cardiac muscle but not in smooth muscle, were the first markers used in the immunohistochemical diagnosis of RMS.[76,123-127] Unfortunately, myoglobin is present in demonstrable amounts in fewer than 50% of RMS[85,126]; it may be identified in nonmyogenous tumor cells that are infiltrating skeletal muscle and phagocytosing myoglobin.[128] Commercially available myoglobin antibodies have a high level of nonspecific, background staining, which may be difficult to distinguish from true myoglobin expression. This is in distinct contrast to desmin and the myogenic regulatory proteins, which do not diffuse. Antibodies to myoglobin are not used in a routine practice. Other muscle markers that have been used for diagnosing RMS include antibodies to myosin,[126] creatine kinase subunit M,[125] and titin,[129] among others. In general, these alternative markers suffer from a lack of sensitivity and/or specificity, and their use cannot be recommended.

Recommendations for the Use of Muscle Markers

In summary, for identifying skeletal muscle differentiation, the myogenic regulatory proteins myogenin and MyoD1 are the most specific; antibodies to desmin and muscle actins (i.e., HHF35) are of high sensitivity but are not skeletal muscle-specific. For identification of smooth muscle differentiation (e.g., in leiomyosarcomas), antibodies to desmin and muscle actins (i.e., antibody HHF35) or smooth muscle α-actin (e.g., antibody 1A4) are the best markers of smooth muscle differentiation. For identifying myofibroblasts (e.g., the type of differentiation present in lesions, such as nodular fasciitis), antibodies to desmin are useful only for distinguishing myofibroblasts from true smooth muscle cells because the former (in contrast to the latter) generally do not express desmin.[130,131] Both cell types express smooth muscle actins, however, although myofibroblasts generally express the latter in a characteristic wispy or tram-track pattern of immunostaining that, upon higher resolution, can be demonstrated to correspond to the peripheral bundles of actin filaments, which are the hallmark of this cell type. Myofibroblasts also manifest little or no expression of the smooth muscle and myoepithelial cell-associated proteins caldesmon and smooth muscle myosin heavy chain, and these markers may assist in the distinction of myofibroblastic and true smooth muscle proliferations.[132-134]

MARKERS OF NERVE SHEATH DIFFERENTIATION

S-100 Protein

The S-100 protein is a 20-kDa acidic calcium-binding protein, so named for its solubility in 100% ammonium sulfate. The protein is composed of two subunits, α and β, which combine to form three isotypes. The α-α isotype is normally found in myocardium, skeletal muscle, and neurons; the α-β isotype is present in melanocytes, glia, chondrocytes, and skin adnexae; and the β-β isotype is seen in Langerhans cells and Schwann cells.[135]

Immunohistochemically, S-100 protein can be demonstrated in a large number of normal tissues, including some neurons and glia; Schwann cells; melanocytes; Langerhans cells; interdigitating reticulum cells of lymph nodes; chondrocytes; myoepithelial cells and ducts of sweat glands, salivary glands, and the breast; serous glands of the lung; fetal neuroblasts; and sustentacular cells of the adrenal medulla and paraganglia (Figs. 7-13 and 7-14).[136] In the immunohistochemical diagnosis of soft tissue neoplasms, S-100 protein is of most value as a marker of benign and malignant nerve sheath tumors and melanoma. S-100 protein is strongly and uniformly expressed in essentially all schwannomas.[136-138] The finding of uniform S-100 immunoreactivity may be a valuable clue to the diagnosis of cellular schwannoma[139,140] because malignant peripheral nerve sheath tumors usually show only patchy, weak expression of S-100,[56,138,141,142] and fibrosarcomas would not be expected to be S-100-positive (Fig. 7-15). S-100 protein expression is much more variable in neurofibromas than in schwannomas.[138] S-100 protein expression is seen in 40% to 80% of malignant peripheral nerve sheath tumors.[56,138,141,142]

However, as may be inferred from the long list of normal tissues that express this protein, significant S-100 protein expression may be seen in a subset of non-neural tumors included in the differential diagnosis of malignant peripheral nerve sheath tumors: synovial sarcoma,[15,143,144] RMS,[43] leiomyosarcoma,[145] and myoepithelioma.[146-148] Other tumors that may express S-100 protein include adipocytic tumors, chondrocytic tumors, ossifying fibromyxoid tumor, and chordoma. Malignant melanomas of all types, including the desmoplastic and sarcomatoid variants, are almost always strongly positive for S-100 protein.[138,149,150] Uniform, strong S-100 protein expression may be a valuable clue that one is dealing with a melanoma rather than a malignant peripheral nerve sheath tumor of skin or soft tissue because, as noted previously, S-100 protein expression in malignant peripheral nerve sheath tumors tends to be weaker and patchier. Approximately 2% to 3% of melanomas (more often in the metastatic setting) are negative for S-100 protein; additional immunostaining for melanosome-specific markers, such as gp100 protein (identified by antibody HMB-45[151]) or Melan-A,[152] is essential for arriving at the correct diagnosis in these cases.

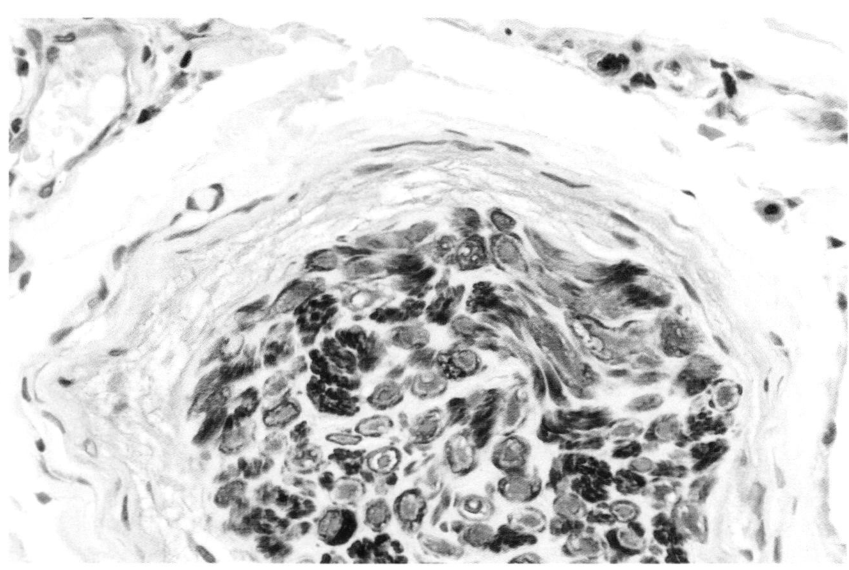

FIGURE 7-13. Nerve illustrating S-100 protein expression in Schwann cells. Note that the perineurial cells do not express S-100.

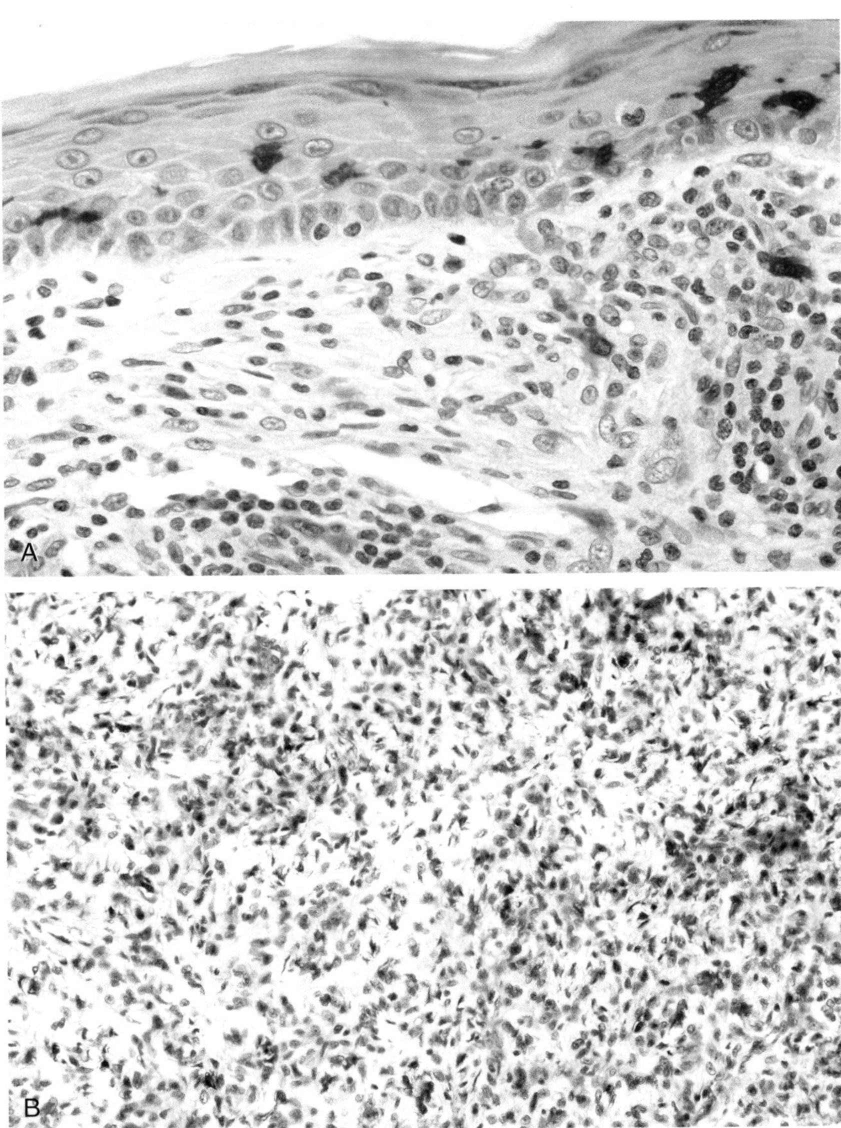

FIGURE 7-14. (A) Skin showing S-100 protein expression in both intraepidermal and dermal Langerhans cells. (B) Some dermal tumors, such as this benign fibrous histiocytoma, have a large number of infiltrating Langerhans cells. It is important to distinguish reactive from neoplastic subpopulations when interpreting immunostains of mesenchymal tumors.

Claudin-1

The claudins are a family of approximately 20 homologous proteins that help determine tight junction structure and permeability, and that appear to be differentially expressed in tissues, with claudin-1 expression, for example, being relatively widespread among epithelia, and claudin-3 expression being confined to lung and liver epithelia.[153] Claudins are integral transmembrane proteins that complex with other transmembrane proteins, such as junctional adhesion molecule and occludin, and interact with scaffolding proteins, such as ZO-1, ZO-2, and ZO-3.[153] Among normal mesenchymal tissues, claudin-1 expression appears to be limited to perineurial cells.[154] In the appropriate histologic context, claudin-1 is a useful marker of perineuriomas, present in 20% to 90% of perineuriomas, but not in other tumors in this differential diagnosis, such as neurofibromas, schwannomas, low-grade fibromyxoid sarcoma, desmoplastic fibroblastoma, dermatofibrosarcoma protuberans, and fibromatosis (Fig. 7-16).[73,154] Aberrant, non-polarized expression of claudin-1 and other tight junction-related proteins is seen in a significant number of synovial sarcomas and EFT.[14,155]

GLUT-1

GLUT-1 is the erythrocyte-type glucose transporter protein, which plays a particular role in transporting glucose across epithelial and endothelial barrier tissues.[156] Expression of GLUT-1 protein has recently been demonstrated to be a consistent feature of normal perineurial cells and benign and malignant perineurial tumors.[157,158] However, in soft tissue and bone tumors, GLUT-1 expression is frequently identified adjacent to foci of necrosis, presumably representing upregulation of this protein within hypoxic zones, secondary to upstream activation of proteins, such as hypoxia-inducible factor 1-α, and, therefore, GLUT-1 is a highly nonspecific marker of perineurial differentiation in malignant-appearing lesions.[159,160] Among vascular tumors, expression of GLUT-1 protein is seen in essentially all juvenile capillary hemangiomas but not in

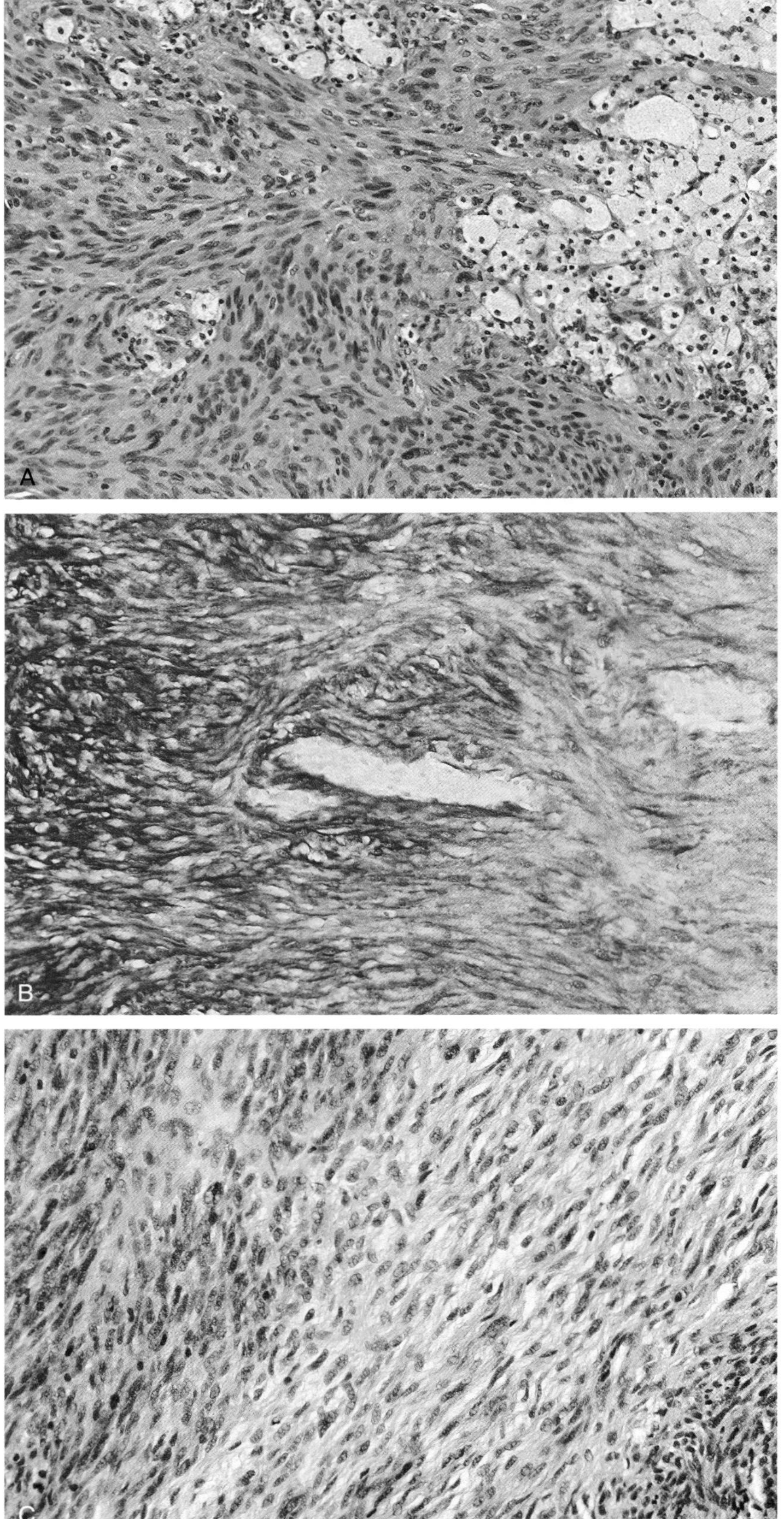

FIGURE 7-15. Cellular schwannoma (A) demonstrating uniform, intense S-100 protein expression (B). Such intense expression is characteristic of schwannomas and melanocytic tumors. In contrast, malignant peripheral nerve sheath tumors (C) typically show only patchy, weak S-100 expression (D).

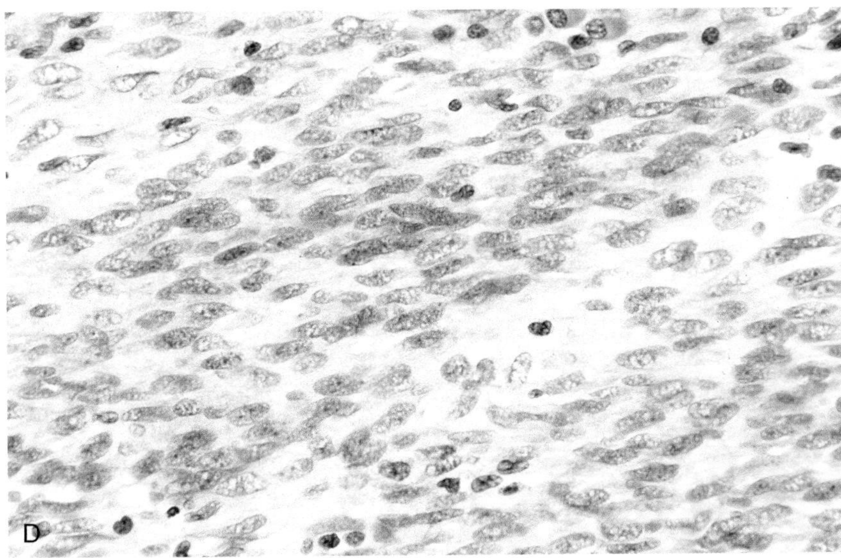

FIGURE 7-15, cont'd

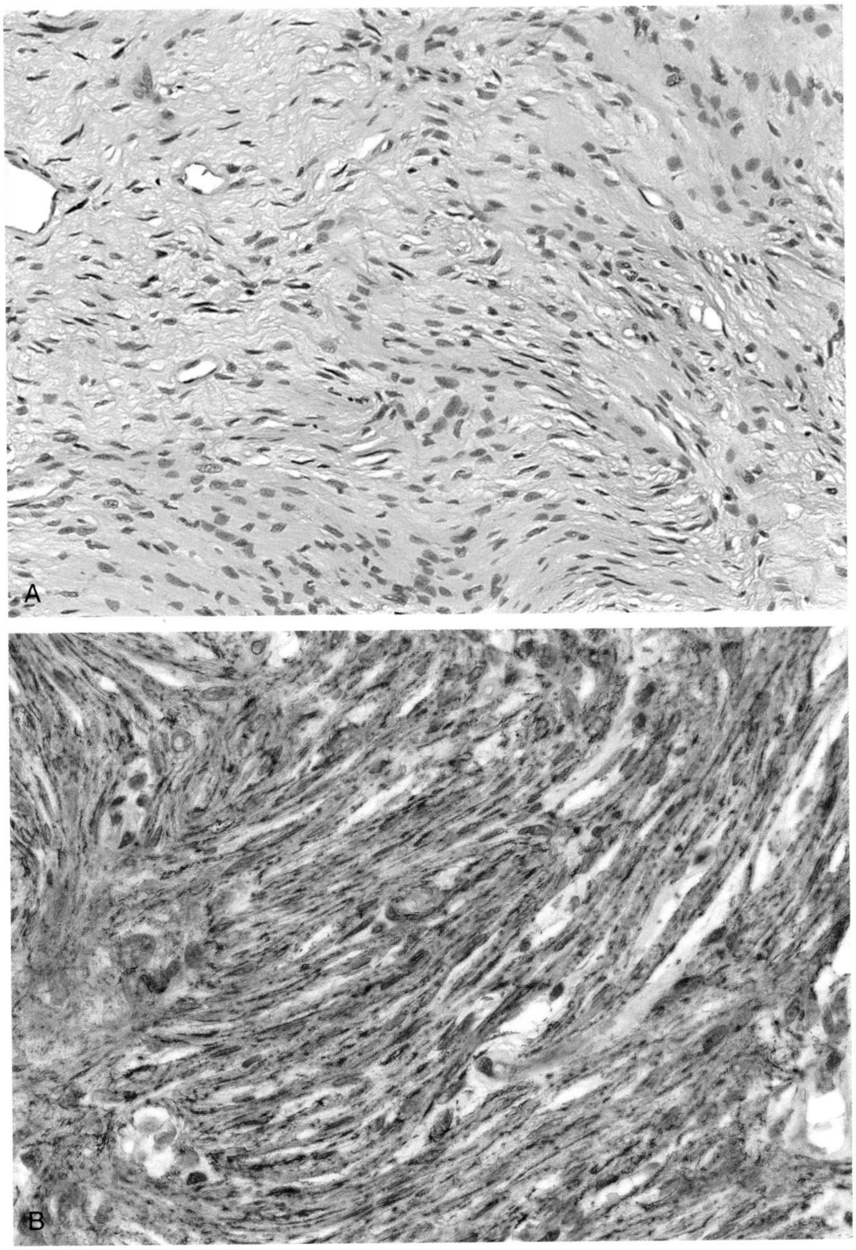

A

B

FIGURE 7-16. Perineurioma (A), showing granular membrane immunoreactivity for claudin-1 (B). Claudin-1 and/or GLUT-1 may be useful additional markers of perineurial differentiation, particularly when EMA is weak or absent.

other pediatric vascular tumors, including vascular malformations[161,162] and kaposiform hemangioendothelioma (Fig. 7-17).[163] Its expression in vascular tumors appears unrelated to the proliferative activity of the lesions.

p75NTR

The nerve growth factor receptor p75NTR, a low-affinity 75-kDa receptor, is normally expressed on neuronal axons, Schwann cells, perineurial cells, perivascular fibroblasts, outer follicular root sheath epithelium, and myoepithelium.[164,165] Expression of p75NTR has been reported in up to 80% of malignant peripheral nerve sheath tumors and nearly all schwannomas, granular cell tumors, and neurofibromas.[166] However, p75NTR expression is not limited to malignant peripheral nerve sheath tumors and may be seen in other sarcomas, including synovial sarcoma and malignant melanoma, particularly spindle cell variants.[165]

NEUROECTODERMAL MARKERS

CD99

The product of the pseudoautosomal MIC2 gene,[167] CD99 is a transmembrane glycoprotein of 30 to 32 kDa (p30/32).[168] Its exact function is unknown, although it appears to play a role in cellular adhesion and regulation of cellular proliferation.[169,170] The MIC2 gene is expressed, and the CD99 antigen

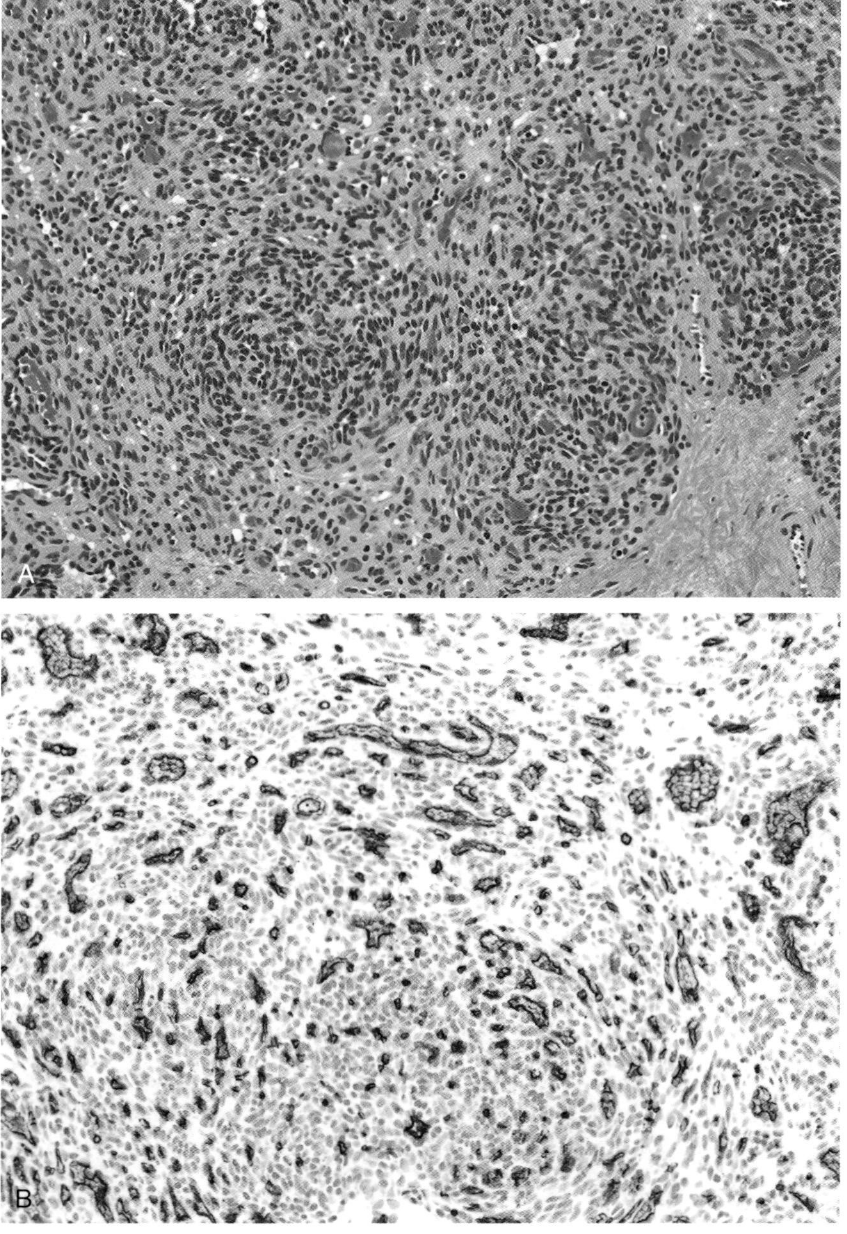

FIGURE 7-17. Kaposiform hemangioendothelioma (A), lacking expression of GLUT-1 protein (B). Erythrocytes serve as a positive internal control. In contrast to juvenile hemangiomas, kaposiform hemangioendotheliomas lack GLUT-1 expression.

is produced in nearly all human tissues, although the level of expression varies significantly. Normal tissues that commonly display strong CD99 expression include cortical thymocytes and Hassall corpuscles, granulosa and Sertoli cells, endothelium, pancreatic islets, adenohypophysis, ependyma, and some epithelium, including urothelium, squamous epithelium, and columnar epithelium.[171,172]

The most important use of antibodies to CD99 is for an immunohistochemical diagnosis of EFT. Many studies have shown that well over 90% of EFT express CD99, with a characteristic membranous pattern (Fig. 7-18).[171,173-178] Despite early claims that CD99 expression was also specific for this tumor, it is clear that this is not true.[171,173-178] It is particularly important to recognize that a significant subset of other small, blue round cell tumors considered in the differential diagnosis of EFT may express this antigen. CD99 expression is seen in more than 90% of lymphoblastic lymphomas,[179,180] 20% to 25% of primitive RMS,[173] more than 75% of PDSS,[15,181,182] approximately 50% of mesenchymal chondrosarcomas,[183,184] and in rare cases of small cell osteosarcomas[185] and intra-abdominal DSRCT.[47,186] CD99 expression has never been reported in neuroblastomas[171,173-178] and has been seen in a single esthesioneuroblastoma only.[187,188]

Immunohistochemical analysis of CD99 expression plays a limited role in the diagnosis of pleomorphic or spindle cell soft tissue neoplasms. As noted previously, many synovial sarcomas express CD99, which may be helpful in discriminating them from malignant peripheral nerve sheath tumors and fibrosarcomas.[15,181,182] Expression of CD99 may also be seen in solitary fibrous tumors, mesotheliomas, leiomyosarcomas, and undifferentiated pleomorphic sarcoma (also known as malignant fibrous histiocytoma).[173,189-191]

CD56 (Neural Cell Adhesion Molecule)

The 140-kDa isoform of the neural cell adhesion molecule, CD56, is an integral membrane glycoprotein that mediates calcium-independent homophilic cell–cell binding.[192,193] CD56 is expressed by many normal cells and tissues, including neurons, astrocytes, and glia of the cerebral cortex and cerebellum, adrenal cortex and medulla, renal proximal tubules, follicular epithelium of the thyroid; gastric parietal cells; cardiac muscle; regenerating and fetal skeletal muscle; pancreatic islet cells, and peripheral nerve.[194] CD56 is also ubiquitously expressed on human natural killer cells and on a subset of T lymphocytes.[195,196]

As might be expected from this long list of CD56-positive normal tissues, CD56 expression is widespread among sarcomas. Soft tissue tumors that often express CD56 include synovial sarcoma, malignant peripheral nerve sheath tumor, schwannoma, RMS, leiomyosarcoma, leiomyoma, chondrosarcoma, and osteosarcoma.[197-199] For this reason, an examination of CD56 expression is not helpful when evaluating spindle-cell soft tissue tumors. CD56 expression may, however, be useful for evaluating primitive small, blue round cell tumors, particularly in combination with CD99. CD56 expression is seen in only 10% to 25% of EFT and in rare lymphoblastic lymphomas, compared with nearly 100% of neuroblastomas, PDSS, alveolar and primitive ERMS, small cell carcinomas, Wilms tumors, and mesenchymal chondrosarcomas.[15,198,199] The absence of CD56 expression may be a clue to the diagnosis of EFT in cases where results with more specific positive markers, such as CD99, CD45, cytokeratin, and desmin, are equivocal. Demonstrating CD56 expression may also be of some value in the diagnosis of ossifying fibromyxoid tumor, particularly when S-100 protein expression is weak or absent.[200]

NB-84

Monoclonal antibody NB-84, raised against two neuroblastoma cell lines, recognizes an as yet uncharacterized 57-kDa molecule.[201] NB-84 is a highly sensitive marker of neuroblastoma, being positive in more than 95% of cases, including undifferentiated and poorly differentiated subtypes.[47,188,201-204] It displays only moderate specificity for neuroblastoma because 16% to 25% of EFT react with NB-84, as do a small number of RMS, esthesioneuroblastomas, Wilms tumors, DSRCT, and small cell osteosarcomas.[47,188,201-204] NB-84 antigen expression has not been examined in other soft tissue neoplasms, although it has recently been shown to be present in 50% of clear cell sarcoma-like tumors of the gastrointestinal tract.[205]

NKX2.2

NKX2.2 is a homeodomain-containing transcription factor that plays an important role in both neuroendocrine and glial differentiation; it has also been identified as a gene necessary for the oncogenic transformation of EFT, and one regulated by the fusion gene, *EWSR1-FLI1*, that results from the t(11;22) characteristic of this tumor.[206] NKX2.2 appears to represent a highly sensitive and specific marker of EFT in the context of small, blue round cell tumors, with a sensitivity and specificity in the range of 90%. Non-EFT tumors positive for NKX2.2 expression include olfactory neuroblastomas and a subset of mesenchymal chondrosarcomas, small cell carcinomas, and melanomas.[207]

MARKERS OF MELANOCYTIC DIFFERENTIATION

HMB-45

Monoclonal antibody HMB-45 identifies the Pmel 17 gene product, gp100.[208] This gene product is a component of the premelanosomal/melanosomal melanogenic oxidoreductive enzymes and, as such, is melanosome-specific but not melanoma-specific.[209] HMB-45 is positive in the unusual myomelanocytic tumors that comprise the perivascular epithelioid cell family of tumors (angiomyolipoma, clear cell tumor of lung, lymphangioleiomyomatosis, soft tissue and bone PEComas)[11,210,211] but has not convincingly been shown to react with any tumor that does not contain melanosomes. Previous reports of HMB-45 positivity in carcinomas were based on the use of contaminated ascites fluid and have been retracted in the literature.[212] HMB-45 is generally negative in nevi and resting melanocytes but is expressed in approximately 85% of melanomas (Fig. 7-19).[208] Fewer than 10% of desmoplastic melanomas are HMB-45 positive.[213]

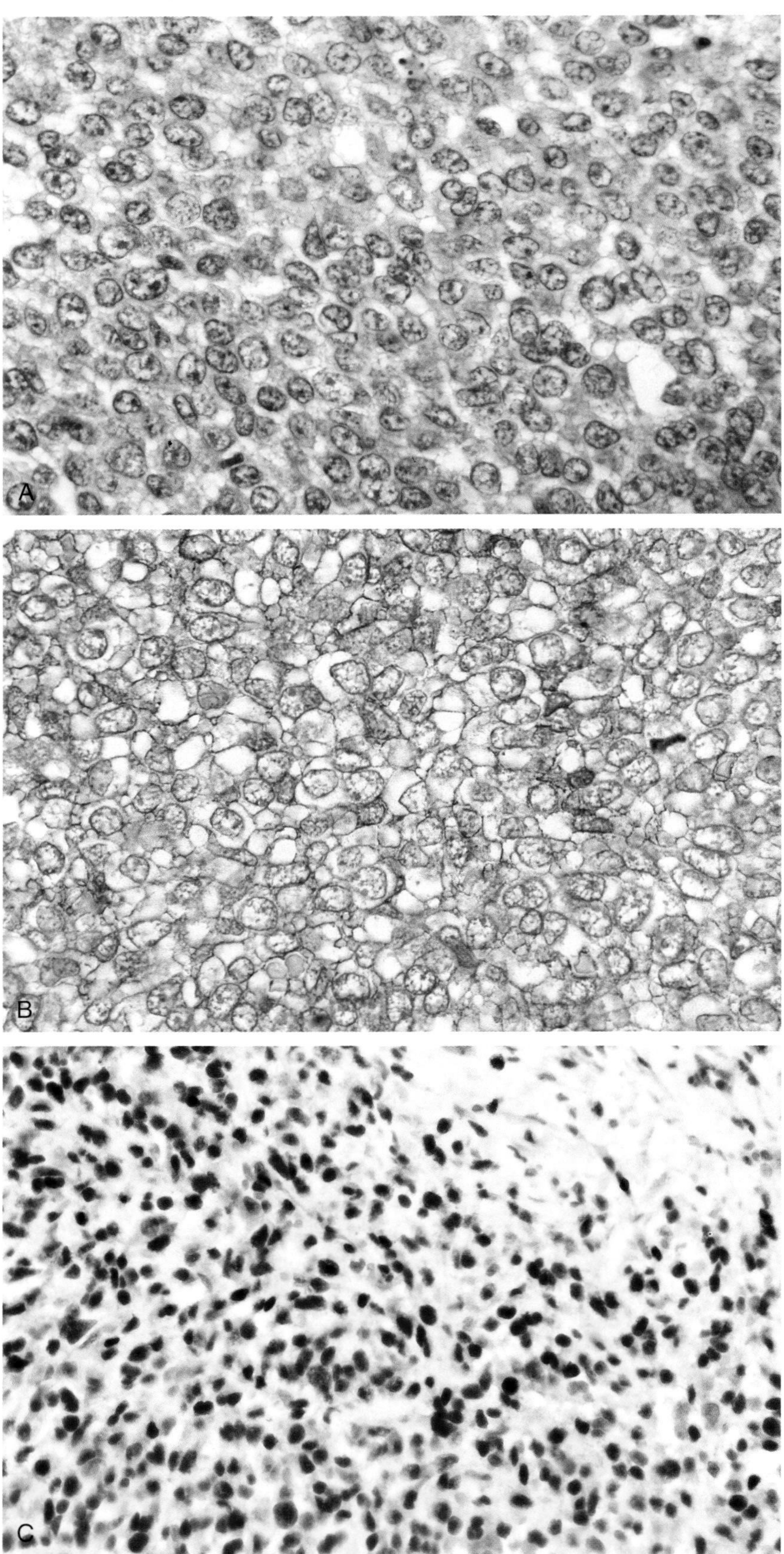

FIGURE 7-18. EFT (A) with intense membranous expression of CD99 (MIC2) (B). Although CD99 expression is highly characteristic of EFT, it is not specific. Detection of nuclear expression of the carboxy-terminus of the FLI-1 or ERG proteins, expressed as a result of the EFT-specific *EWSR1/FLI-1* or *EWSR1-ERG* gene fusions, is a more specific marker of these tumors (C).

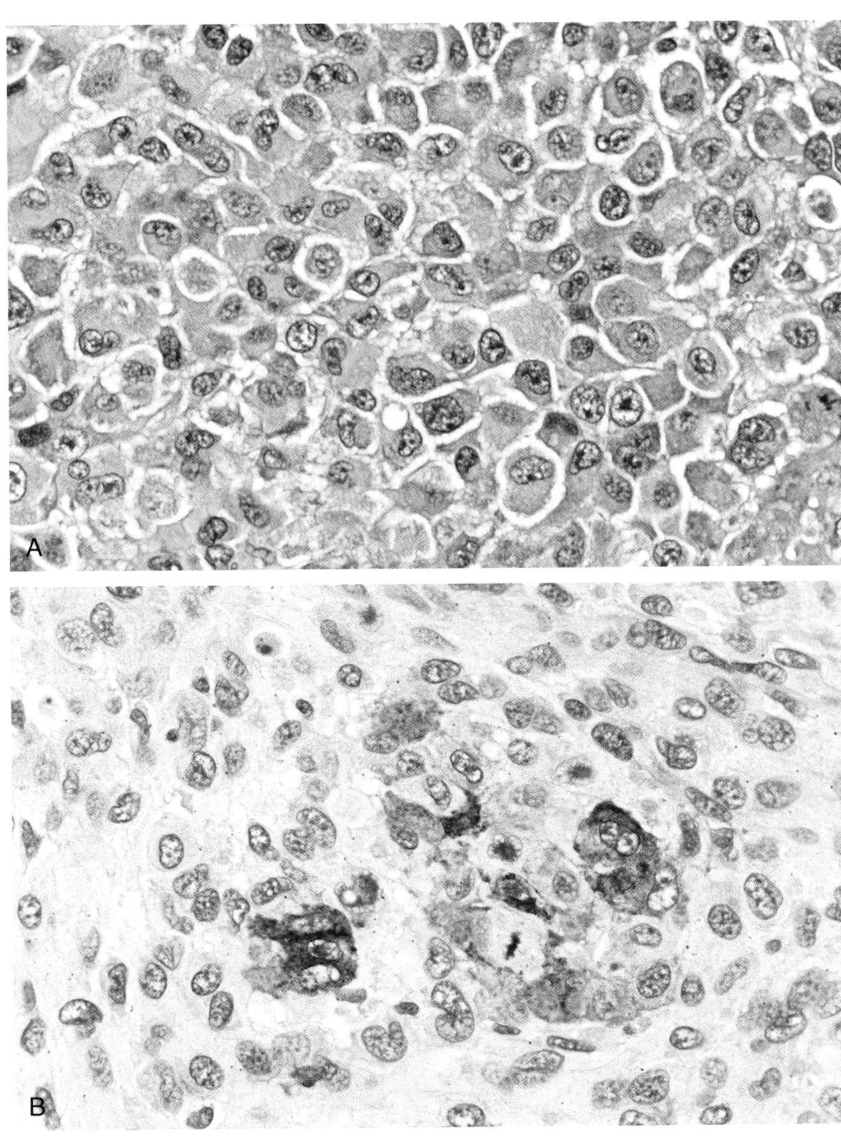

FIGURE 7-19. Malignant melanoma (A) immunostained with monoclonal antibody HMB-45 to gp100 protein (B). HMB-45 is positive in approximately 85% of epithelioid melanomas but in only a small fraction of spindled melanomas.

Melan-A

Melan-A, the product of the MART-1 gene (melanoma antigen recognized by T cells), is a 20- to 22-kDa component of the premelanosomal membrane.[152,214-217] Its function is unknown. Like HMB-45, Melan-A is a marker of melanosomes, not melanomas: it is also present in perivascular epithelioid cell tumors (PEComas) (Fig. 7-20).[11] Unlike HMB-45, Melan-A is positive in resting melanocytes and nevi. Melan-A is expressed by approximately 85% of epithelioid melanomas and has been reported to be present in the upward of 50% of desmoplastic melanomas, although the true rate is almost certainly far lower and is probably similar to that of HMB-45.[152,214-218] Melan-A is present in some HMB-45-negative melanomas, and vice versa. One other interesting application of the most widely used antibody to Melan-A, A103, is for the diagnosis of adrenal cortical and other steroid-producing tumors. A103 has reproducible cross-reactivity with an unknown epitope present in these tumors, and it may be helpful for distinguishing adrenal cortical carcinomas from renal cell carcinoma.[216]

Microphthalmia Transcription Factor

Microphthalmia transcription factor (MiTF), the product of the microphthalmia (*mi*) gene located on chromosome 3p14.1, is a transcription factor critical for melanocyte development.[219-221] Mutations in *mi* were first described in mice in the 1940s, and it was subsequently shown in humans that heterozygous *mi* deficiency results in Waardenburg syndrome type IIa, clinically defined by skin pigmentation abnormalities, bilateral hearing loss, and a white forelock.[222] Biochemical studies have shown that microphthalmia transcription factor, the protein encoded by *mi*, can transactivate several downstream gene promoters, including genes ultimately responsible for melanin biosynthesis, namely tyrosinase and related pigmentation enzymes TRP-1 and TRP-2.[223]

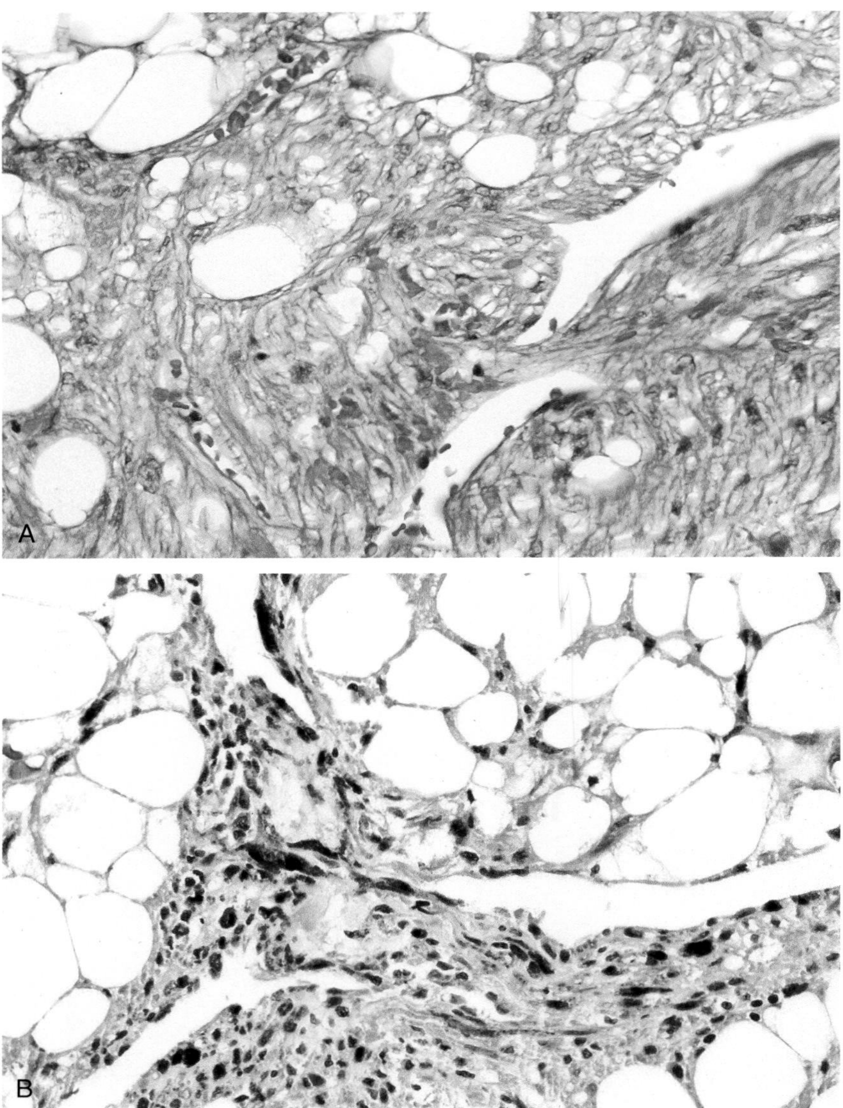

FIGURE 7-20. Angiomyolipoma (A), showing Melan-A expression in epithelioid cells, spindled cells and in the cytoplasm of lipid-distended cells (adipocytes) (B). Co-expression of melanosome-related proteins, such as gp100 and Melan-A, with smooth muscle markers is characteristic of the perivascular epithelioid cell (PEComa) family of tumors.

MiTF is expressed in essentially all resting melanocytes and nevi. Both melanocyte-specific and nonspecific isoforms of this protein exist[224]; however, the commercially available antibodies to MiTF are not specific for the melanocytic isoforms, despite claims to the contrary.

MiTF was initially described as highly sensitive and a specific marker of melanoma, and is expressed in well over 90% of epithelioid melanomas.[225,226] Sarcomatoid melanomas are less often positive (40%), and true desmoplastic melanomas are very infrequently positive (less than 5%).[227,228] MiTF is also expressed in nearly all clear cell sarcomas (melanoma of soft parts) (Fig. 7-21).[227,229] MiTF expression may also be seen in PEComas of all types.[11,230] Because the commercially available antibodies are not specific for the melanocytic MiTF isoforms, MiTF expression is not limited to melanomas and may be seen in leiomyosarcomas, atypical fibroxanthomas, atypical lipomatous neoplasms, and very rare carcinomas.[227,230] Therefore, MiTF is best used for the confirmation of S-100 protein-positive, HMB-45/Melan-A/tyrosinase-negative tumors suspected of being melanomas. MiTF expression in the absence of S-100 protein expression is not diagnostic of melanoma. Demonstration of MiTF expression may be of some value in the diagnosis of cellular neurothekeoma, particularly in its distinction from plexiform fibrohistiocytic tumor.[231]

PNL2

PNL2 is a monoclonal antibody that was generated to a fixative-resistant melanocytic antigen. Initial studies using PNL2 demonstrated it to have sensitivity and specificity for melanoma comparable to that of HMB-45 and antibodies to Melan-A, with the solitary exception of neutrophils, which were also identified with antibody PNL2. Furthermore, like the latter two antibodies, PNL2 did not label desmoplastic melanomas.[232] In a larger and more recent series of over 1000 tumors, PNL2 was demonstrated to be positive in greater than 85% of epithelioid melanomas and also positive in PEComas; all other non-melanocytic tumors were negative. PNL2 seems

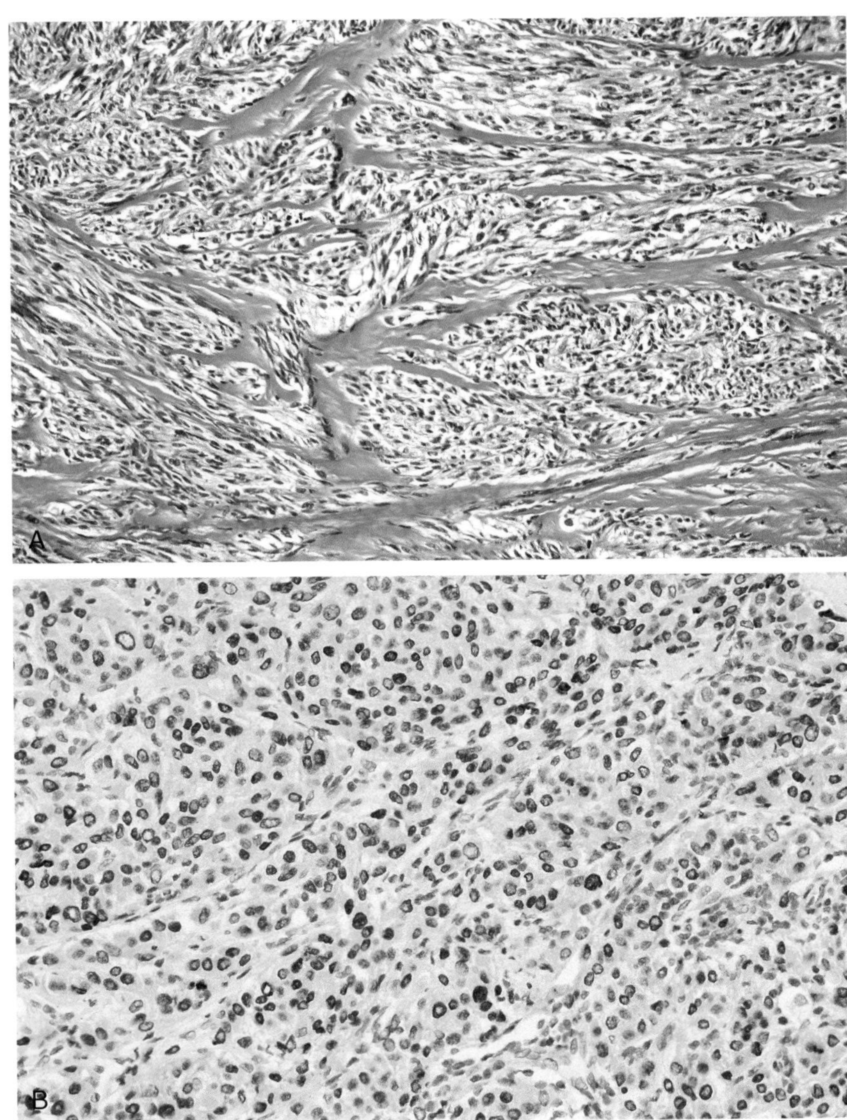

FIGURE 7-21. Clear cell sarcoma (A) with uniform nuclear expression of microphthalmia transcription factor (B). Microphthalmia transcription factor is a highly sensitive marker of melanoma and of mesenchymal tumors with melanocytic differentiation.

to represent a melanoma marker of comparable utility to HMB-45 and antibodies to Melan-A.[233]

Tyrosinase

Tyrosinase is an enzyme involved in the synthesis of melanin.[234] Antibodies to tyrosinase have recently been shown to have a sensitivity and specificity that is roughly equivalent to those of HMB-45 and Melan-A.[214,235] In general, the use of tyrosinase is reserved for cases strongly suspected of representing melanoma, which are negative with HMB-45 or A103.

SOX10

SOX10 is a transcription factor involved in neural crest development, and differentiation of neural crest cells into melanocytic and schwannian lineages.[236] Nonaka et al.[237] first demonstrated SOX10 expression by immunohistochemistry in melanocytic and schwannian neoplasms, noting expression in 85% of melanomas of all subtypes, 60% of clear cell sarcomas, greater than 93% of neurofibromas of all subtypes, 100% of schwannomas, and 30% of malignant peripheral nerve sheath tumors (Fig. 7-22). These authors also noted SOX10 expression in sustentacular cells of various neuroendocrine tumors but in no other epithelial or mesenchymal tumor studied. Similar findings were reported by Karamchanani et al.[238] Therefore, SOX10 shows significant promise as an additional marker for the diagnosis of melanocytic and schwannian neoplasms, although additional studies are necessary to determine whether this marker should be used along with, or in place of, S-100 protein.

MARKERS OF ENDOTHELIAL DIFFERENTIATION

A number of markers have been used to demonstrate endothelial differentiation, paralleling the progression of soft tissue tumors manifesting endothelial differentiation. Endothelial markers include commonly used markers, such as von Willebrand factor (vWF) (factor VIII-associated protein, often

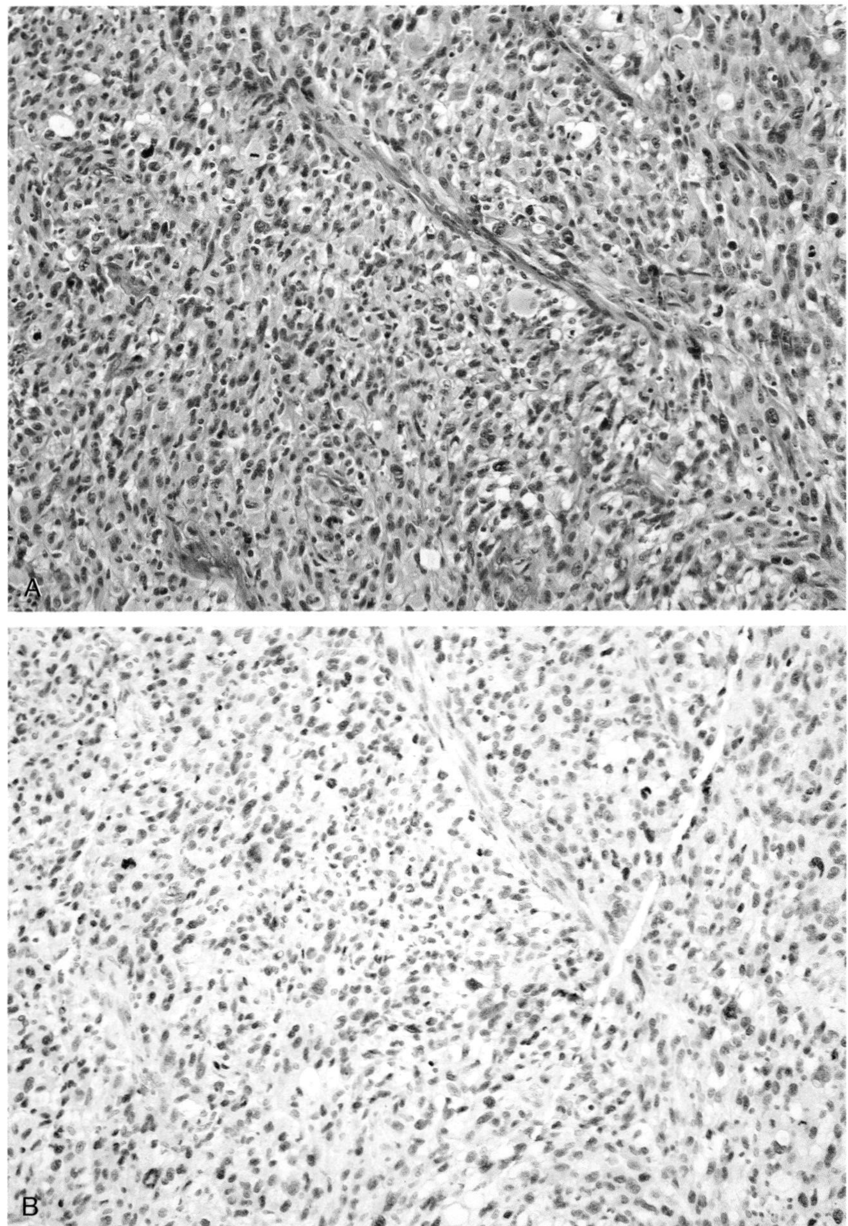

FIGURE 7-22. Malignant peripheral nerve sheath tumor (A), showing strong nuclear expression of SOX10 (B). *(Courtesy of Dr. Andrew Horvai, University of California at San Francisco, San Francisco, CA.)*

erroneously referred to as *factor VIII*), CD34, CD31, as well as more recently described markers such as FLI-1/ERG, human herpesvirus 8 latency associated nuclear antigen (HHV-8 LANA) protein, and podoplanin. The pattern of expression of these markers in endothelial tumors is much like an overlapping Venn diagram, in which most tumors express all of these markers, but some express a subset only. Whereas early studies had suggested that markers such as vWF could differentially identify vascular versus lymphatic endothelium,[239-241] more recent studies have demonstrated that both vascular and lymphatic endothelium express all three markers; and novel markers, such as podoplanin, Prospero homeobox 1 protein (Prox1), and vascular endothelial growth factor receptor-3 (VEGFR-3) (positive on lymphatic endothelium and negative on vascular endothelium), are required to make this distinction.[242-245]

von Willebrand Factor (Factor VIII-Related Antigen)

The vWF was the first endothelium-specific marker used in diagnostic immunohistochemical studies.[240] It was first used to identify the nature of the vinyl chloride-induced sarcomas of liver[246] and has subsequently been demonstrated to be a marker of vascular tumors of multiple sites, including, but not limited to, those of the central nervous system,[247] gastrointestinal tract,[248] and breast.[249] The vWF is the least sensitive of the vascular markers and is positive in 50% to 75% of vascular tumors.[243] Although vWF expression is, in theory, absolutely specific for vascular tumors, technical problems limit its usefulness. The vWF is not only produced by endothelial cells but also circulates in the serum, and, therefore, it can be found often in zones of tumor necrosis and hemorrhage (Fig. 7-23). Given the availability of much better endothelial markers (discussed in the following sections), there is little role for vWF immunohistochemistry in current practice.

CD34 (Human Hematopoietic Progenitor Cell Antigen)

The function of CD34, a 110-kDa transmembrane glycoprotein, is thought to be related to cell-cell adhesion. It is expressed on hematopoietic stem cells, endothelium, the interstitial cells of Cajal, and a group of interesting dendritic cells present in the dermis, around blood vessels, and in the nerve sheath.[250] CD34 is expressed in more than 90% of vascular tumors[251] and is a highly sensitive marker of Kaposi sarcoma (KS).[243] As may be gathered from the previous list of normal tissues, CD34 expression is not limited to vascular tumors. CD34 expression is well documented in dermatofibrosarcoma protuberans,[252] solitary fibrous tumors (Fig. 7-24),[253] malignant peripheral nerve sheath tumors,[254] gastrointestinal stromal tumors (GIST),[255] and epithelioid sarcomas.[16,17,256] CD34 is expressed by approximately 50% to 60% of epithelioid sarcomas, compared with fewer than 2% of carcinomas. CD34 expression may be valuable for distinguishing cytokeratin-positive epithelioid angiosarcomas and epithelioid sarcomas from carcinoma.[16,17,256]

CD31 (Platelet Endothelial Cell Adhesion Molecule-1)

One of the newer of the commonly used vascular markers, CD31 is generally considered to be the most sensitive and specific marker.[251,257] It is expressed in more than 90% of angiosarcomas, hemangioendotheliomas, hemangiomas, and KS and in fewer than 1% of carcinomas (probably much less than 1%) (see Fig. 7-5). CD31 expression is not seen in any nonendothelial tissue or tumor, with the notable exception of macrophages and platelets (Fig. 7-25).[258] CD31 expression in intratumoral macrophages may result in the misdiagnosis of a nonvascular tumor as a vascular tumor, if one is not aware of this potential pitfall.[259] The CD31 expression seen in macrophages is distinctly granular, compared with the intense cytoplasmic and linear membranous staining of endothelium.

FLI-1 and ERG Proteins

Members of the ETS family of transcription factors,[260] FLI-1 and ERG are the best currently available nuclear markers of endothelial differentiation. Both FLI-1 and ERG are positive in greater than 95% of endothelial neoplasms of all types and degrees of malignancy, including hemangiomas, hemangioendotheliomas, angiosarcomas, and KS.[261-263] FLI-1 and ERG are not expressed by epithelioid sarcomas, which is helpful in the distinction of these tumors from epithelioid forms of angiosarcoma.[261-263] Very rare melanomas, adenocarcinomas, and Merkel cell carcinomas have been reported to show focal FLI-1 positivity.[262] ERG expression is present in close to 50% of prostatic adenocarcinoma, reflecting the presence of the prostate cancer-associated *TMPRSS2-ERG* fusion.[264] ERG expression may also be seen in a small minority of EFT, 70% of blastic extramedullary myeloid tumors, and very rare large cell pulmonary carcinomas and mesotheliomas.[263] FLI-1 is commonly present in subsets of mature lymphocytes, whereas ERG is not.[263] It has been suggested that commercially available antibodies to ERG are somewhat more user-friendly than are those to FLI-1, although there are no significant differences.

Claudin-5

As with claudin-1, claudin-5 shows a restricted pattern of normal tissue expression, normally confined to endothelial cells and glomerular podocytes.[265] Antibodies to claudin-5 have recently been shown to be highly sensitive (greater than

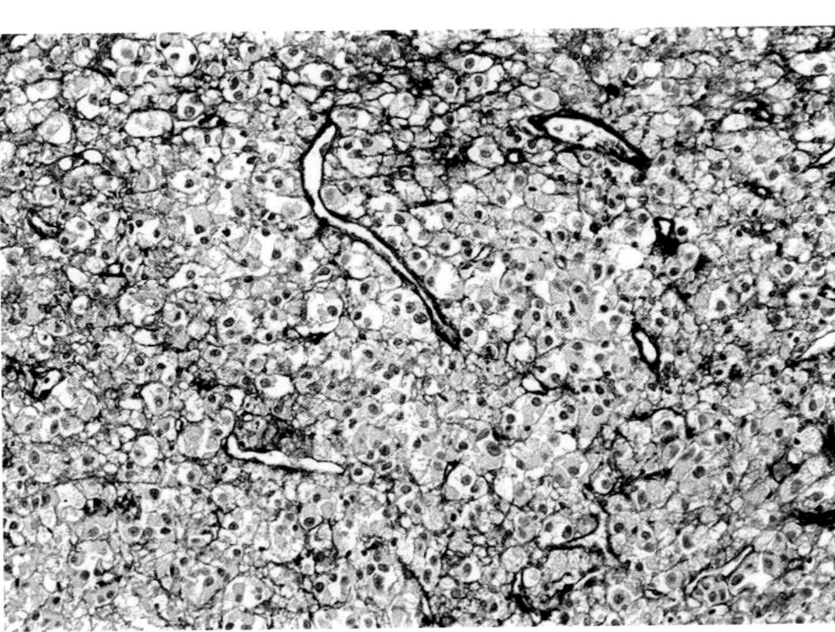

FIGURE 7-23. Immunostain for von Willebrand factor (factor VIII-related protein) showing spurious membranous positivity in a renal cell carcinoma. Staining of circulating vWF in the serum may be extremely difficult to distinguish from true membranous staining in an endothelial neoplasm.

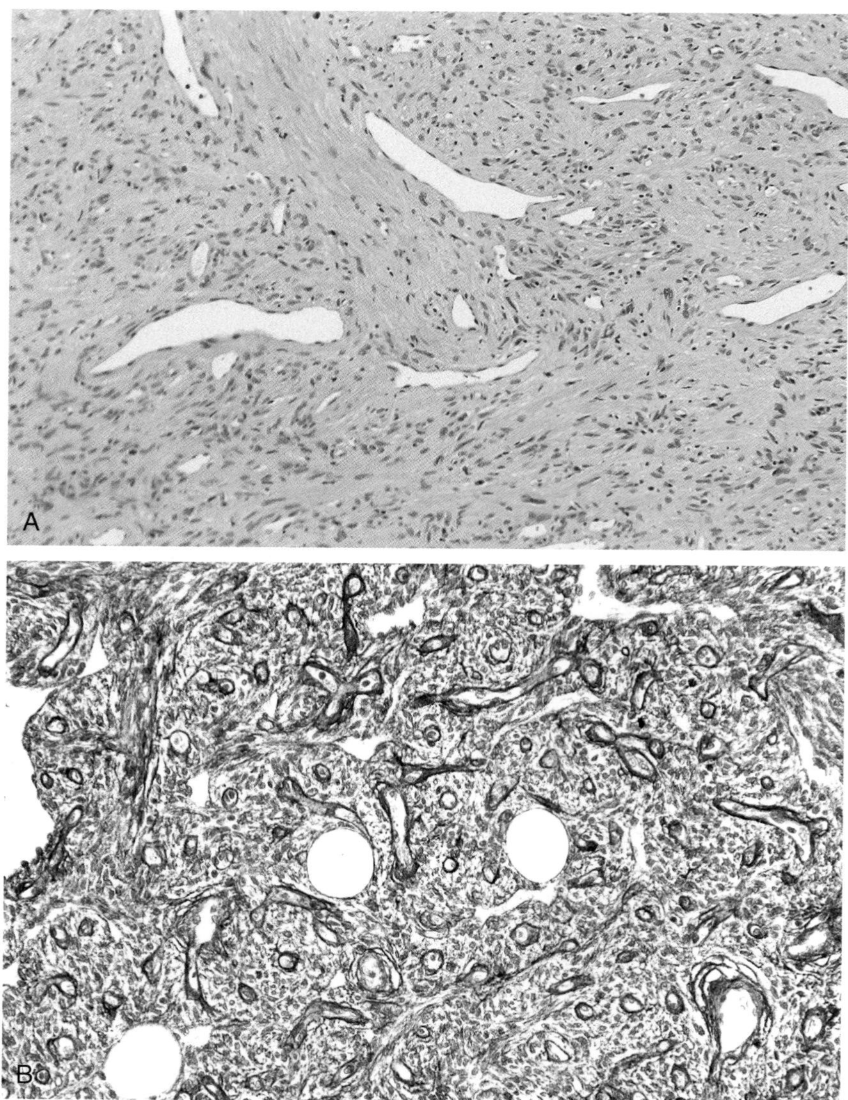

FIGURE 7-24. Solitary fibrous tumor (A) with uniform CD34 expression (B).

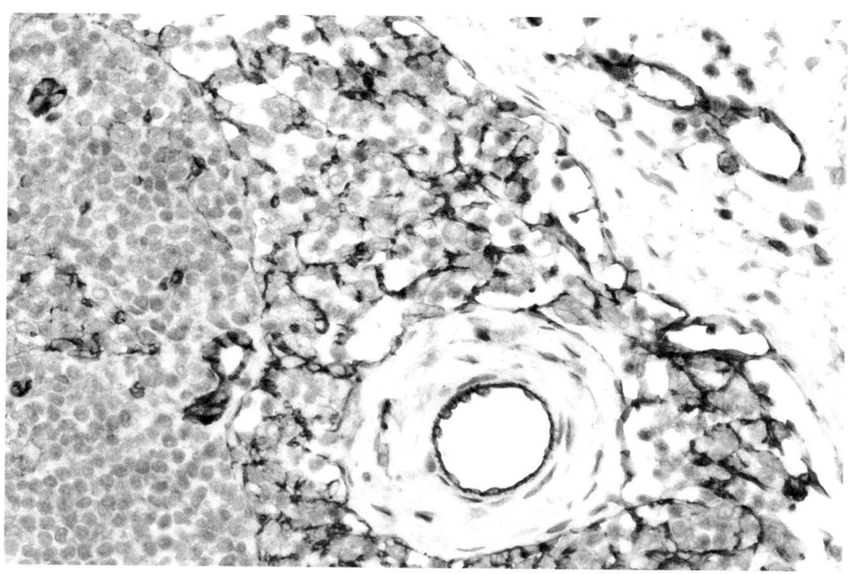

FIGURE 7-25. Granular, membranous CD31 expression in macrophages of the lymph node sinusoid. This granular expression in macrophages infiltrating a tumor may be mistaken for true expression by the tumor cells, leading to an erroneous diagnosis of angiosarcoma. CD31 expression in angiosarcomas is usually stronger and shows a linear, rather than granular, staining pattern (see also Fig. 7-5).

95%) markers of all types of endothelial tumors.[266] However, claudin-5 expression is also commonly found in a wide variety of carcinomas and in synovial sarcoma, and it is difficult to see what, if any, benefits this new marker has over other, more specific endothelial markers.

Putative Markers of Lymphatic Endothelial Differentiation: VEGFR-3, Podoplanin (D2-40), and Prox1

The platelet derived growth factor family, including vascular endothelial growth factor (VEGF), and the closely related molecules VEGF-B, VEGF-C, and VEGF-D play a significant role in angiogenesis and vascular permeability.[267] VEGF-C plays a critical role in lymphangiogenesis; in transgenic mice, VEGF-C has the ability to induce both lymphatic endothelial proliferation and lymphatic vessel formation.[268] Early studies suggested that VEGFR-3 was a highly sensitive and specific marker of KS, normal lymphatics, and lymphangiomas.[244] Two subsequent large studies confirmed its superb (greater than 95%) sensitivity for KS, but also noted expression in close to 50% of angiosarcomas, some of which had features suggestive of lymphatic differentiation, occasional hemangiomas, and almost all cases of kaposiform hemangioendothelioma, Dabska tumor, and retiform hemangioendothelioma.[243,269] It is now generally conceded that VEGFR-3 expression is not specific for lymphatic differentiation in endothelial neoplasms. VEGFR-3 expression has not been extensively studied in nonendothelial neoplasms.

Podoplanin (D2-40)

Podoplanin is a transmembrane glycoprotein normally expressed by lymphatic endothelial cells, glomerular podocytes, choroid plexus epithelium, type 1 alveolar cells, osteoblasts, and mesothelial cells.[242,270] Expression of podoplanin is regulated by the homeobox gene *Prox1* (see the following section).[271] Although, at one time, podoplanin was considered a relatively restricted marker of lymphatic endothelial-derived tumors,[272] subsequent investigations have shown podoplanin expression in a wide variety of endothelial tumors and in many different types of mesenchymal, germ cell, and glial neoplasms.[273] Therefore, podoplanin is of relatively little value as an endothelial marker. Antibodies to podoplanin, however, are of value in the differential diagnosis of mesothelioma (often positive) and adenocarcinoma (usually negative).[274,275]

Prox1

Expression of Prox1 is critical for normal lymphatic differentiation and is seen in the nuclei of developing and mature lymphatic endothelial cells.[271,276,277] A small number of older studies have evaluated Prox1 as a marker of neoplastic endothelial cells, with expression noted in KS,[278] kaposiform hemangioendothelioma,[279] and lymphangiomas.[280] Most recently, Miettinen and Wang[245] have evaluated Prox1 in a very large number of endothelial and nonendothelial tumors, noting expression in close to 100% of KS, 48% of angiosarcomas, 56% of hemangioendotheliomas (including epithelioid, kaposiform, and retiform subtypes), and in 42% of hemangiomas, most notably spindle cell hemangiomas (94%). These investigators also showed Prox1 expression in smaller percentages of EFT, paragangliomas, synovial sarcomas, non-small cell carcinomas of various primary sites, and pancreatic islet cell tumors.[245] Therefore, it is difficult to see a potential role for Prox1 immunohistochemistry in routine surgical pathology practice.

Human Herpesvirus 8 (HHV-8) Latency Associated Nuclear Antigen (LANA)

An infectious etiology for KS has long been suspected, and epidemiologic, serologic, and molecular genetic studies over the past 10 to 15 years have identified a novel herpesvirus, HHV-8, as the presumed causative agent of KS.[281-285] HHV-8 is known to latently infect endothelial cells, as well as peripheral blood monocytes and B lymphocytes in patients with KS. LANA is one of the most highly expressed proteins during latent HHV-8 infection. The LANA protein is encoded by the open reading frame 73 (ORF73) of the HHV-8 genome, where it tethers viral DNA to host heterochromatin and is thereby required for persistence of viral DNA in dividing cells.[286] LANA also has an essential role in the maintenance of the episomal DNA during latent infection and cell division, and also regulates gene expression in infected cells.[287,288] Using a polyclonal antisera, Katano et al.[289] found LANA expression in 100% of KS cases studied. Three separate studies, all using the LNA53 monoclonal antibody, noted LANA expression in well over 90% of KS cases, as compared to 0% of non-KS controls.[290-292] Using the 13B10 clone, four studies have noted LANA expression in very close to 100% of KS, as compared to 0% of non-KS potential mimics (Fig. 7-26).[293-296] LANA expression has not been reported in any non-KS tumor, with the notable exceptions of primary effusion lymphoma and Castleman disease.[290,291]

Type IV Collagen

Type IV collagen, associated with basement membrane expression, is produced by smooth muscle, glomus cells, nerve sheath, and endothelial cells. In selected cases, demonstration of type IV collagen expression around clusters of cells, indicative of primitive vascular channel formation, may be a clue to the diagnosis of angiosarcoma.[297] Demonstration of uniform pericellular type IV collagen may also be a clue to the diagnosis of a glomus tumor (Fig. 7-27). The presence of abundant type IV collagen around individual cells and cell nests may on occasion be helpful in the discrimination of epithelioid malignant peripheral nerve sheath tumor from melanoma, which generally shows lesser amounts of collagen IV production. In general, however, there are relatively few uses for collagen IV immunostains in the diagnosis of soft tissue neoplasms.

Recommendations for the Use of Vascular Markers

As a practical issue, it is best to use a highly specific (e.g., antibodies to CD31) and a highly sensitive (e.g., antibodies to

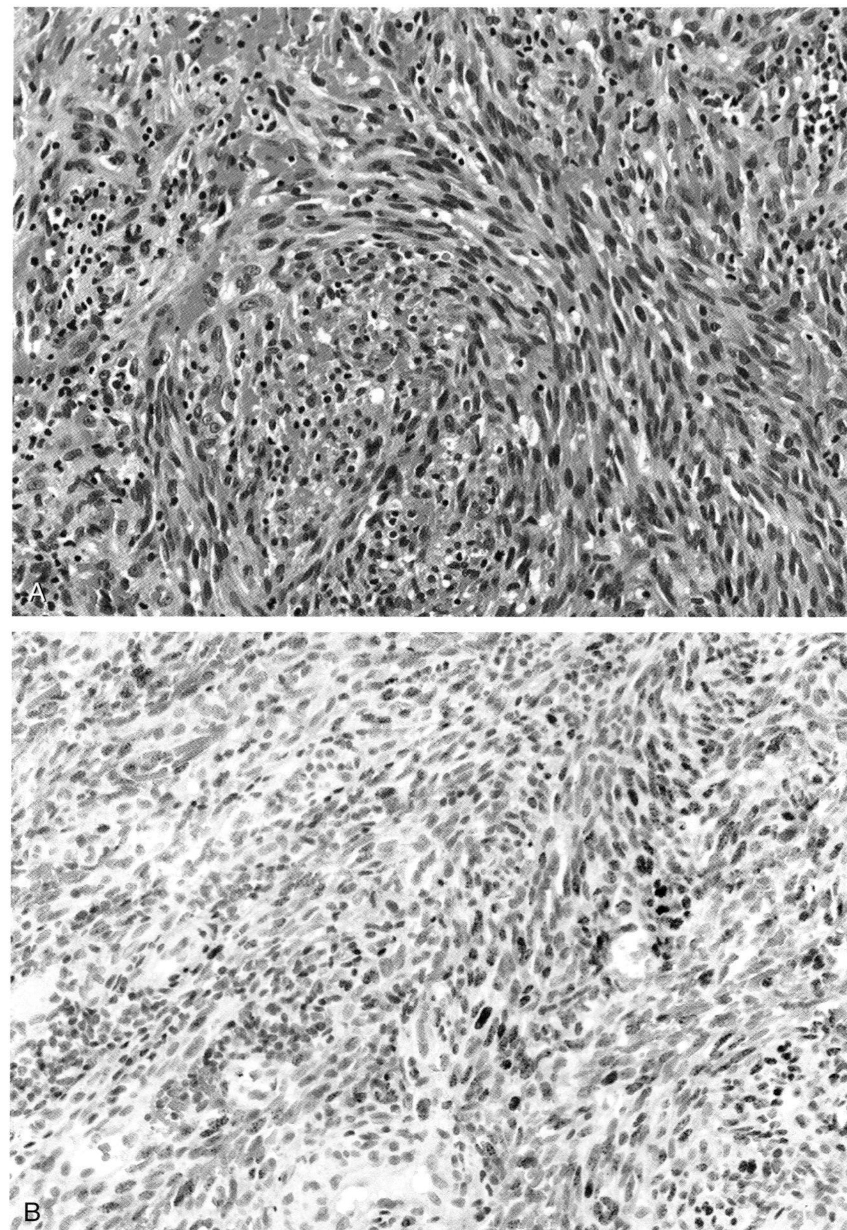

FIGURE 7-26. Kaposi sarcoma (A) showing strong nuclear expression of LANA protein (B).

CD34) marker to assess the presence of endothelial differentiation in histologic and clinical settings in which the diagnosis of angiosarcoma is entertained. The endothelial markers are summarized in Table 7-3.

MARKERS OF GASTROINTESTINAL STROMAL TUMORS

CD117 (C-KIT)

The c-kit proto-oncogene product (CD117), a transmembrane receptor for stem cell factor, is normally expressed by mast cells, melanocytes, germ cells, various subsets of hematopoietic cells, and the interstitial cells of Cajal of the gastrointestinal tract.[255,298] CD117 is expressed by 85% to 95% of GIST.[255,299-302] In the gastrointestinal tract, CD117 is a highly specific marker of GIST; it is not expressed by tumors typically in the differential diagnosis of a gastrointestinal mesenchymal tumor, such as leiomyomas, leiomyosarcomas, and nerve sheath tumors (Fig. 7-28).[255,299-302] CD117 is expressed by melanocytic tumors, however, such as melanoma and clear cell sarcoma.[302] CD117 expression may also be seen in a minority of Ewing sarcoma and PEComas.[11,41,303-306] In any type of tumor, care should be taken not to mistake mast cells in a tumor for scattered CD117-positive tumor cells (Fig. 7-29).

Protein Kinase C-θ

Protein kinase C-θ is a recently described protein kinase involved in T-cell activation, skeletal muscle signal

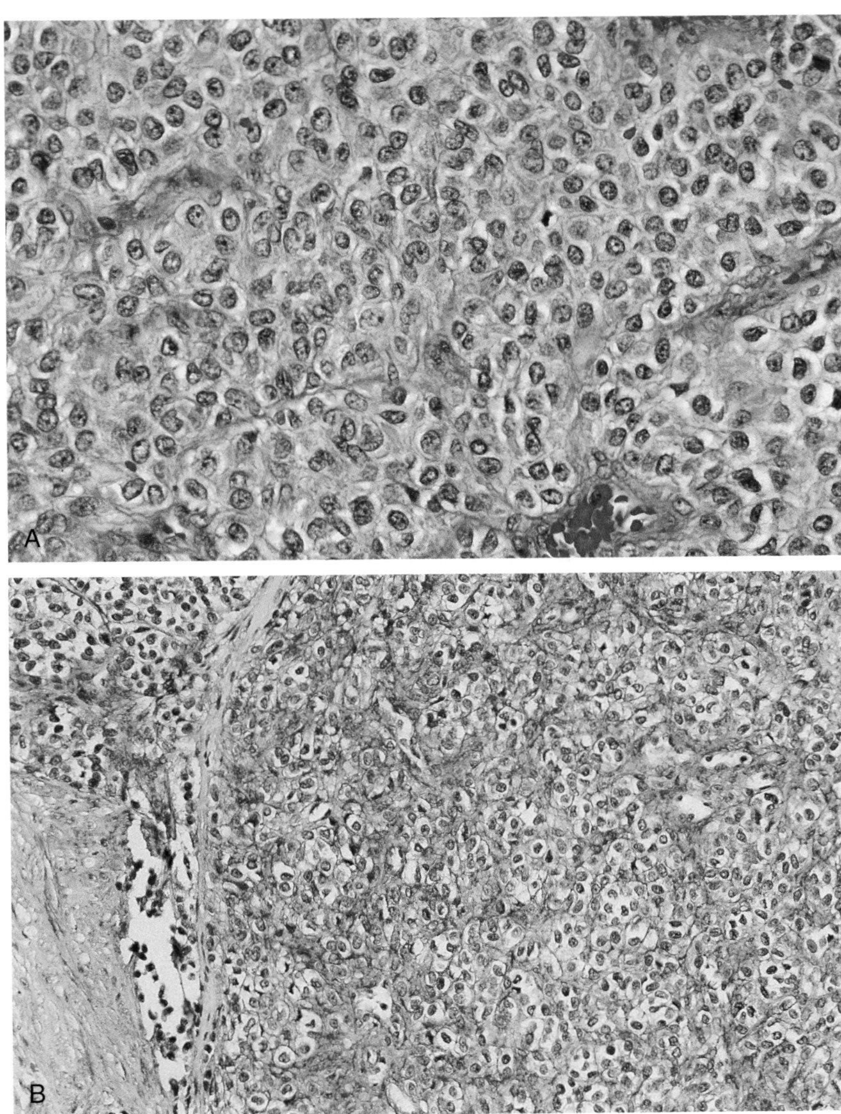

FIGURE 7-27. Malignant glomus tumor (A) with characteristic investment of individual cells by type IV collagen (B). Pericellular type IV collagen is characteristic of tumors with glomus cell, endothelial, schwannian, perineurial, and smooth muscle differentiation.

transduction, and neuronal differentiation.[307-309] Overexpression of the protein kinase C-θ gene in GIST has been identified in two gene expression studies using DNA microarrays.[310,311] Most recently, two studies have shown expression of protein kinase C-θ to be a highly sensitive and specific marker of GIST, including CD117-negative ones, with expression in 85% to 100% of routinely processed GIST, and in essentially no other mesenchymal or non-mesenchymal tumors, with the exception of greater than 15% of schwannomas.[312,313]

Anoctamin-1 (ANO1, DOG1, TMEM16A)

Anoctamin-1, more widely known as DOG1 (discovered on gastrointestinal stromal tumor 1), is a calcium activated chloride channel[314] normally expressed in a wide variety of tissues, including the interstitial cells of Cajal.[315] Using expression profiling, DOG1 was found by West et al.[316] in 2004 to be selectively expressed by GIST, among studied tumors. A subsequent

TABLE 7-3 Endothelial Markers

MARKER	SPECIFICITY	SENSITIVITY	ALSO IDENTIFIES
CD31	High	High	Macrophages
CD34	Moderate	High	Epithelioid sarcoma, solitary fibrous tumor, DFSP, GIST
vWF	High	Low	Megakaryocytes
FLI-1	Moderate	High	Ewing family of tumors, small lymphocytes, lymphoblastic lymphoma
ERG	Moderate	High	Extramedullary myeloid tumor, subset of prostatic adenocarcinoma
Claudin-5	Moderate	High	Epithelium and large subset of carcinomas, synovial sarcoma
Type IV collagen	Moderate*	Moderate	Glomus tumors, nerve sheath tumors, smooth muscle tumors

*von Willebrand factor (vWF).

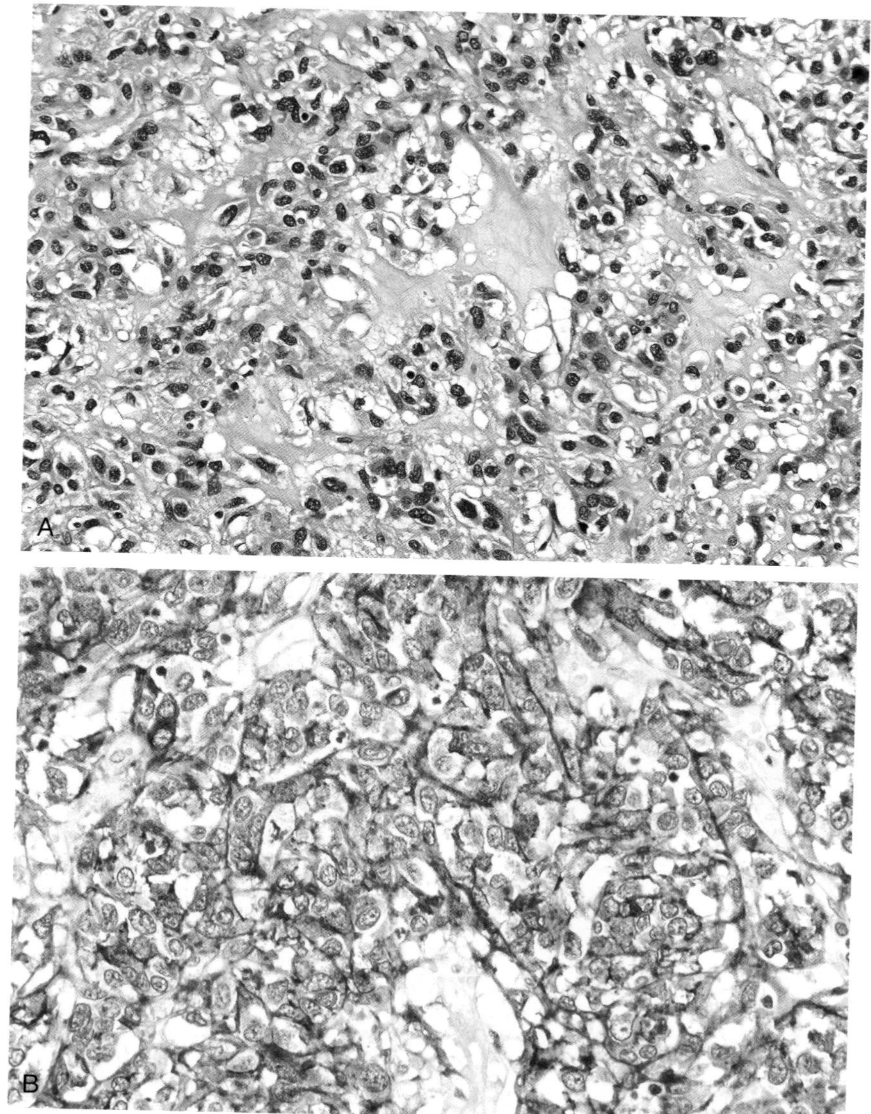

FIGURE 7-28. Gastrointestinal stromal tumor (A) with characteristic CD117 (c-kit) expression (B). Such expression distinguishes stromal tumors from leiomyosarcomas and nerve sheath tumors.

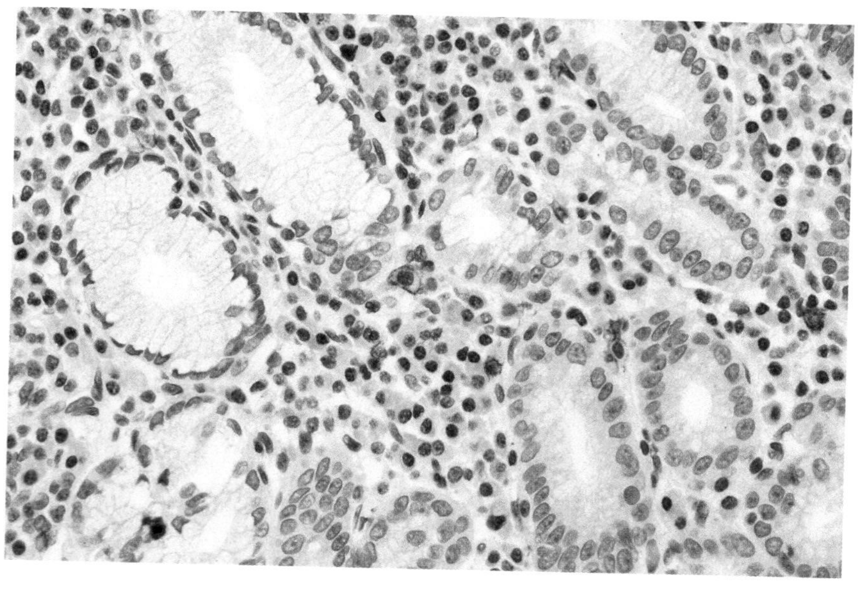

FIGURE 7-29. Mast cells in the lamina propria of the gut, demonstrating CD117 (c-kit) expression. Failure to distinguish CD117 expression by mast cells infiltrating a nongastrointestinal stromal tumor from expression by tumor cells is a potential pitfall.

study of large numbers of GIST, by a number of different investigators, has confirmed the high sensitivity (greater than 94%) and relatively high specificity of DOG1 for GIST, among mesenchymal tumors.[316-327] Near constant DOG1 expression has been shown in GIST from all anatomic locations, irrespective of CD117 expression or *KIT* mutational status (Fig. 7-30),[323,325] and in GIST arising in unusual clinical settings (e.g., pediatric GIST and NF1-associated GIST).[321,323] Expression of DOG1, generally weaker in intensity or in a small number of cells than is typically seen in GIST, has also been reported in a small number of leiomyomas, synovial sarcomas, and adenocarcinomas,[323] including acinar cell carcinomas of salivary gland origin.[328] Patchy and weak DOG1 have been observed in leiomyosarcomas arising in gastrointestinal locations, emphasizing the need to use this antibody as part of a panel of immunohistochemical markers.

USE OF IMMUNOHISTOCHEMISTRY AS A SURROGATE FOR THE PRESENCE OF TUMOR-SPECIFIC MOLECULAR ALTERATIONS

The immunohistochemical studies applied to sarcomas described to this point are used to identify cell-type-specific markers, that is, to identify the normal cell counterpart to the mesenchymal tumor in question. There is an emerging class of soft tissue tumors, however, that does not appear to have a normal cell counterpart and represents a set of tumors that are instead characterized by specific genetic alterations, usually chromosomal translocations. The latter can result in the abnormal juxtaposition of two genes, resulting in the neo-expression of one of the gene products, or a portion thereof. The latter can sometimes be identified by immunohistochemical studies, which, therefore, serve as a surrogate for the

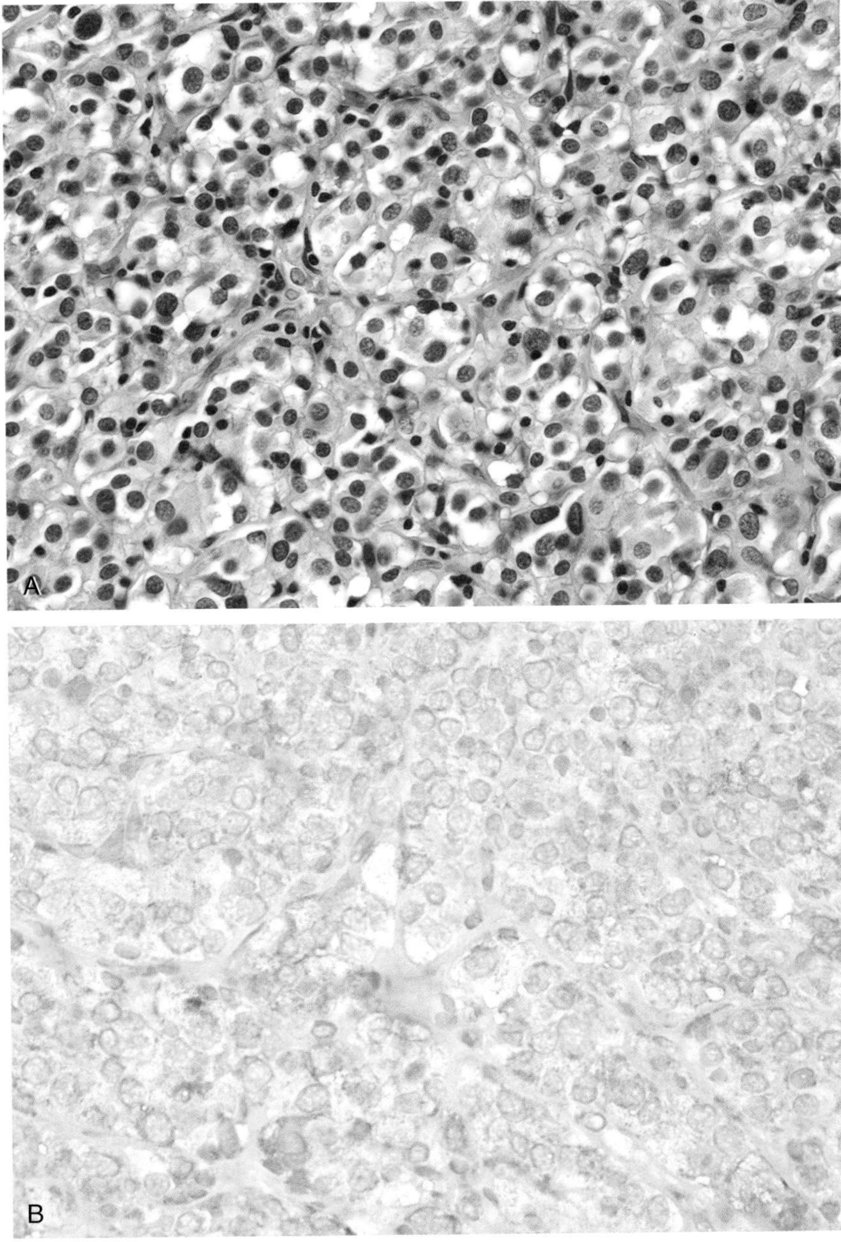

FIGURE 7-30. Typical epithelioid morphology of a PDGFRA D842V gastric GIST (A) showing faint immunoreactivity for KIT (CD117) (B) and diffuse and strong immunoreactivity for DOG1 (C). *(Courtesy of Dr. Brian Rubin, Cleveland Clinic, Cleveland, OH.)* *Continued*

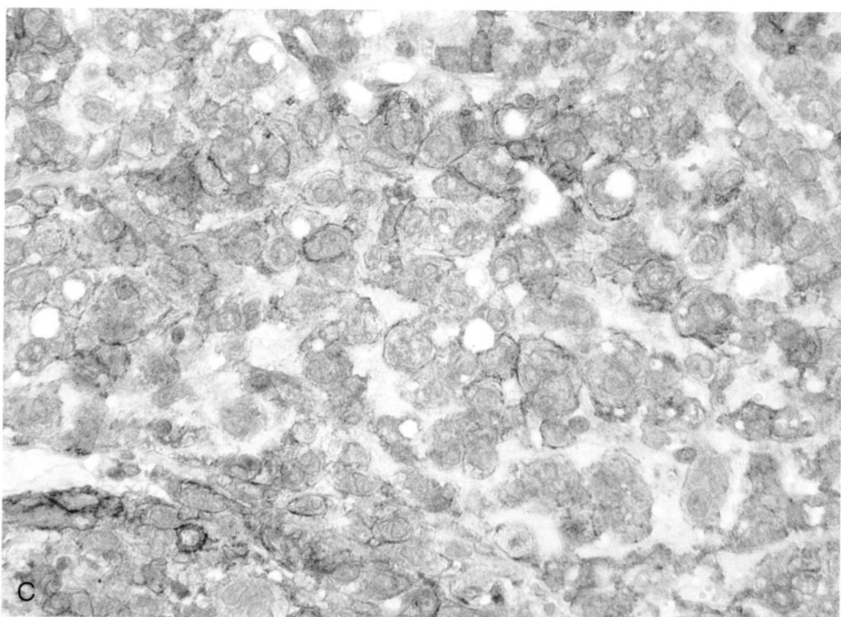

FIGURE 7-30, cont'd

presence of the chromosomal translocation. The following are five applications of this concept to soft tissue tumors.

FLI-1 and ERG as Markers of EFT

EFT is characterized by recurrent translocations involving the *EWSR1* gene on 2q12, most frequently involving the *FLI1* gene located on 11q22 (~85% of cases) or the *ERG* gene located on 21q12 (~5% of cases).[329-334] Polyclonal and monoclonal antibodies to FLI-1 protein are positive in 70% to 90% of genetically confirmed EFT, most often reflecting the presence of the EWSR1-FLI1 fusion protein.[41,262,335,336] Interestingly, antibodies to FLI-1 are positive in a significant percentage of EFT with known *EWSR1-ERG* fusions, reflecting protein homology between FLI-1 and ERG.[41,337] In contrast, antibodies to ERG seem to be much more specific for EFT containing *ERG* rearrangements, showing only weak positivity in rare cases known to have *FLI1* rearrangements.[337] FLI-1 expression is not generally seen in other tumors that enter this differential diagnosis, including RMS, mesenchymal chondrosarcoma, neuroblastoma, and Wilms tumor. However, lymphoblastic lymphomas are routinely FLI-1-positive, as are occasional cases of Merkel cell carcinoma, melanoma, and DSRCT.[262,336] As noted previously, both FLI-1 and ERG are routinely positive in endothelial tumors. ERG expression seems to be somewhat more restricted but may be seen in blastic extramedullary myeloid tumors and in a subset of prostatic adenocarcinomas.[263]

WT-1 as a Marker of the t(11;22)(13;q24) Translocation of DSRCT

DSRCT is characterized in almost all cases by a specific translocation t(11;22)(p13;q24) that fuses the *EWSR1* and *WT1* genes and produces a fusion protein containing the carboxy-terminus of WT-1.[338-340] Antibodies directed against the carboxy-terminus of WT-1 have been shown to be highly sensitive (greater than 90%) and relatively specific markers of DSRCT among small blue round cell tumors.[47,341-343] It is important to realize that many RMS express cytoplasmic wild-type WT-1, which will be identified by both amino- and carboxy-terminus antibodies and should be rigorously distinguished from the nuclear positivity seen in DSRCT.[344] Wild-type WT-1 expression is also seen in Wilms tumor, although this is seldom in the differential diagnosis of DSRCT and is usually easily identified by routine microscopy.[342]

TFE3 as a Marker of the der(17)t(X;17)(p11;q25) Translocation of ASPS

ASPS is characterized in almost all cases by a tumor-specific der(17)t(X;17) (p11;q25) that fuses the *TFE3* gene at Xp11 to the *ASPL* gene at 17q25, creating an ASPL-TFE3 fusion protein.[345] Recently, an antibody directed against the carboxy-terminus of the TFE3 transcription factor has been shown to be a highly sensitive and specific marker of ASPS (Fig. 7-31).[346] Although low levels of TFE3 expression is present in almost all normal tissues, strong nuclear expression of TFE3 is confined to tumors known to harbor TFE3 gene fusions, such as ASPS and rare pediatric renal carcinomas.[346] Only nuclear expression of TFE3 is of diagnostic value; the cytoplasmic staining (possibly nonspecific) is seen in a variety of tumors. Among other soft tissue tumors, TFE3 expression is confined to granular cell tumors[346] and to a small minority of PEComas.[11,347]

SMARCB1 (INI1) Expression Loss as a Marker of Monosomy or Homozygous Deletions of the *hSNF5/INI-1/SMARCB1/BAF47* Gene

The SMARCB1 protein is the product of the *hSNF5/INI-1/SMARCB1/BAF47* gene, located on chromosome 22q11.2.[348-350] Loss of *SMARCB1*, either in the form of

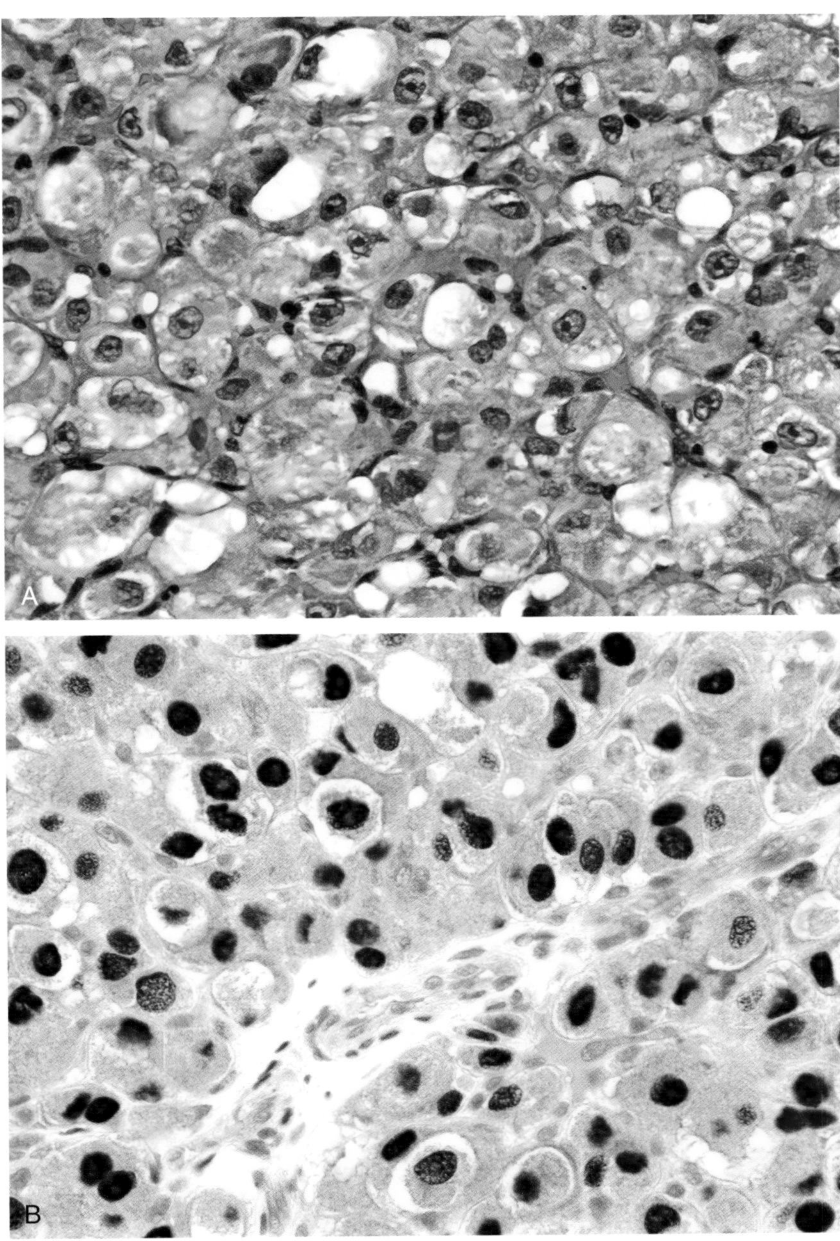

FIGURE 7-31. Alveolar soft part sarcoma (A), showing nuclear positivity with anti-TFE3 antibody (B), indicative of an ASPL-TFE3 fusion protein.

monosomy 22 or as homozygous deletions in the gene itself, has been strongly implicated in the pathogenesis of renal and extrarenal rhabdoid tumors as well as atypical teratoid/rhabdoid tumors of the central nervous system.[351] The SMARCB1 protein is a tumor suppressor and is normally present within all normal tissues. By immunohistochemistry, loss of SMARCB1 protein is seen in essentially all renal/extrarenal rhabdoid tumors (Fig. 7-32) and in greater than 90% of epithelioid sarcomas of both conventional and proximal types.[352-361] Loss of SMARCB1 expression is also seen in approximately 50% of epithelioid malignant peripheral nerve sheath tumors, where it may be a useful marker in the distinction of this tumor from melanoma.[361,362] It is lost in approximately 17% of extraskeletal myxoid chondrosarcoma and in medullary carcinoma of the kidney, a tumor often associated with sickle cell trait.[361] The link between loss of SMARCB1 expression and the presence of rhabdoid histologic features in many (but not all) of these tumors remains undefined. From a practical perspective, it can be least confusing to report SMARCB1 results as retained (normal) and absent (abnormal), rather than positive and negative, respectively.

Anaplastic Lymphoma Kinase

Anaplastic lymphoma kinase (ALK) is a transmembrane tyrosine kinase first identified as part of the characteristic t(2;5) (*NPM-ALK*) translocation seen in anaplastic large cell lymphomas.[363] In normal tissues, expression of ALK protein is restricted to the central nervous system.[364] Inflammatory myofibroblastic tumors frequently contain chromosomal rearrangements that result in activation of the *ALK* gene, with

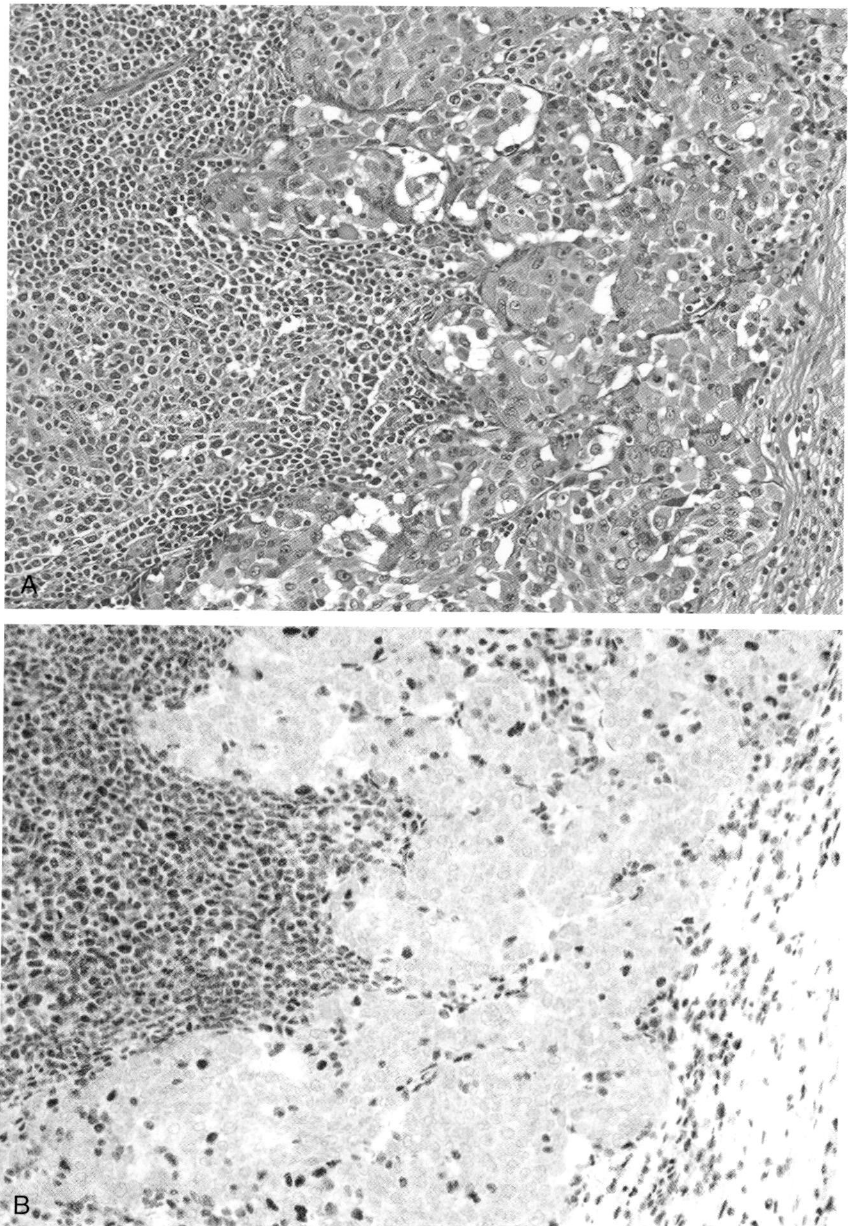

FIGURE 7-32. Malignant extrarenal rhabdoid tumor (A), showing complete loss of expression of SMARCB1 (INI) protein (B).

subsequent overexpression of ALK protein in roughly 40% of cases (Fig. 7-33).[365-368] However, not all molecular alterations in the *ALK* locus may be reflected in immunohistochemistry-detectable ALK protein, and fluorescence in-situ hybridization (FISH) studies may prove more sensitive in this regard.[369] Overexpression of ALK may also be seen in a variety of other soft tissue tumors, including RMS, lipogenic tumors, EFT, undifferentiated pleomorphic sarcoma, leiomyosarcoma, and others.[366,368] In RMS, the presence of cytoplasmic ALK expression, more commonly seen in alveolar versus ERMS, is associated with the presence of increased gene copy number and, less frequently, other gene alterations.[370] ALK expression has been demonstrated to help distinguish inflammatory myofibroblastic tumors from low-grade myofibroblastic sarcoma, which does not express ALK.[371]

OTHER MARKERS

TLE1

Transducin-like enhancer of split 1 (*TLE1*), one of four members of the *TLE* gene family encoding transcriptional corepressors homologous to the *Drosophila groucho* gene, is involved in control of hematopoiesis, neuronal differentiation, and terminal epithelial differentiation.[372-374] *TLE1* also plays an important role in the Wnt/β-catenin signaling pathway, where TLE1 protein competes with and displaces β-catenin, producing TLE1-TCT/LEF complexes that repress transcription.[375-377] The Wnt/β-catenin signaling pathway is known to be associated with synovial sarcoma,[378-380] and *TLE1* has been shown in

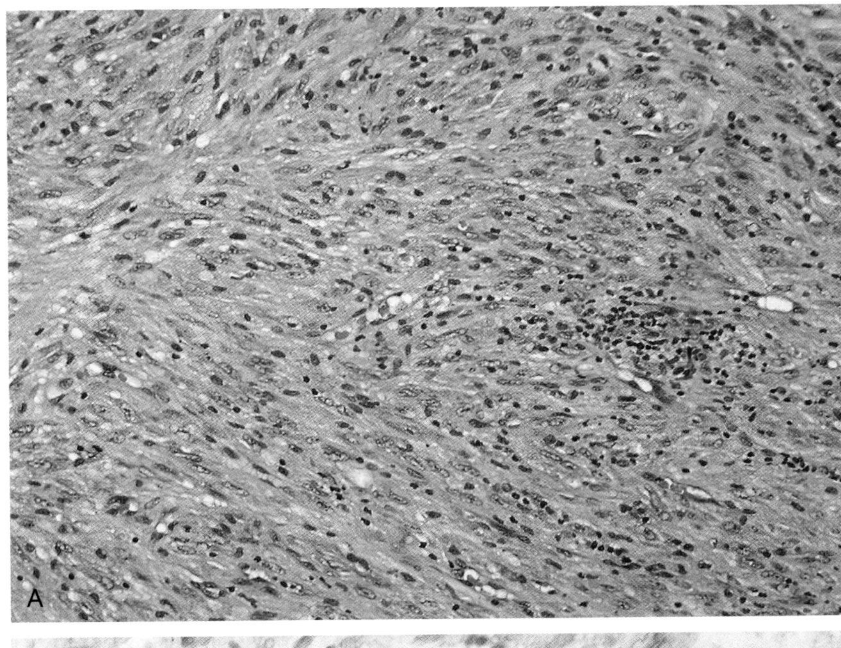

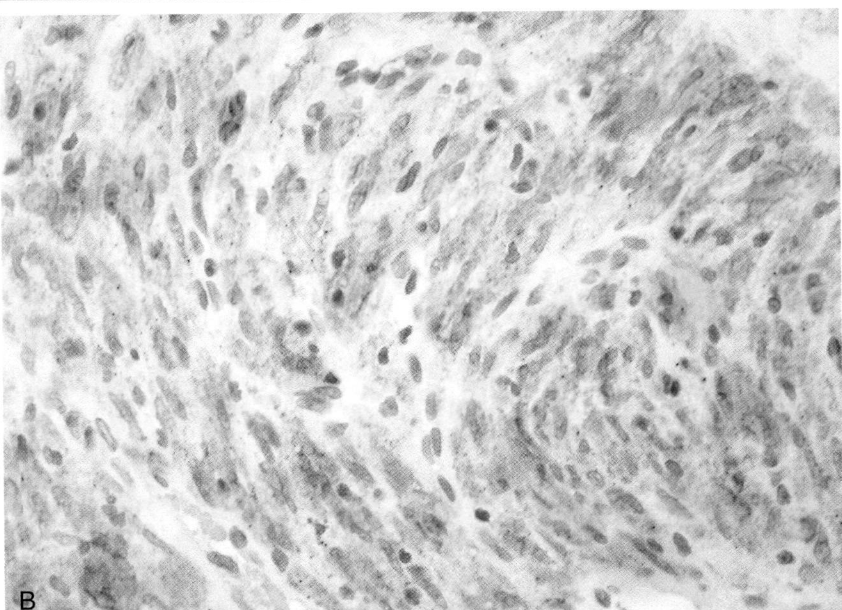

FIGURE 7-33. Inflammatory myofibroblastic tumor (A), showing ALK protein expression (B). This tumor was known to have an *ALK* gene rearrangement. *(Courtesy of Dr. Eunhee Yee, Mayo Clinic, Rochester, MN.)*

a variety of DNA microarray studies to be consistently expressed in synovial sarcomas.[378,380,381] Using tissue microarrays, Terry et al.[382] showed TLE1 protein expression to be a sensitive and relatively specific marker of synovial sarcoma in formalin-fixed, paraffin-embedded tissues. Similar results were reported by Jagdis et al.,[383] who noted TLE1 expression in 100% of synovial sarcomas, and in only isolated cases of malignant peripheral nerve sheath tumor and fibrosarcoma. However, using whole tissue sections rather than tissue microarrays, Kosemehmetoglu et al.[384] noted strong (2-3+) expression of TLE1 in significant subsets of benign and malignant peripheral nerve sheath tumors (including cases from known NF1 patients), solitary fibrous tumors and RMS, strongly suggesting that the specificity of TLE1 is somewhat less than what was originally believed. TLE1 is a superbly sensitive marker of synovial sarcomas, including cytokeratin-negative tumors,[385] and it continues to be used as a screening marker for this diagnosis (Fig. 7-34). Furthermore, recent studies suggest a relationship between TLE1 protein expression and the presence of the SS18-SSX fusion oncogene.[386] Although TLE1 is an unquestionable useful marker, molecular confirmation of the synovial sarcoma-specific t(X;18) remains the gold standard for the discrimination of this tumor from malignant peripheral nerve sheath tumor.

MUC4

MUC4, a transmembrane glycoprotein normally expressed by a variety of epithelia, is thought to play a protective role on the cell surface as well as participate in cell growth signaling through interactions with the ErbB/HER2 family of growth

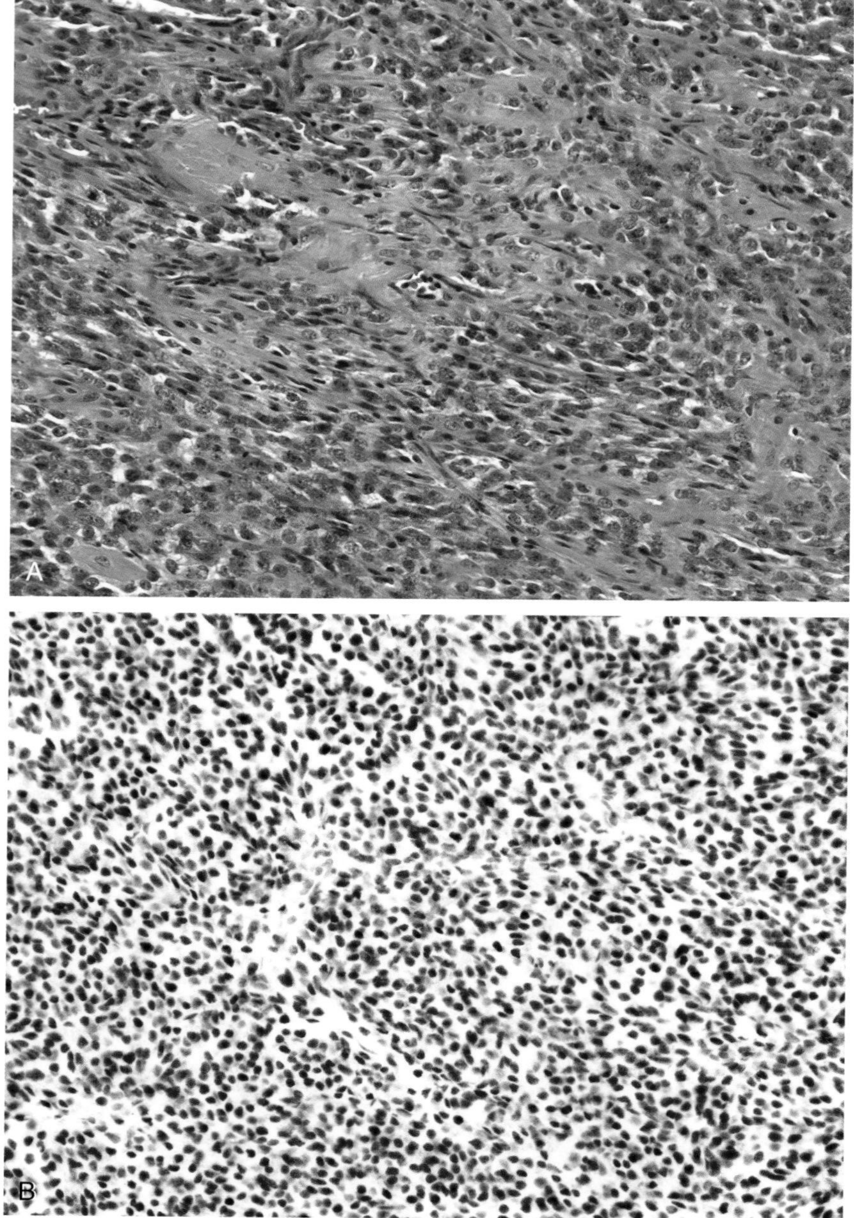

FIGURE 7-34. Poorly differentiated synovial sarcoma (A), showing diffuse nuclear immunoreactivity for TLE1 protein (B). Although TLE1 expression is not entirely specific for synovial sarcoma, it is highly sensitive, being positive even in cytokeratin-negative cases. Definitive diagnosis in such cases, however, requires molecular genetic techniques.

factor receptors.[387] Using gene expression profiling, Moller et al.[388] found upregulated *MUC4* gene expression and MUC4 protein expression by immunohistochemistry in genetically confirmed low-grade fibromyxoid sarcomas. This finding was confirmed in a much larger series by Doyle et al.,[389] who noted MUC4 expression in 100% of studied low-grade fibromyxoid sarcomas (Fig. 7-35), and in only 6 of 260 (2%) potential morphologic mimics. Upregulated *MUC4* gene expression and MUC4 protein expression have also been noted in a minority of cases of ossifying fibromyxoid tumor of soft parts.[200] Although FISH for *FUS* rearrangements continues to be regarded as the gold standard for the diagnosis of low-grade fibromyxoid sarcoma, there is no question that MUC4 immunohistochemistry may be very helpful in establishing this diagnosis, particularly in centers where FISH is not routinely available.

CD68

The 110-kDa glycoprotein recognized by antibodies to CD68 (e.g., KP1, KI-M1P) is closely associated with, or a part of, lysosomes.[390] Although CD68 has been thought of as a marker of histiocytes (owing to the presence of large numbers of lysosomes in these cells), it is important to remember that CD68 is organelle-specific rather than lineage-specific. Although CD68 expression is commonly seen in fibrohistiocytic soft tissue tumors, it may also be seen in a variety of other sarcomas, melanomas, and carcinomas.[391-394] For this reason, antibodies to CD68 play only a limited role in the diagnosis of soft tissue tumors. CD68 is expressed at high levels by lysosome-rich tumors such as granular cell tumors and may also be useful in bringing out the sometimes subtle

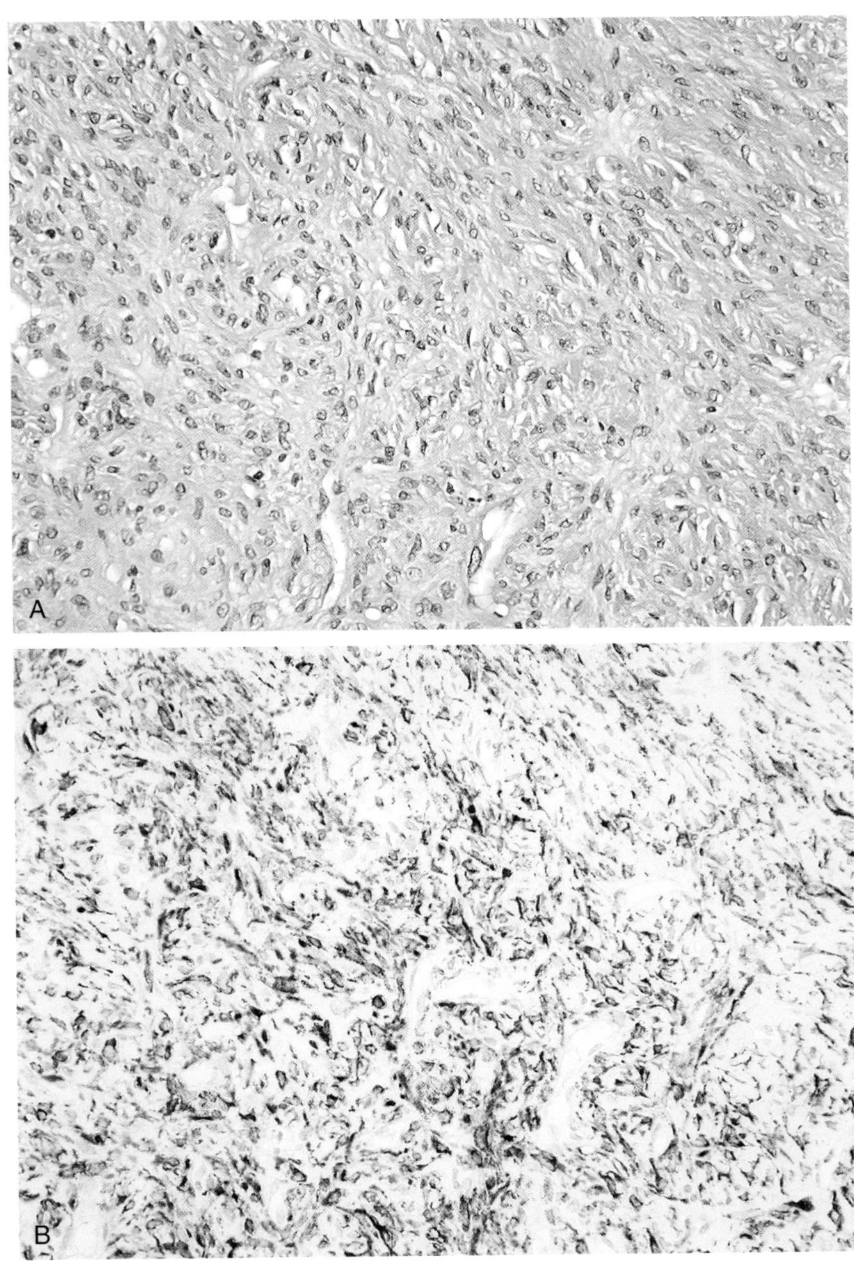

FIGURE 7-35. Low-grade fibromyxoid sarcoma (A), positive for MUC4 (B). Demonstration of MUC4 expression may be a valuable adjunct in the diagnosis of low-grade fibromyxoid sarcoma, particularly when molecular cytogenetic tests for *FUS* gene rearrangement are not available. *(Courtesy of Dr. Jason Hornick, Brigham and Women's Hospital, Boston, MA.)*

round cell population of plexiform fibrohistiocytic tumors (Fig. 7-36).

β-Catenin

β-catenin is a 92-kDa protein involved in both cadherin-mediated cellular cohesion, through binding to the cytoplasmic tail of E-cadherin, and in intracellular signaling, as a component of the Wnt signaling pathway.[395] In normal cells, β-catenin expression is tightly regulated by the *APC* gene and by glycogen synthetase kinase 3-beta.[396-398] Loss of β-catenin regulation may be the result of either mutations in the *APC* genes or in the *β-catenin* gene itself, resulting in accumulation of cytosolic β-catenin protein and eventual translocation to the nucleus.

Essentially, all familial fibromatoses harbor mutation in the *APC* gene, whereas sporadic fibromatoses are more likely to contain *β-catenin* mutations.[399,400] As a consequence of these mutations, nuclear overexpression of β-catenin protein is seen in over 90% of fibromatoses.[381,401-404] Superficial fibromatoses lack *β-catenin* mutations but also express nuclear β-catenin protein in approximately 90% of cases.[401] Nuclear β-catenin expression is relatively specific for fibromatoses, although it may also be seen in a substantial minority of solitary fibrous tumors, synovial sarcomas, and endometrial stromal sarcomas, and in isolated cases of clear cell sarcoma, osteosarcoma, and liposarcoma.[381,405-407] Interestingly, desmoplastic fibromas

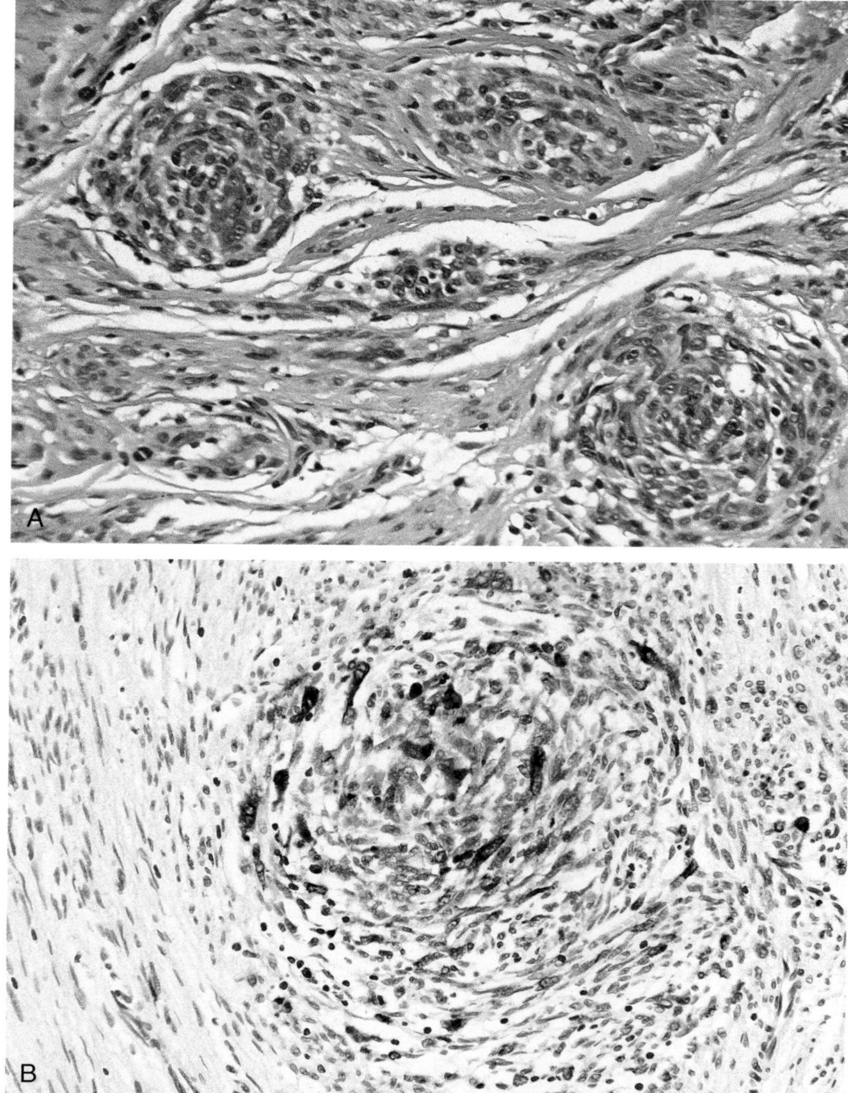

FIGURE 7-36. Plexiform fibrohistiocytic tumor (A) with strong CD68 expression in the histiocytoid nodules but not in the surrounding fibroblastic fascicles (B).

of bone, which have been presumed to represent the bony counterpart of soft tissue fibromatoses, appear to lack β-catenin expression, suggesting a different pathogenesis for these morphologically identical lesions.[408]

MDM2 and cdk4

A nuclear phosphoprotein whose transcription is activated by the p53 gene, MDM2 binds the p53 gene and removes its block on the cell cycle at the G1/S checkpoint.[409,410] The MDM2 marker has also been shown to exert an inhibitory effect through binding retinoblastoma protein[411] and a stimulatory effect on the E2F family of transcription factors.[412] Although overexpression of MDM2 has been previously documented in 33% to 37% of sarcomas, it does not appear to be of prognostic significance.[413-415] Most recently, MDM2 (and cdk4) expression has been shown to be highly characteristic of well-differentiated liposarcoma (atypical lipomatous tumor) and dedifferentiated liposarcoma, and detection of this protein may be useful in the distinction of these tumors from ordinary lipomas and other pleomorphic soft tissue sarcomas, respectively.[416-419] However, FISH studies for *MDM2* gene amplification are much more specific for the diagnosis of well-differentiated liposarcoma than is immunohistochemistry for MDM2 protein.

Bcl-2

The Bcl-2 protein is a mitochondrial and microsomal protein that plays a critical role in the prevention of cellular apoptosis.[420] Bcl-2 is expressed in a variety of normal cell types, including trophoblast, renal tubules, and neurons.[421] Bcl-2 is perhaps best known for its role in the pathogenesis of follicular lymphomas, wherein the translocation t(14;18) results in fusion of the Bcl-2 and immunoglobulin heavy chain genes, with subsequent overexpression of Bcl-2 protein.[422] In soft tissue tumors, Bcl-2 expression is relatively common in synovial sarcoma and solitary fibrous tumors, and some authors have suggested a role for this marker in the diagnosis of these entities.[190,191,423-426] However, careful reading of these same studies suggests that Bcl-2 expression may actually be seen in most of the entities that enter into the differential diagnosis of monophasic synovial sarcoma and solitary fibrous tumor, and, for this reason, the use of Bcl-2 immunostains in the diagnosis of soft tissue tumors is not advocated.

PROGNOSTIC MARKERS

Ki-67

A 395-kDa nuclear antigen, Ki-67 is encoded by a single gene on chromosome 10, the expression of which is confined to late G1, S, M, and G2 growth phases.[427] It appears to be localized to the nucleolus and may be a component of nucleolar preribosomes.[428] In formalin-fixed tissue, the most widely used antibody against this antigen is MIB-1. Several studies have documented a correlation between a high Ki-67 labeling index and poor prognostic features in soft tissue sarcomas.[429-432] Significant associations have been shown between a Ki-67 labeling index of more than 20% with high-grade, shortened overall survival and the development of metastatic disease.[433] In high-grade sarcomas of the extremities, a Ki-67 labeling index of more than 20% has been shown to be an independent predictor of distant metastases and tumor mortality.[434]

p53

The *TP53* gene product, p53, is a nuclear phosphoprotein that appears to regulate transcription by arresting cells with damaged DNA in G1 phase.[435-437] Mutations of the *TP53* gene produce a mutant protein that loses its tumor-suppressing ability and has a longer half-life than wild-type p53[435]; this allows immunohistochemical detection of mutated p53. Overexpression of p53 has been examined in a variety of soft tissue sarcomas, with the incidence ranging from 9% to 41%.[415,434,438-442] Most studies of p53 expression in sarcomas have shown a correlation between p53 overexpression, high tumor grade, and worse outcome; however, p53 overexpression has not been shown to have prognostic significance independent of grade.[430,434,440-443]

p21WAF1

A downstream effector of p53, p21WAF1 is an inhibitor of the cyclin/cyclin-dependent kinase complexes.[444] Loss of normal p21WAF1 expression has been documented in a subset of liposarcomas, including dedifferentiated, myxoid, and round cell liposarcomas, but has not yet been shown to be of prognostic significance.[409,410]

p16 AND p27kip

The p16 and p27kip markers are cyclin-dependent kinase inhibitors (CKIs) of the INK4 and KIP families, respectively.[444] These CKIs have been most extensively studied in malignant peripheral nerve sheath tumors. Loss of p16 expression, secondary to homozygous deletion of *CDKN2A/p16*, has been shown to be present in malignant peripheral nerve sheath tumors but not neurofibromas from patients with neurofibromatosis 1.[445] Loss of p27kip constitutive expression has been implicated in the malignant transformation of neurofibromas.[446]

TABLE 7-4 Basic Antigen Groups for Sarcoma Immunodiagnosis

TUMOR GROUP	MARKERS
Synovial sarcoma, epithelioid sarcoma	Cytokeratin, EMA, CD34, TLE1, SMARCB1
Nerve sheath group	S-100 protein, NGF receptor, SOX10
Muscle group	Desmin, muscle actins, myogenic regulatory proteins
Endothelial group	CD31, CD34, FLI-1, vWF, ERG, claudin-5

vWF, von Willebrand factor.

APPLICATION OF IMMUNOHISTOCHEMISTRY TO SARCOMA DIAGNOSIS: CLINICAL SCENARIOS

In general, it is advisable to have an initial panel of antibodies to analyze a sarcoma that is of uncertain differentiation histologically, including at least a representative of each of the antibody groups listed in Table 7-4. Of course, depending on the histologic setting of the tumor, it may or may not be necessary to include a member of each of the four groups.

Several common histologic scenarios of soft tissue tumors, in which immunohistochemistry can provide valuable clues to the correct diagnosis, are described in the following sections. These histologic settings include the undifferentiated round cell tumor, the monomorphic spindle cell tumor, and the poorly differentiated epithelioid tumor.

A basic principle in diagnostic immunohistochemistry that is illustrated in each of the four scenarios is the utilization of panels of antibodies, rather than single antibodies directed against markers of the suspected correct diagnosis. In general, such a panel should include not only antibodies that one would expect to be positive in a given tumor, but also antibodies that would be expected to be negative. This approach is essential for several reasons. First, many, if not most, antigens are expressed by more than one type of tumor. Second, for technical reasons, antibodies may show false-negative and, occasionally, false-positive results. Last, malignant cells may show unexpected or anomalous expression of antigens, and this may be very confusing if not interpreted within the context of other results.

The Undifferentiated Round Cell Tumor

The differential diagnosis of this case includes both sarcomas and nonsarcomas. As with all other diagnostic scenarios, the first task is to exclude a nonsarcoma. Nonsarcomatous neoplasms that might be legitimately included in this differential diagnosis include lymphoma, melanoma, and in an older patient, small cell carcinoma. Sarcomas that should be included in the differential diagnosis include EFT, RMS, PDSS, and DSRCT. Table 7-5 presents a screening panel of antibodies and the expected results for these tumors. The results of this panel dictate what additional studies are needed to confirm a specific diagnosis.

Small cell carcinoma (poorly differentiated neuroendocrine carcinoma): Confirm with antibodies to chromogranin A or synaptophysin.

Melanoma: Confirm with antibodies to melanosome-specific proteins (gp100, Melan-A, tyrosinase, microphthalmia transcription factor). As noted previously, a small number of melanomas may be S-100 protein negative, and occasional melanomas express cytokeratin or desmin. Small cell melanomas of the sinonasal tract appear to be particularly likely to show the S-100 protein-negative/HMB-45-positive phenotype.

Lymphoma: Lymphoblastic lymphoma in children may be CD45 negative and CD99/FLI-1 positive, which can easily result in a misdiagnosis as EFT. If the clinical or histologic features are suggestive of lymphoma, immunohistochemistry for terminal deoxyribonucleotide transferase, also known as TDT, may be critically important in arriving at the correct diagnosis. In adults and children, anaplastic large cell lymphomas (which have a small cell variant) may also be CD45 negative. In this setting, antibodies to CD30 may be useful.

Ewing family of tumors: As noted previously, EFT is unique among small blue round cell tumors in that the group does not usually express CD56. This negative finding may be useful in cases where CD99 is equivocal or where there is anomalous expression of cytokeratin or desmin. Demonstration of FLI-1/ERG protein or NKX2.2 expression may also be helpful.

Rhabdomyosarcoma: Confirm with myogenin or MyoD1.

Poorly differentiated synovial sarcoma: Cytokeratin expression may be patchy or absent, particularly in some PDSS. The addition of antibodies to EMA and high-molecular-weight cytokeratins may allow the detection of scattered positive cells. Antibodies to TLE1 can be helpful in identifying this tumor; molecular genetic testing for evidence of the t(X;18) is diagnostic.

Desmoplastic small round cell tumor: Confirm with antibodies to carboxy-terminus WT-1 or molecular genetic studies looking for the presence of t(11;22)(p13;q12) (*EWSR1-WT1*).

Monomorphic Spindle Cell Tumors

The differential diagnosis of monomorphic spindle cell tumors often includes entities such as fibrosarcoma, monophasic fibrous synovial sarcoma, malignant peripheral nerve sheath tumor, and malignant solitary fibrous tumor. Table 7-6 presents a screening immunohistochemical panel and the expected result for each tumor.

The following comments should also be borne in mind when immunostaining monomorphic spindle cell tumors.

Synovial sarcoma: As noted previously, cytokeratin and EMA expression may be focal in synovial sarcomas. Expression of CD34 is exceptionally rare in synovial sarcoma, and negative TLE1 studies would argue against this diagnosis, given its very high sensitivity for synovial sarcoma.

Malignant peripheral nerve sheath tumor: S-100 protein expression is often weak and focal. EMA, claudin-1, and Glut-1 expression may be seen in tumors with perineurial differentiation. Nerve sheath differentiation may also be confirmed with antibodies to p75NTR. Patchy TLE1 expression is not uncommon.

Fibrosarcoma: It may show limited actin expression, often in a myofibroblastic pattern.

Solitary fibrous tumor: Occasional cases, particularly those with histologic features of malignancy, can show anomalous cytokeratin expression. Strong CD34 expression is helpful in distinguishing such cases from monophasic synovial sarcoma.

Poorly Differentiated Epithelioid Tumor

The differential diagnosis of poorly differentiated epithelioid tumors includes carcinoma, melanoma, lymphoma (including anaplastic large cell lymphoma), and epithelioid soft tissue tumors such as epithelioid sarcoma and angiosarcoma. The

TABLE 7-5 Screening Panel for Undifferentiated Round Cell Tumor

ANTIBODY TO	SMALL CELL CARCINOMA	MELANOMA	LYMPHOMA	EFT	RMS	PDSS	DSRCT
Cytokeratins	Positive	Variable	Negative	Variable	Rare	Positive	Positive
Melanocytic markers	Negative	Positive	Negative	Negative	Negative	Negative	Negative
CD45	Negative	Negative	Positive*	Negative	Negative	Negative	Negative
Desmin	Negative	Variable	Negative	Rare	Positive	Negative	Positive
FLI1/ERG, NKX2.2	Negative	Negative	Negative	Positive	Negative	Negative	Negative
Synaptophysin	Positive	Negative	Negative	Variable	Rare	Negative	Negative

EFT, Ewing family of tumors; RMS, rhabdomyosarcoma; DSRCT, desmoplastic small round cell tumor; PDSS, poorly differentiated synovial sarcoma.
*Lymphoblastic lymphomas may be CD45 negative. In children, screen with TdT and CD43 instead of CD45.

TABLE 7-6 Screening Panel for Monomorphic Spindle Cell Tumors

ANTIBODY TO	SYNOVIAL SARCOMA	MPNST	FIBROSARCOMA	LEIOMYOSARCOMA	SOLITARY FIBROUS TUMOR
Cytokeratins	Positive	Negative	Negative	Rare	Rare
S-100 protein	Variable	Positive	Negative	Rare	Negative
CD34	Negative	Variable	Negative	Rare	Positive
Smooth muscle actin	Negative	Negative	Variable (myofibroblast pattern)	Positive	Negative

MPNST, malignant peripheral nerve sheath tumor.

TABLE 7-7 Screening Panel for Epithelioid Tumors in Soft Tissue

ANTIBODY TO	CARCINOMA	MELANOMA	B- OR T-CELL LYMPHOMA	ANAPLASTIC LARGE CELL LYMPHOMA	EPITHELIOID SARCOMA	EPITHELIOID ANGIOSARCOMA
Cytokeratin	Positive	Variable	Negative	Negative	Positive	Variable
Melanocytic markers	Negative	Positive	Negative	Negative	Negative	Negative
CD45	Negative	Negative	Positive	Negative	Negative	Negative
CD30	Negative	Negative	Negative	Positive	Negative	Negative
CD31*	Negative	Negative	Negative	Negative	Negative	Positive

*Incomplete sensitivity of CD31 for angiosarcoma may require use of additional endothelial markers.

TABLE 7-8 Discrimination of Carcinoma, Epithelioid Sarcoma, and Epithelioid Angiosarcoma

ANTIBODY TO	CARCINOMA	EPITHELIOID SARCOMA	EPITHELIOID ANGIOSARCOMA
High-molecular-weight cytokeratin	Variable	Variable	Negative
CD34	Negative	Variable	Positive
CD31	Negative	Negative	Positive
FLI-1	Negative	Negative	Positive
SMARCB1 (INI1)	Positive	Negative*	Positive

*Normal tissues and most tumors express SMARCB1. Epithelioid sarcomas lose SMARCB1 expression.

recommended panel of antibodies and their expected reactivities are presented in Table 7-7. This initial screening panel can make a specific diagnosis of melanoma, lymphoma, or anaplastic large cell lymphoma, but, generally, it is not able to discriminate carcinoma from epithelioid sarcoma or epithelioid angiosarcoma. These tumors can be reliably distinguished with the additional panel of antibodies listed in Table 7-8.

Orphan Sarcomas

It should be noted, with the previous discussion notwithstanding, that there remain orphan sarcomas without specific markers. This group includes tumors for which there is no known normal cell counterpart (e.g., undifferentiated pleomorphic sarcoma) and those for which there is a known cell counterpart (e.g., liposarcoma, osteogenic sarcoma, chondrosarcoma) but for which there are no reliable and useful specific markers, at present. Although markers for osteosarcoma have been developed, such as osteocalcin and osteonectin, they have not proved to be more sensitive markers than is the histologic identification of tumor osteoid.[447]

CONCLUSION

Immunohistochemistry continues to be a rapidly evolving field, with a number of exciting new markers having already entered the armamentarium of the diagnostic pathologist, and more to come. In many respects, advances in the immunohistochemical diagnosis of soft tissue neoplasms serve as logical extensions of the groundbreaking cytogenetic and molecular genetic advances in the understanding of these tumors, with new markers such as FLI-1, WT-1, INI1, TFE3, and β-catenin serving as surrogate protein markers of underlying genetic events. It is anticipated that new markers will assist in the diagnosis of tumors with other, more recently described specific genetic events, such as the newly described 6p21 (*PHF1* gene) rearrangements seen in ossifying fibromyxoid tumors of soft parts.[448]

References

1. Damjanov I. Antibodies to intermediate filaments and histogenesis. Lab Invest 1982;47(3):215–17.
2. Denk H, Krepler R, Artlieb U, et al. Proteins of intermediate filaments. An immunohistochemical and biochemical approach to the classification of soft tissue tumors. Am J Pathol 1983;110(2):193–208.
3. Osborn M, Weber K. Tumor diagnosis by intermediate filament typing: a novel tool for surgical pathology. Laboratory Investigation 1983;48(4):372–94.
4. Dahl D. The vimentin-GFA protein transition in rat neuroglia cytoskeleton occurs at the time of myelination. J Neurosci Res 1981;6(6): 741–8.
5. Akhtar M, Tulbah A, Kardar AH, et al. Sarcomatoid renal cell carcinoma: the chromophobe connection. Am J Surg Pathol 1997;21(10): 1188–95.
6. Eckert F, de Viragh PA, Schmid U. Coexpression of cytokeratin and vimentin intermediate filaments in benign and malignant sweat gland tumors. J Cutan Pathol 1994;21(2):140–50.
7. Lopez-Beltran A, Escudero AL, Cavazzana AO, et al. Sarcomatoid transitional cell carcinoma of the renal pelvis. A report of five cases with clinical, pathological, immunohistochemical and DNA ploidy analysis. Pathol Res Pract 1996;192(12):1218–24.
8. Meis JM, Ordonez NG, Gallager HS. Sarcomatoid carcinoma of the breast: an immunohistochemical study of six cases. Virchows Arch A Pathol Anat Histopathol 1987;410(5):415–21.
9. Skalli O, Gabbiani G, Babai F, et al. Intermediate filament proteins and actin isoforms as markers for soft tissue tumor differentiation and origin. II. Rhabdomyosarcomas. Am J Pathol 1988;130(3):515–31.
10. Judkins AR, Montone KT, LiVolsi VA, et al. Sensitivity and specificity of antibodies on necrotic tumor tissue. Am J Clin Pathol 1998;110(5): 641–6.
11. Folpe AL, Mentzel T, Lehr HA, et al. Perivascular epithelioid cell neoplasms of soft tissue and gynecologic origin: a clinicopathologic study of 26 cases and review of the literature. Am J Surg Pathol 2005;29(12): 1558–75.
12. Fanburg-Smith JC, Miettinen M, Folpe AL, et al. Lingual alveolar soft part sarcoma; 14 cases: novel clinical and morphological observations. Histopathology 2004;45(5):526–37.
13. Miettinen M. Keratin subsets in spindle cell sarcomas. Keratins are widespread but synovial sarcoma contains a distinctive keratin polypeptide pattern and desmoplakins. Am J Pathol 1991;138(2):505–13.
14. Billings SD, Walsh SV, Fisher C, et al. Aberrant expression of tight junction-related proteins ZO-1, claudin-1 and occludin in synovial sarcoma: an immunohistochemical study with ultrastructural correlation. Mod Pathol 2004;17(2):141–9.
15. Folpe AL, Schmidt RA, Chapman D, et al. Poorly differentiated synovial sarcoma: immunohistochemical distinction from primitive neuroectodermal tumors and high-grade malignant peripheral nerve sheath tumors. Am J Surg Pathol 1998;22(6):673–82.

16. Miettinen M, Fanburg-Smith JC, Virolainen M, et al. Epithelioid sarcoma: an immunohistochemical analysis of 112 classical and variant cases and a discussion of the differential diagnosis. Hum Pathol 1999;30(8):934–42.
17. Laskin WB, Miettinen M. Epithelioid sarcoma: new insights based on an extended immunohistochemical analysis. Arch Pathol Lab Med 2003;127(9):1161–8.
18. Smith TA, Machen SK, Fisher C, et al. Usefulness of cytokeratin subsets for distinguishing monophasic synovial sarcoma from malignant peripheral nerve sheath tumor. Am J Clin Pathol 1999;112(5):641–8.
19. Fanburg-Smith JC, Hengge M, Hengge UR, et al. Extrarenal rhabdoid tumors of soft tissue: a clinicopathologic and immunohistochemical study of 18 cases. Ann Diagn Pathol 1998;2(6):351–62.
20. Hoefler H, Kerl H, Rauch HJ, et al. New immunocytochemical observations with diagnostic significance in cutaneous neuroendocrine carcinoma. Am J Dermatopathol 1984;6(6):525–30.
21. Miettinen M, Lehto VP, Virtanen I, et al. Neuroendocrine carcinoma of the skin (Merkel cell carcinoma): ultrastructural and immunohistochemical demonstration of neurofilaments. Ultrastruct Pathol 1983;4(2–3):219–25.
22. Jahn L, Fouquet B, Rohe K, et al. Cytokeratins in certain endothelial and smooth muscle cells of two taxonomically distant vertebrate species, Xenopus laevis and man. Differentiation 1987;36(3):234–54.
23. Brown DC, Theaker JM, Banks PM, et al. Cytokeratin expression in smooth muscle and smooth muscle tumours. Histopathology 1987;11(5):477–86.
24. Norton AJ, Thomas JA, Isaacson PG. Cytokeratin-specific monoclonal antibodies are reactive with tumours of smooth muscle derivation. An immunocytochemical and biochemical study using antibodies to intermediate filament cytoskeletal proteins. Histopathology 1987;11(5):487–99.
25. Gown AM, Boyd HC, Chang Y, et al. Smooth muscle cells can express cytokeratins of "simple" epithelium. Immunocytochemical and biochemical studies in vitro and in vivo. Am J Pathol 1988;132(2):223–32.
26. Miettinen M. Immunoreactivity for cytokeratin and epithelial membrane antigen in leiomyosarcoma. Arch Pathol Lab Med 1988;112(6):637–40.
27. Ramaekers FC, Pruszczynski M, Smedts F. Cytokeratins in smooth muscle cells and smooth muscle tumours. Histopathology 1988;12(5):558–61.
28. Tauchi K, Tsutsumi Y, Yoshimura S, et al. Immunohistochemical and immunoblotting detection of cytokeratin in smooth muscle tumors. Acta Pathologica Japonica 1990;40(8):574–80.
29. Gown AM, Vogel AM. Monoclonal antibodies to human intermediate filament proteins. III. Analysis of tumors. Am J Clin Pathol 1985;84(4):413–24.
30. Zarbo RJ, Gown AM, Nagle RB, et al. Anomalous cytokeratin expression in malignant melanoma: one- and two-dimensional Western blot analysis and immunohistochemical survey of 100 melanomas. Mod Pathol 1990;3(4):494–501.
31. Ben-Izhak O, Stark P, Levy R, et al. Epithelial markers in malignant melanoma. A study of primary lesions and their metastases. Am J Dermatopathol 1994;16(3):241–6.
32. Ben-Izhak O, Auslander L, Rabinson S, et al. Epithelioid angiosarcoma of the adrenal gland with cytokeratin expression. Report of a case with accompanying mesenteric fibromatosis. Cancer 1992;69(7):1808–12.
33. Gray MH, Rosenberg AE, Dickersin GR, et al. Cytokeratin expression in epithelioid vascular neoplasms. Hum Pathol 1990;21(2):212–17.
34. O'Connell JX, Kattapuram SV, Mankin HJ, et al. Epithelioid hemangioma of bone. A tumor often mistaken for low-grade angiosarcoma or malignant hemangioendothelioma [see comments]. Am J Surg Pathol 1993;17(6):610–17.
35. van Haelst UJ, Pruszczynski M, ten Cate LN, et al. Ultrastructural and immunohistochemical study of epithelioid hemangioendothelioma of bone: coexpression of epithelial and endothelial markers. Ultrastruct Pathol 1990;14(2):141–9.
36. Wenig BM, Abbondanzo SL, Heffess CS. Epithelioid angiosarcoma of the adrenal glands. A clinicopathologic study of nine cases with a discussion of the implications of finding "epithelial-specific" markers. Am J Surg Pathol 1994;18(1):62–73.
37. Meis-Kindblom JM, Kindblom LG. Angiosarcoma of soft tissue: a study of 80 cases. Am J Surg Pathol 1998;22(6):683–97.
38. Collini P, Sampietro G, Bertulli R, et al. Cytokeratin immunoreactivity in 41 cases of ES/PNET confirmed by molecular diagnostic studies. Am J Surg Pathol 2001;25(2):273–4.
39. Gu M, Antonescu CR, Guiter G, et al. Cytokeratin immunoreactivity in Ewing's sarcoma: prevalence in 50 cases confirmed by molecular diagnostic studies. Am J Surg Pathol 2000;24(3):410–16.
40. Bridge JA, Fidler ME, Neff JR, et al. Adamantinoma-like Ewing's sarcoma: genomic confirmation, phenotypic drift. Am J Surg Pathol 1999;23(2):159–65.
41. Folpe AL, Goldblum JR, Rubin BP, et al. Morphologic and immunophenotypic diversity in Ewing family tumors: a study of 66 genetically confirmed cases. Am J Surg Pathol 2005;29(8):1025–33.
42. Miettinen M, Rapola J. Immunohistochemical spectrum of rhabdomyosarcoma and rhabdomyosarcoma-like tumors. Expression of cytokeratin and the 68-kD neurofilament protein. Am J Surg Pathol 1989;13(2):120–32.
43. Coindre JM, de Mascarel A, Trojani M, et al. Immunohistochemical study of rhabdomyosarcoma. Unexpected staining with S100 protein and cytokeratin. J Pathol 1988;155(2):127–32.
44. Droz D, Rousseau-Merck MF, Jaubert F, et al. Cell differentiation in Wilms' tumor (nephroblastoma): an immunohistochemical study. Hum Pathol 1990;21(5):536–44.
45. Wick MR, Manivel C, O'Leary TP, et al. Nephroblastoma. A comparative immunocytochemical and lectin-histochemical study. Arch Pathol Lab Med 1986;110(7):630–5.
46. Nikolaou I, Barbatis C, Laopodis V, et al. Intra-abdominal desmoplastic small-cell tumours with divergent differentiation. Report of two cases and review of the literature. Pathol Res Pract 1992;188(8):981–8.
47. Ordonez NG. Desmoplastic small round cell tumor: II: an ultrastructural and immunohistochemical study with emphasis on new immunohistochemical markers. Am J Surg Pathol 1998;22(11):1314–27.
48. Weiss SW, Bratthauer GL, Morris PA. Postirradiation malignant fibrous histiocytoma expressing cytokeratin. Implications for the immunodiagnosis of sarcomas [see comments]. Am J Surg Pathol 1988;12(7):554–8.
49. Rosenberg AE, O'Connell JX, Dickersin GR, et al. Expression of epithelial markers in malignant fibrous histiocytoma of the musculoskeletal system: an immunohistochemical and electron microscopic study. Hum Pathol 1993;24(3):284–93.
50. Litzky LA, Brooks JJ. Cytokeratin immunoreactivity in malignant fibrous histiocytoma and spindle cell tumors: comparison between frozen and paraffin-embedded tissues. Mod Pathol 1992;5(1):30–4.
51. Miettinen M, Soini Y. Malignant fibrous histiocytoma. Heterogeneous patterns of intermediate filament proteins by immunohistochemistry. Arch Pathol Lab Med 1989;113(12):1363–6.
52. Abramovici LC, Steiner GC, Bonar F. Myxoid chondrosarcoma of soft tissue and bone: a retrospective study of 11 cases. Hum Pathol 1995;26(11):1215–20.
53. Hasegawa T, Seki K, Yang P, et al. Differentiation and proliferative activity in benign and malignant cartilage tumors of bone. Hum Pathol 1995;26(8):838–45.
54. Dardick I, Schatz JE, Colgan TJ. Osteogenic sarcoma with epithelial differentiation. Ultrastruct Pathol 1992;16(4):463–74.
55. Hasegawa T, Shibata T, Hirose T, et al. Osteosarcoma with epithelioid features. An immunohistochemical study. Arch Pathol Lab Med 1993;117(3):295–8.
56. Hirose T, Hasegawa T, Kudo E, et al. Malignant peripheral nerve sheath tumors: an immunohistochemical study in relation to ultrastructural features. Hum Pathol 1992;23(8):865–70.
57. Battifora H. Misuse of the term 'expression.' Am J Clin Pathol [Comment Letter] 1989;92(5):708–9.
58. Swanson PE. HIERanarchy: the state of the art in immunohistochemistry. Am J Clin Pathol [Editorial Review] 1997;107(2):139–40.
59. Swanson PE. Heffalumps, jagulars, and cheshire cats. A commentary on cytokeratins and soft tissue sarcomas. Am J Clin Pathol [Review] 1991;95(4 Suppl 1):S2–7.
60. Fanburg-Smith JC, Majidi M, Miettinen M. Keratin expression in schwannoma; a study of 115 retroperitoneal and 22 peripheral schwannomas. Mod Pathol 2006;19(1):115–21.
61. Bachi CE, Zarbo RJ, Jiang JJ, et al. Do glioma cells express cytokeratin? Applied Immunohistochemistry 1995;3(1):45–53.
62. Heyderman E, Steele K, Ormerod MG. A new antigen on the epithelial membrane: its immunoperoxidase localisation in normal and neoplastic tissue. J Clin Pathol 1979;32(1):35–9.
63. Pinkus GS, Kurtin PJ. Epithelial membrane antigen–a diagnostic discriminant in surgical pathology: immunohistochemical profile in epithelial, mesenchymal, and hematopoietic neoplasms using paraffin sections and monoclonal antibodies. Hum Pathol 1985;16(9):929–40.

64. Erlandson RA. The enigmatic perineurial cell and its participation in tumors and in tumorlike entities. Ultrastruct Pathol 1991;15(4–5):335–51.
65. Theaker JM, Fletcher CD. Epithelial membrane antigen expression by the perineurial cell: further studies of peripheral nerve lesions. Histopathology 1989;14(6):581–92.
66. Theaker JM, Gatter KC, Puddle J. Epithelial membrane antigen expression by the perineurium of peripheral nerve and in peripheral nerve tumours. Histopathology 1988;13(2):171–9.
67. Theaker JM, Gillett MB, Fleming KA, et al. Epithelial membrane antigen expression by meningiomas, and the perineurium of peripheral nerve. Arch Pathol Lab Med 1987;111(5):409.
68. Theaker JM, Gatter KC, Esiri MM, et al. Epithelial membrane antigen and cytokeratin expression by meningiomas: an immunohistological study. J Clin Pathol 1986;39(4):435–9.
69. Ariza A, Bilbao JM, Rosai J. Immunohistochemical detection of epithelial membrane antigen in normal perineurial cells and perineurioma. Am J Surg Pathol 1988;12(9):678–83.
70. Zamecnik M, Michal M. Malignant peripheral nerve sheath tumor with perineurial cell differentiation (malignant perineurioma). Pathol Int 1999;49(1):69–73.
71. Hirose T, Scheithauer BW, Sano T. Perineurial malignant peripheral nerve sheath tumor (MPNST): a clinicopathologic, immunohistochemical, and ultrastructural study of seven cases. Am J Surg Pathol 1998;22(11):1368–78.
72. Perentes E, Nakagawa Y, Ross GW, et al. Expression of epithelial membrane antigen in perineurial cells and their derivatives. An immunohistochemical study with multiple markers. Acta Neuropathol 1987;75(2):160–5.
73. Hornick JL, Fletcher CD. Soft tissue perineurioma: clinicopathologic analysis of 81 cases including those with atypical histologic features. Am J Surg Pathol 2005;29(7):845–58.
74. Fanburg-Smith JC, Miettinen M. Angiomatoid "malignant" fibrous histiocytoma: a clinicopathologic study of 158 cases and further exploration of the myoid phenotype. Hum Pathol 1999;30(11):1336–43.
75. Guillou L, Benhattar J, Gengler C, et al. Translocation-positive low-grade fibromyxoid sarcoma: clinicopathologic and molecular analysis of a series expanding the morphologic spectrum and suggesting potential relationship to sclerosing epithelioid fibrosarcoma: a study from the French Sarcoma Group. Am J Surg Pathol 2007;31(9):1387–402.
76. Kindblom LG, Seidal T, Karlsson K. Immuno-histochemical localization of myoglobin in human muscle tissue and embryonal and alveolar rhabdomyosarcoma. Acta Pathologica, Microbiologica, et Immunologica ScandinavicassSection A, Pathology 1982;90(3):167–74.
77. Andriko JW, Kaldjian EP, Tsokos M, et al. Reticulum cell neoplasms of lymph nodes: a clinicopathologic study of 11 cases with recognition of a new subtype derived from fibroblastic reticular cells. Am J Surg Pathol 1998;22(9):1048–58.
78. Cho J, Gong G, Choe G, et al. Extrafollicular reticulum cells in pathologic lymph nodes. J Korean Med Sci 1994;9(1):9–15.
79. Van Muijen GN, Ruiter DJ, Warnaar SO. Coexpression of intermediate filament polypeptides in human fetal and adult tissues. Lab Invest 1987;57(4):359–69.
80. Franquemont DW, Frierson HF Jr, Mills SE. An immunohistochemical study of normal endometrial stroma and endometrial stromal neoplasms. Evidence for smooth muscle differentiation. Am J Surg Pathol 1991;15(9):861–70.
81. Altmannsberger M, Weber K, Droste R, et al. Desmin is a specific marker for rhabdomyosarcomas of human and rat origin. Am J Pathol 1985;118(1):85–95.
82. Tsokos M. The role of immunocytochemistry in the diagnosis of rhabdomyosarcoma. Arch Pathol Lab Med [Editorial] 1986;110(9):776–8.
83. Azumi N, Ben-Ezra J, Battifora H. Immunophenotypic diagnosis of leiomyosarcomas and rhabdomyosarcomas with monoclonal antibodies to muscle-specific actin and desmin in formalin-fixed tissue. Mod Pathol 1988;1(6):469–74.
84. Leader M, Collins M, Patel J, et al. Desmin: its value as a marker of muscle derived tumours using a commercial antibody. Virchows Arch A Pathol Anat Histopathol 1987;411(4):345–9.
85. Parham DM, Webber B, Holt H, et al. Immunohistochemical study of childhood rhabdomyosarcomas and related neoplasms. Results of an Intergroup Rhabdomyosarcoma study project. Cancer 1991;67(12):3072–80.
86. Chiles MC, Parham DM, Qualman SJ, et al. Sclerosing rhabdomyosarcomas in children and adolescents: a clinicopathologic review of 13 cases from the Intergroup Rhabdomyosarcoma Study Group and Children's Oncology Group. Pediatr Dev Pathol 2004;7(6):583–94.
87. Folpe AL, McKenney JK, Bridge JA, et al. Sclerosing rhabdomyosarcoma in adults: report of four cases of a hyalinizing, matrix-rich variant of rhabdomyosarcoma that may be confused with osteosarcoma, chondrosarcoma, or angiosarcoma. Am J Surg Pathol 2002;26(9):1175–83.
88. Furlong MA, Mentzel T, Fanburg-Smith JC. Pleomorphic rhabdomyosarcoma in adults: a clinicopathologic study of 38 cases with emphasis on morphologic variants and recent skeletal muscle-specific markers. Mod Pathol 2001;14(6):595–603.
89. Rubin BP, Hasserjian RP, Singer S, et al. Spindle cell rhabdomyosarcoma (so-called) in adults: report of two cases with emphasis on differential diagnosis. Am J Surg Pathol 1998;22(4):459–64.
90. Coffin CM, Rulon J, Smith L, et al. Pathologic features of rhabdomyosarcoma before and after treatment: a clinicopathologic and immunohistochemical analysis. Mod Pathol 1997;10(12):1175–87.
91. Rangdaeng S, Truong LD. Comparative immunohistochemical staining for desmin and muscle-specific actin. A study of 576 cases. Am J Clin Pathol [Comparative Study] 1991;96(1):32–45.
92. Truong LD, Rangdaeng S, Cagle P, et al. The diagnostic utility of desmin. A study of 584 cases and review of the literature. Am J Clin Pathol [Comparative Study Review] 1990;93(3):305–14.
93. Parham DM, Dias P, Kelly DR, et al. Desmin positivity in primitive neuroectodermal tumors of childhood. Am J Surg Pathol 1992;16(5):483–92.
94. Gerald WL, Miller HK, Battifora H, et al. Intra-abdominal desmoplastic small round-cell tumor. Report of 19 cases of a distinctive type of high-grade polyphenotypic malignancy affecting young individuals [see comments]. Am J Surg Pathol 1991;15(6):499–513.
95. Sugimoto T, Ueyama H, Hosoi H, et al. Alpha-smooth-muscle actin and desmin expressions in human neuroblastoma cell lines. Int J Cancer 1991;48(2):277–83.
96. Hurlimann J. Desmin and neural marker expression in mesothelial cells and mesotheliomas. Hum Pathol 1994;25(8):753–7.
97. Folpe AL, Patterson K, Gown AM. Antibodies to desmin identify the blastemal component of nephroblastoma. Mod Pathol 1997;10(9):895–900.
98. Folpe AL, Weiss SW, Fletcher CD, et al. Tenosynovial giant cell tumors: evidence for a desmin-positive dendritic cell subpopulation. Mod Pathol 1998;11(10):939–44.
99. Folpe AL, Weiss SW. Ossifying fibromyxoid tumor of soft parts: a clinicopathologic study of 70 cases with emphasis on atypical and malignant variants. Am J Surg Pathol [Review] 2003;(4):421–31.
100. Hasegawa T, Seki K, Ono K, et al. Angiomatoid (malignant) fibrous histiocytoma: a peculiar low-grade tumor showing immunophenotypic heterogeneity and ultrastructural variations. Pathol Int 2000;50(9):731–8.
101. Lessard JL. Two monoclonal antibodies to actin: one muscle selective and one generally reactive. Cell Motil Cytoskeleton 1988;10(3):349–62.
102. Skalli O, Ropraz P, Trzeciak A, et al. A monoclonal antibody against alpha-smooth muscle actin: a new probe for smooth muscle differentiation. J Cell Biol 1986;103(6 Pt 2):2787–96.
103. Tsukada T, McNutt MA, Ross R, et al. HHF35, a muscle actin-specific monoclonal antibody. II. Reactivity in normal, reactive, and neoplastic human tissues. Am J Pathol 1987;127(2):389–402.
104. Tsukada T, Tippens D, Gordon D, et al. HHF35, a muscle-actin-specific monoclonal antibody. I. Immunocytochemical and biochemical characterization. Am J Pathol 1987;126(1):51–60.
105. Foschini MP, Ceccarelli C, Eusebi V, et al. Alveolar soft part sarcoma: immunological evidence of rhabdomyoblastic differentiation. Histopathology 1988;13(1):101–8.
106. Venuti JM, Morris JH, Vivian JL, et al. Myogenin is required for late but not early aspects of myogenesis during mouse development. J Cell Biol 1995;128(4):563–76.
107. Weintraub H. The MyoD family and myogenesis: redundancy, networks, and thresholds. Cell 1993;75(7):1241–4.
108. Dias P, Dilling M, Houghton P. The molecular basis of skeletal muscle differentiation. Semin Diagn Pathol 1994;11(1):3–14.
109. Rudnicki MA, Jaenisch R. The MyoD family of transcription factors and skeletal myogenesis. Bioessays 1995;17(3):203–9.
110. Dias P, Parham DM, Shapiro DN, et al. Monoclonal antibodies to the myogenic regulatory protein MyoD1: epitope mapping and diagnostic utility. Cancer Res 1992;52(23):6431–9.

111. Wang NP, Marx J, McNutt MA, et al. Expression of myogenic regulatory proteins (myogenin and MyoD1) in small blue round cell tumors of childhood. Am J Pathol 1995;147(6):1799–810.
112. Tonin PN, Scrable H, Shimada H, et al. Muscle-specific gene expression in rhabdomyosarcomas and stages of human fetal skeletal muscle development. Cancer Res 1991;51(19):5100–6.
113. Kumar S, Perlman E, Harris CA, et al. Myogenin is a specific marker for rhabdomyosarcoma: an immunohistochemical study in paraffin-embedded tissues. Mod Pathol 2000;13(9):988–93.
114. Cessna MH, Zhou H, Perkins SL, et al. Are Myogenin and MyoD1 expression specific for rhabdomyosarcoma? A study of 150 cases, with emphasis on spindle cell mimics. Am J Surg Pathol 2001;25(9): 1150–7.
115. Dias P, Chen B, Dilday B, et al. Strong immunostaining for myogenin in rhabdomyosarcoma is significantly associated with tumors of the alveolar subclass. Am J Pathol 2000;156(2):399–408.
116. Mentzel T, Katenkamp D. Sclerosing, pseudovascular rhabdomyosarcoma in adults. Clinicopathological and immunohistochemical analysis of three cases. Virchows Arch 2000;436(4):305–11.
117. Wesche WA, Fletcher CD, Dias P, et al. Immunohistochemistry of MyoD1 in adult pleomorphic soft tissue sarcomas. Am J Surg Pathol 1995;19(3):261–9.
118. Folpe AL. MyoD1 and Myogenin expression in human neoplasia: a review and update. Adv Anat Pathol 2002;9(3):198–203.
119. Rosai J, Dias P, Parham DM, et al. MyoD1 protein expression in alveolar soft part sarcoma as confirmatory evidence of its skeletal muscle nature. Am J Surg Pathol 1991;15(10):974–81.
120. Dias P, Parham DM, Shapiro DN, et al. Myogenic regulatory protein (MyoD1) expression in childhood solid tumors: diagnostic utility in rhabdomyosarcoma. Am J Pathol 1990;137(6):1283–91.
121. Croes R, Debiec-Rychter M, Cokelaere K, et al. Adult sclerosing rhabdomyosarcoma: cytogenetic link with embryonal rhabdomyosarcoma. Virchows Arch 2005;446(1):64–7.
122. Adhikari LA, McCalmont TH, Folpe AL. Merkel cell carcinoma with heterologous rhabdomyoblastic differentiation: the role of immunohistochemistry for Merkel cell polyomavirus large T-antigen in confirmation. J Cutan Pathol 2012;39(1):47–51.
123. Mukai K, Rosai J, Hallaway BE. Localization of myoglobin in normal and neoplastic human skeletal muscle cells using an immunoperoxidase method. Am J Surg Pathol 1979;3(4):373–6.
124. Brooks JJ. Immunohistochemistry of soft tissue tumors. Myoglobin as a tumor marker for rhabdomyosarcoma. Cancer 1982;50(9):1757–63.
125. Tsokos M, Howard R, Costa J. Immunohistochemical study of alveolar and embryonal rhabdomyosarcoma. Lab Invest 1983;48(2):148–55.
126. Jong AS, van Vark M, Albus-Lutter CE, et al. Myosin and myoglobin as tumor markers in the diagnosis of rhabdomyosarcoma. A comparative study. Am J Surg Pathol 1984;8(7):521–8.
127. Seidal T, Kindblom LG, Angervall L. Myoglobin, desmin and vimentin in ultrastructurally proven rhabdomyomas and rhabdomyosarcomas. An immunohistochemical study utilizing a series of monoclonal and polyclonal antibodies. Appl Pathol 1987;5(4):201–19.
128. Eusebi V, Bondi A, Rosai J. Immunohistochemical localization of myoglobin in nonmuscular cells. Am J Surg Pathol 1984;8(1):51–5.
129. Osborn M, Hill C, Altmannsberger M, et al. Monoclonal antibodies to titin in conjunction with antibodies to desmin separate rhabdomyosarcomas from other tumor types. Lab Invest 1986;55(1):101–8.
130. Iwasaki H, Isayama T, Ichiki T, et al. Intermediate filaments of myofibroblasts. Immunochemical and immunocytochemical analyses. Pathol Res Pract 1987;182(2):248–54.
131. Kuhn C, McDonald JA. The roles of the myofibroblast in idiopathic pulmonary fibrosis. Ultrastructural and immunohistochemical features of sites of active extracellular matrix synthesis. Am J Pathol 1991; 138(5):1257–65.
132. Wang NP, Wan BC, Skelly M, et al. Antibodies to novel myoepithelium-associated proteins distinguish benign lesions and carcinoma in situ from invasive carcinoma of the breast. Appl Immunohistochem Mol Morphol 1997;5(3):141–51.
133. Oliva E, Young RH, Amin MB, et al. An immunohistochemical analysis of endometrial stromal and smooth muscle tumors of the uterus: a study of 54 cases emphasizing the importance of using a panel because of overlap in immunoreactivity for individual antibodies. Am J Surg Pathol 2002;26(4):403–12.
134. Nucci MR, O'Connell JT, Huettner PC, et al. h-Caldesmon expression effectively distinguishes endometrial stromal tumors from uterine smooth muscle tumors. Am J Surg Pathol 2001;25(4):455–63.
135. Taylor CR. Immunomicroscopy: a diagnostic tool for the surgical pathologist. Saunders: Philadelphia; 1986.
136. Kahn HJ, Marks A, Thom H, et al. Role of antibody to S100 protein in diagnostic pathology. Am J Clin Pathol 1983;79(3):341–7.
137. Johnson MD, Glick AD, Davis BW. Immunohistochemical evaluation of Leu-7, myelin basic-protein, S100-protein, glial-fibrillary acidic-protein, and LN3 immunoreactivity in nerve sheath tumors and sarcomas. Arch Pathol Lab Med 1988;112(2):155–60.
138. Weiss SW, Langloss JM, Enzinger FM. Value of S-100 protein in the diagnosis of soft tissue tumors with particular reference to benign and malignant Schwann cell tumors. Lab Invest 1983;49(3):299–308.
139. White W, Shiu MH, Rosenblum MK, et al. Cellular schwannoma. A clinicopathologic study of 57 patients and 58 tumors. Cancer 1990; 66(6):1266–75.
140. Casadei GP, Scheithauer BW, Hirose T, et al. Cellular schwannoma. A clinicopathologic, DNA flow cytometric, and proliferation marker study of 70 patients. Cancer 1995;75(5):1109–19.
141. Matsunou H, Shimoda T, Kakimoto S, et al. Histopathologic and immunohistochemical study of malignant tumors of peripheral nerve sheath (malignant schwannoma). Cancer 1985;56(9):2269–79.
142. Meis JM, Enzinger FM, Martz KL, et al. Malignant peripheral nerve sheath tumors (malignant schwannomas) in children. Am J Surg Pathol 1992;16(7):694–707.
143. Fisher C, Schofield JB. S-100 protein positive synovial sarcoma. Histopathology 1991;19(4):375–7.
144. Guillou L, Wadden C, Kraus MD, et al. S-100 protein reactivity in synovial sarcomas—A potentially frequent diagnostic pitfall. Immunohistochemical analysis of 100 cases. Appl Immunohistochem 1996;4(3): 167–75.
145. Kaddu S, Beham A, Cerroni L, et al. Cutaneous leiomyosarcoma. Am J Surg Pathol 1997;21(9):979–87.
146. Kilpatrick SE, Hitchcock MG, Kraus MD, et al. Mixed tumors and myoepitheliomas of soft tissue: a clinicopathologic study of 19 cases with a unifying concept. Am J Surg Pathol 1997;21(1):13–22.
147. Fisher C. Parachordoma exists–but what is it? Adv Anat Pathol 2000;7(3):141–8.
148. Michal M, Miettinen M. Myoepitheliomas of the skin and soft tissues. Report of 12 cases. Virchows Arch 1999;434(5):393–400.
149. Nakajima T, Watanabe S, Sato Y, et al. Immunohistochemical demonstration of S100 protein in human malignant melanoma and pigmented nevi. Gann 1981;72(2):335–6.
150. Nakajima T, Watanabe S, Sato Y, et al. Immunohistochemical demonstration of S100 protein in malignant melanoma and pigmented nevus, and its diagnostic application. Cancer 1982;50(5):912–18.
151. Gown AM, Vogel AM, Hoak D, et al. Monoclonal antibodies specific for melanocytic tumors distinguish subpopulations of melanocytes. Am J Pathol 1986;123(2):195–203.
152. Busam KJ, Chen YT, Old LJ, et al. Expression of melan-A (MART1) in benign melanocytic nevi and primary cutaneous malignant melanoma. Am J Surg Pathol 1998;22(8):976–82.
153. Heiskala M, Peterson PA, Yang Y. The roles of claudin superfamily proteins in paracellular transport. Traffic 2001;2(2):93–8.
154. Folpe AL, Billings SD, McKenney JK, et al. Expression of claudin-1, a recently described tight junction-associated protein, distinguishes soft tissue perineurioma from potential mimics. Am J Surg Pathol 2002; 26(12):1620–6.
155. Schuetz AN, Rubin BP, Goldblum JR, et al. Intercellular junctions in Ewing sarcoma/primitive neuroectodermal tumor: additional evidence of epithelial differentiation. Mod Pathol 2005;18(11):1403–10.
156. Mueckler M. Facilitative glucose transporters. Eur J Biochem/FEBS [Research Support, Non-U.S. Gov't Research Support, U.S. Gov't, P.H.S. Review] 1994;219(3):713–25.
157. Yamaguchi U, Hasegawa T, Hirose T, et al. Sclerosing perineurioma: a clinicopathological study of five cases and diagnostic utility of immunohistochemical staining for GLUT1. Virchows Arch 2003;443(2):159–63.
158. Hirose T, Tani T, Shimada T, et al. Immunohistochemical demonstration of EMA/Glut1-positive perineurial cells and CD34-positive fibroblastic cells in peripheral nerve sheath tumors. Mod Pathol [Comparative Study] 2003;16(4):293–8.
159. Ahrens WA, Ridenour RV 3rd, Caron BL, et al. GLUT-1 expression in mesenchymal tumors: an immunohistochemical study of 247 soft tissue and bone neoplasms. Hum Pathol 2008;39(10):1519–26.
160. Smith ME, Awasthi R, O'Shaughnessy S, et al. Evaluation of perineurial differentiation in epithelioid sarcoma. Histopathology 2005;47(6): 575–81.

161. North PE, Waner M, Mizeracki A, et al. GLUT1: a newly discovered immunohistochemical marker for juvenile hemangiomas. Hum Pathol 2000;31(1):11–22.
162. Leon-Villapalos J, Wolfe K, Kangesu L. GLUT-1: an extra diagnostic tool to differentiate between haemangiomas and vascular malformations. Br J Plast Surg 2005;58(3):348–52.
163. Lyons LL, North PE, Mac-Moune Lai F, et al. Kaposiform hemangioendothelioma: a study of 33 cases emphasizing its pathologic, immunophenotypic, and biologic uniqueness from juvenile hemangioma. Am J Surg Pathol 2004;28(5):559–68.
164. Thompson SJ, Schatteman GC, Gown AM, et al. A monoclonal antibody against nerve growth factor receptor. Immunohistochemical analysis of normal and neoplastic human tissue. Am J Clin Pathol 1989;92(4):415–23.
165. Kanik AB, Yaar M, Bhawan J. P75 nerve growth factor receptor staining helps identify desmoplastic and neurotropic melanoma. J Cutan Pathol 1996;23(3):205–10.
166. Perosio PM, Brooks JJ. Expression of nerve growth factor receptor in paraffin-embedded soft tissue tumors. Am J Pathol 1988;132(1):152–60.
167. Goodfellow PN, Pym B, Pritchard C, et al. MIC2: a human pseudoautosomal gene. Philos Trans R Soc Lond B Biol Sci 1988;322(1208):145–54.
168. Fellinger EJ, Garin-Chesa P, Su SL, et al. Biochemical and genetic characterization of the HBA71 Ewing's sarcoma cell surface antigen. Cancer Res 1991;51(1):336–40.
169. Gelin C, Aubrit F, Phalipon A, et al. The E2 antigen, a 32 kd glycoprotein involved in T-cell adhesion processes, is the MIC2 gene product. EMBO J 1989;8(11):3253–9.
170. Hamilton G, Mallinger R, Hofbauer S, et al. The monoclonal HBA-71 antibody modulates proliferation of thymocytes and Ewing's sarcoma cells by interfering with the action of insulin-like growth factor I. Thymus 1991;18(1):33–41.
171. Fellinger EJ, Garin-Chesa P, Triche TJ, et al. Immunohistochemical analysis of Ewing's sarcoma cell surface antigen p30/32MIC2. Am J Pathol 1991;139(2):317–25.
172. Stevenson A, Chatten J, Bertoni F, et al. CD99 (p30/32MIC2) neuroectodermal/Ewing's sarcoma antigen as an immunohistochemical marker. Review of more than 600 tumors and the literature experience. Appl Immunohistochem Mol Morphol 1994;2(4):231.
173. Stevenson A, Chatten J, Bertoni F, et al. CD99 (p30/32MIC2) Neuroectodermal/Ewing's sarcoma antigen as an immunohistochemical marker. Review of more than 600 tumors and the literature experience. Appl Immunohistochem 1994;2(4):231–40.
174. Ambros IM, Ambros PF, Strehl S, et al. MIC2 is a specific marker for Ewing's sarcoma and peripheral primitive neuroectodermal tumors. Evidence for a common histogenesis of Ewing's sarcoma and peripheral primitive neuroectodermal tumors from MIC2 expression and specific chromosome aberration. Cancer 1991;67(7):1886–93.
175. Ramani P, Rampling D, Link M. Immunocytochemical study of 12E7 in small round-cell tumours of childhood: an assessment of its sensitivity and specificity. Histopathology 1993;23(6):557–61.
176. Riopel M, Dickman PS, Link MP, et al. MIC2 analysis in pediatric lymphomas and leukemias. Hum Pathol 1994;25(4):396–9.
177. Shanfeld RL, Edelman J, Willis JE, et al. Immunohistochemical analysis of neural markers in peripheral primitive neuroectodermal tumors (pPNET) without light microscopic evidence of neural differentiation. Appl Immunohistochem 1997;5(2):78–86.
178. Weidner N, Tjoe J. Immunohistochemical profile of monoclonal antibody O13: antibody that recognizes glycoprotein p30/32MIC2 and is useful in diagnosing Ewing's sarcoma and peripheral neuroepithelioma. Am J Surg Pathol 1994;18(5):486–94.
179. Vartanian RK, Sudilovsky D, Weidner N. Immunostaining of monoclonal antibody O13 [anti-MIC2 gene product (CD99)] in lymphomas. Impact of heat-induced epitope retrieval. Appl Immunohistochem 1996;4(1):43–55.
180. Dorfman DM, Pinkus GS. CD99 (p30/32(MIC2)) immunoreactivity in the diagnosis of thymic neoplasms and mediastinal lymphoproliferative disorders. A study of paraffin sections using monoclonal antibody O13. Appl Immunohistochem 1996;4(1):34–42.
181. Dei AP, Wadden C, Calonje E, et al. Immunohistochemical demonstration of glycoprotein p30/32(MIC2) (CD99) in synovial sarcoma: a potential cause of diagnostic confusion. Appl Immunohistochem 1995;3(3):168–73.
182. Pelmus M, Guillou L, Hostein I, et al. Monophasic fibrous and poorly differentiated synovial sarcoma: immunohistochemical reassessment of 60 t(X;18)(SYT-SSX)-positive cases. Am J Surg Pathol 2002;26(11):1434–40.
183. Granter SR, Renshaw AA, Fletcher CD, et al. CD99 reactivity in mesenchymal chondrosarcoma. Hum Pathol 1996;27(12):1273–6.
184. Devaney K, Abbondanzo SL, Shekitka KM, et al. MIC2 detection in tumors of bone and adjacent soft tissues. Clin Orthop Relat Res 1995;(310):176–87.
185. Devaney K, Vinh TN, Sweet DE. Small cell osteosarcoma of bone: an immunohistochemical study with differential diagnostic considerations. Hum Pathol 1993;24(11):1211–25.
186. Ordi J, de Alava E, Torne A, et al. Intraabdominal desmoplastic small round cell tumor with EWS/ERG fusion transcript. Am J Surg Pathol 1998;22(8):1026–32.
187. Devaney K, Wenig BM, Abbondanzo SL. Olfactory neuroblastoma and other round cell lesions of the sinonasal region. Mod Pathol 1996;9(6):658–63.
188. Folpe AL, Patterson K, Gown AM. Antineuroblastoma antibody NB-84 also identifies a significant subset of other small blue round cell tumors. Appl Immunohistochem 1997;5(4):239–45.
189. Renshaw AA. O13 (CD99) in spindle cell tumors. Reactivity with hemangiopericytoma, solitary fibrous tumor, synovial sarcoma, and meningioma but rarely with sarcomatoid mesothelioma. Appl Immunohistochem 1995;3(4):250–6.
190. Guillou L, Gebhard S, Coindre JM. Orbital and extraorbital giant cell angiofibroma: a giant cell-rich variant of solitary fibrous tumor? Clinicopathologic and immunohistochemical analysis of a series in favor of a unifying concept. Am J Surg Pathol 2000;24(7):971–9.
191. Guillou L, Gebhard S, Coindre JM. Lipomatous hemangiopericytoma: a fat-containing variant of solitary fibrous tumor? Clinicopathologic, immunohistochemical, and ultrastructural analysis of a series in favor of a unifying concept. Hum Pathol 2000;31(9):1108–15.
192. Cunningham BA, Hemperly JJ, Murray BA, et al. Neural cell adhesion molecule: structure, immunoglobulin-like domains, cell surface modulation, and alternative RNA splicing. Science 1987;236(4803):799–806.
193. Edelman GM. Cell adhesion molecules in the regulation of animal form and tissue pattern. Annu Rev Cell Biol 1986;2:81–116.
194. Shipley WR, Hammer RD, Lennington WJ, et al. Paraffin immunohistochemical detection of CD56, a useful marker for neural cell adhesion molecule (NCAM), in normal and neoplastic fixed tissues. Appl Immunohistochem 1997;5(2):87–93.
195. Chan JK, Sin VC, Wong KF, et al. Nonnasal lymphoma expressing the natural killer cell marker CD56: a clinicopathologic study of 49 cases of an uncommon aggressive neoplasm. Blood 1997;89(12):4501–13.
196. Lanier LL, Le AM, Civin CI, et al. The relationship of CD16 (Leu-11) and Leu-19 (NKH-1) antigen expression on human peripheral blood NK cells and cytotoxic T lymphocytes. J Immunol 1986;136(12):4480–6.
197. Mechtersheimer G, Staudter M, Moller P. Expression of the natural killer cell-associated antigens CD56 and CD57 in human neural and striated muscle cells and in their tumors. Cancer Res 1991;51(4):1300–7.
198. Miettinen M, Cupo W. Neural cell adhesion molecule distribution in soft tissue tumors. Hum Pathol 1993;24(1):62–6.
199. Garin-Chesa P, Fellinger EJ, Huvos AG, et al. Immunohistochemical analysis of neural cell adhesion molecules. Differential expression in small round cell tumors of childhood and adolescence. Am J Pathol 1991;139(2):275–86.
200. Graham RP, Dry S, Li X, et al. Ossifying fibromyxoid tumor of soft parts: a clinicopathologic, proteomic, and genomic study. Am J Surg Pathol 2011;35(11):1615–25.
201. Thomas JO, Nijjar J, Turley H, et al. NB84: a new monoclonal antibody for the recognition of neuroblastoma in routinely processed material. J Pathol 1991;163(1):69–75.
202. Miettinen M, Chatten J, Paetau A, et al. Monoclonal antibody NB84 in the differential diagnosis of neuroblastoma and other small round cell tumors. Am J Surg Pathol 1998;22(3):327–32.
203. Bomken SN, Redfern K, Wood KM, et al. Limitations in the ability of NB84 to detect metastatic neuroblastoma cells in bone marrow. J Clin Pathol [Evaluation Studies] 2006;59(9):927–9.
204. Sebire NJ, Gibson S, Rampling D, et al. Immunohistochemical findings in embryonal small round cell tumors with molecular diagnostic confirmation. Appl Immunohistochem Mol Morphol 2005;13(1):1–5.
205. Stockman DL, Miettinen M, Suster S, et al. Malignant gastrointestinal neuroectodermal tumor: clinicopathologic, immunohistochemical, ultrastructural, and molecular analysis of 16 cases with a reappraisal of clear cell sarcoma-like tumors of the gastrointestinal tract. Am J Surg Pathol 2012;36(6):857–68.

206. Smith R, Owen LA, Trem DJ, et al. Expression profiling of EWS/FLI identifies NKX2.2 as a critical target gene in Ewing's sarcoma. Cancer Cell 2006;9(5):405–16.
207. Yoshida A, Sekine S, Tsuta K, et al. NKX2.2 is a useful immunohistochemical marker for Ewing sarcoma. Am J Surg Pathol 2012;36(7): 993–9.
208. Bacchi CE, Bonetti F, Pea M, et al. HMB-45. A review. Appl Immunohistochem 1996;4(2):73–85.
209. Kapur RP, Bigler SA, Skelly M, et al. Anti-melanoma monoclonal antibody HMB45 identifies an oncofetal glycoconjugate associated with immature melanosomes. J Histochem Cytochem 1992;40(2):207–12.
210. Pea M, Martignoni G, Zamboni G, et al. Perivascular epithelioid cell. Am J Surg Pathol [Case Reports Comment Letter Research Support, Non-U.S. Gov't] 1996;20(9):1149–53.
211. Pea M, Martignoni G, Bonetti F, et al. Tumors characterized by the presence of HMB45-positive perivascular epithelioid cell (PEC)—a novel entity in surgical pathology. Electron J Pathol Histol 1997;3(2):28–40.
212. Pea M, Bonetti F, Zamboni G, et al. Melanocyte-marker-HMB-45 is regularly expressed in angiomyolipoma of the kidney. Pathology 1991;23(3):185–8.
213. Longacre TA, Egbert BM, Rouse RV. Desmoplastic and spindle-cell malignant melanoma. An immunohistochemical study. Am J Surg Pathol 1996;20(12):1489–500.
214. Kaufmann O, Koch S, Burghardt J, et al. Tyrosinase, melan-A, and KBA62 as markers for the immunohistochemical identification of metastatic amelanotic melanomas on paraffin sections. Mod Pathol 1998; 11(8):740–6.
215. Busam KJ, Jungbluth AA. Melan-A, a new melanocytic differentiation marker. Adv Anat Pathol 1999;6(1):12–18.
216. Busam KJ, Iversen K, Coplan KA, et al. Immunoreactivity for A103, an antibody to melan-A (Mart-1), in adrenocortical and other steroid tumors. Am J Surg Pathol 1998;22(1):57–63.
217. Jungbluth AA, Busam KJ, Gerald WL, et al. A103: An anti-melan-a monoclonal antibody for the detection of malignant melanoma in paraffin-embedded tissues. Am J Surg Pathol 1998;22(5):595–602.
218. Lim E, Browning J, MacGregor D, et al. Desmoplastic melanoma: comparison of expression of differentiation antigens and cancer testis antigens. Melanoma research [Comparative Study Research Support, Non-U.S. Gov't] 2006;16(4):347–55.
219. Hodgkinson CA, Moore KJ, Nakayama A, et al. Mutations at the mouse microphthalmia locus are associated with defects in a gene encoding a novel basic-helix-loop-helix-zipper protein. Cell 1993;74(2):395–404.
220. Bentley NJ, Eisen T, Goding CR. Melanocyte-specific expression of the human tyrosinase promoter: activation by the microphthalmia gene product and role of the initiator. Mol Cell Biol 1994;14(12): 7996–8006.
221. Hemesath TJ, Steingrimsson E, McGill G, et al. Microphthalmia, a critical factor in melanocyte development, defines a discrete transcription factor family. Genes Dev 1994;8(22):2770–80.
222. Read AP, Newton VE. Waardenburg syndrome. J Med Genet 1997;34(8):656–65.
223. Bertolotto C, Busca R, Abbe P, et al. Different cis-acting elements are involved in the regulation of TRP1 and TRP2 promoter activities by cyclic AMP: pivotal role of M boxes (GTCATGTGCT) and of microphthalmia. Mol Cell Biol 1998;18(2):694–702.
224. Steingrimsson E, Copeland NG, Jenkins NA. Melanocytes and the microphthalmia transcription factor network. Annu Rev Genet 2004;38:365–411.
225. King R, Weilbaecher KN, McGill G, et al. Microphthalmia transcription factor. A sensitive and specific melanocyte marker for Melanoma-Diagnosis. Am J Pathol 1999;155(3):731–8.
226. King R, Googe PB, Weilbaecher KN, et al. Microphthalmia transcription factor expression in cutaneous benign, malignant melanocytic, and nonmelanocytic tumors. Am J Surg Pathol 2001;25(1):51–7.
227. Koch MB, Shih IM, Weiss SW, et al. Microphthalmia transcription factor and melanoma cell adhesion molecule expression distinguish desmoplastic/spindle cell melanoma from morphologic mimics. Am J Surg Pathol 2001;25(1):58–64.
228. Granter SR, Weilbaecher KN, Quigley C, et al. Microphthalmia transcription factor: not a sensitive or specific marker for the diagnosis of desmoplastic melanoma and spindle cell (non-desmoplastic) melanoma. Am J Dermatopathol 2001;23(3):185–9.
229. Granter SR, Weilbaecher KN, Quigley C, et al. Clear cell sarcoma shows immunoreactivity for microphthalmia transcription factor: further evidence for melanocytic differentiation. Mod Pathol 2001;14(1):6–9.
230. Zavala-Pompa A, Folpe AL, Jimenez RE, et al. Immunohistochemical study of microphthalmia transcription factor and tyrosinase in angiomyolipoma of the kidney, renal cell carcinoma, and renal and retroperitoneal sarcomas: comparative evaluation with traditional diagnostic markers. Am J Surg Pathol 2001;25(1):65–70.
231. Page RN, King R, Mihm MC Jr, et al. Microphthalmia transcription factor and NKI/C3 expression in cellular neurothekeoma. Mod Pathol 2004;17(2):230–4.
232. Rochaix P, Lacroix-Triki M, Lamant L, et al. PNL2, a new monoclonal antibody directed against a fixative-resistant melanocyte antigen. Mod Pathol 2003;16(5):481–90.
233. Aung PP, Sarlomo-Rikala M, Lasota J, et al. KBA62 and PNL2: 2 new melanoma markers-immunohistochemical analysis of 1563 tumors including metastatic, desmoplastic, and mucosal melanomas and their mimics. Am J Surg Pathol 2012;36(2):265–72.
234. Sanchez-Ferrer A, Rodriguez-Lopez JN, Garcia-Canovas F, et al. Tyrosinase: a comprehensive review of its mechanism. Biochimica et Biophysica Acta 1995;1247(1):1–11.
235. Hofbauer GF, Kamarashev J, Geertsen R, et al. Tyrosinase immunoreactivity in formalin-fixed, paraffin-embedded primary and metastatic melanoma: frequency and distribution. J Cutan Pathol 1998;25(4): 204–9.
236. Kelsh RN. Sorting out Sox10 functions in neural crest development. Bioessays 2006;28(8):788–98.
237. Nonaka D, Chiriboga L, Rubin BP. Sox10: a pan-schwannian and melanocytic marker. Am J Surg Pathol 2008;32(9):1291–8.
238. Karamchandani JR, Nielsen TO, van de Rijn M, et al. Sox10 and S100 in the diagnosis of soft-tissue neoplasms. Appl Immunohistochem Mol Morphol 2012; 20(5):445–50.
239. Beckstead JH, Wood GS, Fletcher V. Evidence for the origin of Kaposi's sarcoma from lymphatic endothelium. Am J Pathol 1985;119(2): 294–300.
240. Burgdorf WH, Mukai K, Rosai J. Immunohistochemical identification of factor VIII-related antigen in endothelial cells of cutaneous lesions of alleged vascular nature. Am J Clin Pathol 1981;75(2):167–71.
241. Hashimoto H, Muller H, Falk S, et al. Histogenesis of Kaposi's sarcoma associated with AIDS: a histologic, immunohistochemical and enzyme histochemical study. Pathol Res Pract 1987;182(5):658–68.
242. Breiteneder-Geleff S, Matsui K, Soleiman A, et al. Podoplanin, novel 43-kd membrane protein of glomerular epithelial cells, is down-regulated in puromycin nephrosis. Am J Pathol 1997;151(4):1141–52.
243. Folpe AL, Veikkola T, Valtola R, et al. Vascular endothelial growth factor receptor-3 (VEGFR-3): a marker of vascular tumors with presumed lymphatic differentiation, including Kaposi's sarcoma, kaposiform and Dabska-type hemangioendotheliomas, and a subset of angiosarcomas. Mod Pathol 2000;13(2):180–5.
244. Jussila L, Valtola R, Partanen TA, et al. Lymphatic endothelium and Kaposi's sarcoma spindle cells detected by antibodies against the vascular endothelial growth factor receptor-3. Cancer Res 1998;58(8): 1599–604.
245. Miettinen M, Wang ZF. Prox1 transcription factor as a marker for vascular tumors-evaluation of 314 vascular endothelial and 1086 nonvascular tumors. Am J Surg Pathol 2012;36(3):351–9.
246. Fortwengler HP Jr, Jones D, Espinosa E, et al. Evidence for endothelial cell origin of vinyl chloride-induced hepatic angiosarcoma. Gastroenterology 1981;80(6):1415–19.
247. Bohling T, Paetau A, Ekblom P, et al. Distribution of endothelial and basement membrane markers in angiogenic tumors of the nervous system. Acta Neuropathologica 1983;62(1–2):67–72.
248. Ordonez NG, del Junco GW, Ayala AG, et al. Angiosarcoma of the small intestine: an immunoperoxidase study. Am J Gastroenterol 1983; 78(4):218–21.
249. Merino MJ, Carter D, Berman M. Angiosarcoma of the breast. Am J Surg Pathol 1983;7(1):53–60.
250. van de Rijn M, Rouse R. CD34: a review. Appl Immunohistochem 1994;2(2):71–80.
251. Miettinen M, Lindenmayer AE, Chaubal A. Endothelial cell markers CD31, CD34, and BNH9 antibody to H- and Y-antigens–evaluation of their specificity and sensitivity in the diagnosis of vascular tumors and comparison with von Willebrand factor. Mod Pathol 1994;7(1): 82–90.
252. Kutzner H. Expression of the human progenitor cell antigen CD34 (HPCA-1) distinguishes dermatofibrosarcoma protuberans from fibrous histiocytoma in formalin-fixed, paraffin-embedded tissue. J Am Acad Dermatol 1993;28(4):613–17.

253. Westra WH, Gerald WL, Rosai J. Solitary fibrous tumor. Consistent CD34 immunoreactivity and occurrence in the orbit. Am J Surg Pathol 1994;18(10):992–8.
254. Weiss SW, Nickoloff BJ. CD-34 is expressed by a distinctive cell population in peripheral nerve, nerve sheath tumors, and related lesions. Am J Surg Pathol 1993;17(10):1039–45.
255. Kindblom LG, Remotti HE, Aldenborg F, et al. Gastrointestinal pacemaker cell tumor (GIPACT): gastrointestinal stromal tumors show phenotypic characteristics of the interstitial cells of Cajal. Am J Pathol 1998;152(5):1259–69.
256. Sirgi KE, Wick MR, Swanson PE. B72.3 and CD34 immunoreactivity in malignant epithelioid soft tissue tumors. Adjuncts in the recognition of endothelial neoplasms. Am J Surg Pathol 1993;17(2):179–85.
257. De Young BR, Frierson HF Jr, Ly MN, et al. CD31 immunoreactivity in carcinomas and mesotheliomas. Am J Clin Pathol 1998;110(3):374–7.
258. Rizzo M, SivaSai KS, Smith MA, et al. Increased expression of inflammatory cytokines and adhesion molecules by alveolar macrophages of human lung allograft recipients with acute rejection: decline with resolution of rejection [In Process Citation]. J Heart Lung Transplant 2000;19(9):858–65.
259. McKenney JK, Weiss SW, Folpe AL. CD31 expression in intratumoral macrophages: a potential diagnostic pitfall. Am J Surg Pathol 2001; 25(9):1167–73.
260. Meadows SM, Myers CT, Krieg PA. Regulation of endothelial cell development by ETS transcription factors. Semin Cell Dev Biol 2011; 22(9):976–84.
261. Folpe AL, Chand EM, Goldblum JR, et al. Expression of Fli-1, a nuclear transcription factor, distinguishes vascular neoplasms from potential mimics. Am J Surg Pathol 2001;25(8):1061–6.
262. Rossi S, Orvieto E, Furlanetto A, et al. Utility of the immunohistochemical detection of FLI-1 expression in round cell and vascular neoplasm using a monoclonal antibody. Mod Pathol 2004;17(5):547–52.
263. Miettinen M, Wang ZF, Paetau A, et al. ERG transcription factor as an immunohistochemical marker for vascular endothelial tumors and prostatic carcinoma. Am J Surg Pathol 2011;35(3):432–41.
264. Tomlins SA, Rhodes DR, Perner S, et al. Recurrent fusion of TMPRSS2 and ETS transcription factor genes in prostate cancer. Science 2005;310(5748):644–8.
265. Morita K, Sasaki H, Furuse M, et al. Endothelial claudin: claudin-5/TMVCF constitutes tight junction strands in endothelial cells. J Cell Biol 1999;147(1):185–94.
266. Miettinen M, Sarlomo-Rikala M, Wang ZF. Claudin-5 as an immunohistochemical marker for angiosarcoma and hemangioendotheliomas. Am J Surg Pathol 2011;35(12):1848–56.
267. Ferrara N, Davis-Smyth T. The biology of vascular endothelial growth factor. Endocr Rev 1997;18(1):4–25.
268. Jeltsch M, Kaipainen A, Joukov V, et al. Hyperplasia of lymphatic vessels in VEGF-C transgenic mice. Science [Research Support, Non-U.S. Gov't Research Support, U.S. Gov't, P.H.S.] 1997;276(5317):1423–5.
269. Partanen TA, Alitalo K, Miettinen M. Lack of lymphatic vascular specificity of vascular endothelial growth factor receptor 3 in 185 vascular tumors. Cancer 1999;86(11):2406–12.
270. Wetterwald A, Hoffstetter W, Cecchini MG, et al. Characterization and cloning of the E11 antigen, a marker expressed by rat osteoblasts and osteocytes. Bone 1996;18(2):125–32.
271. Hong YK, Harvey N, Noh YH, et al. Prox1 is a master control gene in the program specifying lymphatic endothelial cell fate. Dev Dyn 2002;225(3):351–7.
272. Kahn HJ, Bailey D, Marks A. Monoclonal antibody D2-40, a new marker of lymphatic endothelium, reacts with Kaposi's sarcoma and a subset of angiosarcomas. Mod Pathol [Research Support, Non-U.S. Gov't] 2002;15(4):434–40.
273. Xu Y, Ogose A, Kawashima H, et al. High-level expression of podoplanin in benign and malignant soft tissue tumors: immunohistochemical and quantitative real-time RT-PCR analysis. Oncol Rep 2011;25(3): 599–607.
274. Ordonez NG. D2-40 and podoplanin are highly specific and sensitive immunohistochemical markers of epithelioid malignant mesothelioma. Hum Pathol 2005;36(4):372–80.
275. Chu AY, Litzky LA, Pasha TL, et al. Utility of D2-40, a novel mesothelial marker, in the diagnosis of malignant mesothelioma. Mod Pathol 2005;18(1):105–10.
276. Bixel MG, Adams RH. Master and commander: continued expression of Prox1 prevents the dedifferentiation of lymphatic endothelial cells. Genes Dev 2008;22(23):3232–5.
277. Johnson NC, Dillard ME, Baluk P, et al. Lymphatic endothelial cell identity is reversible and its maintenance requires Prox1 activity. Genes Dev 2008;22(23):3282–91.
278. Hong YK, Foreman K, Shin JW, et al. Lymphatic reprogramming of blood vascular endothelium by Kaposi sarcoma-associated herpesvirus. Nat Genet 2004;36(7):683–5.
279. Le Huu AR, Jokinen CH, Rubin BP, et al. Expression of prox1, lymphatic endothelial nuclear transcription factor, in Kaposiform hemangioendothelioma and tufted angioma. Am J Surg Pathol 2010;34(11):1563–73.
280. Wilting J, Papoutsi M, Christ B, et al. The transcription factor Prox1 is a marker for lymphatic endothelial cells in normal and diseased human tissues. FASEB J 2002;16(10):1271–3.
281. Babal P, Pec J. Kaposi's sarcoma—still an enigma. J Eur Acad Dermatol Venereol 2003;17(4):377–80.
282. Mbulaiteye SM, Parkin DM, Rabkin CS. Epidemiology of AIDS-related malignancies an international perspective. Hematol Oncol Clin North Am 2003;17(3):673–96, v.
283. Dukers NH, Rezza G. Human herpesvirus 8 epidemiology: what we do and do not know. AIDS 2003;17(12):1717–30.
284. Stebbing J, Portsmouth S, Bower M. Insights into the molecular biology and sero-epidemiology of Kaposi's sarcoma. Curr Opin Infect Dis 2003;16(1):25–31.
285. Gandhi M, Greenblatt RM. Human herpesvirus 8, Kaposi's sarcoma, and associated conditions. Clin Lab Med 2002;22(4):883–910.
286. Boshoff C, Schulz TF, Kennedy MM, et al. Kaposi's sarcoma-associated herpesvirus infects endothelial and spindle cells. Nat Med 1995; 1(12):1274–8.
287. Komatsu T, Ballestas ME, Barbera AJ, et al. The KSHV latency-associated nuclear antigen: a multifunctional protein. Front Biosci 2002;7: d726–730.
288. Szekely L, Kiss C, Mattsson K, et al. Human herpesvirus-8-encoded LNA-1 accumulates in heterochromatin-associated nuclear bodies. J Gen Virol 1999;80(Pt 11):2889–900.
289. Katano H, Sato Y, Kurata T, et al. High expression of HHV-8-encoded ORF73 protein in spindle-shaped cells of Kaposi's sarcoma. Am J Pathol 1999;155(1):47–52.
290. Kellam P, Bourboulia D, Dupin N, et al. Characterization of monoclonal antibodies raised against the latent nuclear antigen of human herpesvirus 8. J Virol 1999;73(6):5149–55.
291. Dupin N, Fisher C, Kellam P, et al. Distribution of human herpesvirus-8 latently infected cells in Kaposi's sarcoma, multicentric Castleman's disease, and primary effusion lymphoma. Proc Natl Acad Sci U S A 1999;96(8):4546–51.
292. Courville P, Simon F, Le Pessot F, et al. [Detection of HHV8 latent nuclear antigen by immunohistochemistry. A new tool for differentiating Kaposi's sarcoma from its mimics]. Ann Pathol 2002;22(4):267–76.
293. Cheuk W, Wong KO, Wong CS, et al. Immunostaining for human herpesvirus 8 latetent nuclear antigen-1 helps distinguish Kaposi sarcoma from its mimickers. Am J Clin Pathol 2004;121:335–42.
294. Robin YM, Guillou L, Michels JJ, et al. Human herpesvirus 8 immunostaining: a sensitive and specific method for diagnosing Kaposi sarcoma in paraffin-embedded sections. Am J Clin Pathol 2004; 121(3):330–4.
295. Patel RM, Goldblum JR, Hsi ED. Immunohistochemical detection of human herpes virus-8 latent nuclear antigen-1 is useful in the diagnosis of Kaposi sarcoma. Mod Pathol 2004;17(4):456–60.
296. Hammock L, Reisenauer A, Wang W, et al. Latency-associated nuclear antigen expression and human herpesvirus-8 polymerase chain reaction in the evaluation of Kaposi sarcoma and other vascular tumors in HIV-positive patients. Mod Pathol 2005;18(4):463–8.
297. Leong AS, Vinyuvat S, Suthipintawong C, et al. Patterns of basal lamina immunostaining in soft-tissue and bony tumors. Appl Immunohistochem 1997;5(1):1–7.
298. Hirota S, Isozaki K, Moriyama Y, et al. Gain-of-function mutations of c-kit in human gastrointestinal stromal tumors. Science 1998;279(5350): 577–80.
299. Hornick JL, Fletcher CD. Immunohistochemical staining for KIT (CD117) in soft tissue sarcomas is very limited in distribution. Am J Clin Pathol 2002;117(2):188–93.
300. Fletcher CD, Berman JJ, Corless C, et al. Diagnosis of gastrointestinal stromal tumors: a consensus approach. Hum Pathol 2002;33(5): 459–65.
301. Reith JD, Goldblum JR, Lyles RH, et al. Extragastrointestinal (soft tissue) stromal tumors: an analysis of 48 cases with emphasis on histologic predictors of outcome. Mod Pathol 2000;13(5):577–85.

302. Sarlomo-Rikala M, Kovatich AJ, Barusevicius A, et al. CD117: a sensitive marker for gastrointestinal stromal tumors that is more specific than CD34. Mod Pathol 1998;11(8):728–34.
303. Scotlandi K, Manara MC, Strammiello R, et al. C-kit receptor expression in Ewing's sarcoma: lack of prognostic value but therapeutic targeting opportunities in appropriate conditions. J Clin Oncol 2003;21(10): 1952–60.
304. Smithey BE, Pappo AS, Hill DA. C-kit expression in pediatric solid tumors: a comparative immunohistochemical study. Am J Surg Pathol 2002;26(4):486–92.
305. Makhlouf HR, Remotti HE, Ishak KG. Expression of KIT (CD117) in angiomyolipoma. Am J Surg Pathol 2002;26(4):493–7.
306. Hotfilder M, Lanvers C, Jurgens H, et al. c-KIT-expressing Ewing tumour cells are insensitive to imatinib mesylate (STI571). Cancer Chemother Pharmacol 2002;50(2):167–9.
307. Altman A, Villalba M. Protein kinase C-theta (PKCtheta): it's all about location, location, location. Immunological reviews [Research Support, Non-U.S. Gov't Research Support, U.S. Gov't, P.H.S. Review] 2003; 192:53–63.
308. Altman A, Villalba M. Protein kinase C-theta (PKC theta): a key enzyme in T cell life and death. J Biochem [Research Support, U.S. Gov't, P.H.S. Review] 2002;132(6):841–6.
309. Villalba M, Altman A. Protein kinase C-theta (PKCtheta), a potential drug target for therapeutic intervention with human T cell leukemias. Current cancer drug targets [Research Support, Non-U.S. Gov't Research Support, U.S. Gov't, P.H.S. Review] 2002;2(2):125–37.
310. Allander SV, Nupponen NN, Ringner M, et al. Gastrointestinal stromal tumors with KIT mutations exhibit a remarkably homogeneous gene expression profile. Cancer Res [Research Support, Non-U.S. Gov't] 2001;61(24):8624–8.
311. Nielsen TO, West RB, Linn SC, et al. Molecular characterisation of soft tissue tumours: a gene expression study. Lancet [Research Support, Non-U.S. Gov't Research Support, U.S. Gov't, Non-P.H.S. Research Support, U.S. Gov't, P.H.S.] 2002;359(9314):1301–7.
312. Motegi A, Sakurai S, Nakayama H, et al. PKC theta, a novel immunohistochemical marker for gastrointestinal stromal tumors (GIST), especially useful for identifying KIT-negative tumors. Pathol Int 2005;55(3):106–12.
313. Blay P, Astudillo A, Buesa JM, et al. Protein kinase C theta is highly expressed in gastrointestinal stromal tumors but not in other mesenchymal neoplasias. Clin Cancer Res [Research Support, Non-U.S. Gov't] 2004;10(12 Pt 1):4089–95.
314. Caputo A, Caci E, Ferrera L, et al. TMEM16A, a membrane protein associated with calcium-dependent chloride channel activity. Science 2008;322(5901):590–4.
315. Kunzelmann K, Tian Y, Martins JR, et al. Anoctamins. Pflugers Arch 2011;462(2):195–208.
316. West RB, Corless CL, Chen X, et al. The novel marker, DOG1, is expressed ubiquitously in gastrointestinal stromal tumors irrespective of KIT or PDGFRA mutation status. Am J Pathol 2004;165(1):107–13.
317. Espinosa I, Lee CH, Kim MK, et al. A novel monoclonal antibody against DOG1 is a sensitive and specific marker for gastrointestinal stromal tumors. Am J Surg Pathol 2008;32(2):210–18.
318. Hwang DG, Qian X, Hornick JL. DOG1 antibody is a highly sensitive and specific marker for gastrointestinal stromal tumors in cytology cell blocks. Am J Clin Pathol 2011;135(3):448–53.
319. Kang GH, Srivastava A, Kim YE, et al. DOG1 and PKC-theta are useful in the diagnosis of KIT-negative gastrointestinal stromal tumors. Mod Pathol 2011;24(6):866–75.
320. Lee CH, Liang CW, Espinosa I. The utility of discovered on gastrointestinal stromal tumor 1 (DOG1) antibody in surgical pathology-the GIST of it. Adv Anat Pathol 2010;17(3):222–32.
321. Liegl B, Hornick JL, Corless CL, et al. Monoclonal antibody DOG1.1 shows higher sensitivity than KIT in the diagnosis of gastrointestinal stromal tumors, including unusual subtypes. Am J Surg Pathol 2009;33(3):437–46.
322. Lopes LF, West RB, Bacchi LM, et al. DOG1 for the diagnosis of gastrointestinal stromal tumor (GIST): comparison between 2 different antibodies. Appl Immunohistochem Mol Morphol 2010;18(4):333–7.
323. Miettinen M, Wang ZF, Lasota J. DOG1 antibody in the differential diagnosis of gastrointestinal stromal tumors: a study of 1840 cases. Am J Surg Pathol 2009;33(9):1401–8.
324. Novelli M, Rossi S, Rodriguez-Justo M, et al. DOG1 and CD117 are the antibodies of choice in the diagnosis of gastrointestinal stromal tumours. Histopathology 2010;57(2):259–70.
325. Rios-Moreno MJ, Jaramillo S, Pereira Gallardo S, et al. Gastrointestinal stromal tumors (GISTs): CD117, DOG-1 and PKCtheta expression. Is there any advantage in using several markers? Pathol Res Pract 2012;208(2):74–81.
326. Sui XL, Wang H, Sun XW. Expression of DOG1, CD117 and PDGFRA in gastrointestinal stromal tumors and correlations with clinicopathology. Asian Pac J Cancer Prev 2012;13(4):1389–93.
327. Wong NA, Shelley-Fraser G. Specificity of DOG1 (K9 clone) and protein kinase C theta (clone 27) as immunohistochemical markers of gastrointestinal stromal tumour. Histopathology 2010;57(2):250–8.
328. Chenevert J, Duvvuri U, Chiosea S, et al. DOG1: a novel marker of salivary acinar and intercalated duct differentiation. Mod Pathol 2012;25(7):919–29.
329. Khoury JD. Ewing sarcoma family of tumors: a model for the new era of integrated laboratory diagnostics. Expert Rev Mol Diagn 2008;8(1): 97–105.
330. Shing DC, McMullan DJ, Roberts P, et al. FUS/ERG gene fusions in Ewing's tumors. Cancer Res 2003;63(15):4568–76.
331. de Alava E, Pardo J. Ewing tumor: tumor biology and clinical applications. Int J Surg Pathol 2001;9(1):7–17.
332. Peter M, Couturier J, Pacquement H, et al. A new member of the ETS family fused to EWS in Ewing tumors. Oncogene 1997;14(10): 1159–64.
333. Sorensen PH, Lessnick SL, Lopez-Terrada D, et al. A second Ewing's sarcoma translocation, t(21;22), fuses the EWS gene to another ETS-family transcription factor, ERG. Nat Genet 1994;6(2):146–51.
334. Giovannini M, Biegel JA, Serra M, et al. EWS-erg and EWS-Fli1 fusion transcripts in Ewing's sarcoma and primitive neuroectodermal tumors with variant translocations. J Clin Invest 1994;94(2):489–96.
335. Nilsson G, Wang M, Wejde J, et al. Detection of EWS/FLI-1 by immunostaining. An adjunctive tool in diagnosis of Ewing's sarcoma and primitive neuroectodermal tumor on cytological samples and paraffin-embedded archival material. Sarcoma 1999;3:25–32.
336. Folpe AL, Hill CE, Parham DM, et al. Immunohistochemical detection of FLI-1 protein expression: a study of 132 round cell tumors with emphasis on CD99-positive mimics of Ewing's sarcoma/primitive neuroectodermal tumor. Am J Surg Pathol 2000;24(12):1657–62.
337. Wang WL, Patel NR, Caragea M, et al. Expression of ERG, an Ets family transcription factor, identifies ERG-rearranged Ewing sarcoma. Mod Pathol 2012;25(10):1378–83.
338. Ladanyi M, Gerald W. Fusion of the EWS and WT1 genes in the desmoplastic small round cell tumor. Cancer Res 1994;54(11):2837–40.
339. de Alava E, Ladanyi M, Rosai J, et al. Detection of chimeric transcripts in desmoplastic small round cell tumor and related developmental tumors by reverse transcriptase polymerase chain reaction. A specific diagnostic assay. Am J Pathol 1995;147(6):1584–91.
340. Gerald WL, Ladanyi M, de Alava E, et al. Clinical, pathologic, and molecular spectrum of tumors associated with t(11;22)(p13;q12): desmoplastic small round-cell tumor and its variants. J Clin Oncol 1998;16(9):3028–36.
341. Charles AK, Moore IE, Berry PJ. Immunohistochemical detection of the Wilms' tumour gene WT1 in desmoplastic small round cell tumour. Histopathology 1997;30(4):312–14.
342. Barnoud R, Sabourin JC, Pasquier D, et al. Immunohistochemical expression of WT1 by desmoplastic small round cell tumor: a comparative study with other small round cell tumors. Am J Surg Pathol 2000;24(6):830–6.
343. Hill DA, Pfeifer JD, Marley EF, et al. WT1 staining reliably differentiates desmoplastic small round cell tumor from Ewing sarcoma/primitive neuroectodermal tumor. An immunohistochemical and molecular diagnostic study. Am J Clin Pathol 2000;114(3):345–53.
344. Carpentieri DF, Nichols K, Chou PM, et al. The expression of WT1 in the differentiation of rhabdomyosarcoma from other pediatric small round blue cell tumors. Mod Pathol 2002;15(10):1080–6.
345. Ladanyi M, Lui MY, Antonescu CR, et al. The der(17)t(X;17)(p11;q25) of human alveolar soft part sarcoma fuses the TFE3 transcription factor gene to ASPL, a novel gene at 17q25. Oncogene 2001;20(1):48–57.
346. Argani P, Lal P, Hutchinson B, et al. Aberrant nuclear immunoreactivity for TFE3 in neoplasms with TFE3 gene fusions: a sensitive and specific immunohistochemical assay. Am J Surg Pathol 2003;27(6):750–61.
347. Argani P, Aulmann S, Illei PB, et al. A distinctive subset of PEComas harbors TFE3 gene fusions. Am J Surg Pathol 2010;34(10):1395–406.
348. Biegel JA. Molecular genetics of atypical teratoid/rhabdoid tumor. Neurosurgical focus [Research Support, N.I.H., Extramural Research Support, Non-U.S. Gov't Review] 2006;20(1):E11.

349. Biegel JA, Tan L, Zhang F, et al. Alterations of the hSNF5/INI1 gene in central nervous system atypical teratoid/rhabdoid tumors and renal and extrarenal rhabdoid tumors. Clin Cancer Res: an official journal of the American Association for Cancer Research [Research Support, Non-U.S. Gov't Research Support, U.S. Gov't, P.H.S.] 2002;8(11):3461–7.
350. Biegel JA, Zhou JY, Rorke LB, et al. Germ-line and acquired mutations of INI1 in atypical teratoid and rhabdoid tumors. Cancer Res [Research Support, U.S. Gov't, P.H.S.] 1999;59(1):74–9.
351. Biegel JA, Kalpana G, Knudsen ES, et al. The role of INI1 and the SWI/SNF complex in the development of rhabdoid tumors: meeting summary from the workshop on childhood atypical teratoid/rhabdoid tumors. Cancer Res [Congresses Research Support, Non-U.S. Gov't Research Support, U.S. Gov't, P.H.S.] 2002;62(1):323–8.
352. Hoot AC, Russo P, Judkins AR, et al. Immunohistochemical analysis of hSNF5/INI1 distinguishes renal and extra-renal malignant rhabdoid tumors from other pediatric soft tissue tumors. Am J Surg Pathol [Research Support, Non-U.S. Gov't Research Support, U.S. Gov't, P.H.S.] 2004;28(11):1485–91.
353. Sigauke E, Rakheja D, Maddox DL, et al. Absence of expression of SMARCB1/INI1 in malignant rhabdoid tumors of the central nervous system, kidneys and soft tissue: an immunohistochemical study with implications for diagnosis. Mod Pathol [Research Support, Non-U.S. Gov't] 2006;19(5):717–25.
354. Judkins AR, Burger PC, Hamilton RL, et al. INI1 protein expression distinguishes atypical teratoid/rhabdoid tumor from choroid plexus carcinoma. J Neuropathol Exp Neurol [Comparative Study Research Support, N.I.H., Extramural Research Support, Non-U.S. Gov't Research Support, U.S. Gov't, P.H.S.] 2005;64(5):391–7.
355. Perry A, Fuller CE, Judkins AR, et al. INI1 expression is retained in composite rhabdoid tumors, including rhabdoid meningiomas. Mod Pathol: an official journal of the United States and Canadian Academy of Pathology, Inc [Research Support, N.I.H., Extramural Research Support, U.S. Gov't, P.H.S.] 2005;18(7):951–8.
356. Judkins AR, Mauger J, Ht A, et al. Immunohistochemical analysis of hSNF5/INI1 in pediatric CNS neoplasms. Am J Surg Pathol [Research Support, Non-U.S. Gov't Research Support, U.S. Gov't, P.H.S.] 2004; 28(5):644–50.
357. Kosemehmetoglu K, Kaygusuz G, Bahrami A, et al. Intra-articular epithelioid sarcoma showing mixed classic and proximal-type features: report of 2 cases, with immunohistochemical and molecular cytogenetic INI-1 study. Am J Surg Pathol 2011;35(6):891–7.
358. Hollmann TJ, Hornick JL. INI1-deficient tumors: diagnostic features and molecular genetics. Am J Surg Pathol 2011;35(10):e47–63.
359. Raoux D, Peoc'h M, Pedeutour F, et al. Primary epithelioid sarcoma of bone: report of a unique case, with immunohistochemical and fluorescent in situ hybridization confirmation of INI1 deletion. Am J Surg Pathol 2009;33(6):954–8.
360. Orrock JM, Abbott JJ, Gibson LE, et al. INI1 and GLUT-1 expression in epithelioid sarcoma and its cutaneous neoplastic and nonneoplastic mimics. Am J Dermatopathol 2009;31(2):152–6.
361. Hornick JL, Dal Cin P, Fletcher CD. Loss of INI1 expression is characteristic of both conventional and proximal-type epithelioid sarcoma. Am J Surg Pathol 2009;33(4):542–50.
362. Carter JM, O'Hara C, Dundas G, et al. Epithelioid malignant peripheral nerve sheath tumor arising in a schwannoma, in a patient with "neuroblastoma-like" schwannomatosis and a novel germline SMARCB1 mutation. Am J Surg Pathol 2012;36(1):154–60.
363. Morris SW, Kirstein MN, Valentine MB, et al. Fusion of a kinase gene, ALK, to a nucleolar protein gene, NPM, in non-Hodgkin's lymphoma. Science [Research Support, Non-U.S. Gov't Research Support, U.S. Gov't, P.H.S.] 1994;263(5151):1281–4.
364. Pulford K, Lamant L, Espinos E, et al. The emerging normal and disease-related roles of anaplastic lymphoma kinase. Cell Mol Life Sci [Research Support, Non-U.S. Gov't Research Support, U.S. Gov't, P.H.S. Review] 2004;61(23):2939–53.
365. Griffin CA, Hawkins AL, Dvorak C, et al. Recurrent involvement of 2p23 in inflammatory myofibroblastic tumors. Cancer Res [Case Reports] 1999;59(12):2776–80.
366. Cessna MH, Zhou H, Sanger WG, et al. Expression of ALK1 and p80 in inflammatory myofibroblastic tumor and its mesenchymal mimics: a study of 135 cases. Mod Pathol [Comparative Study] 2002;15(9): 931–8.
367. Cook JR, Dehner LP, Collins MH, et al. Anaplastic lymphoma kinase (ALK) expression in the inflammatory myofibroblastic tumor: a comparative immunohistochemical study. Am J Surg Pathol [Research Support, Non-U.S. Gov't Research Support, U.S. Gov't, P.H.S.] 2001;25(11):1364–71.
368. Li XQ, Hisaoka M, Shi DR, et al. Expression of anaplastic lymphoma kinase in soft tissue tumors: an immunohistochemical and molecular study of 249 cases. Hum Pathol 2004;35(6):711–21.
369. Siminovich M, Galluzzo L, Lopez J, et al. Inflammatory myofibroblastic tumor of the lung in children: anaplastic lymphoma kinase (ALK) expression and clinico-pathological correlation. Pediatr Dev Pathol 2012;15(3):179–86.
370. van Gaal JC, Flucke UE, Roeffen MH, et al. Anaplastic lymphoma kinase aberrations in rhabdomyosarcoma: clinical and prognostic implications. J Clin Oncol 2012;30(3):308–15.
371. Qiu X, Montgomery E, Sun B. Inflammatory myofibroblastic tumor and low-grade myofibroblastic sarcoma: a comparative study of clinicopathologic features and further observations on the immunohistochemical profile of myofibroblasts. Hum Pathol 2008;39(6):846–56.
372. Liu Y, Dehni G, Purcell KJ, et al. Epithelial expression and chromosomal location of human TLE genes: implications for notch signaling and neoplasia. Genomics 1996;31(1):58–64.
373. Chen G, Courey AJ. Groucho/TLE family proteins and transcriptional repression. Gene 2000;249(1–2):1–16.
374. Stifani S, Blaumueller CM, Redhead NJ, et al. Human homologs of a Drosophila Enhancer of split gene product define a novel family of nuclear proteins. Nat Genet 1992;2(2):119–27.
375. Daniels DL, Weis WI. Beta-catenin directly displaces Groucho/TLE repressors from Tcf/Lef in Wnt-mediated transcription activation. Nat Struct Mol Biol 2005;12(4):364–71.
376. Brantjes H, Roose J, van De Wetering M, et al. All Tcf HMG box transcription factors interact with Groucho-related co-repressors. Nucleic Acids Res 2001;29(7):1410–19.
377. Levanon D, Goldstein RE, Bernstein Y, et al. Transcriptional repression by AML1 and LEF-1 is mediated by the TLE/Groucho corepressors. Proc Natl Acad Sci U S A 1998;95(20):11590–5.
378. Pretto D, Barco R, Rivera J, et al. The synovial sarcoma translocation protein SYT-SSX2 recruits beta-catenin to the nucleus and associates with it in an active complex. Oncogene 2006;25(26):3661–9.
379. Bozzi F, Ferrari A, Negri T, et al. Molecular characterization of synovial sarcoma in children and adolescents: evidence of akt activation. Transl Oncol 2008;1(2):95–101.
380. Baird K, Davis S, Antonescu CR, et al. Gene expression profiling of human sarcomas: insights into sarcoma biology. Cancer Res 2005; 65(20):9226–35.
381. Ng TL, Gown AM, Barry TS, et al. Nuclear beta-catenin in mesenchymal tumors. Mod Pathol 2005;18(1):68–74.
382. Terry J, Saito T, Subramanian S, et al. TLE1 as a diagnostic immunohistochemical marker for synovial sarcoma emerging from gene expression profiling studies. Am J Surg Pathol 2007;31(2):240–6.
383. Jagdis A, Rubin BP, Tubbs RR, et al. Prospective evaluation of TLE1 as a diagnostic immunohistochemical marker in synovial sarcoma. Am J Surg Pathol 2009;33(12):1743–51.
384. Kosemehmetoglu K, Vrana JA, Folpe AL. TLE1 expression is not specific for synovial sarcoma: a whole section study of 163 soft tissue and bone neoplasms. Mod Pathol 2009;22(7):872–8.
385. Bahrami A, Folpe AL. Adult-type fibrosarcoma: a reevaluation of 163 putative cases diagnosed at a single institution over a 48-year period. Am J Surg Pathol 2010;34(10):1504–13.
386. Jones KB, Su L, Jin H, et al. SS18-SSX2 and the mitochondrial apoptosis pathway in mouse and human synovial sarcomas. Oncogene 2013;32(18): 2365–71.
387. Bafna S, Kaur S, Batra SK. Membrane-bound mucins: the mechanistic basis for alterations in the growth and survival of cancer cells. Oncogene 2010;29(20):2893–904.
388. Moller E, Hornick JL, Magnusson L, et al. FUS-CREB3L2/L1-positive sarcomas show a specific gene expression profile with upregulation of CD24 and FOXL1. Clin Cancer Res 2011;17(9):2646–56.
389. Doyle LA, Moller E, Dal Cin P, et al. MUC4 is a highly sensitive and specific marker for low-grade fibromyxoid sarcoma. Am J Surg Pathol 2011;35(5):733–41.
390. Holness CL, Simmons DL. Molecular cloning of CD68, a human macrophage marker related to lysosomal glycoproteins. Blood [Research Support, Non-U.S. Gov't] 1993;81(6):1607–13.
391. Cassidy M, Loftus B, Whelan A, et al. KP-1: not a specific marker. Staining of 137 sarcomas, 48 lymphomas, 28 carcinomas, 7 malignant melanomas and 8 cystosarcoma phyllodes. Virchows Arch 1994;424(6): 635–40.

392. Smith ME, Costa MJ, Weiss SW. Evaluation of CD68 and other histiocytic antigens in angiomatoid malignant fibrous histiocytoma. Am J Surg Pathol [Research Support, Non-U.S. Gov't] 1991;15(8):757–63.
393. Dei Tos AP, Doglioni C, Laurino L, et al. KP1 (CD68) expression in benign neural tumours. Further evidence of its low specificity as a histiocytic/myeloid marker. Histopathology 1993;23(2):185–7.
394. Gloghini A, Rizzo A, Zanette I, et al. KP1/CD68 expression in malignant neoplasms including lymphomas, sarcomas, and carcinomas. Am J Clin Pathol 1995;103(4):425–31.
395. Taipale J, Beachy PA. The Hedgehog and Wnt signalling pathways in cancer. Nature 2001;411(6835):349–54.
396. Barth AI, Nathke IS, Nelson WJ. Cadherins, catenins and APC protein: interplay between cytoskeletal complexes and signaling pathways. Curr Opin Cell Biol 1997;9(5):683–90.
397. Rubinfeld B, Albert I, Porfiri E, et al. Binding of GSK3beta to the APC-beta-catenin complex and regulation of complex assembly. Science 1996;272(5264):1023–6.
398. Hart MJ, de los Santos R, Albert IN, et al. Downregulation of beta-catenin by human Axin and its association with the APC tumor suppressor, beta-catenin and GSK3 beta. Curr Biol 1998;8(10):573–81.
399. Alman BA, Li C, Pajerski ME, et al. Increased beta-catenin protein and somatic APC mutations in sporadic aggressive fibromatoses (desmoid tumors). Am J Pathol 1997;151(2):329–34.
400. Miyoshi Y, Iwao K, Nawa G, et al. Frequent mutations in the beta-catenin gene in desmoid tumors from patients without familial adenomatous polyposis. Oncol Res 1998;10(11–12):591–4.
401. Montgomery E, Lee JH, Abraham SC, et al. Superficial fibromatoses are genetically distinct from deep fibromatoses. Mod Pathol 2001;14(7):695–701.
402. Abraham SC, Reynolds C, Lee JH, et al. Fibromatosis of the breast and mutations involving the APC/beta-catenin pathway. Hum Pathol 2002;33(1):39–46.
403. Montgomery E, Torbenson MS, Kaushal M, et al. Beta-catenin immunohistochemistry separates mesenteric fibromatosis from gastrointestinal stromal tumor and sclerosing mesenteritis. Am J Surg Pathol 2002;26(10):1296–301.
404. Bhattacharya B, Dilworth HP, Iacobuzio-Donahue C, et al. Nuclear beta-catenin expression distinguishes deep fibromatosis from other benign and malignant fibroblastic and myofibroblastic lesions. Am J Surg Pathol 2005;29(5):653–9.
405. Iwao K, Miyoshi Y, Nawa G, et al. Frequent beta-catenin abnormalities in bone and soft-tissue tumors. Jpn J Cancer Res 1999;90(2):205–9.
406. Kuhnen C, Herter P, Muller O, et al. Beta-catenin in soft tissue sarcomas: expression is related to proliferative activity in high-grade sarcomas. Mod Pathol 2000;13(9):1005–13.
407. Sato H, Hasegawa T, Kanai Y, et al. Expression of cadherins and their undercoat proteins (alpha-, beta-, and gamma-catenins and p120) and accumulation of beta-catenin with no gene mutations in synovial sarcoma. Virchows Arch 2001;438(1):23–30.
408. Hauben EI, Jundt G, Cleton-Jansen AM, et al. Desmoplastic fibroma of bone: an immunohistochemical study including beta-catenin expression and mutational analysis for beta-catenin. Hum Pathol 2005;36(9):1025–30.
409. Dei Tos AP, Doglioni C, Piccinin S, et al. Molecular abnormalities of the p53 pathway in dedifferentiated liposarcoma. J Pathol [Research Support, Non-U.S. Gov't] 1997;181(1):8–13.
410. Dei Tos AP, Piccinin S, Doglioni C, et al. Molecular aberrations of the G1-S checkpoint in myxoid and round cell liposarcoma. Am J Pathol 1997;151(6):1531–9.
411. Xiao ZX, Chen J, Levine AJ, et al. Interaction between the retinoblastoma protein and the oncoprotein MDM2. Nature 1995;375(6533):694–8.
412. Martin K, Trouche D, Hagemeier C, et al. Stimulation of E2F1/DP1 transcriptional activity by MDM2 oncoprotein. Nature 1995;375(6533):691–4.
413. Leach FS, Tokino T, Meltzer P, et al. p53 Mutation and MDM2 amplification in human soft tissue sarcomas. Cancer Res 1993;53(10 Suppl):2231–4.
414. Oliner JD, Kinzler KW, Meltzer PS, et al. Amplification of a gene encoding a p53-associated protein in human sarcomas. Nature [Comparative Study Research Support, Non-U.S. Gov't Research Support, U.S. Gov't, P.H.S.] 1992;358(6381):80–3.
415. Cordon-Cardo C, Latres E, Drobnjak M, et al. Molecular abnormalities of MDM2 and p53 genes in adult soft tissue sarcomas. Cancer Res 1994;54(3):794–9.
416. Binh MB, Sastre-Garau X, Guillou L, et al. MDM2 and CDK4 immunostainings are useful adjuncts in diagnosing well-differentiated and dedifferentiated liposarcoma subtypes: a comparative analysis of 559 soft tissue neoplasms with genetic data. Am J Surg Pathol [Comparative Study Research Support, Non-U.S. Gov't] 2005;29(10):1340–7.
417. Coindre JM, Hostein I, Maire G, et al. Inflammatory malignant fibrous histiocytomas and dedifferentiated liposarcomas: histological review, genomic profile, and MDM2 and CDK4 status favour a single entity. J Pathol [Research Support, Non-U.S. Gov't] 2004;203(3):822–30.
418. Coindre JM, Mariani O, Chibon F, et al. Most malignant fibrous histiocytomas developed in the retroperitoneum are dedifferentiated liposarcomas: a review of 25 cases initially diagnosed as malignant fibrous histiocytoma. Mod Pathol: an official journal of the United States and Canadian Academy of Pathology, Inc [Research Support, Non-U.S. Gov't] 2003;16(3):256–62.
419. Thway K, Flora R, Shah C, et al. Diagnostic utility of p16, CDK4, and MDM2 as an immunohistochemical panel in distinguishing well-differentiated and dedifferentiated liposarcomas from other adipocytic tumors. Am J Surg Pathol 2012;36(3):462–9.
420. Hockenbery DM. Bcl-2, a novel regulator of cell death. Bioessays [Research Support, Non-U.S. Gov't Review] 1995;17(7):631–8.
421. LeBrun DP, Warnke RA, Cleary ML. Expression of Bcl-2 in fetal tissues suggests a role in morphogenesis. Am J Pathol [Research Support, Non-U.S. Gov't Research Support, U.S. Gov't, P.H.S.] 1993;142(3):743–53.
422. Weiss LM, Warnke RA, Sklar J, et al. Molecular analysis of the t(14;18) chromosomal translocation in malignant lymphomas. N Engl J Med [Research Support, Non-U.S. Gov't Research Support, U.S. Gov't, P.H.S.] 1987;317(19):1185–9.
423. Nakanishi H, Ohsawa M, Naka N, et al. Immunohistochemical detection of Bcl-2 and p53 proteins and apoptosis in soft tissue sarcoma: their correlations with prognosis. Oncology 1997;54(3):238–44.
424. Suster S, Fisher C, Moran CA. Expression of Bcl-2 oncoprotein in benign and malignant spindle cell tumors of soft tissue, skin, serosal surfaces, and gastrointestinal tract. Am J Surg Pathol 1998;22(7):863–72.
425. Hasegawa T, Matsuno Y, Shimoda T, et al. Frequent expression of Bcl-2 protein in solitary fibrous tumors. Jpn J Clin Oncol 1998;28(2):86–91.
426. Chilosi M, Facchettti F, Dei Tos AP, et al. Bcl-2 expression in pleural and extrapleural solitary fibrous tumours. J Pathol 1997;181(4):362–7.
427. Gerdes J, Li L, Schlueter C, et al. Immunobiochemical and molecular biologic characterization of the cell proliferation-associated nuclear antigen that is defined by monoclonal antibody Ki-67. Am J Pathol 1991;138(4):867–73.
428. Isola J, Helin H, Kallioniemi OP. Immunoelectron-microscopic localization of a proliferation-associated antigen Ki-67 in MCF-7 cells. Histochem J 1990;22(9):498–506.
429. Choong PF, Akerman M, Willen H, et al. Prognostic value of Ki-67 expression in 182 soft tissue sarcomas. Proliferation–a marker of metastasis? APMIS 1994;102(12):915–24.
430. Drobnjak M, Latres E, Pollack D, et al. Prognostic implications of p53 nuclear overexpression and high proliferation index of Ki-67 in adult soft-tissue sarcomas. J Natl Cancer Inst 1994;86(7):549–54.
431. Levine EA, Holzmayer T, Bacus S, et al. Evaluation of newer prognostic markers for adult soft tissue sarcomas. J Clin Oncol 1997;15(10):3249–57.
432. Ueda T, Aozasa K, Tsujimoto M, et al. Prognostic significance of Ki-67 reactivity in soft tissue sarcomas. Cancer 1989;63(8):1607–11.
433. Rudolph P, Kellner U, Chassevent A, et al. Prognostic relevance of a novel proliferation marker, Ki-S11, for soft-tissue sarcoma. A multivariate study. Am J Pathol 1997;150(6):1997–2007.
434. Heslin MJ, Cordon-Cardo C, Lewis JJ, et al. Ki-67 detected by MIB-1 predicts distant metastasis and tumor mortality in primary, high grade extremity soft tissue sarcoma. Cancer 1998;83(3):490–7.
435. Finlay CA, Hinds PW, Tan TH, et al. Activating mutations for transformation by p53 produce a gene product that forms an hsc70-p53 complex with an altered half-life. Mol Cell Biol 1988;8(2):531–9.
436. Kastan MB, Onyekwere O, Sidransky D, et al. Participation of p53 protein in the cellular response to DNA damage. Cancer Res 1991;51(23 Pt 1):6304–11.
437. Lane DP. Cancer. p53, guardian of the genome. Nature [Comment News] 1992;358(6381):15–16.
438. Castresana JS, Rubio MP, Gomez L, et al. Detection of TP53 gene mutations in human sarcomas. Eur J Cancer 1995;5:735–8.
439. Golouh R, Bracko M, Novak J. Predictive value of proliferation-related markers, p53, and DNA ploidy for survival in patients with soft tissue spindle-cell sarcomas. Mod Pathol 1996;9(9):919–24.

440. Kawai A, Noguchi M, Beppu Y, et al. Nuclear immunoreaction of p53 protein in soft tissue sarcomas. A possible prognostic factor. Cancer 1994;73(10):2499–505.
441. Latres E, Drobnjak M, Pollack D, et al. Chromosome 17 abnormalities and TP53 mutations in adult soft tissue sarcomas. Am J Pathol 1994;145(2):345–55.
442. Toffoli G, Doglioni C, Cernigoi C, et al. P53 overexpression in human soft tissue sarcomas: relation to biological aggressiveness. Ann Oncol 1994;5(2):167–72.
443. Yang P, Hirose T, Hasegawa T, et al. Prognostic implication of the p53 protein and Ki-67 antigen immunohistochemistry in malignant fibrous histiocytoma. Cancer 1995;76(4):618–25.
444. Sherr CJ. Cancer cell cycles. Science 1996;274(5293):1672–7.
445. Nielsen GP, Stemmer-Rachamimov AO, Ino Y, et al. Malignant transformation of neurofibromas in neurofibromatosis 1 is associated with CDKN2A/p16 inactivation. Am J Pathol 1999;155(6):1879–84.
446. Kourea HP, Cordon-Cardo C, Dudas M, et al. Expression of p27(kip) and other cell cycle regulators in malignant peripheral nerve sheath tumors and neurofibromas: the emerging role of p27(kip) in malignant transformation of neurofibromas. Am J Pathol 1999;155(6):1885–91.
447. Fanburg JC, Rosenberg AE, Weaver DL, et al. Osteocalcin and osteonectin immunoreactivity in the diagnosis of osteosarcoma. Am J Clin Pathol 1997;108(4):464–73.
448. Gebre-Medhin S, Nord KH, Moller E, et al. Recurrent rearrangement of the PHF1 gene in ossifying fibromyxoid tumors. Am J Pathol 2012;181(3):1069–77.

Benign Fibroblastic/ Myofibroblastic Proliferations, Including Superficial Fibromatoses

CHAPTER CONTENTS

Fibrous connective tissue consists principally of fibroblasts and an extracellular matrix containing fibrillary structures (collagen, elastin) and non-fibrillary extracellular matrix, or ground substance. Dense fibrous connective tissue, such as that found in tendons, aponeuroses, and ligaments, is composed predominantly of fibrillar collagen, whereas loose fibrous connective tissue contains a relative abundance of non-fibrillary ground substance.

Fibroblasts are the predominant cells in fibrous connective tissue. These cells are spindle-shaped with pale-staining, smooth-contoured oval nuclei, one- or two-minute nucleoli, and eosinophilic to basophilic cytoplasm, depending on the state of synthetic activity. The cytoplasmic borders are usually indistinct, although fibroblasts deposited in a rich myxoid stroma tend to assume a more stellate shape with multiple slender cytoplasmic extensions. Ultrastructurally, fibroblasts typically contain numerous, often dilated, cisternae of rough endoplasmic reticulum, a large Golgi complex associated with small vesicles filled with granular or flocculent material, scattered mitochondria typically in a perinuclear location, many free ribosomes, occasional fat droplets, and slender microfilaments. Fibroblasts are responsible for the intracellular assembly of various extracellular fibrillary and non-fibrillary products such as procollagen, protoelastin, and glycosaminoglycans, which form the ground substance of connective tissue.

Myofibroblasts share morphologic features with fibroblasts and smooth muscle cells (Table 8-1).[1] These cells are found in variable proportions in diverse processes, including responses to injury and repair phenomena, in quasi-neoplastic proliferative conditions, as part of the stromal response to neoplasia,

TABLE 8-1 Ultrastructural Features of Myofibroblasts Compared with Fibroblasts and Smooth Muscle Cells

FEATURE	FIBROBLASTS	MYOFIBROBLASTS	SMOOTH MUSCLE CELLS
Cell shape	Bipolar/tapered	Bipolar/stellate	Wider
Nucleus	Smooth	Deep marginations	Cigar-shaped
Golgi	+	+	Scanty
Rough endoplasmic reticulum	++	+	Scanty
Pinocytosis	–	+	++
Attachment plaques	–	+	++
Dense bodies	–	+	++
External lamina	–	Interrupted	Continuous
Cell–cell attachments	–	Gap, adherens	Gap, adherens
Cell–stroma attachments (fibronexus)	–	++	Attenuated

Modified from Fisher C. IAP presentation, Nice, France, October 1998.

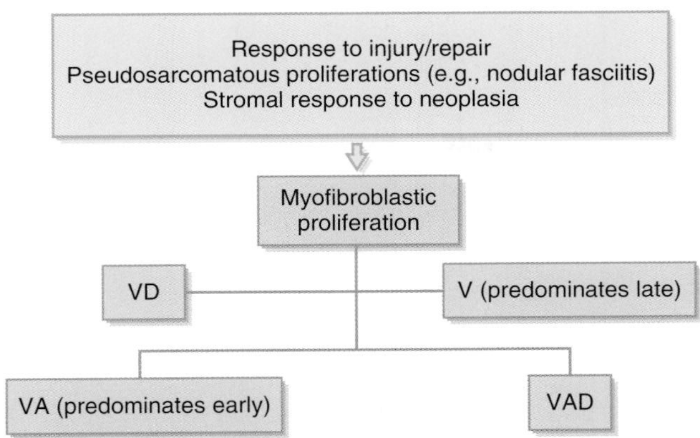

FIGURE 8-1. Immunophenotypes of myofibroblasts. V, vimentin; A, actin; D, desmin.

and in a variety of benign and malignant neoplasms composed, at least in part, of myofibroblasts. Ultrastructurally, myofibroblasts are characterized by indented nuclei with numerous long, cytoplasmic extensions. In the cytoplasm, bundles of microfilaments, which are usually arranged parallel to the long axis of the cell, are present with interspersed dense bodies. Subplasmalemmal plaques and pinocytotic vesicles are also numerous. The cells are partly enveloped by a basal lamina. The fibronexus, transmembrane complexes of intracellular microfilaments in continuity with the extracellular matrix are also characteristic of this cell type.[2] Immunohistochemically, myofibroblasts may have a variable phenotype, including those that express (1) vimentin (V type) only; (2) vimentin, smooth muscle α-actin, and desmin (VAD type); (3) vimentin and smooth muscle α-actin (VA type); and (4) vimentin and desmin (VD type) (Fig. 8-1).[3,4] These immunophenotypes differ depending on the type of myofibroblastic proliferation encountered.

Collagen is the main product of fibroblasts and the major constituent of the extracellular matrix. Up to 11 closely related but genetically distinct types of collagen are found in connective tissue, differing in the amino acid composition of their α chains.[5] Collagen chain polypeptides are synthesized on the ribosomes of the rough endoplasmic reticulum of fibroblasts and a variety of other cell types. These precursor pro-α chains are then transported to the Golgi apparatus, where they coil into a triple helix, forming procollagens. After release from the Golgi apparatus, they are discharged into the pericellular matrix by exocytosis. Following enzymatic cleavage by procollagen peptidases, tropocollagen filaments spontaneously aggregate in a staggered fashion, resulting in the formation of typical banded collagen fibrils with 64-nm periodicity. Long-spacing collagen with 240-nm periodicity is occasionally encountered in both normal and neoplastic tissues.

Type 1 collagen is ubiquitous and consists of parallel arrays of thick, closely packed banded fibrils. This type of collagen is found in the dermis, tendons, ligaments, bone, fascia, corneal tissue, and dentin. It is strongly birefringent and consists of two α_1 chains and one α_2 chain entwined in a helical configuration. *Type 2 collagen*, synthesized by chondroblasts, is found in the extracellular matrix of cartilage and in the notochord, nucleus pulposus, embryonic cornea, and vitreous body of the eye. *Type 3 collagen* is often associated with type 1 collagen, characteristically in loose connective tissue, including the dermis, blood vessel walls, and various glands and parenchymal organs. *Type 4 collagen* is the major component of basal lamina. This collagen type is non-fibrillar and does not undergo any changes following secretion from the cell. *Type 5 collagen* is primarily found in blood vessels and smooth muscle tissue. Other types of collagen (*types 7, 8, 9*) are less common and less well defined. Reticular fibers form a delicate network of fibers that have the same cross-banding as collagen (67 nm) but differ from collagen fibers by their small size (approximately 50 nm in diameter) and their argyrophilia. They are composed of mainly type 3 collagen. Amianthoid fibers are fused, abnormally thick collagen fibers with a typical periodicity but measuring up to 1000 nm in diameter.

Elastic fibers are usually closely associated with collagen fibers and are important components of the extracellular matrix of the dermis, large vessels, and internal organs such as the heart and the lung. Light microscopy reveals them to be slender, branching, highly refractile, weakly birefringent structures that stain with Weigert resorcin-fuchsin, Verhoeff, and aldehyde-fuchsin stains. Ultrastructurally, they have no cross-striations or banding. Elastic fibers are composed of two distinct components: *elastin*, a large amorphous homogeneous or finely granular structure of low electron density, and peripherally located *microfibrils* that are 10 to 12 nm in length.[6] Elastin, the main component of elastic fibers, is synthesized and secreted as tropoelastin by fibroblasts; it typically contains large amounts of glycine, alanine, valine, and desmosine and little hydroxyproline. It is resistant to trypsin digestion but is hydrolyzed by elastase. Altered elastic fibers are found in a variety of heritable and acquired diseases and in the extracellular matrix of both benign and malignant neoplasms.

The extracellular matrix is also composed in part of *glycoproteins*, including fibronectin and laminin. *Fibronectin* is a high-molecular-weight glycoprotein synthesized by fibroblasts and a variety of other cells. It affects cell-to-cell cohesion and the interaction between cells and the extracellular matrix, serving as a molecular glue.[7] *Laminin* is a large glycoprotein distributed throughout the lamina lucida and lamina densa of the basement membrane.[8]

Glycosaminoglycans (*mucopolysaccharides*) form the ground substance of connective tissue. They are intimately associated with fibroblasts and collagen fibers, play an important role in salt and water distribution, and serve as a link in various cellular interactions. These substances are synthesized in fibroblasts or chondroblasts, where they are polymerized and sulfated in the Golgi complex. Chemically, they are linear polysaccharide chains of hexosamines (glycosamino-) and various sugars (-glycans) that are bound to proteins, with the exception of hyaluronic acid. They have a high molecular weight, are negatively charged, and are capable of binding large amounts of fluids. These substances do not stain with hematoxylin and eosin but stain well with Alcian blue, colloidal iron, and toluidine blue.

One of the most important glycosaminoglycans is *hyaluronic acid*, a non-sulfated disaccharide chain composed of glucosamine and glucuronic acid. This substance is abundant in fibrous connective tissue and is the major component of synovial fluid. Histochemically, it is depolymerized and decolorized by hyaluronidase. *Chondroitin sulfates* (types 4 and 6) combine galactosamine and glucuronic acid, and these substances predominate in hyaline and elastic cartilage, nucleus pulposus, and intervertebral disks. Other glycosaminoglycans are *dermatan sulfate* and *heparin sulfate*. Dermatan sulfate is found predominantly in the dermis, tendons, and ligaments, whereas heparin sulfate is found in various structures rich in reticular fibers.[9]

BENIGN FIBROBLASTIC/MYOFIBROBLASTIC PROLIFERATIONS

On the basis of distinct clinical and histologic features, there are four categories of fibroblastic/myofibroblastic lesions: (1) reactive lesions of which nodular fasciitis is the prototype; (2) fibromatoses, locally recurring but nonmetastasizing lesions; (3) sarcomas with fibroblastic and/or myofibroblastic features that range in behavior from low to high grade; and (4) fibroblastic/myofibroblastic proliferations of infancy and childhood. The fourth category is included as a separate category because most fibroblastic/myofibroblastic lesions that occur during the first years of life have characteristic features that differ from those in older children and adults. The chapter will also include the superficial fibromatoses (penile, palmar and plantar fibromatoses, and knuckle pads), whereas the deep fibromatoses will be fully discussed in Chapter 10.

NODULAR FASCIITIS

Nodular fasciitis is a pseudosarcomatous, self-limiting reactive process composed of fibroblasts and myofibroblasts. Despite heightened awareness of this entity over the past 20 years and the topic of innumerable soft tissue seminars, nodular fasciitis is undoubtedly still the most common reactive or benign mesenchymal lesion that is misdiagnosed as a sarcoma given its characteristic rapid growth, rich cellularity, and mitotic activity. It is one of the most common soft tissue lesions and exceeds in frequency any other tumor or tumor-like lesion of fibrous tissue.

Although nodular fasciitis is clearly a benign process, the precise cause of this proliferation is unknown. Histologically, it bears a close resemblance to organizing granulation tissue, supporting a reactive proliferation that may be a result of trauma, inconspicuous or otherwise. Morphologic variants of nodular fasciitis have been described, including intravascular, cranial, and ossifying fasciitis (described in later sections), all of which have overlapping histologic features unified by a proliferation of cytologically bland fibroblasts and myofibroblasts. It is differences in clinical, gross, and light microscopic features that warrant retention of these specific designations, although recognition as a reactive process is far more important than the ability to apply a precise name.

Clinical Findings

Some patients provide a history of a rapidly growing mass or nodule that has been present for only 1 to 2 weeks. In about half of the cases, there is associated soreness, tenderness, or slight pain. Numbness, paresthesia, or shooting pain is rare and develops only when the rapidly growing nodule exerts pressure on a peripheral nerve. Virtually all lesions are solitary; nodular fasciitis at multiple sites is not encountered.

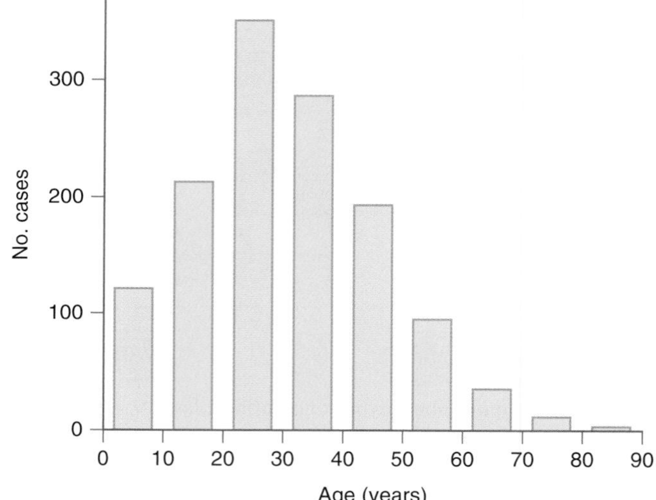

FIGURE 8-2. Age distribution for 1317 cases of nodular fasciitis.

TABLE 8-2 Anatomic Distribution of Nodular Fasciitis (1319 Cases)

ANATOMIC LOCATION	NO. OF PATIENTS	PERCENTAGE (%)
Lower extremities	610	46
Head, neck	269	20
Trunk	235	18
Lower extremities	205	16
TOTAL	1319	100

Although nodular fasciitis may occur in patients of any age, it is most common in adults 20 to 40 years of age (Fig. 8-2). In the series by Allen,[10] only 14% of patients were less than 10 or more than 60 years of age. Males and females are about equally affected. Most of the lesions grow rapidly and have a preoperative duration of 1 month or less. Although nodular fasciitis may occur virtually anywhere on the body, there is a distinct predilection for certain sites, the most common being the upper extremities, especially the volar aspect of the forearm, followed by the trunk, particularly the chest wall and back. Nodular fasciitis in the head and neck is next in frequency and is the most common site in infants and children.[11,12] It is less common in the lower extremities and infrequent in the hands and feet (Table 8-2).[13] This lesion has also been reported in a variety of unusual locations, including the parotid gland (Fig. 8-3),[14] external ear,[15] oral cavity,[16] breast,[17] and lymph node capsule (Fig. 8-4).

Gross Findings

The gross appearance of nodular fasciitis is highly dependent on the relative amounts of myxoid and fibrous stroma and the

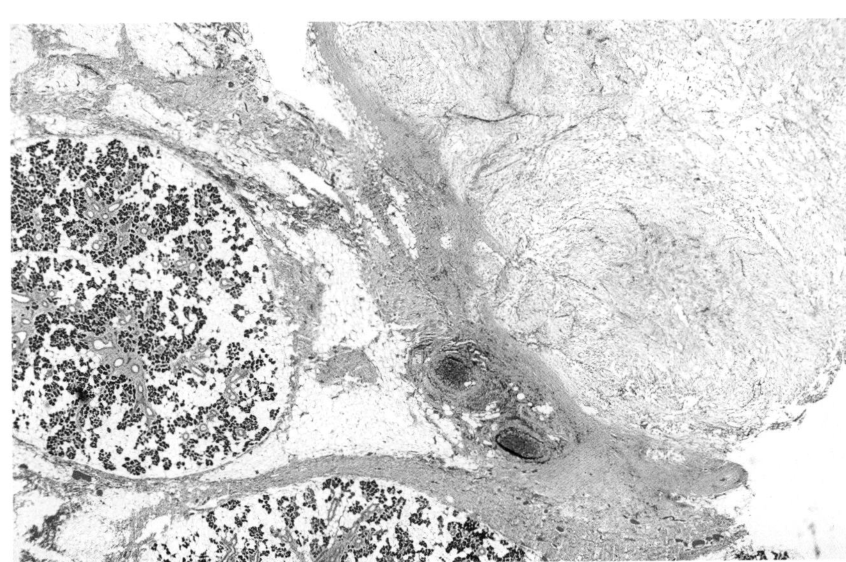

FIGURE 8-3. Nodular fasciitis involving the parotid gland. Note the circumscription and profuse myxoid change in the central portion of the lesion.

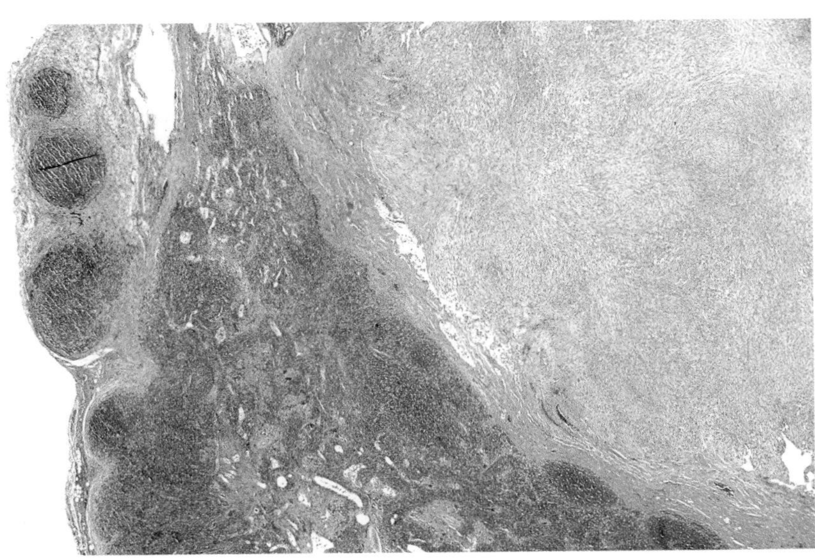

FIGURE 8-4. Rare example of nodular fasciitis involving the lymph node capsule.

cellularity of the lesion. Most are relatively well circumscribed albeit nonencapsulated lesions, although some, particularly those centered around the deep fascia, are poorly circumscribed and appear to infiltrate the surrounding soft tissues. Most are 2 cm or less in greatest dimension when they are excised,[18,19] but occasional cases get as large as 7 cm, although such cases should evoke concern about the diagnosis. Intramuscular lesions tend to be slightly larger than those found in the subcutaneous tissue.

The appearance of the cut surface depends on the relative amounts of myxoid and collagenous material. Those with a predominantly myxoid matrix are soft and gelatinous and grossly resemble other myxoid soft tissue lesions such as myxoma, ganglion, or benign peripheral nerve sheath tumors. Those with a pronounced collagenous stroma are firm and resemble other fibrous lesions such as fibromatosis or fibrosarcoma. Although extravasated erythrocytes are a frequent microscopic feature, these lesions are rarely grossly hemorrhagic.

Microscopic Findings

Nodular fasciitis can be grouped into three subtypes, based on their relation with the fascia. The *subcutaneous type*, the most common form of nodular fasciitis, is a well-circumscribed spherical nodule attached to the fascia but growing upward into the subcutis (Figs. 8-5 and 8-6). The *intramuscular type* is superficially attached to the fascia; it grows as an ovoid intramuscular mass and is often larger than the subcutaneous type. The *fascial type*, which is centered along the fascia, is less well circumscribed than the other forms, growing along the interlobular septa of the subcutaneous fat, resulting in a ray-like or stellate growth pattern. Rare examples of dermal nodular fasciitis have been reported.[20]

All cases of nodular fasciitis, regardless of whether they are predominantly fibrous or myxoid, are composed of plump, immature-appearing fibroblasts and myofibroblasts that bear a close resemblance to the fibroblasts found in

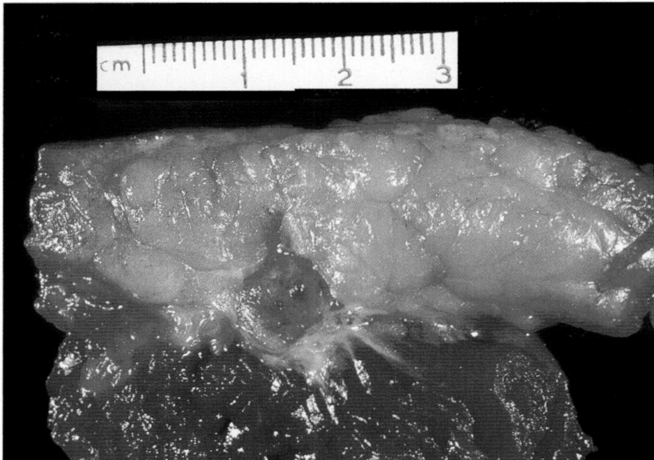

FIGURE 8-5. Gross appearance of the subcutaneous form of nodular fasciitis. The lesion is small and well circumscribed; it is superficially attached to the fascia.

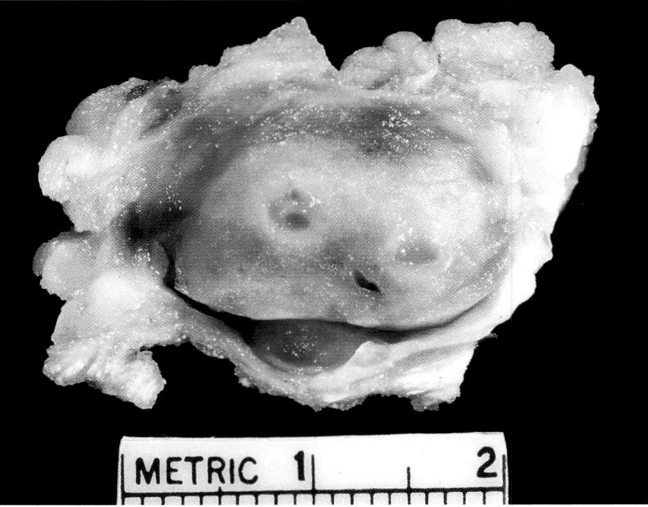

FIGURE 8-6. Nodular fasciitis with central cyst-like spaces, with accumulation of myxoid ground substance.

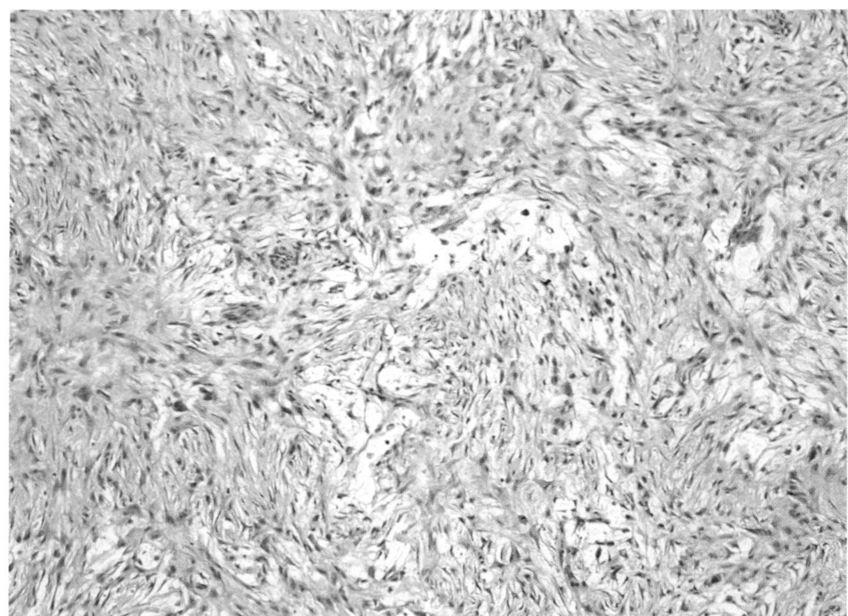

FIGURE 8-7. Area of myxoid degeneration in nodular fasciitis.

tissue culture or granulation tissue (Fig. 8-7). In general, the cells vary little in size and shape and have oval, pale-staining nuclei with prominent nucleoli (Fig. 8-8). Mitotic figures are fairly common, but atypical mitoses are virtually never seen.

Characteristically, the cells are arranged in short, irregular bundles and fascicles and are accompanied by a dense reticulin meshwork and only small amounts of mature birefringent collagen. The intervening matrix is rich in mucopolysaccharides that stain readily with Alcian blue preparation and are depolymerized by hyaluronidase. The abundance of ground substance, in most cases, is responsible for the characteristic loosely textured, feathery pattern of nodular fasciitis; there are also cellular forms with only small amounts of interstitial myxoid material. Intermixed with the spindled cells are scattered lymphoid cells and erythrocytes and, in the more central portion of the lesion, a small number of lipid macrophages and multinucleated giant cells. Occasionally, there are associated areas of microhemorrhage, but siderophages are rare (Fig. 8-9).

There are minor variations in the histologic picture; sometimes the intramuscular form of nodular fasciitis contains residual atrophic muscle fibers and muscle giant cells; this feature, however, is much less pronounced in nodular fasciitis than in fibromatosis. The fascial type of nodular fasciitis may have cells arranged in a radial fashion around a central, poorly cellular, edematous area containing a mixture of mucoid material and fibrin.

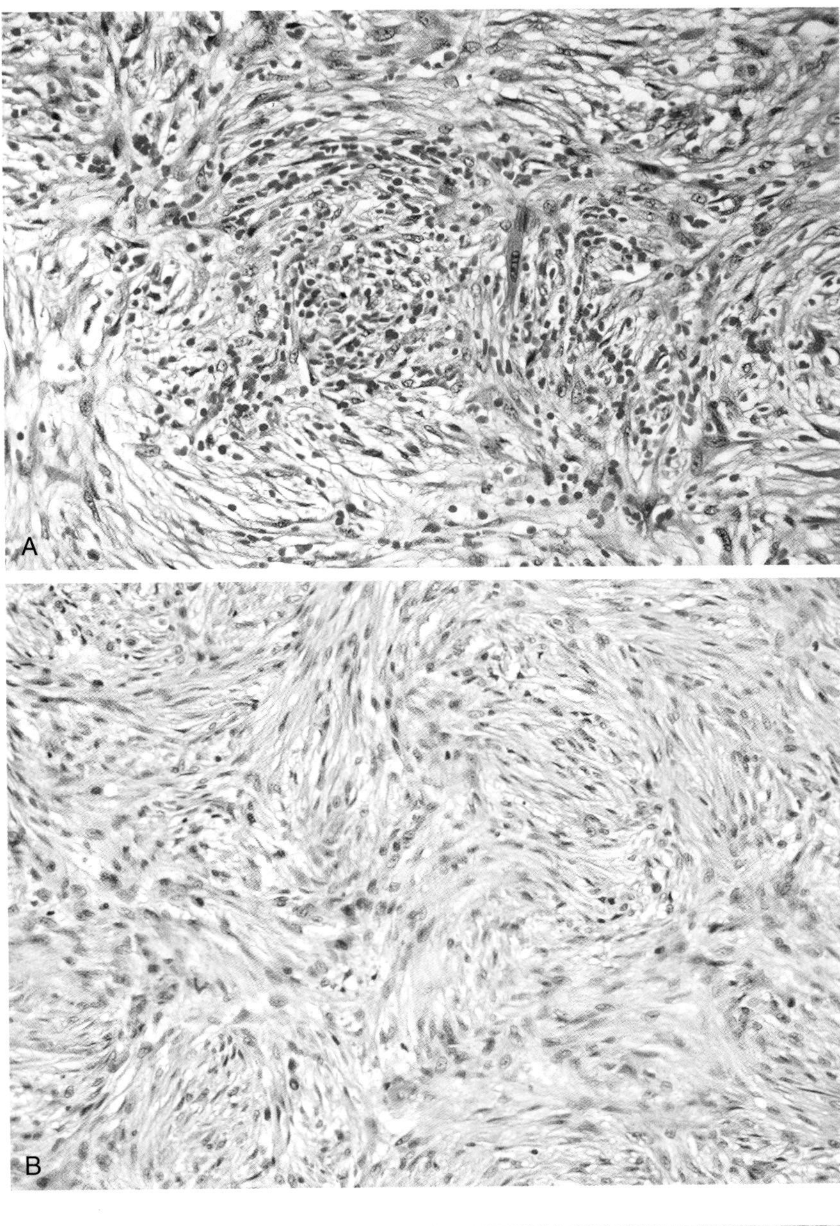

FIGURE 8-8. Nodular fasciitis. (A) Microhemorrhages between bundles of fibroblasts. (B) Storiform growth pattern in nodular fasciitis.

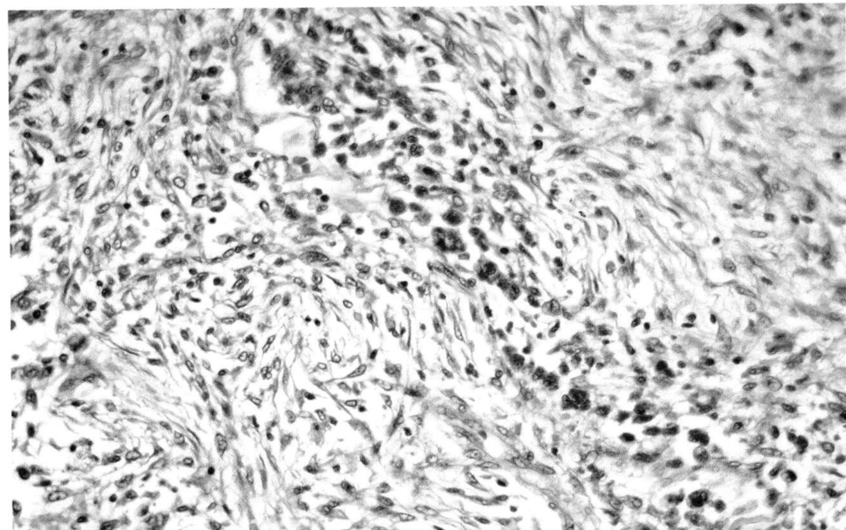

FIGURE 8-9. Nodular fasciitis with focal hemosiderin deposition, a feature rarely seen in this lesion.

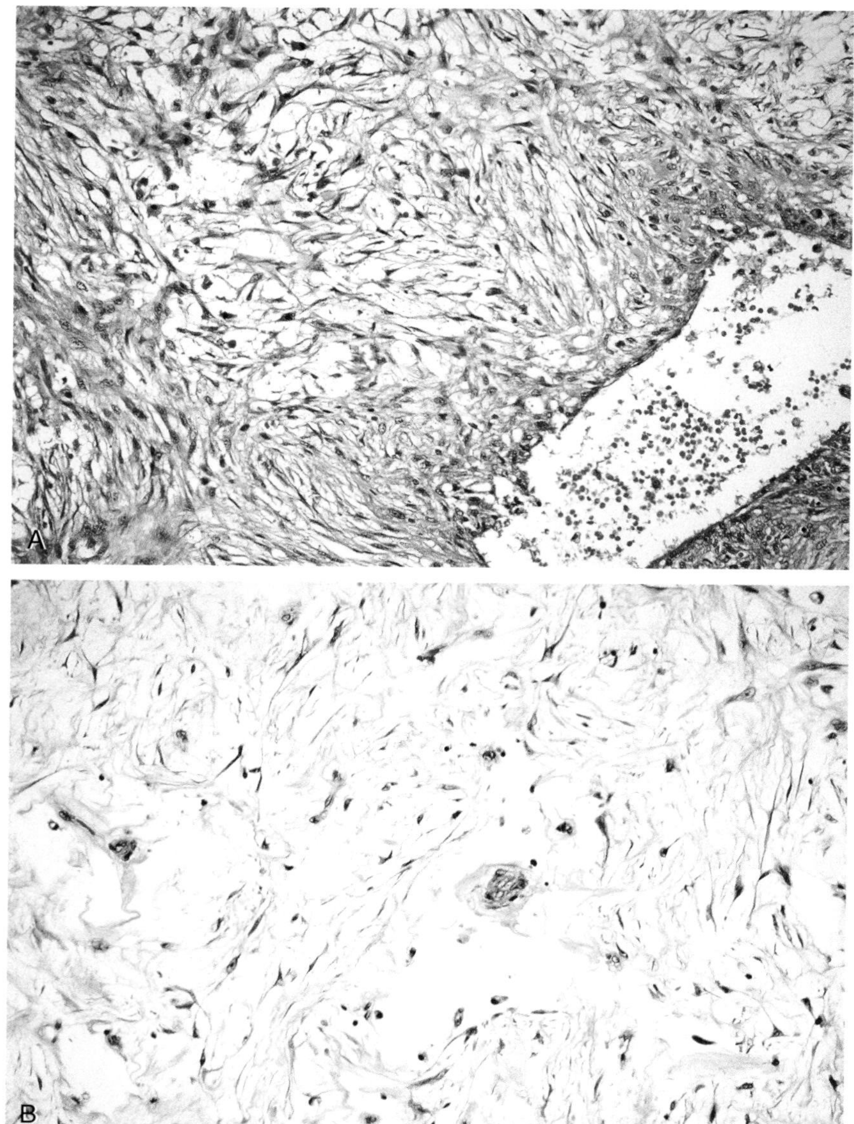

FIGURE 8-10. Nodular fasciitis. (A) Small area of myxoid breakdown imparting a loosely textured arrangement of fibroblasts. (B) More pronounced myxoid matrix with cells widely spaced by mucoid pools.

There is a close correlation between the microscopic picture and the preoperative duration of the lesion. Lesions of short duration tend to have a predominantly myxoid appearance (Fig. 8-10A, B), whereas those of longer duration are characterized by hyaline fibrosis (Fig. 8-10C, D), tissue shrinkage, and formation of minute fluid-filled spaces, or microcysts, a sequence closely paralleling the cicatrization of granulation tissue. In cases of long duration, the microcysts sometimes fuse and form a large centrally located cystic space (*cystic nodular fasciitis*).[21]

Ossifying Fasciitis

On rare occasions, a nodular fasciitis-like lesion has metaplastic bone, a condition described as *ossifying fasciitis*[22] or *fasciitis ossificans*[23] and, when arising from the periosteum, as *parosteal fasciitis* (Fig. 8-11).[24] Most of these lesions have features of both nodular fasciitis and myositis ossificans, but they are less well circumscribed than nodular fasciitis and lack the zonal maturation of myositis ossificans. Occasionally, small foci of metaplastic bone are also found in morphologically typical nodular fasciitis. *Panniculitis ossificans* and *fibro-osseous pseudotumor of the digits* are closely related lesions that have a more irregular pattern and are somewhat akin to myositis ossificans. Rare cases of proliferative fasciitis, proliferative myositis, and cranial fasciitis may also contain foci of metaplastic bone.

Intravascular Fasciitis

Intravascular fasciitis is a rare variant of nodular fasciitis characterized by the involvement of small or medium-size veins or arteries.[25] It has been estimated to account for less than 3% of histologically proven cases of nodular fasciitis.[26] Males and females are equally affected, and most patients are young; very few patients are 30 years or older. The typical presentation is

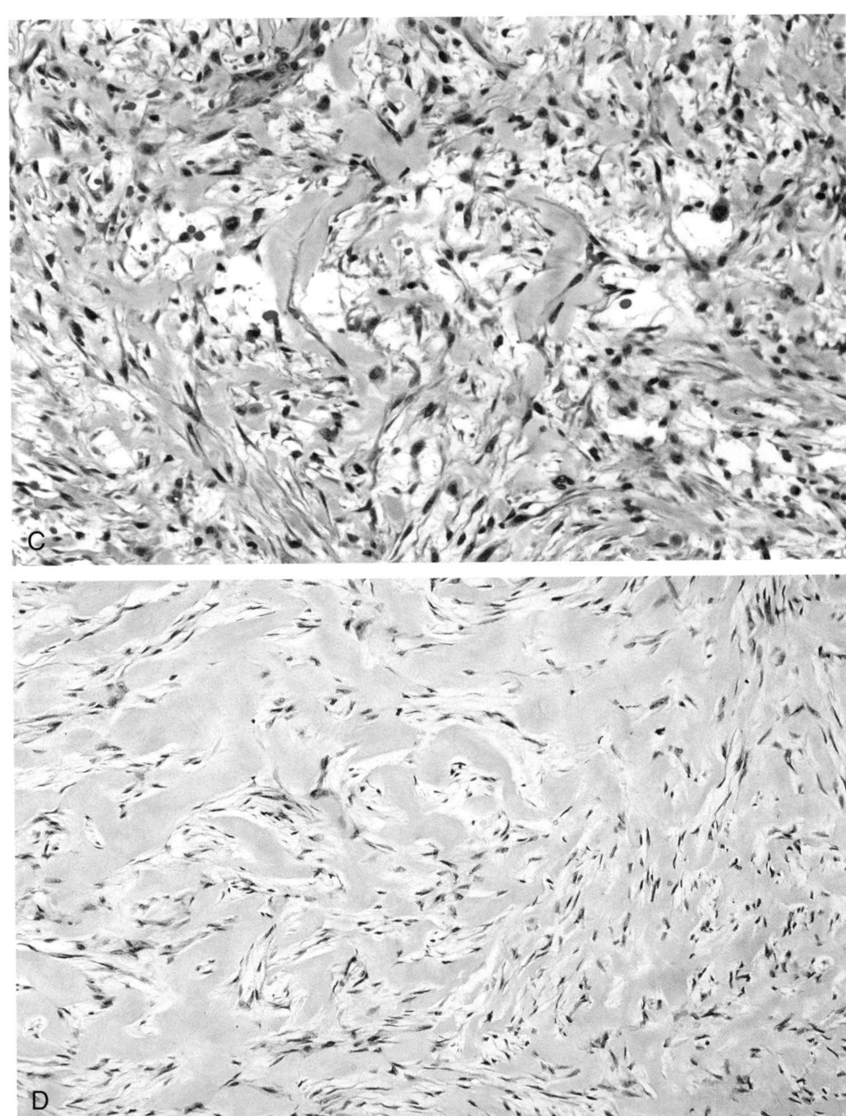

FIGURE 8-10, cont'd. (C) Nodular fasciitis showing hyaline fibrosis between fibroblasts. (D) Nodular fasciitis showing marked hyaline fibrosis, a feature usually encountered in lesions of long duration.

that of a slowly growing, painless, solitary subcutaneous mass usually 2 cm or smaller. The upper extremity is the most common site, followed closely by the head and neck. Less common sites include the trunk, lower extremities, and oral cavity.[27,28] Grossly, the lesions may be round or oval, or they may be elongated, multinodular, or plexiform, particularly those that grow as a predominantly intravascular mass (Fig. 8-12). Small to medium-size veins are most commonly affected, but some lesions involve arteries alone or are seen in conjunction with venous structures. In most cases, there is an involvement of the intima, media, adventitia, and perivascular soft tissue, frequently with a predominantly extravascular component, although some grow as an intraluminal polypoid mass (Fig. 8-13). The association with a vessel may be obscured by the proliferation so that special stains are required to highlight the involved vessel.

Histologically, the intravascular growth closely resembles nodular fasciitis, but it has a less prominent mucoid matrix and a conspicuous number of multinucleated giant cells resulting in a close resemblance to a benign fibrous histiocytoma or a giant-cell tumor of soft parts (Figs. 8-14 and 8-15). Rare examples are predominantly myxoid.[29] Clefts are often present in areas where the proliferation has separated from the vessel wall. Because of the vessel involvement, this lesion may be confused with an organizing thrombus, intravascular capillary hemangioma, intravascular leiomyoma, or a sarcoma; 6 of 15 of the original lesions reported were initially confused with a sarcoma.[25] Despite the intravascular growth, there is no evidence of aggressive clinical behavior, recurrence, or metastasis.

Cranial Fasciitis

Cranial fasciitis is a rapidly growing myofibroblastic proliferation that occurs chiefly, but not exclusively, in infants during the first year of life and involves the soft tissues of the scalp and the underlying skull.[30,31] It usually erodes the outer table

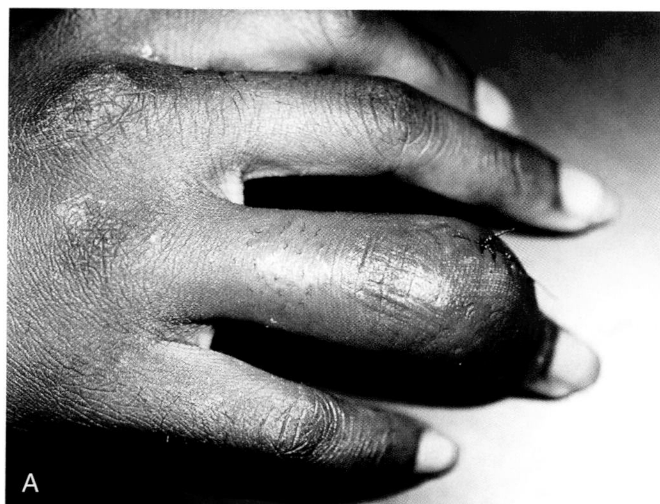

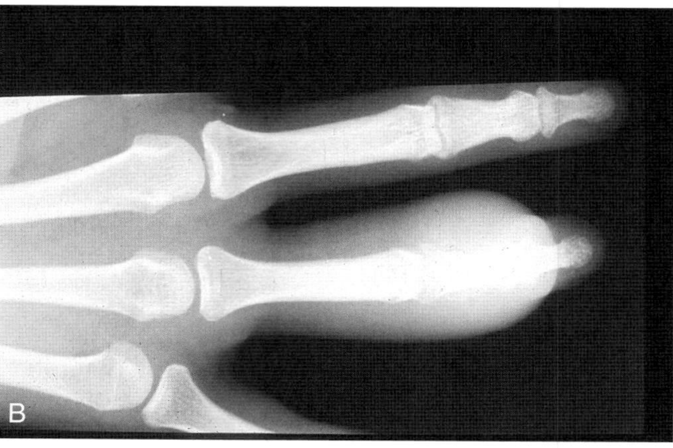

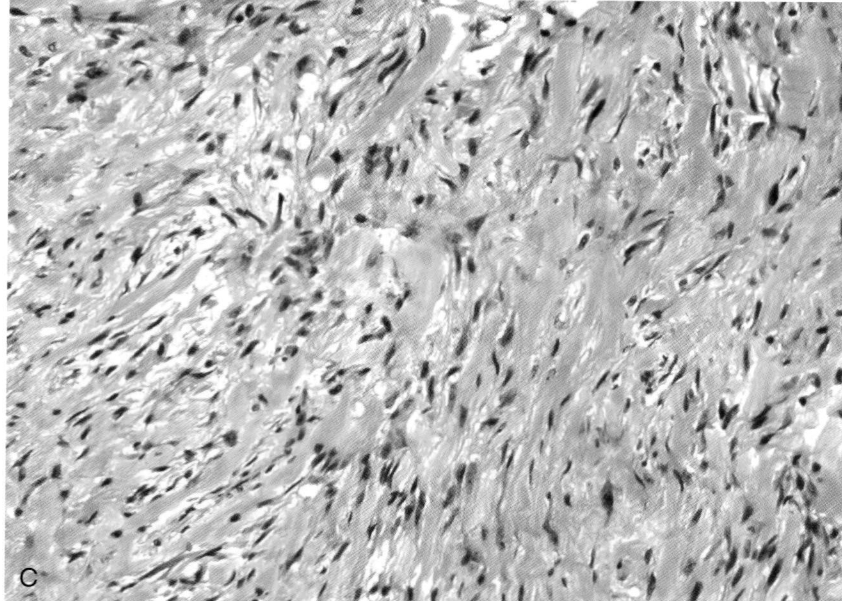

FIGURE 8-11. Parosteal fasciitis. (A) Gross appearance of parosteal fasciitis. (B) Accompanying radiograph of parosteal fasciitis. (C) Histologic appearance of parosteal fasciitis, which is identical to that seen in nodular fasciitis.

of the cranium and frequently also penetrates the inner table, infiltrating the dura and sometimes even the leptomeninges.[32] Radiographically, those that involve the underlying cranium create a lytic defect, often with a sclerotic rim (Fig. 8-16).[33] Histologically, cranial fasciitis exhibits the broad morphologic spectrum of nodular fasciitis; it is composed of a proliferation of fibroblasts and myofibroblasts deposited in a variably myxoid and hyalinized matrix, occasionally with foci of osseous metaplasia. The circumscription and the prominent myxoid matrix help distinguish the lesion from infantile fibromatosis or myofibromatosis.

Birth trauma may play a role in the development of cranial fasciitis; some affected children have been delivered by forceps.[31,34] Interestingly, Rakheja[35] reported a case of cranial fasciitis arising in a child with familial adenomatous polyposis (FAP); this lesion showed strong and diffuse nuclear immunoreactivity for β-catenin, suggesting a dysregulation of the Wnt/β-catenin pathway in a subset of cranial fasciitis. Rare cases also arise at the site of a prior craniotomy.[36] Cranial fasciitis is a benign, probably reactive process that seems to arise from the galea aponeurotica or the epicranial aponeurosis; it infiltrates the incompletely formed cranial bone.

There is no relation between cranial fasciitis and the *head banger's tumor*, a fibrosing lesion of the forehead with pigmentation of the overlying skin. Also, there is no association with an inherited fibrosing lesion of the scalp (*cutis verticis gyrata*) that occurs in adults and is associated with clubbing of the digits, enlargement of the distal extremities, and periosteal bone formation (pachydermoperiostosis).

Immunohistochemical Findings

As one would expect in a lesion composed of myofibroblasts, most cells of nodular, ossifying, intravascular and cranial fasciitis stain for smooth muscle actin and muscle-specific actin

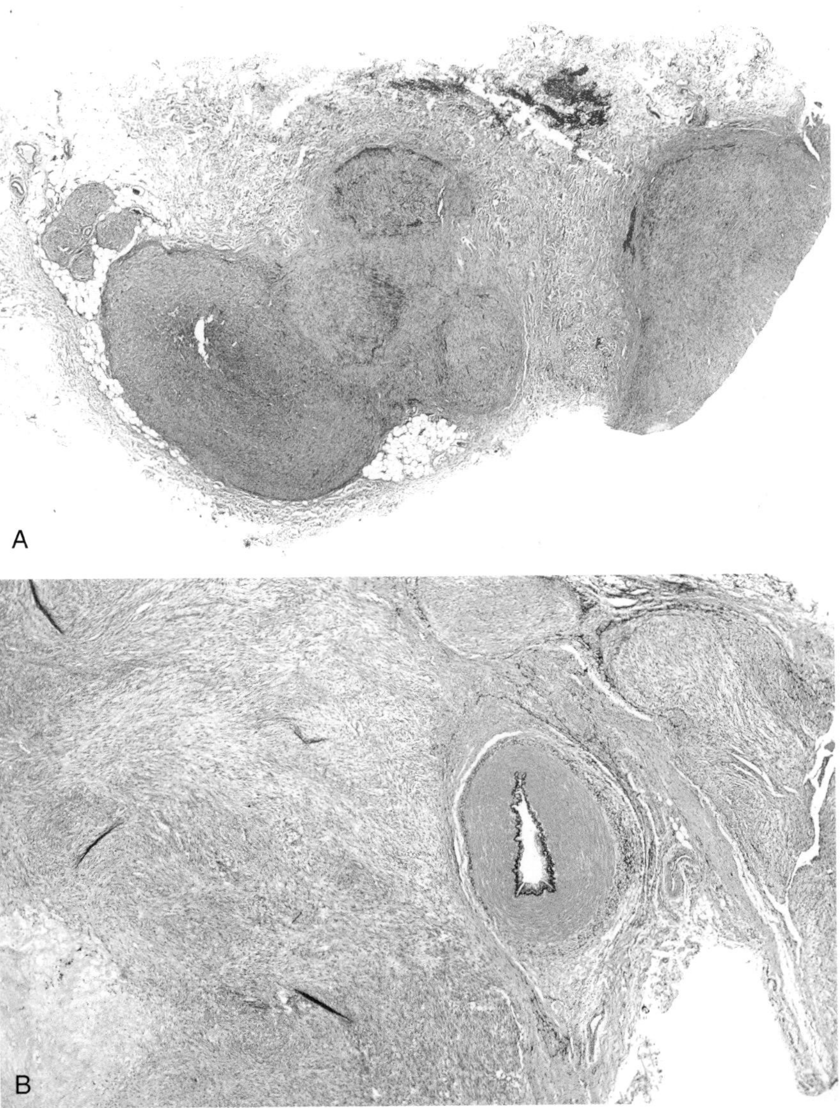

FIGURE 8-12. Intravascular fasciitis. (A) Low-power view showing multinodular growth in several markedly dilated veins. (B) Movat stain of intravascular fasciitis outlining intravascular growth of the spindle-cell proliferation.

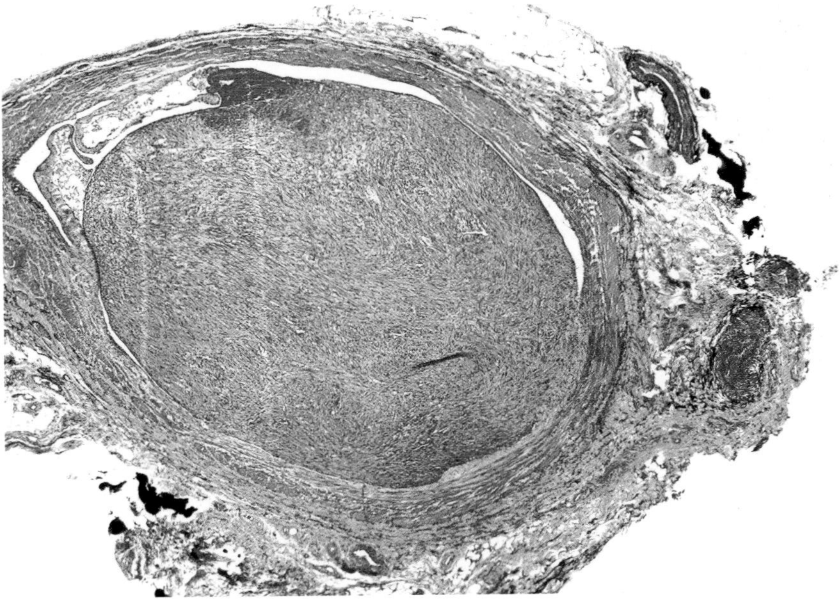

FIGURE 8-13. Movat stain of intravascular fasciitis highlighting the intravascular growth in a markedly dilated vein.

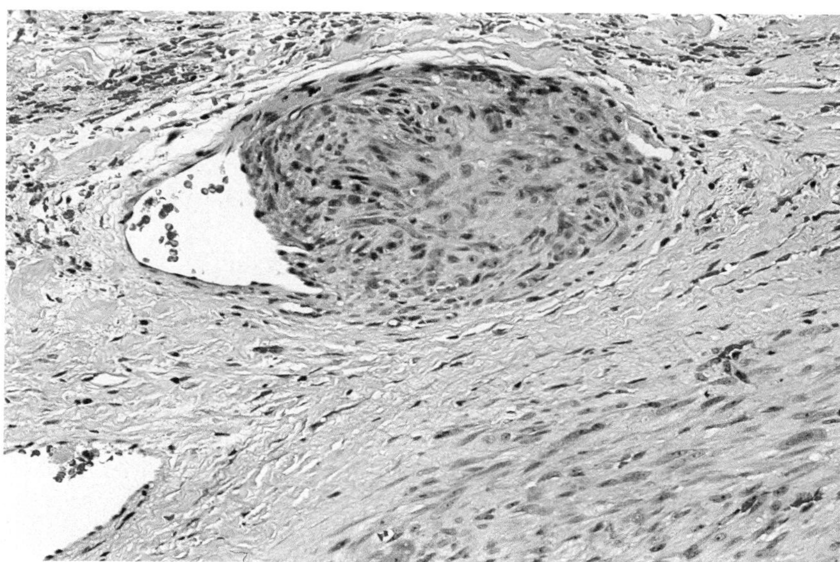

FIGURE 8-14. Small satellite nodule of intravascular fasciitis.

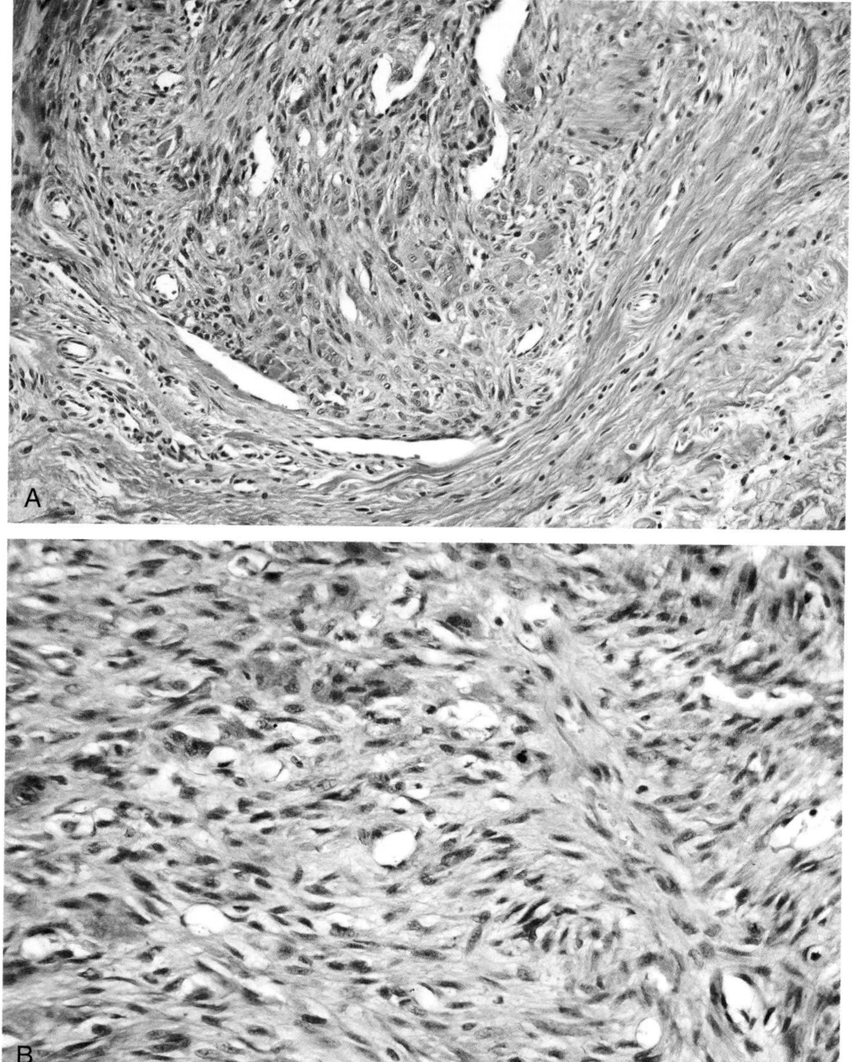

FIGURE 8-15. Intravascular fasciitis. (A) Intravascular proliferation of spindle-shaped cells with a conspicuous number of multinucleated giant cells. (B) Intravascular fasciitis composed of cytologically bland spindle cells similar to those found in nodular fasciitis.

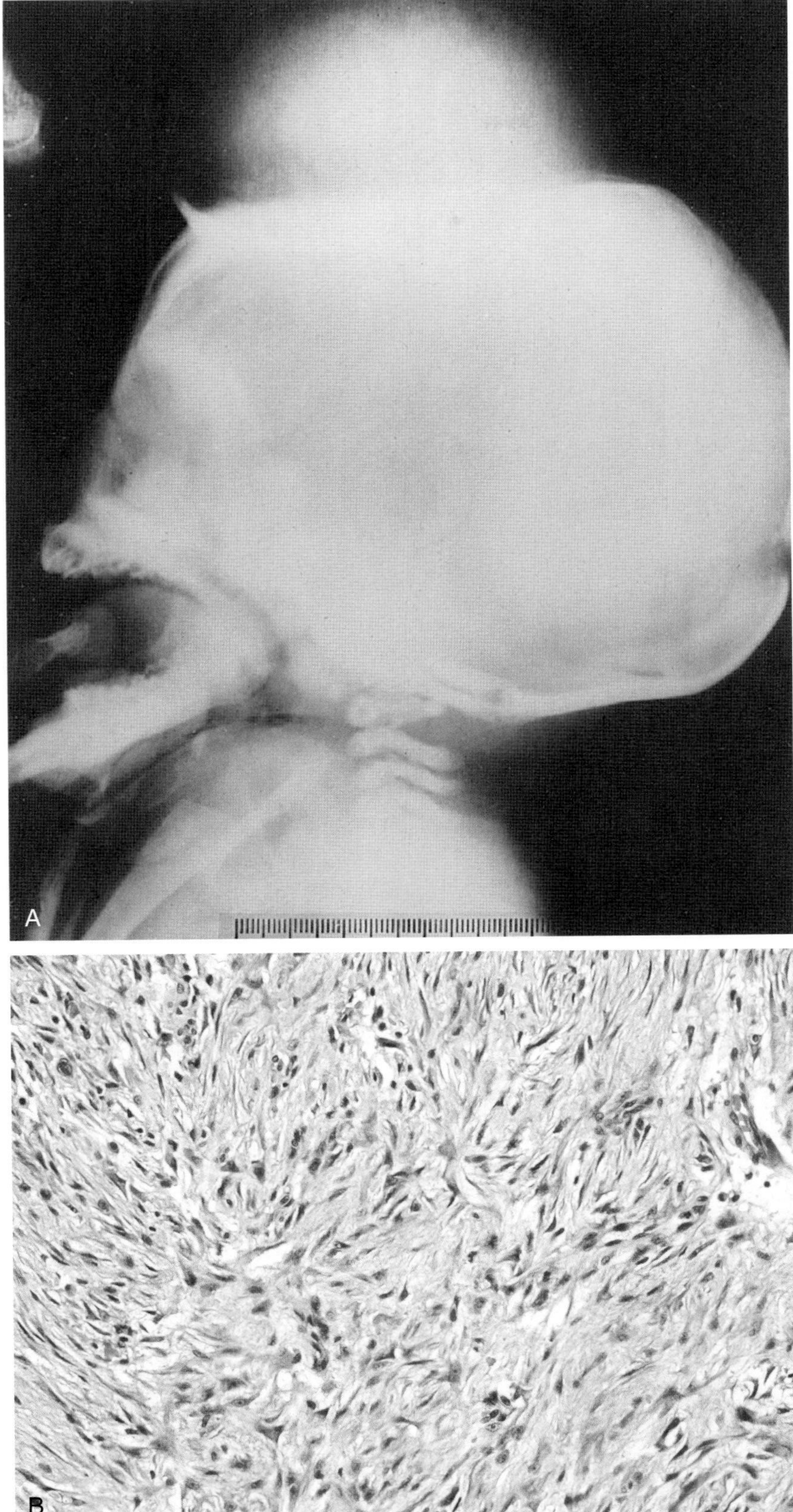

FIGURE 8-16. Cranial fasciitis. (A) Radiograph of large soft tissue mass attached to the inner table of the skull in an infant. (B) Histologic picture of cranial fasciitis.

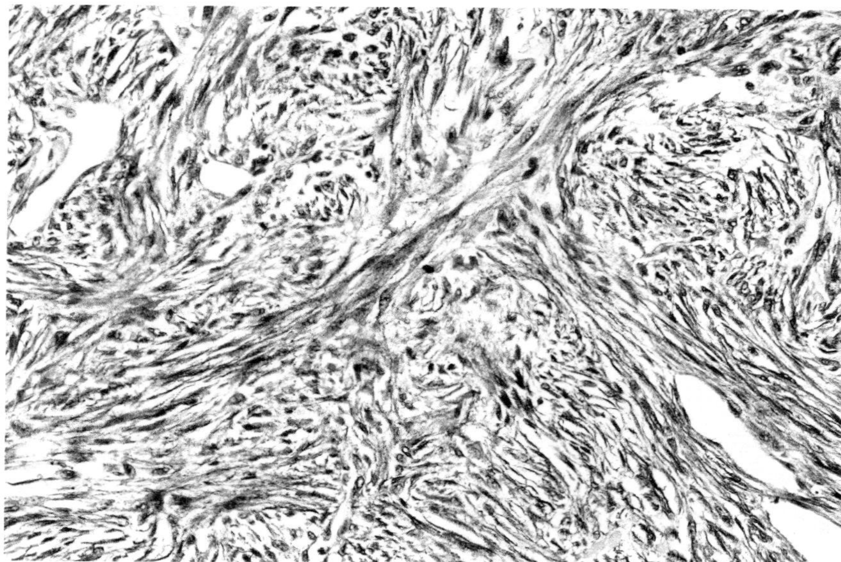

FIGURE 8-17. Nodular fasciitis with diffuse smooth muscle actin immunoreactivity.

(Fig. 8-17).[19] Desmin is rarely expressed by the constituent cells; of the 53 cases stained by Montgomery and Meis,[19] none expressed this antigen. H-caldesmon has been purported to be a useful marker in distinguishing smooth muscle from myofibroblastic proliferations. Ceballos et al.[37] and Perez-Montiel et al.[38] found this marker to be consistently expressed by smooth muscle tumors and absent in nodular fasciitis. In small biopsy specimens, nodular fasciitis may be difficult to distinguish from a fibromatosis. β-catenin may be useful in this regard because the antigen is consistently expressed by the nuclei in fibromatoses and is absent in the myofibroblasts of nodular fasciitis.[39] Immunostains for cytokeratin and S-100 protein are consistently negative. An ultrastructural analysis of the constituent cells shows features expected of a myofibroblastic proliferation, including electron-dense microfilaments and fibronexus junctions.[1]

Cytogenetic and Molecular Genetic Features

Few cases of nodular fasciitis have been evaluated cytogenetically. Rearrangements of 3q21 have been detected on several occasions.[40,41] Another case of nodular fasciitis of the breast exhibited a 2;15 translocation, loss of chromosomes 2 and 13, and several marker chromosomes.[42] A third report by Velagaleti et al.[42] also found a cytogenetic abnormality involving both homologues of chromosome 15, and the authors postulated a possible role for the *NTRK3* gene, a member of the neurotrophin transducing receptor family. Contrary to these findings, using a HUMARA-methylation-specific polymerase chain reaction, Koizumi et al.[43] were unable to document clonality in 24 cases of nodular fasciitis from female patients. In a recent fascinating study from the Mayo Clinic, 44 of 48 (92%) cases of nodular fasciitis were found to have rearrangements of *USP6* (located at 17p13). Further analysis identified *MYH9* (22q13.1) as the translocation partner, a fusion that was not identified in any of the control tissues or tumors.[44] The authors proposed the concept of transient neoplasia, given that this is the first known example of a self-limited process characterized by a recurrent gene fusion.

Differential Diagnosis

Nodular fasciitis may be confused with numerous benign and malignant mesenchymal lesions, and the differential diagnosis depends on the relative amounts of myxoid and fibrous stroma and the cellularity of the lesion in question. As previously mentioned, nodular fasciitis remains the most common benign mesenchymal lesion misdiagnosed as a sarcoma. Therefore, many cases of nodular fasciitis have been treated by unnecessary and excessive radical surgery.

Although nodular fasciitis and *myxoma* may display a prominent myxoid matrix, the latter lesion is readily recognized by its paucity of cells and its poor vascularization. Myxomas also lack the zonal organization and regional heterogeneity of nodular fasciitis. Cellular nodular fasciitis may be confused with *fibrous histiocytoma*, and, in a small number of cases, distinction of these two lesions may be difficult, if not somewhat arbitrary. The typical fibrous histiocytoma is dermis-based, less well circumscribed, and composed of a more polymorphous proliferation of spindle-shaped and round cells arranged in a more consistent storiform pattern. Secondary elements, such as chronic inflammatory cells, xanthoma cells, siderophages, and Touton giant cells, are also common. Peripherally located dense collagen fibers are typical, but similar-appearing fibers may occur in the central portion of nodular fasciitis, particularly in lesions of longer duration. Immunohistochemistry may play an ancillary role in distinguishing between these lesions because most fibrous histiocytomas stain strongly for factor XIIIa, in contrast to nodular fasciitis. Although smooth muscle actin can be focally present in some cases of fibrous histiocytoma, most nodular fasciitis lesions stain diffusely for this antigen. In general, however, the distinction between the two lesions is best made on histologic sections rather than on minor differences in immunophenotype.

Some cases of nodular fasciitis resemble *fibromatosis*. Grossly, fibromatosis is a large, poorly circumscribed lesion that typically infiltrates the surrounding soft tissue, in contrast to the circumscription of nodular fasciitis. Histologically, it is characterized by slender, spindle-shaped fibroblasts arranged in long sweeping fascicles and separated by abundant collagen. Mitotic figures occur in both lesions, but they are much less frequent in musculoaponeurotic fibromatosis than in nodular fasciitis. Both lesions consistently express smooth muscle actin, but nuclear expression of β-catenin is characteristic of fibromatosis and absent in nodular fasciitis.[39]

Distinction from *fibrosarcoma* is primarily a matter of growth pattern and cellularity, and atypia. The cells in fibrosarcoma are nearly always densely packed and are arranged in interweaving bundles, resulting in the characteristic herringbone pattern. Moreover, the individual cells are marked by a greater variation in size and shape, hyperchromatic nuclei, and a more pronounced mitotic rate, including atypical mitotic figures. The deep location, large size, and long duration of most fibrosarcomas also aid in the differential diagnosis.

Of the malignant myxoid lesions, *myxofibrosarcoma* may closely resemble nodular fasciitis. This lesion occurs principally in patients older than 50 years and usually measures more than 3 cm when first excised. Microscopically, the cells show more nuclear pleomorphism, and there is typically a regular arborizing vasculature composed of coarse vessels, often invested with tumor cells. Atypical mitotic figures may be seen, as may areas of transition to a high-grade pleomorphic sarcoma.

Discussion

Although a well-documented history of trauma is present in a small number of cases, nodular fasciitis is clearly a benign process that is likely triggered by local injury or in response to a localized inflammatory process. Regardless of the precise cause, histologic recognition of this reactive pattern is important to avoid misdiagnosing a sarcoma and unnecessary radical surgical treatment. The benign nature and excellent prognosis of nodular fasciitis have been well documented by numerous large clinicopathologic studies (Table 8-3). In the series of 895 cases reported by Allen,[10] only 9 (1%) reappeared after an attempted complete surgical excision. Even those lesions that are incompletely excised rarely recur. Of the 18 cases of recurrent nodular fasciitis in the series by Bernstein and Lattes,[18] a review of the histology and clinical course led to revision of the original diagnosis in all 18 cases. In fact, these authors stated that a recurrence of a lesion initially diagnosed as nodular fasciitis should lead to a reappraisal of the original pathologic findings. Although most cases are surgically excised, there are well-documented cases of regression of these lesions over a period of time.[45]

TABLE 8-3 Recurrence Rates in Large Series of Nodular Fasciitis

	RECURRENCE	PERCENTAGE (%)
Bernstein and Lattes[18]	18/134*	13
Allen[10]	9/895	1

* Upon re-review, all recurrent lesions were reclassified as something other than nodular fasciitis.

PROLIFERATIVE FASCIITIS

Proliferative fasciitis, a term coined by Chung and Enzinger[46] in 1975, is the subcutaneous counterpart of proliferative myositis. Both of these lesions are pseudosarcomatous, myofibroblastic proliferations characterized by the presence of unusual ganglion-like myofibroblasts. The microscopic appearance of the lesion may be suggestive of a sarcoma, and many cases of this type have been misinterpreted in the past as embryonal rhabdomyosarcoma, ganglioneuroblastoma, or some other type of malignant neoplasm.

Clinical Findings

Proliferative fasciitis is a lesion of adult life, with most patients being 40 to 70 years of age (mean, 54 years).[46] Although well recognized, it is quite uncommon for patients younger than 15 years of age to develop proliferative fasciitis.[47] There is no gender or race predilection, and most of the lesions occur in the subcutaneous tissues of the extremities, with the upper extremity (especially the forearm) affected more commonly than the lower extremity. The lesion also occurs with some frequency on the trunk and rarely on the head and neck.[48]

Clinically, most patients present with a firm, palpable subcutaneous nodule that is freely movable and unattached to the overlying skin, although about two-thirds of patients also have complaints of pain or tenderness. Most lesions measure less than 5 cm in greatest diameter, with a median size of 2.5 cm. Like nodular fasciitis, these lesions are typically rapidly growing, most being excised 2 to 6 weeks after their initial discovery. A history of trauma in the vicinity of the mass is elicited in about one-third of cases.[46]

Pathologic Findings

Grossly, proliferative fasciitis is usually poorly circumscribed, forming an elongated or discoid-shaped mass that predominantly involves the subcutaneous tissue, although some involve the superficial fascia. Rare lesions also involve the superficial skeletal muscle, making it difficult to distinguish from proliferative myositis. Cases that arise during childhood tend to be more circumscribed and vaguely lobular, with only an occasional extension along fascial planes.[49]

Microscopically, like nodular fasciitis, proliferative fasciitis is composed of tissue culture-like fibroblastic and myofibroblastic spindle cells that have bland cytologic features and are deposited in a variably myxoid and collagenous stroma. This proliferation extends along the interlobular septa of the subcutaneous tissue, with some extension along the superficial fascia (Fig. 8-18). Very rarely, the lesion can extend to or even be centered in the dermis.[50] Proliferative fasciitis is characterized by the presence of large, basophilic ganglion-like cells with one or two vesicular nuclei and prominent nucleoli. The cells have abundant basophilic, slightly granular cytoplasm but lack cross-striations typical of rhabdomyoblasts

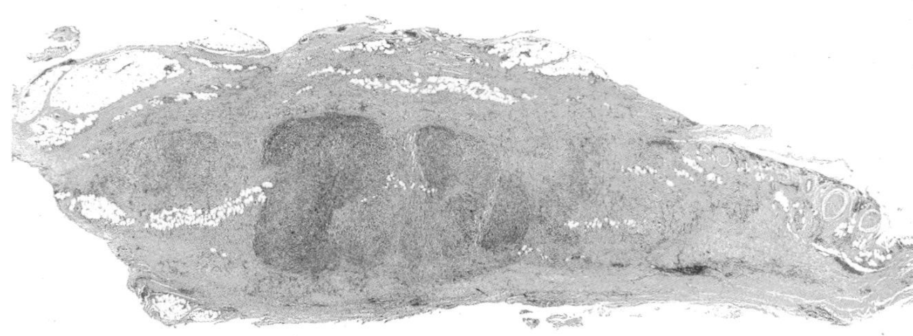

FIGURE 8-18. Proliferative fasciitis involving the subcutis.

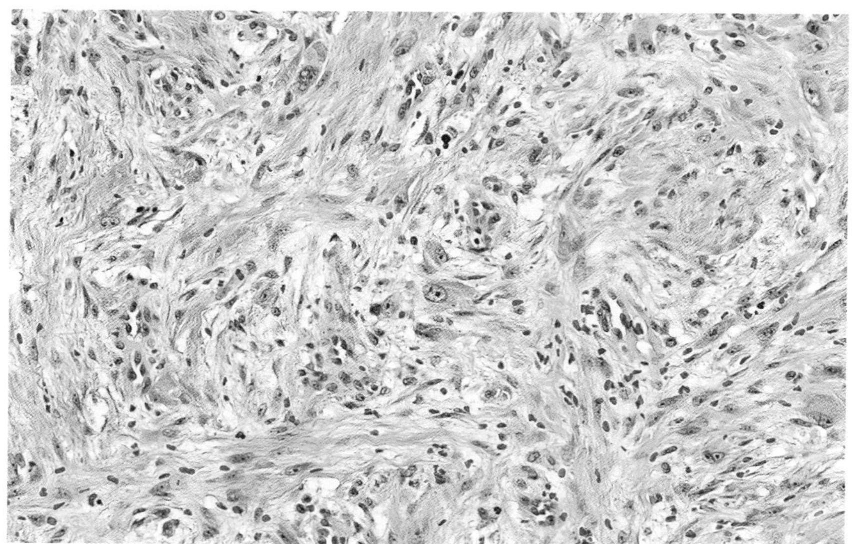

FIGURE 8-19. Proliferative fasciitis composed of a mixture of fibroblasts and giant cells with abundant basophilic cytoplasm bearing some resemblance to ganglion cells.

(Figs. 8-19 to 8-21). Some cells have intracytoplasmic inclusions of collagen. These ganglion-like cells may be packed together or loosely arranged in aggregates. Multinucleated giant cells of the type seen in nodular fasciitis are rare in proliferative fasciitis. Curiously, pediatric lesions tend to be more cellular (Fig. 8-22), have numerous mitoses, and have foci of acute inflammation and necrosis, features that are distinctly unusual in the typical adult form.[51] Childhood cases also tend to have less collagen and a less conspicuous myxoid matrix than their adult counterparts. Some lesions, particularly those that have been present for a long duration before excision, may have abundant hyalinized collagen that surrounds the ganglion-like cells, which could cause confusion with neoplastic osteoid and a misdiagnosis of osteosarcoma.

The immunohistochemical findings of proliferative fasciitis are similar to those of nodular fasciitis. The spindle and stellate-shaped cells stain for muscle-specific and smooth-muscle actin. Some cells stain for CD68 (KP1); immunostains for cytokeratins, S-100 protein, and desmin are usually negative. The ganglion-like cells may also stain for actin, although the staining is often focal and weak and may be membranous in distribution.[51,52] Ultrastructurally, the spindle- and stellate-shaped cells have the typical features of fibroblasts and myofibroblasts.[2,53] The ganglion-like cells are characterized by abundant rough endoplasmic reticulum with dilated cisternae, some of which may contain short-spacing collagen fibrils.[54]

PROLIFERATIVE MYOSITIS

Proliferative myositis is the intramuscular counterpart of proliferative fasciitis. Although Kern[55] is credited with the original description of proliferative myositis, Ackerman[56] probably reported the first cases in his study of extra-osseous non-neoplastic localized bone and cartilage formation. Like proliferative fasciitis, proliferative myositis is a rapidly growing lesion that infiltrates muscle tissue in a diffuse manner and is characterized by bizarre giant cells bearing a close resemblance to ganglion cells.

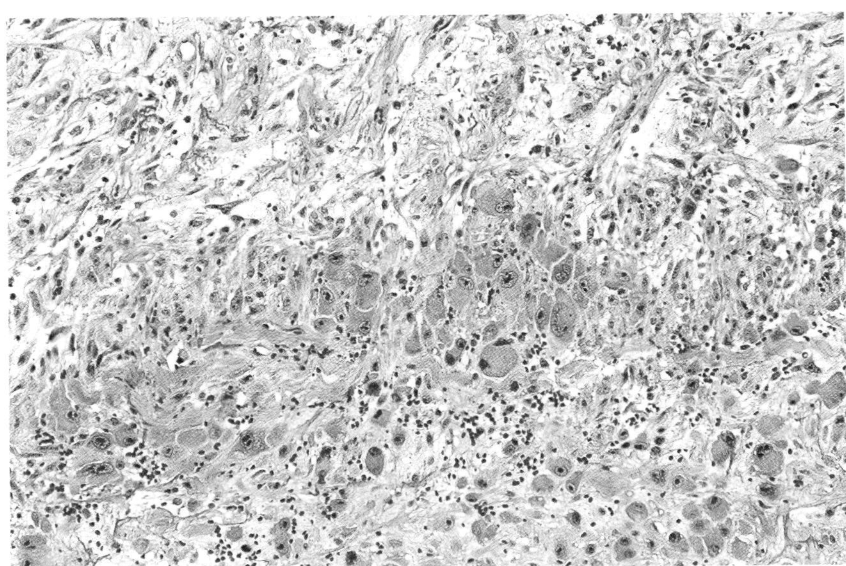

FIGURE 8-20. Peripheral portion of proliferative fasciitis with numerous ganglion-like giant cells.

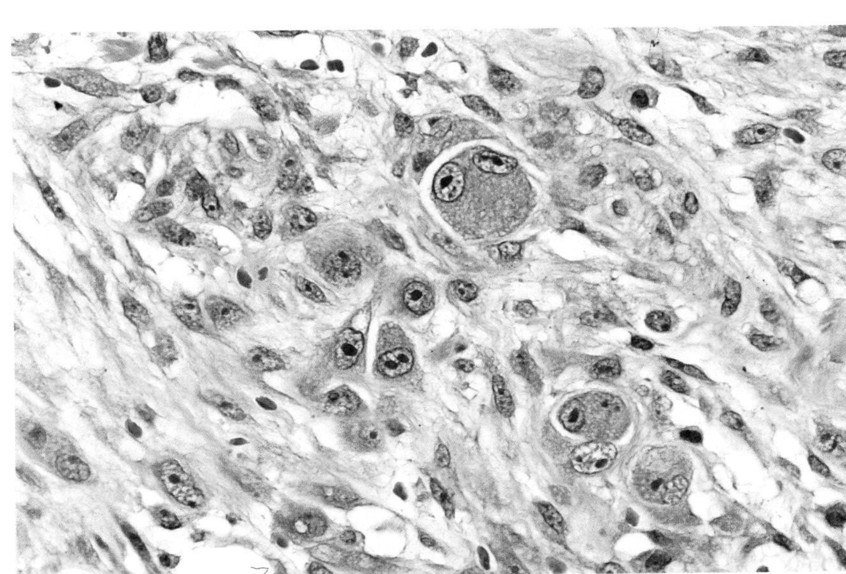

FIGURE 8-21. Proliferative fasciitis with large ganglion-like cells, some of which are multinucleated.

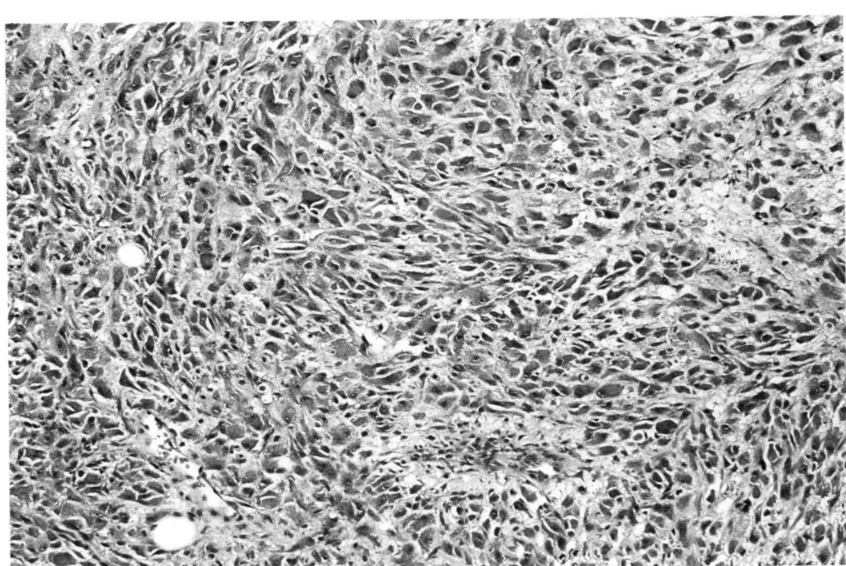

FIGURE 8-22. Proliferative fasciitis of childhood composed of round and polygonal cells with abundant cytoplasm and prominent nucleoli.

Clinical Findings

The symptoms are nonspecific, and the diagnosis always rests on the histologic examination of tissue obtained by fine-needle aspiration cytology,[57,58] biopsy, or excision. In most cases, the lesion is first noted as a palpable, more or less discrete, solitary nodular mass that measures 1 to 6 cm in diameter. It rarely causes tenderness or pain, even though it may double in size within a period of a few days. The duration between onset and excision is usually less than 3 weeks.

The patients tend to be older than those with nodular fasciitis, with a median age of 50 years,[59] although rare cases have been described in children.[51] There seems to be no predilection for either gender or any particular race. The lesion mainly affects the flat muscles of the trunk and shoulder girdle, especially the pectoralis, latissimus dorsi, or serratus anterior muscle. Occasionally, tumors are also found in the muscles of the thigh. Involvement of the head and neck is uncommon.[60,61]

Pathologic Findings

Similar to proliferative fasciitis, proliferative myositis typically appears pale gray or scar-like, resulting in induration of the involved skeletal muscle (Fig. 8-23). When present in small or flat muscles, it often replaces most or all of the involved musculature. When involving large muscles, there is preferential involvement of the skeletal muscle immediately underneath the fascia with a progressive decrease in the central portion of the muscle in a wedge-like fashion.

The cellular components of proliferative myositis are identical to those found in proliferative fasciitis. There is a poorly demarcated proliferation of fibroblast-like cells that involve the epimysium, perimysium, and endomysium. Unlike the intramuscular form of nodular fasciitis and musculoaponeurotic fibromatosis, this cellular proliferation rarely completely replaces large areas of the involved muscle and, rather, is most striking in the subfascial region and interfascicular connective tissue septa. The skeletal muscle fibers are relatively unaffected except for the presence of secondary atrophy, with neither sarcolemmal proliferation nor any evidence of skeletal muscle regeneration. This alternation of proliferating fibrous tissue with persistent atrophic skeletal muscle fibers results in a typical checkerboard pattern that is apparent at low magnification (Fig. 8-24). The other conspicuous histologic feature of proliferative myositis is the presence of large basophilic ganglion-like cells, identical to those found in proliferative fasciitis (Figs. 8-25 and 8-26). Mitotic figures are often easily identified in both the spindle and giant cells, although atypical mitoses are not seen. Rare lesions contain foci of metaplastic bone[62] (Fig. 8-27).

The immunohistochemical and ultrastructural features of proliferative myositis are identical to those of proliferative fasciitis[63] (Fig. 8-28).

Trisomy 2 has been described in both proliferative fasciitis and proliferative myositis.[64,65] McComb et al.[66] reported a single case with a t(6;14)(q23;q32).

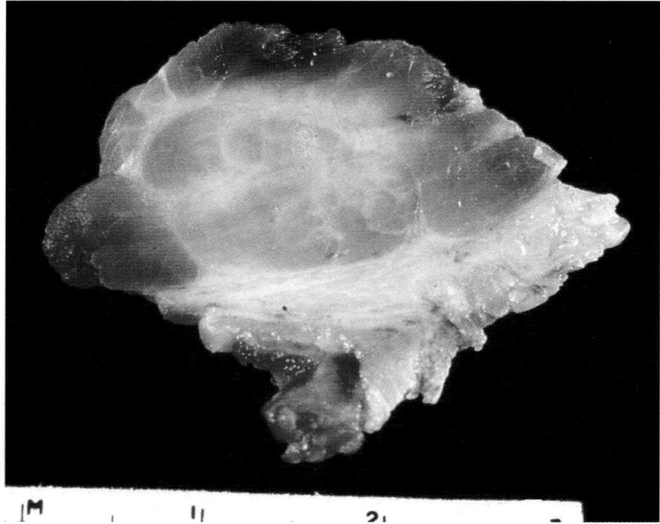

FIGURE 8-23. Proliferative myositis characterized by a poorly circumscribed scar-like fibrosing process involving muscle and muscle fascia.

Differential Diagnosis

Proliferative fasciitis and myositis may be mistaken for a variety of malignant neoplasms, most commonly *rhabdomyosarcoma* or *ganglioneuroblastoma*. In the series of 53 cases of proliferative fasciitis by Chung and Enzinger,[46] 16 were originally diagnosed as a sarcoma. Similarly, 14 of 33 cases of proliferative myositis reported by Enzinger and Dulcey[59] were believed to be some type of sarcoma. Errors are most likely to occur with childhood cases in which rhabdomyosarcoma is a strong diagnostic consideration. The history of a rapidly growing mass of short duration that typically attains a maximum size of less than 3 cm is more consistent with a reactive process than with a sarcoma. Histologically, the ganglion-like cells lack cross-striations and show more cytoplasmic basophilia than is seen in rhabdomyoblasts. Although the immunohistochemical profiles may overlap, stains for desmin, MyoD1, and myogenin are negative in the ganglion-like cells, in contrast to the staining found in true rhabdomyoblasts.

Discussion

Proliferative fasciitis and myositis, like nodular fasciitis, are self-limiting, benign, reactive processes that are probably preceded by some type of fascial or muscular injury resulting in a proliferation of myofibroblasts. However, only a small number of patients report a preceding injury in the exact location of the lesion, raising the possibility that causes other than mechanical trauma play a role in the development of proliferative fasciitis and myositis. Although some have reported the diagnosis of these lesions by fine-needle aspiration cytology, the unusual histologic features of these lesions warrant caution with this technique. Both proliferative fasciitis and myositis are adequately treated by local excision, and recurrence is exceedingly rare. As with some cases of nodular fasciitis, spontaneous resolution in a period of 1 to 16 weeks has been observed in cases of proliferative fasciitis and myositis.[67]

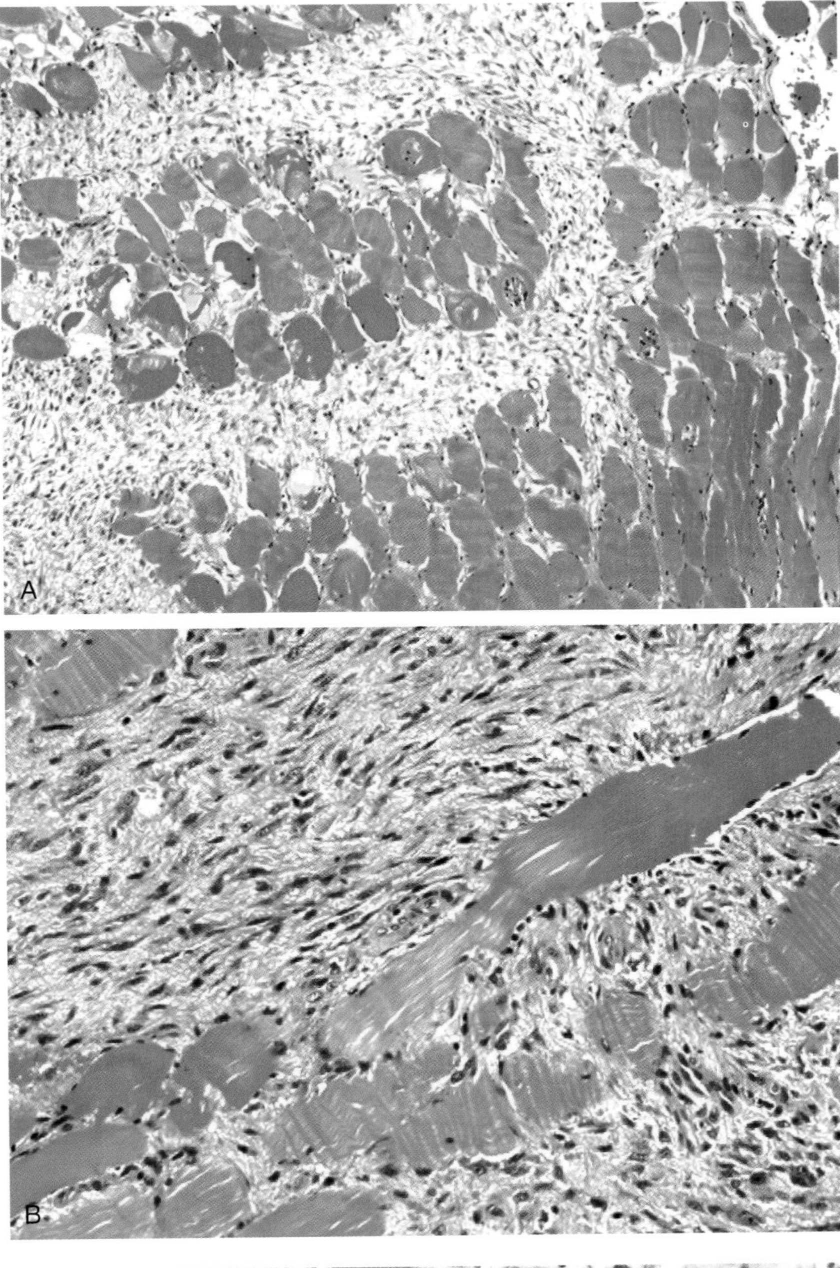

FIGURE 8-24. (A) Low-magnification view of proliferative myositis showing the characteristic checkerboard pattern. (B) Fasciitis-like area surrounding skeletal muscle fibers in a case of proliferative myositis.

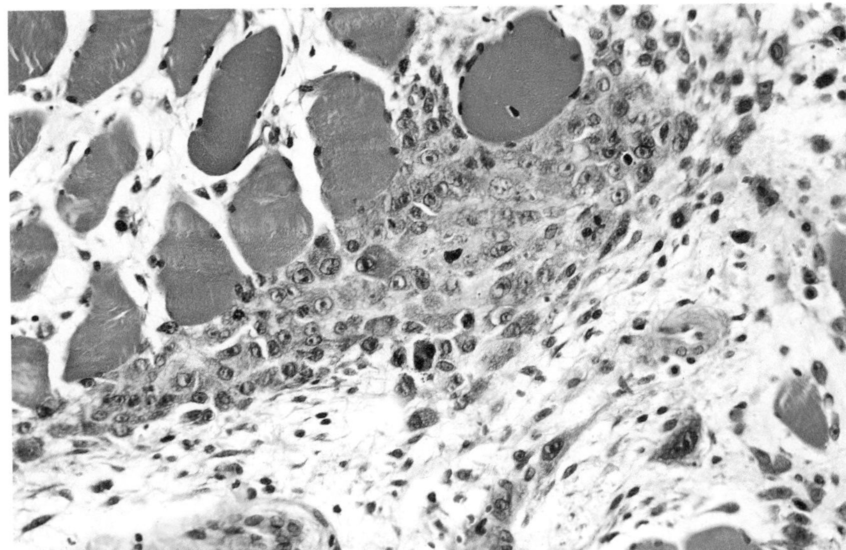

FIGURE 8-25. Proliferative myositis. Ganglion-like giant cells are seen immediately adjacent to and infiltrating skeletal muscle fibers.

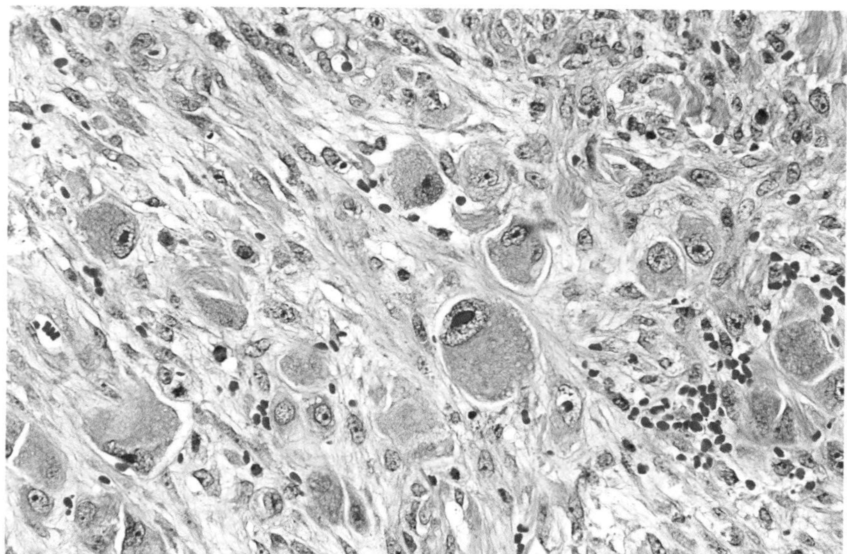

FIGURE 8-26. High-power view of ganglion-like giant cells in proliferative myositis.

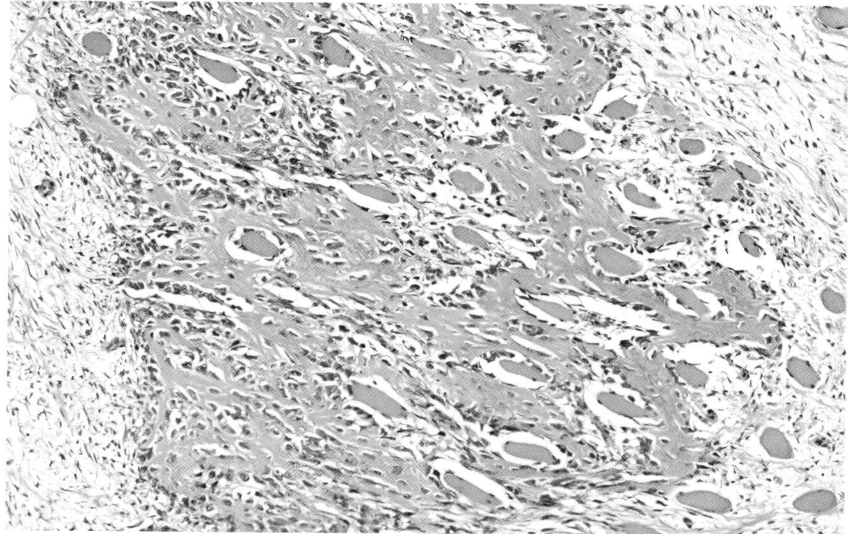

FIGURE 8-27. Unusual case of proliferative myositis with extensive metaplastic bone formation.

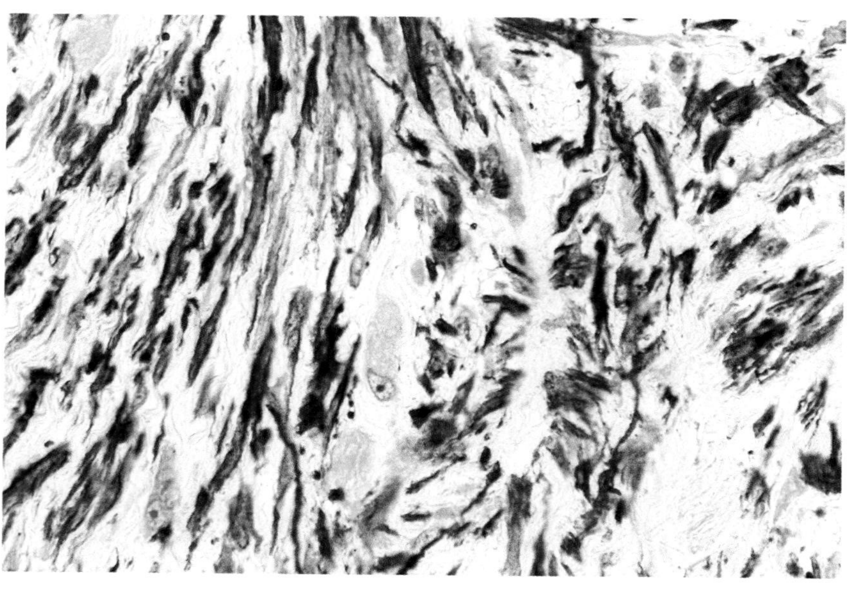

FIGURE 8-28. Proliferative myositis stained for smooth muscle actin. Most spindle cells stain for this antigen, but the ganglion-like cells, in this case, are negative.

ORGAN-ASSOCIATED PSEUDOSARCOMATOUS MYOFIBROBLASTIC PROLIFERATIONS

Organ-associated pseudosarcomatous myofibroblastic proliferations, most of which arise in the genitourinary tract, have been described under an impressive variety of names, including *inflammatory pseudotumor, pseudosarcomatous myofibroblastic tumor, pseudosarcomatous myofibroblastic proliferation, pseudosarcomatous fibromyxoid tumor,* and even *nodular fasciitis.* Most commonly, those arising as a result of preceding trauma or surgical instrumentation have been referred to as *postoperative spindle-cell nodule,*[68,69] whereas those arising spontaneously have often been referred to as *inflammatory pseudotumor.*[70] Certainly, the vast array of names used to describe these proliferations has contributed to some of this confusion. However, the major controversy has focused on whether these lesions are reactive or neoplastic, including whether they are best designated as *inflammatory myofibroblastic tumor,* a term that implies a neoplastic process characterized by alterations of the anaplastic lymphoma kinase (*ALK*) gene on 2p23.[71] Several studies demonstrating *ALK* gene rearrangement and immunostaining for the ALK protein suggest that these lesions are neoplastic, although the two studies differ as to whether the lesions are believed to be identical to inflammatory myofibroblastic tumor.[71,72] Harik et al.[71] consider these lesions to be neoplastic, but distinct from an inflammatory myofibroblastic tumor, and favor the term *pseudosarcomatous myofibroblastic proliferation,* whereas the other group recommends calling them *inflammatory myofibroblastic tumor.*[72] What is clear, however, is that there is no histologic difference between lesions harboring *ALK* gene abnormalities and those that do not. Likewise, there are no significant histologic differences between lesions that arise spontaneously and those that arise following instrumentation.

Clinical Findings

Although these lesions can arise anywhere in the genitourinary tract, including the prostate,[73] vagina,[74] urethra,[75] and ureter,[76] they are most common in the urinary bladder. For example, in the study by Hirsch et al.,[74] 21 of 27 pseudosarcomatous myofibroblastic proliferations of the genitourinary tract arose in the urinary bladder. Similarly, 42 of 46 inflammatory myofibroblastic tumors reported by Montgomery et al.[72] arose in the urinary bladder. Most commonly, patients present with hematuria, although some present with dysuria, abdominal pain, or weight loss. Based upon the larger clinicopathologic studies, it is still unclear whether these lesions are more common in women or men. In the studies by Harik et al.[71] and Montgomery et al.,[72] males outnumbered females by a 2:1 or 3:1 ratio. However, Hirsch et al.[74] found exactly the opposite, because women were affected three times as often as men.[74] Although the age range is broad, lesions most commonly arise in patients in their fourth to fifth decades of life. Approximately 20% to 25% of patients have a history of antecedent trauma or surgical instrumentation. Those that arise secondary to surgical instrumentation usually become clinically apparent between 5 and 12 weeks following the surgical procedure.

Pathologic Findings

Grossly, most lesions present as exophytic, nodular, or polypoid intraluminal lesions that may extend deeply into the visceral organ from which they arise. They range in size from 1.5 cm to up to 12 cm, although most are between 3 and 5 cm at the time of excision. The lesion may be firm or soft, depending upon the relative amounts of fibrous and myxoid stroma present.

On microscopic examination, these lesions are characterized by a proliferation of spindle- to stellate-shaped cells, often with a tissue culture-like appearance reminiscent of nodular fasciitis (Figs. 8-29 to 8-31). The cells lack cytologic atypia or nuclear hyperchromasia and have bipolar or stellate-shaped cytoplasmic processes. Most commonly, the cells are widely separated and haphazardly distributed in a myxoid stroma, but some cases are characterized by more cellular areas in which the cells are arranged in irregular fascicles with variable amounts of intercellular collagen. The cells have oval- to spindle-shaped nuclei with open chromatin, variably sized nucleoli, and eosinophilic to amphophilic cytoplasm. Mitotic figures are present, usually with fewer than 1 to 2 mitotic

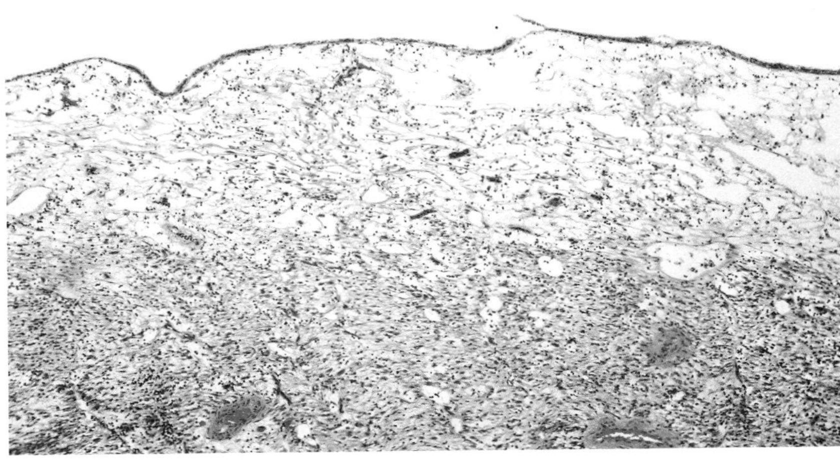

FIGURE 8-29. Pseudosarcomatous myofibroblastic proliferation of urinary bladder. Proliferation of spindle cells in a loose, edematous, myxoid stroma with mixed acute and chronic inflammatory cells.

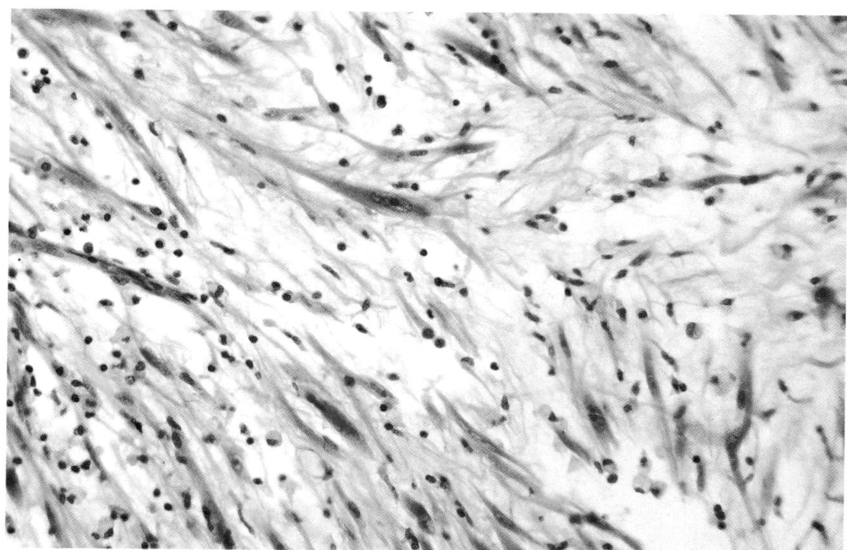

FIGURE 8-30. High-power view of pseudosarcomatous myofibroblastic proliferation of the urinary bladder. Haphazard arrangement of spindle cells with bipolar or stellate-shaped cytoplasmic processes deposited in a myxoid stroma with scattered chronic inflammatory cells.

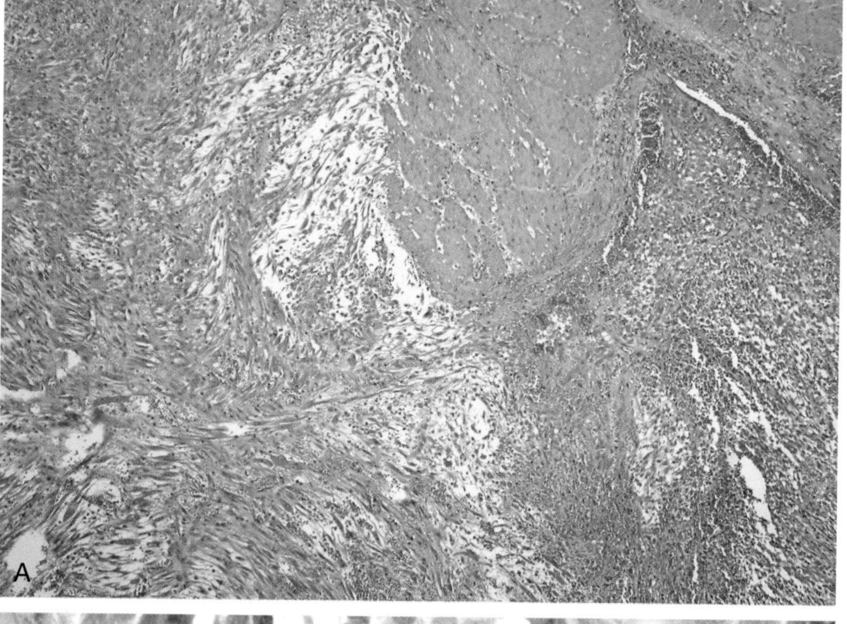

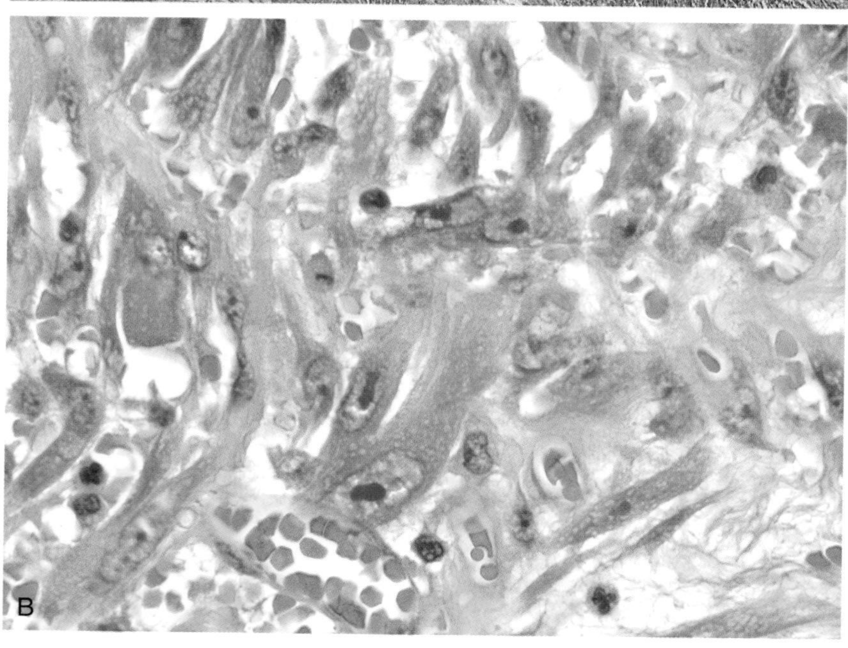

FIGURE 8-31. (A) Low-magnification view of a pseudosarcomatous myofibroblastic proliferation of the urinary bladder with infiltration of the muscularis propria. (B) High-magnification view of reactive-appearing spindled-shaped cells with prominent nucleoli.

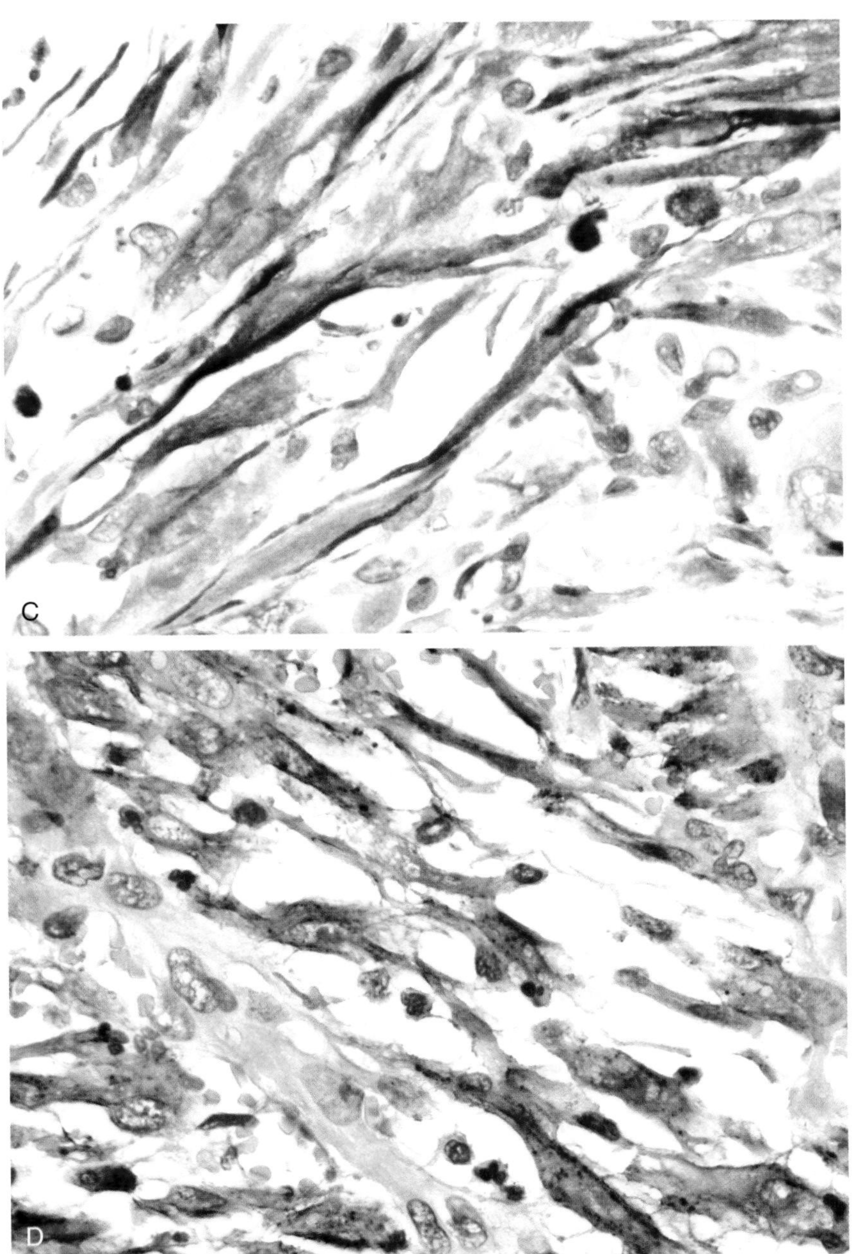

FIGURE 8-31, cont'd. (C) Strong cytokeratin immunoreactivity in the constituent cells of a pseudosarcomatous myofibroblastic proliferation of the urinary bladder. (D) Strong ALK immunoreactivity in the same case as seen in Figure 8-31C.

figures per 10 high-power fields, and they are not atypical. In the more myxoid zones, there is a prominent capillary network often associated with extravasated erythrocytes. A mixed inflammatory infiltrate composed of lymphocytes, plasma cells, eosinophils, and occasional mast cells is usually conspicuous. When present, neutrophils are associated with areas of mucosal ulceration.

Some cases have histologic features that cause great concern for a malignancy. Rare examples have a brisk mitotic rate, with up to 20 mitotic figures per 10 high-power fields. Invasion into the muscularis propria of the urinary bladder is a common finding, and some even infiltrate into the perivesicular adipose tissue. Although necrosis is usually focal and confined to the surface of the lesion and associated with mucosal ulceration, some cases show necrosis of the deeper tissue.

Immunohistochemical Findings

Immunohistochemically, the spindle cells stain strongly for vimentin and various muscle markers, including muscle-specific actin, smooth muscle actin, and desmin. In addition, many cases show focal or often diffuse staining for cytokeratins (see Fig. 8-31C), which obviously can lead to diagnostic confusion.[71,72,74] In the study by Harik et al.,[71] 31 of 35 cases stained for cytokeratins. Similarly, Montgomery et al.[72] found 25 of 34 cases (73%) to stain for AE1/AE3, including 23 cases with strong, diffuse immunoreactivity.

A significant percentage of these lesions also stains for ALK (Fig. 8-31D), but there is an imperfect correlation between ALK immunoreactivity and the detection of an *ALK* gene translocation by fluorescence in-situ hybridization

TABLE 8-4 Frequency of ALK Immunoreactivity and *ALK* Gene Rearrangements by FISH in Pseudosarcomatous Myofibroblastic Proliferations/Inflammatory Myofibroblastic of the Urinary Bladder

STUDY	ALK STAINING	*ALK* GENE REARRANGEMENTS (FISH)
Tsuzuki et al.[78]	10/14	
Hirsch et al.[74]	10/21	0/6*
Harik et al.[71]	12/26	4/10**
Montgomery et al.[72]	20/35	13/18
Total	52/96 (54%)	17/34 (50%)

*All six cases tested stained for ALK.
**Includes four ALK-negative cases (0/4) and six ALK-positive cases (4/6).

TABLE 8-5 Differential Diagnostic Features of Genitourinary Pseudosarcomatous Myofibroblastic Proliferations

FEATURE	PMP	ML	B-RMS	SC
Cellularity	+	+/++	+/++	++
Growth pattern	Loose	Loose	Botryoid	Biphasic
Atypia	+	+/++	++	+++
Electron microscopy	Fibroblast/ myofibroblast	Smooth muscle	Striated muscle	Epithelial
Cytokeratin	Frequent +	Rare	–	+
Desmin	±	+	+	±
SMA	+	+	–	±
ALK	50%	–	–	–

B-RMS, botryoid rhabdomyosarcoma; ML, myxoid leiomyosarcoma; PMP, pseudosarcomatous myofibroblastic proliferation; SC, sarcomatoid urothelial carcinoma.

(FISH) (Table 8-4). In the study by Harik et al.,[71] 12 of 26 (46%) cases stained for this antigen; an analysis by FISH confirmed a translocation of the *ALK* gene in 4 of 6 (67%) ALK-positive tumors. Montgomery et al.[72] found 20 of 35 cases (57%) to stain for ALK, and 13 of 18 ALK-positive cases (72%) showed evidence of an *ALK* gene alteration by FISH. In contrast, of the 6 ALK immunoreactive cases evaluated by Hirsch et al.,[74] none showed evidence of an *ALK* gene translocation by FISH. Sukov et al.[77] found *ALK* gene rearrangements in 14 of 21 cases (67%), with ALK staining in 13 of 21 cases (62%). All cases with *ALK* gene expression harbored *ALK* gene rearrangements; one ALK-negative case exhibited an *ALK* gene rearrangement. All other lesions studied (leiomyosarcomas, sarcomatoid carcinomas, embryonal rhabdomyosarcomas, and lesions felt to be reactive) were negative for *ALK* gene rearrangement and ALK staining.

Differential Diagnosis

Although a pseudosarcomatous myofibroblastic proliferation should be suspected when one encounters a spindle-cell lesion in the genitourinary tract, particularly in a patient who has undergone recent instrumentation at that site, numerous other benign and malignant spindle-cell proliferations must be considered (Table 8-5). *Myxoid leiomyosarcoma* tends to occur in older patients and is quite rare before the age of 20 years. Microscopically, the lesion is composed of spindle cells with densely eosinophilic fibrillar cytoplasm, often with perinuclear vacuoles, deposited in a myxoid stroma. These lesions can also express cytokeratins, but they do not stain for ALK. Pseudosarcomatous myofibroblastic proliferations are characterized by a more prominent vasculature, variable cellularity, and a more conspicuous inflammatory component. Moreover, these lesions characteristically have a zonal quality consisting of superficial (submucosal) myxoid zones juxtaposed to deep cellular zones associated with a prominent arcuate vascular pattern.

Botryoid-type rhabdomyosarcoma is also a diagnostic consideration; this lesion is characterized by the presence of a cambium layer under the epithelium composed of atypical, hyperchromatic cells, occasionally with overt rhabdomyoblastic differentiation. Immunohistochemical (myogenin) analysis reveals evidence of skeletal muscle differentiation.

The immunohistochemical detection of epithelial differentiation in many pseudosarcomatous myofibroblastic proliferations often raises concern for a *sarcomatoid urothelial carcinoma*. The presence of marked cytologic atypia, atypical mitotic figures, non-myxoid zones with markedly increased cellularity, and the identification of an in-situ urothelial carcinoma are useful features in recognizing sarcomatoid urothelial carcinoma. In addition, the expression of ALK in pseudosarcomatous myofibroblastic proliferations is a useful finding in this differential diagnosis.

Discussion

Whether these lesions should be considered true neoplasms or exuberant reactive proliferations is controversial because there is some evidence to support both points of view. The history of prior surgical instrumentation in up to 25% of cases and the bland myofibroblastic appearance of the constituent cells, in association with a myxoinflammatory background, are hallmarks of many reactive soft tissue processes (most notably, nodular fasciitis). However, the majority of cases arise spontaneously without a history of prior surgical instrumentation. These lesions may show extensive mural growth with some infiltrating into the perivesicular adipose tissue. From an immunophenotypic standpoint, they are rather unique when compared to other pseudosarcomatous myofibroblastic proliferations because most express cytokeratins, sometimes diffusely.

Although there are conflicting data, some lesions clearly harbor translocations of the *ALK* gene.[71,72,78] It is possible that some myofibroblastic proliferations of the genitourinary tract are reactive, whereas others are truly neoplastic and associated with *ALK* gene abnormalities. The consensus is that there are some subtle differences that allow one to separate these lesions from the inflammatory myofibroblastic tumor, in most instances. These lesions have a relative paucity of plasma cells, a more prominent edematous stroma, and a lack of the peculiar ganglion-like cells of inflammatory myofibroblastic tumor. It is also possible that pseudosarcomatous myofibroblastic proliferations and inflammatory myofibroblastic tumors represent various points along a single spectrum, as opposed to representing two distinct entities.

Regardless of whether one considers these reactive or neoplastic, the vast majority of these genitourinary lesions follow a benign clinical course. In the study by Harik et al.,[71] follow-up information available in 28 patients with urinary bladder lesions revealed recurrences in three patients only, and none developed metastatic disease. Hirsch et al.[74] found 3 of 17 patients to develop nondestructive recurrences 3 months to 108 months following initial excision. Montgomery et al.[72] found a higher rate of local recurrence, as 10 of 32 patients with clinical follow-up developed local recurrence at a mean of 3 months following initial excision. These authors found no association between the risk of local recurrence and histologic features or the presence or absence of *ALK* gene abnormalities. However, one of the cases in this study, a tumor involving the prostatic urethra and urinary bladder, showed features consistent with a malignant inflammatory myofibroblastic tumor. This patient had a rapid recurrence of his tumor, and the patient died with intra-abdominal metastatic disease at 9 months, despite being treated aggressively with chemotherapy.

ISCHEMIC FASCIITIS (ATYPICAL DECUBITAL FIBROPLASIA)

Ischemic fasciitis and *atypical decubital fibroplasia* are synonyms for a pseudosarcomatous fibroblastic/myofibroblastic proliferation that predominantly involves soft tissues overlying bony prominences and often (but not always) occurs in elderly and physically debilitated or immobilized patients.[79,80] Most patients are elderly, with a peak incidence during the eighth and ninth decades of life, although this lesion has rarely been described in adolescents (Table 8-6).[81] Although there are conflicting data in the literature, the largest study published to date by Liegl and Fletcher[82] showed a male predilection (15 females/29 males). Most patients present with a painless mass of short duration, usually less than 6 months; many, but not all, patients are debilitated or immobilized, bedridden, or wheelchair-bound. In the study of Liegl and Fletcher,[82] only 7 of 44 patients were debilitated. However, nine patients had a history of chronic or malignant disease and another four patients had a history of local trauma to the affected site. The soft tissues in the region of the shoulder are most commonly affected, followed by the soft tissues of the chest wall overlying the ribs, those overlying the sacrococcygeal region, or the greater trochanter.

Pathologic Findings

Grossly, ischemic fasciitis tends to be poorly circumscribed and vaguely multinodular, often with a myxoid quality; it ranges from 1.0 to 10.0 cm in greatest diameter with a medium size of around 5 cm. It typically involves the subcutaneous tissue but may extend into the overlying dermis, with infrequent epidermal ulceration. In addition, the proliferation can involve the underlying skeletal muscles or adjacent periosteum.

Microscopically, ischemic fasciitis has a zonal pattern, often with a central zone of liquefactive or focally coagulative necrosis surrounded by a fringe of proliferating vessels and fibroblasts/myofibroblasts (Figs. 8-32 and 8-33). The peripheral vessels are usually small, thin-walled, and ectatic; they are lined by prominent, occasionally atypical, endothelial cells (Fig. 8-34). In addition, a proliferation of plump cells form perivascular clusters or merge imperceptibly with the peripheral vessels; these cells may be cytologically atypical, with large, eccentric, often smudgy hyperchromatic nuclei, prominent nucleoli, and abundant basophilic cytoplasm. Some

TABLE 8-6 Clinical Features of Ischemic Fasciitis: Summary of Three Series

AUTHORS	YEAR	MALE/FEMALE RATIO	AGE RANGE	RECURRENCE
Perosio et al.[79]	1993	2/4	37-87 (median: 76)	1/5 (20%)
Montgomery et al.[80]	1992	12/16	15-95 (median: 78)	3/21 (14%)
Liegl et al.[82]	2008	29/15	23-96 (median: 74)	1/13 (8%)

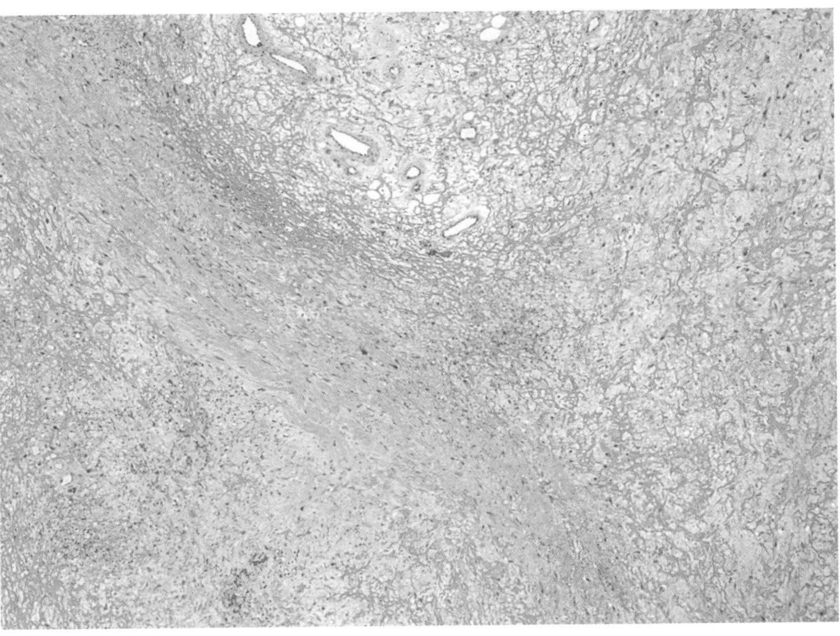

FIGURE 8-32. Low-power appearance showing zonal quality in ischemic fasciitis.

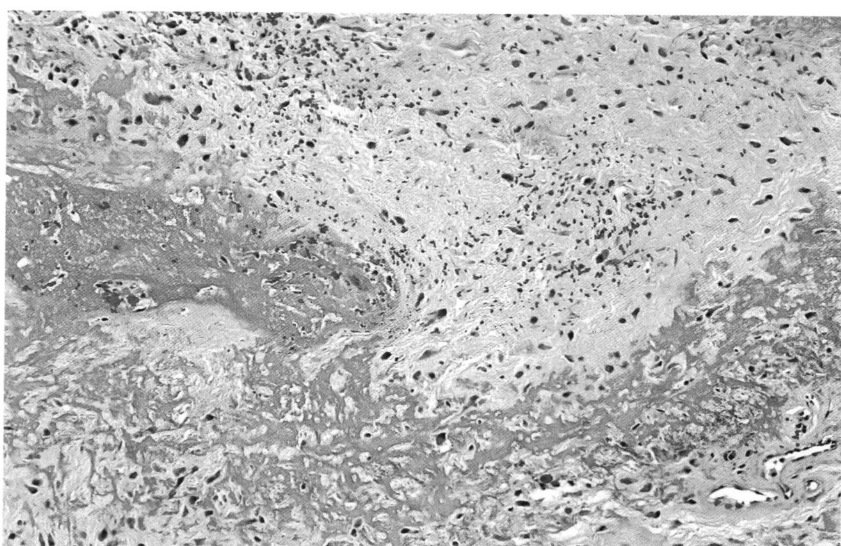

FIGURE 8-33. Interface between a liquefactive zone with fibrinous material and a reactive zone with atypical-appearing fibroblasts. *(Case courtesy of Dr. Elizabeth Montgomery, Johns Hopkins Hospital, Baltimore, Maryland.)*

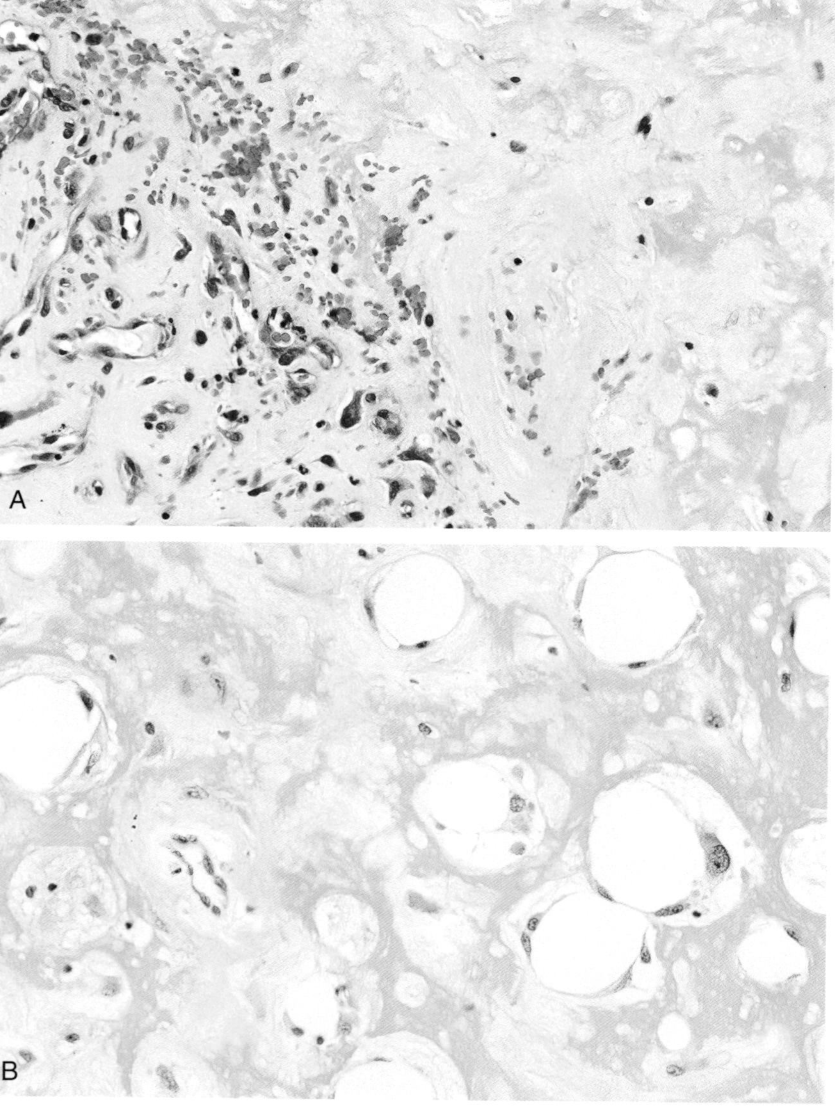

FIGURE 8-34. Ischemic fasciitis. (A) Interface between a zone of liquefactive necrosis and reactive fibroblastic and vascular proliferation. (B) High-power view of residual "ghosted" fat cells in a zone of coagulative necrosis.

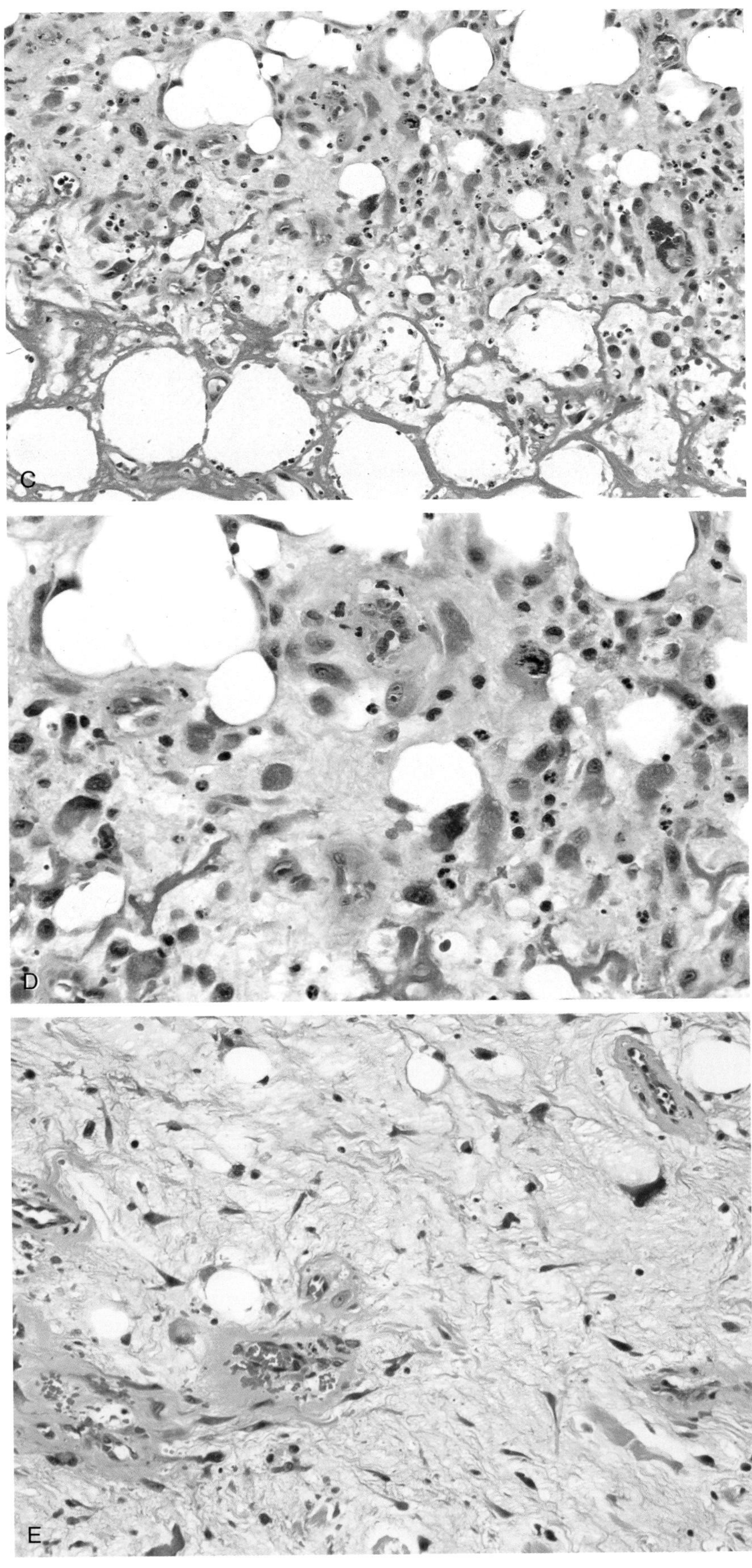

FIGURE 8-34, cont'd. (C) Fibrinous material with an adjacent reactive fibroblastic zone. Some of the fibroblasts are round and similar to those seen in proliferative fasciitis. (D) High-power view of atypical fibroblasts in a reactive zone of ischemic fasciitis. (E) Myxoid zone in ischemic fasciitis.

resemble the ganglion-like cells seen in proliferative fasciitis or myositis. The proliferation is usually paucicellular; although mitotic figures may be numerous, they are not atypical. The peripheral vessels may contain fibrin thrombi and secondary acute inflammation with perivascular hyalinization. Multivacuolated muciphages can be seen in the myxoid zones and may mimic the lipoblasts of myxoid liposarcoma.

Immunohistochemically, the atypical fibroblast-like cells often stain for actin, desmin, or both markers, whereas stains for S-100 protein and cytokeratins are consistently negative.[82]

Differential Diagnosis

In more than one-third of reported cases of ischemic fasciitis, a malignant diagnosis is seriously considered.[79,80,82] Although the multinodular appearance with central necrosis is reminiscent of *epithelioid sarcoma*, the latter typically occurs on the distal extremity of young patients and is composed of cells with prominent cytoplasmic eosinophilia and cytokeratin immunoreactivity with loss of INI1 expression. *Myxoid liposarcoma* is also a consideration, but ischemic fasciitis lacks the organized plexiform vasculature typical of myxoid liposarcoma. Furthermore, although multivacuolated muciphages may be seen, true lipoblasts are not identified. *Myxofibrosarcoma* lacks the zonation of ischemic fasciitis and the degenerative and reactive features, such as cells with smudgy chromatin, fat necrosis, hemosiderin deposition, and fibrin thrombi.

Discussion

Ischemic fasciitis, at least those cases associated with immobility, is probably related to intermittent soft tissue ischemia with subsequent tissue breakdown and regenerative changes. Most lesions develop in areas where the subcutaneous tissue lies in close apposition to bone. Histologically, the zonal quality is similar to that seen in other reactive fibroblastic and myofibroblastic proliferations. As suggested by Perosio and Weiss,[79] the pathogenesis is probably similar to that of a decubitus ulcer, except that the ischemia may be less severe or of an intermittent nature and does not lead to breakdown of the overlying skin. However, alternative mechanisms likely also play a role because not all cases are associated with debilitation or immobility.[82] Although local recurrences have been described (presumably related to incomplete excision and regrowth as a result of the underlying ischemic process), most patients are cured by conservative excision, supporting its benign nature.[79,80,82] Awareness of this entity should allow the pathologist to avert a misdiagnosis of sarcoma and guide the clinical measures necessary to prevent subsequent recurrence or progression.

FIBROMA OF TENDON SHEATH

Fibroma of tendon sheath is a slowly growing, dense, fibrous nodule that is firmly attached to the tendon sheath and is found most frequently in the hands and feet. This lesion seems to evolve by way of a fasciitis-like proliferation that eventually hyalinizes, giving rise to a hypocellular nodule that characterizes the typical case. Its lobular configuration resembles that of a giant-cell tumor of tendon sheath, but it is much less cellular and lacks the polymorphic features of the latter lesion.

TABLE 8-7 Anatomic Distribution of 165 Cases of Fibroma of the Tendon Sheath

SITE	NO. OF PATIENTS	PERCENTAGE (%)
Upper extremities	145	88
Fingers	79	
Hands	41	
Wrist	17	
Forearm	4	
Elbow	3	
Upper arm	1	
Lower extremities	18	11
Knee	7	
Foot	5	
Ankle	3	
Toes	2	
Leg	1	
Trunk	2	1
Chest	1	
Back	1	

Data from Chung and Enzinger[83] and Pulitzer et al.[88]

Fibroma of tendon sheath is usually small (less than 2 cm) and typically has been present for some time and has increased slowly in size, often over many years. It is found most commonly in adults of 20 to 50 years of age and is more than twice as common in men as in women.[83] Almost all of these tumors arise in the extremities; the upper extremity is more commonly affected than the lower extremity (Table 8-7). The most common sites of involvement in the upper extremity are the fingers (especially the thumb, index, and middle fingers), hand, and wrist, with only rare involvement of the forearm, elbow, or upper arm.[84] Sites of involvement in the lower extremity are the knee, foot, ankle, and rarely the toe or leg.[85,86] Some cases arise as an intra-articular mass that can restrict the normal range of motion.[87] As many as one-third of patients have slight tenderness, pain, or limited range of motion of the affected digit. A history of antecedent trauma has been reported in approximately 9% of cases.[83,88]

Pathologic Findings

Most lesions are well circumscribed and have a lobular configuration, similar to that of a giant-cell tumor of tendon sheath. Actual attachment to a tendon or tendon sheath is visible in most but not all cases. On a cut section, the lesions are usually uniform in appearance, with a gray or pearly white color. Occasionally, grossly myxoid and cystic areas are seen.

Microscopically, the lesion appears well circumscribed and lobulated or multilobulated and is composed of spindle-shaped cells resembling fibroblasts with elongated nuclei, fine chromatin, and small basophilic nucleoli. Most lesions lack cytologic atypia, although striking nuclear pleomorphism has been described (so-called pleomorphic fibroma of tendon sheath).[89] In these unusual cases, the mitotic index is not commensurate with the degree of nuclear pleomorphism, suggesting a degenerative phenomenon. Stellate-shaped cells may also

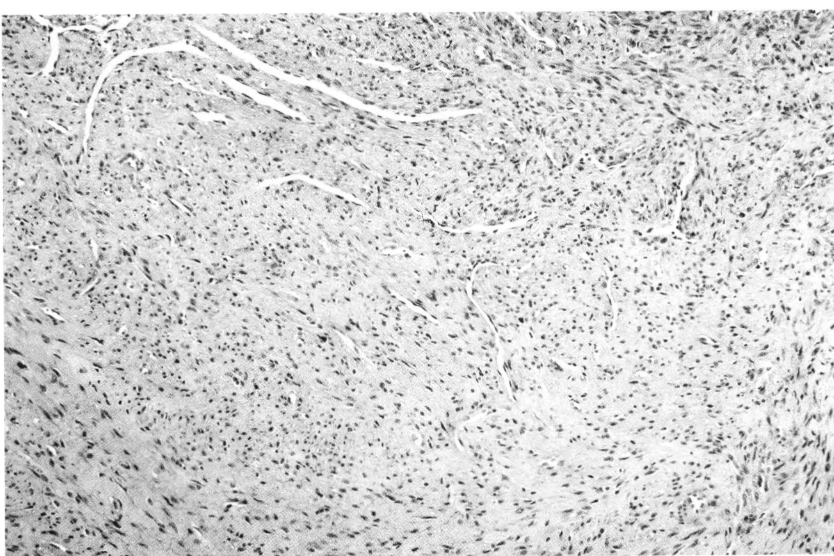

FIGURE 8-35. Cellular zone of a fibroma of the tendon sheath, including cleft-like spaces.

be present, particularly in myxoid zones. Most lesions are hypocellular, with widely spaced cytologically bland cells deposited in a densely eosinophilic hyalinized collagenous stroma. However, some have zones of increased cellularity in which the cells are arranged in either a storiform or fascicular growth pattern closely resembling nodular fasciitis (Figs. 8-35 and 8-36). These cellular areas always blend with less cellular collagenous areas. Not uncommonly, small myxoid zones are interspersed between the densely collagenized zones. A characteristic feature is the presence of elongated cleft-like spaces lined by flattened cells, particularly at the periphery of the lobules. These cells have been reported to stain for von Willebrand factor, suggesting that the spaces are truly vascular.[90] Some lesions contain multinucleated giant cells, but xanthoma cells and hemosiderin deposits are not present. Osteocartilaginous metaplasia may be seen but is not common.[91]

Immunohistochemical Findings

The lesional cells express muscle markers, including muscle-specific and smooth muscle actin, without staining for desmin.[92] In addition, stains for markers (albeit relatively nonspecific) of monocytic-histiocytic differentiation, including CD68 (KP1) and HAM 56, may also be positive in some cases. Given the overlapping immunophenotype with giant-cell tumor of tendon sheath, some authors have proposed that fibroma and giant-cell tumor of tendon sheath represent histogenetically related lesions that are at the extremes in a spectrum of histiocytic-fibroblastic-myofibroblastic differentiation[92,93]; however, this is doubtful given the fact that these tumors rarely contain areas resembling a giant-cell tumor. Fibromas of tendon sheath do not express clusterin, a marker found in almost all examples of giant-cell tumor of tendon sheath.

Differential Diagnosis

The typical fibroma of tendon sheath, composed of a hypocellular proliferation of bland spindle cells deposited in a densely collagenized stroma, is characteristic and unlikely to be confused with other entities; lesions that show more cellular zones may be confused with *fibrous histiocytoma* or *nodular fasciitis*. Pulitzer et al.[88] reported that up to one-fourth of their cases had areas that were indistinguishable from nodular fasciitis. There are, however, minor differences in location and manner of presentation of the two lesions.

Although fibroma of tendon sheath and *giant-cell tumor of tendon sheath* arise in similar locations and resemble each other grossly, the giant-cell tumor of tendon sheath is composed of a proliferation of round cells (in contrast to spindle-shaped cells) and usually contains more multinucleated giant cells as well as xanthoma cells and hemosiderin deposits. Interestingly, translocations involving the long arm of chromosome 2 have been described in fibroma of tendon sheath (t[2;11][q31-32;q12]) as well as giant-cell tumor of tendon sheath, but the breakpoints were found to be different (2q31-32 and 2q35-36, respectively). Sciot et al.[94] also reported a case of fibroma of tendon sheath with an 11q12 alteration. Aberrations of *colony stimulating factor 1*, which are characteristic of giant-cell tumor of tendon sheath, have not been detected in fibroma of tendon sheath.

Rare fibromas of tendon sheath show striking nuclear pleomorphism and may be confused with a pleomorphic sarcoma. However, the latter is characterized by greater cellularity and mitotic activity, including atypical mitoses, as well as a more pronounced storiform growth pattern. Finally, simply based upon location, one could consider an *inflammatory myxohyaline tumor*, but this entity is characterized by an intimate admixture of inflammatory, myxoid, and hyalinized zones as well as bizarre cells resembling Reed-Sternberg cells or cytomegalovirus-infected cells.

Discussion

Fibroma of tendon sheath is a benign process that can recur but does not metastasize. In the series by Chung and Enzinger,[83] 13 of 54 patients (24%) with follow-up information developed local recurrences, including 3 patients with two

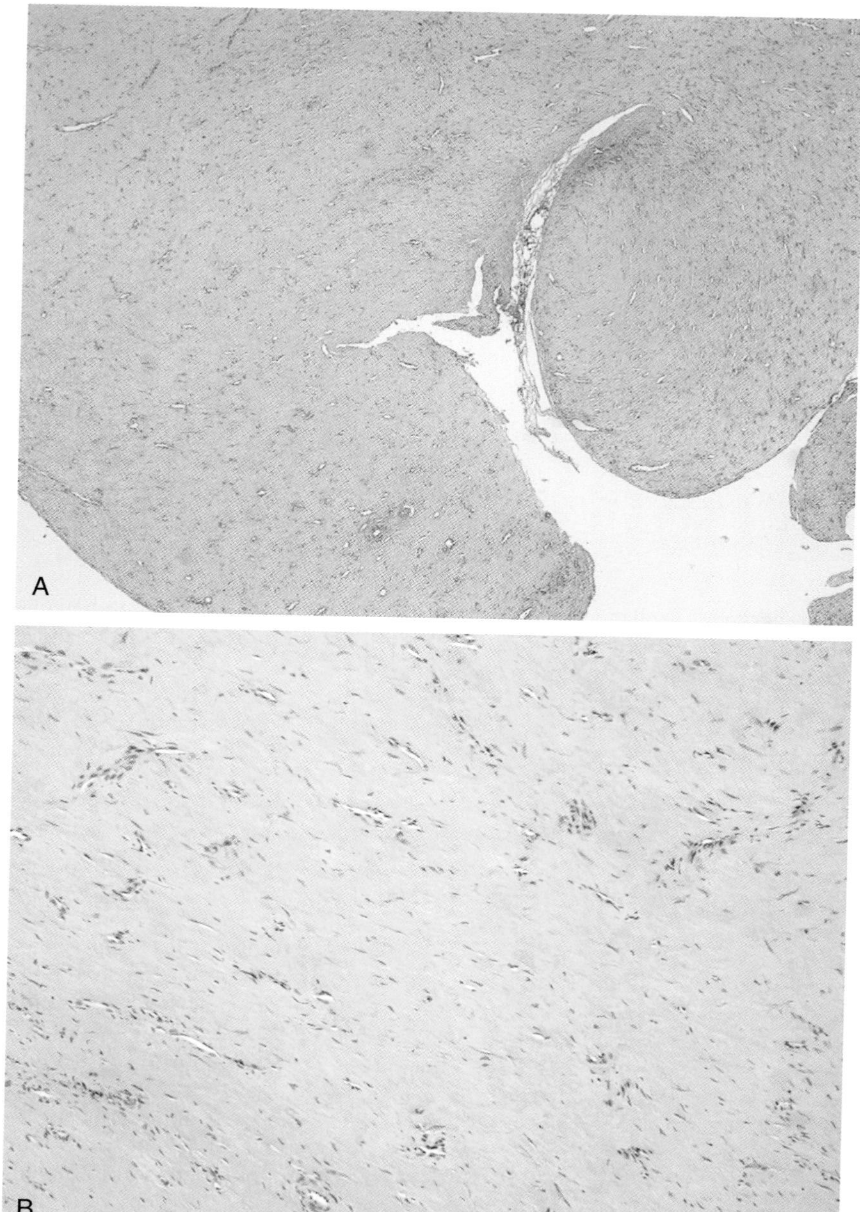

FIGURE 8-36. Fibroma of tendon sheath. (A) Low-power view showing a circumscription. (B) Hypocellular zone typical of this tumor.

recurrences. Local excision and re-excision of recurrences is the treatment of choice.

The initial, transient cellular phase resembling nodular fasciitis strongly suggests that these are reactive lesions. Friction inherent in the location of the lesion or vascular impairment may incite ongoing sclerosis. The possibility that a minority of fibromas arise secondary to hyalinization of benign mesenchymal tumors cannot be totally discounted and might account for the rare reports of clonality.

PLEOMORPHIC FIBROMA OF THE SKIN

Pleomorphic fibroma involving the skin is an uncommon entity that shares histologic features with pleomorphic fibroma of tendon sheath, particularly the presence of large pleomorphic, hyperchromatic cells deposited in a collagenized stroma. Clinically, most patients present with a slowly growing, asymptomatic, solitary lesion that appears as a flesh-colored, non-ulcerated, dome-shaped papule. These lesions most commonly involve the papillary and reticular dermis of the extremities, followed by the trunk and the head and neck.[95-98] Some arise in a subungual location.[99] The tumor usually arises in adults, with a peak incidence during the fifth decade of life; women are affected slightly more commonly than men. The lesion is almost always small (<2 cm) and clinically is often mistaken for a nevus, neurofibroma, or hemangioma.

Grossly, the tumor is well circumscribed and involves the papillary and reticular dermis, resulting in a dome-shaped or polypoid lesion covered by a thin, non-ulcerated epidermis, often associated with an epidermal collarette. Histologically, it is sparsely cellular and composed predominantly of thick, haphazardly arranged collagen. The characteristic feature is the presence of scattered spindle-shaped or stellate cells, including multinucleated giant cells with large pleomorphic, hyperchromatic nuclei and small nucleoli (Fig. 8-37). Mitotic figures are rare, but occasionally an atypical mitotic figure is seen.[96] The stroma may show focal or (rarely) diffuse myxoid change.[99,100] Adnexal structures are generally not found, and there may be a sparse intralesional lymphoplasmacytic infiltrate.

Immunohistochemically, the cells show variable immunoreactivity for smooth muscle and muscle-specific actin, suggesting myofibroblastic differentiation.[97] Some also stain for CD34 and CD99,[101] but immunostains for S-100 protein, desmin, and cytokeratin are negative.[102]

The differential diagnosis includes other cutaneous neoplasms characterized by the presence of pleomorphic cells. *Atypical fibroxanthoma* most commonly occurs as a rapidly growing lesion on sun-damaged skin of the face of elderly patients. It is characterized by a much higher cellularity, cells with foamy cytoplasm, and a large number of typical and atypical mitotic figures. *Dermatofibroma with atypical cells*, also referred to as *dermatofibroma with monster cells*, *atypical cutaneous fibrous histiocytoma*, *pseudosarcomatous dermatofibroma*, and *atypical (pseudosarcomatous) cutaneous histiocytoma*, is a more densely cellular proliferation of pleomorphic cells, including cells with hemosiderin and foamy cytoplasm. In addition, most lesions have foci of typical fibrous histiocytoma. *Giant-cell fibroblastoma* most commonly occurs as an infiltrative lesion on the trunk or extremities of patients less than 10 years of age. It is characterized by pseudovascular or angiectatic spaces lined by atypical spindle cells and floret-like giant cells. The absence of S-100 protein in pleomorphic

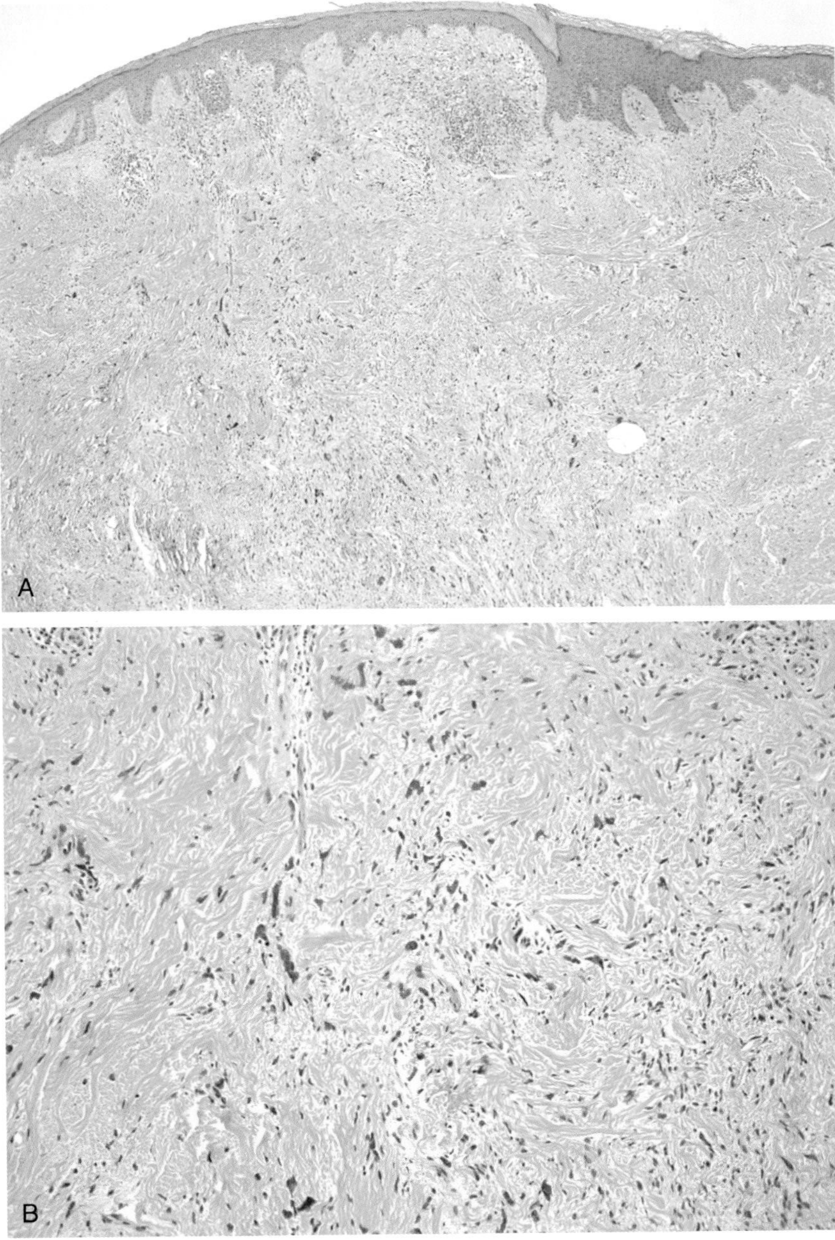

FIGURE 8-37. Pleomorphic fibroma of the skin. (A) Low-power view. (B) Cellular zone with pleomorphic cells deposited in a collagenous matrix. *Continued*

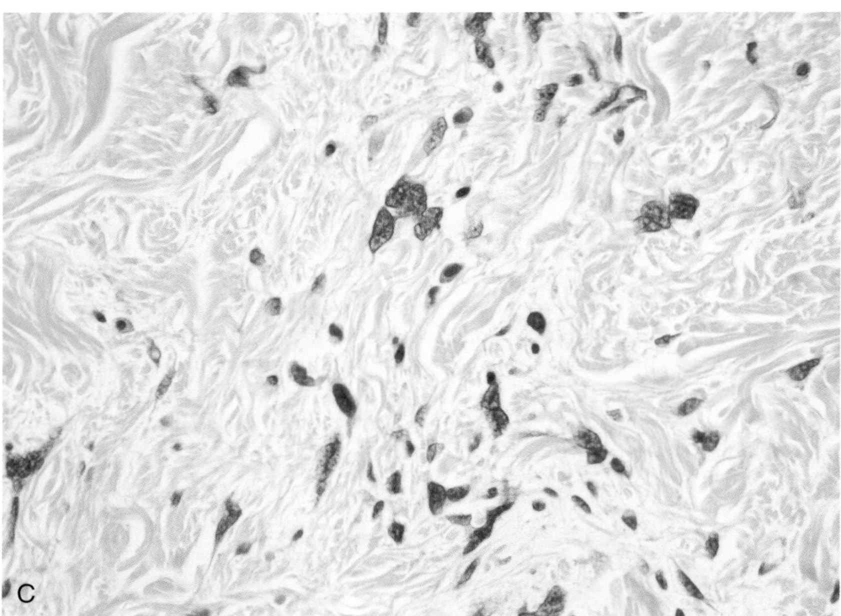

FIGURE 8-37, cont'd. (C) High-power view of pleomorphic cells.

fibroma of skin helps distinguish it from benign peripheral nerve sheath tumors with atypia (*ancient schwannoma* and *neurofibroma with atypia*).

Simple excision of this lesion is generally curative, and local recurrences are quite rare.

NUCHAL-TYPE FIBROMA

Nuchal fibroma is an uncommon fibrocollagenous proliferation that typically arises in the cervicodorsal region in middle-aged adults.[103,104] However, it is increasingly clear that this lesion is not restricted to a nuchal location, and up to 30% arise in an extra-nuchal site (buttocks, extremities, lumbosacral region) and, as such, is preferably referred to as *nuchal-type fibroma*.[104-107] Patients typically present with a solitary unencapsulated subcutaneous mass. Regardless of anatomic site, nuchal-type fibroma is significantly more common in men, with a peak incidence during the third through fifth decades of life.[104] This process is strongly associated with diabetes mellitus because up to 44% of patients with this lesion have diabetes.[104,106,107] Although there are earlier reports of nuchal-type fibroma associated with Gardner syndrome, there are enough clinical and pathologic differences to distinguish nuchal-type fibroma from Gardner-associated fibroma. The latter lesion will be discussed separately in the chapter.

Grossly, nuchal-type fibroma is unencapsulated and arises in the subcutaneous tissue, with minimal extension into the deep dermis, and, occasionally, the superficial skeletal muscle. Most are 1 to 6 cm in greatest dimension at the time of excision, and the mass is usually present for several years before surgical excision.

Microscopically, nuchal-type fibroma is quite bland; it is a hypocellular or almost completely acellular, densely collagenized mass with scattered mature fibroblasts and islands of mature adipose tissue of varying size (Fig. 8-38). The mass is ill-defined, with some radiation of collagenous septa into the subcutaneous fat and deep dermis. Small nerves that are often proliferated are frequently entrapped by this fibrous proliferation, and there is often an encasement of adnexal structures. The spindle cells usually stain for CD34 and CD99 but are negative for smooth muscle actin and desmin.[104]

This lesion most commonly is mistaken for a *fibrolipoma*. Unlike nuchal-type fibroma, fibrolipoma is well circumscribed and encapsulated, has a greater proportion of the lesion composed of mature adipose tissue, and lacks entrapped nerves. The subcutaneous location and paucity of cells permit the exclusion of *extra-abdominal fibromatosis*. The *nuchal fibrocartilaginous pseudotumor* arises in the posterior aspect of the base of the neck at the junction of the nuchal ligament and the deep cervical fascia and probably develops as a reaction to soft tissue injury.[108,109] Unlike the former lesion, nuchal-type fibroma lacks an association with ligaments, occurs superficially to the fascia, and lacks cartilaginous metaplasia. *Elastofibroma* typically occurs in the deep soft tissue in the vicinity of the inferomedial portion of the scapula. Nuchal-type fibroma is benign but may recur if incompletely excised.[104]

GARDNER-ASSOCIATED FIBROMA

As mentioned previously, Gardner-associated fibroma has many features that overlap with nuchal-type fibroma, but there are also enough distinctive features to consider it separately. This lesion was first highlighted in a series of 11 cases in young patients by Wehrli et al.[110] in which an association with Gardner syndrome (FAP) was clearly established. Subsequently, a number of other reports confirmed these initial observations and the association of this benign fibromatous lesion with a polyposis syndrome.[111-113] The largest series was published by Coffin et al.[114] in 2007, which meticulously described 45 patients with 57 fibromas, highlighting the association with desmoids and FAP.

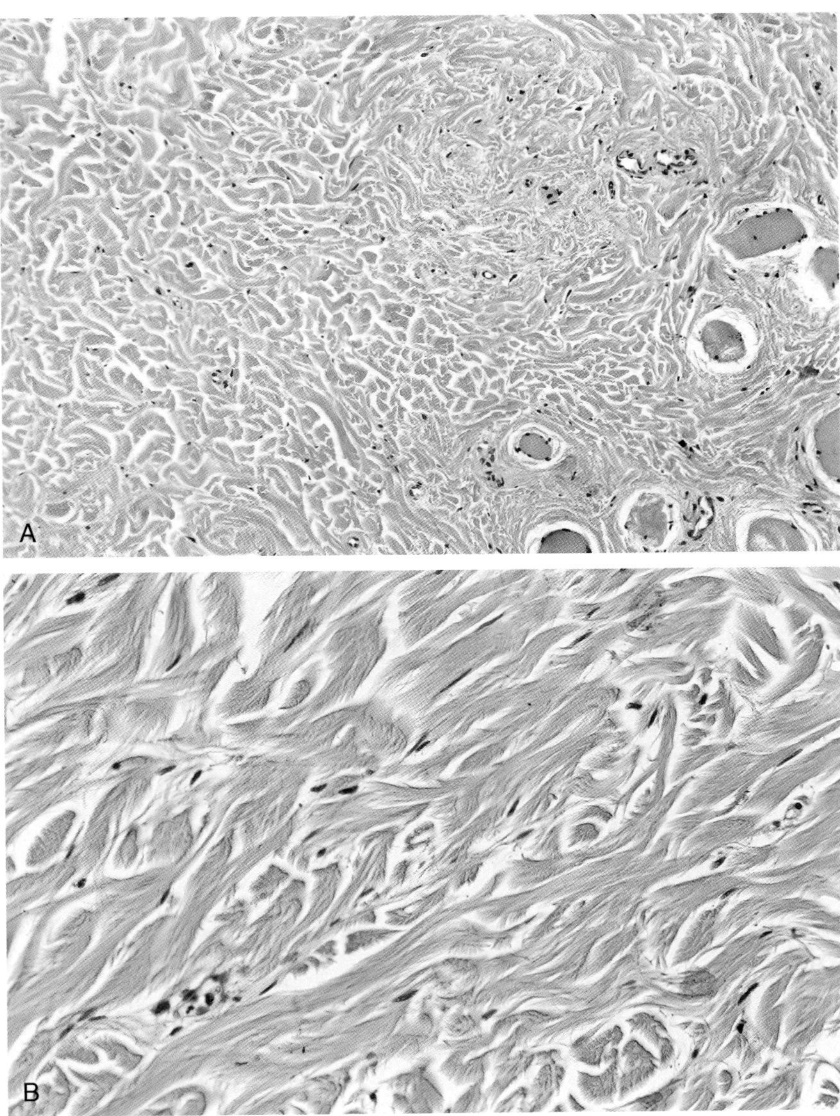

FIGURE 8-38. Nuchal-type fibroma. (A) Low-power view of nuchal-type fibroma, characterized by a hypocellular, densely collagenized mass with scattered fibroblasts among skeletal muscle fibers. (B) Scattered fibroblasts deposited in densely collagenized stroma.

Clinical Findings

Unlike nuchal-type fibroma, which has a peak incidence in the third through fifth decades of life, Gardner-associated fibroma usually arises in much younger patients. In the study by Coffin et al.,[114] patients ranged in age from 2 months to 36 years, but the mean age was 5 years, and 78% presented in the first decade of life. Although nuchal-type fibroma shows a striking predilection for men, there is only a slight male predominance in patients with Gardner-associated fibroma. Most lesions are solitary, but some patients have multiple lesions. For example, in the study by Coffin et al.,[114] 7 of 45 patients had more than one fibroma with a range of two to eight lesions. The most common location is the back and paraspinal region, accounting for about 60% of all cases. The head-and-neck region and extremities each account for approximately 15% of cases, followed by the chest and abdomen.

The close relationship between Gardner-associated fibroma with desmoids and FAP is fascinating and is nicely highlighted by the study by Coffin et al.[114] (Box 8-1). Although there was incomplete follow-up information in a substantial subgroup, at least 69% of patients were found to have FAP, including some in which the fibroma was the sentinel event, an observation previously made by Wehrli et al.[110,114] Desmoids were found in eight patients (19%), including four with known FAP.[114] One other patient had familial desmoids. The desmoids were observed before, subsequent, and concurrently to the Gardner-associated fibromas.

Pathologic Findings

Grossly, Gardner-associated fibromas are poorly demarcated soft tissue masses with a rubbery texture and white cut surface. When adipose tissue is a conspicuous component, the cut surface may have softer yellow areas. In those rare cases where this lesion is associated with a desmoid, the latter area tends to be more circumscribed and has a whorled cut surface. Tumor size can range from less than 1 cm to up to 12 cm, with a mean size of approximately 4 cm. Histologically, sheets of densely collagenized tissue with a sparse population of bland spindle cells interspersed with mature lobules of adipose tissue are seen (Fig. 8-39). There is some entrapment of nerves, blood vessels, and fat at the periphery of the lesion, but increased numbers of small nerve bundles identified in nuchal-type fibroma are not seen.

BOX 8-1 Clinicopathologic Features of 45 Patients with Gardner-Associated Fibromas

Age at diagnosis of GAF: 2 months to 36 years (mean: 5 years)
- 29% ≤1 year
- 78% ≤9 years

Male/female ratio: 25/20

Number of GAF
- Solitary: 38 patients
- Multiple: 7 patients

Sites of GAF
- Back/paraspinal: 61%
- Head and neck: 14%
- Extremities: 14%
- Chest/abdomen: 11%

Desmoids
- Found in 8/45 (18%)
- Known FAP with desmoids and GAF in 4/8 (50%)
- Familial desmoids and GAF in 1/8 (12%)

Modified from Coffin CM, Hornick JL, Zhou H, et al. Gardner fibroma: a clinicopathologic and immunohistochemical analysis of 45 patients with 57 fibromas. *Am J Surg Pathol* 2007;31(3):410–6.

Immunohistochemical Findings

Like nuchal-type fibroma, the lesion usually also stains for CD34 and often CD99.[104,115] Many also express β-catenin. In the study by Coffin et al.,[114] 64% of cases expressed this antigen, including 10 of 16 cases that showed diffuse nuclear immunoreactivity. In their study, the β-catenin immunoreactivity seemed to be far more robust in freshly cut sections when compared to stored unstained sections. Of the 16 β-catenin positive cases, 9 had FAP, and no information about FAP would be ascertained in 6 cases. Among the nine patients whose tumors did not stain for this antigen, one had known FAP. The presence of β-catenin nuclear immunoreactivity reflects either an adenomatous polyposis coli (*APC*) mutation or activating mutations in β-catenin, therefore serving as an adjunct for recognizing an *APC*-associated neoplasm.[116] Interestingly, Coffin et al.[114] also found universal immunoexpression of both cyclin-D1 and *C-MYC*, both of which are *Wnt* target genes activated by nuclear β-catenin.

Discussion

Gardner-associated fibromas are benign but may recur if incompletely excised. These lesions may be associated with not only synchronous or metachronous desmoids, but also, on rare occasion, they may transform into a desmoid imparting an even higher rate of local recurrence.[117] Clearly, the importance of recognizing this lesion lies in its association with FAP, sometimes arising years before other manifestations of this syndrome.

ELASTOFIBROMA

Elastofibroma, an unusual fibroelastic pseudotumor, is most commonly encountered in elderly persons; it arises chiefly from the connective tissue between the inferomedial portion

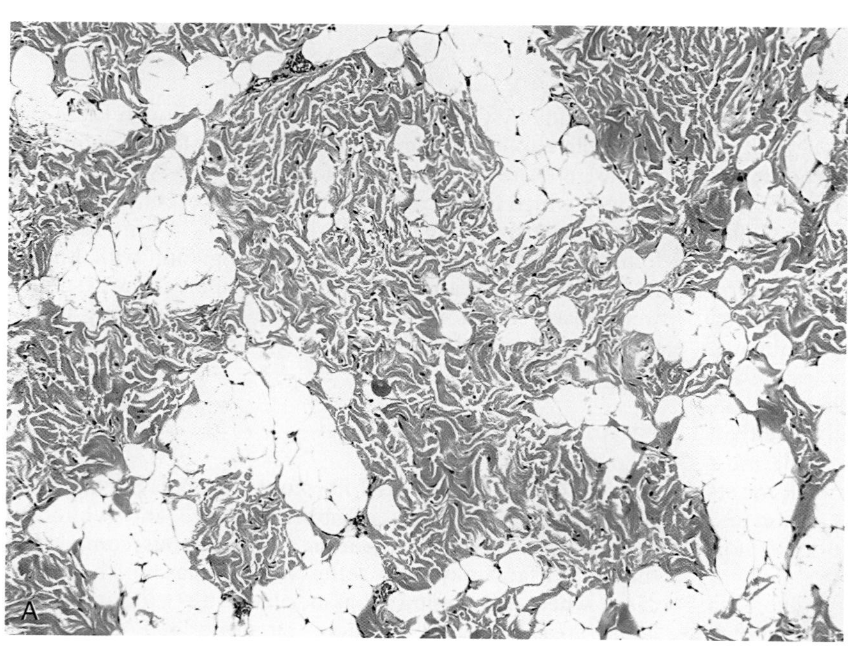

FIGURE 8-39. (A) Low-magnification view of a Gardner-associated fibroma showing interdigitation of mature fat and dense collagen.

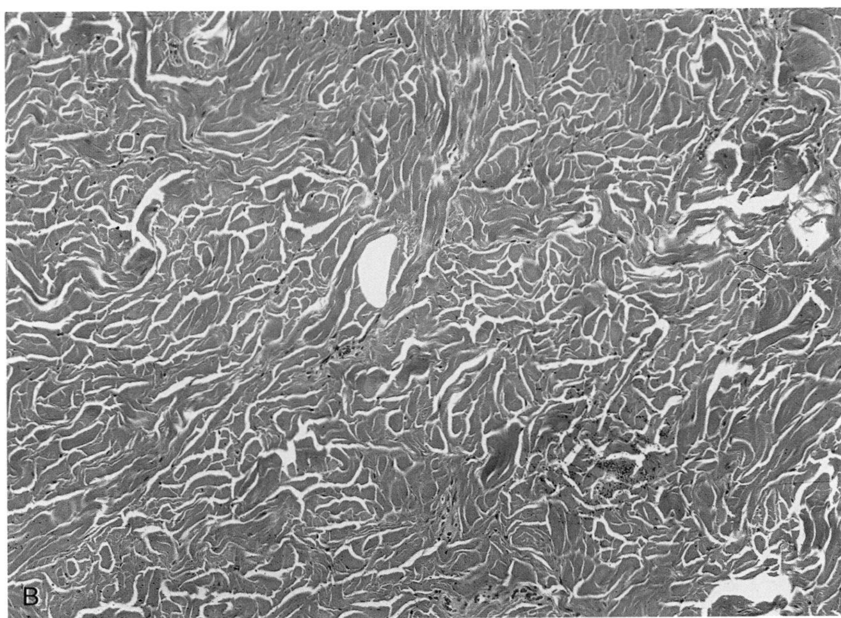

FIGURE 8-39, cont'd. (B) Densely collagenous area of Gardner-associated fibroma.

of the scapula and the chest wall. Originally described by Järvi and Saxén[118] in 1961 as elastofibroma dorsi, it has become increasingly apparent that identical lesions may be found in extrascapular locations; therefore, the term *elastofibroma* is preferred.

Clinical Findings

Most patients are elderly, with a peak incidence during the sixth and seventh decades of life[119]; only rare lesions have been described in children.[120] Women are affected almost four times as often as men. Many patients have a history of intensive, often repetitive manual labor. Although thought to be uncommon, several autopsy studies have shown elastofibroma and pre-elastofibroma-like changes in 13% to 17% of elderly individuals.[121,122] The most common presentation is that of a slowly growing, deep-seated mass that only rarely causes pain, tenderness, limitation of motion, or scapular snapping.[123] Most arise from the connective tissue between the lower portion of the scapula and the chest wall, deep to the rhomboid major and latissimus dorsi muscles, with attachment to the periosteum and ligaments in the region of the sixth, seventh, and eighth ribs. A significant percentage of patients have bilateral lesions[124]; in the review of the literature by Martinez-Hernandez et al.,[124] about 50% of patients had bilateral lesions. Similarly, Naylor et al.[125] described the radiologic findings in 12 patients with elastofibroma; all patients in whom both sides of the chest wall were imaged had bilateral elastofibromas, suggesting subclinical bilateral involvement in many cases. This lesion has been increasingly recognized by radiologists on CT and MRI as a poorly circumscribed, heterogeneous soft tissue mass with attenuation of signal intensity similar to that of skeletal muscle; it is interlaced with fat, allowing a presumptive diagnosis.[126,127] Numerous extrascapular sites have been reported, particularly in the gastrointestinal tract (colon, stomach), where this change may be associated with an array of inflammatory conditions.[128-130]

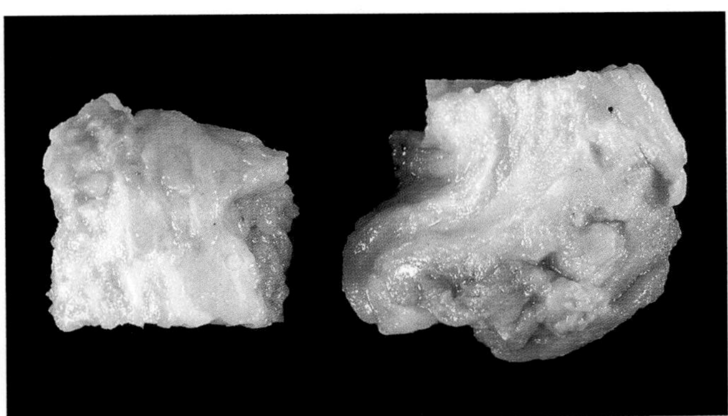

FIGURE 8-40. Elastofibroma. There is an intimate admixture of firm collagenous tissue with fat.

Pathologic Findings

The mass is usually ill-defined, oblong or spherical, firm, and ranges from 5 to 10 cm. The cut surface has a variegated appearance with small areas of adipose tissue interposed between gray-white fibrous areas, occasionally with cystic change (Fig. 8-40). Not infrequently, the surgeon is concerned about the possibility of a sarcoma given the irregular margins and infiltration of skeletal muscle or periosteum.

On microscopic examination, the tumor-like mass consists of a mixture of intertwining swollen, eosinophilic collagen and elastic fibers in about equal proportions associated with occasional fibroblasts, small amounts of interstitial mucoid material, and variably sized aggregates of mature fat cells (Fig. 8-41). Typically, the elastic fibers have a degenerated, beaded appearance or are fragmented into small flower-like, serrated disks or globules (chenille bodies) with a distinct linear arrangement.

Elastic stains reveal deeply staining, branched, and unbranched fibers that have a central dense core and an

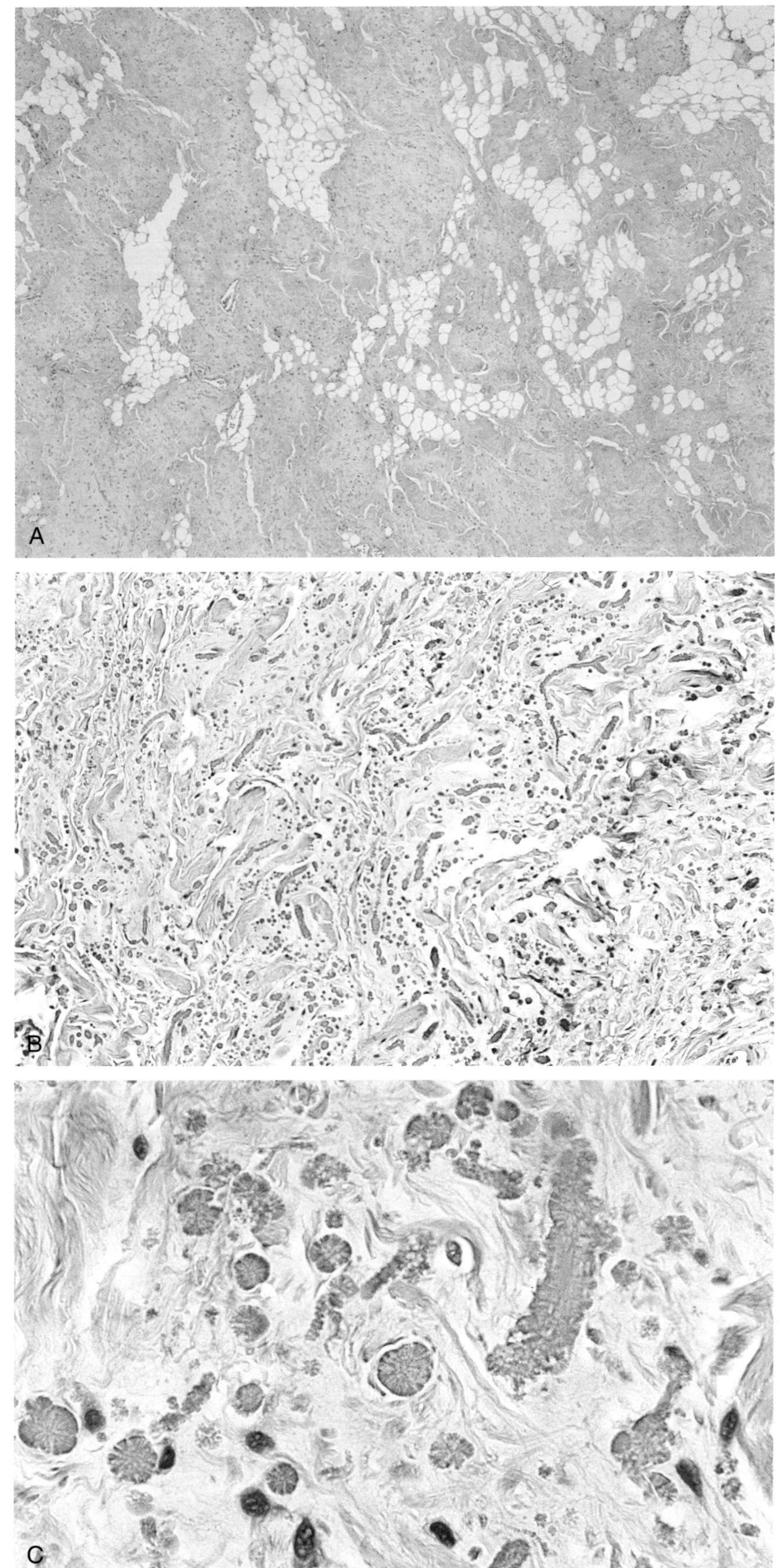

FIGURE 8-41. Low-power view typical of elastofibroma. (A) Low-power view of typical elastofibroma. (B) Altered elastic fibers in a collagenous matrix. (C) Elastic fibers in a cross-section showing a characteristic serrated edge (petaloid globules).

irregular moth-eaten or serrated margin (Figs. 8-42 and 8-43). The few spindle cells that are present are negative for smooth muscle actin, desmin, and S-100 protein.

Ultrastructurally, numerous electron-dense elongated and globular masses corresponding to the elastinophilic material seen on light microscopy are present in the collagenous stroma. A central core of more electron-lucent material resembling mature elastic tissue is surrounded by granular or fibrillary aggregations of electron-dense material resembling immature elastin or pre-elastin. The proximity of these aggregates to fibroblasts further supports a process of abnormal elastogenesis by these cells.[131]

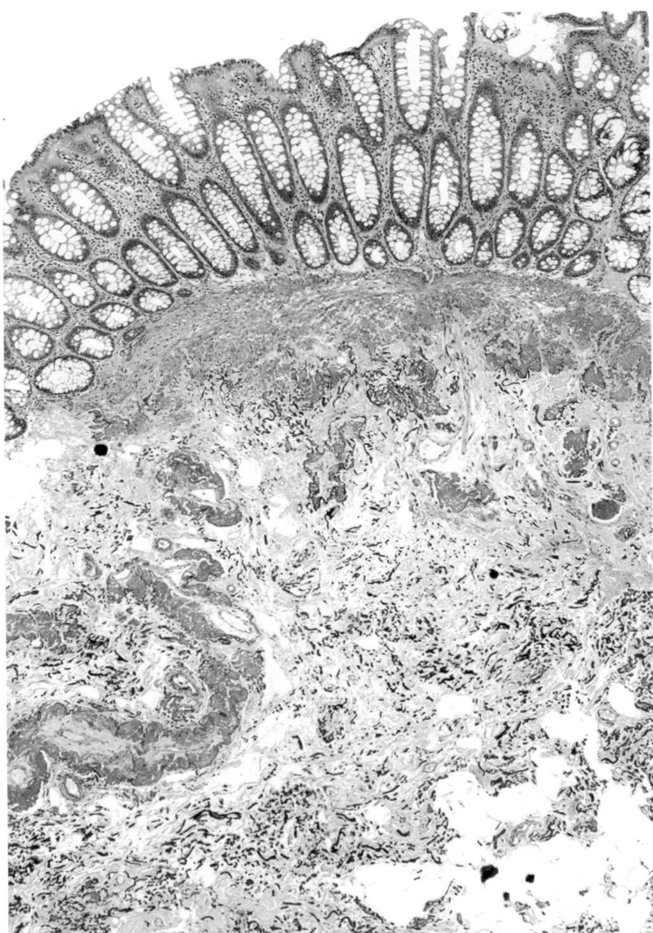

FIGURE 8-42. Verhoeff elastin stain shows elastic fibers in the submucosa of the rectum. This patient had a history of radiation therapy to this area.

Differential Diagnosis

The clinical and histologic features of elastofibroma are characteristic and are unlikely to be confused with those of other fibroblastic proliferations. De Nictolis et al.[132] described a case of an *elastofibrolipoma* arising in the mediastinum. Unlike elastofibroma, the elastofibrolipoma is well circumscribed, is surrounded by a fibrous capsule, and has a more conspicuous adipose component in both the central and peripheral portions of the tumor. In a report of elastofibromatous change of the rectal submucosa,[133] the lesion closely mimicked *amyloidosis*, although elastic and Congo red stains allowed this distinction.

Discussion

The etiology of the abnormal elastic fibers has been debated since its initial description by Järvi and Saxén.[118] Whereas some have suggested that these fibers are derived from the elastotic degeneration of collagen fibers,[134] others believe that they are derived from a degeneration of preexisting elastic fibers or from disturbed elastic fibrillogenesis.[135] The preponderance of evidence suggests that elastofibroma is a degenerative pseudotumor that is the result of excessive formation of collagen and abnormal elastic fibers. Although friction

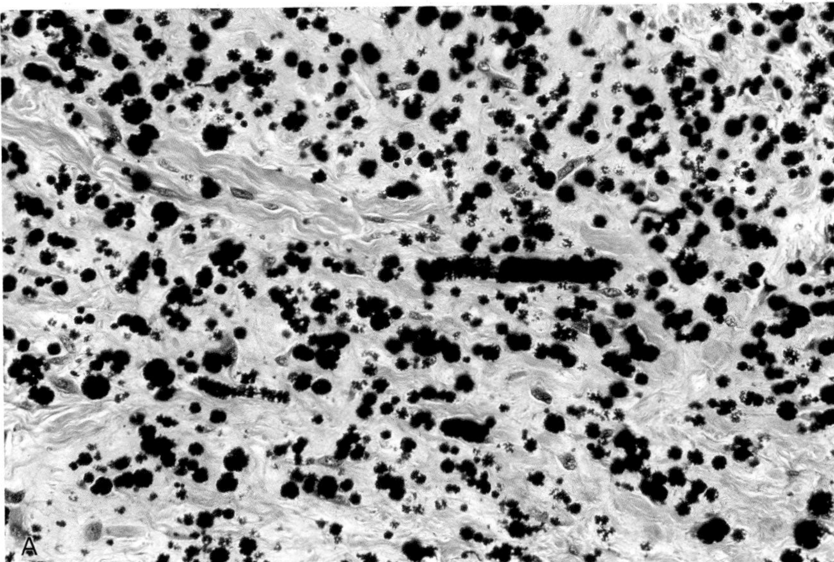

FIGURE 8-43. Elastofibroma. (A) Verhoeff elastin stain shows elongated and globoid elastic fibers.

Continued

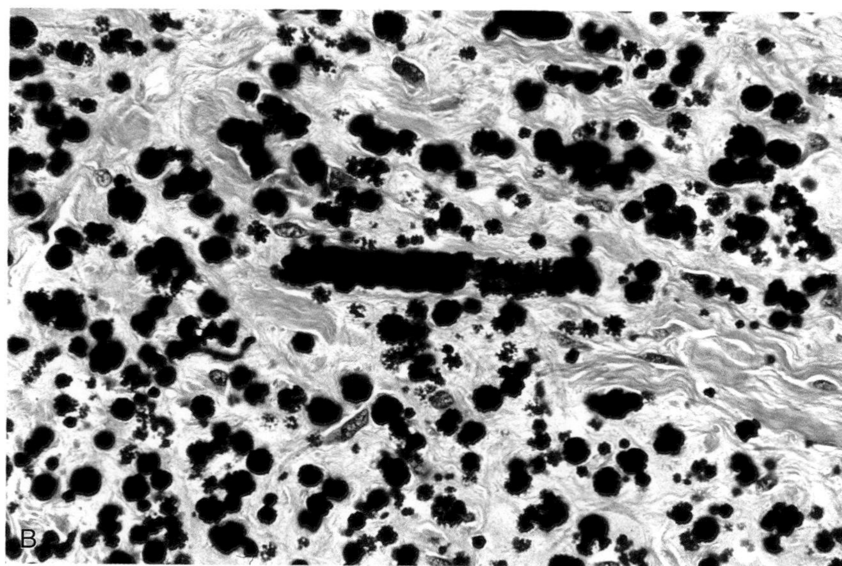

FIGURE 8-43, cont'd. (B) High-power view of Verhoeff elastin stain showing elastic fibers with a dense core.

between the inferior edge of the scapula and the underlying chest wall has been implicated as the cause of this abnormal elastogenesis, other factors may play a role, particularly for lesions arising in extrascapular sites. Interestingly, Nagamine et al.[136] reported that about one-third of the patients with this lesion in Okinawa occurred in patients with a family history of elastofibroma, suggesting a genetic predisposition. Others have found elastofibromas to arise in patients with other family members with this lesion.[137] A high-resolution, genome-wide analysis of two cases of elastofibroma showed losses on 1p, 13q, 19p, and 22q, among other alterations.[138] Others have found alterations of the short arm of chromosome 1[139-141] or gains in the region of Xq.[137]

Elastofibroma is a benign lesion and is best treated by conservative excision given that local recurrence is uncommon. This diagnosis can be made by fine-needle aspiration cytology or a core biopsy in the appropriate clinical and radiographic setting, thereby potentially avoiding additional unnecessary surgery. There are no reports of malignant transformation.[142]

NASOPHARYNGEAL ANGIOFIBROMA

Nasopharyngeal angiofibroma is a relatively uncommon, histologically benign fibrovascular tumor that occurs virtually exclusively in the nasopharynx of adolescent boys.[143] Although originally referred to as *juvenile nasopharyngeal angiofibroma*, some occur in adults, so this lesion is best referred to as simply *nasopharyngeal angiofibroma*.

Clinical Findings

Most of these lesions occur in adolescent boys and young men of 10 to 20 years of age. Almost all of these tumors occur in males, with only a few having been reported in females.[144] As its name implies, virtually all arise in the nasopharynx, although tumors of identical morphology may arise at extranasopharyngeal sites, including the maxillary and ethmoid sinuses and nasal septum.[145] To this point, extranasopharyngeal angiofibromas have been restricted to the head-and-neck region and arise in patients who are slightly older and more likely to be female.[146] Nasopharyngeal angiofibroma may also arise in patients with FAP,[147] although this association has been disputed, and some believe that these rare cases are nothing more than a fortuitous association.[148] Abraham et al.[149,150] have detected frequent β-catenin mutations in nasopharyngeal angiofibromas, resulting in diffuse intranuclear protein accumulation, but mutations in the *APC* gene have not been detected.[151]

Most patients present with nasal obstruction, facial deformity, or repeated epistaxis. In some cases, excessive hemorrhage requires blood transfusions and hospitalization and may even be life-threatening. This can initiate consumptive coagulopathy, although this is an extremely rare complication.[152] Other symptoms include headache, sinusitis, otitis media, mastoiditis, and dacryocystitis.[153]

A physical examination typically reveals a variably sized, red or red-blue, lobulated or polypoid mass that can be easily seen through the nose or underneath the palate with a nasopharyngeal mirror. Most lesions originate from the superolateral nasopharyngeal area and, with growth, extend into the posterior aspect of the nasal cavity and superiorly into the sphenoid sinus. As the tumor enlarges, it extends through the pterygopalatine foramen and grows laterally into the pterygomaxillary and infratemporal fossae. It can extend into the soft tissues of the cheek and the orbit and often erodes bone with extension into the middle or anterior cranial fossae.[154]

Radiologic techniques are useful for diagnostic and staging purposes. MRI and CT scans usually show a well-demarcated soft tissue mass in the nasopharynx with or without extension into the nasal cavity or paranasal sinuses, anterior bowing of the posterior wall of the maxillary sinus, and erosion of adjacent bony structures (Fig. 8-44). MRI appears to be superior to CT for demarcating the margin of the tumor from the surrounding soft tissue.[155] Angiography is useful for demonstrating the tumor's vascularity; transarterial embolization can be performed at the same time.[156] For cases in which the diagnosis remains in question following radiographic evaluation, a transnasal biopsy may be used to confirm the diagnosis, but this procedure should be performed in an operating room because significant hemorrhage requiring nasal packing or cautery may be encountered.[157]

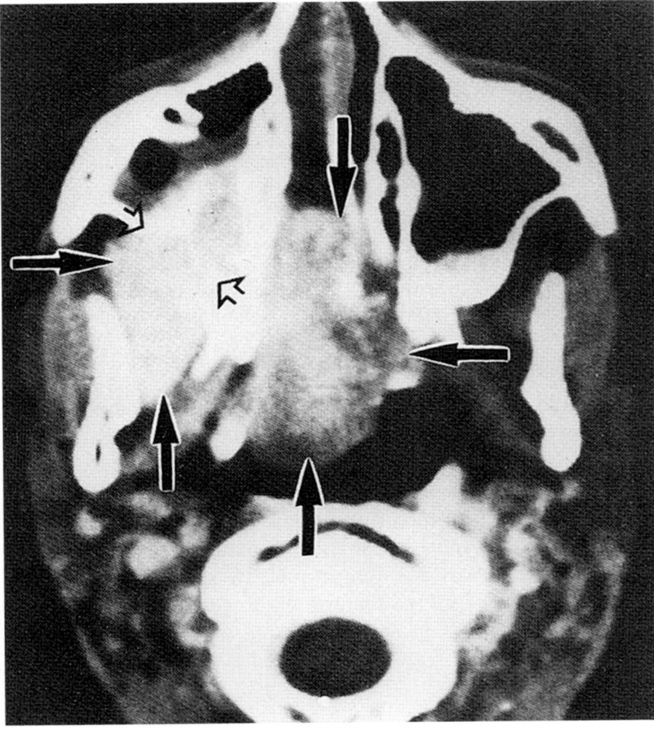

FIGURE 8-44. Nasopharyngeal angiofibroma involving the nasopharynx, nasal cavity, and right infratemporal fossa (large arrows) and eroding through the posterior wall of the right maxillary antrum (small arrows). *(From Chandler JR, Goulding R, Moskowitz L, et al. Nasopharyngeal angiofibromas: staging and management. Ann Otol Rhinol Laryngol 1984;93:322.)*

Pathologic Findings

The tumor is well circumscribed with a lobulated, smooth, glistening mucosal surface that may be focally ulcerated. The tissue is firm and rubbery; on a cut section, it has a spongy appearance as a result of the presence of numerous vascular spaces characteristic of this lesion.

Nasopharyngeal angiofibroma has a very consistent histologic appearance, with little variation from case to case, with numerous vascular channels surrounded by dense paucicellular fibrous tissue (Fig. 8-45). The cells in the fibrous tissue are cytologically bland and may be spindle or stellate in shape with nuclei that lack hyperchromasia and have small nucleoli and little mitotic activity (Fig. 8-46). The dense, fibrous stroma may show hyalinization or focal myxoid change, often with collagen fibers arranged in a parallel fashion. Mature fat entrapped within the lesion can occur but is unusual.[158] The vascular channels are slit-like or dilated and vary in number, configuration, and thickness. Some vessels are surrounded by few, if any, smooth muscle cells, whereas others show focal pad-like thickenings.[159] Peripherally located vessels are often larger and of the arterial type with visible elastic laminae. However, the smaller vessels in the central portion of the tumor typically lack elastic laminae, which may explain the propensity for spontaneous or surgically induced hemorrhage.[159] The nature and organization of the vessels have suggested to some that this lesion could represent a vascular malformation as opposed to a neoplastic process.[153]

Immunohistochemical Findings

Immunohistochemically, the endothelial cells lining the slit-like or dilated vessels stain for endothelial markers, including CD31 and CD34. The immediate perivascular cells show variable staining for smooth muscle actin, depending on the amount of perivascular smooth muscle.[160] The spindle and stellate-shaped cells deposited in the dense fibrous stroma show variable staining for myoid markers. As one might

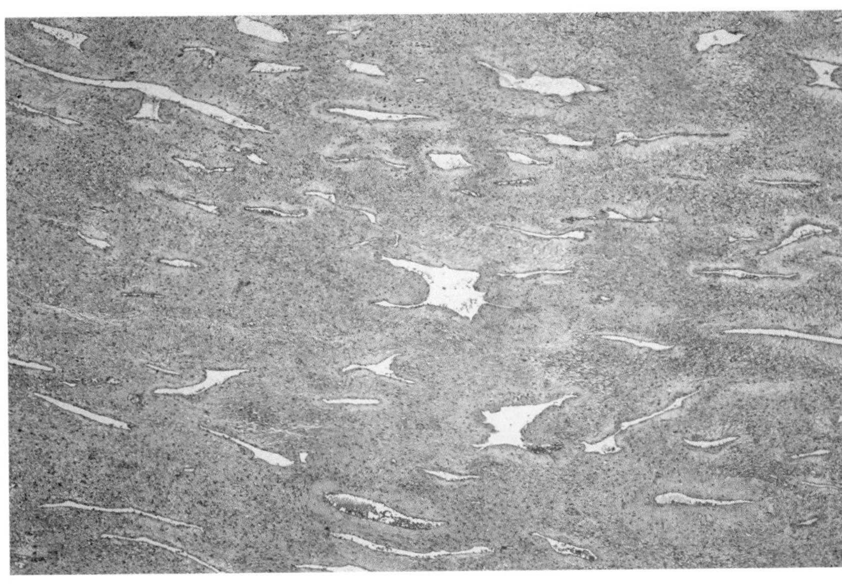

FIGURE 8-45. Nasopharyngeal angiofibroma consisting of dense fibrocollagenous tissue with interspersed vascular channels of varying caliber.

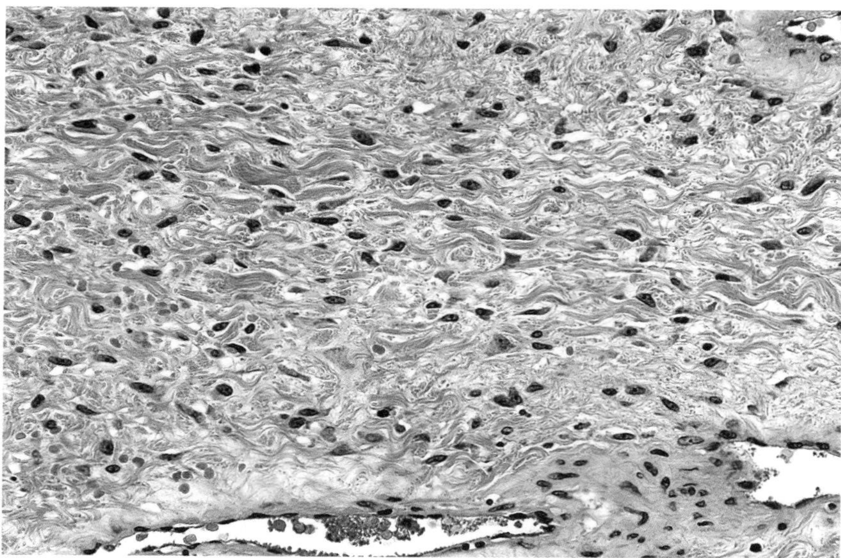

FIGURE 8-46. Nasopharyngeal angiofibroma composed of cytologically bland fibroblasts deposited in a dense collagenous stroma.

expect in a tumor that occurs virtually exclusively in males, androgen receptors have been detected in the nuclei of endothelial and stromal cells.[161] As mentioned previously, strong and diffuse nuclear immunoreactivity for β-catenin is identified in the spindle cells in virtually all cases.[149,162] Whereas some studies have found consistent expression of c-Kit (CD117), others have not.[163]

Discussion

Although nasopharyngeal angiofibroma is histologically benign, it may act in an aggressive fashion characterized by recurrences that can extend into and destroy adjacent bony structures. The likelihood of recurrence is most closely related to the adequacy of the initial surgical excision, which, in turn, depends on the tumor stage.[164] Other predictors of recurrence include tumor size and patient age, with a higher risk of recurrence in patients less than 18 years of age.[164] The type of surgical approach is dictated by the extent of the tumor, as determined by preoperative radiographic studies. For low-stage tumors, most propose a transnasal or intranasal endoscopic approach.[165] A transcranial approach may be more appropriate for tumors that have intracranial extension.[166] Preoperative transarterial embolization has been reported to result in decreased blood loss and a decreased rate of local recurrence.[156] Hormone therapy, including the use of anti-androgenic agents, has generally been ineffective. Some authors advocate the use of radiation therapy, particularly for tumors with intracranial extension,[167] but radiation may cause osteonecrosis and, rarely, postradiation sarcomas.

KELOID

Keloid is a benign dermal fibroproliferative process that occurs at sites of cutaneous injury and forms as a result of an abnormal wound healing process in genetically susceptible individuals.[168] It may be solitary or multiple and has a predilection for dark-skinned individuals.[169] Keloid (Greek: "claw-like") was named for its multiple extensions, which bestow on the lesion an imaginary crab-like appearance. There are, in addition to its common cicatricial forms, spontaneous or idiopathic forms of the condition, but these, too, are likely the result of some minor infection or injury in areas with increased skin tension. *Hypertrophic scars*, lesions that remain confined to the original wound site, should be distinguished from keloids because of their substantially lower recurrence rate.

Clinical Findings

Keloids usually manifest as well-circumscribed round, oval, or linear elevations of the skin and often extend with multiple processes into the surrounding areas. They may be asymptomatic but more often are described by the patient as being itchy, tender, or painful, possibly related to a small nerve fiber neuropathy secondary to the dense collagen.[170] In their earlier phase, keloids tend to be soft and erythematous; later, they become increasingly indurated and turn white. They are found more commonly above than below the waist and have a predilection for the face, shoulders, forearms, and hands. About half of spontaneous keloids occur as a transverse band in the presternal region, probably the result of a minor infection and increased skin tension in this region. In some patients, keloids are limited to one portion of the body; therefore, they may develop after piercing the earlobes for earrings but are absent in an appendectomy scar (Figs. 8-47 and 8-48). Patients who develop keloids at multiple sites are generally younger and more likely to have a positive family history than those with solitary keloids.[171] In addition, women seem to be more likely than men to develop multiple keloids.

Keloids are induced by minor infections (especially acne and furuncles), vaccinations, tattooing and cautery, and laparotomies and various other surgical procedures.[172] Sometimes even minor injuries, such as needle marks or mosquito bites, produce small keloids of pinhead size. In some African countries, keloidal scarification is produced deliberately in a special design and is considered an adornment and mark of beauty. The condition occurs mainly during the late teens and early

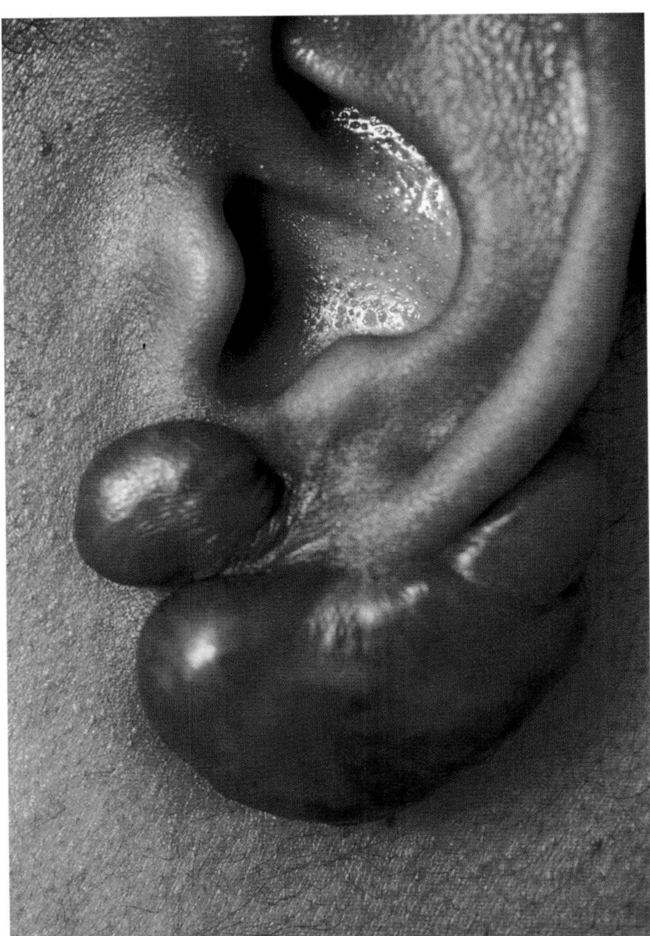

FIGURE 8-47. Keloid in a 25-year-old African-American woman. It appeared after the earlobes were pierced for earrings.

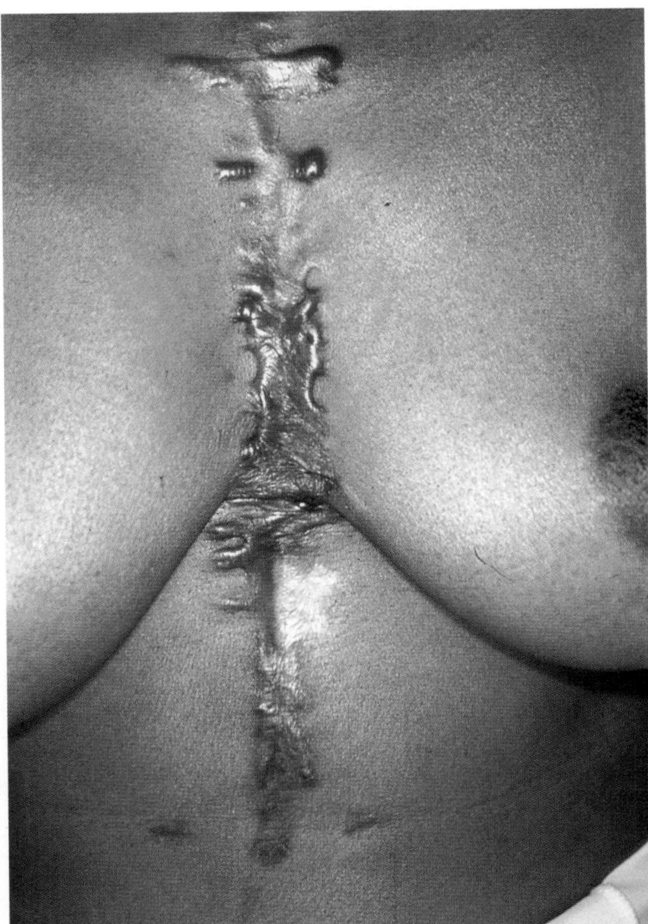

FIGURE 8-48. Keloid in the presternal region. These lesions may develop as the result of minor infection in an area of increased skin tension.

adult life. It is found rarely in infants, small children, or the aged. Although originally reported to be more common in women than men, more recent studies have found no significant difference in incidence between the genders.[173]

Keloids are more commonly encountered in dark-skinned persons, particularly those of African descent.[174] Of the various risk factors, a familial predisposition is clearly of paramount importance because up to 50% of affected individuals report another family member with a keloid.[175] Although an autosomal recessive pattern of inheritance was initially suggested, it is unclear whether the development of keloids is a complex oligogenic condition or inherited as a simple monogenic mendelian disorder.[176] Keloid formation has been reported in association with numerous dermatologic disorders, particularly acne vulgaris,[177] and some connective tissue diseases, including Ehlers-Danlos syndrome, scleroderma, and Rubinstein-Taybi syndrome.[178-180] An association of keloids with palmar, plantar, and penile fibromatosis has also been observed.[181]

Pathologic Findings

Keloids are characterized by a fibrocollagenous proliferation of the dermis with haphazardly arranged thick, glassy, deeply acidophilic collagen fibers (Fig. 8-49). During the early phase, the lesions tend to be vascular, particularly at their periphery, accounting for the clinical appearance of an erythematous lesion. Later, lesions show decreased vascularity and more prominent hyalinization, which may undergo focal calcification or osseous metaplasia. Bland spindle-shaped cells are scattered throughout this hypocellular lesion. As the lesion grows, there is progressive displacement of the normal skin appendages, often with flattening or even atrophy of the overlying epidermis. Immunohistochemically, although smooth-muscle actin decorates the spindle cells of hypertrophic scars, the cells of keloids show minimal or no staining for this antigen.[182] Ultrastructurally, the constituent cells have the features of active fibroblasts, with abundant rough endoplasmic reticulum and prominent Golgi apparatus, although some cells clearly have myofibroblastic features.[183]

Differential Diagnosis

Hypertrophic scars share the macroscopic features of keloids during the early phase of the lesion, but at later stages they flatten and have a less mucoid matrix and few or no glassy collagen fibers. Unlike keloids, hypertrophic scars stay within the confines of the initial wound and increase in size by

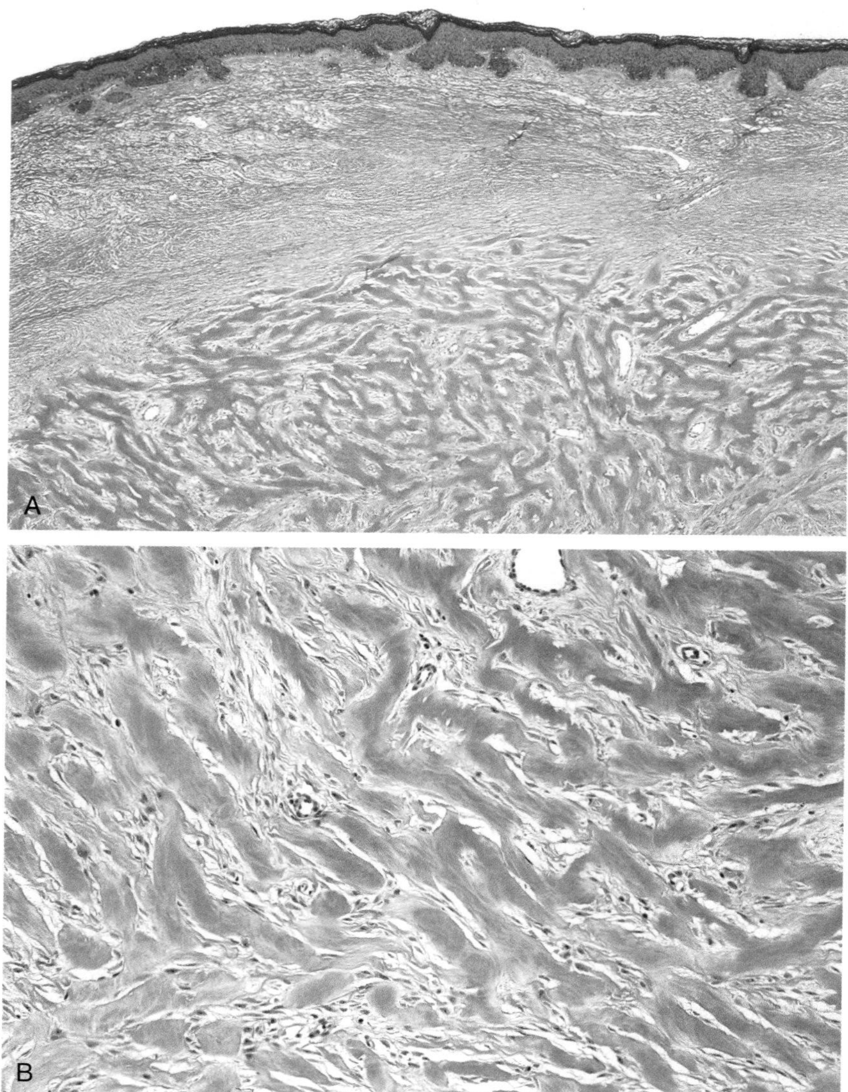

FIGURE 8-49. Keloid. (A) Low-power view. (B) Keloid displaying thick, glassy eosinophilic fibers in fibroblastic tissue.

pushing out the margins of the scar, as opposed to invading the surrounding normal tissues.[168] The initial cellular phase is also marked by a larger proportion of myofibroblasts, which may play a role in the contraction and elevation of the lesion. Features that are more commonly seen in keloids when compared to hypertrophic scars include a lack of flattening, minimal scarring of the papillary dermis, the absence of prominent vertically oriented blood vessels, and the presence of a tongue-like advancing edge beneath a normal-appearing epidermis and papillary dermis.[184]

Collagenoma, a connective tissue nevus, is an intradermal fibrocollagenous nodule that microscopically resembles a hypertrophic scar or keloid, but there is no history of acne or dermal injury. The condition presents clinically as multiple discrete, asymptomatic, skin-colored, small nodules that affect mainly the regions of the trunk and the proximal portion of the upper extremities.[185] In general, they make their first appearance during the postpubertal period and are frequently found in two or more members of the same family. Their number is significantly increased during pregnancy.[186]

Circumscribed storiform collagenoma (sclerotic fibroma) and *fibrous papules of the face* are two other morphologically related lesions. The former presents as a solitary dermal nodule composed of glassy, thickened collagen fibers arranged in a storiform pattern, occasionally with bizarre multinucleated giant cells.[187] It is identical to the fibrous nodules that occur in the multiple hamartoma syndrome or Cowden disease.[188] The term *fibrous papules of the face* has been applied to a small, dome-shaped fibrous nodule of the nose and face with an onion-skin periadnexal or perivascular collagen pattern. This lesion has also been described as perifollicular fibroma and melanocytic angiofibroma.[189]

Scleroderma (morphea) is characterized by thickening and altered staining characteristics of existing collagen fibers. There is no new fiber formation and, consequently, no elevation of the skin.

Keloidal dermatofibroma is a variant of dermatofibroma that may also histologically resemble a keloid.[190] Clinically, these lesions appear similar to ordinary dermatofibromas but are characterized by the presence of keloid-like collagen admixed with elements typically present in the usual dermatofibroma.

Discussion

Numerous treatment modalities have been attempted to minimize local recurrence of keloids; 45% to 100% of keloids locally recur following surgical excision.[191] Surgery combined with topical injection of corticosteroids reduces the local recurrence rate to less than 50%.[192] Postoperative radiation therapy and high-dose-rate brachytherapy have also been reported to have good results, with local recurrence rates of less than 10%. Numerous other therapeutic modalities, including laser therapy,[193] cryosurgery,[194] 5-fluorouracil,[195] and silicone gel or occlusive sheeting,[196] may also be effective. Patients who have a history of keloid formation should also avoid elective cosmetic procedures.

Unlike hypertrophic scars, keloids remain stationary or grow slowly and do not regress spontaneously. Although these lesions have a distinct tendency for local recurrence, the rate is highly dependent on the treatment. Immunohistochemical analyses of the proliferative activity of keloids have consistently found keloids to have a greater proliferative activity than is found in hypertrophic scars or normal skin, accounting for their tendency for continued growth.

DESMOPLASTIC FIBROBLASTOMA (COLLAGENOUS FIBROMA)

Desmoplastic fibroblastoma, also called *collagenous fibroma*, is a distinctive fibrous soft tissue tumor that typically occurs in the subcutaneous tissue or skeletal muscle of adults.[197-200] This tumor is rather nondescript in its morphologic appearance and, undoubtedly, had been diagnosed as fibroma or some other benign mesenchymal lesion for many years before its initial description by Evans[197] in 1995. Most patients are in their fifth or sixth decade of life and present with a slowly growing, painless mass. Few cases have been reported in children.[201] Men are affected three to four times more commonly than women. The most common sites are the soft tissues of the upper extremities, including the shoulder, upper arm, and forearm, followed by the lower extremity; rare lesions arise in other locations, including the head and neck.[202,203] Most are predominantly subcutaneous, but some involve skeletal muscle exclusively, and rare examples even involve the dermis.[204] The vast majority of tumors are 4 cm or smaller at the time of excision.

Pathologic Findings

Grossly, desmoplastic fibroblastoma is a well-circumscribed, firm mass with a white-to-gray cut surface, without hemorrhage or necrosis. Microscopically, the tumor is more or less circumscribed but not infrequently minimally infiltrates the surrounding soft tissues. The lesion is hypocellular and consists of widely spaced bland spindle- to stellate-shaped cells embedded in a collagenous or myxocollagenous stroma (Figs. 8-50 to 8-52). Mitotic figures are rare or absent, and necrosis is not present. Blood vessels are usually inconspicuous but may exhibit perivascular hyalinization.

Immunohistochemically, most show focal staining for smooth muscle actin or muscle-specific actin, consistent with myofibroblastic differentiation,[204,205] but stains for desmin, CD34, S-100 protein, and cytokeratins are typically negative.

Differential Diagnosis

The differential diagnosis includes a variety of benign or low-grade, predominantly fibrous lesions. *Neurofibroma* is composed of cells with a wavy configuration deposited in a

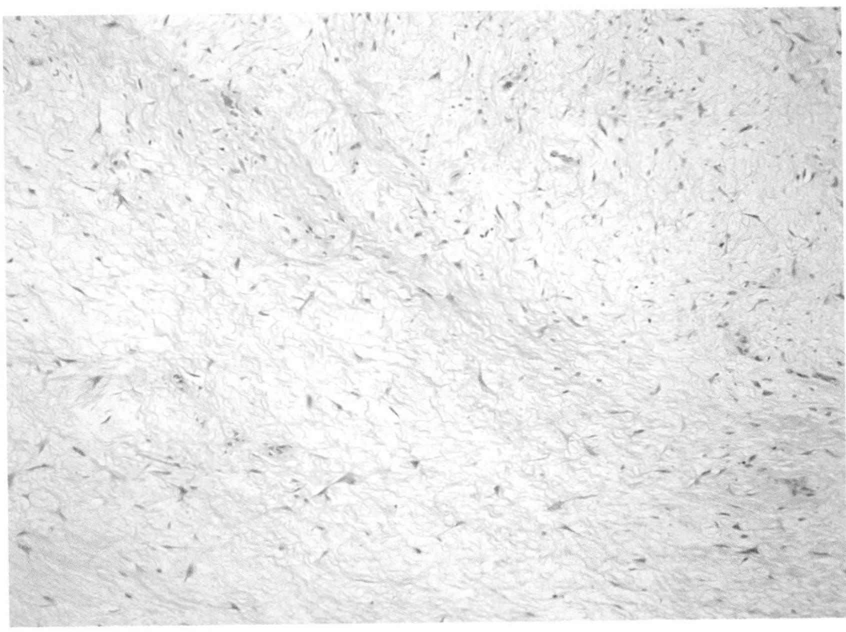

FIGURE 8-50. Myxoid zone in a collagenous fibroma.

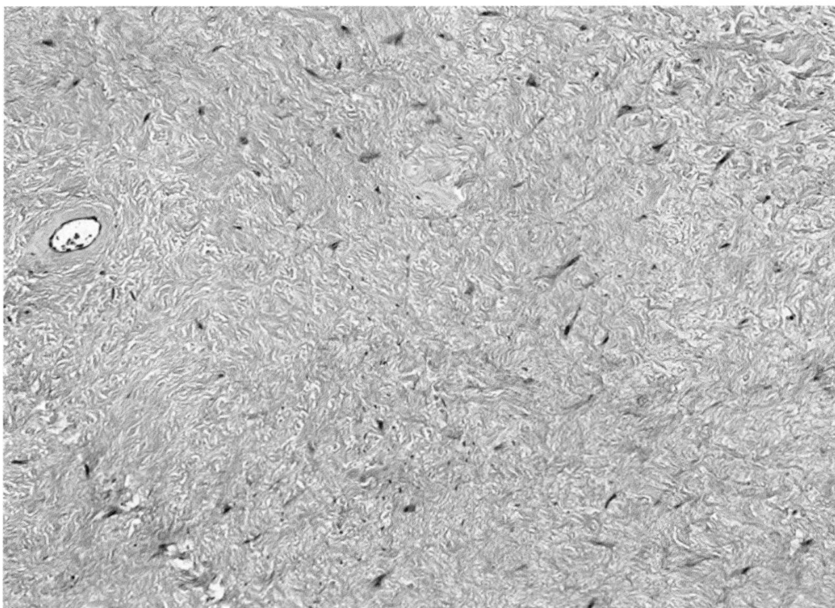

FIGURE 8-51. Desmoplastic fibroblastoma (collagenous fibroma). The lesion is hypocellular with widely spaced spindled and stellate-shaped cells embedded in a fibromyxoid stroma.

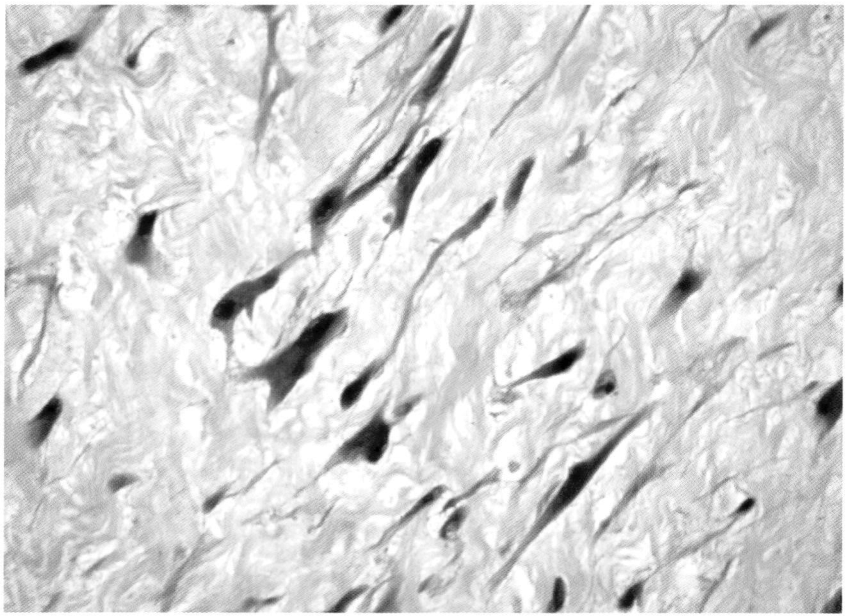

FIGURE 8-52. High-magnification view of bland spindled and stellate-shaped fibroblasts in a desmoplastic fibroblastoma (collagenous fibroma).

myxocollagenous stroma, often with shredded-carrot bundles of collagen. Unlike desmoplastic fibroblastoma, S-100 protein is typically strongly positive in neurofibromas. *Fibromatosis*, even when hypocellular, is more cellular than desmoplastic fibroblastoma, more infiltrative, and the cells tend to be arranged in broad fascicles. *Calcifying fibrous pseudotumor*, which affects children and young adults, is characterized by psammomatous calcifications and a lymphoplasmacytic infiltrate. *Low-grade fibromyxoid sarcoma* is typically more cellular, with cells arranged in whorls and deposited in a variably fibromyxoid stroma. *Elastofibroma*, usually found in the subscapular area, is characterized by wavy elastic fibers that are not present in desmoplastic fibroblastoma. *Nodular fasciitis* of long duration can also resemble this lesion but usually has areas of increased cellularity and other features typical of nodular fasciitis, even if present focally.

Discussion

Most patients have been treated by a conservative simple excision, and neither local recurrence nor metastasis has been reported. Because of the bland hypocellular appearance, it is not certain whether these lesions are the end-stage of a reactive process or a true neoplasm. Sciot et al.[206,207] and others have reported aberrations of 11q12, similar to those described for fibroma of tendon sheath. Bernal et al.[208] reported a case with a t(2;11)(q31;q12), and another case was found to have a t(11;17)(q12;p11.2).[209]

INTRANODAL PALISADED MYOFIBROBLASTOMA

Reported simultaneously by Weiss et al.[210] as palisaded myofibroblastoma and by Suster and Rosai[211] as intranodal hemorrhagic spindle cell tumor with amianthoid fibers, the palisaded myofibroblastoma is a distinctive benign spindle cell tumor arising within lymph nodes and bearing an unmistakable similarity to a schwannoma.[212,213] In fact, so striking is the resemblance that these lesions were originally regarded as schwannoma of the lymph node.[214] Based on immunohistochemistry, the lesions have features of a modified smooth muscle cell or myofibroblast. The tumor may develop at any age but usually arises in middle-aged adults as a localized swelling in the region of the groin.[215] A few cases have been reported in submandibular lymph nodes,[216,217] and a consultation case has also been reviewed in the mediastinal nodes.

Pathologic Findings

On cut section, the tumors are gray-white, focally hemorrhagic masses that obscure the nodal landmarks (Fig. 8-53). It is usually possible to identify a rim of residual node at the periphery of the tumor (Fig. 8-54). The spindle cells are arranged in short intersecting or crisscrossed fascicles with vaguely palisaded nuclei (Figs. 8-55 to 8-57). In some areas, the cells form broad sheets with slit-like extracellular spaces containing erythrocytes similar to those of Kaposi sarcoma (Fig. 8-58). There is minimal, if any, cytologic atypia and a rare mitotic figure only.

The most distinctive feature of the tumor is the amianthoid fibers or thick collagen mats that are almost always present. These structures appear as broad eosinophilic bands, ellipses, or circular profiles, depending on the plane of the section. They contain a central collagen-rich zone surrounded by a paler collagen-poor zone containing actin and other materials extruded from nearby degenerating cells. Although the name *amianthoid* was used by Suster and Rosai[218] for these distinctive bodies, it has been pointed out that these structures do not meet the strict definition of amianthoid fibers. The latter are thick collagen fibers measuring 280 to 600 nm, whereas the fibers in these structures have the width of normal collagen fibers. The mechanism of formation of these unusual bodies is not clear. Some have suggested that they represent a degenerative change around vessels to which the tumor cells and their contents become adherent.[217,218] These lesions appear to arise from modified smooth muscle cells that normally are found in the lymph node capsule and stroma. The predilection of this tumor to occur in the groin probably reflects the relative frequency with which smooth muscle cells are found in this location relative to other lymph-node chains.[210] Immunohistochemically, the cells strongly express smooth-muscle and muscle-specific actin but not desmin.[219,220] Linear striations, which are easily identified in conventional benign smooth muscle cells, cannot be demonstrated with the Masson trichrome stain, although, in many cases, fuchsinophilic bodies representing accumulations of actin are prominent.

Discussion

All of the cases reported in the literature have behaved in a benign fashion, with no recurrence or metastasis. It is important to recognize that this lesion represents a primary benign mesenchymal lesion and not a metastatic sarcoma. These tumors are quite well differentiated and have extremely low levels of mitotic activity, in contrast to most metastatic

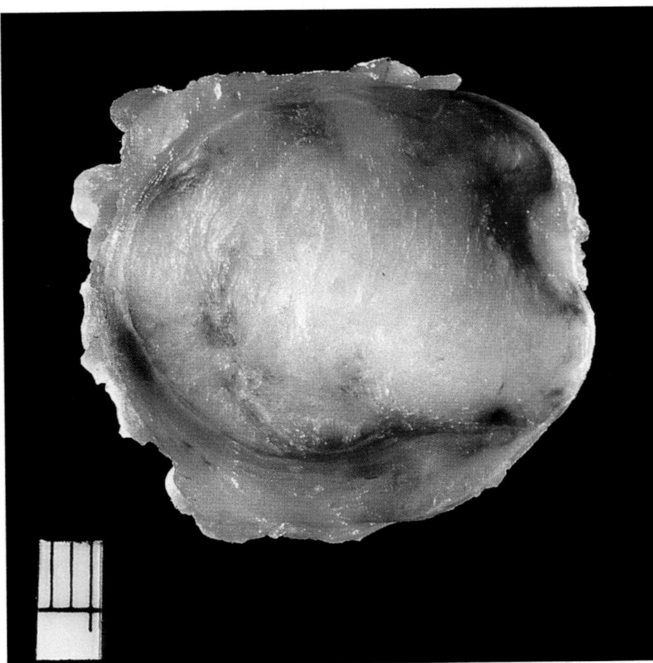

FIGURE 8-53. Gross specimen of a palisaded myofibroblastoma. Note the focal hemorrhages.

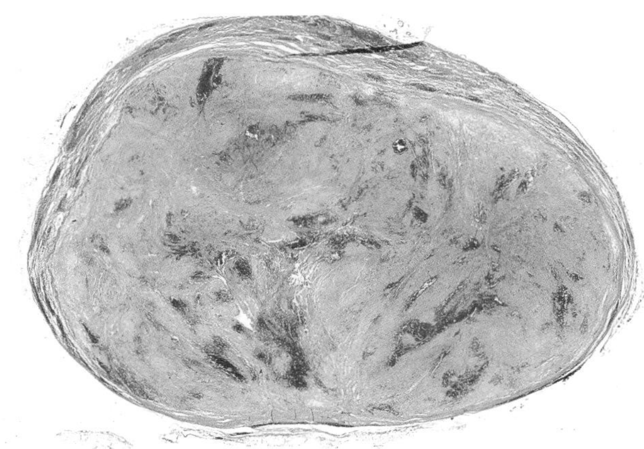

FIGURE 8-54. Palisaded myofibroblastoma with nearly complete effacement of a lymph node.

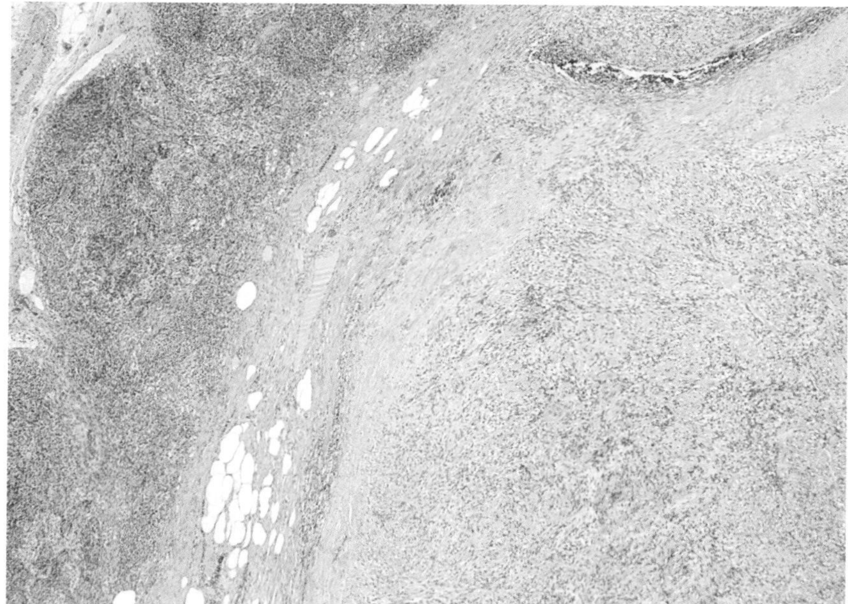

FIGURE 8-55. Low-power view of intranodal palisaded myofibroblastoma. Residual nodal tissue can be seen.

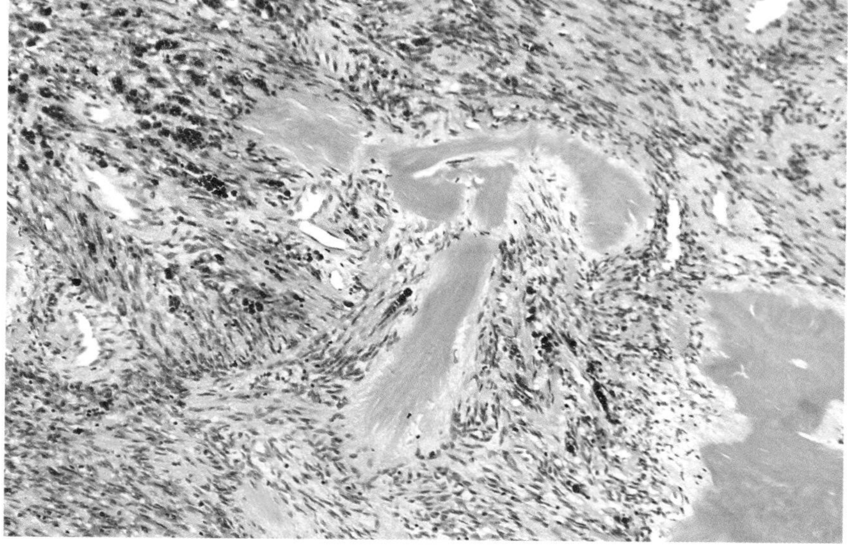

FIGURE 8-56. Palisaded myofibroblastoma with amianthoid fibers. It has a deeply eosinophilic core and lighter periphery.

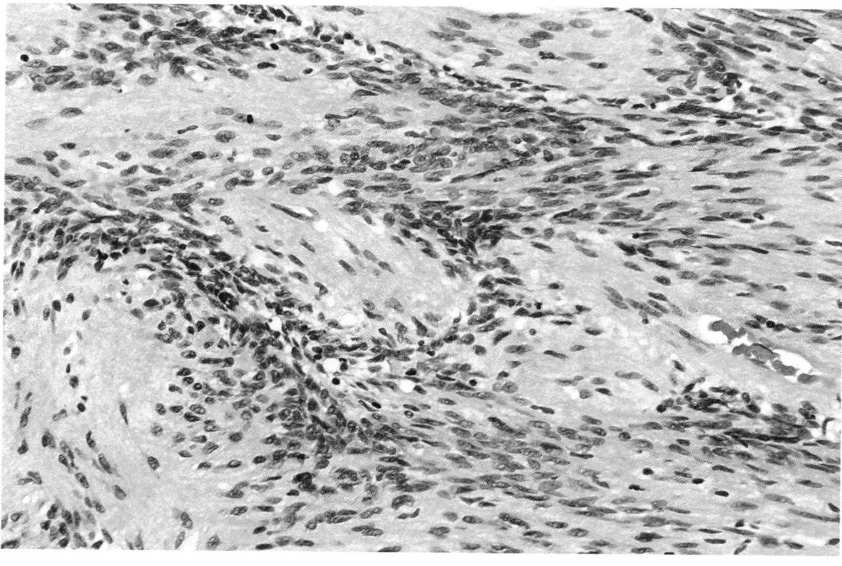

FIGURE 8-57. Palisaded myofibroblastoma with vague palisading of cells.

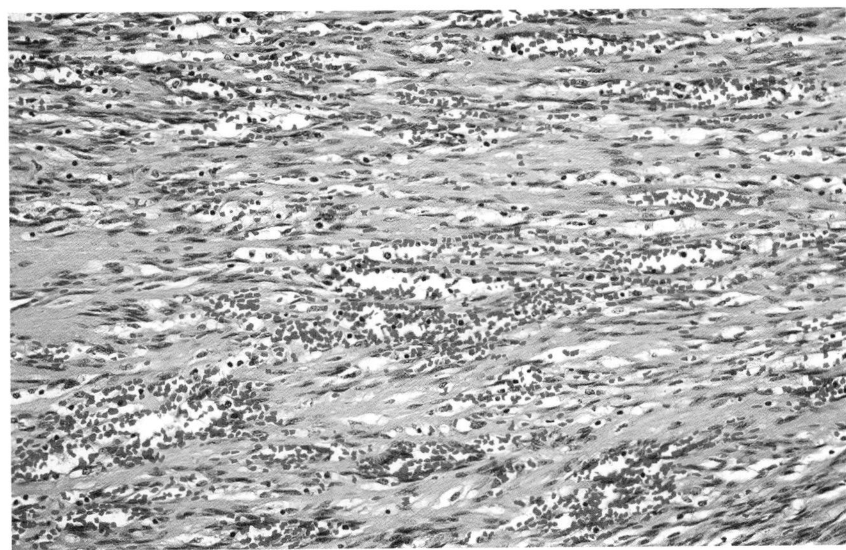

FIGURE 8-58. Kaposi-like areas in a palisaded myofibroblastoma.

sarcomas. Moreover, sarcomas infrequently metastasize to lymph nodes, and, when they do, it is usually an expression of disseminated disease and rarely an initial presentation.

MAMMARY-TYPE MYOFIBROBLASTOMA

Mammary myofibroblastoma is an uncommon but highly characteristic mesenchymal tumor, first reported as a spindle cell tumor of the breast.[221,222] Although originally thought to show a striking predilection for males,[223] these lesions arise with almost equal frequency in females, perhaps because of increased detection from mammographic screening.[224] It has become increasingly apparent that identical lesions arise at extramammary sites[225] and, therefore, the designation mammary-type myofibroblastoma is preferred.

Clinical Findings

Most patients present with a well-circumscribed, slowly growing solitary mass. Mammary lesions most commonly arise in postmenopausal women and older men (Fig. 8-59). In the original study by Wargotz et al.,[223] the mean age at diagnosis was 63 years. Extramammary lesions most commonly arise in older male patients, and cases have been reported in a wide variety of anatomic sites, including the buttocks,[226] vulva,[227] perianal region,[228] paratesticular region,[229] extremities,[230] and head and neck.[231] In the study of nine cases published by McMenamin and Fletcher,[225] the most common site was the inguinal/groin area.

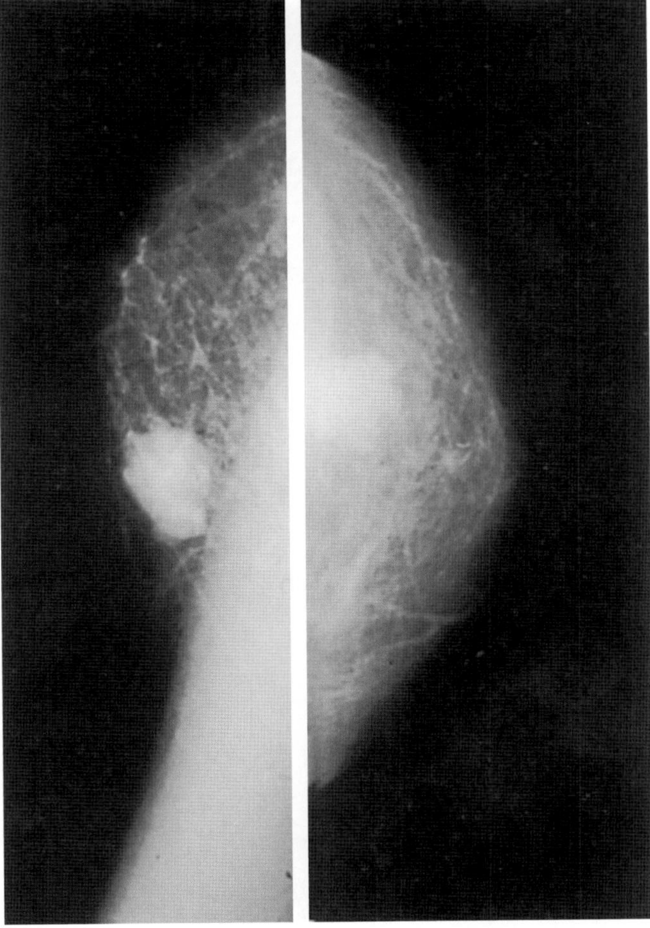

FIGURE 8-59. Mammogram showing a sharply marginated myofibroblastoma.

Pathologic Findings

The tumors, regardless of site, are generally well circumscribed and range in size from 2 cm to up to 13 cm although most are less than 5 cm at the time of excision. The cut surface often has a whorled appearance and is white to gray, occasionally with foci of myxoid change.[232]

Histologically, the tumor is composed of a haphazard arrangement of packets or short fascicles of slender fibroblast-like spindle cells separated by thick collagen bundles (Fig. 8-60). The cells have inconspicuous nucleoli and rare intracytoplasmic inclusions.[225] The cytoplasm is amphophilic or slightly eosinophilic; mitotic activity is variable but usually less than two mitotic figures per high-power field, and atypical forms are not seen. Mast cells are often a conspicuous finding. Mature adipose tissue is not an uncommon finding and can even comprise greater than half the tumor, creating the impression of a primary lipomatous neoplasm, particularly spindle cell lipoma (Fig. 8-61). Blood vessels are usually inconspicuous, but some cases may show focal thick-walled, hyalinized vessels. Other unusual features include a prominent component of epithelioid cells (Fig. 8-62),[233] myxoid change, multinucleated cells, and scattered atypical cells.[225]

Immunohistochemically, the cells typically express desmin and CD34;[225,234] there is variable expression of smooth-muscle actin. There is also consistent expression of CD10[235] that, like CD34, is also consistently expressed in spindle cell lipoma; S-100 protein and cytokeratins are typically negative.

Cytogenetic and Molecular Genetic Findings

Over recent years, mammary-type myofibroblastoma has consistently been found to show aberrations of 13q14,[236] which is also frequently involved in both spindle cell lipoma and cellular angiofibroma.[237] These lesions share a great deal of histologic and immunohistochemical overlap with mammary-type myofibroblastoma, suggesting a histogenetic relationship among these tumors. FISH analysis has shown aberrations of *Rb1* at 13q14, indicating this gene likely plays an important pathogenetic role.[231,237] Aberrations of *RB1* by FISH in mammary-type myofibroblastoma have also been consistently found in spindle cell lipoma and cellular angiofibroma, but not in solitary fibrous tumor, suggesting that the latter lesion is unrelated to the former.[238]

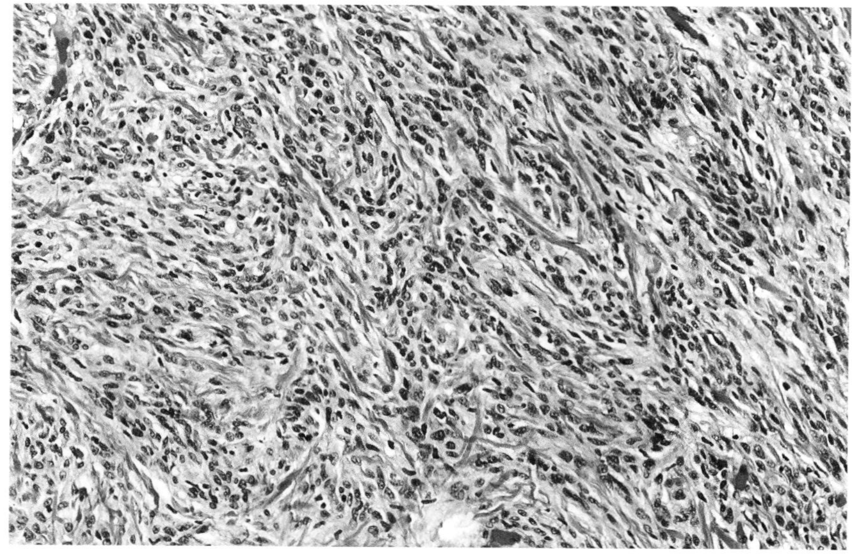

FIGURE 8-60. Mammary-type myofibroblastoma.

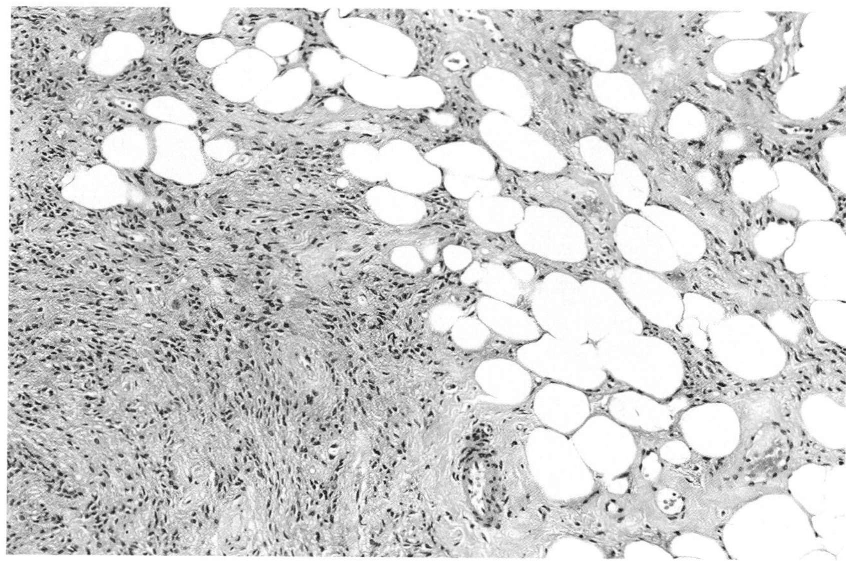

FIGURE 8-61. Fat trapping in a mammary-type myofibroblastoma.

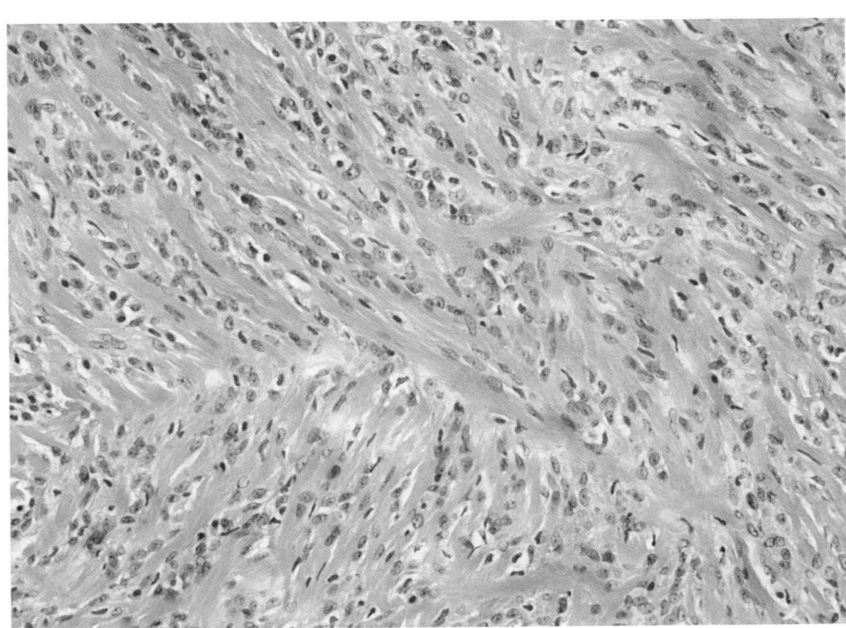

FIGURE 8-62. Epithelioid variant of mammary-type myofibroblastoma.

Differential Diagnosis

After becoming familiar with the pattern of this tumor in the breast, most pathologists have little difficulty making this diagnosis. Those unfamiliar with this lesion may consider *fibromatosis*, *metaplastic carcinoma*, or even a *stromal sarcoma*. Extramammary lesions may be confused with a wide array of mesenchymal neoplasms, especially *spindle cell lipoma*. Both lesions are composed of bland spindled cells admixed with benign-appearing fat, prominent mast cells, and immunoreactivity for CD34 and CD10. However, the pattern of collagen deposition is a bit different in these tumors, and mammary-type myofibroblastoma expresses desmin in addition to CD34 (spindle cell lipomas do not express desmin). Nevertheless, as emphasized by Pauwels et al.,[239] the overlap between these two entities is impressive (including cytogenetic findings) and, in some cases, the distinction between them is somewhat arbitrary. Similarly, mammary-type myofibroblastoma shows features that overlap with those of *cellular angiofibroma*, including a predilection to arise in an inguinal location.[225,240,241] The latter lesion (also reported as an angiomyofibroblastoma-like tumor[240]) is a benign spindle cell tumor with variable cellularity, intralesional fat, hyalinized blood vessels, and usually negative staining for both desmin and smooth-muscle actin, although it is often positive for CD34.

Mammary-type myofibroblastoma may also be confused with *solitary fibrous tumor*, another consistently CD34-positive lesion. In fact, it has been suggested that mammary myofibroblastoma simply represents a solitary fibrous tumor of the breast.[242] Solitary fibrous tumor is characterized by variable cellularity with spindled cells arranged in a patternless pattern, a striking hemangiopericytoma-like vascular pattern, and wire-like collagen. However, desmin staining is quite uncommon in solitary fibrous tumor, and clinical behavior is more unpredictable. In select cases, a number of other entities could be considered, including *spindle cell liposarcoma*, *nodular fasciitis*, *low-grade malignant peripheral nerve sheath tumor*, *perineurioma*, and *dermatofibrosarcoma protuberans (DFSP)*. However, clinical, morphologic, and immunohistochemical findings usually allow easy distinction among these entities.

Discussion

Mammary-type myofibroblastomas are benign. None of the original patients described by Chan et al.[222] and Wargotz et al.[223] developed recurrence or metastases. Similarly, recurrences were not reported in the series of extramammary lesions by McMenamin and Fletcher.[225] Therefore, simple excision is adequate therapy.

SUPERFICIAL ACRAL FIBROMYXOMA (DIGITAL FIBROMYXOMA)

First described in 2001 by Fetsch et al.[243] in a series of 37 cases, superficial acral fibromyxoma (also referred to as *digital fibromyxoma*) is a benign myxoid mesenchymal neoplasm that characteristically arises in the fingers or toes in a subungual or periungual location. Its exact relationship to so-called *cellular digital fibroma* has yet to be fully defined, but it is quite possible that these lesions lie on a histologic spectrum.

Clinical Findings

This lesion arises in patients with a wide age range, although the mean age is in the fourth decade of life.[244] In the original study by Fetsch et al.,[243] patients ranged in age from 14 to 72 years. Prescott et al.[245] reported an age range from 19 to 91 years, whereas the more recent report by Hollman et al.[246] in a study of 124 cases had an age range of 4 to 86 years with a median age of 48 years. Both studies have found a male predilection with a male-to-female ratio of close to 2:1. Most patients present with a slowly enlarging nodule on the fingers or toes, and up to 75% are in a subungual or periungual location.[243,245,247] Rare cases arise in the palm,[243] heel,[247] or ankle/leg.[246] Although most cases do not affect the underlying bone, there are rare examples that can cause a smooth erosion of bone,[248] scalloping,[243] or even true bony invasion.[246]

Pathologic Findings

Grossly, the lesion ranges in size from less than 1 cm to up to 5 cm, but most are smaller than 2 cm at the time of excision.[244] The tumor is dome-shaped and well circumscribed with a firm or gelatinous white-to-gray cut surface.

Histologically, there is a fairly consistent constellation of features with a moderately cellular proliferation of bland spindled to stellate-shaped cells deposited in a myxoid or myxocollagenous matrix with a prominent vascular pattern (Figs. 8-63 and 8-64). Only rare cases show more than mild cytologic atypia.[243] Mitotic figures are infrequent, and atypical mitoses are not seen. Multinucleated stromal cells and mast cells are also common features.[246] The cells are generally arranged in a loose storiform or fascicular growth pattern, but they also may be randomly distributed. The tumor border is often pushing, but there can be an irregular infiltrative margin in some cases.[243] Most lesions are restricted to the dermis, but some extend into the subcutis. Some cases are much more cellular; these examples have features that overlap with cellular digital fibroma.[249]

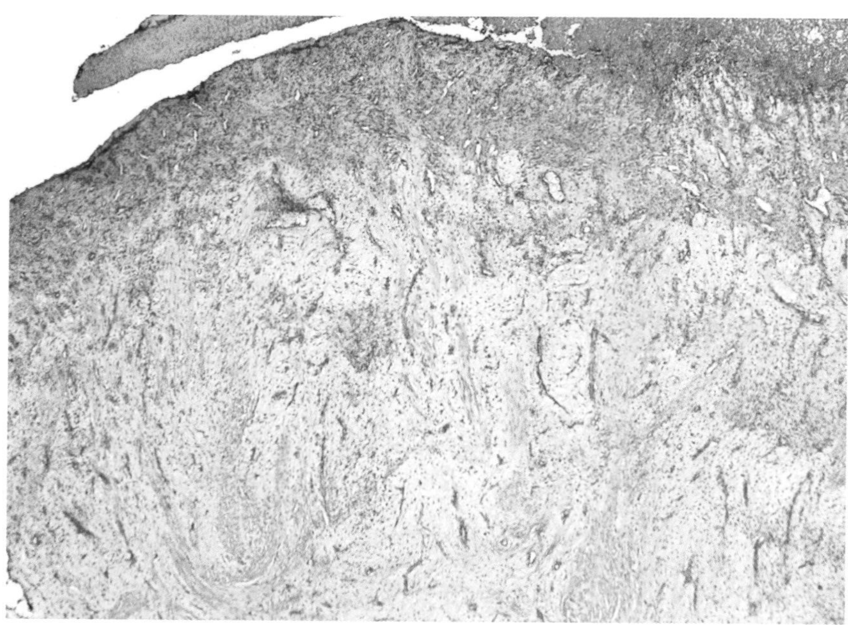

FIGURE 8-63. Low-power view of superficial acral fibromyxoma.

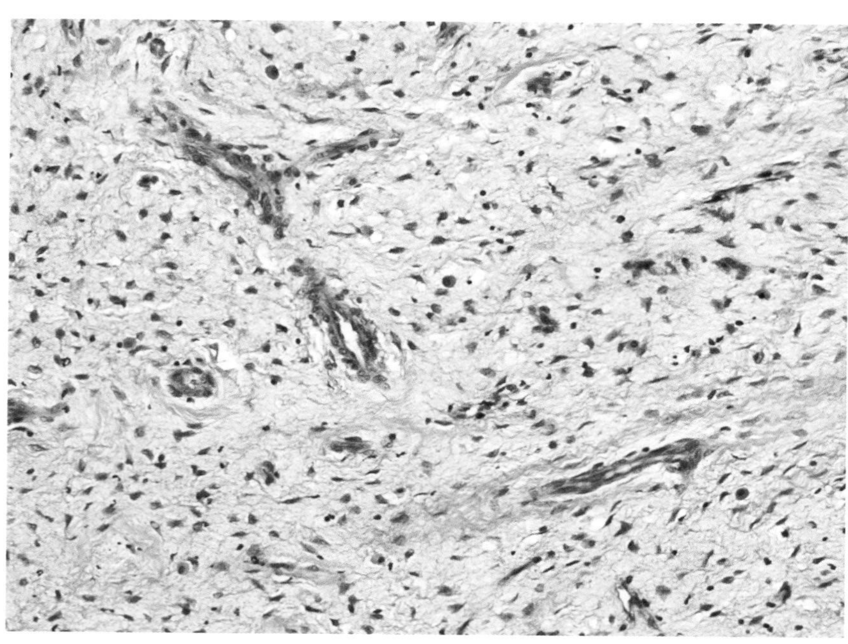

FIGURE 8-64. Superficial acral fibromyxoma. Lobules showing an even distribution of bland spindled cells in a fibrous and myxoid matrix.

Immunohistochemical Findings

The tumor has a fairly consistent immunophenotype with strong and diffuse expression of CD34, in most cases, and frequent but more variable expression of CD99 and EMA[243,245,247,250,251]; many also express CD10.[252,253] The cells are usually negative for S-100 protein, desmin, smooth muscle actin, GFAP, MUC4, claudin-1, and cytokeratins. Ultrastructurally, the cells have features consistent with fibroblastic differentiation.[254]

Differential Diagnosis

This lesion has a large differential diagnosis, which includes a number of benign cutaneous mesenchymal neoplasms that have a myxoid matrix, CD34-positivity, or both. In particular, it may be difficult to distinguish from DFSP, particularly if only a superficial biopsy is obtained. DFSP is rare in an acral location. Histologically, it is characterized by a more consistent, monotonous storiform growth pattern with lace-like infiltration into the subcutis, a feature that may not be seen in a superficial biopsy. In cases of DFSP with prominent myxoid change, the vascular pattern becomes more conspicuous and can resemble that seen in superficial acral fibromyxoma. Both lesions strongly express CD34, adding further to this confusion. Lisovsky et al.[255] found consistent expression of ApoD in DFSP and its absence in superficial acral fibromyxoma. In difficult cases, FISH or other molecular analysis for evidence of the *COL1A1/PDGFB* fusion characteristic of DFSP may be extremely helpful.

Other lesions that enter the differential diagnosis include *myxoid neurofibroma*, which can be recognized by the neural appearance of the spindled cells, shredded-carrot collagen, and strong S-100 protein staining. *Superficial angiomyxomas* are most common in the head and neck and trunk and are exceedingly rare in acral sites. There may be an epithelial component, slit-like clefts, and a prominent neutrophilic infiltrate. Although the cells also stain for CD34, stains for EMA and CD99 are typically negative. *Sclerosing perineurioma* is a variant of perineurioma that occurs on the fingers and palms of young adults. The cells are often epithelioid and arranged into cords and trabeculae, or there is an onion-skin pattern. The cells show EMA staining along their cytoplasmic extensions.

Discussion

Superficial acral fibromyxoma is benign and is best treated by complete surgical excision and clinical follow-up. In the original study from the Armed Forces Institute of Pathology (AFIP), follow-up information in 18 patients revealed one recurrence after local excision and two instances of persistent disease after partial excision.[243] In a study by Al-Daraji and Miettinen,[256] 3 of 14 (22%) patients developed a local recurrence. In the more recent study by Hollman et al.,[246] 24% of cases locally recurred, all of which had positive margins on initial excision.

In 2005, McNiff et al.[249] described 14 CD34-positive acral fibroblastic lesions as cellular digital fibroma. These arose in patients of 33 to 83 years of age with a mean age of 54 years (similar to superficial acral fibromyxoma). Sites of involvement included the fingers (seven cases), toes (four cases), and palms (two cases). Histologically, the lesions were composed of a cellular proliferation of uniform spindled cells forming short, intersecting fascicles oriented in a parallel or haphazard fashion in the upper reticular dermis. However, unlike superficial acral fibromyxoma, there was an absence of a prominent myxoid matrix or organized vascular pattern. All cases were strongly positive for CD34, but none stained for EMA; CD99 was not tested in this series. Although the authors of this study did not raise superficial acral fibromyxoma as a diagnostic consideration, the consensus is that there is significant clinical, morphologic, and immunohistochemical overlap, raising the strong possibility that these are related neoplasms.[256-258]

ANGIOFIBROMA OF SOFT TISSUE

In 2012, Mariño-Enriquez and Fletcher[259] described 37 cases of a distinctive benign fibrovascular tumor that arose most commonly as a soft tissue mass of the extremities and was characterized by a specific cytogenetic aberration. The authors designated these lesions as angiofibroma of soft tissue.

Clinical Findings

In the report of Mariño-Enriquez and Fletcher,[259] the tumors arose in patients of ages 6 to 86 years with a median age of 49 years. Females were affected twice as often as males. Most patients presented with a slowly enlarging, painless mass located in the soft tissues of the extremities, which were equally likely to be subfascial or deep-seated as subcutaneous. The lower limbs were the most common site (62% of cases), followed by the upper limbs (16%), but other sites of involvement included the back, abdominal wall, retromammary soft tissue, and pelvis.

Pathologic Findings

Grossly, the tumors were generally very well circumscribed with only rare infiltration into adjacent tissues (Fig. 8-65). They ranged in size from 1.2 to 12 cm (mean, 4.3 cm) and had a firm, rubbery cut surface, in most cases.

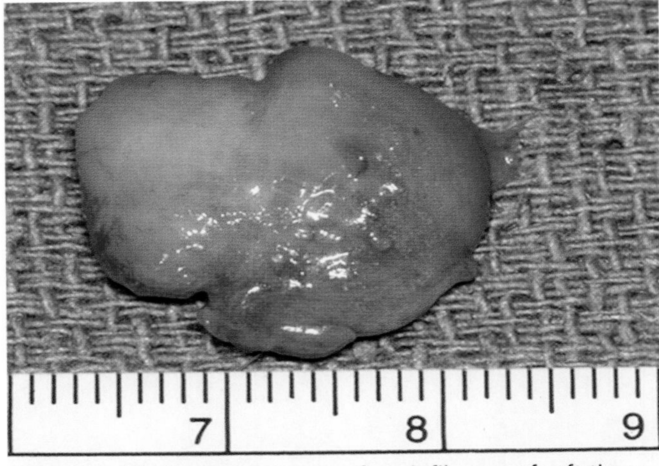

FIGURE 8-65. Gross appearance of angiofibroma of soft tissue.

Histologically, the tumors were characterized by a proliferation of uniform bland spindled cells with inconspicuous cytoplasm and ovoid nuclei deposited in a variably myxoid or collagenous stroma with a prominent network of small thin-walled and finely branched blood vessels (Figs. 8-66 and 8-67). The nuclei were quite uniform, and mitotic figures were infrequently observed (1 to 4 mitotic figures per 10 high-power fields). Rare cases showed what was interpreted as mild degenerative nuclear atypia.

Immunohistochemical Findings

The most frequently expressed antigen was EMA, but this was found in 16 of 36 (44%) cases only and usually in scattered tumor cells only. CD34 and SMA were detected in 14% of cases each; desmin expression was even less common. The S-100 protein was consistently absent.

Cytogenetic and Molecular Genetic Findings

Although this tumor is rather nondistinctive morphologically, Mariño-Enriquez and Fletcher[259] detected a balanced t(5;8)(p15;q12) translocation in four of six cases. A fifth case showed a three-way t(5;8;8)(p15;q13;p11), and another showed gains of 10q24-26, 12q13, and 17p13. Subsequent FISH mapping by Jin et al.[260] suggested the involvement of the aryl hydrocarbon receptor repression gene on 5p15 and the nuclear receptor coactivator 2 gene on 8q13.

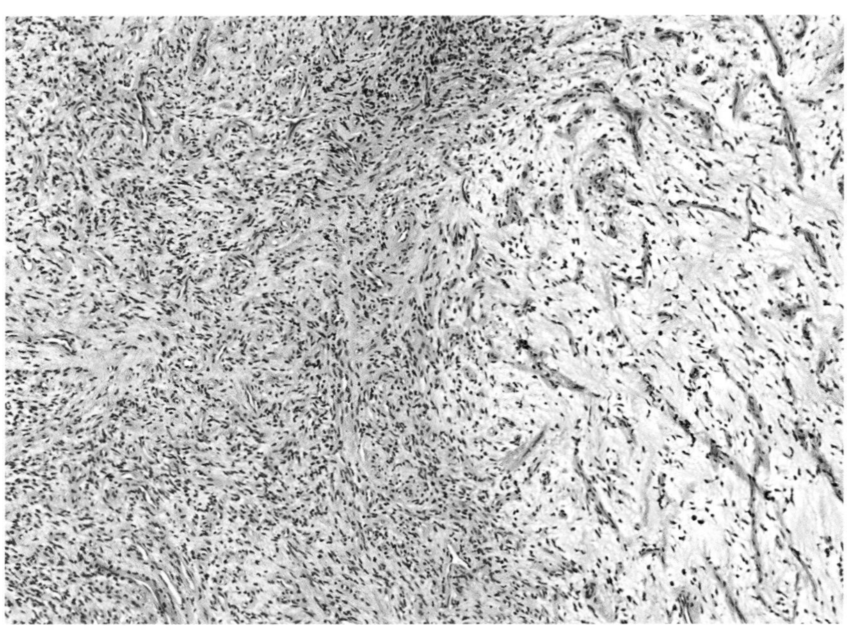

FIGURE 8-66. Angiofibroma of soft tissue showing cellular and myxoid zones.

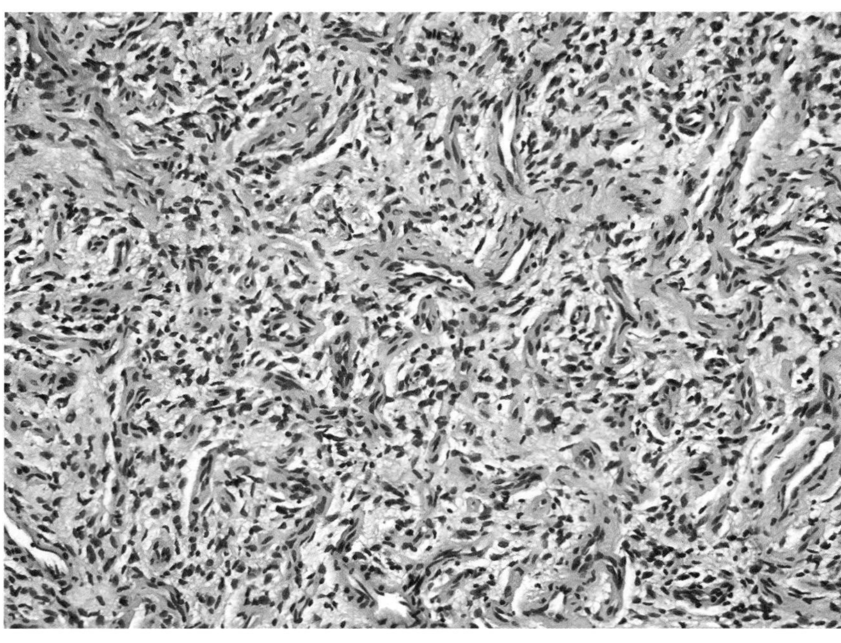

FIGURE 8-67. Cellular zone in angiofibroma of soft tissue.

Differential Diagnosis

The differential diagnosis includes an array of benign/low-grade malignant spindle cell lesions. In extensively myxoid examples, angiofibroma of soft tissue can be confused with *myxoma*, but the latter usually arises as an infiltrative, intramuscular mass that is less cellular and has far fewer blood vessels. *Cellular angiofibroma* is a tumor that most often arises in the perineal or pelvic region and is composed of more rounded, medium-sized, thicker non-branching vessels and a more uniformly cellular proliferation of plumper spindled cells. *Solitary fibrous tumor* may arise in any anatomic location and is characterized by CD34-positive spindled cells arranged in a patternless pattern, wire-like collagen and foci with a hemangiopericytoma-like vascular pattern, which differs from the finely branched, thin-walled vessels seen in angiofibroma of soft tissue. *Low-grade myxofibrosarcoma* usually arises in the subcutis of middle-aged patients and is composed of cells with a greater degree of nuclear hyperchromasia and pleomorphism, as well as thicker walled curvilinear vessels with perivascular hypercellularity. *Myxoid liposarcoma* is composed of fairly uniform plumper spindled cells deposited in a uniformly myxoid matrix, often with cystic spaces (mucin pools). Although there is some resemblance of the vascular pattern between myxoid liposarcoma and angiofibroma of soft tissue, the former has even more delicate arborizing capillaries. Obviously, lipoblasts are a distinguishing feature of myxoid liposarcoma. Finally, *low-grade fibromyxoid sarcoma* bears some resemblance to angiofibroma of soft tissue. The former shows distinct lobularity, alternating fibrous and myxoid zones and bland spindled cells. A prominent vascular pattern is usually seen in the myxoid zones only, and the cells often show a swirling, whorling growth pattern. In difficult cases, molecular analysis for evidence of the *FUS-CREB3L2* (or, rarely, *FUS-CREB3L1*) characteristic of this tumor can resolve diagnostic confusion.

Discussion

Angiofibroma of soft tissue is a benign neoplasm that only rarely recurs, even with incomplete excision. Follow-up information available for 28 patients (mean, 51.9 months) revealed only 4 patients with local recurrence, which did not seem to correlate well with resection margin status.[259] None of the patients developed metastatic disease. Simple local excision seems to be the ideal mode of therapy.

SUPERFICIAL FIBROMATOSES

Fibromatoses comprise a broad group of benign fibroblastic proliferations of similar microscopic appearance characterized by infiltrative growth and a tendency toward recurrence, but they never metastasize.

The various entities that constitute this group occur predominantly in adults and consist of highly differentiated fibroblasts and, to a lesser degree, myofibroblasts that form a firm, poorly circumscribed nodular mass that may be solitary or multiple and have a predilection for certain anatomic sites. The term *fibromatosis* should not be applied to nonspecific reactive fibrous proliferations that are part of an inflammatory process or are secondary to injury or hemorrhage and have no tendency toward infiltrative growth or recurrence.

BOX 8-2 Classification of Fibromatoses

Superficial (fascial) fibromatoses
Palmar fibromatosis (Dupuytren disease)
Plantar fibromatosis (Ledderhose's disease)
Penile fibromatosis (Peyronie disease)
Knuckle pads
Deep (musculoaponeurotic) fibromatoses
Extra-abdominal fibromatosis (extra-abdominal desmoid)
Abdominal fibromatosis (abdominal desmoid)
Intra-abdominal fibromatosis (intra-abdominal desmoid)
Pelvic fibromatosis
Mesenteric fibromatosis
Mesenteric fibromatosis in Gardner syndrome

The fibromatoses can be divided into two major groups with several subdivisions (Box 8-2). *Superficial (fascial) fibromatoses* are small, slowly growing, and arise from the fascia or aponeuroses and only rarely involve deep structures. The clinical course usually can be divided into an early, rather cellular proliferative phase and a late, richly collagenous regressive or contractile phase. *Deep (musculoaponeurotic) fibromatoses* are large, more rapidly growing tumors. Their biologic behavior is more aggressive than that of the superficial (fascial) fibromatoses; they have a high recurrence rate, and, as their name indicates, involve deep structures, particularly the musculature of the trunk and the extremities. The descriptive term *desmoid tumor* is still widely used in the literature as a synonym for this type of fibromatosis.

Because of the benign clinical course of the superficial fibromatoses, they will be included in the chapter. However, because of their more aggressive clinical behavior, the deep/musculoaponeurotic fibromatoses will be fully discussed in Chapter 10, which will focus on borderline and malignant fibroblastic/myofibroblastic tumors.

PALMAR FIBROMATOSIS

Palmar fibromatosis, better known as *Dupuytren disease* or *Dupuytren contracture*, is by far the most common type of fibromatosis. Although it is named for Baron Guillaume Dupuytren, who reported this condition in 1831, there are much earlier descriptions of this lesion.[261] For example, Norse folklore from the twelfth century refers to the MacCrimmons, a Scottish clan famed for its pipers, some of whom were unable to play because of digital contractures.[262] This form of superficial fibromatosis is characterized by a nodular fibroblastic proliferation that occurs on the volar surface of the hand and histologically closely resembles other forms of fibromatosis. The lesion progresses through a series of clinical and histologic stages and, ultimately, results in flexion contracture of the fingers, a complication that usually necessitates surgical therapy.[263]

Clinical Findings

Palmar fibromatosis is a relatively common condition that affects adults, with a rapid increase in incidence with advancing age and an average age of onset of 60 years.[264] It has been estimated that almost 20% of the general population is affected by 65 years of age. Patients younger than 30 years of age, particularly children, are seldom affected.[265,266] The condition is about three or four times more frequent in men than in women, but the difference in gender incidence diminishes with increasing age. There is clearly a genetic susceptibility to this disease, because this form of fibromatosis is found virtually exclusively in Caucasians and is found only sporadically in those of Asian or African descent.[267] The highest prevalence of palmar fibromatosis is found in those of Northern European descent, particularly from Northern Scotland, Norway, and Iceland.[268]

The onset of the disease is slow and insidious, and the initial manifestation is typically an isolated, usually asymptomatic, firm nodule in the palmar surface of the hand. Because of the lack of symptoms at this stage, many patients ignore the presence of the nodule and do not seek medical therapy. There is a slight predilection for the right palmar surface, but almost 50% of cases are bilateral. Although clinical progression does not invariably occur, in many patients, several months or years after the original appearance of the fibrous nodules, cord-like indurations or bands develop between nodules and adjacent fingers, often causing puckering and dimpling of the overlying skin (Fig. 8-68). These changes are usually most prominent on the ulnar side of the palm and are accompanied by flexion contractures that principally affect the fourth and fifth fingers of the hand. The thumb and index finger are least often affected. With increasing severity of the contractures, normal function of the hand becomes greatly impaired, and it is at this point that therapy is usually sought.

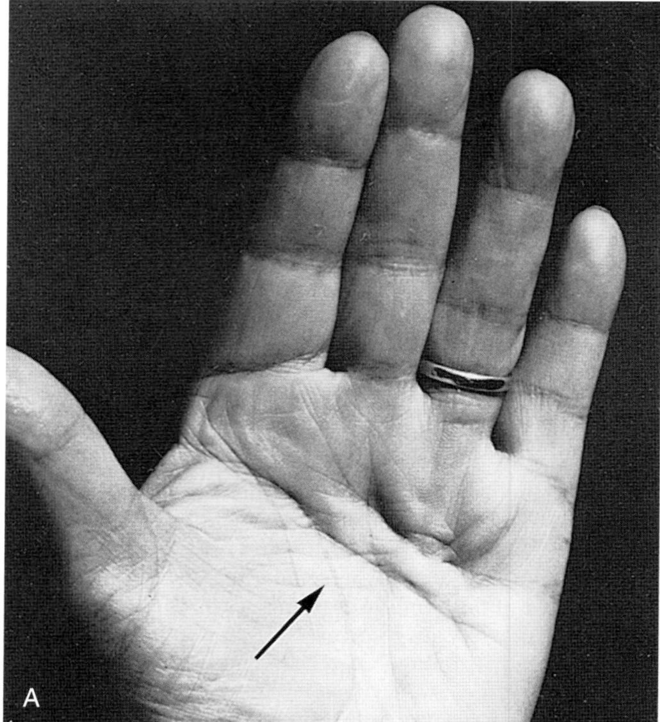

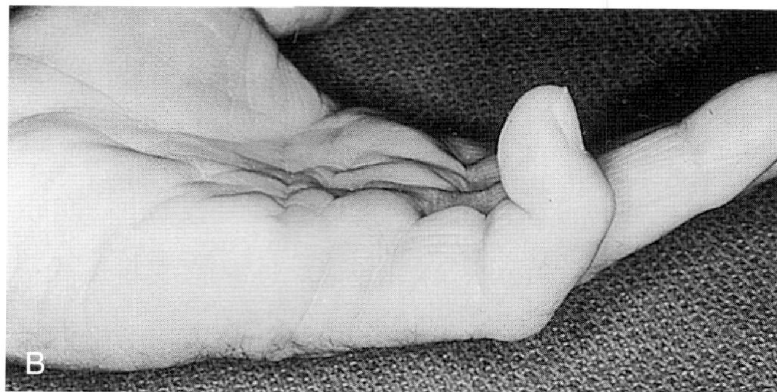

FIGURE 8-68. (A) Palmar fibromatosis with firm cord-like indurations and nodules causing puckering and dimpling (arrow) of the overlying skin. (B) Flexion contracture of the fifth finger (Dupuytren contracture).

Concurrence of Palmar Fibromatosis With Other Diseases

Palmar fibromatosis has been linked with numerous other disease processes, including other forms of fibromatosis. Approximately 5% to 20% of cases of palmar fibromatosis are associated with plantar fibromatosis, and about 2% to 4% of patients also have penile fibromatosis (Peyronie disease).[265,269] Knuckle pads (fibrous thickenings on the dorsal aspect of the proximal interphalangeal or metacarpophalangeal joints) have also been associated with palmar fibromatosis.[265,270] Rare patients have been described with polyfibromatosis syndrome, a condition characterized by the occurrence of several cutaneous fibroproliferative lesions, including Dupuytren contracture and keloids.[271]

Palmar fibromatosis has been consistently linked with seemingly unrelated diseases. For example, approximately 20% of patients with diabetes mellitus have a palmar fibromatosis.[272,273] It is equally common in type 1 and type 2 diabetes mellitus, although it occurs at a younger age in patients with type 1.[274] Interestingly, the disease tends to be quite mild in patients with diabetes and rarely requires surgery.[275] Microvascular changes secondary to diabetes mellitus may result in local hypoxia, stimulating the fibroblastic proliferation. Epilepsy is also an associated disease, possibly related to the use of anticonvulsant drugs as opposed to the underlying disease itself.[276,277] In contrast to those with diabetes, patients with epilepsy who also develop Dupuytren disease often have a severe form that is bilateral and symmetrical. Those who suffer from alcoholism also have a high prevalence of Dupuytren contracture.[273] The prevalence of palmar fibromatosis is far higher in those who suffer from alcoholism with liver disease than in those without it, suggesting that it is the effect of alcohol on the liver (rather than the direct effects of alcohol) that is the causative factor.[278] The effect of alcohol in the development of palmar fibromatosis may be exacerbated by cigarette smoking.[273] There is an equivocal association with HIV infection,[279,280] but the incidence of Dupuytren contracture is actually lower in patients with rheumatoid arthritis.[281]

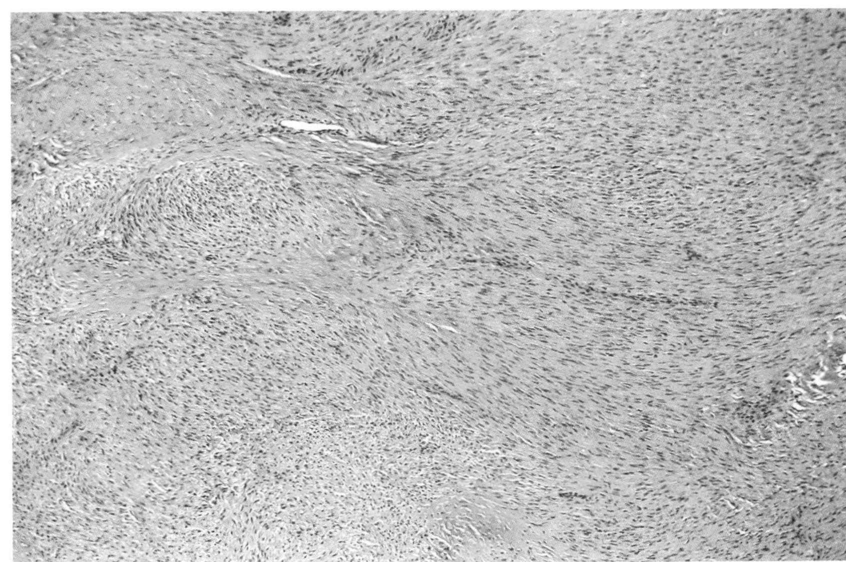

FIGURE 8-69. Palmar fibromatosis composed of parallel fascicles of slender fibroblasts separated by variable amounts of collagen.

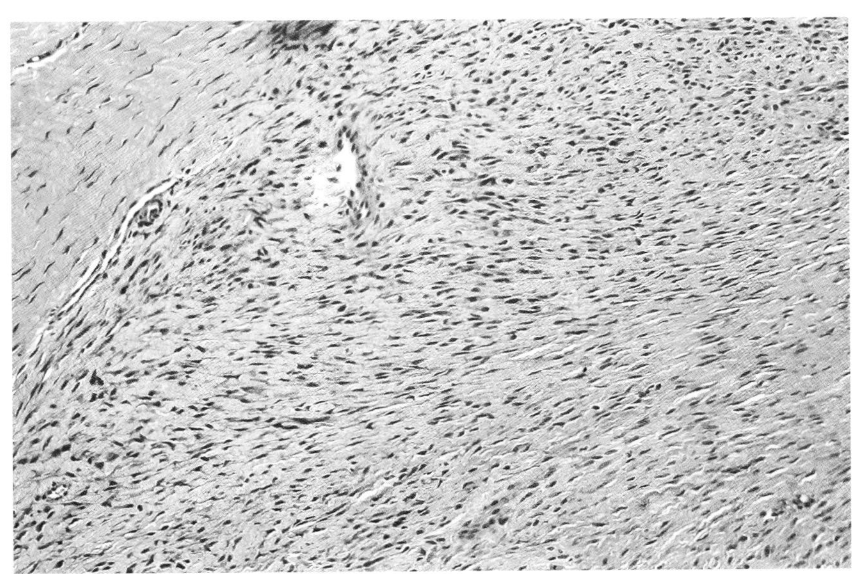

FIGURE 8-70. Uniform fibroblastic proliferation in palmar fibromatosis.

Pathologic Findings

The excised tissue consists of a single small nodule, usually measuring less than 1 cm in diameter or an ill-defined conglomerate of several nodular masses intimately associated with a thickened palmar aponeurosis and subcutaneous fat. The tissue is firm and scar-like on palpation, and on cut section reveals a gray-yellow to gray-white surface, although the color depends on the collagen content, which, in turn, depends on the age of the lesion. The gross specimen may also contain excised skin, and, occasionally, these nodular masses adhere to the overlying skin.

The microscopic findings depend on the age of the lesion. In general, palmar fibromatosis progresses from a proliferative nodular phase with relatively high cellularity, some mitotic activity and minimal collagen deposition to an involutional stage with increased myofibroblastic differentiation, decreased proliferative activity, and increased collagen deposition to an end-stage that is less cellular and more collagenous. The proliferative phase of the disease is characterized by a strikingly cellular proliferation of plump, immature-appearing spindle-shaped fibroblasts that form one or more nodules (Figs. 8-69 and 8-70). The fibroblasts are uniform in size and shape, with normochromatic nuclei and small, pinpoint nucleoli (Fig. 8-71). Mitotic figures may be identified but are usually not numerous. The cells are intimately associated with small to moderate amounts of collagen suspended in a mucopolysaccharide-rich matrix. Upon close examination, multinucleated giant cells are frequently seen.[265] Microhemorrhages with small deposits of hemosiderin and scattered chronic inflammatory cells may be present. The fibrous nodules originate within the palmar aponeurosis and extend into and replace the overlying subcutaneous fat.

Nodules that have been present a long time are less cellular and contain markedly increased amounts of dense birefringent collagen. The fibroblasts are smaller and more slender,

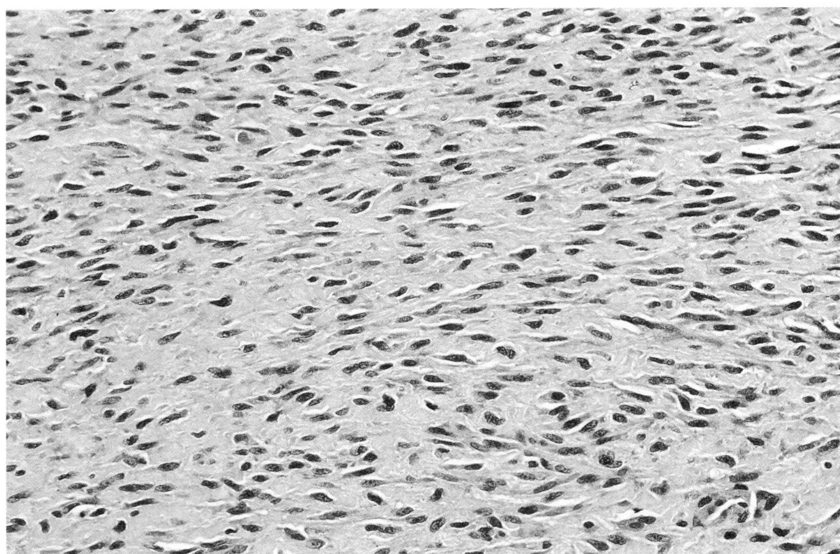

FIGURE 8-71. Early, cellular form of palmar fibromatosis showing uniform spindled cells separated by collagen.

and the fascial or aponeurotic cords between nodules are composed of dense fibrocollagenous tissue that resembles tendons. Osseous and cartilaginous metaplasia of the fibrous nodules may be seen, but it is uncommon.

Immunohistochemical Findings

Gabbiani and Majno,[282] the first to emphasize the presence of myofibroblasts in palmar fibromatosis, suggested that these cells played a role in the pathogenesis of the contraction observed clinically. Since then, numerous reports have confirmed the role of myofibroblasts in this disease.[183] Therefore, it is not surprising that a subset of cells often stain for smooth muscle actin and muscle-specific actin, depending on the stage and the degree of myofibroblastic differentiation.[283] In addition, smooth-muscle-actin-positive cells are often numerous in apparently uninvolved dermis and provide a pool of progenitor cells from which new foci develop, accounting for the high rate of local recurrence.[284] Although the majority of palmar fibromatoses show nuclear β-catenin staining, the percentage of cells that stain is far less than that in deep fibromatoses.[285] Numerous growth factors, including transforming growth factor-β, platelet-derived growth factor, and basic fibroblast growth factor, have been implicated in the pathogenesis of this disease because these growth factors are potent stimulators of collagen production.[286-288]

Cytogenetic and Molecular Genetic Findings

Standard karyotypic analysis of a large series of superficial fibromatoses has revealed clonal chromosomal aberrations in approximately 10% of cases.[289] De Wever et al.[289] from the Chromosomes and Morphology (CHAMP) Collaborative Study Group, comprising cytogeneticists, pathologists, and surgeons, carried out a systematic evaluation of 78 superficial and deep fibromatoses. Of 28 superficial fibromatoses studied, only 3 cases showed cytogenetic aberrations, including 2 palmar fibromatoses with trisomy 8 and 1 plantar fibromatosis with trisomy 8 and loss of the X chromosome. Other studies have also found trisomies of chromosomes 7 and 8.[290,291] Shih et al.[292] found differential expression of several candidate genes in cases of palmar fibromatosis, including *ALDH1A1*, *PRG4*, and *TNC*. Recently, Dolmans et al.[293] detected upregulation of a number of genes that encode proteins in the *Wnt* signaling pathway, strongly suggesting a pathogenetic role.

Differential Diagnosis

In its most cellular phase, palmar fibromatosis may closely resemble *fibrosarcoma*. However, the cells of fibrosarcoma tend to be arranged in long fascicles or a herringbone pattern and show a greater degree of nuclear hyperchromasia, pleomorphism and mitotic activity, and, occasionally, necrosis. Furthermore, fibrosarcoma of the hand is incredibly rare, and, as stated by Fetsch et al.,[265] "a healthy degree of skepticism is warranted whenever the diagnosis is suggested." On those very rare occasions in which a fibrosarcoma does arise in this location, it is usually a deep-seated tumor that affects the aponeurosis and subcutaneous tissue secondarily only. In contrast, the cellular nodules in palmar fibromatosis arise within the aponeurosis and infiltrate the subcutaneous tissue.

The differential diagnosis also includes *cellular benign fibrous histiocytoma*. This is a dermal-based neoplasm that may secondarily involve the subcutaneous tissue. Although the central portion of the lesion may have a fascicular growth pattern reminiscent of palmar fibromatosis, the peripheral portion maintains a characteristic storiform growth pattern and other features that are seen in the usual form of benign fibrous histiocytoma, such as peripherally entrapped dense collagen bundles. *Calcifying (juvenile) aponeurotic fibroma* has a strong predilection for the palmar region of pediatric patients, but, on rare occasions, this lesion may be encountered in adults. Although fibromatosis-like areas are characteristically found, this lesion is also characterized by small foci of cords of epithelioid fibroblasts and distinctive chondroid nodules that frequently calcify. Finally, although *monophasic fibrous synovial sarcoma* can present as a mass in the hands or feet, it is composed of plumper spindled to epithelioid cells, frequently a hemangiopericytoma-like vascular pattern, immunoreactivity for cytokeratins, and TLE1 and evidence of a t(X;18).

Discussion

The pathogenesis of palmar fibromatosis is multifactorial, although there is clearly a genetic component, as documented by twin and family studies.[269] Patients with a family history of palmar fibromatoses often develop a more severe form at a younger age.[294] Although an autosomal dominant pattern of inheritance with variable penetrance has been suggested, the exact pattern of inheritance is still unclear.[295]

In addition to a genetic predisposition, other factors have been implicated, including trauma and microtrauma.[296] Dupuytren himself suggested that repetitive minor trauma may be the major causative factor in this disease. Because of claims for compensation from patients with Dupuytren contractures that the patients believed to be the result of work injuries, Herzog[297] undertook a review of the literature of over 1000 steelworkers, miners, and clerks in 1951. No significant difference was found in the prevalence of this disease between the different groups. Nevertheless, numerous case reports have implicated trauma as an etiologic factor. Liss and Stock[298] reviewed 10 previously published studies and found good support for an association between hand vibration exposure and the development of palmar fibromatosis.

Microvascular changes may also be an etiologic factor in the development of palmar fibromatosis and other fibrosing lesions. Kischer and Speer[299] observed microvascular occlusion in and around areas involved by the fibromatosis and proposed that hypoxia stimulates the excessive collagen production, possibly through a generation of oxygen-free radicals. Such a hypothesis would be attractive for linking hyperlipidemia, diabetes mellitus, and cigarette smoking, all of which affect the microvasculature.

Finally, some have proposed an immunologic basis for this disease. Several studies have found circulating serum antibodies to collagen types 1 to 4 in some patients with palmar fibromatosis,[300] and others have found an increased prevalence of HLA-DR3, a major histocompatibility complex class II antigen that is associated with autoimmune diseases.[301] Although inflammation is usually not a conspicuous component of this disease, most of the inflammatory cells present are $CD3^+$ lymphocytes and express HLA-DR antigen, suggesting a T-cell-mediated autoimmune disorder.[302]

Surgical extirpation remains the treatment of choice in patients with severe flexion contractures that impair normal hand function. Fasciotomy (subcutaneous division of the fibrous bands) leads to good immediate improvement of contractures of the metacarpophalangeal joints. This procedure has no effect on the progression of the disease because it affects the proximal interphalangeal joint only; therefore, long-term results are marginal only.[268] Furthermore, this procedure may result in injury to the digital arteries or nerves. More extensive surgical procedures, including wide or radical fasciectomy or dermofasciectomy, are usually advocated because of the lower risk of local recurrence.[303] The latter technique has been advocated for cases of recurrent Dupuytren contracture requiring reoperation and as a primary procedure when there is significant skin involvement.[304-306] Radiologic evaluation, particularly with an MRI, is useful for determining the extent of the disease process, thereby facilitating the most appropriate surgical therapy.[307] A number of other nonsurgical approaches have been assessed, including injection of *Clostridium histolyticum* collagenase injection,[308] radiotherapy,[309] and injections of corticosteroid[310] and gamma-interferon,[311] with variable success.

Regardless of mode of treatment, there is a high rate of local recurrence; of course, rates vary significantly, depending upon the type of surgery performed. Dermofasciectomy, the most extensive surgical procedure (aside from amputation), has a recurrence rate of approximately 8%.[263]

PLANTAR FIBROMATOSIS

Plantar fibromatosis, sometimes referred to as *Ledderhose's disease*, is characterized by a nodular fibrous proliferation arising within the plantar aponeurosis, usually in non–weight-bearing areas. Although Dupuytren recognized that a process similar to that occurring with palmar aponeurosis could involve plantar aponeurosis, it was Madelung who reported the first isolated case of plantar fibromatosis in 1875, described in more detail by Ledderhose in 1897. This condition is much less common than its palmar counterpart, but, because it rarely produces a contracture and often has few, if any, symptoms, it is probably less frequently brought to the attention of physicians.[312]

Clinical Findings

Like palmar fibromatosis, its incidence increases progressively with advancing age, although there is a much higher incidence in children and young persons. In the recent large study by Fetsch et al.,[265] almost 44% of 501 patients with plantar fibromatosis reviewed at the AFIP were 30 years of age or less. In this same study of 56 cases of palmar or plantar fibromatosis in children and pre-adolescents, only 2 patients had palmar lesions. Overall, plantar fibromatosis affects males and females with similar frequency, but there is a striking female predilection in pediatric cases.[265] Approximately 30% to 35% of cases are bilateral, and, in such cases, the lesions are usually metachronous with one lesion preceding the other by an interval of 2 to 7 years.[313]

Not infrequently, palmar and plantar fibromatoses affect the same patient, but the two lesions rarely occur at the same time; usually one precedes the other by 5 to 10 years.[314] The association with penile fibromatosis (Peyronie disease) is much less common. In a review of the literature by Pickren et al.,[315] only 1 of 104 patients with plantar fibromatosis had penile fibromatosis. Coexistence with dorsal knuckle pads has also been noted in up to 42% of cases.[265,270] Like palmar fibromatosis, this disease appears to be more common among those with epilepsy, diabetes, those suffering from alcoholism

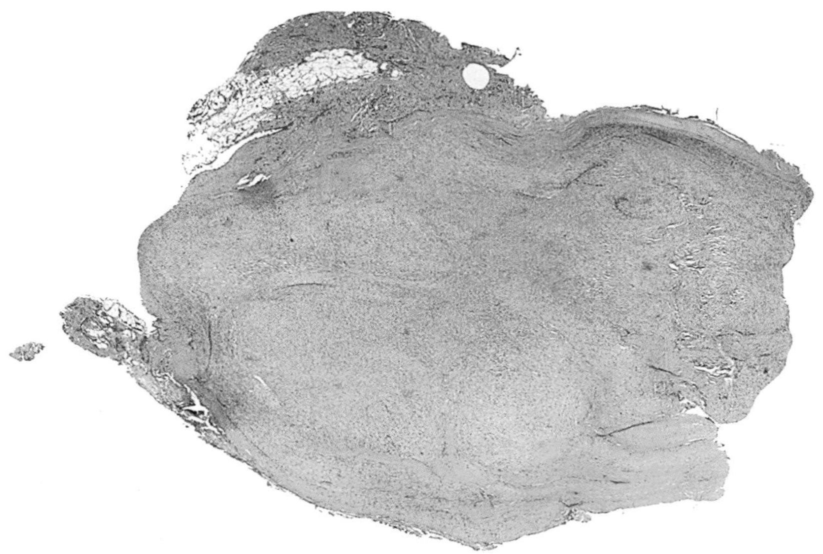

FIGURE 8-72. Plantar fibromatosis showing the characteristic nodular growth pattern.

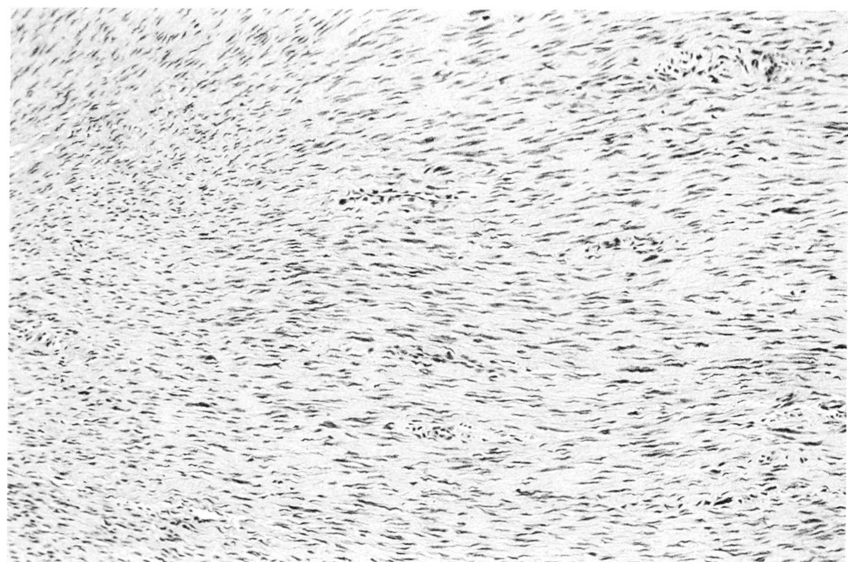

FIGURE 8-73. Plantar fibromatosis composed of uniform spindle-shaped cells arranged in long fascicles.

with liver disease, and those with keloids. Fetsch et al.[265] noted an apparent association with fifth finger clinodactyly, a finding in 3 of 23 (13%) patients with pediatric plantar fibromatosis.

The lesion first appears as a single, firm subcutaneous thickening or nodule that adheres to the skin and is typically located in the medial plantar arch from the region of the navicular bone to the base of the first metatarsal. It may be entirely asymptomatic but not infrequently causes mild pain after prolonged standing or walking.[316] Rarely, paresthesia of the distal portion of the sole of the foot and the undersurface of one or more toes may result when there is entrapment of the superficial plantar nerve.[317] Unlike its palmar counterpart, plantar fibromatosis exceptionally results in contraction of the toes only, presumably because the distal extensions of the plantar aponeurosis to the toes are much less well developed than in the hand. In patients with symptoms, plantar fibromatosis is often treated with a biopsy or excised at an earlier, more cellular stage than palmar fibromatosis and may cause serious diagnostic concern that a sarcoma is present, particularly fibrosarcoma.

Pathologic Findings

Grossly and microscopically, the lesions are virtually indistinguishable from palmar fibromatosis, although they are less often multinodular and only rarely contain the thick cords of fibrocollagenous tissue extending distally from the nodular growth (Fig. 8-72). Many of the lesions are highly cellular, but the cells lack nuclear hyperchromasia or pleomorphism and have small, pinpoint nucleoli (Figs. 8-73 and 8-74). Mitotic figures may also be identified but are few in number and are not atypical. Occasionally, one encounters mild perivascular chronic inflammation and deposits of hemosiderin; scattered lesions of long duration may have focal chondroid or osseous

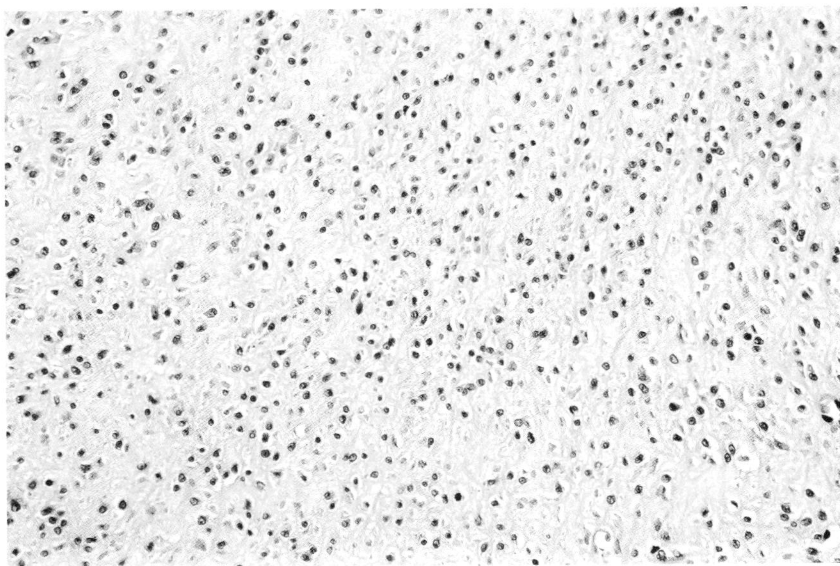

FIGURE 8-74. Plantar fibromatosis. Round-cell pattern caused by a cross-section of spindle-shaped fibroblasts.

metaplasia.[318] Multinucleated giant cells are also a consistent but frequently overlooked feature.

Immunohistochemically, as with palmar fibromatosis, this lesion is characterized by a population of cells that stain for smooth muscle actin, indicating focal myofibroblastic differentiation. In addition, many of the growth factors identified in cases of palmar fibromatosis are also present in the plantar lesions and likely play an important role in stimulating collagen production by fibroblasts.[319,320]

The differential diagnosis is similar to that described for palmar fibromatosis but usually is restricted to *fibrosarcoma*. Although well-documented cases of fibrosarcoma in the foot have been reported, they are exceedingly rare and histologically are characterized by more hyperchromatic nuclei that show greater nuclear pleomorphism and a higher degree of mitotic activity than that found with plantar fibromatosis.

In most cases, surgical therapy is not required unless the nodules cause discomfort or disability. Although intralesional steroid injections have been effective in some cases,[321] surgical excision is the treatment of choice. Radiologic evaluation, particularly with MRI, is useful for determining the extent of the disease process, thereby facilitating the most appropriate surgical therapy.[322] Simple excision of the lesion is associated with a high rate of local recurrence,[323] but complete fasciectomy, with or without skin grafting, is associated with a much lower rate of recurrence.[324] Most lesions recur less than 1 year after initial excision with an increased risk of local recurrence in patients with multiple nodules, bilateral lesions, a positive family history, and those who develop a postoperative neuroma.[312]

Discussion

The etiology of plantar fibromatosis, like palmar fibromatosis, is probably multifactorial; and there seems to be a genetic predisposition. Like its palmar counterpart, cytogenetic aberrations have been reported in these lesions, including trisomies of chromosomes 8 and 14.[325,326] Sawyer et al.[327] reported a reciprocal t(2;7)(p13;p13) in a single case of plantar fibromatosis. Trauma has frequently been considered an important factor in the pathogenesis of this disease. Certainly, the sole of the foot suffers a great variety of minor injuries over the years, and it is not surprising that a history of trauma can be elicited in many cases. There does not appear to be any occupational predilection, and most of these lesions arise in the medial portion of the plantar arch, an area least exposed to traumatic injury. The coexistence of the disease with epilepsy, diabetes, and alcohol-induced liver disease makes it likely that factors other than trauma are etiologically important.

PENILE FIBROMATOSIS (PEYRONIE DISEASE)

Although François de la Peyronie is generally credited with describing the disease that bears his name,[328] descriptions of this disease date back as far as at least the mid-sixteenth century.[329] It is considered a superficial fibromatosis that results in an ill-defined fibrous thickening or plaque-like mass in the penile shaft, frequently resulting in a curvature of the erect penis.

Clinical Findings

Although previously considered rare, this condition is clearly more common today. In a study by Mulhall et al.,[330] Peyronie disease was found in 8.9% of men who were being screened for prostate cancer in the United States. It primarily affects men 45 to 60 years of age; it is uncommon in young adults, and there are no reports of cases in children. Most patients are white; the disease very rarely affects blacks and those of Asian descent.[331]

This condition results in a palpable plaque-like induration typically located on the dorsal or lateral aspect of the shaft of the penis, causing the penis to curve toward the affected side. This curvature is the result of the relatively inelastic plaque-like scar tissue in the normally compliant tunica albuginea of the erectile body of the penis. It restricts expansion of the involved aspect of the penis during tumescence, limiting the extension of that segment of the penile shaft and causing the erection to be bent.[332] Associated symptoms include pain on erection and painful intercourse. Some patients who have penile curvature may have difficulty achieving an erection, presumably because the plaque-like induration impairs the veno-occlusive function of the tunica albuginea.

Penile fibromatosis is more common in patients with palmar and plantar fibromatosis than in the general population; its incidence varies from 2% to 4% in palmar fibromatosis and from 1% to 2% in plantar fibromatosis. There is also an increased incidence in patients with epilepsy and diabetes.[333] Both erectile dysfunction and coital trauma appear to be risk factors for the development of Peyronie disease.[334]

Pathologic Findings

The fibrous mass chiefly involves fascial structures, corpus cavernosum, and rarely corpus spongiosum. It consists of dense, pearly white to gray-brown tissue that glistens on a section; it averages 2 cm in greatest dimension.

There are relatively few descriptions of the pathologic features of Peyronie disease. The most consistent histologic abnormality is the irregular orientation and character of the collagen within the tunica albuginea.[335] There is an increased number of cytologically bland fibroblasts associated with haphazardly arranged collagen bands, irregular collagen plates, or nodules (Fig. 8-75). Elastic stains highlight a marked reduction of elastic fibers in affected areas. Fibrin may or may not be present, and inflammatory cells, particularly lymphocytes

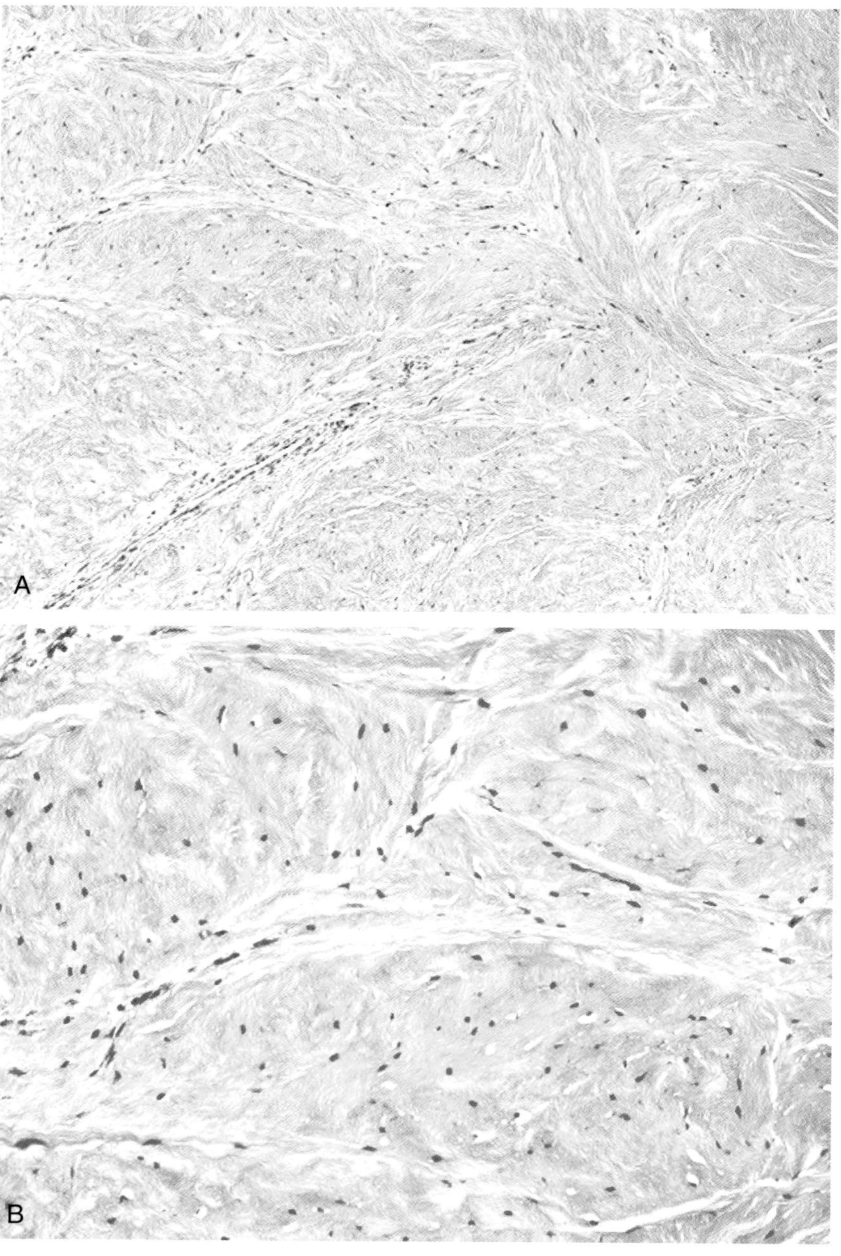

FIGURE 8-75. Peyronie disease. (A) Hypocellular proliferation typical of this lesion. (B) Higher-power view of bland cells entrapped in dense collagen.

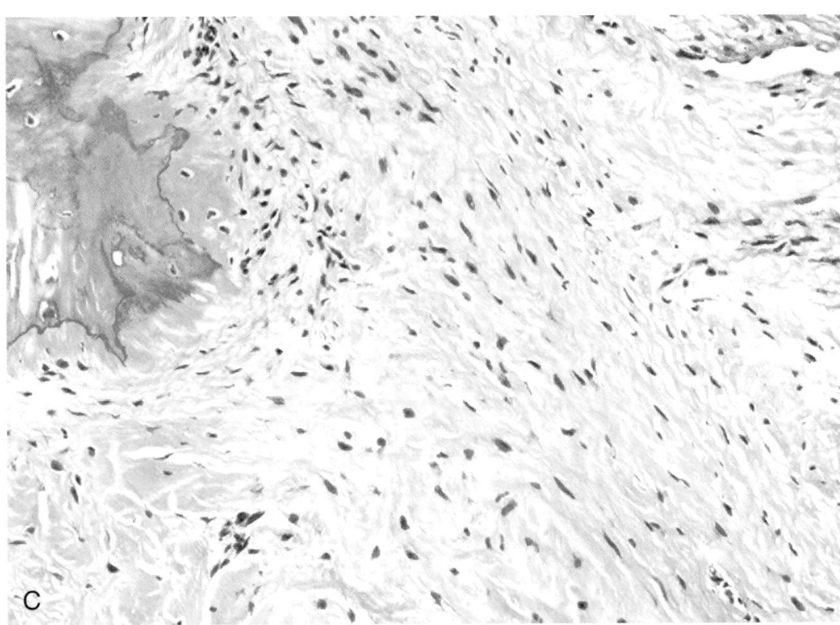

FIGURE 8-75, cont'd. (C) Focus of ossification.

and plasma cells, may be seen in early lesions, predominantly in a perivascular location, both within and external to the tunica albuginea.[335] As the lesions persist, there tends to be a decrease in the amount of chronic inflammation with a progressive increase in fibrosis, often with focal calcification or ossification. Metaplastic cartilage has also been described.[336] There are cases of penile epithelioid sarcoma that clinically mimic Peyronie disease, but the cells of epithelioid sarcoma are cytologically atypical and have densely eosinophilic cytoplasm.

Discussion

The exact cause of Peyronie disease is not clear. As with palmar and plantar fibromatoses, a genetic component has been suggested, perhaps requiring some environmental trigger. An inflammatory/infectious etiology was originally proposed, but more recent evidence makes an infectious etiology highly unlikely. There is some evidence to support an autoimmune etiology, because this disease has been associated with several HLA tissue types, particularly HLA-DQ5,[337] but others have found no such associations.[338] Ralph et al.[339] found that patients with early Peyronie disease had immunoglobulin M (IgM) antibody deposition and a marked T-lymphocytic infiltrate with increased expression of HLA class II antigens.

Trauma may also be an important etiologic factor. Devine et al.[340] suggested that repetitive microvascular injury results in the deposition of fibrin followed by fibroblast activation and proliferation and subsequent collagen deposition. Genes involved in collagen synthesis and myofibroblastic differentiation have also been found to be upregulated in this disease, a similar pattern of gene upregulation and downregulation to that of palmar fibromatoses.[341-343] A number of studies have found inducible nitric oxide synthetase to be upregulated, while constitutive (endothelial) nitric oxide synthetase expression is downregulated.[344] The exact role of nitric oxide synthetase in the pathophysiology of Peyronie disease has yet to be fully elucidated, but it is likely to induce the production of reactive oxygen species and collagen deposition.[333] It is possible that Peyronie disease does not represent a single distinct entity but a common morphologic appearance that occurs secondary to a variety of insults.

The optimal therapy for Peyronie disease remains controversial, because innumerable nonsurgical therapies have been attempted (vitamin E, potassium amino benzoate, colchicine, intralesional injections of corticosteroids, calcium channel blockers, shockwave therapy, and collagenase), all with limited success.[345] Surgery appears to be the most effective treatment, although there is no consensus as to which technique offers the best outcome.[346] Surgical candidates include patients who have erectile dysfunction and those whose penile curvature precludes intercourse. Straightening the penis usually requires at least partial excision of the plaque with surgery or laser therapy, coupled with some type of grafting procedure.[347] There is a significant rate of postoperative erectile dysfunction, and some patients also require placement of a penile prosthesis.[348] Given that about one-third of patients who remain untreated have spontaneous resolution of their symptoms, many urologists choose to observe these patients for a period of time before embarking on definitive therapy.

KNUCKLE PADS

Knuckle pads are flat or dome-shaped noninflammatory fibrous thickenings that occur on the dorsal aspect of the proximal interphalangeal or metacarpophalangeal joints and the paratenon of the extensor tendons (Fig. 8-76).[349] Most patients are asymptomatic, although some have mild tenderness or pain; the lesions rarely require surgical intervention. Knuckle pads comprise yet another fibrous proliferation not

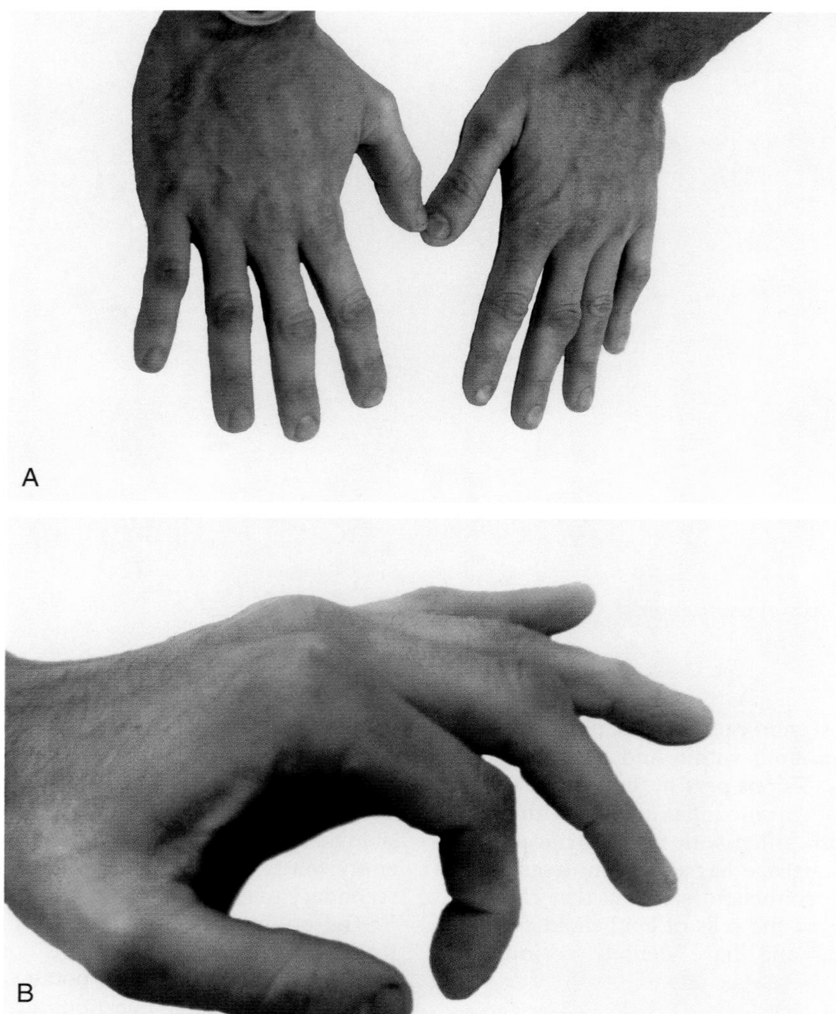

FIGURE 8-76. (A) Knuckle pads is a lesion marked by fibrous thickening over the extensor surfaces of the interphalangeal joints. It may be associated with both palmar and plantar fibromatoses. (B) Side view of knuckle pads.

infrequently encountered in conjunction with palmar or plantar fibromatosis.[265,270] The knuckle pads may precede the onset of palmar or plantar fibromatosis and may disappear spontaneously after these lesions are excised. Like palmar and plantar fibromatoses, the knuckle pad chiefly affects patients during the fourth, fifth, and sixth decades of life and is observed more commonly in men than in women. *Pachydermodactyly* is a rare variant of this condition that occurs mainly in adolescent boys.[350] Microscopically, knuckle pads resemble palmar fibromatosis, but digital contractures do not occur. Grossly, knuckle pads may be confused with pad-like hyperkeratoses that occur secondarily to occupational trauma (e.g., boxing) or self-manipulation.[351]

Bart-Pumphrey syndrome is an autosomal dominant disorder characterized by sensorineural hearing loss, palmoplantar keratoderma, leukonychia, and knuckle pads, although there is considerable phenotypic variability.[352] Recently, this disorder has been associated with missense mutations in the *GJB2* gene, which encodes for a gap junction protein, connexin-26.[352,353] However, abnormalities of this gene have not been found in other superficial fibromatoses.

References

1. Eyden B. The myofibroblast: a study of normal, reactive and neoplastic tissues, with an emphasis on ultrastructure. Part 2—tumours and tumour-like lesions. J Submicrosc Cytol Pathol 2005;37(3-4):231–96.
2. Eyden B. The fibronexus in reactive and tumoral myofibroblasts: further characterisation by electron microscopy. Histol Histopathol 2001;16(1):57–70.
3. Skalli O, Schürch W, Seemayer T, et al. Myofibroblasts from diverse pathologic settings are heterogeneous in their content of actin isoforms and intermediate filament proteins. Lab Invest 1989;60(2):275–85.
4. Mentzel T, Katenkamp D. [Myofibroblastic tumors. Brief review of clinical aspects, diagnosis and differential diagnosis]. Pathologe 1998;19(3):176–86.
5. Canty EG, Kadler KE. Procollagen trafficking, processing and fibrillogenesis. J Cell Sci 2005;118(Pt 7):1341–53.
6. Ushiki T. Collagen fibers, reticular fibers and elastic fibers. A comprehensive understanding from a morphological viewpoint. Arch Histol Cytol 2002;65(2):109–26.
7. Briggs SL. The role of fibronectin in fibroblast migration during tissue repair. J Wound Care 2005;14(6):284–7.
8. Swartz R, Scheel P. Retroperitoneal fibrosis: gaining traction on an enigma. Lancet 2011;378(9788):294–6.
9. Gibbs RV. Cytokines and glycosaminoglycans (GAGs). Adv Exp Med Biol 2003;535:125–43.
10. Allen PW. Nodular fasciitis. Pathology 1972;4(1):9–26.

11. Weinreb I, Shaw AJ, Perez-Ordoñez B, et al. Nodular fasciitis of the head and neck region: a clinicopathologic description in a series of 30 cases. J Cutan Pathol 2009;36(11):1168–73.
12. Bemrich-Stolz CJ, Kelly DR, Muensterer OJ, et al. Single institution series of nodular fasciitis in children. J Pediatr Hematol Oncol 2010;32(5):354–7.
13. Hara H, Fujita I, Fujimoto T, et al. Nodular fasciitis of the hand in a young athlete. A case report. Ups J Med Sci 2010;115(4):291–6.
14. Jaryszak EM, Shah RK, Bauman NM, et al. Unexpected pathologies in pediatric parotid lesions: management paradigms revisited. Int J Pediatr Otorhinolaryngol 2011;75(4):558–63.
15. Abdel-Aziz M, Khattab H, El-bosraty H, et al. Nodular fasciitis of the external auditory canal in six Egyptian children. Int J Pediatr Otorhinolaryngol 2008;72(5):643–6.
16. Leventis M, Vardas E, Gkouzioti A, et al. Oral nodular fasciitis: report of a case of the buccal mucosa. J Craniomaxillofac Surg 2011;39(5):340–2.
17. Ozben V, Aydogan F, Karaca FC. Nodular fasciitis of the breast previously misdiagnosed as breast carcinoma. Breast Care (Basel) 2009;4(6):401–2.
18. Bernstein KE, Lattes R. Nodular (pseudosarcomatous) fasciitis, a nonrecurrent lesion: clinicopathologic study of 134 cases. Cancer 1982;49(8):1668–78.
19. Montgomery EA, Meis JM. Nodular fasciitis. Its morphologic spectrum and immunohistochemical profile. Am J Surg Pathol 1991;15(10):942–8.
20. de Feraudy S, Fletcher CDM. Intradermal nodular fasciitis: a rare lesion analyzed in a series of 24 cases. Am J Surg Pathol 2010;34(9):1377–81.
21. Shimizu S, Hashimoto H, Enjoji M. Nodular fasciitis: an analysis of 250 patients. Pathology 1984;16(2):161–6.
22. Kim JH, Kwon H, Song D, et al. Clinical case of ossifying fasciitis of the hand. J Plast Reconstr Aesthet Surg 2007;60(4):443–6.
23. Sato K, Oda Y, Ueda Y, et al. Fasciitis ossificans of the breast. Pathol Res Pract 2007;203(10):737–9.
24. Park C, Park J, Lee K-Y. Parosteal (nodular) fasciitis of the hand. Clin Radiol 2004;59(4):376–8.
25. Patchefsky AS, Enzinger FM. Intravascular fasciitis: a report of 17 cases. Am J Surg Pathol 1981;5(1):29–36.
26. Samaratunga H, Searle J, O'Loughlin B. Intravascular fasciitis: a case report and review of the literature. Pathology 1996;28(1):8–11.
27. Chi AC, Dunlap WS, Richardson MS, et al. Intravascular fasciitis: report of an intraoral case and review of the literature. Head Neck Pathol 2011. Available at: http://www.ncbi.nlm.nih.gov/pubmed/21779880. Accessed July 23, 2011.
28. Sticha RS, Deacon JS, Wertheimer SJ, et al. Intravascular fasciitis in the foot. J Foot Ankle Surg 1997;36(2):95–9.
29. Wang L, Wang G, Wang L, et al. Myxoid intravascular fasciitis. J Cutan Pathol 2011;38(1):63–6.
30. Hussein MR. Cranial fasciitis of childhood: a case report and review of literature. J Cutan Pathol 2008;35(2):212–4.
31. Lauer DH, Enzinger FM. Cranial fasciitis of childhood. Cancer 1980;45(2):401–6.
32. Takeda N, Fujita K, Katayama S, et al. Cranial fasciitis presenting with intracranial mass: a case report. Pediatr Neurosurg 2008;44(2):148–52.
33. Johnson KK, Dannenbaum MJ, Bhattacharjee MB, et al. Diagnosing cranial fasciitis based on distinguishing radiological features. J Neurosurg Pediatr 2008;2(5):370–4.
34. Oh C-K, Whang S-M, Kim B-G, et al. Congenital cranial fasciitis—"watch and wait" or early intervention. Pediatr Dermatol 2007;24(3):263–6.
35. Rakheja D, Cunningham JC, Mitui M, et al. A subset of cranial fasciitis is associated with dysregulation of the Wnt/beta-catenin pathway. Mod Pathol 2008;21(11):1330–6.
36. Summers LE, Florez L, Berberian ZJM, et al. Postoperative cranial fasciitis. Report of two cases and review of the literature. J Neurosurg 2007;106(6):1080–5.
37. Ceballos KM, Nielsen GP, Selig MK, et al. Is anti-h-caldesmon useful for distinguishing smooth muscle and myofibroblastic tumors? An immunohistochemical study. Am J Clin Pathol 2000;114(5):746–53.
38. Perez-Montiel MD, Plaza JA, Dominguez-Malagon H, et al. Differential expression of smooth muscle myosin, smooth muscle actin, h-caldesmon, and calponin in the diagnosis of myofibroblastic and smooth muscle lesions of skin and soft tissue. Am J Dermatopathol 2006;28(2):105–11.
39. Bhattacharya B, Dilworth HP, Iacobuzio-Donahue C, et al. Nuclear beta-catenin expression distinguishes deep fibromatosis from other benign and malignant fibroblastic and myofibroblastic lesions. Am J Surg Pathol 2005;29(5):653–9.
40. Sawyer JR, Sammartino G, Baker GF, et al. Clonal chromosome aberrations in a case of nodular fasciitis. Cancer Genet Cytogenet 1994;76(2):154–6.
41. Weibolt VM, Buresh CJ, Roberts CA, et al. Involvement of 3q21 in nodular fasciitis. Cancer Genet Cytogenet 1998;106(2):177–9.
42. Velagaleti GVN, Tapper JK, Panova NE, et al. Cytogenetic findings in a case of nodular fasciitis of subclavicular region. Cancer Genet Cytogenet 2003;141(2):160–3.
43. Koizumi H, Mikami M, Doi M, et al. Clonality analysis of nodular fasciitis by HUMARA-methylation-specific PCR. Histopathology 2005;47(3):320–1.
44. Erickson-Johnson MR, Chou MM, Evers BR, et al. Nodular fasciitis: a novel model of transient neoplasia induced by MYH9-USP6 gene fusion. Lab Invest 2011. Available at: http://www.ncbi.nlm.nih.gov/pubmed/21826056. Accessed August 24, 2011.
45. Yanagisawa A, Okada H. Nodular fasciitis with degeneration and regression. J Craniofac Surg 2008;19(4):1167–70.
46. Chung EB, Enzinger FM. Proliferative fasciitis. Cancer 1975;36(4):1450–8.
47. Magro G, Michal M, Alaggio R, et al. Intradermal proliferative fasciitis in childhood: a potential diagnostic pitfall. J Cutan Pathol 2011;38(1):59–62.
48. Honda Y, Oh-i T, Koga M, et al. A case of proliferative fasciitis in the abdominal region. J Dermatol 2001;28(12):753–8.
49. Kiryu H, Takeshita H, Hori Y. Proliferative fasciitis. Report of a case with histopathologic and immunohistochemical studies. Am J Dermatopathol 1997;19(4):396–9.
50. Fleming MG, Sharata HH. Intradermal proliferative fasciitis. J Cutan Pathol 2011. Available at: http://www.ncbi.nlm.nih.gov/pubmed/21592183. Accessed August 23, 2011.
51. Meis JM, Enzinger FM. Proliferative fasciitis and myositis of childhood. Am J Surg Pathol 1992;16(4):364–72.
52. Lundgren L, Kindblom LG, Willems J, et al. Proliferative myositis and fasciitis. A light and electron microscopic, cytologic, DNA-cytometric and immunohistochemical study. APMIS 1992;100(5):437–48.
53. Domínguez-Malagón H. Intracellular collagen and fibronexus in fibromatosis and other fibroblastic tumors. Ultrastruct Pathol 2004;28(2):67–73.
54. Ghadially FN, Thomas MJ, Jabi M, et al. Intracisternal collagen fibrils in proliferative fasciitis and myositis of childhood. Ultrastruct Pathol 1993;17(2):161–8.
55. Kern WH. Proliferative myositis; a pseudosarcomatous reaction to injury: a report of seven cases. Arch Pathol 1960;69:209–16.
56. Ackerman LV. Extra-osseous localized non-neoplastic bone and cartilage formation (so-called myositis ossificans): clinical and pathological confusion with malignant neoplasms. J Bone Joint Surg Am 1958;40-A(2):279–98.
57. Klapsinou E, Despoina P, Dimitra D. Cytologic findings and potential pitfalls in proliferative myositis and myositis ossificans diagnosed by fine needle aspiration cytology: report of four cases and review of the literature. Diagn Cytopathol 2012;40(3):239–44.
58. Wong NL. Fine needle aspiration cytology of pseudosarcomatous reactive proliferative lesions of soft tissue. Acta Cytol 2002;46(6):1049–55.
59. Enzinger FM, Dulcey F. Proliferative myositis. Report of thirty-three cases. Cancer 1967;20(12):2213–23.
60. Fauser C, Nährig J, Niedermeyer HP, et al. Proliferative myositis: a rare pseudomalignant tumor of the head and neck. Arch Otolaryngol Head Neck Surg 2008;134(4):437–40.
61. Brooks JK, Scheper MA, Kramer RE, et al. Intraoral proliferative myositis: case report and literature review. Head Neck 2007;29(4):416–20.
62. Ryś J, Gruchała A, Korobowicz E. Proliferative myositis with bone/osteoid formation. Pol J Pathol 2009;60(3):144–6.
63. el-Jabbour JN, Bennett MH, Burke MM, et al. Proliferative myositis. An immunohistochemical and ultrastructural study. Am J Surg Pathol 1991;15(7):654–9.
64. Dembinski A, Bridge JA, Neff JR, et al. Trisomy 2 in proliferative fasciitis. Cancer Genet Cytogenet 1992;60(1):27–30.
65. Ohjimi Y, Iwasaki H, Ishiguro M, et al. Trisomy 2 found in proliferative myositis cultured cell. Cancer Genet Cytogenet 1994;76(2):157.
66. McComb EN, Neff JR, Johansson SL, et al. Chromosomal anomalies in a case of proliferative myositis. Cancer Genet Cytogenet 1997;98(2):142–4.

67. Wong NL, Di F. Pseudosarcomatous fasciitis and myositis: diagnosis by fine-needle aspiration cytology. Am J Clin Pathol 2009;132(6): 857–65.
68. Garijo MF, Val-Bernal JF, Vega A, et al. Postoperative spindle cell nodule of the breast: pseudosarcomatous myofibroblastic proliferation following endo-surgery. Pathol Int 2008;58(12):787–91.
69. Proppe KH, Scully RE, Rosai J. Postoperative spindle cell nodules of genitourinary tract resembling sarcomas. A report of eight cases. Am J Surg Pathol 1984;8(2):101–8.
70. Young RH. Pseudotumors of the urinary bladder. Int J Surg Pathol 2010;18(3 Suppl):101S–5S.
71. Harik LR, Merino C, Coindre J-M, et al. Pseudosarcomatous myofibroblastic proliferations of the bladder: a clinicopathologic study of 42 cases. Am J Surg Pathol 2006;30(7):787–94.
72. Montgomery EA, Shuster DD, Burkart AL, et al. Inflammatory myofibroblastic tumors of the urinary tract: a clinicopathologic study of 46 cases, including a malignant example inflammatory fibrosarcoma and a subset associated with high-grade urothelial carcinoma. Am J Surg Pathol 2006;30(12):1502–12.
73. Huang WL, Ro JY, Grignon DJ, et al. Postoperative spindle cell nodule of the prostate and bladder. J Urol 1990;143(4):824–6.
74. Hirsch MS, Dal Cin P, Fletcher CDM. ALK expression in pseudosarcomatous myofibroblastic proliferations of the genitourinary tract. Histopathology 2006;48(5):569–78.
75. Young RH, Scully RE. Pseudosarcomatous lesions of the urinary bladder, prostate gland, and urethra. A report of three cases and review of the literature. Arch Pathol Lab Med 1987;111(4):354–8.
76. Harper L, Michel J-L, Riviere J-P, et al. Inflammatory pseudotumor of the ureter. *J Pediatr Surg* 2005;40(3):597–9.
77. Sukov WR, Cheville JC, Carlson AW, et al. Utility of ALK-1 protein expression and ALK rearrangements in distinguishing inflammatory myofibroblastic tumor from malignant spindle cell lesions of the urinary bladder. Mod Pathol 2007;20(5):592–603.
78. Tsuzuki T, Magi-Galluzzi C, Epstein JI. ALK-1 expression in inflammatory myofibroblastic tumor of the urinary bladder. Am J Surg Pathol 2004;28(12):1609–14.
79. Perosio PM, Weiss SW. Ischemic fasciitis: a juxta-skeletal fibroblastic proliferation with a predilection for elderly patients. Mod Pathol 1993;6(1):69–72.
80. Montgomery EA, Meis JM, Mitchell MS, et al. Atypical decubital fibroplasia. A distinctive fibroblastic pseudotumor occurring in debilitated patients. Am J Surg Pathol 1992;16(7):708–15.
81. Baranzelli MC, Lecomte-Houcke M, De Saint Maur P, et al. [Atypical decubitus fibroplasia: a recent entity. Apropos of a case of an adolescent girl]. Bull Cancer 1996;83(1):81–4.
82. Liegl B, Fletcher CDM. Ischemic fasciitis: analysis of 44 cases indicating an inconsistent association with immobility or debilitation. Am J Surg Pathol 2008;32(10):1546–52.
83. Chung EB, Enzinger FM. Fibroma of tendon sheath. Cancer 1979;44(5): 1945–54.
84. Degreef I, Sciot R, De Smet L. Intraarticular fibroma of the tendon sheath in the wrist. J Hand Surg Eur Vol 2007;32(6):723.
85. Moretti VM, de la Cruz M, Lackman RD, et al. Fibroma of tendon sheath in the knee: a report of three cases and literature review. Knee 2010;17(4): 306–9.
86. Ciatti R, Mariani PP. Fibroma of tendon sheath located within the ankle joint capsule. J Orthop Traumatol 2009;10(3):147–50.
87. Kundangar R, Pandey V, Acharya KKV, et al. An intraarticular fibroma of the tendon sheath in the knee joint. Knee Surg Sports Traumatol Arthrosc 2011. Available at: http://www.ncbi.nlm.nih.gov/pubmed/21340629. Accessed July 26, 2011.
88. Pulitzer DR, Martin PC, Reed RJ. Fibroma of tendon sheath. A clinicopathologic study of 32 cases. Am J Surg Pathol 1989;13(6):472–9.
89. Lamovec J, Bracko M, Voncina D. Pleomorphic fibroma of tendon sheath. Am J Surg Pathol 1991;15(12):1202–5.
90. Jablokow VR, Kathuria S. Fibroma of tendon sheath. J Surg Oncol 1982;19(2):90–2.
91. Le Corroller T, Bouvier-Labit C, Sbihi A, et al. Mineralized fibroma of the tendon sheath presenting as a bursitis. Skeletal Radiol 2008;37(12): 1141–5.
92. Maluf HM, DeYoung BR, Swanson PE, et al. Fibroma and giant cell tumor of tendon sheath: a comparative histological and immunohistological study. Mod Pathol 1995;8(2):155–9.
93. Satti MB. Tendon sheath tumours: a pathological study of the relationship between giant cell tumour and fibroma of tendon sheath. Histopathology 1992;20(3):213–20.
94. Sciot R, Samson I, van den Berghe H, et al. Collagenous fibroma (desmoplastic fibroblastoma): genetic link with fibroma of tendon sheath? Mod Pathol 1999;12(6):565–8.
95. Cohen PR, Schulze KE, Cohen SA, et al. Pleomorphic fibroma of the skin. Skinmed 2010;8(2):113–5.
96. Kamino H, Lee JY, Berke A. Pleomorphic fibroma of the skin: a benign neoplasm with cytologic atypia. A clinicopathologic study of eight cases. Am J Surg Pathol 1989;13(2):107–13.
97. García-Doval I, Casas L, Toribio J. Pleomorphic fibroma of the skin, a form of sclerotic fibroma: an immunohistochemical study. Clin Exp Dermatol 1998;23(1):22–4.
98. Aguilar C, Rosai J. Pleomorphic fibroma of the skin, atypical lipomatous tumor, or both? Int J Surg Pathol 2011;19(1):63.
99. Hsieh Y-J, Lin Y-C, Wu Y-H, et al. Subungual pleomorphic fibroma. J Cutan Pathol 2003;30(9):569–71.
100. Pinto-Blázquez J, Velasco-Alonso J, Alonso-de la Campa J, et al. [Myxoid pleomorphic fibroma of the skin]. Actas Dermosifiliogr 2006;97(9): 581–2.
101. Mahmood MN, Salama ME, Chaffins M, et al. Solitary sclerotic fibroma of skin: a possible link with pleomorphic fibroma with immunophenotypic expression for O13 (CD99) and CD34. J Cutan Pathol 2003;30(10): 631–6.
102. Layfield LJ, Fain JS. Pleomorphic fibroma of skin. A case report and immunohistochemical study. Arch Pathol Lab Med 1991;115(10): 1046–9.
103. Balachandran K, Allen PW, MacCormac LB. Nuchal fibroma. A clinicopathological study of nine cases. Am J Surg Pathol 1995;19(3): 313–7.
104. Michal M, Fetsch JF, Hes O, et al. Nuchal-type fibroma: a clinicopathologic study of 52 cases. Cancer 1999;85(1):156–63.
105. Shek TW, Chan AC, Ma L. Extranuchal nuchal fibroma. Am J Surg Pathol 1996;20(7):902–3.
106. Lee GK, Suh KJ, Lee SM, et al. Nuchal-type fibroma of the buttock: magnetic resonance imaging findings. Jpn J Radiol 2010;28(7):538–41.
107. Sraj SA, Lahoud LE, Musharafieh R, et al. Nuchal-type fibroma of the ankle: a case report. J Foot Ankle Surg 2008;47(4):332–6.
108. Laskin WB, Fetsch JF, Miettinen M. Nuchal fibrocartilaginous pseudotumor: a clinicopathologic study of five cases and review of the literature. Mod Pathol 1999;12(7):663–8.
109. Nicoletti GF, Platania N, Cicero S, et al. Nuchal fibrocartilaginous pseudomotor. Case report and review of the literature. J Neurosurg Sci 2003;47(3):173–5; discussion 175.
110. Wehrli BM, Weiss SW, Yandow S, et al. Gardner-associated fibromas (GAF) in young patients: a distinct fibrous lesion that identifies unsuspected Gardner syndrome and risk for fibromatosis. Am J Surg Pathol 2001;25(5):645–51.
111. Linos K, Sedivcová M, Cerna K, et al. Extra nuchal-type fibroma associated with elastosis, traumatic neuroma, a rare APC gene missense mutation, and a very rare MUTYH gene polymorphism: a case report and review of the literature(*). J Cutan Pathol 2011. Available at: http://www.ncbi.nlm.nih.gov/pubmed/21752055. Accessed August 26, 2011.
112. Michal M. Non-nuchal-type fibroma associated with Gardner's syndrome. A hitherto-unreported mesenchymal tumor different from fibromatosis and nuchal-type fibroma. Pathol Res Pract 2000;196(12): 857–60.
113. Michal M, Boudova L, Mukensnabl P. Gardner's syndrome associated fibromas. Pathol Int 2004;54(7):523–6.
114. Coffin CM, Hornick JL, Zhou H, et al. Gardner fibroma: a clinicopathologic and immunohistochemical analysis of 45 patients with 57 fibromas. Am J Surg Pathol 2007;31(3):410–6.
115. Diwan AH, Graves ED, King JA, et al. Nuchal-type fibroma in two related patients with Gardner's syndrome. Am J Surg Pathol 2000;24(11): 1563–7.
116. Montgomery E, Folpe AL. The diagnostic value of beta-catenin immunohistochemistry. Adv Anat Pathol 2005;12(6):350–6.
117. Allen PW. Nuchal-type fibroma appearance in a desmoid fibromatosis. Am J Surg Pathol 2001;25(6):828–9.
118. Jarvi O, Saxen E. Elastofibroma dorse. Acta Pathol Microbiol Scand Suppl 1961;51(Suppl. 144):83–4.
119. Go PH, Meadows MC, Deleon EMB, et al. Elastofibroma dorsi: a soft tissue masquerade. Int J Shoulder Surg 2010;4(4):97–101.
120. Hatano H, Morita T, Kawashima H, et al. Symptomatic elastofibroma in young baseball pitchers: report of three cases. J Shoulder Elbow Surg 2010;19(8):e7–10.
121. Giebel GD, Bierhoff E, Vogel J. Elastofibroma and pre-elastofibroma–a biopsy and autopsy study. Eur J Surg Oncol 1996;22(1):93–6.

122. Järvi OH, Länsimies PH. Subclinical elastofibromas in the scapular region in an autopsy series. Acta Pathol Microbiol Scand A 1975;83(1): 87–108.
123. Hayes AJ, Alexander N, Clark MA, et al. Elastofibroma: a rare soft tissue tumour with a pathognomonic anatomical location and clinical symptom. Eur J Surg Oncol 2004;30(4):450–3.
124. Martínez Hernández NJ, Figueroa Almanzar S, Arnau Obrer A. Bilateral elastofibroma dorsi: a very rare presentation for a rare pathology. Arch Bronconeumol 2011. Available at: http://www.ncbi.nlm.nih.gov/pubmed/21764205. Accessed July 26, 2011.
125. Naylor MF, Nascimento AG, Sherrick AD, et al. Elastofibroma dorsi: radiologic findings in 12 patients. AJR Am J Roentgenol 1996;167(3): 683–7.
126. Nishio J, Isayama T, Iwasaki H, et al. Elastofibroma dorsi: diagnostic and therapeutic algorithm. J Shoulder Elbow Surg 2011. Available at: http://www.ncbi.nlm.nih.gov/pubmed/21524925. Accessed July 26, 2011.
127. Parratt MTR, Donaldson JR, Flanagan AM, et al. Elastofibroma dorsi: management, outcome and review of the literature. J Bone Joint Surg Br 2010;92(2):262–6.
128. Lau KN, Sindram D, Ahrens WA, et al. Gastric elastofibroma. Am Surg 2010;76(12):1446–8.
129. Hobbs CM, Burch DM, Sobin LH. Elastosis and elastofibromatous change in the gastrointestinal tract: a clinicopathologic study of 13 cases and a review of the literature. Am J Clin Pathol 2004;122(2): 232–7.
130. Märkl B, Kerwel TG, Langer E, et al. Elastosis of the colon and the ileum as polyp causing lesions: a study of six cases and review of the literature. Pathol Res Pract 2008;204(6):395–9.
131. Yamazaki K. An ultrastructural and immunohistochemical study of elastofibroma: CD 34, MEF-2, prominin 2 (CD133), and factor XIIIa-positive proliferating fibroblastic stromal cells connected by Cx43-type gap junctions. Ultrastruct Pathol 2007;31(3):209–19.
132. De Nictolis M, Goteri G, Campanati G, et al. Elastofibrolipoma of the mediastinum. A previously undescribed benign tumor containing abnormal elastic fibers. Am J Surg Pathol 1995;19(3):364–7.
133. Goldblum JR, Beals T, Weiss SW. Elastofibromatous change of the rectum. A lesion mimicking amyloidosis. Am J Surg Pathol 1992;16(8): 793–5.
134. Tighe JR, Clark AE, Turvey DJ. Elastofibroma dorsi. J Clin Pathol 1968;21(4):463–9.
135. Kahn HJ, Hanna WM. "Aberrant elastic" in elastofibroma: an immunohistochemical and ultrastructural study. Ultrastruct Pathol 1995;19(1): 45–50.
136. Nagamine N, Nohara Y, Ito E. Elastofibroma in Okinawa. A clinicopathologic study of 170 cases. Cancer 1982;50(9):1794–805.
137. Schepel JA, Wille J, Seldenrijk CA, et al. Elastofibroma: a familial occurrence. Eur J Surg 1998;164(7):557–8.
138. Hernández JLG, Rodríguez-Parets JO, Valero JM, et al. High-resolution genome-wide analysis of chromosomal alterations in elastofibroma. Virchows Arch 2010;456(6):681–7.
139. Batstone P, Forsyth L, Goodlad J. Clonal chromosome aberrations secondary to chromosome instability in an elastofibroma. Cancer Genet Cytogenet 2001;128(1):46–7.
140. McComb EN, Feely MG, Neff JR, et al. Cytogenetic instability, predominantly involving chromosome 1, is characteristic of elastofibroma. Cancer Genet Cytogenet 2001;126(1):68–72.
141. Vanni R, Marras S, Faa G, et al. Chromosome instability in elastofibroma. Cancer Genet Cytogenet 1999;111(2):182–3.
142. Vincent J, Maleki Z. Elastofibroma: cytomorphologic, histologic, and radiologic findings in five cases. Diagn Cytopathol 2011. Available at: http://www.ncbi.nlm.nih.gov/pubmed/21630483. Accessed August 27, 2011.
143. Blount A, Riley KO, Woodworth BA. Juvenile nasopharyngeal angiofibroma. Otolaryngol Clin North Am 2011;44(4):989–1004.
144. Szymańska A, Korobowicz E, Gołabek W. A rare case of nasopharyngeal angiofibroma in an elderly female. Eur Arch Otorhinolaryngol 2006; 263(7):657–60.
145. Mohindra S, Grover G, Bal AK. Extranasopharyngeal angiofibroma of the nasal septum: a case report. Ear Nose Throat J 2009;88(11): E17–19.
146. Tasca I, Compadretti GC. Extranasopharyngeal angiofibroma of nasal septum. A controversial entity. Acta Otorhinolaryngol Ital 2008;28(6): 312–4.
147. Giardiello FM, Hamilton SR, Krush AJ, et al. Nasopharyngeal angiofibroma in patients with familial adenomatous polyposis. Gastroenterology 1993;105(5):1550–2.
148. Klockars T, Renkonen S, Leivo I, et al. Juvenile nasopharyngeal angiofibroma: no evidence for inheritance or association with familial adenomatous polyposis. Fam Cancer 2010;9(3):401–3.
149. Abraham SC, Montgomery EA, Giardiello FM, et al. Frequent beta-catenin mutations in juvenile nasopharyngeal angiofibromas. Am J Pathol 2001;158(3):1073–8.
150. Abraham SC, Wu TT. Nasopharyngeal angiofibroma. Hum Pathol 2001;32(4):455.
151. Guertl B, Beham A, Zechner R, et al. Nasopharyngeal angiofibroma: an APC-gene-associated tumor? Hum Pathol 2000;31(11):1411–3.
152. Baguley C, Sandhu G, O'Donnell J, et al. Consumptive coagulopathy complicating juvenile angiofibroma. J Laryngol Otol 2004;118(11): 835–9.
153. Beham A, Beham-Schmid C, Regauer S, et al. Nasopharyngeal angiofibroma: true neoplasm or vascular malformation? Adv Anat Pathol 2000;7(1):36–46.
154. Liu Z-F, Wang D-H, Sun X-C, et al. The site of origin and expansive routes of juvenile nasopharyngeal angiofibroma (JNA). Int J Pediatr Otorhinolaryngol 2011;75(9):1088–92.
155. Fyrmpas G, Konstantinidis I, Constantinidis J. Endoscopic treatment of juvenile nasopharyngeal angiofibromas: our experience and review of the literature. Eur Arch Otorhinolaryngol 2011. Available at: http://www.ncbi.nlm.nih.gov/pubmed/21789677. Accessed August 27, 2011.
156. Aziz-Sultan MA, Moftakhar R, Wolfe SQ, et al. Endoscopically assisted intratumoral embolization of juvenile nasopharyngeal angiofibroma using Onyx. J Neurosurg Pediatr 2011;7(6):600–3.
157. Radkowski D, McGill T, Healy GB, et al. Angiofibroma. Changes in staging and treatment. Arch Otolaryngol Head Neck Surg 1996;122(2): 122–9.
158. Guo G, Paulino AFG. Lipomatous variant of nasal angiofibroma. Arch Otolaryngol Head Neck Surg 2003;129(4):499.
159. Beham A, Kainz J, Stammberger H, et al. Immunohistochemical and electron microscopical characterization of stromal cells in nasopharyngeal angiofibromas. Eur Arch Otorhinolaryngol 1997;254(4):196–9.
160. Beham A, Fletcher CD, Kainz J, et al. Nasopharyngeal angiofibroma: an immunohistochemical study of 32 cases. Virchows Arch A Pathol Anat Histopathol 1993;423(4):281–5.
161. Hwang HC, Mills SE, Patterson K, et al. Expression of androgen receptors in nasopharyngeal angiofibroma: an immunohistochemical study of 24 cases. Mod Pathol 1998;11(11):1122–6.
162. Zhang PJ, Weber R, Liang H-H, et al. Growth factors and receptors in juvenile nasopharyngeal angiofibroma and nasal polyps: an immunohistochemical study. Arch Pathol Lab Med 2003;127(11):1480–4.
163. Pauli J, Gundelach R, Vanelli-Rees A, et al. Juvenile nasopharyngeal angiofibroma: an immunohistochemical characterisation of the stromal cell. Pathology 2008;40(4):396–400.
164. Sun X-C, Wang D-H, Yu H-P, et al. Analysis of risk factors associated with recurrence of nasopharyngeal angiofibroma. J Otolaryngol Head Neck Surg 2010;39(1):56–61.
165. Wang QY, Chen HH, Lu YY. Comparison of two approaches to the surgical management of juvenile nasopharyngeal angiofibroma stages I and II. J Otolaryngol Head Neck Surg 2011;40(1):14–8.
166. Roche P-H, Paris J, Régis J, et al. Management of invasive juvenile nasopharyngeal angiofibromas: the role of a multimodality approach. Neurosurgery 2007;61(4):768–77; discussion 777.
167. McAfee WJ, Morris CG, Amdur RJ, et al. Definitive radiotherapy for juvenile nasopharyngeal angiofibroma. Am J Clin Oncol 2006;29(2): 168–70.
168. Gauglitz GG, Korting HC, Pavicic T, et al. Hypertrophic scarring and keloids: pathomechanisms and current and emerging treatment strategies. Mol Med 2011;17(1-2):113–25.
169. Bayat A, McGrouther DA. Clinical management of skin scarring. Skinmed 2005;4(3):165–73.
170. Lee S-S, Yosipovitch G, Chan Y-H, et al. Pruritus, pain, and small nerve fiber function in keloids: a controlled study. J Am Acad Dermatol 2004;51(6):1002–6.
171. Liu MF, Yencha M. Cushing's syndrome secondary to intralesional steroid injections of multiple keloid scars. Otolaryngol Head Neck Surg 2006;135(6):960–1.
172. Seifert O, Mrowietz U. Keloid scarring: bench and bedside. Arch Dermatol Res 2009;301(4):259–72.
173. Murray JC. Keloids and hypertrophic scars. Clin Dermatol 1994;12(1): 27–37.
174. Speranza G, Sultanem K, Muanza T. Descriptive study of patients receiving excision and radiotherapy for keloids. Int J Radiat Oncol Biol Phys 2008;71(5):1465–9.

175. Shih B, Bayat A. Genetics of keloid scarring. Arch Dermatol Res 2010;302(5):319–39.
176. Brown JJ, Bayat A. Genetic susceptibility to raised dermal scarring. Br J Dermatol 2009;161(1):8–18.
177. Shapero J, Shapero H. Acne keloidalis nuchae is scar and keloid formation secondary to mechanically induced folliculitis. J Cutan Med Surg 2011;15(4):238–40.
178. Burk CJ, Aber C, Connelly EA. Ehlers-Danlos syndrome type IV: keloidal plaques of the lower extremities, amniotic band limb deformity, and a new mutation. J Am Acad Dermatol 2007;56(2 Suppl):S53–54.
179. Kanitakis J, Claudy A. Clinical quiz. Rubinstein-Taybi syndrome (synonyms: broad thumbs and great toes, characteristic facies, and mental retardation—broad thumb-hallux syndrome). Eur J Dermatol 2002; 12(1):107, 108–9.
180. Wriston CC, Rubin AI, Elenitsas R, et al. Nodular scleroderma: a report of 2 cases. Am J Dermatopathol 2008;30(4):385–8.
181. González-Martínez R, Marín-Bertolín S, Amorrortu-Velayos J. Association between keloids and Dupuytren's disease: case report. Br J Plast Surg 1995;48(1):47–8.
182. Kamath NV, Ormsby A, Bergfeld WF, et al. A light microscopic and immunohistochemical evaluation of scars. J Cutan Pathol 2002;29(1): 27–32.
183. Eyden B. Electron microscopy in the study of myofibroblastic lesions. Semin Diagn Pathol 2003;20(1):13–24.
184. Chen MA, Davidson TM. Scar management: prevention and treatment strategies. Curr Opin Otolaryngol Head Neck Surg 2005;13(4):242–7.
185. Endo Y, Shirase T, Utani A, et al. Isolated collagenoma with a unique appearance on the scalp. Eur J Dermatol 2011. Available at: http://www.ncbi.nlm.nih.gov/pubmed/21768057. Accessed August 27, 2011.
186. McClung AA, Blumberg MA, Huttenbach Y, et al. Development of collagenomas during pregnancy. J Am Acad Dermatol 2005;53(2 Suppl 1):S150–153.
187. Metcalf JS, Maize JC, LeBoit PE. Circumscribed storiform collagenoma (sclerosing fibroma). Am J Dermatopathol 1991;13(2):122–9.
188. Celebi JT, Tsou HC, Chen FF, et al. Phenotypic findings of Cowden syndrome and Bannayan-Zonana syndrome in a family associated with a single germline mutation in PTEN. J Med Genet 1999;36(5): 360–4.
189. Nam J-H, Min JH, Lee G-Y, et al. A case of perifollicular fibroma. Ann Dermatol 2011;23(2):236–8.
190. Kuo TT, Hu S, Chan HL. Keloidal dermatofibroma: report of 10 cases of a new variant. Am J Surg Pathol 1998;22(5):564–8.
191. Chike-Obi CJ, Cole PD, Brissett AE. Keloids: pathogenesis, clinical features, and management. Semin Plast Surg 2009;23(3):178–84.
192. Emad M, Omidvari S, Dastgheib L, et al. Surgical excision and immediate postoperative radiotherapy versus cryotherapy and intralesional steroids in the management of keloids: a prospective clinical trial. Med Princ Pract 2010;19(5):402–5.
193. Scrimali L, Lomeo G, Nolfo C, et al. Treatment of hypertrophic scars and keloids with a fractional CO_2 laser: a personal experience. J Cosmet Laser Ther 2010;12(5):218–21.
194. Har-Shai Y, Brown W, Pallua N, et al. Intralesional cryosurgery for the treatment of hypertrophic scars and keloids. Plast Reconstr Surg 2010;126(5):1798–1800; author reply 1800.
195. Shockman S, Paghdal KV, Cohen G. Medical and surgical management of keloids: a review. J Drugs Dermatol 2010;9(10):1249–57.
196. Sakuraba M, Takahashi N, Akahoshi T, et al. Experience of silicone gel sheets for patients with keloid scars after median sternotomy. Gen Thorac Cardiovasc Surg 2010;58(9):467–70.
197. Evans HL. Desmoplastic fibroblastoma. A report of seven cases. Am J Surg Pathol 1995;19(9):1077–81.
198. Fukunaga M, Ushigome S. Collagenous fibroma (desmoplastic fibroblastoma): a distinctive fibroblastic soft tissue tumor. Adv Anat Pathol 1999;6(5):275–80.
199. Hasegawa T, Shimoda T, Hirohashi S, et al. Collagenous fibroma (desmoplastic fibroblastoma): report of four cases and review of the literature. Arch Pathol Lab Med 1998;122(5):455–60.
200. Nielsen GP, O'Connell JX, Dickersin GR, et al. Collagenous fibroma (desmoplastic fibroblastoma): a report of seven cases. Mod Pathol 1996;9(7):781–5.
201. Nishio J, Iwasaki H, Nishijima T, et al. Collagenous fibroma (desmoplastic fibroblastoma) of the finger in a child. Pathol Int 2002;52(4): 322–5.
202. de Sousa SF, Caldeira PC, Grossmann S, et al. Desmoplastic fibroblastoma (collagenous fibroma): a case identified in the buccal mucosa. Head Neck Pathol 2011;5(2):175–9.
203. Nonaka CF, Carvalho Mde V, de Moraes M, et al. Desmoplastic fibroblastoma (collagenous fibroma) of the tongue. J Cutan Pathol 2010;37(8): 911–4.
204. Takahara M, Ichikawa R, Oda Y, et al. Desmoplastic fibroblastoma: a case presenting as a protruding nodule in the dermis. J Cutan Pathol 2008;35 (Suppl 1):70–3.
205. Huang H-Y, Sung M-T, Eng H-L, et al. Superficial collagenous fibroma: immunohistochemical, ultrastructural, and flow cytometric study of three cases, including one pemphigus vulgaris patient with a dermal mass. APMIS 2002;110(4):283–9.
206. Sciot R, Samson I, van den Berghe H, et al. Collagenous fibroma (desmoplastic fibroblastoma): genetic link with fibroma of tendon sheath? Mod Pathol 1999;12(6):565–8.
207. Sakamoto A, Yamamoto H, Yoshida T, et al. Desmoplastic fibroblastoma (collagenous fibroma) with a specific breakpoint of 11q12. Histopathology 2007;51(6):859–60.
208. Bernal K, Nelson M, Neff JR, et al. Translocation (2;11)(q31;q12) is recurrent in collagenous fibroma (desmoplastic fibroblastoma). Cancer Genet Cytogenet 2004;149(2):161–3.
209. Maghari A, Ma N, Aisner S, et al. Collagenous fibroma (desmoplastic fibroblastoma) with a new translocation involving 11q12: a case report. Cancer Genet Cytogenet 2009;192(2):73–5.
210. Weiss SW, Gnepp DR, Bratthauer GL. Palisaded myofibroblastoma. A benign mesenchymal tumor of lymph node. Am J Surg Pathol 1989;13(5):341–6.
211. Suster S, Rosai J. Intranodal hemorrhagic spindle-cell tumor with "amianthoid" fibers. Report of six cases of a distinctive mesenchymal neoplasm of the inguinal region that simulates Kaposi's sarcoma. Am J Surg Pathol 1989;13(5):347–57.
212. Lee JY, Abell E, Shevechik GJ. Solitary spindle cell tumor with myoid differentiation of the lymph node. Arch Pathol Lab Med 1989;113(5): 547–50.
213. Michal M, Chlumská A, Skálová A, et al. Palisaded intranodal myofibroblastoma. Electron microscopic study. Zentralbl Pathol 1993;139(1): 81–8.
214. Katz DR. Neurilemmoma with calcosiderotic nodules. Isr J Med Sci 1974;10(9):1156–5.
215. Nguyen T, Eltorky MA. Intranodal palisaded myofibroblastoma. Arch Pathol Lab Med 2007;131(2):306–10.
216. Fletcher CD, Stirling RW. Intranodal myofibroblastoma presenting in the submandibular region: evidence of a broader clinical and histological spectrum. Histopathology 1990;16(3):287–93.
217. Alguacil-Garcia A. Intranodal myofibroblastoma in a submandibular lymph node. A case report. Am J Clin Pathol 1992;97(1):69–72.
218. Bigotti G, Coli A, Mottolese M, et al. Selective location of palisaded myofibroblastoma with amianthoid fibres. J Clin Pathol 1991;44(9): 761–4.
219. Kandemir NO, Barut F, Ekinci T, et al. Intranodal palisaded myofibroblastoma (intranodal hemorrhagic spindle cell tumor with amianthoid fibers): a case report and literature review. Diagn Pathol 2010; 5:12.
220. Koseoglu RD, Ozkan N, Filiz NO, et al. Intranodal palisaded myofibroblastoma; a case report and review of the literature. Pathol Oncol Res 2009;15(2):297–300.
221. Toker C, Tang CK, Whitely JF, et al. Benign spindle cell breast tumor. Cancer 1981;48(7):1615–22.
222. Chan KW, Ghadially FN, Alagaratnam TT. Benign spindle cell tumour of breast–a variant of spindled cell lipoma or fibroma of breast? Pathology 1984;16(3):331–6.
223. Wargotz ES, Weiss SW, Norris HJ. Myofibroblastoma of the breast. Sixteen cases of a distinctive benign mesenchymal tumor. Am J Surg Pathol 1987;11(7):493–502.
224. Magro G. Mammary myofibroblastoma: a tumor with a wide morphologic spectrum. Arch Pathol Lab Med 2008;132(11):1813–20.
225. McMenamin ME, Fletcher CD. Mammary-type myofibroblastoma of soft tissue: a tumor closely related to spindle cell lipoma. Am J Surg Pathol 2001;25(8):1022–9.
226. Arsenovic N, Abdulla KE, Shamim KS. Mammary-type myofibroblastoma of soft tissue. Indian J Pathol Microbiol 2011;54(2):391–3.
227. Magro G, Caltabiano R, Kacerovská D, et al. Vulvovaginal myofibroblastoma: expanding the morphological and immunohistochemical spectrum. A clinicopathologic study of 10 cases. Hum Pathol 2011. Available at: http://www.ncbi.nlm.nih.gov/pubmed/21820148. Accessed August 27, 2011.
228. Zhang Y, Jorda M, Goldblum JR. Perianal mammary-type myofibroblastoma. Ann Diagn Pathol 2010;14(5):358–60.

229. Mukonoweshuro P, McCormick F, Rachapalli V, et al. Paratesticular mammary-type myofibroblastoma. Histopathology 2007;50(3):396–7.
230. Scotti C, Camnasio F, Rizzo N, et al. Mammary-type myofibroblastoma of popliteal fossa. Skeletal Radiol 2008;37(6):549–53.
231. Hox V, Vander Poorten V, Delaere PR, et al. Extramammary myofibroblastoma in the head and neck region. Head Neck 2009;31(9):1240–4.
232. Corradi D, Bosio S, Maestri R, et al. A giant myxoid mammary myofibroblastoma: evidence for a myogenic/synthetic phenotype and an extracellular matrix rich in fibronectin. Histopathology 2008;52(3):396–9.
233. Magro G. Epithelioid-cell myofibroblastoma of the breast: expanding the morphologic spectrum. Am J Surg Pathol 2009;33(7):1085–92.
234. Wei Q, Zhu Y. Collision tumor composed of mammary-type myofibroblastoma and eccrine adenocarcinoma of the vulva. Pathol Int 2011;61(3):138–42.
235. Magro G, Amico P, Gurrera A. Myxoid myofibroblastoma of the breast with atypical cells: a potential diagnostic pitfall. Virchows Arch 2007;450(4):483–5.
236. Maggiani F, Debiec-Rychter M, Verbeeck G, et al. Extramammary myofibroblastoma is genetically related to spindle cell lipoma. Virchows Arch 2006;449(2):244–7.
237. Flucke U, van Krieken JH, Mentzel T. Cellular angiofibroma: analysis of 25 cases emphasizing its relationship to spindle cell lipoma and mammary-type myofibroblastoma. Mod Pathol 2011;24(1):82–9.
238. Fritchie KJ, Carver P, Sun Y, et al. Solitary fibrous tumor: is there a molecular relationship with cellular angiofibroma, spindle cell lipoma, and mammary-type myofibroblastoma? Am J Clin Pathol 2012;137(6):963–70.
239. Pauwels P, Sciot R, Croiset F, et al. Myofibroblastoma of the breast: genetic link with spindle cell lipoma. J Pathol 2000;191(3):282–5.
240. Laskin WB, Fetsch JF, Mostofi FK. Angiomyofibroblastomalike tumor of the male genital tract: analysis of 11 cases with comparison to female angiomyofibroblastoma and spindle cell lipoma. Am J Surg Pathol 1998;22(1):6–16.
241. Nucci MR, Granter SR, Fletcher CD. Cellular angiofibroma: a benign neoplasm distinct from angiomyofibroblastoma and spindle cell lipoma. Am J Surg Pathol 1997;21(6):636–44.
242. Damiani S, Miettinen M, Peterse JL, et al. Solitary fibrous tumour (myofibroblastoma) of the breast. Virchows Arch 1994;425(1):89–92.
243. Fetsch JF, Laskin WB, Miettinen M. Superficial acral fibromyxoma: a clinicopathologic and immunohistochemical analysis of 37 cases of a distinctive soft tissue tumor with a predilection for the fingers and toes. Hum Pathol 2001;32(7):704–14.
244. Ashby-Richardson H, Rogers GS, Stadecker MJ. Superficial acral fibromyxoma: an overview. Arch Pathol Lab Med 2011;135(8):1064–6.
245. Prescott RJ, Husain EA, Abdellaoui A, et al. Superficial acral fibromyxoma: a clinicopathological study of new 41 cases from the U.K.: should myxoma (NOS) and fibroma (NOS) continue as part of 21st-century reporting? Br J Dermatol 2008;159(6):1315–21.
246. Hollmann TJ, Bovée JV, Fletcher CD. Digital fibromyxoma (superficial acral fibromyxoma): a detailed characterization of 124 cases. Am J Surg Pathol 2012;36:789–98.
247. Al-Daraji WI, Al-Daraji U, Al-Mahmoud RM. Superficial acral fibromyxoma: report of two cases and discussion of the nomenclature. Dermatol Online J 2008;14(2):27.
248. Oteo-Alvaro A, Meizoso T, Scarpellini A, et al. Superficial acral fibromyxoma of the toe, with erosion of the distal phalanx. A clinical report. Arch Orthop Trauma Surg 2008;128(3):271–4.
249. McNiff JM, Subtil A, Cowper SE, et al. Cellular digital fibromas: distinctive CD34-positive lesions that may mimic dermatofibrosarcoma protuberans. J Cutan Pathol 2005;32(6):413–8.
250. Fanti P, Dika E, Piraccini B, et al. Superficial acral fibromyxoma: a clinicopathological and immunohistochemical analysis of 12 cases of a distinctive soft tissue tumor with a predilection for the fingers and toes. G Ital Dermatol Venereol 2011;146(4):283–7.
251. Cogrel O, Stanislas S, Coindre JM, et al. [Superficial acral fibromyxoma: three cases]. Ann Dermatol Venereol 2010;137(12):789–93.
252. Misago N, Ohkawa T, Yanai T, et al. Superficial acral fibromyxoma on the tip of the big toe: expression of CD10 and nestin. J Eur Acad Dermatol Venereol 2008;22(2):255–7.
253. Tardío JC, Butrón M, Martín-Fragueiro LM. Superficial acral fibromyxoma: report of 4 cases with CD10 expression and lipomatous component, two previously underrecognized features. Am J Dermatopathol 2008;30(5):431–5.
254. Pasquinelli G, Foroni L, Papadopoulos F, et al. Superficial acral fibromyxoma: immunohistochemical and ultrastructural analysis of a case, with literature review. Ultrastruct Pathol 2009;33(6):293–301.
255. Lisovsky M, Hoang MP, Dresser KA, et al. Apolipoprotein D in CD34-positive and CD34-negative cutaneous neoplasms: a useful marker in differentiating superficial acral fibromyxoma from dermatofibrosarcoma protuberans. Mod Pathol 2008;21(1):31–8.
256. Al-Daraji WI, Miettinen M. Superficial acral fibromyxoma: a clinicopathological analysis of 32 tumors including 4 in the heel. J Cutan Pathol 2008;35(11):1020–6.
257. Guitart J, Ramirez J, Laskin WB. Cellular digital fibromas: what about superficial acral fibromyxoma? J Cutan Pathol 2006;33(11):762–3; author reply 764.
258. Lewin MR, Montgomery EA, Barrett TL. New or unusual dermatopathology tumors: a review. J Cutan Pathol 2011;38(9):689–96.
259. Mariño-Enríquez A, Fletcher CD. Angiofibroma of soft tissue: clinicopathologic characterization of a distinctive benign fibrovascular neoplasm in a series of 37 cases. Am J Surg Pathol 2012;36(4):500–8.
260. Jin Y, Möller E, Nord KH, et al. Fusion of the AHRR and NCOA2 genes through a recurrent translocation t(5;8)(p15;q13) in soft tissue angiofibroma results in upregulation of aryl hydrocarbon receptor target genes. Genes Chromosomes Cancer 2012;51(5):510–20.
261. Maravic M, Landais P. Dupuytren's disease in France–1831 to 2001–from description to economic burden. J Hand Surg Br 2005;30(5):484–7.
262. Elliot D. The early history of Dupuytren's disease. Hand Clin 1999;15(1):1–19, v.
263. Shih B, Bayat A. Scientific understanding and clinical management of Dupuytren disease. Nat Rev Rheumatol 2010;6(12):715–26.
264. Stahl S, Calif E. Dupuytren's palmar contracture in women. Isr Med Assoc J 2008;10(6):445–7.
265. Fetsch JF, Laskin WB, Miettinen M. Palmar-plantar fibromatosis in children and preadolescents: a clinicopathologic study of 56 cases with newly recognized demographics and extended follow-up information. Am J Surg Pathol 2005;29(8):1095–105.
266. Usmar S, Peat B. Paediatric Dupuytren's disease. ANZ J Surg 2010;80(4):298–9.
267. Saboeiro AP, Porkorny JJ, Shehadi SI, et al. Racial distribution of Dupuytren's disease in Department of Veterans Affairs patients. Plast Reconstr Surg 2000;106(1):71–5.
268. Bayat A, McGrouther DA. Management of Dupuytren's disease–clear advice for an elusive condition. Ann R Coll Surg Engl 2006;88(1):3–8.
269. Burge P. Genetics of Dupuytren's disease. Hand Clin 1999;15(1):63–71.
270. Mikkelsen OA. Knuckle pads in Dupuytren's disease. Hand 1977;9(3):301–5.
271. Lee YC, Chan HH, Black MM. Aggressive polyfibromatosis: a 10 year follow-up. Australas J Dermatol 1996;37(4):205–7.
272. Al-Matubsi HY, Hamdan F, Alhanbali OA, et al. Diabetic hand syndromes as a clinical and diagnostic tool for diabetes mellitus patients. Diabetes Res Clin Pract 2011. Available at: http://www.ncbi.nlm.nih.gov/pubmed/21831469. Accessed August 28, 2011.
273. Burke FD, Proud G, Lawson IJ, et al. An assessment of the effects of exposure to vibration, smoking, alcohol and diabetes on the prevalence of Dupuytren's disease in 97,537 miners. J Hand Surg Eur Vol 2007;32(4):400–6.
274. Arkkila PE, Kantola IM, Viikari JS. Dupuytren's disease: association with chronic diabetic complications. J Rheumatol 1997;24(1):153–9.
275. Noble J, Heathcote JG, Cohen H. Diabetes mellitus in the aetiology of Dupuytren's disease. J Bone Joint Surg Br 1984;66(3):322–5.
276. Arafa M, Noble J, Royle SG, et al. Dupuytren's and epilepsy revisited. J Hand Surg Br 1992;17(2):221–4.
277. Lucas G, Brichet A, Roquelaure Y, et al. Dupuytren's disease: personal factors and occupational exposure. Am J Ind Med 2008;51(1):9–15.
278. Noble J, Arafa M, Royle SG, et al. The association between alcohol, hepatic pathology and Dupuytren's disease. J Hand Surg Br 1992;17(1):71–4.
279. Bower M, Nelson M, Gazzard BG. Dupuytren's contractures in patients infected with HIV. BMJ 1990;300(6718):164–5.
280. French PD, Kitchen VS, Harris JR. Prevalence of Dupuytren's contracture in patients infected with HIV. BMJ 1990;301(6758):967.
281. Arafa M, Steingold RF, Noble J. The incidence of Dupuytren's disease in patients with rheumatoid arthritis. J Hand Surg Br 1984;9(2):165–6.
282. Gabbiani G, Majno G. Dupuytren's contracture: fibroblast contraction? An ultrastructural study. Am J Pathol 1972;66(1):131–46.

283. Tomasek J, Rayan GM. Correlation of alpha-smooth muscle actin expression and contraction in Dupuytren's disease fibroblasts. J Hand Surg Am 1995;20(3):450–5.
284. McCann BG, Logan A, Belcher H, et al. The presence of myofibroblasts in the dermis of patients with Dupuytren's contracture. A possible source for recurrence. J Hand Surg Br 1993;18(5):656–61.
285. Montgomery E, Lee JH, Abraham SC, et al. Superficial fibromatoses are genetically distinct from deep fibromatoses. Mod Pathol 2001;14(7): 695–701.
286. Badalamente MA, Hurst LC, Grandia SK, et al. Platelet-derived growth factor in Dupuytren's disease. J Hand Surg Am 1992;17(2):317–23.
287. Bisson MA, Beckett KS, McGrouther DA, et al. Transforming growth factor-beta1 stimulation enhances Dupuytren's fibroblast contraction in response to uniaxial mechanical load within a 3-dimensional collagen gel. J Hand Surg Am 2009;34(6):1102–10.
288. Zhang AY, Fong KD, Pham H, et al. Gene expression analysis of Dupuytren's disease: the role of TGF-beta2. J Hand Surg Eur Vol 2008;33(6): 783–90.
289. De Wever I, Dal Cin P, Fletcher CD, et al. Cytogenetic, clinical, and morphologic correlations in 78 cases of fibromatosis: a report from the CHAMP Study Group. Chromosomes and Morphology. Mod Pathol 2000;13(10):1080–5.
290. Dal Cin P, De Smet L, Sciot R, et al. Trisomy 7 and trisomy 8 in dividing and non-dividing tumor cells in Dupuytren's disease. Cancer Genet Cytogenet 1999;108(2):137–40.
291. Bonnici AV, Birjandi F, Spencer JD, et al. Chromosomal abnormalities in Dupuytren's contracture and carpal tunnel syndrome. J Hand Surg Br 1992;17(3):349–55.
292. Shih B, Wijeratne D, Armstrong DJ, et al. Identification of biomarkers in Dupuytren's disease by comparative analysis of fibroblasts versus tissue biopsies in disease-specific phenotypes. J Hand Surg Am 2009;34(1):124–36.
293. Dolmans GH, Werker PM, Hennies HC, et al. Wnt signaling and Dupuytren's disease. N Engl J Med 2011;365(4):307–17.
294. Hindocha S, John S, Stanley JK, et al. The heritability of Dupuytren's disease: familial aggregation and its clinical significance. J Hand Surg Am 2006;31(2):204–10.
295. Ling RS. The genetic factor in Dupuytren's disease. J Bone Joint Surg Br 1963;45:709–18.
296. Gupta R, Allen F, Tan V, et al. The effect of shear stress on fibroblasts derived from Dupuytren's tissue and normal palmar fascia. J Hand Surg Am 1998;23(5):945–50.
297. Herzog EG. The aetiology of Dupuytren's contracture. Lancet 1951; 1(6668):1305–6.
298. Liss GM, Stock SR. Can Dupuytren's contracture be work-related?: review of the evidence. Am J Ind Med 1996;29(5):521–32.
299. Kischer CW, Speer DP. Microvascular changes in Dupuytren's contracture. J Hand Surg Am 1984;9A(1):58–62.
300. Pereira RS, Black CM, Turner SM, et al. Antibodies to collagen types I-VI in Dupuytren's contracture. J Hand Surg Br 1986;11(1): 58–60.
301. Neumüller J, Menzel J, Millesi H. Prevalence of HLA-DR3 and autoantibodies to connective tissue components in Dupuytren's contracture. Clin Immunol Immunopathol 1994;71(2):142–8.
302. Baird KS, Alwan WH, Crossan JF, et al. T-cell-mediated response in Dupuytren's disease. Lancet 1993;341(8861):1622–3.
303. Bayat A, Cunliffe EJ, McGrouther DA. Assessment of clinical severity in Dupuytren's disease. Br J Hosp Med (Lond) 2007;68(11):604–9.
304. Brotherston TM, Balakrishnan C, Milner RH, et al. Long term follow-up of dermofasciectomy for Dupuytren's contracture. Br J Plast Surg 1994;47(6):440–3.
305. Abe Y, Rokkaku T, Kuniyoshi K, et al. Clinical results of dermofasciectomy for Dupuytren's disease in Japanese patients. J Hand Surg Eur Vol 2007;32(4):407–10.
306. Shaw Jr RB, Chong AK, Zhang A, et al. Dupuytren's disease: history, diagnosis, and treatment. Plast Reconstr Surg 2007;120(3): 44e–54e.
307. Yacoe ME, Bergman AG, Ladd AL, et al. Dupuytren's contracture: MR imaging findings and correlation between MR signal intensity and cellularity of lesions. AJR Am J Roentgenol 1993;160(4):813–7.
308. Hurst LC, Badalamente MA, Hentz VR, et al. Injectable collagenase clostridium histolyticum for Dupuytren's contracture. N Engl J Med 2009;361(10):968–79.
309. Betz N, Ott OJ, Adamietz B, et al. Radiotherapy in early-stage Dupuytren's contracture. Long-term results after 13 years. Strahlenther Onkol 2010;186(2):82–90.
310. Meek RM, McLellan S, Reilly J, et al. The effect of steroids on Dupuytren's disease: role of programmed cell death. J Hand Surg Br 2002;27(3): 270–3.
311. Pittet B, Rubbia-Brandt L, Desmoulière A, et al. Effect of gamma-interferon on the clinical and biologic evolution of hypertrophic scars and Dupuytren's disease: an open pilot study. Plast Reconstr Surg 1994; 93(6):1224–35.
312. de Bree E, Zoetmulder FA, Keus RB, et al. Incidence and treatment of recurrent plantar fibromatosis by surgery and postoperative radiotherapy. Am J Surg 2004;187(1):33–8.
313. Griffith JF, Wong TY, Wong SM, et al. Sonography of plantar fibromatosis. AJR Am J Roentgenol 2002;179(5):1167–72.
314. Elhadd TA, Ghosh S, Malik MI, et al. Plantar fibromatosis and Dupuytren's disease: an association to remember in patients with diabetes. Diabet Med 2007;24(11):1305.
315. Pickren JW, Smith AG, Stevenson Jr TW, et al. Fibromatosis of the plantar fascia. Cancer 1951;4(4):846–56.
316. Hafner S, Han N, Pressman MM, et al. Proximal plantar fibroma as an etiology of recalcitrant plantar heel pain. J Foot Ankle Surg 2011;50(3): 366.e1–5.
317. Boc SF, Kushner S. Plantar fibromatosis causing entrapment syndrome of the medial plantar nerve. J Am Podiatr Med Assoc 1994;84(8): 420–2.
318. DeBrule MB, Mott RC, Funk C, et al. Osseous metaplasia in plantar fibromatosis: a case report. J Foot Ankle Surg 2004;43(6):430–2.
319. Alman BA, Naber SP, Terek RM, et al. Platelet-derived growth factor in fibrous musculoskeletal disorders: a study of pathologic tissue sections and in vitro primary cell cultures. J Orthop Res 1995;13(1):67–77.
320. Zamora RL, Heights R, Kraemer BA, et al. Presence of growth factors in palmar and plantar fibromatoses. J Hand Surg Am 1994;19(3): 435–41.
321. Pentland AP, Anderson TF. Plantar fibromatosis responds to intralesional steroids. J Am Acad Dermatol 1985;12(1 Pt 2):212–4.
322. McNally EG, Shetty S. Plantar fascia: imaging diagnosis and guided treatment. Semin Musculoskelet Radiol 2010;14(3):334–43.
323. van der Veer WM, Hamburg SM, de Gast A, et al. Recurrence of plantar fibromatosis after plantar fasciectomy: single-center long-term results. Plast Reconstr Surg 2008;122(2):486–91.
324. Beckmann J, Kalteis T, Baer W, et al. [Plantar fibromatosis: therapy by total plantarfasciectomy]. Zentralbl Chir 2004;129(1):53–7.
325. Breiner JA, Nelson M, Bredthauer BD, et al. Trisomy 8 and trisomy 14 in plantar fibromatosis. Cancer Genet Cytogenet 1999;108(2): 176–7.
326. De Wever I, Dal Cin P, Fletcher CD, et al. Cytogenetic, clinical, and morphologic correlations in 78 cases of fibromatosis: a report from the CHAMP Study Group. Chromosomes and Morphology. Mod Pathol 2000;13(10):1080–5.
327. Sawyer JR, Sammartino G, Gokden N, et al. A clonal reciprocal t(2;7) (p13;p13) in plantar fibromatosis. Cancer Genet Cytogenet 2005; 158(1):67–9.
328. Androutsos G. [François Gigot de La Peyronie(1678-1747), benefactor of surgery and supporter of the fusion of medicine and surgery, and the disease that bears his name]. Prog Urol 2002;12(3):527–33.
329. Dunsmuir WD, Kirby RS. Francois de LaPeyronie (1978-1747): the man and the disease he described. Br J Urol 1996;78(4):613–22.
330. Mulhall JP, Creech SD, Boorjian SA, et al. Subjective and objective analysis of the prevalence of Peyronie's disease in a population of men presenting for prostate cancer screening. J Urol 2004;171(6 Pt 1): 2350–3.
331. Hellstrom WJ. History, epidemiology, and clinical presentation of Peyronie's disease. Int J Impot Res 2003;15 (Suppl 5):S91–92.
332. Kadioglu A, Sanli O, Akman T, et al. Factors affecting the degree of penile deformity in Peyronie disease: an analysis of 1001 patients. J Androl 2011;32(5):502–8.
333. Gonzalez-Cadavid NF. Mechanisms of penile fibrosis. J Sex Med 2009;6 (Suppl 3):353–62.
334. Casabé A, Bechara A, Cheliz G, et al. Risk factors of Peyronie's disease. What does our clinical experience show? J Sex Med 2011;8(2):518–23.
335. Davis Jr CJ. The microscopic pathology of Peyronie's disease. J Urol 1997;157(1):282–4.
336. Anafarta K, Bedük Y, Uluoğlu O, et al. The significance of histopathological changes of the normal tunica albuginea in Peyronie's disease. Int Urol Nephrol 1994;26(1):71–7.
337. Nachtsheim DA, Rearden A. Peyronie's disease is associated with an HLA class II antigen, HLA-DQ5, implying an autoimmune etiology. J Urol 1996;156(4):1330–4.

338. Hauck EW, Hauptmann A, Weidner W, et al. Prospective analysis of HLA classes I and II antigen frequency in patients with Peyronie's disease. J Urol 2003;170(4 Pt 1):1443–6.
339. Ralph DJ, Schwartz G, Moore W, et al. The genetic and bacteriological aspects of Peyronie's disease. J Urol 1997;157(1):291–4.
340. Devine Jr CJ, Somers KD, Jordan SG, et al. Proposal: trauma as the cause of the Peyronie's lesion. J Urol 1997;157(1):285–90.
341. Szardening-Kirchner C, Konrad L, Hauck EW, et al. Upregulation of mRNA expression of MCP-1 by TGF-beta1 in fibroblast cells from Peyronie's disease. World J Urol 2009;27(1):123–30.
342. Sampaio FJ. Comparison of gene expression profiles between Peyronie's disease and Dupuytren's contracture. Int Braz J Urol 2004;30(4): 349–50.
343. Qian A, Meals RA, Rajfer J, et al. Comparison of gene expression profiles between Peyronie's disease and Dupuytren's contracture. Urology 2004; 64(2):399–404.
344. Ferrini MG, Rivera S, Moon J, et al. The genetic inactivation of inducible nitric oxide synthase (iNOS) intensifies fibrosis and oxidative stress in the penile corpora cavernosa in type 1 diabetes. J Sex Med 2010;7(9): 3033–44.
345. Larsen SM, Levine LA. Peyronie's disease: review of nonsurgical treatment options. Urol Clin North Am 2011;38(2):195–205.
346. Ralph D, Gonzalez-Cadavid N, Mirone V, et al. The management of Peyronie's disease: evidence-based 2010 guidelines. J Sex Med 2010;7(7): 2359–74.
347. Ralph DJ. Long-term results of the surgical treatment of Peyronie's disease with plaque incision and grafting. Asian J Androl 2011. Available at: http://www.ncbi.nlm.nih.gov/pubmed/21785446. Accessed August 28, 2011.
348. Kadioglu A, Küçükdurmaz F, Sanli O. Current status of the surgical management of Peyronie's disease. Nat Rev Urol 2011;8(2):95–106.
349. Nenoff P, Woitek G. Images in clinical medicine. Knuckle pads. N Engl J Med 2011;364(25):2451.
350. Prieto D, Gallego E, López-Navarro N, et al. Pachydermodactyly: an uncommon acquired digital fibromatosis. J Clin Rheumatol 2011;17(1): 53–4.
351. Dickens R, Adams BB, Mutasim DF. Sports-related pads. Int J Dermatol 2002;41(5):291–3.
352. Richard G, Brown N, Ishida-Yamamoto A, Krol A. Expanding the phenotypic spectrum of Cx26 disorders: Bart-Pumphrey syndrome is caused by a novel missense mutation in GJB2. J Invest Dermatol 2004; 123(5):856–63.
353. Alexandrino F, Sartorato EL, Marques-de-Faria AP, et al. G59S mutation in the GJB2 (connexin 26) gene in a patient with Bart-Pumphrey syndrome. Am J Med Genet A 2005;136(3):282–4.

Fibrous Tumors of Infancy and Childhood

CHAPTER CONTENTS

Fibrous tumors of infancy and childhood can be divided into two large groups. The first group consists of lesions that correspond to similar lesions in adults in terms of clinical setting, microscopic picture, and behavior. Typical examples of such lesions are nodular fasciitis, palmar or plantar fibromatosis, and abdominal or extra-abdominal fibromatosis. The second group consists of fibrous lesions that are peculiar to infancy and childhood and generally have no clinical or morphologic counterpart in adult life. The latter are less common; because of their unusual microscopic features, they pose a special problem in diagnosis. In fact, the microscopic picture often fails to accurately reflect the biologic behavior, and features such as cellularity and rapid growth may be mistaken for evidence of malignancy, sometimes leading to unnecessary and excessive therapy. Therefore, accurate interpretation and diagnosis of these lesions are of utmost importance for predicting clinical behavior and for selecting the proper forms of therapy (Table 9-1).

FIBROUS HAMARTOMA OF INFANCY

Fibrous hamartoma of infancy is a distinctive, benign, fibrous growth that most frequently occurs during the first 2 years of life.[1-3] This lesion was first reported by Reye[4] in 1956 as a *subdermal fibromatous tumor of infancy*. In 1965, Enzinger[5] reviewed a series of 30 cases from the files of the Armed Forces Institute of Pathology (AFIP) and suggested the term *fibrous hamartoma of infancy* to emphasize its organoid microscopic appearance and its frequent occurrence at birth and during the immediate postnatal period.

Clinical Findings

The lesion virtually always develops during the first 2 years of life (median age 10 months) as a small, rapidly growing mass in the subcutis or reticular dermis. In the literature review by Dickey and Sotelo-Avila,[3] of 197 cases, 91% arose within the first year of life. Rare lesions have been reported in older infants and children. About 23% of cases are present at birth.[3,5] Like other fibrous tumors in children, it is more common in boys than in girls, with boys affected two to three times more often.[3] The mass is often freely movable; occasionally, it is fixed to the underlying fascia but only rarely involves the superficial portion of the musculature. These lesions grow rapidly from the outset up to the age of about 5 years. The growth of the lesion then slows but does not cease or regress spontaneously.[6]

Most occur above the waist, with the most common location being the anterior or posterior axillary fold, followed in frequency by the upper arm, thigh, inguinal, and pubic region, shoulder, back, and forearm. This lesion has also been described in unusual locations, including the scrotum,[7] labium majus,[8] scalp,[9] and gluteal region.[10] Few cases have been described in the feet or hands,[11] a feature that helps distinguish this lesion from infantile digital fibromatosis and calcifying aponeurotic fibroma. Virtually all cases are solitary, with only rare reports of multiple lesions in the same patient.[12] There is no evidence of increased familial incidence or associated malformations or other neoplasms. Antecedent trauma is occasionally reported at the time of presentation but is likely unrelated to its pathogenesis.[13]

Pathologic Findings

The excised lesion tends to be poorly circumscribed and consists of an intimate mixture of firm gray-white tissue and fat. In some cases, the fatty component is inconspicuous, whereas in others it occupies a large portion of the tumor, thereby resembling a fibrolipoma. Most measure 3 to 5 cm in greatest diameter, but tumors as large as 15 cm have been reported.

TABLE 9-1 Clinicopathologic Characteristics of Fibrous Tumors of Infancy and Childhood

HISTOLOGIC DIAGNOSIS	AGE (YEARS)	LOCATION	SOLITARY	MULTIPLE	REGRESSION
Fibrous hamartoma of infancy	B-2	Axilla, inguinal area	+	−	−
Digital fibromatosis	B-2	Fingers, toes	+	+	+
Myofibromatosis	B-A	Soft tissue, bone, viscera	+	+	+
Hyaline fibromatosis	2-A	Dermis, subcutis	−	+	−
Gingival fibromatosis	B-A	Gingiva, hard palate	+	+	+
Fibromatosis colli	B-2	Sternocleidomastoid muscle	+	Bilateral	+
Infantile fibromatosis	B-4	Musculature	+	−	−
Congenital/infantile fibrosarcoma	B-2	Musculature	+	−	−
Calcifying aponeurotic fibroma	2-A	Hands, feet	+	−	+

A, adult life; B, birth.

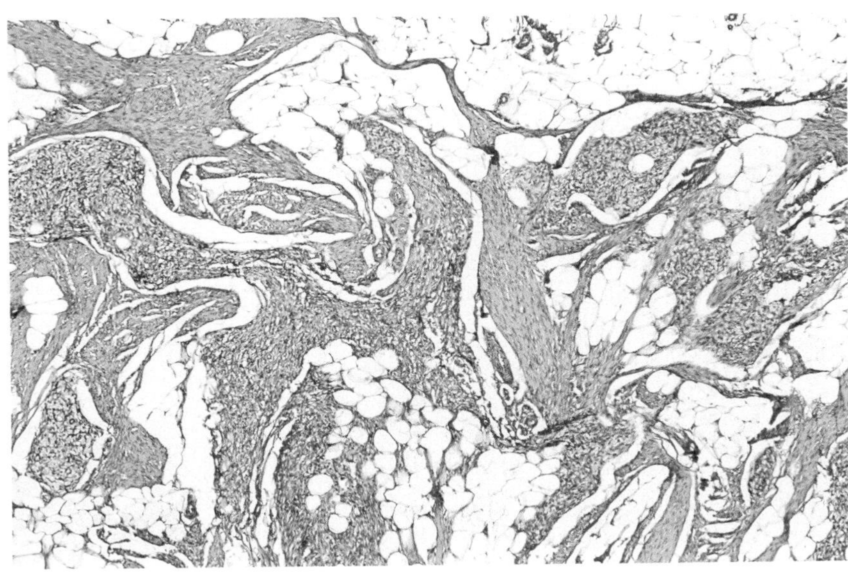

FIGURE 9-1. Fibrous hamartoma of infancy showing a characteristic organoid pattern composed of interlacing fibrous trabeculae, islands of loosely arranged spindle-shaped cells, and mature adipose tissue.

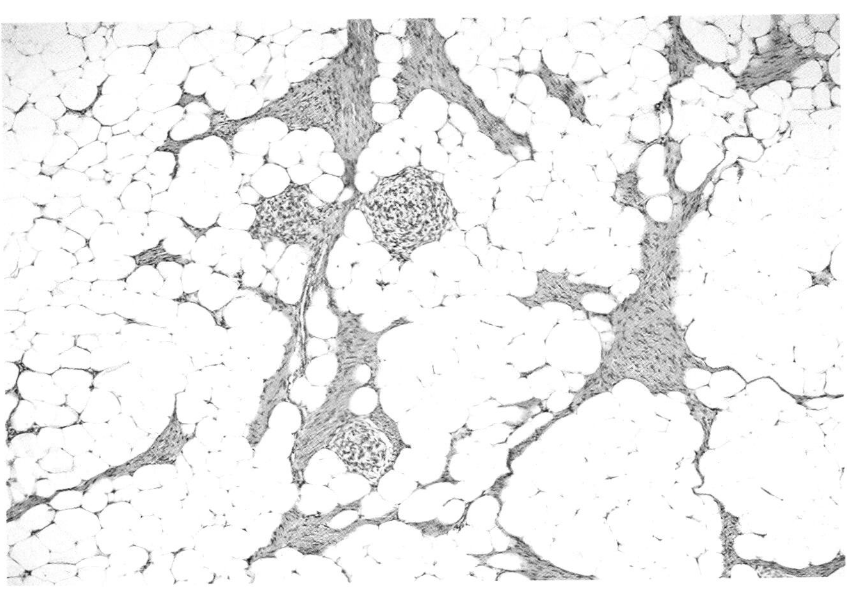

FIGURE 9-2. Fibrous hamartoma of infancy with an organoid pattern but composed predominantly of mature adipose tissue.

Fibrous hamartoma of infancy is characterized by three distinct components forming a vague, irregular, organoid pattern (Figs. 9-1 and 9-2): (1) well-defined intersecting trabeculae of fibrous tissue of varying size and shape and composed of well-oriented spindle-shaped cells (predominantly myofibroblasts) separated by varying amounts of collagen (Figs. 9-3 and 9-4); (2) loosely textured areas consisting chiefly of immature small, round, or stellate cells in a matrix of Alcian blue-positive hyaluronidase sensitive material (Figs. 9-5 to 9-7); and (3) varying amounts of interspersed mature fat, which may be present at only the periphery of the lesion or may be the major component. Despite the lack of clear boundaries between the fat in the tumor and that in the surrounding subcutis, there is little doubt that the fat is an integral part of the lesion. In fact, in many cases, its total amount exceeds many times the amount of fat normally present in the surrounding subcutis. In some cases, the immature small round cells in the myxoid foci are oriented around small veins.[14]

Some tumors show an additional tissue component, a peculiar fibrosing process that has a superficial resemblance to a neurofibroma.[5] It consists of thick collagen fibers and scattered fibroblasts that replace the fat in the loosely textured mesenchymal areas; sometimes it is the principal component of the tumor.

Immunohistochemical Findings

Immunohistochemically, smooth muscle and muscle-specific actin are present in the trabecular component only, and desmin is rarely expressed.[13] In some cases, the spindle cell component stains for CD34, which on occasion can cause confusion with giant cell fibroblastoma.

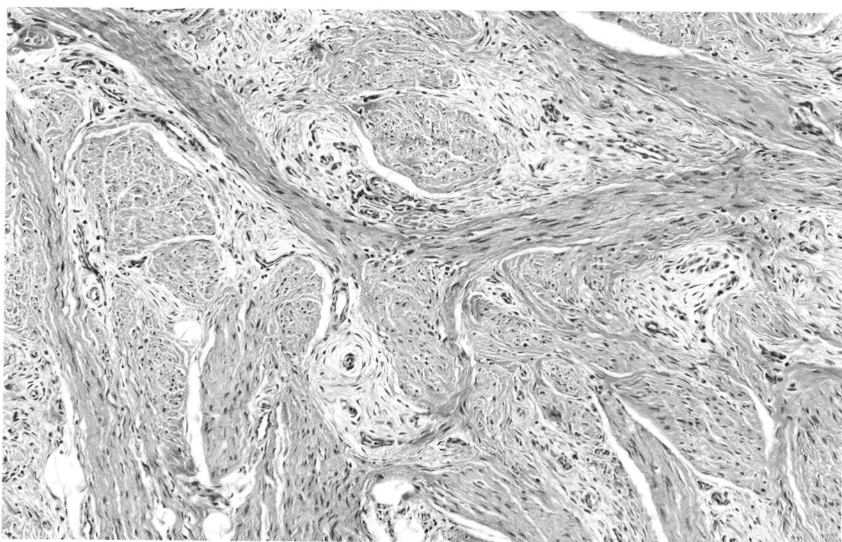

FIGURE 9-3. Fibrous hamartoma of infancy with interlacing fibrous trabeculae and interspersed myxoid zones.

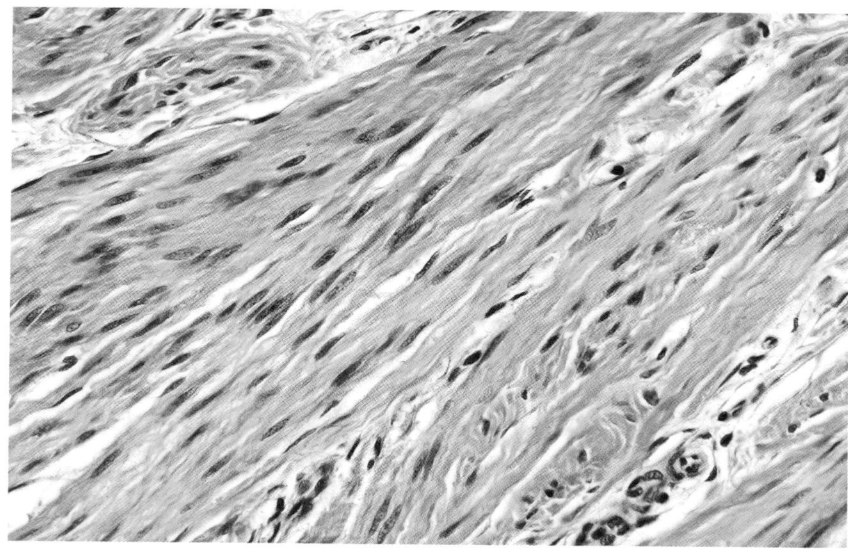

FIGURE 9-4. High-power view of spindle-shaped cells in fibrous trabeculae of a fibrous hamartoma of infancy.

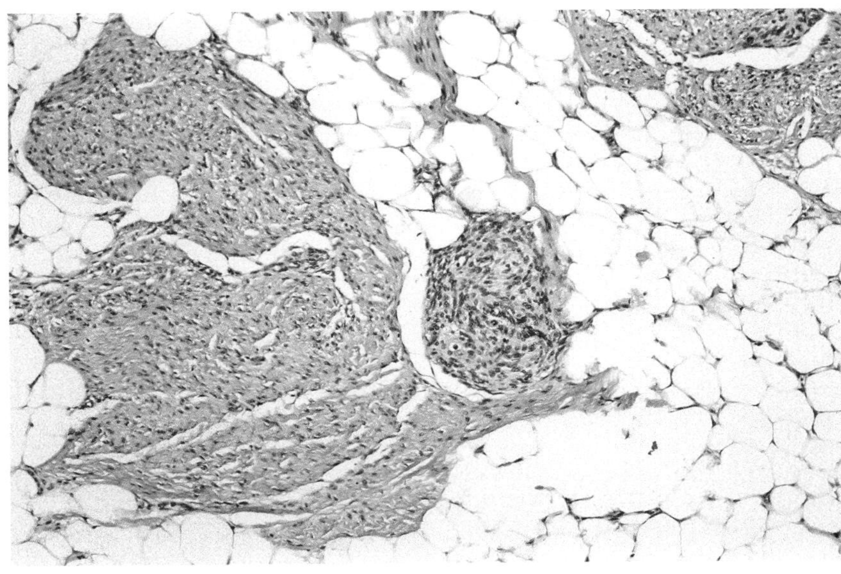

FIGURE 9-5. Fibrous hamartoma of infancy showing an admixture of mature adipose tissue, fibrous trabeculae, and a nodule of spindle-shaped cells.

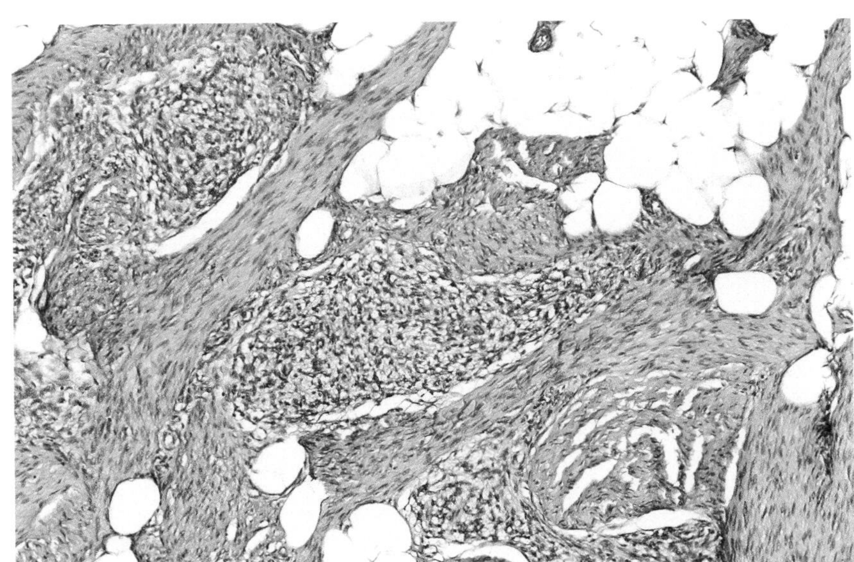

FIGURE 9-6. Organoid pattern with a characteristic arrangement of the three distinct components typical of fibrous hamartoma of infancy.

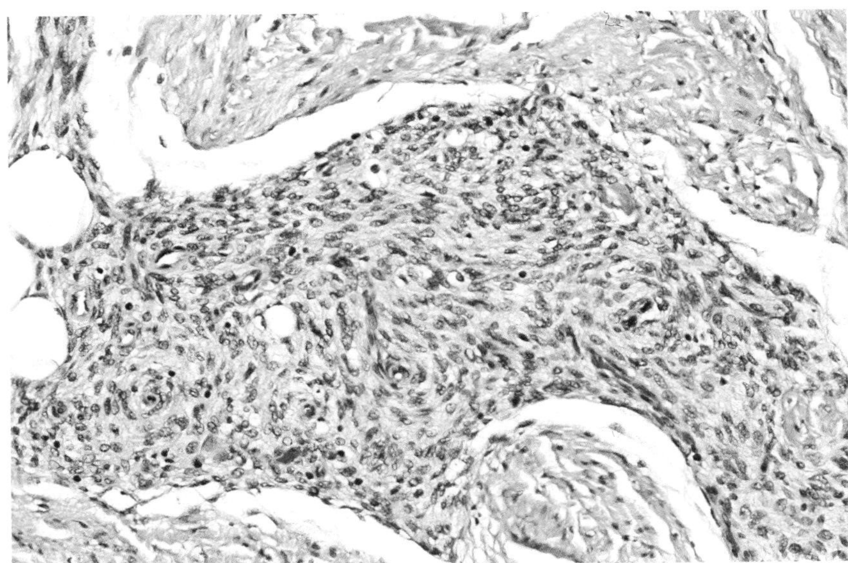

FIGURE 9-7. High-power view of cytologically bland spindle-shaped cells deposited in a myxoid stroma in a fibrous hamartoma of infancy.

Differential Diagnosis

In most cases, the organoid pattern characteristic of fibrous hamartoma of infancy is readily recognized, so the lesion is not difficult to distinguish from other entities. On occasion, when the myofibroblastic areas predominate, the lesion may be difficult to distinguish from infantile fibromatosis (also known as *lipofibromatosis*), diffuse myofibromatosis, and calcifying aponeurotic fibroma. *Infantile fibromatosis/lipofibromatosis* may encroach on the subcutis in a similar trabecular manner, but this tumor arises primarily in muscle rather than in the subcutis and lacks the organoid pattern of fibrous hamartoma. *Diffuse myofibromatosis*, typically nodular or multinodular, is characterized by light-staining nodules separated by or associated with hemangiopericytoma-like vascular areas. *Calcifying aponeurotic fibroma* may grow in the same trabecular manner, especially during its earliest phase, when there is still little or no calcification. However, the older age of the children and the location of the tumor in the palm of the hand permit an unequivocal diagnosis.

Awareness of the characteristic organoid pattern also facilitates distinction from *infantile fibrosarcoma* and *embryonal rhabdomyosarcoma*. Because some fibrous hamartomas of infancy occur in the scrotal region, the *spindle cell form of embryonal rhabdomyosarcoma* enters the differential diagnosis; however, this lesion generally occurs in older children and is composed of cells with more cytologic atypia.

Discussion

It is important to recognize and distinguish fibrous hamartoma of infancy from other forms of fibromatosis because it is a benign lesion that, despite its focal cellularity, is usually cured by local excision. Up to 16% locally recur, but recurrences are nondestructive and are generally cured by local re-excision.[3] Rare cases have been described with cytogenetic aberrations, including a case with a complex (6;12;8)(q25;q24.3;q13),[15] one with a reciprocal translocation t(2;3)(q31;q21),[16] and another with rearrangement of chromosomes 1, 2, 4, and 17.[17]

The true nature of fibrous hamartoma of infancy remains obscure. Although Reye[4] suggested that it might be a reparative process, there are no histologic features that suggest the lesion is a response to local injury. As its name implies, most have advocated the hamartomatous nature of this lesion, but the possibility that this is a benign neoplasm cannot be excluded. A single case of fibrous hamartoma of infancy with a t(2;3)(q31;q21) has been reported.[16]

INFANTILE DIGITAL FIBROMATOSIS

Infantile digital fibromatosis is a distinctive fibrous proliferation of infancy characterized by its occurrence in the fingers and toes, a marked tendency for local recurrence, and the presence of characteristic inclusion bodies in the cytoplasm of the neoplastic fibroblasts. In 1957, Jensen et al.[18] reported seven patients whose presentations were consistent with this entity but referred to these lesions as *digital neurofibrosarcoma in infancy*. Enzinger[19] subsequently reported seven cases in 1965 as *infantile dermal fibromatosis*.

Clinical Findings

Most patients present with a firm, broad-based, hemispheric or dome-shaped, nontender nodule with a smooth, glistening surface that is skin-colored or pale red. It is usually small, rarely exceeding 2 cm in greatest diameter. Almost all lesions are noted within the first 3 years of life, with most recognized by 1 year of age. Up to one-third of cases are already present at birth.[20,21] In the large study of 57 patients by Laskin et al.,[22] patients ranged in age from newborn to 10 years with a median age of 12 months at the time of surgery. Rare examples have been described in older children, adolescents, and even in adults.[23] Unlike most other forms of fibromatosis, the condition has a roughly equal gender distribution, but there is no evidence of any familial tendency. This lesion has been identified in patients with terminal osseous dysplasia and pigmentary defects, a rare, lethal X-linked dominant disease that has been linked with mutations of the *FLNA* gene.[24]

The nodules are more often found in the fingers than in the toes and, in most instances, are located on the sides or dorsum of the distal or middle phalangeal joints, especially of the third, fourth, and fifth digits. Although the thumb can be affected, cases involving the great toe have not been reported. The lesions may be single or multiple and often affect more than one digit of the same hand or foot. Occasionally, they involve both the fingers and toes of the same patient. Very few cases have been described as occurring outside of the hands and feet. Purdy and Colby[25] reported a case with typical eosinophilic perinuclear inclusions in the upper arm of a 2½-year-old child near an old injection site. Pettinato et al.[26] described two cases of extradigital inclusion body fibromatosis in the breasts of 24- and 53-year-old women.

Although pain and tenderness are not typical symptoms, associated functional impairment or joint deformities may be present, including lateral deviation or flexion deformities of the adjacent joints, which typically remain unchanged following surgical removal of the lesions.

Pathologic Findings

The excised lesions are small, firm masses that are covered on one side by intact skin and have a solid white cut surface (Fig. 9-8). They show little variation in their microscopic appearance; they consist of a uniform proliferation of fibroblasts surrounded by a dense collagenous stroma (Fig. 9-9). The lesions are poorly circumscribed and extend from the epidermis into the deeper portions of the dermis and subcutis, typically surrounding the dermal appendages. The overlying epidermis is usually minimally altered, with slight hyperkeratosis or acanthosis.

The most striking feature of the tumor is the presence of small, round inclusions in the cytoplasm of the fibroblasts. The number of inclusions varies from case to case.[22,27] In some, they are numerous and easily detected, whereas in others they are scarce and difficult to find with hematoxylin and eosin-stained slides. Typically, these inclusions are situated close to the nucleus from which a narrow clear zone (Fig. 9-10) often separates them. They are eosinophilic and resemble erythrocytes, except for their more variable size (3 to 15 μm), intracytoplasmic location, and lack of refringence. Numerous histochemical preparations can be used to highlight these

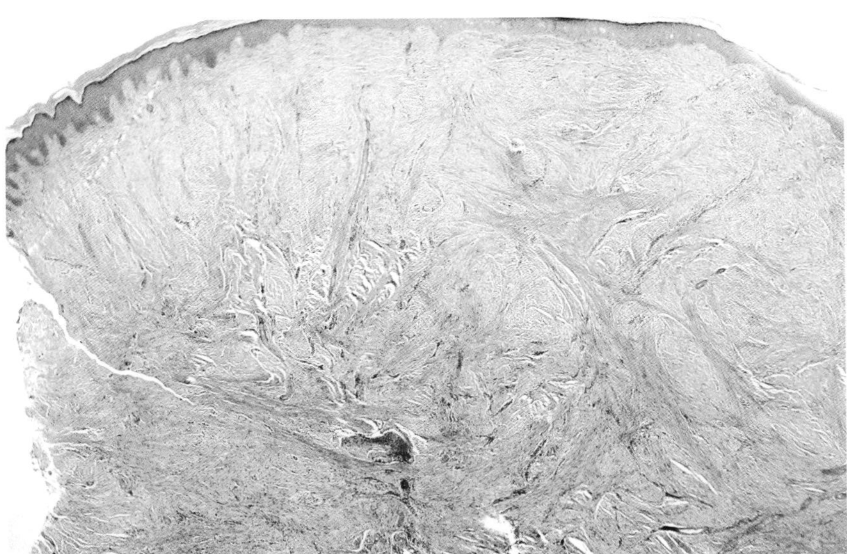

FIGURE 9-8. Low-power view of a broad-based hemispheric dermal nodule composed of spindle-shaped cells, characteristic of infantile digital fibromatosis.

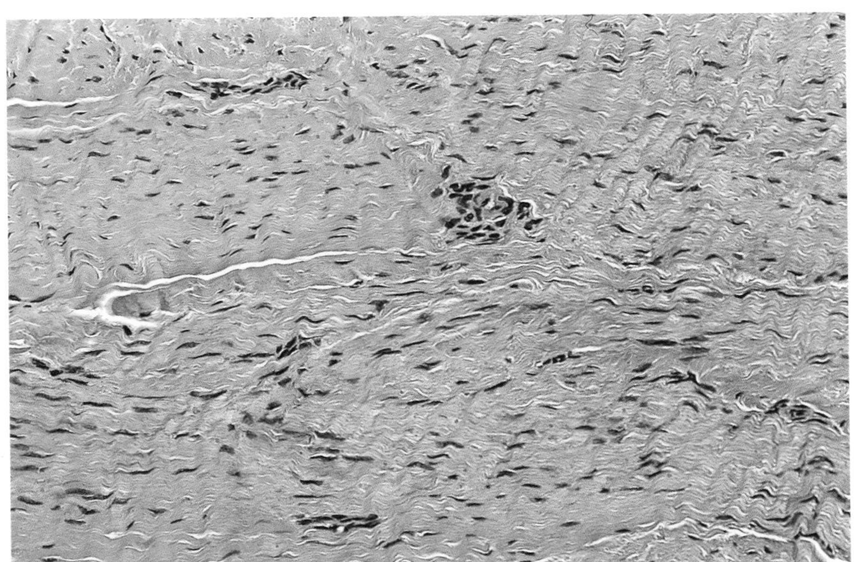

FIGURE 9-9. Infantile digital fibromatosis, composed of a uniform proliferation of fibroblasts surrounded by a dense collagenous stroma.

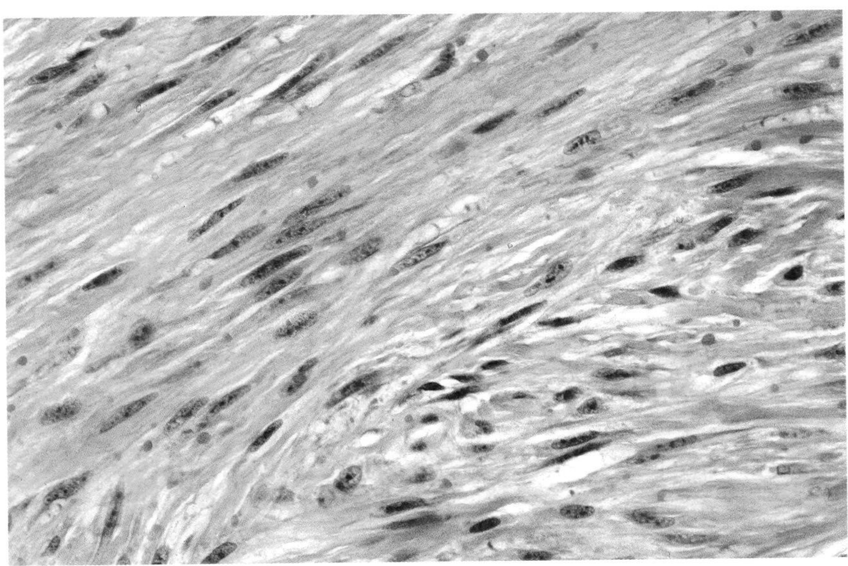

FIGURE 9-10. Infantile digital fibromatosis. Fibroblasts with characteristic intracytoplasmic inclusions separated by a narrow clear zone.

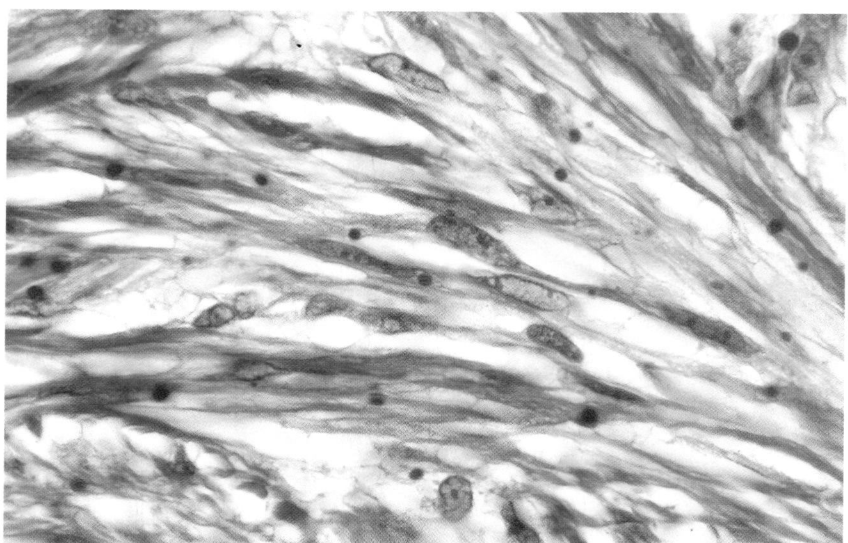

FIGURE 9-11. Masson trichrome stain demonstrating intracytoplasmic inclusions characteristic of infantile digital fibromatosis.

inclusions; they stain a deep red with Masson trichrome stain (Fig. 9-11), but they do not stain with periodic acid-Schiff (PAS), Alcian blue, or colloidal iron stains.

Immunohistochemical Findings

Immunohistochemically, the spindled cells stain consistently for actin, but variable results have been obtained with respect to actin immunoreactivity of the inclusion bodies themselves. Most of the earlier studies using formalin-fixed tissues were unable to demonstrate actin staining of the inclusion bodies.[28] However, actin staining of the inclusion bodies has been demonstrated using alcohol-fixed tissue as well as potassium hydroxide and trypsin-pretreated formalin-fixed tissue.[29] In the study by Laskin et al.,[22] the cells consistently expressed calponin, smooth muscle actin, desmin, and CD99. Most also expressed CD117, but stains for cytokeratins, estrogen, and progesterone receptors were negative. Unlike deep fibromatoses, this lesion does not show nuclear immunoreactivity for β-catenin.[30]

Bhawan et al.[31] were the first to emphasize the myofibroblastic nature of many of the cells in infantile digital fibromatosis and proposed the alternate term *infantile digital myofibroblastoma*. The myofibroblasts contain narrow intracellular bundles of 5 to 7 nm microfilaments with interspersed dense bodies and occasional patches of basal lamina. These strap-like bundles of filaments are continuous with the juxtanuclear inclusion bodies, which also consist of fibrillary and granular material that has no limiting membrane and seems to originate in the endoplasmic reticulum[32] (Fig. 9-12).

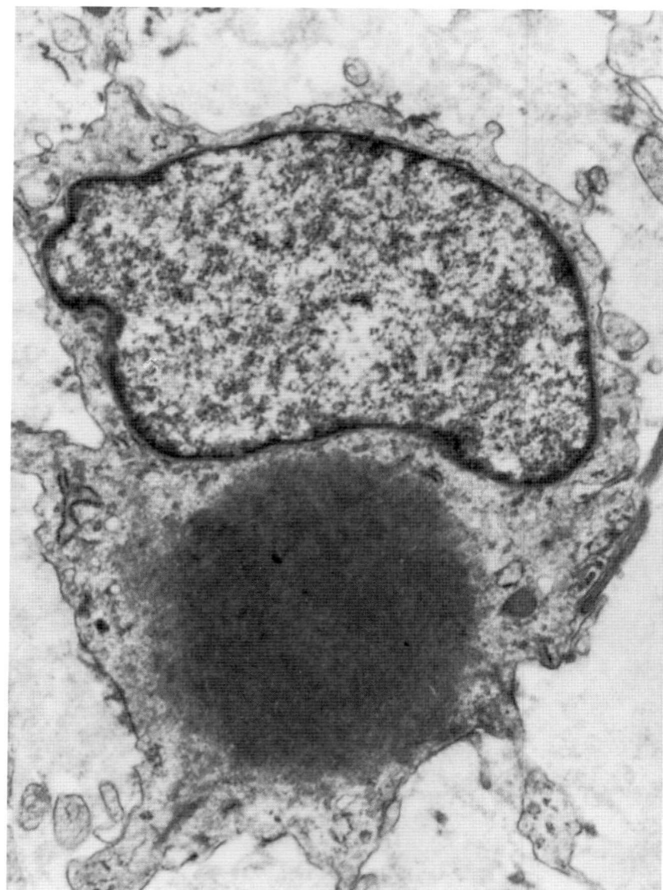

FIGURE 9-12. Infantile digital fibromatosis. Electron microscopy shows an inclusion within the fibroblast. *(From Taxy JB, Battifora H. The electron microscope in the study and diagnosis of soft tissue tumors. In: Trump BF, Jones RT, editors. Diagnostic electron microscopy. New York: Wiley; 1980, with permission.)*

Discussion

The exact nature of the inclusions is not clear. Because of the resemblance of these inclusions to the viroplasm of fibroblasts infected with Shope fibroma virus, Battifora and Hines[33] proposed a possible viral etiology. The immunohistochemical and ultrastructural findings strongly suggest that the inclusions are related to the intracellular bundles of microfilaments and represent densely packed masses of actin microfilaments.[28,32] The occurrence of extradigital posttraumatic lesions that are histologically indistinguishable from those on the digits and antecedent trauma or surgery related to digital lesions suggests that trauma may stimulate development of the lesion.[34,35] Inclusion bodies identical to those found in infantile digital fibromatosis have also been described in a variety of tumors, including benign phyllodes tumor and fibroadenoma of the breast[36,37] and endocervical polyps,[38] among others.

Although a significant percentage of these lesions recur locally, the ultimate prognosis is excellent.[22,39] Recurrences usually appear at the same site within a few weeks or months after the initial excision.[22] Although there is an initial period of growth, if watched for a long enough period of time, many lesions regress spontaneously.[40] In the large study by Laskin et al., 28 of 38 (74%) cases with follow-up information locally recurred a median of 4 months after surgery.[22] Most authors advocate conservative treatment because there is no evidence of aggressive behavior or malignant transformation. Some advocate a watch-and-wait approach following a diagnosis, given the high rate of spontaneous regression.[41] Holmes et al.[42] found only one recurrence amongst seven patients treated with an intralesional injection of corticosteroids. Mohs micrographic surgery may be effective in minimizing the risk of local recurrence.[41] Deformities and contractures develop in some cases, regardless of whether the lesions are removed surgically, and surgical correction of contractures and functional changes are sometimes necessary.

MYOFIBROMA AND MYOFIBROMATOSIS

Myofibromatosis was initially described in 1951 by Williams and Schrum,[43] who designated the lesions *congenital fibrosarcoma*. Three years later, Stout[44] renamed the entity *congenital generalized fibromatosis*, and he described two male infants who died soon after birth with multiple fibrous nodules in soft tissues and internal organs. In 1965, Kauffman and Stout[45] grouped their cases of congenital fibromatosis into two categories: (1) a multiple form, with lesions restricted to skin, subcutaneous tissue, skeletal muscle, and bone and characterized by a good prognosis; and (2) a generalized form, with visceral lesions and a poor prognosis. Following recognition of the myofibroblastic nature of the constituent cells, Chung and Enzinger[46] reported 61 cases of this entity and renamed it *infantile myofibromatosis*. The terms *myofibroma* and *myofibromatosis* for solitary and multiple lesions, respectively, are generally preferred, not only because these lesions occur in infants, children, and adults and have a prominent myofibroblastic component, but also because their behavior distinguishes them from other, more aggressive types of fibromatosis.

Clinical Findings

Myofibroma manifests as a solitary nodule (most commonly in the dermis and subcutis) that measures a few millimeters to several centimeters in diameter. The more superficially located nodules are freely movable, and when skin is involved, the lesion can manifest as a purplish macule giving the impression of a hemangioma. Some lesions are more deeply seated and appear to be fixed. Although Chung and Enzinger[46] found solitary lesions to be almost three times as common as the multicentric form, in a review of the literature of 170 cases by Wiswell et al.,[47] solitary lesions were half as common as the multicentric form. The condition is almost twice as common in males as in females, and both the solitary and multicentric forms occur not only in infants and children, but also in adults.[48,49]

Solitary nodules are found most commonly in the general region of the head and neck, including the scalp, forehead, orbit, parotid region, and oral cavity.[50,51] The trunk is the second most commonly affected site, followed by the lower and upper extremities. There have also been several reports of solitary intraosseous myofibromas, most of which have involved the craniofacial bones.[52,53] Solitary lesions involving the viscera are rare.[54]

In patients with multiple lesions (*myofibromatosis*), the individual nodules have essentially the same appearance as solitary nodules; they occur not only in dermis and subcutis, but also in muscle, the internal organs, and the skeleton. Up to 40% of patients have visceral lesions that are invariably present at birth (Fig. 9-13).[55] The nodules may be numerous, especially when they are in the subcutis, lung, or skeleton.

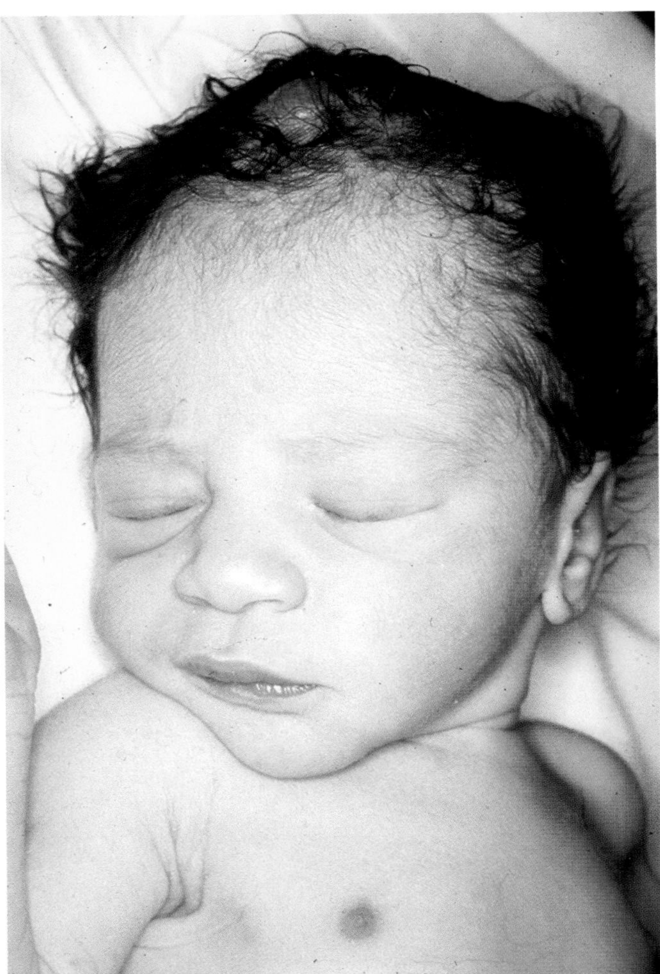

FIGURE 9-13. Newborn infant with myofibromatosis, with numerous dermal and subcutaneous nodules of the head and neck region.

Schaffzin et al.[56] reported a newborn girl who had 59 subcutaneous nodules noted at birth, and Heiple et al.[57] reported an infant who had more than 100 lesions in the skeleton that involved both flat and long bones. In the latter case, the nodules were recognized only after the infant suffered a fracture in a minor fall and underwent a radiographic examination of the injured leg.

Apart from the soft tissues and the skeleton, the most common sites of organ involvement are the lung, heart, gastrointestinal tract, pancreas, and rarely the central nervous system.[49,58,59] Internal lesions often cause symptoms such as severe respiratory distress, vomiting, or diarrhea, which often fail to respond to therapy and prove fatal within a few days or weeks after birth. Others cause few symptoms, making it likely that some internal lesions remain unrecognized. The nodules grow principally during the immediate perinatal period, but enlargement or formation of new nodules may be observed during infancy or even later in life.[60]

Radiographically, the bone lesions are circumscribed lytic areas with marginal sclerosis and without penetration of the cortex, in most cases.[61] Occasionally, however, a soft tissue lesion may extend into the underlying bone. Extraosseous lesions may show weak radiodensity as a result of focal calcification (Fig. 9-14).[62]

Pathologic Findings

As a rule, the nodules in the dermis and subcutis are better delineated than those in the muscle, bone, or viscera. They are rubbery or firm and scar-like in consistency and typically have a white-gray or pink surface; they vary greatly in size, averaging 0.5 to 1.5 cm in greatest diameter. Large lesions may ulcerate the overlying epidermis.

Microscopically, *myofibroma* and *myofibromatosis* have similar features. At low magnification, there is typically a nodular or multinodular growth pattern that appears biphasic owing to the alternation of light- and dark-staining areas. The light-staining areas consist mainly of plump myoid spindle cells with eosinophilic cytoplasm arranged in nodules, short fascicles, or whorls (Figs. 9-15 and 9-16). The nuclei are elongated and tapering or cigar-shaped and lack nuclear atypia. Some foci have extensive hyalinization. These areas are usually located more peripherally, although, in some cases, particularly in older children and adults, they are distributed haphazardly throughout the lesion.

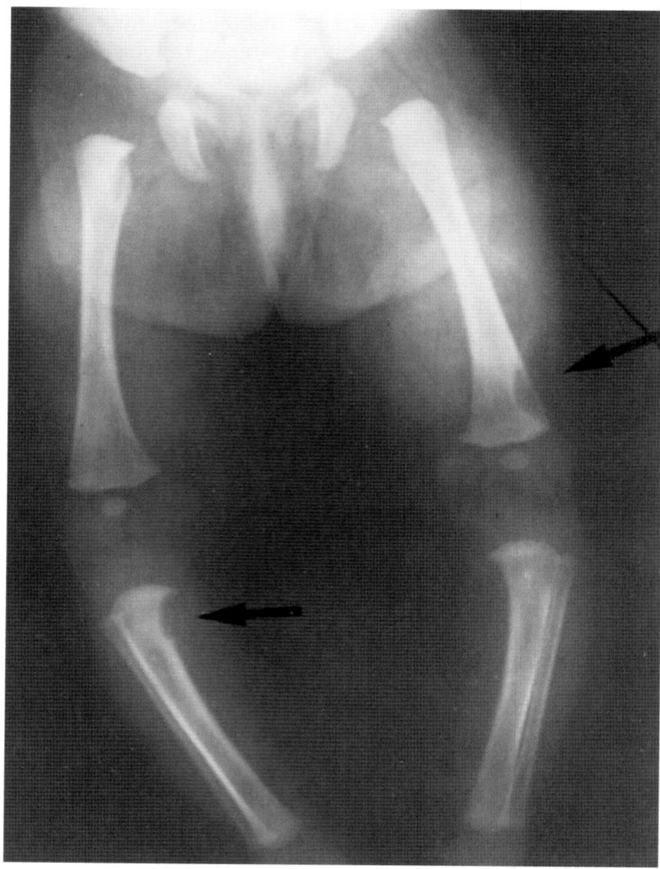

FIGURE 9-14. Infantile myofibromatosis, multicentric type, with multiple bone involvement (arrows). These osseous lesions tend to regress spontaneously and usually are no longer demonstrable after a few years.

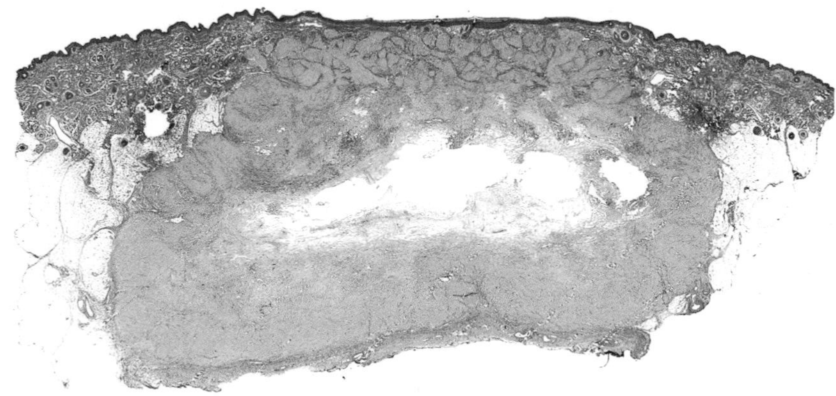

FIGURE 9-15. Low-power view of a solitary myofibroma involving the dermis and subcutis.

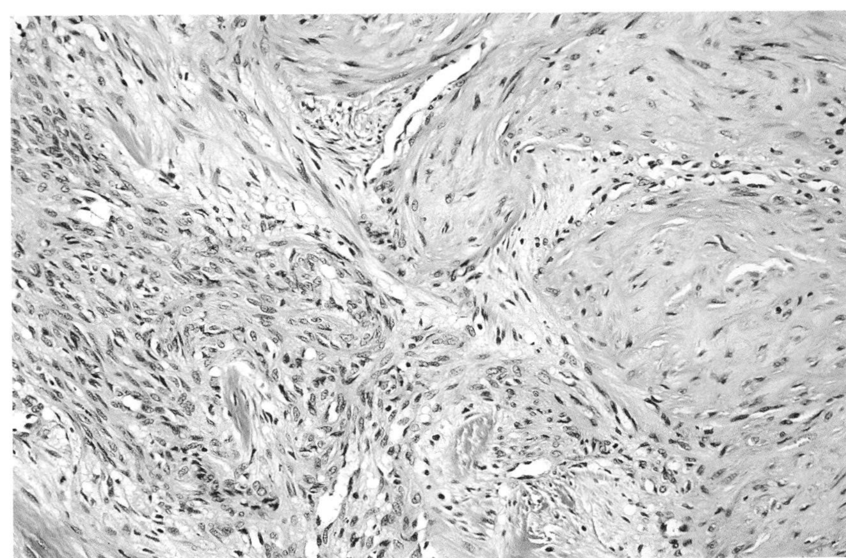

FIGURE 9-16. Infantile myofibromatosis, solitary type, consisting of broad bundles of plump myoid spindle cells with eosinophilic cytoplasm.

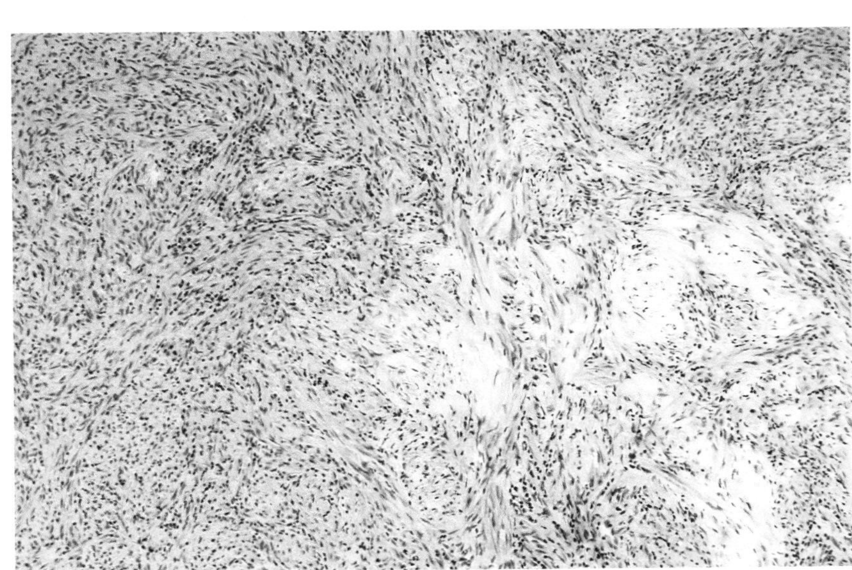

FIGURE 9-17. Infantile myofibromatosis, solitary type, composed predominantly of darkly staining spindle-shaped cells with intermixed plumper myoid-like cells.

The dark-staining areas of the lesion, usually centrally located, are composed of round or polygonal cells with slightly hyperchromatic nuclei or small spindle cells arranged around a distinct hemangiopericytoma-like vascular pattern (Figs. 9-17 and 9-18). These primitive cells have vesicular nuclei, small amounts of eosinophilic cytoplasm, indistinct cell margins, and a low mitotic index. In some cases, focal hemorrhage, cystic degeneration, or coagulative necrosis is present, often with foci of calcification. Peripherally located chronic inflammatory cells, including lymphocytes and plasma cells, may be present. Because of these cellular and richly vascular areas and the extensive necrosis, these lesions can be mistaken for a sarcoma. In addition, the presence of intravascular growth, a feature that is present in up to one-fifth of cases, may also be worrisome but does not seem to have any prognostic significance. Some cases are composed almost exclusively of these cellular areas (so-called monophasic cellular variant of infantile myofibromatosis), which may represent the earliest stage of the disease.[63]

Immunohistochemical Findings

Immunohistochemically, the primitive-appearing cells stain focally and weakly for muscle-specific and smooth muscle actin, but they usually do not express desmin, as is often the case with myofibroblastic proliferations.[64,65]

Differential Diagnosis

The differential diagnosis of this lesion depends in part on whether the eosinophilic myofibroblasts or more primitive small cells predominate in a given lesion. The peripheral areas of myofibroma can resemble nodular fasciitis, fibrous histiocytoma, neurofibroma, or infantile fibromatosis/lipofibromatosis. *Nodular fasciitis* is a rare lesion in newborns and infants but certainly should be considered in the differential diagnosis in adults. Nodular fasciitis arises from the fascia, has a more prominent myxoid matrix, and usually contains scattered

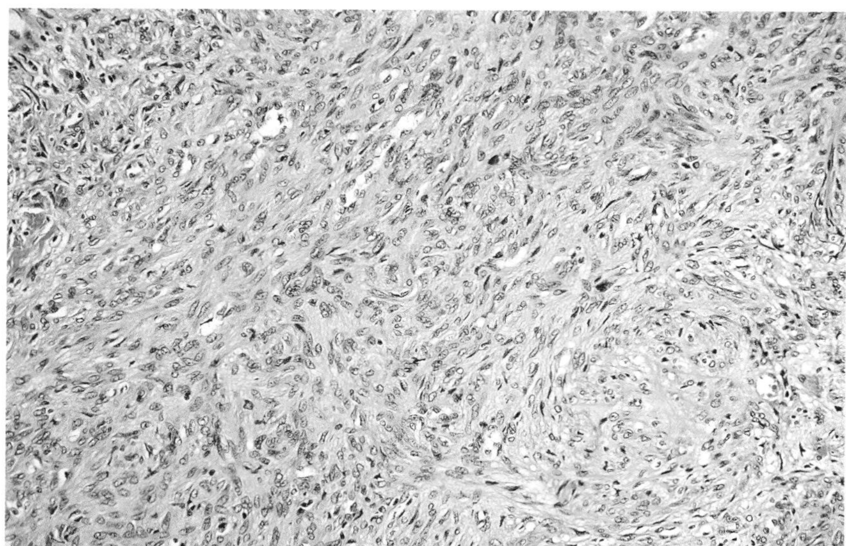

FIGURE 9-18. Infantile myofibromatosis with cellular proliferation of ovoid cells without cytologic atypia.

chronic inflammatory cells and occasional erythrocytes. The hemangiopericytoma-like pattern characteristic of myofibroma is absent in nodular fasciitis. The peripheral areas may also resemble *neurofibroma*, but the myofibroblastic cells lack S-100 protein. Clinically, myofibromatosis should not be confused with *type 1 neurofibromatosis (NF-1)* because myofibromatosis manifests with multiple nodules at birth or within the first few weeks of life, whereas neurofibromatosis affects older children with evidence of multiple café au lait spots and other stigmata of NF-1. *Fibrous histiocytoma* is composed of a polymorphous proliferation of cells arranged in a more pronounced storiform pattern. Although smooth muscle actin may be found in fibrous histiocytoma, the staining is usually focal. Furthermore, the cells of fibrous histiocytoma usually express factor XIIIa. Solitary forms of the disease may be mistaken for *infantile fibromatosis/lipofibromatosis*. The latter tends to be less well circumscribed, arise in muscle, and show a more uniform spindle cell pattern. In addition, infantile fibromatosis/lipofibromatosis shows neither central necrosis nor a central hemangiopericytoma-like vascular pattern.

Myofibromatosis has a number of clinical and morphologic similarities with *infantile hemangiopericytoma*.[66] As in myofibromatosis, most infantile hemangiopericytomas are present at birth or occur early in life, with a predilection for boys. Although most are solitary subcutaneous lesions, multicentricity and visceral involvement have been described. In addition, the main affected sites are similar between these lesions. Histologically, the central immature-appearing areas of myofibromatosis are indistinguishable from those of infantile hemangiopericytoma. Upon review of 11 cases originally diagnosed as infantile hemangiopericytoma, Mentzel et al.[66] found focal mature-appearing, actin-positive, spindle-shaped cells similar to those seen in myofibromatosis in all cases. These authors proposed that infantile hemangiopericytoma and myofibromatosis represent different stages of maturation of a single entity, a contention supported by others,[67,68] but this remains an unresolved issue.

Finally, biopsy specimens obtained from the central portion of this lesion may have features that resemble various types of sarcoma, particularly those composed of small round cells arranged around a hemangiopericytoma-like vasculature. Such lesions include the Ewing family of tumors, mesenchymal chondrosarcoma, malignant solitary fibrous tumor/hemangiopericytoma, and poorly differentiated synovial sarcoma. A battery of immunostains, including those for cytokeratins, S-100 protein, and CD99, can assist in the differential diagnosis, as can select molecular genetic assays. Although not always present, identifying peripheral myoid-appearing cells is the most useful feature for recognizing myofibromatosis.

Discussion

The clinical course seems to be largely determined by the extent of the disease. Solitary and multiple lesions confined to soft tissues and bone (with no evidence of visceral involvement) carry an excellent prognosis; they tend to regress spontaneously and rarely require more than a diagnostic biopsy.[46,69,70] In the review by Wiswell et al.,[47] only 5 of 54 (9%) solitary lesions recurred locally following excision, even after incomplete excision. In addition, 11 of 18 (61%) patients with multicentric lesions without visceral involvement and follow-up of more than 1 year had spontaneous regression of the lesions. Chung and Enzinger[46] found that only 3 of 28 (11%) solitary lesions locally recurred, and several of the multicentric lesions without visceral involvement showed spontaneous regression. Fukasawa et al.[71] documented massive apoptosis in two cases of infantile myofibromatosis and proposed that this mechanism may account for the high rate of spontaneous regression of these lesions.

The prognosis is much less favorable in newborns and infants with multiple visceral lesions, and as many as 75% die with signs of respiratory distress or diarrhea soon after birth.[46,47,72] There are exceptions, however. Hatzidaki et al.[73] reported one case of a child with multicentric visceral involvement with apparent spontaneous regression of the lesions. In some cases, low-dose chemotherapy has been shown to be efficacious in a subset of patients with multicentric visceral involvement.[74,75]

Several studies have documented a familial occurrence, including the presence of this lesion in siblings, and both autosomal recessive and dominant modes of inheritance have been proposed.[76-80] Very few cases have been studied cytogenetically. Stenman et al.[81] reported a case of solitary myofibroma with a del(6)(q12;q15). Monosomy 9q and trisomy 16q have also been reported.[82] Interestingly, Alaggio et al.[83] described a series of cases with morphologic features of both infantile myofibroma and congenital/infantile fibrosarcoma, but none were found to have the *ETV6-NTRK3* fusion characteristic of the latter entity, suggesting that these are unusual and highly cellular variants of myofibroma.

JUVENILE HYALINE FIBROMATOSIS/INFANTILE SYSTEMIC HYALINOSIS

Juvenile hyaline fibromatosis (JHF) is another rare hereditary disease that bears a superficial resemblance to myofibromatosis but differs by its cutaneous distribution of the tumor nodules, the histologic picture, and associated clinical features. The condition was first described by Murray[84] in 1873 as *molluscum fibrosum in children* and was thought to represent an unusual variant of neurofibromatosis. Whitfield and Robinson[85] offered a follow-up report of these three cases in 1903, but, amazingly, no further reports occurred until 1962, when Puretic et al.[86] reported a case under the name *mesenchymal dysplasia*. A variety of terms were used in subsequent reports, but Kitano[87] coined the term *juvenile hyaline fibromatosis*, which has become the preferred term. For many years, the terms *juvenile hyaline fibromatosis* and *infantile systemic hyalinosis (ISH)* were used interchangeably, and the exact relationship between these two entities was unclear. Although they share a number of characteristics in common, there are some significant clinical differences. Recent genetic data (described later) clearly link these two diseases along a spectrum.[30,88-90]

Clinical Findings

A number of clinical findings are common to both JHF and ISH, including joint contractures, gingival hyperplasia, osteopenia, and papular and nodular skin lesions.[91] The skin lesions have been grouped into three types: (1) small pearly papules on the face and neck; (2) small nodules and large plaques with a translucent appearance and a gelatinous consistency developing on fingers and ears and around the nose; and (3) firm, large, subcutaneous tumors with a predilection for the scalp, trunk, and limbs (Fig. 9-19).[92] The lesions vary in size from 1 mm to up to 10 cm; they are slow-growing and painless and have a tendency to recur following excision. The number of cutaneous lesions varies from case to case, but some patients can have more than 100 lesions in various parts of the body.[93] Most patients have extracutaneous findings, including painful flexion contractures of major joints and gingival hypertrophy, which may precede the development of skin lesions.[94] More than 60% of patients reveal multiple osteolytic defects on radiographic examination.[95] Most patients have painful, debilitating flexion contractures of large joints, resulting in marked deformity and generalized stiffness.[96]

As mentioned previously, there are some clinical features that distinguish ISH from JHF. Patients with ISH usually present within the first 6 months of life and often die of intractable diarrhea or infection by the age of 2 years.[97] In contrast, patients with JHF typically present later in infancy or childhood and often live into the third decade of life.[91,98] Features unique to ISH include persistent diarrhea with a protein-losing enteropathy, presumably secondary to intestinal lymphangiectasia,[99] hyperpigmentation over bony prominences, and failure to thrive.

Pathologic Findings

The lesions are poorly circumscribed and consist of cords of spindle-shaped cells embedded in a homogeneous eosinophilic matrix (Figs. 9-20 to 9-22). They are often found in the dermis, subcutis, and gingiva, although the bone and joints may also be involved.[100] Deposition of this amorphous eosinophilic matrix is widespread in some patients; Kitano et al.[101] reported one patient with autopsy-proven deposition of this substance in the tongue, esophagus, stomach, intestine, thymus, spleen, and lymph nodes. Early lesions show increased cellularity and less prominent stroma, whereas the large, older

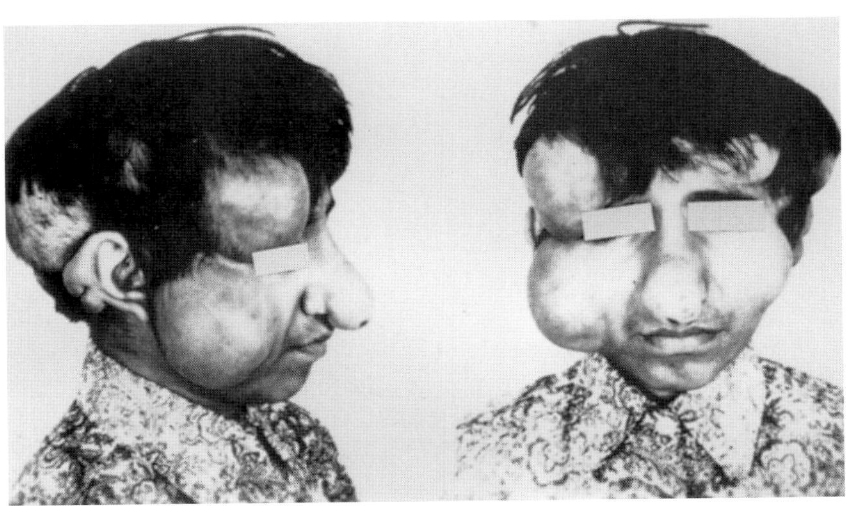

FIGURE 9-19. Juvenile hyaline fibromatosis. Multiple masses involve the scalp and face. *(Courtesy of Prof. Dr. Eduardo Carceres, Director, Instituto Nacional de Enfermades Neoplasicas, Lima, Peru.)*

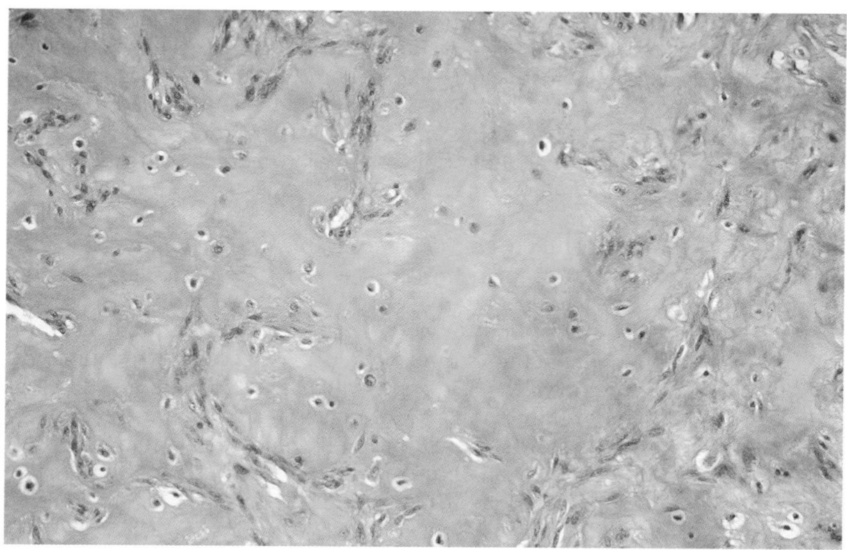

FIGURE 9-20. Hypocellular zone of a juvenile hyaline fibromatosis. Scattered cells with bland nuclei are deposited in a densely hyalinized stroma.

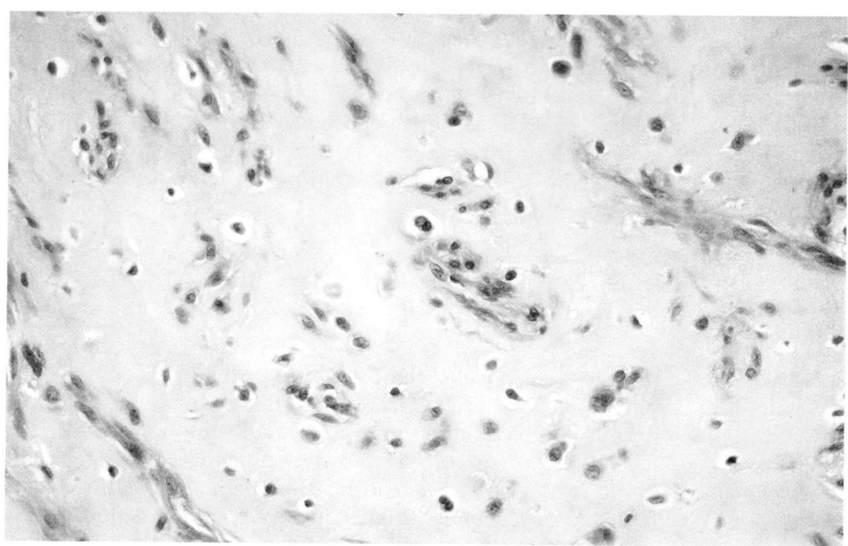

FIGURE 9-21. Juvenile hyaline fibromatosis. High-power view of cytologically bland cells deposited in a densely hyalinized stroma.

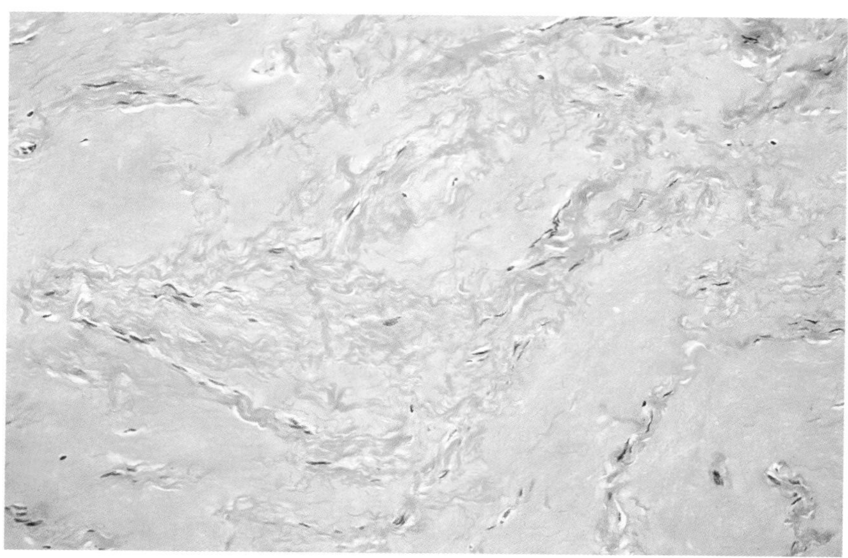

FIGURE 9-22. Juvenile hyaline fibromatosis. This lesion of long duration is almost completely acellular.

lesions are less cellular and contain more ground substance. The matrix stains positively with PAS and Alcian blue but does not stain with Congo red. Elastic tissue is completely absent. Occasional nodules reveal marked calcification, including calcospherites,[102] and multinucleated giant cells may occasionally be seen.[103]

The nature of this amorphous eosinophilic material is not clear. Ultrastructural studies have found this material to have a banding pattern identical to type 2 collagen.[104] By immunohistochemistry, the spindled cells are generally negative for actins,[105] but there is a conspicuous population of CD68-positive macrophages between the spindled cells.[103]

Cytogenetic and Molecular Genetic Findings

In 2003, studies by Dowling et al.[106] and Hanks et al.[107] identified mutations of the capillary morphogenesis gene 2 (*CMG2*) on 4q21 in both JHF and ISH, confirming a long-suspected genetic link. The gene, also known as *ANTXR2*, codes for a protein involved in basement membrane matrix assembly and morphogenesis of endothelial cells.[108] Mutations likely affect normal cell interactions with the extracellular matrix.[106] Both ISH and JHF are associated with distinct mutations of this gene, suggesting a genotypic-phenotypic correlation. Given the clear-cut relationship between JHF and ISH, some prefer the designation of hyaline fibromatosis syndrome.[88-90]

These diseases are inherited in an autosomal recessive manner.[109,110] Interestingly, there seems to be a preponderance of cases reported in patients of Middle Eastern descent, possibly as a result of a higher rate of consanguineous relationships.[91,111]

Differential Diagnosis

Multicentric infantile myofibromatosis is composed of multiple nodules that are almost always present at birth or appear during the first year of life. In general, the nodules are better circumscribed and are found not only in the subcutis, but also in muscle, bone, and viscera. Microscopically, they consist of broad, interlacing bundles of plump myofibroblasts, often with a central hemangiopericytoma-like area composed of primitive-appearing cells. The gums or joints are never involved. *Neurofibromatosis* tends to make its first appearance in slightly older children and is associated with café au lait spots; the tumors are composed of hyperchromatic serpentine nuclei in a fibrillary eosinophilic matrix and are positive for S-100 protein. *Gingival fibromatosis*, a lesion with a similar hereditary pattern, is limited to the gums of the upper and lower jaws and consists of dense, scar-like connective tissue rich in collagen. *Cylindromas*, or turban tumors, are confined to the head.

Winchester syndrome, a rare autosomal hereditary disease, is characterized by densely cellular, poorly demarcated fibrous proliferations in the dermis, subcutis, and joints without deposition of a hyaline matrix; periarticular thickening and limited motion in the limbs and the spine, corneal opacities, and radiographic changes of bones and joints are also part of this disorder.[112] The precise relation between JHF/ISH and Winchester syndrome is unclear, and some believe that these conditions represent different expressions of the same disorder,[98] although mutations in the *CMG2* gene have not been identified in this syndrome.

Discussion

Although most lesions in this condition are formed during childhood, new lesions may continue to appear into adult life. The nodules continue to grow slowly and may ulcerate the overlying skin. Surgical excision of lesions and hypertrophic gingival tissue is the treatment of choice, although the treatment can be as mutilating as the lesions in those patients with innumerable nodules.[113] Most patients with long-term follow-up are severely physically handicapped by joint contractures. Some patients can even develop upper airway obstruction because of the profound gingival hypertrophy that may occur.[114]

GINGIVAL FIBROMATOSIS

Gingival fibromatosis is a rare benign fibroproliferative disorder that is clinically distinct, chiefly affecting young persons of both genders with a tendency for recurrent local growth. Lesions may be idiopathic or familial, and some are associated with a heterogeneous group of hereditary syndromes. Takagi et al.[115] classified gingival fibromatosis into six categories: (1) isolated familial gingival fibromatosis; (2) isolated idiopathic gingival fibromatosis; (3) gingival fibromatosis associated with hypertrichosis; (4) gingival fibromatosis associated with hypertrichosis and mental retardation or epilepsy (or both); (5) gingival fibromatosis with mental retardation, epilepsy, or both; and (6) gingival fibromatosis associated with hereditary syndromes.

Clinical Findings

Patients with gingival fibromatosis present with a slowly growing, ill-defined enlargement or swelling of the gingivae, causing little pain but considerable difficulty in speaking and eating. The gingival overgrowth occurs to such a degree that the teeth are completely covered and the lips are prevented from closing.[116] The lesions may also extend over the hard palate, resulting in a deformity of the contour of the palate;[115] some also have marked swelling of the jaw bone. In some patients, the gingival swelling is minimal and limited to a small portion of the gum (*localized type*), but in most it is extensive and bilateral, involving the gingival tissues of both the upper and lower jaws and the hard palate (*generalized type*). Idiopathic cases are slightly more common than familial cases. Among the idiopathic cases, the generalized type outnumbers the localized type by almost 2 to 1.[117,118] The vast majority of familial cases are generalized. The condition occurs at any age, but most present at the time of eruption of the deciduous or permanent teeth. In fact, it has been postulated that the erupting teeth trigger the fibrous growth, as evidenced by effective treatment with tooth extraction alone, in some cases. Patients with the familial form of the disease tend to be younger than those with the idiopathic form. Up to 8% of cases are found at birth or immediately after delivery.[115]

Hypertrichosis is found in almost 10% of patients with this condition. Some patients also have mental retardation or epilepsy (or both), although the latter features can also be present in the absence of hypertrichosis. The gingival fibromatosis associated with these conditions generally occurs at a younger age than in the idiopathic form and is more common in females.

Gingival fibromatosis may also be associated with a variety of rare syndromes. *Zimmermann-Laband syndrome* is a rare autosomal dominant disorder characterized by gingival fibromatosis; hypertrichosis; intellectual disability; and various skeletal anomalies, including absence or hypoplasia of nails or terminal phalanges of the hands and feet.[119] It appears to be inherited in an autosomal dominant manner. In 2003, Stefanova et al.[120] reported a case with a balanced translocation t(3;8)(p21.2;q24.3), an observation that has been confirmed by others.[121] Gingival fibromatosis has also been found to be associated with cherubism (*Ramon syndrome*),[122] hearing loss and supernumerary teeth,[123,124] *Klippel-Trenaunay-Weber syndrome*,[116] prune-belly syndrome,[125] and growth hormone deficiency.[126]

Pathologic Findings

Grossly, the growth consists of dense scar-like tissue that cuts with difficulty and has a gray-white glistening surface. On microscopic examination, the lesions (which vary little in appearance) consist of poorly cellular, richly collagenous fibrous connective tissue underneath a normal or acanthotic squamous epithelium. Mild perivascular chronic inflammation and small foci of dystrophic calcification may be present.[127] The histologic features of the familial and idiopathic forms are indistinguishable.

Differential Diagnosis

There is a striking resemblance between gingival fibromatosis and hypertrophy of the gums following prolonged therapy with diphenylhydantoin sodium (Dilantin, phenytoin sodium).[128] In epileptic patients treated with this drug, it is difficult, if not impossible, to determine the cause of the gingival overgrowth. However, patients with gingival fibromatosis and epilepsy were described before the use of phenytoin, indicating that the changes are not entirely drug-induced. Other drugs, including immunosuppressive agents (cyclosporin A) and calcium channel blockers (nifedipine), can induce the same changes.[129] Lesions of similar appearance may also be found during pregnancy and as the result of chronic gingivitis. In most of these cases, a detailed clinical and family history permits the correct diagnosis. JHF, a hereditary lesion that may involve the gingiva in a similar manner, can be distinguished by its association with multiple cutaneous tumors and the characteristic microscopic appearance, especially the prominent PAS-positive hyaline matrix.

Discussion

Surgical excision of the hyperplastic tissue is frequently followed by local recurrence. However, the overgrowth may recede or disappear with tooth extraction. Many authors recommend excision of the excess tissue and removal of all teeth in severe cases.[130]

Approximately 35% of cases of gingival fibromatosis are familial; however, there is clearly genetic heterogeneity. Although some cases appear to be inherited in an autosomal recessive manner, most have an autosomal dominant pattern of inheritance. Several genes have been associated with gingival fibromatosis, including mutations of the *SOS-1* gene, located at 2p21-p22,[131] as well as alterations at 5q13-q22.[132] The fibroblasts in this condition have a higher proliferative rate than normal gingival fibroblasts, possibly mediated by autocrine stimulation by transforming growth factor beta 1.

FIBROMATOSIS COLLI

Fibromatosis colli has long been recognized as a peculiar benign fibrous growth of the sternocleidomastoid muscle that usually appears during the first weeks of life and is often associated with muscular torticollis, or wryneck. It bears a close resemblance to other forms of infantile fibromatosis but is sufficiently different in its microscopic appearance and behavior to warrant separation as a distinct entity. This lesion occurs in approximately 0.4% of live births.[133] The finding of torticollis is not synonymous with the presence of fibromatosis colli because nearly 80 entities have been reported to cause torticollis (acquired torticollis).[134] In a retrospective study of 58 patients with infantile torticollis using MRI, Parikh et al.[135] found evidence of fibromatosis colli in 7 patients only.

Clinical Findings

Characteristically, the lesion manifests between the second and fourth weeks of life as a mass lying in or replacing the mid to lower portion of the sternocleidomastoid muscle, especially its sternal or clavicular portion.[136] The lesion is movable only in a horizontal plane and never affects the overlying skin. Rarely, this process may simultaneously involve the trapezius muscle.[137] Most commonly, a 1- to 3-cm long, hard mass, or bulb, is palpable at the base of the sternocleidomastoid muscle 2 to 4 weeks after birth. Almost all cases are unilateral, with a slight predilection for the right side of the neck; rare cases of bilateral fibromatosis colli have been described.[138] Most authors have found a slight predilection for this lesion to occur in boys.[139]

Initially, the mass grows rapidly, but after a few weeks or months the growth slows and becomes stationary. In many cases, spontaneous regression occurs by the age of 1 to 2 years, and the lesion may no longer be palpable. During the initial growth period, torticollis (rotation and tilting of the head to the affected side) occurs in only about one-fourth to one-third of cases and usually is mild and transient. In addition, the face and skull on the affected side may begin to appear smaller, resulting in facial asymmetry and plagiocephaly; there is flattening of the affected side of the face with posterior displacement of the ipsilateral ear.[139] A number of patients with this lesion present with torticollis later in life because the affected sternocleidomastoid muscle is incapable of keeping pace with the growth and elongation of the

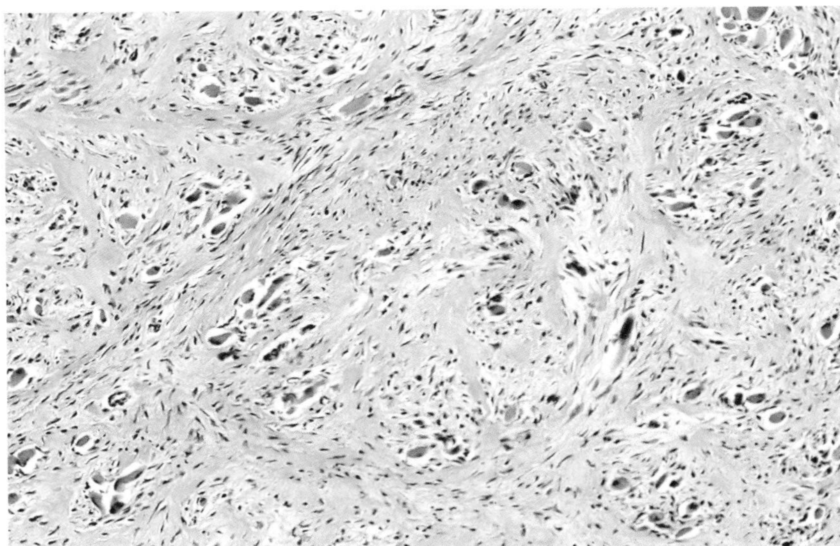

FIGURE 9-23. Fibromatosis colli in a 4-month-old boy. Note the intimate mixture of fibrous tissue and entrapped and partly atrophic muscle fibers.

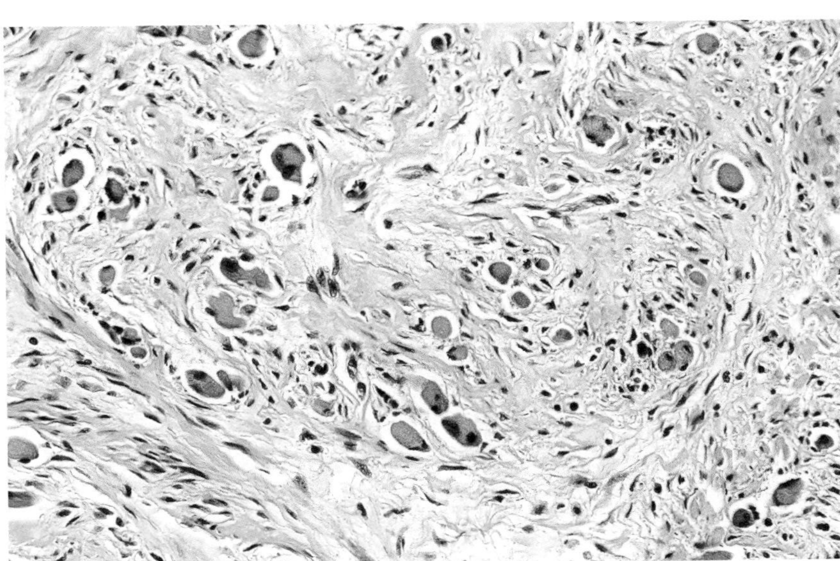

FIGURE 9-24. Fibromatosis colli. Separation of atrophic muscle fibers by dense fibrous tissue.

sternocleidomastoid muscle on the opposite side, causing functional imbalance and torticollis.

Fibromatosis colli is associated with a high incidence of difficult deliveries, including breech (reported in up to 60% of patients) and forceps deliveries.[140] Several reports have noted an association with other congenital anomalies, including rib cage anomalies[141] and ipsilateral congenital dysplasia of the hip.[142] Rare cases of fibromatosis colli appear to be familial.[143] Thompson et al.[144] reported this condition in three sisters who were offspring of consanguineous mating.

Pathologic Findings

When the growth is excised at an early stage, the specimen consists of a small mass of firm tissue averaging 1 to 2 cm in diameter. The cut surface is gray-white and glistening and blends imperceptibly with the surrounding skeletal muscle. Microscopic examination discloses partial replacement of the sternocleidomastoid muscle by a diffuse fibroblastic proliferation of varying cellularity (Figs. 9-23 and 9-24). The constituent cells lack nuclear hyperchromasia, pleomorphism, and mitotic activity. Scattered throughout the lesion are residual muscle fibers that have undergone atrophy or degeneration with swelling, loss of cross-striations, and proliferation of sarcolemmal nuclei. This intimate mixture of proliferated fibroblasts and residual atrophic skeletal muscle fibers is fully diagnostic of the lesion and should not be confused with the infiltrative growth of a malignant neoplasm. Lesions of longer duration typically show less cellularity and more stromal collagen, but there does not appear to be a correlation between the histologic picture and the age of the patient. Although hemosiderin deposits are present in some cases, they are never a prominent feature. Unlike *fibrosing myositis*, there is no inflammatory infiltrate; unlike *fibrodysplasia ossificans progressiva*, there are no associated malformations of the hands or feet. Fine-needle aspiration cytology is a useful diagnostic modality and may obviate the need for further surgery.[140] As one might expect, the aspirate is characterized by bland spindle-shaped fibroblasts of low cellularity admixed with degenerating skeletal muscle fibers. By immunohistochemistry, the cells stain for smooth muscle actin but not for β-catenin.[30]

Discussion

The cause of the growth has been the subject of considerable debate in the literature. In view of the unusually high incidence of breech and forceps deliveries, birth injury likely plays a role. It has been hypothesized that injury to the muscle during labor results in an organizing hematoma with subsequent fibrous replacement. However, microscopic examination reveals little evidence of an organizing hematoma, and few cases exhibit deposition of hemosiderin. The fact that coexistent facial deformities are often present at birth and that these lesions can develop in patients following a cesarean section cast doubt on this hypothesis. Others have postulated that abnormal intrauterine positioning results in vascular occlusion resulting in ischemic necrosis of the sternocleidomastoid muscle. Certainly, contributing genetic factors are suggested by the reports of familial fibromatosis colli and association of the growth with congenital malformations.

After a stationary period of several months, the growth slowly subsides and spontaneously resolves in up to 70% of cases by 1 year of age without surgical treatment.[145] It does not recur, and there is no aggressive growth into the surrounding tissues, although some patients develop a compensatory thoracic scoliosis, persistent head tilt, or obvious cosmetic deformity. Recommendations as to the best type of therapy differ. Most advocate a conservative approach with physiotherapy for patients younger than 1 year of age.[136] Surgery may be a more effective mode of therapy for patients more than 1 year of age.[141] Ferkel et al.[146] reported better surgical results with release of the sternal and clavicular heads of the sternocleidomastoid muscle, but most have not found that one surgical approach is better than another.

INFANTILE FIBROMATOSIS (LIPOFIBROMATOSIS)

Fibromatoses occurring in infancy and early childhood consist of two morphologically distinct types. One type is essentially identical to adult-type fibromatoses. This discussion will focus on the other type, which is unique to childhood and has also been termed *lipofibromatosis*.[147] It affects mainly children from birth to 8 years of age and is slightly more common in boys than girls. There are considerable variations in its morphologic appearance, depending on the stage of differentiation of the constituent fibroblasts.

Stout[44] was the first to identify and describe the childhood form of fibromatosis as a distinct entity, but relatively few cases have since been added to the literature. However, in 2000, Fetsch et al.[147] from the AFIP published a series of 45 cases that significantly contributed to the understanding of this rare entity.

Clinical Findings

Most patients present with a solitary firm, deep-seated mass that is poorly circumscribed and that usually has grown rapidly during the preceding weeks or months. In almost all cases, the mass is noted during the first 8 years of life, most commonly before age 2; some are present at birth. Although most patients are asymptomatic, some report pain or tenderness of the involved site.[147,148] The mass typically originates in skeletal muscle, especially the muscles of the extremities, trunk, and head and neck.[147,149,150] The preferred sites in the head and neck region are the tongue, mandible, maxilla, and mastoid process[144]; rare cases have been described in the orbit.[151] In the study from the AFIP, the majority of cases arose in the extremities, including the hand (18), arm (8), leg (7), and foot (6). Five cases arose in the trunk and one in the head.[147] As the lesion progresses, it may infiltrate adjacent muscles and grow around vessels and nerves, with resultant tenderness, pain, or functional disturbances. Involvement of the joint capsule can lead to contracture and restriction of movement.

Radiographic examination shows a soft tissue mass sometimes associated with bowing or deformation of bone, especially in cases in which the onset was during the first 2 to 3 years of life and has been present for several months or years.[152] Lesions in the regions of the mandible, maxilla, or mastoid frequently involve bone; it may be difficult to determine whether the mass arose in the soft tissues, periosteum, or bone, thereby making the distinction difficult from desmoplastic fibroma of bone, in some cases.[153]

Pathologic Findings

Grossly, the tumor is a firm, ill-defined scar-like mass of gray-white tissue measuring 1 to 10 cm. It is not encapsulated and usually is excised together with portions of the involved muscle and subcutaneous fat.

Microscopically, infantile fibromatosis has a wide morphologic spectrum reflecting progressive stages in the differentiation of the fibroblasts. The more common form of infantile fibromatosis is the *diffuse* (*mesenchymal*) type. This form, found chiefly in infants during the first few months of life, is characterized by small, haphazardly arranged, round or oval cells deposited in a myxoid background (Figs. 9-25 to 9-31). The cells are intermediate in appearance between primitive mesenchymal cells and fibroblasts, and they are often intimately associated with residual muscle fibers and lipocytes. The interspersed lipocytes, which can be extensive in some cases, are probably the result of ex vacuo fatty proliferation secondary to muscular atrophy of the infiltrated and immobilized muscle tissue. Peripherally located lymphocytic inflammation is often present. These areas blend with a more cellular proliferation composed chiefly of plump and spindle-shaped fibroblasts arranged in distinct bundles and fascicles. It may be highly cellular and mitotically active, making the distinction from infantile fibrosarcoma exceedingly difficult, in some cases.

The less common form of infantile fibromatosis (*desmoid type*) is virtually indistinguishable from the adult form of fibromatosis (desmoid tumor). This type usually occurs in children older than 5 years of age, and its behavior appears to

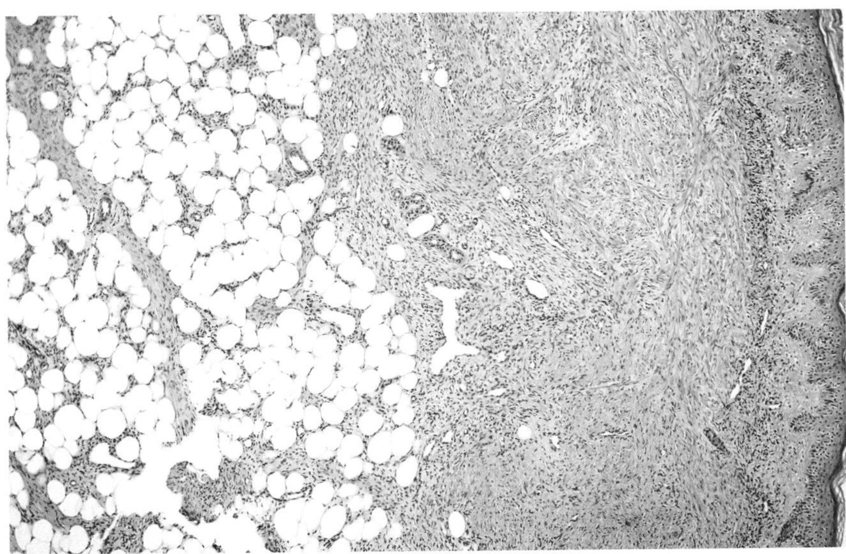

FIGURE 9-25. Infantile fibromatosis. Replacement of muscle tissue by fibrous tissue and mature fat bearing a superficial resemblance to a lipomatous tumor. The lesion was excised from the right arm of a 2-year-old girl.

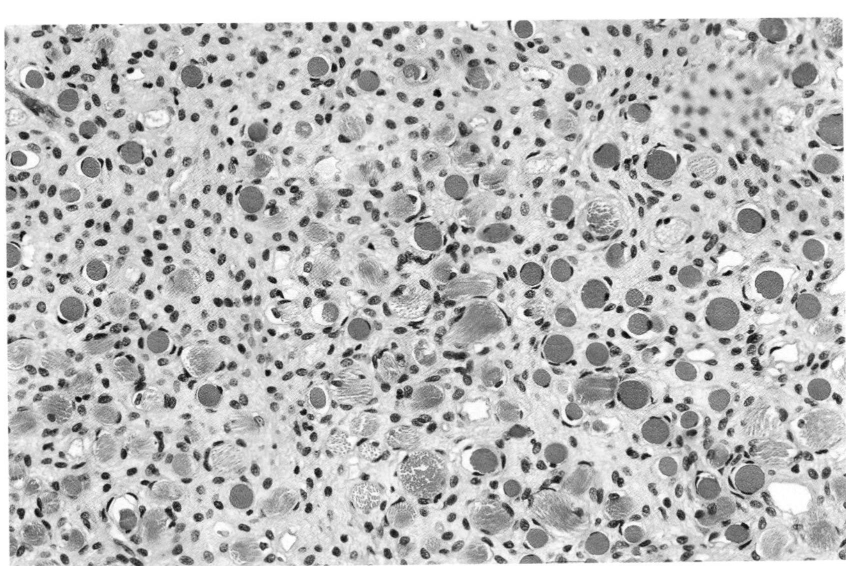

FIGURE 9-26. Infantile fibromatosis, diffuse type, removed from the trapezius muscle of a 5½-month-old girl. The absence of digital malformations helps distinguish it from an early nonossifying stage of fibrodysplasia ossificans progressiva.

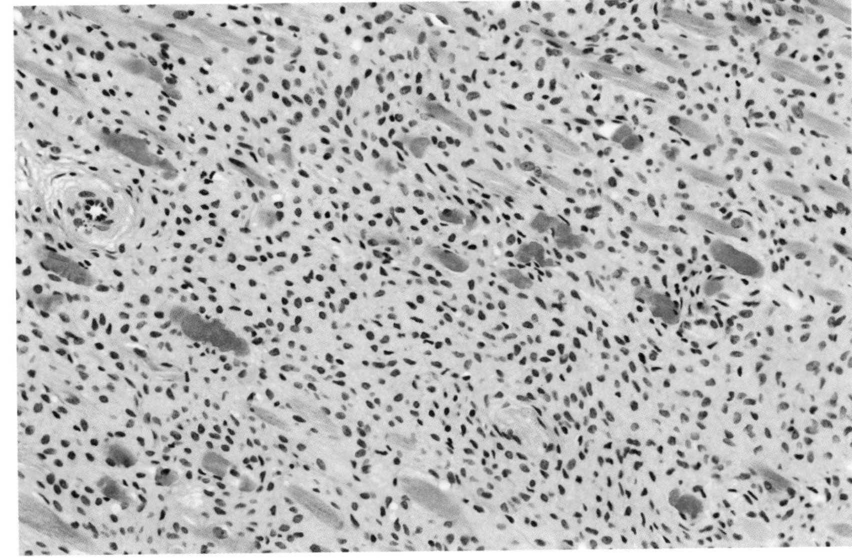

FIGURE 9-27. Infantile fibromatosis, diffuse type. Note the separation of striated muscle fibers by primitive fibroblasts with little variation in size and shape.

be similar to that of the adult form of fibromatosis.[154] Although the morphology is similar to adult lesions, calcification and/or ossification is a feature peculiar to pediatric cases.[155]

Like other forms of fibromatosis, infantile fibromatosis is composed of a mixture of fibroblasts and myofibroblasts. Immunohistochemically, the more primitive-appearing cells characteristic of the diffuse type and the plump spindle-shaped cells of both types show variable staining for muscle markers, including muscle-specific actin and smooth muscle actin, although stains for desmin are typically negative. Although there is no characteristic cytogenetic aberration, Kenney et al.[156] described a case with a three-way t(4;9;6) translocation.

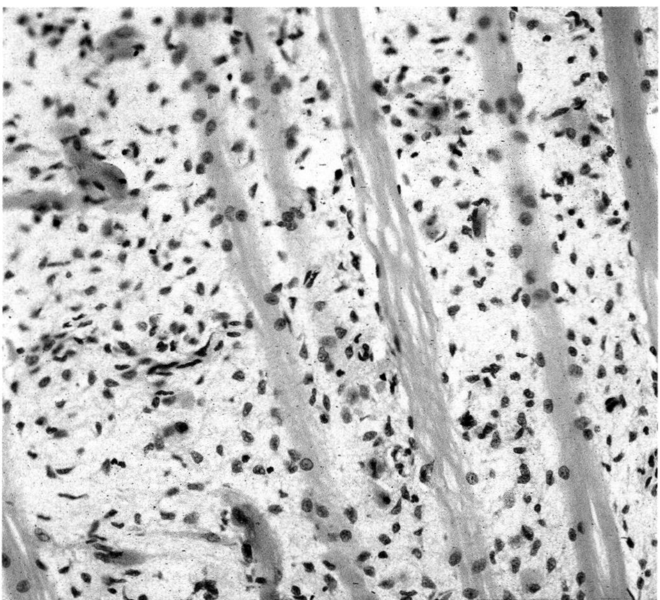

FIGURE 9-28. Higher-magnification view of a diffuse-type infantile fibromatosis. Primitive fibroblasts are seen separating striated muscle fibers.

Differential Diagnosis

The differential diagnosis depends on the type of infantile fibromatosis encountered. The diffuse (mesenchymal) type frequently causes diagnostic problems because it may be confused with a wide variety of myxoid or lipomatous lesions because of the prominent myxoid stroma and the partial replacement of the infiltrated muscle by lipocytes. *Myxoid liposarcoma* is virtually unheard of in children younger than 5 years of age and is characterized by the presence of a uniform plexiform capillary pattern and variable numbers of typical lipoblasts. *Lipoblastomatosis*, the infantile counterpart of lipoma, can be distinguished by its distinctly lobular pattern and the uniform appearance of the constituent adipocytes. There may be some resemblance to *botryoid rhabdomyosarcoma*, which has a similar age incidence; but this lesion is uncommon in the musculature and nearly always occurs in the wall of mucosa-lined cavities, such as the urinary bladder or vagina. *Fibrodysplasia ossificans progressiva* bears some resemblance to the diffuse form of infantile fibromatosis, but patients with this disorder have bilateral malformations and shortening of fingers and toes (microdactylia). Confusion may also occur with the early stages of *calcifying aponeurotic fibroma*, although this lesion is characterized by its location in the palmar and plantar regions as well as foci of linear calcifications and chondroid metaplasia.

The most difficult problem in the differential diagnosis is distinguishing the more cellular variants of infantile fibromatosis from *congenital/infantile fibrosarcoma* (Table 9-2). The latter tumor resembles the adult form of fibrosarcoma, with a characteristic high cellularity, arrangement in a uniform herringbone pattern, and a high mitotic rate. In addition, zones of hemorrhage and necrosis are not uncommon. The distinction between infantile fibromatosis and congenital/infantile

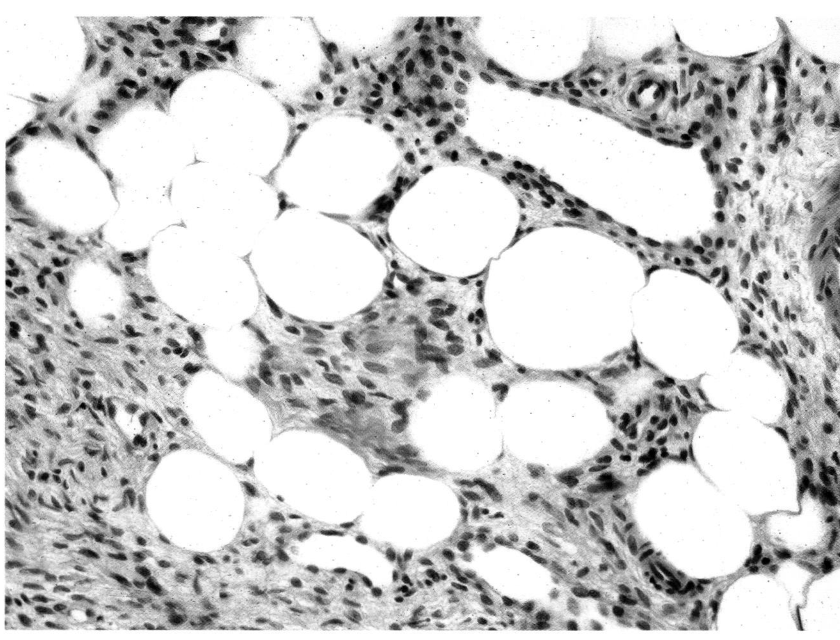

FIGURE 9-29. Infantile fibromatosis, diffuse type. Immature fibroblasts are seen infiltrating between adipocytes.

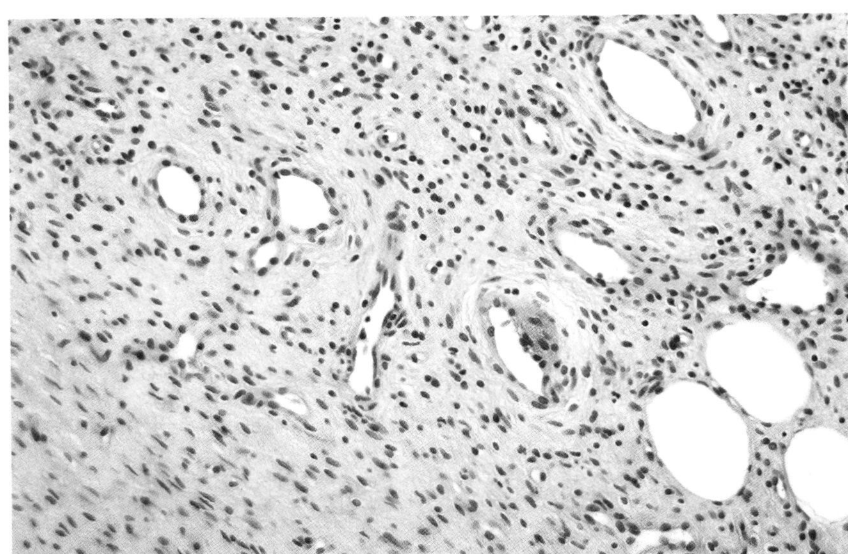

FIGURE 9-30. Infantile fibromatosis, diffuse type. Immature fibroblasts are deposited in a myxoid background.

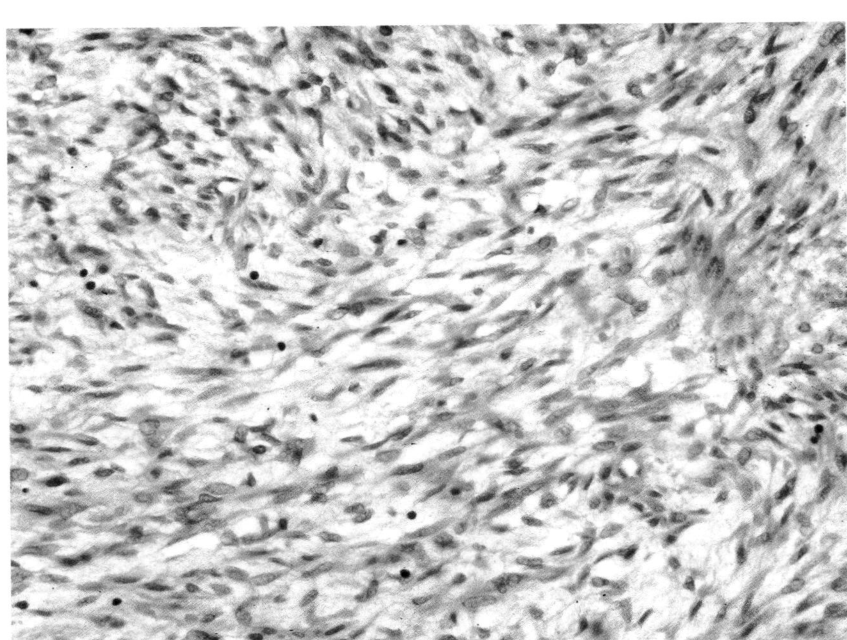

FIGURE 9-31. Infantile fibromatosis closely resembling the adult form of fibromatosis.

TABLE 9-2 Summary of Features Distinguishing Infantile Fibromatosis and Infantile Fibrosarcoma

FEATURE	INFANTILE FIBROMATOSIS	CONGENITAL/INFANTILE FIBROSARCOMA
Cellularity	Variable	Moderate to high
Herringbone pattern	Absent	Usually present
Mitotic figures	Rare	Few to many
Hemorrhage	Absent	Often present
Necrosis	Absent	Often present
t(12;15)(p13;q25)	Absent	Present

fibrosarcoma is usually feasible if one pays attention to the infiltrative growth pattern of fibromatosis and its variation in the degree of cellularity, often with alternating cellular and more collagenous areas, resembling the desmoid form. Yet, in some cases, reliable distinction between these entities is exceedingly difficult. Cytogenetic and molecular genetic analyses are highly reliable in this distinction. By traditional cytogenetics, congenital/infantile fibrosarcoma is characterized by gains of chromosomes 8, 11, 17, and 20.[157] These alterations are not found in infantile fibromatosis, although gains in chromosome 17 have been reported in some cases.[158] As described in greater detail in Chapter 10, congenital/infantile fibrosarcoma is characterized by a t(12;15)(p13;q25), resulting in the fusion of the *ETV6* gene (chromosome 12) with the *NTRK3* gene (chromosome 15), which can be reliably detected by a variety of molecular techniques.[159]

Discussion

Although infantile fibromatosis does not metastasize, it may reach a large size and, like other forms of fibromatosis, tends to recur locally when inadequately excised. In the series by Faulkner et al.[160] of desmoid-type lesions, none of the patients developed metastatic disease or died as a direct result of their tumor, but 41 of 63 patients (65%) developed local recurrences, with 51% recurring less than 1 year after initial excision, and 90% recurring within 3 years. The status of the resection margins was the only significant prognostic factor because those patients who had undergone a wide local excision with tumor-free margins were significantly less likely to develop a local recurrence. Unfortunately, histologic features do not allow accurate prediction of the clinical course, although some have found a correlation between a large number of slit-like blood vessels and increased numbers of undifferentiated mesenchymal cells and risk of recurrence.[161] In rare cases, encroachment on critical structures, particularly those arising in the head and neck, may result in the patient's death.[162]

Complete excision with ample margins is the treatment of choice, although it is difficult in some anatomic locations and may be impossible without disfigurement or dysfunction. There is relatively little information as to the efficacy of adjuvant chemotherapy (including imatinib) or radiotherapy, but some have found these modalities to be of therapeutic benefit.[163]

The cause of infantile fibromatosis is not clear. As with other forms of fibromatosis, trauma has been implicated as an inciting factor. In the series by Faulkner et al.,[160] 17% of patients had a history of antecedent trauma in the vicinity of the lesion. Coffin and Dehner[164] reported two cases that arose at sites of previous surgery. Unlike many other fibrous lesions, increased familial incidence has not been observed with this type of fibromatosis.

CALCIFYING APONEUROTIC FIBROMA

Originally described in juvenile and adolescent patients as *juvenile aponeurotic fibroma* by Keasbey[165] in 1953, it has subsequently become apparent that this lesion affects a much wider age range than other forms of juvenile fibromatosis.[166] Keasbey described its characteristic histologic picture, its predilection for the palm and fingers of the hand, and its propensity to locally recur after excision. In view of the wide age range of patients, the term *calcifying aponeurotic fibroma* is now the preferred name for this entity.

Clinical Findings

Most patients present with a slowly growing, painless mass in the hands or feet of several months' or even years' duration. The mass is usually poorly circumscribed and causes neither discomfort nor limitation of movement, although some patients do have complaints of mild tenderness.[167] Grossly, lesions that have been present for several years are often more sharply circumscribed and distinctly nodular than those of shorter duration.

Most lesions occur in children, with a peak incidence of 8 to 14 years. Although most small series have not reported a distinct gender predilection, 70% of the patients in the series by Allen and Enzinger[167] were male. There is no record of increased familial incidence. The two principal sites of growth are the hands and feet. In the hand, the most common sites are the palm and fingers with only rare involvement of the dorsum of the hand. Fewer lesions occur on the plantar surface of the foot or ankle region and rarely the toes. Isolated tumors have been observed at other sites, including the elbow, scalp, and gluteal region, among others.[168-170] They may be found in the subcutaneous tissue or attached to the aponeurosis, tendons, or fascia. Preoperative radiographic examination reveals a faint mass, frequently with calcific stippling, especially in the more heavily calcified tumors. MRI is more precise at outlining the anatomic extent of the process and is useful in planning the surgical excision.[171]

Pathologic Findings

Grossly, most lesions are ill-defined, firm or rubbery, and gray-white, usually less than 3 cm in greatest diameter. Older lesions are more grossly well circumscribed, although there is typically microscopic infiltration of the surrounding soft tissues even in these cases. Portions of the surrounding fat, skeletal muscle, and fibrous tissue frequently merge with the tumor. In some cases, calcifications are evident as small white flecks (Fig. 9-32), but, in heavily calcified cases, they may be more grossly apparent. On sectioning, the lesion often has a gritty sensation as a result of these calcifications.

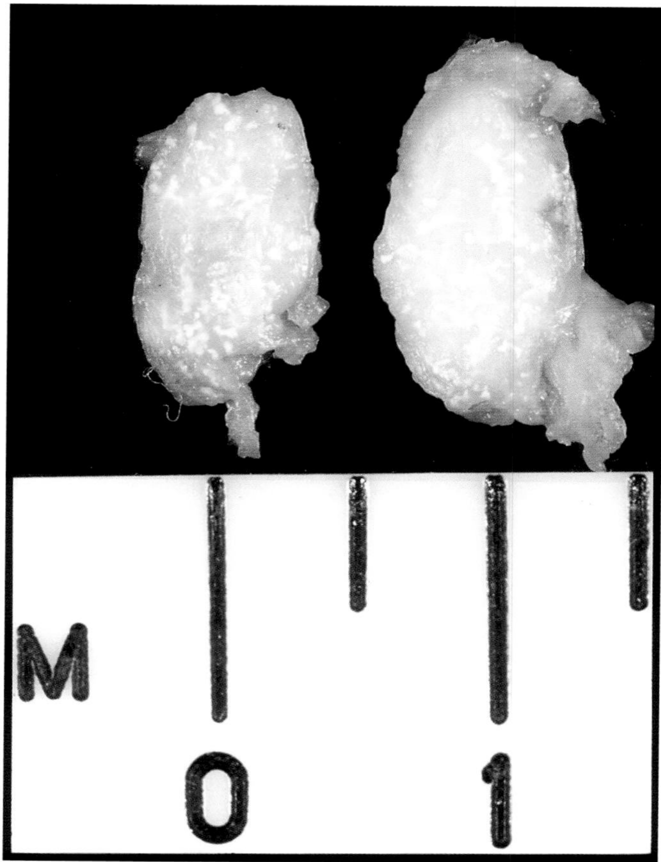

FIGURE 9-32. Calcifying aponeurotic fibroma in the palm of a 4-year-old boy. Note the small white flecks, indicative of calcification.

The histologic picture varies little from case to case. It reveals a fibrous growth that extends with multiple processes into the surrounding tissue with more centrally located foci of calcification and cartilage formation. The cellularity of the lesion varies from region to region and is composed of plump fibroblasts with round or ovoid nuclei and indistinctly outlined cytoplasm separated by a densely collagenous stroma (Figs. 9-33 to 9-37). Despite the focal cellularity of the lesion, mitotic figures are scarce. Not infrequently, the fibrous growth is attached to a tendon or aponeurosis and encircles blood vessels and nerves. Unlike other forms of fibromatosis, there tends to be orientation of the stromal cells. There may be a vague cartwheel or whorled pattern, or the nuclei may line up in columns, occasionally resulting in marked nuclear palisading.

Calcification and cartilage formation are much more pronounced in lesions removed from older children and young adults. The calcifications are usually small and vary from fine granules or string-like deposits to large amorphous masses. In many cases, these calcified foci are surrounded by radiating columns of cells that resemble chondrocytes, with rounded nuclei lying in lacunae (see Fig. 9-35). These cartilage-like cells are often aligned in linear columns that radiate from the center of the calcified areas, although there may be a circumferential arrangement as well. Occasionally, multinucleated giant cells resembling osteoclasts are present adjacent to the calcific foci (Fig. 9-38), but they may also be seen adjacent to noncalcified fibrocartilage-like tissue. Ossification occurs but is rare, and even hematopoiesis has been observed within the bony elements.[172]

Differential Diagnosis

The differential diagnosis differs from case to case, depending on the age of the patient at the time that the lesion is excised. In infants and small children, when there is still little or no calcification, this lesion may be difficult to distinguish from

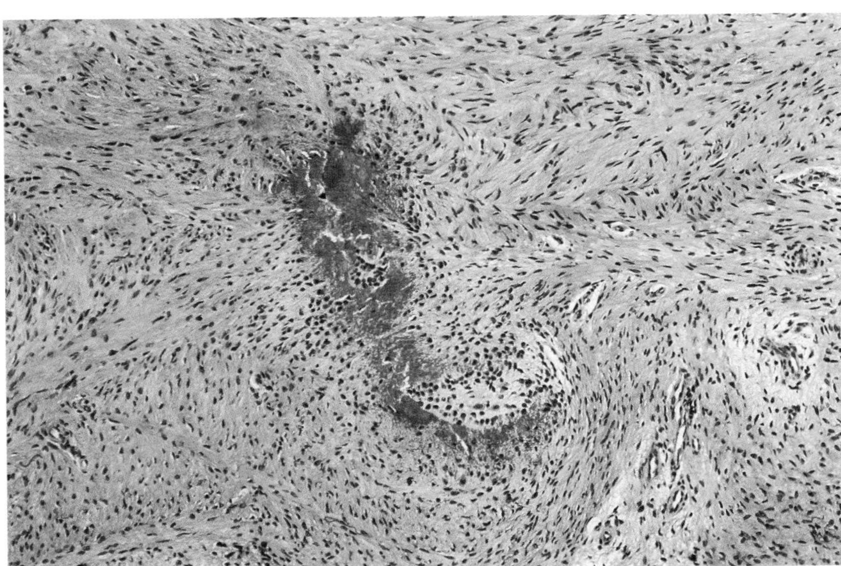

FIGURE 9-33. Calcifying aponeurotic fibroma with early focal calcification.

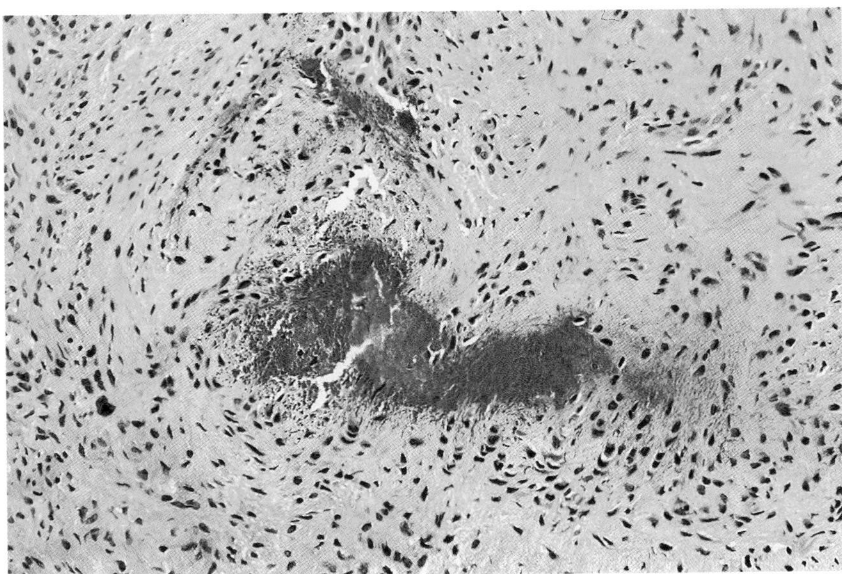

FIGURE 9-34. Calcifying aponeurotic fibroma showing hyalinization of the fibrous tissue in the vicinity of heavily calcified areas.

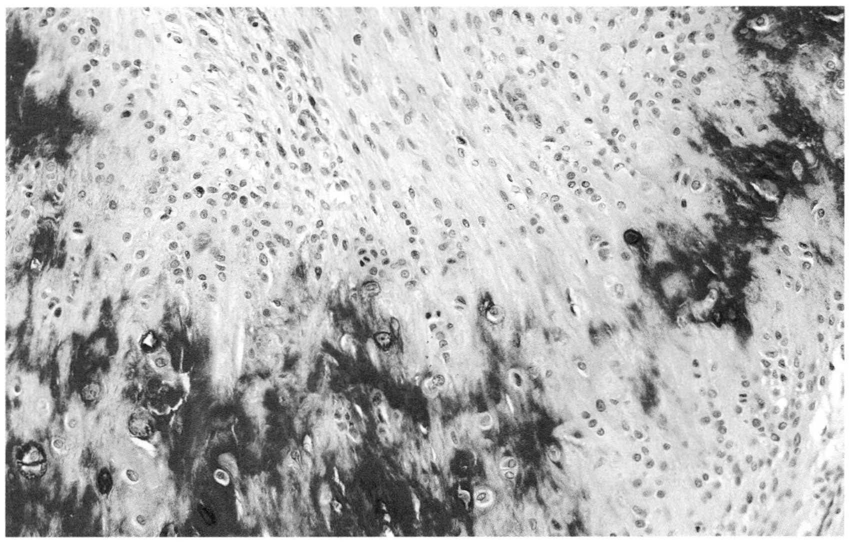

FIGURE 9-35. Calcifying aponeurotic fibroma with small round cells radiating from the calcified areas and arranged in linear arrays.

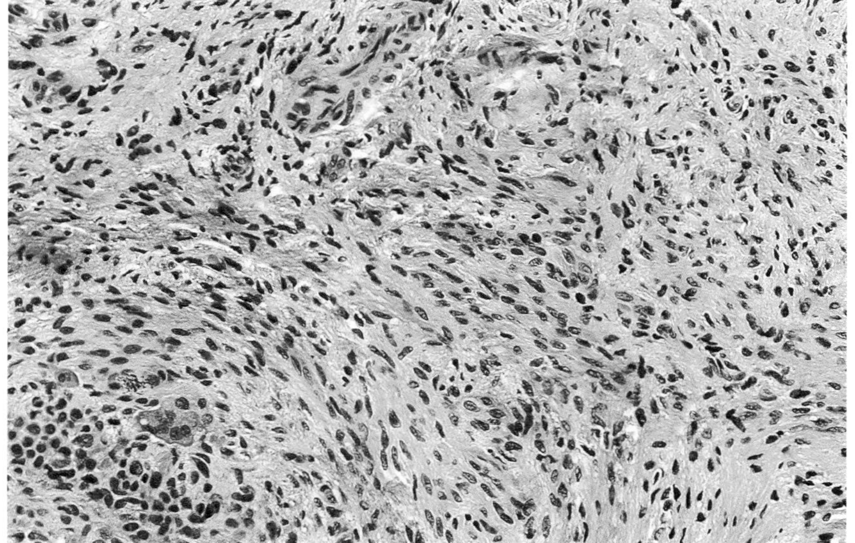

FIGURE 9-36. High-power view of the cellular portion of a calcifying aponeurotic fibroma.

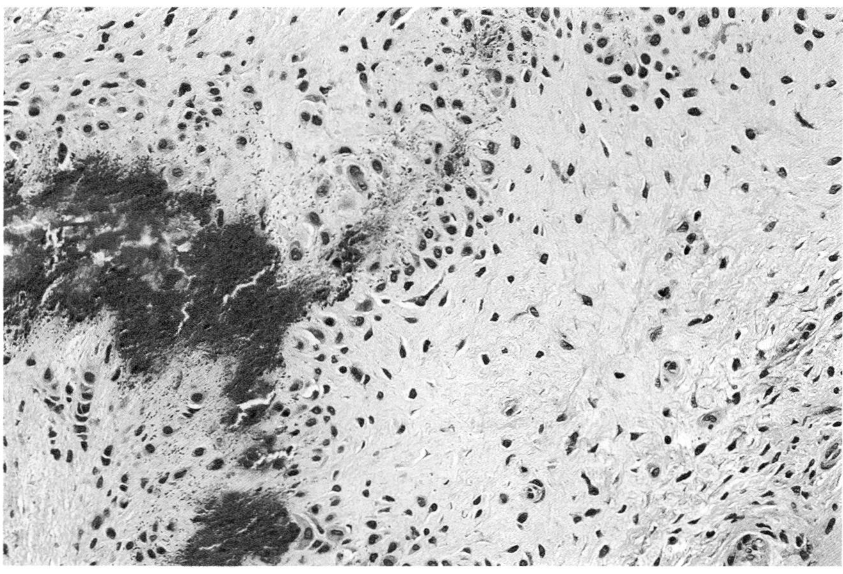

FIGURE 9-37. Calcifying aponeurotic fibroma with focal cartilaginous metaplasia in an area of calcification.

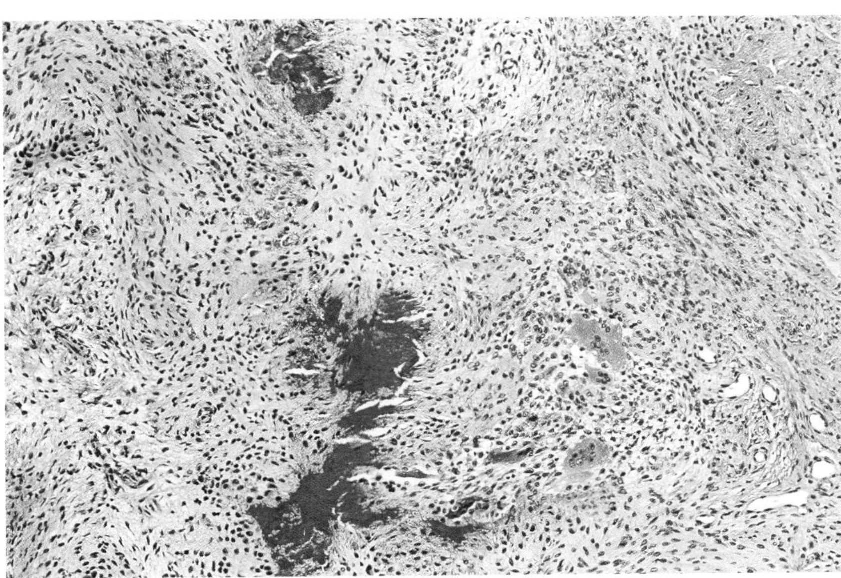

FIGURE 9-38. Calcifying aponeurotic fibroma with multinucleated giant cells adjacent to an area of calcification.

infantile fibromatosis. However, infantile fibromatosis most commonly presents as a soft tissue mass in the extremities or head and neck, and the fibroblasts of infantile fibromatosis are more elongated and are often deposited in a myxoid background; foci of calcification and ossification are uncommon. Giant cells, a common feature of calcifying aponeurotic fibroma, are not typical of fibromatosis. *Palmar* and *plantar fibromatoses* may occur in children but are not common, especially palmar lesions. They are more nodular in appearance and lack calcification or chondroid differentiation. Malignant spindle cell tumors, such as *monophasic fibrous-type synovial sarcoma*, may rarely be mistaken for calcifying aponeurotic fibroma with a prominent spindle cell pattern. Immunoreactivity for epithelial markers and analysis for *SYT* gene aberrations allow for recognition of synovial sarcoma.

In older patients, distinction of the growth from a *soft part chondroma* may cause considerable difficulty, especially because both lesions are most common in the hands. However, soft part chondromas more frequently affect older adults and have a lower rate of local recurrence than aponeurotic fibromas. Histologically, soft part chondromas are well-circumscribed, lobulated masses that are sharply demarcated from the surrounding soft tissues. Furthermore, the extent of chondroid differentiation is far better developed in soft tissue chondromas than in aponeurotic fibromas.

Discussion

Because of its infiltrative nature, the calcifying aponeurotic fibroma is characterized by a high rate of local recurrence. In the series by Allen and Enzinger,[167] 10 of 19 lesions recurred 1 month to 11 years after the initial excision. The authors did not identify any histologic features that predicted recurrence but did note that young patients, particularly those under 5 years of age, had a higher risk of recurrence. Very few cases of malignant transformation have been reported.[173] Lafferty et al.[174] reported a calcifying aponeurotic fibroma of the palm in a 3-year-old girl that metastasized as a metastatic fibrosarcoma to the lungs and bones 5 years after a second local excision. Sharon W. Weiss has also reviewed a single case of malignant transformation of a calcifying aponeurotic fibroma.

Surgical management should be conservative. In fact, excision and re-excision, if necessary, are preferable to radical or mutilating surgical procedures to maintain function of the extremity.

There seem to be two phases in the development of this tumor: (1) an initial phase, which is more common in infants and small children, in which the tumor grows diffusely, often lacks calcification, and bears a resemblance to infantile fibromatosis; and (2) a late phase, in which the tumor is more compact and nodular and shows a more prominent degree of calcification and cartilage formation. In some of the latter cases, calcification and cartilage formation are so prominent it may be difficult to distinguish this lesion from a calcifying soft part chondroma.

CONGENITAL AND ACQUIRED MUSCULAR FIBROSIS

Since its initial description, numerous examples of muscular fibrosis have been reported in the literature; most affected the quadriceps muscle,[175] although a few have been reported in the gluteus,[176] deltoid,[177] triceps,[178] and gastrocnemius muscles.[179] Both congenital and acquired lesions of this type have been described.

Clinical Findings

Although the onset of the lesion usually dates back to the first year of life, the mass develops slowly and often does not become apparent before the second or third year of life. Clinically, most patients present with a progressive, painless mass or cord-like induration of the involved muscle. Lesions are generally poorly circumscribed and may occur on one or both sides. Progressive fibrosis results in a shortening and contracture of the involved muscle, which leads to various functional disturbances depending on the extent of the fibrosis and the muscle involved. Concomitant dimpling or depressions of the overlying skin are observed occasionally; they are most likely a result of fatty atrophy and extension of the fibrosing process into the adjacent fascia and subcutaneous fat.

The fibrosing process is most commonly encountered in the quadriceps muscle, where it usually affects the distal portion of the vastus intermedius and vastus lateralis. It severely limits the range of active and passive flexion of the knee joint and causes difficulty squatting and sitting straight as well as an abnormal gait. In some cases, the patella dislocates laterally every time the knee is flexed. Involvement of the gluteus muscle may lead to external rotation and abduction contracture of the hip in a seated position and a waddling gait. Involvement of the deltoid muscle may cause an abduction contracture of the shoulder and lateral elevation of the arms.[180]

Pathologic Findings

Grossly, the involved muscle shows patchy, firm, scar-like, gray or gray-yellow areas that consist microscopically of a conglomerate of collagenous fibrous tissue, residual partly degenerated atrophic muscle fibers, and replacement of atrophic muscle by mature fat. Not infrequently, the fibrosis extends into the muscle fascia or aponeurosis and even into the subcutaneous fat. There is no evidence of a foreign body reaction or significant inflammation.

Discussion

Various concepts have been suggested as to the most likely cause of the fibrosing process. Certainly, some cases are associated with intramuscular injections of antibiotics or other medications.[181] No single drug has been incriminated as the cause of the fibrosis, although antibiotics are most frequently implicated.[180] It has been proposed that the intramuscular injection results in chemical myositis or pressure ischemia with subsequent fibrosis.[180] Given the fact that only a small number of infants who undergo this type of therapy develop intramuscular fibrosis, other predisposing factors are certainly at play. There are reports of muscle fibrosis in children who have had the lesions since birth, with no history of intramuscular injections. There is no clear hereditary pattern, but the condition has been observed in four pairs of siblings[182] and several pairs of identical twins.[183]

To regain a normal range of function, tenotomy (rather than physical therapy or other conservative measures) is the treatment of choice. Most patients regain full range of motion, although a subset of patients continue to have functional impairment of the involved extremity.

CEREBRIFORM FIBROUS PROLIFERATION (PROTEUS SYNDROME)

Proteus syndrome, a rare entity, is included here because the cerebriform or gyriform fibrous proliferation characteristically found on the volar surfaces may be mistaken for fibromatosis. Although isolated or localized cerebriform fibrous proliferations have been described,[184] they occur more commonly in conjunction with a complex group of lesions involving the skin, soft tissue, and skeleton. Proteus syndrome was first described by Cohen and Hayden[185] in 1979 and named by Wiedemann[186] in 1983 after the Greek ocean deity, Proteus (the polymorphous), because of the broad range of its features. Although "the elephant man," Joseph Merrick, was originally believed to have neurofibromatosis, evidence indicates that he suffered from Proteus syndrome.[187]

Patients with the Proteus syndrome exhibit a constellation of congenital and developmental defects that cannot be classified into previously defined disorders, and these patients demonstrate wide morphologic variability.[188] Manifestations include gigantism of the hands or feet (macrodactyly); asymmetry; skeletal abnormalities, including hemihypertrophy and exostoses (particularly cranial exostoses); pulmonary abnormalities (bulla, varicosities); and a variety of cutaneous abnormalities, including epidermal nevi and lipomatous and hemangiomatous tumors.[189-192] The lipomatous proliferations may be present in the subcutis but may also affect the abdomen, pelvis, and mesentery.[193,194] The cerebriform fibrous changes affect the plantar surfaces and, to a lesser degree, the palmar surfaces, and they are associated with unilateral or bilateral macrodactyly or hypertrophy of long bones (partial gigantism).[195]

Proteus syndrome has been reported in discordant monozygomatic twins,[196] and evidence suggests that this disease is caused by a somatic mutation that is lethal when constitutive.[197] Recently, Lindhurst et al.[198] identified mosaic activating mutations in *AKT1* in 26 of 29 patients with Proteus syndrome. Interestingly, this syndrome has also been associated with somatic *PTEN* mutations,[199,200] although mutations in *PTEN* are identified in a syndrome with significant morphologic overlap with Proteus syndrome, called segmental overgrowth, lipomatosis, arteriovenous malformation, and epidermal nevus syndrome (SOLAMEN) or type 2 segmental Cowden syndrome.[201,202] Because *AKT1* is activated by *PTEN* mutations, it is not surprising that these syndromes have significant morphologic overlap.[203]

Grossly, there is marked thickening of the skin in the volar areas, resulting in a coarse cerebriform or gyriform pattern (Fig. 9-39). Microscopically, the plantar and palmar lesions consist of dense fibrosis involving both the dermis and subcutis, with hyperkeratosis of the overlying skin (Figs. 9-40 to 9-42).[204,205]

CALCIFYING FIBROUS PSEUDOTUMOR

Originally reported as *childhood fibrous tumor with psammoma bodies*,[206] calcifying fibrous pseudotumor is uncommon; it is a hypocellular, fibrous lesion that most often affects patients during the second or third decade of life.[207,208] Females are affected slightly more commonly than males. Most patients present with a slowly growing, painless mass in the subcutaneous or deep soft tissues that may be associated with systemic symptoms. The lesions most commonly arise in the extremities, followed by the trunk, inguinal and scrotal regions, and head and neck. Rare lesions have also been described in virtually every anatomic location, including the gastrointestinal tract,[209] oral cavity,[210] omentum/mesentery,[211] pleura,[212] and peritoneum,[213] among others. Most are 3 to 5 cm at the time of excision, but the lesions can be as large as 15 cm.

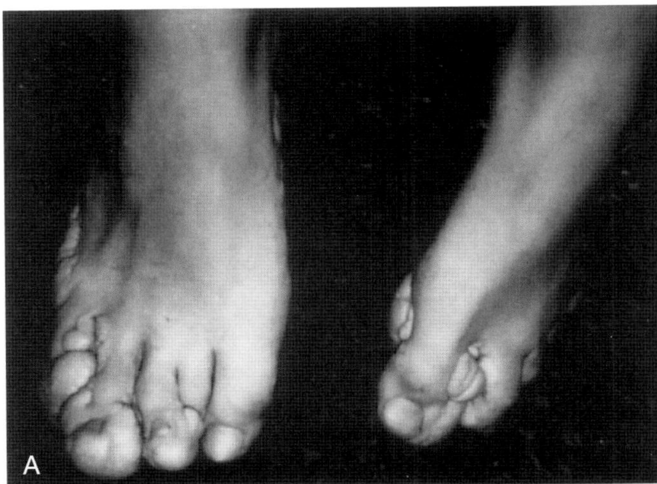

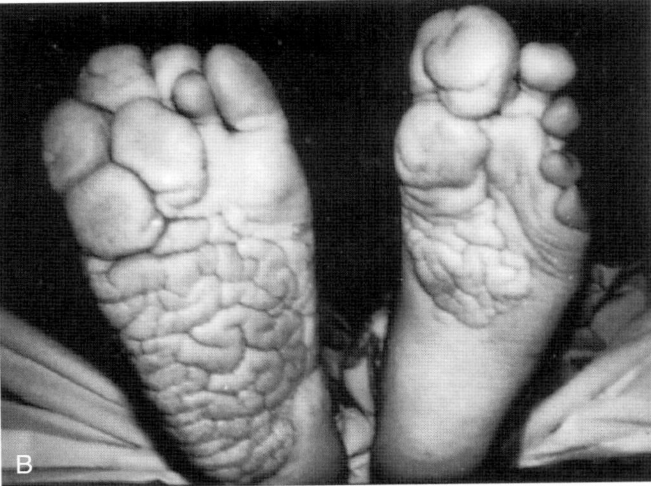

FIGURE 9-39. Bilateral cerebriform (gyriform) fibrous proliferation of toes (A) and plantar surfaces (B). This process may occur alone or in conjunction with lipomatous and hemangiomatous tumors and various skeletal changes, including scoliosis, multiple exostoses, and craniofacial asymmetry (Proteus syndrome).

On gross examination, the mass is well circumscribed, somewhat lobulated, and solid or firm; it has a uniform gray-white fibrous appearance on a cross-section. It often cuts with a gritty sensation as a result of the extensive calcifications that are typically present. Histologically, the mass is well circumscribed, nonencapsulated, and composed chiefly of hyalinized birefringent fibrosclerotic tissue with a variable inflammatory infiltrate composed of lymphocytes and plasma cells, with the formation of occasional germinal centers. The lesions are hypocellular, with scattered cytologically bland, fibroblastic, or myofibroblastic spindle cells.[207,208] A characteristic feature is the presence of dystrophic, frequently psammomatous calcifications that may be focally present or comprise most of the tumor (Fig. 9-43). Immunohistochemically, these cells show variable immunoreactivity for muscle-specific actin, smooth muscle actin, and desmin.[208] Generally, scattered cells express these markers, but they are never diffusely positive. Many of the lesional cells also express CD34 and/or factor XIIIa.[208,214] However, stains for anaplastic lymphoma kinase (ALK), a marker found in many (but not all) inflammatory myofibroblastic tumors, is consistently negative in calcifying fibrous pseudotumor.[215]

Recently, Kuo et al.[216] described a fascinating series of five cases of disseminated intra-abdominal calcifying fibrous pseudotumors associated with sclerosing angiomatoid nodular transformation of the spleen, an unusual vascular lesion that has features that overlap with other IgG4-related sclerosing diseases. These authors found consistent IgG4 staining in the plasma cells in both lesions. A similar case was reported by Aceñero et al.[217] in 2010. These studies raise the possibility that calcifying fibrous pseudotumor, at least in some cases, is part of the spectrum of IgG4 sclerosing diseases.

The differential diagnosis includes inflammatory myofibroblastic tumor, reactive nodular fibrous pseudotumor, fibromatosis, nodular fasciitis, fibroma of the tendon sheath, calcifying aponeurotic fibroma, and amyloidoma. *Inflammatory myofibroblastic tumor* is generally more cellular, less hyalinized, and typically lacks calcifications. However, clearly there is histologic overlap of these lesions, and it has been proposed that

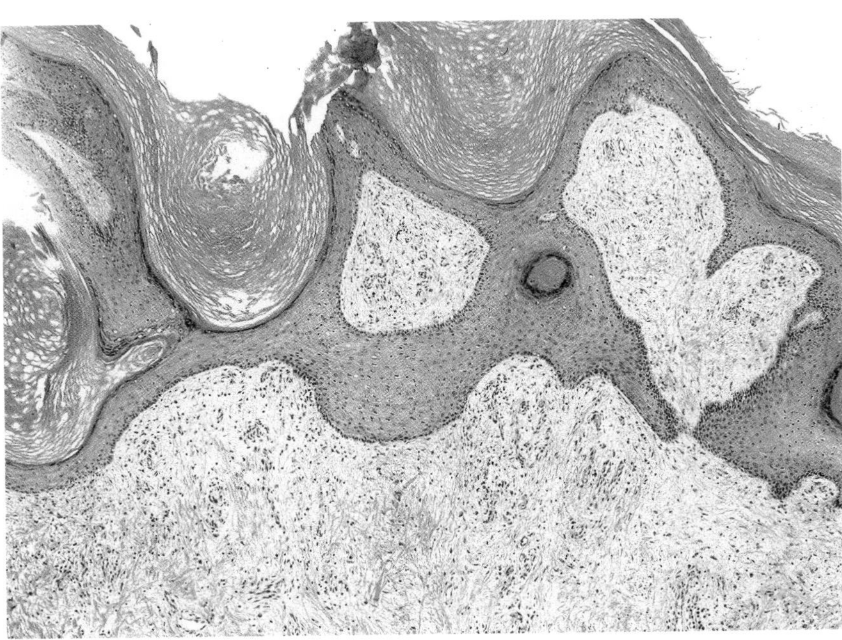

FIGURE 9-40. Proteus syndrome. The lesion shows evidence of acanthosis and hyperkeratosis of the overlying epithelium associated with dermal fibrosis and mild chronic inflammation.

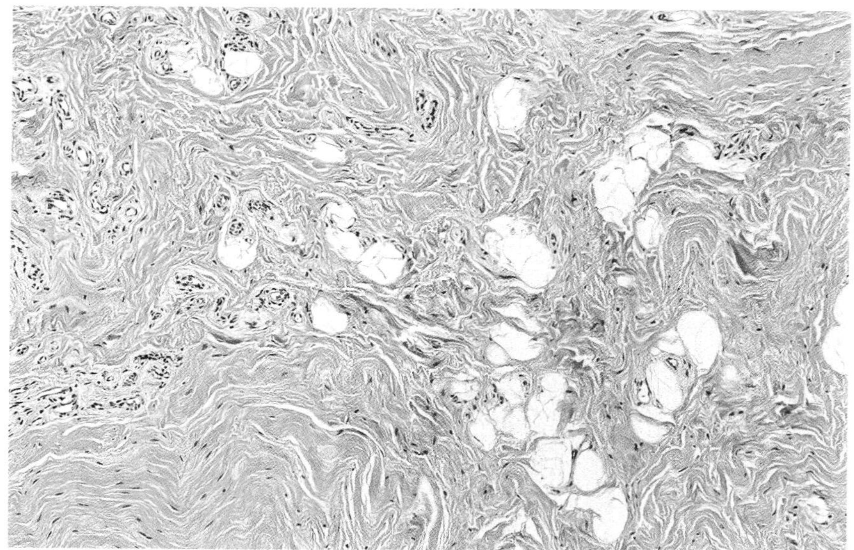

FIGURE 9-41. Proteus syndrome. Hypocellular dense collagen with admixed adipocytes.

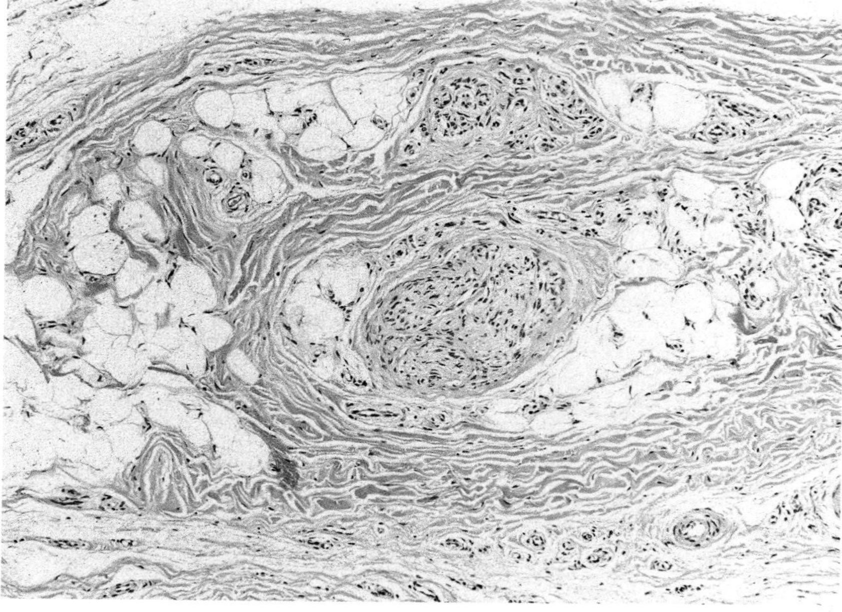

FIGURE 9-42. Benign lipomatous lesion with entrapped nerves in a patient with Proteus syndrome.

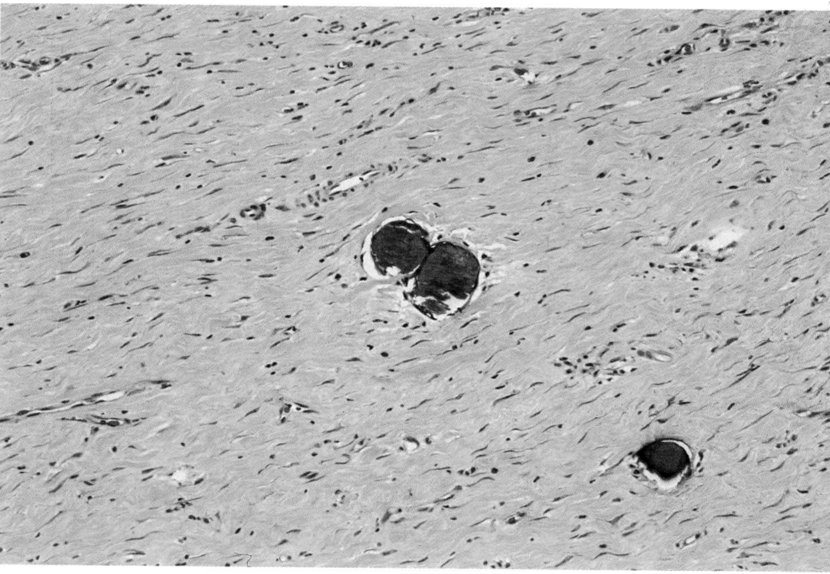

FIGURE 9-43. Calcifying fibrous pseudotumor chiefly composed of a uniform dense collagenous matrix with psammomatous calcifications and scattered spindle-shaped and inflammatory cells.

calcifying fibrous pseudotumor represents a late sclerosing phase of inflammatory myofibroblastic tumor.[207,218,219] Van Dorpe et al.[219] described an intra-abdominal tumor that arose in a 17-year-old female with features overlapping those seen in these two entities, as well as transitional stages between calcifying fibrous pseudotumor and inflammatory myofibroblastic tumor. However, as mentioned previously, calcifying fibrous pseudotumor is consistently negative for ALK, and there is no evidence to suggest that alterations of the *ALK* gene are involved in its pathogenesis.

Yantiss et al.[220] described a fibroinflammatory lesion that typically arises in the mesentery and coined the term *reactive nodular fibrous pseudotumor*. Although there are some similarities to calcifying fibrous pseudotumor, the authors argued that this entity is distinct, based upon histologic and immunohistochemical grounds. In contrast to reactive nodular fibrous pseudotumor, calcifying fibrous pseudotumor is usually more cellular, the infiltrate contains lymphocytes, plasma cells and granulocytes, and calcifications are characteristic. The lesional cells of reactive nodular fibrous pseudotumor express actins, desmin, and CD117, and are negative for CD34.[220,221]

Fibromatosis is less well circumscribed, and, histologically, the spindle cells typically infiltrate the surrounding soft tissues. In addition, fibromatosis is characterized by greater cellularity with arrangement in a prominent fascicular growth pattern. Microcalcifications are extremely uncommon in fibromatosis. *Nodular fasciitis* is composed of tissue culture-like spindle cells deposited in a myxoid stroma that lacks microcalcifications. Unlike calcifying fibrous pseudotumor, *fibroma of the tendon sheath* typically arises in the distal extremities. It is composed chiefly of densely sclerotic collagen, but there are frequently areas of increased cellularity, some of which resemble nodular fasciitis. In addition, elongated slit-like spaces are typical, and calcifications are not present. *Calcifying aponeurotic fibroma* usually arises in the hands or feet, is less well circumscribed than calcifying fibrous pseudotumor, and is characterized by band-like calcifications frequently surrounded by cartilaginous metaplasia and multinucleated giant cells. Unlike the amyloid tumor (*amyloidoma*), calcifying fibrous pseudotumor is devoid of giant cells or demonstrable amyloid because Congo red stains are negative.

Although metastases have not been reported, some lesions locally recur.[207,222] In the study by Nascimento et al.,[208] 3 of the 10 cases with clinical follow-up recurred, including 2 cases that recurred more than once. Nevertheless, this lesion is clearly benign, and conservative excision is the ideal mode of therapy.

References

1. Sotelo-Avila C, Bale PM. Subdermal fibrous hamartoma of infancy: pathology of 40 cases and differential diagnosis. Pediatr Pathol 1994; 14(1):39–52.
2. Scott DM, Peña JR, Omura EF. Fibrous hamartoma of infancy. J Am Acad Dermatol 1999;41(5 Pt 2):857–9.
3. Dickey GE, Sotelo-Avila C. Fibrous hamartoma of infancy: current review. Pediatr Dev Pathol 1999;2(3):236–43.
4. Reye RD. A consideration of certain subdermal fibromatous tumours of infancy. J Pathol Bacteriol 1956;72(1):149–54.
5. Enzinger FM. Fibrous hamartoma of infancy. Cancer 1965;18:241–8.
6. Efem SE, Ekpo MD. Clinicopathological features of untreated fibrous hamartoma of infancy. J Clin Pathol 1993;46(6):522–4.
7. Thami GP, Jaswal R, Kanwar AJ. Fibrous hamartoma of infancy in the scrotum. Pediatr Dermatol 1998;15(4):326.
8. Stock JA, Niku SD, Packer MG, et al. Fibrous hamartoma of infancy: a report of two cases in the genital region. Urology 1995;45(1): 130–1.
9. Eppley BL, Harruff R, Shah M, et al. Fibrous hamartomas of the scalp in infancy. Plast Reconstr Surg 1994;94(1):195–7.
10. Imaji R, Goto T, Takahashi Y, et al. A case of recurrent and synchronous fibrous hamartoma of infancy. Pediatr Surg Int 2005;21(2):119–20.
11. Ashwood N, Witt JD, Hall-Craggs MA. Fibrous hamartoma of infancy at the wrist and the use of MRI in preoperative planning. Pediatr Radiol 2001;31(6):450–2.
12. McGowan J 4th, Smith CD, Maize Jr J, et al. Giant fibrous hamartoma of infancy: a report of two cases and review of the literature. J Am Acad Dermatol 2011;64(3):579–86.
13. German DS, Paletta CE, Gabriel K. Fibrous hamartoma of infancy. Orthopedics 1996;19(3):258–60.
14. Fletcher CD, Powell G, van Noorden S, et al. Fibrous hamartoma of infancy: a histochemical and immunohistochemical study. Histopathology 1988;12(1):65–74.
15. Rougemont AL, Fetni R, Murthy S, et al. A complex translocation (6;12;8)(q25;q24.3;q13) in a fibrous hamartoma of infancy. Cancer Genet Cytogenet 2006;171(2):115–8.
16. Lakshminarayanan R, Konia T, Welborn J. Fibrous hamartoma of infancy: a case report with associated cytogenetic findings. Arch Pathol Lab Med 2005;129(4):520–2.
17. Tassano E, Nozza P, Tavella E, et al. Cytogenetic characterization of a fibrous hamartoma of infancy with complex translocations. Cancer Genet Cytogenet 2010;201(1):66–9.
18. Jensen AR, Martin LW, Longino LA. Digital neurofibrosarcoma in infancy. J Pediatr 1957;51(5):566–70.
19. Enzinger FM. Dermal fibromatosis. In: Tumors of Bone and Soft Tissue. Year Book Medical Publishers Inc, Chicago: 1965. p. 375.
20. Heymann WR. Infantile digital fibromatosis. J Am Acad Dermatol 2008;59(1):122–3.
21. Kang SK, Chang SE, Choi JH, et al. A case of congenital infantile digital fibromatosis. Pediatr Dermatol 2002;19(5):462–3.
22. Laskin WB, Miettinen M, Fetsch JF. Infantile digital fibroma/fibromatosis: a clinicopathologic and immunohistochemical study of 69 tumors from 57 patients with long-term follow-up. Am J Surg Pathol 2009;33(1):1–13.
23. Rimareix F, Bardot J, Andrac L, et al. Infantile digital fibroma–report on eleven cases. Eur J Pediatr Surg 1997;7(6):345–8.
24. Sun Y, Almomani R, Aten E, et al. Terminal osseous dysplasia is caused by a single recurrent mutation in the FLNA gene. Am J Hum Genet 2010;87(1):146–53.
25. Purdy LJ, Colby TV. Infantile digital fibromatosis occurring outside the digit. Am J Surg Pathol 1984;8(10):787–90.
26. Pettinato G, Manivel JC, Gould EW, et al. Inclusion body fibromatosis of the breast. Two cases with immunohistochemical and ultrastructural findings. Am J Clin Pathol 1994;101(6):714–8.
27. Grenier N, Liang C, Capaldi L, et al. A range of histologic findings in infantile digital fibromatosis. Pediatr Dermatol 2008;25(1):72–5.
28. Mukai M, Torikata C, Iri H, et al. Immunohistochemical identification of aggregated actin filaments in formalin-fixed, paraffin-embedded sections. I. A study of infantile digital fibromatosis by a new pretreatment. Am J Surg Pathol 1992;16(2):110–5.
29. Choi KC, Hashimoto K, Setoyama M, et al. Infantile digital fibromatosis. Immunohistochemical and immunoelectron microscopic studies. J Cutan Pathol 1990;17(4):225–32.
30. Thway K, Gibson S, Ramsay A, et al. Beta-catenin expression in pediatric fibroblastic and myofibroblastic lesions: a study of 100 cases. Pediatr Dev Pathol 2009;12(4):292–6.
31. Bhawan J, Bacchetta C, Joris I, et al. A myofibroblastic tumor. Infantile digital fibroma (recurrent digital fibrous tumor of childhood). Am J Pathol 1979;94(1):19–36.
32. Mukai M, Torikata C, Iri H, et al. Infantile digital fibromatosis. An electron microscopic and immunohistochemical study. Acta Pathol Jpn 1986;36(11):1605–15.
33. Battifora H, Hines JR. Recurrent digital fibromas of childhood. An electron microscope study. Cancer 1971;27(6):1530–6.
34. Miyamoto T, Mihara M, Hagari Y, et al. Posttraumatic occurrence of infantile digital fibromatosis. A histologic and electron microscopic study. Arch Dermatol 1986;122(8):915–8.
35. Taylor HO, Gellis SE, Schmidt BA, et al. Infantile digital fibromatosis. Ann Plast Surg 2008;61(4):472–6.

36. Dey D, Nicol A, Singer S. Benign phyllodes tumor of the breast with intracytoplasmic inclusion bodies identical to infantile digital fibromatosis. Breast J 2008;14(2):198–9.
37. Shin SJ, Rosen PP. Bilateral presentation of fibroadenoma with digital fibroma-like inclusions in the male breast. Arch Pathol Lab Med 2007; 131(7):1126–9.
38. Yusoff KL, Spagnolo DV, Digwood KI. Atypical cervical polyp with intracytoplasmic inclusions. Pathology 1998;30(2):215–7.
39. Spingardi O, Zoccolan A, Venturino E. Infantile digital fibromatosis: our experience and long-term results. Chir Main 2011;30(1):62–5.
40. Ishii N, Matsui K, Ichiyama S, et al. A case of infantile digital fibromatosis showing spontaneous regression. Br J Dermatol 1989;121(1): 129–33.
41. Campbell LB, Petrick MG. Mohs micrographic surgery for a problematic infantile digital fibroma. Dermatol Surg 2007;33(3):385–7.
42. Holmes WJ, Mishra A, McArthur P. Intra-lesional steroid for the management of symptomatic infantile digital fibromatosis. J Plast Reconstr Aesthet Surg 2011;64(5):632–7.
43. Williams JO, Schrum D. Congenital fibrosarcoma; report of a case in a newborn infant. AMA Arch Pathol 1951;51(5):548–52.
44. Stout AP. Juvenile fibromatoses. Cancer 1954;7(5):953–78.
45. Kauffman SL, Stout AP. Congenital mesenchymal tumors. Cancer 1965; 18:460–76.
46. Chung EB, Enzinger FM. Infantile myofibromatosis. Cancer 1981;48(8): 1807–18.
47. Wiswell TE, Davis J, Cunningham BE, et al. Infantile myofibromatosis: the most common fibrous tumor of infancy. J Pediatr Surg 1988;23(4): 315–8.
48. Konishi E, Mazaki T, Urata Y, et al. Solitary myofibroma of the lumbar vertebra: adult case. Skeletal Radiol 2007;36(Suppl 1):S86–90.
49. Xiao HL, Eyden B, Yan XC, et al. Intraparenchymal myofibromatosis of the brain in an adult: report of an unusual case. Neuropathology 2010;30(3):288–93.
50. Calsina M, Philipone E, Patwardhan M, et al. Solitary orbital myofibroma: clinical, radiographic, and histopathologic findings. A report of two cases. Orbit 2011;30(4):180–2.
51. Vered M, Allon I, Buchner A, et al. Clinico-pathologic correlations of myofibroblastic tumors of the oral cavity. II. Myofibroma and myofibromatosis of the oral soft tissues. J Oral Pathol Med 2007;36(5): 304–14.
52. Merciadri P, Pavanello M, Nozza P, et al. Solitary infantile myofibromatosis of the cranial vault: case report. Childs Nerv Syst 2011;27(4): 643–7.
53. Souza DP, Loureiro CC, Rejas RA, et al. Intraosseous myofibroma simulating an odontogenic lesion. J Oral Sci 2009;51(2):307–11.
54. Wang S, Huang H, Ruan Z, et al. A rare case of adult pulmonary myofibromatosis. Asian Cardiovasc Thorac Ann 2009;17(2):199–202.
55. Jones MA, Young RH, Scully RE. Benign fibromatous tumors of the testis and paratesticular region: a report of 9 cases with a proposed classification of fibromatous tumors and tumor-like lesions. Am J Surg Pathol 1997;21(3):296–305.
56. Schaffzin EA, Chung SM, Kaye R. Congenital generalized fibromatosis with complete spontaneous regression. A case report. J Bone Joint Surg Am 1972;54(3):657–62.
57. Heiple KG, Perrin E, Aikawa M. Congenital generalized fibromatosis: a case limited to osseous lesions. J Bone Joint Surg Am 1972;54(3): 663–9.
58. Dhall D, Frykman PK, Wang HL. Colorectal infantile myofibromatosis: an unusual cause of rectal prolapse and sigmoid colo-colonic intussusception: a case report. Cases J 2008;1(1):397.
59. Thomas-de-Montpréville V, Nottin R, Dulmet E, et al. Heart tumors in children and adults: clinicopathological study of 59 patients from a surgical center. Cardiovasc Pathol 2007;16(1):22–8.
60. Hogan SF, Salassa JR. Recurrent adult myofibromatosis. A case report. Am J Clin Pathol 1992;97(6):810–4.
61. Murphey MD, Ruble CM, Tyszko SM, et al. From the archives of the AFIP: musculoskeletal fibromatoses: radiologic-pathologic correlation. Radiographics 2009;29(7):2143–73.
62. Ben Haj Amor M, Nectoux E, Basraoui D, et al. [Solitary calcified myofibroma of the leg: a case report]. J Radiol 2011;92(3):243–6.
63. Zelger BW, Calonje E, Sepp N, et al. Monophasic cellular variant of infantile myofibromatosis. An unusual histopathologic pattern in two siblings. Am J Dermatopathol 1995;17(2):131–8.
64. Beham A, Badve S, Suster S, et al. Solitary myofibroma in adults: clinicopathological analysis of a series. Histopathology 1993;22(4): 335–41.
65. Hausbrandt PA, Leithner A, Beham A, et al. A rare case of infantile myofibromatosis and review of literature. J Pediatr Orthop B 2010;19(1): 122–6.
66. Mentzel T, Calonje E, Nascimento AG, et al. Infantile hemangiopericytoma versus infantile myofibromatosis. Study of a series suggesting a continuous spectrum of infantile myofibroblastic lesions. Am J Surg Pathol 1994;18(9):922–30.
67. Dictor M, Elner A, Andersson T, et al. Myofibromatosis-like hemangiopericytoma metastasizing as differentiated vascular smooth-muscle and myosarcoma. Myopericytes as a subset of "myofibroblasts." Am J Surg Pathol 1992;16(12):1239–47.
68. Variend S, Bax NM, van Gorp J. Are infantile myofibromatosis, congenital fibrosarcoma and congenital haemangiopericytoma histogenetically related? Histopathology 1995;26(1):57–62.
69. Zhou DB, Zhao JZ, Zhang D, et al. Multicentric infantile myofibromatosis: a rare disorder of the calvarium. Acta Neurochir (Wien) 2009; 151(6):641–5; discussion 645–6.
70. Miwa T, Oi S, Nonaka Y, et al. Rapid spontaneous regression of multicentric infantile myofibromatosis in the posterior fossa and lumbar vertebra. Childs Nerv Syst 2011;27(3):491–6.
71. Fukasawa Y, Ishikura H, Takada A, et al. Massive apoptosis in infantile myofibromatosis. A putative mechanism of tumor regression. Am J Pathol 1994;144(3):480–5.
72. Pelluard-Nehmé F, Coatleven F, Carles D, et al. Multicentric infantile myofibromatosis: two perinatal cases. Eur J Pediatr 2007;166(10): 997–1001.
73. Hatzidaki E, Korakaki E, Voloudaki A, et al. Infantile myofibromatosis with visceral involvement and complete spontaneous regression. J Dermatol 2001;28(7):379–82.
74. Brasseur B, Chantrain CF, Godefroid N, et al. Development of renal and iliac aneurysms in a child with generalized infantile myofibromatosis. Pediatr Nephrol 2010;25(5):983–6.
75. Azzam R, Abboud M, Muwakkit S, et al. First-line therapy of generalized infantile myofibromatosis with low-dose vinblastine and methotrexate. Pediatr Blood Cancer 2009;52(2):308.
76. Bracko M, Cindro L, Golouh R. Familial occurrence of infantile myofibromatosis. Cancer 1992;69(5):1294–9.
77. Narchi H. Four half-siblings with infantile myofibromatosis: a case for autosomal-recessive inheritance. Clin Genet 2001;59(2):134–5.
78. Smith A, Orchard D. Infantile myofibromatosis: Two families supporting autosomal dominant inheritance. Australas J Dermatol 2011;52(3): 214–7.
79. Puzenat E, Marioli S, Algros MP, et al. [Familial infantile myofibromatosis]. Ann Dermatol Venereol 2009;136(4):346–9.
80. Zand DJ, Huff D, Everman D, et al. Autosomal dominant inheritance of infantile myofibromatosis. Am J Med Genet A 2004;126A(3):261–6.
81. Stenman G, Nadal N, Persson S, et al. del(6)(q12q15) as the sole cytogenetic anomaly in a case of solitary infantile myofibromatosis. Oncol Rep 1999;6(5):1101–4.
82. Sirvent N, Perrin C, Lacour JP, et al. Monosomy 9q and trisomy 16q in a case of congenital solitary infantile myofibromatosis. Virchows Arch 2004;445(5):537–40.
83. Alaggio R, Barisani D, Ninfo V, et al. Morphologic overlap between infantile myofibromatosis and infantile fibrosarcoma: a pitfall in diagnosis. Pediatr Dev Pathol 2008;11(5):355–62.
84. Murray J. On three peculiar cases of molluscum fibrosum in children in which one or more of the following conditions were observed: hypertrophy of the gums, enlargement of the ends of the fingers and toes, numerous connective-tissue tumours on the scalp, &c. Med Chir Trans 1873;56:235–54.1.
85. Whitfield A, Robinson AH. A further report on the remarkable series of cases of molluscum fibrosum in children communicated to the society by Dr. John Murray in 1873. Med Chir Trans 1903;86:293–302.
86. Puretic S, Puretic B, Fiser-Herman M, et al. A unique form of mesenchymal dysplasia. Br J Dermatol 1962;74:8–19.
87. Kitano Y. Juvenile hyalin fibromatosis. Arch Dermatol 1976;112(1): 86–8.
88. Nofal A, Sanad M, Assaf M, et al. Juvenile hyaline fibromatosis and infantile systemic hyalinosis: a unifying term and a proposed grading system. J Am Acad Dermatol 2009;61(4):695–700.
89. Denadai R, Bertola DR, Raposo-Amaral CE. Systemic hyalinosis: new terminology, severity grading system, and surgical approach. J Pediatr 2012;161(1):173.
90. Denadai R, Bertola DR, Stelini RF, et al. Additional thoughts about juvenile hyaline fibromatosis and infantile systemic hyalinosis. Adv Anat Pathol 2012;19(3):191–2; author reply 192.

91. Lindvall LE, Kormeili T, Chen E, et al. Infantile systemic hyalinosis: case report and review of the literature. J Am Acad Dermatol 2008;58(2): 303–7.
92. Finlay AY, Ferguson SD, Holt PJ. Juvenile hyaline fibromatosis. Br J Dermatol 1983;108(5):609–16.
93. Woyke S, Domagala W, Markiewicz C. A 19-year follow-up of multiple juvenile hyaline fibromatosis. J Pediatr Surg 1984;19(3):302–4.
94. El-Maaytah M, Jerjes W, Shah P, et al. Gingival hyperplasia associated with juvenile hyaline fibromatosis: a case report and review of the literature. J Oral Maxillofac Surg 2010;68(10):2604–8.
95. Kan AE, Rogers M. Juvenile hyaline fibromatosis: an expanded clinicopathologic spectrum. Pediatr Dermatol 1989;6(2):68–75.
96. Bedford CD, Sills JA, Sommelet-Olive D, et al. Juvenile hyaline fibromatosis: a report of two severe cases. J Pediatr 1991;119(3):404–10.
97. Al-Mubarak L, Al-Makadma A, Al-Khenaizan S. Infantile systemic hyalinosis presenting as intractable infantile diarrhea. Eur J Pediatr 2009;168(3):363–5.
98. Urbina F, Sazunic I, Murray G. Infantile systemic hyalinosis or juvenile hyaline fibromatosis? Pediatr Dermatol 2004;21(2):154–9.
99. Aghighi Y, Bahremand S, Nematollahi LR. Infantile systemic hyalinosis: report of three Iranian children and review of the literature. Clin Rheumatol 2007;26(1):128–30.
100. Shin HT, Paller A, Hoganson G, et al. Infantile systemic hyalinosis. J Am Acad Dermatol 2004;50(Suppl 2):S61–4.
101. Kitano Y, Horiki M, Aoki T, et al. Two cases of juvenile hyalin fibromatosis. Some histological, electron microscopic, and tissue culture observations. Arch Dermatol 1972;106(6):877–83.
102. Ko CJ, Barr RJ. Calcospherules associated with juvenile hyaline fibromatosis. Am J Dermatopathol 2003;25(1):53–6.
103. Haleem A, Al-Hindi HN, Juboury MA, et al. Juvenile hyaline fibromatosis: morphologic, immunohistochemical, and ultrastructural study of three siblings. Am J Dermatopathol 2002;24(3):218–24.
104. Glover MT, Lake BD, Atherton DJ. Clinical, histologic, and ultrastructural findings in two cases of infantile systemic hyalinosis. Pediatr Dermatol 1992;9(3):255–8.
105. Uğraş S, Akpolat N, Metin A. Juvenile hyaline fibromatosis in one Turkish child. Turk J Pediatr 2000;42(3):264–6.
106. Dowling O, Difeo A, Ramirez MC, et al. Mutations in capillary morphogenesis gene-2 result in the allelic disorders juvenile hyaline fibromatosis and infantile systemic hyalinosis. Am J Hum Genet 2003;73(4): 957–66.
107. Hanks S, Adams S, Douglas J, et al. Mutations in the gene encoding capillary morphogenesis protein 2 cause juvenile hyaline fibromatosis and infantile systemic hyalinosis. Am J Hum Genet 2003;73(4): 791–800.
108. Bell SE, Mavila A, Salazar R, et al. Differential gene expression during capillary morphogenesis in 3D collagen matrices: regulated expression of genes involved in basement membrane matrix assembly, cell cycle progression, cellular differentiation and G-protein signaling. J Cell Sci 2001;114(Pt 15):2755–73.
109. Mancini GM, Stojanov L, Willemsen R, et al. Juvenile hyaline fibromatosis: clinical heterogeneity in three patients. Dermatology (Basel) 1999;198(1):18–25.
110. Stucki U, Spycher MA, Eich G, et al. Infantile systemic hyalinosis in siblings: clinical report, biochemical and ultrastructural findings, and review of the literature. Am J Med Genet 2001;100(2):122–9.
111. Al-Mayouf SM, AlMehaidib A, Bahabri S, et al. Infantile systemic hyalinosis: a fatal disorder commonly diagnosed among Arabs. Clin Exp Rheumatol 2005;23(5):717–20.
112. Vanatka R, Rouzier C, Lambert JC, et al. Winchester syndrome: the progression of radiological findings over a 23-year period. Skeletal Radiol 2011;40(3):347–51.
113. Quintal D, Jackson R. Juvenile hyaline fibromatosis. A 15-year follow-up. Arch Dermatol 1985;121(8):1062–3.
114. Karabulut AB, Ozden BC, Onel D, et al. Management of airway obstruction in a severe case of juvenile hyaline fibromatosis. Ann Plast Surg 2005;54(3):328–30.
115. Takagi M, Yamamoto H, Mega H, et al. Heterogeneity in the gingival fibromatoses. Cancer 1991;68(10):2202–12.
116. Hallett KB, Bankier A, Chow CW, et al. Gingival fibromatosis and Klippel-Trénaunay-Weber syndrome. Case report. Oral Surg Oral Med Oral Pathol Oral Radiol Endod 1995;79(5):578–82.
117. Martelli Jr H, Santos SM, Guimarães AL, et al. Idiopathic gingival fibromatosis: description of two cases. Minerva Stomatol 2010;59(3): 143–8.
118. Santosham K, Suresh R, Malathi N. A case report of idiopathic gingival fibromatosis: diagnosis and treatment. J Int Acad Periodontol 2009;11(4): 258–63.
119. Chacon-Camacho OF, Vázquez J, Zenteno JC. Expanding the phenotype of gingival fibromatosis-mental retardation-hypertrichosis (Zimmermann-Laband) syndrome. Am J Med Genet A 2011;155A(7): 1716–20.
120. Stefanova M, Atanassov D, Krastev T, et al. Zimmermann-Laband syndrome associated with a balanced reciprocal translocation t(3;8) (p21.2;q24.3) in mother and daughter: molecular cytogenetic characterization of the breakpoint regions. Am J Med Genet A 2003;117A(3): 289–94.
121. Abo-Dalo B, Kim HG, Roes M, et al. Extensive molecular genetic analysis of the 3p14.3 region in patients with Zimmermann-Laband syndrome. Am J Med Genet A 2007;143A(22):2668–74.
122. Suhanya J, Aggarwal C, Mohideen K, et al. Cherubism combined with epilepsy, mental retardation and gingival fibromatosis (Ramon syndrome): a case report. Head Neck Pathol 2010;4(2):126–31.
123. Holzhausen M, Gonçalves D, Corrêa F de OB, et al. A case of Zimmermann-Laband syndrome with supernumerary teeth. J Periodontol 2003;74(8):1225–30.
124. Kasaboğlu O, Tümer C, Balci S. Hereditary gingival fibromatosis and sensorineural hearing loss in a 42-year-old man with Jones syndrome. Genet Couns 2004;15(2):213–8.
125. Harrison M, Odell EW, Agrawal M, et al. Gingival fibromatosis with prune-belly syndrome. Oral Surg Oral Med Oral Pathol Oral Radiol Endod 1998;86(3):304–7.
126. Radhakrishnan S, Rajan P. Gingival fibromatosis and growth hormone deficiency syndrome–report of a rare case and review of literature. Indian J Dent Res 2003;14(3):170–2.
127. Sakamoto R, Nitta T, Kamikawa Y, et al. Histochemical, immunohistochemical, and ultrastructural studies of gingival fibromatosis: a case report. Med Electron Microsc 2002;35(4):248–54.
128. Yu DS, Lee YB. Images in clinical medicine. Medication-induced gingival hypertrophy. N Engl J Med 2009;360(2):e2.
129. Ciancio SG. Medications' impact on oral health. J Am Dent Assoc 2004;135(10):1440–8; quiz 1468–9.
130. Odessey EA, Cohn AB, Casper F, et al. Hereditary gingival fibromatosis: aggressive 2-stage surgical resection in lieu of traditional therapy. Ann Plast Surg 2006;57(5):557–60.
131. Jang SI, Lee EJ, Hart PS, et al. Germ line gain of function with SOS1 mutation in hereditary gingival fibromatosis. J Biol Chem 2007;282(28): 20245–55.
132. Xiao S, Bu L, Zhu L, et al. A new locus for hereditary gingival fibromatosis (GINGF2) maps to 5q13-q22. Genomics 2001;74(2):180–5.
133. Coventry MB, Harris LE, Bianco Jr AJ, et al. Congenital muscular torticollis (wryneck). Postgrad Med 1960;28:383–92.
134. Kiwak KJ. Establishing an etiology for torticollis. Postgrad Med 1984;75(7):126–34.
135. Parikh SN, Crawford AH, Choudhury S. Magnetic resonance imaging in the evaluation of infantile torticollis. Orthopedics 2004;27(5): 509–15.
136. Lowry KC, Estroff JA, Rahbar R. The presentation and management of fibromatosis colli. Ear Nose Throat J 2010;89(9):E4–8.
137. Vajramani A, Witham FM, Richards RH. Congenital unilateral absence of sternocleidomastoid and trapezius muscles: a case report and literature review. J Pediatr Orthop B 2010;19(5):462–4.
138. Kumar V, Prabhu BV, Chattopadhayay A, et al. Bilateral sternocleidomastoid tumor of infancy. Int J Pediatr Otorhinolaryngol 2003;67(6): 673–5.
139. Blythe WR, Logan TC, Holmes DK, et al. Fibromatosis colli: a common cause of neonatal torticollis. Am Fam Physician 1996;54(6): 1965–7.
140. Kumar B, Pradhan A. Diagnosis of sternomastoid tumor of infancy by fine-needle aspiration cytology. Diagn Cytopathol 2011;39(1):13–7.
141. Canale ST, Griffin DW, Hubbard CN. Congenital muscular torticollis. A long-term follow-up. J Bone Joint Surg Am 1982;64(6):810–6.
142. Minihane KP, Grayhack JJ, Simmons TD, et al. Developmental dysplasia of the hip in infants with congenital muscular torticollis. Am J Orthop 2008;37(9):E155–8; discussion E158.
143. Hosalkar H, Gill IS, Gujar P, et al. Familial torticollis with polydactyly: manifestation in three generations. Am J Orthop 2001;30(8):656–8.
144. Thompson DH, Khan A, Gonzalez C, et al. Juvenile aggressive fibromatosis: report of three cases and review of the literature. Ear Nose Throat J 1991;70(7):462–8.

145. Binder H, Eng GD, Gaiser JF, et al. Congenital muscular torticollis: results of conservative management with long-term follow-up in 85 cases. Arch Phys Med Rehabil 1987;68(4):222–5.
146. Ferkel RD, Westin GW, Dawson EG, et al. Muscular torticollis. A modified surgical approach. J Bone Joint Surg Am 1983;65(7):894–900.
147. Fetsch JF, Miettinen M, Laskin WB, et al. A clinicopathologic study of 45 pediatric soft tissue tumors with an admixture of adipose tissue and fibroblastic elements, and a proposal for classification as lipofibromatosis. Am J Surg Pathol 2000;24(11):1491–500.
148. Rao BN, Horowitz ME, Parham DM, et al. Challenges in the treatment of childhood fibromatosis. Arch Surg 1987;122(11):1296–8.
149. Pontes HA, Pontes FS, E Silva BT, et al. Congenital infantile fibromatosis of the cheek: report of a rare case and differential diagnosis. Int J Oral Maxillofac Surg 2011.
150. Greene AK, Karnes J, Padua HM, et al. Diffuse lipofibromatosis of the lower extremity masquerading as a vascular anomaly. Ann Plast Surg 2009;62(6):703–6.
151. Nuruddin M, Osmani M, Mudhar HS, et al. Orbital lipofibromatosis in a child: a case report. Orbit 2010;29(6):360–2.
152. Walton JR, Green BA, Donaldson MM, et al. Imaging characteristics of lipofibromatosis presenting as a shoulder mass in a 16-month-old girl. Pediatr Radiol 2010;40(Suppl 1):S43–6.
153. Wilkins Jr SA, Waldron CA, Mathews WH, et al. Aggressive fibromatosis of the head and neck. Am J Surg 1975;130(4):412–5.
154. McCarville MB, Hoffer FA, Adelman CS, et al. MRI and biologic behavior of desmoid tumors in children. AJR Am J Roentgenol 2007; 189(3):633–40.
155. Fromowitz FB, Hurst LC, Nathan J, et al. Infantile (desmoid type) fibromatosis with extensive ossification. Am J Surg Pathol 1987;11(1): 66–75.
156. Kenney B, Richkind KE, Friedlaender G, et al. Chromosomal rearrangements in lipofibromatosis. Cancer Genet Cytogenet 2007;179(2): 136–9.
157. Mandahl N, Heim S, Rydholm A, et al. Nonrandom numerical chromosome aberrations (+8, +11, +17, +20) in infantile fibrosarcoma. Cancer Genet Cytogenet 1989;40(1):137–9.
158. Flores-Stadler EM, Chou PM, Barquin N, et al. Fibrous tumors in children—a morphologic and interphase cytogenetic analysis of problematic cases. Int J Oncol 2000;17(3):433–7.
159. Knezevich SR, McFadden DE, Tao W, et al. A novel ETV6-NTRK3 gene fusion in congenital fibrosarcoma. Nat Genet 1998;18(2):184–7.
160. Faulkner LB, Hajdu SI, Kher U, et al. Pediatric desmoid tumor: retrospective analysis of 63 cases. J Clin Oncol 1995;13(11):2813–8.
161. Schmidt D, Klinge P, Leuschner I, et al. Infantile desmoid-type fibromatosis. Morphological features correlate with biological behaviour. J Pathol 1991;164(4):315–9.
162. Ayala AG, Ro JY, Goepfert H, et al. Desmoid fibromatosis: a clinicopathologic study of 25 children. Semin Diagn Pathol 1986;3(2): 138–50.
163. Chugh R, Wathen JK, Patel SR, et al. Efficacy of imatinib in aggressive fibromatosis: results of a phase II multicenter Sarcoma Alliance for Research through Collaboration (SARC) trial. Clin Cancer Res 2010;16(19):4884–91.
164. Coffin CM, Dehner LP. Fibroblastic-myofibroblastic tumors in children and adolescents: a clinicopathologic study of 108 examples in 103 patients. Pediatr Pathol 1991;11(4):569–88.
165. Keasbey LE. Juvenile aponeurotic fibroma (calcifying fibroma); a distinctive tumor arising in the palms and soles of young children. Cancer 1953;6(2):338–46.
166. Sferopoulos NK, Kotakidou R. Calcifying aponeurotic fibroma: a report of three cases. Acta Orthop Belg 2001;67(4):412–6.
167. Allen PW, Enzinger FM. Juvenile aponeurotic fibroma. Cancer 1970;26(4):857–67.
168. Takaku M, Hashimoto I, Nakanishi H, et al. Calcifying aponeurotic fibroma of the elbow: a case report. J Med Invest 2011;58(1-2): 159–62.
169. Arora S, Sabat D, Arora SK, et al. Giant intramuscular calcifying aponeurotic fibroma of gluteus maximus: case report. Ann Trop Paediatr 2010;30(3):259–63.
170. Oruç M, Uysal A, Kankaya Y, et al. A case of calcifying aponeurotic fibroma of the scalp: case report and review of the literature. Dermatol Surg 2007;33(11):1380–3.
171. Murphey MD, Ruble CM, Tyszko SM, et al. From the archives of the AFIP: musculoskeletal fibromatoses: radiologic-pathologic correlation. Radiographics 2009;29(7):2143–73.
172. Kramer JM, Doscher JC, Ruvinsky M, et al. Calcifying aponeurotic fibroma with bone islands exhibiting hematopoiesis: a case report and review of the literature. Oral Surg Oral Med Oral Pathol Oral Radiol Endod 2010;109(6):878–82.
173. Amaravati R. Rare malignant transformation of a calcifying aponeurotic fibroma. J Bone Joint Surg Am 2002;84-A(10):1889; author reply 1889.
174. Lafferty KA, Nelson EL, Demuth RJ, et al. Juvenile aponeurotic fibroma with disseminated fibrosarcoma. J Hand Surg Am 1986;11(5): 737–40.
175. Ozdemir O, Atalay A, Celiker R, et al. Congenital contracture of the quadriceps muscle: confirming the diagnosis with magnetic resonance imaging. Joint Bone Spine 2006;73(5):554–6.
176. Aggarwal A, Singh S, Singh M, et al. Idiopathic bilateral gluteus maximus contracture: a case report and review of literature. Acta Orthop Belg 2005;71(4):493–5.
177. Ngoc HN. Fibrous deltoid muscle in Vietnamese children. J Pediatr Orthop B 2007;16(5):337–44.
178. Midroni G, Moulton R. Radial entrapment neuropathy due to chronic injection-induced triceps fibrosis. Muscle Nerve 2001;24(1):134–7.
179. Matsusue Y, Yamamuro T, Ohta H, et al. Fibrotic contracture of the gastrocnemius muscle. A case report. J Bone Joint Surg Am 1994; 76(5):739–43.
180. Groves RJ, Goldner JL. Contracture of the deltoid muscle in the adult after intramuscular injections. J Bone Joint Surg Am 1974;56(4): 817–20.
181. Lloyd-Roberts GC, Thomas TG. The etiology of quadriceps contracture in children. J Bone Joint Surg Br 1964;46:498–517.
182. Shen YS. Abduction contracture of the hip in children. J Bone Joint Surg Br 1975;57(4):463–5.
183. Chiu SS, Furuya K, Arai T, et al. Congenital contracture of the quadriceps muscle. Four case reports in identical twins. J Bone Joint Surg Am 1974;56(5):1054–8.
184. Smeets E, Fryns JP, Cohen Jr MM. Regional Proteus syndrome and somatic mosaicism. Am J Med Genet 1994;51(1):29–31.
185. Cohen Jr MM, Hayden PW. A newly recognized hamartomatous syndrome. Birth Defects Orig Artic Ser 1979;15(5B):291–6.
186. Wiedemann HR, Burgio GR, Aldenhoff P, et al. The proteus syndrome. Partial gigantism of the hands and/or feet, nevi, hemihypertrophy, subcutaneous tumors, macrocephaly or other skull anomalies and possible accelerated growth and visceral affections. Eur J Pediatr 1983;140(1): 5–12.
187. Tibbles JA, Cohen Jr MM. The Proteus syndrome: the Elephant Man diagnosed. Br Med J (Clin Res Ed) 1986;293(6548):683–5.
188. Biesecker L. The challenges of Proteus syndrome: diagnosis and management. Eur J Hum Genet 2006;14(11):1151–7.
189. Pazzaglia UE, Beluffi G, Bonaspetti G, et al. Bone malformations in Proteus syndrome: an analysis of bone structural changes and their evolution during growth. Pediatr Radiol 2007;37(8):829–35.
190. Lim GY, Kim OH, Kim HW, et al. Pulmonary manifestations in Proteus syndrome: pulmonary varicosities and bullous lung disease. Am J Med Genet A 2011;155A(4):865–9.
191. Juergens P, Beinemann J, Zandbergen M, et al. A computer-assisted diagnostic and treatment concept to increase accuracy and safety in the extracranial correction of cranial vault asymmetries. J Oral Maxillofac Surg 2011.
192. Macedo Jr A, Ottoni SL, Barroso Jr U, et al. Bladder hemangiomas and Proteus syndrome: a rare clinical association. J Pediatr Urol 2010;6(4): 429–31.
193. Nakayama Y, Kusuda S, Nagata N, et al. Excision of a large abdominal wall lipoma improved bowel passage in a Proteus syndrome patient. World J Gastroenterol 2009;15(26):3312–4.
194. Cohen Jr MM. Proteus syndrome: an update. Am J Med Genet C Semin Med Genet 2005;137C(1):38–52.
195. Di Stefani A, Gabellini M, Ferlosio A, et al. Cerebriform plantar hyperplasia: the clinico-pathological hallmark of Proteus syndrome. Acta Derm Venereol 2011;91(5):580–1.
196. Brockmann K, Happle R, Oeffner F, et al. Monozygotic twins discordant for Proteus syndrome. Am J Med Genet A 2008;146A(16):2122–5.
197. Happle R. Lethal genes surviving by mosaicism: a possible explanation for sporadic birth defects involving the skin. J Am Acad Dermatol 1987;16(4):899–906.
198. Lindhurst MJ, Sapp JC, Teer JK, et al. A mosaic activating mutation in AKT1 associated with the Proteus syndrome. N Engl J Med 2011; 365(7):611–9.

199. Eng C, Thiele H, Zhou XP, et al. PTEN mutations and proteus syndrome. Lancet 2001;358(9298):2079–80.
200. Zhou X, Hampel H, Thiele H, et al. Association of germline mutation in the PTEN tumour suppressor gene and Proteus and Proteus-like syndromes. Lancet 2001;358(9277):210–1.
201. Caux F, Plauchu H, Chibon F, et al. Segmental overgrowth, lipomatosis, arteriovenous malformation and epidermal nevus (SOLAMEN) syndrome is related to mosaic PTEN nullizygosity. Eur J Hum Genet 2007;15(7):767–73.
202. Happle R. Type 2 segmental Cowden disease vs. Proteus syndrome. Br J Dermatol 2007;156(5):1089–90.
203. Cantley LC, Neel BG. New insights into tumor suppression: PTEN suppresses tumor formation by restraining the phosphoinositide 3-kinase/AKT pathway. Proc Natl Acad Sci USA 1999;96(8):4240–5.
204. Hoey SE, Eastwood D, Monsell F, et al. Histopathological features of Proteus syndrome. Clin Exp Dermatol 2008;33(3):234–8.
205. Nguyen D, Turner JT, Olsen C, et al. Cutaneous manifestations of Proteus syndrome: correlations with general clinical severity. Arch Dermatol 2004;140(8):947–53.
206. Rosenthal NS, Abdul-Karim FW. Childhood fibrous tumor with psammoma bodies. Clinicopathologic features in two cases. Arch Pathol Lab Med 1988;112(8):798–800.
207. Fetsch JF, Montgomery EA, Meis JM. Calcifying fibrous pseudotumor. Am J Surg Pathol 1993;17(5):502–8.
208. Nascimento AF, Ruiz R, Hornick JL, et al. Calcifying fibrous "pseudotumor": clinicopathologic study of 15 cases and analysis of its relationship to inflammatory myofibroblastic tumor. Int J Surg Pathol 2002;10(3):189–96.
209. Agaimy A, Bihl MP, Tornillo L, et al. Calcifying fibrous tumor of the stomach: clinicopathologic and molecular study of seven cases with literature review and reappraisal of histogenesis. Am J Surg Pathol 2010;34(2):271–8.
210. Lewis CM, Bell DM, Lai SY. Pathology quiz case 2. Calcifying fibrous pseudotumor (CFT) of the oral cavity. Arch Otolaryngol Head Neck Surg 2010;136(8):841, 843–4.
211. Liang HH, Chai CY, Lin YH, et al. Jejunal and multiple mesenteric calcifying fibrous pseudotumor induced jejunojejunal intussusception. J Formos Med Assoc 2007;106(6):485–9.
212. Jang KS, Oh YH, Han HX, et al. Calcifying fibrous pseudotumor of the pleura. Ann Thorac Surg 2004;78(6):e87–8.
213. Jain A, Maheshwari V, Alam K, et al. Calcifying fibrous pseudotumor of peritoneum. J Postgrad Med 2007;53(3):189–90.
214. Hill KA, Gonzalez-Crussi F, Omeroglu A, et al. Calcifying fibrous pseudotumor involving the neck of a five-week-old infant. Presence of factor XIIIa in the lesional cells. Pathol Res Pract 2000;196(7):527–31.
215. Sigel JE, Smith TA, Reith JD, et al. Immunohistochemical analysis of anaplastic lymphoma kinase expression in deep soft tissue calcifying fibrous pseudotumor: evidence of a late sclerosing stage of inflammatory myofibroblastic tumor? Ann Diagn Pathol 2001;5(1):10–4.
216. Kuo TT, Chen TC, Lee LY. Sclerosing angiomatoid nodular transformation of the spleen (SANT): clinicopathological study of 10 cases with or without abdominal disseminated calcifying fibrous tumors, and the presence of a significant number of IgG4+ plasma cells. Pathol Int 2009;59(12):844–50.
217. Aceñero MJ, Vorwald PW, Yamauchi SC. Calcifying fibrous pseudotumor affecting the retroperitoneum: could it be a new entity within the spectrum of IgG-4 sclerosing disease? Virchows Arch 2010;456(6):719–21.
218. Jiménez-Heffernan JA, Urbano J, Tobio R, et al. Calcifying fibrous pseudotumor: a rare entity related to inflammatory pseudotumor. Acta Cytol 2000;44(5):932–4.
219. Van Dorpe J, Ectors N, Geboes K, et al. Is calcifying fibrous pseudotumor a late sclerosing stage of inflammatory myofibroblastic tumor? Am J Surg Pathol 1999;23(3):329–35.
220. Yantiss RK, Nielsen GP, Lauwers GY, et al. Reactive nodular fibrous pseudotumor of the gastrointestinal tract and mesentery: a clinicopathologic study of five cases. Am J Surg Pathol 2003;27(4):532–40.
221. Gauchotte G, Bressenot A, Serradori T, et al. Reactive nodular fibrous pseudotumor: a first report of gastric localization and clinicopathologic review. Gastroenterol Clin Biol 2009;33(12):1076–81.
222. Maeda A, Kawabata K, Kusuzaki K. Rapid recurrence of calcifying fibrous pseudotumor (a case report). Anticancer Res 2002;22(3):1795–7.

Borderline and Malignant Fibroblastic/ Myofibroblastic Tumors

CHAPTER CONTENTS

In prior editions of this textbook, both superficial and deep fibromatoses were grouped together within a comprehensive chapter on fibromatoses. However, because of distinct differences in clinical behavior, the superficial fibromatoses have been included in the chapter describing benign fibroblastic/myofibroblastic proliferations (Chapter 8). Deep fibromatoses are included in this chapter, which focuses on fibroblastic/myofibroblastic tumors of borderline and malignant behaviors. Also included in this chapter are congenital/infantile fibrosarcoma and inflammatory myofibroblastic tumor, which had been discussed in the chapter on fibrous tumors of infancy and childhood in previous editions of this textbook. However, because these entities are variants of fibrosarcoma with borderline clinical features, they are now discussed in this chapter.

DEEP (DESMOID-TYPE) FIBROMATOSES

These lesions (whether they arise from the abdominal wall, mesentery, or other extra-abdominal locations) share overlapping clinical, morphologic, immunohistochemical, and molecular genetic features, although there are attributes that are unique to each. This discussion will focus on those features that are shared by the deep fibromatoses and will elaborate on features that distinguish these entities from one another.

Extra-Abdominal Fibromatosis

Extra-abdominal fibromatosis arises principally from the connective tissue of muscle and the overlying fascia or aponeurosis (*musculoaponeurotic fibromatosis*); it chiefly affects the muscles of the shoulder, pelvic girdle, and thigh of adolescents and young adults. Other terms used to describe this condition include *extra-abdominal desmoid*, *desmoid tumor*, and *aggressive fibromatosis*. Despite its relatively common occurrence, this tumor continues to present a problem in recognition and management, especially because of the striking discrepancy between its deceptively bland microscopic appearance and its propensity to recur locally and infiltrate neighboring soft tissues.

Clinical Findings

Extra-abdominal fibromatosis is most common in patients between puberty and 40 years of age, with a peak incidence between the ages of 25 and 35 years. In the large study by Mankin et al.[1] of 234 patients, the mean age was 36.7 years and 61% were female. Children are uncommonly affected. In the series by Rock et al.,[2] only 5% of the patients were 10 years of age or less, the youngest being 9 months old. Almost all large studies have found a definite female predilection.[1-4] In a study of 89 cases of desmoid tumor by Reitamo et al.,[5] four major age groups were delineated in which the site of the tumor, the gender of the patient, or both were non randomly distributed. *Juvenile* tumors occurred predominantly in an extra-abdominal location, with a distinct predilection for girls younger than 15 years of age. *Fertile* tumors occurred nearly exclusively as abdominal tumors in fertile females. *Menopausal* tumors occurred predominantly in the abdomen, with an approximately equal gender distribution. *Senescent* tumors were equally distributed between abdominal and extra-abdominal locations and showed no gender predilection.

Most patients present with a deeply situated, firm, poorly circumscribed mass that has grown insidiously and causes little or no pain. Decreased mobility of an adjacent joint may occur. Neurologic symptoms, including numbness, tingling, a stabbing or shooting pain, or motor weakness, may occur when the lesion compresses nearby nerves.

Radiographically, the lesion appears as a soft tissue mass that interrupts the adjacent intermuscular and soft tissue planes; it may encroach on adjacent bone, resulting in pressure erosion or superficial cortical defects. Up to 80% of affected patients have multiple minor bony anomalies of the mandible, chest, and long bones, including cortical thickening, exostoses, and areas of cystic translucence or compact islands in the femur (or both).[6] As with other soft tissue tumors, CT and MRI are helpful in the diagnosis and assessment of tumor extent before surgery.[7] Pritchard et al.[4] found a lower local recurrence rate after the introduction of these improved imaging techniques compared to the recurrence rate before their routine use, presumably as a result of better surgical planning.

Anatomic Location

The principal site of extra-abdominal fibromatosis is the musculature of the shoulder, followed by the chest wall and back, thigh, and head and neck.

In the shoulder region, the growth presents most often in the deltoid, scapular region, supraclavicular fossa, or posterior cervical triangle where it may extend into the anterior or posterior portion of the axilla and upper arm. Because of the numerous vital structures at this site, including nerves of the brachial plexus and large vessels, complete surgical excision of tumors in this location is often difficult, if not impossible.

Fibromatoses in the region of the pelvic girdle primarily affect the gluteus muscle, whereas those in the region of the thigh affect the quadriceps muscle and muscles of the popliteal fossa.

The head and neck is not an unusual location for these lesions. As many as 23% of all extra-abdominal fibromatoses occur in this location.[8-11] In children, more than one-third of extra-abdominal fibromatoses are located in the head and neck.[12] The soft tissue of the neck is most commonly involved, followed by the face, oral cavity, scalp, paranasal sinuses, and orbit.[13] Clinically, fibromatoses arising in this location are often more aggressive than extra-abdominal fibromatoses arising elsewhere and are capable of massive destruction of adjacent bone and erosion of the base of the skull; they occasionally encroach on the trachea, sometimes with a fatal outcome.[13]

Fibromatosis of the breast may arise in the mammary gland or from extension of a lesion arising in the aponeurosis of the chest wall or shoulder girdle.[14,15] Occasional fibromatoses of the breast have been associated with breast implants. The differential diagnosis in this location includes metaplastic carcinoma, malignant phyllodes tumor, and benign reactive processes such as nodular fasciitis and keloid.

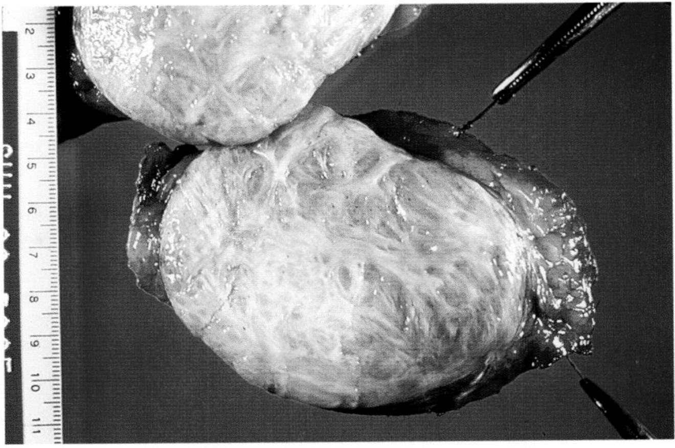

FIGURE 10-1. Extra-abdominal fibromatosis (desmoid tumor) involving the chest wall. The cut surface reveals a trabecular appearance reminiscent of that seen in uterine leiomyomas.

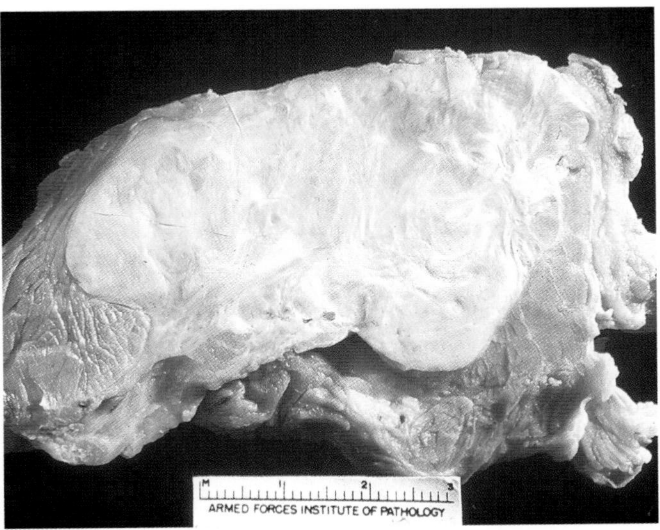

FIGURE 10-2. Extra-abdominal fibromatosis (desmoid tumor) involving the pectoralis muscle.

Multicentric Fibromatoses

Extra-abdominal fibromatoses may be multicentric.[16,17] Fong et al.[18] found almost 5% of these lesions to be multicentric, typically involving one anatomic region of the body. In most cases, the second growth develops proximal to the primary lesion. Rarely, coexistence of abdominal and extra-abdominal fibromatoses has been observed in the same patient.[19]

Pathologic Findings

Grossly, the tumor is almost always confined to the musculature and the overlying aponeurosis or fascia. Large tumors may extend along the fascial plane or infiltrate the overlying subcutaneous tissue. Occasional lesions involve the periosteum and may lead to bone erosion, thereby closely resembling desmoplastic fibroma of bone. Most tumors measure 5 to 10 cm in greatest dimension, although lesions as large as 20 cm have been reported. The tumor is firm, cuts with a gritty sensation, and on a cross-section reveals a glistening white, coarsely trabeculated surface resembling scar tissue (Figs. 10-1 and 10-2) and, as such, surgeons may have difficulty distinguishing recurrent fibromatosis from scar tissue related to a prior excision.

Histologically, the lesion is poorly circumscribed and infiltrates the surrounding tissue, usually skeletal muscle (Fig. 10-3). The proliferation consists of elongated, slender, spindle-shaped cells of uniform appearance surrounded and separated from one another by collagen, with little or no cell-to-cell contact (Fig. 10-4). The cells lack nuclear hyperchromasia, but the cellularity varies from area to area. The nuclei are small, pale-staining, and sharply defined, with one to three minute nucleoli (Figs. 10-5, 10-6, and 10-7). Clearly defined cellular boundaries can be discerned in cases with a prominent myxoid matrix and relatively small amounts of collagen (Fig. 10-8).[20]

Cells and collagen fibers are usually arranged in sweeping bundles that are less well defined than those of fibrosarcoma. Glassy keloid-like collagen fibers or extensive hyalinization may be present and may obscure the basic pattern of the lesion (Fig. 10-9). At the periphery of the growth where the tumor has infiltrated muscle tissue, remnants of striated muscle fibers are frequently entrapped and undergo atrophy or form multinucleated giant cells that may be mistaken for malignancy (Fig. 10-10). Microhemorrhages and focal aggregates of lymphocytes are common. In rare instances, there is calcification or chondroid or osseous metaplasia, but this is never a prominent feature of the tumor.

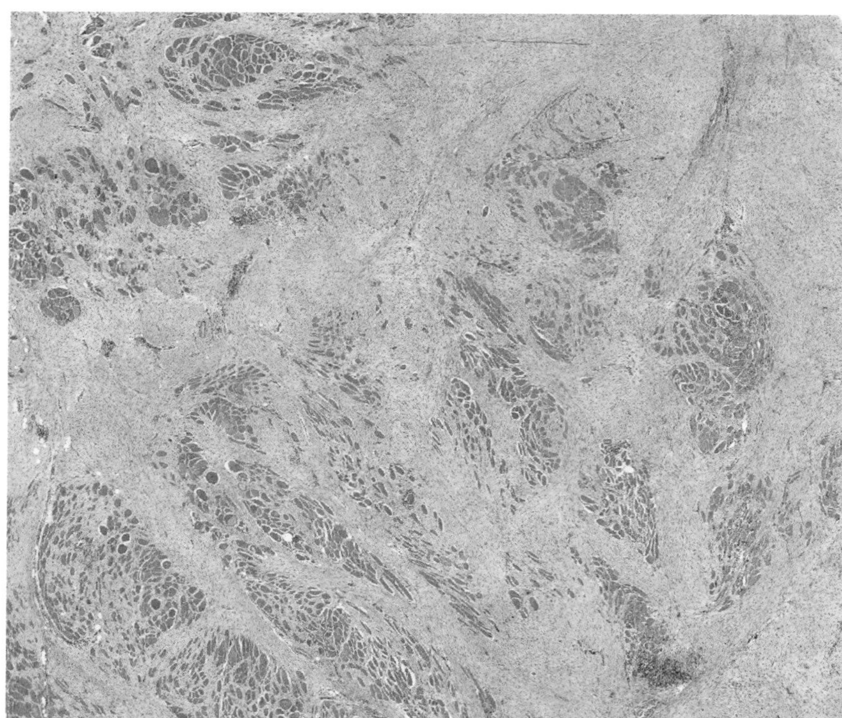

FIGURE 10-3. Extra-abdominal fibromatosis (extra-abdominal desmoid) invading striated muscle tissue.

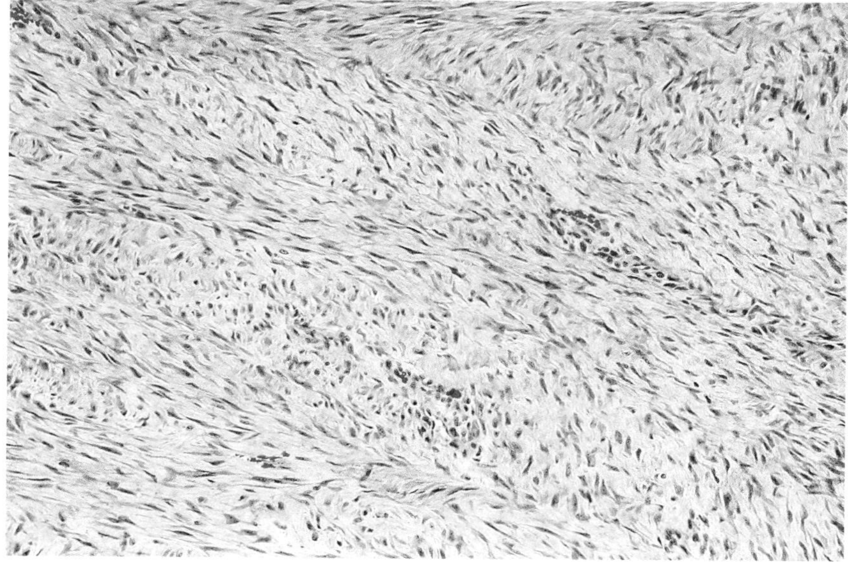

FIGURE 10-4. Interlacing bundles of fibroblasts separated by variable amounts of collagen in extra-abdominal fibromatosis.

Differential Diagnosis

Fibromatosis most closely resembles fibrosarcoma on the one extreme and reactive processes on the other. *Fibrosarcoma* is more uniformly cellular, and the cells are arranged in a more consistent sweeping fascicular (herringbone) growth pattern. Unlike fibromatosis, the cells are often overlapping and separated by less collagen. The nuclei are more hyperchromatic and atypical and have more prominent nucleoli than those found in fibromatosis. Although it is important to remember that there can be considerable overlap in levels of mitotic activity between fibromatosis and fibrosarcoma, high mitotic counts (>1 per 10 high-power fields [HPF]) throughout a tumor should arouse suspicion of fibrosarcoma. A small biopsy specimen may lead to a misdiagnosis because some examples of fibrosarcoma have areas that are indistinguishable from fibromatosis, and vice versa.

Fibromatosis can also be difficult to distinguish from *reactive fibroblastic/myofibroblastic proliferations* following injuries such as trauma, minor muscle tear, or intramuscular injection. Cytologically, these reactive proliferations are composed of

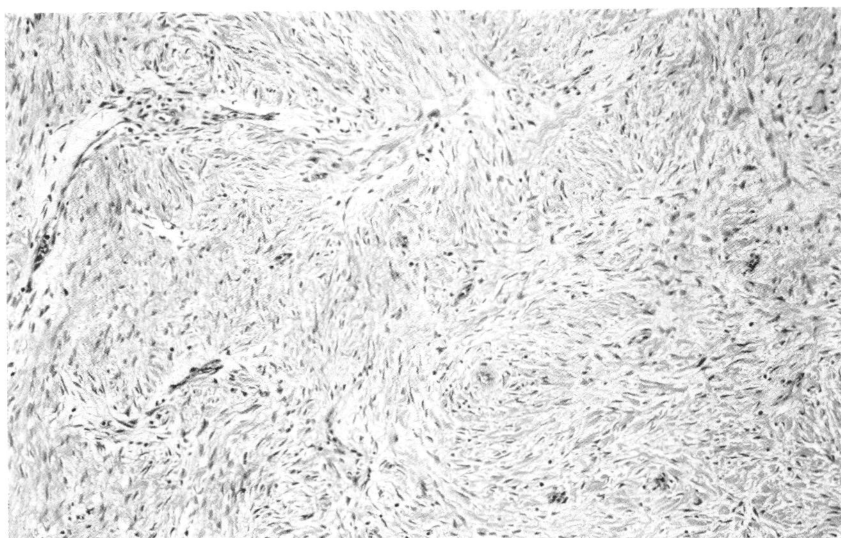

FIGURE 10-5. Extra-abdominal fibromatosis in which the cells are arranged in a focal storiform growth pattern.

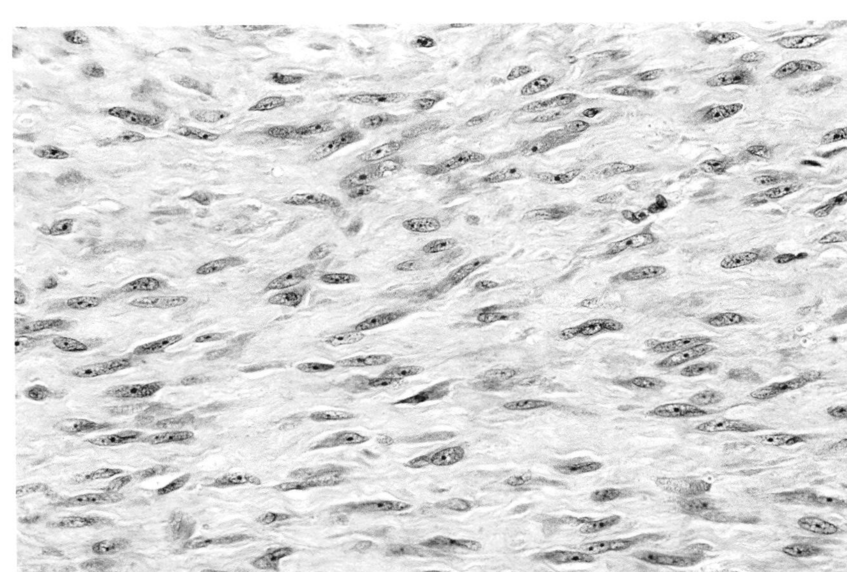

FIGURE 10-6. High-power view of extra-abdominal fibromatosis showing vesicular nuclei with minute nucleoli, rather indistinct cytoplasm, and interstitial collagen.

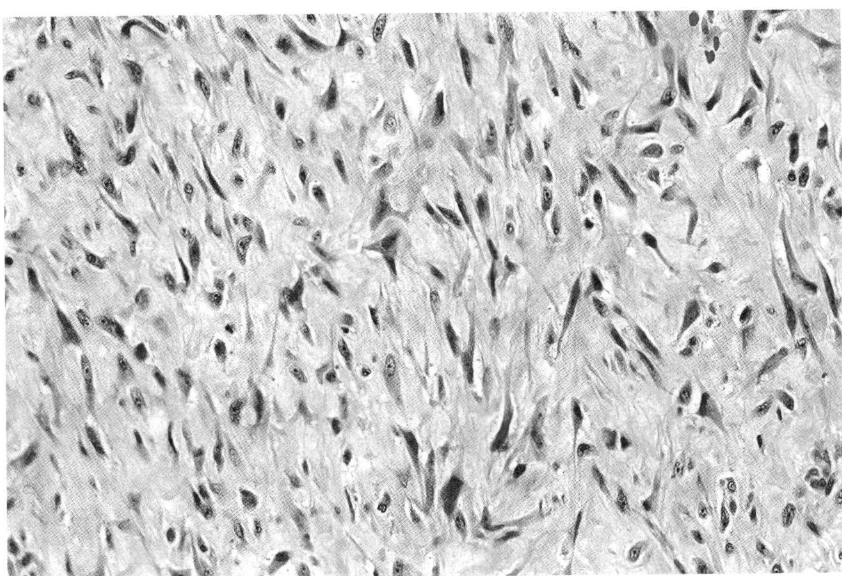

FIGURE 10-7. Stellate-shaped cells with uniform cytologic features in extra-abdominal fibromatosis.

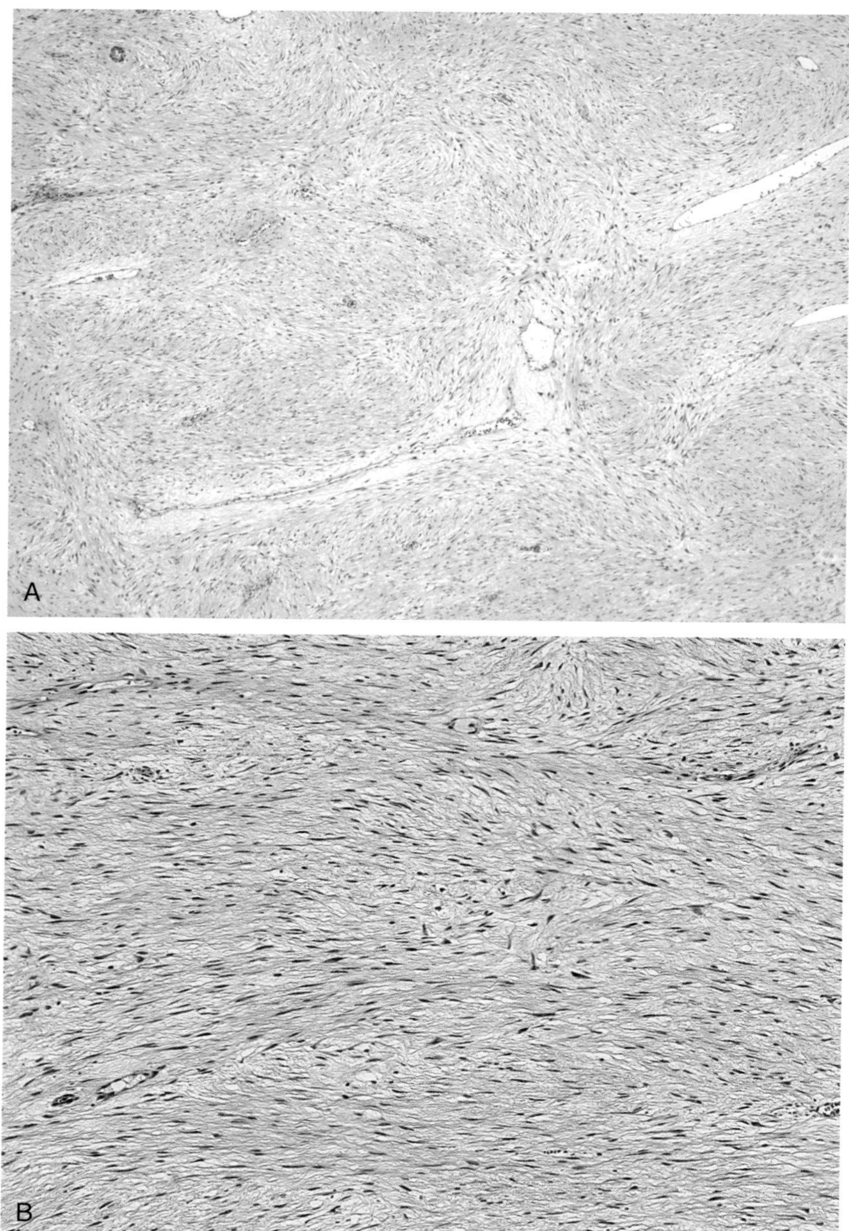

FIGURE 10-8. (A) Extra-abdominal fibromatosis with a partially myxoid matrix. Regularly distributed blood vessels are conspicuous. (B) High-magnification view of extra-abdominal fibromatosis with bland-appearing spindled cells arranged into short intersecting fascicles.

cells indistinguishable from those found in fibromatosis. The low-magnification appearance is more useful for distinguishing these two entities because reactive processes have a more variable growth pattern and frequently have focal hemorrhage or hemosiderin deposition, often situated along vascular structures. In some cases, iron stains are useful for highlighting hemosiderin that is difficult to identify on hematoxylin and eosin-stained sections. In addition, an infiltrative growth pattern is much more characteristic of fibromatosis.

Desmoplastic fibroma of bone is histologically indistinguishable from fibromatosis, especially when it presents as a soft tissue mass after breaking through the thinned or expanded cortex of the involved bone. This lesion predominates in the metaphyseal or diaphyseal portions of long bones (e.g., the femur) or in the jaw, and radiographic studies are essential for distinguishing between these lesions.

Confusion with *myxoma* is possible, particularly if only a small biopsy is available for examination. Myxoma is usually paucicellular, with the cells separated from one another by abundant myxoid matrix. In contrast, fibromatosis always displays a greater degree of cellularity and more interstitial collagen than myxoma.

Fibrosarcomatous transformation of fibromatosis is exceedingly rare. Soule and Scanlon[21] described and illustrated a case of typical fibromatosis of the inguinal region that evolved into a fibrosarcoma 10 years after initial excision and 9 years after radiotherapy. Mooney et al.[22] reported a case of metastasizing fibrosarcoma of the thigh that appeared 28 years after excision of a fibromatosis from the same region. However, following a review of the slides from this reported case, Allen[23] thought that the cells from the initial excision had too much nuclear hyperchromasia and atypia for fibromatosis and believed the

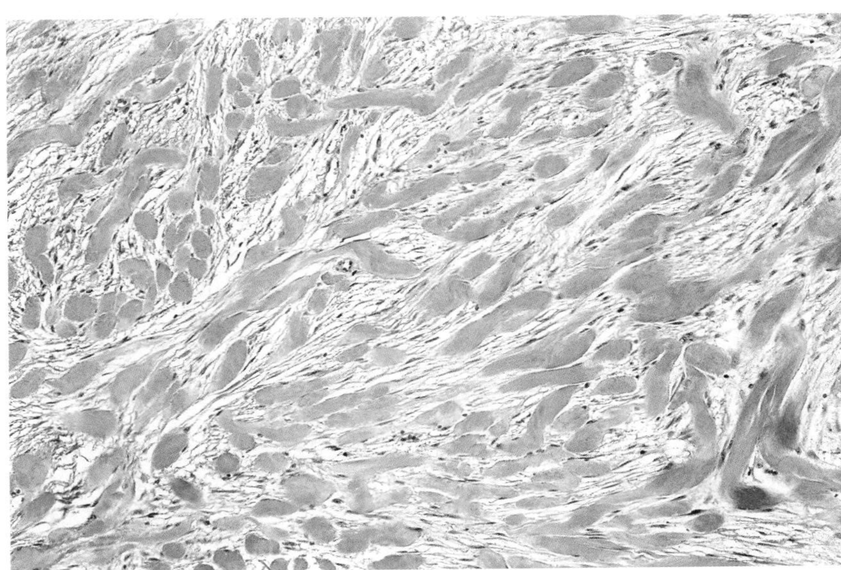

FIGURE 10-9. Fibromatosis with glassy hyalinized collagen fibers reminiscent of keloid, a rare feature of this tumor.

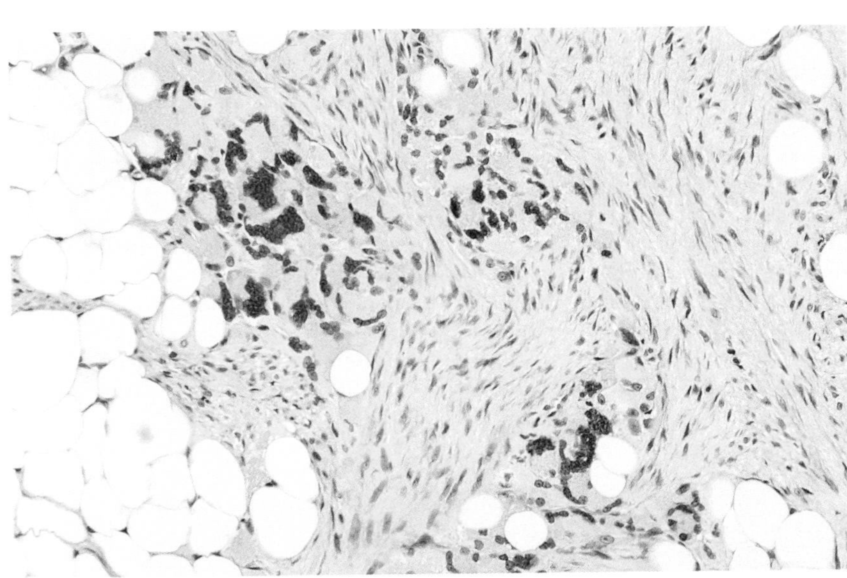

FIGURE 10-10. Peripheral portion of extra-abdominal fibromatosis with entrapped muscle giant cells.

lesion was a low-grade fibrosarcoma at the time of initial excision. He went on to state that, "In my experience, all cases of metastasizing 'desmoid tumors' have proved to differ histologically from aggressive fibromatosis when the sections have been reviewed." Malignant transformation of fibromatosis may be erroneously suggested by occasional foci of increased cellularity and by exceptionally well-differentiated fibromatosis-like areas in some fibrosarcomas. A convincing case of fibrosarcomatous transformation of a fibromatosis has not been reviewed.

Discussion

Like other forms of fibromatosis, the etiology of extra-abdominal fibromatosis is almost certainly multifactorial because genetic, endocrine, and physical factors seem to play an important role in its pathogenesis. Features suggesting an underlying genetic basis are the occasional occurrence in siblings,[24,25] the presence of multiple bony abnormalities (in up to 80% of patients),[5] and the occurrence of extra-abdominal fibromatosis in patients with familial adenomatous polyposis (FAP)[26,27] (described later in greater detail), as mutations of the adenomatous polyposis coli (APC)/β-catenin pathway are identified in the majority of sporadic and FAP-associated deep fibromatoses.[28-30]

Although clearly implicated in the development of abdominal fibromatosis (discussed in the following section), endocrine factors may also play a role in the development and growth of extra-abdominal fibromatoses. Physical factors such as trauma or irradiation likely serve as a trigger mechanism because examples of extra-abdominal fibromatosis have been reported in the chest wall following trauma and reconstructive mammoplasty.[31,32] Large studies of extra-abdominal fibromatosis have reported an antecedent history of trauma in 16% to 28% of cases.[4,33]

Abdominal Fibromatosis

Although abdominal fibromatosis is indistinguishable grossly and microscopically from extra-abdominal fibromatosis, it deserves separate consideration because of its characteristic location and its tendency to occur in women of childbearing age during or following pregnancy. The tumor arises from musculoaponeurotic structures of the abdominal wall, especially the rectus and internal oblique muscles and their fascial coverings.

Clinical Findings

Abdominal fibromatosis occurs in young, gravid, or parous women during gestation or, more frequently, during the first year following childbirth. Rare examples have been reported in children of both genders (especially boys) and adult men. The relative frequency of abdominal and extra-abdominal desmoid tumors varies from one study to another. In a study carried out in Finland by Reitamo et al.,[5] abdominal fibromatoses (49%) outnumbered extra-abdominal (43%) and mesenteric (8%) fibromatoses. Most lesions are solitary, but patients with both abdominal and extra-abdominal fibromatoses have been described.[34]

Pathologic Findings

The gross and microscopic appearances are virtually identical to those described for extra-abdominal fibromatosis, except that the average tumor is smaller and behaves less destructively than those in extra-abdominal locations. Most tumors measure 3 to 10 cm in greatest dimension, and, when arising in the rectus muscle or its fascia, they usually remain at the site of origin and do not cross the abdominal midline.

Microscopically, these lesions are variably cellular and often predominantly hypocellular; they are composed of cells with normochromatic nuclei with small, pinpoint nucleoli (Figs. 10-11 and 10-12). The cells lack nuclear pleomorphism, and only rare mitotic figures can be identified. Cells are arranged into ill-defined fascicles with dense collagen separating the individual tumor cells with infiltration of the surrounding muscle tissue. Immunohistochemical features are also similar to those of other deep fibromatoses (described later in the chapter).

Discussion

Like extra-abdominal fibromatosis, genetic, endocrine, and physical factors seem to play an important role in the development of these tumors. Some arise in the setting of FAP, often at the site of previous abdominal surgery.[35-37] Endocrine factors are clearly implicated by the frequent occurrence of this tumor during or after pregnancy, and there are reports of these tumors regressing with menopause.[38] The reported inhibitory effect of antiestrogenic agents, such as tamoxifen and raloxifene, supports the role of hormonal factors in the development of this disease.[39,40]

Similar to extra-abdominal lesions, trauma may serve as a contributory cause because some tumors have been reported to arise in the scars of radical nephrectomy sites, the site of insertion of peritoneal dialysis catheters, and other abdominal operations (*cicatricial fibromatosis*).[41,42] Because most patients with abdominal fibromatosis have no history of gross injury to this region, minor and undetected trauma, such as minute muscle tears, may conceivably serve as a contributing etiologic factor that triggers the fibrous growth in a hormonally or genetically predisposed individual.

Intra-Abdominal Fibromatosis

The intra-abdominal fibromatoses are a group of closely related lesions (rather than a single entity) that pose similar problems for the histologic diagnosis but can be distinguished from one another by the clinical setting and location. This

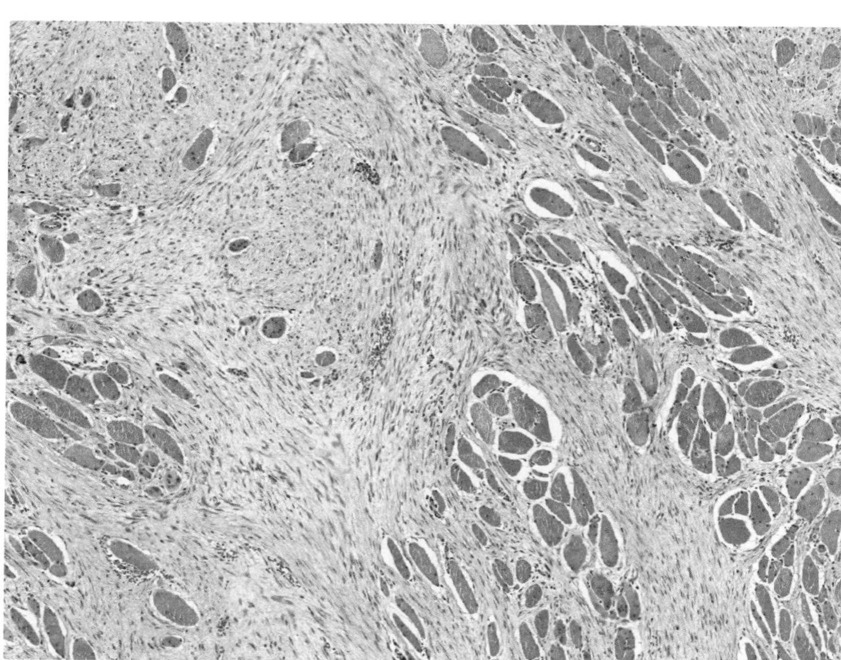

FIGURE 10-11. Fibromatosis of the abdominal wall showing infiltration of skeletal muscle.

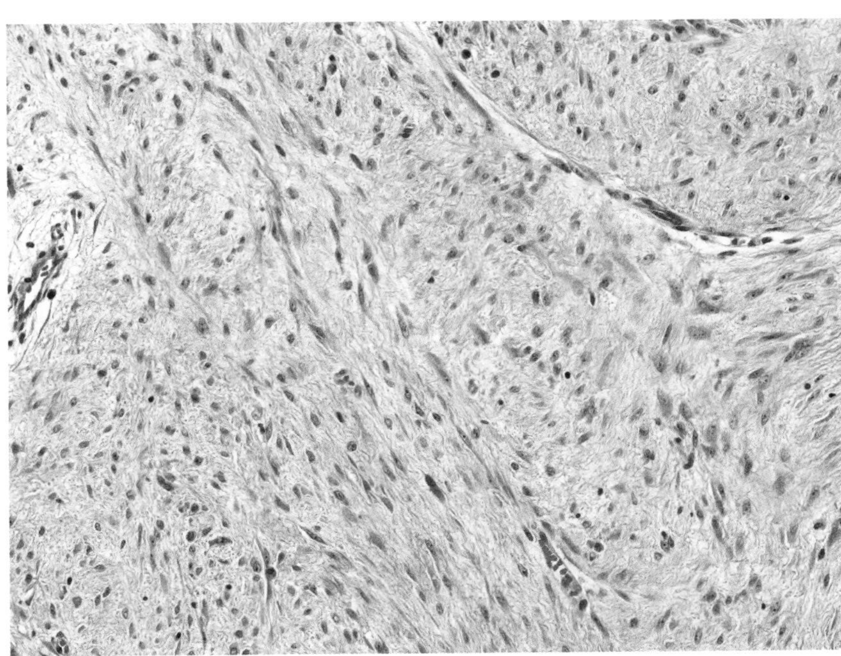

FIGURE 10-12. High-power view of an abdominal wall fibromatosis showing bland cytologic features.

category includes pelvic fibromatoses and mesenteric fibromatoses, including those associated with FAP/Gardner syndrome.

Pelvic Fibromatosis

Pelvic fibromatosis is a variant of intra-abdominal fibromatosis, differing from the latter by its location in the iliac fossa and lower portion of the pelvis, where it manifests as a slowly growing palpable mass that is asymptomatic or causes slight pain only. Clinically, it is often mistaken for an ovarian neoplasm or a mesenteric cyst. Large tumors in this location may encroach on the urinary bladder, vagina, or rectum—or they may cause hydronephrosis or compress the iliac vessels.[43-45] As with fibromatosis of the abdominal wall, the tumor arises from the aponeurosis or muscle tissue and occurs chiefly in young women 20 to 35 years of age; in most cases, it is unrelated to gestation or childbirth. Grossly and microscopically, the tumor is indistinguishable from other forms of extra-abdominal or abdominal fibromatosis and requires similar modes of therapy.

Mesenteric Fibromatosis

Fibromatosis is the most common primary tumor of the mesentery and accounts for approximately 8% of all fibromatoses. Although most cases are sporadic, some are associated with FAP/Gardner syndrome, trauma, or hyperestrogenic states. Most commonly, these tumors are located in the mesentery of the small bowel, but some originate from the ileocolic mesentery, gastrocolic ligament, omentum, or retroperitoneum. In the absence of a history of FAP, distinguishing this lesion from other fibrosing processes that occur in this location, such as idiopathic retroperitoneal fibrosis or sclerosing mesenteritis, may be difficult, especially if the biopsy specimen is limited.

As with pelvic fibromatosis, most patients present with an asymptomatic abdominal mass, although some have mild abdominal pain. Less commonly, patients present with gastrointestinal bleeding or an acute abdomen secondary to bowel perforation.[46] Occasionally, the tumor is found incidentally at laparotomy performed for some other reason, including patients undergoing a bowel resection for FAP.[47] Data on age and gender vary; Burke et al.[48] noted that the tumor was more commonly encountered in males, and the mean age was 41 years.

Like many other neoplasms in the abdomen and retroperitoneum, most mesenteric fibromatoses are quite large at the time of excision, with the majority measuring 10 cm or more. Many have an initial phase of rapid growth, and complications may be caused by compression of the ureter, development of a ureteral fistula, or compression of the small or large intestines, sometimes complicated by intestinal perforation.[47,48]

Pathologic Findings

Grossly, most lesions appear circumscribed, but like other forms of fibromatosis, there is microscopic infiltration into the surrounding soft tissues, including the bowel wall.

Microscopically, the lesions are composed of cytologically bland spindle-shaped or stellate cells evenly deposited in a densely collagenous stroma. Typically, there is variable cellularity, with some areas showing almost complete replacement by dense fibrous tissue. In others, the stroma shows marked myxoid change. Scattered keloid-type collagen fibers may be present, including prominent dilated thin-walled veins and muscular hyperplasia of small arteries. Nodular lymphoid aggregates may be present at the advancing edge of the tumor.

Differential Diagnosis

The differential diagnosis includes *sclerosing mesenteritis*, a lesion also sometimes referred to as *mesenteric panniculitis* and *mesenteric lipodystrophy*.[49] Like mesenteric fibromatosis, sclerosing mesenteritis typically involves the small bowel mesentery and presents as a large solitary mass, although multiple lesions or diffuse mesenteric thickening may also be seen.

Histologically, sclerosing mesenteritis is composed of variable amounts of fibrosis, chronic inflammation, and fat necrosis. Any of these three components may predominate in a given lesion. In difficult cases, immunohistochemical staining for β-catenin can be useful because mesenteric fibromatosis consistently shows strong nuclear β-catenin staining, whereas sclerosing mesenteritis does not express this antigen (Table 10-2).[50] We, however, have found this immunostain to be difficult to interpret.

Inflammatory myofibroblastic tumor (also known as *inflammatory fibrosarcoma*) of the mesentery and retroperitoneum is also a diagnostic consideration, but this lesion is more cellular, has more pronounced cytologic atypia, and is more inflamed than mesenteric fibromatosis. Moreover, many, but not all, cases of inflammatory myofibroblastic tumor/inflammatory fibrosarcoma stain for anaplastic lymphoma kinase (ALK)-1 protein, which is not found in mesenteric fibromatosis.

Also included in the differential diagnosis is *idiopathic retroperitoneal fibrosis*, also known as *Ormond's disease*. This is a rare fibroinflammatory process characterized by diffuse or localized fibroblastic proliferation and a chronic lymphoplasmacytic infiltrate in the retroperitoneum causing compression or obstruction of the ureters, aorta, or other vascular structures. It is more common in men, and most patients present in the fifth or sixth decade of life.[51] Most patients present with vague, nonspecific abdominal symptoms, but some have weight loss, nausea and vomiting, anorexia, or fever.[52] Although most cases are idiopathic, some are clearly drug-related (methysergide, pergolide),[53] and others are related to malignancy.[54]

Grossly, the mass is dense, white, and plaque-like, usually arising at or just below the aortic bifurcation. With progression, it surrounds the aorta and inferior vena cava and spreads through the retroperitoneum in a perivascular distribution. Histologically, there are broad anastomosing bands of hyalinized collagen associated with a fibroblastic proliferation and lymphoplasmacytic infiltrate with occasional germinal centers. The aorta, which is surrounded by the proliferation, usually shows severe atherosclerosis, with protrusion of atherosclerotic debris through the media into the adventitia with intramural chronic inflammation.[55] Recent studies have shown a large number of IgG4 immunoreactive cells within the infiltrate, suggesting that it is part of a larger group of IgG4-related sclerosing diseases.[56,57] Immunosuppressive agents have been found to be effective in the treatment of this rare condition.[58]

Over the past several years, there have been several studies that have focused on distinguishing mesenteric fibromatosis from mesenteric *gastrointestinal stromal tumors* (GIST).[59-62] Distinguishing between these lesions is of clinical significance because of their vastly different therapeutic and prognostic implications. In a study of 25 cases of mesenteric fibromatosis, Rodriguez et al.[59] found that GIST was by far the most common misdiagnosis, occurring in 52% of the cases. Histologically, mesenteric fibromatosis is composed of a monotonous proliferation of cytologically bland spindle-shaped cells that are arranged into broad, sweeping fascicles and deposited in a finely collagenous stroma. Mitotic activity is typically low, and there is no evidence of necrosis. Keloidal-like collagen, an infiltrative growth pattern, and prominent muscular arteries and dilated, thin-walled veins are also characteristic features. The histologic features of GIST are heterogeneous and can range from bland spindle-cell tumors to highly cellular and overtly malignant epithelioid tumors (see Table 10-1). The confusion between these entities is compounded by and, in large part, may have arisen as a result of reports of KIT (CD117) expression in mesenteric fibromatosis. For example, in the study by Yantiss et al.,[60] CD117 was expressed in 88% of the GIST but was also found in 75% of fibromatoses. Similarly, 6 of 10 mesenteric fibromatoses reported by Montgomery et al.[63] expressed CD117. In both of these studies, CD34 was common in GIST but was not detected in mesenteric fibromatoses. Generally, mesenteric fibromatoses are consistently negative for CD117, and reports to the contrary may be a result of technical issues or antibody quality. Nuclear β-catenin staining characteristic of mesenteric fibromatosis (but absent in GIST) is also a useful finding.[63] Finally, DOG1 is a consistently positive marker in GIST, including those arising in the mesentery, whereas mesenteric fibromatoses do not stain for this antigen.[64] Regardless of the immunophenotypic findings, mesenteric fibromatosis is sufficiently distinct from GIST on a morphologic basis so that immunohistochemistry does not necessarily have to be performed for diagnostic purposes, in most cases (see Table 10-2).

TABLE 10-1 Features Useful in Distinguishing Between Mesenteric Fibromatosis and Gastrointestinal Stromal Tumor

FEATURE	MESENTERIC FIBROMATOSIS	GIST
Cell shape	Wavy, spindled	Spindled and/or epithelioid
Atypia	None	Variable
Growth pattern	Uniform, fascicular	Organoid, fascicles (variable)
Cellularity	Low to moderate	Moderate to high
Blood vessels	Regular, dilated, and thin-walled	Hyalinized
Keloidal collagen	Frequent	Absent
Skeinoid fibers	Absent	May be present
Necrosis	Absent	May be present
Margins	Infiltrative	Often pushing
CD117	–	+
DOG1	–	+
CD34	–	+
β-catenin	+ (nuclear)	–

Modified from Rodriguez JA, Guarda LA, Rosai J. Mesenteric fibromatosis with involvement of the gastrointestinal tract. Am J Clin Pathol 2004;121:93.

GIST, gastrointestinal stromal tumor.

TABLE 10-2 Immunophenotypic Features of Mesenteric Fibromatosis Compared to Gastrointestinal Stromal Tumor and Sclerosing Mesenteritis

	GIST	SCLEROSING MESENTERITIS	MESENTERIC FIBROMATOSIS
CD117	+	–	–
DOG1	+	–	–
β-catenin	–	–	+
CD34	+	–	–
SMA	±	+	±
Desmin	–	–	Rare
S-100 protein	–	–	–

GIST, gastrointestinal stromal tumor.

Mesenteric Fibromatosis in FAP/Gardner Syndrome

In 1951, Gardner[65] reported the familial occurrence of intestinal polyposis, osteomas, fibromas, and epidermal or sebaceous cysts; the term *Gardner syndrome* was coined by Smith[66] in 1958. This syndrome is inherited as an autosomal dominant trait that occurs in approximately half of the children of afflicted parents. It is more common in women than in men and is usually diagnosed in adults of 25 to 35 years of age. Essentially, this syndrome is simply FAP with extra-abdominal tumors. Approximately 10% to 15% of patients with FAP/Gardner syndrome develop intra-abdominal fibromatoses, an estimated 800-fold increased risk of developing such lesions.[27,35,67]

Mesenteric or retroperitoneal fibromatosis usually has its onset 1 to 2 years after excision of the diseased portion of the intestinal tract, and these lesions are the most common cause of death in polyposis patients after colectomy is performed.[68] In the study by Gurbuz et al.,[67] almost 70% of FAP patients who developed these lesions had abdominal surgery before the discovery of the fibromatosis. Compared to sporadic lesions, FAP-associated mesenteric fibromatoses arise in slightly younger patients (36 versus 42 years, according to a large study in the Netherlands).[27,67] In a meta-analysis of 10 published studies, Sinha et al.[69] found that a positive family history of a desmoid tumor was the only factor predictive of development of this lesion in patients with FAP/Gardner syndrome. Durno et al.[70] found that early colectomy, especially in female patients, significantly increased the risk of developing mesenteric fibromatosis.

Clinically, the fibromatosis may be asymptomatic or may cause mild abdominal pain or intestinal obstruction as a result of infiltrative growth into the wall of the small or large bowel. Histologically, the fibromatosis is virtually indistinguishable from those at other sites, and one cannot distinguish polyposis-related cases from sporadic cases by morphology alone. These tumors tend to have a prominent myxoid matrix (Figs. 10-13 to 10-16), and the cells may be arranged in a vague storiform pattern, in addition to sweeping fascicles.

Mesenteric fibromatoses with or without associated FAP/Gardner syndrome frequently recur, an observation that is not surprising given the central location and difficulty of complete surgical extirpation. There is significant morbidity associated with attempted resection, including ischemia, fistula formation, obstruction, and additional small bowel resections, which can result as short bowel syndrome and necessitate small bowel transplantation.[35]

Discussion

As previously mentioned, Gardner syndrome is a genetically determined, autosomal dominant disease caused by a germline abnormality of the *APC* gene on the long arm of chromosome 5.[71,72] Tumors arising in the setting of FAP/Gardner syndrome harbor inactivating mutations of the *APC* gene.[25] Up to 85% of sporadic lesions harbor mutations in the gene that codes for β-catenin (*CTNNB1*).[30] In fact, molecular assays for *CTNNB1* mutations using paraffin-embedded tissue may be extremely useful in difficult-to-diagnose lesions, particularly distinguishing recurrent/residual fibromatosis from scar tissue.[73] Mutations of this gene have not been detected in the spindle cell lesions likely to enter the diagnosis. These mutations result in the intranuclear accumulation of β-catenin protein, which can also be used as a diagnostic adjunct, as mentioned later.

Other cytogenetic alterations that have been found in both FAP/Gardner syndrome and sporadic fibromatoses include trisomies of chromosomes 8 and 20[74-78] and loss of the Y chromosome.[79]

Immunohistochemical Findings in Deep Fibromatoses

The immunohistochemical features of all subtypes of deep fibromatoses are similar and will be discussed as a group. The spindle cells show variable staining for smooth muscle actin and muscle-specific actin, consistent with fibroblastic/myofibroblastic differentiation, as confirmed by ultrastructural findings.[80] Virtually all deep fibromatoses show strong nuclear accumulation of β-catenin, although this stain clearly lacks specificity (Fig. 10-17).[50,81-84] In the study by Amary et al.,[81] all deep fibromatoses stained for this antigen, although 72% of the lesions that can mimic fibromatosis also stained,

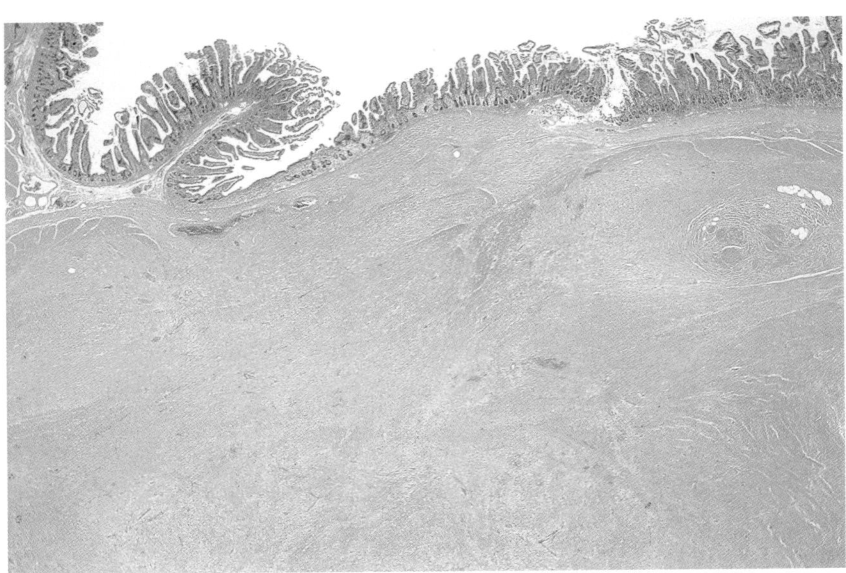

FIGURE 10-13. Low-power view of mesenteric fibromatosis in Gardner syndrome showing uniform fibrocollagenous growth infiltrating the wall of the small bowel.

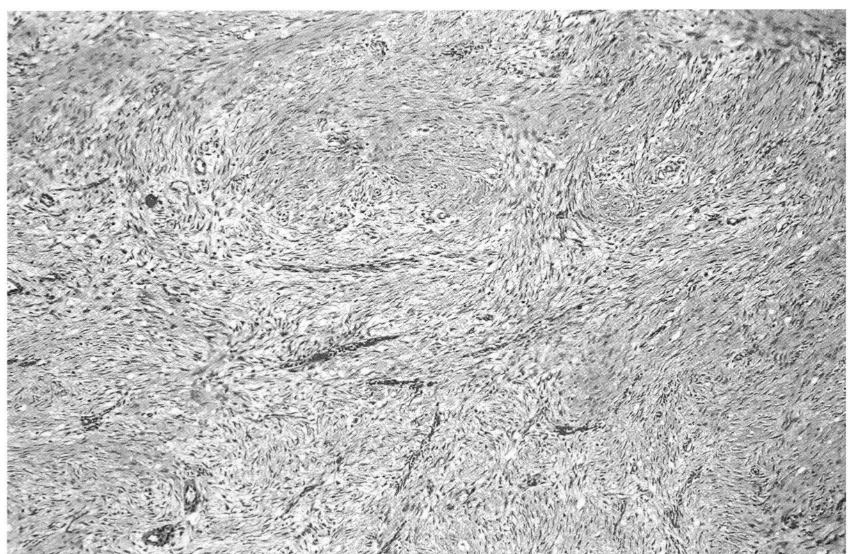

FIGURE 10-14. Orderly arrangement of uniform fibroblasts associated with moderate amounts of collagen and mucoid material in mesenteric fibromatosis.

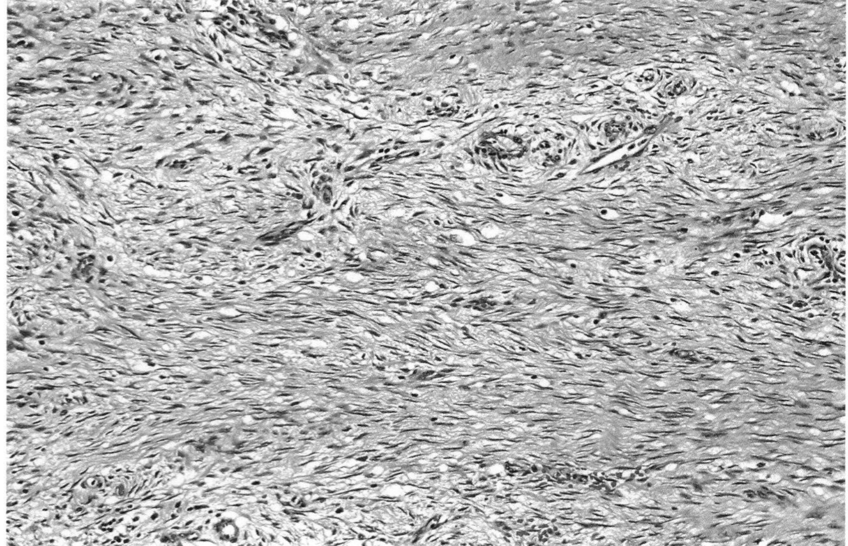

FIGURE 10-15. Uniform spindled proliferation in mesenteric fibromatosis.

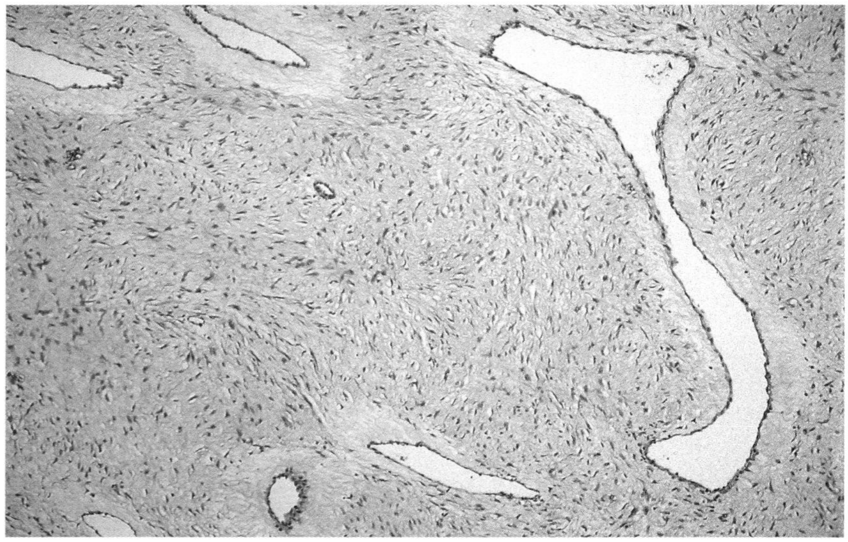

FIGURE 10-16. Prominent dilated blood vessels with perivascular hyalinization, a common feature of intra-abdominal fibromatosis.

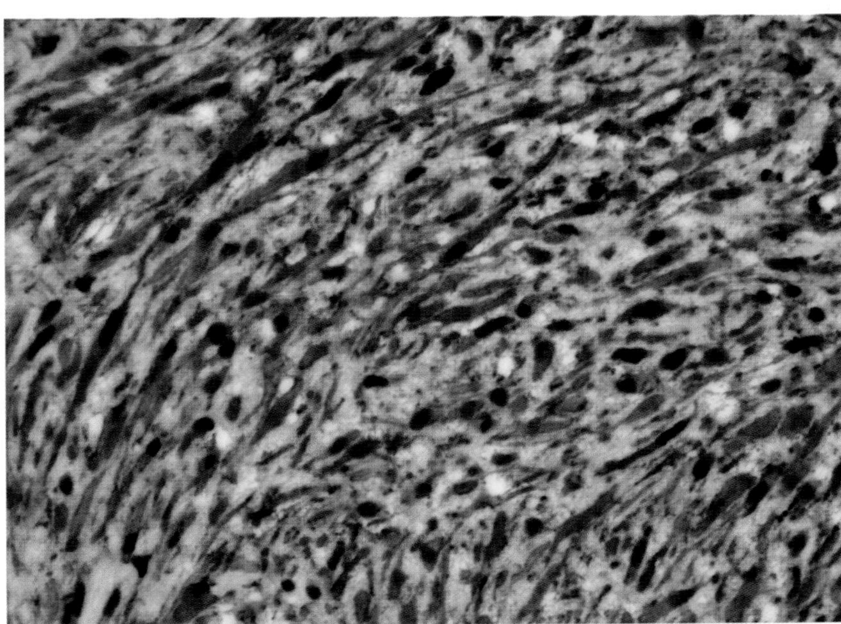

FIGURE 10-17. Nuclear beta-catenin immunoreactivity in an extra-abdominal fibromatosis.

indicating a complete lack of specificity. This stain is difficult to interpret because of background/nonspecific staining.

Clinical Behavior of Deep Fibromatoses

As a group, deep fibromatoses share the common feature of frequent local recurrence, although there are some differences between subtypes. Despite its bland microscopic appearance, extra-abdominal fibromatoses frequently behave in an aggressive manner. Although incapable of metastasizing, there is a high rate of local recurrence, although the frequency varies significantly in the literature. In the study from the Armed Forces Institute of Pathology, also known as AFIP, by Enzinger and Shiraki[20] with a minimum of 10 years of follow-up, 57% of these tumors recurred. In another large series of extra-abdominal desmoid tumors, Rock et al.[2] found that 68% of patients experienced a recurrence on an average of 1.4 years after the initial treatment. In a more recent study of 203 consecutive patients with extra-abdominal fibromatoses and treated with surgery over a 35-year period at a single referral center, Gronchi et al.[85] reported a local recurrence rate of 76% at 10 years. Although tumor size was associated with risk of local recurrence, microscopically positive surgical margins did not predict recurrence risk, as one might anticipate. However, other studies have found the extent and adequacy of initial excision to be prognostically significant.[4,44,86,87]

Spontaneous regression of these tumors has been observed in sporadic cases, particularly in menarchal and menopausal patients. McDougall and McGarrity[19] reported two cases of extra-abdominal fibromatoses that spontaneously regressed after menopause. Enzinger and Shiraki[20] reported a 36-year-old man with an extensive tumor involving the supraclavicular fossa, scalenus muscles, and brachial plexus that apparently resolved 9.5 years after the initial presentation. A second patient, an elderly man with a large recurrent tumor of the axilla and chest wall, declined further treatment; 15 years later, the tumor had substantially decreased in size and was no longer palpable.

Like their extra-abdominal counterparts, abdominal lesions also have a propensity to recur locally, although the rate of local recurrence (15% to 30%) is slightly lower than that of extra-abdominal lesions (35% to 65%).[88,89] In most cases, the lesions recur within the first 2 years after the initial excision or in connection with subsequent gestations or deliveries. Multiple recurrences are not uncommon.

Intra-abdominal lesions, not unexpectedly, also have a propensity for local recurrence, although data on the recurrence rates differ greatly. In the study by Burke et al.,[48] 23% of all tumors recurred, although there was a striking difference in recurrence rates between patients with (90%) and without (12%) FAP/Gardner syndrome. In fact, none of the patients with sporadic mesenteric fibromatosis had more than one recurrence, and none of those patients died as a direct result of their tumor. In contrast, most of the patients with FAP/Gardner syndrome had more than one recurrence, and four patients died of their tumor. Similar findings of aggressive behavior of mesenteric fibromatosis in this setting have been reported by others.[90]

Treatment of Deep Fibromatoses

A number of different modalities have been attempted in the treatment of deep fibromatoses, including surgery, chemotherapy, radiation therapy, and even observation. The optimum treatment for any given patient depends upon a number of tumor and patient-related factors, including tumor size, tumor site, the patient's medical status, and comorbidities, among others. Observation is an acceptable mode of therapy for asymptomatic tumors.[91] However, for symptomatic tumors, treatment of some kind is indicated, particularly if vital structures are at risk. Surgical excision with negative microscopic margins is one of the mainstays of therapy, but local recurrences do occur following what appears to be complete surgical excision. Incomplete excisions are associated with an even higher rate of recurrence. The goal of surgery is complete removal while preserving function and minimizing morbidity.

In situations where a wide local excision cannot be performed, postoperative radiation therapy is often used. Gluck et al.[92] found equivalent local control for patients treated with surgery, radiation, or both.

As one might expect, imatinib mesylate (Gleevec) therapy has been attempted in the salvage setting in patients with deep fibromatoses.[93-95] Similarly, sorafenib, a closely related tyrosine kinase inhibitor, has also been assessed as a mode of therapy.[96] Both drugs have shown some activity, with evidence of tumor shrinkage, in some cases.

Cytotoxic and noncytotoxic drug therapy has also been attempted for the treatment of these tumors. Chemotherapeutic agents and nonsteroidal antiinflammatory prostaglandin-inhibiting drugs, such as sulindac and indomethacin, have been reported to cause stabilization or regression of both primary and recurrent tumors.[97,98] The efficacy of antiestrogenic therapy, including tamoxifen, progesterone, or the luteinizing hormone-releasing hormone analogue goserelin acetate, is not fully established but appears to be promising.[99,100]

CONGENITAL/INFANTILE FIBROSARCOMA

Fibrosarcoma in newborns, infants, and small children bears some resemblance to adult fibrosarcoma but is considered a separate entity because of its markedly different clinical behavior as well as its distinctive molecular alterations. On one hand, it must be distinguished from richly cellular forms of infantile fibromatosis, a lesion that lacks metastatic capability; on the other hand, it must be separated from more aggressive childhood sarcomas (e.g., embryonal rhabdomyosarcoma), which are prone to metastasize and require more radical therapy. Fibrosarcomas in older children behave similarly to those seen in adults.

Congenital/infantile fibrosarcoma is relatively rare. The first detailed clinicopathologic study of this entity was reported by Stout[101] in 1962. He reviewed 31 cases from the literature and added 23 new cases of juvenile fibrosarcoma, 11 of which developed during the first 5 years of life and 4 of which were present at birth. He suggested that fibrosarcomas arising in this group of patients were more indolent than their adult counterparts. Although several subsequent smaller series of congenital/infantile fibrosarcoma were reported, it was not until Chung and Enzinger's[102] series of 53 cases (reported in 1976) that conclusive evidence supported this tumor as a distinct entity. Similar conclusions were reached by Soule and Pritchard[103] in their report of 110 cases, including 70 previously published cases and 40 new cases from the files of the Mayo Clinic.

Clinical Findings

The principal manifestation of the disease is a nontender, painless swelling or mass that ranges from 1 to 20 cm. Up to one-third of the tumors are present at birth; in most cases, the mass becomes evident during the first year of life. In the

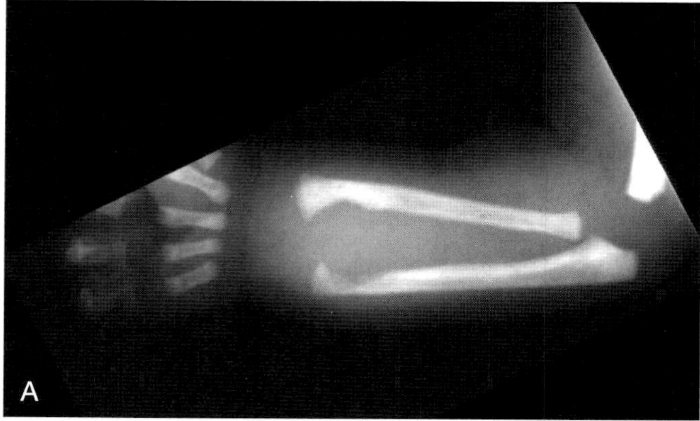

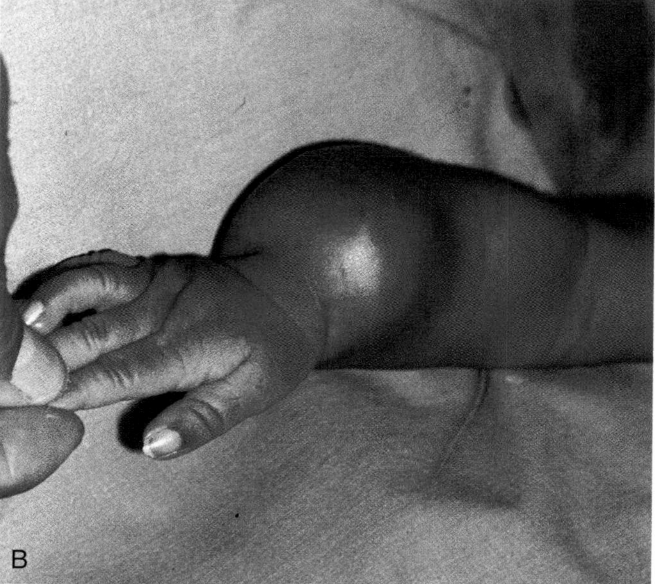

FIGURE 10-18. Radiograph (A) and gross photomicrograph (B) of a congenital fibrosarcoma in a 1-day-old infant.

series by Chung and Enzinger,[102] 20 of 53 (38%) tumors were present at birth, and 27 (51%) were noted before 3 months of life. Similarly, 40 of 110 (36%) cases reported by Soule and Pritchard[103] were congenital. Males are affected slightly more commonly than females. The principal sites of involvement are the extremities, especially the regions of the foot, ankle, and lower leg and the hand, wrist, and forearm. The next most common sites of involvement are the trunk and head and neck regions, although these tumors have also been reported in locations such as the retroperitoneum,[104] colon,[105] and heart.[106]

Radiographic examination may show, in addition to a soft tissue mass, cortical thickening, bending deformities, and rarely extensive destruction of the underlying bone (Fig. 10-18).[102] Both the MRI and ultrasound are useful in the evaluation of these tumors, including the detection of congenital tumors in utero.[107,108]

Pathologic Findings

The tumors vary considerably in size. Some are only a few centimeters when first detected, whereas others are extremely

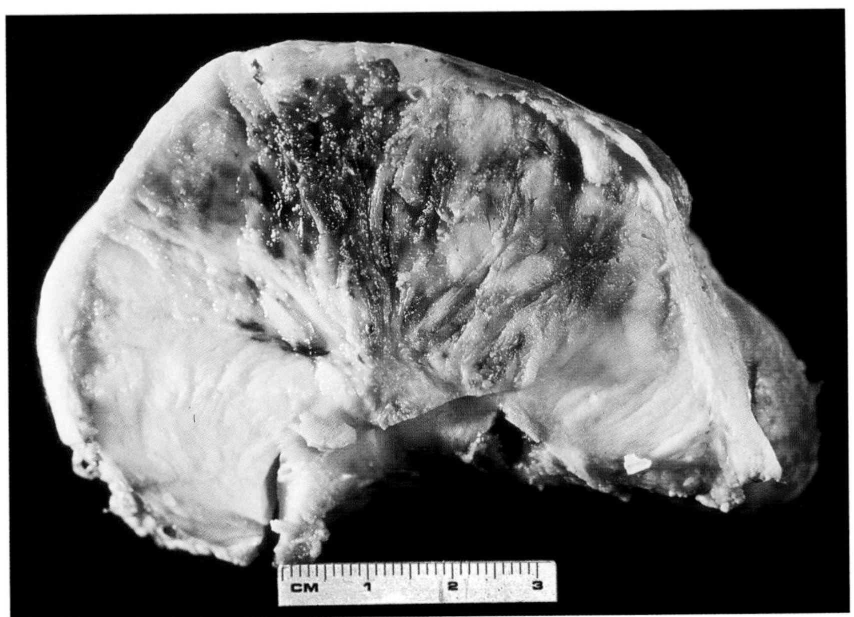

FIGURE 10-19. Infantile fibrosarcoma of the right shoulder in a 1-month-old boy, showing marked interstitial hemorrhage.

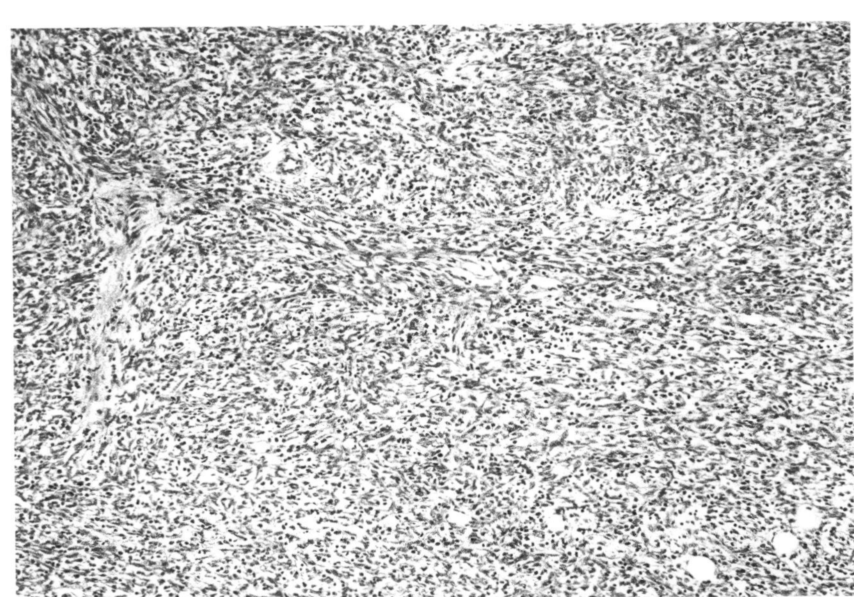

FIGURE 10-20. Infantile fibrosarcoma composed of uniform, well-oriented fibroblasts arranged in a fascicular growth pattern.

large and may replace the entire distal portion of the involved limb. Some patients present with a large exophytic mass that ulcerates the overlying skin. Most are poorly circumscribed, fusiform or disk-shaped, and have a gray-white or pale pink cut surface. Large tumors may be markedly distorted by central necrosis or hemorrhage (Fig. 10-19), whereas others show extensive myxoid or cystic change.

Histologically, most examples closely resemble their adult counterparts and are composed of sheets of solidly packed, spindle-shaped cells that are relatively uniform in appearance and arranged in bundles or fascicles, imparting a herringbone appearance. The cells show little nuclear pleomorphism and are mitotically active, but their numbers vary from area to area in the same tumor. Tumors with abundant collagen tend to be more fasciculated and often approach the appearance of an adult fibrosarcoma (sometimes referred to as the *desmoplastic* type). Tumors with minimal amounts of collagen, on the other hand, show a lesser degree of cellular polarity and consist of small, more rounded, immature-appearing cells with only focal evidence of fibroblastic differentiation (medullary type) (Figs. 10-20 to 10-22).[109] Bizarre cells and multinucleated giant cells are rare. Scattered chronic inflammatory cells, particularly lymphocytes, are another common, sometimes striking feature that distinguishes infantile from adult fibrosarcoma. A hemangiopericytoma-like vascular pattern may be prominent (Fig. 10-23).

Immunohistochemical Findings

Immunohistochemically, the spindle cells of congenital/infantile fibrosarcoma stain variably for muscle markers, including

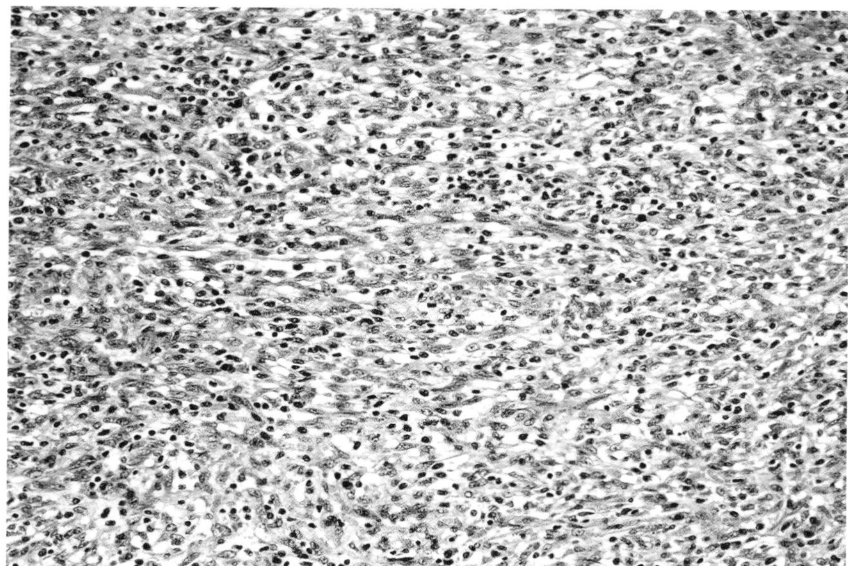

FIGURE 10-21. Characteristic microscopic view of an infantile fibrosarcoma with immature-appearing fibroblasts associated with small round cells, probably lymphocytes.

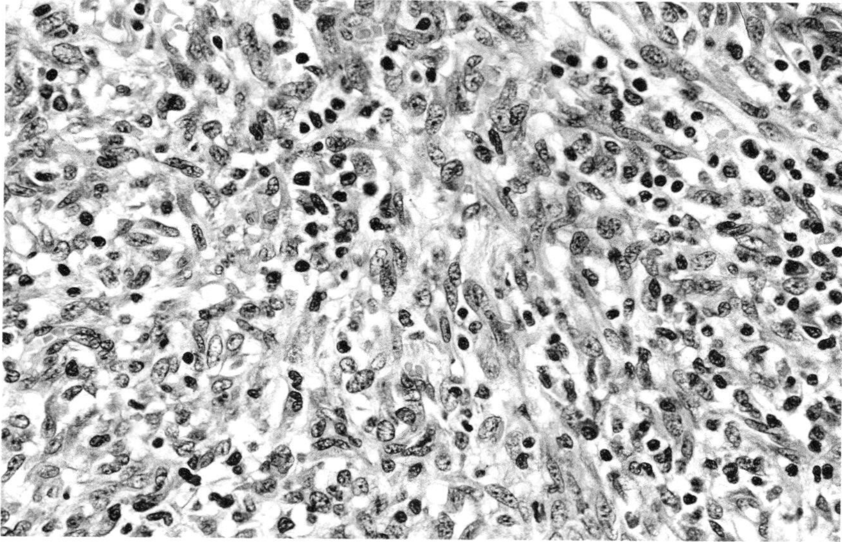

FIGURE 10-22. High-power view of immature-appearing fibroblasts with a prominent lymphocytic infiltrate, characteristic of infantile fibrosarcoma.

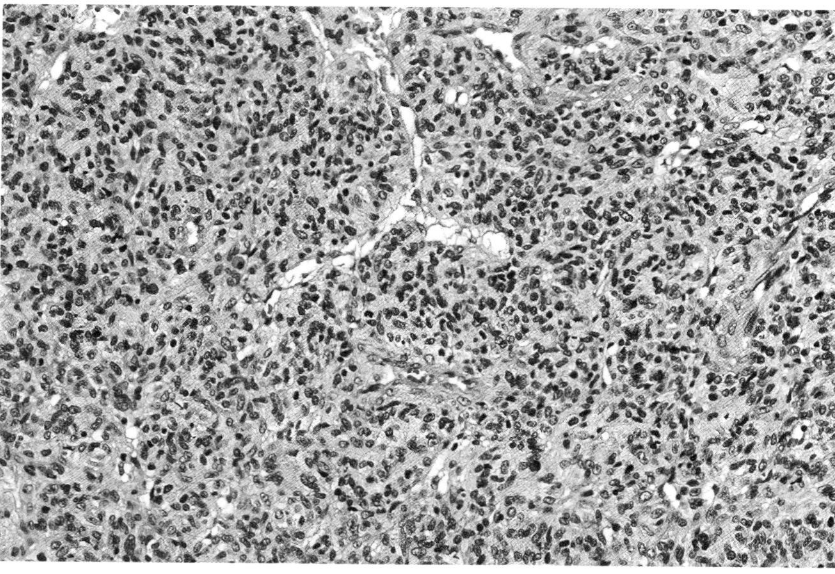

FIGURE 10-23. Infantile fibrosarcoma composed of immature-appearing fibroblasts arranged around a prominent hemangiopericytoma-like vascular pattern.

muscle-specific actin, smooth muscle actin, and h-caldesmon.[110,111] The more primitive-appearing ovoid cells tend not to express these muscle markers.

Cytogenic and Molecular Genetic Findings

Numerous studies have noted a nonrandom gain of chromosomes 11, 20, 17, and 8 (in descending order of frequency).[112-114] Using fluorescence in-situ hybridization (FISH), Schofield et al.[113] found gains of these chromosomes (in various combinations) in 11 of 12 infantile fibrosarcomas in patients less than 2 years of age. In contrast, alterations of these chromosomes were not found in four fibrosarcomas in patients of 6 to 17 years of age. Interestingly, one of three cases of cellular fibromatosis also showed the above cytogenetic abnormalities, suggesting that "these two entities constitute a spectrum and that their distinction may not be clear-cut."[113]

Most congenital/infantile fibrosarcomas and cellular mesoblastic nephromas have the same diagnostic chromosomal translocation: t(12;15)(p13;q25).[115,116] This translocation results in a fusion of the *ETV6* gene on chromosome 12 with the neurotrophin-3 receptor *NTRK3* (also known as *TRKC*) gene on chromosome 15. Although this translocation is difficult to detect by conventional cytogenetics, it can be readily demonstrated by reverse transcription polymerase chain reaction (RT-PCR) or FISH.[117-119] Given the similar histologic and cytogenetic findings in congenital/infantile fibrosarcoma and cellular mesoblastic nephroma, it has been suggested that these two lesions are histogenetically related entities arising in soft tissue and renal locations, respectively.[116,118] Interestingly, secretory breast carcinoma and rare subtypes of acute myeloid leukemia also harbor this same translocation.[120,121]

Differential Diagnosis

The microscopic picture may be confused with that of other mesenchymal neoplasms, but, in most cases, the uniformity of the spindle-shaped tumor cells, the solid growth pattern, the fascicular arrangement, and the lack of any other form of cellular differentiation permit a reliable diagnosis.

Spindle cell rhabdomyosarcoma is a subtype of embryonal rhabdomyosarcoma that may be difficult to distinguish from congenital/infantile fibrosarcoma. This tumor is most often encountered in the paratesticular region and the head and neck, but it may also be present at other sites, including the extremities. Histologically, it is composed of uniform spindled cells often with eosinophilic fibrillar cytoplasm and elongated hyperchromatic nuclei separated by abundant, partly hyalinized collagen. Immunohistochemically, this tumor characteristically expresses desmin and myogenin, which are absent in congenital/infantile fibrosarcoma.

In 1993, Lundgren et al.[122] described three cases of *infantile rhabdomyofibrosarcoma*, each of which was initially diagnosed as congenital/infantile fibrosarcoma. This tumor, which was observed in children from 3 months to 3 years of age, has features that overlap spindle cell rhabdomyosarcoma and desmoplastic portions of congenital/infantile fibrosarcoma. Immunohistochemically, the cells express smooth muscle actin and desmin; Mentzel et al.[123] found focal MyoD1 staining as well. By ultrastructure, the cells have the features of rhabdomyoblasts, fibroblasts, and myofibroblasts. Two of the three cases reported by Lundgren et al.[122] showed monosomy of chromosome 19 and 22, among other abnormalities; a case reported by Miki et al.[124] showed der(2) t(2;11)(q37;q13). Two of the patients developed metastases and died within 2 years of the primary operation; the third patient was alive with a local recurrence. The exact nature of this tumor is still not clear. It may represent an intermediate form between a congenital/infantile fibrosarcoma and a spindle cell rhabdomyosarcoma.[125] The authors also raised the possibility that some tumors reported as congenital/infantile fibrosarcoma that have metastasized and followed a fatal course may actually be examples of this very rare entity.

Congenital/infantile fibrosarcoma with a marked degree of vascularity may be difficult to distinguish from *infantile hemangiopericytoma*. The latter is marked by a distinct lobulated arrangement and more regularly distributed dilated vascular channels that form a branching, or staghorn, pattern. In some cases, a clear distinction is difficult and mandates an examination of multiple sections from different portions of the tumor. Some authors have reported tumors with overlapping histologic features and have proposed that these two entities represent a histologic continuum.[126]

Perhaps the most difficult lesion to distinguish from congenital/infantile fibrosarcoma is the cellular form of *infantile fibromatosis* (Table 10-3). Some authors have reported cases in which the primary tumor had the appearance and growth pattern of infantile fibromatosis, whereas the recurrent tumor showed more cellularity and was virtually indistinguishable from fibrosarcoma,[102] On the other hand, tumors with a fibrosarcoma-like appearance in the primary neoplasm and a fibromatosis-like appearance in the recurrence have also been observed. Detection of the t(12;15) by cytogenetic or molecular techniques allows for distinction between these lesions.

TABLE 10-3 Summary of Features Distinguishing Infantile Fibromatosis and Infantile Fibrosarcoma

FEATURE	INFANTILE FIBROMATOSIS	CONGENITAL/INFANTILE FIBROSARCOMA
Cellularity	Variable	Moderate to high
Herringbone pattern	Absent	Usually present
Mitotic figures	Rare	Few to many
Hemorrhage	Absent	Often present
Necrosis	Absent	Often present
t(12;15)(p13;q25)	Absent	Present

Discussion

Compared with adult-type fibrosarcoma, the clinical course of congenital/infantile fibrosarcoma is a favorable one. Of the 48 patients with follow-up in the study by Chung and Enzinger,[102] only 8 (17%) developed one or more local recurrences from 6 weeks to 10 years after the initial excision. Only 4 of the 48 (8%) patients died of metastatic disease, and 1 patient was living 6.5 years after a lobectomy for a metastatic tumor. The 5-year survival rate in this series was 84%. The recurrent and nonrecurrent groups showed no demonstrable differences in

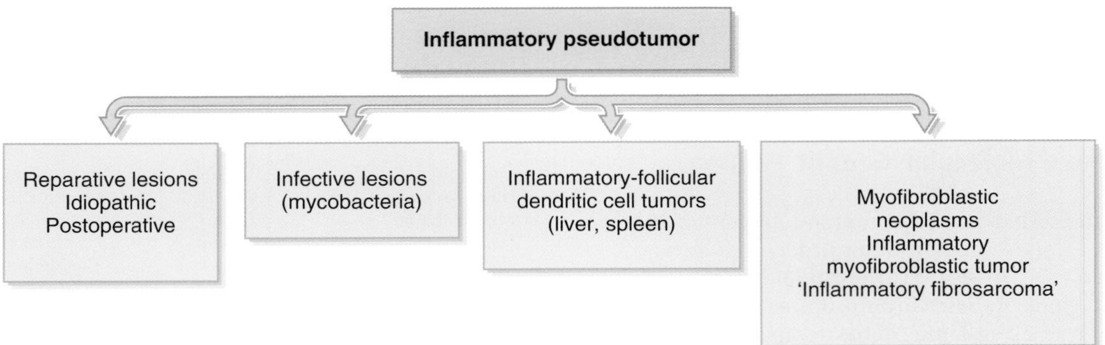

FIGURE 10-24. Inflammatory pseudotumor. A variety of lesions of differing etiologies have been referred to as *inflammatory pseudotumor*.

regard to tumor site, age at onset, or size of the tumor. However, the initial therapy was more radical for the tumors that neither recurred nor metastasized. Most studies have found that neither cellularity, mitotic counts, nor the extent of tumor necrosis correlates well with clinical behavior.[102,127] Blocker et al.[128] found that tumors located in the axial skeleton behaved more aggressively than those found peripherally. There are reports of incompletely excised infantile fibrosarcomas that have not recurred or metastasized after several years,[129] as well as sporadic reports of spontaneous regression.[130]

Despite rapid growth and a high degree of cellularity, most congenital/infantile fibrosarcomas are cured by wide local excision. A number of reports have indicated that preoperative chemotherapy is useful for decreasing tumor bulk, enabling a more conservative surgical approach.[131] There are also reports of success with postoperative chemotherapy and with chemotherapy alone as a mode of treatment for inoperable tumors.[132] In view of the generally favorable clinical course, it appears that adjuvant radiotherapy and chemotherapy should be reserved for congenital/infantile fibrosarcomas that are unresectable or have recurred or metastasized.

INFLAMMATORY MYOFIBROBLASTIC TUMOR

Inflammatory myofibroblastic tumor is a histologically distinctive lesion that occurs primarily in the viscera and soft tissue of children and young adults. It is considered a tumor of borderline malignancy because of its tendency to recur locally (at least at certain sites) and its ability to rarely metastasize. Although original descriptions of this lesion focused on its occurrence in the lung, inflammatory myofibroblastic tumor has been described in virtually every anatomic location and under many appellations, including plasma cell granuloma, plasma cell pseudotumor, inflammatory myofibrohistiocytic proliferation, omental-mesenteric myxoid hamartoma, inflammatory fibrosarcoma, and, most commonly, inflammatory pseudotumor. The term *inflammatory myofibroblastic tumor* is preferred because inflammatory pseudotumor has been applied to diverse entities, including pseudosarcomatous myofibroblastic proliferations of the lower genitourinary tract, infectious lesions (including those secondary to *Mycobacterium avium intracellulare*),[133] Epstein-Barr virus-associated follicular dendritic cell tumors usually found in the liver or spleen,[134] and reactive inflammatory pseudotumors of lymph nodes (Fig. 10-24).[135] This discussion focuses on extrapulmonary inflammatory myofibroblastic tumors.

Clinical Findings

Inflammatory myofibroblastic tumors have been reported in virtually every anatomic site. The most common sites of extrapulmonary inflammatory myofibroblastic tumor are the mesentery and omentum.[136,137] In a seminal study by Coffin et al.,[137] 36 of 84 (43%) extrapulmonary lesions arose at these sites. Unusual sites of involvement include the head and neck,[138] brain,[139] female genital tract,[140] pancreas,[141] heart,[142] and sites attached to various parts of the gastrointestinal tract.[143-145] Although the age range is broad, extrapulmonary inflammatory myofibroblastic tumors show a predilection for children, with a mean age of approximately 10 years. Females are affected slightly more commonly than males.

Presenting symptoms depend on the site of primary tumor involvement. Patients with intra-abdominal tumors most commonly complain of abdominal pain or an abdominal mass with increased girth, occasionally with signs and symptoms of gastrointestinal obstruction. Some patients have prominent systemic manifestations, including fever, night sweats, weight loss, and malaise, possibly related to the secretion of cytokines, including interleukin-6.[146] Laboratory abnormalities are present in a small number of patients and include an elevated erythrocyte sedimentation rate, anemia, thrombocytosis, and hypergammaglobulinemia, which often resolve when the lesion is excised.[137,147]

Pathologic Findings

Grossly, most lesions are lobular, multinodular, or bosselated with a hard or rubbery cut surface that appears white, gray, tan-yellow, or red (Fig. 10-25). Some cut with a gritty sensation because of the presence of calcifications. Although most are solitary tumors, multiple nodules generally restricted to the same anatomic location are found in almost one-third of cases.[137,148] The tumors range in size from 2 to 20 cm, but most are 5 to 10 cm.

A variety of histologic patterns may be seen, and different patterns may be found in the same tumor. Some tumors are composed predominantly of cytologically bland spindle- or

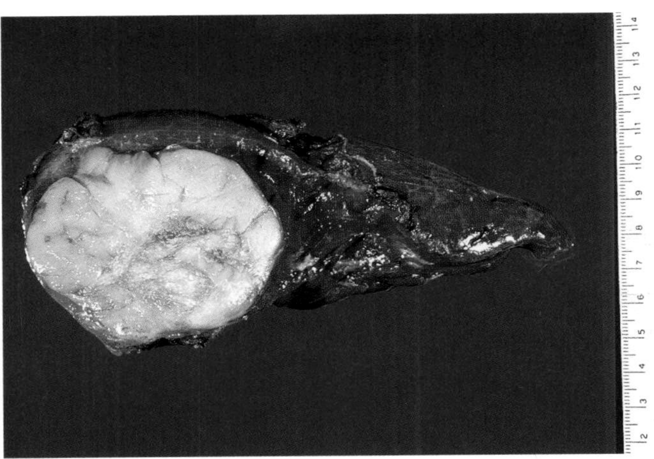

FIGURE 10-25. Gross appearance of an inflammatory myofibroblastic tumor in the left upper lobe of the lung of a 21-year-old woman.

stellate-shaped cells loosely arranged in a myxoid or hyaline stroma with scattered inflammatory cells, somewhat resembling nodular fasciitis. Others are composed of a compact proliferation of spindle-shaped cells arranged in a storiform or fascicular growth pattern (Figs. 10-26 to 10-30). In these foci, the nuclei tend to be elongated but lack significant hyperchromasia or cytologic atypia. Mitotic figures are variable but not atypical. These foci are usually associated with a prominent lymphoplasmacytic infiltrate, occasionally with formation of germinal centers. Other foci may be sparsely cellular, with cytologically bland cells deposited in a sclerotic stroma resembling a scar. Lymphocytes and plasma cells are often seen in these foci, and small punctate areas of calcification or metaplastic bone may be observed.

In some lesions, there is pronounced cytologic atypia, with cells containing large nuclei and distinct nucleoli. Some tumors have large histiocytoid cells resembling ganglion cells or Reed-Sternberg cells.[149] Recently, Mariño-Enriques et al.[150]

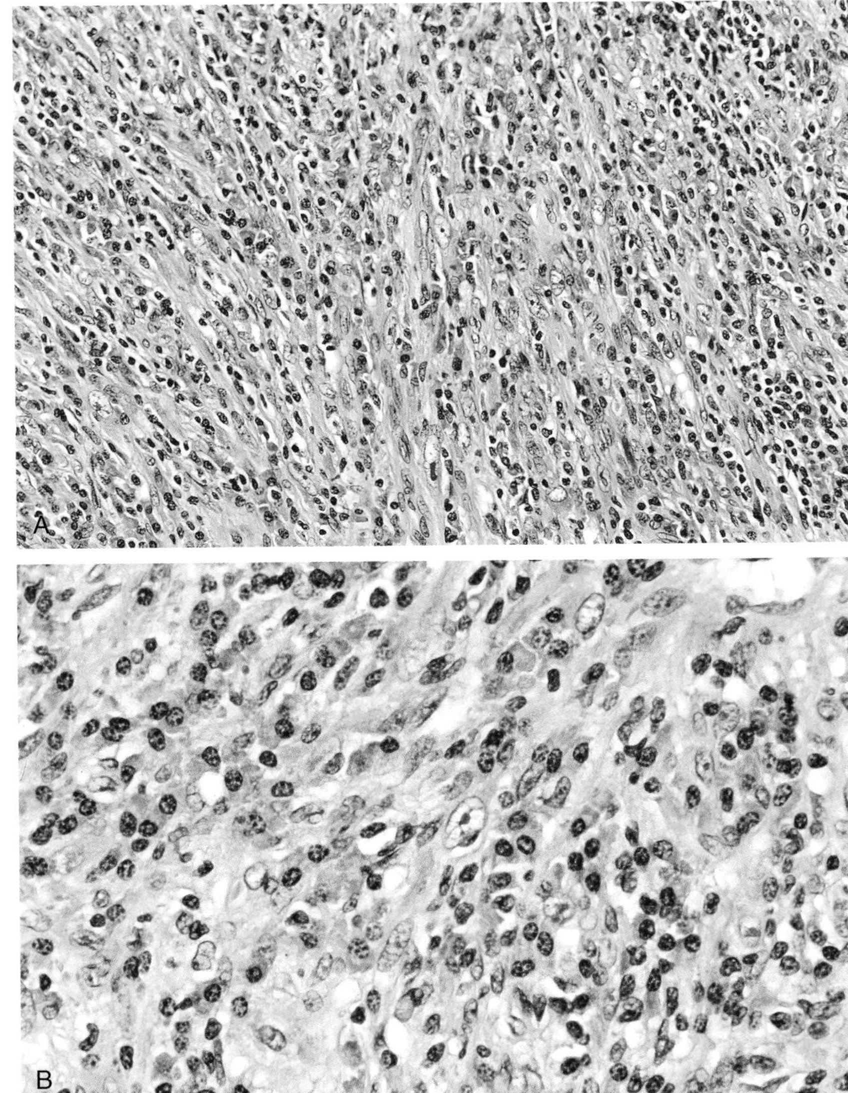

FIGURE 10-26. Inflammatory myofibroblastic tumor. (A) Low-power view showing an admixture of spindle-shaped and ovoid cells with a prominent inflammatory infiltrate. (B) High-power view of an inflammatory myofibroblastic tumor. Note the conspicuous admixture of lymphocytes and plasma cells.

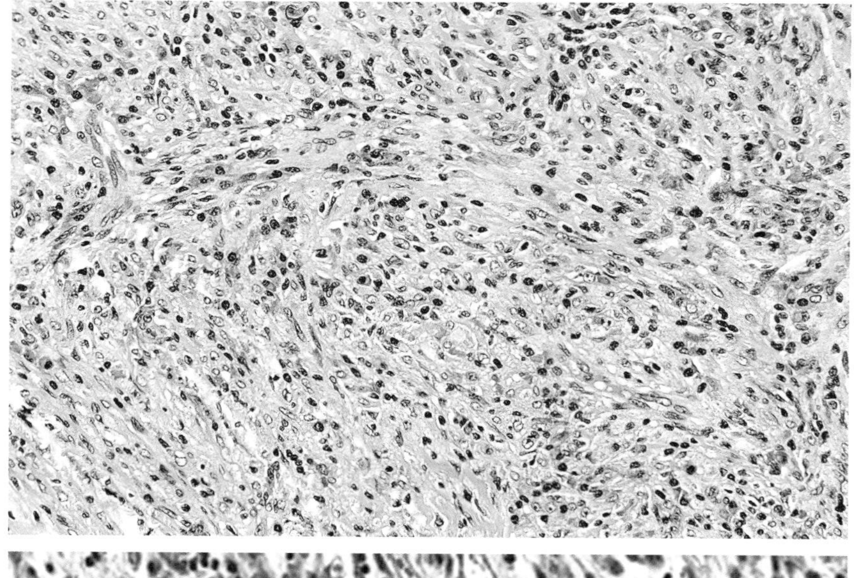

FIGURE 10-27. Inflammatory myofibroblastic tumor. Cytologically bland spindle-shaped cells are intimately admixed with a predominantly plasmacytic infiltrate.

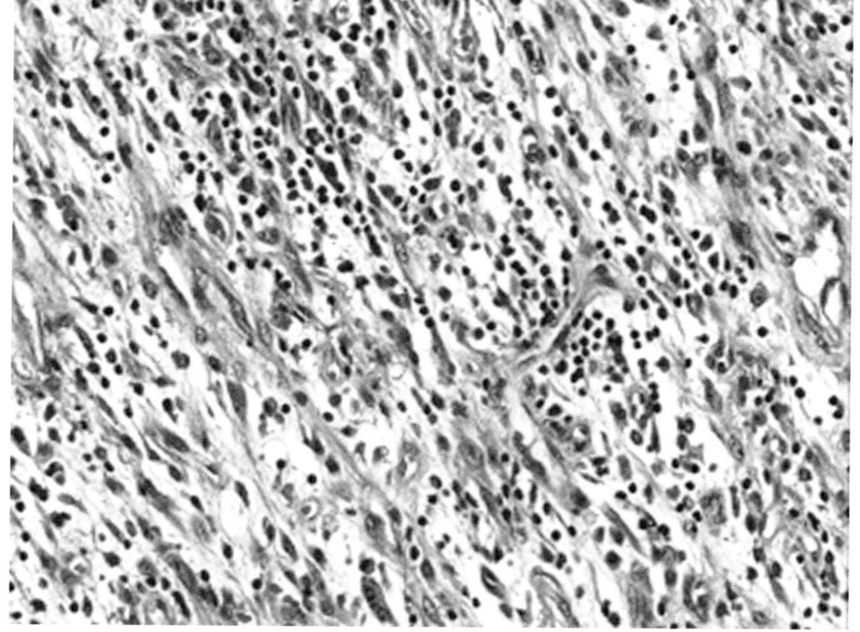

FIGURE 10-28. High-power view of plump spindle-shaped cells admixed with inflammatory cells in an inflammatory myofibroblastic tumor.

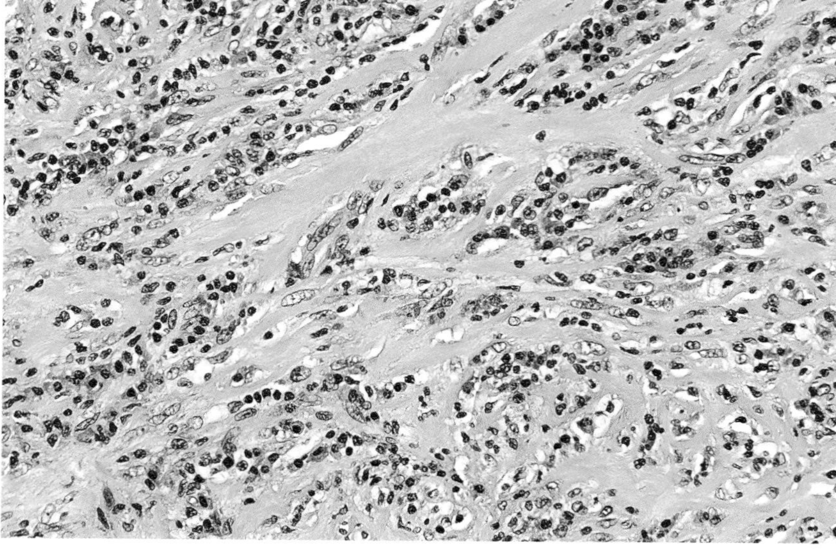

FIGURE 10-29. Less cellular inflammatory myofibroblastic tumor than that depicted in Figures 10-26 and 10-27. Plate-like collagen is present.

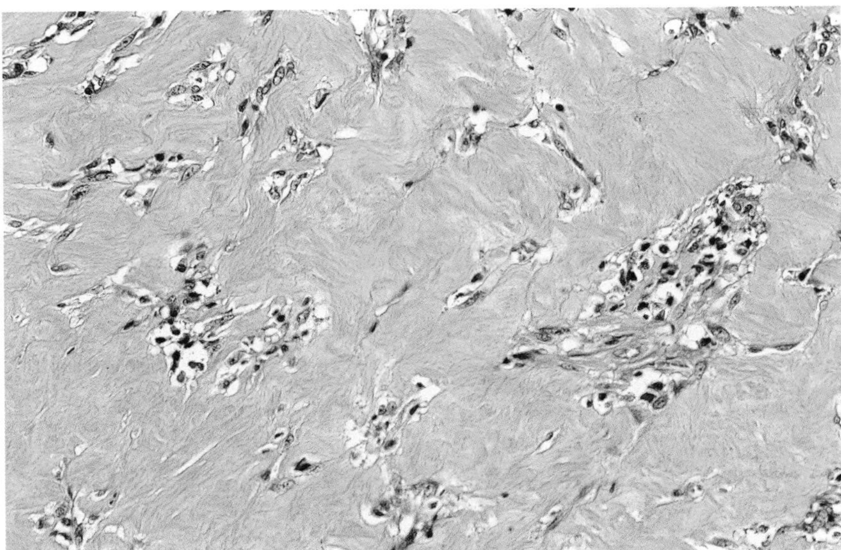

FIGURE 10-30. Hypocellular inflammatory myofibroblastic tumor composed of predominantly sclerotic fibrous tissue with scattered spindle-shaped and inflammatory cells.

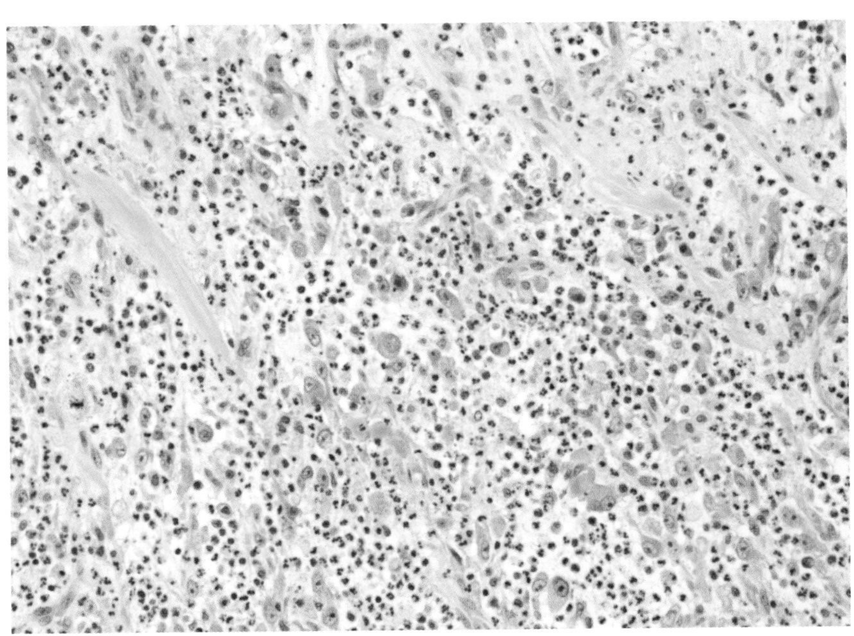

FIGURE 10-31. Low-power view of epithelioid inflammatory myofibroblastic sarcoma with an admixture of neutrophils and enlarged atypical epithelioid cells. *(Case courtesy of Dr. Jason Hornick, Brigham and Women's Hospital.)*

described 11 cases of inflammatory myofibroblastic tumor, all arising within the abdomen (mesentery or omentum) with prominent epithelioid morphology, a unique pattern of nuclear membrane or perinuclear ALK immunoreactivity and aggressive clinical behavior, coining the term *epithelioid inflammatory myofibroblastic sarcoma* (Figs. 10-31 and 10-32).

Immunohistochemical Findings

The tumor cells stain variably with myoid markers, including smooth muscle actin (Fig. 10-33), muscle-specific actin, and desmin. In the study by Meis and Enzinger,[148] smooth muscle actin and muscle-specific actin marked 90% and 83% of cases, respectively. On the other hand, there was equivocal desmin staining in only 1 of 11 (9%) cases. Coffin et al.[137] found staining for smooth muscle actin, muscle-specific actin, and desmin in 92%, 89%, and 69% of cases, respectively. Focal cytokeratin immunoreactivity was noted in 36% of the cases in the study by Coffin et al.[137] and 77% of the cases in the study by Meis and Enzinger,[148] predominantly in portions of the tumor that were in a submesothelial location.

As discussed in the section on cytogenetics and molecular genetic findings, a high percentage of inflammatory myofibroblastic tumors are associated with *ALK* mutations and, as such, many are also immunoreactive for ALK. There was a wide range of ALK positivity reported in the literature, ranging from 36% to 60% of cases.[151-153] Therefore, this marker lacks specificity and sensitivity, and there is an imperfect correlation with *ALK* mutations. There is evidence to suggest that different fusion partners result in different patterns of ALK immunoreactivity. For example, Chen et al.[154] described an inflammatory myofibroblastic tumor with a *RANBP2-ALK* fusion that was associated with round cell transformation and

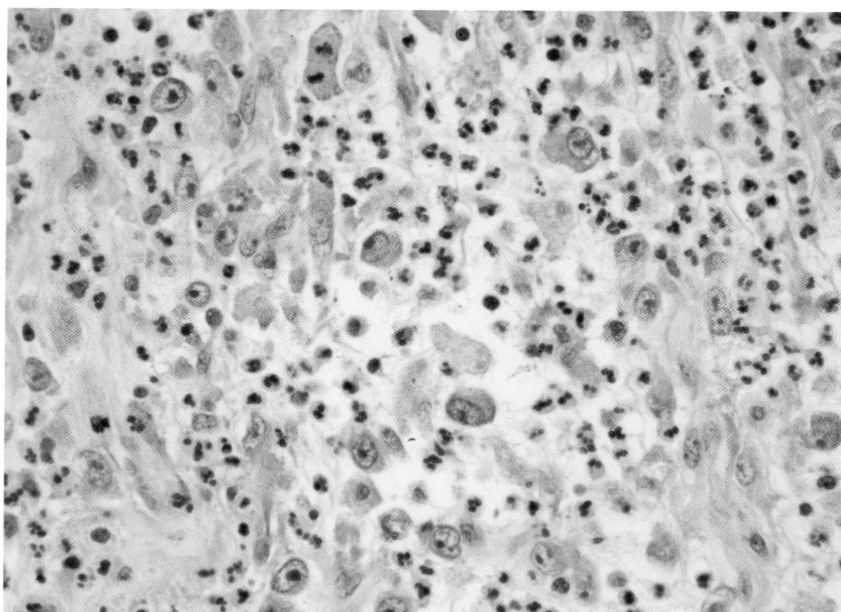

FIGURE 10-32. High-power view of atypical epithelioid cells in epithelioid inflammatory myofibroblastic sarcoma. *(Case courtesy of Dr. Jason Hornick, Brigham and Women's Hospital.)*

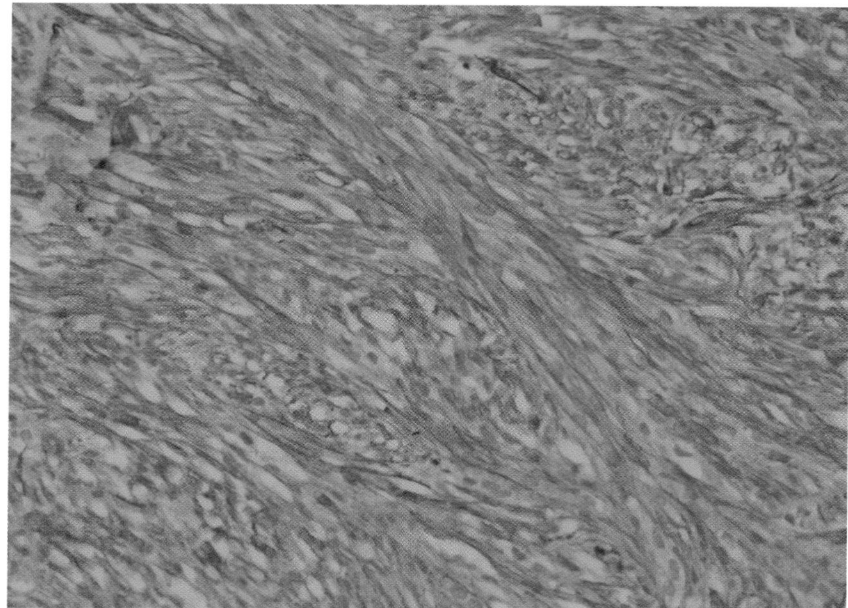

FIGURE 10-33. Strong smooth muscle actin positivity in inflammatory myofibroblastic tumor.

an unusual pattern of nuclear membrane ALK expression. Similarly, Mariño-Enriques[150] reported cases with *RANBP2-ALK* fusions associated with a high-grade epithelioid morphology that also showed nuclear membrane staining for ALK, although some showed perinuclear ALK staining. Others have also noted this correlation between a fusion partner (in this case, *RANBP2*) and pattern of ALK staining.[155,156] Diffuse cytoplasmic staining for ALK is typically seen with *TPM3*, *TPM4*, *ATIC*, *SEC31L1*, and *CARS* fusions, whereas granular cytoplasmic staining is seen with a *CLTC* fusion.[150,157]

Cytogenetic and Molecular Genetic Findings

Approximately 50% of inflammatory myofibroblastic tumors harbor clonal rearrangements of the *ALK* gene at 2p23.[158] This gene codes for a tyrosine kinase receptor that is a member of the insulin growth factor receptor superfamily. *ALK* rearrangements result in constitutive expression and activation of this gene with abnormal phosphorylation of cellular substrates. This gene has a variety of fusion partners, including *TPM3*, *TPM4*, *CLTC*, *CARS*, ATIC, *SEC31L1*, and *RANBP2* (Table 10-4).[153,159-162]

Differential Diagnosis

The differential diagnosis of this lesion depends on the clinicopathologic setting, including the patient's age, gender, tumor location, and number of lesions. For tumors composed of elongated spindle cells with eosinophilic cytoplasm arranged in a focal fascicular growth pattern, differentiation from

TABLE 10-4 Reported *ALK* Fusion Partners in Inflammatory Myofibroblastic Tumor

GENE	LOCUS
TPM3	1q21
TPM4	19p13
CLTC	17q23
CARS	11p15
ATIC	2q35
SEC31L1	4q21
RANBP2	2q12

inflammatory leiomyosarcoma may pose a problem. However, the nuclei in leiomyosarcoma are cigar-shaped and arranged in a more regular fascicular growth pattern. Rare inflammatory myofibroblastic tumors have a conspicuous population of large multinucleated tumor cells with prominent nucleoli bearing a resemblance to the Reed-Sternberg cells of *Hodgkin's disease*. The immunohistochemical reactivity of the spindle and ganglion-like cells for actins and ALK and negativity for CD15 and CD30 assist in distinguishing these two entities. Inflammatory myofibroblastic tumor can occasionally arise in the gastrointestinal tract and can be confused with an *inflammatory fibroid polyp*. The latter is a benign lesion that most often occurs in the stomach and ileum as a solitary submucosal polyp. Histologically, this lesion is dominated by stellate-shaped cells deposited in a myxoid stroma with reactive blood vessels and mixed inflammatory cells, particularly eosinophils. GIST may occasionally closely resemble an inflammatory myofibroblastic tumor, but GIST consistently stain for CD117 and DOG1 and are ALK negative. Although they share some histologic similarities, inflammatory myofibroblastic tumors can be distinguished from the group of inflammatory fibrosclerosing lesions, including *sclerosing mediastinitis*, *idiopathic retroperitoneal fibrosis*, and *Riedel thyroiditis*, by paying close attention to the clinical setting and gross and microscopic findings. These lesions tend to occur in older patients and, although mass-forming, are usually ill-defined, entrapping the normal tissues in the vicinity. They tend to have more prominent sclerosis and phlebitis than the typical inflammatory myofibroblastic tumor. Recently, a number of studies have found IgG4-positive plasma cells in inflammatory myofibroblastic tumors.[163,164] Yamamoto et al.[164] found significantly fewer IgG4-positive plasma cells and a lower IgG4/IgG ratio than that found in IgG4-related sclerosing diseases, but Saab et al.[163] found IgG4/IgG ratios that overlapped between these entities, suggesting that this ratio does not reliably distinguish them. Other fibroinflammatory processes that occur in this location, including *xanthogranulomatous inflammation secondary to Erdheim-Chester disease* and *pseudotumor resulting from atypical mycobacterial infection*, also may be in the differential diagnosis and can be distinguished by virtue of their distinct clinicopathologic setting.

Finally, the question as to whether inflammatory myofibroblastic tumor and *inflammatory fibrosarcoma* are the same tumor, distinct entities, or represent a spectrum has been debated.[136,148,165] Certainly, these two entities share clinical and pathologic features; as stated by Coffin et al.,[137] the distinction of inflammatory fibrosarcoma "from inflammatory myofibroblastic tumor may be more semantic than real." The consensus is that the two lesions are the same, and, therefore, these terms are synonymous, although the term *inflammatory myofibroblastic tumor* is preferred because of its more universal usage.

Discussion

There have been a number of controversial issues with respect to these lesions over the years, such as whether the lesions are a homogeneous entity, whether they are neoplastic, and, if neoplastic, their level of malignancy. The general consensus is that it is not possible to make histologic distinctions between lesions reported by some authors as inflammatory fibrosarcoma and by others as inflammatory myofibroblastic tumor. In support of this statement is that there is overlap in case material reported in the two largest studies under the two preceding terms.[137,148] There is also compelling evidence that these lesions are true neoplasms rather than pseudotumors. Many have been associated with aggressive local behavior that has resulted in patient death. In addition, as previously mentioned, some (but not all) tumors show aberrations of the *ALK* gene, supportive evidence of a neoplastic process.

Based on the two largest studies of abdominal and retroperitoneal lesions, it is clear that tumors in this location have a propensity for more aggressive behavior than their extra-abdominal counterparts, with recurrence rates of 23% to 37%.[137,148] The major question seems to be whether these lesions have metastatic potential or whether multiple lesions in a single patient represent multifocal disease. Coffin et al.,[137] in a series of 53 cases with follow-up, reported no instances of metastasis, whereas 3 of 27 patients reported by Meis and Enzinger[148] developed metastasis to the lung and brain. The reasons for this discrepancy are not clear. In at least one case reported by Meis and Enzinger[148] (case 26), the simultaneous presentation of histologically bland mediastinal and cerebral lesions with no evidence of disease nearly 4 years after surgery raises the possibility that these lesions may be multifocal. However, there are other reports that clearly indicate that some examples of this tumor metastasize and can result in patient death.[149,150] Debelenko et al.[162] reported a primary lesion and metastasis with identical *CARS-ALK* fusions, supporting a metastasis as opposed to multifocal disease.

There is certainly an imperfect correlation between clinicopathologic features of these tumors and prognosis. Traditional features, including tumor size, nuclear atypia, mitotic activity, and necrosis, do not correlate well with outcome. There are rare examples of inflammatory myofibroblastic tumors with usual features that have behaved aggressively.[137,166,167] There is also a group of tumors that have undergone histologic progression with so-called *round cell transformation*, characterized by highly atypical spindled or epithelioid cells with vesicular nuclei, prominent nucleoli, and increased mitotic activity, including atypical mitotic figures.[149,154,155,166,168] Interestingly, as mentioned earlier in the chapter, a subgroup of these tumors with *RANBP2-ALK* fusion and a distinctive pattern of ALK nuclear membrane immunoreactivity behave aggressively.[150,154-156] In the study by Mariño-Enriques et al.,[150] a distinctive morphologic variant of intra-abdominal inflammatory myofibroblastic tumor composed predominantly of sheets of highly atypical round/epithelioid cells with prominent myxoid stroma and neutrophilic infiltrate were described, all of which stained for ALK, had *ALK* gene rearrangements by FISH and, in the three cases tested, a *RANBP2-ALK* fusion. The ALK staining was distinctive, either showing a nuclear membrane or perinuclear pattern of positivity. Five of eight patients with follow-up died of disease 3 to 36 months after diagnosis, indicating that this constellation of findings is a homogeneous and highly aggressive variant of inflammatory myofibroblastic tumor.

The mainstay of therapy is surgical resection with re-excision of recurrent tumors. Some have advocated chemotherapy and radiation therapy in recurrent or metastatic cases.[169] Recently, a novel *ALK*-targeted inhibitor, crizotinib, has been found to be efficacious in the treatment of aggressive inflammatory myofibroblastic tumors. Therefore, accurate recognition of the aggressive variant mentioned previously has become increasingly important.

BOX 10-1 Classification of Fibrosarcoma

- Adult-type fibrosarcoma
- Myxoid type (myxofibrosarcoma)
- Fibromyxoid type (low-grade fibromyxoid sarcoma/hyalinizing spindle cell tumor with giant rosettes)
- Sclerosing epithelioid type
- Juvenile/infantile fibrosarcoma

ADULT-TYPE FIBROSARCOMA

Definitionally, the cells of fibrosarcoma recapitulate the appearance of the normal fibroblast. This admittedly broad definition has resulted in a great deal of subjectivity as to which spindle cell, collagen-forming tumors are appropriately termed *fibrosarcoma* and which are better classified as another form of sarcoma. Depending on the era and the accepted criteria at that time, the incidence and behavior of this neoplasm have varied greatly. This trend is well illustrated by a series of studies from the Mayo Clinic over a period of 50 years. In 1974 Pritchard et al.[169a] reported that 12% of all soft tissue sarcomas were fibrosarcomas (down from 65% in an earlier Mayo Clinic study), which was revised by Scott et al.[170] to an even lower percentage by 1989. More recently, Bahrami and Folpe[171] revised this number to less than 1% of all adult soft tissue sarcomas, a fascinating evolution of diagnostic criteria.

On closer scrutiny, several factors are probably responsible for the apparent decline in the incidence of what will be referred to as *adult-type fibrosarcoma*. The categorization by many pathologists of high-grade, pleomorphic spindle cell tumors with fibroblastic and myofibroblastic differentiation as malignant fibrous histiocytoma (MFH) or, more recently, undifferentiated pleomorphic sarcoma, as opposed to fibrosarcoma, certainly has contributed to this trend. Second, a refinement of histologic criteria resulted in the segregation of fibromatosis (desmoid tumors) as a unique group of tumors distinct from fibrosarcoma. Last, with the advent of immunohistochemistry, cytogenetics, and, more recently, molecular genetic techniques, it became possible to more reproducibly recognize monophasic fibrous synovial sarcomas and malignant peripheral nerve sheath tumors, which were undoubtedly frequently misclassified as fibrosarcomas. Despite significant progress in this area, the differential diagnosis of spindle cell tumors remains a difficult, challenging, and sometimes unsolvable problem, especially when only a small biopsy specimen is available for microscopic examination.

As a result of the foregoing trends, a number of general statements can be made concerning the diagnosis of fibrosarcoma:

1. Adult-type fibrosarcoma has become, in large part, a diagnosis of exclusion. It presupposes that diagnoses such as monophasic fibrous synovial sarcoma and malignant peripheral nerve sheath tumor (MPNST) have been excluded by the appropriate immunohistochemical or cytogenetic/molecular genetic studies.
2. Adult-type fibrosarcoma, like other fibroblastic tumors (e.g., fibromatosis), may have a variable component of neoplastic cells with features of myofibroblasts. Therefore, the finding of various actin isoforms within these tumors does not mitigate against the diagnosis of fibrosarcoma. On the other hand, there are some spindle cell sarcomas that are composed predominantly of cells with myofibroblastic differentiation, and the entity of myofibrosarcoma (myofibroblastic sarcoma) has become increasingly accepted.
3. Collagen-forming, spindle cell tumors of high nuclear grade showing fibroblastic differentiation are, by convention, classified as undifferentiated pleomorphic sarcomas (see Chapter 13). Consequently, lesions diagnosed as adult-type fibrosarcoma, for the most part, occupy the low-grade end (grades 1 and 2) of a spectrum that includes undifferentiated pleomorphic sarcoma at the high-grade end.

Despite the fact that the incidence of adult-type fibrosarcoma has markedly decreased in recent years, there have been renewed efforts to identify unique subsets or variants within this group of lesions. Although it is still not clear to what extent these variants are biologically different from one another, they certainly have distinct histologic and sometimes molecular genetic features that allow their identification in a consistent fashion. These variants include myxoid fibrosarcoma (myxofibrosarcoma), low-grade fibromyxoid sarcoma, and sclerosing epithelioid fibrosarcoma (Box 10-1). This discussion will also include those sarcomas that are composed of predominantly myofibroblasts (myofibrosarcoma), an entity that has only begun to gain acceptance over the past 10 years.

Clinical Findings

Like most other sarcomas, adult-type fibrosarcoma causes no characteristic symptoms and is difficult to diagnose clinically. Most patients present with a solitary palpable mass ranging from 3 to 8 cm in greatest dimension. It is slowly growing and usually painless; pain is encountered more commonly with synovial sarcoma and MPNST than with fibrosarcoma.

The skin overlying the tumor is generally intact, although more superficially located neoplasms that grow rapidly or have been traumatized may result in ulceration of the skin. Such tumors, particularly when clinically neglected, may form large fungating masses in the areas of ulceration. The preoperative duration of symptoms varies greatly and ranges from as little as a few weeks to as long as 20 years. Adult-type fibrosarcoma is most common in the third through fifth decades of life. In

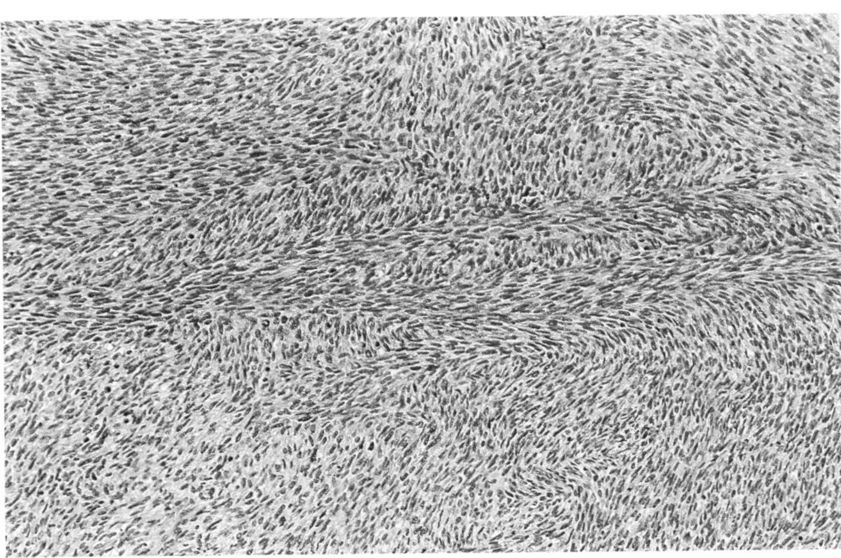

FIGURE 10-34. Low-power view of a fibrosarcoma exhibiting a distinct fascicular (herringbone) pattern.

the study by Bahrami and Folpe,[171] patients ranged in age from 6 to 74 years, with a median age of 50 years. In the other recent study of fibrosarcomas that took great pains to exclude other lesions and seems to be a uniform group of tumors, the median age was 56.3 years.[172]

The tumor may occur in any soft tissue site but is most common in the deep soft tissues of the lower extremities, particularly the thigh and knee, followed by the trunk and upper extremities, although some arise in the head and neck. Rare examples of this tumor have been reported in virtually every anatomic site.

Fibrosarcoma predominantly involves deep structures, where it tends to originate from the intramuscular and intermuscular fibrous tissue, fascial envelopes, aponeuroses, and tendons. Deeply situated tumors may even encircle bone and cause radiographically demonstrable periosteal and cortical thickening; in such cases, distinction from parosteal osteosarcoma may be difficult. Other radiographic findings, in addition to a soft tissue mass, include occasional foci of calcification and ossification, although this feature is much more common with synovial sarcoma than fibrosarcoma. Fibrosarcomas arising from the subcutis, excluding those that arise in dermatofibrosarcoma protuberans (DFSP), are less common and tend to originate in tissues damaged by radiation, heat, or scarring (described later). In the study by Bahrami and Folpe,[171] only 5 of 26 tumors arose in a suprafascial location.

Pathologic Findings

Generally, the excised tumor consists of a solitary, soft to firm, fleshy, rounded or lobulated mass that is gray-white to tan-yellow and measures 3 to 8 cm in greatest dimension. Small tumors are usually well circumscribed and are partly or completely encapsulated. Large tumors are less well defined; they often extend with multiple processes into the surrounding tissues or grow in a diffusely invasive or destructive manner. The frequent circumscription of small fibrosarcomas can be misleading and may result in an erroneous diagnosis of a benign tumor and inadequate surgical therapy.

Although there are minor variations in the histologic picture, most adult-type fibrosarcomas have in common a rather uniform fasciculated growth pattern consisting of fusiform or spindle-shaped cells that vary little in size and shape, have scanty cytoplasm with indistinct cell borders, and are separated by interwoven collagen fibers arranged in a parallel fashion. Mitotic activity varies, but caution should be exercised when diagnosing fibrosarcoma in the absence of mitotic figures. Multinucleated giant cells or giant cells of bizarre size and shape are rarely a feature of this tumor.

Histologic grading of adult-type fibrosarcomas is based on the cellularity and differentiation, mitotic activity, and necrosis. *Low-grade fibrosarcomas* are characterized by a uniform, orderly appearance of the spindle cells associated with abundant collagen (Figs. 10-34 to 10-37). In some cases, the cells are oriented in curving or interlacing fascicles, forming a classic herringbone pattern. In others, the cells are separated by thick, wire-like collagen fibers. Secondary features may be seen, including focal chondro-osseous differentiation. Some tumors have areas that are less cellular or extensively myxoid (Fig. 10-38) and closely mimic portions of fibromatosis, thereby making distinction of these two lesions difficult, in some cases, particularly when only a small sample is available for evaluation.

High-grade fibrosarcomas are characterized by closely packed, less well-oriented tumor cells that are small, ovoid or rounded, and associated with less collagen (Fig. 10-39). The fascicular or herringbone growth pattern is less distinct, the nuclei are more pleomorphic, mitotic figures are more numerous, and there are areas of necrosis and/or hemorrhage.

Immunohistochemical Findings

Fibrosarcomas by definition do not exhibit any lineage-specific markers such as cytokeratin or S-100 protein. The lack of cytokeratin immunoreactivity aids in distinction from monophasic fibrous synovial sarcoma. Negative immunostaining for S-100 protein distinguishes fibrosarcoma from spindle cell or desmoplastic malignant melanomas but not necessarily

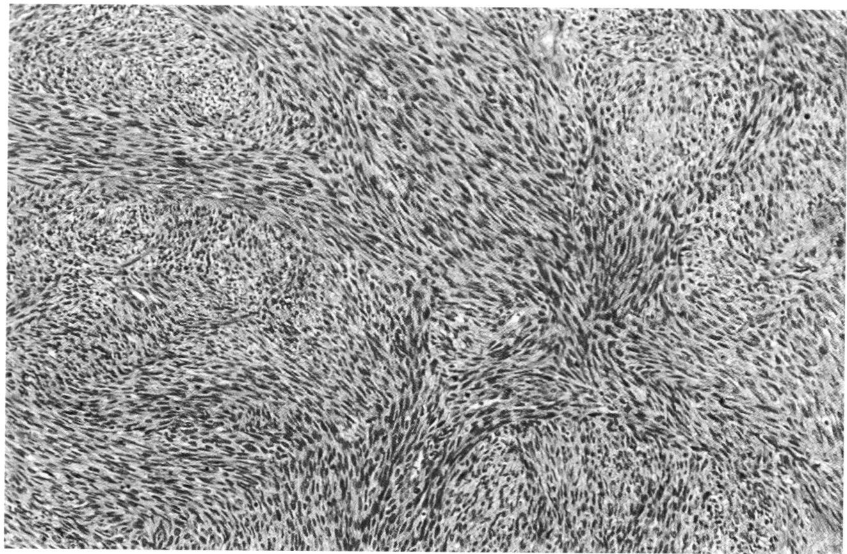

FIGURE 10-35. Fibrosarcoma consisting of uniform spindle cells showing little variation in size and shape and a distinct fascicular pattern.

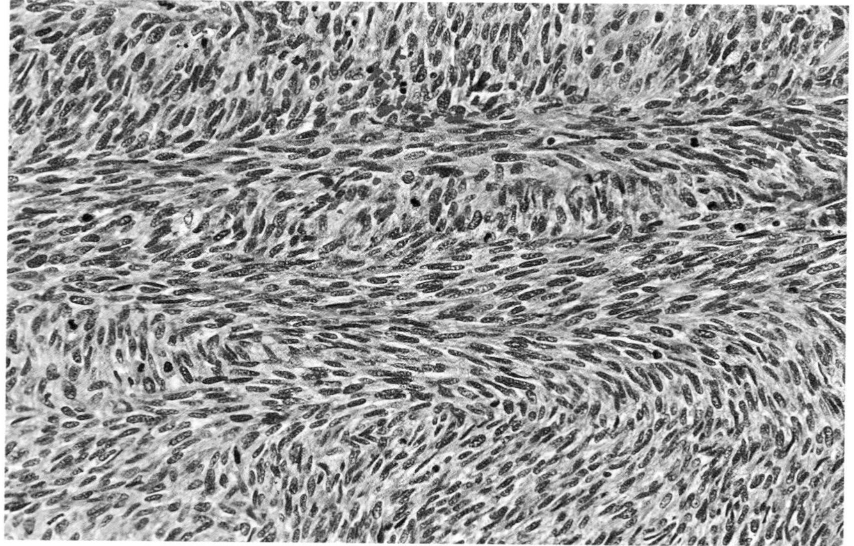

FIGURE 10-36. Fibrosarcoma showing arrangement of the fibroblasts in distinct intersecting fascicles (herringbone pattern).

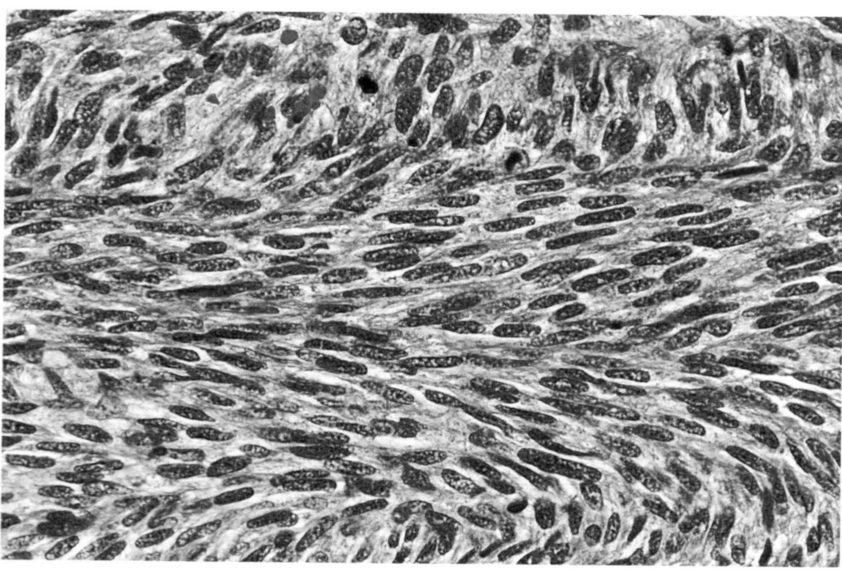

FIGURE 10-37. High-power view of fibrosarcoma showing uniformity of the tumor cells and the characteristic fascicular pattern.

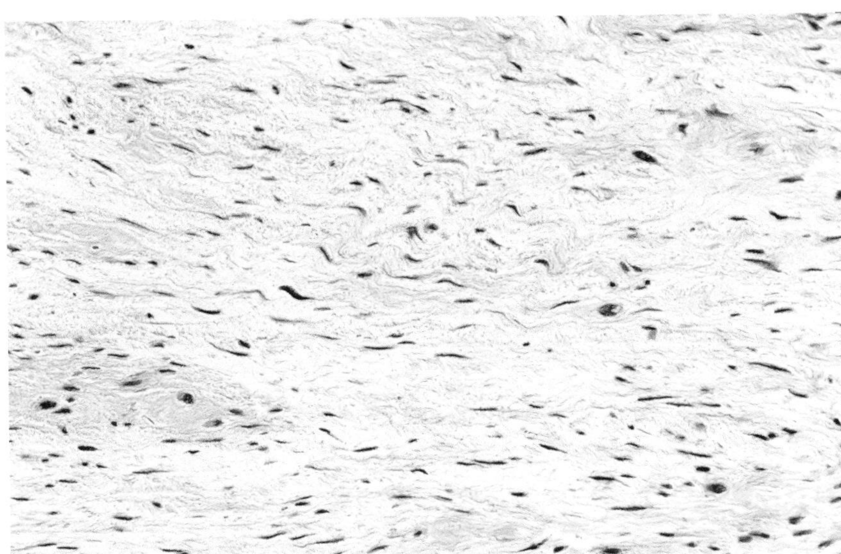

FIGURE 10-38. Fibrosarcoma with extensive myxoid change. The fibroblasts are widely separated by abundant myxoid stroma, making the fascicular pattern less conspicuous.

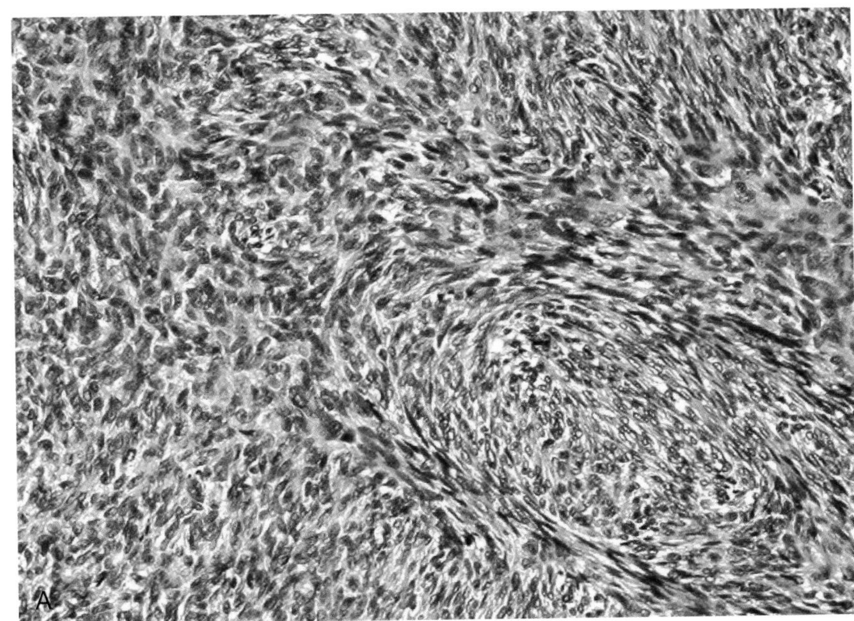

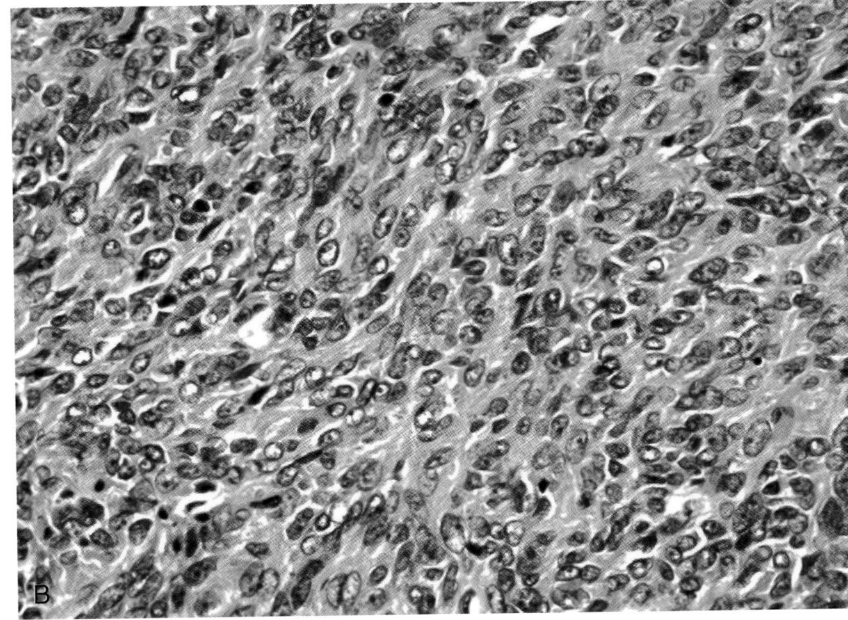

FIGURE 10-39. (A,B) High-grade fibrosarcoma characterized by closely packed, less well-oriented, rounded tumor cells with high-grade nuclear features.

from malignant peripheral nerve sheath tumors because only 50% to 60% of the latter stain focally for this antigen. In some fibrosarcomas, scattered cells stain for smooth muscle or muscle-specific actin, reflecting focal myofibroblastic differentiation.[171]

Cytogenetic and Molecular Genetic Findings

Little is known about the cytogenetic and molecular genetic alterations in adult-type fibrosarcoma. In contrast to congenital/infantile fibrosarcoma, this tumor does not appear to have a characteristic cytogenetic abnormality, although multiple complex chromosomal rearrangements have been reported.[173,174] Limon et al.[173] reported a nonrandom chromosomal change involving t(2;19) with involvement of 2q21-qter.

Differential Diagnosis

It is often difficult to distinguish adult-type fibrosarcoma from other spindle cell tumors, and, in many instances, only careful examination of multiple sections and ancillary studies permit a correct diagnosis, which is always a diagnosis of exclusion. *Benign processes* likely to be mistaken for fibrosarcoma range from nodular fasciitis to cellular benign fibrous histiocytoma and fibromatosis. *Malignant neoplasms* considered in the differential diagnosis are much more numerous and include malignant peripheral nerve sheath tumor, pleomorphic undifferentiated sarcoma, and monophasic fibrous synovial sarcoma. Other tumors that tend to simulate fibrosarcoma include sarcomatoid mesothelioma, clear cell sarcoma, epithelioid sarcoma, DFSP, desmoplastic leiomyosarcoma, spindle cell forms of rhabdomyosarcoma, malignant melanoma, and spindle cell carcinoma. Because the differential diagnosis of most of these tumors is discussed elsewhere, the following comments are limited to lesions most frequently confused with fibrosarcoma.

Nodular fasciitis, a pseudosarcomatous reactive myofibroblastic proliferation that grows rapidly and is marked by its cellularity and immature cellular appearance, differs from fibrosarcoma by its smaller size and microscopically by its more irregular growth pattern; characteristically, its cells are arranged in short bundles—never in long, sweeping fascicles or a herringbone pattern as in fibrosarcoma. The cells lack nuclear hyperchromasia, and there is usually a prominent myxoid matrix and scattered chronic inflammatory cells.

Cellular benign fibrous histiocytoma may be difficult to distinguish from fibrosarcoma because this lesion is characteristically cellular and often forms fascicles. However, the fascicles are usually not as regular or as long and sweeping as those seen in fibrosarcoma. Areas of more conventional benign fibrous histiocytoma may be present and are extremely useful in this distinction. In most cases, cellular benign fibrous histiocytoma is situated in the dermis or subcutis; unlike fibrosarcoma, it is rarely found in deep soft tissue structures. Mitotic figures are present in cellular benign fibrous histiocytoma, but the presence of atypical mitotic figures lends strong support to a diagnosis of malignancy. The cells also characteristically express factor XIIIa antigen, although this lacks specificity.

Musculoaponeurotic fibromatosis (desmoid tumor) has a growth pattern similar to that of fibrosarcoma but is less cellular and contains more collagen. The cells are uniformly spindled, with delicate chromatin and one or two minute nucleoli. In general, the cells do not touch one another but, rather, are separated by collagen, whereas the cells of fibrosarcoma frequently overlap with closely spaced hyperchromatic nuclei. Low levels of mitotic activity may be present in fibromatosis so that considerable overlap in mitotic activity between fibromatosis and fibrosarcoma may be encountered (Table 10-5). Therefore, mitotic activity is not a reliable discriminant between fibromatosis and fibrosarcoma when dealing with low levels of mitotic activity but might become useful when higher levels of mitotic activity are present. Because fibromatosis-like areas may be present in low-grade fibrosarcoma, careful sampling of the tumor is mandatory. Clinical considerations are of little help for distinguishing these tumors because they may occur at the same location and in patients of similar age. As mentioned earlier in the chapter, deep fibromatoses typically show strong nuclear β-catenin immunoreactivity.

Undifferentiated pleomorphic sarcoma (so-called *malignant fibrous histiocytoma*) has been included in many of the earlier reports of poorly differentiated or pleomorphic fibrosarcomas. Clinically, these tumors principally arise in elderly persons, with a peak during the seventh decade; microscopically, they are characterized by a storiform to haphazard growth pattern and the presence of multinucleated bizarre giant cells, often with eosinophilic cytoplasm and containing delicate droplets of lipid material. Siderophages and xanthoma cells are also common features that assist in the diagnosis. Transitions between fibrosarcoma and pleomorphic undifferentiated sarcoma do occur, suggesting a form of tumor progression, in some cases. Admittedly, where one draws the line between a high-grade fibrosarcoma and an undifferentiated pleomorphic sarcoma is, at times, quite subjective.

MPNST may display areas that are virtually indistinguishable from fibrosarcoma. However, by definition, some evidence of nerve sheath differentiation must be present to support the diagnosis of MPNST. For example, cells showing neural differentiation often have a wavy or buckled appearance, rather than the finely tapered fibroblasts of fibrosarcoma. Although the cells can be arranged into an irregular fascicular growth pattern, the long, sweeping fascicles characteristic of fibrosarcoma are usually not present. Moreover, the cells of MPNST tend to show perivascular cuffing and may be arranged in distinct whorls or palisades. At low magnification, MPNST often shows a marbled appearance with alternating myxoid

TABLE 10-5 Comparison of Histologic Features of Low-Grade Fibrosarcoma and Fibromatosis

PARAMETER	LOW-GRADE FIBROSARCOMA	FIBROMATOSIS
Cellularity	Low to moderate	Low to moderate
Nuclear overlap	Present	Usually absent
Nuclear hyperchromasia	Present	Absent
Nucleoli	More prominent	Inconspicuous
Mitotic figures	1+ to 3+	1+
Necrosis	Rare	Absent
Vessel wall infiltration	Rare	Absent

and cellular zones. In addition, MPNST may show transitions between malignant and benign neurofibroma-like areas. The finding of S-100 protein in scattered tumor cells supports a diagnosis of MPNST, although up to 50% of cases do not stain for this antigen, and S-100 protein staining is not specific for MPNST.

Monophasic fibrous synovial sarcoma may also closely simulate a fibrosarcoma, although it is generally composed of more ovoid-appearing cells arranged in an irregular fascicular growth pattern. Moreover, many of these sarcomas have areas in which the cells contain more eosinophilic cytoplasm with a suggestion of cellular cohesion, even if well-formed glands are not present. Immunohistochemically, almost all cases of synovial sarcoma express at least one epithelial marker, a feature not found in fibrosarcoma. In addition, TLE1 is found to be a reliable marker of synovial sarcoma, although admittedly there have been only rare opportunities to stain adult-type fibrosarcomas for this antigen. The identification of t(X;18) by FISH or RT-PCR is a highly sensitive and specific method for identifying a tumor as a synovial sarcoma.

Discussion

It is difficult to compare the results of published studies because many of the tumors included in older series probably represent entities other than fibrosarcoma. Few studies have used immunohistochemistry and/or molecular genetics to exclude other lesions in the differential diagnosis. As such, the rate of local recurrence varies significantly among studies. For example, Mackenzie[175] noted a recurrence in 93 of 190 (49%) cases and Pritchard et al.[176] in 113 of 199 (57%) cases. In the study by Scott et al.,[170] the overall rate of recurrence was 42% at 5 years. In that study, although neither tumor grade nor tumor stage was associated with an increased risk of local recurrence, the status of the surgical margins was strongly predictive; the 5-year cumulative probability of local recurrence was 79% in tumors with inadequate surgical margins and 18% in tumors treated by wide or radical excision. To gain more reliable information about the true clinical behavior of adult-type fibrosarcoma, it seems reasonable to focus on modern studies that have used ancillary techniques in an attempt to exclude tumors that mimic fibrosarcoma. In the study by Bahrami and Folpe[171] of 26 adult-type fibrosarcomas (after starting with 163 putative tumors diagnosed as fibrosarcoma over a 48-year period at Mayo Clinic), 12 of 24 (50%) patients with follow-up died of locally aggressive and/or metastatic disease; only 6 patients were alive without disease and 6 died of other causes. In the 2006 study by Hansen et al.,[172] local recurrences were reported in 7 of 21 (33%) patients with follow-up, and 3 of 21 (14.3%) patients developed metastases and died of a tumor. Unfortunately, there were insufficient data in either study to determine prognostic parameters.

Metastasis of fibrosarcoma occurs almost exclusively by way of the bloodstream. The lung is the principal metastatic site, followed by the skeleton, especially the vertebrae and skull. Most metastases are noted within the first 2 years after diagnosis, although some patients, particularly those with low-grade fibrosarcomas, develop metastasis late in their course. Lymph node metastasis is rare; as such, regional lymph node excision is not a necessary part of the initial therapeutic regimen.

Considering the prominent role of fibroblasts in posttraumatic repair, it is not surprising that trauma has been implicated repeatedly as a possible and even likely causative factor.[177] Stout,[101] for example, reported 36 cases of fibrosarcoma arising in scar tissue (*cicatricial fibrosarcoma*) or at the site of a former injury. One patient had suffered an injury at age 9 years and developed a fibrosarcoma in the scar at age 35. Ivins et al.[178] noted a history of preceding trauma in 19 of 78 cases of fibrosarcoma but concluded that "only in one an etiologic significance was remotely possible." Fibrosarcoma has also been reported to arise in a draining sinus of long duration.[179] Evaluation of the significance of these cases is difficult. In some of them, trauma may be a contributing factor, whereas, in others, trauma may merely serve to alert the patient or the physician to the presence of the disease and may be an incidental finding rather than a tumor-provoking factor.

Factors other than trauma have also been implicated to induce or contribute to the development of fibrosarcoma. Burns et al.[180] reported a tumor arising in a 31-year-old man 10 years after a plastic Teflon-Dacron prosthetic vascular graft was placed for a lacerated femoral artery. Eckstein et al.[181] reported a fibrosarcoma that arose in the vicinity of a total knee joint prosthesis. Finally, it is clear that fibrosarcomas can arise following radiation therapy; 2 of 26 cases in the recent Mayo Clinic study arose in this setting.[171]

As mentioned earlier in the chapter, the evolution of concepts and diagnostic criteria has resulted in this once commonly diagnosed sarcoma to become a relative rarity. This is beautifully exemplified by the recent Mayo Clinic study that evaluated 163 cases diagnosed as fibrosarcoma over a 48-year period (Table 10-6).[171] In the end, after applying rigid diagnostic criteria and using both immunohistochemistry and molecular techniques, only 26 (16%) cases met the diagnostic criteria of fibrosarcoma. Specifically, the authors required the tumor to be composed of hyperchromatic spindled cells with mild or moderate nuclear pleomorphism with arrangement into a fascicular herringbone growth pattern with a variable degree of interstitial collagen. In addition, there had to be an absence

TABLE 10-6 Summary of Re-Analysis of 163 Cases Diagnosed as Fibrosarcoma at Mayo Clinic Over a 48-Year Period

FINAL DIAGNOSIS	NUMBER OF CASES
True fibrosarcoma	26 (16%)
Pleomorphic undifferentiated sarcoma	32 (20%)
Synovial sarcoma	21 (13%)
Solitary fibrous tumor	14 (9%)
Myxofibrosarcoma	11 (7%)
MPNST	8 (5%)
Low-grade fibromyxoid sarcoma	3 (2%)
Sclerosing epithelioid fibrosarcoma	2 (1%)
Fibrosarcomatous DFSP	4 (3%)
Myofibroblastic sarcoma	3 (2%)
Misc./other mesenchymal tumors	21
Non-mesenchymal tumors	7
Sarcomatoid carcinoma	3 (2%)
Spindle cell melanoma	4 (3%)

Modified from Bahrami A, Folpe AL. Adult-type fibrosarcoma: a reevaluation of 163 putative cases diagnosed at a single institution over a 48-year period. Am J Surg Pathol 2010;34(10):1504–13.

DFSP, dermatofibrosarcoma protuberans; MPNST, malignant peripheral nerve sheath tumor.

of morphologic features of myxofibrosarcoma, low-grade fibromyxoid sarcoma (with or without rosettes), sclerosing epithelioid fibrosarcoma, or fibrosarcoma arising in DFSP. Immunohistochemically, the cells could express only vimentin or focal smooth muscle actin.[171]

Of the 137 non-fibrosarcomas, most were reclassified as undifferentiated pleomorphic sarcoma (32 [20%] cases). Twenty cases (12%) were classified as specific variants of fibrosarcoma, including low-grade fibromyxoid sarcoma (3 cases), myxofibrosarcoma (11 cases), fibrosarcoma arising in DFSP (4 cases), and sclerosing epithelioid fibrosarcoma (2 cases). The largest group were reclassified as non-fibrosarcoma mesenchymal tumors (78 [48%] cases), including, most commonly, monophasic synovial sarcoma (21 cases), solitary fibrous tumor (14 cases), and MPNST (8 cases), among others. Finally, 7 cases (4%) were reclassified as non-mesenchymal tumors, including desmoplastic melanoma (4 cases) and sarcomatoid carcinoma (3 cases).

FIBROSARCOMA VARIANTS

Fibrosarcoma, Sclerosing Epithelioid Type (Sclerosing Epithelioid Fibrosarcoma)

Sclerosing epithelioid fibrosarcoma is an unusual but distinctive variant of fibrosarcoma composed of epithelioid cells arranged in nests and cords and deposited in a densely hyalinized collagenous matrix. Since the initial description of this tumor by Meis-Kindblom et al.[182] in 1995, fewer than 120 cases of this neoplasm have appeared in the literature.

Clinical Findings

Most patients present with a deep-seated mass that is painful in up to one-third of cases. The age range is wide, with a median age of approximately 45 years; there does not seem to be any striking gender predilection.[182,183] The most common location is the deep soft tissues of the lower extremity/limb girdle followed by the trunk, upper extremities/limb girdle, and head and neck region.[182-184] Other unusual locations include intraosseous tumors,[185] the liver,[186] and colon,[187] among others.

Pathologic Findings

Grossly, the tumor is usually well circumscribed and lobulated, bosselated, or multinodular; most are 5 to 10 cm in greatest diameter. Occasional tumors show cystic or myxoid change, and some have a gritty sensation upon sectioning as a result of focal calcifications. Most arise within the skeletal muscles of the extremities, deep fascia, or periosteum; some invade adjacent bone or the deep subcutaneous tissue.

Although grossly well circumscribed, there is characteristically infiltration of the surrounding soft tissues. At low magnification, the tumor is hypocellular with extensive areas of densely hyalinized stroma (Figs. 10-40 and 10-41). The neoplastic cells are predominantly epithelioid in appearance and are arranged in a variety of patterns, including nests, cords, strands, and occasionally acini or alveoli. The cells have oval to round angulated nuclei with finely stippled or vesicular chromatin, small basophilic nucleoli, and scanty cleared-out or faintly eosinophilic cytoplasm. Mitotic figures are generally inconspicuous, but occasional tumors are characterized by a high mitotic rate (>5 mitotic figures/10 HPF). Necrosis may be seen in up to one-third of cases. The stroma is composed of predominantly deeply acidophilic collagen, which, in some foci, nearly completely obliterates the neoplastic cells, resulting in hypocellular occasionally calcified zones. Myxoid and chondro-osseous areas may be present. Branching vessels, which are frequently hyalinized and organized in a hemangiopericytoma-like pattern, may also be present. Peripherally located cleft-like spaces filled with tumor, suggesting true angiolymphatic invasion, may be seen. In almost all cases, the tumor shows foci of spindle-shaped sarcoma similar to conventional fibrosarcoma. Occasionally, there are areas that closely resemble low-grade fibromyxoid sarcoma with or without rosettes.[188-190]

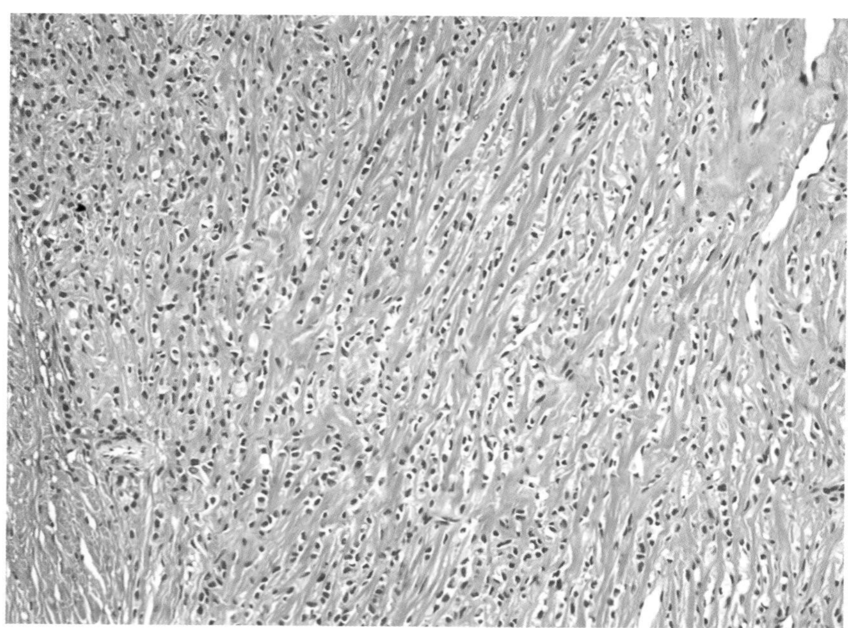

FIGURE 10-40. Medium poster view of sclerosing epithelioid fibrosarcoma with cords of cells separated by dense collagen. *(Photograph courtesy of Dr. Alex Lazar, MD Anderson Cancer Center.)*

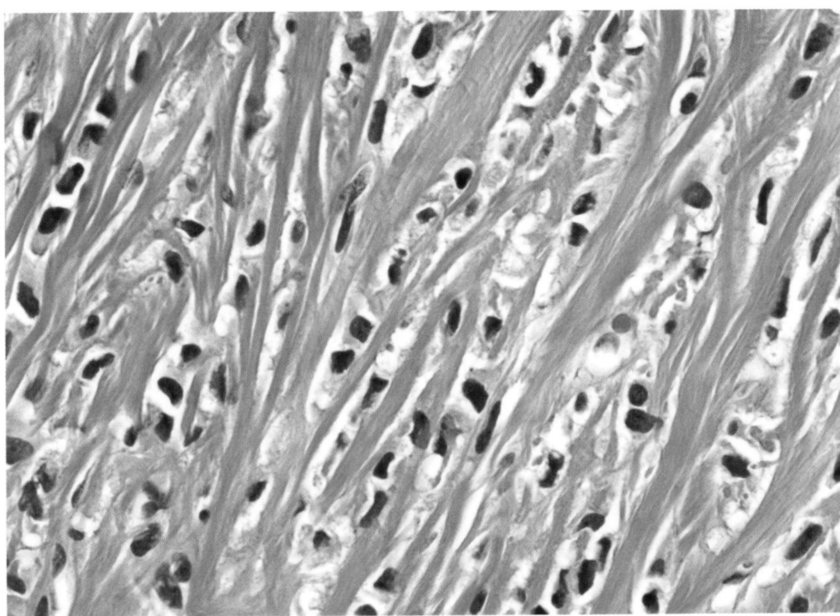

FIGURE 10-41. High-power view of epithelioid cells in sclerosing epithelioid fibrosarcoma. *(Photograph courtesy of Dr. Alex Lazar, MD Anderson Cancer Center.)*

Immunohistochemical Findings

There is no pathognomonic immunoprofile for this difficult to diagnose neoplasm. Up to 50% have a membranous pattern of immunoreactivity to epithelial membrane antigen (EMA), contributing to confusion with carcinoma, epithelioid sarcoma, and synovial sarcoma.[191,192] However, cytokeratins are typically not expressed by the neoplastic cells. Neural markers, including S-100 protein and neuron-specific enolase, are positive in a small number of cases. Stains for desmin, smooth muscle actin, HMB-45, CD68, leukocyte common antigen, and CD34 are typically negative. Ultrastructurally, the neoplastic cells have the features of fibroblasts and sometimes myofibroblasts.[188,193]

Cytogenetic and Molecular Genetic Findings

Gisselsson et al.[194] reported a case arising in a 14-year-old boy with a complex karyotype with amplification of 12q13 and 12q15 (including the *HMGIC* gene) as well as 9q13 rearrangement. Donner et al.[191] described a tumor arising in the calf of a 55-year-old man with involvement of 6q15,22q13 and Xq13. Another case was found to have a der t(10;17)(p11;q11).

Since 2007, a number of studies have cited a possible relationship between sclerosing epithelioid fibrosarcoma and low-grade fibromyxoid sarcoma. In 2007, in a large study of the latter entity, Guillou et al.[189] noted several cases with distinct foci of epithelioid cells reminiscent of that seen in sclerosing epithelioid fibrosarcoma. Others have also noted cases with overlapping morphologic features.[190,195,196] Tumors comprising predominantly sclerosing epithelioid fibrosarcoma with smaller areas resembling low-grade fibromyxoid sarcoma, and vice versa, have also been observed. There are also rare cases of apparently pure sclerosing epithelioid fibrosarcoma with evidence of *FUS* translocations, as one typically sees in low-grade fibromyxoid sarcoma. In the study by Wang et al.,[197] only 2 of 22 (9%) cases of sclerosing epithelioid fibrosarcoma showed *FUS* rearrangements.

Therefore, it seems possible that at least some tumors with sclerosing epithelioid fibrosarcomatous features are related to low-grade fibromyxoid sarcoma.

Differential Diagnosis

The differential diagnosis includes a wide range of both benign and malignant lesions composed, at least in part, of epithelioid cells. In the series by Meis-Kindblom et al.,[182] many of the cases were submitted in consultation with a diagnosis of a benign lesion, including nodular fasciitis, fibrous histiocytoma, myositis ossificans, hyalinized leiomyoma, or desmoid tumor, perhaps accounting for the large number of cases treated with inadequate surgical excision in that series.

The most difficult differential diagnostic considerations are other malignant epithelioid neoplasms, particularly *infiltrating lobular carcinoma* and *infiltrating signet ring adenocarcinoma*. This distinction is made more difficult by the immunohistochemical expression of EMA in up to one-half of cases of sclerosing epithelioid fibrosarcoma. Identification of conventional areas of fibrosarcoma and ultrastructural features indicative of fibroblastic or myofibroblastic differentiation allows this distinction. The absence of leukocyte common antigen is helpful for distinguishing this tumor from a *sclerosing lymphoma*. *Clear cell sarcoma* is characterized by a more uniform pattern of nested cells with vesicular nuclei and macronucleoli. Although S-100 protein is present in a few cases of sclerosing epithelioid fibrosarcoma, the absence of HMB-45 or Melan A helps distinguish between these lesions. The more nested and cord-like areas of sclerosing epithelioid fibrosarcoma may resemble *ossifying fibromyxoid tumor of soft parts*, but the latter entity is characterized by a peripherally located incomplete shell of lamellar bone, in most cases, and is composed of cells of lower nuclear grade. *Synovial sarcoma*, particularly those with poorly differentiated areas, may be composed of round cells often arranged around a hemangiopericytoma-like vascular pattern, with the immunohistochemical expression of epithelial markers. All of these features are similar to those of sclerosing epithelioid fibrosarcoma, and, therefore, the recognition of lower-grade biphasic or monophasic synovial sarcoma is useful for this distinction. Cytogenetic or molecular genetic identification of the t(X;18) characteristic of synovial sarcoma is extremely helpful. Distinction from MPNST may be difficult, particularly because both tumors may express S-100 protein and neuron-specific enolase. Recognizing that the tumor originated from a nerve or a surrounding benign peripheral nerve sheath tumor is useful in this regard. Finally, *sclerosing rhabdomyosarcoma* may closely resemble sclerosing epithelioid fibrosarcoma.[198] The former may show overt rhabdomyoblastic differentiation in the form of strap cells, and the cells typically express desmin, often in a peculiar dot-like pattern. MyoD1 is strongly expressed by the neoplastic cells, but myogenin staining is less impressive.

Discussion

Comparing the clinical behavior of this variant of fibrosarcoma to conventional adult-type fibrosarcoma is difficult, particularly because the latter is a diagnosis of exclusion. In the study by Meis-Kindblom et al.,[182] 8 of 15 (53%) patients in whom follow-up information was available developed local recurrence during a median of 4.8 years after diagnosis. Metastases, most commonly to the lungs, followed by the pleura/chest wall, bones, and brain, were detected in 43% of patients. Of the six patients with metastatic disease, four died and two were alive with pulmonary metastases 14 years after the initial diagnosis. Patients with tumors on the trunk, those with large tumors, and those of male gender may have a worse prognosis. In the study by Antonescu et al.,[188] of 14 patients with more than 1 year of follow-up, 12 (86%) patients developed distant metastases, and 8 (57%) patients died as a direct result of their tumor. In the literature review of 89 cases by Ossendorf et al.,[199] 13% of reported cases had metastases at diagnosis, and an additional 31% developed metastases after diagnosis. Almost 40% developed local recurrences, and 34% died of their tumor during a mean of 46 months after diagnosis. Tumors located in the head and neck seemed to have a particularly aggressive clinical course. Wide surgical excision is the mainstay of therapy, and long-term follow-up is indicated, because some patients develop local recurrence or metastatic disease late in their course.

Myxofibrosarcoma (Fibrosarcoma, Myxoid Type)

The term *myxofibrosarcoma* was originally proposed by Angervall et al.[200] to describe a group of fibroblastic lesions that show a spectrum of cellularity, nuclear pleomorphism, and mitotic activity ranging from a hypocellular lesion with minimal cytologic atypia to a more cellular lesion with features bordering on those of so-called pleomorphic-storiform MFH. Historically, these tumors have been subdivided into three or four grades based on the degree of cellularity, nuclear pleomorphism, and mitotic activity. There is a continuum between low- and high-grade variants, as indicated by the presence of low-grade areas in high-grade lesions and a histologic progression of low-grade to high-grade tumors in recurrences.[201-204] Comparing data among these studies is difficult because the proportion of myxoid areas in the tumor required for inclusion has varied. For example, all of the tumors reported by Merck et al.[205] and Angervall et al.[200] were "wholly, or almost wholly, myxomatous in appearance," whereas Mentzel et al.[206] required only 10% of the tumor to show prominent myxoid change to be included in their study and be considered within the myxofibrosarcoma spectrum. In their seminal description of the *myxoid variant of MFH*, Weiss and Enzinger[207] required at least 50% of the tumor to be composed of myxoid areas. The current WHO definition of myxofibrosarcoma includes tumors with a broad range of cellularity, nuclear atypia and amount of myxoid stroma unified by the multinodular growth pattern and characteristic curvilinear vasculature. The following discussion focuses on the low-grade tumors in the myxofibrosarcoma spectrum. Myxofibrosarcomas of intermediate and high nuclear grade (analogous to so-called myxoid MFH) are discussed in Chapter 13.

Clinical Findings

The tumor most commonly arises as a slowly enlarging, painless mass in the extremities of elderly patients. Although the age range is broad, most patients are in their fifth to seventh decades of life, and men are affected slightly more often than women. The most common site is the extremities, with a predilection for the lower extremities. The tumor is found less commonly on the upper extremities, trunk, and head and neck region. Rare examples have also been described in the skin,[208] breast,[209] heart,[210] and paratesticular region,[211] among others. This tumor is very uncommon in the abdominal cavity and retroperitoneum, and, in fact, extensive sampling and/or molecular genetic analysis usually reveals the myxofibrosarcoma to be a component of a dedifferentiated liposarcoma.[212]

Pathologic Findings

Myxofibrosarcoma is usually centered in the subcutaneous tissue and is composed of multiple gelatinous nodules that have a tendency to spread in a longitudinal manner (Fig. 10-42). In almost one-third of cases, the tumor involves underlying skeletal muscle. Deep-seated lesions tend to be less nodular, demonstrate a more infiltrative growth pattern, and are usually larger than their superficial counterparts. Some cases also involve the dermis, and such lesions can be easily confused for a variety of cutaneous myxoid neoplasms.[208]

Histologically, low magnification reveals a multinodular tumor of low cellularity. The constituent cells are generally spindle or stellate shaped and are deposited in a myxoid matrix composed of predominantly hyaluronic acid. The cells have slightly eosinophilic cytoplasm and indistinct cell borders; the nuclei are hyperchromatic, are mildly pleomorphic, and have rare mitotic figures only. Most tumors have elongated, curvilinear capillaries; there is a tendency for the tumor cells to align themselves along the vessel periphery (Fig. 10-43 to Fig. 10-44). Occasional tumor cells resemble lipoblasts as a result of cytoplasmic vacuolization, but these vacuoles contain acid mucin rather than neutral fat (pseudolipoblasts, Fig. 10-45). This vacuolization seems to be the result of a dilatation of endoplasmic reticulum and the formation of pseudocanaliculi by delicate cytoplasmic processes.

Immunohistochemically, the cells may show focal staining for muscle-specific actin and smooth muscle actin, indicative of myofibroblastic differentiation.

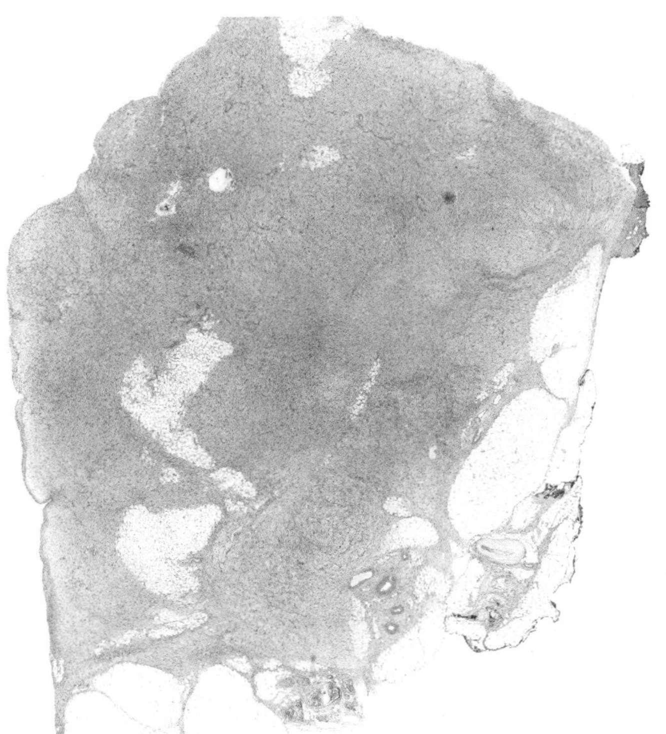

FIGURE 10-42. Low-power view of myxofibrosarcoma showing an infiltrative growth pattern into the surrounding subcutaneous tissue.

Cytogenetic and Molecular Genetic Findings

Most cases of myxofibrosarcoma with cytogenetic aberrations have shown a highly complex karyotype, often with triploid or tetraploid alterations.[213,214] A study of several cases by comparative genomic hybridization has revealed genomic imbalances, including losses of 6p and 13q, with gains of 7p, 9q, and 12q.[215,216] Sawyer et al.[217] reported a reciprocal t(10;17)(p11.2;q23) in a single case of myxofibrosarcoma, whereas another case was found to have a t(2;15)(p23;q21.2) and an interstitial deletion of 7q.[218]

Willems et al.[213] evaluated the karyotype and clinicopathologic features of 32 cases of myxofibrosarcoma. Most cases showed complex cytogenetic anomalies, and such alterations were found in tumors of all grades. However, no tumor-specific chromosomal abnormalities were identified. Interestingly, those cases that locally recurred showed more complex cytogenetic aberrations than those that did not. The authors proposed the concept of progression of myxofibrosarcoma as a multistep genetic process governed by genetic instability.

Differential Diagnosis

The differential diagnosis includes a wide array of benign and malignant myxoid soft tissue neoplasms. Tumors that are uniformly low grade and lack a transition to a higher-grade lesion may be easily mistaken for a benign lesion. *Nodular fasciitis* is characterized by a proliferation of fibroblasts and myofibroblasts that lack nuclear hyperchromasia, although mitotic figures are often easily seen. Other features, such as the presence of slit-like spaces, extravasated erythrocytes, and keloid-like collagen, help distinguish nodular fasciitis from myxofibrosarcoma. *Myxoma* typically presents as a large, painless, fluctuant intramuscular mass composed of oval-shaped cells deposited in an abundant hyaluronic acid-rich myxoid matrix. The cellularity of a myxoma may overlap with that of low-grade myxofibrosarcoma, but the cells show less atypia and mitotic activity. Furthermore, myxoma is hypovascular and lacks the curvilinear vessels characteristically found in myxofibrosarcoma. *Spindle cell lipoma* is a benign lipomatous tumor typically found in the subcutaneous tissue of the posterior neck, shoulder, or back region of elderly people, mostly men. The spindle cells lack cytologic atypia and mitotic activity, and they stain for CD34. Mature lipocytes and ropey collagen fibers are also characteristic of this lesion. *Nerve sheath myxoma* is typically a small, solitary, intradermal or subcutaneous multinodular tumor often located on the fingers. Although some show nuclear pleomorphism, most are composed of cells with less atypia than those found in myxofibrosarcoma; this tumor also lacks the curvilinear vessels found in the latter lesion. In addition, the cells typically stain strongly for S-100 protein.

Myxofibrosarcoma must also be distinguished from other myxoid sarcomas that tend to be more clinically aggressive. *Myxoid liposarcoma* has less cytologic atypia, a fine plexiform vascular pattern without perivascular tumor cell condensation, and scattered lipoblasts. Clinically, myxoid liposarcoma is almost always deep-seated and occurs predominantly in the thigh or popliteal fossa of middle-aged adults. *Extraskeletal myxoid chondrosarcoma* is a multinodular neoplasm composed of rounded cells arranged in strands and cords deposited in a chondroitin sulfate-rich myxoid stroma. These lesions tend to show prominent hemorrhage and lack the curvilinear vessels of myxofibrosarcoma. An analysis by FISH for evidence of a *DDIT3* or *EWSR1* translocation has been found to be useful in this differential diagnosis because these aberrations can be detected in myxoid liposarcoma and extraskeletal myxoid chondrosarcoma, respectively.

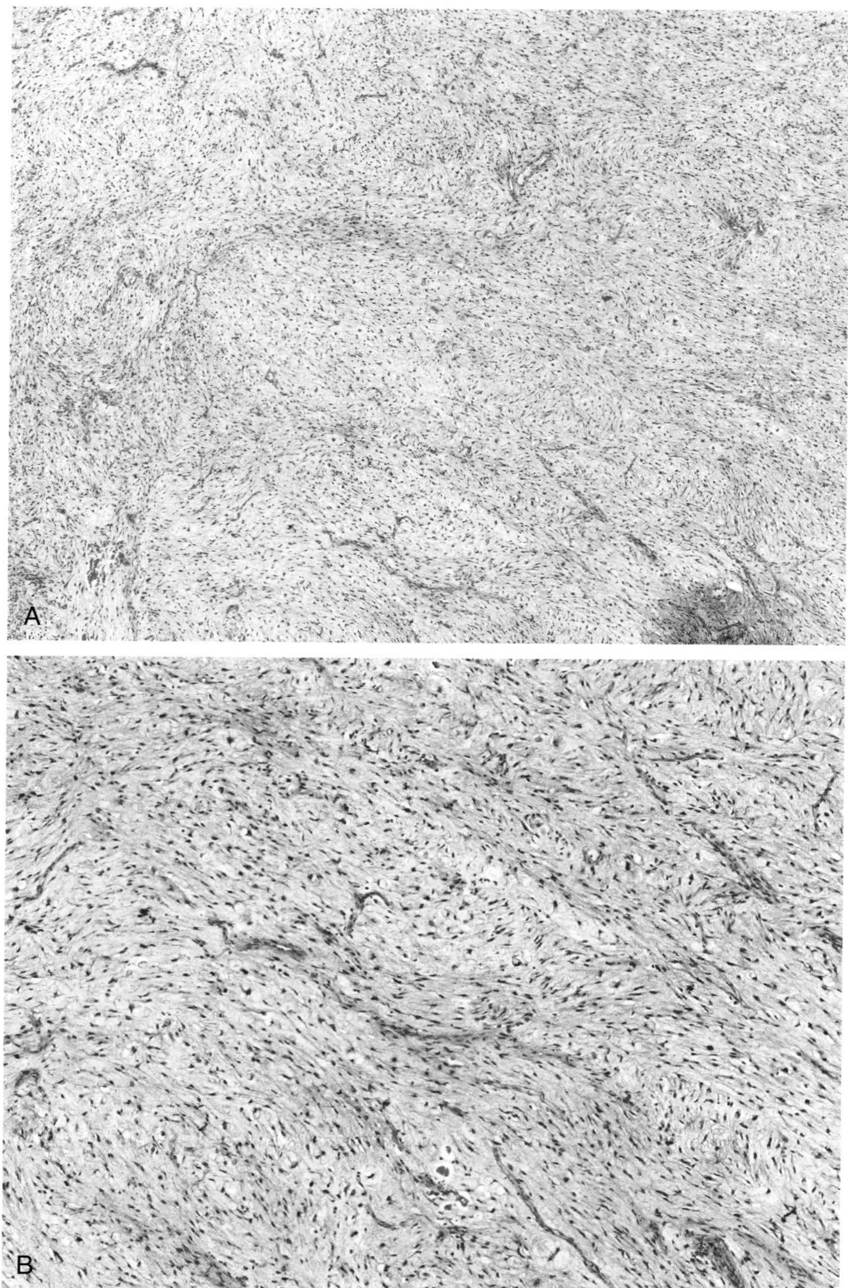

FIGURE 10-43. Myxofibrosarcoma. (A) At low power, the tumor shows low cellularity, mild atypia, and elongated blood vessels. (B) At higher power, vasculature becomes more apparent.

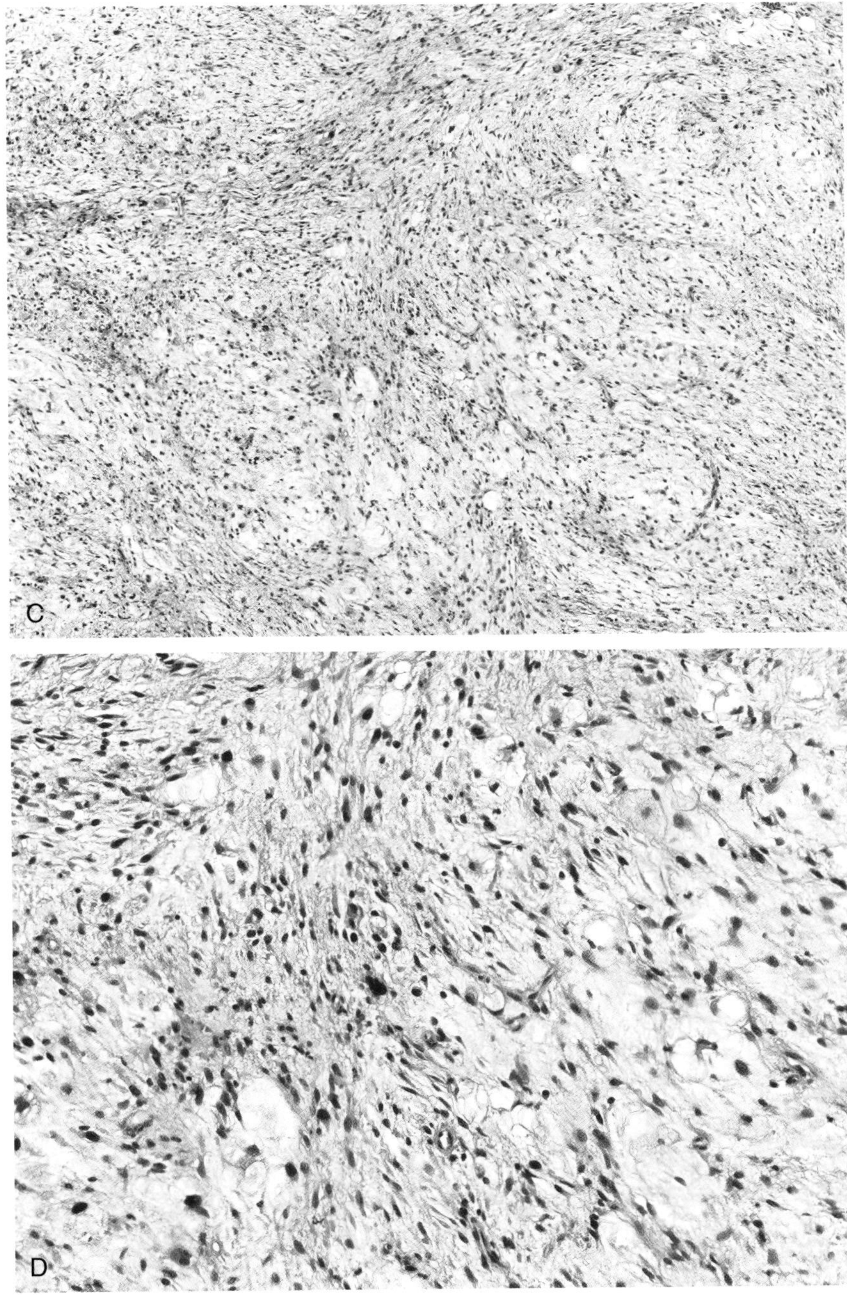

FIGURE 10-43, cont'd. (C) More cellular areas of the same myxofibrosarcoma. (D) Higher power view of scattered hyperchromatic nuclei.

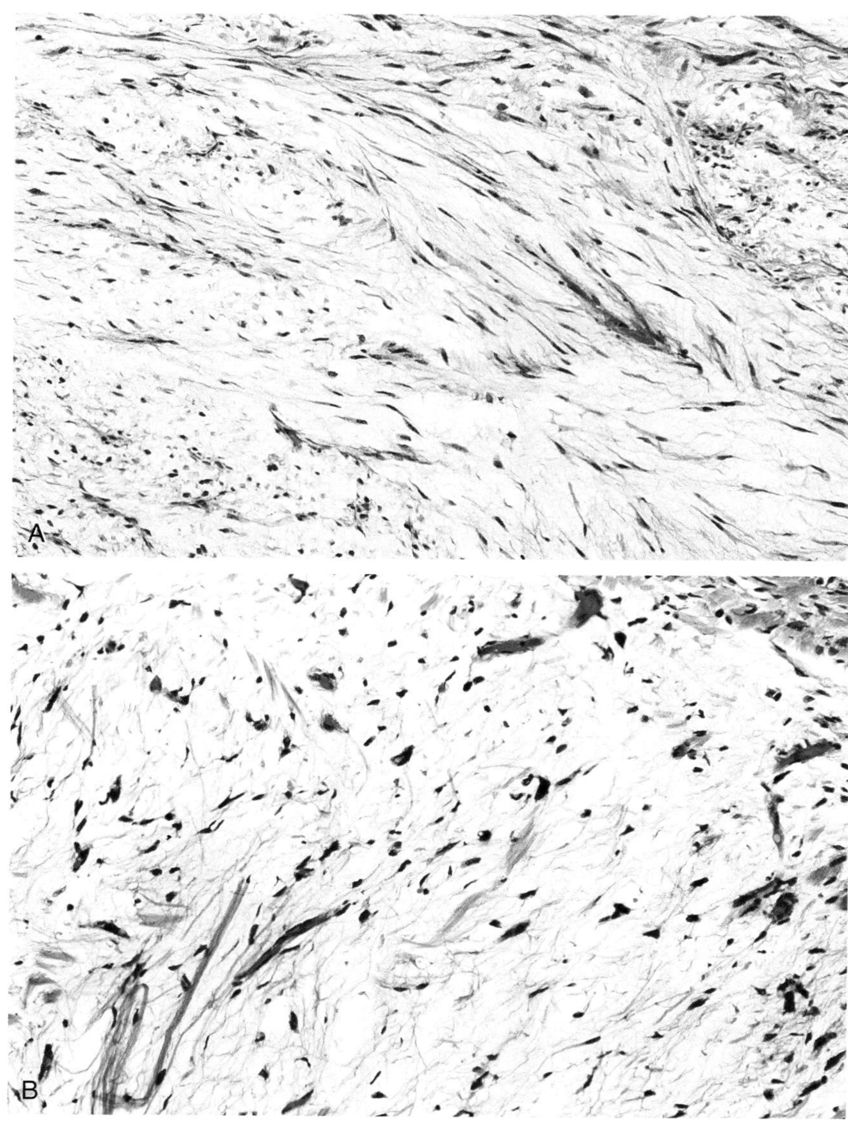

FIGURE 10-44. Myxofibrosarcoma composed of spindled, stellate, and pleomorphic cells arranged in vague fascicles (A) or haphazardly (B) around curvilinear vessels. B shows a greater degree of nuclear atypia.

Perhaps the most difficult distinction is from *low-grade fibromyxoid sarcoma* (Table 10-7), which is also discussed in this chapter. Clinically, this tumor occurs in young patients and has a tendency for multiple recurrences, with a risk of metastasis if the lesion is incompletely excised. Histologically, it is composed of cytologically bland spindle cells arranged in a whorled pattern in a variably myxoid and fibrous stroma. In contrast, myxofibrosarcoma is always predominantly myxoid, and the cells show more cytologic atypia than those found in low-grade fibromyxoid sarcoma. Detection of a *FUS* translocation is a strong confirmatory finding for low-grade fibromyxoid sarcoma.

Discussion

It can be challenging to cull through the literature on myxofibrosarcoma in an attempt to determine the true behavior of low-grade lesions, because many studies have grouped lesions of different grades, and precise boundaries between these grades are often vague. Nevertheless, it is clear from these older studies that the clinical behavior of the spectrum of myxofibrosarcoma is closely related to the tumor grade. For example, Merck et al.[205] found the risk of local recurrence to be 38%, 48%, 51%, and 61% for grade 1, 2, 3, and 4 tumors, respectively. In contrast, in the study by Mentzel et al.,[206] the rate of local recurrence was independent of histologic grade, because 6 of 12 (50%) low-grade lesions recurred; one patient developed 8 recurrences (Table 10-8). Two subcutaneous low-grade lesions recurred as higher-grade lesions with increased cellularity, nuclear pleomorphism, and mitotic activity. Adequate initial surgical therapy is necessary to limit the rate of local recurrence and the subsequent risk of histologic progression. The risk of metastasis is minimal for pure low-grade tumors. In the study by Merck et al.,[205] although 35% of patients developed metastases, none of the eight patients with grade 1 tumors did so. Similarly, Angervall et al.[200] found that no patient with a grade 1 tumor developed metastatic disease, although two of seven patients with grade 2 tumors eventually did so (Tables 10-9 and 10-10).

Huang et al.[219] evaluated 49 myxofibrosarcomas of varying grades treated and followed up at a single institution. With a

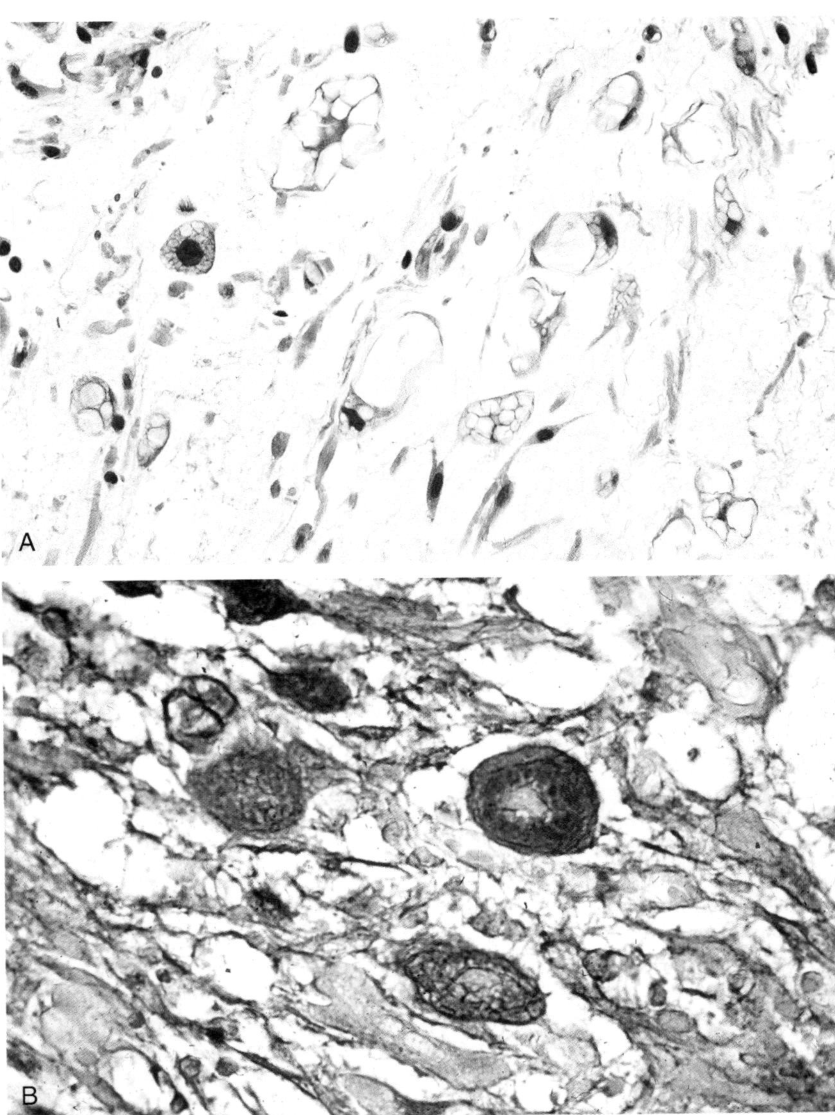

FIGURE 10-45. Pseudolipoblasts in a myxofibrosarcoma. Tumor cells become distended with hyaluronic acid and resemble lipoblasts. Note, however, that the vacuoles are ill-defined and do not cause the sharp indentation of the nucleus seen in true lipoblasts (A). Vacuoles stain positively for hyaluronic acid with Alcian blue (B).

TABLE 10-7 Distinction of Low-Grade Fibromyxoid Sarcoma from Myxofibrosarcoma

FEATURE	LGFMS	MYXOFIBROSARCOMA
Peak age	Young to middle age	Elderly
Depth	Skeletal muscle	Subcutaneous tissue
Stroma	Alternating myxoid and fibrous	Usually uniformly myxoid
Atypia	Absent to minimal	More prominent

LGFMS, low-grade fibromyxoid sarcoma.

TABLE 10-8 Relation Between Histologic Grade and Rate of Local Recurrence for Myxofibrosarcoma

	LOCAL RECURRENCE			
Study	Grade 1	Grade 2	Grade 3	Grade 4
Mentzel et al.[206]*	6/12 (50%)	9/13 (69%)	18/33 (55%)	
Angervall et al.[200]	0/2	2/7 (29%)	6/10 (60%)	7/11 (64%)
Merck et al.[205]	3/8 (38%)	13/27 (48%)	21/41 (51%)	17/28 (61%)

*Used only a three-grade scale.

TABLE 10-9 Relation Between Histologic Grade and Rate of Metastasis for Myxofibrosarcoma

	METASTASIS			
Study	Grade 1	Grade 2	Grade 3	Grade 4
Mentzel et al.[206]*	0/12	5/13 (38%)	10/34 (29%)	
Angervall et al.[200]	0/2	2/7 (29%)	2/11 (18%)	3/11 (27%)
Merck et al.[205]	0/8	6/28 (21%)	21/45 (47%)	11/29 (38%)

*Used only a three-grade scale.

TABLE 10-10 Rates of Local Recurrence and Metastasis for Grade 1 (Low-Grade) Myxofibrosarcoma

STUDY	RECURRENCE	METASTASIS
Mentzel et al.[206]	6/12 (50%)	0/12
Angervall et al.[200]*	0/2	0/2
Merck et al.[205]*	3/8 (38%)	0/8

*Used a four-grade scale; data include only tumors designated as grade 1.

median follow-up period of 55 months, local recurrence and distant metastases were detected in 28 (57%) and 7 (14%) patients, respectively. Only one patient developed metastasis without having had a prior local recurrence. The 5-year recurrence-free survival, metastasis-free survival, and disease-specific mortality rates were 41%, 90%, and 4.4%, respectively. Tumor size larger than 5 cm, tumor necrosis, and <75% myxoid areas were significantly associated with disease-specific mortality, the former two factors being the most predictive of metastasis. There are no large clinicopathologic studies that have evaluated the clinical behavior of only low-grade myxofibrosarcoma.

Fibrosarcoma, Fibromyxoid Type (Low-Grade Fibromyxoid Sarcoma/Hyalinizing Spindle Cell Tumor with Giant Rosettes)

The low-grade fibromyxoid sarcoma was first recognized by Evans[220] in 1987, when he reported bland fibromyxoid neoplasms arising in the deep soft tissue of two young women. Although initially diagnosed as benign, both tumors eventually metastasized; subsequent reports have verified the metastatic potential of this histologically deceptive neoplasm. Although there was a great deal of skepticism as to whether this tumor was a specific entity, subsequent clinicopathologic, cytogenetic, and molecular genetic studies have confirmed this lesion as a distinct variant of fibrosarcoma. This sarcoma is probably more common than the literature would lead one to believe because some have undoubtedly been diagnosed as myxofibrosarcoma, low-grade myxoid sarcoma, not otherwise specified, or a variety of other benign or malignant fibrous or myxoid neoplasms.

Hyalinizing spindle cell tumor with giant rosettes is an unusual fibrous tumor of deep soft tissues first delineated in 1997 by Lane et al.[221] in a series of 19 cases. Since its initial description, many reports have noted the histologic and molecular genetic overlap with low-grade fibromyxoid sarcoma, and there is now irrefutable evidence to support the contention that this tumor represents a variant of the latter.[222,223]

Clinical Findings

Most patients with low-grade fibromyxoid sarcoma are young to middle-aged adults, but this tumor may arise in patients as young as 3 years and as old as 78 years.[223] Males are affected more commonly than females. The usual presentation is that of a slowly growing, painless, deep soft tissue mass that ranges from 1 to 18 cm in greatest diameter, although most are 8 to 10 cm. The tumor most commonly arises in the deep soft tissue of the lower extremities, particularly the thigh, followed, in decreasing order of frequency, by the chest wall/axilla, shoulder region, inguinal region, buttock, and neck. Rare cases have also been described in unusual sites, including the prostate,[224] mediastinum,[225] gastrointestinal tract,[226] and perineum,[227] although there are rare reports of this tumor at virtually every site.

Similarly, most patients with hyalinizing spindle cell tumor with giant rosettes are in their third or fourth decade of life, and men are affected twice as often as women. The overlapping clinical features and anatomic sites of involvement with low-grade fibromyxoid sarcoma are further evidence that these neoplasms are related.

Pathologic Findings

Most examples of low-grade fibromyxoid sarcoma arise in the skeletal muscle, although some appear to be centered in the subcutaneous tissue, with minimal or no muscle involvement. Occasionally, these tumors can be more superficially located and involve the dermis.[228,229] Although typically grossly well circumscribed, there is often extensive microscopic infiltration into the surrounding soft tissues. On a cut section, the tumor often has a yellow-white appearance with focal areas with a glistening appearance secondary to the accumulation of myxoid ground substance; some exhibit cystic degeneration.

Histologically, low-grade fibromyxoid sarcoma is of low or moderate cellularity and is composed of bland spindle-shaped cells with small hyperchromatic oval nuclei, finely clumped chromatin, and one to several small nucleoli. The cells have indistinct pale eosinophilic cytoplasm and show only mild nuclear pleomorphism with little mitotic activity. The cells are deposited in a fibrous and myxoid stroma that tends to vary in different areas of the tumor (Figs. 10-46 to 10-48). In general, the lesions appear more fibrous than myxoid. The myxoid zones may abut abruptly with the fibrous zones, or there may be a gradual transition between these areas. Cells with a stellate configuration are often present in the myxoid zones, and they are generally arranged in a whorled or random fashion (Figs. 10-49 and 10-50). There is often a prominent network of curvilinear and branching capillary-sized blood vessels in the myxoid zones, somewhat reminiscent (although thicker walled) of that seen in myxoid liposarcoma (Figs. 10-51 and 10-52), sometimes with perivascular hypercellularity. Epithelioid cells may also be present focally, and there are areas of intermediate-grade fibrosarcoma in about 15% to 20% of cases.[223] As mentioned previously in the chapter, some cases have foci that are indistinguishable from sclerosing epithelioid fibrosarcoma.[190]

Although this neoplasm is characterized by a deceptively bland appearance, recurrences may show areas of increased cellularity and mitotic activity, sometimes with the formation of hypercellular nodules (Fig. 10-53).[230-232] Evans[233] reported one case that progressed to a neoplasm composed of sheets of anaplastic round cells 30 years after the initial excision. Rare cases have been reviewed that show areas of transition to a high-grade pleomorphic spindle cell sarcoma. In most cases, recurrences and metastases resemble the primary lesions, although there is a known case in which the metastasis had a predominantly primitive round cell appearance.

Cases previously diagnosed as hyalinizing spindle cell tumor with giant rosettes are characterized by the presence of a variable number of large rosette-like structures that merge abruptly or imperceptibly with a spindle cell tumor that looks indistinguishable from typical low-grade fibromyxoid sarcoma. The rosettes, which tend to cluster together, are composed of a central core of brightly eosinophilic birefringent collagen arranged centrifugally from the center surrounded by rounded to ovoid cells that have clear to eosinophilic cytoplasm and little to no nuclear atypia or mitotic activity (Figs. 10-54 to 10-59). Occasional cells show intranuclear cytoplasmic inclusions (Fig. 10-60). Other features include the presence of hemosiderin deposition, cystic degeneration, calcification, osseous and chondroid metaplasia, and peripheral chronic

Text continued on p. 330

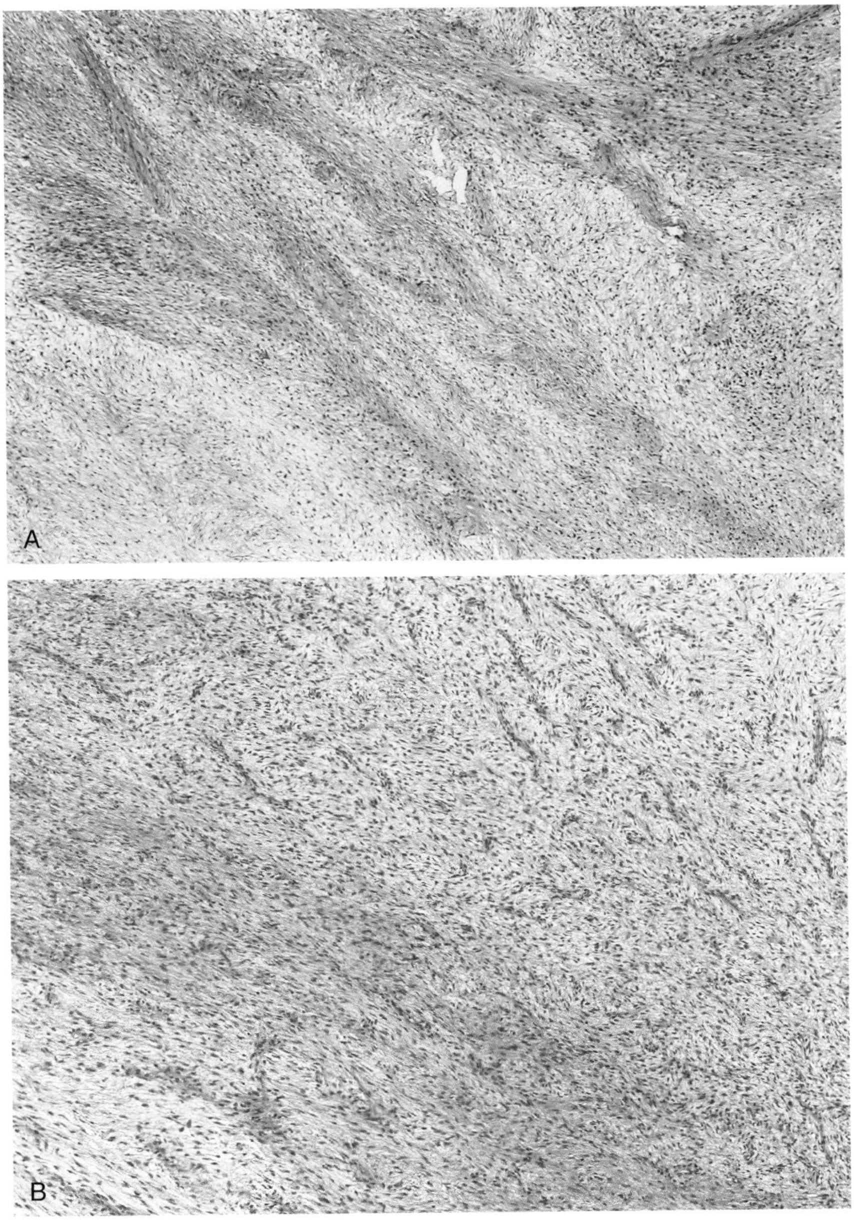

FIGURE 10-46. (A) Low-grade fibromyxoid sarcoma. At low power, alternating areas with a fibrous and myxoid stroma are apparent. (B) Medium power view of alternating myxoid and fibrous zones of a low-grade fibromyxoid sarcoma.

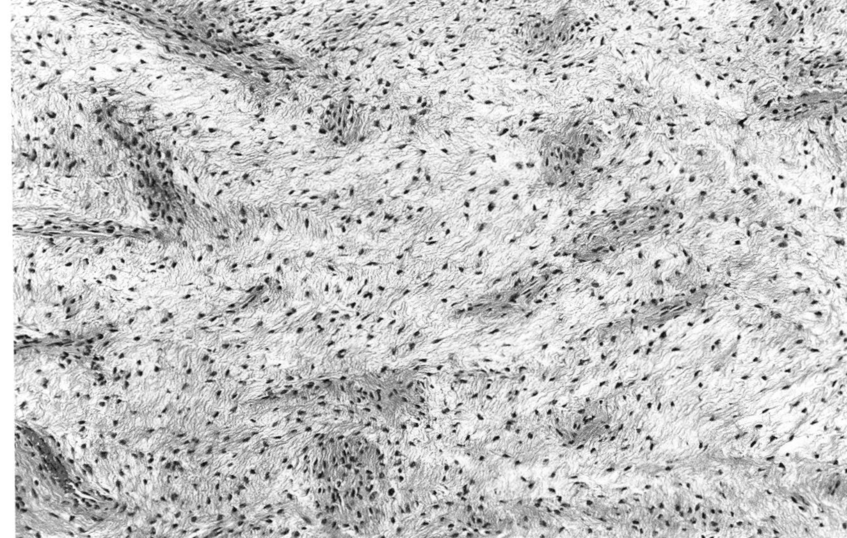

FIGURE 10-47. Low-grade fibromyxoid sarcoma with alternating fibrous and myxoid areas. The cells commonly show a whorled pattern of growth.

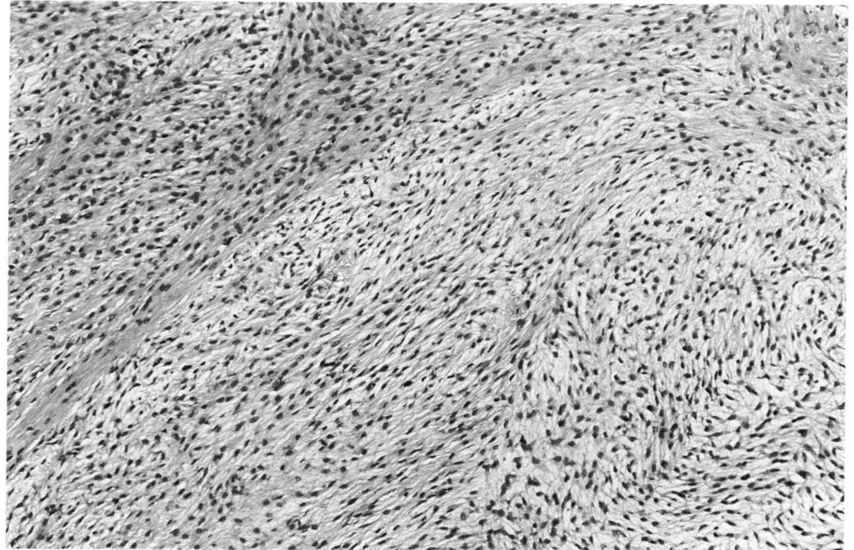

FIGURE 10-48. Junction between fibrous and myxoid zones in low-grade fibromyxoid sarcoma.

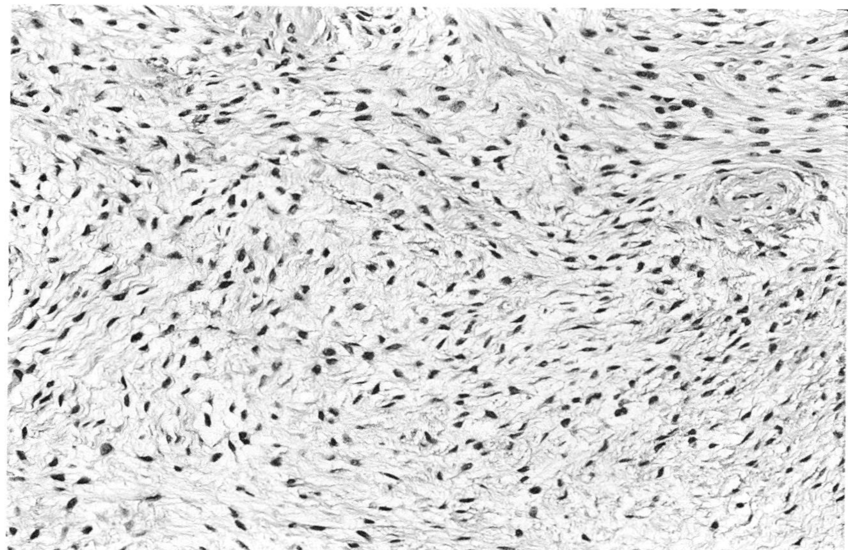

FIGURE 10-49. Myxoid zone of low-grade fibromyxoid sarcoma. The lesion is of low cellularity and composed of bland spindle-shaped cells.

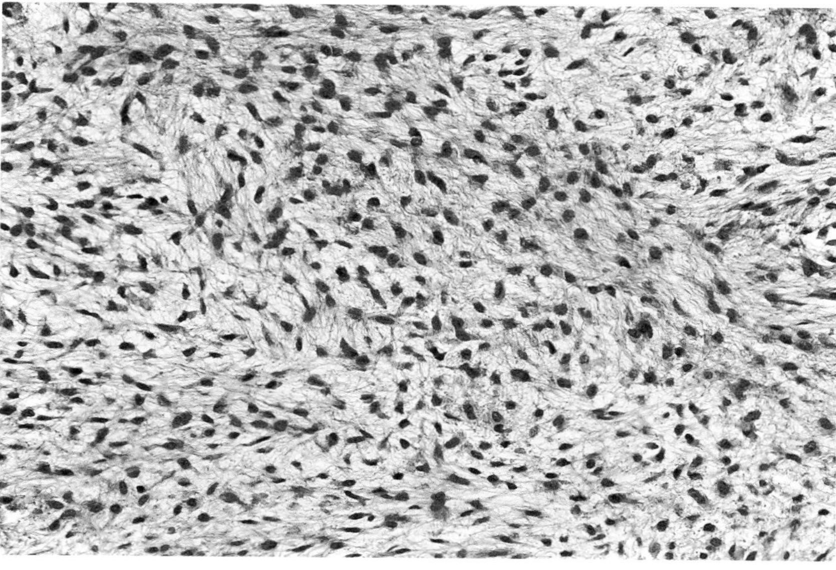

FIGURE 10-50. More cellular area of a low-grade fibromyxoid sarcoma. The cells have a stellate appearance and are evenly distributed within a fibromyxoid stroma.

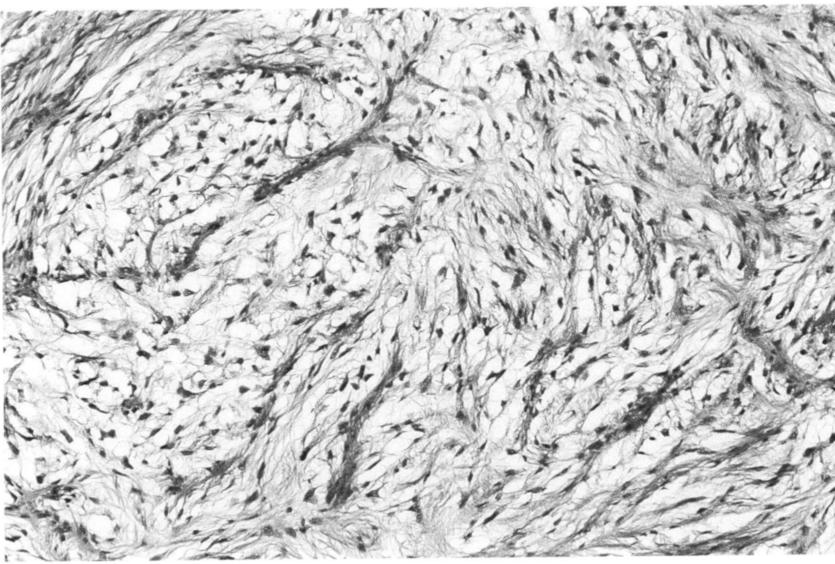

FIGURE 10-51. Low-grade fibromyxoid sarcoma showing a prominent network of branching capillary-sized blood vessels reminiscent of myxoid liposarcoma.

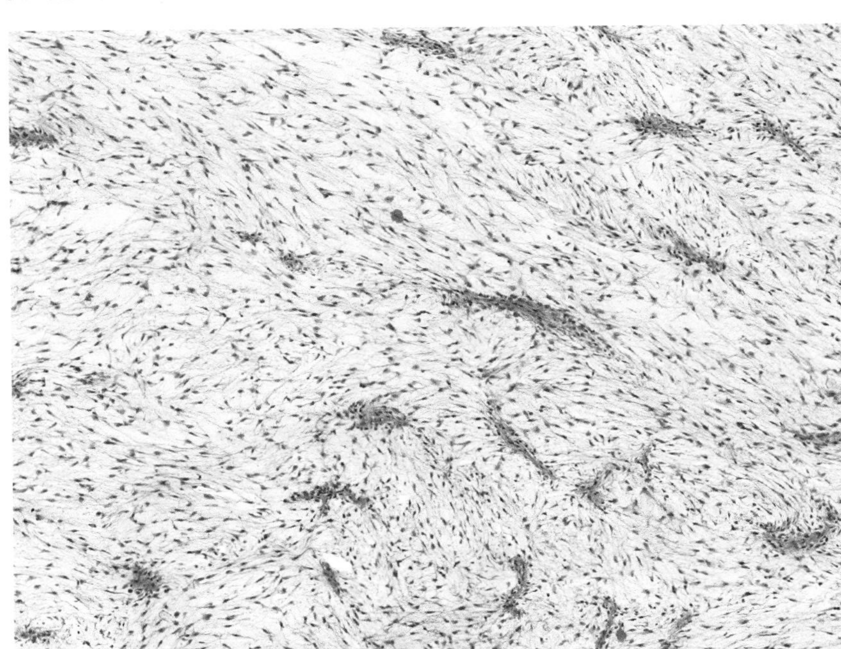

FIGURE 10-52. Prominent blood vessels and low-grade cytology in a low-grade fibromyxoid sarcoma.

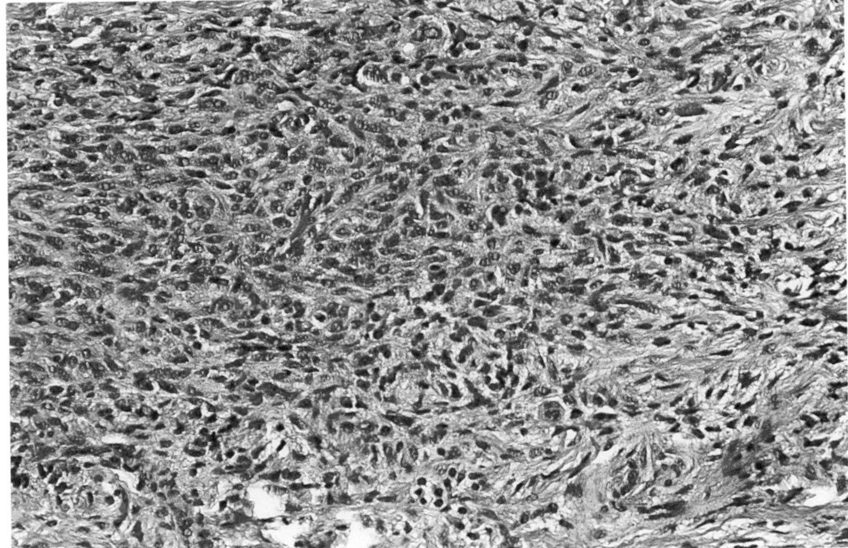

FIGURE 10-53. Recurrent low-grade fibromyxoid sarcoma showing an area of increased cellularity and nuclear pleomorphism.

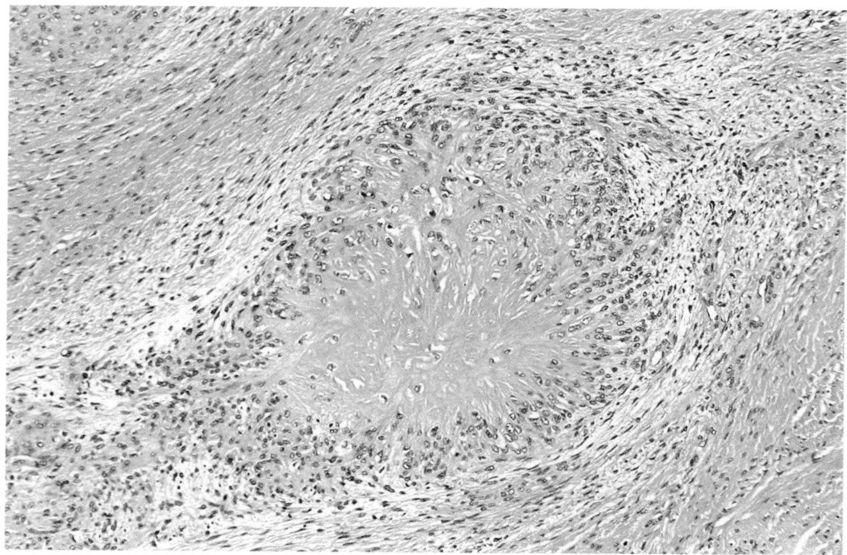

FIGURE 10-54. Hyalinizing spindle cell tumor with giant rosettes. The most characteristic feature is the presence of large collagen rosettes.

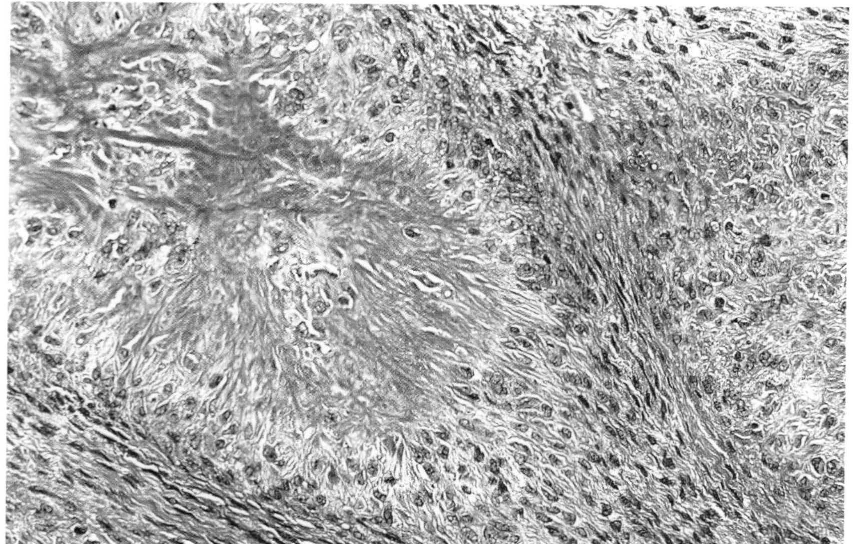

FIGURE 10-55. Trichrome stain of collagen rosette in a case of hyalinizing spindle cell tumor demonstrating that the central eosinophilic portion of the rosette is composed of collagen.

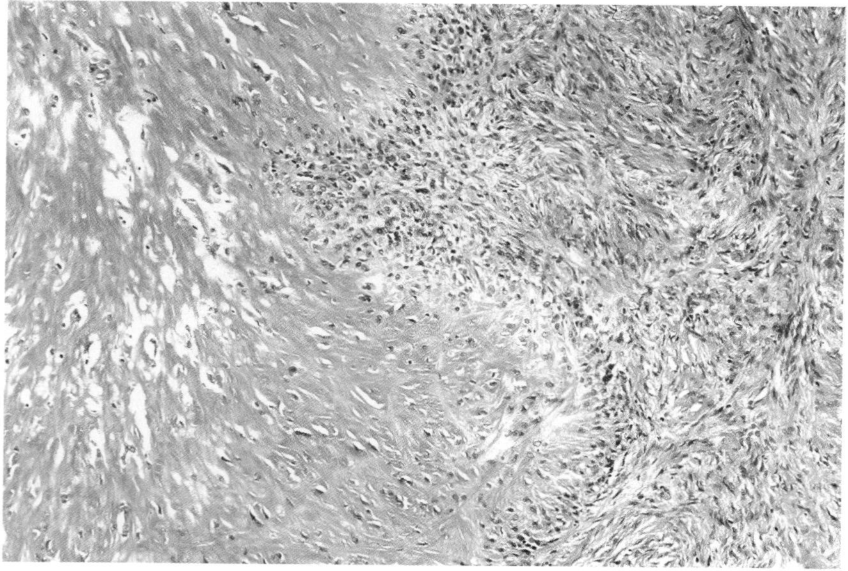

FIGURE 10-56. Hyalinizing spindle cell tumor with giant rosettes showing transition between a collagen rosette and a more cellular fibrosarcoma-like area.

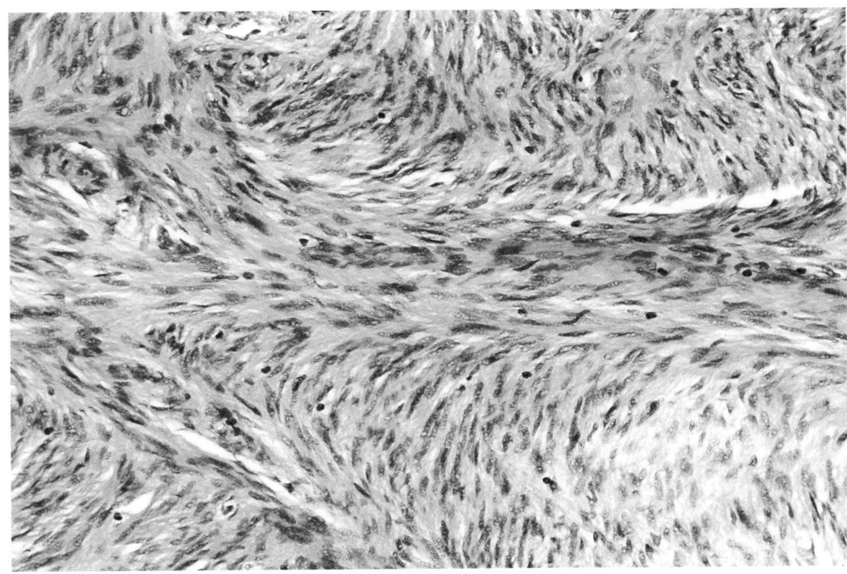

FIGURE 10-57. Fibrosarcoma-like area in a case of hyalinizing spindle cell tumor with giant rosettes. The cells are arranged into irregular crisscrossing fascicles.

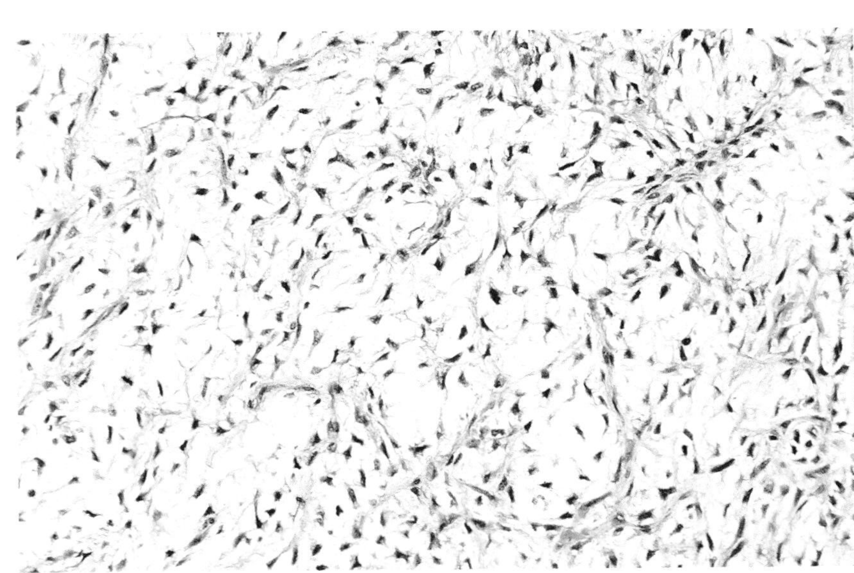

FIGURE 10-58. Myxoid zone of hyalinizing spindle cell tumor with giant rosettes. The neoplastic cells are widely separated by myxoid stroma, and a plexiform vasculature is apparent.

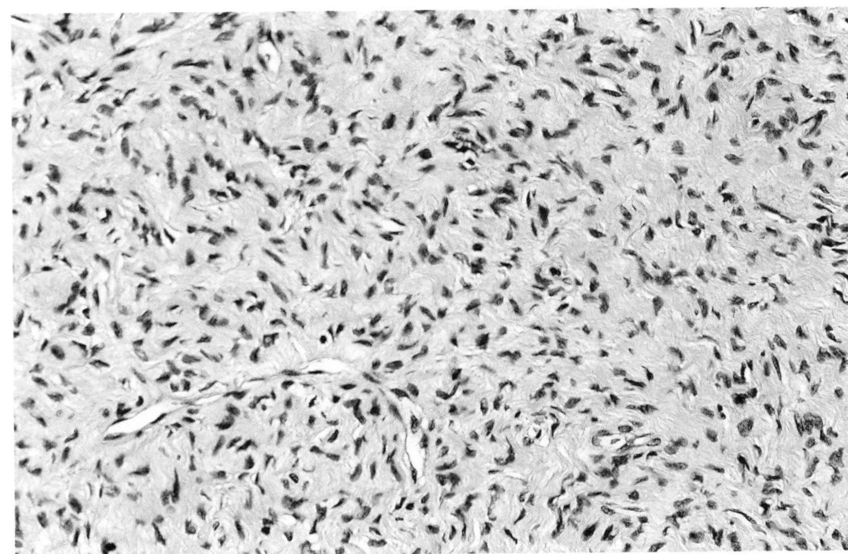

FIGURE 10-59. Hyalinizing spindle cell tumor with giant rosettes. Spindled stroma shows greater cellularity than that in Figure 10-58. Cells have an irregular wavy shape somewhat reminiscent of cells in neurofibroma.

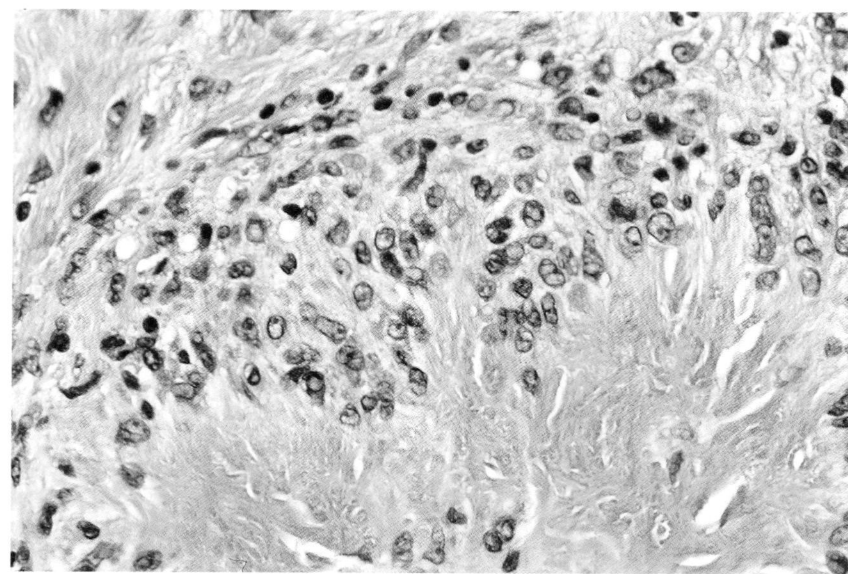

FIGURE 10-60. Rounded cells comprising the periphery of a rosette in a case of hyalinizing spindle cell tumor with giant rosettes. A few of the cells have intranuclear cytoplasmic inclusions.

inflammation.[234,235] At this point, these lesions are diagnosed as simply low-grade fibromyxoid sarcoma with collagen rosettes.

Immunohistochemical Findings

Immunohistochemically, the neoplastic cells in low-grade fibromyxoid sarcoma may show focal immunoreactivity for muscle markers, including smooth muscle actin, muscle-specific actin, and desmin, but most cases are negative for these antigens. Other markers that are usually negative include CD34, S-100 protein, and cytokeratins, although a proportion of the rounded cells in those cases with collagen rosettes can stain for S-100 protein. In a large series of molecularly proven tumors, Guillou et al.[236] found the majority of these tumors to express EMA, CD99, and BCL2. More recently, Doyle et al.[237] found consistent expression of MUC4, a transmembrane glycoprotein that plays a role in cell growth signaling pathways. In this study, all 49 low-grade fibromyxoid sarcomas, including 3 with epithelioid morphology and 3 with collagen rosettes (all *FUS* gene rearrangement positive by FISH), showed strong and diffuse expression of this antigen. Aside from 30% of monophasic synovial sarcomas, all other tumors in the differential diagnosis that were tested were negative for this marker (including 40 soft tissue perineuriomas, 40 myxofibrosarcomas, 20 cellular myxomas, 20 solitary fibrous tumors, 20 neurofibromas, and 20 desmoid fibromatoses). Finally, it should be noted that these tumors may also express claudin1, which may cause confusion with soft tissue perineurioma, especially because both tumors often express EMA.[238]

Cytogenetic and Molecular Genetic Findings

Cytogenetically, early studies of low-grade fibromyxoid sarcoma revealed evidence of a supernumerary ring chromosome containing material from chromosomes 7 and 16.[239,240] Subsequently, studies confirmed the presence of a characteristic translocation involving the *FUS* gene on chromosome 7 and the *CREB3L2* gene on chromosome 16.[241,242] This same translocation was subsequently identified in hyalinizing spindle cell tumor with giant rosettes, supporting the identity of these two tumors.[243] Mertens et al.[244] reported the presence of a *FUS-CREB3L2* fusion in 22 of 23 (96%) cases of low-grade fibromyxoid sarcoma; none of the other fibrous or myxoid neoplasms tested showed evidence of this fusion transcript, supporting the sensitivity and specificity of this translocation. Matsuyama et al.[245] found evidence of a *FUS-CREB3L2* fusion in 14 of 16 (88%) cases of low-grade fibromyxoid sarcoma using a DNA-based polymerase chain reaction (PCR) on formalin-fixed, paraffin-embedded tissue. FISH is found to be a more sensitive technique than PCR-based assays for detecting this aberration.[246] A fixed, paraffin-embedded tissue is used with a break-apart probe for the *FUS* gene to support this diagnosis, which can be difficult to make on morphologic and immunohistochemical grounds, particularly in a small biopsy specimen. It should be noted that a small subgroup showed evidence of a t(11;16) resulting in a *FUS-CREB3L1* fusion.[236]

Differential Diagnosis

The differential diagnosis of low-grade fibromyxoid sarcoma includes numerous benign and malignant soft tissue lesions characterized by a variably fibrous and myxoid stroma. *Myxoid neurofibroma* is composed of cells with more slender and wavy nuclei that consistently express S-100 protein. *Perineurioma* may resemble the fibrous whorled areas seen in low-grade fibromyxoid sarcoma. Given the overlap in immunoprofiles with EMA and claudin1, molecular assays may be necessary, in some cases, to distinguish between these two entities. Some areas of low-grade fibromyxoid sarcoma may resemble *nodular fasciitis*, but the latter lesion is characterized by cells that resemble tissue culture fibroblasts. Other features of fasciitis, such as cleft-like spaces, extravasation of erythrocytes, and the presence of multinucleated giant cells, are not found in low-grade fibromyxoid sarcoma. Occasionally, *cellular myxoma* can resemble low-grade fibromyxoid sarcoma. However, the lesion lacks the abrupt transition between fibrous and myxoid zones and lacks evidence of a *FUS* translocation. *Desmoid fibromatoses* are composed of nuclei that tend to be plumper and more vesicular and are arranged in a fascicular growth pattern. The cells consistently show nuclear β-catenin staining. The *myxoid variant of DFSP* may resemble the myxoid zones of low-grade fibromyxoid sarcoma. Given that low-grade fibromyxoid sarcoma can arise in a superficial location, the distinction between these tumors can be challenging. However, the cells of DFSP are arranged in a monotonous storiform pattern, consistently stain for CD34, and lack *FUS* rearrangements.

Malignant peripheral nerve sheath tumors may contain myxoid foci, but the cells are more elongated or wavy, are typically arranged in an irregular fascicular growth pattern, and stain for S-100 protein in up to 60% of cases. *Spindle cell liposarcoma* usually arises in the subcutaneous tissue of adults and always contains an atypical lipomatous component that includes the presence of lipoblasts. The myxoid zones of low-grade fibromyxoid sarcoma may also resemble *myxoid liposarcoma*, particularly the cases with a well-developed plexiform vascular pattern. However, low-grade fibromyxoid sarcoma lacks lipoblasts, and adequate sampling always reveals fibrous areas. Cytogenetically, myxoid liposarcoma is characterized by t(12;16)(q13;p11). Like low-grade fibromyxoid sarcoma, aberrations of the *FUS* gene on 16p11 are characteristic. Therefore, a strategy to assess for *DDIT3* rearrangements by FISH is used because this rearrangement is found in myxoid liposarcoma only, not in low-grade fibromyxoid sarcoma.

The lesion with which low-grade fibromyxoid sarcoma is most easily confused is *myxofibrosarcoma.* Unlike low-grade fibromyxoid sarcoma, which typically arises in the skeletal muscle of young patients, myxofibrosarcoma commonly arises in the subcutaneous tissues of the extremities of elderly patients. Histologically, myxofibrosarcoma is uniformly myxoid, lacks alternating fibrous zones, and always has a greater degree of nuclear pleomorphism and hyperchromasia.

Those cases that have collagen rosettes may be confused with other tumors with collagen-containing rosettes, including *neuroblastoma-like neurilemmoma*, in which the rosettes are made up of a core of collagen flanked by small, rounded, differentiated S-100 protein-positive Schwann cells. Rare cases of *osteosarcoma* have been reported to contain similar rosettes, but, in these cases, the central core is composed of an osteoid-like material, often with central calcification, and surrounded by cells with more nuclear pleomorphism than those encountered in the hyalinizing spindle cell tumor.

Discussion

Although originally considered distinctive entities, low-grade fibromyxoid sarcoma and hyalinizing spindle cell tumor with giant rosettes are now regarded as part of a histologic spectrum. The reasons for believing them to be the same are as follows: similarity in age and location, virtual identity of the spindled stroma (Fig. 10-61), including the occasional presence of intermediate-grade fibrosarcoma and the presence of the same characteristic translocation [t(7;16)].

Despite its deceptively bland histologic appearance, low-grade fibromyxoid sarcoma was originally thought to have a high rate of local, often repeated recurrence as well as pulmonary metastases in a significant percentage of cases. Before 2000, approximately 65% of cases reported in the literature had locally recurred 6 months to 50 years after initial excision, with many patients developing multiple recurrences. In fact, Evans[233] reported one case in which the patient developed 17 recurrences over a 29-year period. Metastases were reported to be present at the time of initial excision or developed late in the clinical course. Evans[232] described another case that metastasized 45 years after the initial presentation. The lung has been involved in virtually all cases with metastatic disease.

In 2000, Folpe et al.[223] reported the clinicopathologic features of 73 cases of low-grade fibromyxoid sarcoma with and without rosettes. Follow-up information was obtained in 54 cases, with a median follow-up period of 24 months. Of this group, five patients developed local recurrences, three developed metastatic disease, and only one patient died as a direct result of the tumor. Importantly, the diagnosis of low-grade fibromyxoid sarcoma was made prospectively in 51 patients, and none of these patients developed metastatic disease. Therefore, the significantly better prognosis in this study compared with prior studies was felt to reflect that all were initially diagnosed as sarcomas and treated with aggressive surgery. This is in stark contrast to patients reported in the earlier

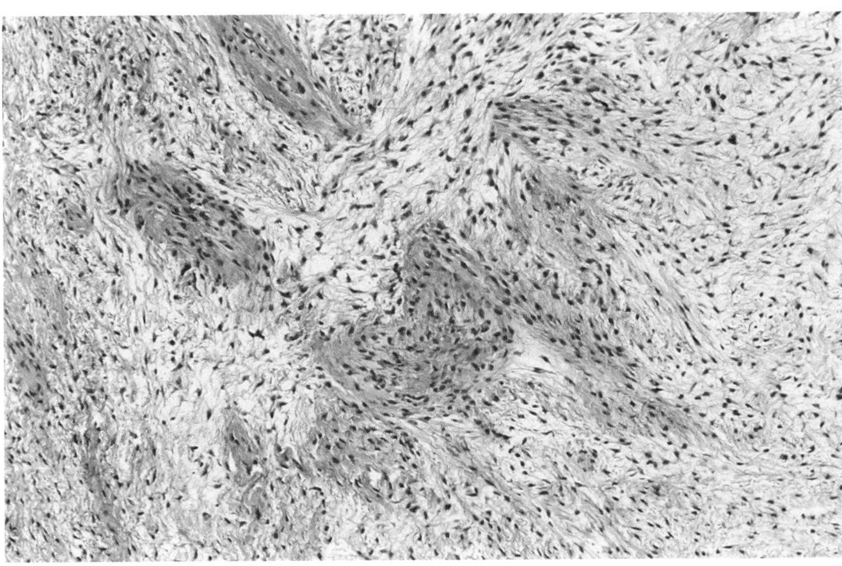

FIGURE 10-61. Alternating fibrous and myxoid zones in a hyalinizing spindle cell tumor with giant rosettes. Such zones are reminiscent of low-grade fibromyxoid sarcoma.

studies, most of whom were originally diagnosed with and treated for a benign neoplasm.

Recently, Evans[232] reported a series of 33 cases with at least 5 years of clinical follow-up. In contrast to the results reported by Folpe et al.,[223] 14 of 33 (42%) patients ultimately died of tumor from 3 to 42 years after initial excision (median, 15 years). Twenty-one (64%) patients had local recurrences, and 15 (45%) patients developed metastases, mostly to the lungs and pleura, some up to 45 years after initial diagnosis. Except for the presence of dedifferentiation, no histologic features correlated with tumor behavior or patient survival. Evans did emphasize the generally short follow-up period in prior studies, suggesting that only studies with long-term follow-up could give a true indication of clinical behavior. Therefore, this tumor is best treated with wide excision and long-term clinical follow-up.

Fibrosarcomatous Change Arising in Dermatofibrosarcoma Protuberans

Up to 10% of cases of DFSP have fascicular areas of increased cellularity, nuclear pleomorphism, and mitotic activity, and resemble conventional soft tissue fibrosarcoma. The significance of fibrosarcomatous change in DFSP is discussed in greater detail in Chapter 12.

Postradiation Fibrosarcoma

Although high-grade pleomorphic sarcomas are by far the most common postradiation sarcoma, there is clearly a higher incidence of fibrosarcoma in patients who have been exposed to radiation than in the general population. There are numerous reports in which a fibrosarcoma originated at the site of therapeutic irradiation for various benign and malignant neoplasms[247,248] and for non-neoplastic disorders such as psoriasis and hypertrichosis.[101]

The latency period between irradiation and tumor development is of significance when evaluating these cases. The tumor usually develops 4 to 15 years following irradiation, although periods as short as 15 months have been reported.[249] Tumors appearing less than 2 years following irradiation are unlikely to be radiation-induced. Opinions vary as to the significance of the radiation dose for tumor development, and both small and large doses have been implicated as being more likely to produce radiation-related neoplasms. In general, the prognosis for patients developing postradiation fibrosarcoma is poor because most patients die within 2 years of the development of the tumor. Rearrangements of the *RET* oncogene have been implicated in the development of postradiation fibrosarcoma.[250]

Fibrosarcoma Arising in Burn Scars

Although less common than postradiation fibrosarcoma, there are rare cases of fibrosarcoma arising in scars formed at sites of thermal injury. Nearly all of the affected patients have suffered extensive burns as children and developed tumors after an interval of 30 years or more.[251,252] Carcinomas are more common than sarcomas as a late sequence of thermal injury (Marjolin ulcer) and usually develop after a 30- to 40-year latent period.[253] Immunohistochemical analysis with cytokeratins (including high-molecular-weight cytokeratins) and p63 are useful for excluding the possibility of a desmoplastic or spindle cell carcinoma before rendering a diagnosis of fibrosarcoma arising in a burn scar.

Low-Grade Myofibroblastic Sarcoma (Myofibrosarcoma)

As mentioned earlier in the chapter, scattered cells in typical cases of adult-type fibrosarcoma may stain for smooth muscle or muscle-specific actin, and ultrastructural data support the presence of cells with myofibroblastic differentiation in otherwise typical fibrosarcoma. The issue as to whether there are sarcomas composed predominantly or exclusively of myofibroblasts remains a contentious one, primarily because the diagnostic criteria for recognizing such tumors remain obscure. Schürch et al.[254] and Lagacé et al.[255] contended that benign and malignant neoplasms composed of myofibroblasts reported in the literature lack specific myofibroblastic features. According to these authors, myofibroblasts can be recognized by only the ultrastructural identification of stress fibers, well-developed microtendons (fibronexus), and intercellular intermediate-type, end-gap junctions.[256] Because of the heterogeneous immunophenotype of myofibroblasts with regard to intermediate filaments and actin isoforms, these authors argued that categorizing a cell as a myofibroblast by its immunohistochemical staining pattern alone is imprecise.[255] Others have argued that myofibroblastic sarcomas are recognizable even in the absence of the aforementioned ultrastructural features.[257-259] Myofibroblastic sarcomas do exist but are uncommon. Although one may suspect a myofibrosarcoma on the basis of routine morphology, confirmation of myofibroblastic differentiation requires at least supportive immunohistochemical analysis. Because high-grade myofibroblastic sarcomas likely get grouped with other high-grade pleomorphic sarcomas or so-called MFH,[260,261] this discussion will focus on low-grade myofibrosarcomas.

Clinical Findings

Low-grade myofibrosarcoma can arise in patients of virtually any age, but the peak incidence is in the fourth decade of life, and there is a slight predilection for males. In the study by Mentzel et al.[262] describing 18 such tumors (5 of which had supportive ultrastructural findings), these tumors occurred in 10 men and 7 women between 19 and 72 years. In the study of 15 cases of myofibrosarcoma reported by Montgomery et al.,[263] the tumors arose in 11 men and 4 women ages 33 to 73 years, with a median age of 54 years. Most patients present with a slowly enlarging, painless mass with tumor size ranging from 1.5 to 12 cm. The most common site of involvement is the head and neck region (especially the oral cavity and tongue),[264,265] followed by the extremities and trunk.[262,263] Rare cases involving the breast,[266] bone,[267] and abdominal cavity[268] have also been described.

Pathologic Findings

Grossly, most tumors are firm and have a pale fibrous-appearing cut surface with ill-defined margins, although some are well circumscribed and have pushing margins.

Histologically, this tumor is characterized by a proliferation of spindled to stellate-shaped cells arranged into intersecting fascicles, sheets, or storiform whorls, with variable collagenous or myxoid stroma and scanty inflammation. Some tumors closely resemble nodular fasciitis (Figs. 10-62 to 10-64). The cells have ill-defined, pale eosinophilic cytoplasm. The nuclei are usually fusiform in shape, and most have an evenly dispersed chromatin pattern, although at least focal nuclear hyperchromasia is always seen. Mitotic activity is typically low, and necrosis is absent in low-grade lesions. The cells often infiltrate the surrounding soft tissue structures, an important feature that helps distinguish this lesion from a reactive process.

Immunohistochemical Findings

The cells usually show a delicate tram-track pattern of actin staining, especially with smooth muscle actin (Table 10-11). Fewer than 50% of cases express desmin, usually in a small percentage of cells.[259,263,269] These antigens can be expressed together or separately, but more commonly low-grade myofibrosarcoma reveals a smooth muscle actin-positive/desmin-negative immunophenotype. In addition, calponin is usually diffusely positive, whereas h-caldesmon shows only focal expression in occasional cases.[258] These immunophenotypic findings, which are quite similar to those of nodular fasciitis, are potentially useful in distinguishing low-grade myofibrosarcoma from leiomyosarcoma, which usually expresses both

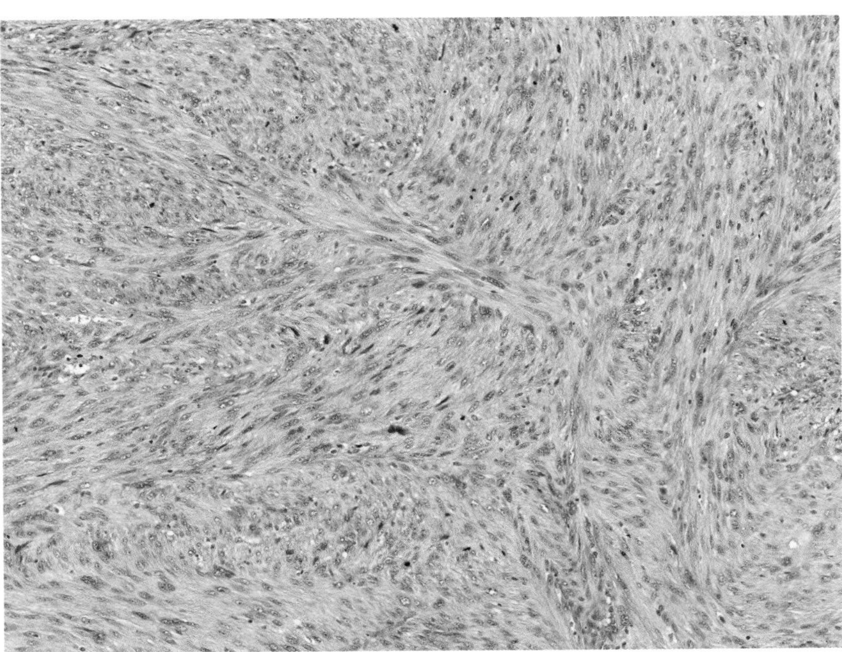

FIGURE 10-62. Myofibrosarcoma with short intersecting fascicles of spindled cells with palely eosinophilic cytoplasm.

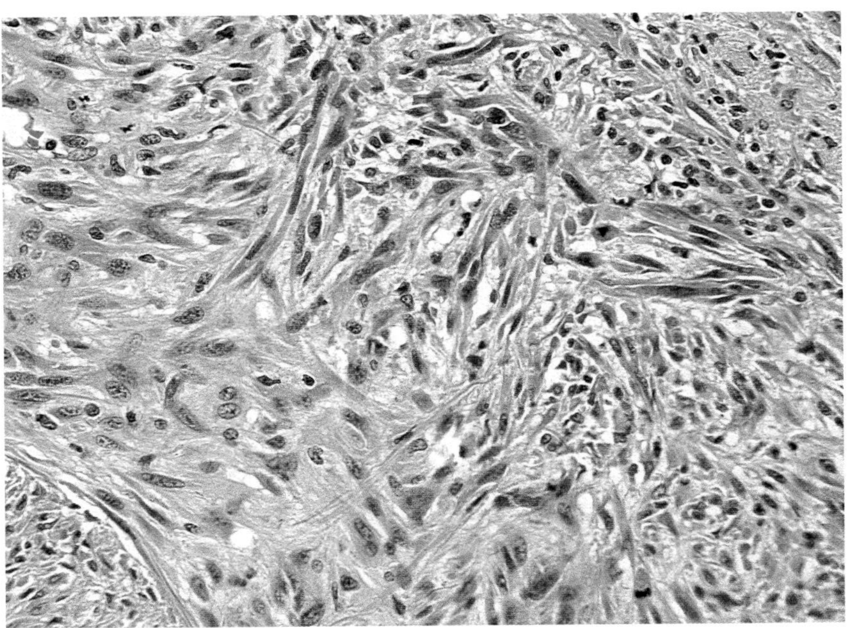

FIGURE 10-63. Myofibrosarcoma composed of spindled to stellate-shaped cells resembling nodular fasciitis. *(Case courtesy of Dr. Cyril Fisher, Royal Marsden Hospital, London, England.)*

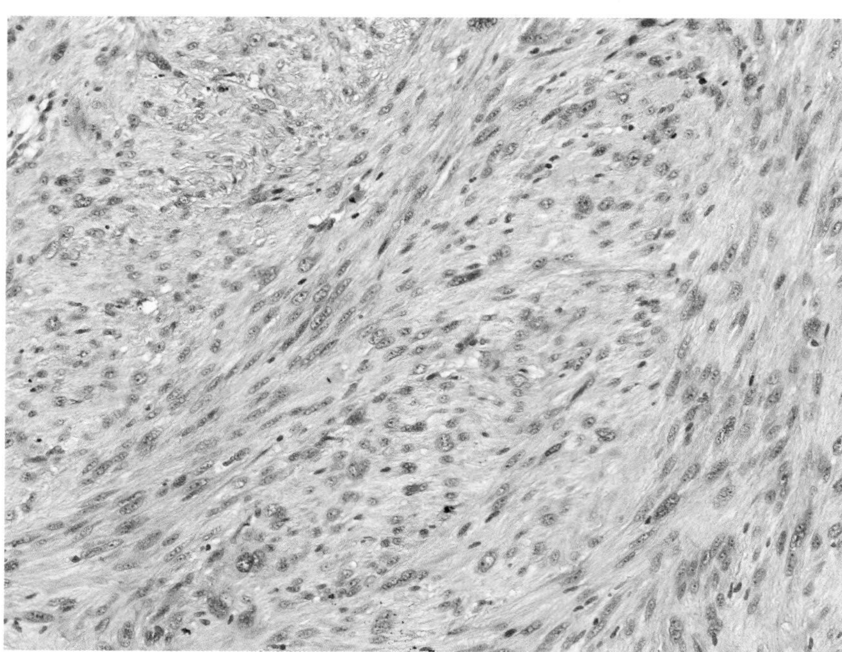

FIGURE 10-64. High-power view of myofibrosarcoma composed of plump spindled cells with palely eosinophilic cytoplasm and mild nuclear atypia.

TABLE 10-11 Immunophenotypic Features of Myofibrosarcoma Compared to Fibrosarcoma and Leiomyosarcoma

	MYOFIBROSARCOMA	FIBROSARCOMA	LEIOMYOSARCOMA
Desmin	±	−	+
Smooth muscle actin	+	±	+
Muscle-specific actin	±	−	+
Calponin	+	−	+
h-caldesmon	−	−	+

Modified from Fisher C. Myofibrosarcoma. Virchows Arch 2004;445(3):215–23.

calponin and h-caldesmon. Some low-grade myofibrosarcomas also express fibronectin but not collagen IV or laminin.[268] The neoplastic cells are typically negative for S-100 protein, CD34, CD99, ALK, epithelial markers, and myogenin. Ultrastructurally, the neoplastic cells show myofibroblastic features, including fibronexus junctions.[270]

Cytogenetic and Molecular Genetic Findings

Given the difficulty in recognizing this tumor and the lack of uniformly accepted criteria, it is not surprising that very few examples of this tumor have been studied by cytogenetics. The few cases that have been studied have shown a moderate number of non-characteristic chromosomal aberrations and a far simpler karyotype than that typically seen in high-grade pleomorphic sarcomas.[271] Comparative genomic hybridization reveals a number of DNA copy number changes, including gains of 1p11, 12p12.2, and 5p13.2.[272]

Differential Diagnosis

Low-grade myofibrosarcoma can resemble reactive processes or benign myofibroblastic neoplasms on the one hand and spindle cell sarcomas on the other. Some cases very closely resemble *nodular fasciitis*, a reactive pseudosarcomatous proliferation that typically appears suddenly and grows rapidly. Nodular fasciitis rarely exceeds 5 cm and is most often located in the subcutis. Regional heterogeneity with zonation is a characteristic feature, and the constituent cells lack nuclear hyperchromasia. Invariably, low-grade myofibrosarcoma shows at least scattered hyperchromatic nuclei, which are not seen in nodular fasciitis. Any case of recurrent nodular fasciitis should engender reconsideration of that diagnosis, and such cases are sometimes better classified as low-grade myofibrosarcoma.

Leiomyosarcoma is also frequently a diagnostic consideration. However, leiomyosarcoma typically has alternating fascicles of cells that are less tapered and have blunt-ended nuclei with perinuclear vacuoles. The cells also have more densely eosinophilic fibrillar cytoplasm. Although the immunophenotype overlaps with that seen in low-grade myofibrosarcoma, leiomyosarcoma usually coexpresses calponin and h-caldesmon, whereas low-grade myofibrosarcoma does not express h-caldesmon. *Fibrosarcoma* is composed of more uniformly hyperchromatic and atypical cells arranged into longer sweeping fascicles with the characteristic herringbone growth pattern. At most, fibrosarcoma shows only focal myofibroblastic differentiation by immunohistochemistry.

Discussion

Low-grade myofibrosarcoma is usually an indolent tumor, although there is a propensity for local recurrence if the lesion is incompletely excised. Occasionally, the tumor can progress to a higher-grade sarcoma in a recurrence. Overall, approximately 33% of these tumors locally recur, and fewer than 10% have been reported to metastasize. In the study by Montgomery et al.,[263] four of nine grade 1 tumors recurred, as did three of four grade 2 tumors. However, many of these tumors were initially incompletely excised, and prospective studies of well-characterized tumors that have been appropriately treated have not been reported. In this same study, although none of the grade 1 tumors metastasized, one of four grade 2 tumors metastasized to the lungs. Others have confirmed the capacity of this tumor to metastasize.[273] Increased proliferative activity and necrosis may portend a more aggressive clinical behavior.[263] Surgery is the mainstay of therapy.[265] For those rare examples that are more superficially located, Mohs micrographic surgery seems to minimize the risk of local recurrence.[274]

References

1. Mankin HJ, Hornicek FJ, Springfield DS. Extra-abdominal desmoid tumors: a report of 234 cases. J Surg Oncol 2010;102(5):380–4.
2. Rock MG, Pritchard DJ, Reiman HM, et al. Extra-abdominal desmoid tumors. J Bone Joint Surg Am 1984;66(9):1369–74.
3. Pignatti G, Barbanti-Bròdano G, Ferrari D, et al. Extraabdominal desmoid tumor. A study of 83 cases. Clin Orthop Relat Res 2000;375:207–13.
4. Pritchard DJ, Nascimento AG, Petersen IA. Local control of extra-abdominal desmoid tumors. J Bone Joint Surg Am 1996;78(6):848–54.
5. Reitamo JJ, Scheinin TM, Häyry P. The desmoid syndrome. New aspects in the cause, pathogenesis and treatment of the desmoid tumor. Am J Surg 1986;151(2):230–7.
6. Häyry P, Reitamo JJ, Vihko R, et al. The desmoid tumor. III. A biochemical and genetic analysis. Am J Clin Pathol 1982;77(6):681–5.
7. Oka K, Yakushiji T, Sato H, et al. Usefulness of diffusion-weighted imaging for differentiating between desmoid tumors and malignant soft tissue tumors. J Magn Reson Imaging 2011;33(1):189–93.
8. Min R, Zun Z, Lizheng W, et al. Oral and maxillofacial desmoid-type fibromatoses in an eastern Chinese population: a report of 20 cases. Oral Surg Oral Med Oral Pathol Oral Radiol Endod 2011;111(3):340–5.
9. Sun G, Xu M, Huang X. Treatment of aggressive fibromatosis of the head and neck. J Craniofac Surg 2010;21(6):1831–3.
10. Kruse AL, Luebbers HT, Grätz KW, et al. Aggressive fibromatosis of the head and neck: a new classification based on a literature review over 40 years (1968-2008). Oral Maxillofac Surg 2010;14(4):227–32.
11. Abikhzer G, Bouganim N, Finesilver A. Aggressive fibromatosis of the head and neck: case report and review of the literature. J Otolaryngol 2005;34(4):289–94.
12. Sharma A, Ngan BY, Sándor GK, et al. Pediatric aggressive fibromatosis of the head and neck: a 20-year retrospective review. J Pediatr Surg 2008;43(9):1596–604.
13. Gnepp DR, Henley J, Weiss S, et al. Desmoid fibromatosis of the sinonasal tract and nasopharynx. A clinicopathologic study of 25 cases. Cancer 1996;78(12):2572–9.
14. Abbas AE, Deschamps C, Cassivi SD, et al. Chest-wall desmoid tumors: results of surgical intervention. Ann Thorac Surg 2004;78(4):1219–23; discussion 1219–23.
15. Brown CS, Jeffrey B, Korentager R, et al. Desmoid tumors of the bilateral breasts in a patient without Gardner syndrome: a case report and review of the literature. Ann Plast Surg 2012;69(2): 220–2.
16. Wagstaff MJ, Raurell A, Perks AG. Multicentric extra-abdominal desmoid tumours. Br J Plast Surg 2004;57(4):362–5.
17. Shimoyama T, Hiraoka K, Shoda T, et al. Multicentric extra-abdominal desmoid tumors arising in bilateral lower limbs. Rare Tumors 2010; 2(1):e12.
18. Fong Y, Rosen PP, Brennan MF. Multifocal desmoids. Surgery 1993; 114(5):902–6.
19. McDougall A, McGarrity G. Extra-abdominal desmoid tumours. J Bone Joint Surg Br 1979;61-B(3):373–7.
20. Enzinger FM, Shiraki M. Musculo-aponeurotic fibromatosis of the shoulder girdle (extra-abdominal desmoid). Analysis of thirty cases followed up for ten or more years. Cancer 1967;20(7):1131–40.
21. Soule EH, Scanlon PW. Fibrosarcoma arising in an extraabdominal desmoid tumor: report of case. Proc Staff Meet Mayo Clin 1962;37:443–51.
22. Mooney EE, Meagher P, Edwards GE, et al. Fibrosarcoma of the thigh 28 years after excision of fibromatosis. Histopathology 1993;23(5):498–500.
23. Allen PW. The fibromatoses: a clinicopathologic classification based on 140 cases. Am J Surg Pathol 1977;1(3):255–70.
24. Gaches C, Burke J. Desmoid tumour (fibroma of the abdominal wall) occurring in siblings. Br J Surg 1971;58(7):495–8.
25. Miyaki M, Konishi M, Kikuchi-Yanoshita R, et al. Coexistence of somatic and germ-line mutations of APC gene in desmoid tumors from patients with familial adenomatous polyposis. Cancer Res 1993;53(21):5079–82.
26. Nieuwenhuis MH, Mathus-Vliegen EM, Baeten CG, et al. Evaluation of management of desmoid tumours associated with familial adenomatous polyposis in Dutch patients. Br J Cancer 2011;104(1):37–42.
27. Nieuwenhuis MH, Casparie M, Mathus-Vliegen LM, et al. A nationwide study comparing sporadic and familial adenomatous polyposis-related desmoid-type fibromatoses. Int J Cancer 2011;129(1):256–61.
28. Alman BA, Li C, Pajerski ME, et al. Increased beta-catenin protein and somatic APC mutations in sporadic aggressive fibromatoses (desmoid tumors). Am J Pathol 1997;151(2):329–34.
29. Clark SK, Phillips RK. Desmoids in familial adenomatous polyposis. Br J Surg 1996;83(11):1494–504.
30. Lazar AJ, Tuvin D, Hajibashi S, et al. Specific mutations in the beta-catenin gene (CTNNB1) correlate with local recurrence in sporadic desmoid tumors. Am J Pathol 2008;173(5):1518–27.
31. Icard P, Le Rochais JP, Galateau F, et al. Desmoid fibromatosis of the shoulder and of the upper chest wall following a clavicular fracture. Eur J Cardiothorac Surg 1999;15(5):723–5.
32. Aaron AD, O'Mara JW, Legendre KE, et al. Chest wall fibromatosis associated with silicone breast implants. Surg Oncol 1996;5(2):93–9.
33. Häyry P, Reitamo JJ, Tötterman S, et al. The desmoid tumor. II. Analysis of factors possibly contributing to the etiology and growth behavior. Am J Clin Pathol 1982;77(6):674–80.
34. Eccles DM, van der Luijt R, Breukel C, et al. Hereditary desmoid disease due to a frameshift mutation at codon 1924 of the APC gene. Am J Hum Genet 1996;59(6):1193–201.
35. Escobar C, Munker R, Thomas JO, et al. Update on desmoid tumors. Ann Oncol 2012;23(3):562–9.
36. Elayi E, Manilich E, Church J. Polishing the crystal ball: knowing genotype improves ability to predict desmoid disease in patients with familial adenomatous polyposis. Dis Colon Rectum 2009;52(10):1762–6.
37. Wanjeri JK, Opeya CJ. A massive abdominal wall desmoid tumor occurring in a laparotomy scar: a case report. World J Surg Oncol 2011; 9:35.
38. Durkin AJ, Korkolis DP, Al-Saif O, et al. Full-term gestation and transvaginal delivery after wide resection of an abdominal desmoid tumor during pregnancy. J Surg Oncol 2005;89(2):86–90.
39. Bocale D, Rotelli MT, Cavallini A, et al. Anti-oestrogen therapy in the treatment of desmoid tumours. A systematic review. Colorectal Dis 2011;13(12):e388–95.
40. Altomare DF, Rotelli MT, Rinaldi M, et al. Potential role of the steroid receptor pattern in the response of inoperable intra-abdominal desmoid to toremifene after failure of tamoxifen therapy. Int J Colorectal Dis 2010;25(6):787–9.
41. Fujita K, Sugao H, Tsujikawa K, et al. Desmoid tumor in a scar from radical nephrectomy for renal cancer. Int J Urol 2003;10(5):274–5.
42. Mall JW, Philipp AW, Zimmerling M, et al. Desmoid tumours following long-term Tenckhoff peritoneal dialysis catheters. Nephrol Dial Transplant 2002;17(5):945–6.
43. Seoud M, Abbas J, Kaspar H, et al. Long-term survival following aggressive surgery and radiotherapy for pelvic fibromatosis. Int J Gynecol Cancer 2005;15(6):1112–4.
44. Huang GS, Lee HS, Lee CH, et al. Pelvic fibromatosis with massive ossification. AJR Am J Roentgenol 2005;184(3):1029–30.
45. Joyce M, Winter DC, Leader M, et al. Aggressive angiomyxoma of the perineum. Ir J Med Sci 2001;170(4):265–6.
46. Tan KK, Yan Z, Liau KH. Emergency surgery for a ruptured intra-abdominal desmoid tumour. Ann Acad Med Singap 2010;39(6):497–8.
47. Hartley JE, Church JM, Gupta S, et al. Significance of incidental desmoids identified during surgery for familial adenomatous polyposis. Dis Colon Rectum 2004;47(3):334–8; discussion 339–40.

48. Burke AP, Sobin LH, Shekitka KM. Mesenteric fibromatosis. A follow-up study. Arch Pathol Lab Med 1990;114(8):832–5.
49. Emory TS, Monihan JM, Carr NJ, et al. Sclerosing mesenteritis, mesenteric panniculitis and mesenteric lipodystrophy: a single entity? Am J Surg Pathol 1997;21(4):392–8.
50. Montgomery E, Folpe AL. The diagnostic value of beta-catenin immunohistochemistry. Adv Anat Pathol 2005;12(6):350–6.
51. Swartz RD. Idiopathic retroperitoneal fibrosis: a review of the pathogenesis and approaches to treatment. Am J Kidney Dis 2009;54(3): 546–53.
52. Palmisano A, Vaglio A. Chronic periaortitis: a fibro-inflammatory disorder. Best Pract Res Clin Rheumatol 2009;23(3):339–53.
53. Cai FZ, Tesar P, Klestov A. Methysergide-induced retroperitoneal fibrosis and pericardial effusion. Intern Med J 2004;34(5):297–8.
54. Hammer ST, Jentzen JM, Lim MS. Anaplastic lymphoma kinase-positive anaplastic large cell lymphoma presenting as retroperitoneal fibrosis. Hum Pathol 2011. Available at: http://www.ncbi.nlm.nih.gov/pubmed/21658744. Accessed September 8, 2011.
55. Parums DV. The spectrum of chronic periaortitis. Histopathology 1990;16(5):423–31.
56. Deshpande V, Zen Y, Chan JK, et al. Consensus statement on the pathology of IgG4-related disease. Mod Pathol 2012;25(9):1181–92.
57. Zen Y, Nakanuma Y. IgG4-related disease: a cross-sectional study of 114 cases. Am J Surg Pathol 2010;34(12):1812–9.
58. Swartz R, Scheel P. Retroperitoneal fibrosis: gaining traction on an enigma. Lancet 2011;378(9788):294–6.
59. Rodriguez JA, Guarda LA, Rosai J. Mesenteric fibromatosis with involvement of the gastrointestinal tract. A GIST simulator: a study of 25 cases. Am J Clin Pathol 2004;121(1):93–8.
60. Yantiss RK, Spiro IJ, Compton CC, et al. Gastrointestinal stromal tumor versus intra-abdominal fibromatosis of the bowel wall: a clinically important differential diagnosis. Am J Surg Pathol 2000;24(7): 947–57.
61. Miettinen M, Monihan JM, Sarlomo-Rikala M, et al. Gastrointestinal stromal tumors/smooth muscle tumors (GISTs) primary in the omentum and mesentery: clinicopathologic and immunohistochemical study of 26 cases. Am J Surg Pathol 1999;23(9):1109–18.
62. Barros A, Linhares E, Valadão M, et al. Extragastrointestinal stromal tumors (EGIST): a series of case reports. Hepatogastroenterology 2011; 58(107–108):865–8.
63. Montgomery E, Torbenson MS, Kaushal M, et al. Beta-catenin immunohistochemistry separates mesenteric fibromatosis from gastrointestinal stromal tumor and sclerosing mesenteritis. Am J Surg Pathol 2002;26(10):1296–301.
64. West RB, Corless CL, Chen X, et al. The novel marker, DOG1, is expressed ubiquitously in gastrointestinal stromal tumors irrespective of KIT or PDGFRA mutation status. Am J Pathol 2004;165(1):107–13.
65. Gardner EJ. A genetic and clinical study of intestinal polyposis, a predisposing factor for carcinoma of the colon and rectum. Am J Hum Genet 1951;3(2):167–76.
66. Smith WG. Multiple polyposis, Gardner's syndrome and desmoid tumors. Dis Colon Rectum 1958;1(5):323–32.
67. Gurbuz AK, Giardiello FM, Petersen GM, et al. Desmoid tumours in familial adenomatous polyposis. Gut 1994;35(3):377–81.
68. Parc Y, Piquard A, Dozois RR, et al. Long-term outcome of familial adenomatous polyposis patients after restorative coloproctectomy. Ann Surg 2004;239(3):378–82.
69. Sinha A, Tekkis PP, Gibbons DC, et al. Risk factors predicting desmoid occurrence in patients with familial adenomatous polyposis: a meta-analysis. Colorectal Dis 2010. Available at: http://www.ncbi.nlm.nih.gov/pubmed/20528895. Accessed September 7, 2011.
70. Durno C, Monga N, Bapat B, et al. Does early colectomy increase desmoid risk in familial adenomatous polyposis? Clin Gastroenterol Hepatol 2007;5(10):1190–4.
71. Nakamura Y, Nishisho I, Kinzler KW, et al. Mutations of the adenomatous polyposis coli gene in familial polyposis coli patients and sporadic colorectal tumors. Int Symp Princess Takamatsu Cancer Res Fund 1991;22:285–92.
72. Kinzler KW, Nilbert MC, Su LK, et al. Identification of FAP locus genes from chromosome 5q21. Science 1991;253(5020):661–5.
73. Colombo C, Bolshakov S, Hajibashi S, et al. "Difficult to diagnose" desmoid tumours: a potential role for CTNNB1 mutational analysis. Histopathology 2011;59(2):336–40.
74. Mayer M, Kulig A, Sygut J, et al. Molecular cytogenetic analysis of chromosome aberrations in desmoid tumors. Pol J Pathol 2007;58(3): 167–71.
75. Salas S, Chibon F, Noguchi T, et al. Molecular characterization by array comparative genomic hybridization and DNA sequencing of 194 desmoid tumors. Genes Chromosomes Cancer 2010;49(6):560–8.
76. Fletcher JA, Naeem R, Xiao S, et al. Chromosome aberrations in desmoid tumors. Trisomy 8 may be a predictor of recurrence. Cancer Genet Cytogenet 1995;79(2):139–43.
77. Qi H, Dal Cin P, Hernández JM, et al. Trisomies 8 and 20 in desmoid tumors. Cancer Genet Cytogenet 1996;92(2):147–9.
78. Dal Cin P, Sciot R, Van Damme B, et al. Trisomy 20 characterizes a second group of desmoid tumors. Cancer Genet Cytogenet 1995; 79(2):189.
79. Bridge JA, Sreekantaiah C, Mouron B, et al. Clonal chromosomal abnormalities in desmoid tumors. Implications for histopathogenesis. Cancer 1992;69(2):430–6.
80. Eyden B. The myofibroblast: a study of normal, reactive and neoplastic tissues, with an emphasis on ultrastructure. Part 2—tumours and tumour-like lesions. J Submicrosc Cytol Pathol 2005;37(3–4): 231–96.
81. Amary MF, Pauwels P, Meulemans E, et al. Detection of beta-catenin mutations in paraffin-embedded sporadic desmoid-type fibromatosis by mutation-specific restriction enzyme digestion (MSRED): an ancillary diagnostic tool. Am J Surg Pathol 2007;31(9):1299–309.
82. Bhattacharya B, Dilworth HP, Iacobuzio-Donahue C, et al. Nuclear beta-catenin expression distinguishes deep fibromatosis from other benign and malignant fibroblastic and myofibroblastic lesions. Am J Surg Pathol 2005;29(5):653–9.
83. Carlson JW, Fletcher CD. Immunohistochemistry for beta-catenin in the differential diagnosis of spindle cell lesions: analysis of a series and review of the literature. Histopathology 2007;51(4):509–14.
84. Ng TL, Gown AM, Barry TS, et al. Nuclear beta-catenin in mesenchymal tumors. Mod Pathol 2005;18(1):68–74.
85. Gronchi A, Casali PG, Mariani L, et al. Quality of surgery and outcome in extra-abdominal aggressive fibromatosis: a series of patients surgically treated at a single institution. J Clin Oncol 2003;21(7): 1390–7.
86. Sherman NE, Romsdahl M, Evans H, et al. Desmoid tumors: a 20-year radiotherapy experience. Int J Radiat Oncol Biol Phys 1990;19(1): 37–40.
87. Salas S, Dufresne A, Bui B, et al. Prognostic factors influencing progression-free survival determined from a series of sporadic desmoid tumors: a wait-and-see policy according to tumor presentation. J Clin Oncol 2011;29(26):3553–8.
88. Stojadinovic A, Hoos A, Karpoff HM, et al. Soft tissue tumors of the abdominal wall: analysis of disease patterns and treatment. Arch Surg 2001;136(1):70–9.
89. Sørensen A, Keller J, Nielsen OS, et al. Treatment of aggressive fibromatosis: a retrospective study of 72 patients followed for 1-27 years. Acta Orthop Scand 2002;73(2):213–9.
90. Sturt NJ, Gallagher MC, Bassett P, et al. Evidence for genetic predisposition to desmoid tumours in familial adenomatous polyposis independent of the germline APC mutation. Gut 2004;53(12):1832–6.
91. Barbier O, Anract P, Pluot E, et al. Primary or recurring extra-abdominal desmoid fibromatosis: assessment of treatment by observation only. Orthop Traumatol Surg Res 2010;96(8):884–9.
92. Gluck I, Griffith KA, Biermann JS, et al. Role of radiotherapy in the management of desmoid tumors. Int J Radiat Oncol Biol Phys 2011;80(3):787–92.
93. Mace J, Sybil Biermann J, Sondak V, et al. Response of extraabdominal desmoid tumors to therapy with imatinib mesylate. Cancer 2002;95(11): 2373–9.
94. Penel N, Le Cesne A, Bui BN, et al. Imatinib for progressive and recurrent aggressive fibromatosis (desmoid tumors): an FNCLCC/French Sarcoma Group phase II trial with a long-term follow-up. Ann Oncol 2011;22(2):452–7.
95. Dufresne A, Bertucci F, Penel N, et al. Identification of biological factors predictive of response to imatinib mesylate in aggressive fibromatosis. Br J Cancer 2010;103(4):482–5.
96. Gounder MM, Lefkowitz RA, Keohan ML, et al. Activity of Sorafenib against desmoid tumor/deep fibromatosis. Clin Cancer Res 2011; 17(12):4082–90.
97. Hansmann A, Adolph C, Vogel T, et al. High-dose tamoxifen and sulindac as first-line treatment for desmoid tumors. Cancer 2004;100(3): 612–20.
98. Nishida Y, Tsukushi S, Shido Y, et al. Successful treatment with meloxicam, a cyclooxygenase-2 inhibitor, of patients with extra-abdominal desmoid tumors: a pilot study. J Clin Oncol 2010;28(6):e107–9.

99. Picariello L, Tonelli F, Brandi ML. Selective oestrogen receptor modulators in desmoid tumours. Expert Opin Investig Drugs 2004;13(11):1457–68.
100. Bonvalot S, Eldweny H, Haddad V, et al. Extra-abdominal primary fibromatosis: aggressive management could be avoided in a subgroup of patients. Eur J Surg Oncol 2008;34(4):462–8.
101. Stout AP. Fibrosarcoma the malignant tumor of fibroblasts. Cancer 1948;1(1):30–63.
102. Chung EB, Enzinger FM. Infantile fibrosarcoma. Cancer 1976;38(2):729–39.
103. Soule EH, Pritchard DJ. Fibrosarcoma in infants and children: a review of 110 cases. Cancer 1977;40(4):1711–21.
104. Steelman C, Katzenstein H, Parham D, et al. Unusual presentation of congenital infantile fibrosarcoma in seven infants with molecular-genetic analysis. Fetal Pediatr Pathol 2011;30(5):329–37.
105. Islam S, Soldes OS, Ruiz R, et al. Primary colonic congenital infantile fibrosarcoma presenting as meconium peritonitis. Pediatr Surg Int 2008;24(5):621–3.
106. Kogon B, Shehata B, Katzenstein H, et al. Primary congenital infantile fibrosarcoma of the heart: the first confirmed case. Ann Thorac Surg 2011;91(4):1276–80.
107. Dumont C, Monforte M, Flandrin A, et al. Prenatal management of congenital infantile fibrosarcoma: unexpected outcome. Ultrasound Obstet Gynecol 2011;37(6):733–5.
108. Canale S, Vanel D, Couanet D, et al. Infantile fibrosarcoma: magnetic resonance imaging findings in six cases. Eur J Radiol 2009;72(1):30–7.
109. Dahl I, Save-Soderbergh J, Angervall L. Fibrosarcoma in early infancy. Pathol Eur 1973;8(3):193–209.
110. Buccoliero AM, Castiglione F, Degl'Innocenti DR, et al. Congenital/infantile fibrosarcoma of the colon: morphologic, immunohistochemical, molecular, and ultrastructural features of a relatively rare tumor in an extraordinary localization. J Pediatr Hematol Oncol 2008;30(10):723–7.
111. Coffin CM, Dehner LP. Fibroblastic-myofibroblastic tumors in children and adolescents: a clinicopathologic study of 108 examples in 103 patients. Pediatr Pathol 1991;11(4):569–88.
112. Mariño-Enríquez A, Li P, Samuelson J, et al. Congenital fibrosarcoma with a novel complex 3-way translocation t(12;15;19) and unusual histologic features. Hum Pathol 2008;39(12):1844–8.
113. Schofield DE, Fletcher JA, Grier HE, et al. Fibrosarcoma in infants and children. Application of new techniques. Am J Surg Pathol 1994;18(1):14–24.
114. Mandahl N, Heim S, Rydholm A, et al. Nonrandom numerical chromosome aberrations (+8, +11, +17, +20) in infantile fibrosarcoma. Cancer Genet Cytogenet 1989;40(1):137–9.
115. Knezevich SR, Garnett MJ, Pysher TJ, et al. ETV6-NTRK3 gene fusions and trisomy 11 establish a histogenetic link between mesoblastic nephroma and congenital fibrosarcoma. Cancer Res 1998;58(22):5046–8.
116. Rubin BP, Chen CJ, Morgan TW, et al. Congenital mesoblastic nephroma t(12;15) is associated with ETV6-NTRK3 gene fusion: cytogenetic and molecular relationship to congenital (infantile) fibrosarcoma. Am J Pathol 1998;153(5):1451–8.
117. Adem C, Gisselsson D, Dal Cin P, et al. ETV6 rearrangements in patients with infantile fibrosarcomas and congenital mesoblastic nephromas by fluorescence in situ hybridization. Mod Pathol 2001;14(12):1246–51.
118. Argani P, Fritsch M, Kadkol SS, et al. Detection of the ETV6-NTRK3 chimeric RNA of infantile fibrosarcoma/cellular congenital mesoblastic nephroma in paraffin-embedded tissue: application to challenging pediatric renal stromal tumors. Mod Pathol 2000;13(1):29–36.
119. Argani P, Fritsch MK, Shuster AE, et al. Reduced sensitivity of paraffin-based RT-PCR assays for ETV6-NTRK3 fusion transcripts in morphologically defined infantile fibrosarcoma. Am J Surg Pathol 2001;25(11):1461–4.
120. Makretsov N, He M, Hayes M, et al. A fluorescence in situ hybridization study of ETV6-NTRK3 fusion gene in secretory breast carcinoma. Genes Chromosomes Cancer 2004;40(2):152–7.
121. Kralik JM, Kranewitter W, Boesmueller H, et al. Characterization of a newly identified ETV6-NTRK3 fusion transcript in acute myeloid leukemia. Diagn Pathol 2011;6:19.
122. Lundgren L, Angervall L, Stenman G, et al. Infantile rhabdomyofibrosarcoma: a high-grade sarcoma distinguishable from infantile fibrosarcoma and rhabdomyosarcoma. Hum Pathol 1993;24(7):785–95.
123. Mentzel T, Mentzel HJ, Katenkamp D. [Infantile rhabdomyofibrosarcoma. An aggressive tumor in the spectrum of spindle cell tumors in childhood]. Pathologe 1996;17(4):296–300.
124. Miki H, Kobayashi S, Kushida Y, et al. A case of infantile rhabdomyofibrosarcoma with immunohistochemical, electronmicroscopical, and genetic analyses. Hum Pathol 1999;30(12):1519–22.
125. Rao SI, Uppin SG, Ratnakar KS, et al. Infantile rhabdomyofibrosarcoma: a distinct variant or a missing link between fibrosarcoma and rhabdomyosarcoma? Indian J Cancer 2006;43(1):39–42.
126. Variend S, Bax NM, van Gorp J. Are infantile myofibromatosis, congenital fibrosarcoma and congenital haemangiopericytoma histogenetically related? Histopathology 1995;26(1):57–62.
127. Cecchetto G, Carli M, Alaggio R, et al. Fibrosarcoma in pediatric patients: results of the Italian Cooperative Group studies (1979-1995). J Surg Oncol 2001;78(4):225–31.
128. Blocker S, Koenig J, Ternberg J. Congenital fibrosarcoma. J Pediatr Surg 1987;22(7):665–70.
129. Wilson MB, Stanley W, Sens D, et al. Infantile fibrosarcoma–a misnomer? Pediatr Pathol 1990;10(6):901–7.
130. Spicer RD. Re: "Chemotherapy for infantile fibrosarcoma." Med Pediatr Oncol 1993;21(1):80.
131. Russell H, Hicks MJ, Bertuch AA, et al. Infantile fibrosarcoma: clinical and histologic responses to cytotoxic chemotherapy. Pediatr Blood Cancer 2009;53(1):23–7.
132. Demir HA, Akyüz C, Varan A, et al. Right foot congenital infantile fibrosarcoma treated only with chemotherapy. Pediatr Blood Cancer 2010;54(4):618–20.
133. Yeh I, Evan G, Jokinen CH. Cutaneous mycobacterial spindle cell pseudotumor: a potential mimic of soft tissue neoplasms. Am J Dermatopathol 2011;33(6):e66–9.
134. Shek TW, Ho FC, Ng IO, et al. Follicular dendritic cell tumor of the liver. Evidence for an Epstein-Barr virus-related clonal proliferation of follicular dendritic cells. Am J Surg Pathol 1996;20(3):313–24.
135. Davis RE, Warnke RA, Dorfman RF. Inflammatory pseudotumor of lymph nodes. Additional observations and evidence for an inflammatory etiology. Am J Surg Pathol 1991;15(8):744–56.
136. Coffin CM, Dehner LP, Meis-Kindblom JM. Inflammatory myofibroblastic tumor, inflammatory fibrosarcoma, and related lesions: an historical review with differential diagnostic considerations. Semin Diagn Pathol 1998;15(2):102–10.
137. Coffin CM, Watterson J, Priest JR, et al. Extrapulmonary inflammatory myofibroblastic tumor (inflammatory pseudotumor). A clinicopathologic and immunohistochemical study of 84 cases. Am J Surg Pathol 1995;19(8):859–72.
138. Chen YF, Zhang WD, Wu MW, et al. Inflammatory myofibroblastic tumor of the head and neck. Med Oncol 2011;28(Suppl. 1):S349–53.
139. Kato K, Moteki Y, Nakagawa M, et al. Inflammatory myofibroblastic tumor of the cerebellar hemisphere–case report. Neurol Med Chir (Tokyo) 2011;51(1):79–81.
140. Fuehrer NE, Keeney GL, Ketterling RP, et al. ALK-1 protein expression and ALK gene rearrangements aid in the diagnosis of inflammatory myofibroblastic tumors of the female genital tract. Arch Pathol Lab Med 2012;136(6):623–6.
141. Schütte K, Kandulski A, Kuester D, et al. Inflammatory myofibroblastic tumor of the pancreatic head: an unusual cause of recurrent acute pancreatitis—case presentation of a palliative approach after failed resection and review of the literature. Case Rep Gastroenterol 2010;4(3):443–51.
142. Shamszad P, Morales DL, Slesnick TC. Right ventricular inflammatory myofibroblastic tumor characterization by cardiovascular magnetic resonance. J Am Coll Cardiol 2011;57(15):e205.
143. Zhou X, Luo C, Lv S, et al. Inflammatory myofibroblastic tumor of the rectum in a 13-month-old girl: a case report. J Pediatr Surg 2011;46(7):E1–4.
144. Lee YK, Wang HY, Shyung LR, et al. Inflammatory myofibroblastic tumor: an unusual submucosal lesion of the stomach. Endoscopy 2011;43(Suppl. 2):E151–2.
145. Chen Y, Tang Y, Li H, et al. Inflammatory myofibroblastic tumor of the esophagus. Ann Thorac Surg 2010;89(2):607–10.
146. Fukano R, Matsubara T, Inoue T, et al. Time lag between the increase of IL-6 with fever and NF-kappaB activation in the peripheral blood in inflammatory myofibroblastic tumor. Cytokine 2008;44(2):293–7.
147. Souid AK, Ziemba MC, Dubansky AS, et al. Inflammatory myofibroblastic tumor in children. Cancer 1993;72(6):2042–8.
148. Meis JM, Enzinger FM. Inflammatory fibrosarcoma of the mesentery and retroperitoneum. A tumor closely simulating inflammatory pseudotumor. Am J Surg Pathol 1991;15(12):1146–56.

149. Coffin CM, Hornick JL, Fletcher CD. Inflammatory myofibroblastic tumor: comparison of clinicopathologic, histologic, and immunohistochemical features including ALK expression in atypical and aggressive cases. Am J Surg Pathol 2007;31(4):509–20.
150. Mariño-Enríquez A, Wang WL, Roy A, et al. Epithelioid inflammatory myofibroblastic sarcoma: An aggressive intra-abdominal variant of inflammatory myofibroblastic tumor with nuclear membrane or perinuclear ALK. Am J Surg Pathol 2011;35(1):135–44.
151. Cessna MH, Zhou H, Sanger WG, et al. Expression of ALK1 and p80 in inflammatory myofibroblastic tumor and its mesenchymal mimics: a study of 135 cases. Mod Pathol 2002;15(9):931–8.
152. Chan JK, Cheuk W, Shimizu M. Anaplastic lymphoma kinase expression in inflammatory pseudotumors. Am J Surg Pathol 2001;25(6):761–8.
153. Cook JR, Dehner LP, Collins MH, et al. Anaplastic lymphoma kinase (ALK) expression in the inflammatory myofibroblastic tumor: a comparative immunohistochemical study. Am J Surg Pathol 2001;25(11): 1364–71.
154. Chen ST, Lee JC. An inflammatory myofibroblastic tumor in liver with ALK and RANBP2 gene rearrangement: combination of distinct morphologic, immunohistochemical, and genetic features. Hum Pathol 2008;39(12):1854–8.
155. Ma Z, Hill DA, Collins MH, et al. Fusion of ALK to the Ran-binding protein 2 (RANBP2) gene in inflammatory myofibroblastic tumor. Genes Chromosomes Cancer 2003;37(1):98–105.
156. Patel AS, Murphy KM, Hawkins AL, et al. RANBP2 and CLTC are involved in ALK rearrangements in inflammatory myofibroblastic tumors. Cancer Genet Cytogenet 2007;176(2):107–14.
157. Gleason BC, Hornick JL. Inflammatory myofibroblastic tumours: where are we now? J Clin Pathol 2008;61(4):428–37.
158. Griffin CA, Hawkins AL, Dvorak C, et al. Recurrent involvement of 2p23 in inflammatory myofibroblastic tumors. Cancer Res 1999;59(12): 2776–80.
159. Lawrence B, Perez-Atayde A, Hibbard MK, et al. TPM3-ALK and TPM4-ALK oncogenes in inflammatory myofibroblastic tumors. Am J Pathol 2000;157(2):377–84.
160. Bridge JA, Kanamori M, Ma Z, et al. Fusion of the ALK gene to the clathrin heavy chain gene, CLTC, in inflammatory myofibroblastic tumor. Am J Pathol 2001;159(2):411–5.
161. Panagopoulos I, Nilsson T, Domanski HA, et al. Fusion of the SEC31L1 and ALK genes in an inflammatory myofibroblastic tumor. Int J Cancer 2006;118(5):1181–6.
162. Debelenko LV, Arthur DC, Pack SD, et al. Identification of CARS-ALK fusion in primary and metastatic lesions of an inflammatory myofibroblastic tumor. Lab Invest 2003;83(9):1255–65.
163. Saab ST, Hornick JL, Fletcher CD, et al. IgG4 plasma cells in inflammatory myofibroblastic tumor: inflammatory marker or pathogenic link? Mod Pathol 2011;24(4):606–12.
164. Yamamoto H, Yamaguchi H, Aishima S, et al. Inflammatory myofibroblastic tumor versus IgG4-related sclerosing disease and inflammatory pseudotumor: a comparative clinicopathologic study. Am J Surg Pathol 2009;33(9):1330–40.
165. Coffin CM, Humphrey PA, Dehner LP. Extrapulmonary inflammatory myofibroblastic tumor: a clinical and pathological survey. Semin Diagn Pathol 1998;15(2):85–101.
166. Cook JR, Dehner LP, Collins MH, et al. Anaplastic lymphoma kinase (ALK) expression in the inflammatory myofibroblastic tumor: a comparative immunohistochemical study. Am J Surg Pathol 2001;25(11): 1364–71.
167. Coffin CM, Hornick JL, Zhou H, et al. Gardner fibroma: a clinicopathologic and immunohistochemical analysis of 45 patients with 57 fibromas. Am J Surg Pathol 2007;31(3):410–6.
168. Coffin CM, Lowichik A, Zhou H. Treatment effects in pediatric soft tissue and bone tumors: practical considerations for the pathologist. Am J Clin Pathol 2005;123(1):75–90.
169. Bertocchini A, Lo Zupone C, Callea F, et al. Unresectable multifocal omental and peritoneal inflammatory myofibroblastic tumor in a child: revisiting the role of adjuvant therapy. J Pediatr Surg 2011;46(4): e17–21.
169a. Pritchard DJ, Soule EH, Taylor WF, et al. Fibrosarcoma—a clinicopathologic and statistical study of 199 tumors of the soft tissues of the extremities and trunk. Cancer 1974;33(3):888–97.
170. Scott SM, Reiman HM, Pritchard DJ, et al. Soft tissue fibrosarcoma. A clinicopathologic study of 132 cases. Cancer 1989;64(4):925–31.
171. Bahrami A, Folpe AL. Adult-type fibrosarcoma: a reevaluation of 163 putative cases diagnosed at a single institution over a 48-year period. Am J Surg Pathol 2010;34(10):1504–13.
172. Hansen T, Katenkamp K, Brodhun M, et al. Low-grade fibrosarcoma–report on 39 not otherwise specified cases and comparison with defined low-grade fibrosarcoma types. Histopathology 2006;49(2):152–60.
173. Limon J, Szadowska A, Iliszko M, et al. Recurrent chromosome changes in two adult fibrosarcomas. Genes Chromosomes Cancer 1998;21(2): 119–23.
174. Dal Cin P, Pauwels P, Sciot R, et al. Multiple chromosome rearrangements in a fibrosarcoma. Cancer Genet Cytogenet 1996;87(2):176–8.
175. Mackenzie DH. Fibroma: a dangerous diagnosis. A review of 205 cases of fibrosarcoma of soft tissues. Br J Surg 1964;51:607–12.
176. Pritchard DJ, Sim FH, Ivins JC, et al. Fibrosarcoma of bone and soft tissues of the trunk and extremities. Orthop Clin North Am 1977;8(4):869–81.
177. Tanz SS. Fibrosarcoma following single trauma; report of a case. J Int Coll Surg 1957;27(5 Part 1):620–6.
178. Ivins JC, Dockerty MB, Ghormley RK. Fibrosarcoma of the soft tissues of the extremities; a review of 78 cases. Surgery 1950;28(3): 495–508.
179. Morris JM, Lucas DB. Fibrosarcoma within a sinus tract of chronic draining osteomyelitis. Case report and review of literature. J Bone Joint Surg Am 1964;46:853–7.
180. Burns WA, Kanhouwa S, Tillman L, et al. Fibrosarcoma occurring at the site of a plastic vascular graft. Cancer 1972;29(1):66–72.
181. Eckstein FS, Vogel U, Mohr W. Fibrosarcoma in association with a total knee joint prosthesis. Virchows Arch A Pathol Anat Histopathol 1992;421(2):175–8.
182. Meis-Kindblom JM, Kindblom LG, Enzinger FM. Sclerosing epithelioid fibrosarcoma. A variant of fibrosarcoma simulating carcinoma. Am J Surg Pathol 1995;19(9):979–93.
183. Antonescu CR, Baren A. Spectrum of low-grade fibrosarcomas: a comparative ultrastructural analysis of low-grade myxofibrosarcoma and fibromyxoid sarcoma. Ultrastruct Pathol 2004;28(5-6):321–32.
184. Folk GS, Williams SB, Foss RB, et al. Oral and maxillofacial sclerosing epithelioid fibrosarcoma: report of five cases. Head Neck Pathol 2007;1(1):13–20.
185. Grunewald TG, von Luettichau I, Weirich G, et al. Sclerosing epithelioid fibrosarcoma of the bone: a case report of high resistance to chemotherapy and a survey of the literature. Sarcoma 2010;2010: 431627.
186. Tomimaru Y, Nagano H, Marubashi S, et al. Sclerosing epithelioid fibrosarcoma of the liver infiltrating the inferior vena cava. World J Gastroenterol 2009;15(33):4204–8.
187. Frattini JC, Sosa JA, Carmack S, et al. Sclerosing epithelioid fibrosarcoma of the cecum: a radiation-associated tumor in a previously unreported site. Arch Pathol Lab Med 2007;131(12):1825–8.
188. Antonescu CR, Rosenblum MK, Pereira P, et al. Sclerosing epithelioid fibrosarcoma: a study of 16 cases and confirmation of a clinicopathologically distinct tumor. Am J Surg Pathol 2001;25(6):699–709.
189. Guillou L, Benhattar J, Gengler C, et al. Translocation-positive low-grade fibromyxoid sarcoma: clinicopathologic and molecular analysis of a series expanding the morphologic spectrum and suggesting potential relationship to sclerosing epithelioid fibrosarcoma: a study from the French Sarcoma Group. Am J Surg Pathol 2007;31(9): 1387–402.
190. Rekhi B, Folpe AL, Deshmukh M, et al. Sclerosing epithelioid fibrosarcoma—a report of two cases with cytogenetic analysis of FUS gene rearrangement by FISH technique. Pathol Oncol Res 2011;17(1): 145–8.
191. Donner LR, Clawson K, Dobin SM. Sclerosing epithelioid fibrosarcoma: a cytogenetic, immunohistochemical, and ultrastructural study of an unusual histological variant. Cancer Genet Cytogenet 2000;119(2): 127–31.
192. Hindermann W, Katenkamp D. [Sclerosing epithelioid fibrosarcoma]. Pathologe 2003;24(2):103–8.
193. Eyden BP, Manson C, Banerjee SS, et al. Sclerosing epithelioid fibrosarcoma: a study of five cases emphasizing diagnostic criteria. Histopathology 1998;33(4):354–60.
194. Gisselsson D, Andreasson P, Meis-Kindblom JM, et al. Amplification of 12q13 and 12q15 sequences in a sclerosing epithelioid fibrosarcoma. Cancer Genet Cytogenet 1998;107(2):102–6.
195. Rekhi B, Deshmukh M, Jambhekar NA. Low-grade fibromyxoid sarcoma: a clinicopathologic study of 18 cases, including histopathologic relationship with sclerosing epithelioid fibrosarcoma in a subset of cases. Ann Diagn Pathol 2011;15(5):303–11.
196. Elkins CT, Wakely Jr PE. Sclerosing epithelioid fibrosarcoma of the oral cavity. Head Neck Pathol 2011;5(4):428–31.

197. Wang WL, Evans HL, Meis JM, et al. FUS rearrangements are rare in "pure" sclerosing epithelioid fibrosarcoma. Mod Pathol 2012;25(6): 846–53.
198. Folpe AL, McKenney JK, Bridge JA, et al. Sclerosing rhabdomyosarcoma in adults: report of four cases of a hyalinizing, matrix-rich variant of rhabdomyosarcoma that may be confused with osteosarcoma, chondrosarcoma, or angiosarcoma. Am J Surg Pathol 2002;26(9): 1175–83.
199. Ossendorf C, Studer GM, Bode B, et al. Sclerosing epithelioid fibrosarcoma: case presentation and a systematic review. Clin Orthop Relat Res 2008;466(6):1485–91.
200. Angervall L, Kindblom LG, Merck C. Myxofibrosarcoma. A study of 30 cases. Acta Pathol Microbiol Scand A 1977;85A(2):127–40.
201. Sanfilippo R, Miceli R, Grosso F, et al. Myxofibrosarcoma: prognostic factors and survival in a series of patients treated at a single institution. Ann Surg Oncol 2011;18(3):720–5.
202. Haglund KE, Raut CP, Nascimento AF, et al. Recurrence patterns and survival for patients with intermediate- and high-grade myxofibrosarcoma. Int J Radiat Oncol Biol Phys 2012;82(1):361–7.
203. Mutter RW, Singer S, Zhang Z, et al. The enigma of myxofibrosarcoma of the extremity. Cancer 2012;118(2):518–27.
204. Kaya M, Wada T, Nagoya S, et al. Bone and/or joint attachment is a risk factor for local recurrence of myxofibrosarcoma. J Orthop Sci 2011;16(4): 413–7.
205. Merck C, Angervall L, Kindblom LG, et al. Myxofibrosarcoma. A malignant soft tissue tumor of fibroblastic-histiocytic origin. A clinicopathologic and prognostic study of 110 cases using multivariate analysis. Acta Pathol Microbiol Immunol Scand Suppl 1983;282:1–40.
206. Mentzel T, Calonje E, Wadden C, et al. Myxofibrosarcoma. Clinicopathologic analysis of 75 cases with emphasis on the low-grade variant. Am J Surg Pathol 1996;20(4):391–405.
207. Weiss SW, Enzinger FM. Myxoid variant of malignant fibrous histiocytoma. Cancer 1977;39(4):1672–85.
208. Clarke LE, Zhang PJ, Crawford GH, et al. Myxofibrosarcoma in the skin. J Cutan Pathol 2008;35(10):935–40.
209. Klopcic U, Lamovec J, Luzar B. Fine needle aspiration biopsy of primary breast myxofibrosarcoma: a case report. Acta Cytol 2009;53(1): 109–12.
210. Heletz I, Abramson SV. Large obstructive cardiac myxofibrosarcoma is nearly invisible on transthoracic echocardiogram. Echocardiography 2009;26(7):847–51.
211. Ozkan B, Ozgüroğlu M, Ozkara H, et al. Adult paratesticular myxofibrosarcoma: report of a rare entity and review of the literature. Int Urol Nephrol 2006;38(1):5–7.
212. Huang HY, Brennan MF, Singer S, et al. Distant metastasis in retroperitoneal dedifferentiated liposarcoma is rare and rapidly fatal: a clinicopathological study with emphasis on the low-grade myxofibrosarcoma-like pattern as an early sign of dedifferentiation. Mod Pathol 2005;18(7): 976–84.
213. Willems SM, Debiec-Rychter M, Szuhai K, et al. Local recurrence of myxofibrosarcoma is associated with increase in tumour grade and cytogenetic aberrations, suggesting a multistep tumour progression model. Mod Pathol 2006;19(3):407–16.
214. Willems SM, Mohseny AB, Balog C, et al. Cellular/intramuscular myxoma and grade I myxofibrosarcoma are characterized by distinct genetic alterations and specific composition of their extracellular matrix. J Cell Mol Med 2009;13(7):1291–301.
215. Ohguri T, Hisaoka M, Kawauchi S, et al. Cytogenetic analysis of myxoid liposarcoma and myxofibrosarcoma by array-based comparative genomic hybridisation. J Clin Pathol 2006;59(9):978–83.
216. Simons A, Schepens M, Jeuken J, et al. Frequent loss of 9p21 (p16(INK4A)) and other genomic imbalances in human malignant fibrous histiocytoma. Cancer Genet Cytogenet 2000;118(2):89–98.
217. Sawyer JR, Binz RL, Gilliland JC, et al. A novel reciprocal (10;17) (p11.2;q23) in myxoid fibrosarcoma. Cancer Genet Cytogenet 2001; 124(2):144–6.
218. Clawson K, Donner LR, Dobin SM. Translocation (2;15)(p23;q21.2) and interstitial deletion of 7q in a case of low-grade myxofibrosarcoma. Cancer Genet Cytogenet 2001;127(2):140–2.
219. Huang HY, Lal P, Qin J, et al. Low-grade myxofibrosarcoma: a clinicopathologic analysis of 49 cases treated at a single institution with simultaneous assessment of the efficacy of 3-tier and 4-tier grading systems. Hum Pathol 2004;35(5):612–21.
220. Evans HL. Low-grade fibromyxoid sarcoma. A report of two metastasizing neoplasms having a deceptively benign appearance. Am J Clin Pathol 1987;88(5):615–9.
221. Lane KL, Shannon RJ, Weiss SW. Hyalinizing spindle cell tumor with giant rosettes: a distinctive tumor closely resembling low-grade fibromyxoid sarcoma. Am J Surg Pathol 1997;21(12):1481–8.
222. Kim L, Yoon YH, Choi SJ, et al. Hyalinizing spindle cell tumor with giant rosettes arising in the lung: report of a case with FUS-CREB3L2 fusion transcripts. Pathol Int 2007;57(3):153–7.
223. Folpe AL, Lane KL, Paull G, et al. Low-grade fibromyxoid sarcoma and hyalinizing spindle cell tumor with giant rosettes: a clinicopathologic study of 73 cases supporting their identity and assessing the impact of high-grade areas. Am J Surg Pathol 2000;24(10):1353–60.
224. Baydar DE, Aki FT. Low-grade fibromyxoid sarcoma metastatic to the prostate. Ann Diagn Pathol 2011;15(1):64–8.
225. Higuchi M, Suzuki H, Shio Y, et al. Successfully resected intrathoracic low-grade fibromyxoid sarcoma. Gen Thorac Cardiovasc Surg 2010; 58(7):348–51.
226. Laurini JA, Zhang L, Goldblum JR, et al. Low-grade fibromyxoid sarcoma of the small intestine: report of 4 cases with molecular cytogenetic confirmation. Am J Surg Pathol 2011;35(7):1069–73.
227. Lee AF, Yip S, Smith AC, et al. Low-grade fibromyxoid sarcoma of the perineum with heterotopic ossification: case report and review of the literature. Hum Pathol 2011;42(11):1804–9.
228. Billings SD, Giblen G, Fanburg-Smith JC. Superficial low-grade fibromyxoid sarcoma (Evans tumor): a clinicopathologic analysis of 19 cases with a unique observation in the pediatric population. Am J Surg Pathol 2005;29(2):204–10.
229. Patel RM, Downs-Kelly E, Dandekar MN, et al. FUS (16p11) gene rearrangement as detected by fluorescence in-situ hybridization in cutaneous low-grade fibromyxoid sarcoma: a potential diagnostic tool. Am J Dermatopathol 2011;33(2):140–3.
230. Périgny M, Dion N, Couture C, et al. [Low grade fibromyxoid sarcoma: a clinico-pathologic analysis of 7 cases]. Ann Pathol 2006;26(6): 419–25.
231. Goodlad JR, Mentzel T, Fletcher CD. Low grade fibromyxoid sarcoma: clinicopathological analysis of eleven new cases in support of a distinct entity. Histopathology 1995;26(3):229–37.
232. Evans HL. Low-grade fibromyxoid sarcoma: a clinicopathologic study of 33 cases with long-term follow-up. Am J Surg Pathol 2011;35(10): 1450–62.
233. Evans HL. Low-grade fibromyxoid sarcoma. A report of 12 cases. Am J Surg Pathol 1993;17(6):595–600.
234. Scolyer RA, McCarthy SW, Wills EJ, et al. Hyalinising spindle cell tumour with giant rosettes: report of a case with unusual features including original histological and ultrastructural observations. Pathology 2001;33(1):101–7.
235. Nielsen GP, Selig MK, O'Connell JX, et al. Hyalinizing spindle cell tumor with giant rosettes: a report of three cases with ultrastructural analysis. Am J Surg Pathol 1999;23(10):1227–32.
236. Guillou L, Benhattar J, Gengler C, et al. Translocation-positive low-grade fibromyxoid sarcoma: clinicopathologic and molecular analysis of a series expanding the morphologic spectrum and suggesting potential relationship to sclerosing epithelioid fibrosarcoma: a study from the French Sarcoma Group. Am J Surg Pathol 2007;31(9): 1387–402.
237. Doyle LA, Möller E, Dal Cin P, et al. MUC4 is a highly sensitive and specific marker for low-grade fibromyxoid sarcoma. Am J Surg Pathol 2011;35(5):733–41.
238. Thway K, Fisher C, Debiec-Rychter M, et al. Claudin-1 is expressed in perineurioma-like low-grade fibromyxoid sarcoma. Hum Pathol 2009; 40(11):1586–90.
239. Bartuma H, Möller E, Collin A, et al. Fusion of the FUS and CREB3L2 genes in a supernumerary ring chromosome in low-grade fibromyxoid sarcoma. Cancer Genet Cytogenet 2010;199(2):143–6.
240. Mezzelani A, Sozzi G, Nessling M, et al. Low grade fibromyxoid sarcoma: a further low-grade soft tissue malignancy characterized by a ring chromosome. Cancer Genet Cytogenet 2000;122(2): 144–8.
241. Storlazzi CT, Mertens F, Nascimento A, et al. Fusion of the FUS and BBF2H7 genes in low grade fibromyxoid sarcoma. Hum Mol Genet 2003;12(18):2349–58.
242. Panagopoulos I, Möller E, Dahlén A, et al. Characterization of the native CREB3L2 transcription factor and the FUS/CREB3L2 chimera. Genes Chromosomes Cancer 2007;46(2):181–91.
243. Reid R, de Silva MV, Paterson L, et al. Low-grade fibromyxoid sarcoma and hyalinizing spindle cell tumor with giant rosettes share a common t(7;16)(q34;p11) translocation. Am J Surg Pathol 2003;27(9): 1229–36.

244. Mertens F, Fletcher CD, Antonescu CR, et al. Clinicopathologic and molecular genetic characterization of low-grade fibromyxoid sarcoma, and cloning of a novel FUS/CREB3L1 fusion gene. Lab Invest 2005;85(3):408–15.
245. Matsuyama A, Hisaoka M, Shimajiri S, et al. DNA-based polymerase chain reaction for detecting FUS-CREB3L2 in low-grade fibromyxoid sarcoma using formalin-fixed, paraffin-embedded tissue specimens. Diagn Mol Pathol 2008;17(4):237–40.
246. Rose B, Tamvakopoulos GS, Dulay K, et al. The clinical significance of the FUS-CREB3L2 translocation in low-grade fibromyxoid sarcoma. J Orthop Surg Res 2011;6(1):15.
247. Thijssens KM, van Ginkel RJ, Suurmeijer AJ, et al. Radiation-induced sarcoma: a challenge for the surgeon. Ann Surg Oncol 2005;12(3): 237–45.
248. Kirova YM, Vilcoq JR, Asselain B, et al. Radiation-induced sarcomas after radiotherapy for breast carcinoma: a large-scale single-institution review. Cancer 2005;104(4):856–63.
249. Aydin F, Ghatak NR, Leshner RT. Possible radiation-induced dural fibrosarcoma with an unusually short latent period: case report. Neurosurgery 1995;36(3):591–4; discussion 594–5.
250. Ito T, Seyama T, Iwamoto KS, et al. In vitro irradiation is able to cause RET oncogene rearrangement. Cancer Res 1993;53(13):2940–3.
251. Zindanci I, Zemheri E, Kavala M, et al. Fibrosarcoma arising from a burn scar. Eur J Dermatol 2011;21(6):996–7.
252. Ozyazgan I, Kontaş O. Burn scar sarcoma. Burns 1999;25(5):455–8.
253. Sharma A, Schwartz RA, Swan KG. Marjolin's warty ulcer. J Surg Oncol 2011;103(2):193–5.
254. Schürch W. The myofibroblast in neoplasia. Curr Top Pathol 1999;93: 135–48.
255. Lagacé R, Seemayer TA, Gabbiani G, et al. Myofibroblastic sarcoma. Am J Surg Pathol 1999;23(11):1432–5.
256. Schürch W, Seemayer TA, Gabbiani G. The myofibroblast: a quarter century after its discovery. Am J Surg Pathol 1998;22(2):141–7.
257. Fisher C. Myofibroblastic malignancies. Adv Anat Pathol 2004;11(4): 190–201.
258. Fisher C. Myofibrosarcoma. Virchows Arch 2004;445(3):215–23.
259. Mentzel T, Katenkamp D. [Myofibroblastic tumors. Brief review of clinical aspects, diagnosis and differential diagnosis]. Pathologe 1998;19(3): 176–86.
260. Watanabe K. Leiomyosarcoma versus myofibrosarcoma. Am J Surg Pathol 2002;26(3):393–4; author reply 394–6.
261. Montgomery E, Fisher C. Myofibroblastic differentiation in malignant fibrous histiocytoma (pleomorphic myofibrosarcoma): a clinicopathological study. Histopathology 2001;38(6):499–509.
262. Mentzel T, Dry S, Katenkamp D, et al. Low-grade myofibroblastic sarcoma: analysis of 18 cases in the spectrum of myofibroblastic tumors. Am J Surg Pathol 1998;22(10):1228–38.
263. Montgomery E, Goldblum JR, Fisher C. Myofibrosarcoma: a clinicopathologic study. Am J Surg Pathol 2001;25(2):219–28.
264. Demarosi F, Bay A, Moneghini L, et al. Low-grade myofibroblastic sarcoma of the oral cavity. Oral Surg Oral Med Oral Pathol Oral Radiol Endod 2009;108(2):248–54.
265. Keller C, Gibbs CN, Kelly SM, et al. Low-grade myofibrosarcoma of the head and neck: importance of surgical therapy. J Pediatr Hematol Oncol 2004;26(2):119–20.
266. Stark M, Hoffmann A, Xiong Z. Mammary myofibrosarcoma: case report and literature review. Breast J 2011;17(3):300–4.
267. Arora R, Gupta R, Sharma A, Dinda AK. A rare case of low-grade myofibroblastic sarcoma of the femur in a 38-year-old woman: a case report. J Med Case Reports 2010;4:121.
268. Agaimy A, Wünsch PH, Schroeder J, et al. Low-grade abdominopelvic sarcoma with myofibroblastic features (low-grade myofibroblastic sarcoma): clinicopathological, immunohistochemical, molecular genetic and ultrastructural study of two cases with literature review. J Clin Pathol 2008;61(3):301–6.
269. Bisceglia M, Tricarico N, Minenna P, et al. Myofibrosarcoma of the upper jawbones: a clinicopathologic and ultrastructural study of two cases. Ultrastruct Pathol 2001;25(5):385–97.
270. Eyden B. The myofibroblast: a study of normal, reactive and neoplastic tissues, with an emphasis on ultrastructure. Part 2—tumours and tumour-like lesions. J Submicrosc Cytol Pathol 2005;37(3-4):231–96.
271. Fletcher CD, Dal Cin P, de Wever I, et al. Correlation between clinicopathological features and karyotype in spindle cell sarcomas. A report of 130 cases from the CHAMP study group. Am J Pathol 1999;154(6): 1841–7.
272. Meng GZ, Zhang HY, Zhang Z, et al. Myofibroblastic sarcoma vs nodular fasciitis: a comparative study of chromosomal imbalances. Am J Clin Pathol 2009;131(5):701–9.
273. Watanabe K, Ogura G, Tajino T, et al. Myofibrosarcoma of the bone: a clinicopathologic study. Am J Surg Pathol 2001;25(12):1501–7.
274. Chiller K, Parker D, Washington C. Myofibrosarcoma treated with Mohs micrographic surgery. Dermatol Surg 2004;30(12 Pt 2):1565–7.

Benign Fibrohistiocytic and Histiocytic Tumors

CHAPTER CONTENTS

The concept of fibrohistiocytic neoplasms has been challenged largely because the malignant forms (i.e., malignant fibrous histiocytoma) consistently lack histiocytic features and because some, but not all, when carefully studied, show a subtle degree of differentiation. Nonetheless, many benign fibrohistiocytic lesions are, in fact, truly derived from histiocytes (e.g., solitary xanthogranuloma, xanthoma), and, for this reason, there remains some merit in retaining this category. This has been recently endorsed by the World Health Organization,[1] recognizing that use of the term *fibrohistiocytic* is descriptive and merely denotes a lesion composed of cells that resemble normal histiocytes and fibroblasts.

Benign fibrohistiocytic tumors, however, are a pathogenetically diverse group of lesions. Xanthoma is a pseudotumor that usually arises in response to a disturbance in serum lipids. The preponderance of evidence suggests that fibrous histiocytoma is a true neoplasm with a definite growth potential but a limited capacity for aggressive behavior. Between these extremes are lesions of an indeterminate nature, exemplified by solitary xanthogranuloma. Although solitary xanthogranuloma resembles a tumor morphologically, it usually regresses with time, thereby raising the question of its proper position in the spectrum between hyperplasia and neoplasia. The present classification represents a practical, rather than a conceptual, approach aimed at defining differences among several histologically similar lesions (Box 11-1).

BOX 11-1 Classification of Histiocytic Syndromes in Children

Class I: Langerhans cell histiocytosis
- Forms of histiocytosis X (including eosinophilic granuloma and Hand–Schüller–Christian disease, among others)

Class II: Mononuclear phagocytes other than Langerhans cells
- Hemophagocytic lymphohistiocytosis
- Infection-associated hemophagocytic syndrome
- Sinus histiocytosis with massive lymphadenopathy
- Solitary xanthogranuloma
- Reticulohistiocytoma

Class III: Malignant histiocytic disorders
- Acute monocytic leukemia
- Malignant histiocytosis
- True histiocytic lymphomas

Data from the Writing Group of the Histiocyte Society. Favara BE, Feller AC, Pauli M, et al. Contemporary classification of histiocytic disorders. The WHO Committee on Histiocytic/Reticulum Cell Proliferations. Reclassification Working Group of the Histiocyte Society. Med Pediatr Oncol [Review] 1997;29(3):157–66.

FIBROUS HISTIOCYTOMA

Fibrous histiocytoma is a neoplastic or quasi-neoplastic lesion composed of a mixture of fibroblastic and histiocytic cells that are arranged in sheets or short fascicles and accompanied by varying numbers of inflammatory cells, foam cells, and siderophages. Most commonly, this tumor occurs in the dermis and superficial subcutis and rarely in deep soft tissues. When located in the skin, fibrous histiocytoma is also referred to as *dermatofibroma*.[2,3] In this chapter, the all-inclusive term *fibrous histiocytoma* is used to refer to lesions of the dermis and soft tissue. The terms *histiocytoma cutis*, *nodular subepidermal fibrosis*, and *sclerosing hemangiomas*, once used as synonyms for fibrous histiocytomas, are now archaic.

Clinical Findings

Cutaneous fibrous histiocytoma is a solitary, slowly growing nodule that usually makes its appearance during early or mid-adult life. A subset occurs following minor trauma or insect bites. Although any part of the skin surface may be affected, it is most common on the extremities.[4] Roughly one-third of these tumors are multiple and present metachronously. Synchronous development can occur in the setting of immunosuppression, particularly systemic lupus erythematosus,[5] but is not associated with human herpesvirus 8, also known as HHV8,[6] as has been demonstrated for other multifocal tumors such as Kaposi sarcoma. Cutaneous fibrous histiocytomas are elevated or pedunculated lesions measuring from a few millimeters to a few centimeters in diameter (Figs. 11-1 to 11-3). Rarely, they result in a depressed area in the skin (atrophic dermatofibroma).[7] They impart a red to red-brown to blue-black color to the overlying skin. Although usually ascribed to the presence of hemosiderin, epidermal hyperpigmentation has recently been attributed to lesional expression of stem cell factor and an increase in tyrosinase-positive melanocytes.[8] Such lesions may be confused clinically with malignant melanoma. The presence of a central dimple on lateral compression is regarded as a useful clinical sign for distinguishing it from melanoma.[9] Deeply situated fibrous histiocytomas are less common than cutaneous ones. The relative incidence is difficult to determine because the latter are less likely to be subjected to a biopsy or excised than the former. In a study by Fletcher,[10] only three cases of fibrous histiocytoma involving skeletal muscle were culled from more than 1000 fibrohistiocytic tumors. Like their cutaneous counterparts, they present as painless masses, usually on an extremity. Rarely deep fibrous histiocytomas may occur in retroperitoneal, mediastinal, and pelvic soft tissue.[11] Although they develop at any age, most occur between the ages of 20 and 40 years. They tend to be larger than the cutaneous tumors. Fibrous histiocytomas involving skeletal muscle and visceral soft tissue locations are often large, measuring 5 cm or more, in contrast to their cutaneous and subcutaneous counterparts, which usually measure 3 cm or less.[11] Grossly, they are circumscribed, yellow or white masses that may have focal areas of hemorrhage.

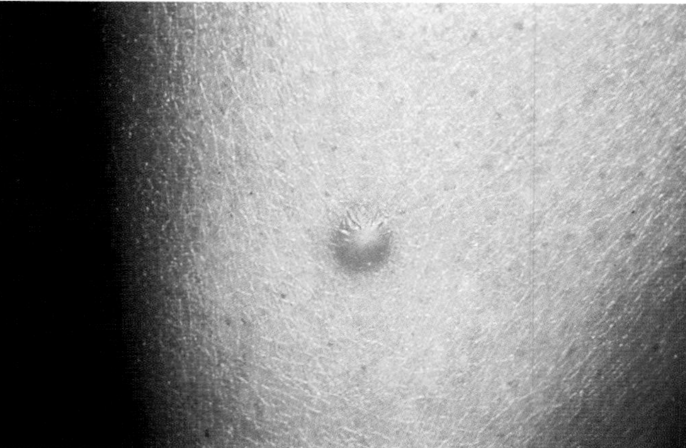

FIGURE 11-1. Red nodular appearance of a benign fibrous histiocytoma. *(Case courtesy of Dr. John T. Headington.)*

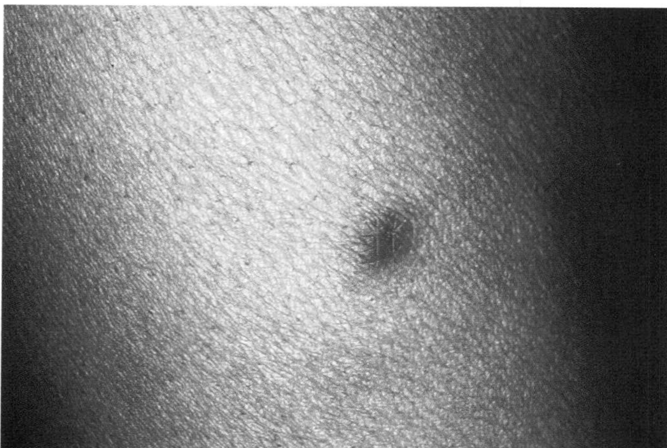

FIGURE 11-2. Benign fibrous histiocytoma with a pigmented appearance. *(Case courtesy of Dr. John T. Headington.)*

Microscopic Findings

The cutaneous fibrous histiocytoma consists of a nodular cellular proliferation involving dermis and occasionally subcutis (Fig. 11-4). The tumor is not sharply defined laterally and

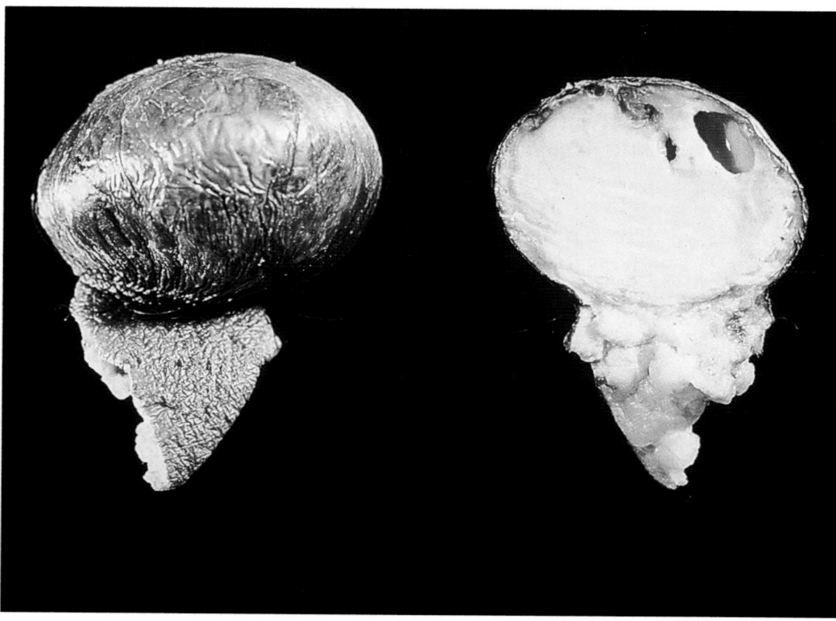

FIGURE 11-3. Gross appearance of a pedunculated cutaneous fibrous histiocytoma. The light color of the lesion is a result of the presence of large amounts of lipid. Focal cyst formation is also present.

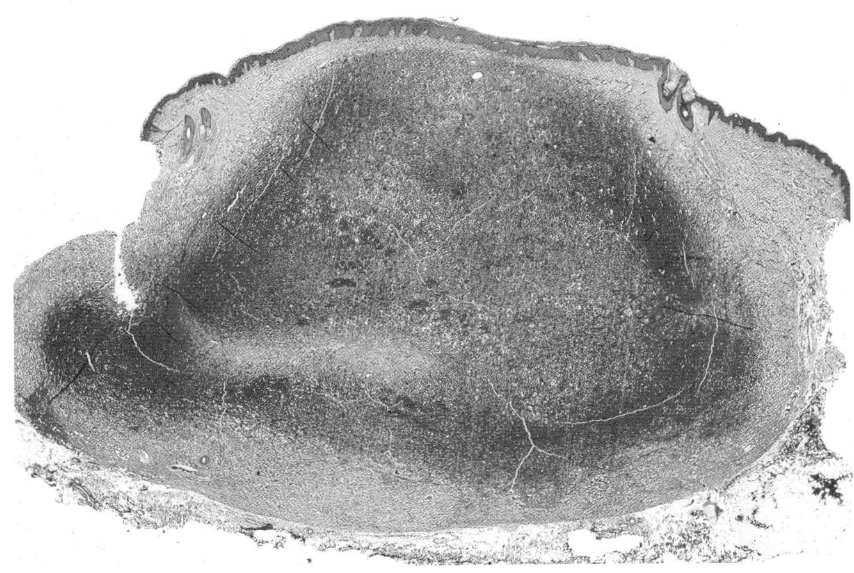

FIGURE 11-4. Low-power view of a cutaneous fibrous histiocytoma. The lesion is confined to the dermis and has a smooth, bulging deep margin.

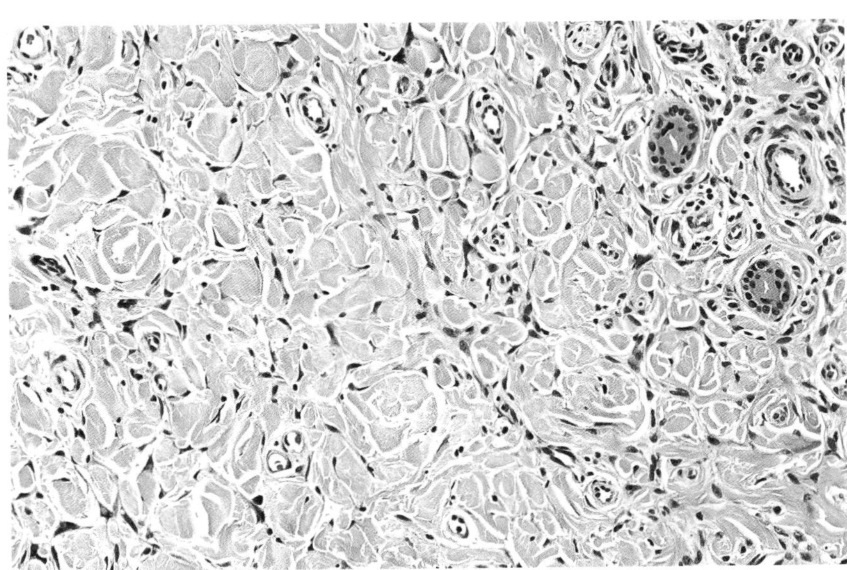

FIGURE 11-5. Lateral border of a fibrous histiocytoma illustrating entrapment of collagen.

typically interdigitates with dermal collagen (*collagen trapping*) (Fig. 11-5). The overlying epidermis frequently shows some degree of hyperplasia, including acanthosis or elongation and widening of the rete pegs (Fig. 11-6). Hyperplasia of other adnexal structures may also be seen, sometimes forming intralesional epithelial cysts. The presence of a rim of normal dermis between the epidermis and tumor is variable. At the deep margin, the tumor extends small tentacles for short distances into the subcutis (Fig. 11-7) or, less commonly, has a smoothly contoured margin (Fig. 11-8). Both patterns contrast with the diffusely infiltrating border of dermatofibrosarcoma protuberans. Most cutaneous fibrous histiocytomas consist of short, intersecting fascicles of lightly eosinophilic fibroblastic cells (Figs. 11-9 to 11-15). The fascicles usually form a loose crisscross pattern or a vague storiform pattern (see Fig. 11-9). Occasional rounded histiocytic cells accompany the spindle cells, but they rarely predominate. Multinucleated giant cells of the foreign body or Touton type are a typical feature of this form of fibrous histiocytoma and often contain phagocytosed lipid and hemosiderin (see Fig. 11-14). Inflammatory cells, particularly lymphocytes and xanthoma cells, are scattered randomly throughout the tumors but vary greatly in number. The stroma consists of a delicate collagen network surrounding individual cells. In a small number of cases, the vessels and stroma exhibit striking hyalinization (see Figs. 11-12 and 11-13). Cystic areas of hemorrhage are common and, when prominent, result in large accumulations of hemosiderin in the tumor cells (see Figs. 11-30 to 11-32). When this feature is striking, some have used the term *aneurysmal* fibrous histiocytoma (see Differential Diagnosis).[12-14] A number of other unusual features are seen in these lesions, including clear-cell change, granular cell change, nuclear palisading, extensive hyalinization, and lipidization (see the following paragraphs). Recently, it was pointed

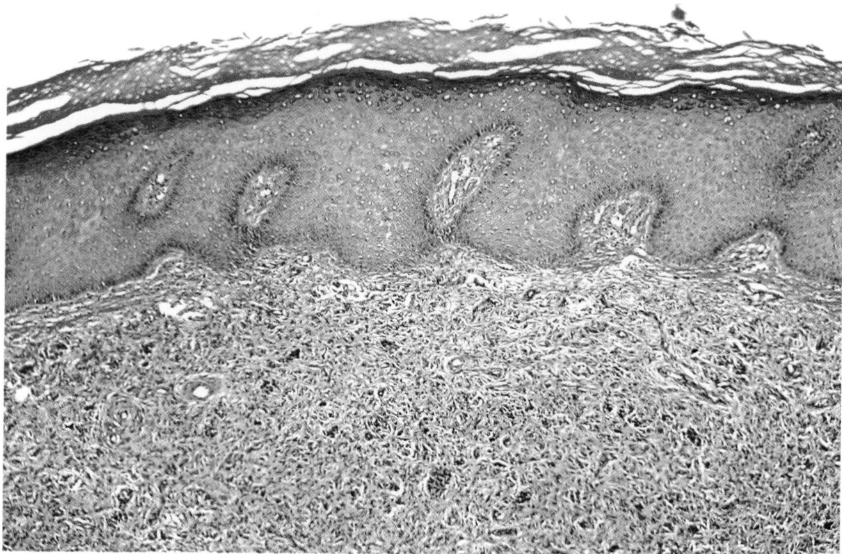

FIGURE 11-6. Epithelial hyperplasia overlying a fibrous histiocytoma.

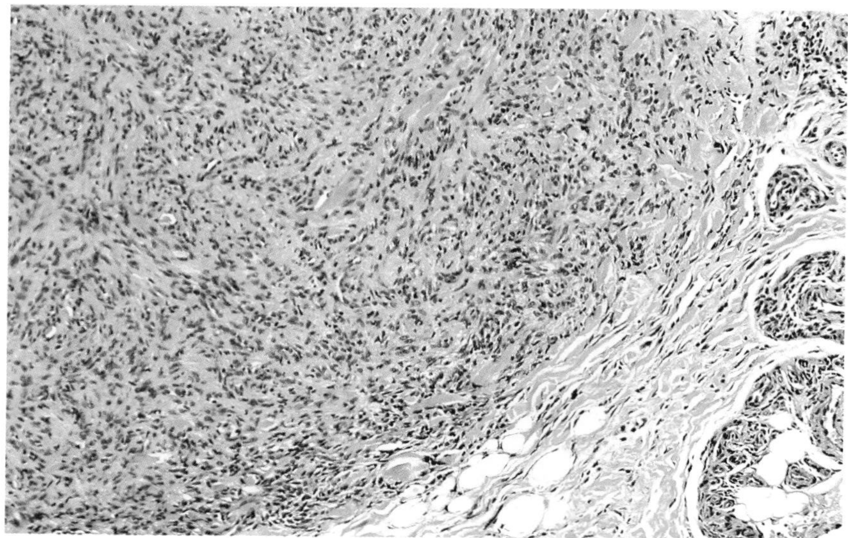

FIGURE 11-7. Smoothly contoured deep border of a fibrous histiocytoma.

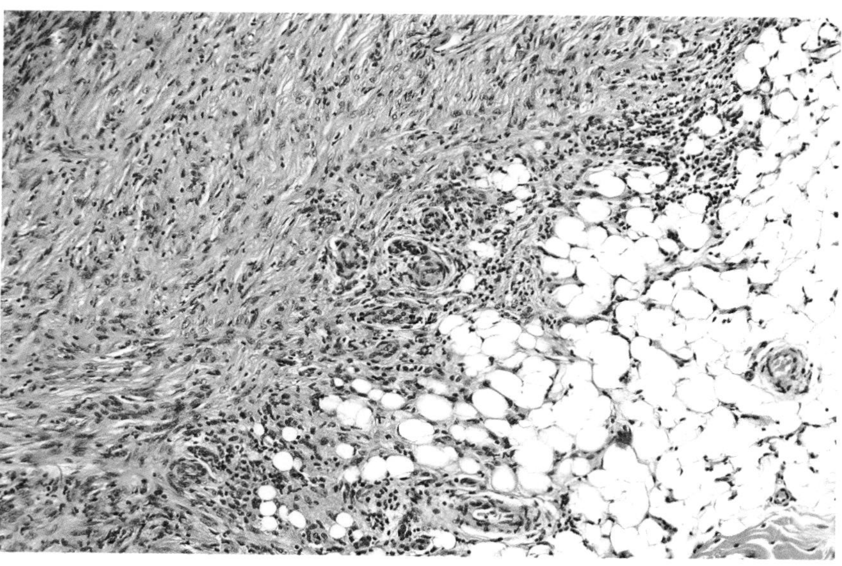

FIGURE 11-8. Minimal irregular penetration of the subcutis at the deep border of a fibrous histiocytoma contrasts with the more infiltrative border of dermatofibrosarcoma protuberans.

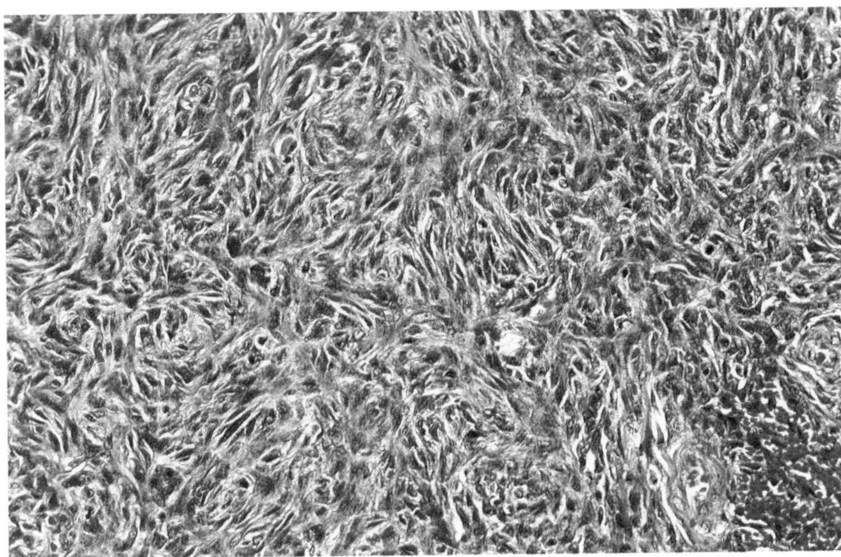

FIGURE 11-9. Fibrous histiocytoma with a predominantly spindled appearance.

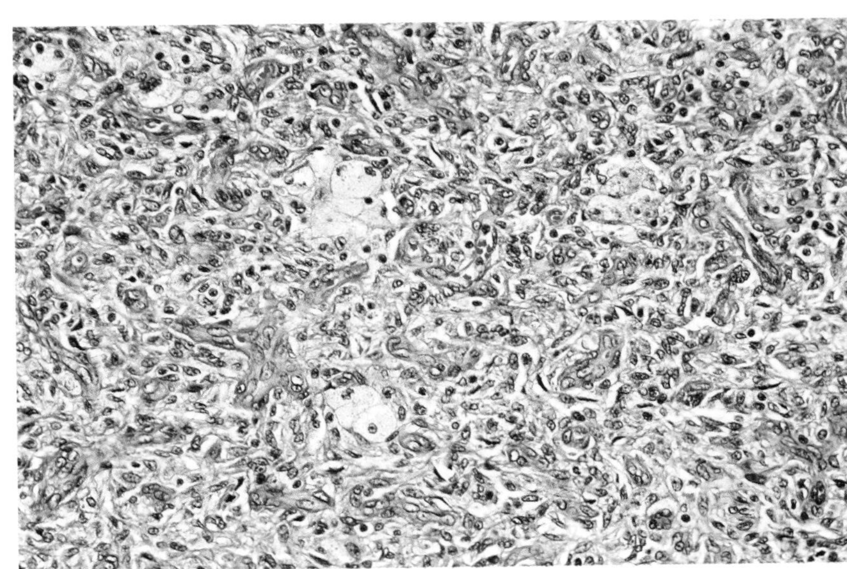

FIGURE 11-10. Fibrous histiocytoma with a mixture of spindled and xanthomatous cells.

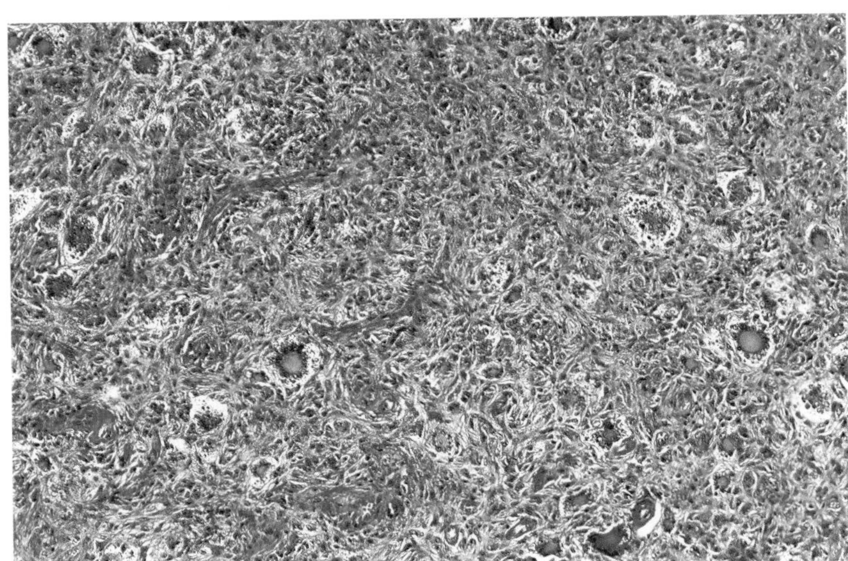

FIGURE 11-11. Fibrous histiocytoma with numerous Touton giant cells.

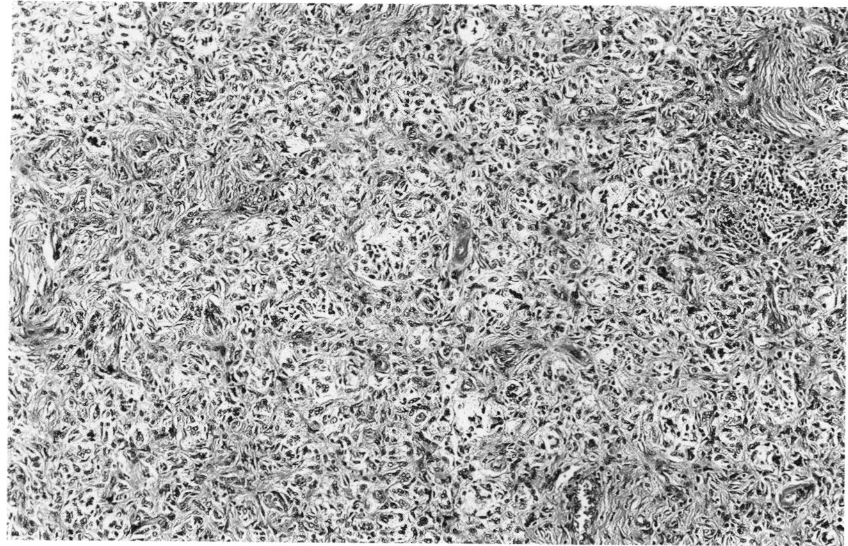

FIGURE 11-12. Fibrous histiocytoma with a lipidized appearance and some nuclear atypia.

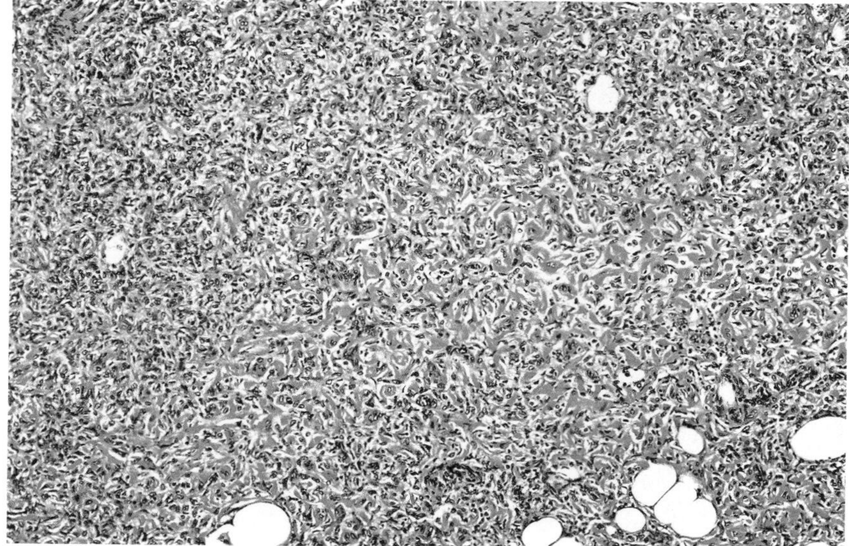

FIGURE 11-13. Fibrous histiocytoma with interstitial and perivascular hyalinization.

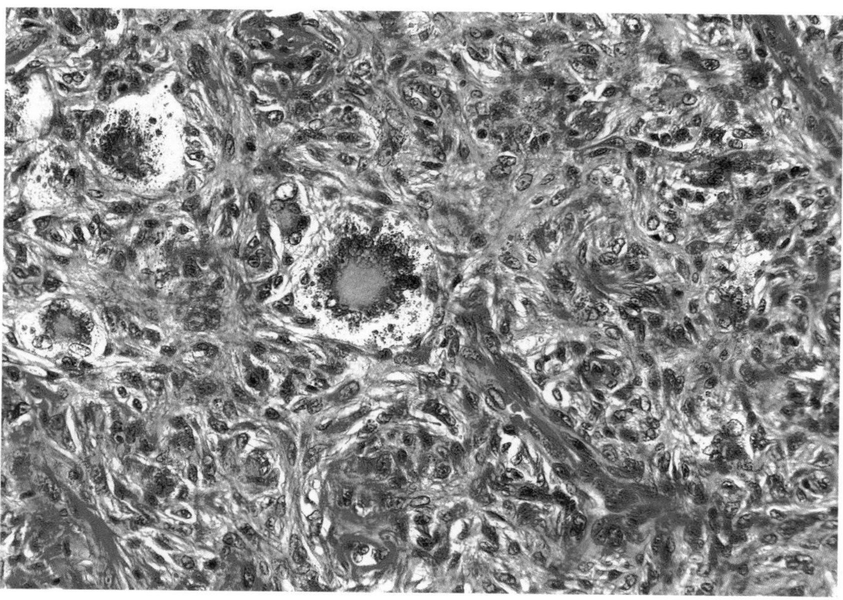

FIGURE 11-14. Touton giant cells containing lipid and hemosiderin.

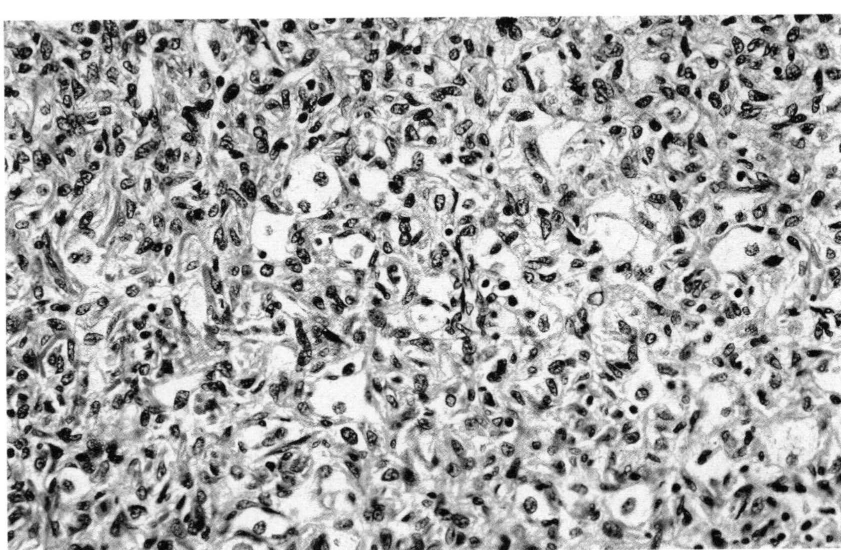

FIGURE 11-15. Xanthoma cells within fibrous histiocytoma.

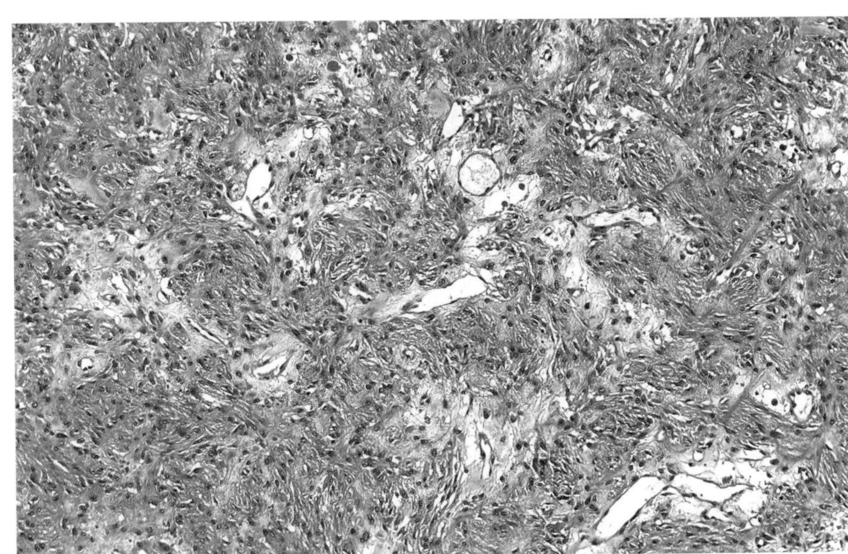

FIGURE 11-16. Fibrous histiocytoma of soft tissue. In contrast to cutaneous fibrous histiocytomas, these lesions have a more distinct storiform pattern but lack the variety of secondary elements such as xanthoma cells and siderophages.

out that fibrous histiocytomas occasionally evoke an unusual mesenchymal response around them, usually in the form of proliferation of mature smooth muscle.[15]

Deep fibrous histiocytomas are similar to their cutaneous counterparts, but they usually have a more prominent storiform pattern and fewer secondary elements such as xanthoma cells (Figs. 11-16 to 11-18). The stroma often undergoes myxoid change (see Fig. 11-17) or hyalinization. In unusual cases, dense bundles of collagen (amianthoid fibers) and even metaplastic osteoid are detected. Not infrequently, deep fibrous histiocytomas blend with areas indistinguishable from a benign solitary fibrous tumor/hemangiopericytoma (see Fig. 11-18). This combination of hemangiopericytic and fibrohistiocytic areas is particularly characteristic of fibrous histiocytomas of the orbit.

The benign nature of fibrous histiocytoma is usually apparent histologically. The cells are well differentiated and exhibit little pleomorphism and usually little or no mitotic activity (Fig. 11-19). The occasional pleomorphic cells with hyperchromatic nuclei and clear to eosinophilic cytoplasm (Fig. 11-20), referred to by some as *monster cells*,[16] within an otherwise typical fibrous histiocytoma seem to be a degenerative phenomenon and do not adversely affect the prognosis.[16,17] However, the presence of both pleomorphism and mitotic activity suggests a more aggressive lesion, either atypical fibrous histiocytoma (see Atypical Fibrous Histiocytoma) or superficial undifferentiated pleomorphic sarcoma. A small subset of fibrous histiocytomas known as *cellular fibrous histiocytomas* is characterized by somewhat longer, cellular fascicles of spindle cells bereft of other cellular elements (e.g., siderophages, giant cells). Although benign, these lesions have a high local recurrence rate and are discussed later.

Immunohistochemical Findings

The majority of fibrous histiocytomas displays immunostaining for factor XIIIa in a significant population of cells, leading

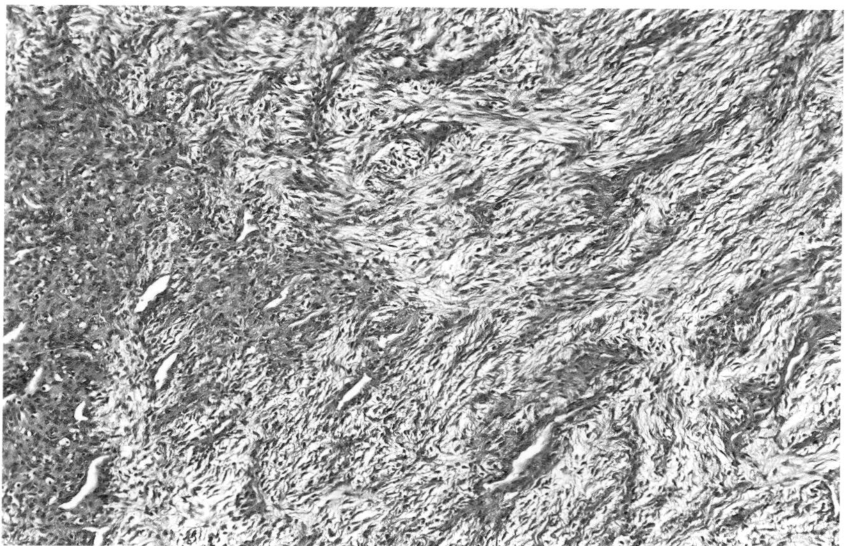

FIGURE 11-17. Fibrous histiocytoma of soft tissue with myxoid areas.

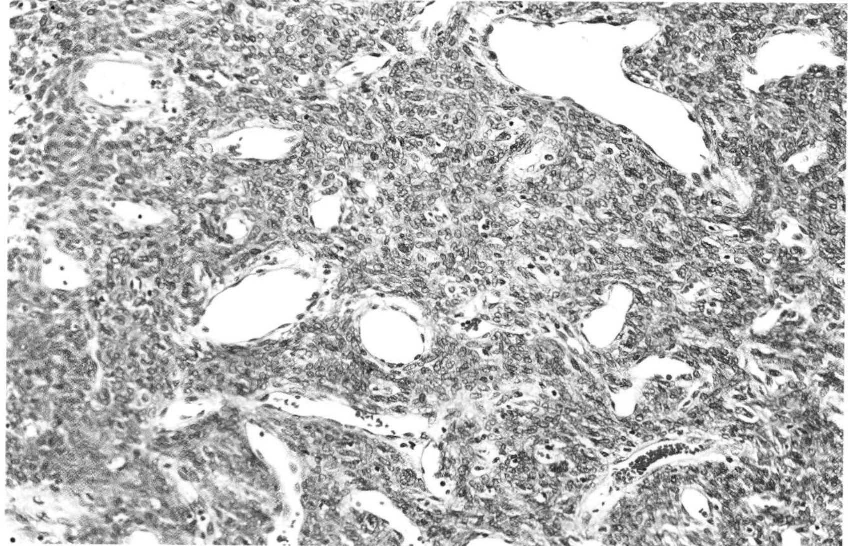

FIGURE 11-18. Hemangiopericytoma-like area within a fibrous histiocytoma of soft tissue.

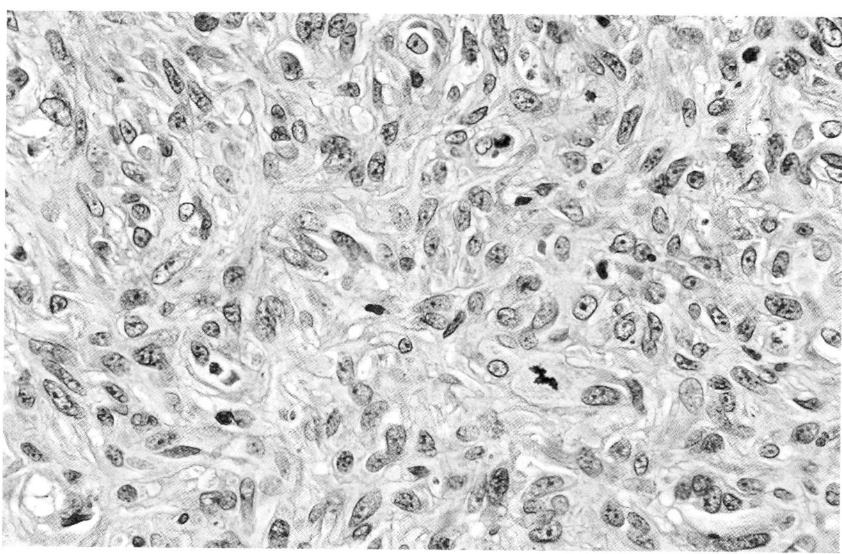

FIGURE 11-19. Plump spindle cells with benign fibrous histiocytoma displaying an occasional mitotic figure.

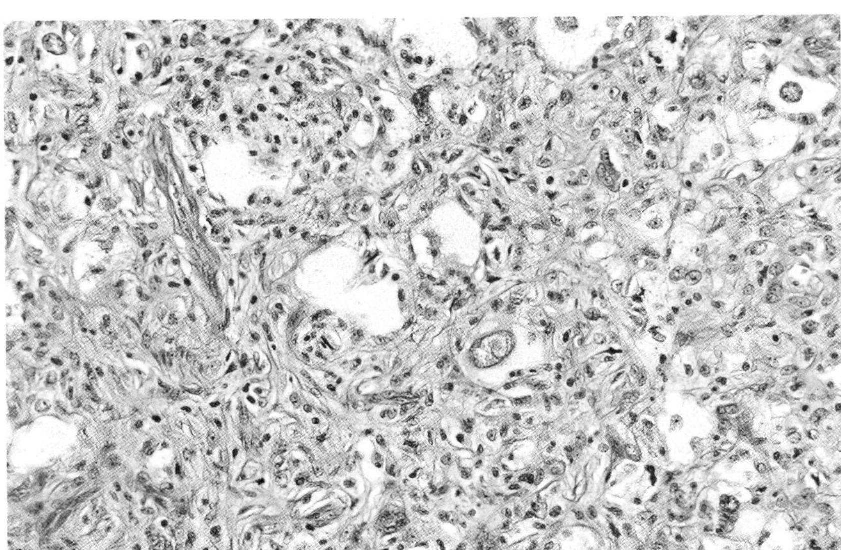

FIGURE 11-20. Pleomorphic (monster) cell within an otherwise benign fibrous histiocytoma of the skin.

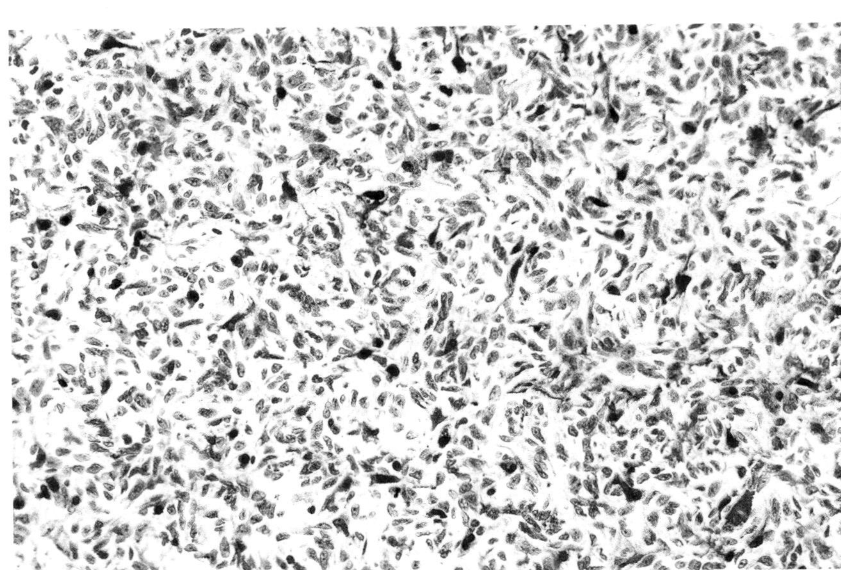

FIGURE 11-21. Factor XIIIa immunostain of a fibrous histiocytoma showing numerous positively staining dendritic cells.

some to conclude that these tumors arise from dermal dendrocytes[18] (Fig. 11-21). Whether factor XIIIa stains tumor elements or reactive dermal dendrocytes that populate benign fibrous histiocytomas is a matter of debate.[19] Factor XIIIa immunolabeling is frequently absent in the neoplastic cells in fibrous histiocytomas, in particular cellular fibrous histiocytomas, and the practical utility of this marker is questionable. Furthermore, factor XIIIa is present in many other mesenchymal lesions, and its presence per se is not diagnostic of fibrous histiocytomas. However, the combination of factor XIIIa and CD34 is commonly used to distinguish benign fibrous histiocytoma from dermatofibrosarcoma protuberans (see Differential Diagnosis). Myoid markers (e.g., desmin, smooth muscle myosin[20]) are occasionally present in fibrous histiocytomas and are significant only to point out that their sporadic presence should not be construed as evidence of a smooth muscle neoplasm. In particular, cellular fibrous histiocytomas commonly express smooth muscle actins in a myofibroblastic (tram-track) pattern. Fibrous histiocytomas also tend to contain other cell types, including dermal interstitial cells (CD34-positive), Langerhans cells (S-100 protein-positive) and macrophages (CD68 and CD163 positive), and the presence of multiple cell types is perhaps the most characteristic immunohistochemical aspect of these tumors.

Electron microscopic studies have shown a spectrum of cell types in these tumors. Cells resembling fibroblasts represent one end of this spectrum. They contain organized lamellae of rough endoplasmic reticulum but few or no lipid droplets and no phagolysosomes.[21] Depending on the functional state of these cells, they may acquire features of myofibroblasts. The other end of the spectrum is represented by rounded cells resembling histiocytes with numerous cell processes, mitochondria, and phagolysosomes.

Differential Diagnosis

Fibrous histiocytomas are most frequently confused with other benign lesions, notably nodular fasciitis, neurofibroma, and leiomyoma. Although nodular fasciitis may display a storiform pattern, it is distinguished from fibrous histiocytoma by its loosely arranged bundles of fibroblasts. Cellular areas containing proliferating fibroblasts alternate with loose myxoid zones containing extravasated red blood cells and inflammatory cells. The vasculature in fasciitis is seldom as orderly or as uniform as that of fibrous histiocytoma. Finally, because most cases of fasciitis are excised during the period of active growth, they usually manifest much more mitotic activity than a fibrous histiocytoma of comparable cellularity. It is difficult, if not impossible, to distinguish the early (cellular) phase of nodular fasciitis from a benign fibrous histiocytoma. Fortunately, from a practical point of view, this diagnostic imprecision has little adverse effect on patient care. The distinction between a fibrous histiocytoma and a neurofibroma is usually not difficult. Neurofibromas contain a population of Schwann cells expressing S-100 protein and having serpentine nuclei. Additional features of neural differentiation may include organoid structures reminiscent of sensory receptors or vague nuclear palisading. The usual lack of any storiform pattern or significant inflammation in the neurofibroma further underscores the difference between the two tumors. Sclerotic forms of leiomyoma may resemble a fibrous histiocytoma. However, smooth muscle tumors have a more distinct fascicular growth pattern. Their blunt-ended nuclei are plumper, and the cytoplasm typically has longitudinal striations corresponding to the presence of myofilamentous material, which can be accentuated with Masson trichrome stain. They strongly express smooth muscle actin and muscle-specific actin in a diffuse pattern, unlike the focal immunoreactivity noted in benign fibrous histiocytomas reflective of myofibroblastic differentiation.

Most important, fibrous histiocytoma must be distinguished from dermatofibrosarcoma protuberans. Like fibrous histiocytoma, dermatofibrosarcoma protuberans occurs in the dermis and subcutis but typically displays extensive subcutaneous involvement in the form of long, penetrating tentacles of tumor. It is also characterized by a more uniform cellular population and lacks overlying epidermal hyperplasia, giant cells, inflammatory cells, and xanthomatous elements. Its fascicles, composed of slender attenuated cells, are longer and arranged in a distinct storiform pattern, unlike the short curlicue fascicles of fibrous histiocytoma. Its margins are highly infiltrative, in contrast to the better defined margins of fibrous histiocytoma. Although fibrous histiocytomas may occasionally show limited extension into the subcutis, it is in the form of bulbous protrusions, rather than the diffuse, honeycomb pattern seen in dermatofibrosarcoma protuberans. Immunostaining reveals distinct differences in the cellular composition of these tumors as well. In contrast to fibrous histiocytomas, which typically consist of an admixture of factor XIIIa, CD34, S-100 protein, smooth muscle actin, and CD68-positive cells, dermatofibrosarcoma protuberans is essentially composed entirely of CD34-positive spindled cells (Fig. 11-22). Many fibrous histiocytomas, in particular cellular fibrous histiocytomas, also show a reactive component of CD34-positive cells, frequently present at the deep and lateral borders of the lesion, and care should be taken not to misinterpret this as evidence of a dermatofibrosarcoma protuberans. Those lesions previously described as indeterminate fibrohistiocytic lesions of the skin likely represent such cases, rather than a distinct entity.[22,23] Careful histologic evaluation and CD34 immunostaining (sometimes with the addition of factor XIIIa) should be sufficient for the distinction of fibrous histiocytoma and dermatofibrosarcoma protuberans in the great majority of cases. Other markers that have been reported to be of value in this differential diagnosis include podoplanin (D2-40),[24] HMGA1 and HMGA2[25] (positive in fibrous histiocytoma but not in dermatofibrosarcoma), and ApoD1 (positive in dermatofibrosarcoma but not in fibrous histiocytoma).[26]

The difference between benign fibrous histiocytomas and superficially located undifferentiated pleomorphic sarcomas is usually apparent because the latter is a pleomorphic, predominantly subcutaneous tumor with numerous typical and atypical mitotic figures and prominent areas of hemorrhage and necrosis. Less apparent is the difference between aneurysmal forms of fibrous histiocytoma and angiomatoid (malignant) fibrous histiocytoma. The latter is a distinctive, pediatric, translocation-associated mesenchymal tumor of uncertain lineage, characterized by sheets of histiocytic cells interrupted by cystic areas of hemorrhage. They are surrounded by a dense cuff of lymphocytes and plasma cells but almost never have giant cells or xanthoma cells as does the aneurysmal variant of fibrous histiocytoma.

Discussion

Whether benign fibrous histiocytomas are reactive or neoplastic is still debated. The most frequently cited arguments in favor of a reactive condition include the frequency with which minor trauma antedates the lesions, the accompanying inflammatory component, and the evolutionary stages of this disease. On the other hand, there is growing and reasonably compelling evidence that at least a subset is neoplastic. In general, benign fibrous histiocytomas do not involute and, in fact, are associated with a definable rate of local recurrence—in exceptional instances, metastases. Clonality, furthermore, has been documented in 30% to 100% of cases examined.[27-30] There seems to be some preliminary evidence suggesting a correlation between clonality and the appearance of the fibrous histiocytoma. For example, in the study by Vanni et al.,[28] clonality was slightly more common in cellular as opposed to conventional fibrous histiocytomas, and Hui et al.[30] noted that histiocytic-appearing lesions were more often clonal. Considering that the incidence of clonality varies from study to study and perhaps even amongst the various types of fibrous histiocytoma lends credence to the idea that fibrous histiocytomas may be a heterogeneous group of lesions, only some of which are neoplastic. The very rare occurrence of metastatic disease in well-documented fibrous histiocytomas also supports a neoplastic etiology, in some instances. A variety of chromosomal translocations have been identified in fibrous histiocytomas, most commonly in cellular variants, although a consistent abnormality has not yet been recognized.[28,29,31]

Regardless of the debate, generalizations can be made concerning behavior. Fewer than 5% of cutaneous fibrous histiocytomas recur following local excision.[3,19] The overall recurrence rate of cutaneous and soft tissue fibrous histiocytomas is approximately 10% following conservative therapy. Those located in deep soft tissue have a recurrence rate that is somewhat higher and is reflective of the larger size and incompleteness of the surgical excision. In this regard,

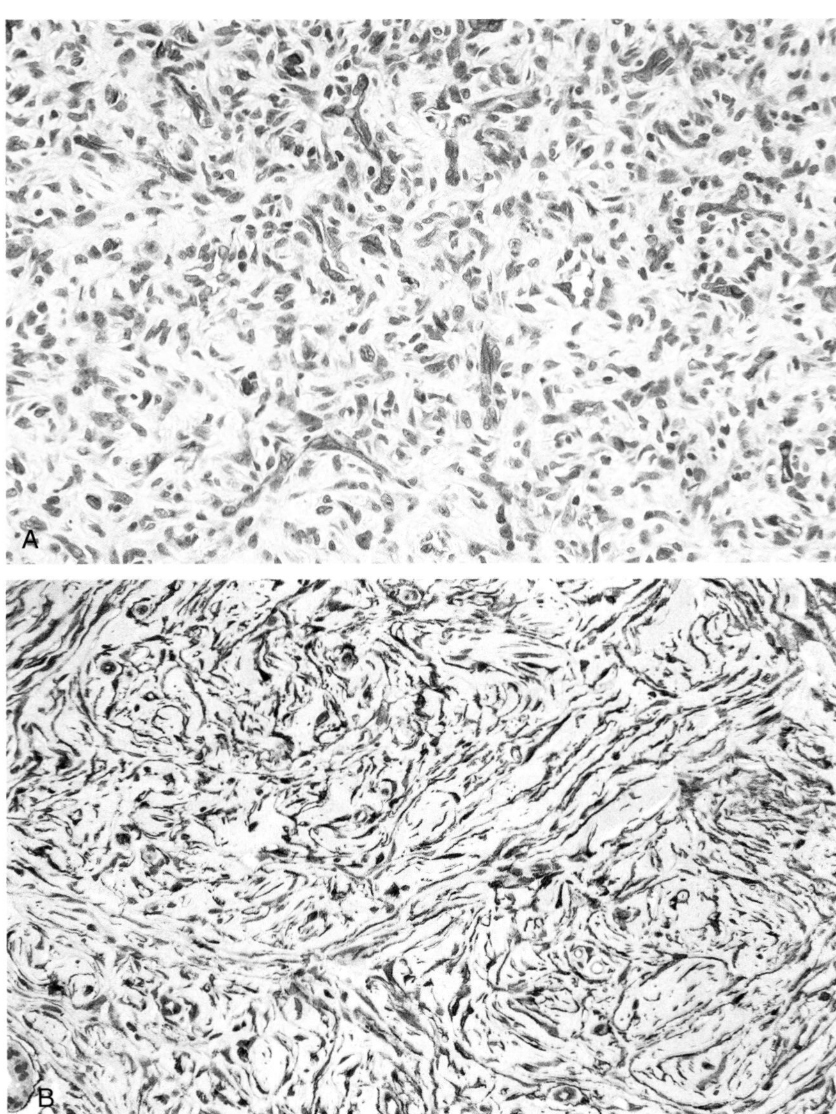

FIGURE 11-22. CD34 immunostains of benign fibrous histiocytoma and dermatofibrosarcoma protuberans. (A) CD34 immunostain of fibrous histiocytoma decorates normal vessels. (B) CD34 immunostain of a dermatofibrosarcoma protuberans in which the majority of tumor cells is decorated.

Franquemont et al.[32] reported a recurrence rate of nearly 50% for fibrous histiocytomas (eight cases) that extended into the subcutis or grew in a multinodular fashion (or both); and Font and Kidayat[33] noted that 57% of orbital fibrous histiocytomas with infiltrative margins or hypercellular zones (or both) recurred compared to 31% of those without these features. Mentzel et al.[34] likewise have commented that facial fibrous histiocytomas, which frequently invade subcutis and muscle, have a high rate of recurrence. Most recently, Gleason et al.[11] have documented a 22% local recurrence rate in deep fibrous histiocytomas.

Nearly every histologic feature used to assess malignancy of tumors in general has been recorded in clinically benign fibrous histiocytomas as an isolated finding (i.e., increased cellularity,[19] necrosis,[10] vascular invasion,[3,10] mitotic activity, atypia[16,17]) and sometimes even in company with one another without adverse consequences. Therefore, it is important to recognize the underlying nature of the lesion to know what significance to place on many of these features. A useful guideline is that benign fibrous histiocytomas may show enhanced cellularity and some level of mitotic activity (e.g., cellular fibrous histiocytoma) and still be considered benign. Likewise, benign fibrous histiocytomas may display nuclear atypia on a degenerative basis in the form of large monster cells set amidst the typical backdrop of banal neoplastic cells. Such lesions also are clinically benign. The presence of both mitotic activity and atypia (especially atypical mitotic figures) in the same lesion should be a cause for concern and raise the question of the so-called *atypical fibrous histiocytomas* (see Atypical Fibrous Histiocytoma) or more ominous lesions such as atypical fibroxanthoma or superficial undifferentiated pleomorphic sarcoma.

Some examples of histologically benign fibrous histiocytomas have produced metastases. Two cases were reported by Colome-Grimmer and Evans.[35] Both were small (2 cm) cutaneous lesions that recurred, producing regional lymph node (and ultimately pulmonary) metastasis. The metastases appeared similar to the primary lesions, and both patients

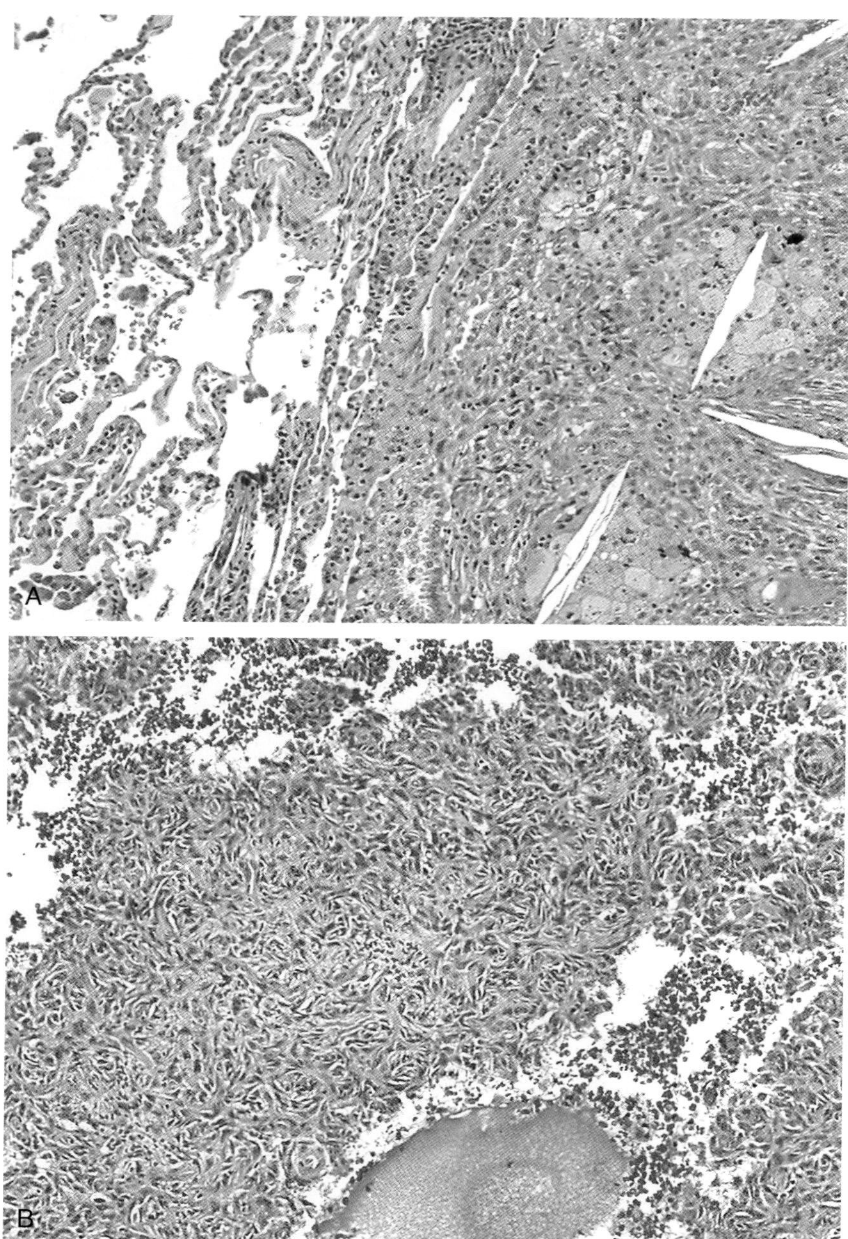

FIGURE 11-23. Pulmonary metastasis from otherwise-typical aneurysmal benign fibrous histiocytoma (A). The primary dermal tumor showed typical features of aneurysmal fibrous histiocytoma (B).

were alive 4 and 8 years after resection of the pulmonary deposits. Guillou et al.[36] described three patients with fibrous histiocytomas of the aneurysmal, cellular, or atypical type who developed regional lymph node metastases but who had a protracted course and favorable outcome.[36] Rare metastases have also been reported in association with otherwise-typical deep fibrous histiocytomas.[11] Cases described in the pulmonary pathology literature as *cystic fibrohistiocytic lesions* of the lung also appear to represent examples of metastasizing fibrous histiocytoma.[37] Instances of pulmonary metastasis from benign cutaneous fibrous histiocytomas have been seen in which the metastases also appeared histologically benign (Fig. 11-23). Fortunately, such cases are exceedingly rare, and the prognosis for these patients appears to be favorable. As such, a discussion of this potential complication in the routine sign-out of cases of fibrous histiocytoma is not recommended.

VARIANTS OF BENIGN FIBROUS HISTIOCYTOMA

There are a number of histologic variants of benign fibrous histiocytoma. With the exception of the cellular and epithelioid forms, these designations are of minor importance. Cellular fibrous histiocytoma appears to have a higher risk of local recurrence and often poses a diagnostic challenge to distinguish it from more aggressive lesions such as fibrosarcoma,

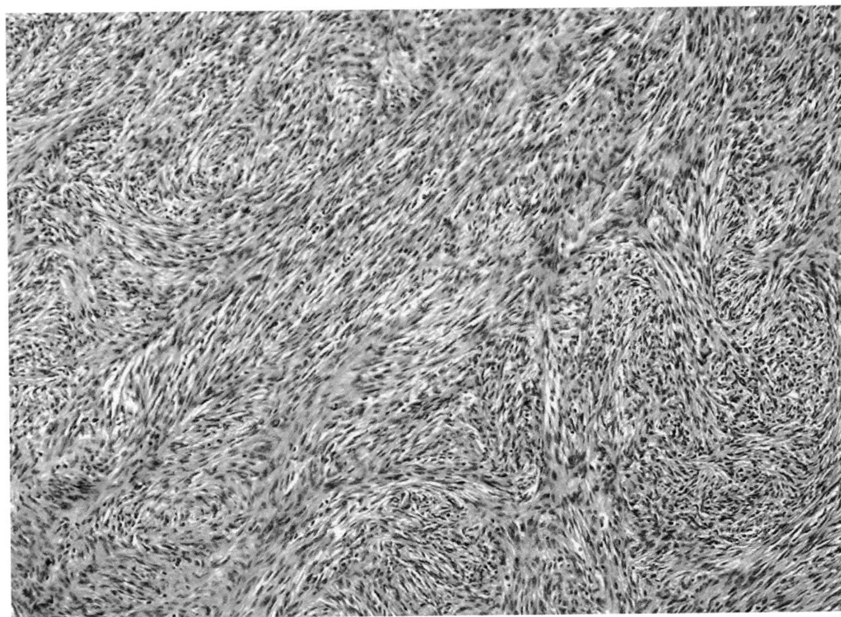

FIGURE 11-24. Cellular fibrous histiocytoma illustrating monomorphic spindle cells arranged in short and long fascicles.

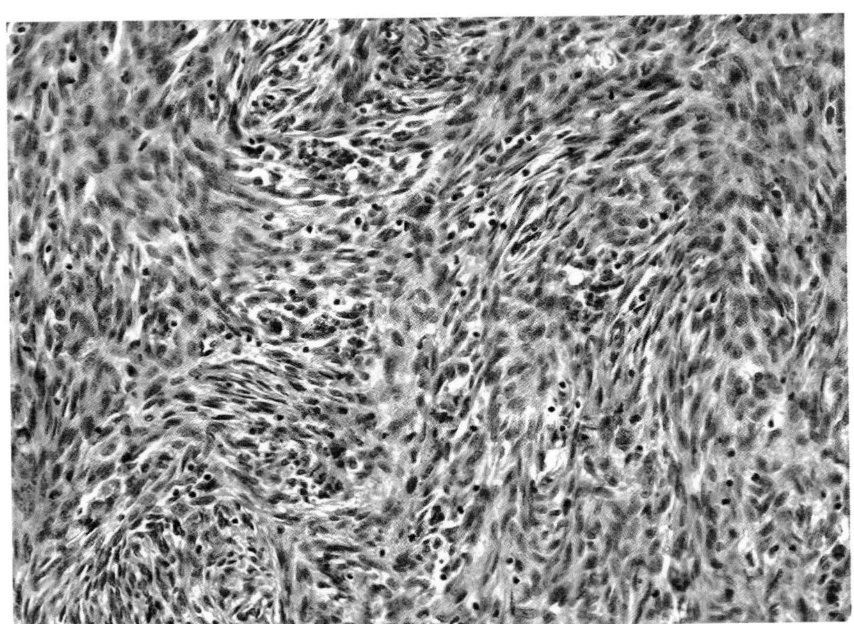

FIGURE 11-25. Cellular fibrous histiocytoma.

whereas the epithelioid fibrous histiocytoma can be confused with tumors of melanocytic lineage.

Cellular Fibrous Histiocytoma

Cellular fibrous histiocytoma is a designation used for lesions characterized by increased cellularity and a more fascicular (and less storiform) growth pattern. Some cases of dermatofibroma with subcutaneous extension[38,39] and dermatofibroma with potential for local recurrence[32] are examples of this variant. Occurring in an age range and anatomic location similar to those for ordinary benign fibrous histiocytoma, these lesions are composed of a relatively monomorphic population of plump spindle cells arranged in longer fascicles with fewer inflammatory cells and giant cells (Figs. 11-24 and 11-25). In addition, mitotic activity is usually somewhat higher (mean 3 mitoses/10 high-power fields [HPF]) and subcutaneous extension more common (30%) than in the usual fibrous histiocytoma. About 10% undergo spontaneous central necrosis, a phenomenon that seems to be particularly common in tumors in younger patients. Although the local recurrence rate of 25% for this form of fibrous histiocytoma seemingly contrasts with that of the ordinary form, it has not been demonstrated that cellularity is an independent predictor of recurrence. The high incidence of extension into the subcutis by this form of fibrous histiocytoma suggests that this feature might be equally significant. Nonetheless, it is still useful to recognize the cellular form of fibrous histiocytoma as a distinct variant, but it is also important to comment on extensive subcutaneous extension when present in fibrous histiocytomas of the usual type as a possible predictor of recurrence.

Epithelioid Fibrous Histiocytoma

Epithelioid fibrous histiocytoma is defined as a fibrous histiocytoma in which one-half or more of the cells assume a rounded epithelioid shape.[40-42] It presents as a solitary, red cutaneous nodule with an epidermal collarette similar to that of a pyogenic granuloma. The cells, large and polygonal with abundant eosinophilic cytoplasm, resemble those of a reticulohistiocytoma. Transitions to areas of conventional fibrous histiocytoma are frequent (Figs. 11-26 to 11-28). Epithelioid fibrous histiocytoma contains a variable population of CD34-positive dermal fibroblasts and factor XIIIa-positive dendritic histiocytes, which supports the idea that these tumors arise from the dermal microvascular unit.[43] The unusual appearance of this variant of fibrous histiocytoma often raises the possibility of a number of other lesions, Spitz nevus being a prime consideration. However, epithelioid fibrous histiocytomas are S-100 protein negative.

Aneurysmal Fibrous Histiocytoma

Approximately 1% to 2% of benign fibrous histiocytomas undergo extensive cystic hemorrhage. Dubbed "aneurysmal fibrous histiocytomas," their significance resides in that they can evolve rapidly as a result of spontaneous intralesional hemorrhage.[12-14,44] Their blue to black color suggests the clinical diagnosis of a vascular or melanocytic tumor. At low power, these lesions are seen to contain large blood-filled spaces lined by discohesive fragments of tumor rather than endothelium (Figs. 11-29 to 11-32). Hemosiderin may be abundant, and mitotic activity is often noted in the immediate vicinity of the hemorrhage. The cells of aneurysmal fibrous histiocytomas are typically plump and grow in tight storiform

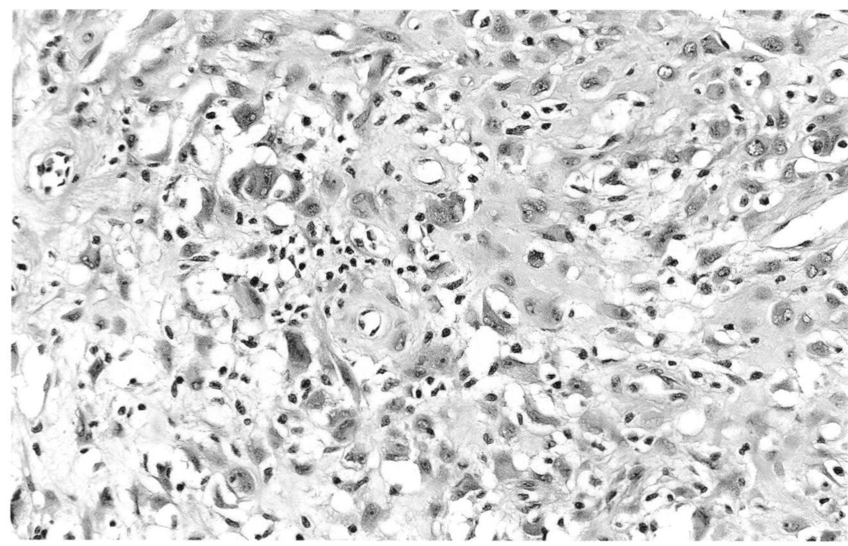

FIGURE 11-26. Epithelioid fibrous histiocytoma.

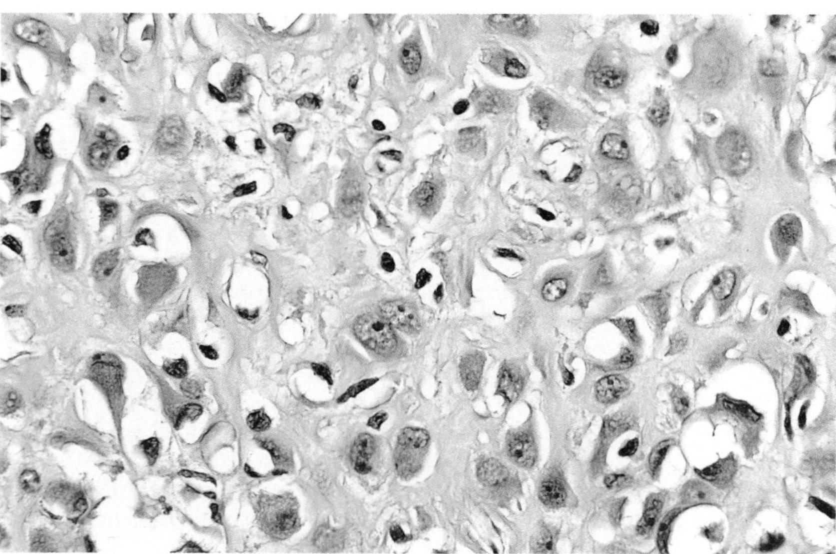

FIGURE 11-27. High-power view of an epithelioid fibrous histiocytoma.

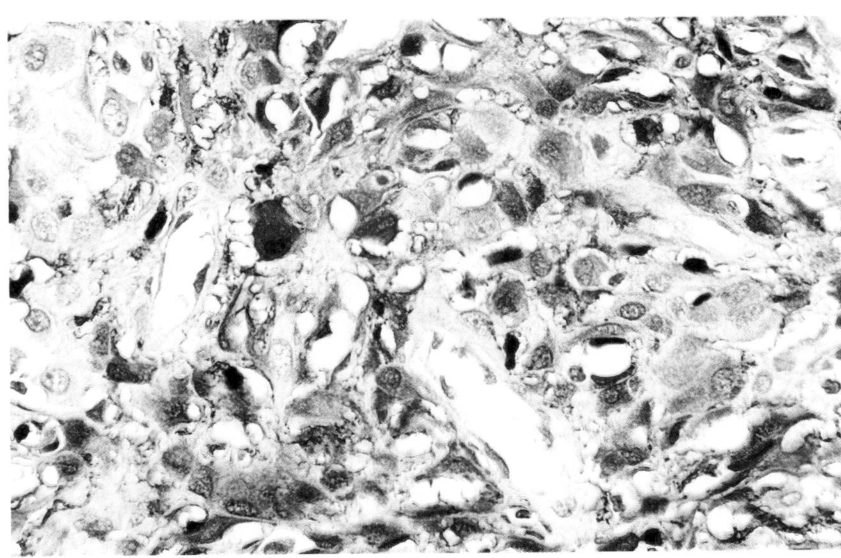

FIGURE 11-28. Factor XIIIa immunostain decorates cells of an epithelioid fibrous histiocytoma.

arrays. A 20% recurrence rate has been reported for these tumors, but there are too few reported cases to know whether this is meaningful. Despite the similarity of names, the aneurysmal fibrous histiocytoma should be clearly distinguished from the angiomatoid (malignant) fibrous histiocytoma of childhood, a subcutaneous lesion often associated with systemic symptoms (see Chapter 12).

Minor Histologic Variants

There are a number of rare and minor variants of benign fibrous histiocytoma.[16,34,45-47] They are principally important in that they evoke a somewhat different list of diagnostic considerations. Zelger et al.[48] described a clear cell dermatofibroma in which most of the cells underwent a translucent clear-cell change (Fig. 11-33). This lesion must be distinguished from clear cell carcinomas or melanocytic tumors involving the skin. The cells are positive for factor XIIIa but not for melanocytic antigens. Lipidized (ankle-type) fibrous histiocytoma, typically a lesion of the lower leg, particularly ankle, is usually larger than the usual fibrous histiocytomas and is characterized by foamy histiocytes situated within a hyalinized collagenous or osteoid-like stromal backdrop (Fig. 11-34).[49] Fortuitous palisading of nuclei (palisaded fibrous histiocytoma[46]), extensive myxoid change (myxoid dermatofibroma[47]), and granular cell change have also been noted in fibrous histiocytomas.

ATYPICAL FIBROUS HISTIOCYTOMA

A very small number of fibrous histiocytomas have borderline histologic features that include significantly more atypia and mitotic activity than are encountered in the usual type. Kaddu et al.[50] coined the term *atypical fibrous histiocytomas* for these lesions. They differ from atypical fibroxanthoma/superficial undifferentiated pleomorphic sarcomas in their predilection for younger individuals (mean, 38 years) and in a distribution that favors the extremities as opposed to the sun-exposed

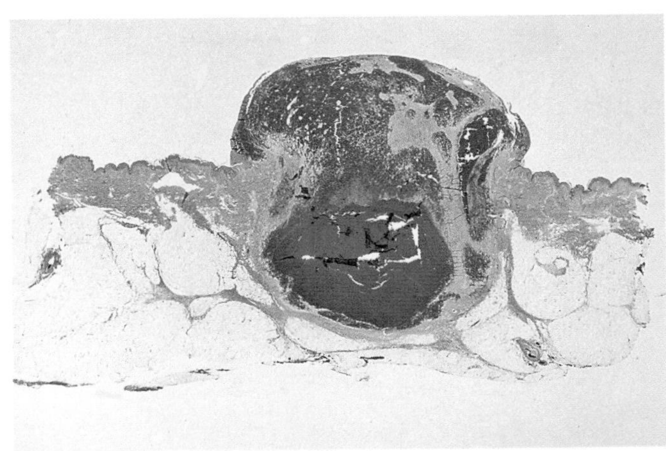

FIGURE 11-29. Aneurysmal fibrous histiocytoma.

surfaces of the face and neck. The average size is less than 2 cm. The majority are restricted to the dermis with superficial subcutaneous involvement in one-third of cases. The diagnosis of atypical fibrous histiocytoma needs to be made judiciously and should be applied only to those cases in which there is a clear-cut background of classic fibrous histiocytoma and that display areas of more generalized atypia than the occasional monster cell described previously and increased mitotic activity, including atypical forms (Figs. 11-35 and 11-36). Follow-up information in 21 patients[50] followed for approximately 4 years disclosed local recurrences in 3 patients and distant metastases in 2, one of whom died.

DERMATOMYOFIBROMA

Dermatomyofibroma, originally described as *haemorrhagic dermatomyofibroma* (plaque-like dermal fibromatosis),[51] is an uncommon benign cutaneous tumor showing fibroblastic and myofibroblastic differentiation. Fewer than 100 cases have been reported.[34,45,51-55]

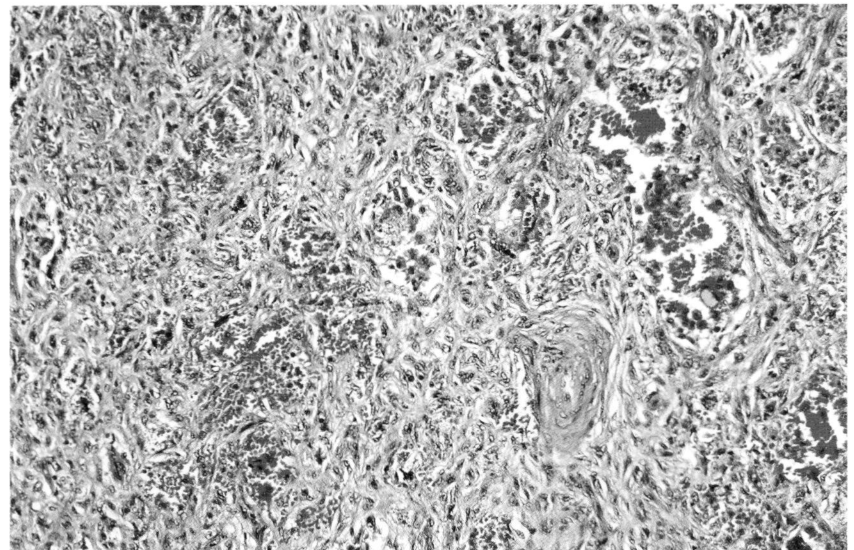

FIGURE 11-30. Cystic hemorrhage in an aneurysmal fibrous histiocytoma.

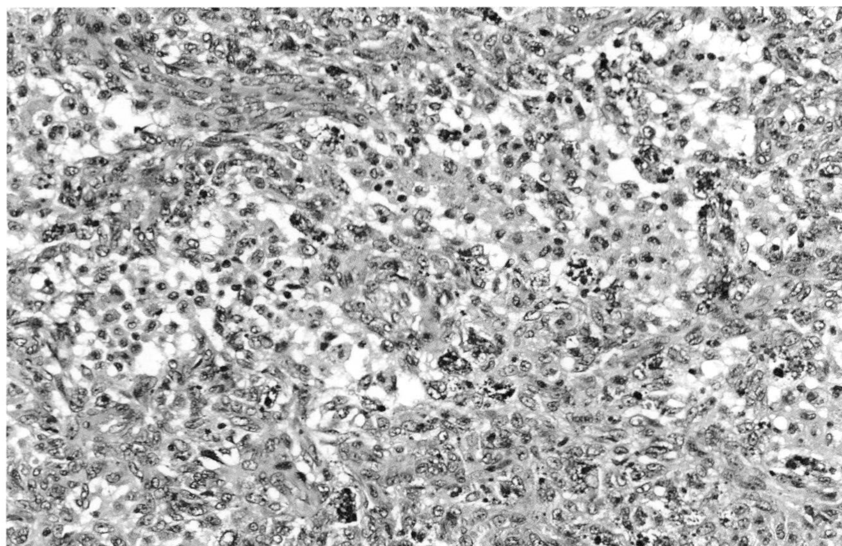

FIGURE 11-31. Hemosiderin deposits in an aneurysmal fibrous histiocytoma.

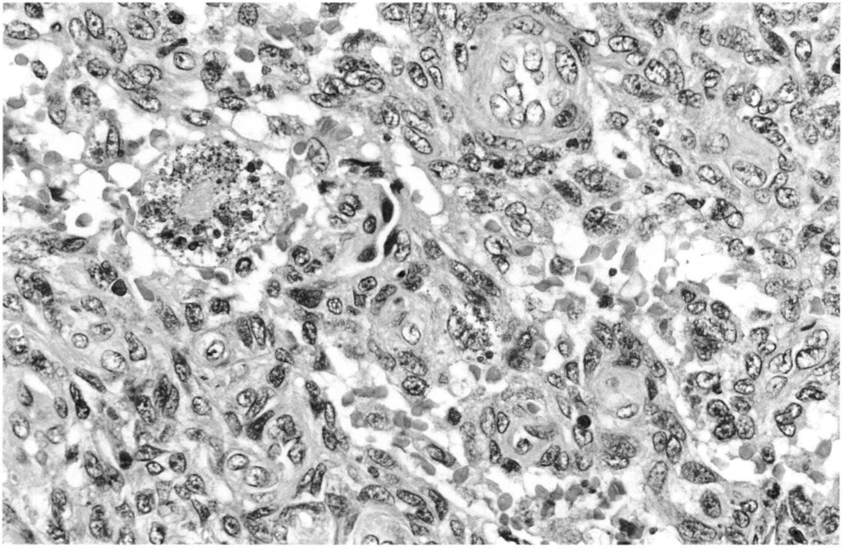

FIGURE 11-32. Hemosiderin deposits and cystic hemorrhage in an aneurysmal fibrous histiocytoma.

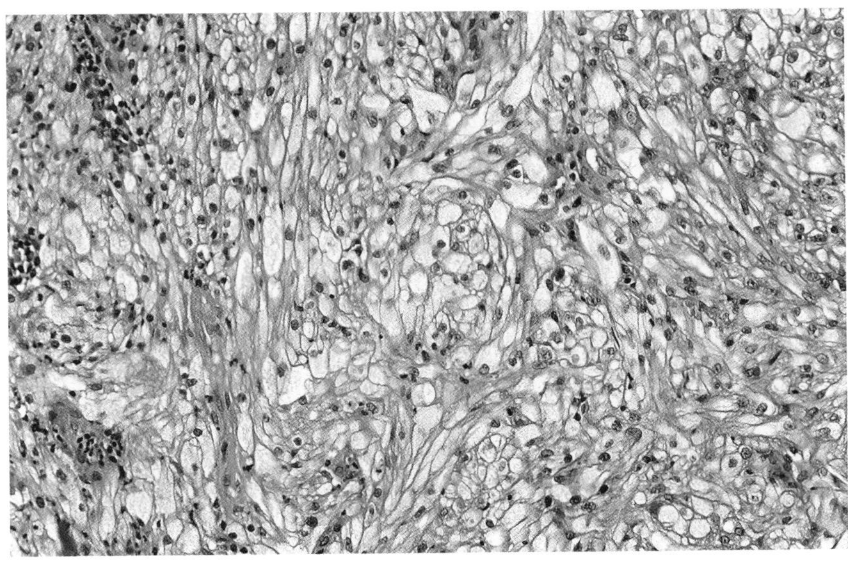

FIGURE 11-33. Clear cell fibrous histiocytoma (dermatofibroma).

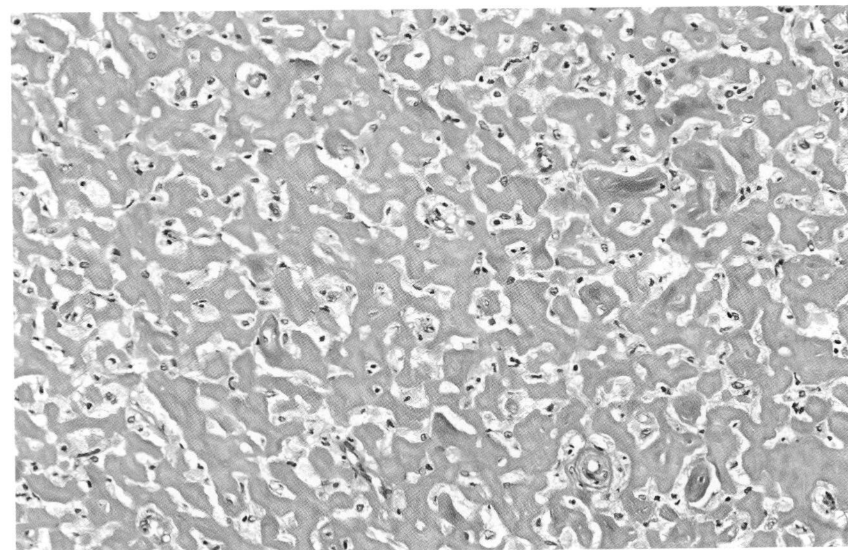

FIGURE 11-34. Lipidized fibrous histiocytoma.

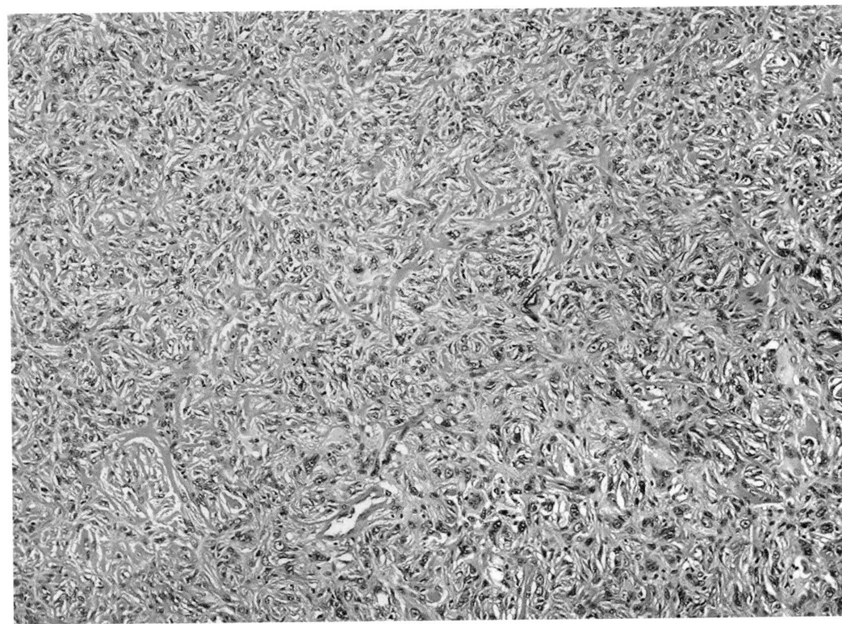

FIGURE 11-35. Atypical fibrous histiocytoma showing interface between classic benign fibrous histiocytoma (upper left) and more atypical areas (lower right).

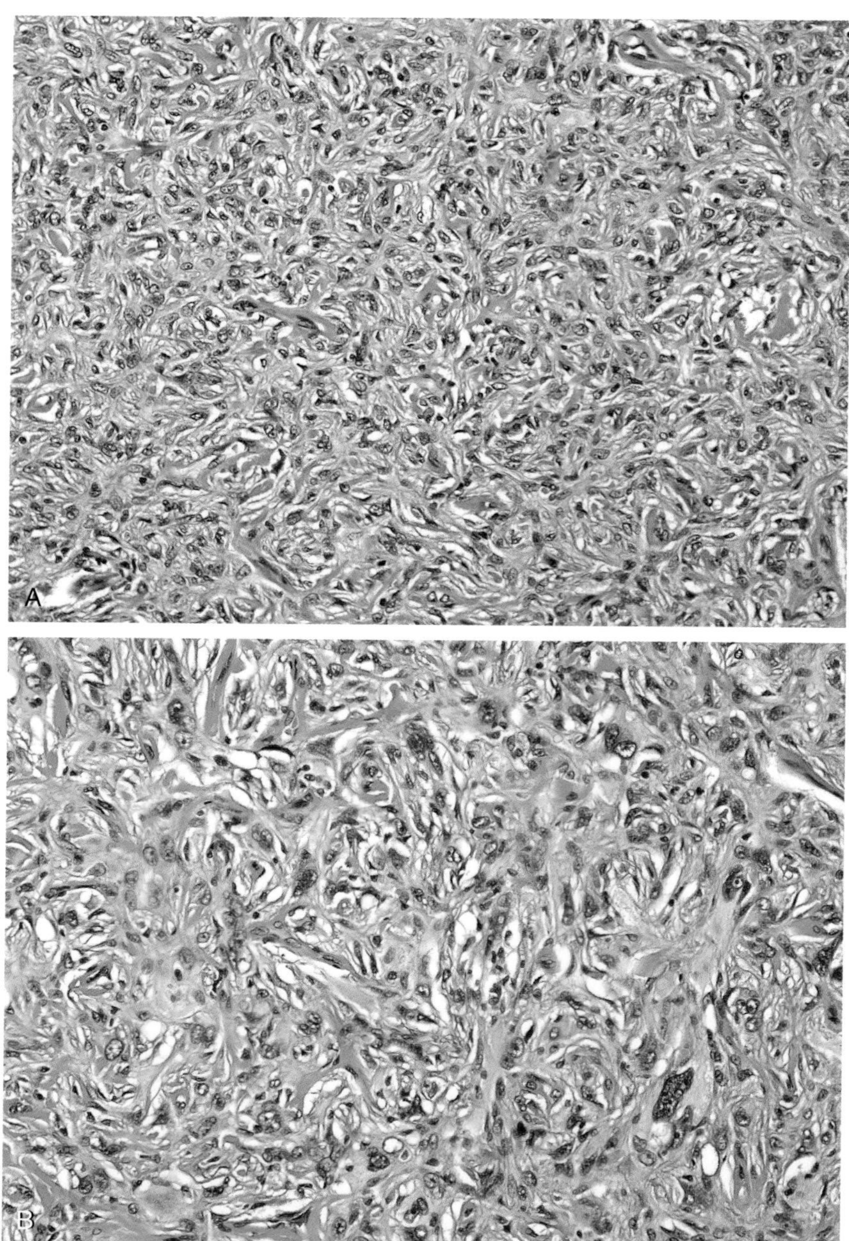

FIGURE 11-36. Atypical fibrous histiocytoma showing areas of classic benign fibrous histiocytoma (A) and more atypical areas (B). Same case as Figure 11-35.

Dermatomyofibroma occurs much more often in women than in men, with a mean patient age of roughly 30 years.[53] Cases occurring in pediatric patients have been reported as well.[53,55] The tumors most often involve the shoulder, neck, and trunk, but may occur in a wide variety of locations. Clinically, dermatomyofibromas present as linear, plaque-like, and sometimes hemorrhagic lesions, mimicking a wide variety of neoplastic and non-neoplastic diseases of the skin. Microscopically, the lesions consist of an ill-defined, plaque-like proliferation of well-differentiated, cytologically bland (myo) fibroblastic spindled cells, typically oriented parallel to the overlying epidermis (Fig. 11-37). Most tumors are confined to the dermis, although limited subcutaneous involvement can be seen as well. Nuclear atypia and mitotic activity are absent. Despite their name, dermatomyofibromas show myofibroblastic differentiation in the form of smooth muscle actin expression in only a minority of cases, with only 11 of 48 cases expressing this marker in the largest reported series to date.[53] Dermatomyofibromas are entirely benign, with only rare local recurrences.

Dermatomyofibromas differ from typical fibrous histiocytomas (dermatofibromas) in that they lack epidermal hyperplasia, peripheral collagen trapping, and siderophages/giant cells, consist of a more uniform proliferation of spindled cells oriented parallel to the epidermis, and contain increased amounts of dermal elastic fibers.[53] Although dermatomyofibromas may show limited CD34 expression, they lack the storiform growth pattern and infiltrative growth pattern seen in dermatofibrosarcoma protuberans. Cutaneous involvement is very rare in desmoid-type fibromatoses, which typically

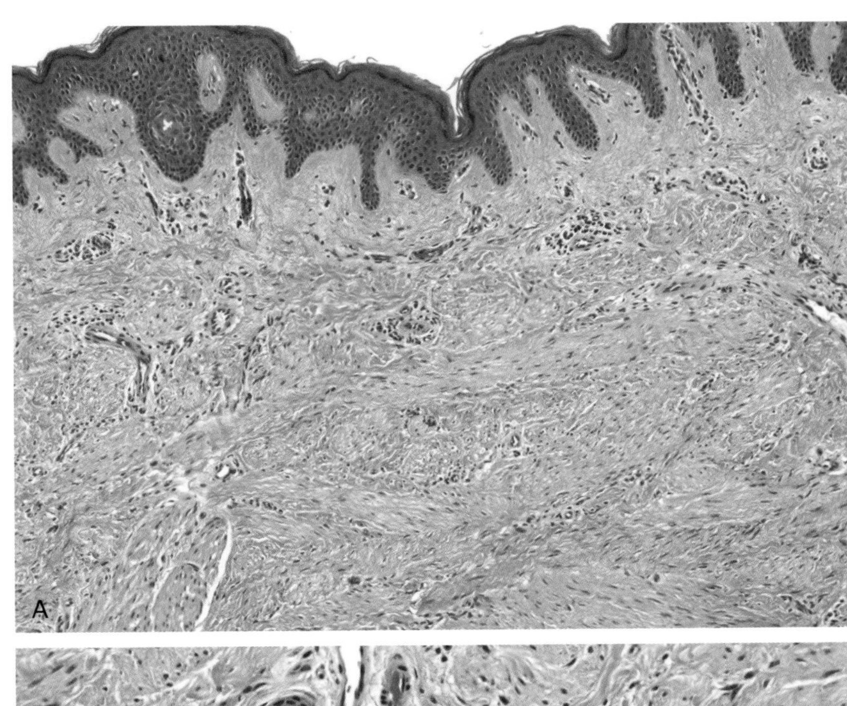

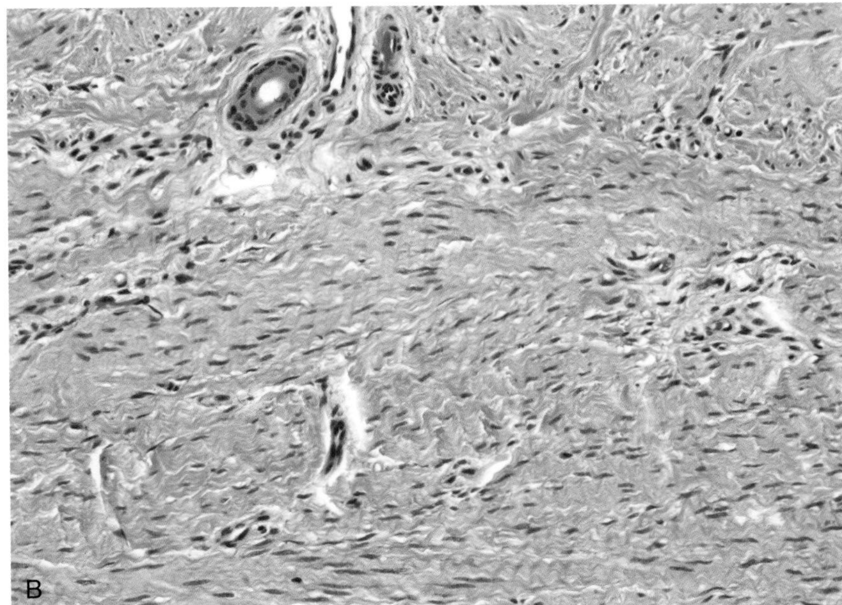

FIGURE 11-37. Dermatomyofibroma, showing moderately cellular fascicles of well-differentiated fibroblastic cells, arranged parallel to the overlying epidermal surface (A). Higher power view of dermatomyofibroma, showing very bland fibroblastic cells and increased dermal elastin fibers (B).

present as larger, deeply situated lesions, showing longer fascicles of myofibroblastic cells.

CELLULAR NEUROTHEKEOMA

Neurothekeoma, originally termed *cellular neurothekeoma*, was described by Barnhill and Mihm,[56] who considered it to represent the cellular, S-100 protein-negative end of the neurothekeoma spectrum of tumors. It has since become abundantly clear that classical, myxoid neurothekeoma (now better termed *nerve sheath myxoma*) and cellular neurothekeoma are entirely unrelated.[24,57-62] Nerve sheath myxoma, a true schwannian neoplasm, is discussed in Chapter 27. Although the terms *neurothekeoma* and *cellular neurothekeoma* are clearly misnomers, they are well-embedded in the literature, and they are retained for the time being. Although the line of differentiation taken by neurothekeoma is unclear, the best available evidence, including very recent gene profiling data,[63] suggests that this tumor falls within the spectrum of fibrohistiocytic tumors.

Clinical Features

Neurothekeomas usually occur in young patients, with a peak incidence in the second decade of life (median age, 17 years); 85% occur in patients younger than 40 years of age.[57,59] The tumors are roughly twice as common in women as in men and most commonly involve the head/neck, upper

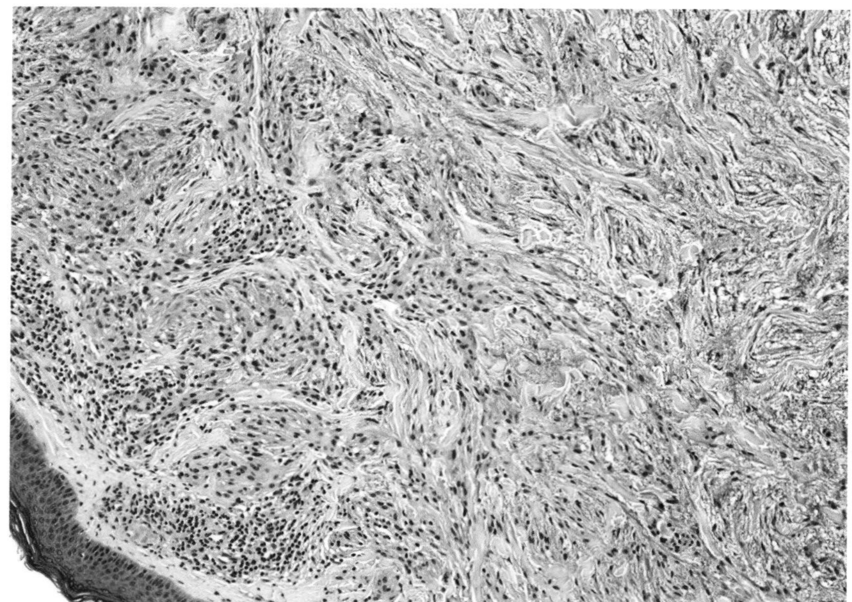

FIGURE 11-38. Cellular neurothekeoma, consisting of a dermal-based, partially myxoid, nested proliferation of bland, histiocytoid cells.

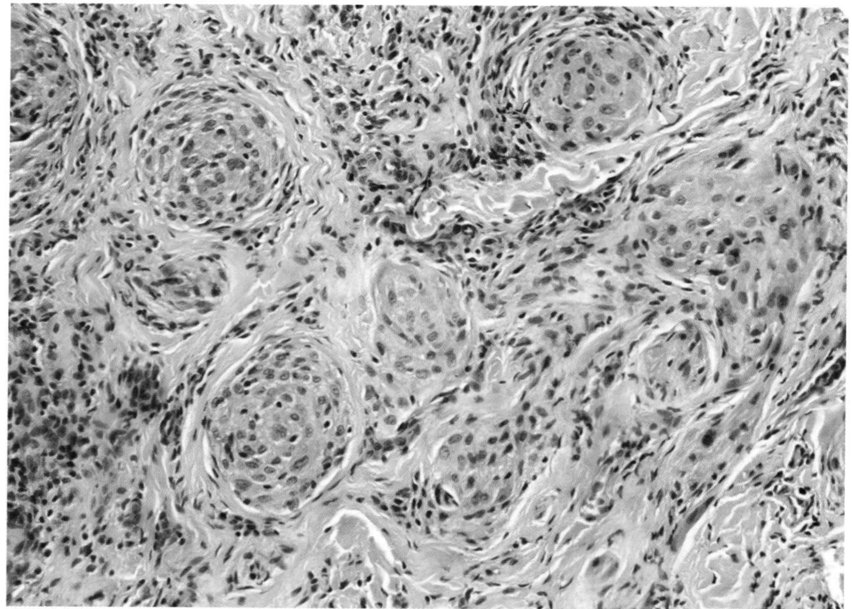

FIGURE 11-39. Nests of histiocytoid cells with a whorled growth pattern in cellular neurothekeoma.

extremities, and shoulder region.[57,59] Neurothekeomas are dermal-based lesions that may extend to involve the subcutis in nearly 50% of cases; involvement of subjacent skeletal muscle is extremely rare. Most tumors are small at the time of diagnosis (<1.5 cm), although very rare examples may be up to 3 cm in size.

Pathologic Features

Cellular neurothekeomas grow in multinodular, lobular, or plexiform patterns and consist of nests of tumor cells of varying sizes, circumscribed by bands of densely hyaline collagen (Fig. 11-38). A whorling growth pattern is frequently present within individual tumor nodules (Fig. 11-39). Rarely, the tumor may grow in a solid, sheetlike pattern within the subcutis (Fig. 11-40). Myxoid stromal change is frequently present and may be so prominent as to mimic nerve sheath myxoma or other myxoid soft tissue tumors, including myxofibrosarcoma (Fig. 11-41). In the past, these myxoid areas were often interpreted as showing a relationship between cellular neurothekeoma and nerve sheath myxoma (so-called *mixed type neurothekeoma*); it is now clear that no such relationship exists. The neoplastic cells are epithelioid to slightly

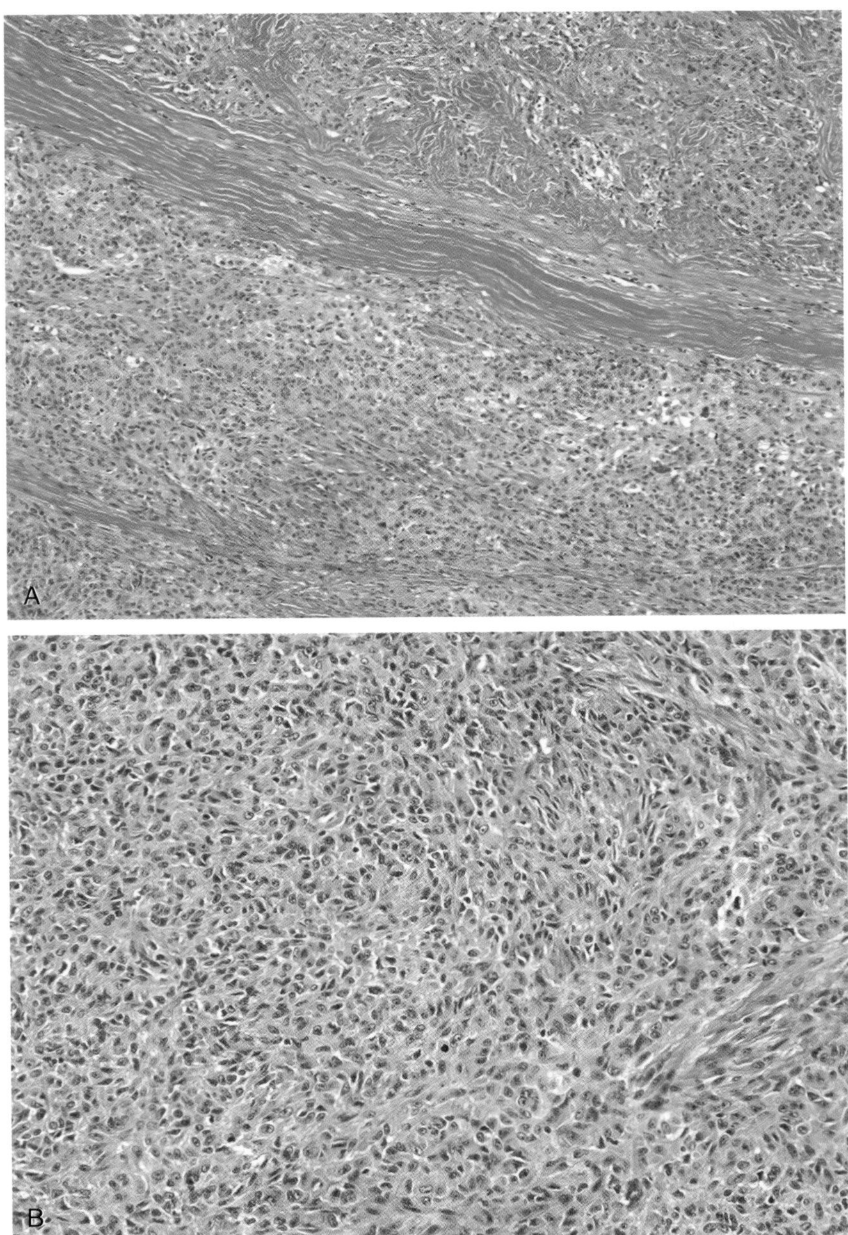

FIGURE 11-40. Cellular neurothekeoma with nested (top) and solid, sheet-like growth patterns (bottom) (A). Higher power view of solid area in cellular neurothekeoma (B).

spindled, contain a moderate amount of lightly eosinophilic cytoplasm, and have generally bland, ovoid nuclei with indistinct nucleoli. Some cases display moderate nuclear variability, and, in rare instances, marked cytologic atypia is focally present (Fig. 11-42). Mitotic activity is usually less than 5/10 HPF, although a significant subset of cases (20%) shows higher mitotic activity.[57,59] Atypical mitotic figures may rarely be identified. Osteoclast-like giant cells are seen in up to 39% of cases.[57,59]

Immunohistochemistry

Neurothekeomas are negative for S-100 protein, emphasizing their lack of relationship to nerve sheath myxoma and other true nerve sheath tumors. They are essentially always positive for NKI/C3, a highly nonspecific marker originally described as a marker of melanoma,[64] and for neuron-specific enolase.[57,59] Immunoreactivity for a wide variety of other markers has been reported, including CD10, microphthalmia transcription factor, PGP9.5, smooth muscle actin, vimentin, and CD68.[57,59] In general, immunohistochemistry is of relatively little use in the differential diagnosis of neurothekeoma.

Outcome

Neurothekeomas are benign tumors with limited capacity for local recurrence. The risk for local recurrence is higher for incompletely excised tumors and tumors located on the face.[59]

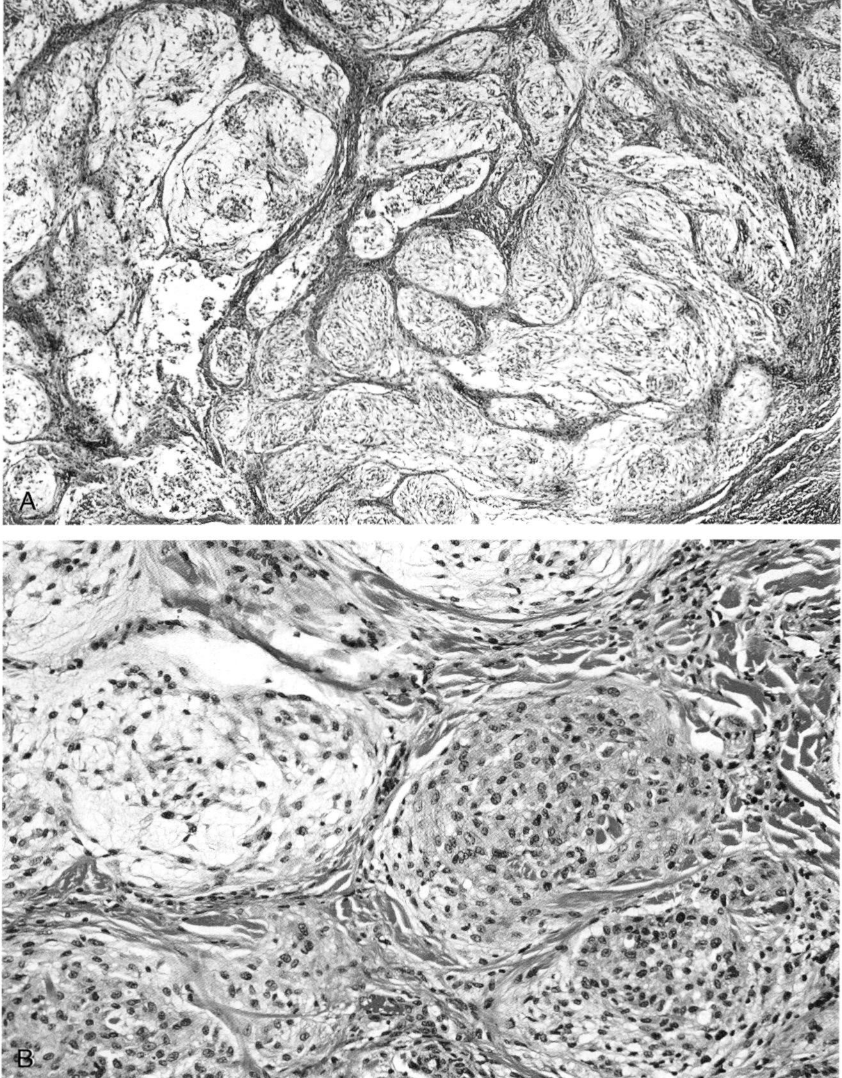

FIGURE 11-41. Cellular neurothekeoma with extensive stromal myxoid change (A). Although the lobular growth pattern and myxoid stroma shown by such tumors is reminiscent of nerve sheath myxoma (classical neurothekeoma), it is now clear that these are unrelated lesions. Transition from typical to myxoid areas in cellular neurothekeoma (B).

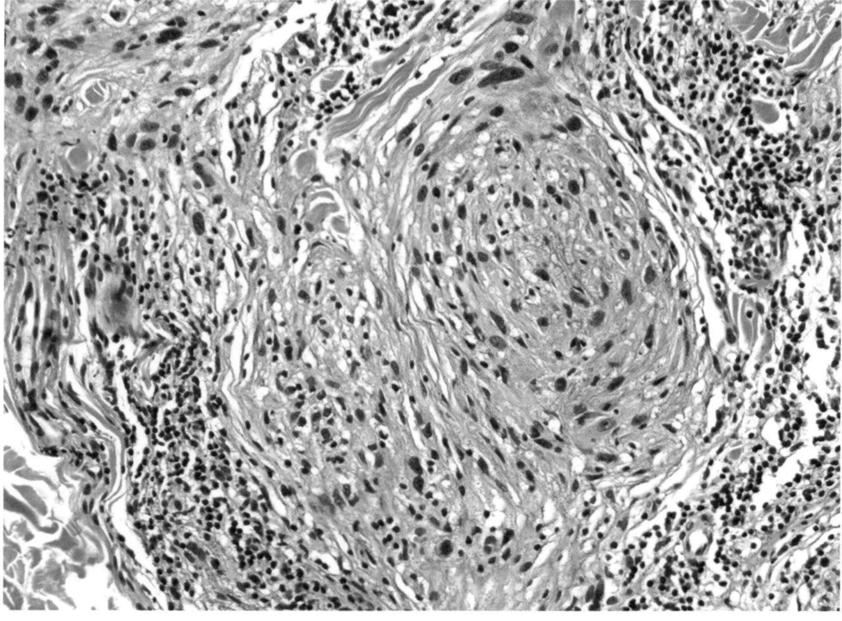

FIGURE 11-42. Cytologic atypia in cellular neurothekeoma. This is not thought to be of clinical significance.

Atypical histologic features, including cytologic atypia, high mitotic activity, atypical mitotic figures, and subcutaneous involvement, have not been associated with worst patient outcome.

Differential Diagnosis

The differential diagnosis of neurothekeoma is relatively broad, depending on the amount of myxoid change present. Neurothekeomas lacking myxoid change should be distinguished from plexiform fibrohistiocytic tumors, reticulohistiocytoma, epithelioid fibrous histiocytoma, and melanocytic tumors. In their classic form, plexiform fibrohistiocytic tumors are biphasic tumors, showing fibromatosis-like fascicles of spindled cells circumscribing nodules of histiocytes and osteoclast-like giant cells. This biphasic growth pattern is perhaps the most useful feature distinguishing plexiform fibrohistiocytic tumor from neurothekeoma, particularly because the round cell areas of these two tumors may be essentially indistinguishable. Indeed, the clinical features of these two tumors overlap significantly, and these may be closely related entities. Expression of microphthalmia transcription factor, seen in neurothekeoma but not in plexiform fibrohistiocytic tumor, has been reported to be of value in this differential diagnosis.[65] As compared with neurothekeoma, reticulohistiocytoma occurs in older patients and lacks plexiform and whorling growth patterns. Epithelioid fibrous histiocytoma more often occurs on the leg and typically shows an epidermal collarette. Melanocytic neoplasms, including Spitz nevus, differ from neurothekeoma by virtue of S-100 protein and melanocytic marker (e.g., HMB45, Melan-A) expression. Extensively myxoid neurothekeomas may be confused with nerve sheath myxomas but lack the S-100 protein expression invariably seen in the latter tumor. Superficial angiomyxomas are lobulated tumors showing a well-developed vasculature, stromal neutrophils, and uniformly spindled to stellate cells. Myxofibrosarcoma (undifferentiated pleomorphic sarcoma with myxoid change) occurs in much older patients, typically involves the extremities, and displays much greater cytologic atypia, in almost all instances.

SOLITARY (JUVENILE) XANTHOGRANULOMA

Solitary xanthogranuloma is a stable or regressing histiocytic lesion that usually occurs during childhood.[66-76] It has recently been reclassified from a non-X form of histiocytosis to a dendritic cell-related histiocytic proliferation. This nosological change places it conceptually closer to Langerhans cell histiocytosis and distinct from the macrophage-related histiocytic proliferations, which include Rosai-Dorfman disease. The lesion(s) usually develop during infancy and is (are) characterized by one or more cutaneous nodules and less often by additional lesions in deep soft tissue or organs.[66,67] As a rule, those that develop after the age of 2 years or in adults are usually solitary.[69] Tahan et al.[69] noted that 15% to 30% of these lesions occur in individuals older than 20 years of age and proposed the use of the term *xanthogranuloma*, rather than *juvenile xanthogranuloma*. Use of this term alone could be problematic because xanthogranuloma has been used for a variety of tumorous and reactive conditions whose pathogenesis varies. Therefore, these lesions are referred to as *solitary xanthogranulomas*.

Clinical Findings and Gross Appearance

This disease may occur exclusively as a cutaneous lesion or a disease affecting deep soft tissue or parenchymal organs. In the more common cutaneous form, one or more nodules develop shortly after birth, although approximately one-third of patients have lesions at birth.[67] Two-thirds of patients develop the lesions by the age of 6 months. Depending on the series, 10% to 40% of patients develop the lesion after the age of 20 years. There is no underlying lipid abnormality and no well-established familial incidence, although rare reports have documented the disease in parent and offspring.

About half of the lesions develop on the head and neck, followed by the trunk and extremities. They measure a few millimeters to a few centimeters in diameter. The early lesions are red papules (Fig. 11-43), and the older lesions are brown or yellow. Following a limited period of growth, most nodules regress spontaneously, leaving a depressed, sometimes hyperpigmented area of skin. In patients with numerous skin nodules, the tumors may appear in crops. Older lesions begin

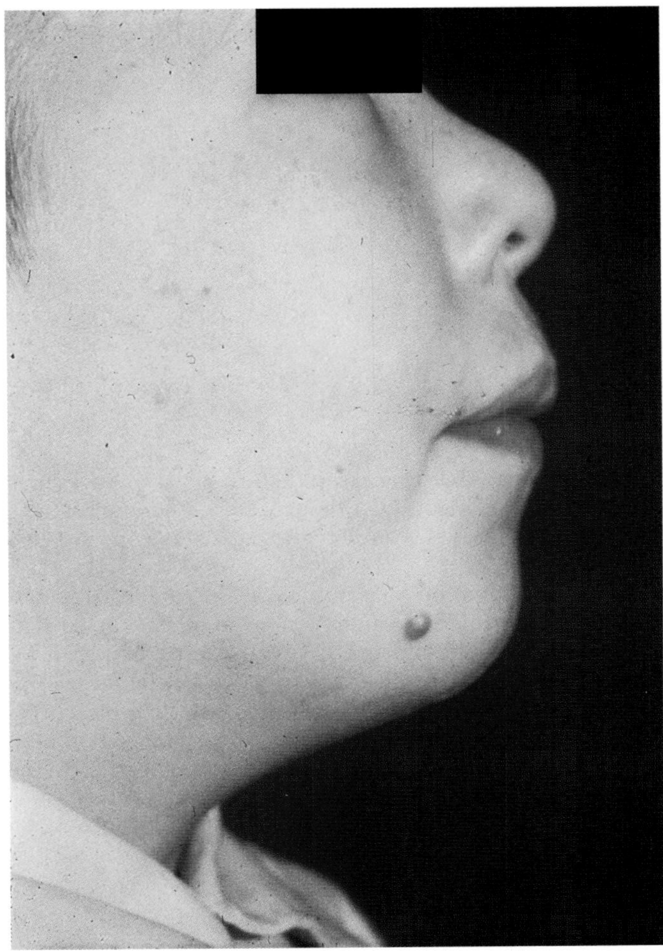

FIGURE 11-43. Clinical appearance of a solitary xanthogranuloma. *(Case courtesy of Dr. Elson Helwig.)*

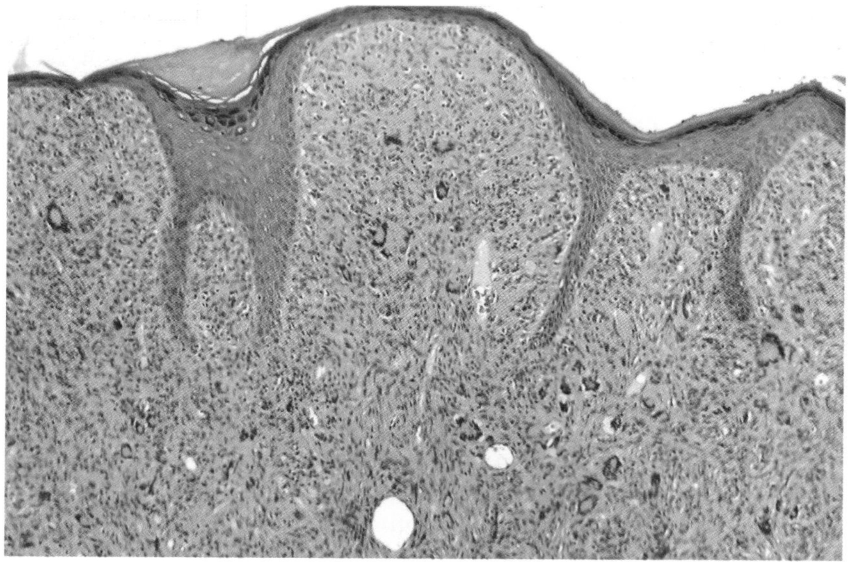

FIGURE 11-44. Solitary xanthogranuloma.

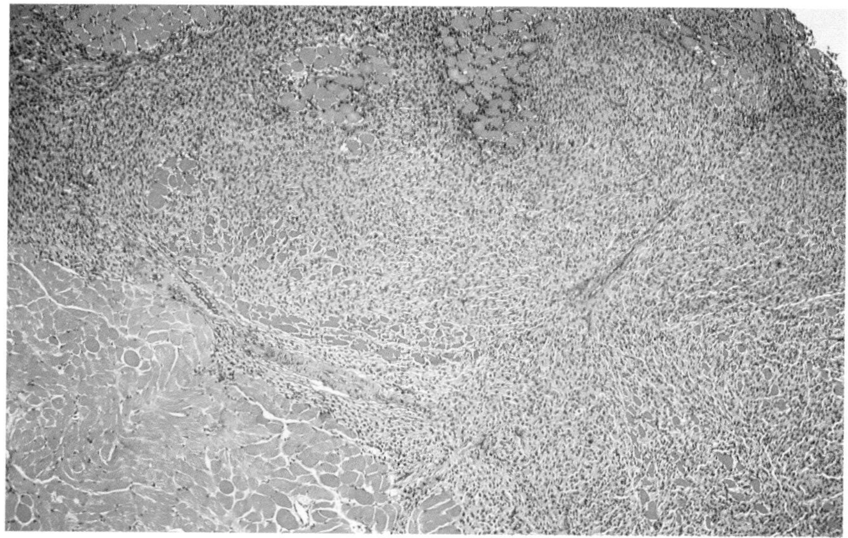

FIGURE 11-45. Deep solitary xanthogranuloma infiltrating muscle.

to regress as new ones emerge, so lesions of various ages may be present simultaneously. Although most lesions subside by adolescence, those that develop after age 20 may persist in a stable form.

In the less common form of the disease, cutaneous lesions may be accompanied by similar lesions in other sites, such as the eye, lung, epicardium, oral cavity, and testis. Less than 5% of cases occur in deep soft tissue (usually skeletal muscle) or parenchymal organs.[66,67] In such patients, the presenting symptoms are often referable to the extracutaneous tumor, and the skin lesions may be overlooked or appear later. The eye is the most common extracutaneous site, and patients may present with anterior chamber hemorrhage and glaucoma.

Microscopic Findings

Solitary xanthogranulomas are similar whether they occur in children or adults.[68] There is a tendency, however, for deep lesions to appear more monomorphic and less lipidized (Figs. 11-44 and 11-45).[72] Lesions consist of sheets of histiocytes involving the dermis and extending to, but not invading, the flattened epidermis (see Fig. 11-8). The infiltrate closely apposes adnexal structures and extends into the subcutis. Deeply situated solitary xanthogranulomas appear circumscribed but blend with or infiltrate skeletal muscle at their periphery (see Fig. 11-45). In both forms of the disease, the histiocytes are well differentiated and exhibit little pleomorphism and only rare mitoses. The appearance of the lesions varies in a more or less time-dependent fashion and with the amount of lipid present. Early lesions have little lipid; therefore, the cells have a homogeneous amphophilic or eosinophilic cytoplasm (Fig. 11-46). In the older, more classic lesions, the cells have a finely vacuolated or even xanthomatous cytoplasm (Figs. 11-47 and 11-48). Giant cells, including Touton giant cells, are typical of this lesion (Figs. 11-49 and 11-50) but may vary considerably in number from one area to another or from lesion to lesion. Usually, a modest number of

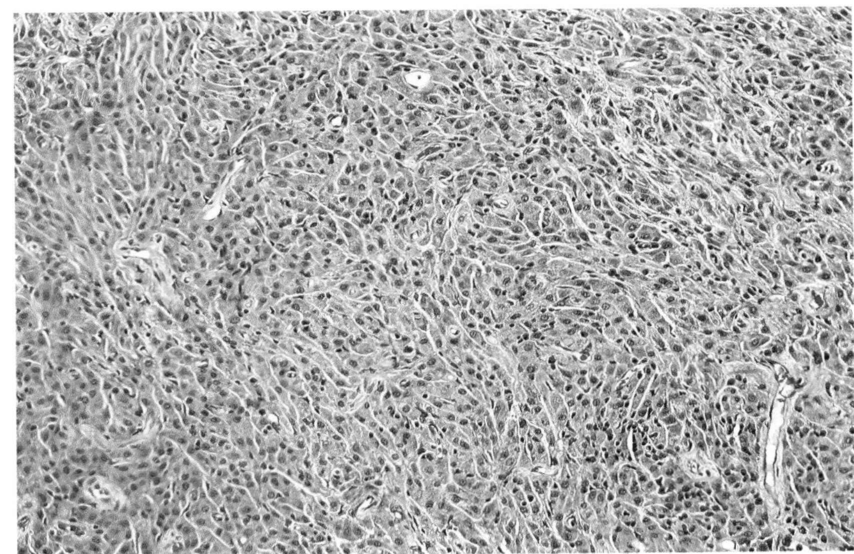

FIGURE 11-46. Early solitary xanthogranuloma composed of nonlipidized histiocytes.

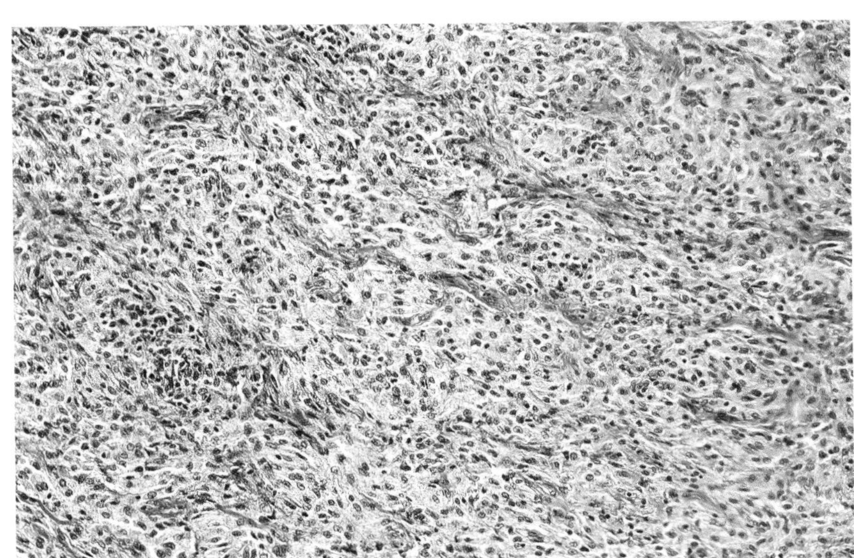

FIGURE 11-47. Lipidized solitary xanthogranuloma.

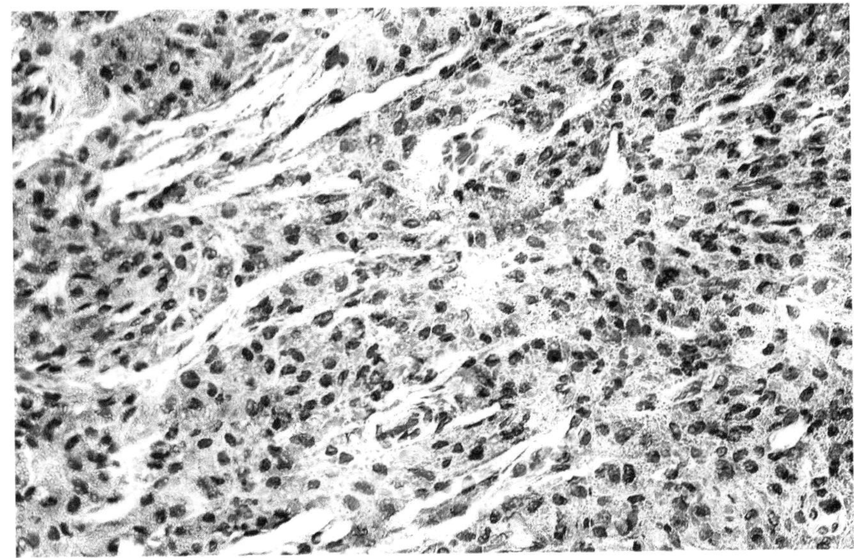

FIGURE 11-48. Fat stain showing extensive lipid within a solitary xanthogranuloma.

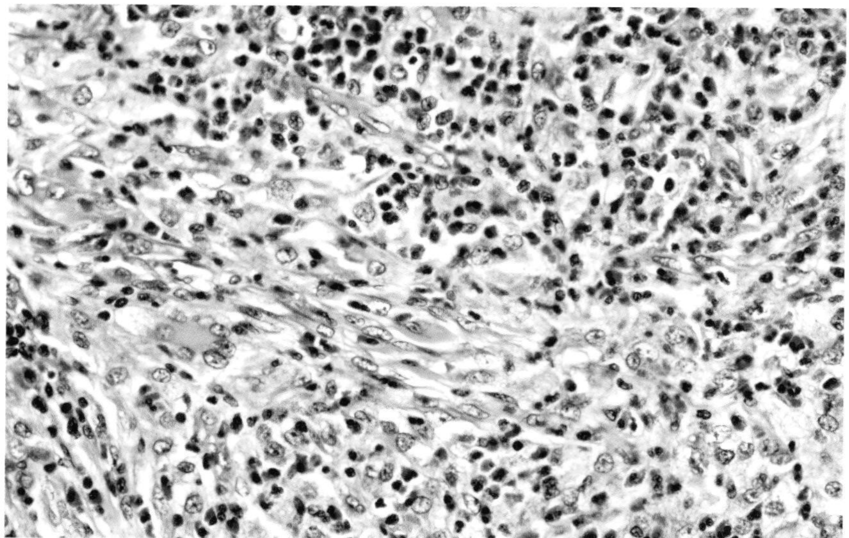

FIGURE 11-49. Solitary xanthogranuloma with an eosinophilic infiltrate.

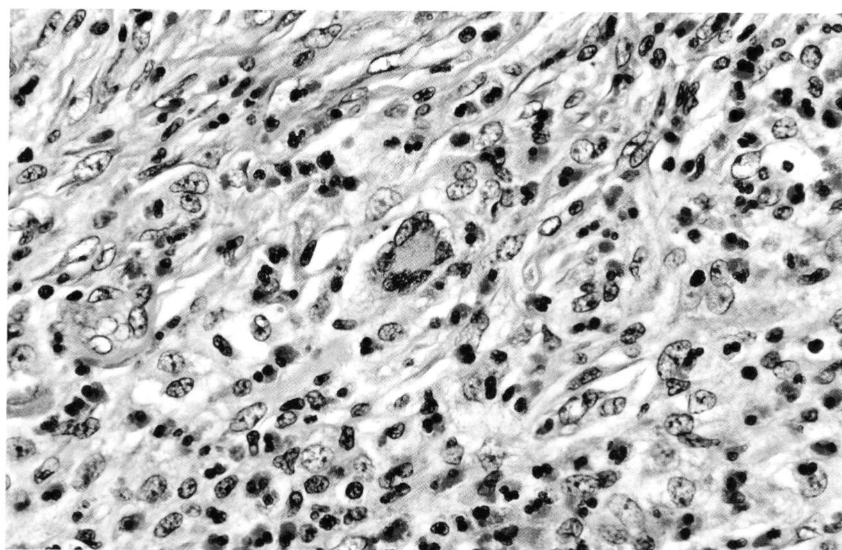

FIGURE 11-50. Solitary xanthogranuloma with eosinophils and Touton giant cells.

inflammatory cells are present, consisting of both acute and chronic inflammatory cells, especially eosinophils. Long-standing or regressive lesions eventually develop interstitial fibrosis and even a vague storiform pattern (Fig. 11-51), so they may resemble the more conventional fibrous histiocytoma seen in adults.

Electron microscopic studies show that the cells have characteristics of histiocytes.[72,73] They have numerous pseudopodia, lipid droplets, and lysosomes. Lipid, however, is not present to any extent within vessel walls, in contrast to certain types of eruptive xanthoma. Langerhans granules, tubular organelles associated with forms of histiocytosis X, have not been demonstrated. The cells express CD68, α1-antitrypsin, α1-antichymotrypsin, lysozyme,[68,71] CD31, and factor XIIIa.[67,74] Factor XIIIa expression is typically diffusely present, in contrast to the patchier pattern of expression seen in cutaneous fibrous histiocytomas. They are consistently negative for CD1a and usually negative for S-100 protein,[67] both of which can be used to distinguish this lesion from Langerhans cell histiocytosis (see the following section).

Differential Diagnosis

Even though solitary xanthogranuloma and Langerhans cell histiocytosis are both considered dendritic cell-related histiocytic proliferations, there are still compelling biologic reasons to distinguish between these two disorders. In contrast to Langerhans cell histiocytosis involving the skin, solitary xanthogranuloma does not generally invade the epidermis and shows greater cellular cohesion and fewer eosinophils. Touton giant cells, a feature of solitary xanthogranuloma, are typically absent in Langerhans cell histiocytosis; when these cells are scarce, distinction of the two diseases may be difficult. In these situations, ultrastructural studies documenting the presence or absence of Langerhans' granules and immunostaining for S-100 protein may be required. The latter is strongly positive in Langerhans cell histiocytosis but is negative or present in scattered cells in solitary xanthogranuloma. Usually, solitary xanthogranuloma can be easily distinguished histologically from xanthomas because the latter contain a more uniform population of foamy cells and lack Touton giant cells and acute

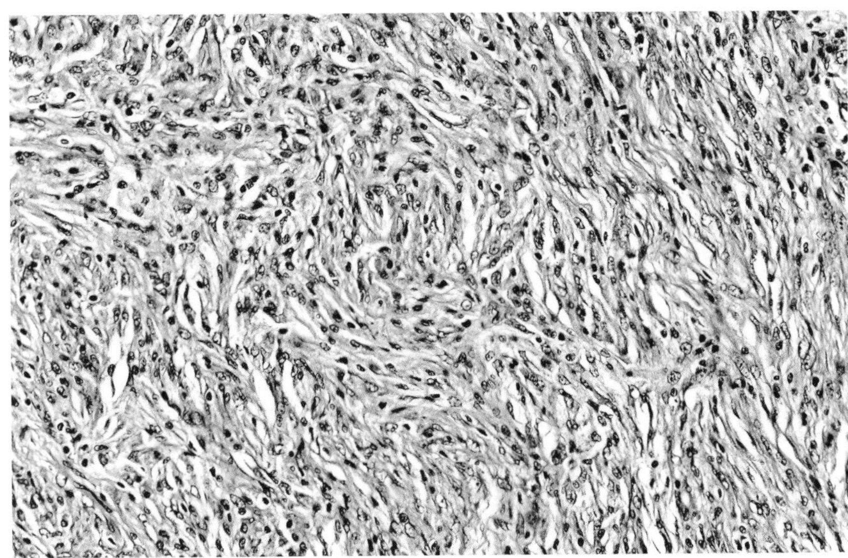

FIGURE 11-51. Late solitary xanthogranuloma with fibrosis.

inflammation. Moreover, xanthomas associated with hypercholesterolemia often have large extracellular cholesterol deposits. The greater uniformity of solitary xanthogranuloma, the usual lack of a storiform pattern, and the distinctive clinical setting distinguish it from fibrous histiocytoma of adults.

Clinical Behavior

The prognosis for patients with this disease is excellent. The skin lesions usually regress (or at least stabilize) with time, and even large, deeply located tumors pursue a favorable course. In the recent experience reported from the Kiel Registry, 83% of patients were cured following excision, 10% experienced recurrence, and 7% developed additional lesion(s) in the same general vicinity as the original tumor.[67] Death from disease may occur in systemic cases. Dehner[74] documented two deaths among eight patients with systemic disease. Surgical excision is the mainstay of treatment for patients with solitary or limited disease, whereas multimodal chemotherapy is the treatment of choice for the rare patient with systemic disease.[67]

SOLITARY RETICULOHISTIOCYTOMA

Reticulohistiocytoma is a distinctive but rare lesion of adult life. It consists of nodules of eosinophilic histiocytes, often exhibiting multinucleation. It has been suggested that the solitary forms of reticulohistiocytoma are similar to adult xanthogranulomas, the distinction being largely based on whether there is a predominance of multinucleated eosinophilic histiocytes. On the other hand, solitary reticulohistiocytoma appears to be a fundamentally different disease from multicentric reticulohistiocytomas, both clinically and immunophenotypically.[77]

Solitary reticulohistiocytoma is a nodular dermatosis[77,78] that develops at any body site. Most patients are adult men, and fewer than one-fifth have multiple tumors.[77,79] The lesions are yellow-brown papules composed of dense circumscribed dermal nodules of deeply eosinophilic histiocytes (Figs. 11-52 to 11-54). Multinucleated forms, often 20 to 30 times larger than their mononuclear counterparts, with abundant nuclei are common. The so-called *oncocytic histiocytes* may display some degree of nuclear atypia, and, occasionally, mitotic figures are noted. In some areas, there is a subtle degree of spindling of the histiocytes, although frankly spindled areas and Touton giant cells such as those seen in fibrous histiocytomas are absent. Occasional lymphocytes are present. Immunohistochemically, the lesions express several markers associated with the non-X forms of histiocytosis. They consistently express CD163, CD68, variably α1-antitrypsin, and lysozyme, but they lack S-100 protein.[79,80] They also express muscle-specific actin, an antigen that has been identified in the mononuclear cells of giant cell tumors of bone and soft tissue giant cell tumors of low malignant potential (see Chapter 12). Microphthalmia transcription factor may be positive.[79]

Isolated cutaneous lesions with some degree of pleomorphism must be distinguished from superficial forms of undifferentiated pleomorphic sarcoma with osteoclast-like giant cells (malignant giant cell tumor of soft parts), carcinoma, and melanoma. In contrast to superficial forms of undifferentiated pleomorphic sarcoma, these tumors are smaller and have fewer mitotic figures, less prominent spindling, and no necrosis. Unlike melanoma, there is no junctional activity, more interstitial collagen, and a less distinct organoid growth pattern. The frequent accompaniment of acute inflammatory cells and numerous multinucleated cells also aids in this distinction.

The lesions pursue a benign or self-limiting course. In one study,[77] most patients with follow-up information were cured by simple excision; two patients developed a recurrence, and three had a nodule elsewhere. Several patients with multiple nodules noted spontaneous regression of a lesion. Similar findings were noted by Miettinen and Fetsch[79] in a more recent series of 44 solitary reticulohistiocytomas retrieved from the Armed Forces Institute of Pathology (AFIP) archives.

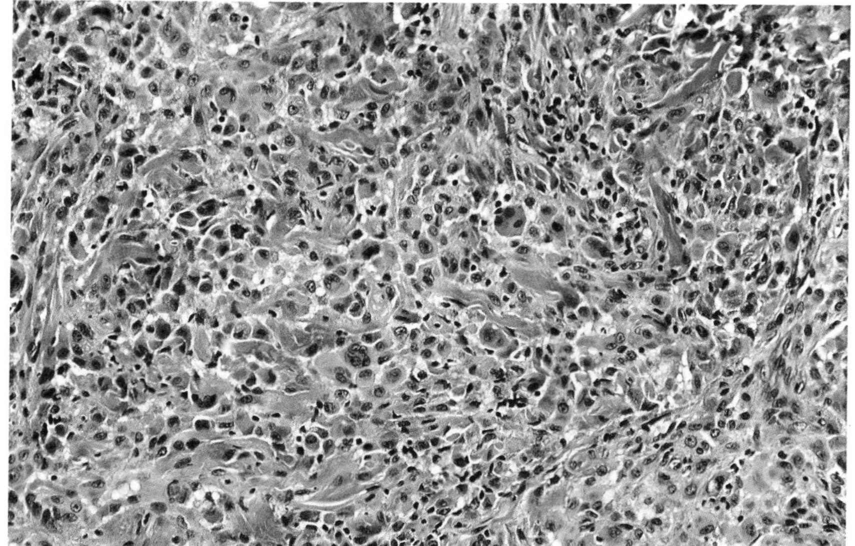

FIGURE 11-52. Reticulohistiocytoma.

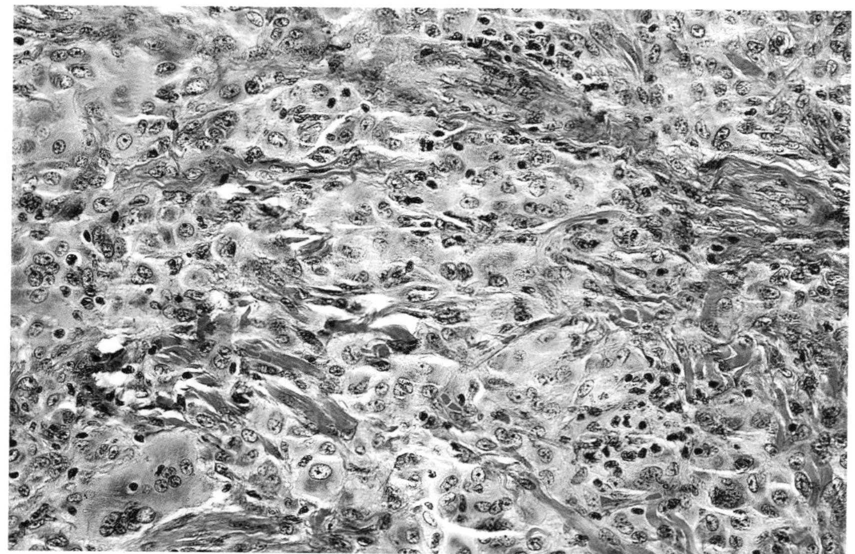

FIGURE 11-53. Reticulohistiocytoma.

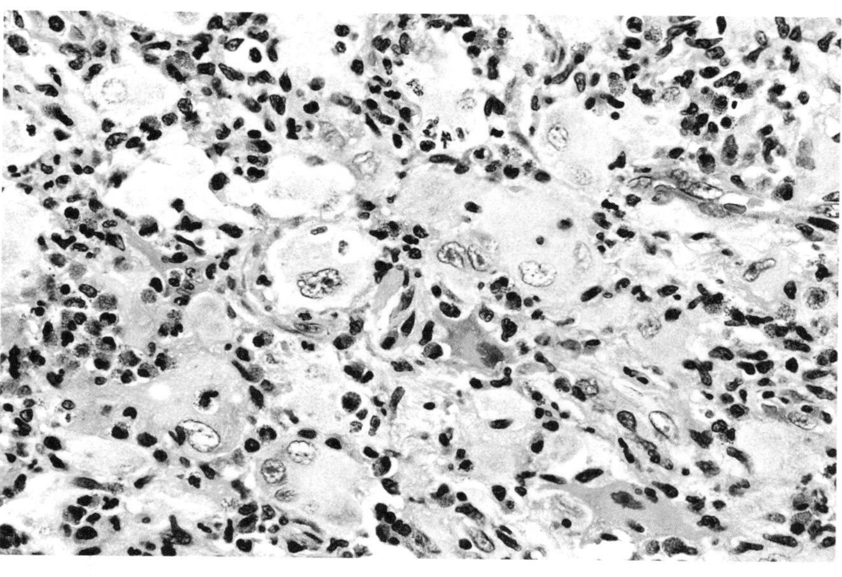

FIGURE 11-54. High-power view of a reticulohistiocytoma.

MULTICENTRIC RETICULOHISTIOCYTOSIS

In contrast to the cutaneous disease, multicentric reticulohistiocytosis is a systemic, occasionally paraneoplastic disease characterized by myriad symptoms, including progressive symmetric, erosive arthritis, episodes of pyrexia, and weight loss.[81-87] Multiple cutaneous and mucosal nodules follow the arthritis within a period of months to years, although, occasionally, the skin lesions initiate the disease. The disease may be associated with a number of other conditions, including tuberculosis, diabetes, Sjögren syndrome, hypothyroidism, Wegener granulomatosis, polyarteritis,[82,88,89] celiac disease, and systemic lupus erythematosus.[80] In addition, malignancies of various types (e.g., carcinoma of the colon, breast, lung, ovary, and cervix; sarcoma; lymphoma) develop in about 30% of patients.[81,90] In one dramatic case, the constitutional symptoms regressed when the underlying neoplasm was treated.[78] Despite that various lipid materials accumulate within lesional cells, no consistent or specific serum lipid abnormality has been identified. The disease is usually marked by a waxing and waning course over a period of several years, eventually leaving most patients with a disfiguring, crippling arthritis that most severely affects the distal interphalangeal joint and bears some similarity to rheumatoid arthritis (Fig. 11-55).

Pathologic Findings

The cutaneous lesions consist of circumscribed collections of histiocytes confined to the dermis or extending to the epidermis and subcutis. Delicate reticulin fibers are present around individual cells, and, occasionally, acute and chronic inflammatory cells are present. Although multinucleated eosinophilic histiocytes characterize this disease and solitary reticulohistiocytoma, these histiocytes tend to be smaller, are less eosinophilic, and show only a minor degree of multinucleation. Similar deposits may be seen in other involved organs such as synovium, bone, and lymph nodes. In most cases, they stain strongly with Sudan black B fat stain, oil red O, and periodic acid-Schiff (PAS) after diastase digestion and are believed to contain a mixture of phospholipid, mucoprotein or glycoprotein, and neutral fat.[81] Immunohistochemically, these cells contrast slightly with those of solitary reticulohistiocytoma in that they lack muscle-specific actin and factor XIIIa, but they express CD68, α1-antitrypsin, and lysozyme. Electron microscopy shows that the histiocytes have numerous lipid droplets and a dilated rough endoplasmic reticulum filled with granular material.[85] Langerhans granules, tubular structures present in certain normal and neoplastic histiocytes, are usually not identified in multicentric reticulohistiocytosis,[91,92] although there have been some reports to the contrary.[93,94]

Discussion

Usually, this disease poses few diagnostic problems for the pathologist because evaluation of the skin lesions is aided immeasurably by the clinical history and, in some cases, by a confirmatory biopsy of synovium or other tissue. However, the etiology of this condition remains obscure. Because a disproportionately large number of patients with multicentric reticulohistiocytosis have associated malignancies or other systemic disease, some have suggested that the disease is a reflection of an altered immune state. Furthermore, it appears that the histiocytes in these lesions have the ability to secrete a wide variety of substances that may be responsible for many of the manifestations of the disease.[92,95,96] β-interleukin-1β and platelet-derived growth factor-β, both of which promote synovial proliferation, can be identified immunohistochemically in the histiocytes.[95] Urokinase is elevated in synovial tissue and could account for the destruction of articular tissue, by activation of collagenase. Although in the past there was little or no therapy for the disease, a number of reports have attested to alleviation of the condition with the use of chemotherapeutic agents, including alkylating agents.[97-99]

XANTHOMA

Xanthoma is a localized collection of tissue histiocytes containing lipid.[100-104] It is not a true tumor but, rather, a reactive

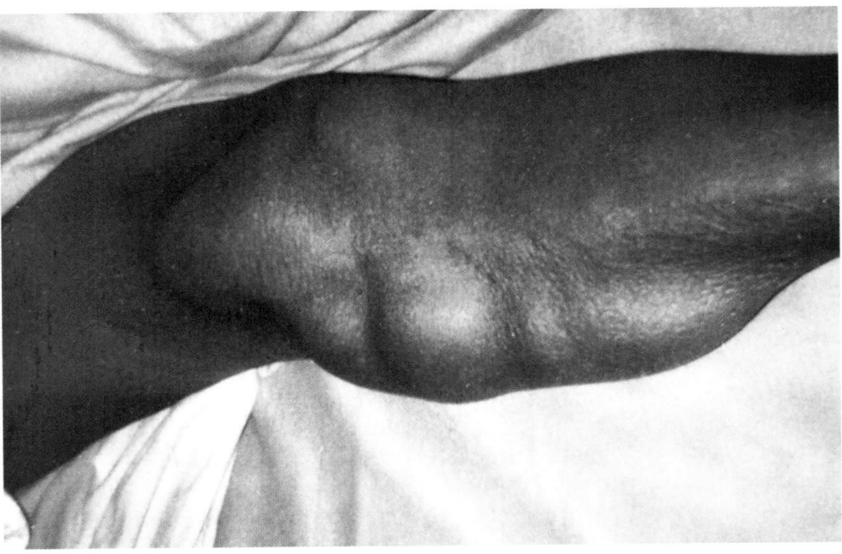

FIGURE 11-55. Deforming arthritis of the elbow in a patient with multicentric reticulohistiocytosis.

TABLE 11-1 Plasma Lipoprotein Phenotypes

DISORDER	I	IIa	IIb	III	IV	V
Lipoprotein elevation	Chylomicrons	LDL	LDL, VLDL	Chylomicrons, VLDL remnants	VLDL	Chylomicrons, VLDL
Xanthoma	Eruptive	Tendon, tuberous	None	Palmar, tuberous, eruptive	None	Eruptive
Molecular defect	Lipoprotein lipase, apoC-II	LDL receptor, apoB-100	Unknown	ApoE	Unknown	Unknown

*Modified from Rader DJ. Disorders of lipid metabolism. In: Kelley WN, editor. Textbook of internal medicine. 3rd ed. Philadelphia: Lippincott-Raven; 1997.

LDL, low density lipoproteins; VLDL, very low density lipoproteins; apo/Apo, apolipoprotein.

TABLE 11-2 Comparison of Clinical Types of Xanthoma

TYPE OF XANTHOMA	ASSOCIATION WITH LIPOPROTEIN PHENOTYPE	LOCATION	HISTOLOGIC APPEARANCE
Eruptive	I, III, V	Predilection for buttocks	Foamy and nonfoamy histiocytes
Tuberous	IIa, III	Elbows, buttocks, knees, fingers	Foamy histiocytes, extracellular cholesterol deposits, fibrosis, inflammation
Tendinous	IIa, cerebrotendinous xanthomatosis	Tendons of hands and feet, Achilles tendon	Similar to tuberous xanthoma
Xanthelasma	IIa, III	Eyelids	Foamy histiocytes
Plane	Primary biliary cirrhosis III, normolipemic states	Skin creases of palms	Foamy histiocytes

histiocytic proliferation that occurs in response to alterations in serum lipids. Xanthomas develop in most primary and some secondary (e.g., primary biliary cirrhosis, diabetes mellitus) hyperlipoproteinemias and, occasionally, in the normolipemic state. A brief synopsis of the various primary hyperlipidemias and their associated defects is provided in Table 11-1. Usually, xanthomas occur in the skin and subcutis,[105-108] but, occasionally, they involve deep soft tissue such as tendons (xanthoma of the tendon sheath)[106,109-111] or synovium.[112]

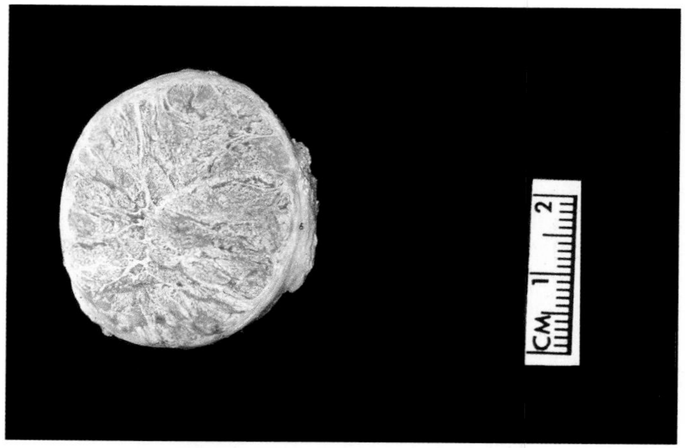

FIGURE 11-56. Xanthoma of the Achilles tendon cut in cross-section. White bands correspond to residual tendinous tissue that has been spread apart by xanthomatous infiltration.

Clinical Findings and Gross Appearance

Cutaneous xanthomas are designated according to their gross appearance and clinical presentation (Table 11-2). Eruptive xanthomas are small, yellow papules with a predilection for the gluteal surfaces. They develop in individuals with hyperlipoproteinemia types I, III, and V. Tuberous xanthomas, large plaque-like lesions of the subcutis, are usually located on the buttocks, elbows, knees, and fingers and are seen with type IIa or III hyperlipoproteinemia. Plane xanthomas occur in skinfolds, such as the palmar creases, and are characteristic of type III hyperlipoproteinemia; they may also be associated with primary biliary cirrhosis. Occasionally, they occur in normolipemic persons, and, in this setting, they have a high association with hematolymphoid malignancies.[107,113] Xanthelasmas are xanthomas of the eyelid and usually are observed in normolipemic persons, although they also occur in those with type IIa or III hyperlipoproteinemia. These last three types of xanthoma contain large amounts of cholesterol and its esters, which may be demonstrated under polarized light in fresh tissue as birefringent crystals.

Deep xanthomas occur most frequently in tendon or synovium, and rarely bone. Most tendinous xanthomas occur in the setting of hypercholesterolemia associated with type IIa hyperlipoproteinemia (Fig. 11-56). Usually, the severity of the xanthoma is roughly proportional to the severity and duration of the increased cholesterol levels. A rare inherited disease known as cerebrotendinous xanthomatosis is now also recognized as a cause of bilateral xanthomas occurring exclusively in the Achilles tendon.[114-116] This disease is an autosomal recessive disorder caused by mutations in the gene for sterol 27-hydroxylase, an enzyme important for hepatic bile acid synthesis. As a result, bile acids are synthesized to the end product cholestanol, which accumulates systemically, producing multiple signs and symptoms, including dementia, ataxia, cataracts, and tendinous xanthomas. Recognition of this disease is important because early treatment with chenodeoxycholic acid can prevent progression of clinical symptoms.

Most tendinous xanthomas present as painless, slowly growing masses that produce few symptoms unless joint function is compromised. The lesions may be solitary or multiple, and they occur in sites subjected to minor trauma such as the finger, wrist, and ankle. They are usually a few centimeters in diameter, although large lesions in excess of 20 cm have been reported in the Achilles tendon (see Fig. 11-56). Xanthomas may be circumscribed or diffuse and are firmly attached to tendon but not to overlying skin. On a cut section, they have a variegated color ranging from yellow to brown to white, depending on the amount of lipid, hemorrhage, and fibrosis present from area to area. Like tuberous and plane xanthomas, they also have a high cholesterol content.

Microscopic Findings

The various types of xanthoma differ in histologic appearance. Eruptive xanthoma, which represents an acute, evanescent lesion, contains a large proportion of nonfoamy histiocytes in addition to occasional foam cells and inflammatory cells. Tuberous and tendinous xanthomas are essentially identical (Figs. 11-57 to 11-59). Although in their early stages they may contain some nonfoamy histiocytes, the typical appearance is that of sheets of foamy histiocytes interspersed with occasional inflammatory cells. The histiocytes are bland with small pyknotic nuclei. Some cells contain fine granules of hemosiderin. Collections of extracellular cholesterol (cholesterol clefts) flanked by giant cells are conspicuous. Varying amounts of fibrosis may be present but are most marked in long-standing lesions. Plane xanthoma and xanthelasma are characterized by sheets of xanthoma cells, but they rarely exhibit the degree of fibrosis present in the foregoing two lesions. Ultrastructurally, xanthoma cells of all of these lesions are similar and contain numerous clear vacuoles, presumably representing cholesterol or its esters. Eruptive xanthomas, in addition, have fat in the vessel walls and tissue macrophages.

Discussion

Cutaneous xanthomas usually present few problems in diagnosis or management. The superficial location, gross appearance, and associated clinical findings leave little doubt as to

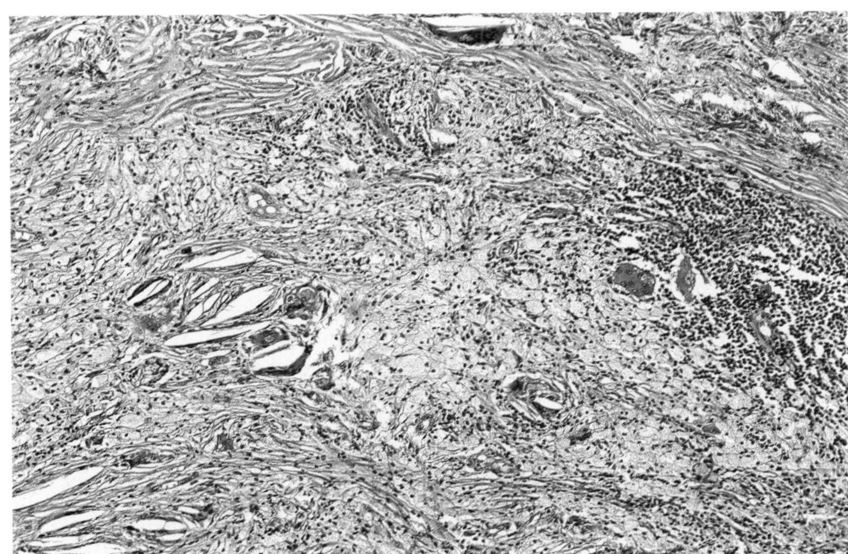

FIGURE 11-57. Tuberous xanthoma of the leg consisting of xanthoma cells admixed with inflammatory cells and giant cells surrounding cholesterol-containing clefts.

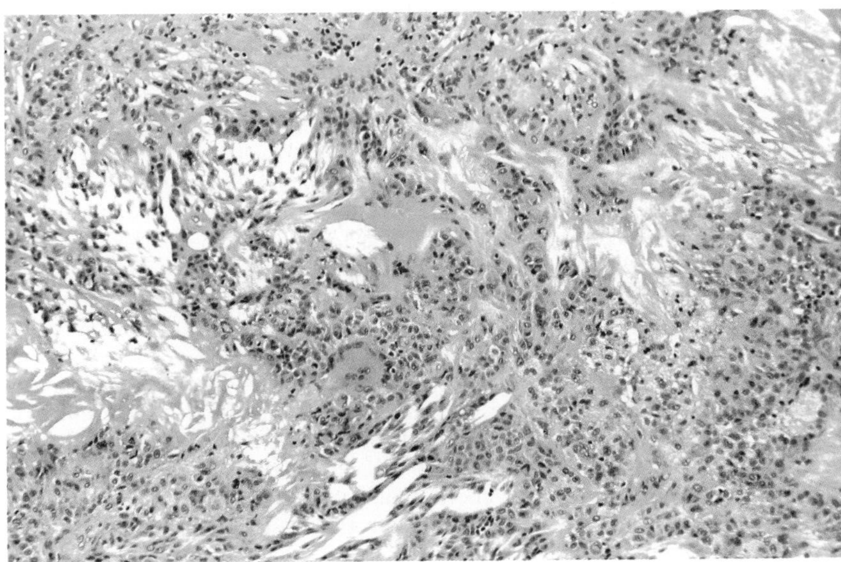

FIGURE 11-58. Tuberous xanthoma with xanthoma cells but without fibrosis or inflammation.

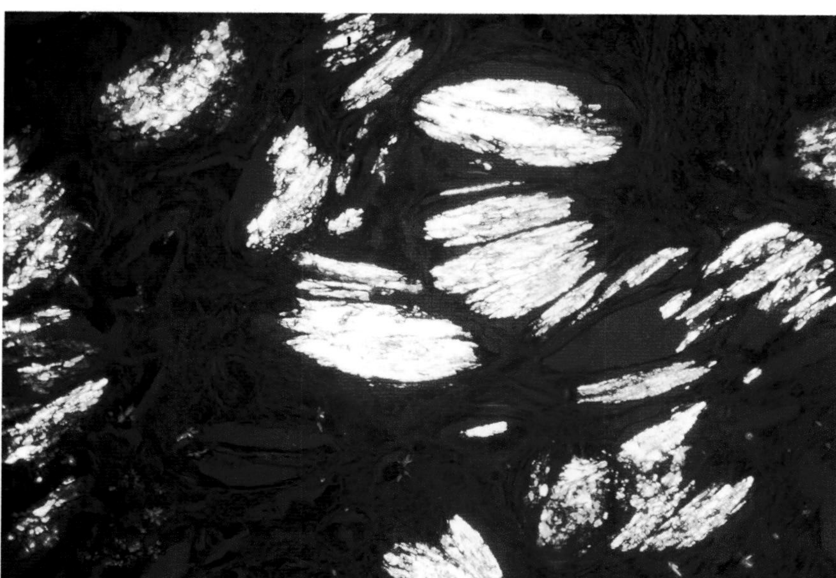

FIGURE 11-59. Frozen section of a xanthoma viewed under polarized light to illustrate numerous birefringent cholesterol crystals.

the diagnosis. Xanthomas of the tendon sheath may be more problematic. The deep location and slow, persistent growth occasionally raise the question of sarcoma. When a biopsy is done, such lesions should be adequately sampled because giant cell tumors of the tendon sheath, pigmented villonodular synovitis, or sarcomas with xanthomatous change may focally resemble this lesion. The diagnosis of xanthoma of the tendon sheath should always be considered in a patient with hypercholesterolemia, especially if the lesions are multiple.

Because of the non-neoplastic nature of these lesions, conservative therapy is generally recommended. In fact, xanthelasmas and tuberous xanthomas have regressed on medical therapy alone,[108,117] although months or years may be required before tangible benefits are appreciated. Surgery, including excision with tendon reconstruction, has been reserved for large or symptomatic xanthomas. Surgically treated xanthomas may slowly recur, although reoperation is generally not necessary.[109] Irradiation has also been used as therapy for these lesions, but there are few data to support its efficacy. Long-term treatment of cerebrotendinous xanthomatosis with chenodeoxycholic acid has resulted in alleviation of some of the neurologic symptoms but has not affected the tendinous xanthomas.[118]

Although xanthomas were formerly considered neoplastic, their association with hyperlipidemic states leaves little doubt that they are reactive lesions. Current evidence suggests that the lipid in them is derived from blood.[119-121] It has been demonstrated experimentally that serum lipoproteins leave the vascular compartment, traverse small vessels, and enter the macrophages of soft tissue.[119] This series of events can be confirmed ultrastructurally by the sequential finding of lipoprotein between endothelium and basement membrane and, finally, in the pericytes. Once ingested by macrophages, the lipoprotein is degraded to a lipid, and the lipid is released to the extracellular space. The fibrosis characteristic of mature or long-standing xanthomas is believed to be related to the fibrogenic properties of extracellular cholesterol.[68] Although xanthomas can potentially occur at any soft tissue site, the localization stimulus seems directly related to the vascular permeability because agents that increase permeability (e.g., histamine) can accelerate xanthoma formation at a given site.[119] Likewise, minor trauma or injury that results in a histamine release also accelerates xanthoma formation.[122] This observation provides an explanation for the common occurrence of such lesions in the tendons of the hands and feet.

MISCELLANEOUS HISTIOCYTIC REACTIONS RESEMBLING A NEOPLASM

Histiocytic reactions may be difficult to distinguish from neoplasms when they are localized lesions with few inflammatory cells. In these cases, it is necessary to obtain detailed clinical data, perform special staining procedures for microorganisms, and examine the specimen under polarized light for foreign material before rendering a diagnosis. Even under the best circumstances, the etiology of some histiocytic proliferations remains enigmatic. The more distinctive histiocytic reactions with known etiologies are discussed in the following sections.

Infectious Disease

Gram-positive and Gram-negative bacteria can induce inflammatory changes similar to those of xanthogranuloma. The lesions are composed of sheets of foamy histiocytes set against a mixed background of inflammatory cells. They differ from a neoplastic xanthogranuloma by the presence of focal abscesses and numerous microorganisms in the histiocytes. There are several cases of chronic staphylococcal infection with this appearance, and there is a similar lesion of the retroperitoneum secondary to *Arizona hinshawii*, a Gram-negative bacillus.[123]

Histoid leprosy, a rare form of lepromatous leprosy described by Wade[124,125] in 1963, grossly and microscopically resembles fibrous histiocytoma (Figs. 11-60 to 11-62). Unlike the usual type of lepromatous leprosy, which spreads in an

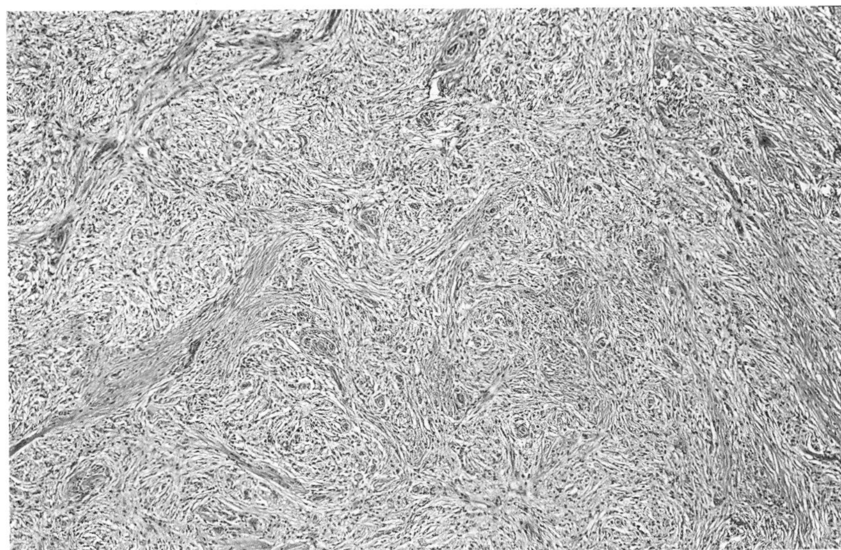

FIGURE 11-60. Histoid leprosy with a pattern similar to that of a fibrous histiocytoma.

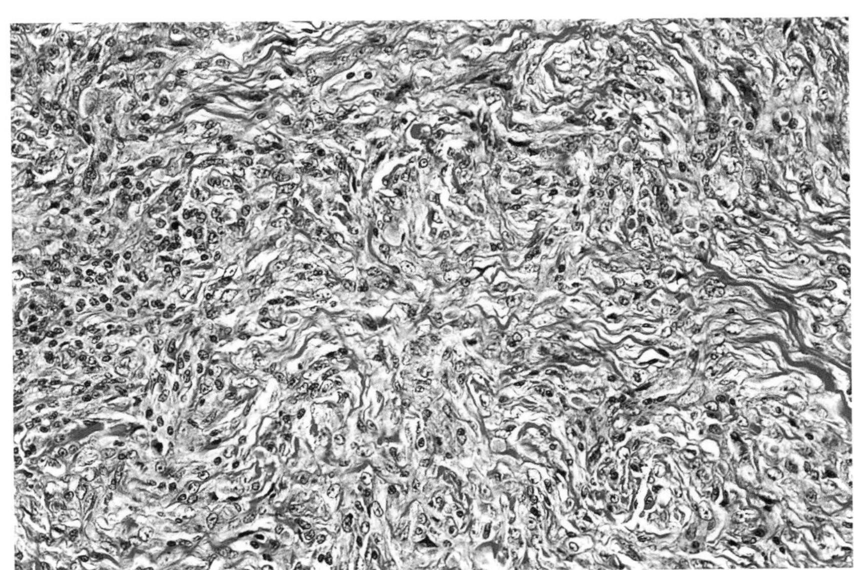

FIGURE 11-61. Medium-power view of histoid leprosy.

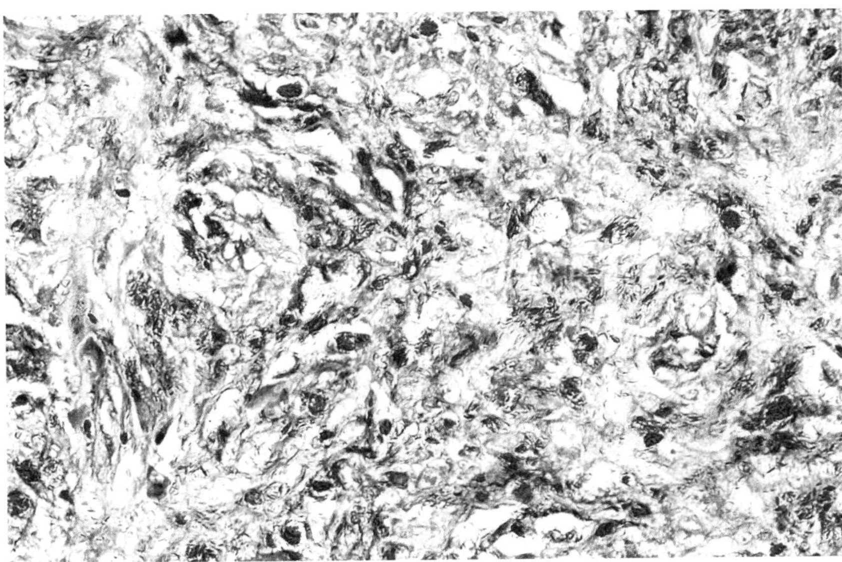

FIGURE 11-62. Fite-Faraco stain demonstrates numerous intracellular acid-fast bacilli in histoid leprosy.

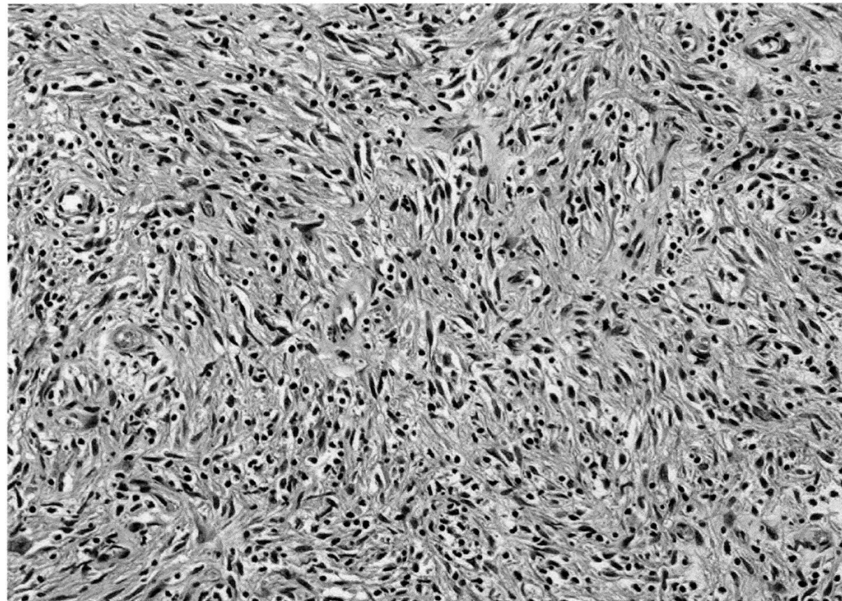

FIGURE 11-63. Atypical mycobacterial pseudotumor.

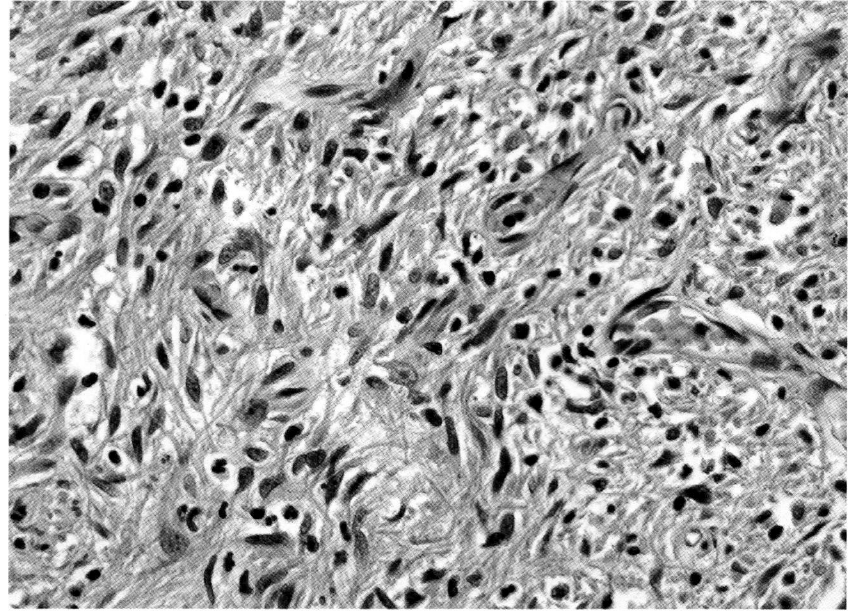

FIGURE 11-64. Atypical mycobacterial pseudotumor.

infiltrative manner, this disease develops as an expansile nodule of the subcutis and dermis. The cells resemble fibroblasts rather than histiocytes and are often arranged in a storiform pattern. Although the similarity of this disease to a true fibrous histiocytoma is striking, numerous intracellular acid-fast bacilli can be demonstrated with special stains (e.g., Fite-Faraco) (see Fig. 11-62). Because this form of leprosy occurs in patients with long-standing lepromatous leprosy treated with sulfones, it has been suggested that these lesions are the result of the emergence of sulfone-resistant bacilli.

Mycobacterial pseudotumors, first recognized by Wood et al.[126] in an immunosuppressed patient, have been reported most recently in AIDS patients in a variety of sites, most commonly lymph nodes but also skin/subcutis.[127] The lesions are analogous to those of histoid leprosy in that they consist of a tumorous proliferation of spindled and epithelioid histiocytes arranged in vague fascicles and associated with occasional chronic inflammatory cells (Figs. 11-63 and 11-64). The cells are laden with numerous acid-fast bacilli easily demonstrable with appropriate stains (Fig. 11-65). The lesional cells are CD68 positive, confirming their histiocytic lineage. In some cases, desmin has been demonstrated but has been attributed to antigenic cross-reactivity with the bacilli.[128]

Malacoplakia

Malacoplakia is a rare inflammatory disease believed to represent an unusual host response to infection with a variety of organisms, including *Escherichia coli*, *Klebsiella*, and acid-fast

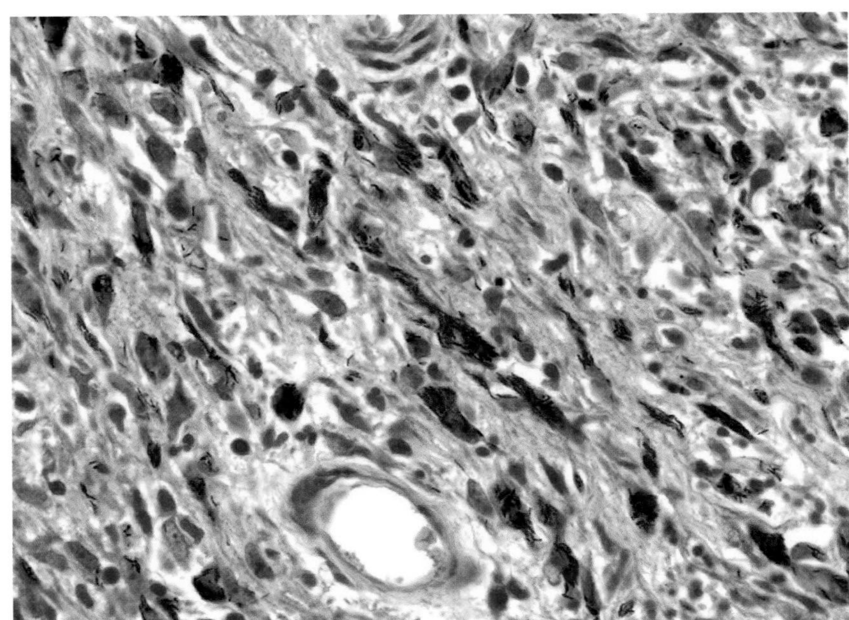

FIGURE 11-65. Acid-fast stain in atypical mycobacterial pseudotumor demonstrating organisms in spindled histiocytes.

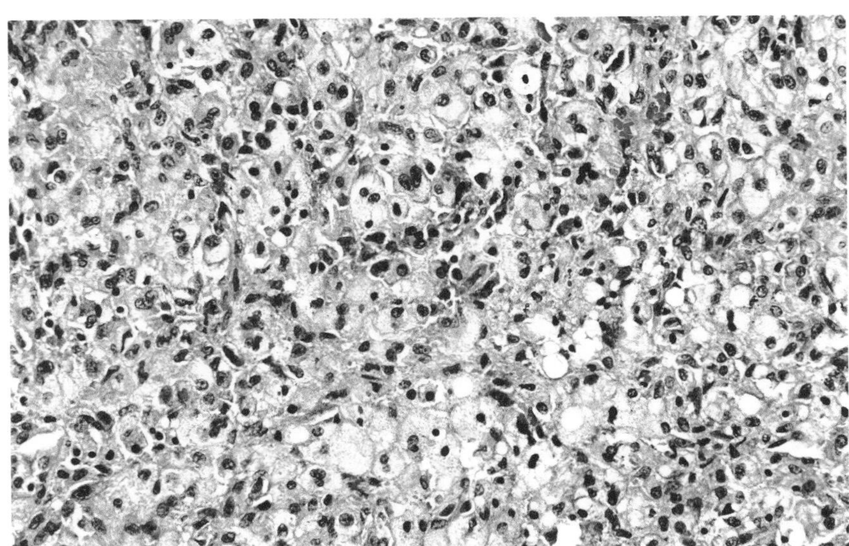

FIGURE 11-66. Malacoplakia of the retroperitoneum with solid sheets of histiocytes admixed with inflammatory cells.

bacilli. The reaction results in the formation of yellow plaque-like lesions on the mucosal surface of the affected organs.[129] The disease typically develops in the genitourinary tract, particularly the bladder, although it may affect the soft tissues of the retroperitoneum as well. It is characterized by sheets of pale, slightly granular, or vacuolated histiocytes (von Hansemann cells) containing PAS-positive, diastase-resistant inclusions in the cytoplasm (Fig. 11-66). Lymphocytes, plasma cells, and neutrophils are typically abundant. The distinctive Michaelis-Gutmann bodies, small calcospherites that consist of a mixture of organic and inorganic materials, including calcium and phosphate, can be identified within the histiocytes and extracellularly (Fig. 11-67). Electron microscopic studies show that the von Hansemann histiocytes contain numerous phagolysosomes, occasional bacterial forms, and lamellated crystalline bodies representing the early stage of Michaelis-Gutmann bodies.[130]

Extranodal (Soft Tissue) Rosai-Dorfman Disease

Rosai-Dorfman disease is a polyclonal histiocytic disorder of uncertain etiology, which, although originally described as a lymph node disease,[131] occurs in sundry locations, including soft tissue. Although the nature of the proliferating histiocyte is still unknown, its appearance and immunophenotype most closely approximate an activated macrophage.[132] Approximately 10% of all cases of Rosai-Dorfman disease are associated with soft tissue involvement, and, in some cases, it is the sole manifestation of the disorder.[133,134] However, the actual incidence of associated lymphadenopathy in patients with soft tissue lesions depends greatly on the bias of the study. In the study by Foucar et al.,[133] most had lymphadenopathy, whereas in the study by Montgomery et al.,[134] only a few did (4 of 23). The former study was based on a referral of all cases

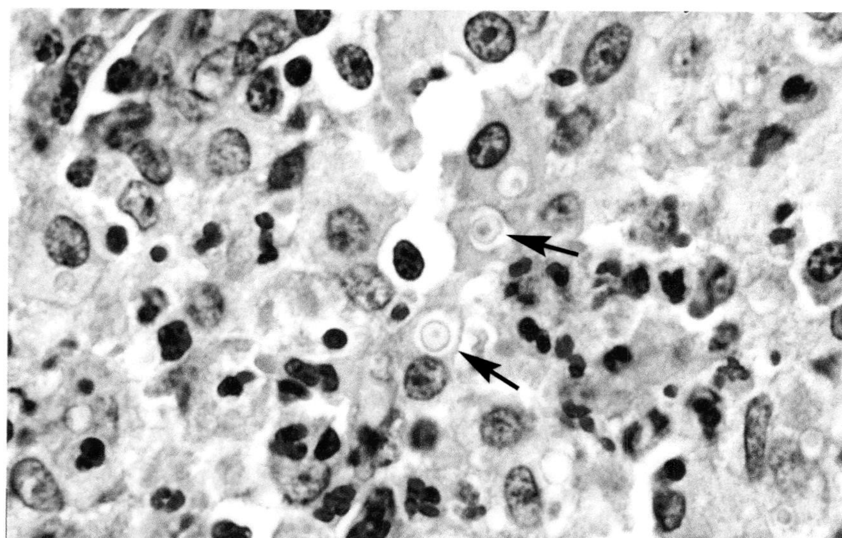

FIGURE 11-67. High-power view of malacoplakia showing Michaelis-Gutmann bodies (arrows) in occasional cells.

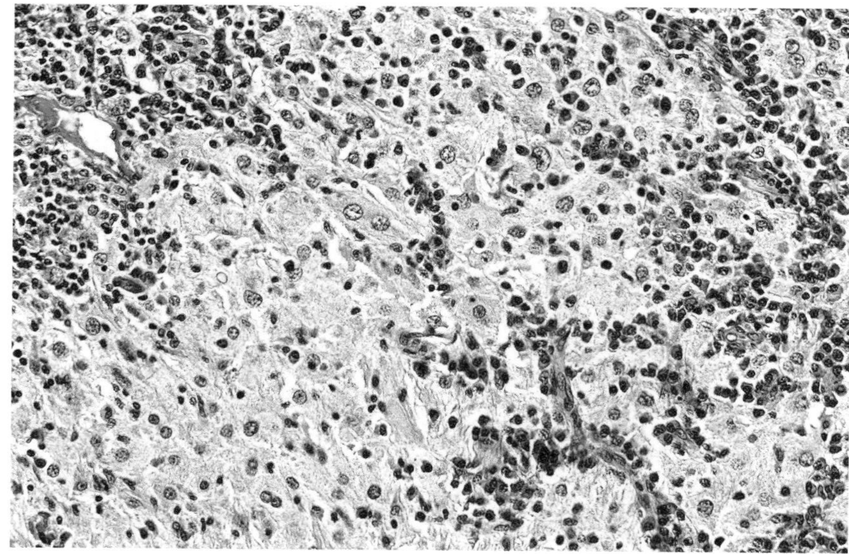

FIGURE 11-68. Extranodal Rosai-Dorfman disease characterized by sheets of pale histiocytes with voluminous cytoplasm.

to the National Sinus Histiocytosis with Massive Lymphadenopathy Registry at Yale University, whereas the latter represented referral cases to the Soft Tissue Registry of the AFIP. Patients with soft tissue Rosai-Dorfman disease tend to be older than those with lymph-node-based disease. Patients with Rosai-Dorfman disease of the skin are more often female, present at an older age than do patients with noncutaneous disease and are less likely to have disease involvement in other locations.[135]

Microscopically, the lesions consist of sheets or syncytia of large, pale histiocytes with large, round, vesicular nuclei with some degree of atypia (Figs. 11-68 and 11-69). Mitotic figures are usually difficult to detect or are absent altogether. The cytoplasm of the histiocytes may contain lymphocytes (emperipolesis), although this is seldom as striking as in the lesions of lymph nodes. Microabscesses, when present, suggest the possibility of an infectious process. The feature that tends to complicate the diagnosis of these unusual lesions is the presence of fibrosis, which distorts the sheet-like growth pattern, creating instead a storiform pattern. Predictably, the latter pattern, in association with atypical histiocytes, is often construed as evidence that one is dealing with a fibrohistiocytic tumor. The histiocytes of Rosai-Dorfman disease consistently and strongly express S-100 protein and, occasionally, other histiocytic antigens,[136] including CD1a. However, they do not contain Birbeck granules.

The presence of S-100 protein is useful for discriminating these lesions from undifferentiated pleomorphic sarcomas and histiocytic proliferations of infectious etiology. Clearly, this antigen does not discriminate examples of soft tissue Rosai-Dorfman disease from Langerhans cell histiocytosis, although usually the cytologic differences between the proliferating histiocytes in the two conditions and the differences in the inflammatory cells accompanying them readily permit

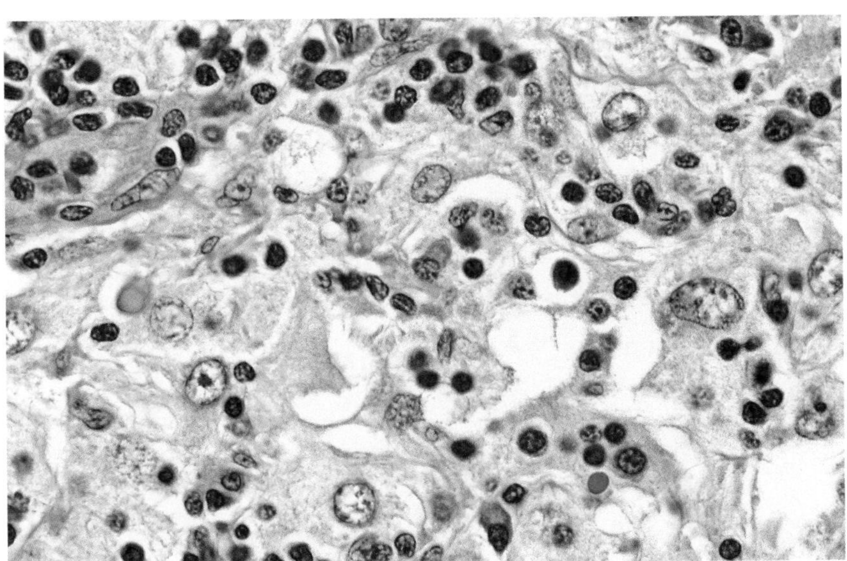

FIGURE 11-69. High-power view of Rosai-Dorfman disease illustrating mild nuclear atypia and emperipolesis.

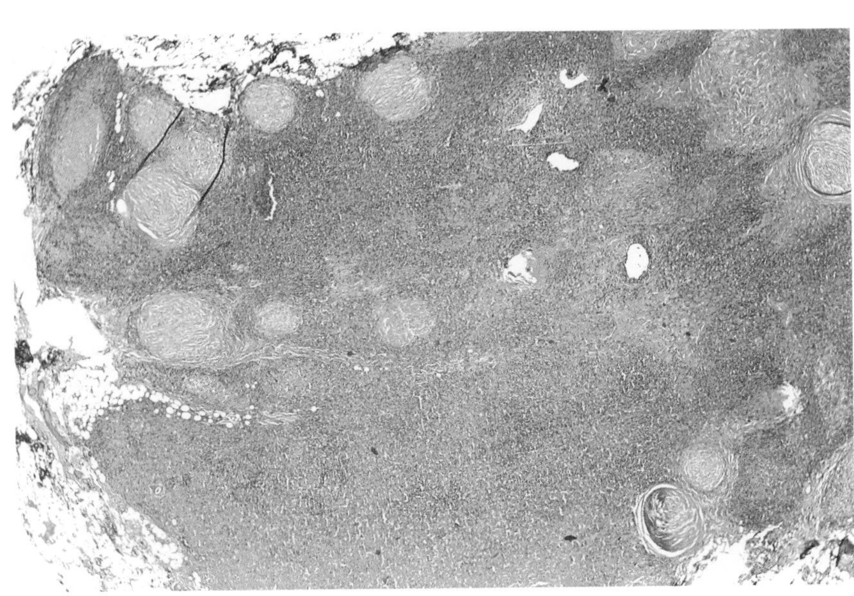

FIGURE 11-70. Silica reaction in the inguinal region. Lesion is composed of sheets of well-differentiated histiocytes interlaced with fibrous bands.

this distinction. The data, at present, suggest that the prognosis of soft tissue Rosai-Dorfman disease is excellent. Most patients with isolated soft tissue masses appeared well following surgery, although some developed recurrent disease. A significant number of patients with isolated cutaneous disease resolve spontaneously.[135]

Histiocytic Reactions to Endogenous and Exogenous Material

Silica Reaction

Although the usual response to silica in soft tissue is a localized foreign body reaction, exuberant reactions to the material simulate a fibrohistiocytic neoplasm (Figs. 11-70 and 11-71). The latter form of soft tissue silicosis is probably related to the presence of large amounts of silica. It seems principally to be an iatrogenic disease secondary to the now obsolete injection therapy for hernias.[137] Clinically, these lesions present as slowly enlarging tumorous masses, usually in the inguinal region or abdominal wall. Typically, they occur many years after the injection of silica, so the causal relation of the injection is minimized or overlooked. Grossly, the lesions are ill-defined, gray-yellow masses with a gritty consistency on cutting. They consist of sheets of histiocytes with a clear or amphophilic cytoplasm. Although usually well differentiated, the histiocytes occasionally display moderate pleomorphism. Mitotic figures are rare. PAS-positive, diastase-resistant bodies may be present in the histiocytes and probably represent large phagolysosomes, organelles involved in the intracellular storage of silica. Numerous silica crystals can be identified under polarized light. A striking feature of the lesion is the large amount of fibrosis. The collagen varies from delicate interstitial or perivascular fibers in the early stages to broad

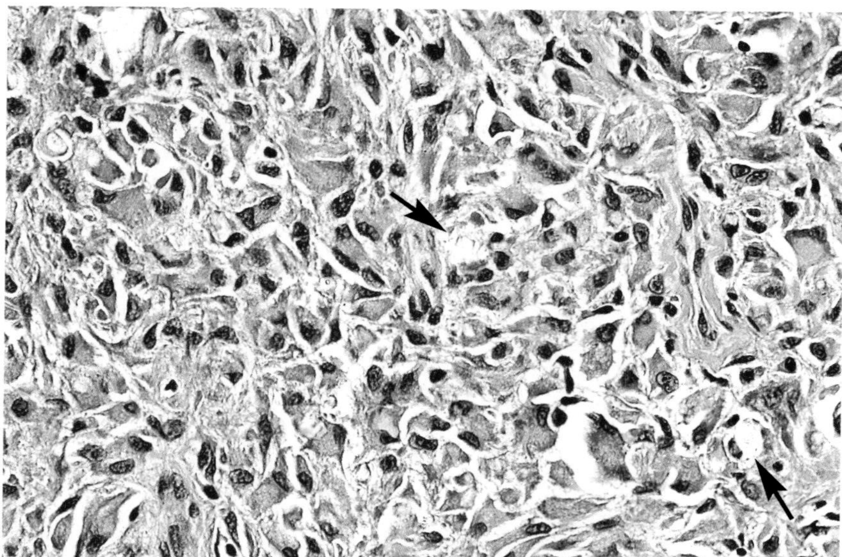

FIGURE 11-71. Silica reaction in the inguinal region showing well-differentiated histiocytes. Spicules of foreign material can be seen in the cytoplasm of some histiocytes, but full elucidation requires polarization.

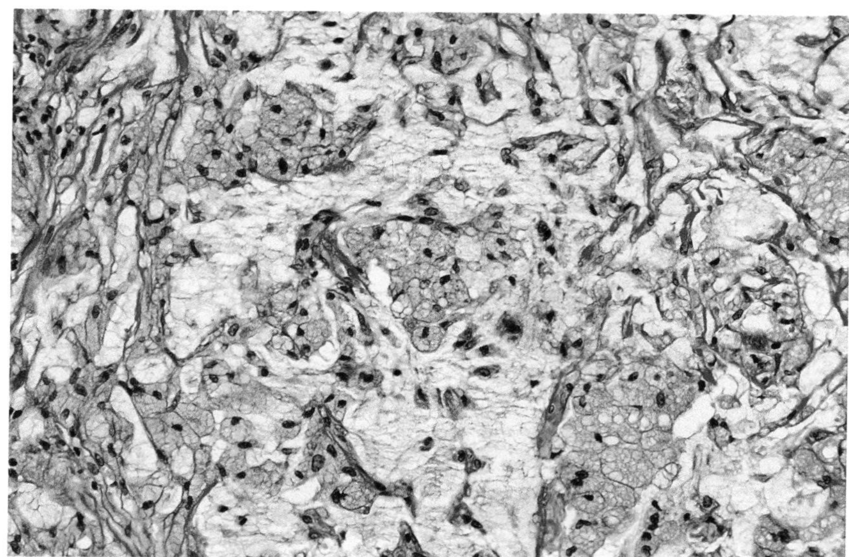

FIGURE 11-72. Polyvinylpyrrolidone (PVP) granuloma. Clusters of bubbly histiocytes are suspended in pools of basophilic-appearing PVP.

bands and, finally, mats or large nodules. The presence of silica, extensive fibrosis, scarcity of mitotic figures, and poorly developed vasculature all serve to distinguish these lesions from fibrous histiocytomas and undifferentiated pleomorphic sarcomas.

Polyvinylpyrrolidone Granuloma

Polyvinylpyrrolidone (PVP) is a polymer of vinylpyrrolidone, which was used notably as a plasma expander during wartime and until recently was used in various intravenous preparations in Asia. It has been marketed under various names, including Plasgen, Periston, Plasmagel, Biseko, Blutogen, and Subplasm. Because of its hydroscopic properties, it has also been used as a retardant in various injectable medicines (hormones, antihypertensives, local anesthetics), as a clarifier in fruit juices, and as a resin in hair sprays.[138] The molecular weight of PVP varies depending on its chain length (MW 10,000 to 200,000 daltons). Low molecular-weight PVP is filtered by the glomerulus and cleared by the kidney, whereas high molecular-weight PVP (MW 50,000 daltons or more) is retained indefinitely by the body and is stored throughout the reticuloendothelial system. The common appearance of PVP disease following intravenous injection of the substance is that of blue-gray histiocytes lining the sinusoids of the liver, spleen, and lymph nodes. A second form of PVP disease presumably occurs following inhalation of the substance from hair spray.[139] The alveolar walls are thickened, and macrophages fill the alveolar spaces. An uncommon form of PVP disease is a localized pseudotumor, [140-142] presumably caused by local injection of the material. Cases reported in the literature have documented PVP pseudotumors secondary to the anesthetic Depot-Impletol[143] and vasopressin.[142]

Histologically, these lesions are composed of numerous histiocytes massively engorged with PVP (Figs. 11-72 to 11-74). The material appears glassy blue or blue-gray in sections stained with hematoxylin-eosin. The histiocytes form

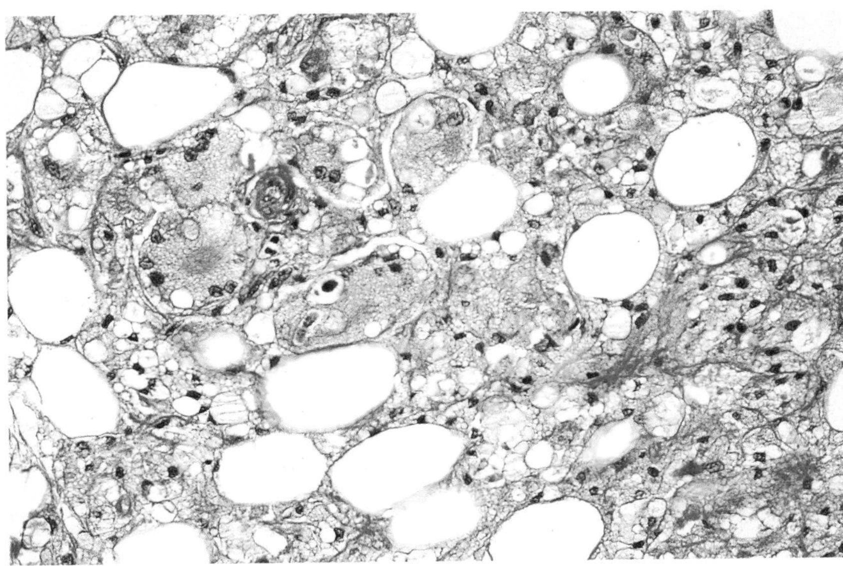

FIGURE 11-73. Multinucleated histiocytes filled with PVP.

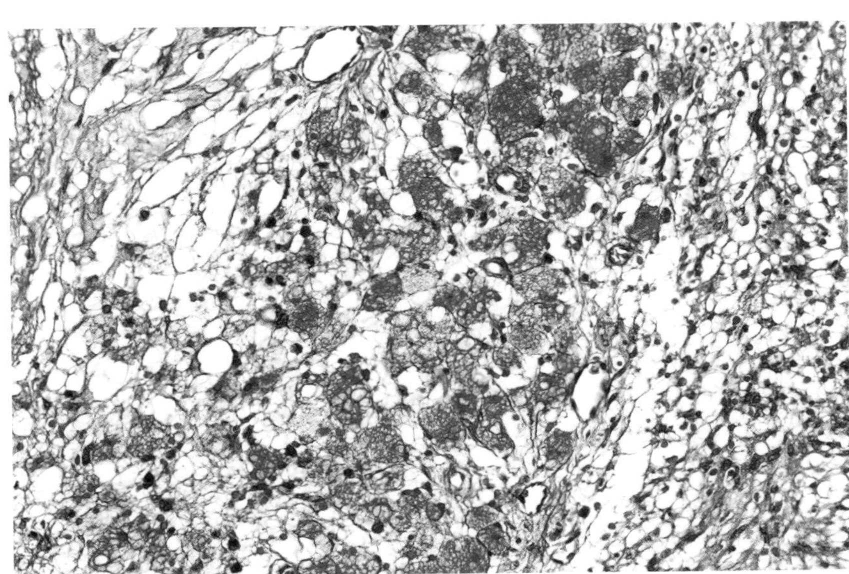

FIGURE 11-74. Congo red staining of PVP.

sheets or small clusters in a matrix containing copious amounts of foreign material. Giant cells are occasionally present and may be helpful in suggesting the diagnosis of a foreign body reaction. Another feature suggesting a reactive process is the manner in which the histiocytes percolate around the adnexal structures, nerves, and vessels. Typically, there are few, if any, inflammatory cells and no necrosis. The tinctorial properties of PVP have been well documented and serve to distinguish this lesion from other myxoid lesions (Box 11-2).[144] PVP characteristically does not stain with Alcian blue and, therefore, stains differently from all myxoid tumors of soft tissue, such as liposarcoma, chondrosarcoma, and chordoma. It does not stain blue with Giemsa stain and, therefore, should not be confused with the syndrome of sea-blue histiocytes. PVP is carminophilic, and this fact should be kept in mind because

BOX 11-2 Staining Reactions of Polyvinylpyrrolidone

Positive
- Congo red
- Sirius red
- Mucicarmine
- Colloidal iron

Negative
- Periodic acid-Schiff (PAS)
- Alcian blue

occasional cases of PVP granuloma have been mistaken for infiltrating carcinomas of the signet-ring type.[144] The best stains for demonstrating the cytoplasmic material are Congo red or Sirius red. Ultrastructurally, the material is contained in large membrane-limited vacuoles believed to be distended lysosomes. Dense bodies, probably composed of ferritin, are condensed at the periphery of the vacuoles.

Granular Cell Reaction

Collections of histiocytes with granular eosinophilic cytoplasm occasionally accumulate at the site of surgical trauma.[145] These peculiar histiocytic reactions bear a close similarity to the granular cell tumor (Figs. 11-75 to 11-77) but can usually be differentiated from the foregoing because the nuclei in these reactions are rather small and inconspicuous, and the granules are large and coarsely textured (see Fig. 11-77). Furthermore, the cells often surround nodules of granular, amorphous debris similar to the cytoplasmic granular material (see Figs. 11-75 and 11-76). Sobel et al.[145] pointed out that the staining reactions serve to distinguish the two lesions. The ceroid-lipofuscin substance in these histiocyte reactions is usually acid fast and autofluorescent compared with that of the granular cell tumor.

Crystal-Storing Histiocytosis Resembling Rhabdomyoma

Crystal-storing histiocytosis is a rare condition in which tumorous deposits of histiocytes containing crystalline immunoglobulin occur in soft tissue.[146,147] A small number of cases have been reported, all of which were associated with a lymphoplasmacytic neoplasm and monoclonal immunoglobulin production. It appears that the immunoglobulin is crystallized locally and phagocytosed by histiocytes, which become massively distorted by the material. The histiocytes are large, rounded to angular cells that occasionally appear multinucleated (Figs. 11-78 and 11-79). The crystalline material varies in size, but the largest deposits can be visualized easily by light microscopy. The histiocytic cells can be few in number or so abundant that the underlying lymphoplasmacytic neoplasm is overlooked, resulting in an erroneous diagnosis of rhabdomyoma.[147] However, the cells can be clearly identified as histiocytic by strong immunostaining for CD68. Ultrastructurally, the crystalline material displays a lattice pattern with a periodicity of 45 to 60 angstroms consistent with immunoglobulin (Fig. 11-80).

Cellular Spindled Histiocytic Pseudotumor Complicating Fat Necrosis

Very recently, Sciallis et al.[148] have reported a distinctive, cellular proliferation of histiocytes showing spindled morphology, arising in the setting of mammary fat necrosis. Identical proliferations in omental/mesenteric fat necrosis have been observed, although not in fat necrosis in other locations. Cellular spindled histiocytic pseudotumor typically occurs in women, often with a history of prior breast carcinoma and therapeutic irradiation. These lesions may closely mimic a new breast carcinoma clinically and radiographically, and many cases were submitted in consultation to rule out a malignant process, in particular spindle cell (metaplastic) carcinoma.[148] Microscopically, these lesions consist of a moderately cellular, fascicular proliferation of mitotically active, normochromatic, lightly eosinophilic spindled cells with mild nuclear variability, folded or grooved nuclei and indistinct nucleoli (Fig. 11-81). Chronic inflammatory cells and multinucleated giant cells are often admixed with the spindled cells, with more typical features of fat necrosis frequently present at the periphery (Fig. 11-82). By immunohistochemistry, the spindled cells show a true histiocytic phenotype, with expression of CD163 and CD11c (Fig. 11-83). Cytokeratins and S-100 protein are negative, as are histochemical stains for acid-fast and fungal organisms.[148] Clinical follow-up on all patients has shown benign behavior, without local recurrences. This process appears to represent an exaggerated histiocytic reaction to fat necrosis in the breast.

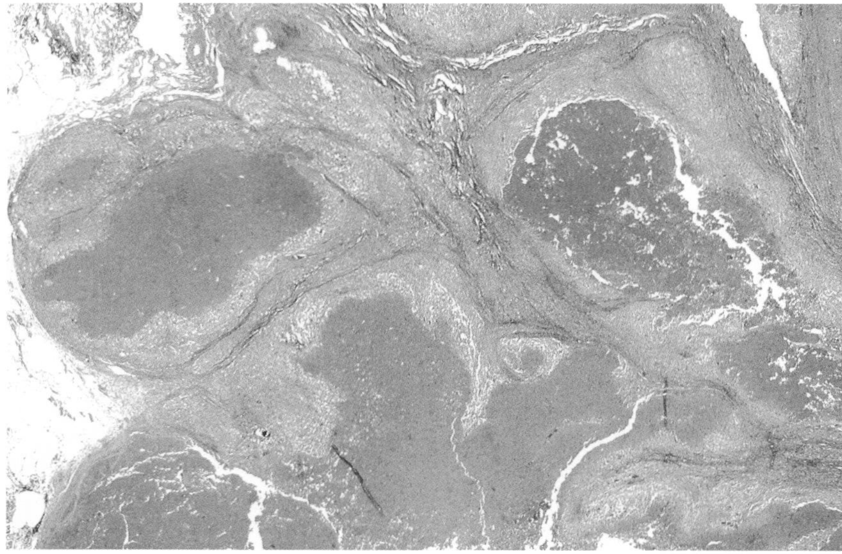

FIGURE 11-75. Granular cell reaction showing a fringe of histiocytes surrounding the core of the granuloamorphous material.

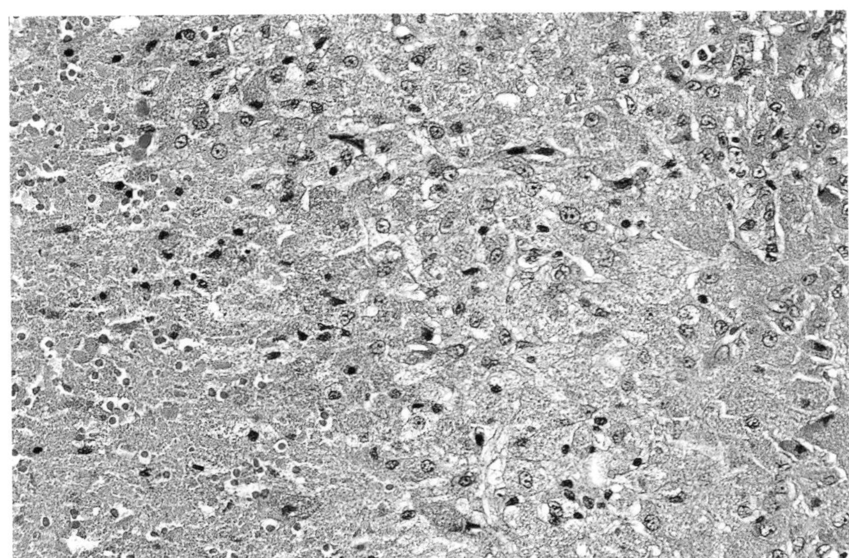

FIGURE 11-76. Histiocytic reaction with "granular cell" features at the site of previous surgery.

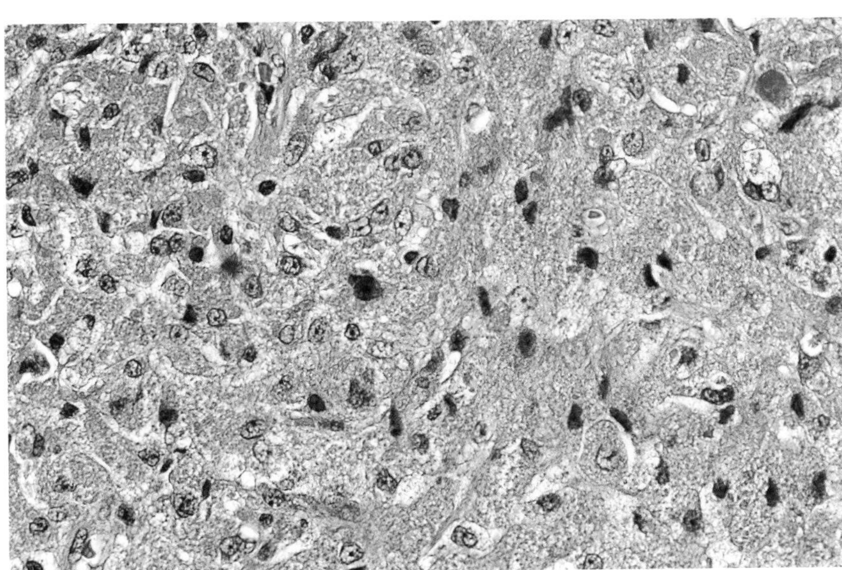

FIGURE 11-77. High-power view of granular-appearing histiocytes in granular cell reactions.

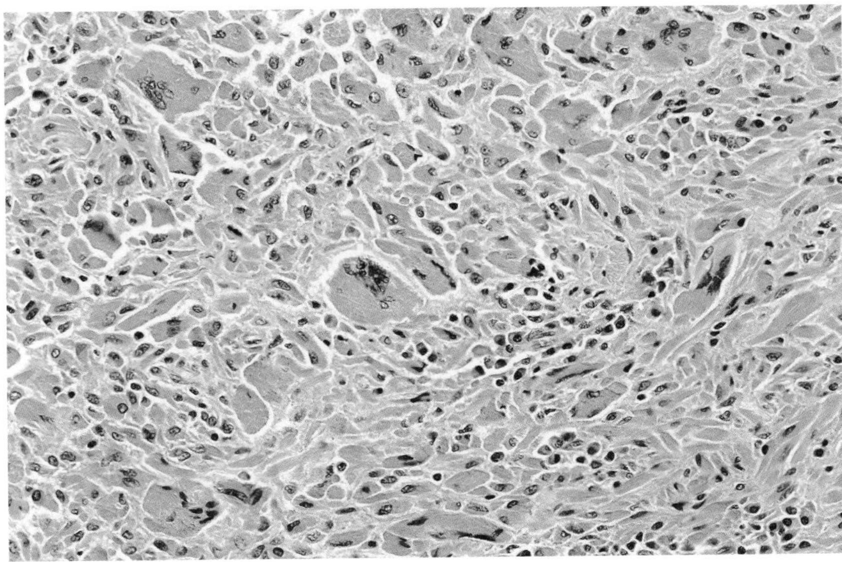

FIGURE 11-78. Crystalline storing histiocytosis in a patient with lymphoplasmatic lymphoma.

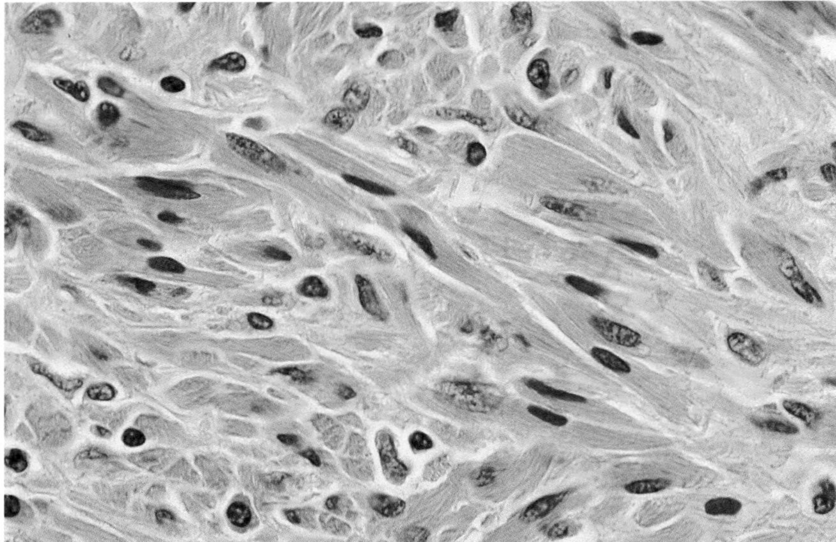

FIGURE 11-79. High-power view of crystal-containing histiocytes from Figure 11-78 showing massive distortion and spindling as a result of intracytoplasmic crystalline immunoglobulin.

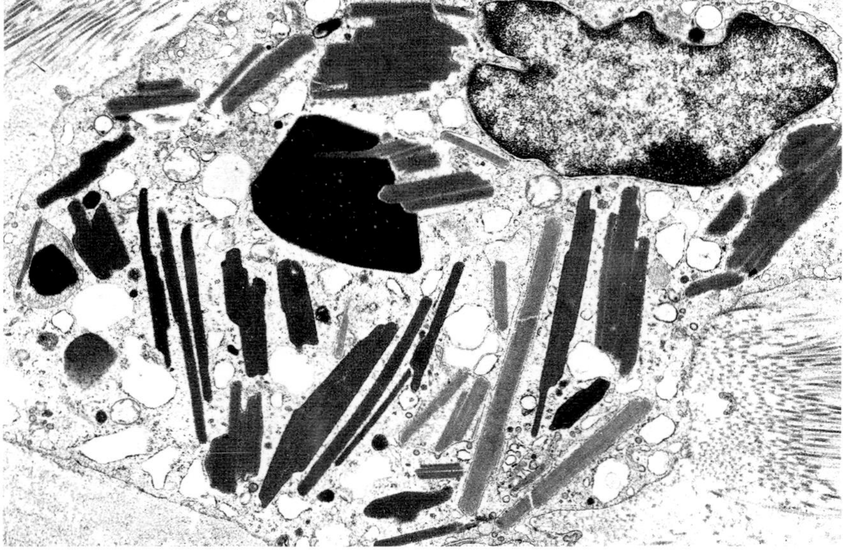

FIGURE 11-80. Electron micrograph of crystalline immunoglobulin from Figure 11-79 showing periodicity.

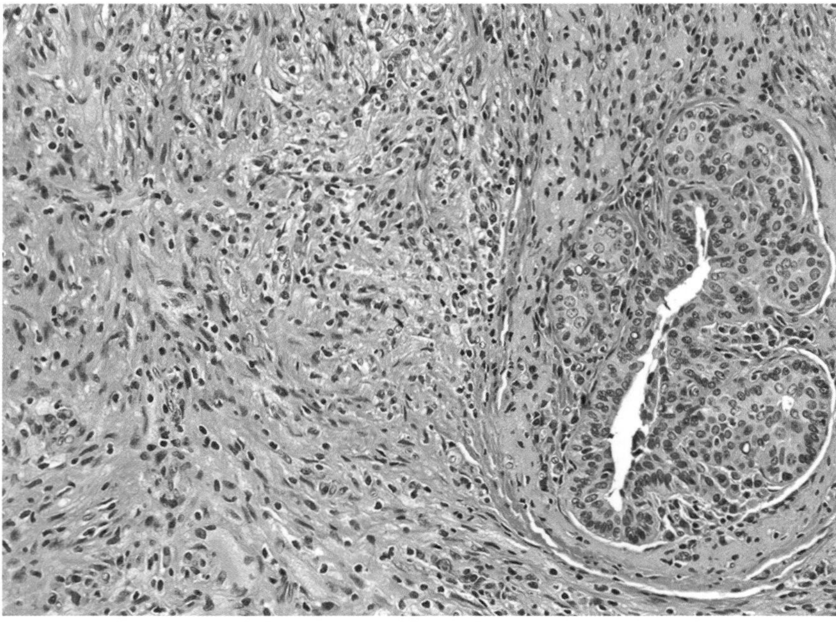

FIGURE 11-81. Cellular spindle histiocytic pseudotumor complicating mammary fat necrosis, showing a cellular, fascicular proliferation of bland spindled cells surrounding a breast lobule.

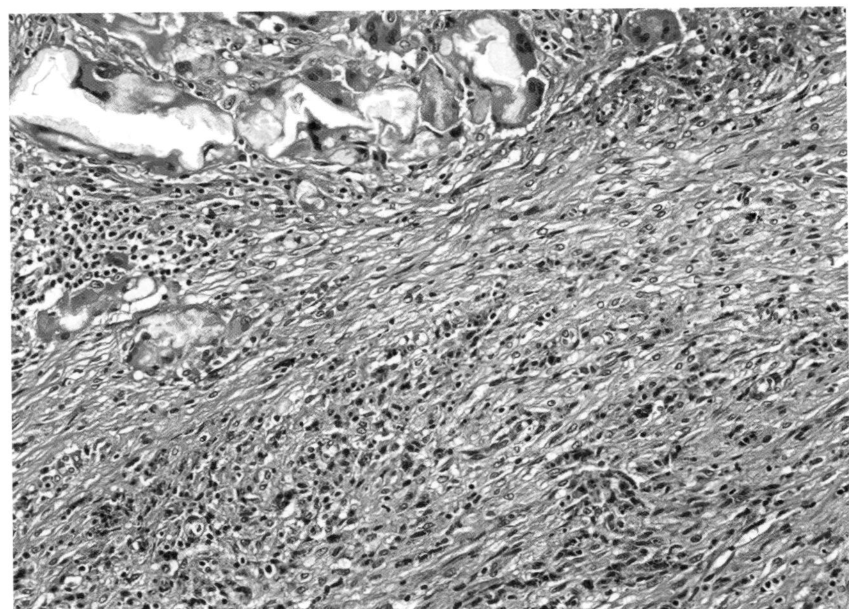

FIGURE 11-82. The presence of more typical features of fat necrosis, such as a foreign body giant-cell reaction to degenerating fat, is a useful clue in the distinction of cellular histiocytic pseudotumor of the breast from other mammary spindle cell neoplasms.

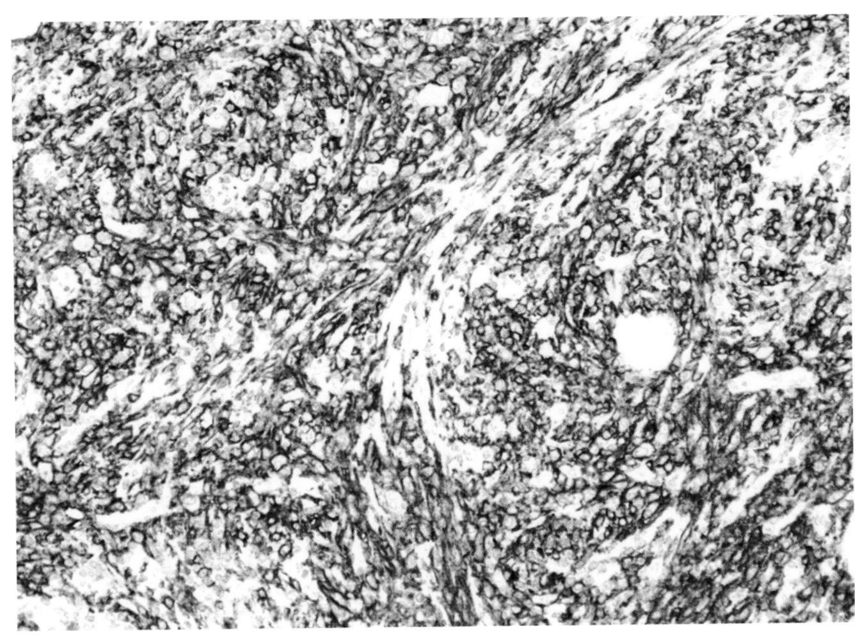

FIGURE 11-83. CD11c, a highly specific marker of macrophages, is typically positive in a cellular histiocytic pseudotumor.

References

1. Fletcher CD, Unni KK, Mertens F. Pathology and genetics of tumors of soft tissue and bone. Lyon, France: IARC Press; 2002.
2. Katenkamp D, Stiller D. Cellular composition of the so-called dermatofibroma (histiocytoma cutis). Virchows Arch A Pathol Anat Histol 1975;367(4):325–36.
3. Niemi KM. The benign fibrohistiocytic tumours of the skin. Acta dermato-venereologica Supplementum 1970;50(Suppl 63):1–6.
4. Gonzalez S, Duarte I. Benign fibrous histiocytoma of the skin. A morphologic study of 290 cases. Pathol Res Pract 1982;174(4):379–91.
5. Newman DM, Walter JB. Multiple dermatofibromas in patients with systemic lupus erythematosus on immunosuppressive therapy. N Engl J Med 1973;289(16):842–3.
6. Foreman K, Bonish B, Nickoloff B. Absence of human herpesvirus 8 DNA sequences in patients with immunosuppression-associated dermatofibromas. Arch Dermatol [Letter] 1997;133(1):108–9.
7. Beer M, Eckert F, Schmoeckel C. The atrophic dermatofibroma. J Am Acad Dermatol 1991;25(6 Pt 1):1081–2.
8. Shishido E, Kadono S, Manaka I, et al. The mechanism of epidermal hyperpigmentation in dermatofibroma is associated with stem cell factor and hepatocyte growth factor expression. J Invest Dermatol 2001;117(3):627–33.
9. Fitzpatrick TB, Gilchrest BA. Dimple sign to differentiate benign from malignant pigmented cutaneous lesions. N Engl J Med 1977;296(26):1518.
10. Fletcher CD. Benign fibrous histiocytoma of subcutaneous and deep soft tissue: a clinicopathologic analysis of 21 cases. Am J Surg Pathol 1990;14(9):801–9.
11. Gleason BC, Fletcher CD. Deep "benign" fibrous histiocytoma: clinicopathologic analysis of 69 cases of a rare tumor indicating occasional metastatic potential. Am J Surg Pathol 2008;32(3):354–62.
12. Calonje E, Fletcher CD. Aneurysmal benign fibrous histiocytoma: clinicopathological analysis of 40 cases of a tumour frequently misdiagnosed as a vascular neoplasm. Histopathology 1995;26(4):323–31.
13. McKenna DB, Kavanagh GM, McLaren KM, et al. Aneurysmal fibrous histiocytoma: an unusual variant of cutaneous fibrous histiocytoma. J Eur Acad Dermatol Venereol [Case Reports] 1999;12(3):238–40.

14. Santa Cruz DJ, Kyriakos M. Aneurysmal ("angiomatoid") fibrous histiocytoma of the skin. Cancer 1981;47(8):2053–61.
15. Argenyi ZB, Cain C, Bromley C, et al. S-100 protein-negative malignant melanoma: fact or fiction? A light-microscopic and immunohistochemical study. Am J Dermatopathol 1994;16(3):233–40.
16. Tamada S, Ackerman AB. Dermatofibroma with monster cells. Am J Dermatopathol 1987;9(5):380–7.
17. Beham A, Fletcher CD. Atypical 'pseudosarcomatous' variant of cutaneous benign fibrous histiocytoma: report of eight cases. Histopathology 1990;17(2):167–9.
18. Cerio R, Spaull J, Jones EW. Histiocytoma cutis: a tumour of dermal dendrocytes (dermal dendrocytoma). Br J Dermatol 1989;120(2):197–206.
19. Calonje E, Mentzel T, Fletcher CD. Cellular benign fibrous histiocytoma. Clinicopathologic analysis of 74 cases of a distinctive variant of cutaneous fibrous histiocytoma with frequent recurrence. Am J Surg Pathol 1994;18(7):668–76.
20. Bruecks AK, Trotter MJ. Expression of desmin and smooth muscle myosin heavy chain in dermatofibromas. Arch Pathol Lab Med [Research Support, Non-U.S. Gov't] 2002;126(10):1179–83.
21. Mihatsch-Konz B, Schaumburg-Lever G, Lever WF. Ultrastructure of dermatofibroma. Archiv fur dermatologische Forschung 1973;246(3):181–92.
22. Horenstein MG, Prieto VG, Nuckols JD, et al. Indeterminate fibrohistiocytic lesions of the skin: is there a spectrum between dermatofibroma and dermatofibrosarcoma protuberans? Am J Surg Pathol 2000;24(7):996–1003.
23. Wang WL, Patel KU, Coleman NM, et al. COL1A1:PDGFB chimeric transcripts are not present in indeterminate fibrohistiocytic lesions of the skin. Am J Dermatopathol 2010;32(2):149–53.
24. Kaddu S, Leinweber B. Podoplanin expression in fibrous histiocytomas and cellular neurothekeomas. Am J Dermatopathol 2009;31(2):137–9.
25. Li N, McNiff J, Hui P, et al. Differential expression of HMGA1 and HMGA2 in dermatofibroma and dermatofibrosarcoma protuberans: potential diagnostic applications, and comparison with histologic findings, CD34, and factor XIIIa immunoreactivity. Am J Dermatopathol [Comparative Study] 2004;26(4):267–72.
26. West RB, Harvell J, Linn SC, et al. Apo D in soft tissue tumors: a novel marker for dermatofibrosarcoma protuberans. Am J Surg Pathol 2004;28(8):1063–9.
27. Chen TC, Kuo T, Chan HL. Dermatofibroma is a clonal proliferative disease. J Cutan Pathol 2000;27(1):36–9.
28. Vanni R, Marras S, Faa G, et al. Cellular fibrous histiocytoma of the skin: evidence of a clonal process with different karyotype from dermatofibrosarcoma. Genes Chromosomes Cancer 1997;18(4):314–7.
29. Vanni R, Fletcher CD, Sciot R, et al. Cytogenetic evidence of clonality in cutaneous benign fibrous histiocytomas: a report of the CHAMP study group. Histopathology 2000;37(3):212–7.
30. Hui P, Glusac EJ, Sinard JH, et al. Clonal analysis of cutaneous fibrous histiocytoma (dermatofibroma). J Cutan Pathol 2002;29(7):385–9.
31. Frau DV, Erdas E, Caria P, et al. Deep fibrous histiocytoma with a clonal karyotypic alteration: molecular cytogenetic characterization of a t(16;17)(p13.3;q21.3). Cancer Genet Cytogenet 2010;202(1):17–21.
32. Franquemont DW, Cooper PH, Shmookler BM, et al. Benign fibrous histiocytoma of the skin with potential for local recurrence: a tumor to be distinguished from dermatofibroma. Mod Pathol 1990;3(2):158–63.
33. Font RL, Hidayat AA. Fibrous histiocytoma of the orbit. A clinicopathologic study of 150 cases. Hum Pathol [Research Support, U.S. Gov't, P.H.S.] 1982;13(3):199–209.
34. Mentzel T, Calonje E, Fletcher CD. Dermatomyofibroma: additional observations on a distinctive cutaneous myofibroblastic tumour with emphasis on differential diagnosis. Brit J Dermatol 1993;129(1):69–73.
35. Colome-Grimmer MI, Evans HL. Metastasizing cellular dermatofibroma. A report of two cases. Am J Surg Pathol 1996;20(11):1361–7.
36. Guillou L, Gebhard S, Salmeron M, et al. Metastasizing fibrous histiocytoma of the skin: a clinicopathologic and immunohistochemical analysis of three cases. Mod Pathol 2000;13(6):654–60.
37. Osborn M, Mandys V, Beddow E, et al. Cystic fibrohistiocytic tumours presenting in the lung: primary or metastatic disease? Histopathology 2003;43(6):556–62.
38. Kamino H, Jacobson M. Dermatofibroma extending into the subcutaneous tissue. Differential diagnosis from dermatofibrosarcoma protuberans. Am J Surg Pathol 1990;14(12):1156–64.
39. Zelger B, Sidoroff A, Stanzl U, et al. Deep penetrating dermatofibroma versus dermatofibrosarcoma protuberans. A clinicopathologic comparison. Am J Surg Pathol [Comparative Study] 1994;18(7):677–86.
40. Glusac EJ, Barr RJ, Everett MA, et al. Epithelioid cell histiocytoma. A report of 10 cases including a new cellular variant. Am J Surg Pathol 1994;18(6):583–90.
41. Singh Gomez C, Calonje E, Fletcher CD. Epithelioid benign fibrous histiocytoma of skin: clinico-pathological analysis of 20 cases of a poorly known variant. Histopathology 1994;24(2):123–9.
42. Jones EW, Cerio R, Smith NP. Epithelioid cell histiocytoma: a new entity. Br J Dermatol 1989;120(2):185–95.
43. Silverman JS, Glusac EJ. Epithelioid cell histiocytoma–histogenetic and kinetics analysis of dermal microvascular unit dendritic cell subpopulations. J Cutan Pathol 2003;30(7):415–22.
44. Zelger BW, Zelger BG, Steiner H, et al. Aneurysmal and haemangiopericytoma-like fibrous histiocytoma. J Clin Pathol 1996;49(4):313–8.
45. Kamino H, Reddy VB, Gero M, et al. Dermatomyofibroma. A benign cutaneous, plaque-like proliferation of fibroblasts and myofibroblasts in young adults. J Cutan Pathol 1992;19(2):85–93.
46. Schwob VS, Santa Cruz DJ. Palisading cutaneous fibrous histiocytoma. J Cutan Pathol 1986;13(6):403–7.
47. Zelger BG, Calonje E, Zelger B. Myxoid dermatofibroma. Histopathology 1999;34(4):357–64.
48. Zelger BW, Steiner H, Kutzner H. Clear cell dermatofibroma. Case report of an unusual fibrohistiocytic lesion. Am J Surg Pathol [Case Reports Review] 1996;20(4):483–91.
49. Iwata J, Fletcher CD. Lipidized fibrous histiocytoma: clinicopathologic analysis of 22 cases. Am J Dermatopathol [Research Support, Non-U.S. Gov't] 2000;22(2):126–34.
50. Kaddu S, McMenamin ME, Fletcher CD. Atypical fibrous histiocytoma of the skin: clinicopathologic analysis of 59 cases with evidence of infrequent metastasis. Am J Surg Pathol 2002;26(1):35–46.
51. Mentzel T, Kutzner H. Haemorrhagic dermatomyofibroma (plaque-like dermal fibromatosis): clinicopathological and immunohistochemical analysis of three cases resembling plaque-stage Kaposi's sarcoma. Histopathology 2003;42(6):594–8.
52. Hugel H. Plaque-like dermal fibromatosis/dermatomyofibroma. J Cutan Pathol 1993;20(1):94.
53. Mentzel T, Kutzner H. Dermatomyofibroma: clinicopathologic and immunohistochemical analysis of 56 cases and reappraisal of a rare and distinct cutaneous neoplasm. Am J Dermatopathol 2009;31(1):44–9.
54. Ng WK, Cheung MF, Ma L. Dermatomyofibroma: further support of its myofibroblastic nature by electronmicroscopy. Histopathology 1996;29(2):181–3.
55. Tardio JC, Azorin D, Hernandez-Nunez A, et al. Dermatomyofibromas presenting in pediatric patients: clinicopathologic characteristics and differential diagnosis. J Cutan Pathol 2011;38(12):967–72.
56. Barnhill RL, Mihm Jr MC. Cellular neurothekeoma. A distinctive variant of neurothekeoma mimicking nevomelanocytic tumors. Am J Surg Pathol 1990;14(2):113–20.
57. Fetsch JF, Laskin WB, Hallman JR, et al. Neurothekeoma: an analysis of 178 tumors with detailed immunohistochemical data and long-term patient follow-up information. Am J Surg Pathol 2007;31(7):1103–14.
58. Laskin WB, Fetsch JF, Miettinen M. The "neurothekeoma": immunohistochemical analysis distinguishes the true nerve sheath myxoma from its mimics. Hum Pathol 2000;31(10):1230–41.
59. Hornick JL, Fletcher CD. Cellular neurothekeoma: detailed characterization in a series of 133 cases. Am J Surg Pathol 2007;31(3):329–40.
60. Busam KJ, Mentzel T, Colpaert C, et al. Atypical or worrisome features in cellular neurothekeoma: a study of 10 cases. Am J Surg Pathol 1998;22(9):1067–72.
61. Calonje E, Wilson-Jones E, Smith NP, et al. Cellular 'neurothekeoma': an epithelioid variant of pilar leiomyoma? Morphological and immunohistochemical analysis of a series. Histopathology 1992;20(5):397–404.
62. Page RN, King R, Mihm Jr MC, et al. Microphthalmia transcription factor and NKI/C3 expression in cellular neurothekeoma. Mod Pathol 2004;17(2):230–4.
63. Sheth S, Li X, Binder S, et al. Differential gene expression profiles of neurothekeomas and nerve sheath myxomas by microarray analysis. Mod Pathol 2011;24(3):343–54.
64. Sachdev R, Sundram UN. Frequent positive staining with NKI/C3 in normal and neoplastic tissues limits its usefulness in the diagnosis of cellular neurothekeoma. Am J Clin Pathol 2006;126(4):554–63.
65. Fox MD, Billings SD, Gleason BC, et al. Expression of MiTF may be helpful in differentiating cellular neurothekeoma from plexiform fibrohistiocytic tumor (histiocytoid predominant) in a partial biopsy specimen. Am J Dermatopathol 2012;34(2):157–60.

66. Helwig EB, Hackney VC. Juvenile xanthogranuloma (nevoxanthoendothelioma). Am J Pathol 1954;30:625.
67. Janssen D, Harms D. Juvenile xanthogranuloma in childhood and adolescence: a clinicopathologic study of 129 patients from the kiel pediatric tumor registry. Am J Surg Pathol 2005;29(1):21–8.
68. Zelger B, Cerio R, Orchard G, et al. Juvenile and adult xanthogranuloma. A histological and immunohistochemical comparison. Am J Surg Pathol 1994;18(2):126–35.
69. Tahan SR, Pastel-Levy C, Bhan AK, et al. Juvenile xanthogranuloma. Clinical and pathologic characterization. Arch Pathol Lab Med 1989;113(9):1057–61.
70. Cohen BA, Hood A. Xanthogranuloma: report on clinical and histologic findings in 64 patients. Pediatr Dermatol 1989;6(4):262–6.
71. Nascimento AG. A clinicopathologic and immunohistochemical comparative study of cutaneous and intramuscular forms of juvenile xanthogranuloma. Am J Surg Pathol 1997;21(6):645–52.
72. Esterly NB, Sahihi T, Medenica M. Juvenile xanthogranuloma. An atypical case with study of ultrastructure. Arch Dermatol 1972;105(1): 99–102.
73. Gonzalez-Crussi F, Campbell RJ. Juvenile xanthogranuloma: ultrastructural study. Arch Pathol 1970;89(1):65–72.
74. Dehner LP. Juvenile xanthogranulomas in the first two decades of life: a clinicopathologic study of 174 cases with cutaneous and extracutaneous manifestations. Am J Surg Pathol 2003;27(5):579–93.
75. Kraus MD, Haley JC, Ruiz R, et al. "Juvenile" xanthogranuloma: an immunophenotypic study with a reappraisal of histogenesis. Am J Dermatopathol 2001;23(2):104–11.
76. Zelger BW, Cerio R. Xanthogranuloma is the archetype of non-Langerhans cell histiocytoses. Br J Dermatol [Comment Letter] 2001; 145(2):369–71.
77. Purvis 3rd WE, Helwig EB. Reticulohistiocytic granuloma (reticulohistiocytoma) of the skin. Am J Clin Pathol 1954;24(9):1005–15.
78. Montgomery H, Polley HF, Pugh DG. Reticulohistiocytoma (reticulohistiocytic granuloma). AMA Arch Derm [Case Reports] 1958;77(1): 61–72.
79. Miettinen M, Fetsch JF. Reticulohistiocytoma (solitary epithelioid histiocytoma): a clinicopathologic and immunohistochemical study of 44 cases. Am J Surg Pathol 2006;30(4):521–8.
80. Zelger B, Cerio R, Soyer HP, et al. Reticulohistiocytoma and multicentric reticulohistiocytosis. Histopathologic and immunophenotypic distinct entities. Am J Dermatopathol [Comparative Study] 1994;16(6):577–84.
81. Barrow MV, Holubar K. Multicentric reticulohistiocytosis. A review of 33 patients. Medicine (Baltimore) [Review] 1969;48(4):287–305.
82. Conaghan P, Miller M, Dowling JP. A unique presentation of multicentric reticulohistiocytosis in pregnancy. Arthritis Rheum 2003;36:269.
83. Davies BT, Wood SR. The so-called reticulohistiocytoma of the skin; a comparison of two distinct types. Br J Dermatol 1955;67(6): 205–11.
84. Davies NE, Roenigk Jr HH, Hawk WA, et al. Multicentric reticulohistiocytosis. Report of a case with histochemical studies. Arch Dermatol 1968;97(5):543–7.
85. Flam M, Ryan SC, Mah-Poy GL, et al. Multicentric reticulohistiocytosis. Report of a case, with atyphical features and electron microscopic study of skin lesions. Am J Med 1972;52(6):841–8.
86. Orkin M, Goltz RW, Good RA, et al. A study of multicentric reticulohistiocytosis. Arch Dermatol 1964;89:640–54.
87. Taylor DR. Multicentric reticulohistiocytosis. Arch Dermatol [Case Reports] 1977;113(3):330–2.
88. Oliver GF, Umbert I, Winkelmann RK, et al. Reticulohistiocytoma cutis–review of 15 cases and an association with systemic vasculitis in two cases. Clin Exp Dermatol [Case Reports] 1990;15(1):1–6.
89. Shiokawa S, Shingu M, Nishimura M, et al. Multicentric reticulohistiocytosis associated with subclinical Sjogren's syndrome. Clin Rheumatol 1991;10(2):201–5.
90. Kuramoto Y, Iizawa O, Matsunaga J, et al. Development of Ki-1 lymphoma in a child suffering from multicentric reticulohistiocytosis. Acta Derm Venereol [Case Reports] 1991;71(5):448–9.
91. Kuwabara H, Uda H, Tanaka S. Multicentric reticulohistiocytosis. Report of a case with electron microscopic studies. Acta Pathol Jpn [Case Reports] 1992;42(2):130–5.
92. Lotti T, Santucci M, Casigliani R, et al. Multicentric reticulohistiocytosis. Report of three cases with the evaluation of tissue proteinase activity. Am J Dermatopathol [Case Reports] 1988;10(6):497–504.
93. Ehrlich GE, Young I, Nosheny SZ, et al. Multicentric reticulohistiocytosis (lipoid dermatoarthritis). A multisystem disorder. Am J Med 1972;52(6):830–40.
94. Hashimoto K, Pritzker MS. Electron microscopic study of reticulohistiocytoma. An unusual case of congenital, self-healing reticulohistiocytosis. Arch Dermatol 1973;107(2):263–70.
95. Nakajima Y, Sato K, Morita H, et al. Severe progressive erosive arthritis in multicentric reticulohistiocytosis: possible involvement of cytokines in synovial proliferation. J Rheumatol [Case Reports] 1992;19(10): 1643–6.
96. Zagala A, Guyot A, Bensa JC, et al. Multicentric reticulohistiocytosis: a case with enhanced interleukin-1, prostaglandin E2 and interleukin-2 secretion. J Rheumatol [Case Reports] 1988;15(1):136–8.
97. Ginsburg WW, O'Duffy JD, Morris JL, et al. Multicentric reticulohistiocytosis: response to alkylating agents in six patients. Ann Intern Med 1989;111(5):384–8.
98. Kenik JG, Fok F, Huerter CJ, et al. Multicentric reticulohistiocytosis in a patient with malignant melanoma: a response to cyclophosphamide and a unique cutaneous feature. Arthritis Rheum [Case Reports] 1990;33(7):1047–51.
99. Lambert CM, Nuki G. Multicentric reticulohistiocytosis with arthritis and cardiac infiltration: regression following treatment for underlying malignancy. Ann Rheum Dis [Case Reports] 1992;51(6):815–7.
100. Crocker AC. Skin xanthomas in childhood. Pediatrics 1951;8(4): 573–97.
101. Fredrickson DS, Lees RS. A system for phenotyping hyperlipoproteinemia. Circulation 1965;31:321–7.
102. Marcoval J, Moreno A, Bordas X, et al. Diffuse plane xanthoma: clinicopathologic study of 8 cases. J Am Acad Dermatol 1998;39(3): 439–42.
103. Wilkes LL. Tendon xanthoma in type IV hyperlipoproteinemia. South Med J [Case Reports] 1977;70(2):254–5.
104. Wilson DE, Floweres CM, Hershgold EJ, et al. Multiple myeloma, cryoglobulinemia and xanthomatosis. Distinct clinical and biochemical syndromes in two patients. Am J Med [Case Reports Research Support, U.S. Gov't, P.H.S.] 1975;59(5):721–9.
105. Beerman H. Lipid diseases as manifested in the skin. Med Clin N Am 1951;35(2):433–56.
106. Cristol DS, Gill AB. Xanthoma of tendon sheath. JAMA 1943;122:1013.
107. Montgomery H. Cutaneous xanthomatosis. Ann Intern Med 1939;13:671.
108. Montgomery H, Osterberg AE. Xanthomatosis: correlation of clinical histopathologic and chemical studies of cutaneous xanthoma. Arch Dermatol Syph 1938;37:373.
109. Fahey JJ, Stark HH, Donovan WF, et al. Xanthoma of the achilles tendon. Seven cases with familial hyperbetalipoproteinemia. J Bone Joint Surg Am 1973;55(6):1197–211.
110. Friedman MS. Xanthoma of the Achilles tendon. J Bone Joint Surg Am 1947;29(3):760–6.
111. McWhorter JE, Weeks C. Multiple xanthoma of the tendons. Surg Gynecol Obstet 1925;40:199.
112. DeSanto DA, Wilson PD. Xanthomatous tumors of joints. J Bone Joint Surg 1939;21:531.
113. Lynch PJ, Winkelmann RK. Generalized plane xanthoma and systemic disease. Arch Dermatol [Case Reports In Vitro] 1966;93(6):639–46.
114. Hughes JD, Meriwether 3rd TW. Familial pseudohypertrophy of tendoachillis with multisystem disease. South Med J 1971;64(3):311–6.
115. Kearns WP, Wood WS. Cerebrotendinous xanthomatosis. Arch Ophthalmol [Case Reports] 1976;94(1):148–50.
116. Sloan HR, Frederickson DS. Rare familial diseases with neutral lipid storage: Wolman's disease, cholesterol ester storage disease, and cerebrotendinous xanthomatosis. In: Stanbury JB, Wyngaarden JB, Frederickson DS, editors. The metabolic basis of inherited disease. 3rd ed. New York: McGraw-Hill; 1972.
117. Buxtorf JC, Beaumont V, Jacotot B, et al. [Regression of xanthomas and hypolipidemic drugs]. Atherosclerosis 1974;19(1):1–11.
118. Berginer VM, Salen G, Shefer S. Long-term treatment of cerebrotendinous xanthomatosis with chenodeoxycholic acid. N Engl J Med [Research Support, Non-U.S. Gov't Research Support, U.S. Gov't, P.H.S.] 1984;311(26):1649–52.
119. Parker F, Odland GF. Electron microscopic similarities between experimental xanthomas and human eruptive xanthomas. J Invest Dermatol 1969;52(2):136–47.
120. Parker F, Odland GF. Experimental xanthoma. A correlative biochemical, histologic, histochemical, and electron microscopic study. Am J Pathol 1968;53(4):537–65.
121. Walton KW, Thomas C, Dunkerley DJ. The pathogenesis of xanthomata. J Pathol 1973;109(4):271–89.
122. Scott PJ, Winterbourn CC. Low-density lipoprotein accumulation in actively growing xanthomas. J Atheroscler Res 1967;7(2):207–23.

123. Keren DF, Rawlings Jr W, Murray HW, et al. Arizona hinshawii osteomyelitis with antecedent enteric fever and sepsis. A case report with a review of the literature. Am J Med [Case Reports] 1976;60(4):577–82.
124. Mansfield RE. Histoid leprosy. Arch Pathol 1969;87(6):580–5.
125. Wade HW. The histoid variety of lepromatous leprosy. Int J Lepr 1963;31:129–42.
126. Wood C, Nickoloff BJ, Todes-Taylor NR. Pseudotumor resulting from atypical mycobacterial infection: a "histoid" variety of Mycobacterium avium-intracellulare complex infection. Am J Clin Pathol [Case Reports] 1985;83(4):524–7.
127. Logani S, Lucas DR, Cheng JD, et al. Spindle cell tumors associated with mycobacteria in lymph nodes of HIV-positive patients: 'Kaposi sarcoma with mycobacteria' and 'mycobacterial pseudotumor'. Am J Surg Pathol [Review] 1999;23(6):656–61.
128. Umlas J, Federman M, Crawford C, et al. Spindle cell pseudotumor due to Mycobacterium avium-intracellulare in patients with acquired immunodeficiency syndrome (AIDS). Positive staining of mycobacteria for cytoskeleton filaments. Am J Surg Pathol 1991;15(12):1181–7.
129. Damjanov I, Katz SM. Malakoplakia. Pathol Annu [Research Support, U.S. Gov't, P.H.S. Review] 1981;16(Pt 2):103–26.
130. Font RL, Bersani TA, Eagle Jr RC. Malakoplakia of the eyelid. Clinical, histopathologic, and ultrastructural characteristics. Ophthalmology [Case Reports Research Support, Non-U.S. Gov't Review] 1988;95(1):61–8.
131. Rosai J, Dorfman RF. Sinus histiocytosis with massive lymphadenopathy: a pseudolymphomatous benign disorder. Analysis of 34 cases. Cancer 1972;30(5):1174–88.
132. Favara BE, Feller AC, Pauli M, et al. Contemporary classification of histiocytic disorders. The WHO Committee on Histiocytic/Reticulum Cell Proliferations. Reclassification Working Group of the Histiocyte Society. Med Pediatr Oncol [Review] 1997;29(3):157–66.
133. Foucar E, Rosai J, Dorfman R. Sinus histiocytosis with massive lymphadenopathy (Rosai-Dorfman disease): review of the entity. Semin Diagn Pathol 1990;7(1):19–73.
134. Montgomery EA, Meis JM, Frizzera G. Rosai-Dorfman disease of soft tissue. Am J Surg Pathol 1992;16(2):122–9.
135. Brenn T, Calonje E, Granter SR, et al. Cutaneous rosai-dorfman disease is a distinct clinical entity. Am J Dermatopathol 2002;24(5):385–91.
136. Eisen RN, Buckley PJ, Rosai J. Immunophenotypic characterization of sinus histiocytosis with massive lymphadenopathy (Rosai-Dorfman disease). Semin Diagn Pathol 1990;7(1):74–82.
137. Weiss SW, Enzinger FM, Johnson FB. Silica reaction simulating fibrous histiocytoma. Cancer 1978;42(6):2738–43.
138. Wessel W, Schoog M, Winkler E. Polyvinylpyrrolidone (PVP), its diagnostic, therapeutic and technical application and consequences thereof. Arzneimittel-Forschung [Review] 1971;21(10):1468–82.
139. Bergmann M, Flance IJ, Cruz PT, et al. Thesaurosis due to inhalation of hair spray. Report of twelve new cases, including three autopsies. N Engl J Med 1962;266:750–5.
140. Bubis JJ, Cohen S, Dinbar J, et al. Storage of polyvinylpyrrolidone mimicking a congenital mucolipid storage disease in a patient with Munchausen's syndrome. Isr J Med Sci 1975;11(10):999–1004.
141. Hizawa K, Inaba H, Nakanishi S, et al. Subcutaneous pseudosarcomatous polyvinylpyrrolidone granuloma. Am J Surg Pathol [Case Reports] 1984;8(5):393–8.
142. Reske-Nielsen E, Bojsen-Moller M, Vetner M, et al. Polyvinylpyrrolidone-storage disease. Light microscopical, ultrastructural and chemical verification. Acta Pathol Microbiol Scand A [Case Reports] 1976;84(5):397–405.
143. Gille J, Brandau H. [Foreign body granulation in the breast after injection of a polyvinylpyrrolidone containing preparation. A case report (author's transl)]. Geburtshilfe und Frauenheilkunde [Case Reports] 1975;35(10):799–801.
144. Kuo TT, Hsueh S. Mucicarminophilic histiocytosis. A polyvinylpyrrolidone (PVP) storage disease simulating signet-ring cell carcinoma. Am J Surg Pathol 1984;8(6):419–28.
145. Sobel HJ, Avrin E, Marquet E, et al. Reactive granular cells in sites of trauma. A cytochemical and ultrastructural study. Am J Clin Pathol 1974;61(2):223–34.
146. Harada M, Shimada M, Fukayama M, et al. Crystal-storing histiocytosis associated with lymphoplasmacytic lymphoma mimicking Weber-Christian disease: immunohistochemical, ultrastructural, and gene-rearrangement studies. Hum Pathol 1996;27(1):84–7.
147. Kapadia SB, Enzinger FM, Heffner DK, et al. Crystal-storing histiocytosis associated with lymphoplasmacytic neoplasms. Report of three cases mimicking adult rhabdomyoma. Am J Surg Pathol 1993;17(5):461–7.
148. Sciallis AP, Chen B, Folpe AL. Cellular spindled histiocytic pseudotumor complicating mammary fat necrosis: a potential diagnostic pitfall. Am J Surg Pathol 2012;36(10):1571–8.

Fibrohistiocytic Tumors of Intermediate Malignancy

CHAPTER CONTENTS

Fibrohistiocytic tumors of intermediate malignancy originally included only dermatofibrosarcoma protuberans and the closely related giant cell fibroblastoma. This category now embraces a number of other lesions such as plexiform fibrohistiocytic tumor and angiomatoid fibrous histiocytoma. All are characterized by a significant risk of local recurrence but a limited risk of regional and distant metastasis. They differ from fully malignant sarcomas in this important respect. They also occur in a decidedly younger population than do most sarcomas; indeed, some seem to occur almost exclusively in children. Although there is a general consensus that these lesions do not display true histiocytic differentiation, the term *fibrohistiocytic* remains a useful and widely understood descriptive term for this group of neoplasms. Their present classification, therefore, should be considered a tentative one, pending a general consensus on reclassification. On the one hand, dermatofibrosarcoma protuberans and its juvenile counterpart, giant cell fibroblastoma, seem to be most closely related to fibroblasts, and indeed the presence of CD34 immunoreactivity in these two lesions provides a linkage to the CD34+ dendritic cells that populate the dermis. On the other hand, plexiform fibrohistiocytic tumor seems to most closely approach the spirit of the term *fibrohistiocytic* because it has a bimodal population of cells, one of which has the histologic and immunophenotypic properties of a histiocyte and the other resembling a fibroblast or myofibroblast. The cells of many angiomatoid fibrous histiocytomas have a striking histiocytic appearance, contain phagocytosed particles of hemosiderin, and occasionally express the histiocyte-associated marker CD68; however, the cells show an unusual desmin and epithelial membrane antigen-positive immunophenotype, as well as specific translocations.

DERMATOFIBROSARCOMA PROTUBERANS

Dermatofibrosarcoma protuberans, first described in 1924 by Darier and Ferrand[1] as "progressive and recurring dermatofibroma," is a nodular cutaneous tumor characterized by a prominent storiform pattern. Over the years, it has been considered a fibroblastic, histiocytic, and neural tumor. It bears some histologic similarity to benign fibrous histiocytoma; on this basis, along with its pigmented counterpart (Bednar tumor), it is classified with the fibrohistiocytic neoplasms. In contrast to fibrous histiocytoma, dermatofibrosarcoma protuberans grows in a more infiltrative fashion and has a greater capacity for local recurrence. Moreover, in unusual instances, it metastasizes, although distant metastasis is usually a late event.

Clinical Findings

Dermatofibrosarcoma protuberans typically presents during early or middle adult life as a nodular cutaneous mass. Although early studies reflected its rarity in children,[2-5] there is an increasing number of reports of dermatofibrosarcoma protuberans in the pediatric age group. In fact, given the indolent growth and long preclinical duration, it is likely that many begin during childhood and become apparent during young adulthood only.[3] Males are affected more frequently than females. Although these tumors occur at almost any site, they are seen most frequently on the trunk and proximal extremities (Table 12-1). Unusual sites for this tumor are the vulva and parotid. Antecedent trauma, reported in about 10% to 20% of cases, is probably coincidental.[4-6]

In most cases, this tumor is characterized by slow but persistent growth over a long period, often several years. The clinical and gross appearances, then, are determined to a great extent by the stage of the disease. The initial manifestation is usually the development of a firm, plaque-like lesion of the skin, often with surrounding red to blue discoloration.[5] These lesions have been compared with the morphea of scleroderma or morphea-like basal cell carcinoma. Rarely, the lesions appear as an area of atrophy (so-called *atrophic variant*). Less often, multiple small subcutaneous nodules appear initially rather than a plaque. The plaque may grow slowly or remain stationary for a variable period, eventually entering a more rapid growth phase and giving rise to one or more nodules. Therefore, the typical protuberant appearance is manifested in only the fully developed lesion. Neglected tumors may achieve enormous proportions and have multiple satellite nodules. Although, despite the large size of many of these tumors, the

TABLE 12-1 Anatomic Distribution of Dermatofibrosarcoma Protuberans (1960-1979)

ANATOMIC LOCATION	NO. OF CASES	%
Head and neck	124	14.5
Upper extremity	155	18.2
Trunk	404	47.4
Lower extremity	170	19.9
Total	853	100

Data are from the Armed Forces Institute of Pathology (AFIP).

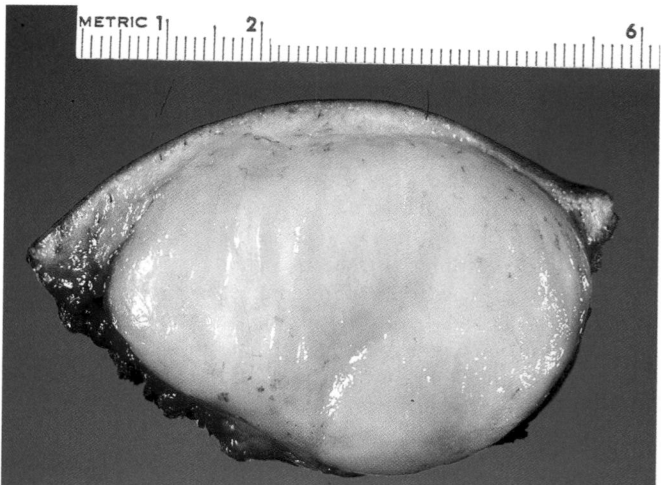

FIGURE 12-1. Typical dermatofibrosarcoma protuberans involving the dermis and subcutis in a nodular fashion.

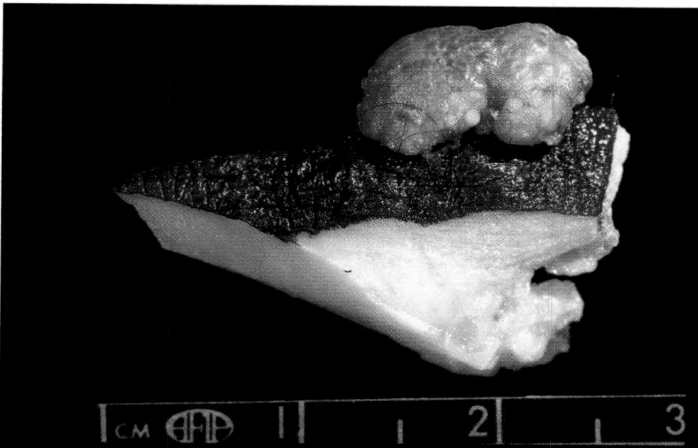

FIGURE 12-2. Small dermatofibrosarcoma displaying protuberant growth.

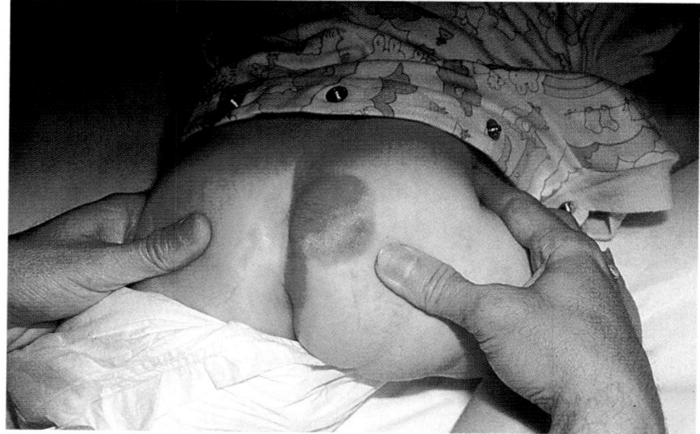

FIGURE 12-3. Dermatofibrosarcoma protuberans from the buttock of young child. It has the red color that some of these lesions exhibit.

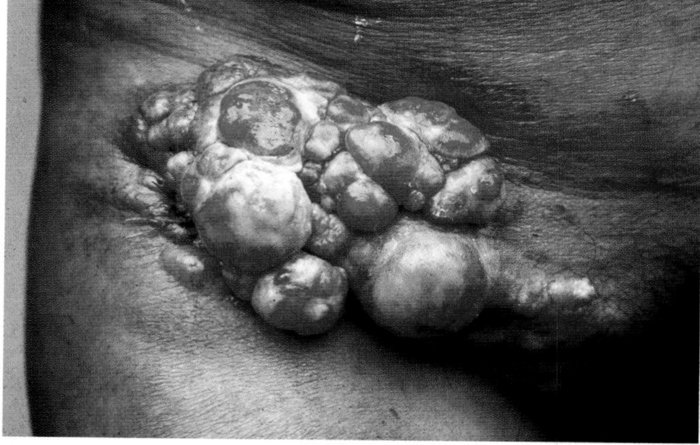

FIGURE 12-4. Gross appearance of an advanced case of dermatofibrosarcoma protuberans with multiple tumor nodules.

patients appear surprisingly well and lack the signs of cachexia associated with malignancies.

Gross Findings

Most of these tumors are removed and examined during the nodular stage; therefore, the specimen consists of a solitary, protuberant, gray-white mass involving subcutis and skin (Figs. 12-1 to 12-3). The average size at surgery is approximately 5 cm.[5] Multiple discrete masses are usually not seen in the original tumor but are more characteristic of recurrent lesions (Fig. 12-4).[5] The skin overlying these tumors is taut or even ulcerated. Skeletal muscle extension is uncommon except in large or recurrent lesions. Rarely, this tumor is confined to the subcutis and lacks dermal involvement altogether.[7] Occasionally, areas of the tumor have a translucent or gelatinous appearance corresponding microscopically to myxoid change. Hemorrhage and cystic change are sometimes seen in the tumors, but necrosis, a common feature of undifferentiated pleomorphic sarcomas, is rare.

Microscopic Findings

Despite the apparent gross circumscription of these lesions, the tumor diffusely infiltrates the dermis and subcutis (Fig. 12-5). The tumor may reach the epidermis or leave an uninvolved zone of dermis just underneath the epidermis. In either event, the overlying epidermis does not usually display the hyperplasia that characterizes some cutaneous fibrous histiocytomas (dermatofibromas).[5] The peripheral portions of the tumor have a deceptively bland appearance, in part, as a result of the marked attenuation of the cells at their advancing edge. This is especially true in superficial areas, where the spread of slender cells between preexisting collagen is easily mistaken for cutaneous fibrous histiocytoma (Fig. 12-6A). In deep

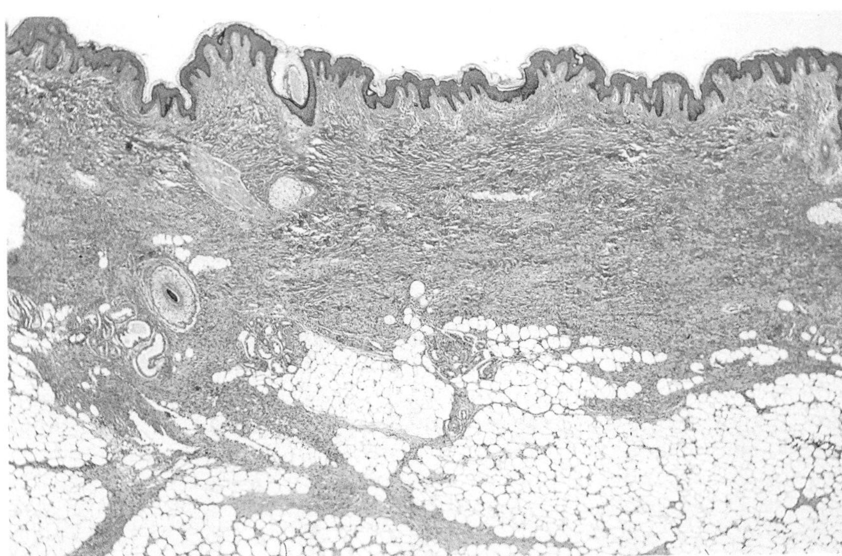

FIGURE 12-5. Plaque form of dermatofibrosarcoma protuberans illustrating the expansion of the interface between dermis and subcutis and the extension into subcutaneous fat.

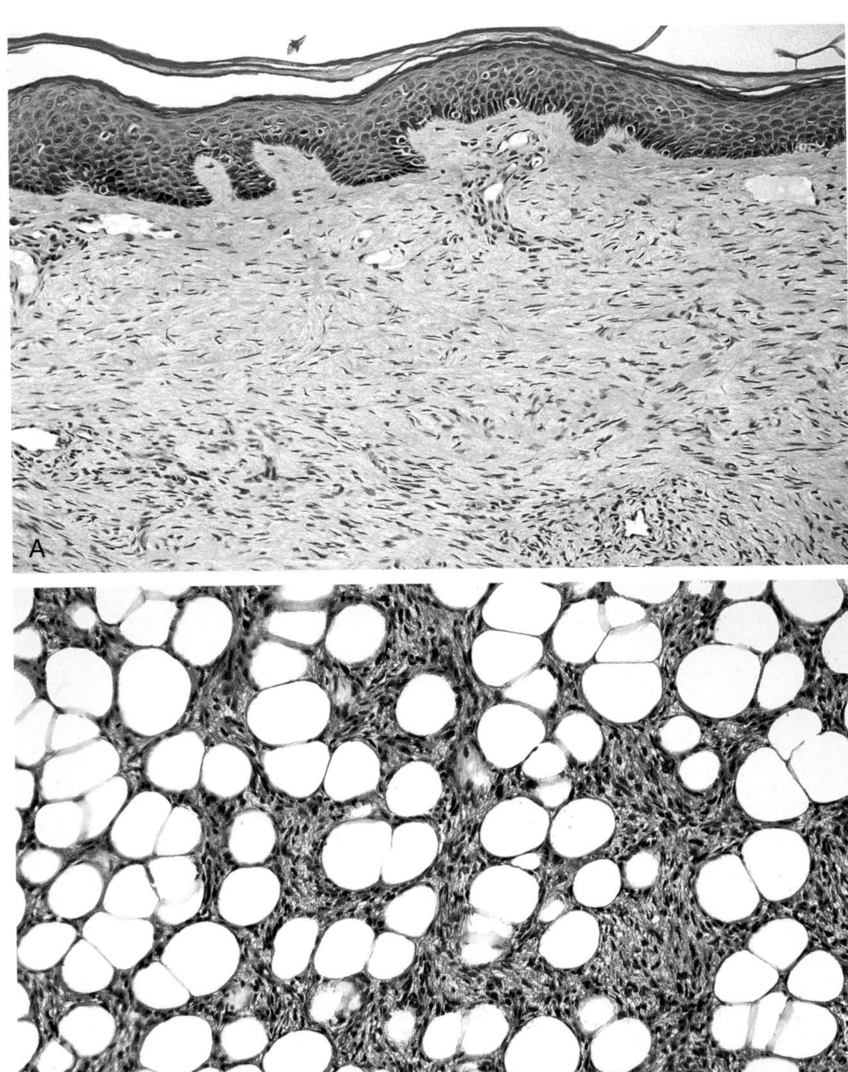

FIGURE 12-6. Superficial (A) and deep (B) extensions of dermatofibrosarcoma protuberans. Spread of the tumor between preexisting collagen of the dermis may simulate the appearance of a cutaneous fibrous histiocytoma (A). At the deep margin, the tumor intricately interdigitates with normal fat (B).

regions, the tumor spreads along connective tissue septa and between adnexae (Fig. 12-7), or it intricately interdigitates with lobules of subcutaneous fat, creating a lace-like or honeycomb effect (see Fig. 12-6B).

The central or main portion of the tumor is composed of a uniform population of slender fibroblasts arranged in a distinct, often monotonous, storiform pattern around an inconspicuous vasculature (Figs. 12-8 and 12-9). There is usually little nuclear pleomorphism and only low to moderate mitotic activity. Secondary elements such as giant cells, xanthoma cells, and inflammatory elements are few in number or absent altogether. In this respect, dermatofibrosarcoma protuberans displays remarkable uniformity compared to other fibrohistiocytic neoplasms. Although most tumors are characterized by these highly ordered cellular areas, occasional tumors contain myxoid areas (Fig. 12-10). These myxoid areas occur in both primary and recurrent lesions and are characterized by the interstitial accumulation of ground substance material. As myxoid change of the stroma becomes more pronounced, the storiform pattern becomes less distinct and the vascular pattern more apparent. By virtue of these features, such tumors can resemble myxoid liposarcoma (see Fig. 12-10B). A confident diagnosis of highly myxoid dermatofibrosarcomas usually requires identification of more typical areas.

Giant cells, similar to those in giant cell fibroblastoma, can be identified in a small percentage of otherwise typical dermatofibrosarcomas. An unusual feature of dermatofibrosarcoma protuberans is the myoid nodule (Fig. 12-11). Originally construed as evidence of myofibroblastic differentiation,[8] these structures seem to be centered, in some cases, around blood vessels[9,10] and likely represent an unusual non-neoplastic vascular response to the tumor. Infrequently, dermatofibrosarcoma protuberans contains areas that are indistinguishable from fibrosarcoma (Figs. 12-12 to 12-14). Characterized by long fascicles of spindle cells with more nuclear atypia and mitotic activity, these areas usually sharply abut conventional

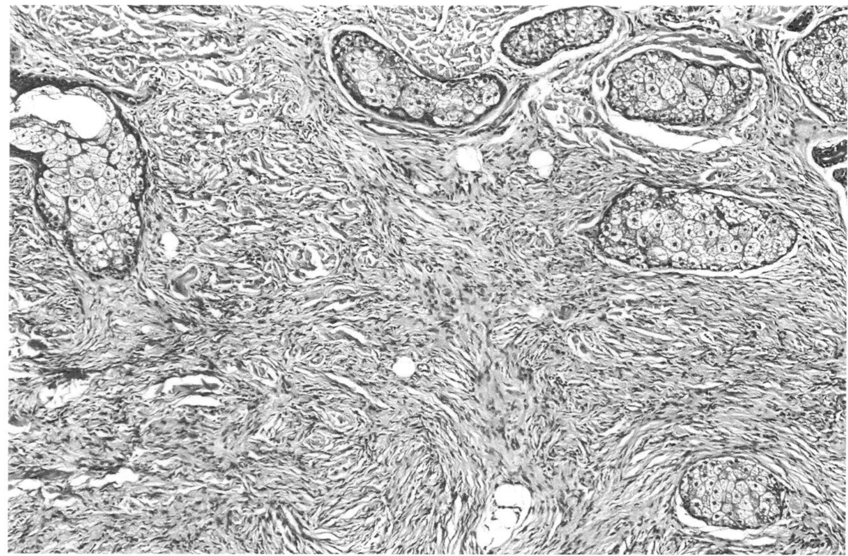

FIGURE 12-7. Dermatofibrosarcoma protuberans infiltrating between adnexal structures.

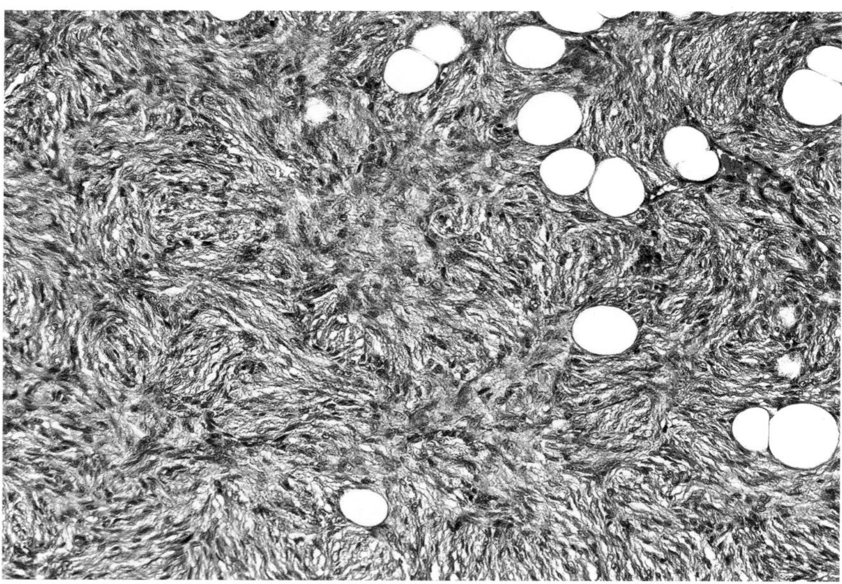

FIGURE 12-8. Slender spindle cells arranged in a distinct storiform pattern characterize most of these tumors.

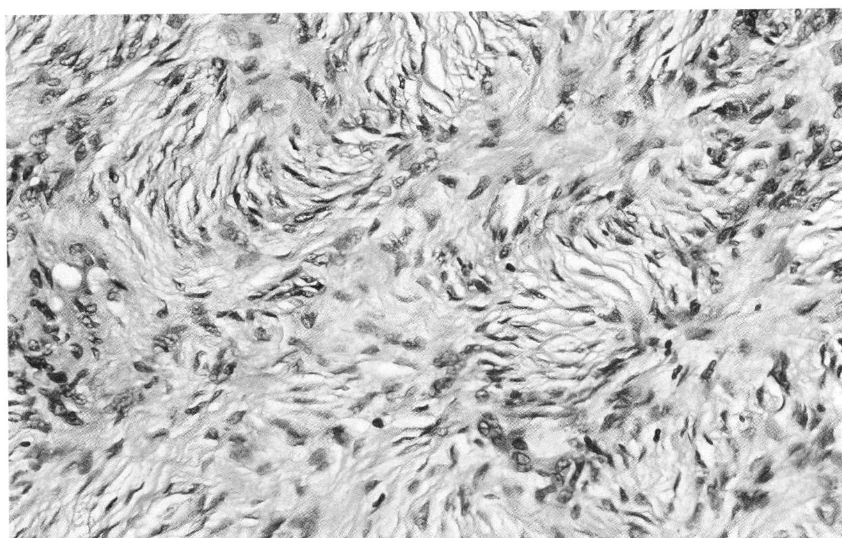

FIGURE 12-9. Dermatofibrosarcoma protuberans showing greater interstitial collagenization.

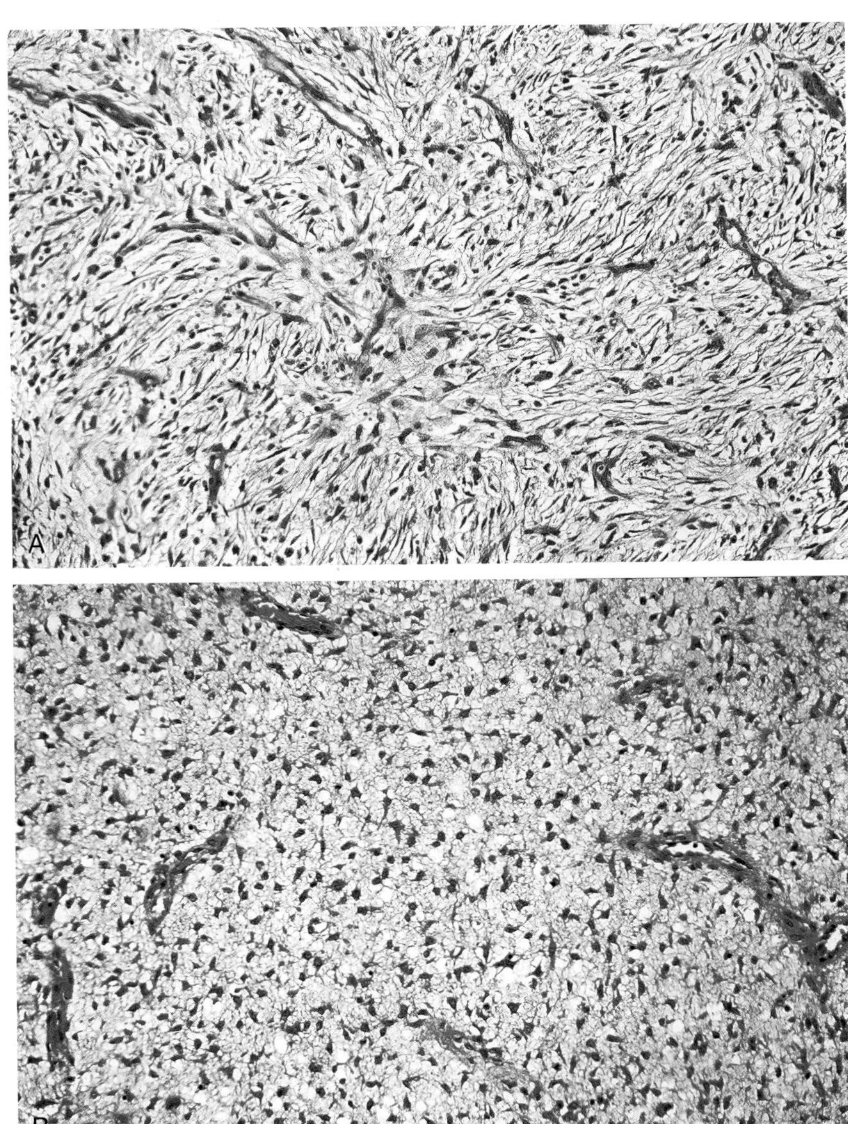

FIGURE 12-10. (A) Myxoid change in dermatofibrosarcoma protuberans. (B) When the myxoid change is prominent, the storiform pattern may be lacking altogether, and the tumor may resemble a myxoid liposarcoma.

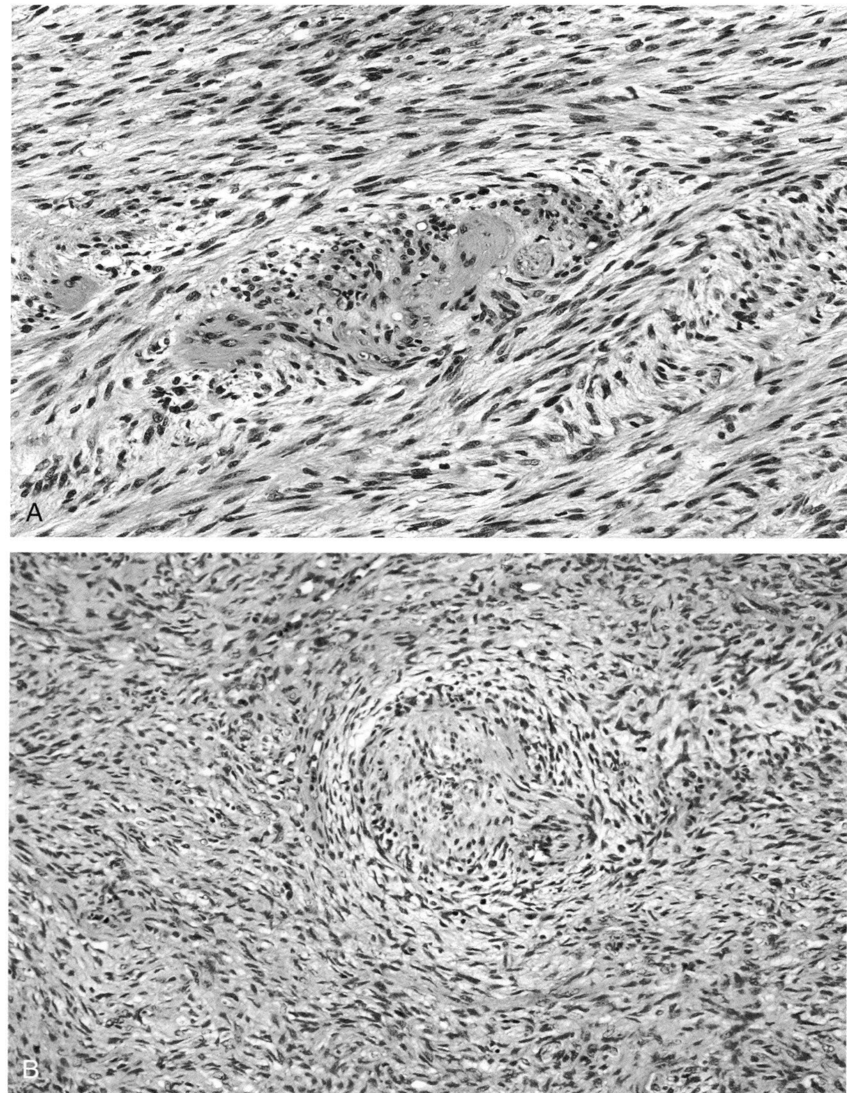

FIGURE 12-11. (A) Myoid balls within dermatofibrosarcoma protuberans. (B) Myoid ball centered around a small vessel.

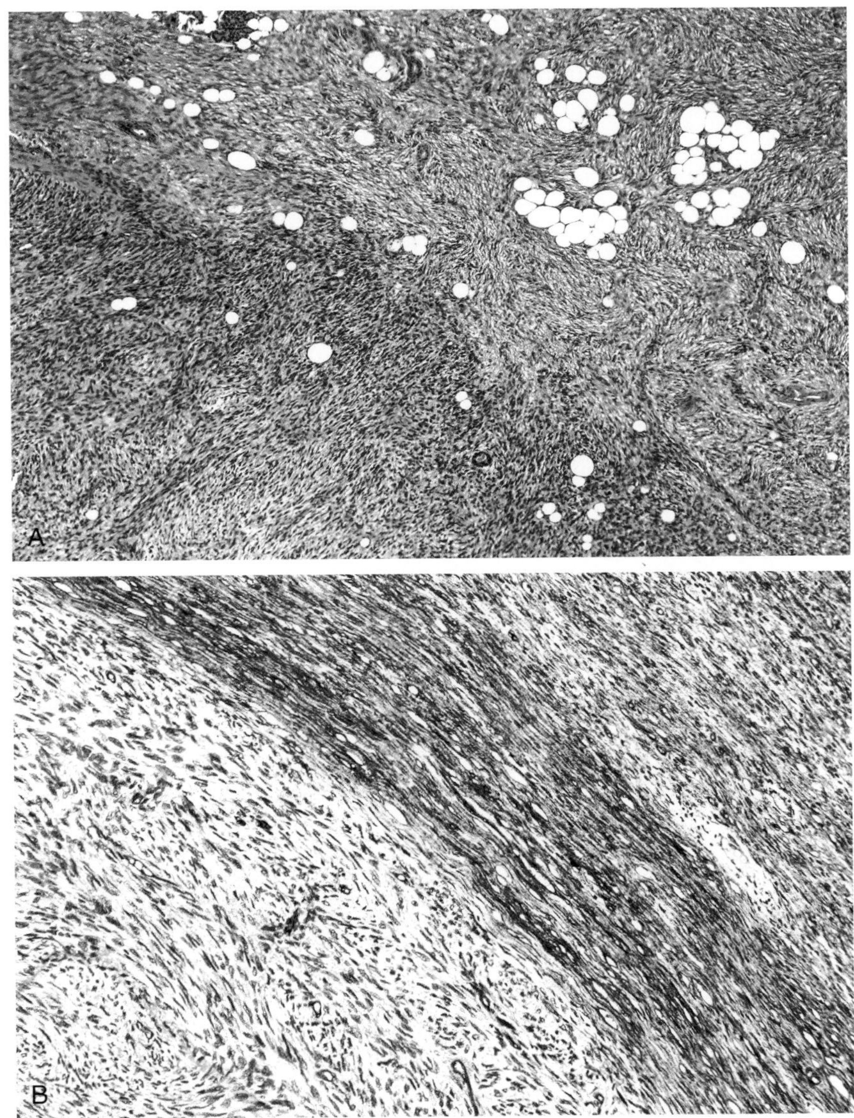

FIGURE 12-12. (A) Dermatofibrosarcoma protuberans showing the transition to fibrosarcoma (lower left corner). (B) CD34 immunostain in a dermatofibrosarcoma (upper right) with fibrosarcomatous areas. Note the marked diminution of CD34 immunostain in the fibrosarcomatous portion of the tumor (lower left).

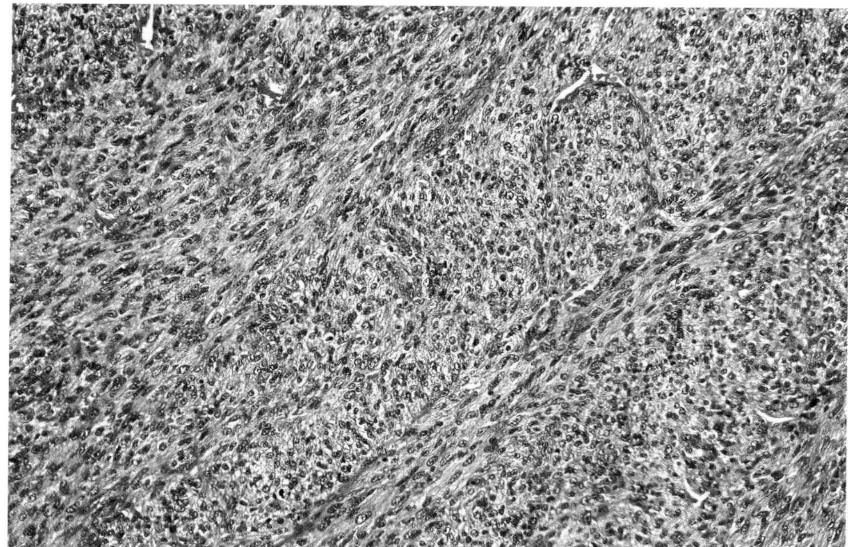

FIGURE 12-13. Fibrosarcomatous areas within dermatofibrosarcoma protuberans.

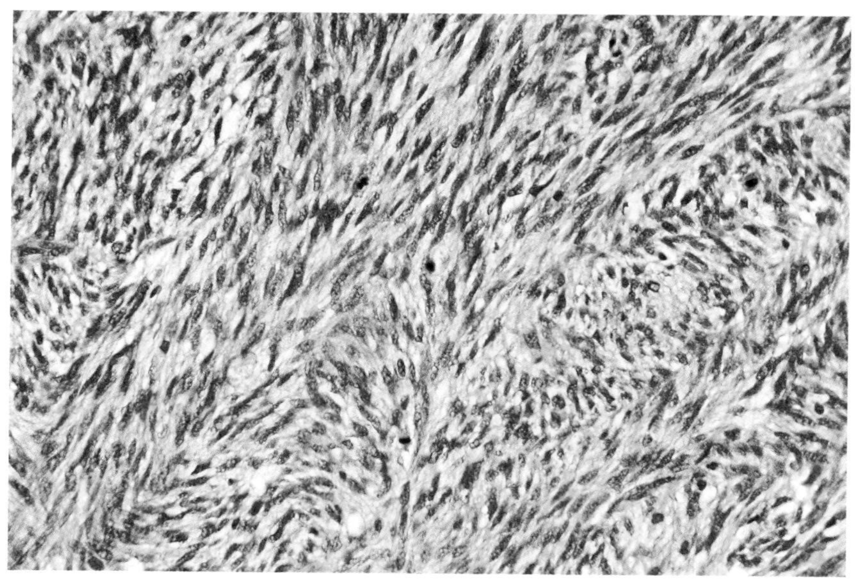

FIGURE 12-14. Fibrosarcomatous areas showing increased cellularity and mitotic activity.

low-grade areas. Mitotic activity usually averages more than 5 mitotic figures/10 high-power fields (HPF), in contrast to areas of conventional dermatofibrosarcoma protuberans, which usually have fewer than 5 mitotic figures/10 HPF. In exceptional instances, dermatofibrosarcoma protuberans contains areas resembling undifferentiated pleomorphic sarcoma (Figs. 12-15 and 12-16).[11,12] Fibrosarcomatous areas were originally believed to be more common in recurrent lesions, but recent studies have documented that the contrary is true.[11] The biologic significance of sarcomatous areas in dermatofibrosarcoma protuberans is discussed later in the chapter. Metastatic deposits from this tumor occur most commonly in the lung and secondly in regional lymph nodes, where they may resemble the parent tumor or may appear more pleomorphic (Fig. 12-17).

Immunohistochemical and Ultrastructural Findings

Dermatofibrosarcoma protuberans is characterized by the nearly consistent presence of CD34 (Fig. 12-18), the human progenitor cell antigen, in a significant proportion of its cells.[11,13,14] Although this antigen has been identified in a growing number of soft tissue tumors, its presence in dermatofibrosarcoma protuberans suggests a close linkage to the normal CD34+ dendritic cells of the dermis, including those that ensheath the adnexae, nerves, and vessels.[14] The nearly consistent expression of this antigen has also proved useful for distinguishing dermatofibrosarcoma protuberans from benign fibrous histiocytoma, especially when dealing with small biopsies. Although cutaneous fibrous histiocytomas may contain

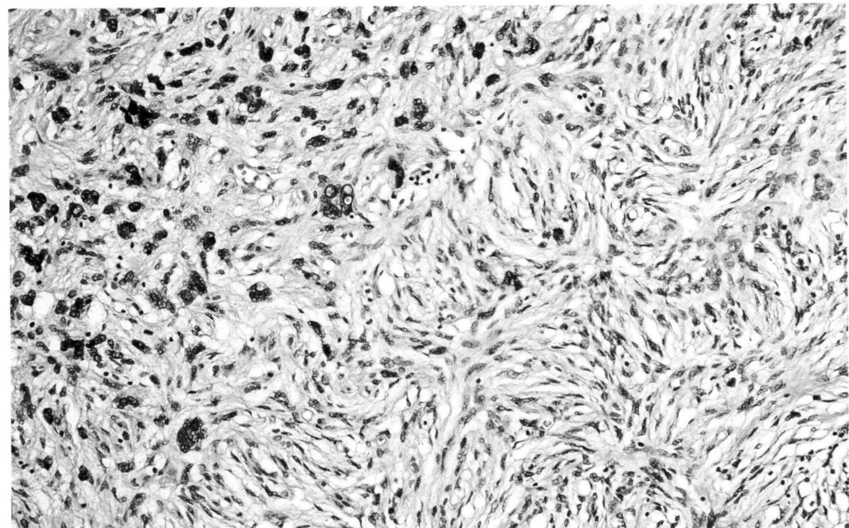

FIGURE 12-15. Dermatofibrosarcoma protuberans with transformation to undifferentiated pleomorphic sarcoma.

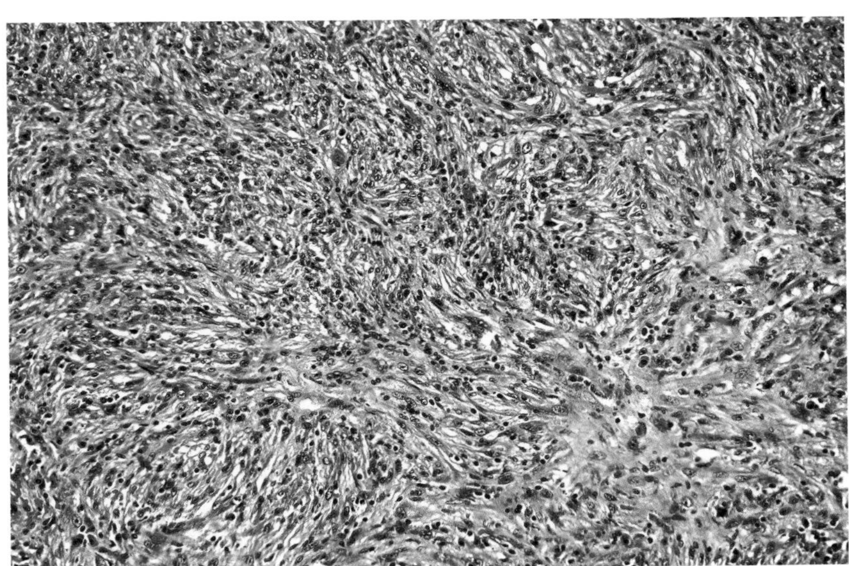

FIGURE 12-16. Undifferentiated pleomorphic sarcoma-like areas in dermatofibrosarcoma protuberans.

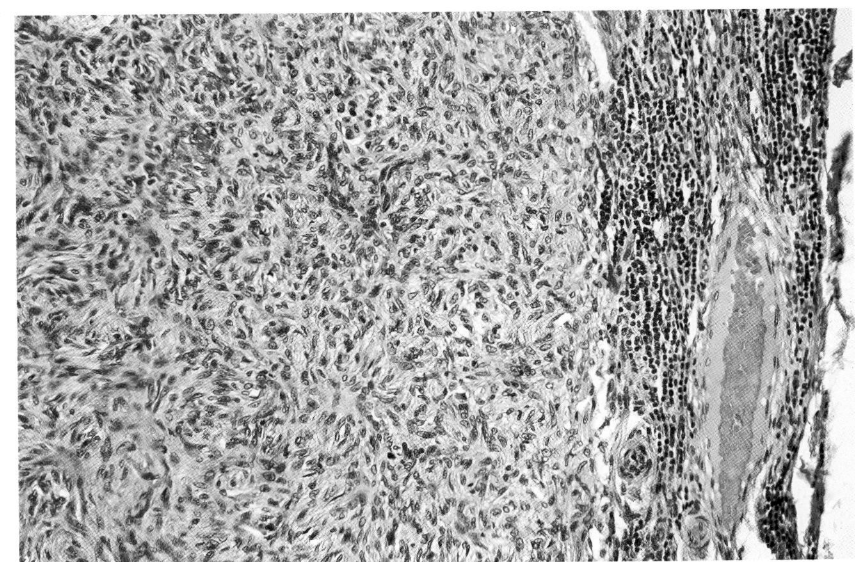

FIGURE 12-17. Lymph node metastasis from dermatofibrosarcoma protuberans.

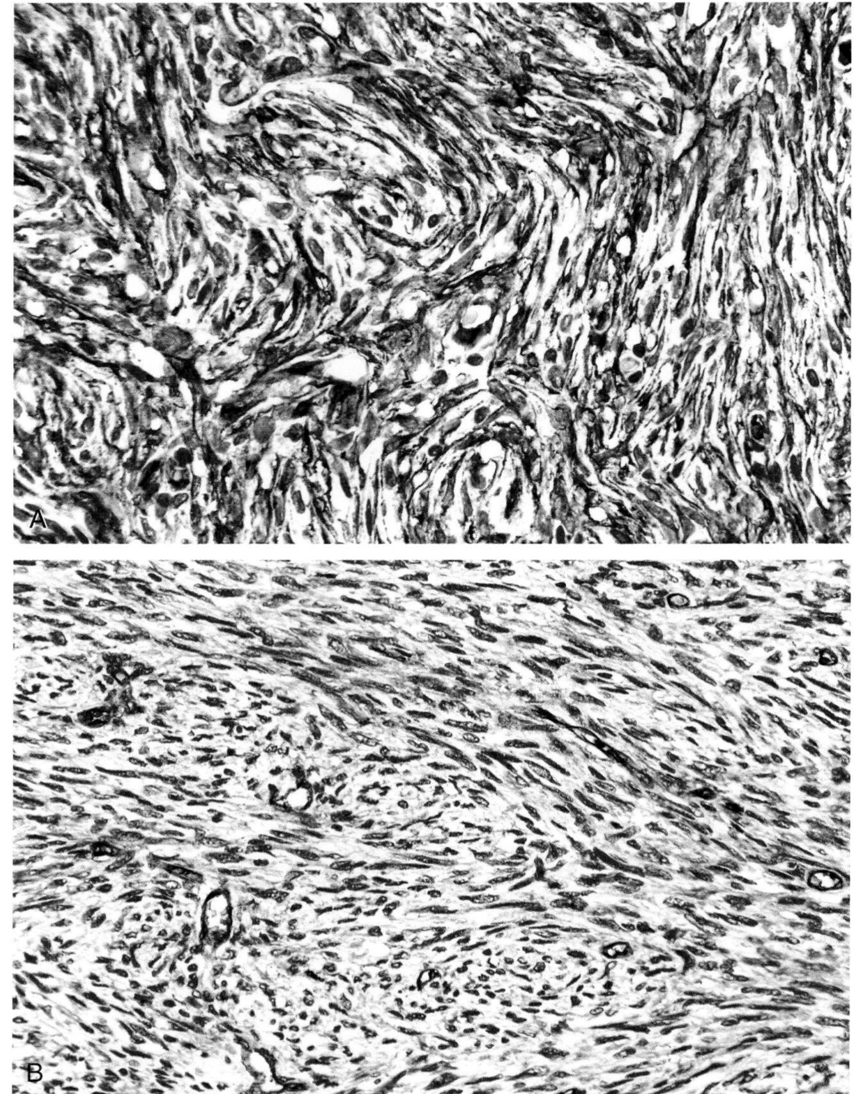

FIGURE 12-18. CD34 immunoreactivity within a conventional dermatofibrosarcoma (A) compared to markedly reduced immunoreactivity within a fibrosarcomatous area of dermatofibrosarcoma protuberans (B).

CD34 positive cells, these frequently account for only a minority of the tumor cell population and are often found at the deep border of the tumor.[11] Caution should be used when interpreting CD34 immunostains in spindle cell tumors of the skin to be certain that positively staining cells are neoplastic, not entrapped normal dermal dendritic cells. Apolipoprotein D has been identified immunohistochemically within a significant percentage of dermatofibrosarcomas and seems to discriminate them well from benign fibrous histiocytomas.[15] Because of the sensitivity of CD34 in the diagnosis of dermatofibrosarcoma protuberans, there has been little recent interest in studying these lesions ultrastructurally. Earlier studies indicated that the cells resemble fibroblasts,[16] although some have noted certain modifications that suggest perineural differentiation.[17,18] These features included convoluted nuclei, elaborate cell processes, moderate numbers of desmosomes, and incomplete basal lamina (Fig. 12-19).

Cytogenetic and Molecular Genetic Features

Both dermatofibrosarcoma and giant cell fibroblastoma are characterized by either the presence of a supernumerary ring chromosome[19] consisting of low-level amplification of sequences from chromosomes 17 and 22[20,21] and 8[22] (uncommonly) or alternatively linear translocation derivatives. The presence of a ring versus a linear translocation may be related to age.[19,22] Specifically, adult cases typically possess the ring chromosome, whereas pediatric cases have the linear translocation derivative.[19] Either event fuses exon 2 of the platelet-derived growth factor β-chain (PDGF β) gene to various exons of the collagen type 1 α1 gene (COL1A1), resulting in a fusion transcript that places PDGF β under the control of the COL1A1 promotor.[23,24] The fusion protein is processed to an end product that is indistinguishable from normal PDGF β.[24] Overproduction of PDGF β by dermatofibrosarcoma

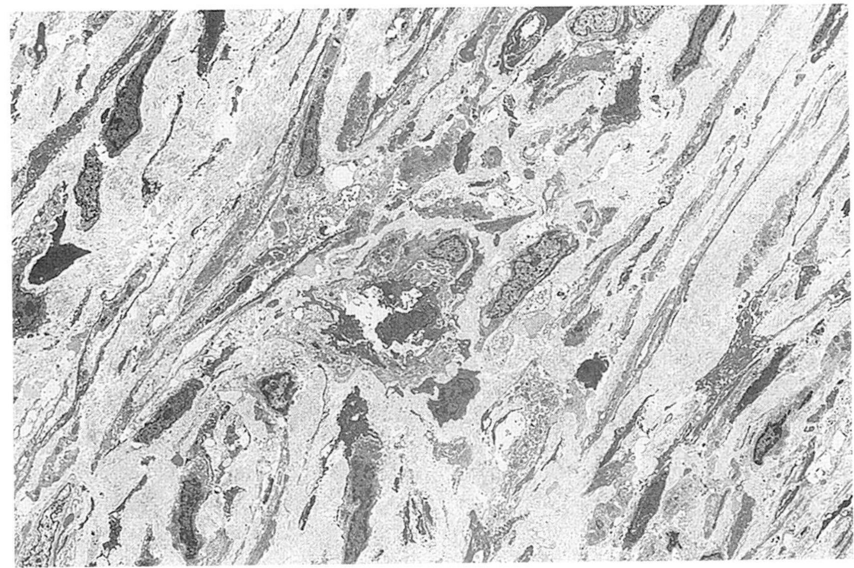

FIGURE 12-19. Electron micrograph of dermatofibrosarcoma protuberans showing the center of a storiform area occupied by a small vessel. Fibroblast-like cells spin out from the vessel and have numerous slender processes that may join each other by means of specialized cell contacts. *(From Taxy JB, Battifora H. The electron microscope in the study and diagnosis of soft tissue tumors. In: Trump BF, Jones RT, editors.* Diagnostic electron microscopy. *New York: Wiley; 1980.)*

TABLE 12-2 Comparison of Fibrous Histiocytoma and Dermatofibrosarcoma Protuberans

PARAMETER	BENIGN FIBROUS HISTIOCYTOMA	DERMATOFIBROSARCOMA
Common locations	Extremities	Trunk; groin
Size	Usually small	Small to large
Growth pattern	Short fascicles, haphazard	Monotonous storiform
Cell population	Plump spindle cells often admixed with inflammatory cells, siderophages, giant cells	Slender spindle cells with few, if any, secondary elements
Hemorrhage	Occasional	No
Subcutaneous extension	Occasional and limited	Consistent and extensive
CD34	Focal staining in occasional cases; cuff of CD34-positive cells at deep border	Diffuse and extensive staining in most cases
Local recurrence	5%-10%	20%-50%
Metastasis	Anecdotal cases only	Rare in conventional form; potentially higher if fibrosarcoma is present with inadequate local control
Malignant transformation	Anecdotal cases only	Fibrosarcoma in occasional cases

results in autocrine stimulation and cell proliferation, a sequence of events that can be interrupted by specific tyrosine kinase inhibitors (see later discussion). Approximately 8% of dermatofibrosarcoma cases are fusion-negative; it remains to be seen whether these rare cases contain cryptic rearrangements of COL1A1 and PDGFB or are altogether different genetic abnormalities.

Differential Diagnosis

The most common problem in the differential diagnosis is distinguishing this tumor from other fibrohistiocytic neoplasms. Dermatofibrosarcoma protuberans has a more uniform appearance, more distinct storiform pattern, and fewer secondary elements (i.e., giant cells, inflammatory cells) than either a benign fibrous histiocytoma or a superficially located undifferentiated pleomorphic sarcoma. The distinction between benign fibrous histiocytoma and dermatofibrosarcoma occasionally proves difficult when only the superficial portion of the dermatofibrosarcoma is present in a biopsy specimen, because these areas appear so well differentiated (Table 12-2). Under these circumstances, knowledge of the size and configuration of the lesion in question suggests the diagnosis, and a biopsy of a deeper portion confirms it. In addition, because CD34 is almost always expressed by dermatofibrosarcoma and is far less often positive in benign fibrous histiocytoma, CD34 is an extremely useful antigen for solving this problem.[13,14] A potential role for HMGA1 and HMBA2 (positive in fibrous histiocytoma, negative in dermatofibrosarcoma) immunohistochemistry in this differential diagnosis has been suggested; however, this is not widely used.[25] Undifferentiated pleomorphic sarcoma is not often confused with this tumor because it is characterized by far greater pleomorphism, mitotic activity, and necrosis. Moreover, its typical deep location in muscle and more rapid growth are at variance with the indolent course of this tumor. Rarely, one encounters dermatofibrosarcoma protuberans with areas of undifferentiated pleomorphic sarcoma (see Figs. 12-15 and 12-16). As indicated earlier, when such areas represent more than just a microscopic focus, they should be diagnosed as "sarcoma arising in dermatofibrosarcoma protuberans."

A second common problem is the confusion of this tumor with benign neural tumors, specifically a diffuse form of neurofibroma. This is most likely to occur when dermatofibrosarcoma is in the plaque stage or when a biopsy is done on only the periphery of the tumor. However, neurofibroma usually contains tactoid structures or other features of neural differentiation, and it lacks the highly cellular areas with mitotic figures that characterize the central portion of a dermatofibrosarcoma. The presence of S-100 protein in virtually all neurofibromas and its absence in dermatofibrosarcoma is an additional point of contrast.

Highly myxoid forms of dermatofibrosarcoma may resemble myxoid liposarcoma by virtue of the prominent vasculature and bland stellate or fusiform cells. However, the superficial location, gross configuration, CD34 immunoreactivity, and complete absence of lipoblasts should raise serious questions concerning the diagnosis of liposarcoma. In such cases, additional sampling of the tumor or review of the original material in a recurrent lesion may reveal the diagnostic cellular areas.

Superficial acral fibromyxoma (cellular digital fibroma), another CD34-positive spindle cell tumor of the dermis, typically occurs in the fingers and toes, unusual locations for dermatofibrosarcomas, contains wiry collagen, and lacks a storiform growth pattern.

Discussion

Unlike benign fibrous histiocytoma, dermatofibrosarcoma protuberans is a locally aggressive neoplasm that recurs in up to one-half of patients.[5,26,27] The high recurrence rate, in part, reflects the extensive infiltration of the tumor compared with fibrous histiocytoma and failure to appreciate this phenomenon at the time of surgery. It is clear that prompt wide local excision (2 to 3 cm), the standard of practice for this lesion, can markedly alter the recurrence rate. Average recurrence rates reported in the literature for patients treated by a wide local excision range from 10% to 20% compared to 43% when the excision was undefined or conservative.[28] In addition, recurrence rates in cases treated primarily at large referral centers are low (1.75% to 33%),[4,6,29] again suggesting that adequate initial surgery is essential for minimizing recurrences. The risk of local recurrence, furthermore, correlates well with the extent of the wide excision. If the excision margin is 3 cm or more, the recurrence rate is 20%, compared to 41% if the margin is 2 cm or less.[30] If local recurrence develops, it is usually within 3 years of the initial surgery,[26] although about one-third of patients will develop recurrences after 5 years, attesting to the need for long-term follow-up. In patients who develop multiple recurrences, progressively shorter intervals between successive recurrences have been noted.[5]

Mohs micrographic surgery has been met with growing enthusiasm for treatment of this disease.[31-35] Those who advocate this approach point out that dermatofibrosarcoma protuberans occasionally grows in an asymmetric fashion from its epicenter so that a traditional wide local excision fails to remove all tumor in a subset of cases.[36] Mohs surgery offers the potential to achieve clear margins with minimum removal of normal tissue, an advantage particularly attractive for sites such as the head and neck. Local recurrence rates following Mohs surgery are less than 10% and, in some studies, approach 0%.[27,33,34]

Despite its locally aggressive behavior, this tumor infrequently metastasizes and, therefore, should be clearly distinguished from conventional sarcomas. The incidence of metastasis is difficult to assess because of the bias introduced when selectively reporting metastasizing tumors, the inability to determine whether sarcomatous areas were noted in a subset of reported cases, and the lack of uniform treatment. In general, however, for the ordinary dermatofibrosarcoma protuberans uncomplicated by areas of fibrosarcoma, metastasis appears to be an uncommon event. In one large study of 115 patients, no metastases were observed,[5] whereas, in two other studies, 5 of 86 patients[26] and 4 of 96 patients[4] developed metastases. In the latter study, the follow-up period was 15 years. Therefore, long-term follow-up may reveal higher metastatic rates than previously reported. Of the 471 patients reported in the literature, 16 (3.4%) developed metastatic disease.[4] About three-fourths of patients with metastases have hematogenous spread to the lungs, and one-fourth have lymphatic spread to regional lymph nodes. Metastases to other sites, such as the brain, bones, and heart, have also been documented. Although some metastasizing cases have clearly originated from tumors with areas of sarcoma (see later discussion), some have not.[37]

Metastasizing lesions share some common clinical features. They are almost always recurrent lesions, and there is usually an interval of several years between diagnosis and metastasis. The low incidence of regional lymph node metastasis and the negative findings in a small series of blind lymph node dissections do not warrant routine node dissection. Resection of isolated pulmonary metastases has been advocated because of the overall low-grade behavior of the tumor. Radiotherapy has been recommended for large, unresectable tumors or postoperatively for margin-positive tumors.[38] Molecular targeting of dermatofibrosarcoma protuberans with imatinib mesylate has been used recently in patients with advanced or metastatic disease with significant reductions in tumor burden.[39-41]

SARCOMA ARISING IN DERMATOFIBROSARCOMA PROTUBERANS (FIBROSARCOMATOUS VARIANT OF DERMATOFIBROSARCOMA PROTUBERANS)

There has been increasing awareness that a small subset of dermatofibrosarcomas contain areas indistinguishable from conventional fibrosarcoma (and rarely undifferentiated pleomorphic sarcoma).[9,11,12,42,43] This has led to the use of the term *fibrosarcomatous variant of dermatofibrosarcoma* and the suggestion that these lesions pursue a more aggressive course, although the risk of distant metastasis is debated. These tumors share the same general clinical properties as ordinary dermatofibrosarcoma protuberans, and, in most cases, the sarcomatous foci are noted in the original tumor.

To diagnose sarcoma arising in dermatofibrosarcoma protuberans, a constellation of features is generally used: the sarcomatous foci should constitute at least 5% to 10% of the tumor, in contrast to simply a rare to occasional microscopic focus. These zones are characterized by a fascicular (rather than storiform) architectural pattern and are composed of plump spindle cells of high nuclear grade. Mitotic activity is increased in these areas, whereas CD34 immunoreactivity is often diminished (see Fig. 12-18B), compared to the surrounding dermatofibrosarcoma. In addition, fibrosarcomatous areas are also characterized by a higher MIB-1 labeling index and increased p53 immunostaining than the classic

TABLE 12-3 Sarcoma Arising in Dermatofibrosarcoma Protuberans

STUDY	NO. OF PATIENTS*	RECURRENCE RATE (%)	METASTATIC RATE (%)
Mentzel et al.[42]	34	58	14.7
Pizarro et al.[46]	19	42	33.0
Goldblum et al.[11]	18	22	0

*Patients with follow-up information.

TABLE 12-4 Sarcomas Arising in Dermatofibrosarcoma Protuberans Treated with Wide Local Excision, with Follow-Up Information

STUDY	NO. OF PATIENTS	METASTASIS
Goldblum et al.[11]	18	0/18
Mentzel et al.[42]	6	0/6
Diaz-Cascajo et al.[50]	3	1/3
O'Connell et al.[51]	2	0/2
Total	29	1/29

areas. Although an absolute level of mitotic activity is not required to diagnose sarcomatous change, mitotic activity within these sarcomatous areas averages 7 to 15/10 HPF [11,42] compared to 1 to 3/10 HPF in dermatofibrosarcoma.

The significance of sarcomatous forms of dermatofibrosarcoma protuberans has been the subject of a number of studies. Although it seems logical that high-grade areas within a low-grade lesion would adversely affect behavior, early studies failed to confirm this hypothesis in a statistically meaningful fashion.[44] Ding and Enjoji[44] suggested that fibrosarcomatous areas within dermatofibrosarcoma protuberans are associated with a higher local recurrence rate and therefore a more aggressive course, but the status and adequacy of surgical excisions in these cases were not made clear. Connelly and Evans[45] reported no difference in the local recurrence rate or in time to recurrence compared to conventional dermatofibrosarcoma protuberans but noted that two of their six patients with fibrosarcomatous areas developed metastatic disease. Two large studies by Mentzel et al.[42] and Pizarro et al.,[46] on the other hand, revealed higher local recurrence rates (58% and 42%, respectively) and metastatic rates (13.7% and 33.0%, respectively) (Table 12-3). However, in either study, a wide local excision with clear margins was not achieved in most cases. A more recent study of 41 patients has documented a 10% incidence of metastasis in fibrosarcomatous dermatofibrosarcoma protuberans, but, again, patients in that study appear not to have received optimal surgical therapy.[47] All received local excisions that often left positive margins, and three of four patients with metastasis also experienced local recurrences, again suggesting inadequate primary surgery. Because the ability to eradicate tumor locally arguably affects the risk of subsequent dissemination, none of these studies addressed the behavior of this neoplasm in the context of the current standard of practice. Of 18 patients treated by wide local excision and clear margins and with a minimum follow-up of 5 years, local recurrence rates are essentially identical to those of ordinary dermatofibrosarcoma protuberans—and no instance of metastasis is noted.[11] Similarly, culling cases from the literature of sarcomatous dermatofibrosarcoma in which wide local excisions were performed, only one instance of metastasis was noted (Table 12-4).[11,42,50,51] To clearly resolve the issue of metastasis in fibrosarcomatous dermatofibrosarcoma protuberans, follow-up of a larger cohort of patients treated with adequate surgery and who achieve negative margins is needed.

In summary, although dermatofibrosarcoma protuberans containing fibrosarcoma may well be an inherently more aggressive neoplasm, this behavior can be favorably influenced by wide local excision to the extent that there may be little increased risk of distant metastasis over that of conventional dermatofibrosarcoma protuberans. Therefore, wide local excision should be even more forcefully encouraged than for conventional dermatofibrosarcoma protuberans.

BEDNAR TUMOR (PIGMENTED DERMATOFIBROSARCOMA PROTUBERANS, STORIFORM NEUROFIBROMA)

In 1957, Bednar[52] described a group of nine cutaneous tumors characterized by indolent growth and a prominent storiform pattern and, in four cases, by the presence of melanin pigment. He regarded these tumors as variants of neurofibroma (storiform neurofibroma) and cited as evidence the presence of similar areas within neural nevi[53] and the presence of melanin. The term *Bednar tumor* is reserved for tumors that resemble dermatofibrosarcoma protuberans but that, in addition, have melanin pigment. These tumors are uncommon,[44,52,54-57] as evidenced by the fact that Bednar gleaned only four cases from among 100,000 biopsy specimens; these tumors account for fewer than 5% of all cases of dermatofibrosarcoma protuberans. The genetic features of Bednar tumor are identical to those of ordinary dermatofibrosarcomas, and it is now clear that these represent simply morphologic variants of this tumor, rather than neural neoplasms.[58] Furthermore, their clinical, gross, and histologic features (with the exception of melanin pigment) are virtually identical to dermatofibrosarcoma protuberans. Most are slowly growing cutaneous masses that extend to the epidermis and advance into the deep subcutis. The number of melanin-bearing cells varies widely within these tumors. In some, large numbers of melanin-containing cells cause black discoloration of the tumor (Fig. 12-20), whereas, in others, melanin is so sparse it can be appreciated microscopically only. These cells are scattered irregularly throughout the tumor (Fig. 12-21A). Their tentacle-like processes emanating from a central nucleus-containing zone give them a characteristic bipolar or multipolar shape, depending on the plane of the section (see Fig. 12-21B). They stain with conventional melanin stains and ultrastructurally contain mature membrane-bound melanosomes. Electron microscopic studies reveal that most areas of Bednar tumors are composed of slender fibroblastic cells arranged in a delicate collagen matrix, although other areas have cells more suggestive of Schwann cell differentiation. The cells have numerous interlocking processes elaborately invested with basal laminae. Mature and immature melanosomes can be identified within the tumor cells. It has been suggested that this finding indicates that the tumor synthesizes rather than phagocytoses melanin, although others have suggested that the tumor is simply colonized by melanin-bearing cells.[57]

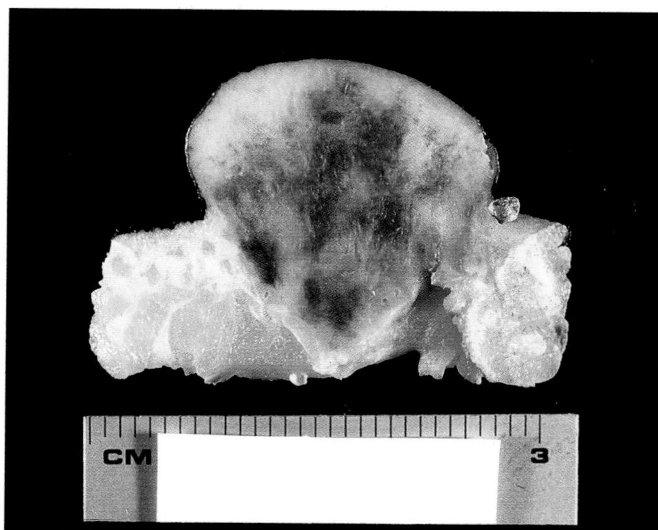

FIGURE 12-20. Bednar tumor. Gross appearance of the tumor is identical to conventional dermatofibrosarcoma protuberans, but the substance of the tumor is flecked with melanin pigment.

S-100 protein, present in many neural tumors, is absent in Bednar tumors.[54]

Because of the rarity of this tumor, there are few collective data in the literature concerning its behavior, although, overall, it appears to be similar to dermatofibrosarcoma protuberans. In addition, these tumors may display fibrosarcomatous areas.[59] There are also rare examples of metastasis, some with areas of fibrosarcoma,[59,60] including one report in the literature of a Bednar tumor with pulmonary metastasis.[61]

GIANT CELL FIBROBLASTOMA

Giant cell fibroblastoma was first described in 1982 by Shmookler and Enzinger,[60] who suggested that it represents a juvenile form of dermatofibrosarcoma protuberans, a view reinforced in their seminal publication in 1989.[62] Subsequent reports reaffirmed it as an entity [63-70] and embraced this notion for describing tumors with hybrid features or lesions that evolved from one pattern to the other.[63,65,66,71-75]

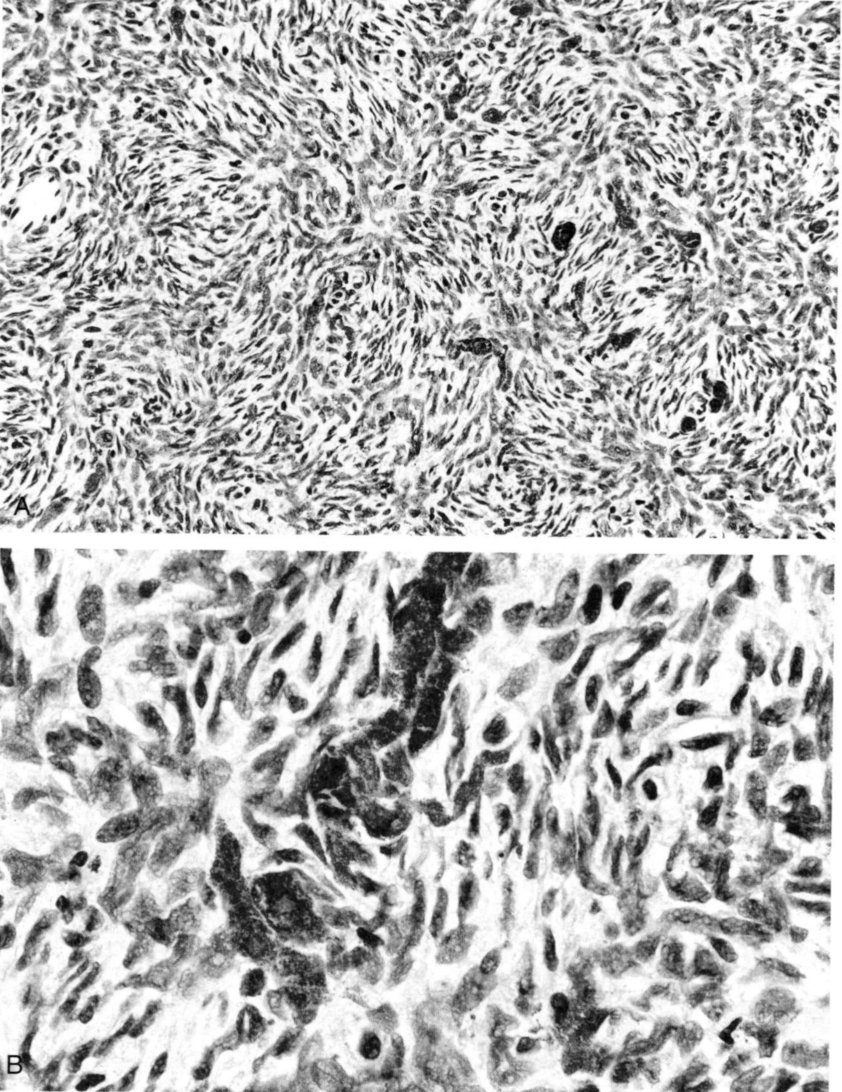

FIGURE 12-21. Pigmented dermatofibrosarcoma protuberans (Bednar tumor) (A) showing dendritic pigmented cells (B).

Finally, the two lesions have been shown to have the same cytogenetic abnormality (supernumerary ring chromosome derived from chromosomes 17 and 22),[76] although there is some evidence that the ring chromosome occurs in cases of dermatofibrosarcoma, whereas the linear derivative chromosome occurs in giant cell fibroblastoma.[19] Both, however, result in the same molecular event (see previous discussion).

Clinical Findings

Giant cell fibroblastoma develops as a painless nodule or mass in the dermis or subcutis, with a predilection for the back of the thigh, inguinal region, and chest wall. It affects predominantly infants and children, being encountered only infrequently in adults.[62,75] About two-thirds of the children are younger than 5 years of age when brought to medical attention, and the median age is 3 years. About two-thirds of patients are male.

Pathologic Findings

Grossly, the lesions consist of gray to yellow mucoid masses that are poorly circumscribed and measure 1 to 8 cm. They are composed of loosely arranged, wavy spindle cells with a moderate degree of nuclear pleomorphism that infiltrate the deep dermis and subcutis and encircle adnexal structures in a fashion similar to dermatofibrosarcoma protuberans (Figs. 12-22 to 12-29). The tumors vary in cellularity from those approximating the cellularity of dermatofibrosarcoma protuberans (see Figs. 12-24 and 12-28) to those that are hypocellular with a myxoid or hyaline stroma (see Figs. 12-25 to 12-27). The characteristic feature of the tumor is the peculiar pseudovascular spaces that seem to reflect a loss of cellular cohesion. Large and irregular in shape, the pseudovascular spaces are lined by a discontinuous row of multinucleated cells that represent variants of the basic proliferating tumor cell (see Figs. 12-23 and 12-29). Although these cells appear to contain multiple overlapping nuclei, as seen by light microscopy, they

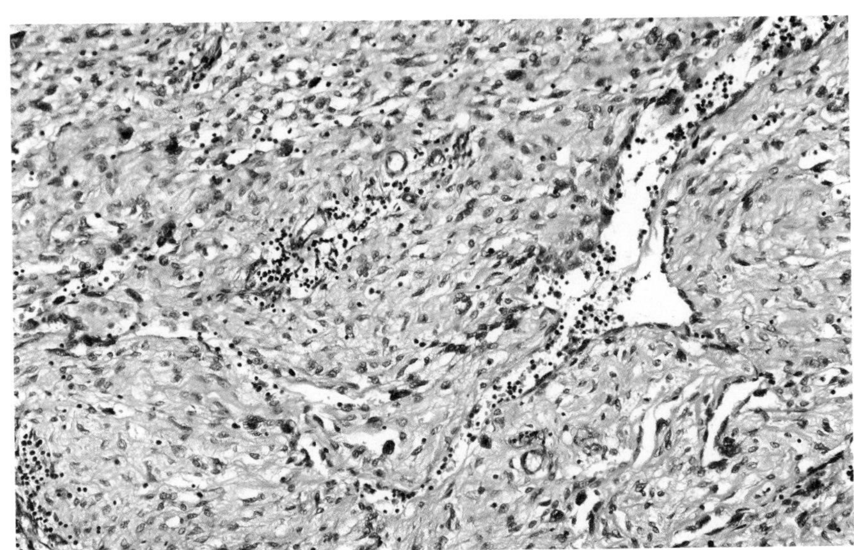

FIGURE 12-22. Classic appearance of a giant cell fibroblastoma showing pseudovascular spaces lined by giant cells.

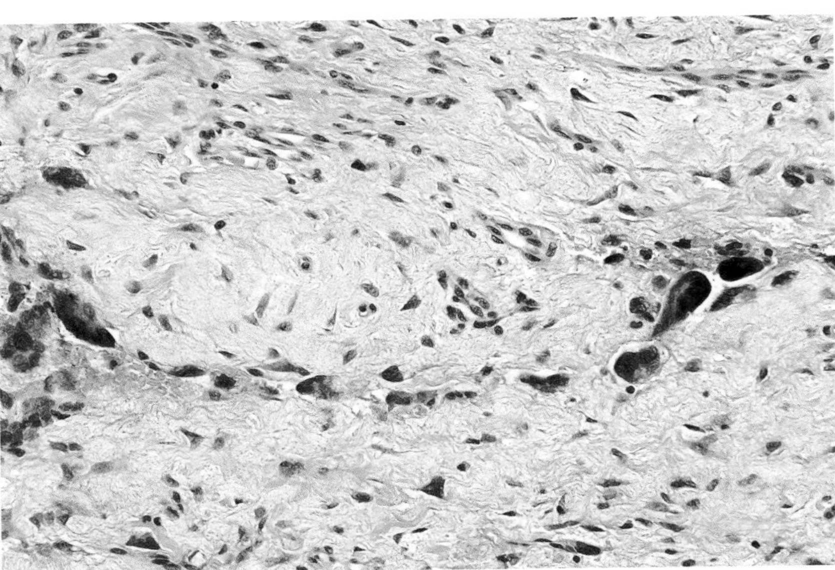

FIGURE 12-23. Hyperchromatic giant cells lining pseudovascular spaces in a giant cell fibroblastoma.

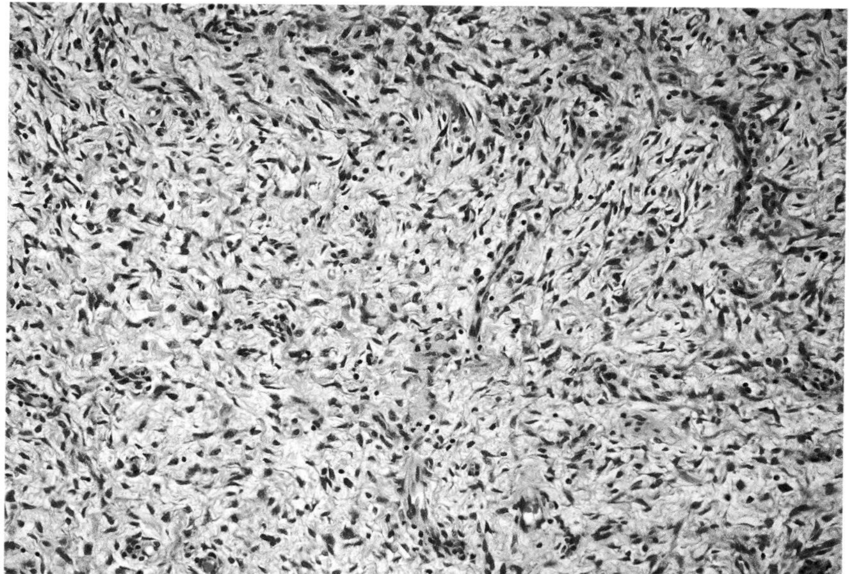

FIGURE 12-24. Cellular areas in a giant cell fibroblastoma.

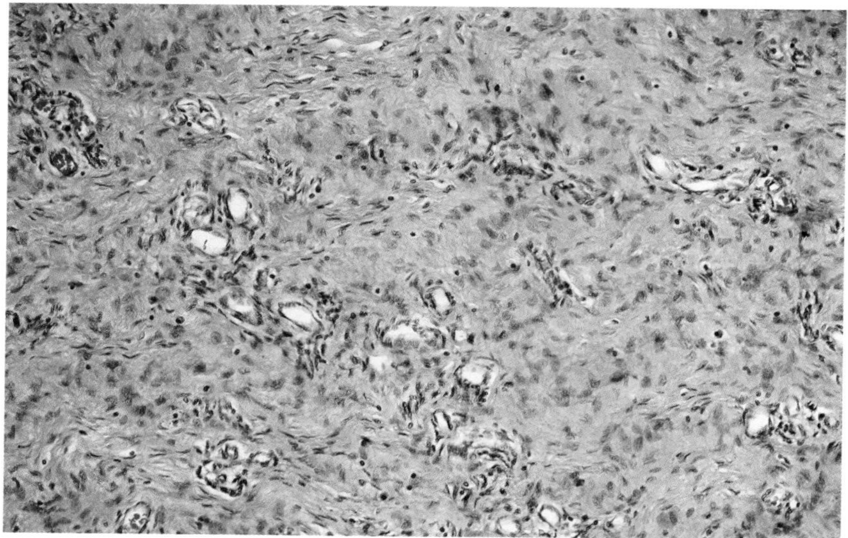

FIGURE 12-25. Hypocellular hyalinized zones in a giant cell fibroblastoma.

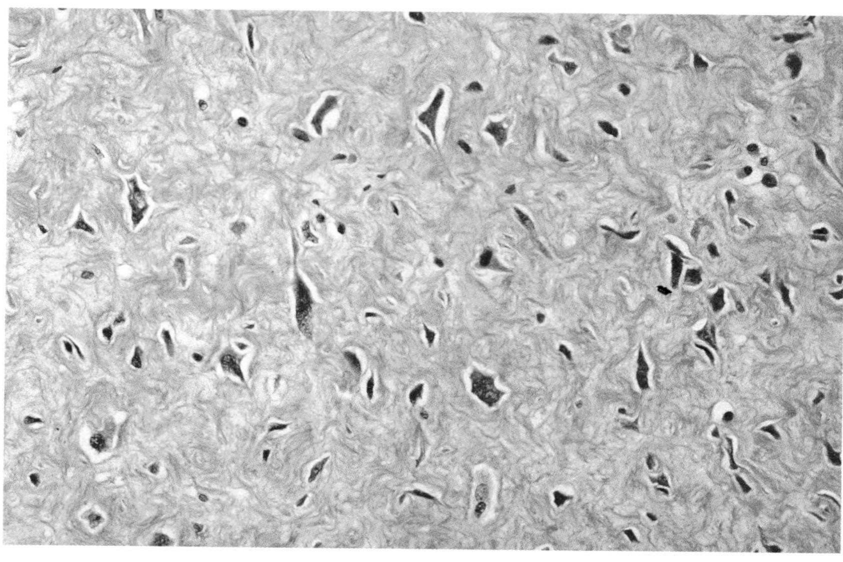

FIGURE 12-26. Markedly hyalinized area in a giant cell fibroblastoma.

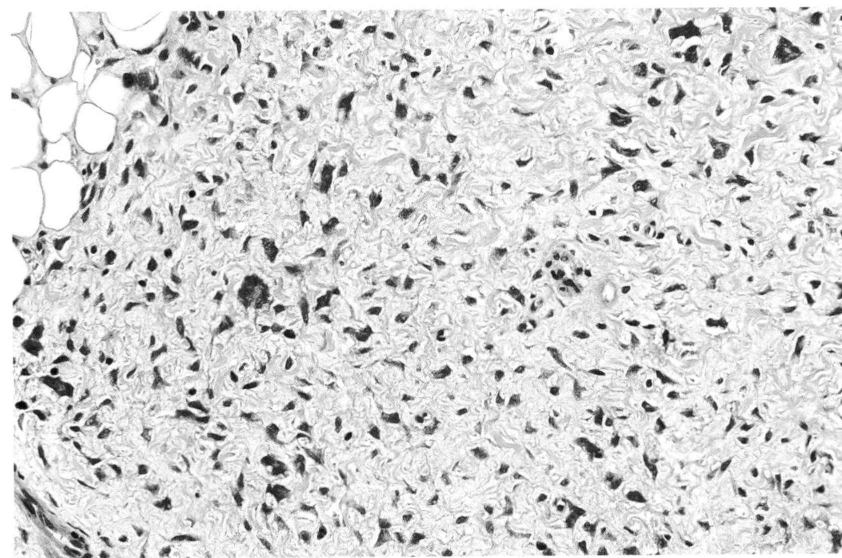

FIGURE 12-27. Hypocellular area in a giant cell fibroblastoma with giant cells not associated with pseudovascular spaces.

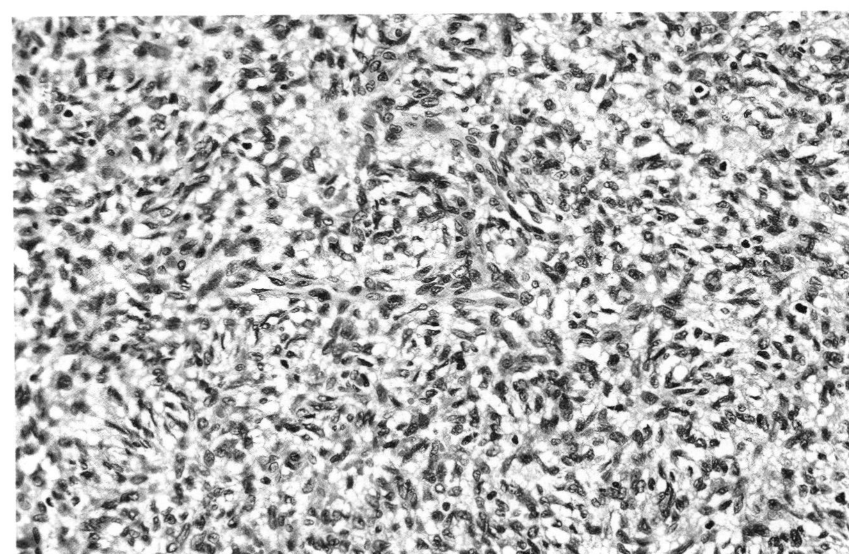

FIGURE 12-28. Dermatofibrosarcoma protuberans-like area in a giant cell fibroblastoma.

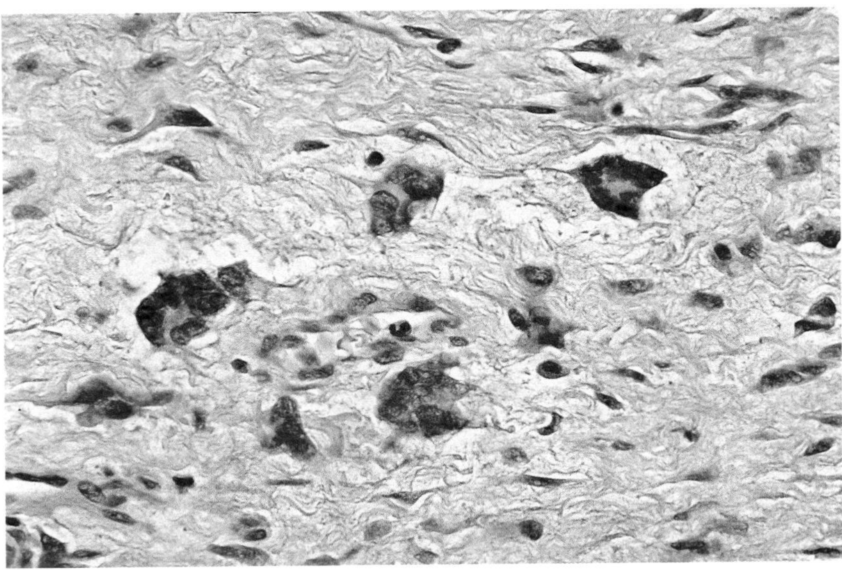

FIGURE 12-29. Giant cells in a giant cell fibroblastoma.

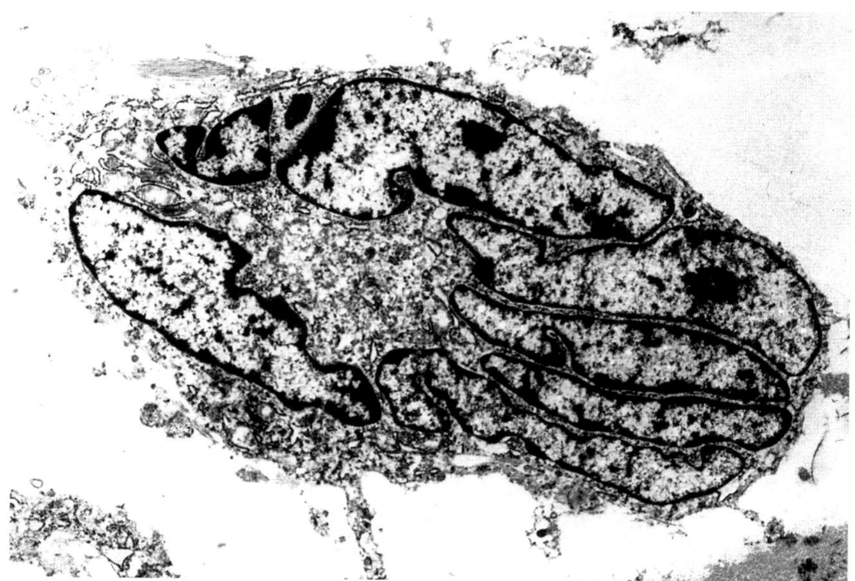

FIGURE 12-30. Electron micrograph of giant cells illustrating a hypersegmented nucleus. *(Courtesy of Dr. Barry Schmookler.)*

actually represent multiple sausage-like lobations of a single nucleus when studied ultrastructurally (Fig. 12-30).[62] Immunohistochemical studies indicate that these tumors express vimentin but lack S-100 protein and vascular markers.[77] Most giant cell fibroblastomas express CD34, a feature that they share with dermatofibrosarcoma protuberans.

Differential Diagnosis

About 40% of giant cell fibroblastomas are misdiagnosed as sarcoma. Because of the myxoid areas and hyperchromatic giant cells, there is a tendency to assume that they represent examples of myxoid liposarcoma or myxoid undifferentiated pleomorphic sarcoma occurring in an unusually young individual. Important clues to the diagnosis include the superficial location, lack of an intricate vasculature, and the presence of hyperchromatic cells lying preferentially along the pseudovascular spaces.

Discussion

There have been fewer reports of giant cell fibroblastoma than dermatofibrosarcoma protuberans in the literature. Recurrences have developed in about one-half of cases, but metastases have not been reported. Treatment of these tumors ideally is wide local excision. If limited therapy is contemplated, conscientious follow-up is advisable to document and treat recurrences.

It is well accepted that giant cell fibroblastoma and dermatofibrosarcoma are slightly different expressions of the same neoplasm. Like dermatofibrosarcoma protuberans, giant cell fibroblastoma occurs in superficial soft tissues, with a strong predilection for the abdominal wall, back, and groin. Even more compelling is the observation that hybrid tumors occur. For example, occasional dermatofibrosarcomas of adults contain giant cells or foci similar to those of giant cell fibroblastoma.[73] Less frequently, otherwise typical giant cell fibroblastomas of childhood contain areas of dermatofibrosarcoma protuberans. There have also been a number of recorded instances in which either dermatofibrosarcoma protuberans or giant cell fibroblastoma has recurred and recapitulated the pattern of the other tumor in the recurrence.[69,72,74] Finally, the giant cell fibroblastoma displays cytogenetic and molecular genetic changes identical to those of dermatofibrosarcoma protuberans (see previous discussion).

ANGIOMATOID FIBROUS HISTIOCYTOMA

Previously termed *angiomatoid malignant fibrous histiocytoma*,[78] this distinctive tumor of children and young adults has been renamed *angiomatoid fibrous histiocytoma*, a designation that reflects the relative rarity of metastasis and the overall excellent clinical course.

Clinical Findings

Angiomatoid fibrous histiocytoma, a tumor that occurs primarily in children and young adults, is rarely encountered in adults over age 40. It develops as a slowly growing nodular, multinodular, or cystic mass of the hypodermis or subcutis. It most often occurs on the extremities. Local symptoms such as pain and tenderness are uncommon, but systemic symptoms such as anemia, pyrexia, and weight loss are occasionally encountered and have been shown to be related to the production of cytokines such as TNF-α, IL-6, and IL-2 by the neoplasm.[79] In some instances, particularly in children, the tumor may present clinically as a recurrent hematoma, and it is important to carefully sample such masses for small nodules of angiomatoid fibrous histiocytoma.

Gross and Microscopic Findings

The tumors are firm, circumscribed lesions that usually measure a few centimeters in diameter and vary in color from gray-tan to red-brown, depending on the amount of hemosiderin present. One of the most characteristic features is the presence of irregular blood-filled cystic spaces best appreciated on cross section (Fig. 12-31). This feature may be so striking as to give the impression of a hematoma, hemangioma, or a thrombosed vessel.

These lesions are characterized by three features: irregular solid masses of histiocyte-like cells, cystic areas of hemorrhage, and chronic inflammation. In general, the solid masses of histiocyte-like cells interspersed with areas of hemorrhage occupy the central portion of the tumor, and the inflammatory cells form a dense peripheral cuff that blends with the surrounding pseudocapsule (Figs. 12-32 to 12-40).

The histiocyte-like cells are usually quite uniform; they have a round or oval nucleus and a faintly staining eosinophilic cytoplasm often containing finely particulate hemosiderin. In most instances, the cells are bland, so that some may be confused with the histiocytes of granulomas (see Figs. 12-38 and 12-39). In about one-fifth of cases, significant nuclear atypia or hyperchromatic giant cells are present (see

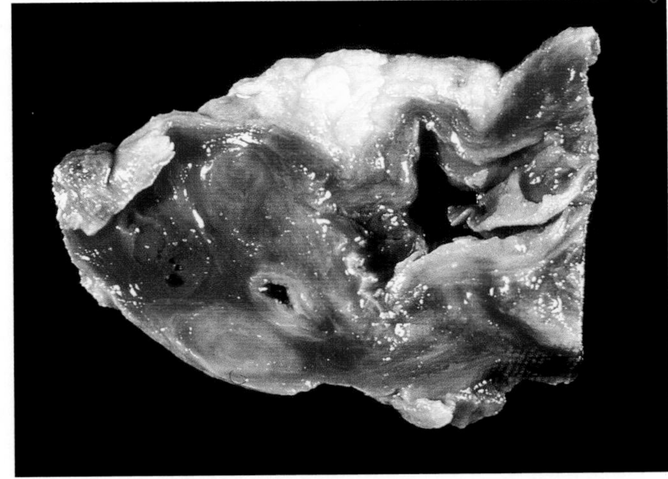

FIGURE 12-31. Gross specimen of an angiomatoid fibrous histiocytoma illustrating cystic change and a hemosiderin-stained tumor. Normal fat is present at the periphery.

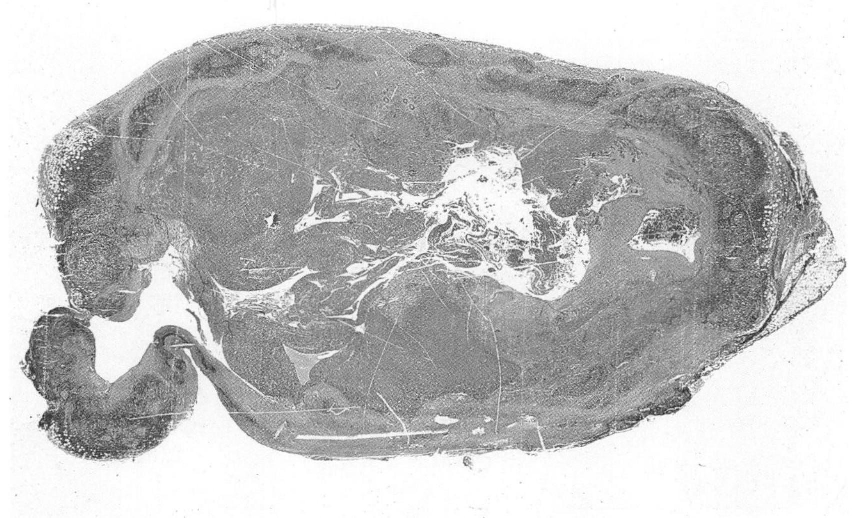

FIGURE 12-32. Angiomatoid fibrous histiocytoma shows a partially cystic tumor mass surrounded by a dense fibrous pseudocapsule and prominent lymphoid cuff.

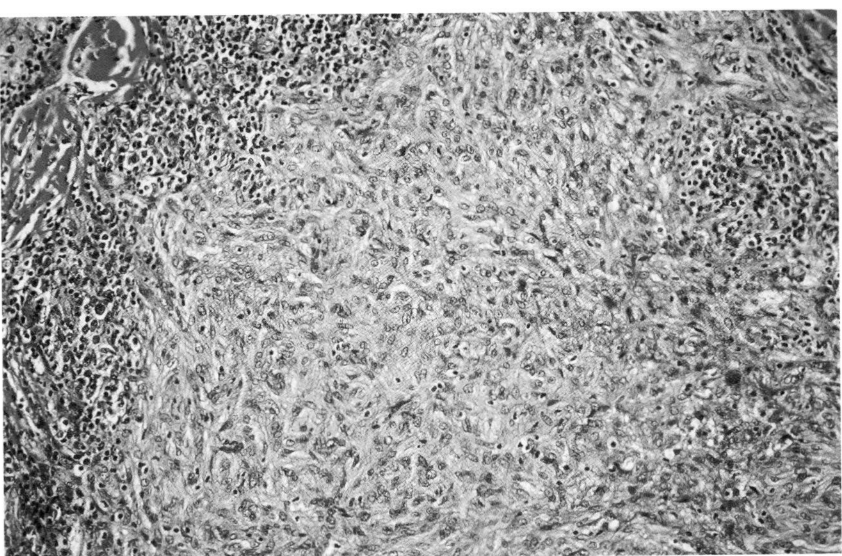

FIGURE 12-33. Angiomatoid fibrous histiocytoma. Histiocyte-like cells are arranged in solid sheets. Lymphoid infiltrate surrounds the tumor nodule.

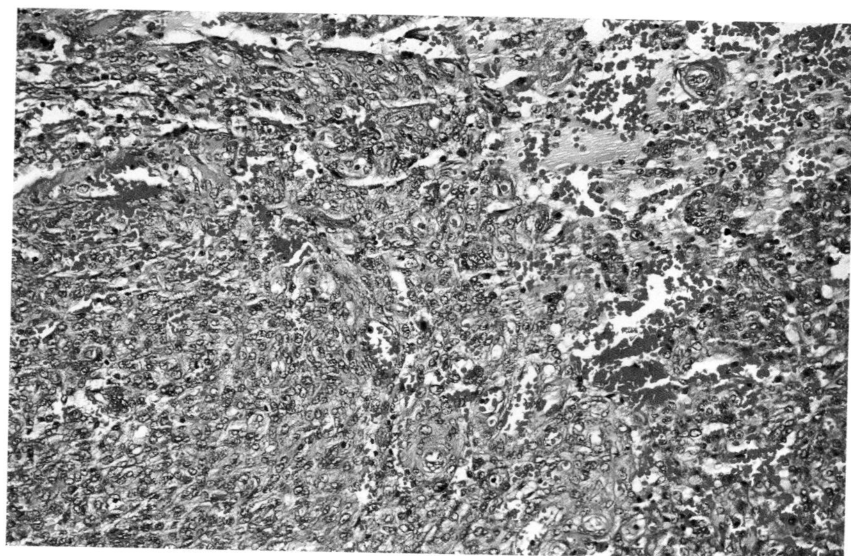

FIGURE 12-34. Areas of microscopic hemorrhage and cystic change in an angiomatoid fibrous histiocytoma.

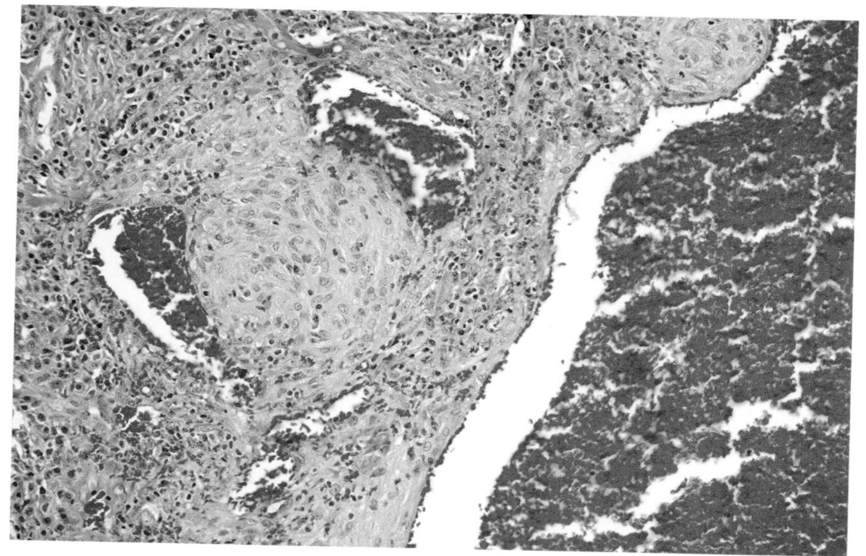

FIGURE 12-35. Cystic hemorrhage in an angiomatoid fibrous histiocytoma.

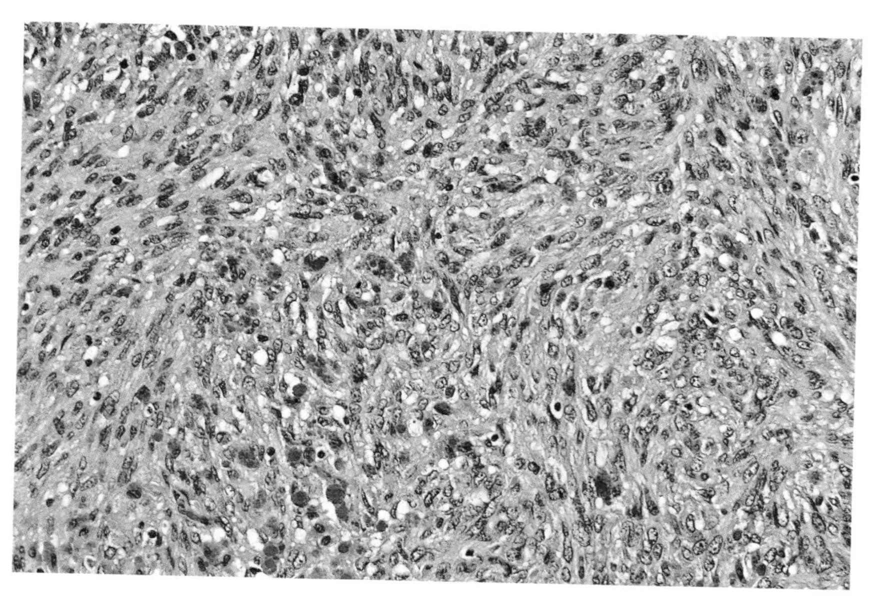

FIGURE 12-36. Spindle cell area in an angiomatoid fibrous histiocytoma.

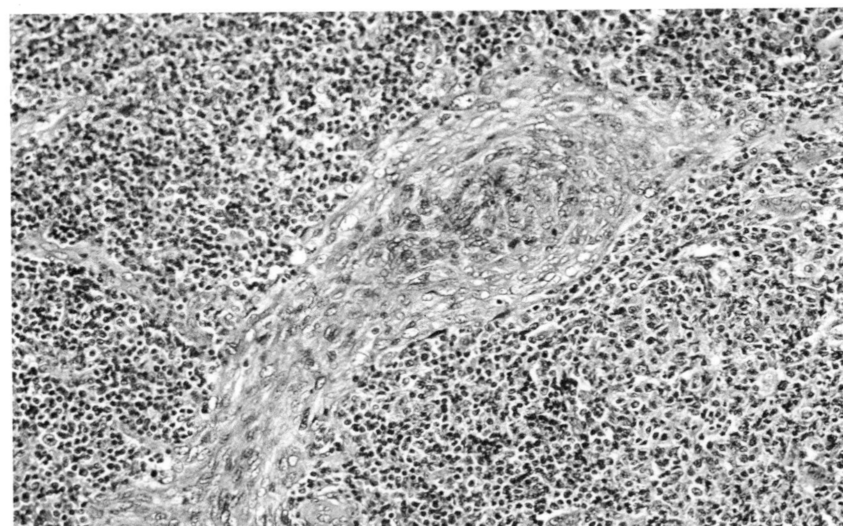

FIGURE 12-37. Tentacle-like extension of tumor in an angiomatoid fibrous histiocytoma surrounded by a chronic inflammatory response.

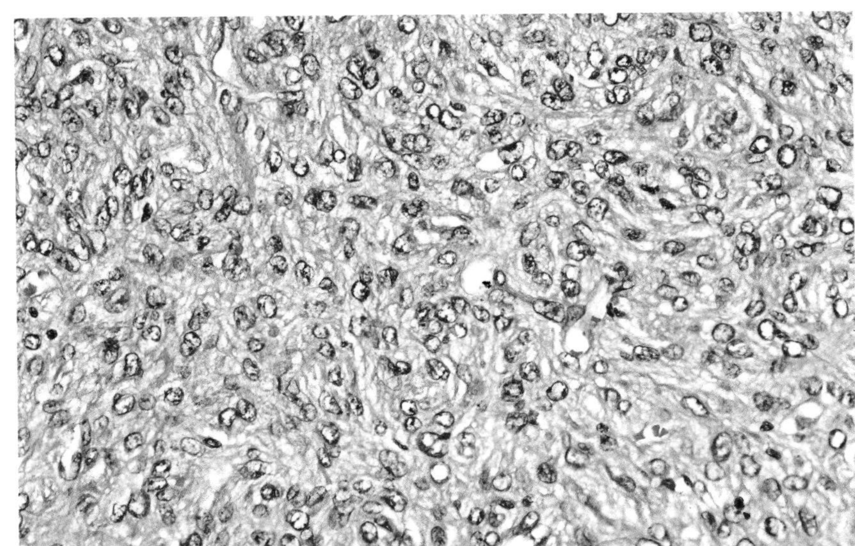

FIGURE 12-38. Histiocyte-like cells in an angiomatoid fibrous histiocytoma.

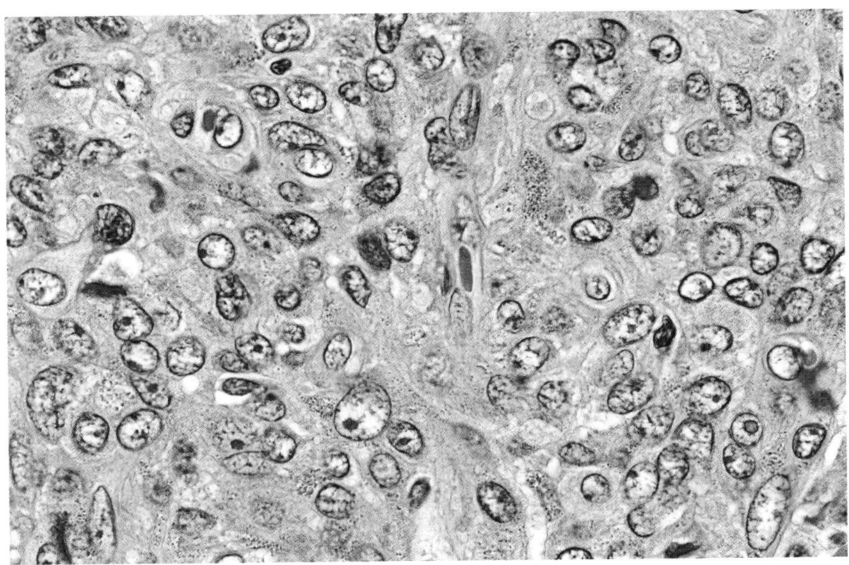

FIGURE 12-39. Histiocyte-like cells in an angiomatoid fibrous histiocytoma.

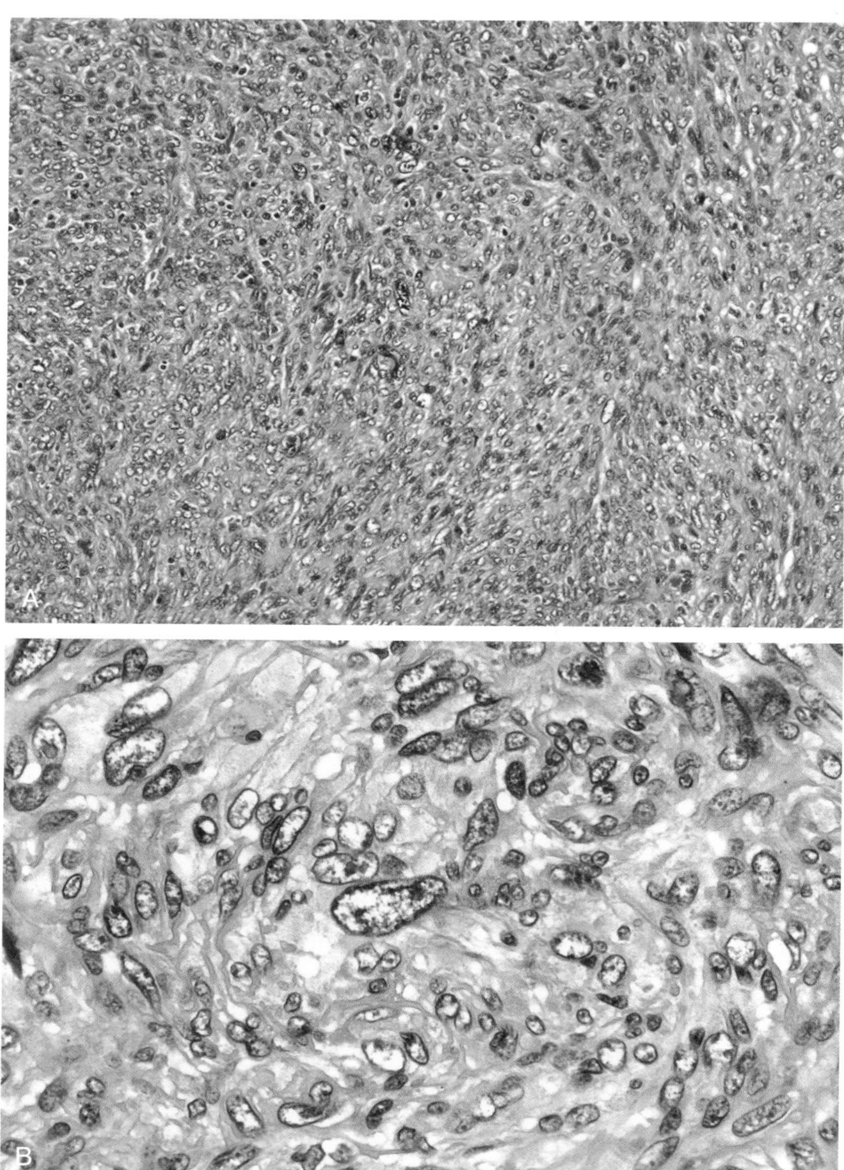

FIGURE 12-40. Angiomatoid fibrous histiocytoma showing diffuse cytological atypia (A). High-power view of pleomorphic cells in angiomatoid fibrous histiocytoma (B). This finding does not seem to be of clinical significance.

Fig. 12-40), a feature that does not correlate with aggressive behavior.[80] In a small number of cases, myxoid change may develop in the tumor (Fig. 12-41). Rarely, angiomatoid fibrous histiocytomas may show a small-cell pattern suggestive of a round cell sarcoma such as Ewing sarcoma (Fig. 12-42), a potentially serious pitfall, especially as both tumors may show CD99 expression and *EWSR1* gene rearrangements (see later discussion). Lipid and especially hemosiderin are present in the cells, but xanthoma cells are usually absent. Multifocal hemorrhage is a striking feature in all cases and results in the formation of irregular cystic spaces (see Figs. 12-37 and 12-38). Although these spaces resemble vascular spaces, they are not lined by endothelium but, rather, by flattened tumor cells. Small vessels may be present at the periphery of the nodules, but they do not seem to be the major components of these tumors. Inflammatory cells consist of a mixture of lymphocytes and plasma cells. Germinal center formation is occasionally observed, a feature suggesting lymph node metastasis, especially if the tumor represents a recurrence. The resemblance to a lymph node is further heightened by the thick pseudocapsule, a structure often interpreted as a lymph node capsule. However, unlike a true lymph node, there are no subcapsular or medullary sinuses, and germinal center formation occurs randomly around the tumor, without a predilection for the subcapsular zone. Long-standing lesions may consist largely of reactive fibrosis and hemosiderin and hematoidin pigment, with only very small, sometimes difficult to identify scattered islands of neoplastic cells. Differentiation of angiomatoid fibrous histiocytomas from aneurysmal and hemosiderotic benign fibrous histiocytomas is discussed in Chapter 11.

Immunohistochemical Features

Since the original description of this tumor in 1979, a number of views have been espoused concerning the line of differentiation. Although the lesions have a decidedly histiocytic

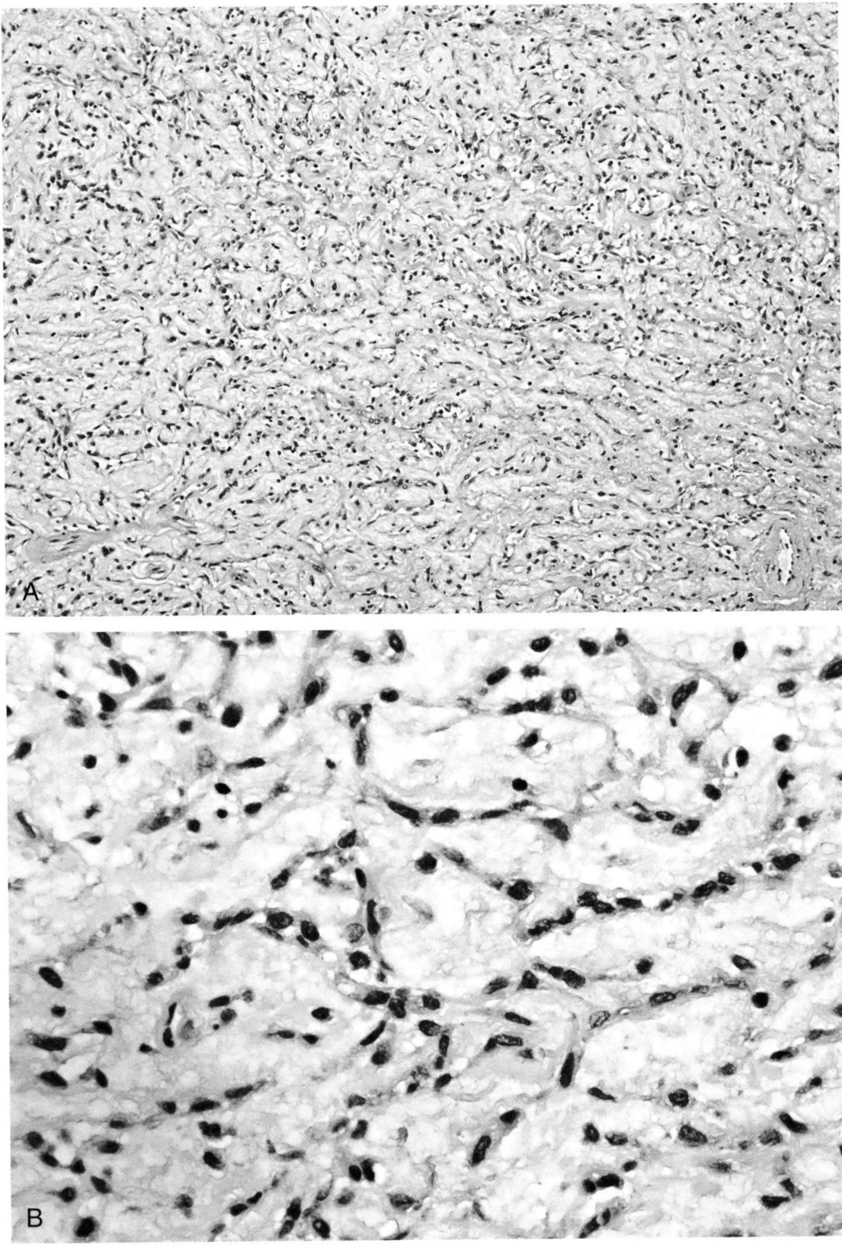

FIGURE 12-41. Extensively myxoid angiomatoid fibrous histiocytoma (A). Higher-power view showing bland cells arranged in a cord-like pattern within an abundantly myxoid matrix (B). This case was known to harbor the fusion gene *EWSR1-CREB1*. *(Courtesy of Dr. André Oliveira, Mayo Clinic, Rochester, MN.)*

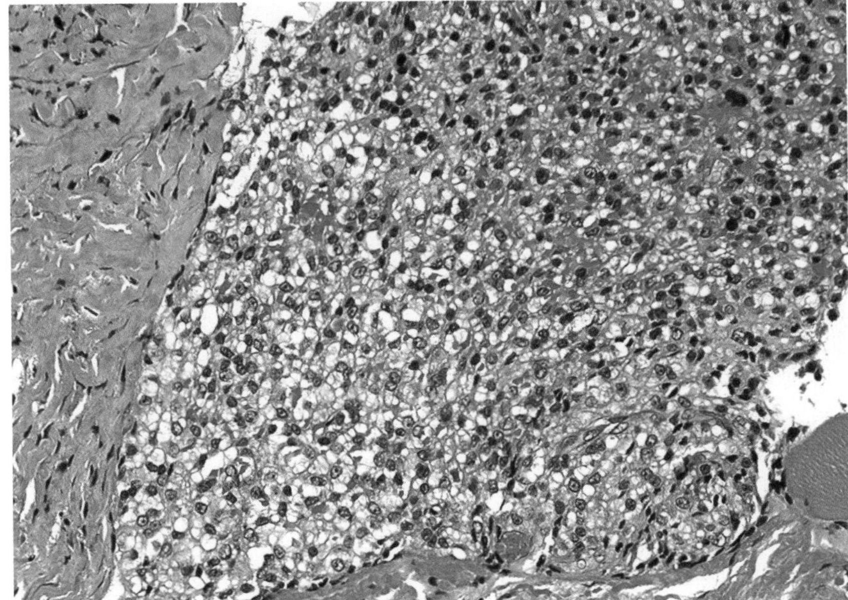

FIGURE 12-42. Small-cell pattern in angiomatoid fibrous histiocytoma. Such tumors may easily be confused with other CD99 and *EWSR1*-positive tumors of childhood, such as Ewing sarcoma.

appearance and show ample evidence of phagocytosis of hemosiderin, immunohistochemical analysis of histiocytic antigens has been disappointing.[81] The tumors do not express muramidase or L-1. About half express CD68 (KP-1),[81] reflecting the presence of a high density of phagolysosomes. An intriguing observation is the finding of desmin and/or epithelial membrane antigen within half of these cases[82-84] (Fig. 12-43) and other muscle markers within a smaller percentage (muscle-specific actin, heavy-caldesmon, smooth muscle actin, and calponin).[83] CD99 is also present in about one-half of cases.[82] The close association of these tumors with lymphoid tissue as well as this myoid phenotype has led to the suggestion that these cells may be related to the desmin-positive stromal cells of lymph node, although this is unlikely to be true.[82] Because these lesions are now known to be translocation-associated (see later discussion), it is more likely that they lack a normal cellular counterpart.

Cytogenetic and Molecular Genetic Features

In 2000, Waters et al.[83] reported the first cytogenetic characterization of angiomatoid fibrous histiocytoma, noting the presence of the translocation t(12;16)(q13;p11) and production of a *FUS-ATF1* fusion gene. This was quickly followed by other reports of *FUS-ATF1* and *EWSR1-ATF1* fusion transcripts in cases of angiomatoid fibrous histiocytoma.[86,87] More recently, two large retrospective studies of angiomatoid fibrous histiocytoma have identified *EWSR1-CREB1* as another fusion gene in angiomatoid fibrous histiocytoma.[88,89] It now appears

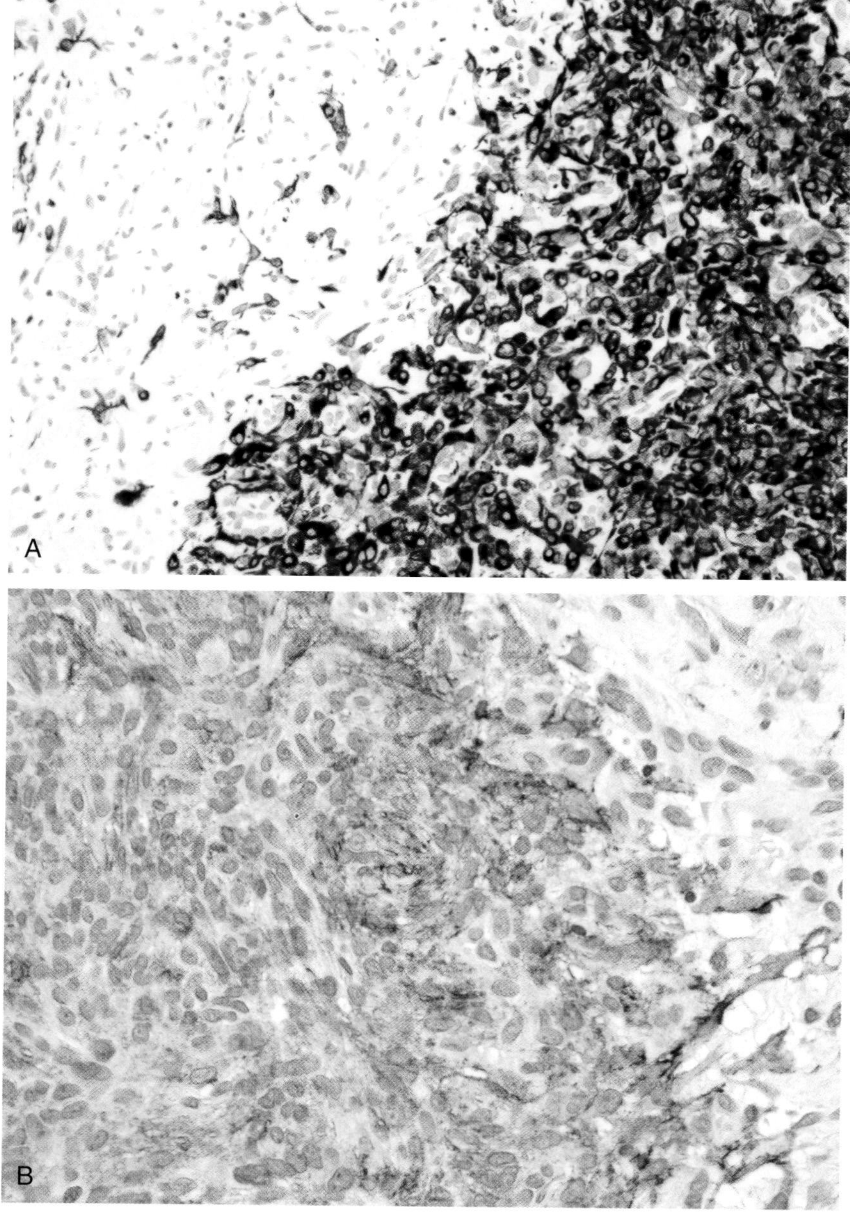

FIGURE 12-43. Desmin (A) and epithelial membrane antigen (B) co-expression, an unusual, characteristic immunophenotype, is seen in many angiomatoid fibrous histiocytomas.

that *EWSR1-CREB1* is the most common fusion transcript in angiomatoid fibrous histiocytoma, with *EWSR1-ATF1* representing the second most common genetic event, and *FUS-ATF1* the least common. Very rare angiomatoid fibrous histiocytomas contain rearrangements involving *EWSR1* without involvement of *CREB1* or *ATF1*, suggesting the existence of additional, yet unknown, fusion partners (Dr. André Oliveira, personal communication). There does not appear to be an association between the type of fusion transcript and other clinical or pathologic parameters in angiomatoid fibrous histiocytoma. Surprisingly, identical *EWSR1-ATF1* and *EWSR1-CREB1* fusion transcripts are also seen in clear cell sarcoma of soft parts, so-called *gastrointestinal clear cell sarcoma-like tumor*, and in a rare salivary gland tumor, hyalinizing clear cell carcinoma.[90] Downstream activation of the microphthalmia transcription factor (MiTF) pathway, leading to melanogenesis, is seen in clear cell sarcoma but not in angiomatoid fibrous histiocytoma bearing these fusion genes.[86]

Discussion

Angiomatoid fibrous histiocytoma was originally believed to be a reasonably aggressive neoplasm, based on follow-up of a small number of cases ascertained retrospectively.[78] Subsequent investigation has, however, proven the generally indolent behavior of this tumor. In the study of Costa and Weiss,[78] of 108 cases, local recurrences were seen in only 12% of patients, all of whom had initially positive margins and who were subsequently cured by excision of the recurrence. Similarly, metastatic disease was seen in only five cases (5%); four of these patients had metastases to regional lymph nodes only and were disease-free at the time of publication, whereas the last patient died of pulmonary and cerebral metastases. Similarly, Fanburg-Smith et al.[80] noted only a 1% metastatic rate in another very large study of angiomatoid (malignant) fibrous histiocytoma. A number of factors can be correlated with the risk of local recurrence, including infiltrating margins, location on the head and neck, and involvement of skeletal muscle rather than the subcutis.[81] Complete surgical excision without adjuvant therapy is the appropriate treatment for these low-grade tumors. Metastectomy may greatly prolong the survival of, or even cure, patients with metastatic angiomatoid fibrous histiocytoma.

PLEXIFORM FIBROHISTIOCYTIC TUMOR

Clinical Findings

Plexiform fibrohistiocytic tumor, like giant cell fibroblastoma and angiomatoid fibrous histiocytoma, occurs almost exclusively in children and young adults and is rarely encountered after the age of 30 years.[91] It typically presents as a slowly growing mass of the deep dermis and subcutaneous tissues. The most common location is the upper extremity (63%) followed by the lower extremity (14%).

Gross and Microscopic Findings

The lesions are relatively small (1 to 3 cm), ill-defined masses with a gray-white trabecular appearance. In its most typical form (about 40% of cases), the lesion contains a mixture of two components: a differentiated fibroblastic component and a round cell histiocytic component containing multinucleated giant cells. At low-power microscopy, one is impressed by the numerous tiny cellular nodules that occupy the dermis and subcutaneous tissue (Figs. 12-44 and 12-45). These nodules are composed of nests of histiocytic cells that often contain multinucleated, osteoclast-like giant cells and occasionally undergo focal hemorrhage (Figs. 12-46 to 12-50). The cells in these nodules are well differentiated and in almost all instances do not display atypia or significant levels of mitotic activity. The nodules, in turn, are circumscribed by short fascicles of fibroblastic cells (see Figs. 12-47 to 12-49) that intersect slightly or ramify in the soft tissue, creating a plexiform growth pattern. The fascicles of spindle cells, to some extent, resemble fibromatosis, except that the cells are usually plumper and the

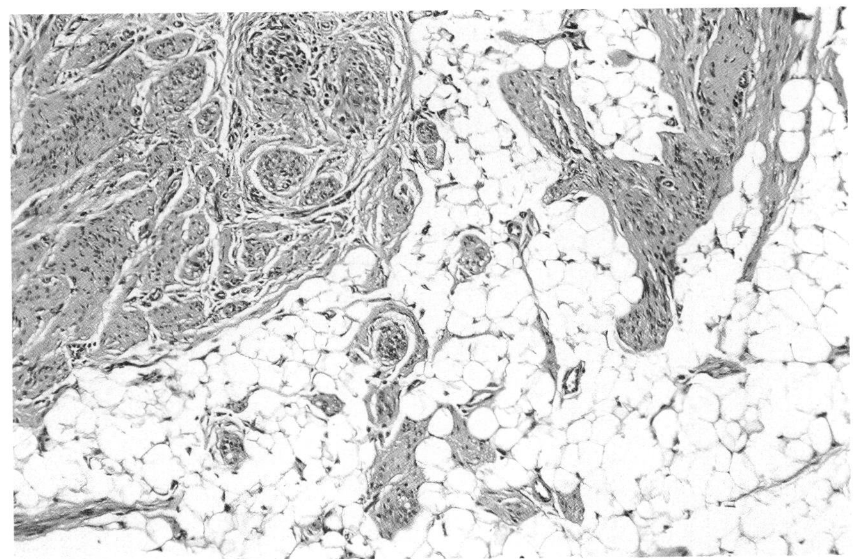

FIGURE 12-44. Plexiform fibrohistiocytic tumor showing ramifying fascicles of tumor in the subcutis.

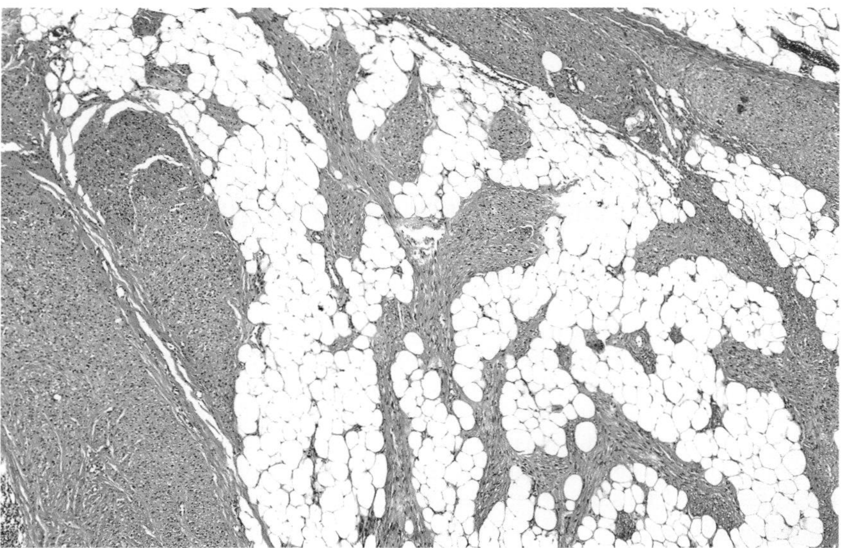

FIGURE 12-45. Plexiform fibrohistiocytic tumor showing relatively acellular ramifying fascicles in the subcutis.

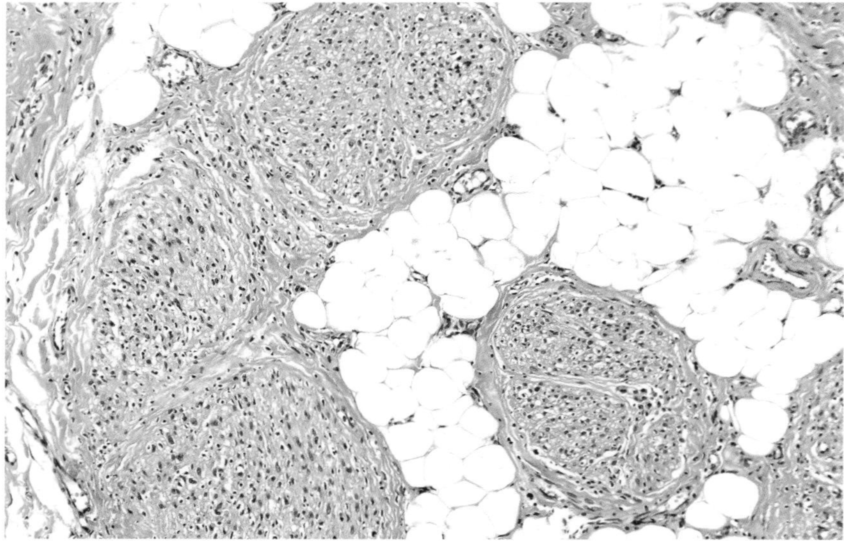

FIGURE 12-46. Irregular fascicles and nodules of a plexiform fibrohistiocytic tumor.

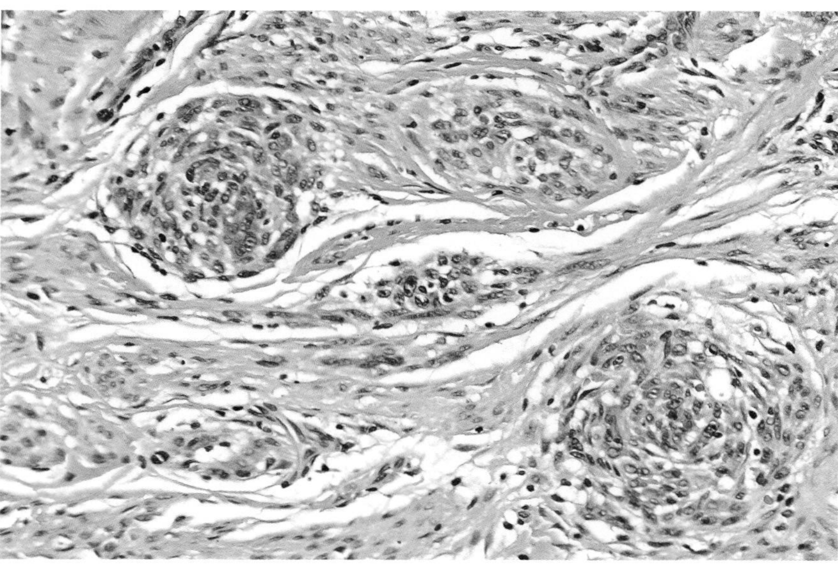

FIGURE 12-47. Typical biphasic appearance of a plexiform fibrohistiocytic tumor. Histiocyte-like nodules circumscribed by fibromatosis-like areas.

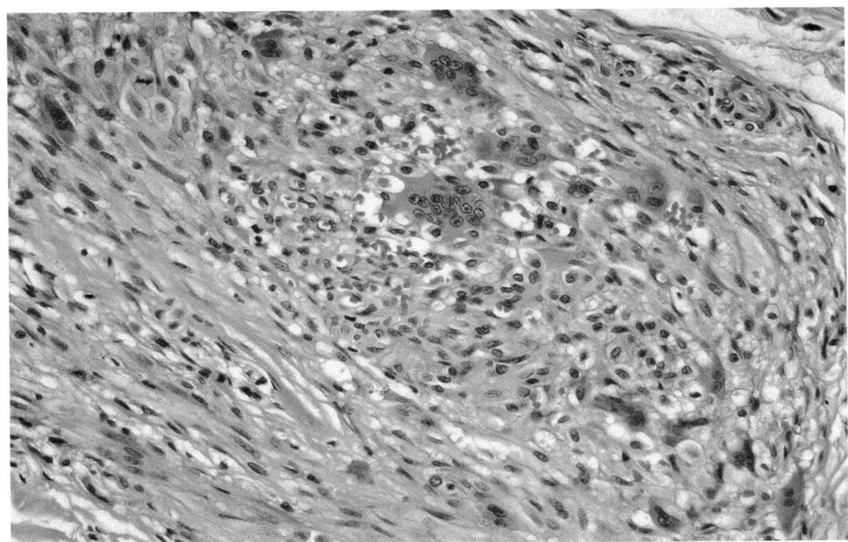

FIGURE 12-48. Nodules of histiocyte-like cells in a plexiform fibrohistiocytic tumor.

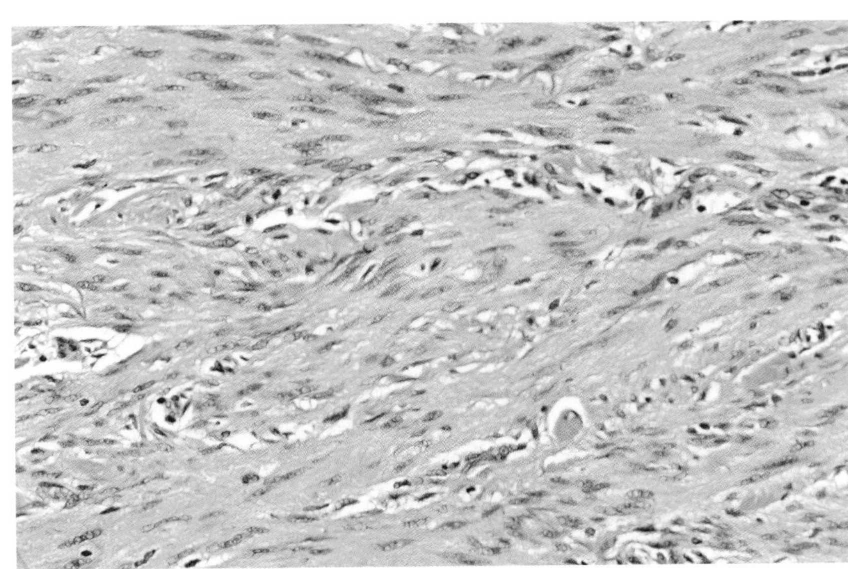

FIGURE 12-49. Plexiform fibrohistiocytic tumor with areas of short, ramifying fascicles of fibroblasts without histiocytes.

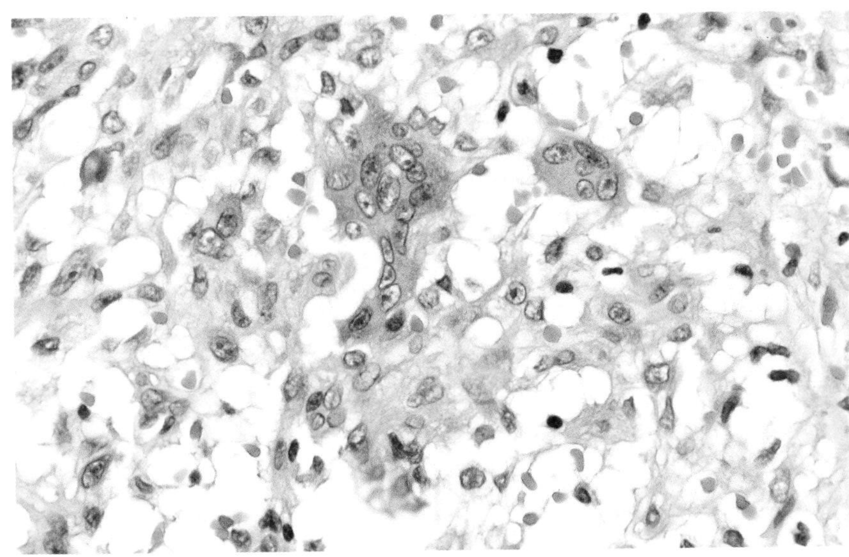

FIGURE 12-50. Plexiform fibrohistiocytic tumor with a high-power view of histiocyte-like cells comprising tumor nodules.

fascicles shorter than those of fibromatosis. In the less typical case, the two components described previously may not be equally represented. For example, in a few cases, the nodules of giant cells are rare or absent, and only short intersecting fascicles of plump spindle cells are seen. In other cases, there may be a blending of the nodules and fascicles, and the cells in these two zones may appear to be in an intermediate stage between fibroblasts and histiocytes.

Ancillary Studies

Immunohistochemically, the multinucleated giant cells and many of the mononuclear cells express CD68, suggesting true histiocytic differentiation, whereas the spindle cells express smooth muscle actin, as one would expect of myofibroblasts (Fig. 12-51). The cells do not contain other histiocytic markers such as HLA-DR, lysozyme, or L-2, and S-100 protein, keratin, desmin, and factor XIIIa are not present.

Ultrastructural studies have identified cells with features of histiocytes and myofibroblasts.[92] In a large series reported by Remstein et al.,[91] all cases were diploid with an S-phase fraction of 0.93% to 7.22%. Cytogenetic analysis has been carried out in a few cases. One patient had a complex karyotype with numerous deletions, whereas the other had a t(4;15)(q21;q15).[94,95]

Differential Diagnosis

A variety of benign diagnoses that includes granuloma, fibrous hamartoma, fibrous histiocytoma, giant cell tumor, cellular neurothekeoma, and fibromatosis is entertained in these cases. The most important distinctions are those that materially affect the management of the patient. It is essential to distinguish the lesion from an infectious granulomatous process. In the typical case, the presence of associated fibroblastic cuffing of the histiocytic nodules is usually sufficient

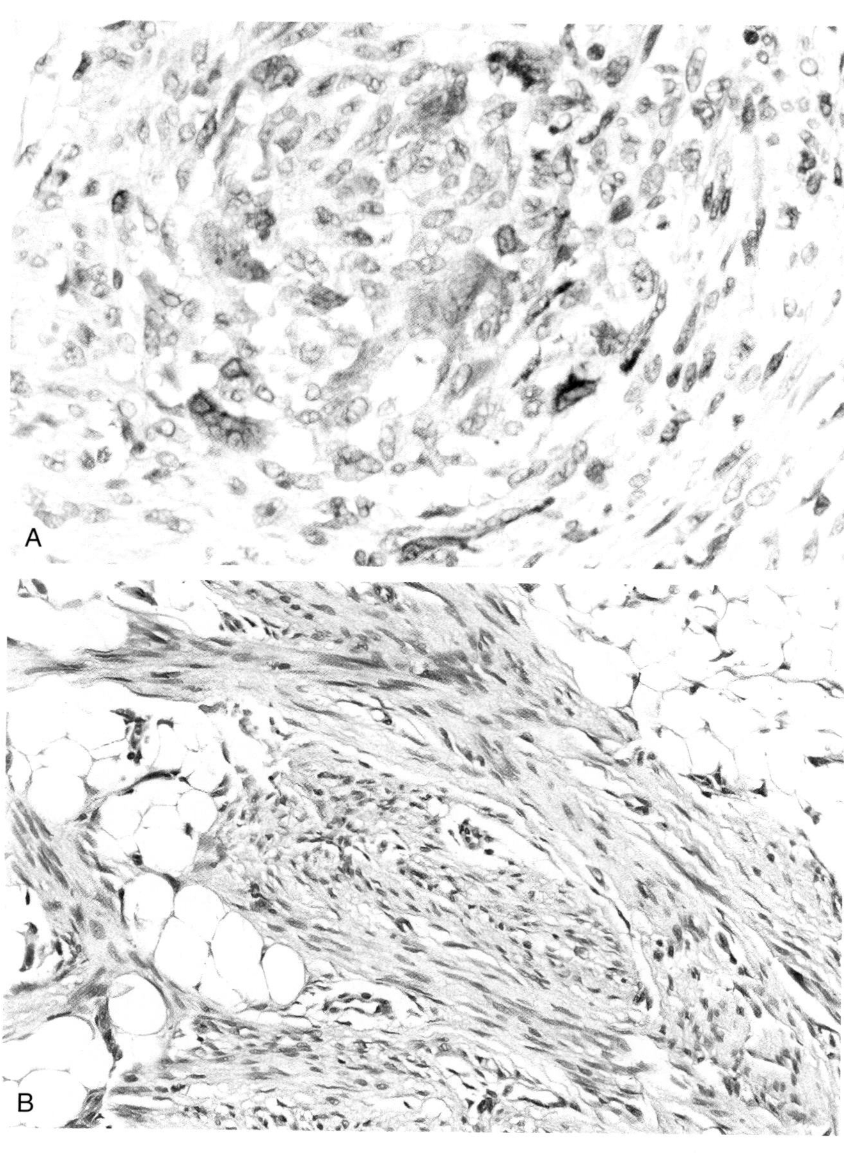

FIGURE 12-51. CD68 immunostain of a plexiform fibrohistiocytic tumor showing positivity of histiocytic giant cell nodules (A) and no positivity of fibroblastic areas (B).

to suggest an alternative diagnosis. In tumors that are predominantly histiocytic, the important observations include that these tumors do not have a surrounding inflammatory infiltrate, and the histiocytic nodules do not undergo central necrosis. Cellular neurothekeomas typically show a greater degree of cytologic variability than do plexiform fibrohistiocytic tumors and often contain prominent bands of hyalinized collagen, a feature typically lacking in the latter tumor. Predominantly fibroblastic forms of plexiform fibrohistiocytic tumor may resemble fibromatosis, but in fibromatosis, the fascicles are wider, longer, and composed of more slender fibroblastic cells.

Discussion

Based on three series, these tumors appear to be low-grade neoplasms that frequently recur (12.5% to 40%) within 1 to 2 years of the original diagnosis.[94,96,97] Lymph node metastases have been observed in two cases only,[94,96] and only three patients in the literature have had histologically proven pulmonary metastases, one of whom died of the disease. It should be noted that there may be pulmonary metastases at the time of presentation, emphasizing the need for careful initial evaluation. Unfortunately, no histologic parameters (e.g., mitotic activity, vascular invasion) have been correlated with aggressive behavior. Ideally, these lesions are completely, if not widely, excised. It does not seem appropriate to commit the patient to adjuvant therapy, based on the limited risk of regional or distant disease.

SOFT TISSUE GIANT CELL TUMOR OF LOW MALIGNANT POTENTIAL

In 1999, the term *soft tissue giant cell tumors of low malignant potential* was proposed for a group of lesions that represents the benign end of the spectrum of malignant giant cell tumor of soft parts (undifferentiated pleomorphic sarcoma, giant cell type) and that seems to be the soft tissue analogue of giant cell tumor of bone.[98] These lesions were first described in two nearly simultaneous publications during the 1970s.[99,100] Salm and Sissons[98] reported a group of 10 giant cell tumors of soft parts that they likened to giant cell tumors of bone, and Guccion and Enzinger[97] noted a subset of malignant giant cell tumors of soft parts characterized by "less atypia and mitotic activity" and that did not give rise to metastatic disease. Two additional studies were subsequently published.

Although seemingly a new entity, these lesions were probably grouped with a number of other lesions in the past, such as tenosynovial giant cell tumor, malignant giant cell tumor of soft parts, plexiform fibrohistiocytic tumor, and even epithelioid sarcoma. Although to date there has not been an instance of metastasis from any of these lesions, logically one might expect to encounter rare instances of metastasis similar to those seen with giant cell tumor of bone.

Clinical and Pathologic Features

These lesions tend to occur in all age groups and may develop in superficial or deep soft tissue, most commonly on the arm or hand. They consist of multiple tumor nodules that diffusely infiltrate soft tissue. The nodules are composed of bland mononuclear cells, short spindle cells, and osteoclasts (Figs. 12-52 to 12-54). By definition, the mononuclear and giant cells in these lesions lack the striking atypia that is the hallmark of giant cell forms of undifferentiated pleomorphic sarcoma (see Fig. 12-53). Despite the lack of nuclear atypia, they often have brisk mitotic activity; about one-half display vascular invasion (as may be seen with giant cell tumor of bone), although necrosis is not seen. Metaplastic bone and angiectatic spaces reminiscent of the changes of aneurysmal bone cysts can be seen (Figs. 12-55 and 12-56). Soft tissue giant cell tumors have an immunophenotypic profile similar to that of giant cell tumor of bone in that they express CD68 and smooth muscle actin, and the osteoclastic giant cells express the osteoclast-specific marker tartrate-resistant acid phosphatase, also known as TRAP. However, they lack CD45, S-100 protein, desmin, and lysozyme.

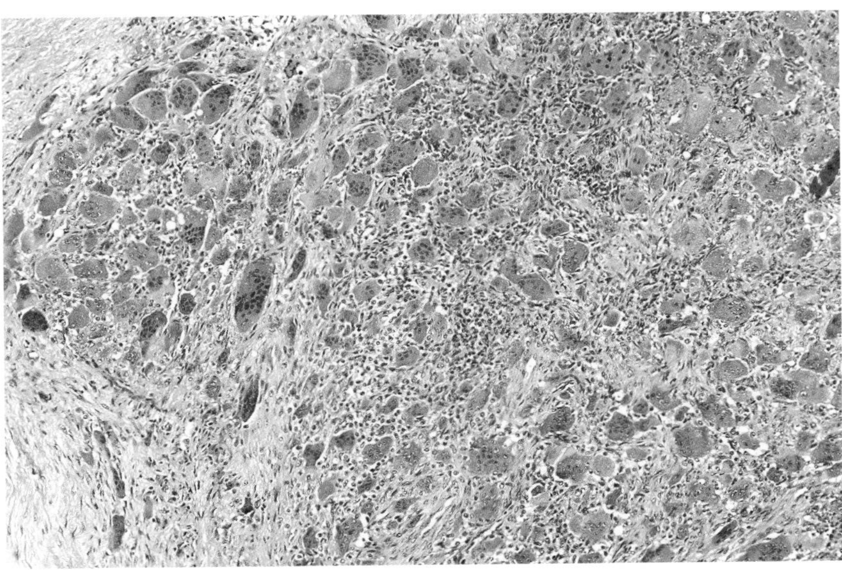

FIGURE 12-52. Giant cell tumor of low malignant potential with coarse nodular architecture.

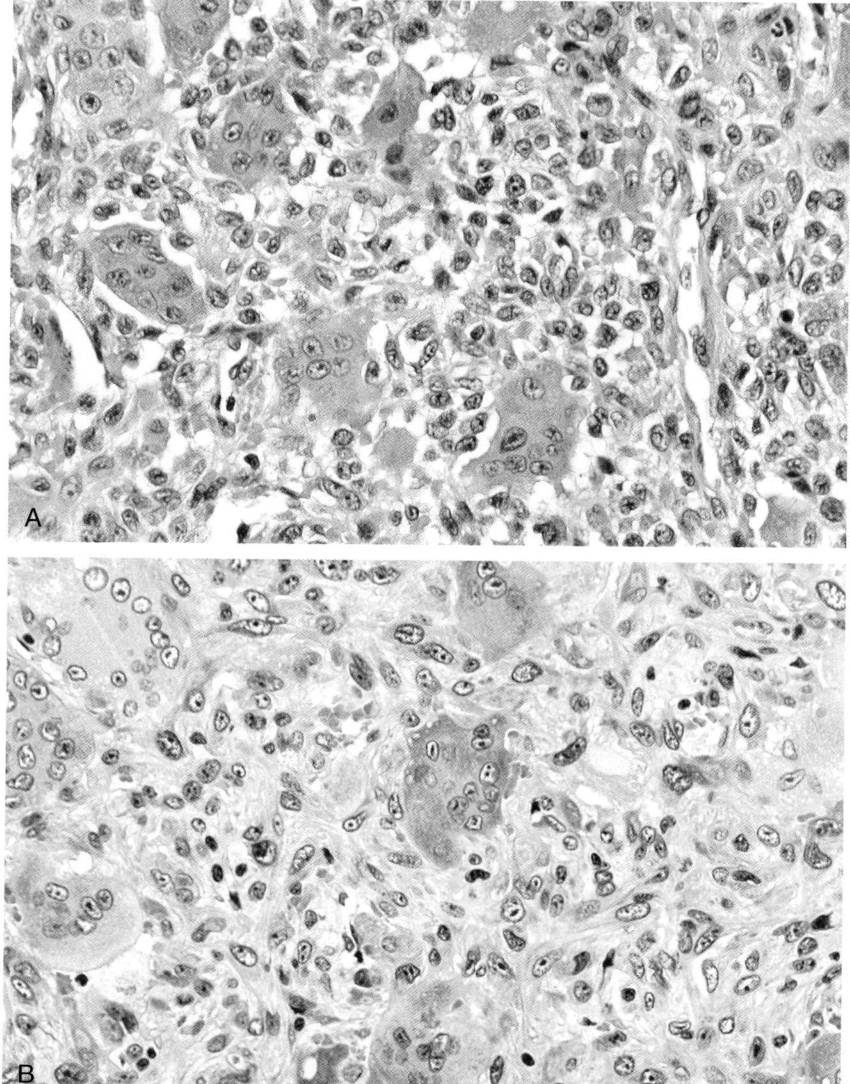

FIGURE 12-53. Giant cell tumor of low malignant potential with mild (A) and moderate (B) atypia of the mononuclear tumor cells. This contrasts with the marked atypia of classic undifferentiated pleomorphic sarcoma, giant cell type.

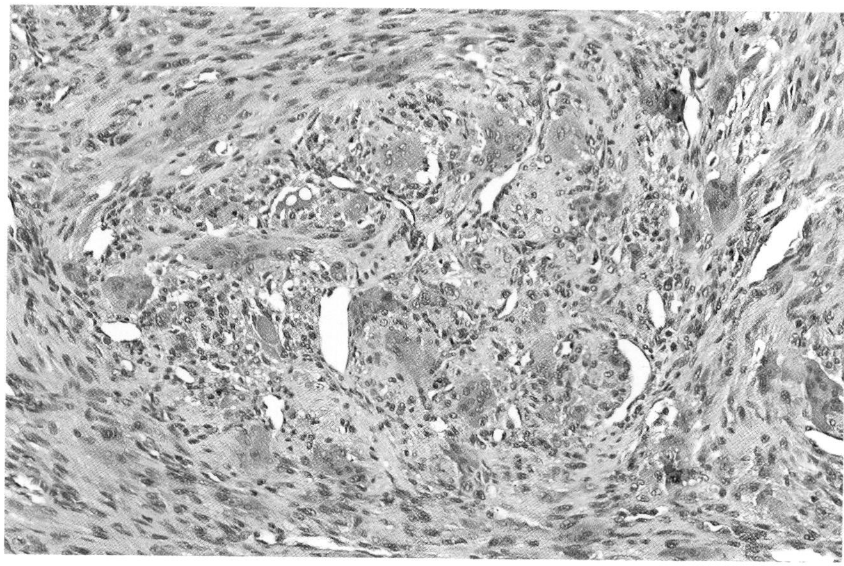

FIGURE 12-54. Giant cell tumor of low malignant potential showing spindling of cells.

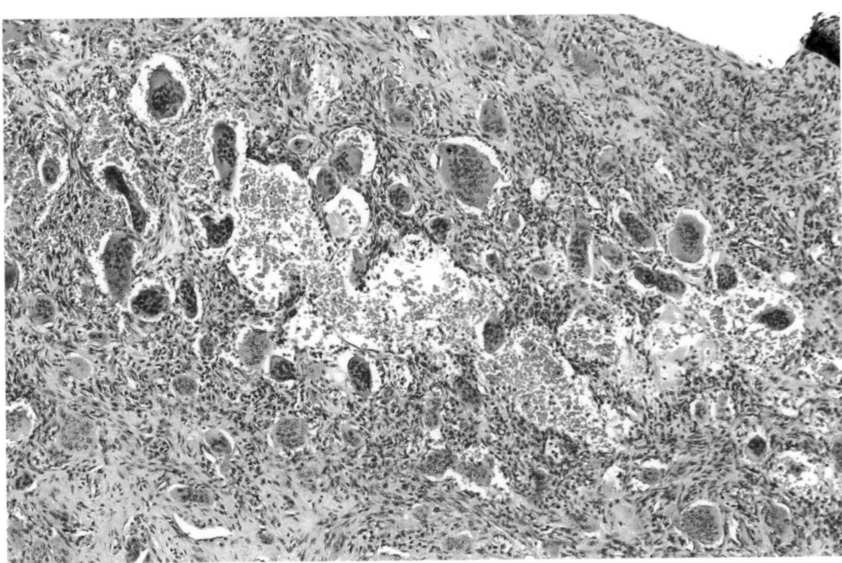

FIGURE 12-55. Aneurysmal bone cyst-like changes in a giant cell tumor of low malignant potential.

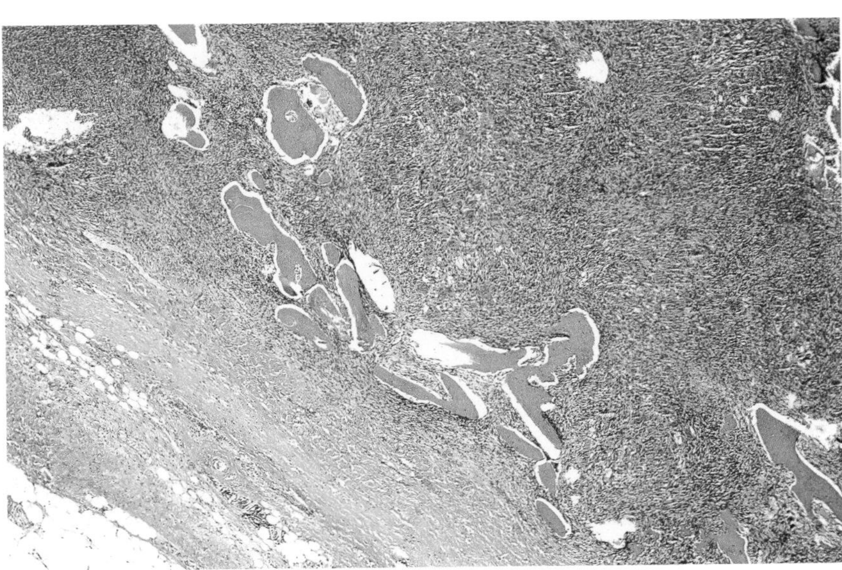

FIGURE 12-56. Metaplastic bone formation in a giant cell tumor of low malignant potential.

Differential Diagnosis

These tumors are most often confused with tenosynovial giant cell tumor or malignant giant cell tumor of soft parts (undifferentiated pleomorphic sarcoma, giant cell type). Apart from the rather significant difference in location, tenosynovial giant cell tumor usually has prominent stromal hyalinization and a more heterogeneous population of cells, including xanthoma cells, siderophages, and lymphocytes. Giant cell forms of undifferentiated pleomorphic sarcoma, by definition, contain mononuclear and giant cells with significant levels of atypia. In addition, necrosis and atypical mitotic figures are often present. Areas of plexiform fibrohistiocytic tumor bear a startling resemblance to these tumors, and identification of the characteristic bimodal growth pattern seen in that tumor may be required for confident distinction. Last, epithelioid sarcomas and nodular fasciitis with giant cells should always be excluded before diagnosing a soft tissue giant cell tumor of low malignant potential. Cytokeratins, present in epithelioid sarcoma, are absent in these tumors.

Clinical Behavior

The clinical behavior of this group of tumors is considerably better than that reported for malignant giant cell tumor of soft parts. Of 17 patients, 4 developed recurrences, but none had metastasis.[98] Metastases are exceedingly rare.[98]

References

1. Darier J, Ferrand M. Dermatofibromas progressifs et recidivants ou fibrosarcomes de la peau. Ann Dermatol Syph 1924;5:545.
2. Degos R, Mouly R, Civatte J, et al. Dermatofibro-sarcome de Darier-Ferrand, datant de 70 ans, opere au stade ultime de tumeur monstrueuse. Bull Soc Fr Derm Syph 1967;74:190.
3. McKee PH, Fletcher CD. Dermatofibrosarcoma protuberans presenting in infancy and childhood. J Cutan Pathol 1991;18(4):241–6.

4. Petoin DS, Verola O, Banzet P, et al. Dermatofibrosarcome de Darier et Ferrand. Etude de 96 cas sur 15 ans. Chirurgie; mémoires de l'Académie de chirurgie 1985;111(2):132–8.
5. Taylor HB, Helwig EB. Dermatofibrosarcoma protuberans. A study of 115 cases. Cancer 1962;15:717–25.
6. Pack GT, Tabah EJ. Dermato-fibrosarcoma protuberans. A report of 39 cases. AMA archives of surgery 1951;62(3):391–411.
7. Bague S, Folpe AL. Dermatofibrosarcoma protuberans presenting as a subcutaneous mass: a clinicopathological study of 15 cases with exclusive or near-exclusive subcutaneous involvement. Am J Dermatopathol 2008;30(4):327–32.
8. Calonje E, Fletcher CD. Myoid differentiation in dermatofibrosarcoma protuberans and its fibrosarcomatous variant: clinicopathologic analysis of 5 cases. J Cutan Pathol 1996;23(1):30–6.
9. Morimitsu Y, Hisaoka M, Okamoto S, et al. Dermatofibrosarcoma protuberans and its fibrosarcomatous variant with areas of myoid differentiation: a report of three cases. Histopathology [Case Reports Research Support, Non-U.S. Gov't] 1998;32(6):547–51.
10. Sanz-Trelles A, Ayala-Carbonero A, Rodrigo-Fernandez I, et al. Leiomyomatous nodules and bundles of vascular origin in the fibrosarcomatous variant of dermatofibrosarcoma protuberans. J Cutan Pathol 1998; 25(1):44–9.
11. Goldblum JR, Reith JD, Weiss SW. Sarcomas arising in dermatofibrosarcoma protuberans: a reappraisal of biologic behavior in eighteen cases treated by wide local excision with extended clinical follow up. Am J Surg Pathol 2000;24(8):1125–30.
12. O'Dowd J, Laidler P. Progression of dermatofibrosarcoma protuberans to malignant fibrous histiocytoma: report of a case with implications for tumor histogenesis. Hum Pathol [Case Reports] 1988;19(3): 368–70.
13. Goldblum JR, Tuthill RJ. CD34 and factor-XIIIa immunoreactivity in dermatofibrosarcoma protuberans and dermatofibroma. Am J Dermatopathol 1997;19(2):147–53.
14. Weiss SW, Nickoloff BJ. CD-34 is expressed by a distinctive cell population in peripheral nerve, nerve sheath tumors, and related lesions. Am J Surg Pathol 1993;17(10):1039–45.
15. West RB, Harvell J, Linn SC, et al. Apo D in soft tissue tumors: a novel marker for dermatofibrosarcoma protuberans. Am J Surg Pathol 2004; 28(8):1063–9.
16. Gutierrez G, Ospina JE, de Baez NE, et al. Dermatofibrosarcoma protuberans. Int J Dermatol [Comparative Study] 1984;23(6):396–401.
17. Alguacil-Garcia A, Unni KK, Goellner JR. Histogenesis of dermatofibrosarcoma protuberans. An ultrastructural study. Am J Clin Pathol 1978; 69(4):427–34.
18. Hashimoto K, Brownstein MH, Jakobiec FA. Dermatofibrosarcoma protuberans. A tumor with perineural and endoneural cell features. Arch Dermatol 1974;110(6):874–85.
19. Sirvent N, Maire G, Pedeutour F. Genetics of dermatofibrosarcoma protuberans family of tumors: from ring chromosomes to tyrosine kinase inhibitor treatment. Genes Chromosomes Cancer 2003;37(1):1–19.
20. Mandahl N, Heim S, Willen H, et al. Supernumerary ring chromosome as the sole cytogenetic abnormality in a dermatofibrosarcoma protuberans. Cancer Genet Cytogenet 1990;49(2):273–5.
21. Simon MP, Pedeutour F, Sirvent N, et al. Deregulation of the platelet-derived growth factor B-chain gene via fusion with collagen gene COL1A1 in dermatofibrosarcoma protuberans and giant-cell fibroblastoma. Nat Genet 1997;15(1):95–8.
22. Nishio J, Iwasaki H, Ohjimi Y, et al. Supernumerary ring chromosomes in dermatofibrosarcoma protuberans may contain sequences from 8q11.2-qter and 17q21-qter: a combined cytogenetic and comparative genomic hybridization study. Cancer Genet Cytogenet [Case Reports] 2001;129(2):102–6.
23. O'Brien KP, Seroussi E, Dal Cin P, et al. Various regions within the alpha-helical domain of the COL1A1 gene are fused to the second exon of the PDGFB gene in dermatofibrosarcomas and giant-cell fibroblastomas. Genes Chromosomes Cancer 1998;23(2):187–93.
24. Shimizu A, O'Brien KP, Sjoblom T, et al. The dermatofibrosarcoma protuberans-associated collagen type I alpha1/platelet-derived growth factor (PDGF) B-chain fusion gene generates a transforming protein that is processed to functional PDGF-BB. Cancer Res [Research Support, Non-U.S. Gov't] 1999;59(15):3719–23.
25. Li N, McNiff J, Hui P, et al. Differential expression of HMGA1 and HMGA2 in dermatofibroma and dermatofibrosarcoma protuberans: potential diagnostic applications, and comparison with histologic findings, CD34, and factor XIIIa immunoreactivity. Am J Dermatopathol [Comparative Study] 2004;26(4):267–72.
26. McPeak CJ, Cruz T, Nicastri AD. Dermatofibrosarcoma protuberans: an analysis of 86 cases–five with metastasis. Ann Surg 1967;166(5): 803–16.
27. Fiore M, Miceli R, Mussi C, et al. Dermatofibrosarcoma protuberans treated at a single institution: a surgical disease with a high cure rate. J Clin Oncol [Comparative Study Review] 2005;23(30):7669–75.
28. Gloster HM Jr., Harris KR, Roenigk RK. A comparison between Mohs micrographic surgery and wide surgical excision for the treatment of dermatofibrosarcoma protuberans. J Am Acad Dermatol 1996; 35(1):82–7.
29. Burkhardt BR, Soule EH, Winkelmann RK, et al. Dermatofibrosarcoma protuberans. Study of fifty-six cases. Am J Surg [Case Reports] 1966; 111(5):638–44.
30. Roses DF, Valensi Q, LaTrenta G, et al. Surgical treatment of dermatofibrosarcoma protuberans. Surg Gynecol Obstet 1986;162(5):449–52.
31. Robinson JK. Dermatofibrosarcoma protuberans resected by Mohs' surgery (chemosurgery). A 5-year prospective study. J Am Acad Dermatol [Case Reports Research Support, Non-U.S. Gov't] 1985;12(6): 1093–8.
32. Nouri K, Lodha R, Jimenez G, et al. Mohs micrographic surgery for dermatofibrosarcoma protuberans: University of Miami and NYU experience. Dermatol Surg 2002;28(11):1060–4; discussion 1064.
33. Wacker J, Khan-Durani B, Hartschuh W. Modified Mohs micrographic surgery in the therapy of dermatofibrosarcoma protuberans: analysis of 22 patients. Ann Surg Oncol 2004;11(4):438–44.
34. Snow SN, Gordon EM, Larson PO, et al. Dermatofibrosarcoma protuberans: a report on 29 patients treated by Mohs micrographic surgery with long-term follow-up and review of the literature. Cancer 2004; 101(1):28–38.
35. Ah-Weng A, Marsden JR, Sanders DS, et al. Dermatofibrosarcoma protuberans treated by micrographic surgery. Br J Cancer [Comparative Study Review] 2002;87(12):1386–9.
36. Ratner D, Thomas CO, Johnson TM, et al. Mohs micrographic surgery for the treatment of dermatofibrosarcoma protuberans. Results of a multiinstitutional series with an analysis of the extent of microscopic spread. J Am Acad Dermatol 1997;37(4):600–13.
37. Kahn LB, Saxe N, Gordon W. Dermatofibrosarcoma protuberans with lymph node and pulmonary metastases. Arch Dermatol [Case Reports] 1978;114(4):599–601.
38. Suit H, Spiro I, Mankin HJ, et al. Radiation in management of patients with dermatofibrosarcoma protuberans. J Clin Oncol 1996;14(8): 2365–9.
39. Rubin BP, Schuetze SM, Eary JF, et al. Molecular targeting of platelet-derived growth factor B by imatinib mesylate in a patient with metastatic dermatofibrosarcoma protuberans. J Clin Oncol 2002;20(17):3586–91.
40. McArthur GA, Demetri GD, van Oosterom A, et al. Molecular and clinical analysis of locally advanced dermatofibrosarcoma protuberans treated with imatinib: Imatinib Target Exploration Consortium Study B2225. J Clin Oncol 2005;23(4):866–73.
41. Labropoulos SV, Fletcher JA, Oliveira AM, et al. Sustained complete remission of metastatic dermatofibrosarcoma protuberans with imatinib mesylate. Anticancer Drugs 2005;16(4):461–6.
42. Mentzel T, Beham A, Katenkamp D, et al. Fibrosarcomatous ("high-grade") dermatofibrosarcoma protuberans: clinicopathologic and immunohistochemical study of a series of 41 cases with emphasis on prognostic significance. Am J Surg Pathol 1998;22(5):576–87.
43. Wrotnowski U, Cooper PH, Shmookler BM. Fibrosarcomatous change in dermatofibrosarcoma protuberans. Am J Surg Pathol 1988;12(4): 287–93.
44. Ding J, Hashimoto H, Enjoji M. Dermatofibrosarcoma protuberans with fibrosarcomatous areas. A clinicopathologic study of nine cases and a comparison with allied tumors. Cancer [Comparative Study] 1989;64(3): 721–9.
45. Connelly JH, Evans HL. Dermatofibrosarcoma protuberans. A clinicopathologic review with emphasis on fibrosarcomatous areas. Am J Surg Pathol 1992;16(10):921–5.
46. Pizarro GB, Fanburg JC, Miettinen M. Dermatofibrosarcoma protuberans (DFSP) with fibrosarcomatous transformation: re-explored. Mod Pathol 1997;10.
47. Abbott JJ, Oliveira AM, Nascimento AG. The prognostic significance of fibrosarcomatous transformation in dermatofibrosarcoma protuberans. Am J Surg Pathol 2006;30(4):436–43.

48. Diaz-Cascajo C, Weyers W, Borrego L, et al. Dermatofibrosarcoma protuberans with fibrosarcomatous areas: a clinico-pathologic and immunohistochemic study in four cases. Am J Dermatopathol 1997;19(6):562–7.
49. O'Connell JX, Trotter MJ. Fibrosarcomatous dermatofibrosarcoma protuberans with myofibroblastic differentiaion: a histologically distinctive variant [corrected]. Mod Pathol [Case Reports] 1996;9(3):273–8.
50. Bednar B. Storiform neurofibromas of the skin, pigmented and nonpigmented. Cancer 1957;10(2):368–76.
51. Bednar B. Storiform neurofibroma in the core of naevocellular naevi. J Pathol 1970;101(2):199–201.
52. Ding JA, Hashimoto H, Sugimoto T, et al. Bednar tumor (pigmented dermatofibrosarcoma protuberans). An analysis of six cases. Acta Pathol Jpn [Case Reports Research Support, Non-U.S. Gov't] 1990;40(10):744–54.
53. Dupree WB, Langloss JM, Weiss SW. Pigmented dermatofibrosarcoma protuberans (Bednar tumor). A pathologic, ultrastructural, and immunohistochemical study. Am J Surg Pathol 1985;9(9):630–9.
54. Fletcher CD, Theaker JM, Flanagan A, et al. Pigmented dermatofibrosarcoma protuberans (Bednar tumour): melanocytic colonization or neuroectodermal differentiation? A clinicopathological and immunohistochemical study. Histopathology 1988;13(6):631–43.
55. Tsuneyoshi M, Ding JA, Hashimoto H, et al. Bednar tumor (pigmented dermatofibrosarcoma protuberans). An analysis of six cases. Acta Pathol Jpn [Case Reports Research Support, Non-U.S. Gov't] 1990;40(10):744–54.
56. Wang J, Hisaoka M, Shimajiri S, et al. Detection of COL1A1-PDGFB fusion transcripts in dermatofibrosarcoma protuberans by reverse transcription-polymerase chain reaction using archival formalin-fixed, paraffin-embedded tissues. Diagn Mol Pathol 1999;8(3):113–9.
57. Bisceglia M, Vairo M, Calonje E, et al. [Pigmented fibrosarcomatous dermatofibrosarcoma protuberans (Bednar tumor). 3 case reports, analogy with the "conventional" type and review of the literature]. Pathologica [Case Reports Review] 1997;89(3):264–73.
58. Onoda N, Tsutsumi Y, Kakudo K, et al. Pigmented dermatofibrosarcoma protuberans (Bednar tumor). An autopsy case with systemic metastasis. Acta Pathol Jpn [Case Reports] 1990;40(12):935–40.
59. Ozawa A, Niizuma K, Onkido M, et al. Pigmented dermatofibrosarcoma protuberans: an analysis of six cases. Acta Pathol Jpn 1990;40:935.
60. Shmookler BM, Enzinger FM, Weiss SW. Giant cell fibroblastoma. A juvenile form of dermatofibrosarcoma protuberans. Cancer 1989;64(10):2154–61.
61. Abdul-Karim FW, Evans HL, Silva EG. Giant cell fibroblastoma: a report of three cases. Am J Clin Pathol [Case Reports] 1985;83(2):165–70.
62. Barr RJ, Young EM Jr., Liao SY. Giant cell fibroblastoma: an immunohistochemical study. J Cutan Pathol [Case Reports] 1986;13(4):301–7.
63. Chou P, Gonzalez-Crussi F, Mangkornkanok M. Giant cell fibroblastoma. Cancer [Case Reports Review] 1989;63(4):756–62.
64. Dymock RB, Allen PW, Stirling JW, et al. Giant cell fibroblastoma. A distinctive, recurrent tumor of childhood. Am J Surg Pathol 1987;11(4):263–71.
65. Kanai Y, Mukai M, Sugiura H, et al. Giant cell fibroblastoma. A case report and immunohistochemical comparison with ten cases of dermatofibrosarcoma protuberans. Acta Pathol Jpn [Case Reports Comparative Study] 1991;41(7):552–60.
66. Michal M, Zamecnik M. Giant cell fibroblastoma with a dermatofibrosarcoma protuberans component. Am J Dermatopathol 1992;14(6):549–52.
67. Nair R, Kane SV, Borges A, et al. Giant cell fibroblastoma. J Surg Oncol [Case Reports Review] 1993;53(2):136–9.
68. Rosen LB, Amazon K, Weitzner J, et al. Giant cell fibroblastoma. A report of a case and review of the literature. Am J Dermatopathol [Review] 1989;11(3):242–7.
69. Alguacil-Garcia A. Giant cell fibroblastoma recurring as dermatofibrosarcoma protuberans. Am J Surg Pathol 1991;15(8):798–801.
70. Allen PW, Zwi J. Giant cell fibroblastoma transforming into dermatofibrosarcoma protuberans. Am J Surg Pathol [Case Reports Letter] 1992;16(11):1127–9.
71. Beham A, Fletcher CD. Dermatofibrosarcoma protuberans with areas resembling giant cell fibroblastoma: report of two cases. Histopathology 1990;17(2):165–7.
72. Coyne J, Kaftan SM, Craig RD. Dermatofibrosarcoma protuberans recurring as a giant cell fibroblastoma. Histopathology [Case Reports] 1992;21(2):184–7.
73. Maeda T, Hirose T, Furuya K, et al. Giant cell fibroblastoma associated with dermatofibrosarcoma protuberans: a case report. Mod Pathol 1998;11(5):491–5.
74. Dal Cin P, Sciot R, de Wever I, et al. Cytogenetic and immunohistochemical evidence that giant cell fibroblastoma is related to dermatofibrosarcoma protuberans. Genes Chromosomes Cancer [Research Support, Non-U.S. Gov't] 1996;15(1):73–5.
75. Fletcher CD. Giant cell fibroblastoma of soft tissue: a clinicopathological and immunohistochemical study. Histopathology 1988;13(5):499–508.
76. Enzinger FM. Angiomatoid malignant fibrous histiocytoma: a distinct fibrohistiocytic tumor of children and young adults simulating a vascular neoplasm. Cancer 1979;44(6):2147–57.
77. Davies KA, Cope AP, Schofield JB, et al. A rare mediastinal tumour presenting with systemic effects due to IL-6 and tumour necrosis factor (TNF) production. Clin Exp Immunol 1995;99(1):117–23.
78. Costa MJ, Weiss SW. Angiomatoid malignant fibrous histiocytoma. A follow-up study of 108 cases with evaluation of possible histologic predictors of outcome. Am J Surg Pathol 1990;14(12):1126–32.
79. Pettinato G, Manivel JC, De Rosa G, et al. Angiomatoid malignant fibrous histiocytoma: cytologic, immunohistochemical, ultrastructural, and flow cytometric study of 20 cases. Mod Pathol [Research Support, Non-U.S. Gov't] 1990;3(4):479–87.
80. Fanburg-Smith JC, Miettinen M. Angiomatoid "malignant" fibrous histiocytoma: a clinicopathologic study of 158 cases and further exploration of the myoid phenotype. Hum Pathol 1999;30(11):1336–43.
81. el-Naggar AK, Ro JY, Ayala AG, et al. Angiomatoid malignant fibrous histiocytoma: flow cytometric DNA analysis of six cases. J Surg Oncol 1989;40(3):201–4.
82. Fletcher CD. Angiomatoid "malignant fibrous histiocytoma": an immunohistochemical study indicative of myoid differentiation. Hum Pathol 1991;22(6):563–8.
83. Waters BL, Panagopoulos I, Allen EF. Genetic characterization of angiomatoid fibrous histiocytoma identifies fusion of the FUS and ATF-1 genes induced by a chromosomal translocation involving bands 12q13 and 16p11. Cancer Genet Cytogenet 2000;121(2):109–16.
84. Hallor KH, Mertens F, Jin Y, et al. Fusion of the EWSR1 and ATF1 genes without expression of the MITF-M transcript in angiomatoid fibrous histiocytoma. Genes Chromosomes Cancer 2005;44(1):97–102.
85. Raddaoui E, Donner LR, Panagopoulos I. Fusion of the FUS and ATF1 genes in a large, deep-seated angiomatoid fibrous histiocytoma. Diagn Mol Pathol 2002;11(3):157–62.
86. Rossi S, Szuhai K, Ijszenga M, et al. EWSR1-CREB1 and EWSR1-ATF1 fusion genes in angiomatoid fibrous histiocytoma. Clin Cancer Res 2007;13(24):7322–8.
87. Antonescu CR, Dal Cin P, Nafa K, et al. EWSR1-CREB1 is the predominant gene fusion in angiomatoid fibrous histiocytoma. Genes Chromosomes Cancer 2007;46(12):1051–60.
88. Antonescu CR, Katabi N, Zhang L, et al. EWSR1-ATF1 fusion is a novel and consistent finding in hyalinizing clear-cell carcinoma of salivary gland. Genes Chromosomes Cancer 2011;50(7):559–70.
89. Enzinger FM, Zhang RY. Plexiform fibrohistiocytic tumor presenting in children and young adults. An analysis of 65 cases. Am J Surg Pathol 1988;12(11):818–26.
90. Hollowood K, Holley MP, Fletcher CD. Plexiform fibrohistiocytic tumour: clinicopathological, immunohistochemical and ultrastructural analysis in favour of a myofibroblastic lesion. Histopathology 1991;19(6):503–13.
91. Remstein ED, Arndt CA, Nascimento AG. Plexiform fibrohistiocytic tumor: clinicopathologic analysis of 22 cases. Am J Surg Pathol 1999;23(6):662–70.
92. Redlich GC, Montgomery KD, Allgood GA, et al. Plexiform fibrohistiocytic tumor with a clonal cytogenetic anomaly. Cancer Genet Cytogenet 1999;108(2):141–3.
93. Smith S, Fletcher CD, Smith MA, et al. Cytogenetic analysis of a plexiform fibrohistiocytic tumor. Cancer Genet Cytogenet 1990;48(1):31–4.
94. Angervall L, Kindblom LG, Lindholm K, et al. Plexiform fibrohistiocytic tumor. Report of a case involving preoperative aspiration cytology and immunohistochemical and ultrastructural analysis of surgical specimens. Pathol Res Pract 1992;188(3):350–6; discussion 356–359.
95. Giard F, Bonneau R, Raymond GP. Plexiform fibrohistiocytic tumor. Dermatologica [Case Reports Research Support, Non-U.S. Gov't] 1991;183(4):290–3.

96. Folpe AL, Morris RJ, Weiss SW. Soft tissue giant cell tumor of low malignant potential: a proposal for the reclassification of malignant giant cell tumor of soft parts. Mod Pathol 1999;12(9):894–902.
97. Guccion JG, Enzinger FM. Malignant giant cell tumor of soft parts. An analysis of 32 cases. Cancer 1972;29(6):1518–29.
98. Salm R, Sissons HA. Giant-cell tumours of soft tissues. J Pathol 1972;107(1):27–39.
99. O'Connell JX, Wehrli BM, Nielsen GP, et al. Giant cell tumors of soft tissue: a clinicopathologic study of 18 benign and malignant tumors. Am J Surg Pathol 2000;24(3):386–95.
100. Oliveira AM, Dei Tos AP, Fletcher CD, et al. Primary giant cell tumor of soft tissues: a study of 22 cases. Am J Surg Pathol 2000;24(2):248–56.

Undifferentiated Pleomorphic Sarcoma

CHAPTER CONTENTS

The concept of malignant fibrous histiocytoma (MFH) has undergone significant change over the past five decades. The term was first introduced in 1963 to refer to a group of soft tissue tumors, characterized by a storiform or cartwheel-like growth pattern, which were believed to be derived from histiocytes on the basis of early tissue culture studies demonstrating ameboid movement and phagocytosis of explanted tumor cells.[1,2] Ultrastructural studies both endorsed and refuted the histiocytic origin of these tumors, however. With the advent of immunohistochemistry and the accessibility of numerous monoclonal antibodies directed against various structural proteins of specific cell types, the phenotype of this tumor was shown to be more closely aligned with a fibroblast than a histiocyte.[3-6] Furthermore, many, but not all, lesions labeled as *malignant fibrous histiocytoma* could, upon close scrutiny, be subclassified as lineage-specific sarcomas, an observation that led some to question the existence of MFH as a distinct entity.[7] The extent to which such lesions can be subclassified as sarcomas of alternative type is, in large part, dependent on definitional criteria and the number of ancillary studies that a pathologist is willing to bring to bear on the evaluation of a pleomorphic sarcoma. There is still no general agreement as to what percentage of pleomorphic sarcomas, when subjected to rigorous evaluation, remain unclassified. Recent studies report percentages from 20% to 70%.[8-11] The largest study to date, published by the Swedish Sarcoma Group, indicates that of the 338 cases referred centrally with a diagnosis of MFH, the diagnosis was confirmed in 70% after reevaluation and additional immunohistochemistry.[11] These discrepancies, nonetheless, underscore that the criteria by which a pleomorphic tumor is provisionally labeled as an undifferentiated pleomorphic sarcoma (UPS/MFH) as well as the criteria by which some are reclassified differ from institution to institution.

Whatever the true incidence of this lesion, there is agreement that the term *MFH* should be used synonymously with *UPS* which, by a combination of sampling and immunohistochemistry, shows no definable line of differentiation and, by electron microscopy, manifests fibroblastic/myofibroblastic features.[10,12,13] As increasingly more advanced technologies are brought to bear on the evaluation of pleomorphic sarcomas, this definition may well change. In this regard, it has been shown with comparative genomic hybridization studies that most, if not all, retroperitoneal MFH of the storiform and inflammatory type are actually dedifferentiated liposarcomas.[14-16]

At this point, the term *undifferentiated pleomorphic sarcoma* is used in diagnostic reports, but it is synonymous with so-called MFH, which may be given in parentheses to avert any misunderstanding with clinicians who continue to be familiar with that term.

PLEOMORPHIC SARCOMA WITH A SPECIFIC LINE OF DIFFERENTIATION

A variety of pleomorphic sarcomas may have areas that resemble UPS. In some cases, determining the specific line of differentiation may rely on random sampling of a small area within a large tumor. Although a specific type of pleomorphic sarcoma may be suggested by histologic features, immunohistochemical stains are often required to confirm the diagnosis. Although it could be argued that subtyping pleomorphic sarcomas is nothing more than an academic exercise, there is some evidence to suggest that pleomorphic sarcomas with myoid differentiation are more clinically aggressive than those without myoid differentiation.[8,9]

The only criterion for rendering a diagnosis of *pleomorphic liposarcoma* is the recognition of multivacuolated pleomorphic lipoblasts. The major difficulty in such cases is separating pleomorphic sarcomas that infiltrate fat and isolate individual cells from those with true lipoblasts. *Pleomorphic leiomyosarcoma* is composed of cells with distinct cytoplasmic eosinophilia. At least focally, most cases have areas with a fascicular arrangement and cells with blunt-ended nuclei with a perinuclear vacuole and deeply eosinophilic cytoplasm. *Pleomorphic rhabdomyosarcoma* is recognized by the presence of large cells with eosinophilic cytoplasm and cross striations that can be confirmed by the immunohistochemical demonstration of skeletal muscle differentiation (desmin, MyoD1, myogenin). A definitive diagnosis of *pleomorphic malignant peripheral nerve sheath tumor* can be difficult unless the pleomorphic sarcoma clearly arises from a benign nerve sheath tumor or arises from a peripheral nerve in a patient with type 1 neurofibromatosis. The only criterion for recognizing *extraskeletal osteosarcoma* is the production of osteoid or bone by cytologically malignant cells.

The process of tumor progression or dedifferentiation involves the transformation of a low-grade sarcoma to a higher-grade sarcoma, which usually (but not always) resembles a UPS. The most common scenario is the progression of a low-grade, well-differentiated liposarcoma to a pleomorphic sarcoma (dedifferentiated liposarcoma). Other low-grade neoplasms can also dedifferentiate, including chondrosarcomas, chordomas, and parosteal osteosarcomas. Certainly in a limited biopsy specimen, it can be impossible to prove that a pleomorphic sarcoma is part of a dedifferentiated sarcoma if the low-grade component is not represented. However, in a retroperitoneal sarcoma where dedifferentiated liposarcoma is always a strong consideration, it can often be suggested that the high-grade sarcoma could be part of a dedifferentiated liposarcoma. Unfortunately, even *MDM2* or *CDK4* amplification does not prove that a given lesion is part of a dedifferentiated liposarcoma because other types of pleomorphic sarcomas can show amplification of these genes.[17,18] The clinical significance of distinguishing a dedifferentiated liposarcoma from a *de novo* pleomorphic sarcoma is not clear, but some have suggested that the former is a more indolent tumor than the latter.[19]

It can be exceedingly difficult to distinguish a UPS from a *sarcomatoid carcinoma*. A reasonable approach would be to assume that a pleomorphic malignant neoplasm arising in the skin, mucosal surface, or parenchymal organ is a sarcomatoid carcinoma, until proven otherwise. A battery of epithelial markers, including broad-spectrum, low- and high- molecular weight cytokeratins is required, but equivocal results are not uncommon for several reasons. First, not all sarcomatoid carcinomas show the immunohistochemical expression of epithelial markers. Second, virtually any type of sarcoma, including UPS, can, on occasion, express cytokeratins. Strong and diffuse cytokeratin expression, especially with multiple antibodies, strongly supports a diagnosis of sarcomatoid carcinoma, as does the recognition of an intraepithelial/intramucosal dysplastic component. In the end, some cases are not resolvable and can be diagnosed as only a pleomorphic malignant neoplasm, sarcoma versus carcinoma. It should also be kept in mind that, on occasion, *sarcomatoid mesothelioma, melanoma,* and *anaplastic lymphoma* can mimic UPS; a panel of markers, including CAM5.2, S-100 protein, melanocytic markers such as HMB45 and Melan A, CD30 and ALK1 can help resolve these issues. Following the exclusion of the aforementioned scenarios, one is left with UPS as a diagnosis of exclusion, the details of which are described in the following sections.

ATYPICAL FIBROXANTHOMA (UNDIFFERENTIATED PLEOMORPHIC SARCOMA OF THE SKIN)

Atypical fibroxanthoma is a cutaneous UPS that typically occurs on sun-damaged, actinic skin of the elderly.[20,21] Its superficial location has generally been credited with its excellent clinical outcome. The diagnosis of atypical fibroxanthoma needs to be strictly defined so that it does not include other pleomorphic tumors of the skin (e.g., melanoma) or deeply invasive sarcomas that are well known to have metastatic potential.

Clinical Findings

Atypical fibroxanthomas typically occur on the exposed surface of the head and neck, particularly the nose, cheek, and ear of elderly individuals. Those rare atypical fibroxanthomas thought to occur on the extremities of young individuals are now thought to be examples of atypical fibrous histiocytomas (see Chapter 11). Solar and therapeutic radiations are strong predisposing factors in the pathogenesis of this disease. This belief is supported by the common occurrence of the tumor on sun-damaged skin, its frequent association with other actinic lesions (e.g., basal cell carcinoma, squamous carcinoma), and the identification of both ultraviolet related mutations and photoproducts within these lesions.[22-24] The incidence of previous irradiation varies from less than 5% in some series[21] to more than 50% in others.[25] In most instances, the latent period between the previous radiation exposure and the appearance of the atypical fibroxanthoma is more than 10 years and, therefore, well in keeping with the accepted interval for a radiation-induced tumor. Some cases arise in immunosuppressed patients; this tumor has been reported in HIV-positive patients[26] and transplant patients taking immunosuppressive agents.[27]

Pathologic Findings

Grossly, the lesions are solitary nodules or ulcers usually measuring less than 2 cm in diameter (Figs. 13-1 and 13-2). Their appearance is not distinctive, and, for this reason, a variety of preoperative diagnoses is considered, including basal cell carcinoma, squamous cell carcinoma, pyogenic granuloma, and sebaceous cyst.

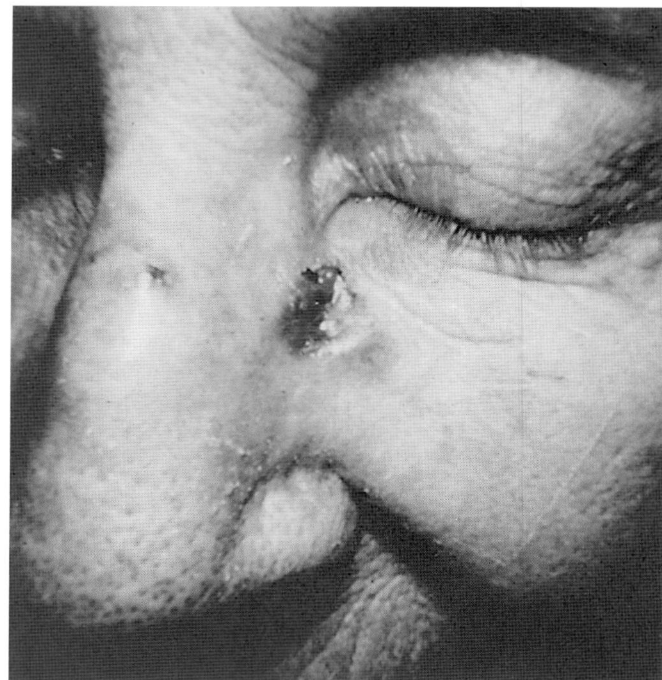

FIGURE 13-1. Ulcerating atypical fibroxanthoma from the nose of an 80-year-old woman. Grossly, the tumor resembled a basal cell carcinoma. *(From Fretzin DF, Helwig EB. Atypical fibroxanthoma of the skin. Cancer 1973;31(6):1541.)*

These tumors are expansile dermal nodules that abut the epidermis, causing pressure atrophy or ulceration (Fig. 13-3). Alternatively, a *grenz* zone of uninvolved dermis is present. The tumor compresses the skin appendages laterally and extends into the subcutis. By definition, the tumor does not extensively involve the subcutis, and it does not invade deeper structures such as fascia or muscle. Areas adjacent to these lesions typically display solar elastosis, vascular dilatation, and capillary proliferation.

Histologically, these tumors resemble UPS, although some can have a more monomorphic fascicular appearance resembling a fibrosarcoma. Most are characterized by bizarre cells arranged in a haphazard or vaguely fascicular pattern (Fig. 13-4). Rarely, a storiform pattern is evident. The cells are spindle-shaped or round, and they exhibit multinucleation, pleomorphism, and numerous typical and atypical mitotic figures. The cells occasionally have small droplets of neutral fat and periodic acid-Schiff (PAS)-positive, diastase-resistant material, two features that probably reflect, in part, degenerative changes. Hemorrhage is occasionally prominent and may lead to extensive hemosiderin deposits that should be distinguished from melanin. Secondary changes, which may rarely be present, include chronic inflammatory cells, prominent stromal myxoid change, osteoclast-like giant cells, osteoid deposition,[28-30] prominent clear cell,[31,32] or granular cell change (Fig. 13-5).[33] Keloidal collagen may be present,[34,35] and some cases show extensive stromal hyalinization, suggesting tumor regression.[36]

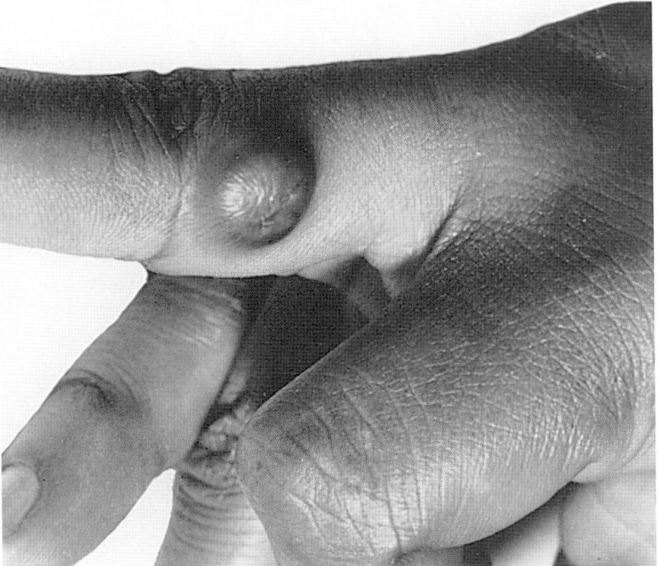

FIGURE 13-2. Nodular atypical fibroxanthoma from the finger of a 36-year-old woman. Atypical fibroxanthomas in young patients typically occur on the extremities, in contrast to those in elderly patients, which are located on sun-exposed or actinic-damaged surfaces. *(From Fretzin DF, Helwig EB. Atypical fibroxanthoma of the skin. Cancer 1973;31(6):1541.)*

Immunohistochemically, atypical fibroxanthoma is typically negative for both S-100 protein and cytokeratins, allowing distinction from melanoma and spindled squamous cell carcinoma. However, rare cases can show scattered cytokeratin-positive cells,[37] although they are usually negative for high-molecular-weight cytokeratins (e.g., CK5/6) and p63, both markers that are frequently expressed in spindled squamous cell carcinomas.[38,39] Most cases of atypical fibroxanthoma also show strong expression of CD10,[40,41] but this marker lacks specificity; most cases of benign fibrous histiocytoma also express this antigen, as do rare cases of spindled squamous cell carcinoma. Other markers that may be expressed in some cases of atypical fibroxanthoma include CD99,[42,43] CD163,[44] and CD117,[45] although none of these markers is specific in distinguishing it from its histologic mimics. Some cases express smooth muscle actin, although desmin is usually negative,[46] consistent with focal myofibroblastic differentiation.

Differential Diagnosis

Because the diagnosis of atypical fibroxanthoma implies a biologically innocuous lesion, it is important that it be carefully distinguished from superficial forms of other pleomorphic sarcoma that have some capacity for distant metastasis. If a

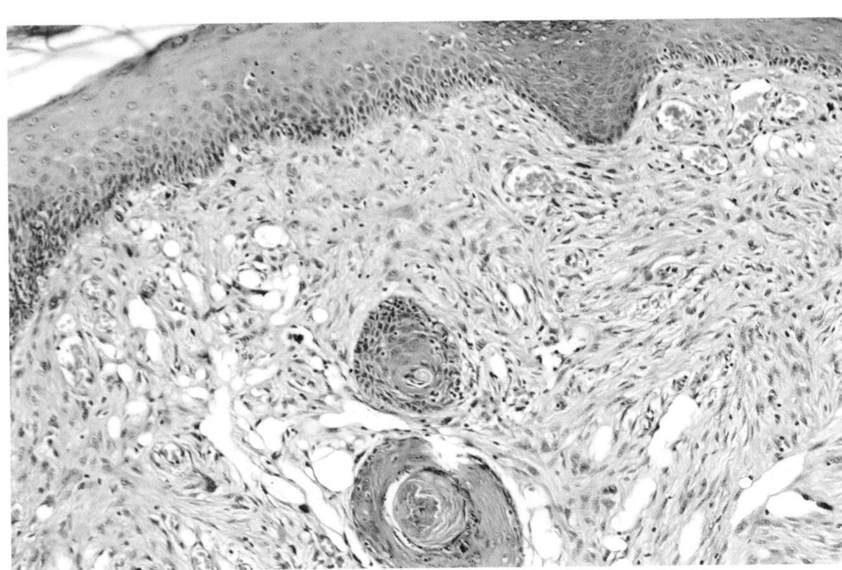

FIGURE 13-3. Atypical fibroxanthoma abutting epidermis. Dilated capillaries are commonly seen adjacent to and in the tumor.

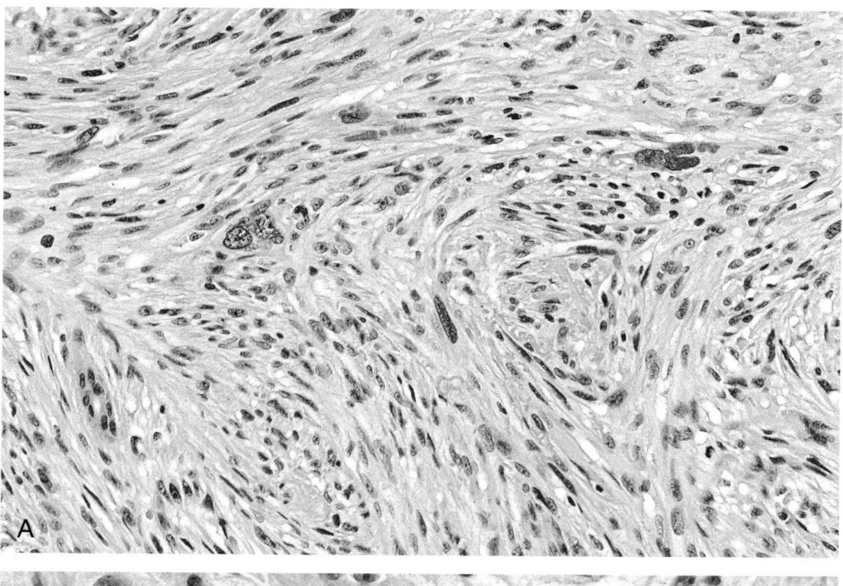

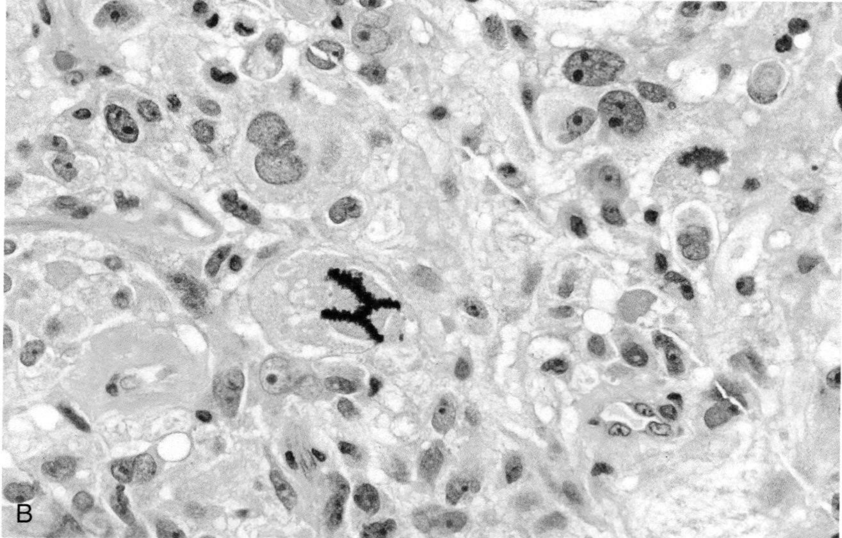

FIGURE 13-4. Bizarre cells comprising atypical fibroxanthoma vary from plump spindled cells to large round cells. (A) Pleomorphism is marked; and mitotic figures, including atypical forms, are common (B).

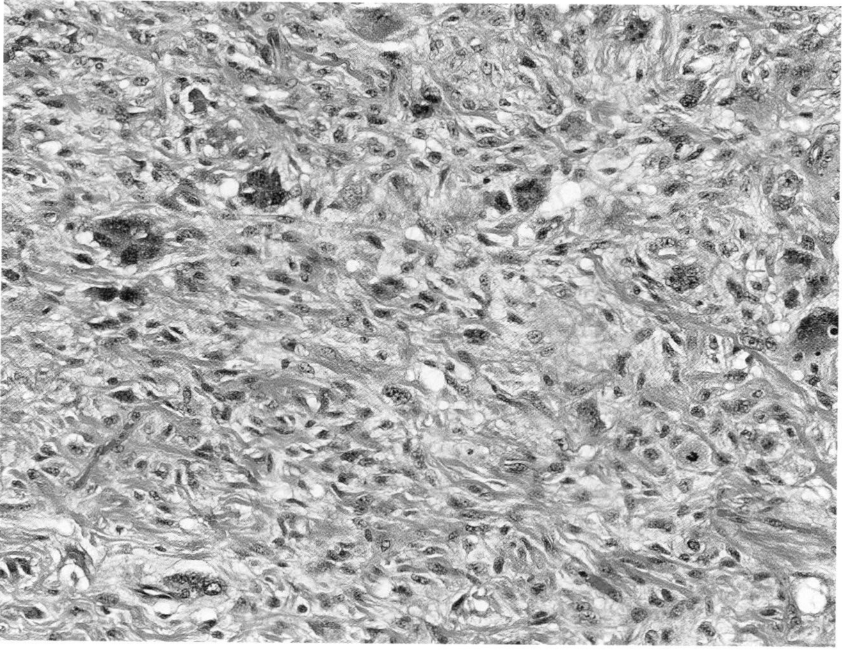

FIGURE 13-5. High-magnification view of atypical fibroxanthoma with multinucleated cells and xanthoma cells.

tumor is large (greater than 2 cm), extensively involves the subcutis, penetrates fascia and muscle, or displays necrosis or vascular invasion, it should be diagnosed as a UPS because such tumors run a definite risk of recurrence and metastasis. Most cases of so-called metastasizing atypical fibroxanthoma are likely lesions more appropriately diagnosed as *superficial undifferentiated pleomorphic sarcoma*.

In assessing a pleomorphic tumor of the skin, immunostains are essential to rule out a carcinoma, melanoma, angiosarcoma, and pleomorphic leiomyosarcoma. The usual primary immunohistochemical panel includes pancytokeratin and high-molecular-weight cytokeratins (CK5/6) and S-100 protein, whereas a secondary panel might include actin, desmin, CD31 and ERG (vascular markers), and melanocytic markers, depending on the appearance of the lesion and the results of the first panel. One should be reminded that S-100 protein-positive dendritic cells and CD31-positive histiocytes may be encountered in atypical fibroxanthomas and should be carefully distinguished from the lesional cells.

Discussion

Although this tumor is histologically indistinguishable from a superficial UPS, it deserves a special designation because of its almost uniformly excellent prognosis following conservative therapy. In one of the largest series in the literature, only 9 of 140 patients had a recurrence, and none developed metastasis.[21] A slightly smaller series documented no recurrences or metastasis among 89 patients.[47] In a recent large series of 171 cases from Australia, Beer et al.[48] found local recurrences in 2 cases only, and no patient developed metastatic disease. Although wide local excision is typically effective in most patients, there does appear to be a lower rate of local recurrence in those patients treated with Mohs micrographic surgery.[49,50]

UNDIFFERENTIATED PLEOMORPHIC SARCOMA

Depending on definitional criteria, UPS still accounts for a significant proportion of sarcomas occurring in late adult life.[11,51] It manifests a broad range of histologic appearances, although the most common form consists of a mixture of storiform and pleomorphic areas. Up to 25% show prominent myxoid stroma. These tumors were formerly referred to as *myxoid MFH* but now are more appropriately diagnosed as high-grade myxofibrosarcoma.

Much of the remainder of the chapter will focus on the approach to a pleomorphic malignant neoplasm which, at first glance, might be easily classified as a UPS. There are three major considerations when one encounters such a lesion. First, the lesion in question may well be a pleomorphic sarcoma, but, with close inspection of routine-stained sections and/or immunohistochemical studies, can be more precisely classified as a specific type of pleomorphic sarcoma (e.g., pleomorphic leiomyosarcoma, pleomorphic liposarcoma). Second, the MFH-like lesion may be part of a dedifferentiated sarcoma. The most common scenario is that of a well-differentiated liposarcoma (often retroperitoneal) that progresses to a pleomorphic sarcoma without an identifiable line of differentiation. Third, and most important, the pleomorphic neoplasm in question may represent a nonsarcoma, most commonly a sarcomatoid carcinoma, but rarely a sarcomatoid mesothelioma, melanoma, or even an anaplastic lymphoma. This distinction of course has major therapeutic and prognostic implications and, as such, consideration of a pseudosarcomatous neoplastic process should be given in every case. Finally, if all of the previous scenarios are excluded, then one can arrive at a diagnosis of UPS.

Clinical Findings

UPS is characteristically a tumor of late adult life, with most cases occurring in persons between the ages of 50 and 70 years.[51] Tumors in children are exceedingly rare, and this diagnosis should always be made with caution in patients under 20 years of age. Approximately two-thirds occur in men, and whites are affected more often than blacks or Asians. The tumor occurs most frequently on the lower extremity (Figs. 13-6 and 13-7), especially the thigh, followed by the upper extremity, usually as a painless, slowly enlarging mass. As with other sarcomas, growth rate acceleration has been observed during pregnancy.[52] In contrast to patients with lesions of the extremity, patients with retroperitoneal tumors develop constitutional symptoms, including anorexia, malaise, weight loss, and signs of increasing abdominal pressure. As mentioned previously, careful sampling and microscopic observation is necessary in retroperitoneal lesions to exclude dedifferentiated liposarcoma, a lesion that is far more common than de novo UPS in this location.

Occasionally, fever and leukocytosis with neutrophilia or eosinophilia dominate the clinical presentation of this disease. This unusual constellation of symptoms has been documented for the inflammatory type of UPS, a lesion formerly referred to as *inflammatory MFH*. Given that the inflammatory variant

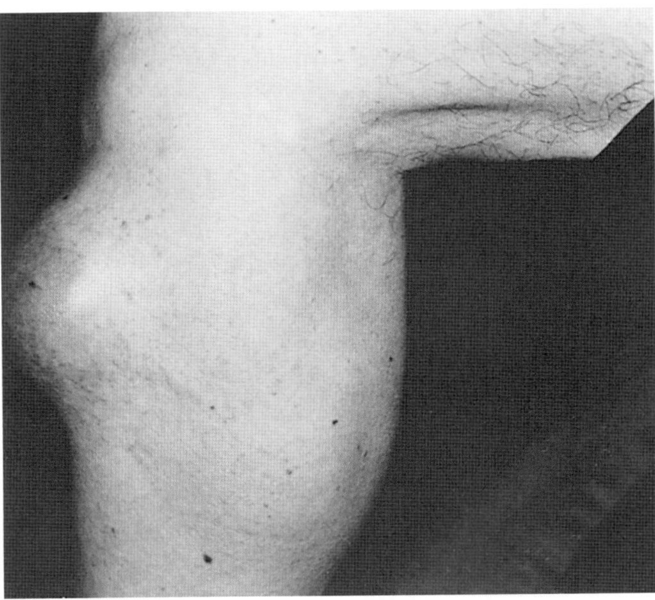

FIGURE 13-6. Undifferentiated pleomorphic sarcoma of the lower leg of a 62-year-old man. *(From Guccion JG, Enzinger FM. Malignant giant cell tumor of soft parts: an analysis of 32 cases. Cancer 1972;29(6): 1518.)*

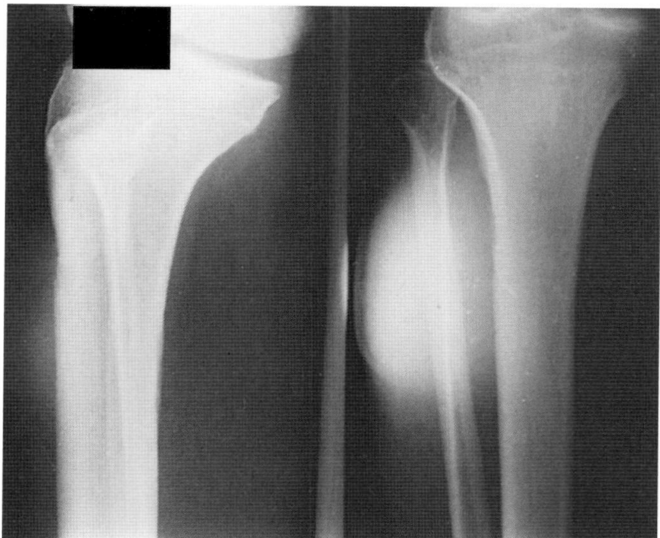

FIGURE 13-7. Radiograph showing an undifferentiated pleomorphic sarcoma of the lower leg (same case as in Figure 13-6). Ill-defined soft tissue mass has eroded a portion of the tibial cortex.

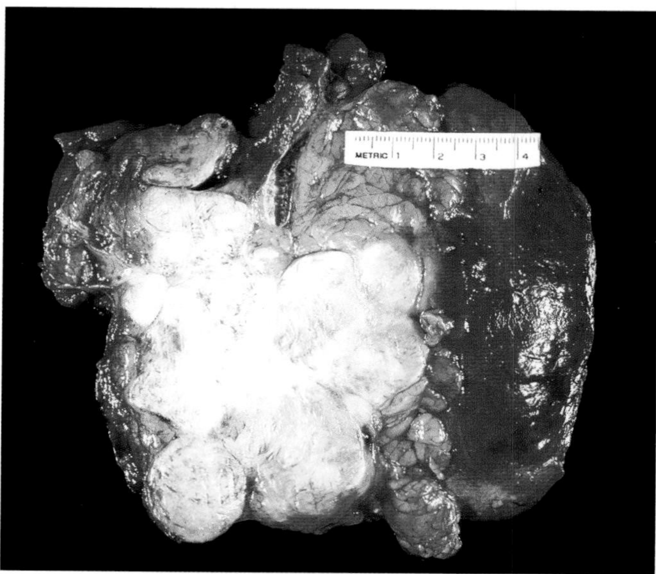

FIGURE 13-8. Gross appearance of an undifferentiated pleomorphic sarcoma of the retroperitoneum. The tumor is a multinodular white mass arising adjacent to the kidney.

of this condition virtually always arises in the retroperitoneum, a similar principle applies as was mentioned previously—that is, to assume the lesion represents the dedifferentiated component of a dedifferentiated liposarcoma until proven otherwise.[14] These paraneoplastic signs and symptoms appear to be the result of a tumor-related production of cytokines, including interleukins (IL-6 and IL-8) and tumor necrosis factor.[53] The symptoms usually remit following removal of the tumor. Rarely, hypoglycemia occurs in association with this disease and may be secondary to tumor production of insulin-like growth factor.[54] UPS rarely presents as a metastatic tumor without a clinically evident primary lesion, although a small percentage of patients presents with synchronous primary and metastatic disease.

Etiologic Factors

Like atypical fibroxanthomas, there is strong circumstantial evidence that some of these tumors are radiation-induced. Aside from these iatrogenic tumors, there are few data on etiologic factors for this disease. About 10% of patients have had or subsequently develop a second neoplasm. This does not seem statistically meaningful in view of the generally older age of these patients and the accepted risk of a second neoplasm complicating the course of a first.

Gross Findings

Typically, the lesions are solitary, multilobulated, fleshy masses of 5 to 10 cm in diameter when first detected (Fig. 13-8), although retroperitoneal lesions are much larger than lesions in the extremities.[55] About two-thirds are located in skeletal muscle, and fewer than 10% are confined to the subcutis. Tumors located adjacent to bone may induce mild degrees of periosteal reaction or cortical erosion. Although UPS has a grossly circumscribed appearance, it often spreads for a considerable distance along fascial planes (Fig. 13-9) or microscopically between muscle fibers, which accounts for its high rate of local recurrence.

On a cut section, most tumors are gray to white (Fig. 13-10), but this pattern may be modified by an abundance of one or more elements. For example, those with a prominent inflammatory component may have a yellow hue because of the predominance of xanthoma cells, whereas hemorrhagic tumors appear brown. Myxoid lesions, depending upon the extent, show a translucent mucoid appearance. Hemorrhage and necrosis are common features; in fact, about 5% of tumors undergo such extensive hemorrhage that they present clinically as fluctuant masses and are diagnosed as cystic hematomas.[51] Nonetheless, residual tumor cells can be identified microscopically in the wall of such cysts, leaving no doubt as to the correct diagnosis.

Microscopic Findings

Microscopically, the classic form of UPS has a highly variable morphologic pattern and shows frequent transitions from storiform to pleomorphic areas (Figs. 13-11 to 13-18), although the emphasis in most tumors is on haphazardly arranged pleomorphic zones. Storiform areas consist of plump spindle cells arranged in short fascicles in a cartwheel, or storiform, pattern around slit-like vessels. Although such tumors resemble dermatofibrosarcoma protuberans, they differ by a less distinctive storiform pattern and by the presence of occasional plump histiocytic cells, numerous typical and atypical mitotic figures, and secondary elements, including xanthoma cells and chronic inflammatory cells. Although this pattern is easily recognized,

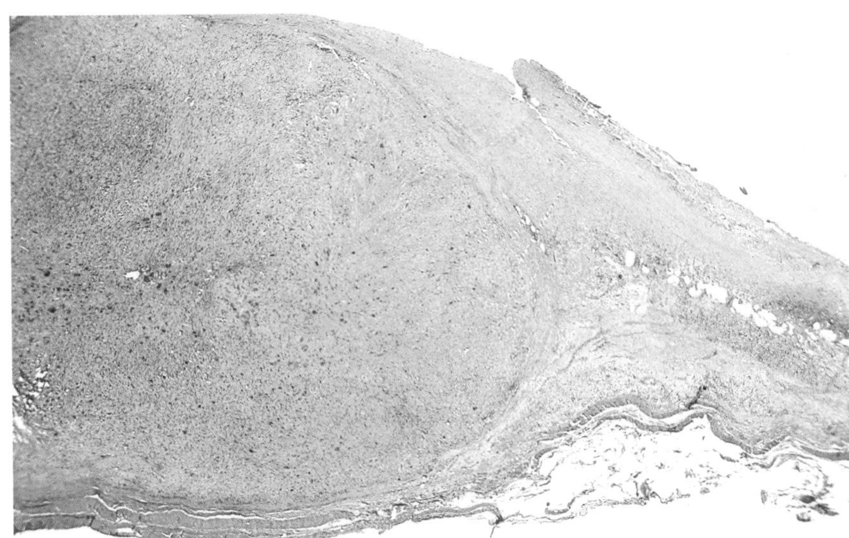

FIGURE 13-9. Undifferentiated pleomorphic sarcoma arising in and extending along superficial fascia.

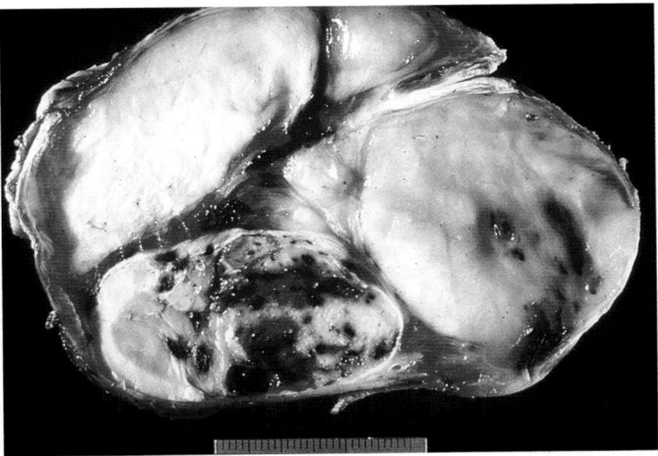

FIGURE 13-10. Typical gross appearance of an undifferentiated pleomorphic sarcoma showing a multinodular white mass with areas of hemorrhage and necrosis.

it is seldom seen throughout the entire tumor. Instead, most tumors have a combination of storiform and pleomorphic areas, with a preponderance on the latter. Least often, tumors have a fascicular growth pattern and resemble fibrosarcomas, except for scattered giant cells, and it may be an arbitrary distinction, in some cases, as to whether a given tumor should be designated as a UPS or fibrosarcoma. In contrast to the storiform areas, pleomorphic areas contain plumper fibroblastic cells and more rounded histiocyte-like cells arranged haphazardly with no particular orientation to vessels. Pleomorphism and mitotic activity are usually more prominent. A characteristic feature of these areas is the presence of large numbers of giant cells with multiple hyperchromatic irregular nuclei. The intense eosinophilia of these giant cells often suggests cells with rhabdomyoblastic differentiation. Although small droplets of neutral fat and PAS-positive, diastase-resistant droplets may be seen in mononuclear cells in this tumor, they are especially prominent in the giant cells and probably reflect a degenerative change.

The stroma and secondary elements vary considerably in the storiform and pleomorphic areas. Usually, the stroma consists of delicate collagen fibrils encircling individual cells, but, occasionally, collagen deposition is extensive and widely separates cells. Rarely, the stroma contains metaplastic osteoid or chondroid material. If, however, bone or cartilage is extensive and/or appears immature, the tumor should be classified as an osteochondrosarcoma or chondrosarcoma. The vasculature, although elaborate, is seldom appreciated unless it becomes dilated and resembles that of a hemangiopericytoma (see Fig. 13-17).

Some examples of this tumor have numerous giant cells, a lesion formerly referred to as the *giant cell type of MFH* or *malignant giant cell tumor of soft parts*.[56,57] These tumors tend to be distinctly multinodular and composed of a mixture of spindled, rounded, and osteoclast-type giant cells. Dense fibrous bands containing vessels often encircle the nodules, which frequently show secondary hemorrhage and necrosis. The cells display pleomorphism and prominent mitotic activity and may contain ingested material, such as lipid or hemosiderin. The nuclei of the osteoclast-type giant cells tend also to be of high nuclear grade. Focal osteoid or mature bone is present in up to 50% of these cases and is usually located at the periphery of the tumor nodules.

As previously mentioned, some examples of UPS have a prominent xanthomatous and neutrophilic infiltrate, possibly related to the elaboration of cytokines, which have chemotactic activity.[58] The neoplastic cells display phagocytosis of neutrophils, a feature that helps distinguish this tumor from an anaplastic lymphoma. There are frequent transitions to spindled areas with a fascicular or storiform growth pattern, which facilitates its recognition as a neoplastic process.

Some examples show prominent stromal myxoid change, although the proportion of myxoid and cellular areas can vary in different portions of the tumor. The myxoid areas appear either as small foci blending with the adjacent cellular areas or as large areas abutting cellular zones with little transition. The storiform pattern becomes less evident and the vasculature more prominent in the myxoid zones; the vessels form arcs along which tumor cells and inflammatory cells

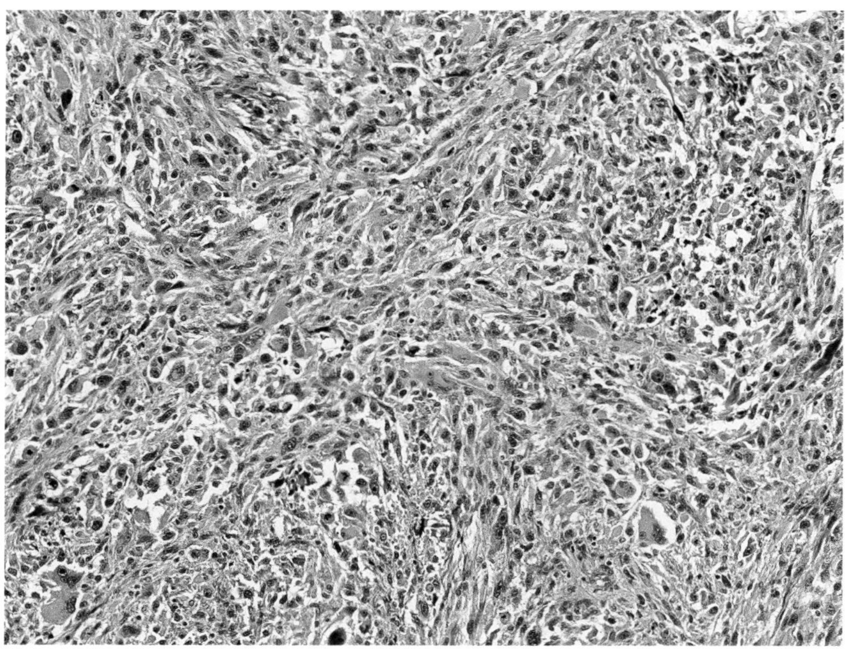

FIGURE 13-11. Undifferentiated pleomorphic sarcoma showing obvious pleomorphic spindled cells arranged in a vague storiform pattern.

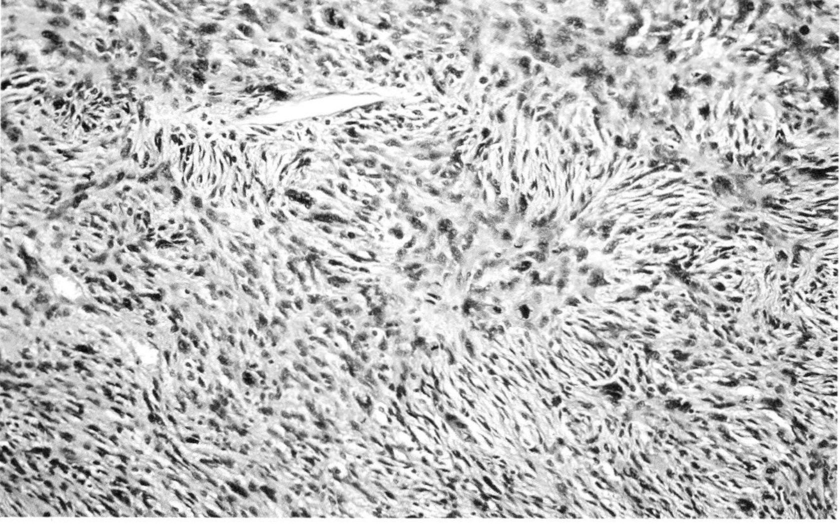

FIGURE 13-12. Undifferentiated pleomorphic sarcoma with a more prominent storiform pattern. Tumors may resemble dermatofibrosarcoma at low power but are distinguished from them by the greater degree of nuclear atypia and mitotic activity.

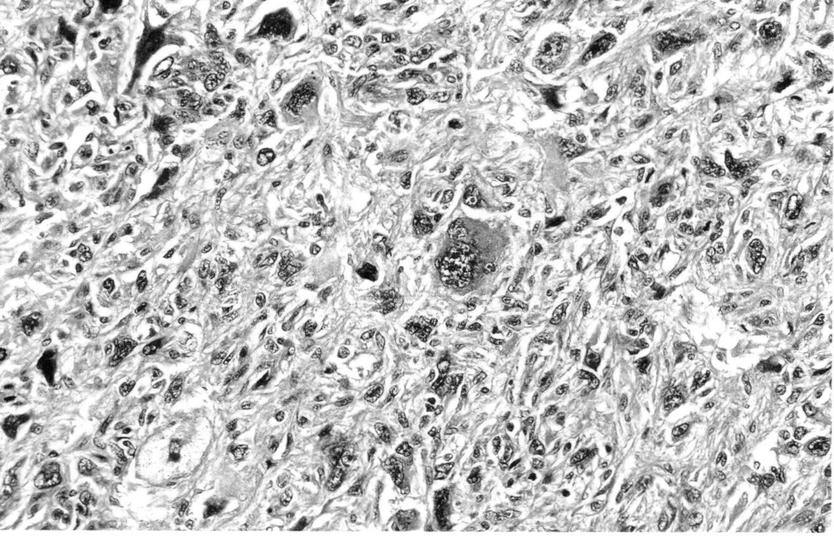

FIGURE 13-13. Undifferentiated pleomorphic sarcoma with anaplastic tumor cells arranged haphazardly in sheets.

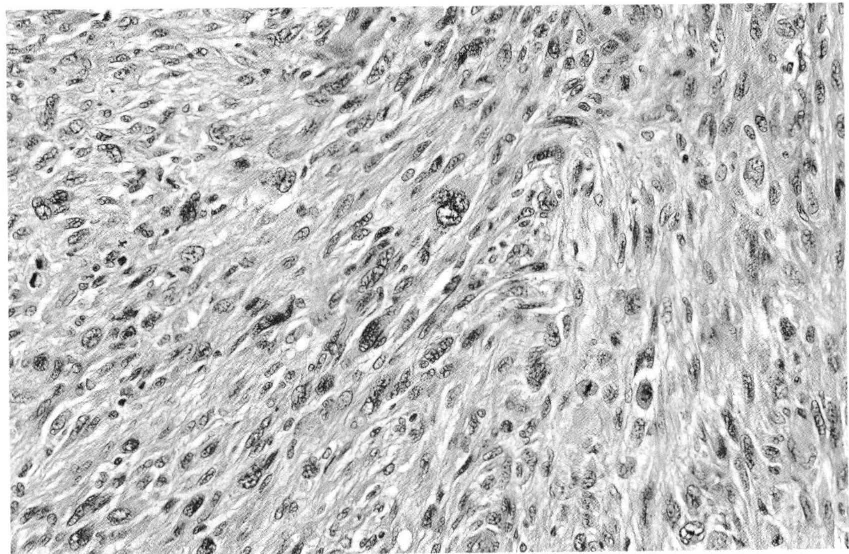

FIGURE 13-14. Undifferentiated pleomorphic sarcoma with a predominantly fascicular pattern. Tumors of this type are classified by some as pleomorphic (high-grade) fibrosarcomas.

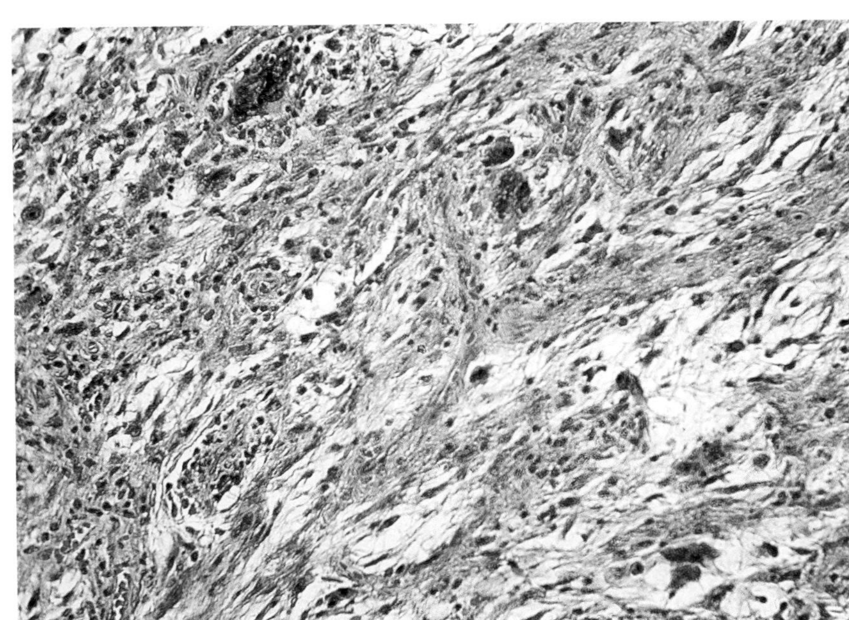

FIGURE 13-15. Undifferentiated pleomorphic sarcoma with focal (microscopic) areas of myxoid change.

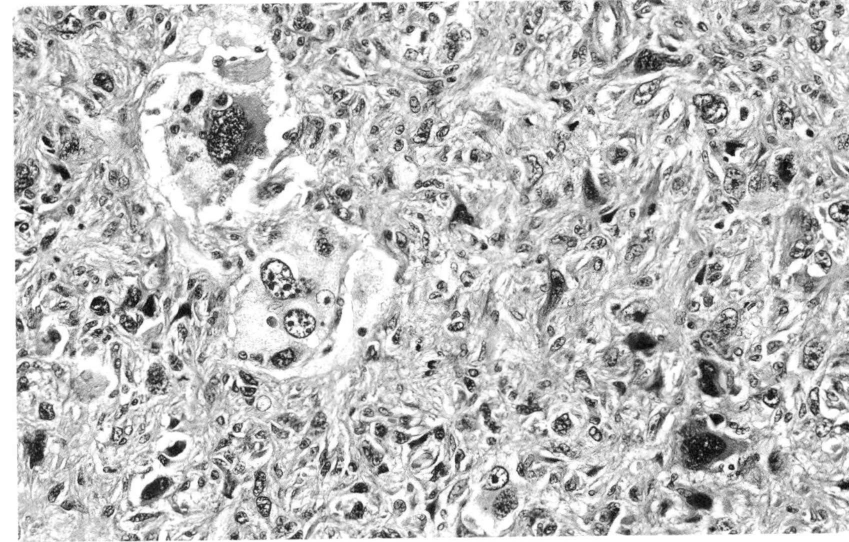

FIGURE 13-16. Cells in an undifferentiated pleomorphic sarcoma are characterized by an extreme degree of pleomorphism and occasional multinucleation. Bizarre cells may vary from deeply eosinophilic to xanthomatous.

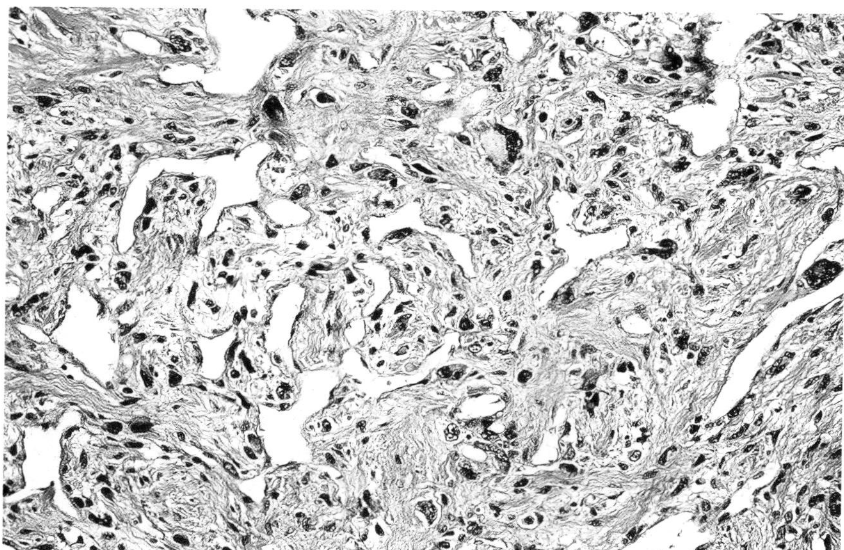

FIGURE 13-17. Hemangiopericytoma-like vascular pattern in an undifferentiated pleomorphic sarcoma.

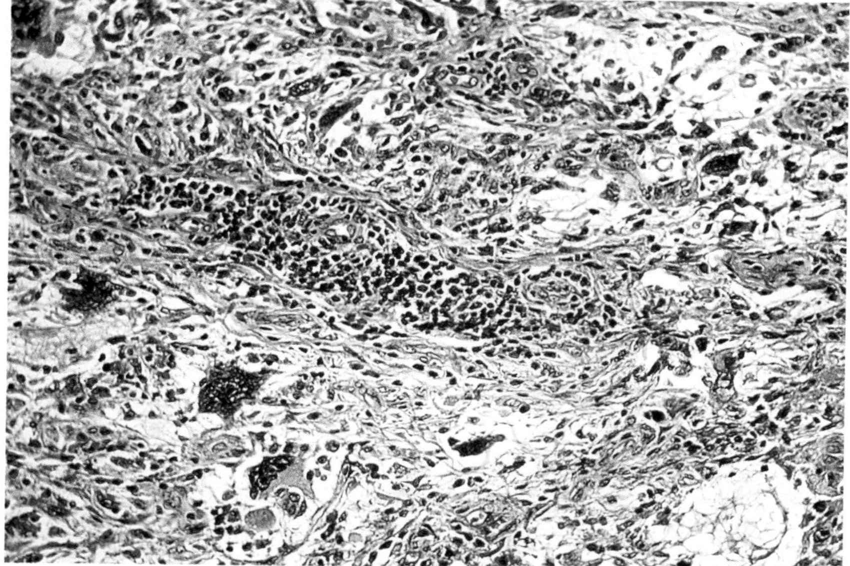

FIGURE 13-18. Undifferentiated pleomorphic sarcoma with a focally dense lymphocytic infiltrate.

condense. Formerly, if greater than 50% of the tumor had prominent myxoid stroma, the lesion was considered a myxoid MFH.[52] However, many lesions of this kind are now diagnosed as high-grade myxofibrosarcoma provided that the distinctive features of myxofibrosarcoma, such as multinodular growth pattern and prominent curvilinear vasculature, are at least focally present (Figs. 13-19 to 13-22). As stated in chapter 10, extensively myxoid lesions with low-grade cytologic atypia are considered low-grade myxofibrosarcomas. Nascimento et al.[59] described an epithelioid variant of myxofibrosarcoma, which accounted for only 3% of all myxofibrosarcomas seen in their consultation material. Some have also seen this rare variant.[60] These tumors are composed predominantly of epithelioid cells resembling carcinoma or malignant melanoma (Fig. 13-23), but conventional areas of myxofibrosarcoma are typically seen, even if focally present only. These tumors are often of a higher grade with prominent mitotic activity and necrosis. Examples of undifferentiated pleomorphic sarcoma with stromal myxoid change but without other classic features of myxofibrosarcoma can be referred to more generally as UPS with myxoid stroma.

Immunohistochemical Findings

The role of immunohistochemistry in the diagnosis of UPS has traditionally been an ancillary one, primarily serving as a means to exclude other pleomorphic tumors. Therefore, the diagnosis continues to presuppose excellent sampling and evaluation of hematoxylin-eosin-stained sections. Despite the limited diagnostic applications of immunohistochemistry aside from excluding other lesions, there is ample evidence that these tumors do not display features of monocytes or macrophages; rather, they display features of fibroblasts/myofibroblasts.[10,61,62] Many of these tumors show focal immunoreactivity for smooth muscle actin, but stains for desmin and h-caldesmon are typically negative.[63] Some examples also show rare cytokeratin-positive cells, which

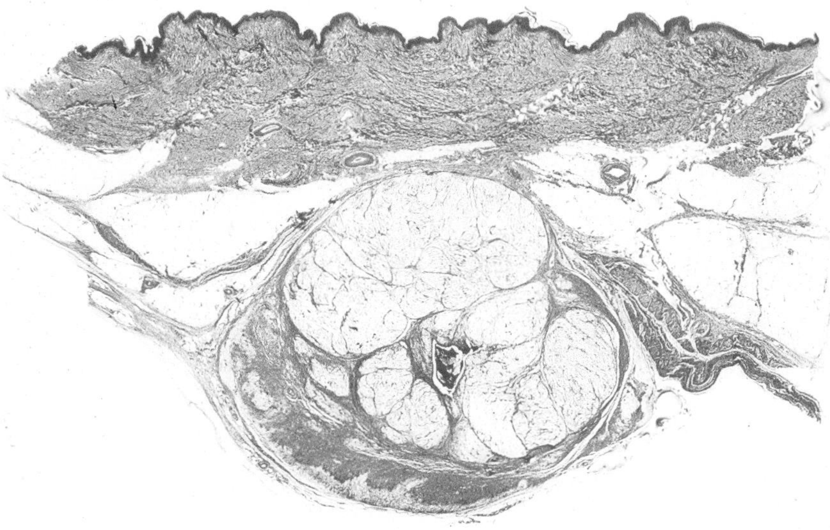

FIGURE 13-19. Low-power view of a superficial (subcutaneous) myxofibrosarcoma. Most of the tumor is myxoid, but, at the deep border, there is a rim of typical (nonmyxoid) undifferentiated pleomorphic sarcoma.

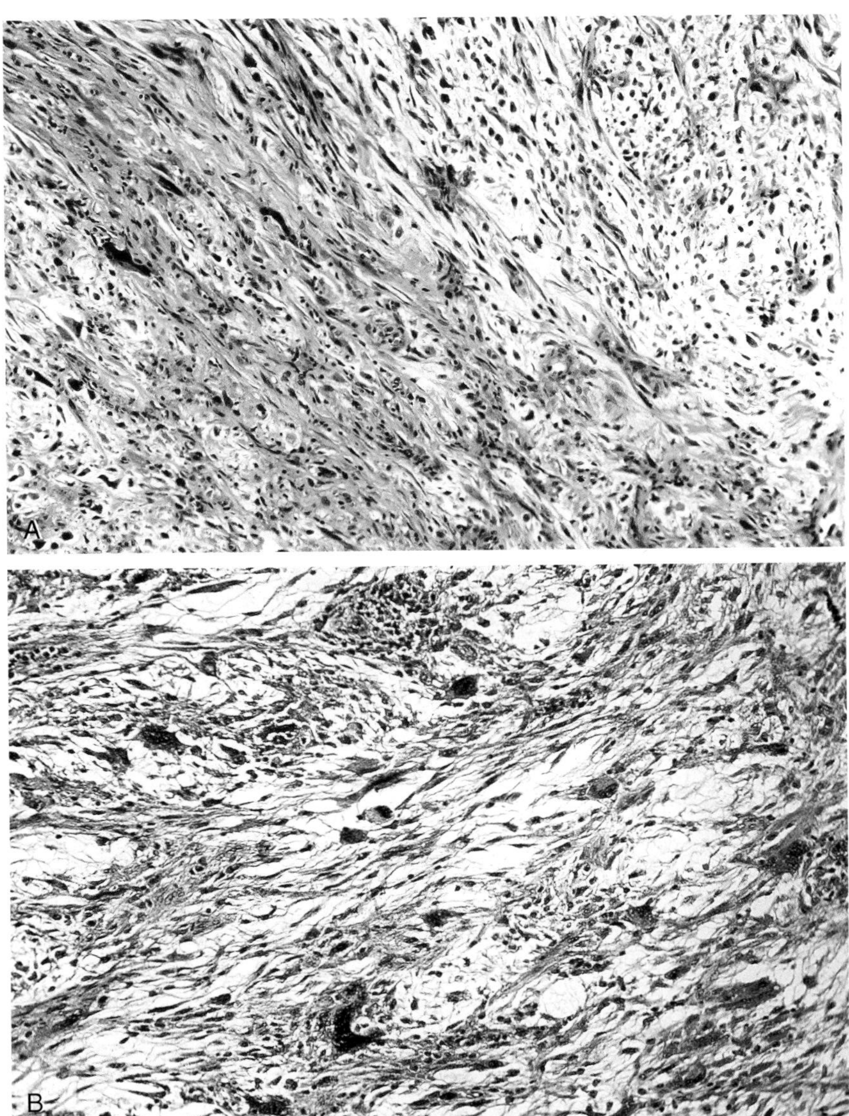

FIGURE 13-20. Broad myxoid zones may sharply abut cellular areas (A) or may be scattered in small microscopic foci (B) throughout the myxofibrosarcoma.

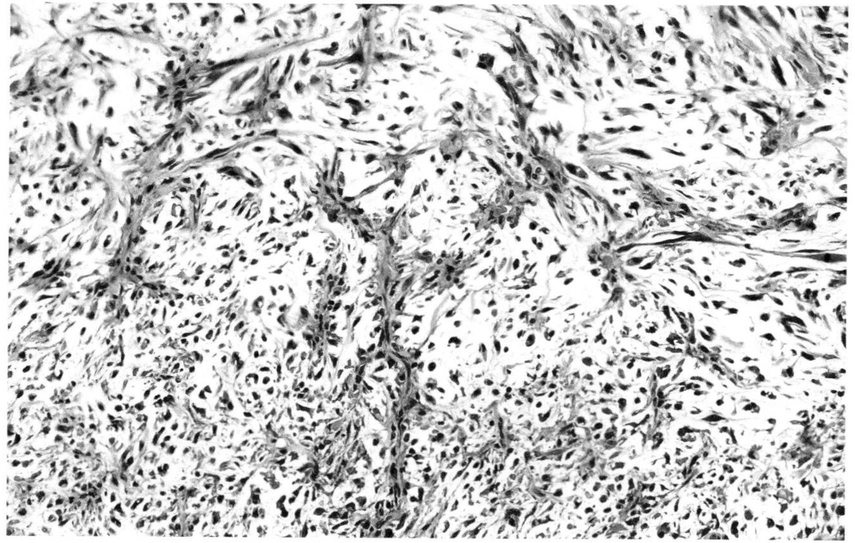

FIGURE 13-21. Prominent arborizing curvilinear blood vessels in a myxofibrosarcoma.

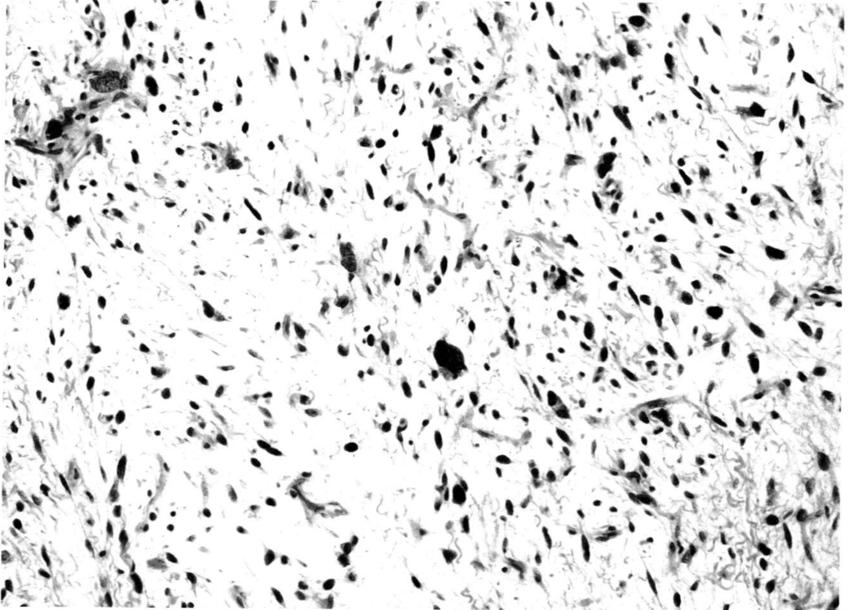

FIGURE 13-22. High-power view of pleomorphic cells in a myxofibrosarcoma.

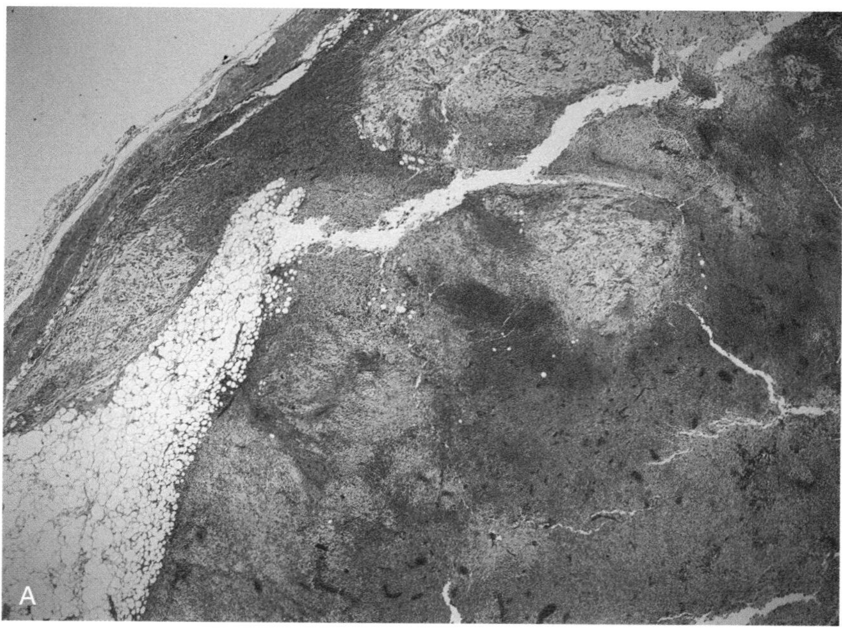

FIGURE 13-23. Epithelioid myxofibrosarcoma. (A) Low-power view showing a typical infiltrative growth pattern. Necrosis is present.

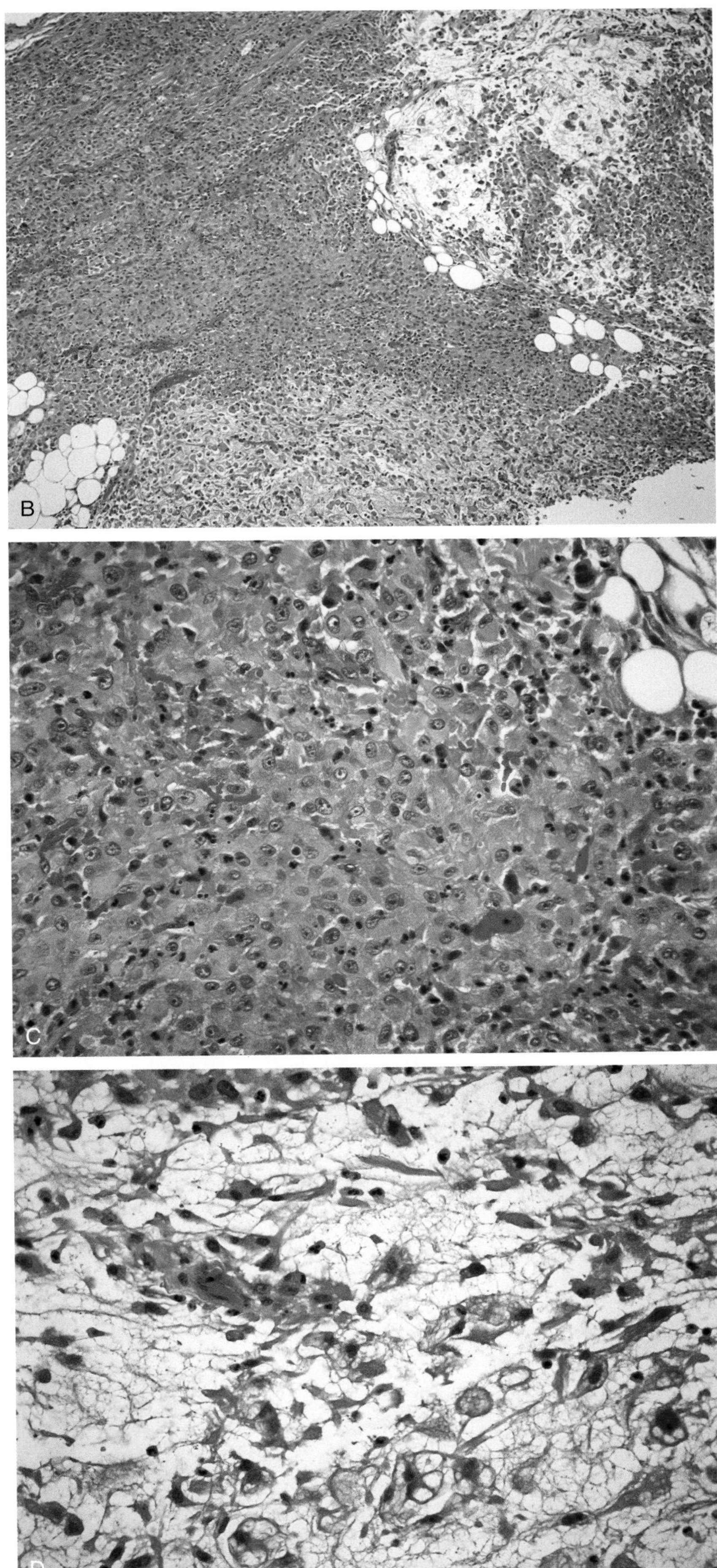

FIGURE 13-23, cont'd (B) Epithelioid myxofibrosarcoma. The tumor is composed of sheets of epithelioid cells alternating with hypocellular myxoid zones. (C) High-power view of epithelioid cells with round or oval nuclei, prominent nucleoli, and eosinophilic cytoplasm resembling carcinoma or malignant melanoma. (D) The myxoid zones show pleomorphic spindle cells, pseudolipoblasts and prominent vasculature typical of a conventional myxofibrosarcoma.

can cause confusion with those tumors in which a sarcomatoid carcinoma is a real consideration.[64-66] Therefore, focal immunoreactivity for any number of intermediate filaments is insufficient evidence of a specific line of differentiation and should not dissuade one from rendering a diagnosis of UPS. On the other hand, diffuse immunoreactivity is far more likely to reflect a specific line of differentiation. Ultrastructural analysis is more useful in ruling out the presence of organelles indicating specific differentiation. Most cells show features of fibroblasts, but up to one-third of cases show evidence of myofibroblastic differentiation.[10]

Cytogenetic and Molecular Genetic Findings

Over the past several decades, studies have reported a variety of cytogenetic abnormalities in MFH; clearly, however, the utility of this information is limited by the varying criteria for making this diagnosis.[67,68] In general, pleomorphic sarcomas of all types are characterized by complex but nonspecific cytogenetic aberrations; therefore, this technique is not useful in distinguishing among these pleomorphic sarcomas.[69]

More recently, a number of studies using comparative genomic hybridization have evaluated UPS and compared the findings to those of other pleomorphic sarcomas.[54,70-72] Interestingly, several studies have found striking similarities between UPS and pleomorphic leiomyosarcoma, suggesting a shared lineage.[70,72] Carneiro et al.[72] found loss of 4q31 (encompassing the *SMAD1* gene), and loss of 18q22 were independent predictors of metastasis.

Differential Diagnosis

As previously discussed, the most common problem in the differential diagnosis is separating UPS from other malignant tumors that display a comparable degree of cellular pleomorphism, such as sarcomatoid carcinoma and pleomorphic forms of liposarcoma, leiomyosarcoma, and rhabdomyosarcoma. Careful sampling in conjunction with a targeted panel of immunostains is the mainstay of diagnosis. Pleomorphic liposarcoma, in particular, may have areas that closely simulate UPS but, ultimately, is diagnosed by the presence of pleomorphic lipoblasts. Dedifferentiated liposarcomas are identified by virtue of areas of well-differentiated liposarcoma. It is especially important that retroperitoneal lesions be well sampled because evidence suggests that the majority of these tumors are dedifferentiated liposarcomas.[15] The distinction between pleomorphic leiomyosarcoma and UPS is probably the most problematic and controversial area in differential diagnosis (Figs. 13-24 to 13-26). Unless there are light microscopic areas that are diagnostic of smooth muscle differentiation, one is usually forced to decide the extent to which immunoreactivity for various myogenic markers (smooth muscle actin, desmin, h-caldesmon) is reflective of smooth muscle differentiation. In evaluating actin immunoreactivity, it is important to distinguish the peripheral actin immunoreactivity of myofibroblasts occurring in UPS from the diffuse actin immunoreactivity of smooth muscle cells in leiomyosarcomas. The diagnosis of pleomorphic rhabdomyosarcoma is often suggested by intense cytoplasmic eosinophilia, cell-to-cell molding, and the presence of strap cells. Because they also express the nuclear regulatory proteins specific for skeletal muscle differentiation, MyoD1 and myogenin, this diagnosis can be definitively made by immunohistochemistry.

Depending on the clinical situation, the differential diagnosis of UPS should also include sarcomatoid carcinoma (Fig. 13-27). This is especially true for lesions based in or around epithelial organs, or those occurring in patients known to have a previous carcinoma. Immunostains for pancytokeratin are invaluable in this distinction, although, as noted previously, keratin is expressed focally in a small percentage of UPS. Electron microscopy may also aid in this distinction by detecting

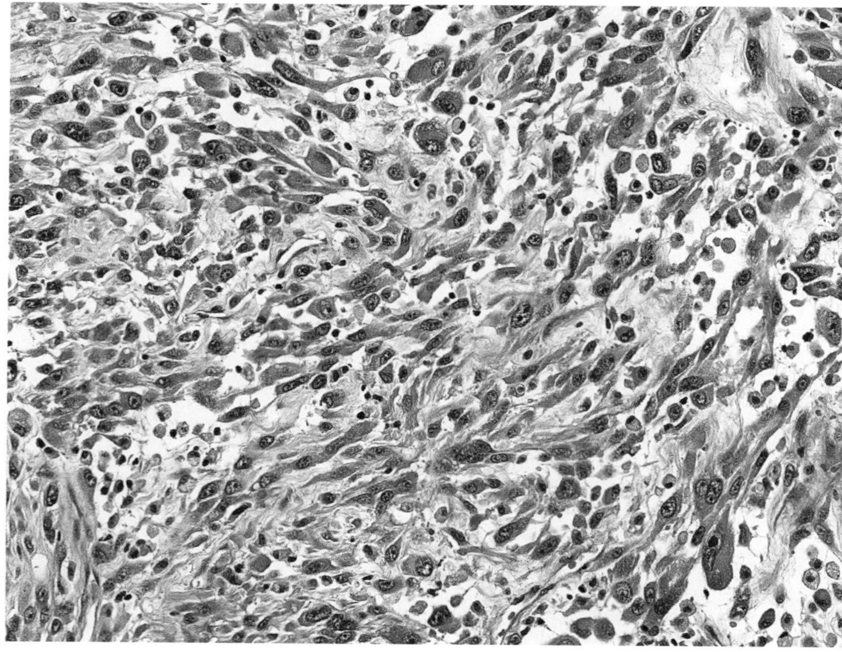

FIGURE 13-24. Pleomorphic leiomyosarcoma with pleomorphic spindled cells with cytoplasmic eosinophila.

minor degrees of epithelial differentiation not readily apparent by light microscopy, such as numerous large intercellular junctions or tonofibrils.

There are also specific differential diagnostic considerations for myxofibrosarcoma and for those cases of UPS with prominent inflammation or giant cells. The differential diagnosis of myxofibrosarcoma includes other myxoid sarcomas such as myxoid liposarcoma. However, myxofibrosarcoma is far more cytologically atypical than the other myxoid sarcomas and is characterized by multinodular growth pattern and arborizing curvilinear blood vessels with perivascular hypercellularity. The differential diagnosis of myxofibrosarcoma is discussed in greater detail in Chapter 10. For those cases of UPS with prominent inflammation, it can be challenging to rule out a non-neoplastic xanthomatous process (Figs. 13-28 to 13-33). Although xanthogranulomatous pyelonephritis may involve the retroperitoneal soft tissue, it first and foremost affects the kidneys and is accompanied by the usual constellation of symptoms of urinary tract infection. Xanthogranulomatous inflammatory processes may be seen in other settings, some of which are secondary to infection, and, therefore, culture and bacterial stains are extremely helpful. Ultimately, the distinction of this tumor from xanthogranulomatous inflammation rests on the documentation of atypia. Therefore,

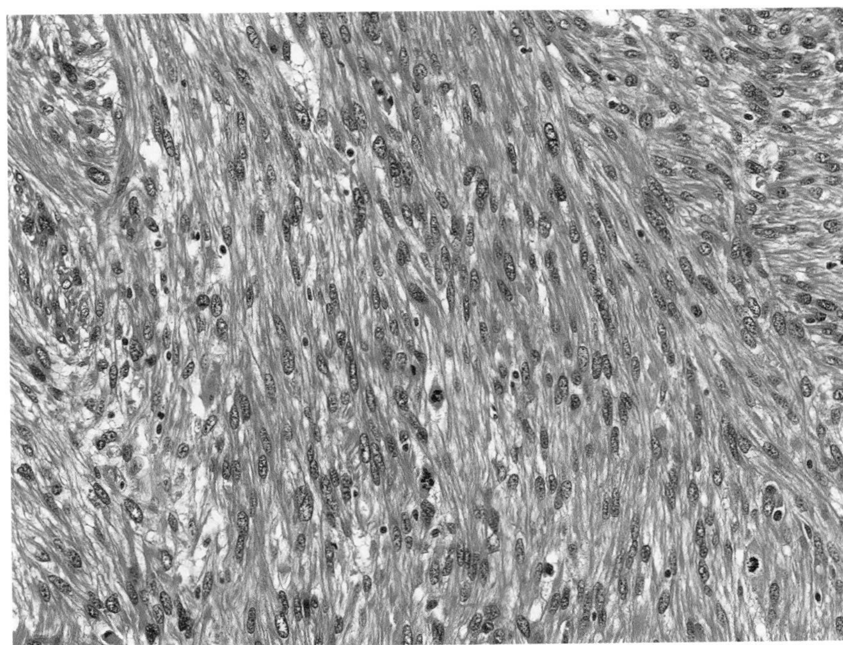

FIGURE 13-25. Low-grade leiomyosarcoma from a different area of the same case, as depicted in Figure 13-24.

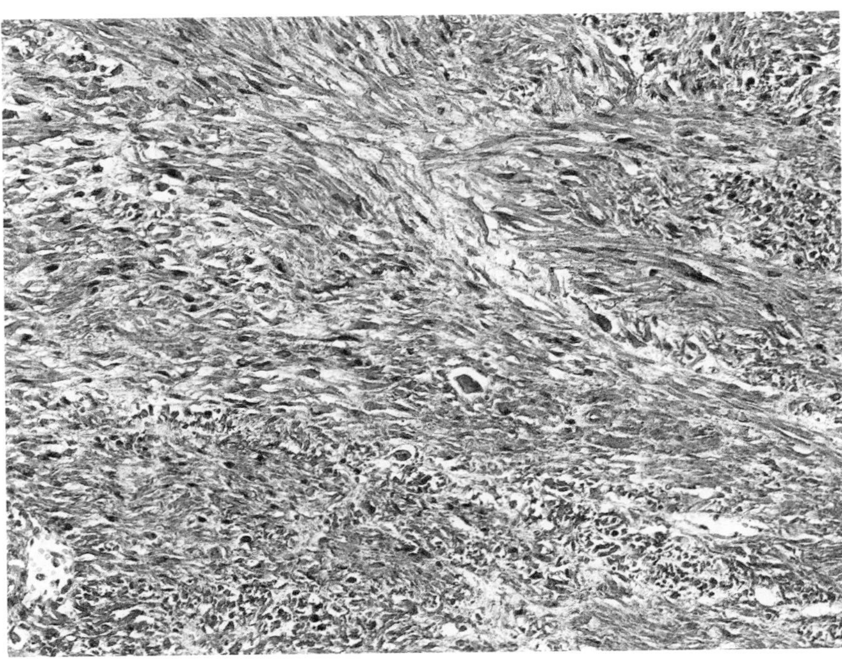

FIGURE 13-26. Strong smooth muscle actin staining in the same leiomyosarcoma as that depicted in Figures 13-24 and 13-25.

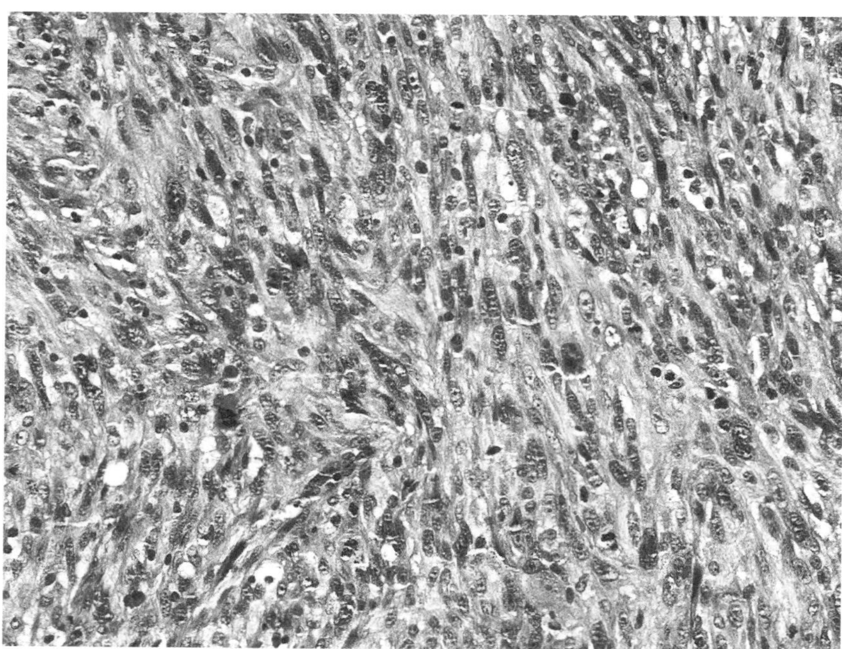

FIGURE 13-27. Sarcomatoid carcinoma that originally was diagnosed as MFH. This lesion showed striking cytokeratin immunopositivity.

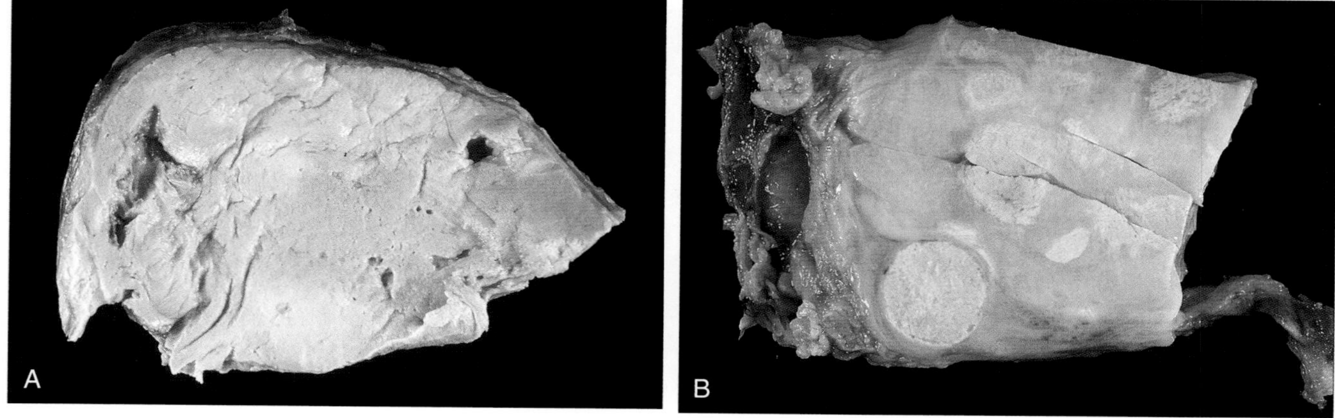

FIGURE 13-28. Gross appearance of an undifferentiated pleomorphic sarcoma with a tawny yellow color (A). In some portions of the tumor, there are areas of conventional undifferentiated pleomorphic sarcoma. (B) Interface of conventional undifferentiated pleomorphic sarcoma (white areas) with inflammatory areas.

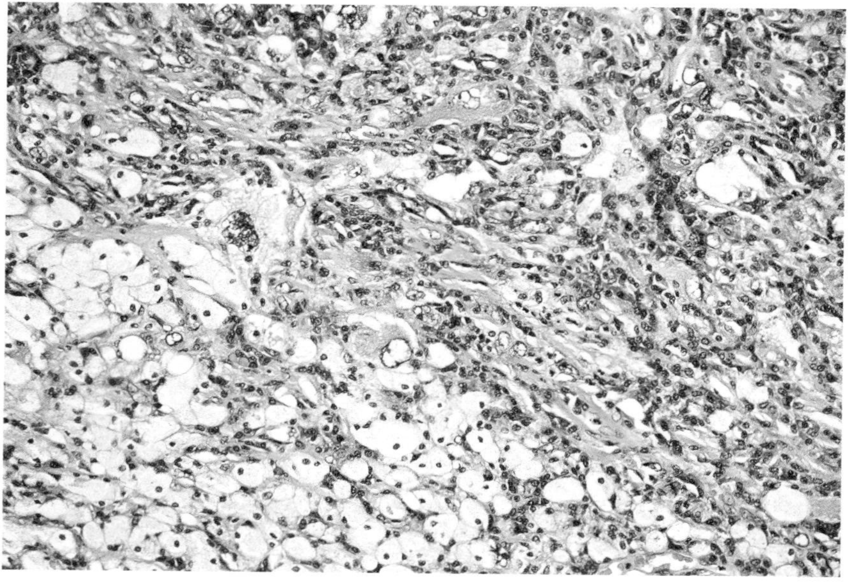

FIGURE 13-29. Undifferentiated pleomorphic sarcoma, inflammatory type, showing transition to a conventional undifferentiated pleomorphic sarcoma (top right).

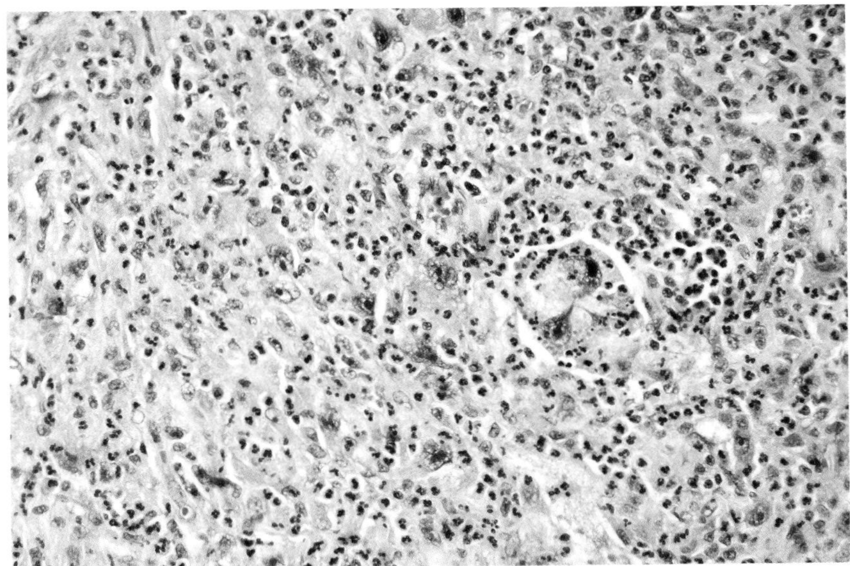

FIGURE 13-30. Undifferentiated pleomorphic sarcoma, inflammatory type, with a predominance of neutrophils, some in tumor cells.

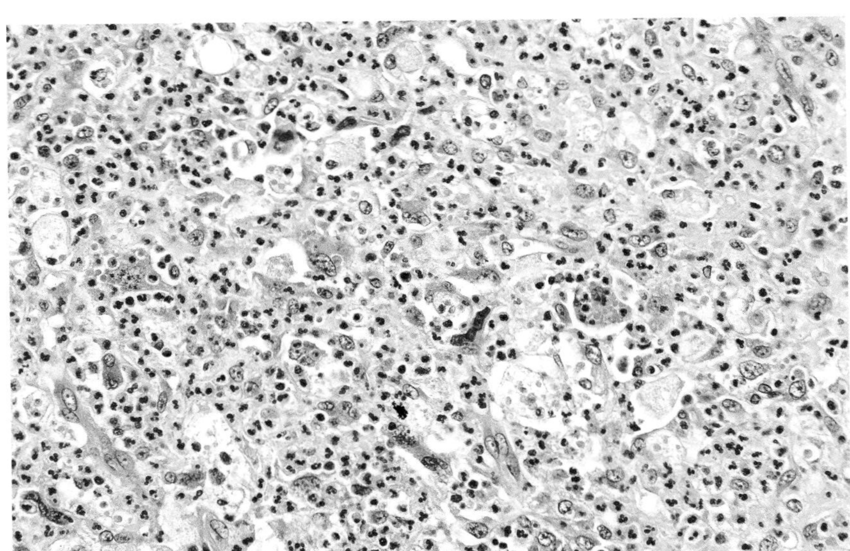

FIGURE 13-31. Undifferentiated pleomorphic sarcoma, inflammatory type.

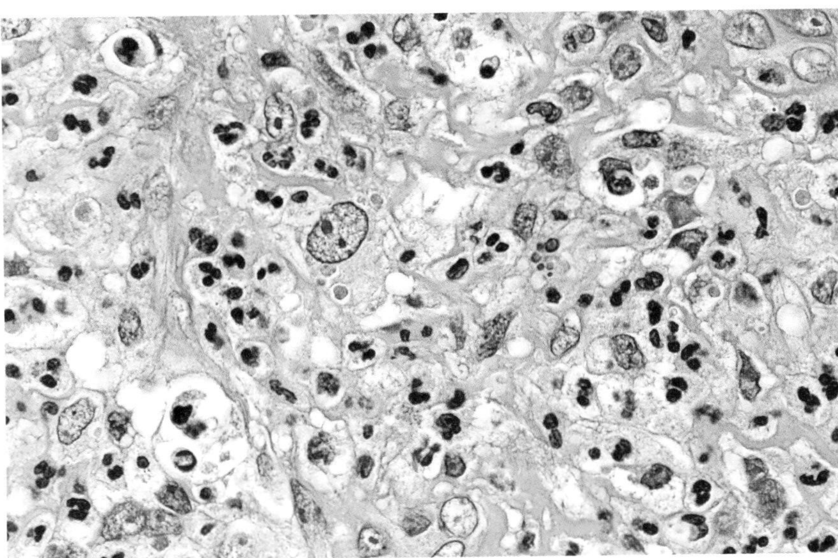

FIGURE 13-32. High-power view of cells in an undifferentiated pleomorphic sarcoma, inflammatory type. The round neoplastic cells sometimes resemble the cells in anaplastic large cell lymphomas or Hodgkin disease.

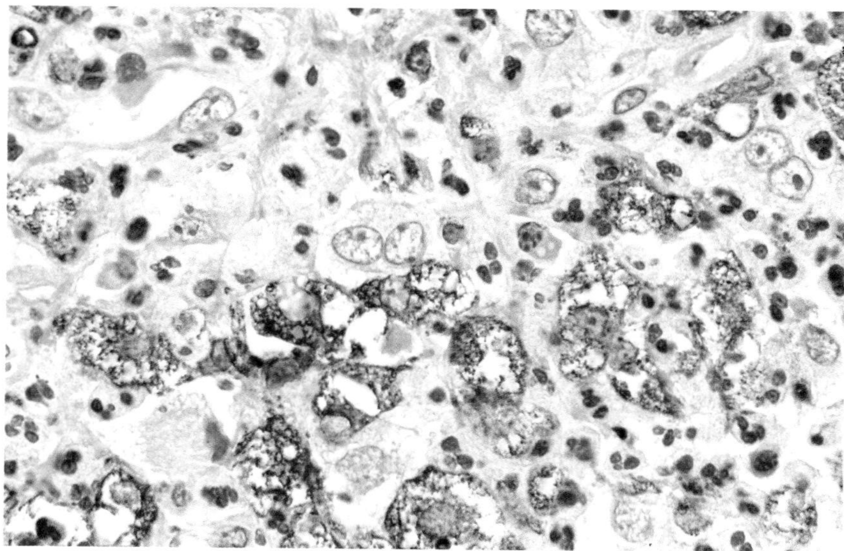

FIGURE 13-33. CD68 stain of an undifferentiated pleomorphic sarcoma, inflammatory type, with staining of benign xanthoma cells. Some phagocytic tumor cells also stain. Other leukocyte lineage markers are not present in the neoplastic cells in the tumor.

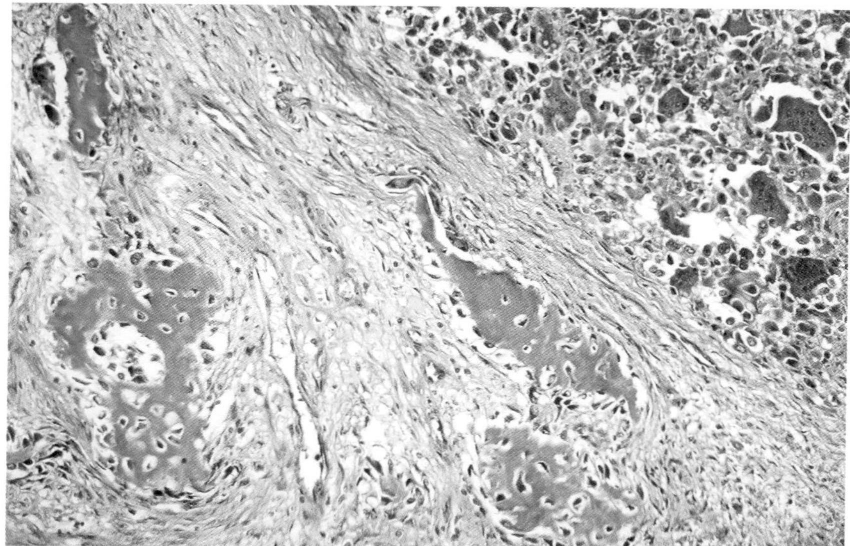

FIGURE 13-34. Giant cell form of undifferentiated pleomorphic sarcoma showing a shell of woven bone at the periphery.

careful sampling of large xanthomatous lesions, especially in the retroperitoneum, is mandatory. Lymphoma is also a major diagnostic consideration, and a panel of immunohistochemical stains is usually necessary to establish the diagnosis, including negative staining for LCA, CD15, CD30, ALK1, CD3, and CD20. CD68 may be identified in neoplastic cells that have evidence of phagocytic activity.[58] For those lesions with numerous giant cells that are deeply situated, giant cell tumor of soft tissue may be a consideration (Figs. 13-34 to 13-37). However, the latter tumor has a greater degree of multinodularity and lacks the cytologic atypia seen in UPS with prominent giant cells.

Discussion

The vast majority of UPS are high-grade lesions having a local recurrence rate ranging from 19% to 31%, a metastatic rate of 31% to 35%, and a 5-year survival rate of 65% to 70% (Table 13-1).[11,73-77] Both local recurrence and distant metastases often develop within 12 to 24 months of diagnosis. Only a minority of patients develop metastases after 5 years, with the common metastatic sites being lung (90%), bone (8%), and liver (1%). Regional lymph node metastases are decidedly uncommon.

The factors that correlate consistently with metastasis, survival, or both are depth, tumor size, grade, necrosis, and local recurrence, although they are not necessarily independent variables (Box 13-1). For example, size and depth appear to co-vary because large tumors tend to be deep tumors. In the study by Engellau et al.,[11] necrosis and local recurrence were significant predictors of metastasis within the first 2 years of diagnosis and throughout a longitudinal follow-up period, whereas only tumor depth and local recurrence were significant predictors beyond 2 years.

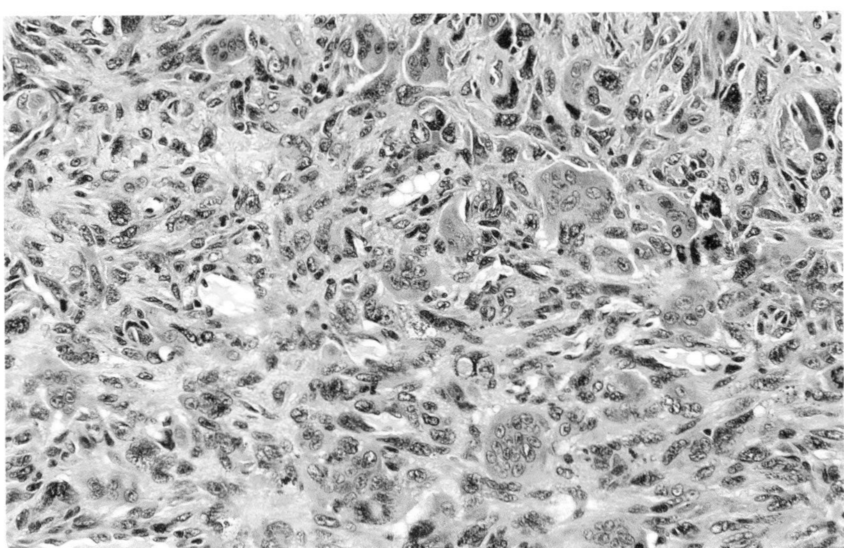

FIGURE 13-35. Giant cell form of undifferentiated pleomorphic sarcoma.

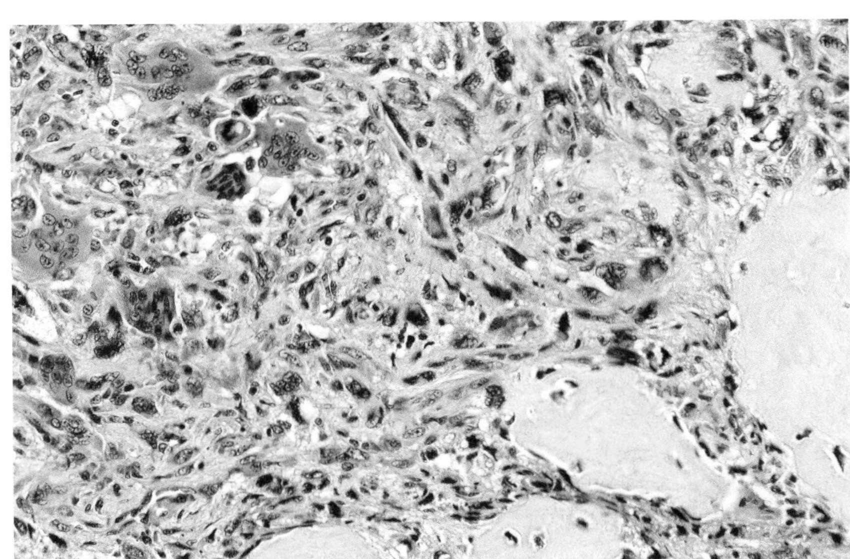

FIGURE 13-36. Giant cell form of undifferentiated pleomorphic sarcoma containing less mature bone in the tumor.

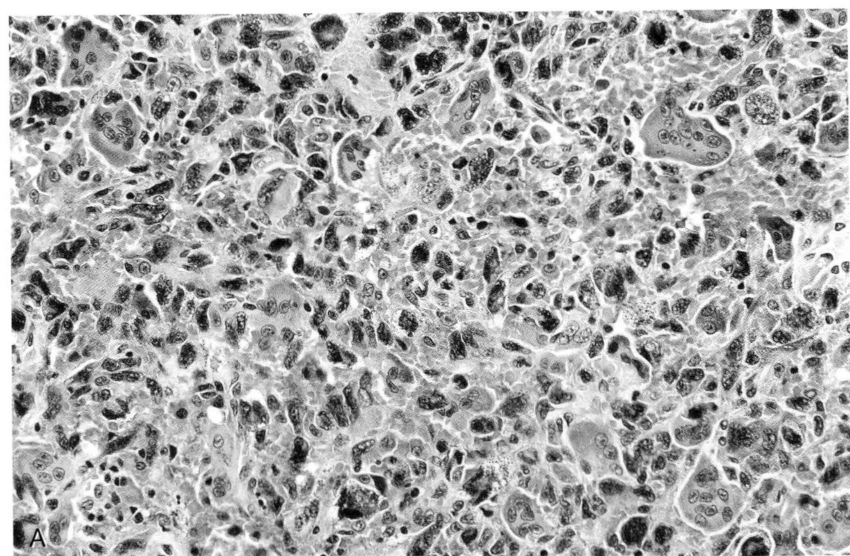

FIGURE 13-37. Hemorrhagic areas in a giant cell form of undifferentiated pleomorphic sarcoma that vary from having a predominantly round cell population with numerous osteoclast-like giant cells with high-grade nuclear atypia (A) to a spindled population (B). *Continued*

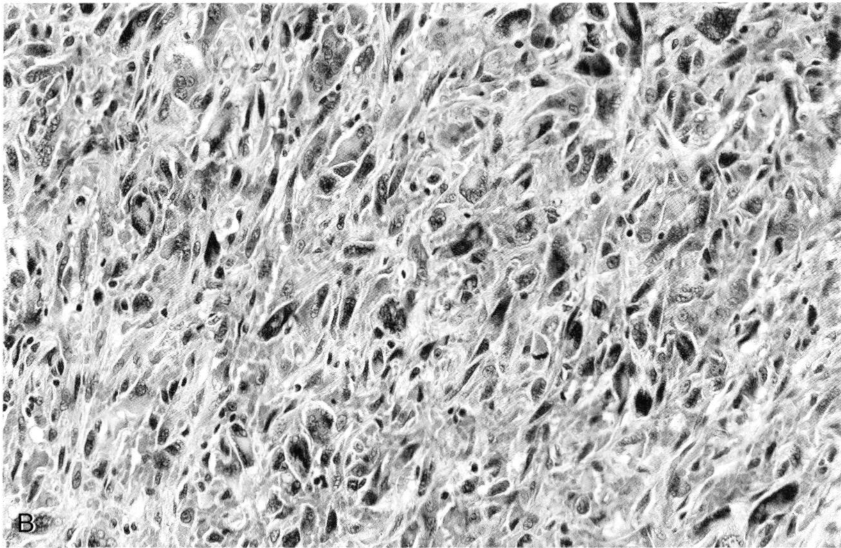

FIGURE 13-37, cont'd

TABLE 13-1 Behavior of Undifferentiated Pleomorphic Sarcoma (So-Called Malignant Fibrous Histiocytoma)

AUTHOR	NO. OF PATIENTS	LOCAL RECURRENCE (%)	METASTASIS (%)	5-YEAR SURVIVAL (%)
Salo et al.[63]	239	19	35	65
Le Doussal et al.[62]	216	31	33	70
Zagars et al.[65]	271	21	31	68
Engellau[10]	338	29	33	

BOX 13-1 Independent Favorable Prognostic Factors With Respect to Disease-Specific Survival in Undifferentiated Pleomorphic Sarcoma (So-Called Malignant Fibrous Histiocytoma)

UICC/AJCC stage I or II
- Freedom from gross disease following initial treatment
- Superficial location
- Myxoid subtype
- Age less than 50 years

Modified from Le Doussal V, Coindre JM, Leroux A, et al. Prognostic factors for patients with localized primary malignant fibrous histiocytoma: a multicenter study of 216 patients with multivariate analysis. Cancer 1996;77(9):1823-1830.

References

1. Ozzello L, Stout AP, Murray MR. Cultural characteristics of malignant histiocytomas and fibrous xanthomas. Cancer 1963;16:331–44.
2. O'Brien JE, Stout AP. Malignant fibrous xanthomas. Cancer 1964;17:1445–55.
3. Iwasaki H, Isayama T, Johzaki H, et al. Malignant fibrous histiocytoma. Evidence of perivascular mesenchymal cell origin immunocytochemical studies with monoclonal anti-MFH antibodies. Am J Pathol 1987;128(3):528–37.
4. Iwasaki H, Isayama T, Ohjimi Y, et al. Malignant fibrous histiocytoma. A tumor of facultative histiocytes showing mesenchymal differentiation in cultured cell lines. Cancer 1992;69(2):437–47.
5. Roholl PJ, Kleyne J, Elbers H, et al. Characterization of tumour cells in malignant fibrous histiocytomas and other soft tissue tumours in comparison with malignant histiocytes. I. Immunohistochemical study on paraffin sections. J Pathol 1985;147(2):87–95.
6. Roholl PJ, Kleyne J, Van Unnik JA. Characterization of tumor cells in malignant fibrous histiocytomas and other soft-tissue tumors, in comparison with malignant histiocytes. II. Immunoperoxidase study on cryostat sections. Am J Pathol 1985;121(2):269–74.
7. Fletcher CD. Pleomorphic malignant fibrous histiocytoma: fact or fiction? A critical reappraisal based on 159 tumors diagnosed as pleomorphic sarcoma. Am J Surg Pathol 1992;16(3):213–28.
8. Deyrup AT, Haydon RC, Huo D, et al. Myoid differentiation and prognosis in adult pleomorphic sarcomas of the extremity: an analysis of 92 cases. Cancer 2003;98(4):805–13.
9. Fletcher CD, Gustafson P, Rydholm A, et al. Clinicopathologic re-evaluation of 100 malignant fibrous histiocytomas: prognostic relevance of subclassification. J Clin Oncol 2001;19(12):3045–50.
10. Montgomery E, Fisher C. Myofibroblastic differentiation in malignant fibrous histiocytoma (pleomorphic myofibrosarcoma): a clinicopathological study. Histopathology 2001;38(6):499–509.
11. Engellau J, Anderson H, Rydholm A, et al. Time dependence of prognostic factors for patients with soft tissue sarcoma: a Scandinavian Sarcoma Group Study of 338 malignant fibrous histiocytomas. Cancer 2004;100(10):2233–9.
12. Kindblom LG, Widéhn S, Meis-Kindblom JM. The role of electron microscopy in the diagnosis of pleomorphic sarcomas of soft tissue. Semin Diagn Pathol 2003;20(1):72–81.
13. Suh CH, Ordóñez NG, Mackay B. Malignant fibrous histiocytoma: an ultrastructural perspective. Ultrastruct Pathol 2000;24(4):243–50.
14. Coindre JM, Hostein I, Maire G, et al. Inflammatory malignant fibrous histiocytomas and dedifferentiated liposarcomas: histological review, genomic profile, and MDM2 and CDK4 status favour a single entity. J Pathol 2004;203(3):822–30.
15. Coindre JM, Mariani O, Chibon F, et al. Most malignant fibrous histiocytomas developed in the retroperitoneum are dedifferentiated liposarcomas: a review of 25 cases initially diagnosed as malignant fibrous histiocytoma. Mod Pathol 2003;16(3):256–62.
16. Fabre-Guillevin E, Coindre JM, Somerhausen N de SA, et al. Retroperitoneal liposarcomas: follow-up analysis of dedifferentiation after clinicopathologic reexamination of 86 liposarcomas and malignant fibrous histiocytomas. Cancer 2006;106(12):2725–33.
17. Binh MB, Sastre-Garau X, Guillou L, et al. MDM2 and CDK4 immunostainings are useful adjuncts in diagnosing well-differentiated and dedifferentiated liposarcoma subtypes: a comparative analysis of 559 soft tissue neoplasms with genetic data. Am J Surg Pathol 2005;29(10):1340–7.

18. Chung L, Lau SK, Jiang Z, et al. Overlapping features between dedifferentiated liposarcoma and undifferentiated high-grade pleomorphic sarcoma. Am J Surg Pathol 2009;33(11):1594–600.
19. McCormick D, Mentzel T, Beham A, et al. Dedifferentiated liposarcoma. Clinicopathologic analysis of 32 cases suggesting a better prognostic subgroup among pleomorphic sarcomas. Am J Surg Pathol 1994; 18(12):1213–23.
20. Dahl I. Atypical fibroxanthoma of the skin. A clinico-pathological study of 57 cases. Acta Pathol Microbiol Scand A 1976;84(2):183–97.
21. Fretzin DF, Helwig EB. Atypical fibroxanthoma of the skin. A clinicopathologic study of 140 cases. Cancer 1973;31(6):1541–52.
22. Dei Tos AP, Maestro R, Doglioni C, et al. Ultraviolet-induced p53 mutations in atypical fibroxanthoma. Am J Pathol 1994;145(1):11–17.
23. Sakamoto A, Oda Y, Itakura E, et al. Immunoexpression of ultraviolet photoproducts and p53 mutation analysis in atypical fibroxanthoma and superficial malignant fibrous histiocytoma. Mod Pathol 2001;14(6): 581–8.
24. Sakamoto A. Atypical fibroxanthoma. Clin Med Oncol 2008;2:117–27.
25. Hudson AW, Winkelmann RK. Atypical fibroxanthoma of the skin: a reappraisal of 19 cases in which the original diagnosis was spindle-cell squamous carcinoma. Cancer 1972;29(2):413–22.
26. Perrett CM, Macedo C, Francis N, et al. Atypical fibroxanthoma in an HIV-infected individual. J Cutan Pathol 2011;38(4):357–9.
27. Ferri E, Iaderosa GA, Armato E. Atypical fibroxanthoma of the external ear in a cardiac transplant recipient: case report and the causal role of the immunosuppressive therapy. Auris Nasus Larynx 2008;35(2): 260–3.
28. Khan ZM, Cockerell CJ. Atypical fibroxanthoma with osteoclast-like multinucleated giant cells. Am J Dermatopathol 1997;19(2):174–9.
29. Patton A, Page R, Googe PB, et al. Myxoid atypical fibroxanthoma: a previously undescribed variant. J Cutan Pathol 2009;36(11):1177–84.
30. Chen KT. Atypical fibroxanthoma of the skin with osteoid production. Arch Dermatol 1980;116(1):113–14.
31. Kemmerling R, Dietze O, Müller S, et al. Aspects of the differential diagnosis of clear-cell lesions of the skin in connection with the rare case of a clear-cell atypical fibroxanthoma. Pathol Res Pract 2009;205(5): 365–70.
32. Suárez-Vilela D, Izquierdo-García F, Domínguez-Iglesias F, et al. Combined papillated Bowen disease and clear cell atypical fibroxanthoma. Case Rep Dermatol 2010;2(2):69–75.
33. Wright NA, Thomas CG, Calame A, et al. Granular cell atypical fibroxanthoma: case report and review of the literature. J Cutan Pathol 2010;37(3):380–5.
34. Fussell JN, Cooke ER, Florentino F, et al. Atypical fibroxanthoma with keloidal collagen. Am J Dermatopathol 2010;32(7):713–15.
35. Kim J, McNiff JM. Keloidal atypical fibroxanthoma: a case series. J Cutan Pathol 2009;36(5):535–9.
36. Stefanato CM, Robson A, Calonje JE. The histopathologic spectrum of regression in atypical fibroxanthoma. J Cutan Pathol 2010;37(3): 310–15.
37. Bansal C, Sinkre P, Stewart D, et al. Two cases of cytokeratin positivity in atypical fibroxanthoma. J Clin Pathol 2007;60(6):716–17.
38. Gleason BC, Calder KB, Cibull TL, et al. Utility of p63 in the differential diagnosis of atypical fibroxanthoma and spindle cell squamous cell carcinoma. J Cutan Pathol 2009;36(5):543–7.
39. Suárez-Vilela D, Izquierdo FM, Escobar-Stein J, et al. Atypical fibroxanthoma with T-cytotoxic inflammatory infiltrate and aberrant expression of cytokeratin. J Cutan Pathol 2011;38(11):930–2.
40. de Feraudy S, Mar N, McCalmont TH. Evaluation of CD10 and procollagen 1 expression in atypical fibroxanthoma and dermatofibroma. Am J Surg Pathol 2008;32(8):1111–122.
41. Kanner WA, Brill LB 2nd, Patterson JW, et al. CD10, p63 and CD99 expression in the differential diagnosis of atypical fibroxanthoma, spindle cell squamous cell carcinoma and desmoplastic melanoma. J Cutan Pathol 2010;37(7):744–50.
42. Nakamura Y, Abe Y, Ichimiya M, et al. Atypical fibroxanthoma presenting immunoreactivity against CD10 and CD99. J Dermatol 2010;37(4): 387–9.
43. Bull C, Mirzabeigi M, Laskin W, et al. Diagnostic utility of low-affinity nerve growth factor receptor (P 75) immunostaining in atypical fibroxanthoma. J Cutan Pathol 2011;38(8):631–5.
44. Pouryazdanparast P, Yu L, Cutlan JE, et al. Diagnostic value of CD163 in cutaneous spindle cell lesions. J Cutan Pathol 2009;36(8): 859–64.
45. Mathew RA, Schlauder SM, Calder KB, et al. CD117 immunoreactivity in atypical fibroxanthoma. Am J Dermatopathol 2008;30(1):34–6.
46. Luzar B, Calonje E. Morphological and immunohistochemical characteristics of atypical fibroxanthoma with a special emphasis on potential diagnostic pitfalls: a review. J Cutan Pathol 2010;37(3):301–9.
47. Mirza B, Weedon D. Atypical fibroxanthoma: a clinicopathological study of 89 cases. Australas J Dermatol 2005;46(4):235–8.
48. Beer TW, Drury P, Heenan PJ. Atypical fibroxanthoma: a histological and immunohistochemical review of 171 cases. Am J Dermatopathol 2010; 32(6):533–40.
49. Ang GC, Roenigk RK, Otley CC, et al. More than 2 decades of treating atypical fibroxanthoma at mayo clinic: what have we learned from 91 patients? Dermatol Surg 2009;35(5):765–72.
50. Wollina U, Schönlebe J, Koch A, et al. Atypical fibroxanthoma: a series of 25 cases. J Eur Acad Dermatol Venereol 2010;24(8):943–6.
51. Weiss SW, Enzinger FM. Malignant fibrous histiocytoma: an analysis of 200 cases. Cancer 1978;41(6):2250–66.
52. Weiss SW, Enzinger FM. Myxoid variant of malignant fibrous histiocytoma. Cancer 1977;39(4):1672–85.
53. Hamada T, Komiya S, Hiraoka K, et al. IL-6 in a pleomorphic type of malignant fibrous histiocytoma presenting high fever. Hum Pathol 1998;29(7):758–61.
54. Kageyama K, Moriyama T, Hizuka N, et al. Hypoglycemia associated with big insulin-like growth factor II produced during development of malignant fibrous histiocytoma. Endocr J 2003;50(6):753–8.
55. Pezzi CM, Rawlings MS Jr, Esgro JJ, et al. Prognostic factors in 227 patients with malignant fibrous histiocytoma. Cancer 1992;69(8):2098–103.
56. Guccion JG, Enzinger FM. Malignant giant cell tumor of soft parts. An analysis of 32 cases. Cancer 1972;29(6):1518–29.
57. van Haelst UJ, de Haas van Dorsser AH. Giant cell tumor of soft parts. An ultrastructural study. Virchows Arch A Pathol Anat Histol 1976; 371(3):199–217.
58. Khalidi HS, Singleton TP, Weiss SW. Inflammatory malignant fibrous histiocytoma: distinction from Hodgkin's disease and non-Hodgkin's lymphoma by a panel of leukocyte markers. Mod Pathol 1997;10(5): 438–42.
59. Nascimento AF, et al. Epithelioid variant of myxofibrosarcoma: expanding the clinicomorphologic spectrum of myxofibrosarcoma in a series of 17 cases. Am J Surg Pathol 2007;31(1):99–105.
60. Weber MH, et al. The cytologic diagnosis of epithelioid myxofibrosarcoma: a case report. Diagn Cytopathol 2012;40(Suppl. 2):E140–3.
61. Brecher ME, Franklin WA. Absence of mononuclear phagocyte antigens in malignant fibrous histiocytoma. Am J Clin Pathol 1986;86(3):344–8.
62. Wood GS, Beckstead JH, Turner RR, et al. Malignant fibrous histiocytoma tumor cells resemble fibroblasts. Am J Surg Pathol 1986;10(5):323–35.
63. Agaimy A, Gaumann A, Schroeder J, et al. Primary and metastatic high-grade pleomorphic sarcoma/malignant fibrous histiocytoma of the gastrointestinal tract: an approach to the differential diagnosis in a series of five cases with emphasis on myofibroblastic differentiation. Virchows Arch 2007;451(5):949–57.
64. Lawson CW, Fisher C, Gatter KC. An immunohistochemical study of differentiation in malignant fibrous histiocytoma. Histopathology 1987; 11(4):375–83.
65. Litzky LA, Brooks JJ. Cytokeratin immunoreactivity in malignant fibrous histiocytoma and spindle cell tumors: comparison between frozen and paraffin-embedded tissues. Mod Pathol 1992;5(1):30–4.
66. Weiss SW, Bratthauer GL, Morris PA. Postirradiation malignant fibrous histiocytoma expressing cytokeratin. Implications for the immunodiagnosis of sarcomas. Am J Surg Pathol 1988;12(7):554–8.
67. Gazziola C, Cordani N, Wasserman B, et al. Malignant fibrous histiocytoma: a proposed cellular origin and identification of its characterizing gene transcripts. Int J Oncol 2003;23(2):343–51.
68. Al-Agha OM, Igbokwe AA. Malignant fibrous histiocytoma: between the past and the present. Arch Pathol Lab Med 2008;132(6): 1030–5.
69. Mertens F, Fletcher CD, Dal Cin P, et al. Cytogenetic analysis of 46 pleomorphic soft tissue sarcomas and correlation with morphologic and clinical features: a report of the CHAMP Study Group. Chromosomes and MorPhology. Genes Chromosomes Cancer 1998;22(1):16–25.
70. Larramendy ML, Gentile M, Soloneski S, et al. Does comparative genomic hybridization reveal distinct differences in DNA copy number sequence patterns between leiomyosarcoma and malignant fibrous histiocytoma? Cancer Genet Cytogenet 2008;187(1):1–11.
71. Nishio J, Iwasaki H, Nabeshima K, et al. Establishment of a new human pleomorphic malignant fibrous histiocytoma cell line, FU-MFH-2: molecular cytogenetic characterization by multicolor fluorescence in situ hybridization and comparative genomic hybridization. J Exp Clin Cancer Res 2010;29:153.

72. Carneiro A, Francis P, Bendahl PO, et al. Indistinguishable genomic profiles and shared prognostic markers in undifferentiated pleomorphic sarcoma and leiomyosarcoma: different sides of a single coin? Lab Invest 2009;89(6):668–75.
73. Le Doussal V, Coindre JM, Leroux A, et al. Prognostic factors for patients with localized primary malignant fibrous histiocytoma: a multicenter study of 216 patients with multivariate analysis. Cancer 1996;77(9): 1823–30.
74. Salo JC, Lewis JJ, Woodruff JM, et al. Malignant fibrous histiocytoma of the extremity. Cancer 1999;85(8):1765–72.
75. Gibbs JF, Huang PP, Lee RJ, et al. Malignant fibrous histiocytoma: an institutional review. Cancer Invest 2001;19(1):23–7.
76. Zagars GK, Mullen JR, Pollack A. Malignant fibrous histiocytoma: outcome and prognostic factors following conservation surgery and radiotherapy. Int J Radiat Oncol Biol Phys 1996;34(5):983–94.
77. Belal A, Kandil A, Allam A, et al. Malignant fibrous histiocytoma: a retrospective study of 109 cases. Am J Clin Oncol 2002;25(1): 16–22.

Chapter 14 Benign Lipomatous Tumors

CHAPTER CONTENTS

The significance and multiple functions of fat are not always fully appreciated. Fat serves not only as one of the principal and most readily available sources of energy in the body, but also functions as a barrier for the conservation of heat and as mechanical protection of the underlying tissues against physical injury. Two basic forms of adipose tissue can be distinguished: *white fat* and *brown fat*.

WHITE FAT

White fat makes its first appearance at a relatively late stage of development; it is rarely encountered before the third or fourth month of intrauterine life. In its earliest stages, after 10 to 14 weeks' gestation, it consists of aggregates of mesenchymal cells that are condensed around proliferating primitive blood vessels.[1] Following this stage, the stellate-shaped preadipocytes are organized into lobules that contain a rich network of proliferating capillaries. At later stages (14 to 24 weeks' gestation), small lipid droplets appear in these cells, gradually converting them to rounded or spherical, multivacuolated lipoblasts. Intracellular glycogen is usually present at this stage of development. The multiple lipid droplets then fuse to form a single vacuole and displace the nucleus marginally, forming the mature fat cell, or lipocyte. Small aggregates of lipocytes form lobules that make their first appearance in the regions of the face, neck, breast, and abdominal wall followed by the back and shoulders. The lobules multiply and enlarge, and, by the end of the fifth month, a continuous subcutaneous layer of fat is formed in the extremities.[2]

Postnatally, white fat cells enlarge significantly during the first 6 months of life without a significant increase in cell number. This phase is followed by a progressive increase in adipocyte number, although the cell size remains fairly constant. At puberty, there is a marked increase in adipocyte size and number. After puberty, new adipocytes continue to form throughout adult life, although at a much slower rate.[3]

Histologically, differentiated white fat consists of spherical or polygonal cells in which most of the cytoplasm has been replaced by a single large lipid droplet, leaving only a narrow rim of cytoplasm at the periphery. The eccentrically placed nucleus is flattened and is crescent-shaped on a cross-section; not infrequently it contains one small lipid invagination (Lochkern). Like any metabolically active tissue, white fat is highly vascularized, a feature that is more evident in atrophic fat than in normal fat. In the subcutis and, to a lesser extent, in deeper tissues, the fat cells are arranged in distinct lobules separated by a thin membrane of fibrous connective tissue. The lobular architecture of white fat is most prominent in areas subjected to pressure and probably has a cushioning effect.

Continued accumulation of cytoplasm and increasing amounts of intracellular lipid lead to more-rounded cells, which are characterized by a large, centrally located lipid droplet, a thin rim of cytoplasm, and a peripherally placed, flattened, or crescent-shaped nucleus. There is a membrane separating the central lipid inclusion from the surrounding cytoplasm. This signet-ring stage of cellular development represents the lipocyte of mature adipose tissue.

BROWN FAT

The precursors of brown fat are spindle-shaped cells that are closely related to a network of capillaries.[4] Subsequently, there is a proliferation of capillaries and brown adipocytes, with organization into lobules by fibrous connective tissue septa. As the cells accumulate lipid, they are initially unilocular; but, with further lipid accumulation, multiple cytoplasmic lipid vacuoles appear. Brown fat is found mainly in infants and children and gradually disappears from most sites with increasing age. In children, brown fat deposits are most conspicuous in the interscapular region, around the blood vessels and muscles of the neck, around the structures of the mediastinum, adjacent to the lung hila, on the anterior abdominal wall, and surrounding intra-abdominal and retroperitoneal structures, including the kidneys, pancreas, and spleen. During adulthood, deposits of brown fat persist around the kidneys, adrenal glands, and aorta and within the mediastinum and neck.

The term *brown fat* refers to its gross appearance, which results from its abundant vascularity and numerous mitochondria. Compared to white fat, brown fat tends to have a more prominent lobulated growth pattern. Its cells are smaller (25 to 40 μm in diameter), are round or polygonal, and contain a large amount of deeply eosinophilic cytoplasm. The cells are mostly multivacuolated, with distinctly granular cytoplasm between the individual lipid droplets. Intermixed with these cells are nonvacuolated, purely granular cells and cells with a single large lipid vacuole, resembling lipocytes. The nuclei are rounded and situated in a central position, although the nucleus may be displaced to the periphery in cells with large lipid vacuoles, as in white fat. The cells are arranged in distinct lobular aggregates and are intimately associated with a prominent vascular network and numerous nerves.[5]

MOLECULAR BIOLOGY OF BENIGN LIPOMATOUS TUMORS

The *DDIT3* gene (formerly known as *CHOP*), located on the long arm of chromosome 12, appears to be involved in adipocytic differentiation.[6] This gene encodes a member of the CCAAT/enhancer binding protein (C/EBP) family, which may be an inhibitor of other C/EBP transcription factors known to be important in cell proliferation. Members of the C/EBP group are highly expressed in fat and are involved in the growth arrest of terminally differentiated adipocytes.[7]

IMMUNOHISTOCHEMISTRY OF BENIGN LIPOMATOUS TUMORS

Adipocytes and benign and malignant fatty tumors stain positively for vimentin and S-100 protein.[8] An antibody to the adipocyte lipid-binding protein p422 (also known as *aP2*), a protein expressed exclusively in preadipocytes late in adipogenesis, has been found to stain only lipoblasts and brown fat cells, as well as liposarcomas.[9] The diagnostic utility of this antibody has yet to be proven.

CLASSIFICATION OF BENIGN LIPOMATOUS TUMORS

It is widely assumed that benign lipomatous tumors represent a common group of neoplasms that cause few complaints or complications and present little diagnostic difficulty. This may be largely true for the ordinary subcutaneous lipoma, but it does not take into account the enormous variety of benign tumors and tumor-like lesions of adipose tissue that are well defined but often have received little attention in the medical literature. In fact, benign lipomatous tumors are among the most frequently received in a consultation practice.

The bulk of lipomatous tumors may be grouped into four categories, including:

1. *Superficial lipoma*, a tumor composed of mature fat and arising in the superficial (subcutaneous) soft tissues, represents by far the most common mesenchymal neoplasm.
2. *Deep lipomas* arise from or are intimately associated with tissues deep to the subcutis or arise in specific anatomic sites. The main subdivisions of this group are angiomyolipoma (a member of the PEComa family of tumors), intramuscular and intermuscular lipoma, lipoma of the tendon sheath, neural fibrolipoma with and without macrodactyly (fibrolipomatous hamartoma), and lumbosacral lipoma.
3. *Infiltrating* or *diffuse neoplastic* or *non-neoplastic proliferations of mature fat* may cause compression of vital structures or may be confused with atypical lipomatous neoplasm/well-differentiated liposarcoma. This group is composed of six entities: diffuse lipomatosis, pelvic lipomatosis, symmetric lipomatosis (Madelung disease), adiposis dolorosa (Dercum disease), steroid lipomatosis, and nevus lipomatosus.
4. *Variants of lipoma* are much less common and differ from ordinary lipoma by a characteristic microscopic picture and specific clinical setting. These include angiolipoma, myolipoma, myelolipoma, chondroid lipoma, spindle cell/pleomorphic lipoma, hibernoma, and lipoblastoma/lipoblastomatosis.

When describing these entities, no attempt has been made to distinguish between true neoplasms, hamartomatous processes, and localized overgrowth of fat, because it would be largely speculative and of little practical consequence. In the past 20 years, cytogenetic data have contributed significantly to the understanding of the pathogenesis of both benign and malignant lipomatous tumors. Although cytogenetic analysis is of limited diagnostic utility in this group of benign lipomatous tumors, the knowledge gained by such analyses has allowed a better understanding of how these lipomatous tumors are related to one another (Table 14-1).

TABLE 14-1 Principal Chromosomal Aberrations of Benign Lipomatous Tumors

TUMOR	CHROMOSOMAL ABERRATION
Lipoma (ordinary)	Translocations involving 12q13-15
	Interstitial deletions of 13q
	Rearrangements involving 6p21-23
Angiolipoma	None
Spindle cell/pleomorphic lipoma	Loss of 16q13
	Unbalanced 13q alterations
Lipoblastoma/lipoblastomatosis	Translocations involving 8q11-13
Hibernoma	Translocations involving 11q13
	Translocations involving 10q22
Chondroid lipoma	t(11;16)(q13;p12-13)

LIPOMA

Solitary lipomas, consisting entirely of mature fat, have been largely ignored in the literature, because they grow insidiously and cause few problems other than those of a localized mass. Many lipomas remain unrecorded or are brought to the attention of a physician only if they reach a large size or cause cosmetic problems or complications because of their anatomic site. As a consequence, the reported incidence of lipoma is certainly much lower than the actual incidence. Even if only the recorded data were considered, however, lipomas outnumber other benign or malignant soft tissue tumors by a considerable margin.

Age and Gender Incidence

Lipoma is rare during the first two decades of life and usually makes its appearance when fat begins to accumulate in inactive individuals. Most become clinically apparent in patients 40 to 60 years of age. When not excised, the lipoma persists for the remainder of life, although they hardly increase in size after the initial growth period. Statistics vary as to gender incidence, but most report a higher incidence in men.[10] There seems to be no difference in regard to race; in the United States, whites and African-Americans are affected in proportion to their distribution in the general population.

Localization

Two types of solitary lipoma can be distinguished. *Subcutaneous (superficial) lipomas* are most common in the regions of the upper back and neck, shoulder, and abdomen, followed in frequency by the proximal portions of the extremities, chiefly the upper arms, buttocks, and upper thigh. They are seldom encountered in the face, hands, lower legs, or feet.

Deep lipomas are far rarer. They are often detected at a relatively late stage of development and consequently tend to be larger than superficial lipomas. When in the extremities, they often arise from the subfascial tissues of the hands and feet. They may also arise from juxta-articular regions or the periosteum (*parosteal lipoma*), sometimes causing nerve compression, erosion of bone, or focal cortical hyperostosis.[11] Deep lipomas in the region of the head occur chiefly in the forehead and scalp;[12] those in the trunk are found principally in the thorax and mediastinum, chest wall and pleura, and pelvis and paratesticular region.[13]

Deep or subfascial lipomas tend to be less well circumscribed than superficial ones, and their contours are usually determined by the space that they occupy. Intrathoracic lipomas, for instance, may extend from the upper mediastinum, neck, or subpleural region (*cervicomediastinal lipoma*) into the subcutis of the chest wall, sometimes assuming an hourglass configuration. Deep-seated lipomas of the hand or wrist form irregular masses with multiple processes underneath fascia or aponeuroses; they may attain a large size and, on rare occasions, extend from the palm to the dorsal surface of the hand. These tumors must be distinguished from lipomas growing in the tendon sheath (*endovaginal lipomas*) and those involving major nerves in the regions of the hand and wrist (*neural fibrolipomas* or *fibrolipomatous hamartomas*), which usually occur in young patients and may be associated with macrodactyly.

There are also rare lipoma-like fatty proliferations in the region of the umbilicus and inguinal ring (*hernial lipoma*) that may be associated with direct or indirect hernias or merely simulate a hernia clinically. A similar overgrowth of fat arising from surgical scars has been termed *incisional lipoma*.

Clinical Findings

The usual clinical history of lipoma is that of an asymptomatic, slowly growing, round or discoid mass with a soft consistency. Pain is rare with ordinary lipomas; when it occurs, it is a late symptom generally confined to large angiolipomas or lipomas that compress peripheral nerves. Although this may seem intuitive, lipomas are more common in obese persons and often increase in size during a period of rapid weight gain. In contrast, severe weight loss in cachectic patients or during periods of prolonged starvation rarely affects the size of a lipoma, suggesting that the fatty tissue of lipomas (or liposarcomas) is largely unavailable for general metabolism.

Deep lipomas may cause a variety of symptoms, depending on their site and size. The symptoms range from a feeling of fullness and discomfort on motion and, rarely, restriction of movement with lipomas of the hand to dyspnea or palpitation with mediastinal tumors. Although some benign lipomatous tumors have been described in the retroperitoneum, most reported in the early literature probably represent well-differentiated liposarcomas rather than lipomas. However, it is clear that retroperitoneal lipomas do exist but can only be diagnosed following extensive sampling and molecular analysis revealing an absence of *MDM2* amplification.[14] This topic is more thoroughly discussed in Chapter 15.

Imaging studies are extremely helpful for diagnosis; lipomas present as globular radiolucent masses clearly outlined by the greater density of the surrounding tissue. CT scans reveal a mass having the appearance of subcutaneous fat and, like fat, having a much more uniform density than liposarcomas. On MRI, both benign and malignant lipomatous tumors exhibit a high signal intensity on T1-weighted images.[15]

Gross Findings

Subcutaneous lipoma usually manifests as a soft, well-circumscribed, thinly encapsulated, rounded mass varying in size from a few millimeters to 5 cm or more (median: 3 cm); lipomas larger than 10 cm are uncommon. On a cross-section, the lipoma is pale yellow to orange and has a uniform greasy surface and an irregular lobular pattern (Fig. 14-1A). Lipomas of deeper structures vary much more in shape, but they also tend to be well delineated from the surrounding tissues by a thin capsule. Focal discoloration caused by hemorrhage or fat necrosis occurs, but it is much less common than in liposarcomas.

Microscopic Findings

Lipomas differ little in microscopic appearance from the surrounding fat because they are composed of mature fat cells,

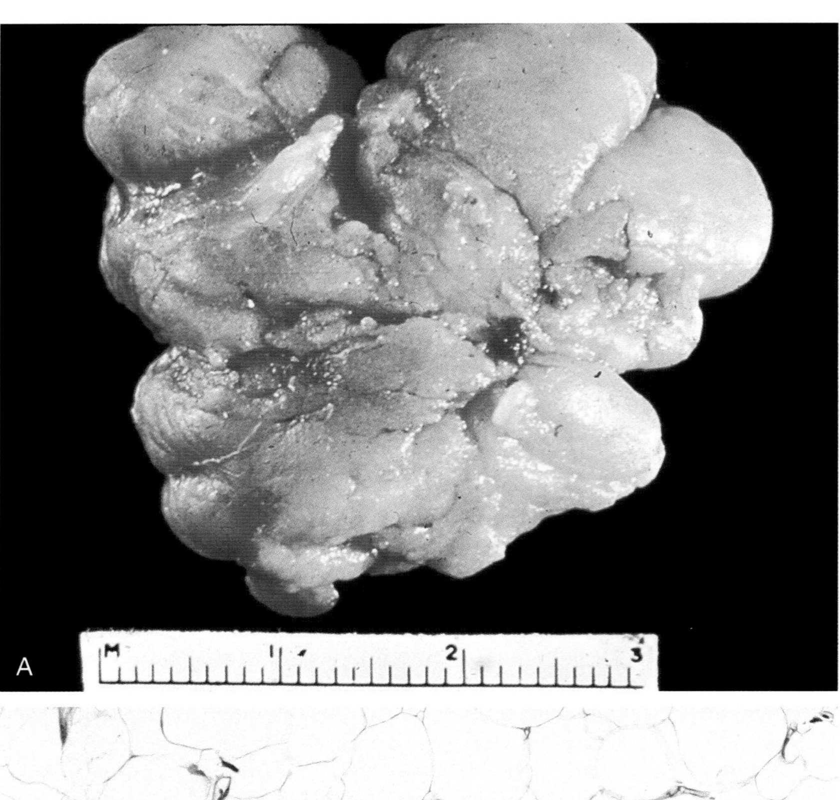

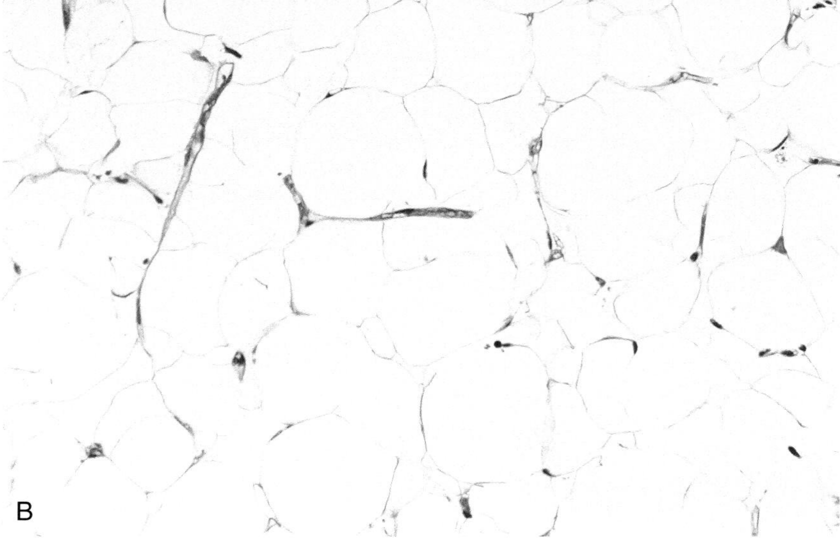

FIGURE 14-1. (A) Lipoma showing a distinct multilobular pattern and uniform yellow color. (B) Lipoma consisting throughout of mature fat cells has only a slight variation in cellular size and shape.

but the cells vary slightly in size and shape and are somewhat larger (Fig. 14-1B). The nuclei are uniform, and it is important to note that there is an absence of nuclear hyperchromasia. Subcutaneous lipomas are usually thinly encapsulated and have a distinct lobular configuration. All are well vascularized, but, under normal conditions, the vascular network is compressed by the distended lipocytes and is not clearly discernible. The rich vascularity of these tumors becomes apparent in atrophic lipomas in which the markedly reduced volume of the lipocytes reveals the intricate vascular network in the interstitial space.

Lipomas are occasionally altered by an admixture of other mesenchymal elements that comprise an intrinsic part of the tumor. The most common of these elements is fibrous connective tissue, which is often hyalinized and may or may not be associated with the capsule or the fibrous septa (*fibrolipomas*). *Sclerotic lipomas* have a predilection to occur on the scalp or hands of young men and are composed predominantly of sclerotic fibrous tissue with only focal lipocytic areas.[16] Some lipomas show extensive myxoid change (*myxolipomas*); such cases may be difficult to distinguish from spindle cell lipomas (Fig. 14-2).[17] Some of these lesions have an abundance of thin- and thick-walled blood vessels and have been termed *vascular myxolipoma* or *angiomyxolipoma,*[18] but these are merely descriptive terms, and they are not used as a distinctive diagnostic category of lipoma. Distinction of these tumors from *myxomas* and *myxoid liposarcomas* may on occasion be difficult. In general, however, the presence of transitional zones between fat and myxoid areas helps rule out myxoma, and the absence of lipoblasts and a diffuse plexiform capillary pattern militates against myxoid liposarcoma. Vacuolated cells containing mucoid material are occasionally seen in myxolipomas and angiomyxolipomas; but, unlike neoplastic lipoblasts, these cells lack hyperchromatic nuclei and distinctly outlined

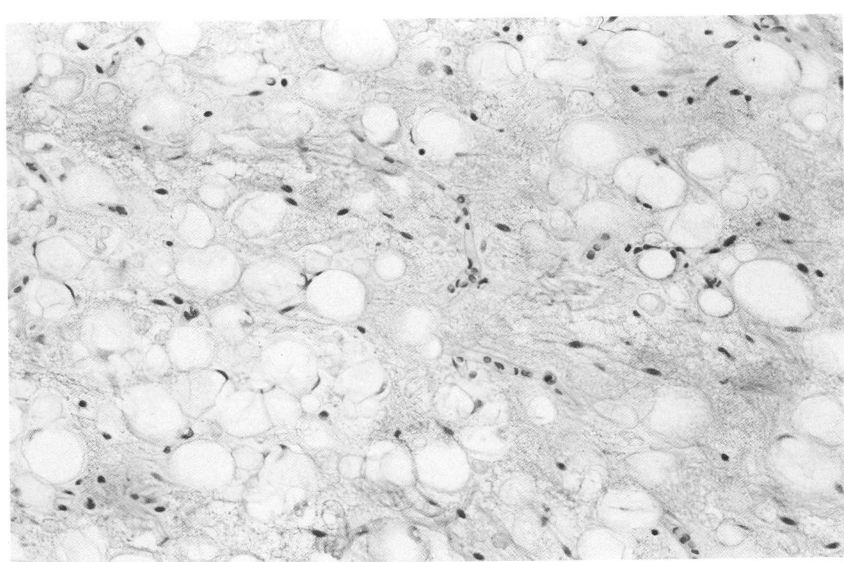

FIGURE 14-2. Lipoma with myxoid change.

lipid droplets within the cytoplasm. In difficult cases, molecular analysis to show an absence of alterations of *DDIT3* (formerly known as *CHOP*) can be extremely helpful. Cartilaginous or osseous metaplasia (*chondrolipoma, osteolipoma*) is rare and is mainly encountered in lipomas of large size and long duration.[19]

Secondary changes occur occasionally as the result of impaired blood supply or traumatic injury.[20] Prolonged ischemia may lead to infarction, hemorrhage, and calcification and may result in cyst-like changes. Similarly, infection or trauma may cause fat necrosis and local liquefaction of fat, a process marked by phagocytic activity and formation of lipid cysts. Characteristically, nests of foamy macrophages are found in the intercellular spaces or around lipocytes that have ruptured or have been traumatized (Fig. 14-3). This process is sometimes accompanied by multinucleated giant cells and scattered inflammatory elements, chiefly lymphocytes or plasma cells. In some cases, cystic spaces are lined by an eosinophilic, hyaline membrane with pseudopapillary luminal projections (membranous fat necrosis).[21]

Cytogenetic and Molecular Findings

Approximately 55% to 75% of lipomas have chromosomal aberrations.[22-24] Of these, approximately 75% show a balanced karyotype, and most have 46 chromosomes. Cytogenetic aberrations seem to increase in prevalence with increasing patient age.[24] There are essentially three major subgroups of cytogenetic aberrations. Approximately two-thirds of tumors with an abnormal karyotype have 12q13-15 aberrations. Although 12q13-15 can combine with many different bands in virtually all chromosomes, the most common is a t(3;12)(q27-28;q13-15), found in approximately 20% of cases with an aberration of 12q13-15. Less than 10% of cases with 12q13-15 aberrations involve 1p36, 1p32-34, 2p22-24, 2q35-37, 5q33, 11q13, and 12p11-12, among others.

Approximately one-third of lipomas with an abnormal karyotype do not harbor aberrations of 12q13-15. Of these, the most commonly involved loci include 6p21-23, 13q11-12, and 12q22-24. The only recurrent translocation involving 6p21-23 is a t(3;6)(q27-28;p21-23). Various combinations can occur in the same tumor, including simultaneous 13q11-12 and 6p21-23 rearrangements or 13q11-12 and 12q13-15 rearrangements, but aberrations of 6p and 12q rarely occur together.

At the molecular level, the *HMGIC* (*HMGA2*) gene, which encodes for a member of the high mobility group of proteins and is located on 12q15, seems to be affected, in some cases, with 12q13-15 rearrangements.[25,26] The t(3;12) results in a fusion of the *HMGIC* gene on 12q15 with the *LPP* gene on 3q27-28.[27,28] This fusion gene has also been detected in some parosteal lipomas and pulmonary chondroid hamartomas.[29] Aberrations of 6p21-23 may involve the *HMGIY* gene (*HMGA1B*).[30] Tallini et al.[31] developed monoclonal antibodies to *HMGIC* and *HMGIY*, and immunoreactivity with these antibodies was found to correlate very well with cytogenetic alterations.

Behavior and Treatment

Lipomas are completely benign, but they may recur locally (fewer than 5%). Malignant change is virtually unheard of, and only a few cases have been reported in the literature. It is likely, however, that some of them are actually pleomorphic lipomas, and others are atypical lipomatous neoplasms (well-differentiated liposarcomas) in which the malignant characteristics were absent or missed when the tumor was first examined. Deep lipomas have a greater tendency to recur, presumably because of the increased difficulty for complete surgical removal.

Discussion

Aside from the relatively small number of patients in whom an increased familial incidence of lipomas can be demonstrated, little is known about the pathogenesis of these tumors. Certainly, lipomas are more common in obese than in slender persons and perhaps, as a consequence, are more frequently encountered in patients older than 45 years. An increased

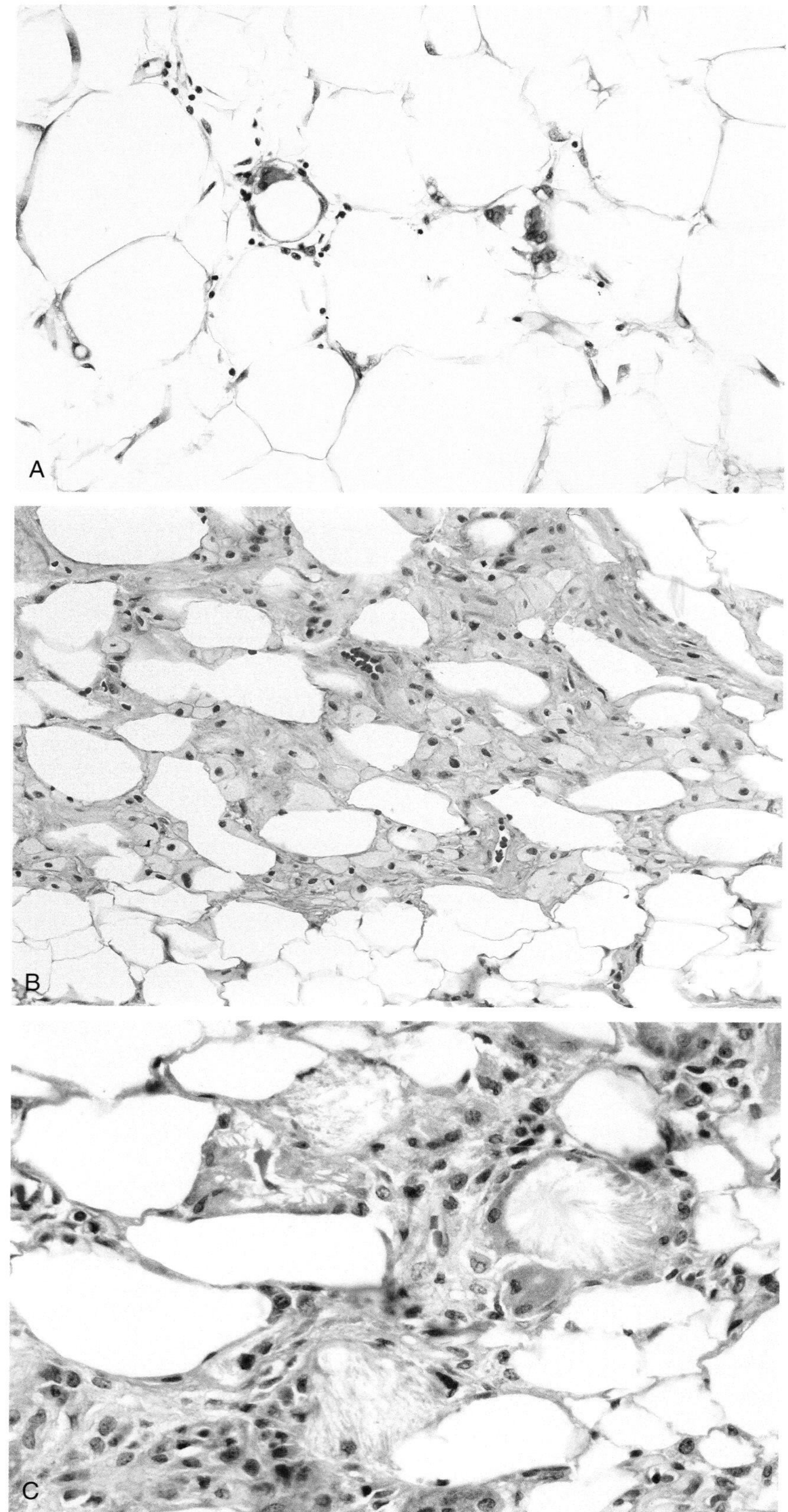

FIGURE 14-3. (A) Lipoma with focal fat necrosis with rare macrophage nuclei and vacuolated cytoplasm between mature fat cells. (B) Lipoma with a more extensive area of fat necrosis. Numerous macrophage nuclei with granular cytoplasm are seen between mature adipocytes. (C) Rare example of fat necrosis in a newborn infant.

incidence of lipomas is also claimed for diabetic patients and those with elevated serum cholesterol. Trauma or irradiation may lead to overgrowth of fat indistinguishable from a lipoma (posttraumatic pseudolipoma). In particular, such lesions, often exceeding 10 cm in diameter, have been observed to develop secondary to blunt, bruising injuries, often preceded by a large hematoma.[32]

MULTIPLE LIPOMAS

Approximately 5% to 8% of all patients with lipomas have multiple tumors that are grossly and microscopically indistinguishable from solitary lipomas. The term *lipomatosis* has been used to describe this lesion, but it is preferred that the name is used to describe a diffuse overgrowth of mature adipose tissue (described later in the chapter).

Multiple lipomas vary in number from a few to several hundred lesions, and they occur predominantly in the upper half of the body, with a predilection for the back, shoulder, and upper arms. Not infrequently, the lipomas are arranged in a symmetric distribution, with a slight predilection for the extensor surfaces of the extremities. They are about three times as common in men as in women. Most have their onset during the fifth and sixth decades, although occasional lesions appear as early as puberty.

There is a definite hereditary trait in about one-third of patients with this condition (*familial multiple lipomas*).[33] Most cases seem to be inherited in an autosomal dominant manner. Mutation in the tRNA gene of mitochondrial DNA has been implicated in this syndrome.[34]

The question of a relationship between multiple lipomas and neurofibromatosis has been raised repeatedly in the literature, but there is no convincing proof of this association.[35] In fact, given the frequency of lipomas and the relative frequency among inherited syndromes of neurofibromatosis, these entities probably occur together fortuitously.

There are several syndromes with multiple lipomatous lesions: *Bannayan-Zonana syndrome* is characterized by the congenital association of multiple lipomas (including lipomatosis of the thoracic and abdominal cavity, in some cases), hemangiomas, and macrocephaly.[36] *Cowden syndrome* consists of multiple lipomas and hemangiomas associated with goiter and lichenoid, papular, and papillomatous lesions of the skin and mucosae. Mutations in the *PTEN* gene have been identified in both of these inherited hamartoma syndromes.[37] *Fröhlich syndrome*, also known as *prune-belly syndrome*, is defined by multiple lipomas, obesity, and sexual infantilism.[38] *Proteus syndrome* is marked by multiple lipomatous lesions, including pelvic lipomatosis, fibroplasia of the feet and hands, skeletal hypertrophy, exostoses and scoliosis, and various pigmented lesions of the skin.[39]

ANGIOLIPOMA

Angiolipoma occurs chiefly as a subcutaneous nodule in young adults, often making its first appearance when the patient is in the late teens or early twenties; it is rare in children and in patients older than 50 years (unlike solitary or multiple subcutaneous lipomas). It also seems to be more common in males. About 5% of cases are familial.[40] The forearm is by far the most common site; almost two-thirds of all angiolipomas are found in this location. Next in frequency are the trunk and upper arm. Like all lipomas, it seldom occurs in the face, scalp, hands, and feet. Spinal angiolipoma is a specific entity that should be distinguished from cutaneous angiolipoma.[41] In addition, intramuscular hemangiomas, sometimes referred to as *infiltrating angiolipoma*, is distinct from cutaneous angiolipoma. Interestingly, angiolipomas are being detected more frequently in the vicinity of the breast, presumably as a result of the increased use of mammography.

Multiple angiolipomas are much more common than solitary ones and account for about two-thirds of all angiolipomas.[42] Characteristically, angiolipomas are tender to painful (often on touch only or palpation), particularly during the initial growth period; frequently, pain becomes less severe or ceases entirely when the tumor reaches its final size, which is rarely more than 2 cm. There seems to be no correlation between the degree of vascularity and the occurrence or intensity of pain, and the pain is not intensified by heat, cold, or venous occlusion.

Angiolipomas are always located in the subcutis, where they present as encapsulated yellow nodules with a more or less pronounced reddish tinge. They consist of mature fat cells separated by a branching network of small vessels (Fig. 14-4); the proportion of fatty tissue and vascular channels varies, but, usually, the vascularity is more prominent in the subcapsular areas (Figs. 14-5 and 14-6). Late forms of this tumor frequently undergo perivascular and interstitial fibrosis. Characteristically, the vascular channels contain fibrin thrombi (Fig. 14-7), a feature that is absent in ordinary lipomas. Mast cells are often conspicuous in angiolipomas, another feature that distinguishes this tumor from the usual lipoma. Some examples are highly cellular and composed almost entirely of vascular channels (cellular angiolipoma) (Fig. 14-8).[43]

Unlike ordinary lipomas, which usually have karyotypic abnormalities involving 12q, 6p, and 13q (described previously), most angiolipomas have been reported to show a normal karyotype.[44,45] Sciot et al.[45] argued that the normal karyotype characteristic of this tumor is more in keeping with a non-neoplastic lesion, possibly a hamartoma. Furthermore, because hemangiomas also usually have a normal karyotype, it raises the possibility that the vascular component is the primary proliferation.

The differential diagnosis of this lesion, in part, depends on the density of vessels. The hypovascular lesions may be difficult to distinguish from *ordinary lipomas*, although the identification of microthrombi allows this distinction. *Intramuscular hemangioma*, at one time referred to as *cellular* or *infiltrating angiolipoma*, should not be difficult to distinguish from the more superficially located angiolipoma; despite similarities in name, the latter can be correctly diagnosed if attention is paid to the encapsulation of the lesion, the presence of microthrombi, and the small size, multiplicity, and subcutaneous location of the lesion. The cellular angiolipoma may be difficult to distinguish from *Kaposi sarcoma*. Like cellular angiolipoma, Kaposi sarcoma can be found as multiple subcutaneous nodules in young men. However, Kaposi sarcoma has slit-like vascular spaces and periodic acid-Schiff-positive globules in the cytoplasm of some of the cells, and it lacks microthrombi. Moreover, this lesion is characterized by immunoreactivity for human herpesvirus HHV-8.

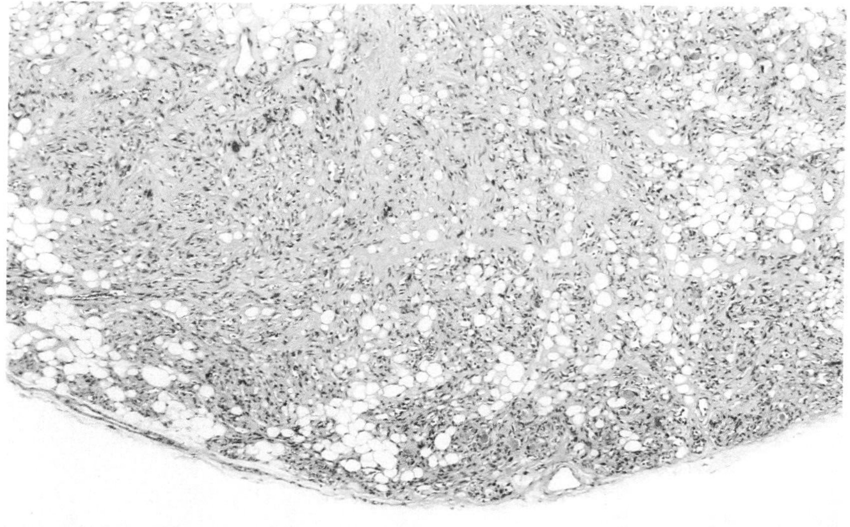

FIGURE 14-4. Angiolipoma showing sharp circumscription and proliferation of numerous vascular channels between mature fat cells.

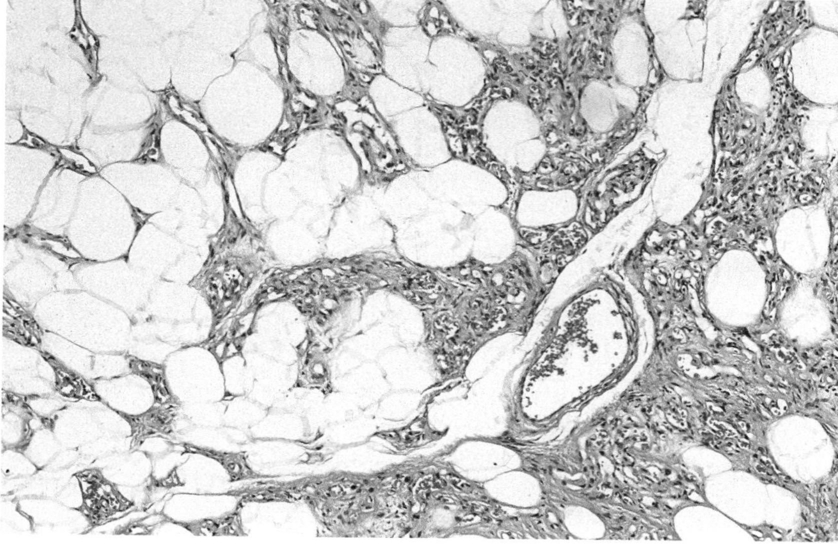

FIGURE 14-5. Angiolipoma consisting of a mixture of fat cells and narrow vascular channels. The vascularity is more prominent in the subcapsular areas.

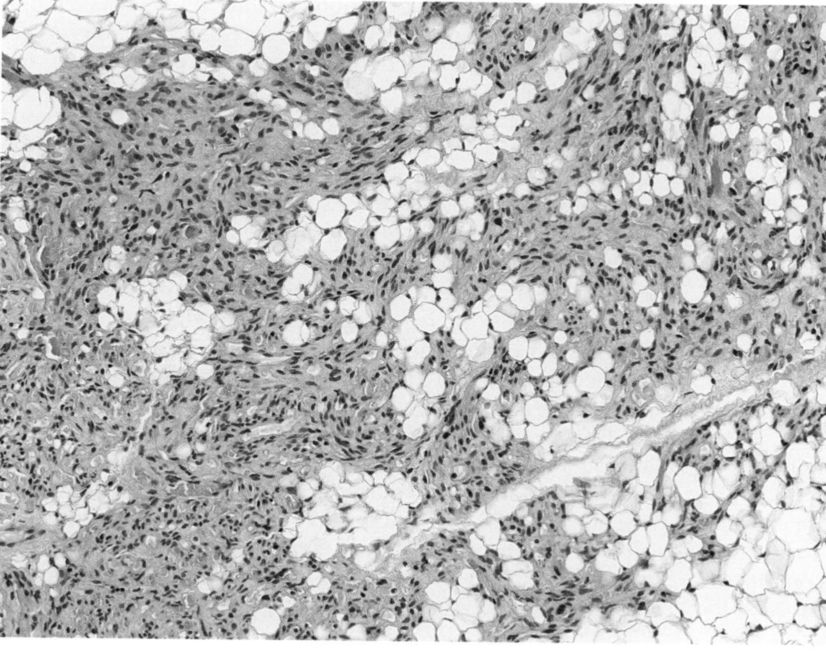

FIGURE 14-6. Angiolipoma with small vessels with an infiltrative-like appearance between mature fat cells.

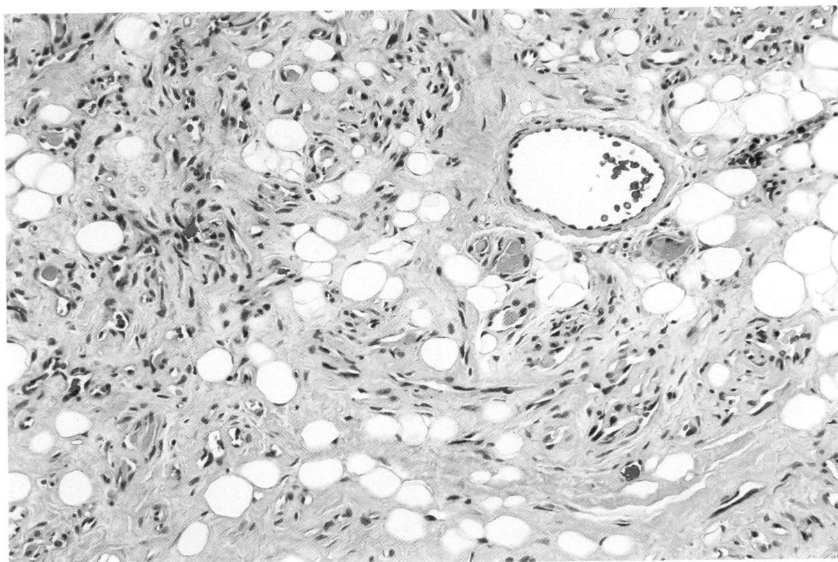

FIGURE 14-7. Angiolipoma with fibrin thrombi, a characteristic feature of this tumor.

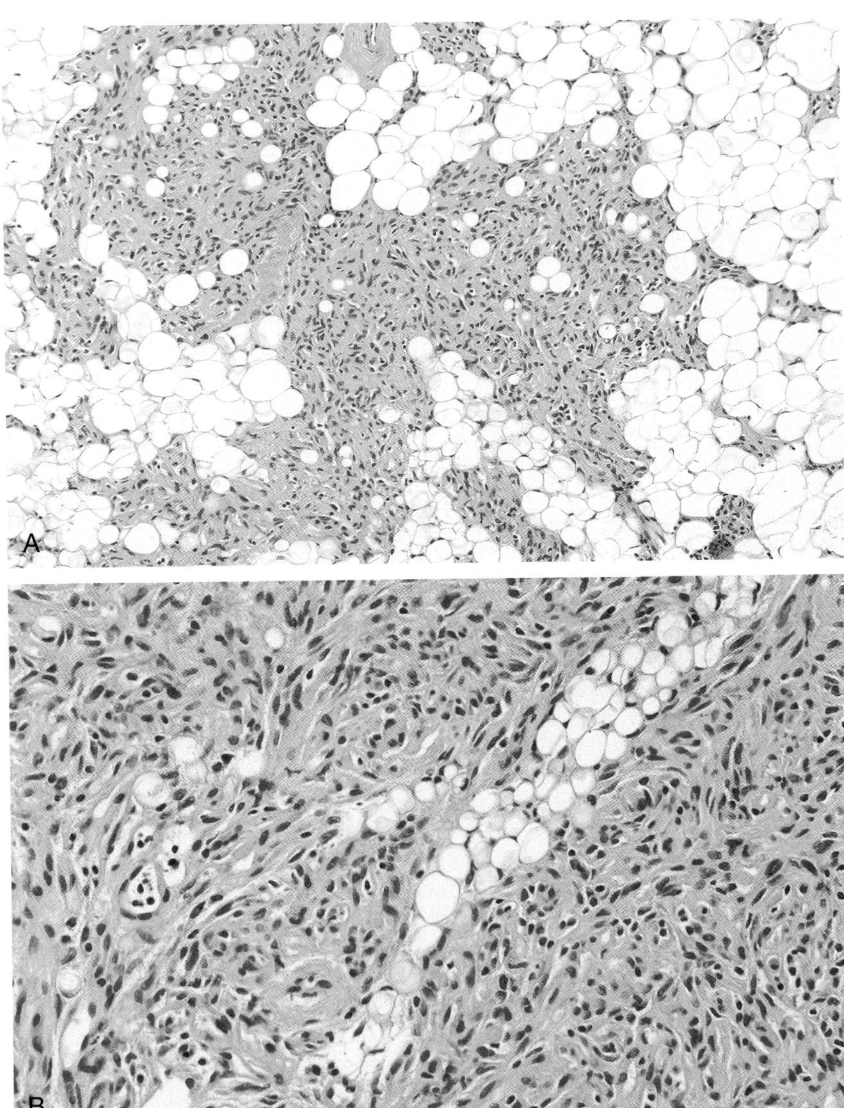

FIGURE 14-8. (A) Low-power appearance of an angiolipoma with increased cellularity. (B) High-power view of a cellular area of the angiolipoma, with virtually complete replacement by proliferating small vessels. Lesions of this type have been mistaken for Kaposi sarcoma or spindle cell angiosarcoma. *Continued*

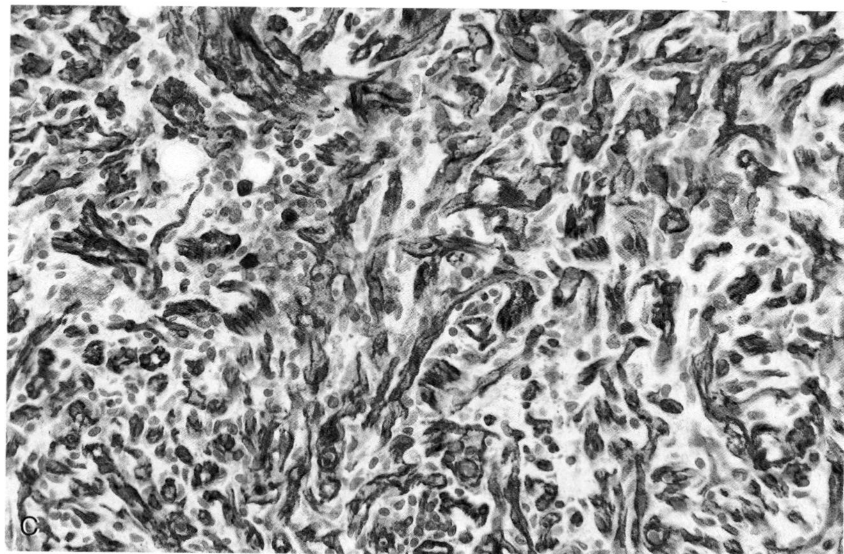

FIGURE 14-8, cont'd. (C) Cellular angiolipoma stained for CD31, indicating that virtually all of the spindle cells are endothelial cells.

Angiolipomas are benign. There is no evidence that these lesions ever undergo malignant transformation.

MYOLIPOMA

Myolipoma is a rare variant of lipoma marked by the proliferation of mature fat and mature smooth-muscle tissue. The alternate term *extrauterine lipoleiomyoma* may also be used, but the preferred term is *myolipoma* because the former implies some relationship to uterine smooth muscle tumors. The tumor occurs in adults, most commonly during the fifth and sixth decades of life, with a predilection for women. Myolipoma is most often found in the retroperitoneum, abdomen, pelvis, inguinal region, or abdominal wall.[46,47] The extremities may also be involved, usually as a subcutaneous mass that can also involve the superficial muscular fascia.[46] Most patients present with a painless mass, but, in some cases, the tumor is found incidentally because of its propensity to arise in deep locations. Deep-seated tumors are often quite large, obtaining an average size of 15 cm, whereas subcutaneous lesions tend to be much smaller.

Grossly, the tumors are completely or partially encapsulated with a glistening, yellow-white cut surface; tumors with a prominent smooth muscle component have large areas of white or gray firm tissue with a whorled appearance. Histologically, myolipoma consists of a variable admixture of mature adipose tissue and bundles or sheets of well-differentiated smooth muscle, both of which lack nuclear atypia (Fig. 14-9), although one case of myolipoma with bizarre, presumably degenerative, nuclei has been described. Generally, the smooth muscle component is regularly interspersed with the adipose tissue, imparting a sieve-like appearance at low magnification. The smooth muscle bundles are typically arranged in short interweaving fascicles and are characterized by cytologically bland oval nuclei with longitudinally oriented deeply eosinophilic fibrillar cytoplasm. The adipose tissue component is entirely mature and lacks floret-like giant cells or lipoblasts.[48] Some lesions have prominent stromal sclerosis and chronic inflammation. Medium-caliber arteries with thick muscular walls, characteristic of angiomyolipoma, are absent.

The smooth muscle element stains strongly for smooth muscle actin and desmin (Fig. 14-10). Estrogen receptor positivity has also been noted, but very few cases have been evaluated for the expression of this antigen.[49]

The differential diagnosis includes spindle cell lipoma, angiolipoma, angiomyolipoma, leiomyoma with fatty degeneration, and dedifferentiated liposarcoma. *Spindle cell lipoma* is composed of cytologically bland, non-myoid spindle-shaped cells that express CD34 but not smooth muscle markers. Furthermore, spindle cell lipoma is exceedingly rare in the retroperitoneum, abdomen, and pelvis. *Angiomyolipoma* often presents as a large retroperitoneal mass, as does myolipoma. It differs from myolipoma by the presence of medium-sized arteries with thick muscular walls, as well as epithelioid smooth muscle cells that are immunoreactive for melanocytic markers. Unlike angiomyolipoma, myolipoma is not associated with tuberous sclerosis. *Leiomyoma with fatty degeneration* lacks the regular distribution of fat that is present in myolipoma (Fig. 14-11). Furthermore, fatty degeneration of smooth muscle tumors of soft tissue is rare. Finally, *dedifferentiated liposarcoma* can be distinguished from myolipoma by the presence of atypical hyperchromatic cells in the adipocytic component and cytologic atypia with mitotic activity in the dedifferentiated component.

Myolipoma, despite its frequently large size and occurrence in deep soft tissue locations, is a benign neoplasm, with no reported recurrence or metastasis.

CHONDROID LIPOMA

Chondroid lipoma is a rare, benign fatty tumor found in the subcutaneous tissue or in deeper soft tissues predominantly in the limbs and limb girdles of adult women. Although it is clinically benign, it is another example of a pseudosarcoma in that it may be mistaken for a myxoid liposarcoma or chondrosarcoma. Although first recognized as a distinct entity in 1993 by

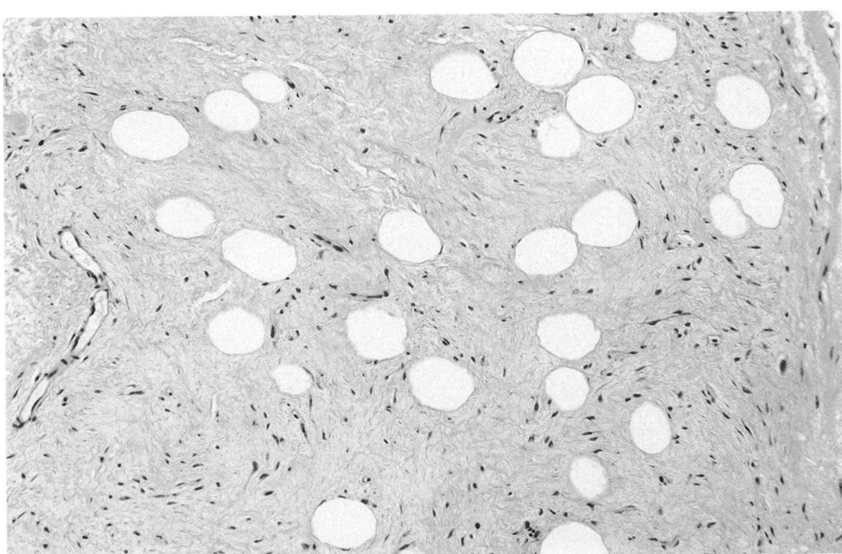

FIGURE 14-9. Myolipoma with a mixture of elongated eosinophilic smooth muscle cells and adipocytes.

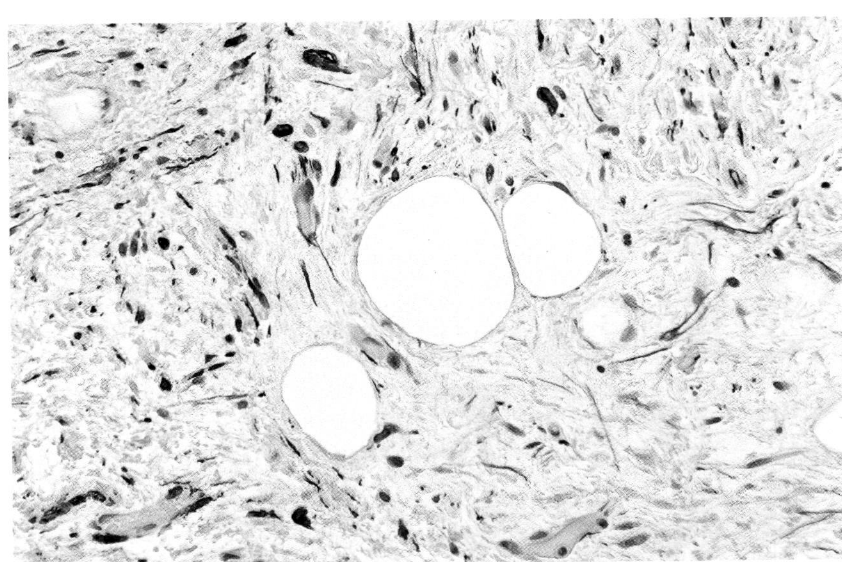

FIGURE 14-10. Myolipoma stained for desmin, showing that virtually all of the spindle cells are smooth muscle cells.

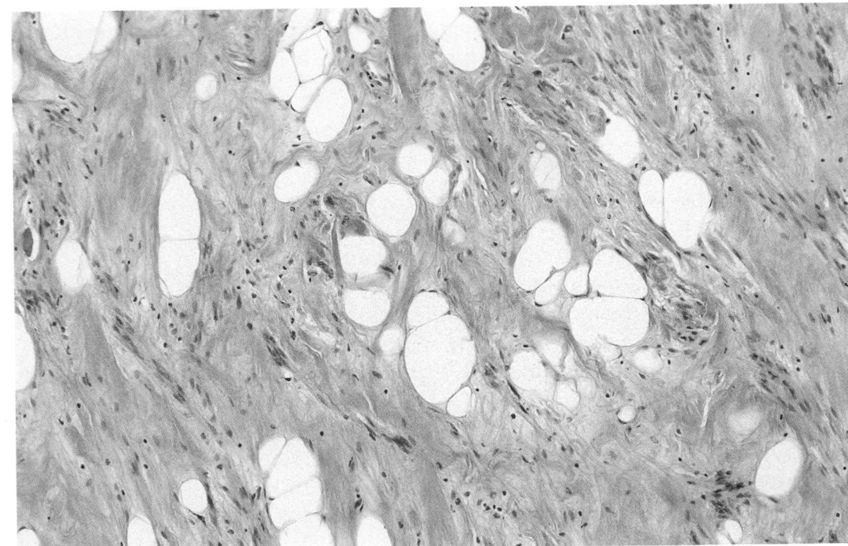

FIGURE 14-11. Uterine leiomyoma with fatty degeneration. This lesion is composed predominantly of mature smooth-muscle cells, with only focal areas of mature fat cells. Fatty degeneration of smooth muscle tumors of soft tissue is rare.

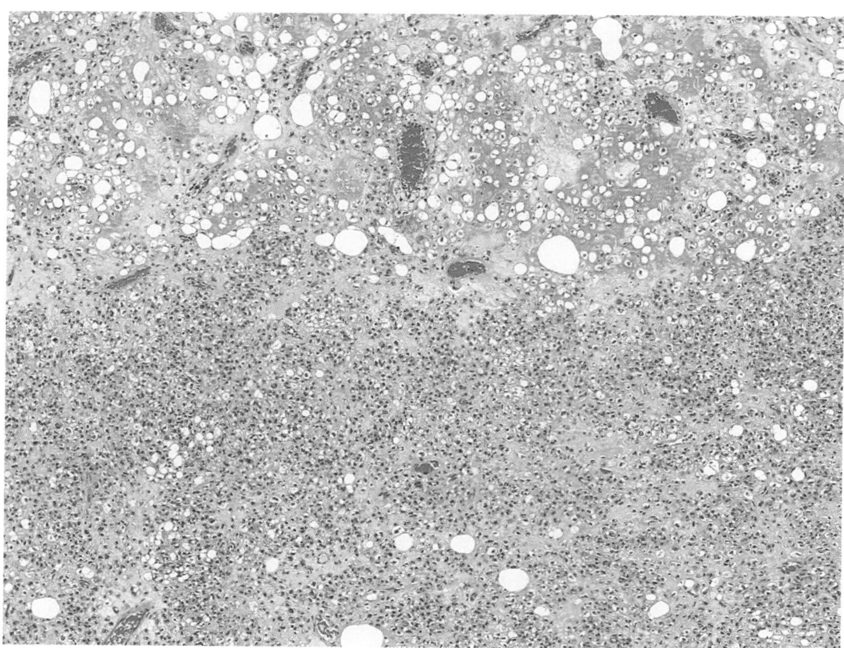

FIGURE 14-12. Low-power view of chondroid lipoma.

Meis and Enzinger,[50] it was probably first described by Chan et al.[51] as an "extraskeletal chondroma with lipoblast-like cells."

Clinical Findings

Although the age range is broad, most patients are in the third or fourth decade of life, and there is a striking predilection for women. In the largest series to date from the Armed Forces Institute of Pathology (AFIP) (20 cases), there were 16 females and 4 males ranging in age from 14 to 70 years, with a median age of 35 years.[50] Most patients present with a slowly growing painless mass that is often present for several years before excision. This lesion most commonly arises in the proximal extremity or limb girdle. Less common sites include the distal extremities, trunk, and the head and neck region, especially the oral cavity.[52,53] Radiologic studies show a heterogeneous soft tissue mass that has features different than typical lipoma, but not distinctive enough to be diagnostic.[54] The diagnosis can be suggested by fine-needle aspiration in the hands of a skilled cytopathologist with some experience with this rare tumor.[55]

Pathologic Findings

Grossly, the tumor is well demarcated and often encapsulated with a yellow, white, or pink-tan cut surface. It ranges in size from 1 to 11 cm (mean: 4 cm). Some lesions are located entirely within the subcutaneous tissue, whereas others involve the superficial fascia or skeletal muscle, and some are entirely intramuscular.

Microscopically, chondroid lipoma has a lobular pattern and consists of strands and nests of round cells deposited in a myxochondroid or hyalinized fibrous background. Some cells have eosinophilic, granular cytoplasm, whereas others have lipid vacuoles indicative of lipoblastic differentiation (Figs. 14-12 to 14-15). Most commonly, these multivacuolated cells predominate, although, in some cases, they may be less conspicuous. The cells are not pleomorphic, and they do not show significant mitotic activity. A mature adipose tissue component may be present focally only, or it may be the predominant component of the tumor. The extracellular matrix is often extensively myxoid and may be intermingled with zones of hyalinization and fibrin deposition reminiscent of serous atrophy of fat. Most lesions are vascular, with thick-walled blood vessels and cavernous thin-walled vascular spaces. Other changes include the presence of hemorrhage, hemosiderin deposition, calcification or even ossification, and hyalinized zones.[56]

By immunohistochemistry, the tumor cells stain positively for S-100 protein with focal staining for CD68 in the vacuolated tumor cells. Some lesions also show focal cytokeratin immunoreactivity, although immunostains for epithelial membrane antigen are negative. Interestingly, Nielson et al.[57] found no evidence of true cartilaginous differentiation by ultrastructural analysis. On the other hand, Kindblom and Meis-Kindblom[58] found a spectrum of differentiation, ranging from primitive cells sharing features of chondroblasts and prelipoblasts, to lipoblasts, preadipocytes, and mature adipocytes.

Cytogenetic and Molecular Genetic Findings

Chondroid lipoma has been found to harbor a consistent balanced translocation t(11;16)(q13;p12-13), which involves the fusion of *C11orf95* and *MKL2*.[59,60]

Differential Diagnosis

The differential diagnosis of chondroid lipoma is broad and includes myxoid liposarcoma, extraskeletal myxoid chondrosarcoma, soft tissue chondroma, and myoepithelial tumors.

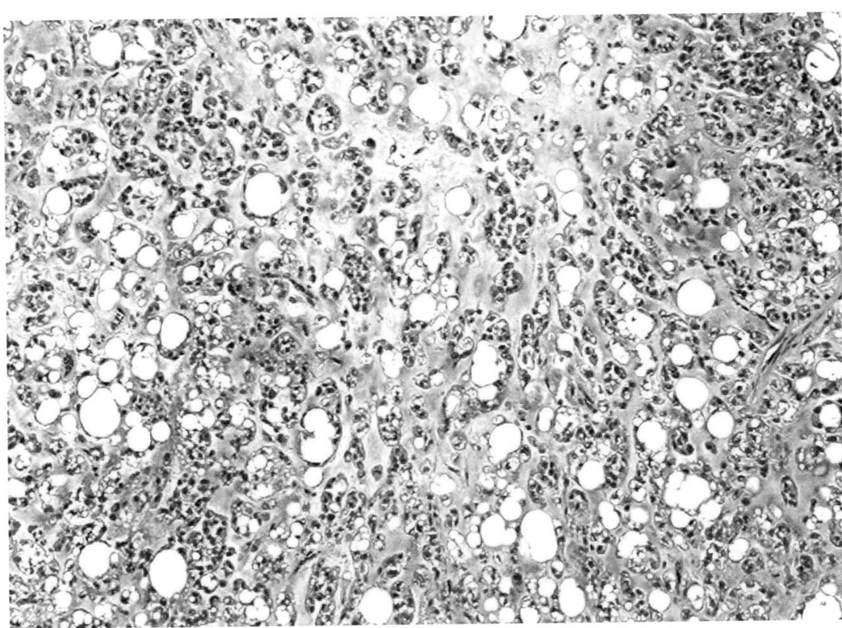

FIGURE 14-13. Chondroid lipoma showing nests of vacuolated cells deposited in a chondroid-like matrix associated with mature fat cells.

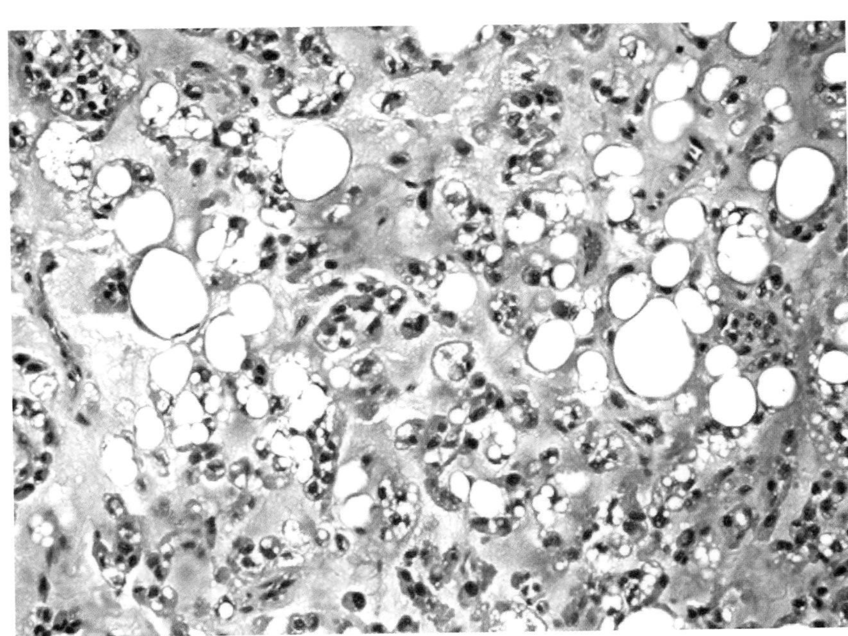

FIGURE 14-14. High-power view of a chondroid lipoma showing vacuolated cells associated with mature fat cells. Some of the vacuolated cells closely simulate lipoblasts.

Myxoid liposarcoma may have hibernoma-like cells deposited in a myxoid matrix that, on occasion, shows chondroid metaplasia. However, unlike chondroid lipoma, this tumor is composed predominantly of mildly atypical spindled cells deposited around a delicate, plexiform vascular pattern. *Extraskeletal myxoid chondrosarcoma* typically has fibrous septa that impart a distinct lobulated appearance. The cells of extraskeletal myxoid chondrosarcoma are more uniformly round or oval, have eosinophilic cytoplasm, and few, if any, intracytoplasmic vacuoles. *Soft tissue chondroma* occurs in the hands and feet and often contains multinucleated giant cells and true hyaline cartilage. *Myoepithelial tumors*, including mixed tumor, tend to be more superficially located and typically display epithelial areas. The myoepithelial cells may have cytoplasmic vacuoles, but they are usually not multivacuolated. Immunohistochemically, myoepithelial cells stain more uniformly for cytokeratins and are marked by antibodies to epithelial membrane antigen and actins.

Discussion

Chondroid lipoma, despite its worrisome histologic appearance, is clearly benign; the lesion does not recur or metastasize. All available evidence supports a neoplastic origin.

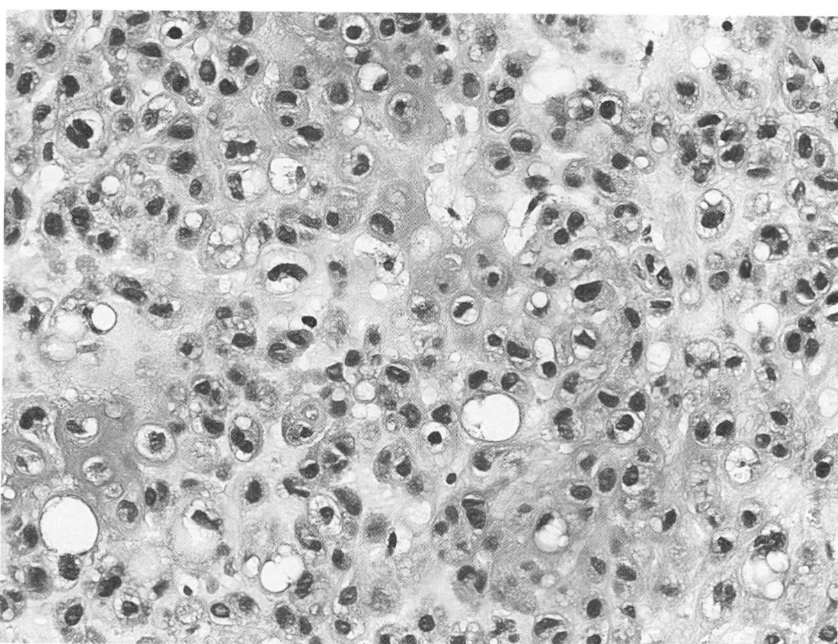

FIGURE 14-15. Cytologic atypia in a chondroid lipoma.

SPINDLE CELL/PLEOMORPHIC LIPOMA

Although spindle cell lipoma and pleomorphic lipoma were described as separate but related entities in the first four editions of this textbook, given the clear-cut overlapping clinical, histologic, immunohistochemical, and cytogenetic features, these lesions are best considered as one entity, although there is considerable histologic range within this family of tumors. Some cases may be pure spindle cell or pleomorphic lipomas, but many show overlapping features of spindle cell and pleomorphic lipoma within the same tumor.

Spindle cell lipoma was originally described as a distinct entity by Enzinger and Harvey[61] in 1975. Several years later (1981), Shmookler and Enzinger[62] described a series of 48 cases of pleomorphic lipoma. Although spindle cell and pleomorphic lipomas, at one time, were grouped under the term *atypical lipoma* by some authors,[63,64] it is clear that this family of tumors is sufficiently characteristic to justify consideration as an entity distinct from atypical lipoma/atypical lipomatous neoplasm/well-differentiated liposarcoma.

Clinical Findings

Spindle cell/pleomorphic lipoma occurs in a characteristic clinical setting, arising mainly in men 45 to 60 years of age in the subcutaneous tissue of the posterior neck, shoulder, and back.[61,62] Approximately 80% of these tumors arise in this characteristic location, but 20% arise in unusual locations, thereby making these cases more difficult to diagnose. For example, a significant number of cases arising outside of the usual location occur in the oral cavity.[65] Similarly, pleomorphic lipoma has also been described in a myriad of unusual locations. In general, spindle cell/pleomorphic lipoma is not encountered in adolescents or children. There is a striking predilection for men. For example, 91% of patients with spindle cell lipoma in the study from the AFIP were men,[61] and 30 of 48 patients with pleomorphic lipoma were men.[62] Like ordinary lipomas, spindle cell/pleomorphic lipoma manifests as a slowly growing, typically solitary, circumscribed or encapsulated, painless, firm nodule, usually centered in the subcutaneous tissue. It is often present for years before excision. Very rarely, these lesions can arise in multiple sites, either as synchronous or metachronous lesions.[66] Fanburg-Smith et al.[67] reported 18 patients with multiple spindle cell lipomas, including 7 familial cases. Most of these patients presented with their initial tumors on the posterior neck or upper back, with subsequent lesions developing bilaterally on the upper neck, shoulders, arms, chest, and then axillae; spread is in a predominantly caudal direction. Some cases involve the dermis or have predominantly dermal involvement.[68] Interestingly, Reis-Filho et al.[69] found these dermal lesions to arise more frequently in women, and they tended to be less circumscribed than their subcutaneous counterparts. Moreover, there seemed to be a wider anatomic distribution. Other rare examples involve the superficial skeletal muscle or are located exclusively in an intramuscular location.[70]

Pathologic Findings

Grossly, spindle cell/pleomorphic lipoma resembles the usual type of lipoma, except for gray-white gelatinous foci, representing the areas of increased cellularity (Fig. 14-16). Some tumors show extensive myxoid change, whereas others are predominantly lipomatous. Although some tumors are quite large (up to 14 cm), most are between 3 and 5 cm. The tumor is usually well circumscribed and easily distinguished from the surrounding subcutaneous tissue (Fig. 14-17). Rare examples have a plexiform architecture and are composed of multiple small nodules separated by collagen.[71]

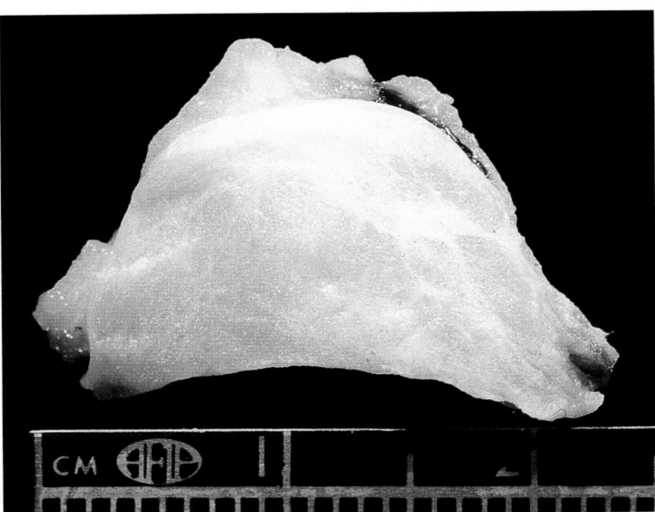

FIGURE 14-16. Gross appearance of a spindle cell lipoma showing a well-circumscribed mass with gray-white foci between areas that resemble the usual type of lipoma.

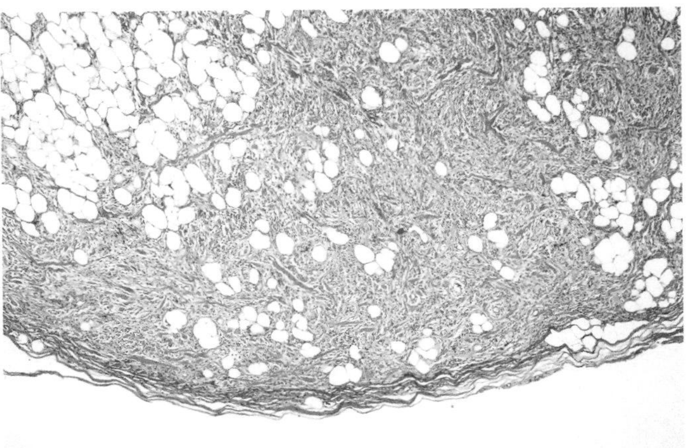

FIGURE 14-17. Spindle cell lipoma. Note the circumscription of the lesion and irregular distribution of the spindle cell areas between mature fat cells.

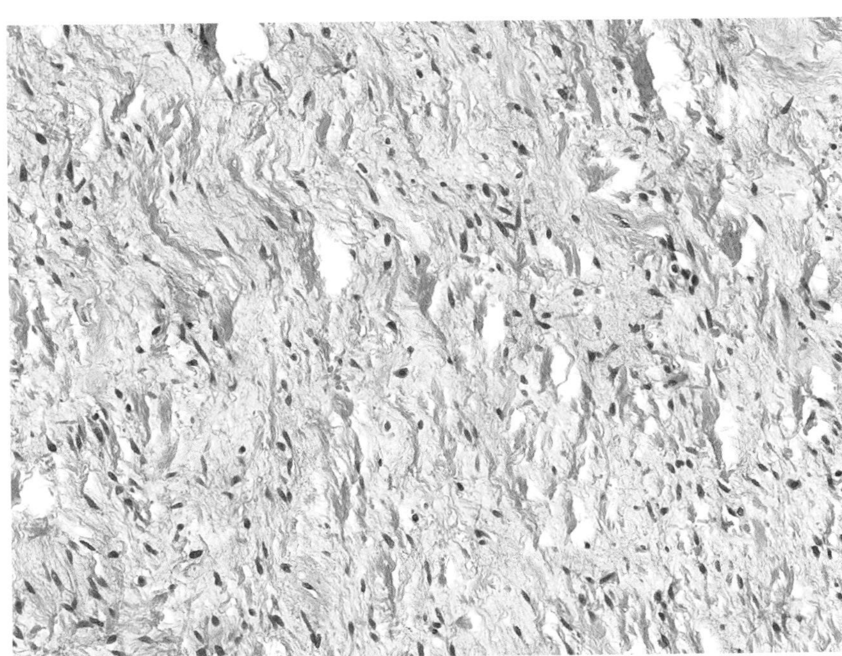

FIGURE 14-18. Fat-free spindle cell lipoma with extensive myxoid change.

Microscopically, spindle cell/pleomorphic lipoma can vary widely in its appearance. Some tumors are predominantly composed of mature adipose tissue with only scattered spindle cell or pleomorphic elements (described later in the chapter). Other tumors are predominantly or even exclusively solid and lack any significant lipomatous component (so-called *fat-free* spindle cell/pleomorphic lipoma) (Fig. 14-18).[72,73] Such cases are obviously quite challenging because the lipomatous nature of the neoplasm is not obvious. Finally, although some examples are purely spindled or purely pleomorphic, many show overlapping features, and either cell type can predominate.

The classic spindle cell lipoma consists of a relative equal mixture of mature fat and spindle cells. The spindle cells are uniform with a single elongated nucleus and narrow, bipolar cytoplasmic processes (Fig. 14-19). Nucleoli are inconspicuous, as are mitotic figures. The cells may be haphazardly distributed but tend to be arranged in short, parallel bundles, often with striking nuclear palisading reminiscent of a neural tumor. The cells are deposited in a mucoid matrix composed of hyaluronic acid and mixed with a varying number of characteristic birefringent collagen fibers (Fig. 14-20). In some cases, the tumors are highly myxoid and hypocellular with haphazardly arranged spindled cells; such cases may be easily confused with a myxoma. The vascular pattern is usually inconspicuous and consists of a few small or intermediate-sized, thick-walled vessels, although some examples have a prominent plexiform vascular pattern reminiscent of myxoid liposarcoma (Fig. 14-21), and others show a predominantly

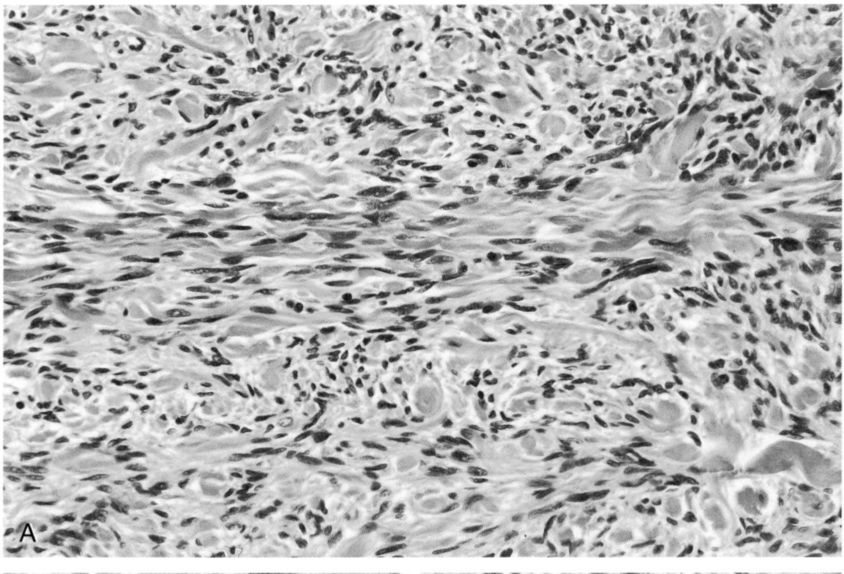

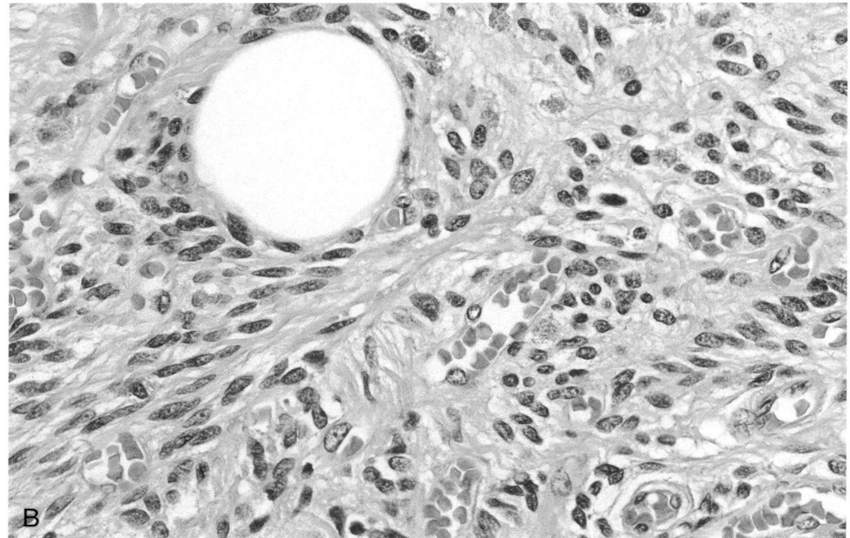

FIGURE 14-19. (A) Cellular area of a spindle cell lipoma showing spindle cells arranged in short bundles and separated by dense collagen. (B) High-power view of cytologically bland spindle cells in a spindle cell lipoma. The cells are uniform, with an elongated nucleus and bipolar cytoplasmic processes.

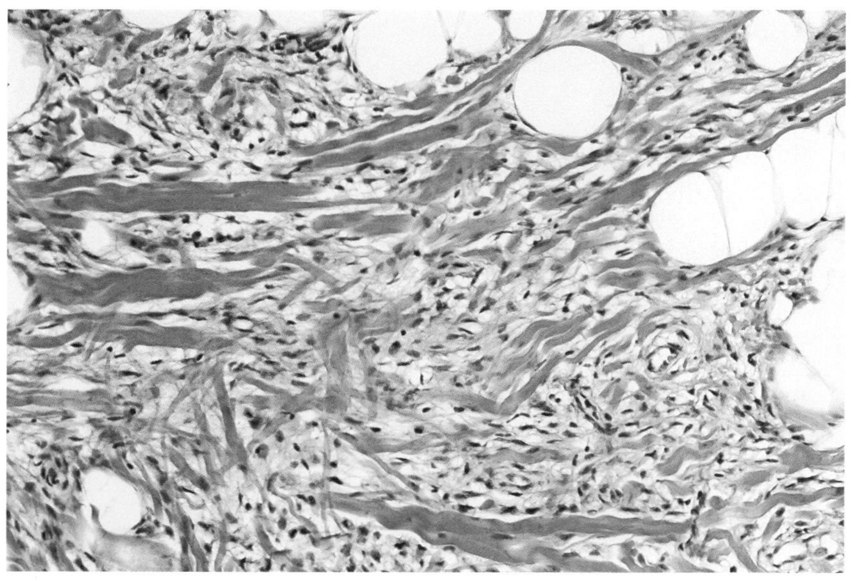

FIGURE 14-20. Spindle cell lipoma with characteristic ropey collagen bundles between bland spindle cells.

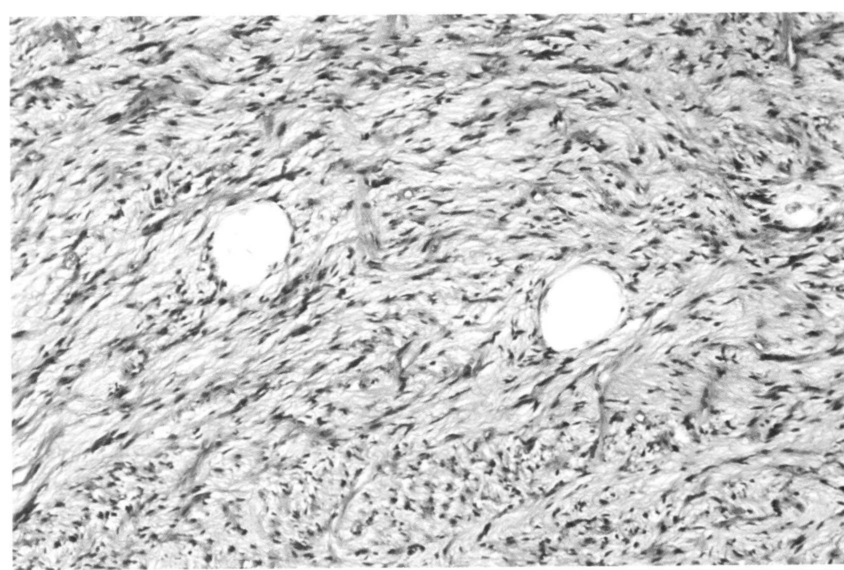

FIGURE 14-21. Spindle cell lipoma with extensive myxoid change. Such areas may resemble myxoid liposarcoma.

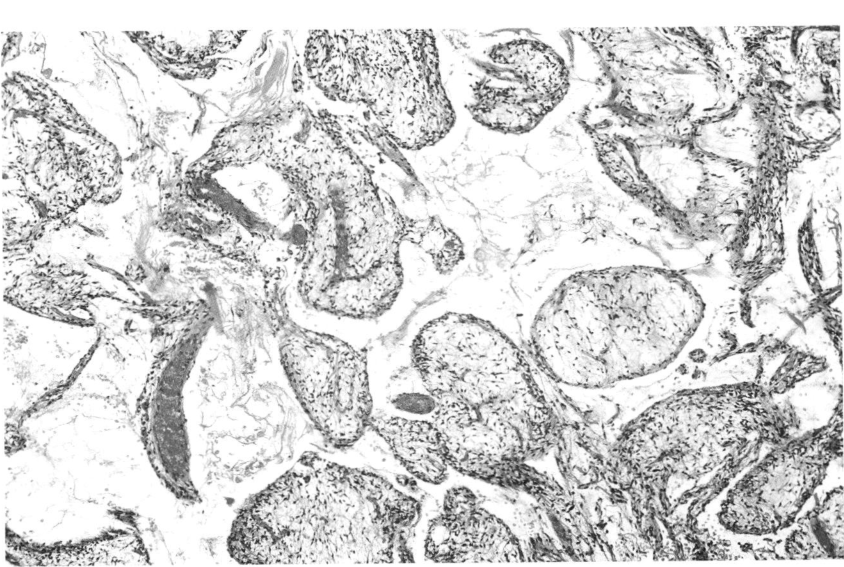

FIGURE 14-22. Spindle cell lipoma with pseudoangiomatous features characterized by irregular branching spaces with well-formed connective tissue projections.

hemangiopericytoma-like vascular pattern.[74,75] A pseudoangiomatous variant, characterized by irregular branching spaces with well-formed connective tissue projections, has also been described (Figs. 14-22 and 14-23),[76] although a close analysis of the cells lining the spaces suggests that these may be lined by endothelial cells and, therefore, are really examples of angiomatous spindle cell lipoma.[77,78] Mast cells are a conspicuous feature in almost all cases. Rare tumors show small foci of osseous or cartilaginous metaplasia.[74]

The classic pleomorphic lipoma is characterized by the presence of scattered, bizarre giant cells that frequently have a concentric floret-like arrangement of multiple hyperchromatic nuclei about a deeply eosinophilic cytoplasm (Figs. 14-24 to 14-26). Ropey collagen bundles identical to those found in spindle cell lipoma are also characteristic. Some tumors also have extensive myxoid change, and mast cells are usually prominent. A pseudoangiomatous variant of pleomorphic lipoma has also been described.[79]

Immunohistochemical Findings

Immunohistochemically, the cells in spindle cell/pleomorphic lipoma stain strongly for CD34 (Figs. 14-27 and 14-28), but they are not immunoreactive for actin or desmin. Although S-100 protein stains the nuclei of mature lipocytes, neither the spindled cells nor the atypical or floret-like giant cells stain for this antigen. BCL-2 is also frequently positive in spindle cell/pleomorphic lipoma, but this marker has not been found to be particularly helpful in distinguishing this lesion from other lesions in the differential diagnosis, because many of those lesions also stain for this antigen.[80] Similarly,

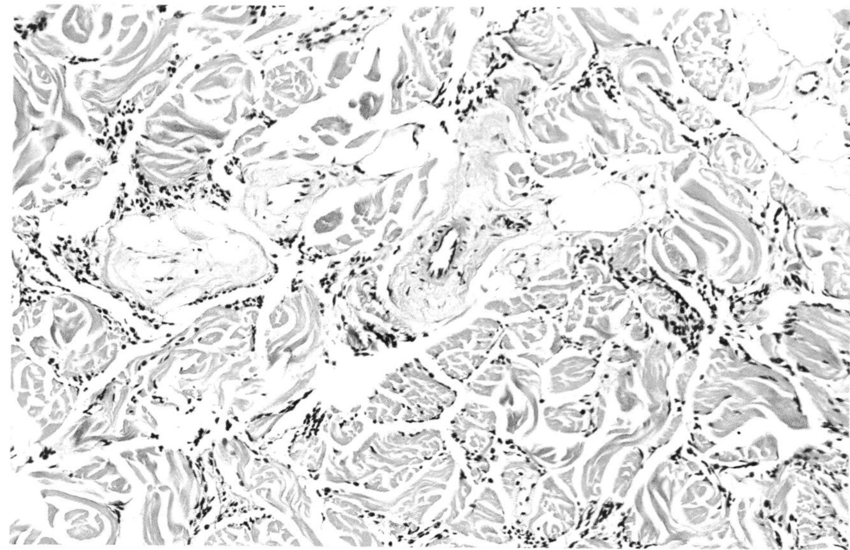

FIGURE 14-23. Pseudoangiomatous variant of a spindle cell lipoma closely resembling angiosarcoma. Short bundles of cytologically bland spindle cells are separated by dense connective tissue projections, simulating the dissecting pattern of angiosarcoma.

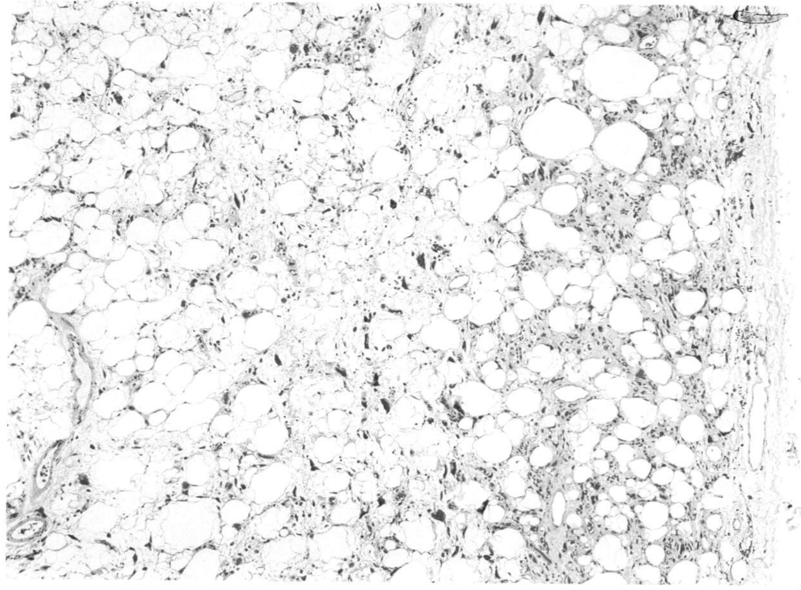

FIGURE 14-24. Pleomorphic lipoma. The lesion is typically well circumscribed and separated from the surrounding subcutaneous tissue.

many examples stain for CD10, but this marker also lacks specificity.[81]

Cytogenetic and Molecular Genetic Findings

Aside from the overlapping clinical, morphologic, and immunohistochemical findings that link spindle cell and pleomorphic lipoma, these lesions also share the same cytogenetic aberrations—that is, most show loss of 16q material and, less frequently, material from 13q.[82,83] These unique cytogenetic abnormalities, coupled with the usual absence of giant marker and ring chromosomes that are typically seen in atypical lipomatous neoplasm/well-differentiated liposarcoma, support the relation between spindle cell and pleomorphic lipoma as well as their distinction from atypical lipomatous neoplasm/well-differentiated liposarcoma.[84] A number of studies have found a consistent monoallelic deletion of *RB1* on 13q14 in spindle cell lipoma. Interestingly, this same deletion has been found in examples of cellular angiofibroma and mammary-type myofibroblastoma, suggesting a histogenetic link between these entities.[85-88]

Differential Diagnosis

The differential diagnosis of spindle cell/pleomorphic lipoma depends upon which elements predominate. Classic spindle cell lipoma can be confused with *dermatofibrosarcoma protuberans* (DFSP). However, DFSP typically arises in the dermis and is composed of a proliferation of plump CD34-positive spindled cells arranged in a monotonous storiform pattern

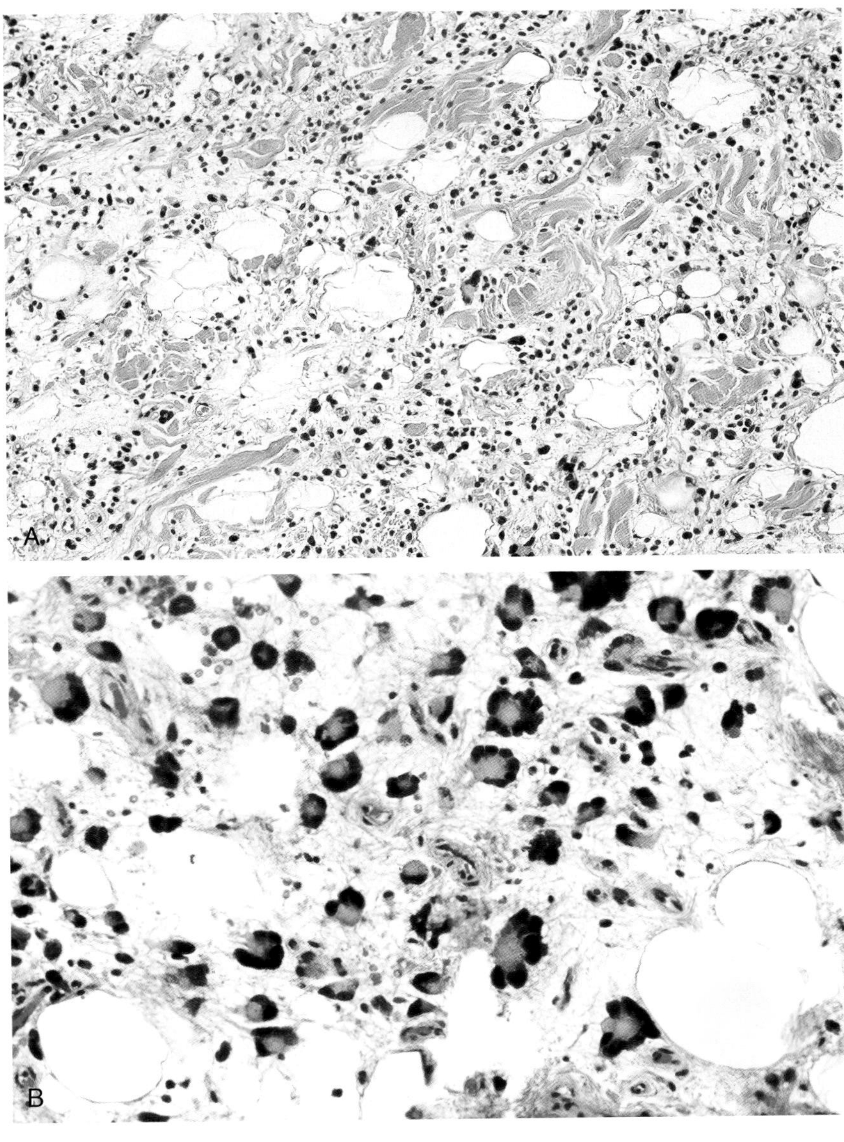

FIGURE 14-25. (A) Pleomorphic lipoma, characterized by a mixture of mature fat cells, multinucleated giant cells, and ropey collagen bundles similar to those found in spindle cell lipoma. (B) Pleomorphic lipoma with numerous multinucleated floret-like giant cells deposited in a myxoid stroma.

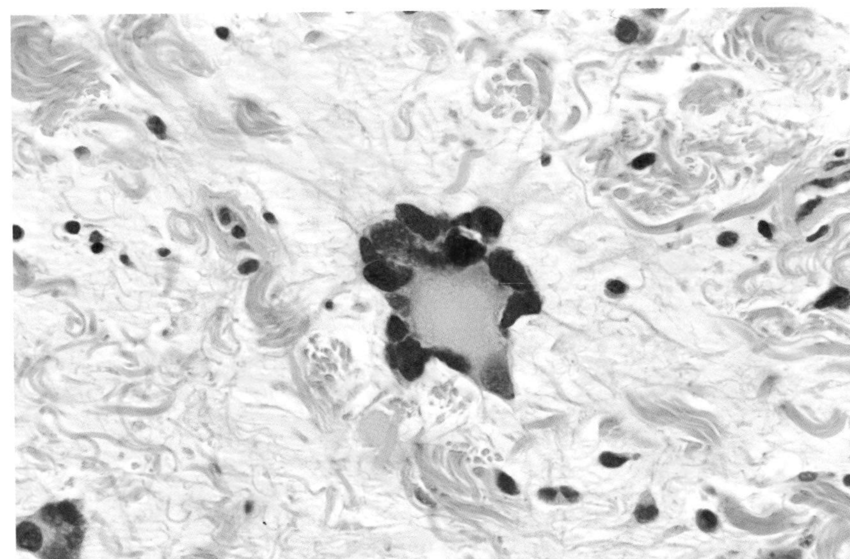

FIGURE 14-26. High-power view of a typical multinucleated floret-like giant cell as seen in pleomorphic lipomas. There is a wreath-like arrangement of hyperchromatic nuclei about a deeply eosinophilic cytoplasm.

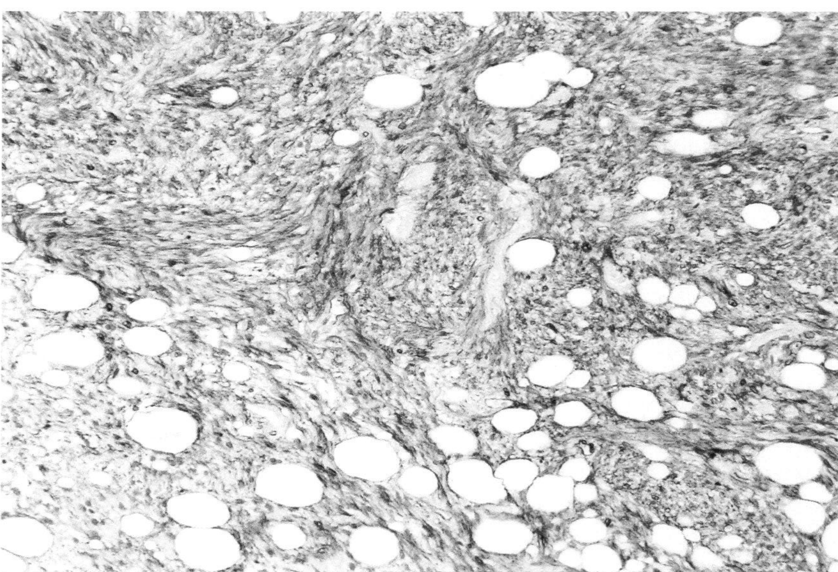

FIGURE 14-27. Diffuse CD34 immunoreactivity in a spindle cell lipoma.

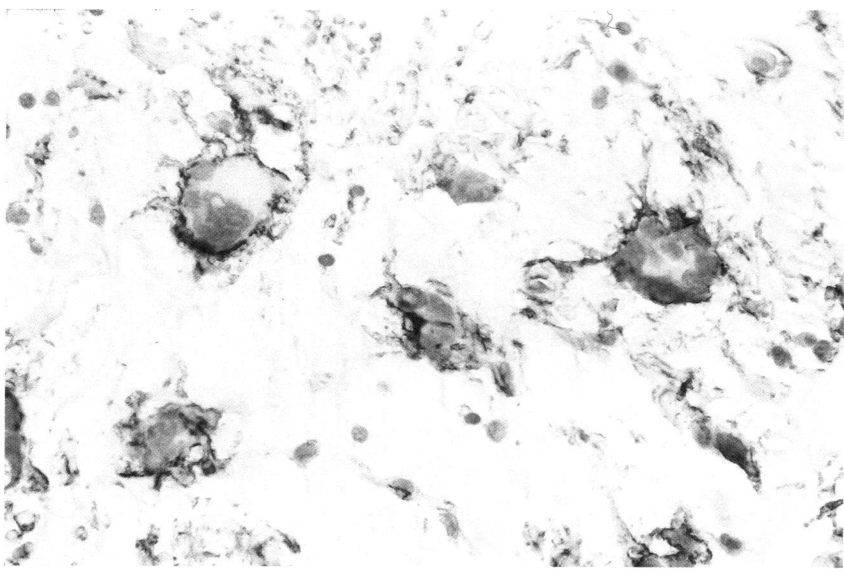

FIGURE 14-28. CD34 immunoreactivity in the multinucleated giant cells of a pleomorphic lipoma.

with infiltration into the underlying subcutaneous tissue. DFSP tends to arise in younger patients and lacks the characteristic ropey collagen of spindle cell/pleomorphic lipoma. *Nodular fasciitis* has a more variable appearance, with tissue culture fibroblast-like cells characterized by smooth muscle actin positivity and an absence of CD34 staining. Spindle cell lipoma has histologic features that overlap with those seen in *angiomyofibroblastoma*, a superficially located vulvar tumor, which, on occasion, can also arise in the male genital tract. Both lesions may contain variable amounts of mature adipose tissue, and both are characteristically CD34 positive. Histologically, angiomyofibroblastoma tends to have a more prominent vascular pattern consisting of uniformly distributed thick-walled blood vessels as well as a predominance of epithelioid (as opposed to spindled) cells. As previously mentioned, a histogenetic link has been suggested between spindle cell/pleomorphic lipoma and *cellular angiofibroma* and *mammary-type myofibroblastoma*, two lesions that share significant morphologic overlap with spindle cell/pleomorphic lipoma. Distinction among these lesions is largely arbitrary, in some cases, and probably lacks any real clinical significance. There is also histologic overlap with *solitary fibrous tumor*, another CD34-positive neoplasm. Interestingly, however, a recent analysis failed to detect *RB1* deletions by fluorescence in-situ hybridization (FISH) in a large number of solitary fibrous tumors, suggesting that this lesion is distinct from the other entities mentioned previously. It is possible that these tumors are derived from a CD34-positive perivascular stem cell with the capacity for lipocytic and fibroblastic/myofibroblastic differentiation, but this theory has yet to be proven.

Given the striking nuclear palisading present in some spindle cell lipomas as well as the conspicuous mast cell infiltrate, *schwannoma* and *neurofibroma* are sometimes

TABLE 14-2 Comparison of Pleomorphic Lipoma, Well-Differentiated Liposarcoma, and Pleomorphic Liposarcoma

FEATURE	PLEOMORPHIC LIPOMA	WELL-DIFFERENTIATED LIPOSARCOMA	PLEOMORPHIC LIPOSARCOMA
Favored site(s)	Subcutis of posterior neck, back, and shoulders	Deep soft tissue of extremities, retroperitoneum	Extremities
Peak age (years)	45-60	50-70	50-70
Floret-like cells	Characteristic	Present	Rare
Pleomorphic lipoblasts	Absent	Present	Characteristic
Cytogenetics	Loss of 16q, 13q	Giant marker and ring chromosomes	Varied complex abnormalities
MDM2 amplification	Absent	Present	May be present
Metastasis	None	Extremely rare, except in dedifferentiated cases	Common

diagnostic considerations. The cells of these benign peripheral nerve sheath tumors tend to be more wavy or buckled in appearance, and, although the cells may express CD34, they invariably express S-100 protein, a marker that is negative in spindle cell lipoma.

Spindle cell lipoma may also be mistaken for several sarcomas, including *myxoid liposarcoma* or *spindle cell liposarcoma*. Some examples of spindle cell lipoma are diffusely myxoid and have a prominent plexiform vascular pattern reminiscent of that seen in myxoid liposarcoma. However, spindle cell lipoma is more circumscribed and superficially located than myxoid liposarcoma, lacks lipoblasts, and is characterized by ropey collagen bundles. Although some CD34 immunoreactivity may be seen in myxoid liposarcoma, it is not the diffuse, strong CD34 staining that one sees in spindle cell lipoma. In difficult cases, FISH analysis for aberrations of *DDIT3* and/or *FUS* genes can be helpful. Spindle cell liposarcoma is characterized by a highly vascularized background resembling a well-differentiated fibrosarcoma in which typical univacuolar or bivacuolar lipoblasts are dispersed. Classic pleomorphic lipoma may be difficult to distinguish from the *sclerosing type of atypical lipomatous neoplasm/well-differentiated liposarcoma*. This distinction can usually be accomplished on the basis of the typical setting of pleomorphic lipoma on the shoulder or head and neck region, its location in subcutaneous tissue, and its circumscription. Although multinucleated floret-like giant cells are characteristic of pleomorphic lipoma, they are not pathognomonic, because such cells are occasionally also seen in atypical lipomatous neoplasm/well-differentiated liposarcoma (as well as a variety of other nonlipogenic neoplasms) (Table 14-2). The ropey collagen bundles characteristic of pleomorphic lipoma are an extremely useful distinguishing feature because this collagen pattern is typically not seen in atypical lipomatous neoplasm/well-differentiated liposarcoma. Ultimately, detection of characteristic cytogenetic aberrations in each of these lipomatous neoplasms can serve as a useful diagnostic adjunct. Paraffin-based FISH analysis for *MDM2* amplification can be a critical discriminant in difficult cases.

Discussion

Spindle cell/pleomorphic lipoma is a completely benign lesion. Even if incompletely excised, the tumor recurs very exceptionally only, and neither dedifferentiation nor metastasis has been reported. Even those cases of pleomorphic lipoma with lipoblasts and atypical mitotic figures have behaved in a clinically benign fashion.

TABLE 14-3 Age Distribution of Lipoblastoma/Lipoblastomatosis Patients at the Time of Operation

AGE (MONTHS)	NO. OF PATIENTS	PERCENTAGE (%)
0-11	26	36
12-23	19	26
24-35	10	14
36-47	4	5
48-59	5	7
60-70	3	4
71-83	2	3
≥84	4	5
Total	73	100

From Collins MH, Chatten J. Lipoblastoma/lipoblastomatosis: a clinicopathologic study of 25 tumors. Am J Surg Pathol 1997;21(10):1131–7; Coffin CM, Lowichik A, Putnam A. Lipoblastoma (LPB): a clinicopathologic and immunohistochemical analysis of 59 cases. Am J Surg Pathol 2009;33(11):1705–12; and Jeong TJ, Oh YJ, Ahn JJ, et al. Lipoblastoma-like tumour of the lip in an adult woman. Acta Derm Venereol 2010;90(5):537–8.

BENIGN LIPOBLASTOMA AND LIPOBLASTOMATOSIS

Benign lipoblastoma and lipoblastomatosis refer, respectively, to the circumscribed and diffuse forms of the same tumor. This tumor is a peculiar variant of lipoma and lipomatosis occurring almost exclusively during infancy and early childhood. The lesions differ from lipoma and lipomatosis by their cellular immaturity and their close resemblance to fetal adipose tissue.

Lipoblastomatosis was named in 1958 by Vellios et al.,[89] who reported an infiltrating lipoblastoma in the region of the anterior chest wall, axilla, and supraclavicular region of an 8-month-old girl. The tumor had not recurred after 30 months. Earlier, Van Meurs[90] reported a similar tumor as embryonic lipoma. He demonstrated its transformation (or maturation) to a common lipoma with repeated biopsies.

Clinical Findings

Lipoblastoma is a tumor of infancy. It is usually noted during the first 3 years of life and occasionally at birth.[91-93] Sporadic examples have also been described in older children and very uncommonly in adults (Table 14-3).[94] In the large series of lipoblastomas published in 2009 by Coffin et al.,[93] the patients ranged in age from 3 months to 16 years. Sixty-eight percent of patients were between 1 and 9 years of age. Most studies

TABLE 14-4 Anatomic Distribution of Lipoblastoma/ Lipoblastomatosis

ANATOMIC SITE	NO. OF PATIENTS	PERCENTAGE (%)
Head and neck	**10**	**14**
Mediastinum	**1**	**2**
Upper extremity	**19**	**26**
Hand	8	
Elbow	1	
Upper arm	2	
Shoulder	3	
Axilla	4	
Forearm	1	
Lower extremity	**29**	**40**
Buttock	8	
Groin	4	
Thigh	11	
Lower leg	6	
Trunk	**10**	**14**
Back	5	
Labia	2	
Chest wall	3	
Retroperitoneum	**3**	**4**
Total	72	100

From Collins MH, Chatten J. Lipoblastoma/lipoblastomatosis: a clinicopathologic study of 25 tumors. Am J Surg Pathol 1997;21(10):1131–7; Coffin CM, Lowichik A, Putnam A. Lipoblastoma (LPB): a clinicopathologic and immunohistochemical analysis of 59 cases. Am J Surg Pathol 2009;33(11):1705–12; and Jeong TJ, Oh YJ, Ahn JJ, et al. Lipoblastoma-like tumour of the lip in an adult woman. Acta Derm Venereol 2010; 90(5):537–8.

have found a predilection for this tumor to occur in boys. It is found most commonly in the trunk or upper and lower extremities as a painless nodule or mass. Less common sites of involvement include the head and neck area,[95,96] mediastinum,[97] mesentery,[98] omentum,[99] scrotum,[100] and retroperitoneum[101] (Table 14-4). Two types of lipoblastoma have been described: circumscribed (*benign lipoblastoma*) and diffuse (*diffuse lipoblastomatosis*). The more common circumscribed form, located in the superficial soft tissues, clinically simulates a lipoma. The diffuse type tends to infiltrate not only the subcutis, but also the underlying muscle tissue, has an infiltrative growth pattern, and a greater tendency to recur.[93,102,103] Most patients present with a slowly growing soft tissue mass, although some report tumors with a rapid period of growth.[104] Depending on the tumor size and location, the mass may compress adjacent structures and interfere with function. For example, tumors arising in the head and neck may cause airway obstruction and respiratory insufficiency.[95] Tumors can also involve the spinal canal, resulting in hemiparesis or even quadriparesis. Radiologic studies typically show a well-delineated soft tissue mass with the density of adipose tissue, although neither CT nor MRI reliably distinguishes this lesion from lipoma or liposarcoma.[105] There are also rare reports of prenatal detection of this lesion by ultrasound.[106]

Recently, Coffin et al.[93] unexpectedly found that 17% of their patients with lipoblastomas had disorders of the central nervous system, including seizures, autism, developmental delay, congenital anomalies, and Sturge-Weber syndrome. Hill and Rademaker[107] reported an unusual case of a newborn with abdominal lipoblastoma associated with multiple digital glomuvenous malformations, temporal alopecia, heterochromia, and an epidermal nevus.

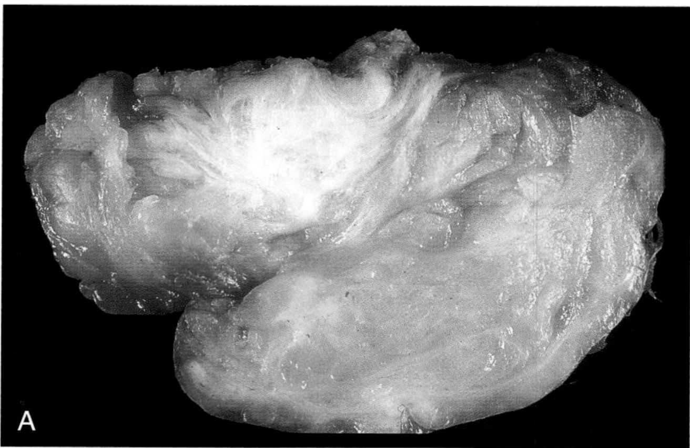

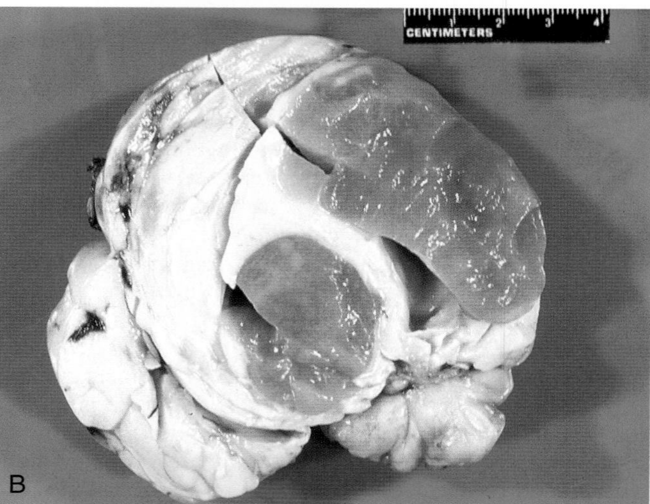

FIGURE 14-29. (A) Gross appearance of a lipoblastoma. This lesion is well circumscribed and has a predominantly fatty appearance, although focal cartilaginous metaplasia (white to gray area) is present. (B) Lipoblastoma with multinodular appearance and foci with extensive myxoid change.

Pathologic Findings

On sectioning, lipoblastoma is paler than the ordinary lipoma, and its cut surfaces are distinctly myxoid or gelatinous (Fig. 14-29). Most tumors are 3 to 5 cm in diameter, although some are much larger and, occasionally, weigh as much as 1 kg.[108]

Histologically, this tumor is composed of irregular small lobules of immature fat cells separated by connective tissue septa of varying thickness and mesenchymal areas with a loose myxoid appearance (Fig. 14-30). The individual lobules are composed of lipoblasts in different stages of development, ranging from primitive, stellate, and spindle-shaped mesenchymal cells (preadipocytes) to lipoblasts approaching the univacuolar signet-ring picture of a mature fat cell. The degree of cellular differentiation may be the same throughout the tumor, or it may vary in different tumor lobules. There are occasional examples in which the cells are more rounded and finely vacuolated with intracellular eosinophilic granules, resembling the cells of brown fat.[93]

Some examples with prominent myxoid change show a plexiform vascular pattern quite reminiscent of myxoid

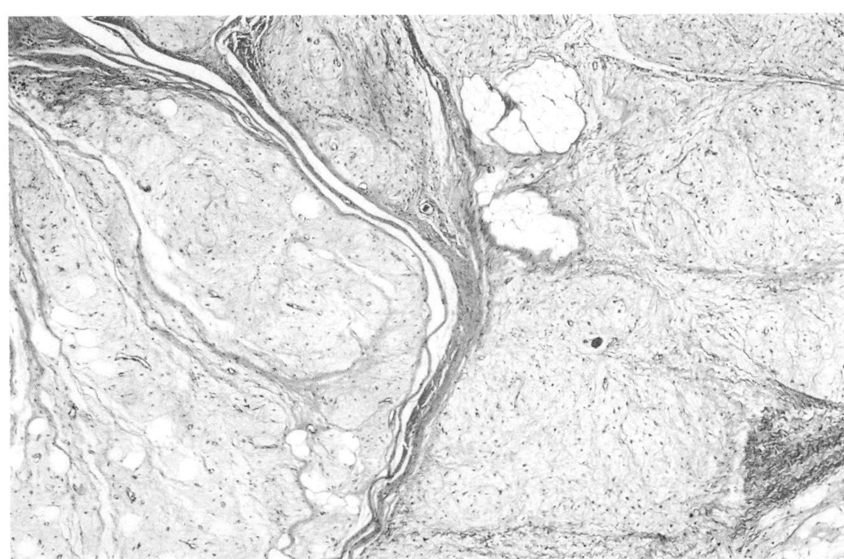

FIGURE 14-30. Lipoblastoma with the characteristic multilobular pattern. Many of the nodules show extensive myxoid change.

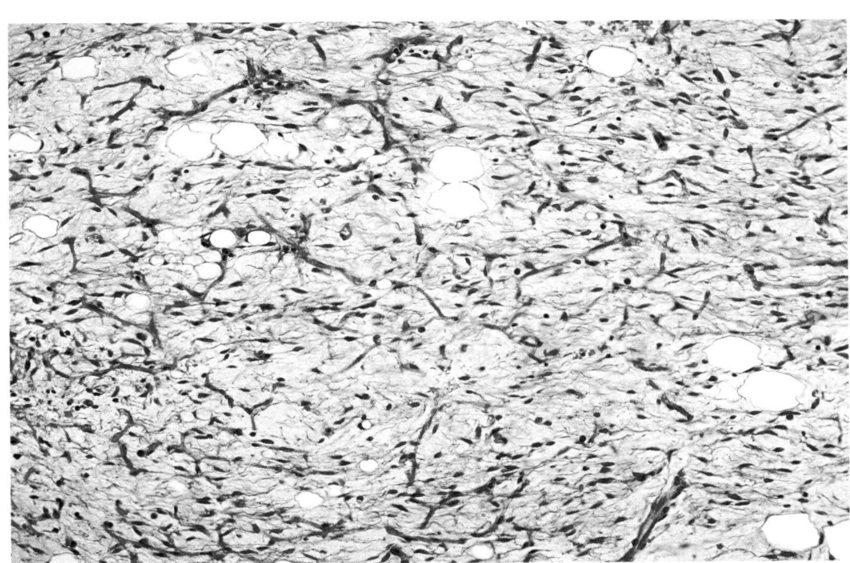

FIGURE 14-31. A 1-year-old child with lipoblastoma composed of lipoblasts and a prominent mucoid matrix. A plexiform vasculature reminiscent of myxoid liposarcoma is also apparent.

liposarcoma (Fig. 14-31). Some examples of lipoblastoma, at least in areas, are indistinguishable from myxoid liposarcoma. The cellular composition is the same regardless of whether the tumor is circumscribed or diffuse. Diffuse tumors (*diffuse lipoblastomatosis*), however, have a less pronounced lobular pattern and usually contain an admixture of residual muscle fibers similar to intramuscular lipoma. Cases with sheets of primitive mesenchymal cells or broad fibrous septa may be mistaken for infantile fibromatosis. Cellular maturation of lipoblastoma has been observed in multiple follow-up biopsies (Fig. 14-32).[92,93]

Cytogenetic and Molecular Genetic Findings

The most characteristic cytogenetic alteration is rearrangement of 8q11-13.[109] In the study by Gisselsson et al.,[110] 11 of 16 cases had rearrangement of 8q12 involving the *PLAG1* gene. Fusion genes have been identified resulting from *PLAG1* rearrangements, including *HAS2/PLAG1* and *COL1A2/PLAG1*.[111,112] The *HAS2* gene is located on 8q24, and the *COL1A2* gene is on 7q22. Interestingly, *PLAG1* alterations have been detected by FISH in all cell types within lipoblastoma, including primitive mesenchymal cells, suggesting origin from a primitive mesenchymal precursor cell.[110] Polysomy of chromosome 8 might represent an alternative oncogenic mechanism, because this was found in 3 of 16 cases of lipoblastoma without a *PLAG1* rearrangement.[110]

Differential Diagnosis

The principal differential diagnostic consideration is *myxoid liposarcoma*. Unlike lipoblastoma, which is a tumor of infancy

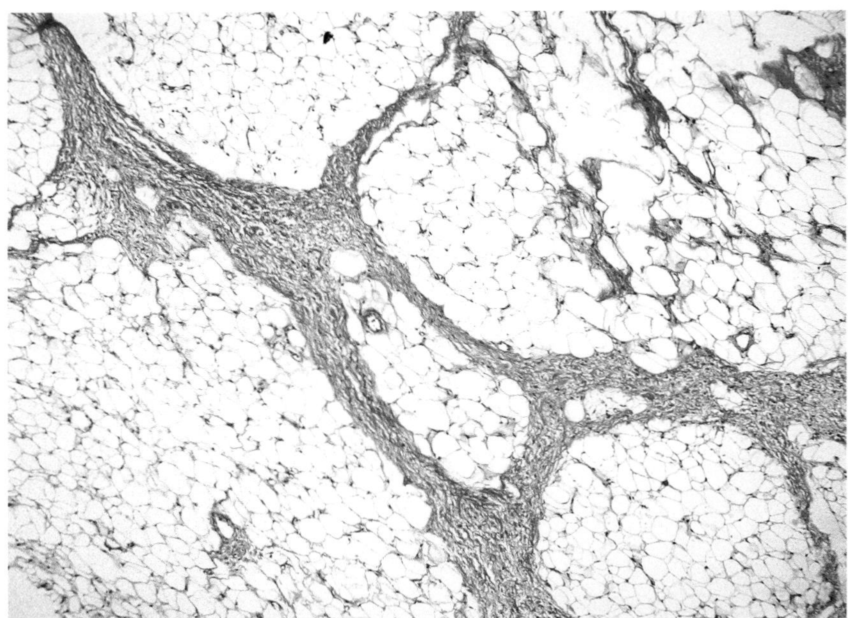

FIGURE 14-32. Recurrent lipoblastoma composed of multiple lobules of mature-appearing fat cells separated by fibrous septa. Some examples of lipoblastoma show maturation in recurrent lesions.

and early childhood predominantly occurring in patients less than 5 years of age, myxoid liposarcoma has a peak incidence during the third through sixth decades of life. Occasional myxoid liposarcomas have been reported during adolescence, but such cases are exceedingly rare under the age of 10 years. Histologically, both lesions may be lobulated, contain lipoblasts, and spindled cells deposited in a myxoid stroma with a prominent plexiform capillary network. However, lipoblastoma is more lobulated than most myxoid liposarcomas. Although myxoid liposarcoma lacks marked nuclear atypia or hyperchromasia, such features are usually present focally, whereas lipoblastoma lacks nuclear atypia altogether. Foci of hypercellularity may be found in myxoid liposarcoma but are not found in extraseptal loci in lipoblastoma. Microcystic spaces may be present in lipoblastoma but are more often found and are more pronounced in myxoid liposarcoma. Finally, lipoblastoma is characterized cytogenetically by deletions of 8q11-13 (*PLAG1*) and lacks the characteristic t(12;16) translocation in myxoid liposarcoma. Several highly myxoid lipoblastomas by FISH have been evaluated and the absence of *DDIT3* and *FUS* alterations documented.

Lipoblastoma may also be confused with other benign adipose tissue tumors, including *ordinary lipoma* and *hibernoma*. Ordinary lipoma is less cellular than lipoblastoma and lacks lipoblasts, whereas hibernoma consists, at least in part, of brown fat cells with mitochondria-rich, eosinophilic, granular cytoplasm. The latter two entities have cytogenetic abnormalities distinct from those found in lipoblastoma.

Discussion

The prognosis is excellent, although local recurrence occurs in a significant number of patients. In the study by Coffin et al.,[93] 46% of patients had one or more local recurrence. Recurrence is not related to any morphologic features such as lobulation, myxoid change, or degree of adipocytic differentiation. Recurrences, for the most part, develop in patients with diffuse rather than circumscribed lipoblastomas, particularly those whose tumors are incompletely excised. Therefore, wide local excision of the diffuse or infiltrating type of lipoblastomatosis is well advised.

ANGIOMYOLIPOMA

Angiomyolipoma is a member of an ever-expanding family of neoplasms with perivascular epithelioid cell differentiation (PEComas). Other members of this family of tumors include clear cell sugar tumor of the lung, lymphangioleiomyomatosis, clear cell myomelanocytic tumor of the falciform ligament/ligamentum teres, and clear cell tumors of the pancreas, uterus, and other soft tissue sites. Rather than discuss angiomyolipoma in this chapter, it is more appropriately described in the chapter on PEComas (Chapter 29).

MYELOLIPOMA

Although myelolipoma, a tumor-like growth of mature fat and bone marrow elements, is most common in the adrenal glands, it also rarely occurs in extra-adrenal sites, including the thoracic,[113] retroperitoneum[114] and presacral region,[115] mediastinum,[116] liver,[117] and bone.[118] It must be distinguished from *extramedullary hematopoietic tumors*, which are more often multiple than solitary, are frequently associated with splenomegaly and hepatomegaly, and are secondary to severe anemia (thalassemia, hereditary spherocytosis), various myeloproliferative diseases, myelosclerosis, and skeletal disorders.[119]

Myelolipomas are quite rare in young patients, and most are encountered in persons older than 40 years. Small tumors tend to be asymptomatic and often are detected as incidental findings during radiologic studies or surgery for some unrelated disease or at autopsy. Some of these tumors can grow to

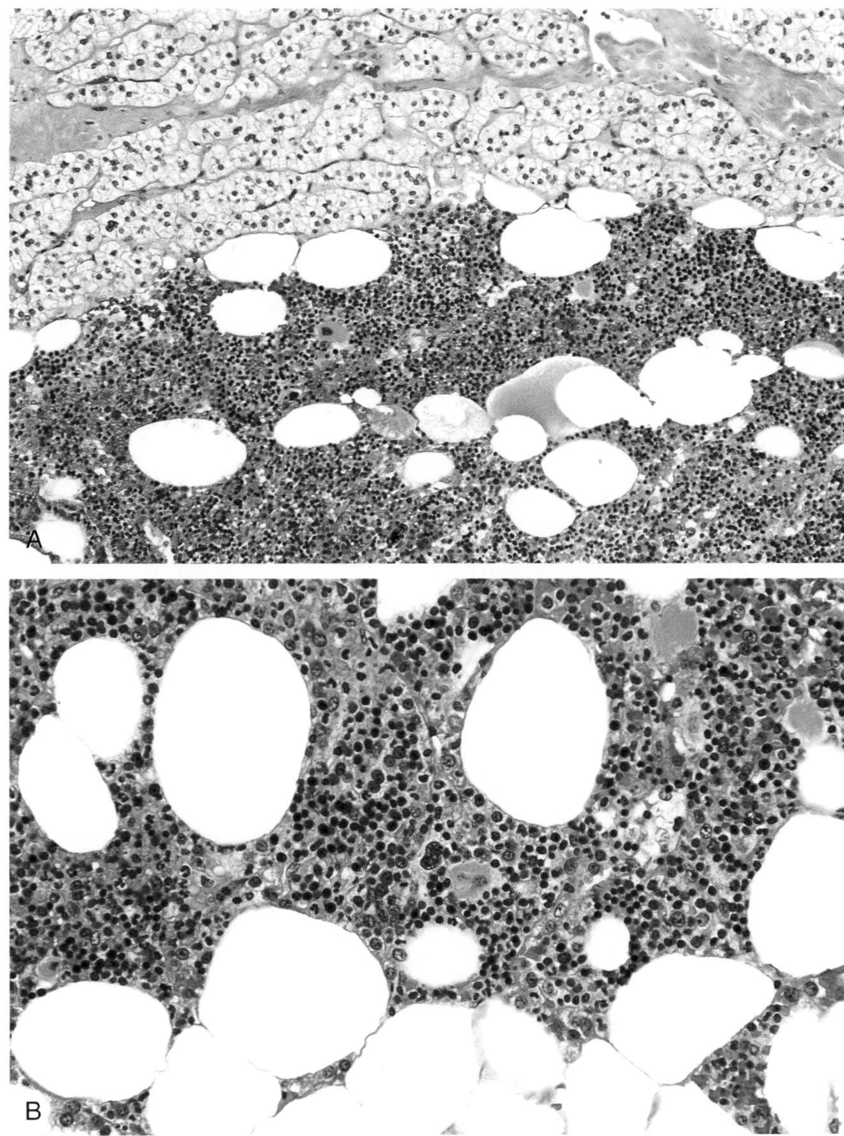

FIGURE 14-33. (A) Low-power view of a myelolipoma with an admixture of adrenal cortical cells, mature fat cells, and myeloid elements. (B) High-power view of a myelolipoma with a mixture of mature fat cells and bone marrow elements, including megakaryocytes.

enormous sizes, and there are innumerable case reports of giant myelolipomas, including one tumor weighing 6000 g.[120] These large tumors tend to cause symptoms, including abdominal pain, constipation, or nausea. Very uncommonly, these tumors can even spontaneously rupture and cause massive retroperitoneal hemorrhage.[121]

Radiologically, myelolipoma presents as a well-circumscribed radiolucent mass, usually in the adrenal gland, where it causes inferior renal displacement that can be seen on intravenous urography. A confident diagnosis can often be made using CT and MRI scans,[122] but endoscopic ultrasound or CT-guided needle biopsy of the lesion may be required for a definitive diagnosis.[123]

Grossly, myelolipoma has the features of a lipoma; however, when the myeloid elements prevail, the tumor assumes a more grayish or grayish-red appearance. Most are between 3 and 7 cm, but, as previously mentioned, some can become enormous. Microscopically, the lesion is composed of a mixture of bone marrow elements and lipocytes in varying proportions (Fig. 14-33). Some exhibit extensive myxoid change.

The histogenesis of this lesion is not clear. Many of the reported tumors have been associated with hormonally active neoplasms, including adrenocortical adenomas,[124] adrenocortical carcinomas,[125] and pheochromocytomas.[126] Others have been described in association with adrenocortical hyperplasia,[127] or 21-hydroxylase deficiency,[128] and Conn syndrome.[129] It has been proposed that these lesions arise by hormonally driven metaplasia of undifferentiated adrenal stromal cells or, in the case of extra-adrenal myelolipomas, from choristomatous hematopoietic stem cell rests.[130] Several cases of myelolipoma have been studied by cytogenetics, revealing a t(3;21)(q25;p11), suggesting a neoplastic process.[131] More recently, Bishop et al.[132] found the majority of myelolipomas to have nonrandom X-chromosome inactivation, further supporting a clonal origin.

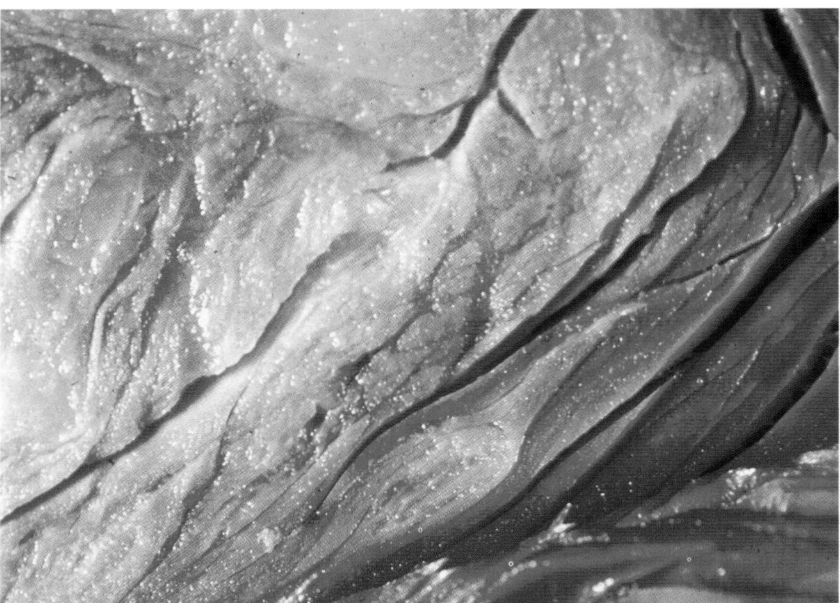

FIGURE 14-34. Partial replacement of muscle tissue by fat in an intramuscular lipoma.

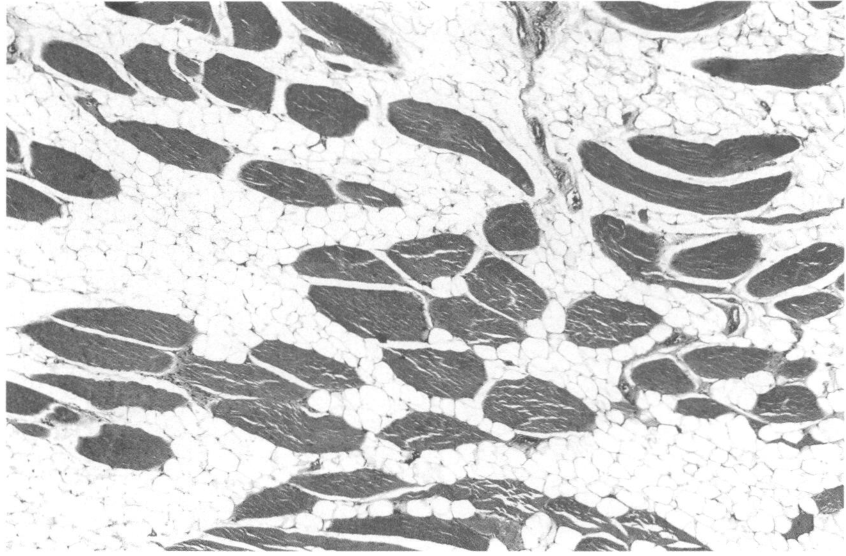

FIGURE 14-35. Intramuscular lipoma with entrapped striated muscle fibers in a cross-section. There is some atrophy of the fat cells but no lipoblasts or cells with hyperchromatic nuclei as in well-differentiated liposarcoma.

INTRAMUSCULAR AND INTERMUSCULAR LIPOMAS

Intramuscular and intermuscular lipomas are relatively common. They concern both clinicians and pathologists because of their large size, deep location, and infiltrating growth. Intramuscular lipomas outnumber intermuscular lipomas by a considerable margin, but many lesions involve both muscular and intermuscular tissues.[133] The condition has also been described in the literature as *infiltrating lipoma*.[134]

The tumor arises at all ages, but most occur in adults of 30 to 60 years of age with a predilection for men. Occasionally, it is encountered in children.[135,136] In such cases, distinction from diffuse lipomatosis and lipoblastomatosis may be difficult, if not impossible. The most common sites of involvement are the large muscles of the extremities, especially those of the thigh, shoulder, and upper arm. Most are slowly growing, painless masses that often become apparent only during muscle contraction when the tumor is converted to a firm spherical mass. On occasion, movement causes aching or pain, but the pain is rarely severe. Their size ranges from minute lesions to tumors of 20 cm or more in diameter. Occasional tumors are found on routine radiologic examination because intramuscular lipomas, like other forms of lipoma, are radiolucent and are readily demonstrated radiographically.[137]

Grossly, cross-sections of the intramuscular lipoma reveal gradual replacement of the muscle tissue by fat that may extend beyond the muscle fascia into the intermuscular connective tissue spaces. On a longitudinal section, it often assumes a striated appearance as a result of the proliferation of fat cells between muscle fibers (Fig. 14-34).

Microscopic examination reveals lipocytes that infiltrate muscle in a diffuse manner. The entrapped muscle fibers usually show few changes other than various degrees of muscular atrophy (Figs. 14-35 and 14-36). Characteristically, the lipocytes are mature; there are no lipoblasts or cells with

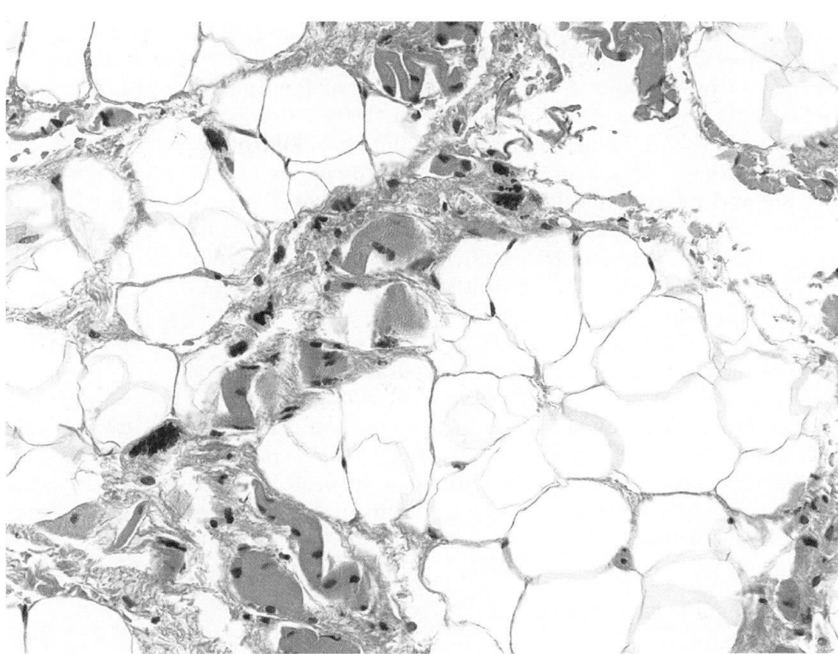

FIGURE 14-36. Atrophic skeletal muscle in an intramuscular lipoma.

atypical nuclei as in *atypical lipomatous neoplasm (well-differentiated liposarcoma)*. Nonetheless, careful sampling of these tumors is mandatory because portions of an intramuscular atypical lipomatous neoplasm may be indistinguishable from intramuscular lipoma. Generally recommended is submitting at least one section per centimeter of tumor for histologic evaluation. *Diffuse lipoblastomatosis and lipomatosis*, lesions that occur mostly in infants and children, affect the subcutis and muscle, and generally more than one muscle is involved. Furthermore, these lesions tend to be more distinctly lobulated than intramuscular lipoma, with connective tissue septa of varying thickness and lobules composed of lipoblasts in different stages of development. On occasion, however, these lesions can be indistinguishable. In some *intramuscular hemangiomas*, ex-vacuo growth of fat may simulate the picture of an intramuscular lipoma; such cases have been misinterpreted as infiltrating angiolipoma. It can be quite easy to mistake an intramuscular hemangioma with fat for an intramuscular lipoma with a few blood vessels.

Very few cases of intramuscular lipoma have been studied by cytogenetics. Heim et al.[138] reported a t(3;12)(q27;q13), whereas Bao and Miles[135] reported a case with a t(1;4;12)(q25,q27;q15). An interesting case of an intramuscular lipoma arising in a 5-year-old boy was found to have a t(9;12)(p22;q14) resulting in a fusion of *HMGA2* and *NFIB*.[136] FISH analysis for *MDM2* amplification can be helpful in distinguishing intramuscular lipoma from atypical lipomatous neoplasm, because these alterations are frequently detected in the latter and not in the former.

The prospect of cure is excellent if the tumor is completely removed. Overall, the recurrence rate reported in the literature has varied from as little as 3.0%[133] to as much as 62.5%,[134] undoubtedly depending on the completeness of the excision and on the criteria used for diagnosis and particularly the distinction from an intramuscular atypical lipomatous neoplasm.

LIPOMAS OF TENDON SHEATHS AND JOINTS

Lipomas of the tendon sheaths and joints are rare. There are two types: (1) solid fatty masses that extend along tendons for varying distances; and (2) *lipoma-like* lesions that consist chiefly of hypertrophic synovial villi distended by fat, most commonly seen in the region of the knee joint (*lipoma arborescens*). When they occur in tendon sheaths, these lesions have been described as *endovaginal* tumors, in contrast to *epivaginal* tumors (e.g., deep lipomas arising outside of the tendon sheath).

Lipoma of the tendon sheath occurs with about equal frequency in both genders and chiefly in young persons (15 to 35 years)[139]; it chiefly affects the wrist and hand and, less commonly, the ankle and foot. About half are bilateral and show a symmetric distribution. Occasionally, they involve both the hands and feet of the same individual. By the time the patient seeks treatment, most of the lesions have been present for several years. Symptoms include severe pain, trigger finger,[140] or symptoms of carpal tunnel syndrome.[141] As with other types of lipoma, radiologic examination shows a mass of less density than the surrounding tissue, which may be helpful for the diagnosis.[142]

Lipoma in joints (*lipoma arborescens*) is far more common than lipoma of the tendon sheath. The condition most commonly affects the knee joint, particularly the suprapatellar pouch[143]; rare cases occur in the shoulder,[144] hip,[145] and elbow.[146] Most patients are adults, and men are affected more commonly than women. The typical presentation is insidious swelling of the knee with intermittent effusions followed by progressive pain and debilitation.[147] Although most patients have only one joint affected (usually the knee), this process can occasionally be bilateral or even affect multiple joints.[148,149] Arthrography reveals irregular, nonspecific filling defects, most commonly in the posteromedial aspect of the suprapatellar pouch. CT, MRI, and high-resolution ultrasonography are extremely useful in making a diagnosis.[150] Using MRI, Vilanova et al.[151] found this lesion to be associated with a number of other types of chronic pathology of the joint in virtually all cases, including joint effusion (100%), degenerative changes (87%), meniscal tear (72%), synovial cysts (38%), bone erosions (25%), and synovial chondromatosis (13%). Grossly and microscopically, the lesion consists of fibrofatty tissue or thickened, grape-like or finger-like villi infiltrated by fat and lined by synovium, sometimes associated with osseous or chondroid metaplasia.[152] Arthroscopy with synovectomy is adequate therapy, in most cases.

Lipoma arborescens is probably a reactive process, given its close association with other types of chronic joint pathology. Hallel et al.[153] proposed the alternate term *villous lipomatous proliferation of the synovial membrane* to avoid confusion with a neoplastic process. It is likely that some of the symmetric lipoma arborescens-like lesions of the tendon sheath are also reactive hyperplastic lesions associated with various forms of chronic tenosynovitis.

LUMBOSACRAL LIPOMA

Lumbosacral lipoma is another curious type of lipomatous growth that deserves recognition because of its close relation to the spinal cord and its coverings. It is characterized by a diffuse proliferation of mature fat overlying the lumbosacral spine. The lesion is always associated with spina bifida or a similar laminar defect (lipomyeloschisis), and there is a stalk-like connection (tethered cord) between the fatty growth and a portion of the spinal cord that often also harbors an intradural or extradural lipoma. The stalk may cause traction and ischemia. Lipomas extending from the middle to one side are more likely to contain a meningocele or a myelocele.

Clinically, lumbosacral lipoma is asymptomatic initially and is noted only because of the presence of a large soft tissue mass or because of a sinus, skin tag, hemangioma, or excessive hair associated with a soft swelling in the lumbosacral region. Later, in about two-thirds of cases, progressive myelopathy or radiculopathy causes motor or sensory disturbances in the lower legs, bladder, or bowel.[154]

The lesion affects females almost twice as often as males and is encountered mainly in infants or children between birth and 10 years of age. Occasional cases in adults have been reported.[155] In the series of Lassman and James,[156] all 19 patients had evidence of spina bifida, and 9 had evidence of progressive neuropathy. The authors also found 26 cases of lumbosacral lipoma among 100 cases of occult spina bifida.

Sonography, CT scans, or MRI are essential for diagnosis and for planning therapy; these procedures show not only the exact position of the cord and its relation to the lipoma, but also the association of the mass with spina bifida or sacral dysgenesis.[157]

At operation, the lipomatous growth is usually unencapsulated and consists of lobulated adipose tissue microscopically indistinguishable from lipoma. In some cases, vascular proliferation and smooth muscle tissue are present in addition to the adipocytes. Unusual elements may rarely be found within the adipose tissue, including islets of neuroglia, ependyma-lined tubular structures, primitive neural tissue, teratomatous elements, and even a neuromuscular choristoma.[158]

Surgical exploration—laminectomy and division of the stalk and fibrous bands that have formed at the upper margin of the spinal defect—should be performed as early as possible, preferably before the onset of neurologic symptoms.[159] Early treatment, however, does not prevent the development of neurologic defects in the long term, because a significant percentage of patients ultimately develop urinary bladder dysfunction and other signs of neurologic deterioration.[160]

NEURAL FIBROLIPOMA (LIPOFIBROMATOUS HAMARTOMA OF NERVES)

Neural fibrolipoma is a tumor-like lipomatous process that involves principally the volar aspects of the hands, wrists, and forearms of young persons. It usually manifests as a soft, slowly growing mass consisting of proliferating fibrofatty tissue surrounding and infiltrating major nerves and their branches. Other terms applied to this condition include *lipofibromatous hamartoma of nerves*[161] and *neural lipofibromatous hamartoma.*[162] About one-third of these lesions are associated with overgrowth of bone and macrodactyly of the digits innervated by the affected nerve. In the series of 26 cases reported from the AFIP, seven were associated with macrodactyly.[163] Lesions of this type have also been described as *macrodystrophia lipomatosa*,[164] but the preferred term is *neural fibrolipoma with macrodactyly.*

The lesion is almost always seen during the first three decades of life, usually because of increasing pain, tenderness, diminished sensation, or paresthesia associated with a gradually enlarging mass causing compression neuropathy. Growth is usually slow and, in most patients, has been noted for many years. Lesions present at birth or infancy far outnumber those recognized later in childhood or adult life. Females predominate when macrodactyly is present, but males are affected more commonly when macrodactyly is absent. There may be a genetic predisposition, but there is no history of any hereditary disorders. Carpal tunnel syndrome is a late complication of some lesions.[165] Findings on MRI are virtually pathognomonic and reveal a fusiform enlargement of the affected nerve secondary to fatty infiltration.[166,167]

At operation, neural fibrolipoma presents as a soft, gray-yellow, fusiform, sausage-shaped mass that has diffusely infiltrated and replaced portions of a large nerve and its branches (Figs. 14-37 and 14-38). The median nerve and its digital branches are affected, in most cases, but other nerves, including the ulnar, radial, peroneal, and cranial nerves, may be involved. Histologically, fibrofatty tissue grows along the epineurium and perineurium and surrounds and infiltrates the nerve trunk (Fig. 14-39). Masses of fibrofatty tissue may also be found outside of the involved nerves, unattached to either the overlying skin or neighboring tendons and indistinguishable from a deep-seated lipoma. There is also marked, often concentric thickening of the perineurium and the perivascular fibrous tissue. Sometimes the affected nerve may show a pseudo-onion bulb formation, thereby mimicking an intraneural perineurioma. The diffuse infiltrative character of the lesion distinguishes it from localized and circumscribed lipomas of nerves occurring elsewhere in the body, including lipomas originating in the spinal canal. Unlike *neuromas* and *neurofibromas*, there is atrophy rather than proliferation of neural elements. Clear distinction from *diffuse lipomatosis with overgrowth of bone* is not always possible, but diffuse lipomatosis is primarily a lesion of the subcutis and muscle and only secondarily affects nerves.

There is no completely effective therapy for neural fibrolipoma. Complete excision of the fibrofatty growth is contraindicated because it may cause severe sensory or motor disturbances. Pain and sensory loss may be partially or completely relieved by dividing the transverse carpal ligament and decompressing the median nerve.[168]

DIFFUSE LIPOMATOSIS

Diffuse lipomatosis may be defined as a rare, diffuse overgrowth of mature adipose tissue that usually affects large portions of an extremity or the trunk. Although it simulates liposarcoma by its size and aggressive growth, it is histologically indistinguishable from lipoma. Like lipoma, it consists entirely of mature fat and lacks lipoblasts or cellular pleomorphism.

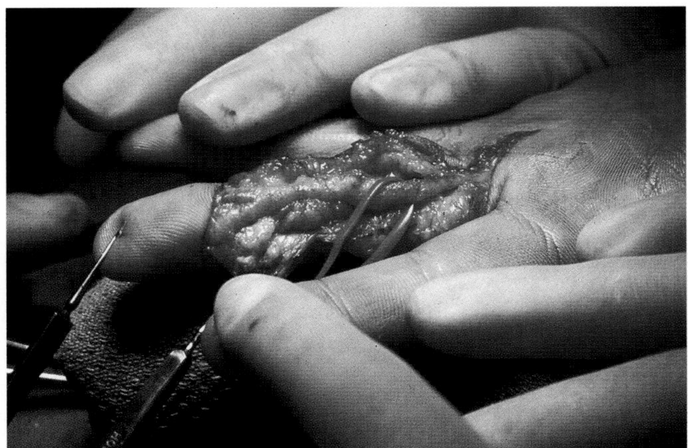

FIGURE 14-37. Neural fibrolipoma with a fusiform, sausage-shaped mass caused by diffuse infiltration of a digital nerve.

The condition is not limited to the panniculus, and, in nearly all cases, subcutis and muscle are diffusely involved. Many lesions are associated with osseous hypertrophy, leading to macrodactyly or giantism of a digit or limb (Fig. 14-40).[169] Unlike neural fibrolipoma, there is no involvement of nerves, and the process is not limited to the extremities. Association with lipomas or angiomas in other portions of the body is by no means rare. In addition to the extremities and trunk, the lesion occurs in the head and neck, intestinal tract, and abdominal cavity.[170,171] Most cases have their onset during the first 2 years of life, but typical examples of this tumor in adolescents and adults have also been observed (Fig. 14-41).[172] This lesion has rarely been associated with tuberous sclerosis.[173]

Arriving at a precise diagnosis may be difficult. *Intramuscular lipomas* exhibit a similar microscopic picture, but these

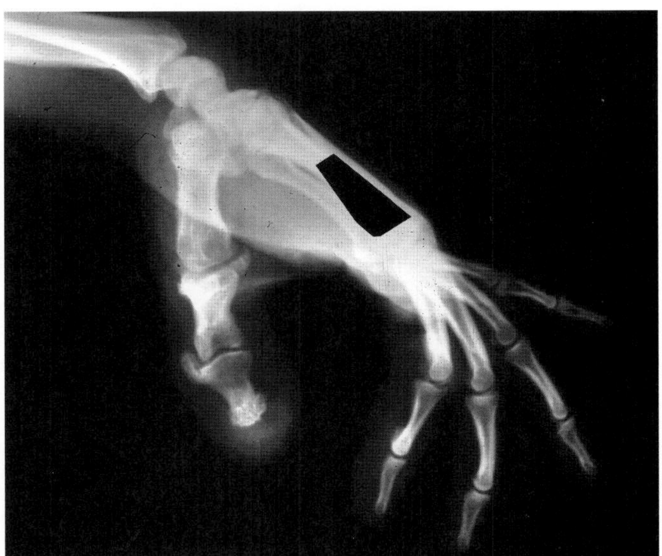

FIGURE 14-38. Radiograph displaying macrodactyly in a patient with an associated neural fibrolipoma.

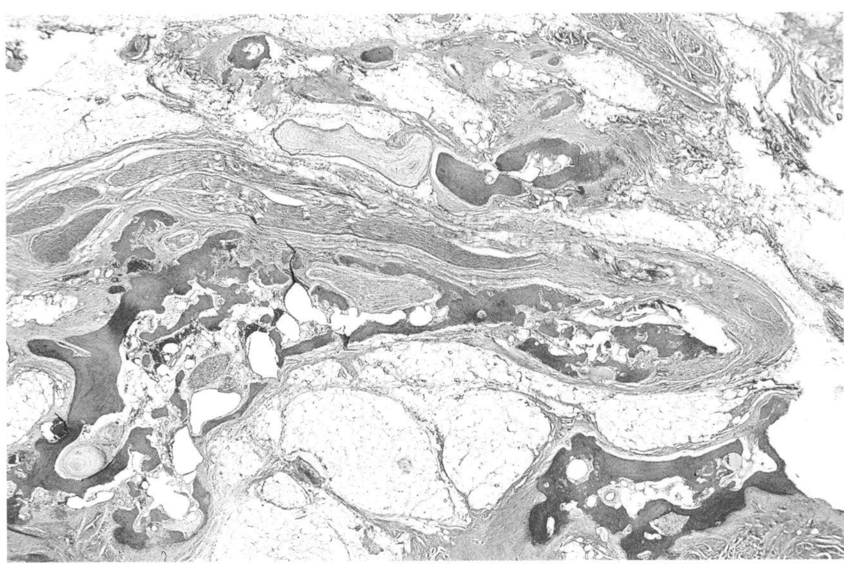

FIGURE 14-39. Low-power view of a neural fibrolipoma with extensive osseous metaplasia.

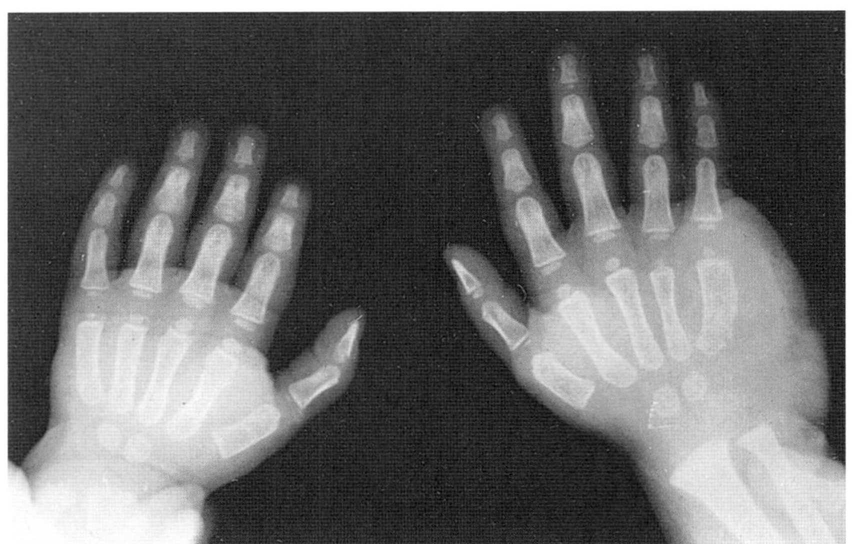

FIGURE 14-40. Diffuse lipomatosis of the right hand with slight overgrowth of phalangeal bones.

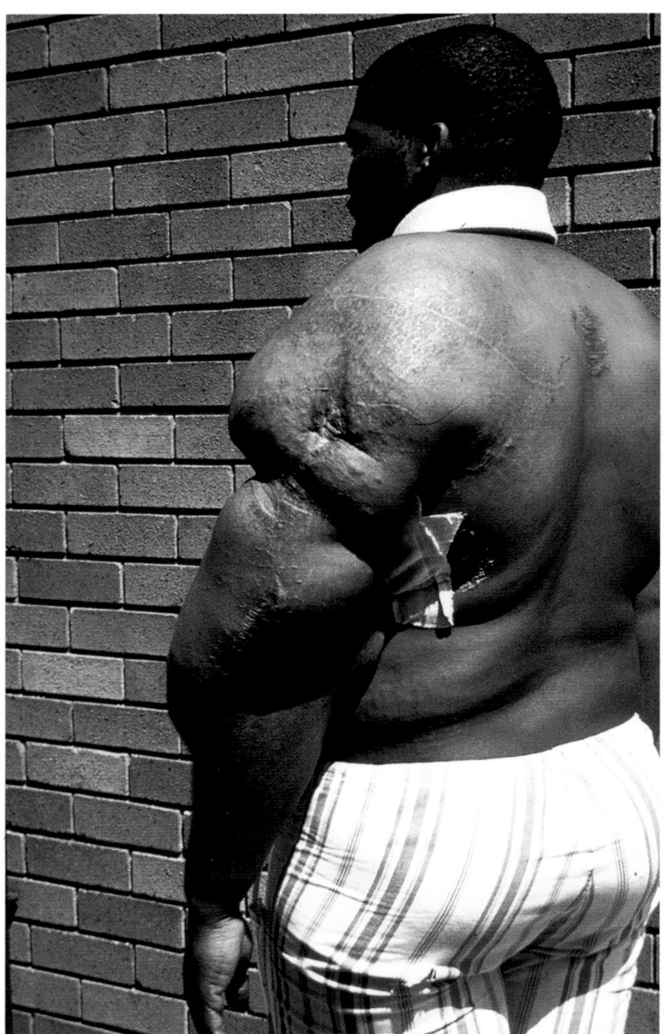

FIGURE 14-41. Diffuse lipomatosis confined to the left arm.

tumors are always confined to muscle or intermuscular tissue spaces and usually contain a larger number of entrapped muscle fibers. *Diffuse angiomatosis* may be accompanied by considerable fatty and osseous overgrowth, but it is always recognizable by its more pronounced vascular pattern. *Atypical lipomatous neoplasm* (*well-differentiated liposarcoma*) is usually less of a problem if the tumor is carefully sampled for evidence of enlarged hyperchromatic nuclei. Distinction is also facilitated by the age of the patient. Liposarcomas are exceedingly rare during infancy.

Not surprisingly, diffuse lipomatosis tends to recur, often repeatedly over many years. It may reach an enormous size and, in rare instances, causes severely impaired function, necessitating drastic surgery.

SYMMETRIC LIPOMATOSIS

Symmetric lipomatosis, also known under the eponyms *Madelung disease* and *Launois-Bensaude syndrome*, is a rare, fascinating disease first described as far back as 1846. Patients with this condition suffer from massive symmetric deposition of mature fat in the region of the neck, so the head appears to be pushed forward by a hump that has been likened to a horse collar or doughnut-shaped ring (*lipoma annulare colli*) (Fig. 14-42).

The disease affects middle-aged men almost exclusively, particularly those of Mediterranean origin.[174] Excessive alcohol intake or liver disease has been reported in up to 90% of patients in various series.[175] The fatty deposits grow insidiously, frequently over many years; and, in contrast to Dercum disease (adiposis dolorosa), they are nontender and painless. They are chiefly located bilaterally in the region of the neck but also may involve the cheeks, breast, upper arm, and axilla. The distal portions of the forearm and leg remain unaffected. The majority of patients have a predominantly axonal sensorimotor neuropathy, and up to 50% have central nervous system involvement, including hearing loss, atrophy of the optic nerve, and cerebellar ataxia.[176] Most cases are sporadic,

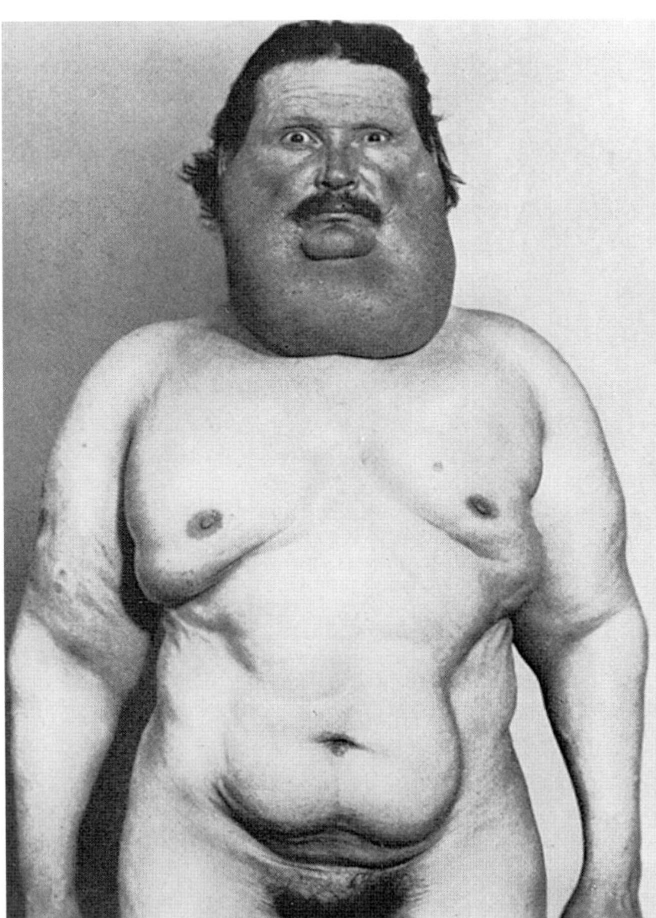

FIGURE 14-42. Symmetric lipomatosis (Madelung disease). *(From Saalfeld E, Saalfeld U. Klinic der gutartigen tumoren; handbuch der haut und geschlechtskrankheiten, geschwuelst der haut. Berlin: Julius Springer; 1932, with permission.)*

but a few are familial, possibly in an autosomal dominant mode of inheritance.[177] It has also been suggested that occult malignancy is found with increased frequency in patients with symmetric lipomatosis.[174]

The fatty deposits are poorly circumscribed and affect both the subcutis and deep soft tissue spaces, frequently extending in tongue-like projections between the cervical and thoracic muscles. Massive deposits in the deep portion of the neck, larynx, and mediastinum may cause dysphagia, stridor, and respiratory embarrassment or progressive vena caval compression.[178] As a rule, patients with this condition are not particularly obese, a fact that adds to the striking appearance of the fatty deposits in the neck. Both CT and MRI are useful for determining the extent of fat accumulation, particularly in deep soft tissue sites.[179] Grossly and microscopically, the accumulated fat is indistinguishable from mature fat, except for varying degrees of fibrosis and, rarely, calcification and ossification.

The exact cause of the condition remains obscure. A variety of metabolic disturbances, such as hyperuricemia and gout, hyperlipidemia, and diabetes, have been associated with symmetric lipomatosis, but these findings are inconsistent.[174] It has been suggested that the increased synthesis of fat is the result of a defect in catecholamine-stimulated lipolysis.[180] Others have proposed that functional sympathetic denervation results in the hypertrophy of embryologic brown fat.[181] A mitochondrial cytopathy with point mutations at the myoclonus epilepsy and ragged-red fibers syndrome (also known as MERRF syndrome) locus of the human mitochondrial genes has been implicated in the pathogenesis.[182-184]

Although conservative surgery and liposuction have been used effectively to treat the disease, it may not be necessary because, in some cases, the deposited fat recedes with abstinence from alcohol and correction of nutritional deficiencies.[185] In a study of 31 patients with follow-up, 8 (25.8%) patients died during this period, including 3 with sudden death; all 3 patients had severe autonomic neuropathy, and none had coronary artery disease.[186]

Symmetric lipomatosis must be distinguished from *adiposis dolorosa* (*Dercum disease*). The latter condition is marked by tender or painful, diffuse or nodular accumulation of subcutaneous fat. It occurs predominantly in postmenopausal women and primarily affects the regions of the pelvic girdle and the thigh. The lesion is associated with marked asthenia (e.g., loss of strength and fatigue with the least amount of effort), depression, and psychic disturbances.

PELVIC LIPOMATOSIS

Pelvic lipomatosis is characterized by an overgrowth of fat in the perirectal and perivesical regions, causing compression of the lower urinary tract and rectosigmoid colon. The condition chiefly affects black men during the third and fourth decades of life. In a review of the literature, Heyns[187] found a male to female ratio of 18 : 1. In this same review, 67% of patients were black and 78% were 20 to 60 years old. The only clinical complaints during the early stages of the disease are mild perineal pain and increased urinary frequency. At later stages, patients often complain of hematuria, constipation, nausea, lower abdominal pain, or backache of increasing severity. Rarely, pelvic lipomatosis causes venous obstruction resulting in recurrent deep venous thrombosis.[188] Hypertension is present in about one-third of patients, and some can even develop uremia secondary to renal failure.[189] Pelvic lipomatosis also has an unusual association with cystitis cystica or cystitis glandularis in up to 75% of cases, and rare cases have been associated with adenocarcinoma of the urinary bladder.[190,191]

Radiographically (excretory urography and CT scan), the typical findings include a pear- or gourd-shaped urinary bladder with an elevated base, a high-lying prostate gland, and straightening and tubular narrowing of the rectosigmoid as the result of extrinsic pressure by a radiolucent mass (Fig. 14-43). The mass may cause dilatation and medial displacement of one or both ureters and, occasionally, unilateral or bilateral hydronephrosis. CT and MRI reveal a homogeneous perivesical mass with linear densities, reflecting fibrous bands within the proliferated fatty tissue.[192]

The fatty growth is diffuse rather than nodular and consists entirely of mature fat grossly and microscopically indistinguishable from fatty tissue elsewhere in the body. Increased vascularity, fibrosis, and inflammatory changes may be present but are rare.

The cause of this overgrowth is unknown, but it appears that it is a hyperplastic rather than a neoplastic process that

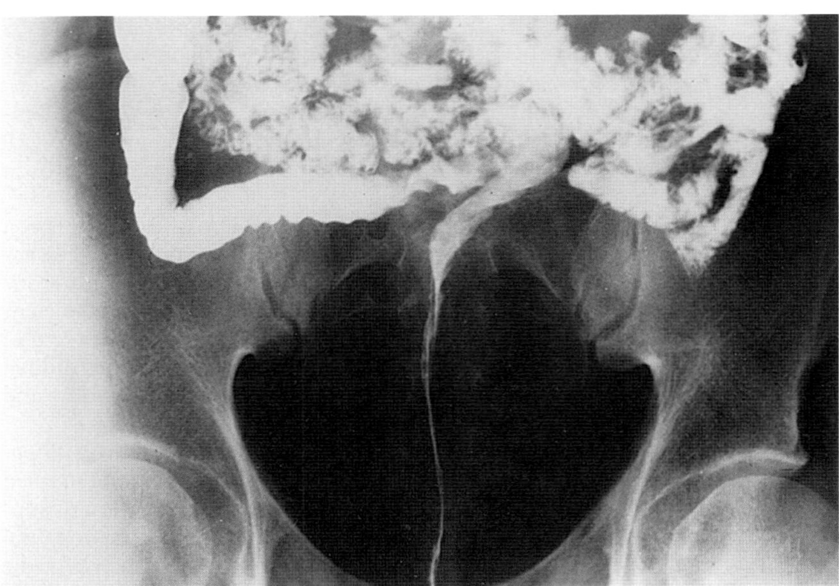

FIGURE 14-43. Radiograph of pelvic lipomatosis with marked compression of the rectum by the accumulated radiolucent fat.

almost always is limited to the pelvic region. *Lipomatosis of the ileocecal region* (submucosal, polypoid fatty infiltration of the ileocecal valve) and *renal replacement lipomatosis* (secondary to long-standing inflammation and calculi with severe atrophy and destruction of the renal parenchyma) should not be confused with this lesion. The symmetric diffuse growth and absence of atypical nuclei help rule out liposarcoma.

Prediction of the clinical course is difficult in the individual case. Frequently, pelvic lipomatosis is a slowly progressive process that may cause vesicoureteric obstruction, hydronephrosis, and uremia requiring surgical intervention, mainly urinary diversion and attempts to excise the accumulated fat.

STEROID LIPOMATOSIS

The term *steroid lipomatosis* is used here to describe a benign, diffuse fatty overgrowth caused by prolonged stimulation by adrenocortical hormones. The condition may be endogenous, as in Cushing disease and adrenal cortical hyperplasia, or the result of prolonged corticosteroid therapy or steroid immunosuppression in transplant patients. As with Cushing disease, the newly formed fat is unevenly distributed and tends to be concentrated in certain portions of the body. In some cases, the accumulation of fat is found mainly in the face (moon face), episternal region (dewlap), or interscapular region (buffalo hump); in others, it is limited to the mediastinum, pericardium, paraspinal region, mesentery, retroperitoneum, or epidural space.[193-195] Symptoms vary depending on the location of the fatty deposition but are usually the result of compression of vital structures in a confined space, such as compression of the trachea in the mediastinum or the spinal cord in the spinal canal. CT scans or MRI and demonstration of increased serum and urine cortisol levels are essential for diagnosis. Steroid lipomatosis tends to resolve when the steroid concentration is lowered. In HIV patients, the use of protease inhibitors is associated with abdominal obesity, buffalo hump, decreased facial and subcutaneous fat, hyperlipidemia, and type 2 diabetes mellitus (so-called HAART-associated dysmetabolic syndrome or HIV-associated lipodystrophy).[196]

NEVUS LIPOMATOSUS CUTANEOUS SUPERFICIALIS

Nevus lipomatosus cutaneous superficialis is an uncommon lesion characterized by groups of ectopic fat cells in the papillary or reticular dermis. Two clinical forms have been identified. The multiple form (classic type) is characterized by multiple soft nontender skin-colored or yellow papules, nodules, or plaques that usually develop shortly after birth or during the first two decades of life (Figs. 14-44 and 14-45).[197] The distribution of these lesions is usually linear or along the lines of the skinfolds with a predilection for the pelvic girdle, most commonly the buttock, sacrococcygeal region, and upper portion of the posterior thigh. Less commonly, these lesions arise as solitary nodules that usually develop after the age of 20 years. There is no site predilection for the solitary form because they have been described in many anatomic sites (scalp, face, back, among others).[198,199] There is no gender predilection, and patients are otherwise in good health.

Microscopically, the nodules are composed of aggregates of mature fat cells in the mid and upper dermis, sometimes with keratotic plugs, increased vascularity, and scattered lymphocytes, mast cells, and histiocytes (Fig. 14-46).

Like other connective tissue nevi, this lesion should be considered a developmental anomaly or hamartomatous growth. Treatment is not necessary other than for cosmetic reasons, and the lesion does not generally recur following a simple excision.

Another peculiar variant of this condition is marked by excessive symmetric, circumferential folds of skin with underlying nevus lipomatosus that affects the neck, forearms, and lower legs and resolves spontaneously during childhood; it has been aptly described as the *Michelin tire baby syndrome*. The syndrome is inherited as an autosomal dominant trait and is characterized by the deletion of chromosome 11. Association

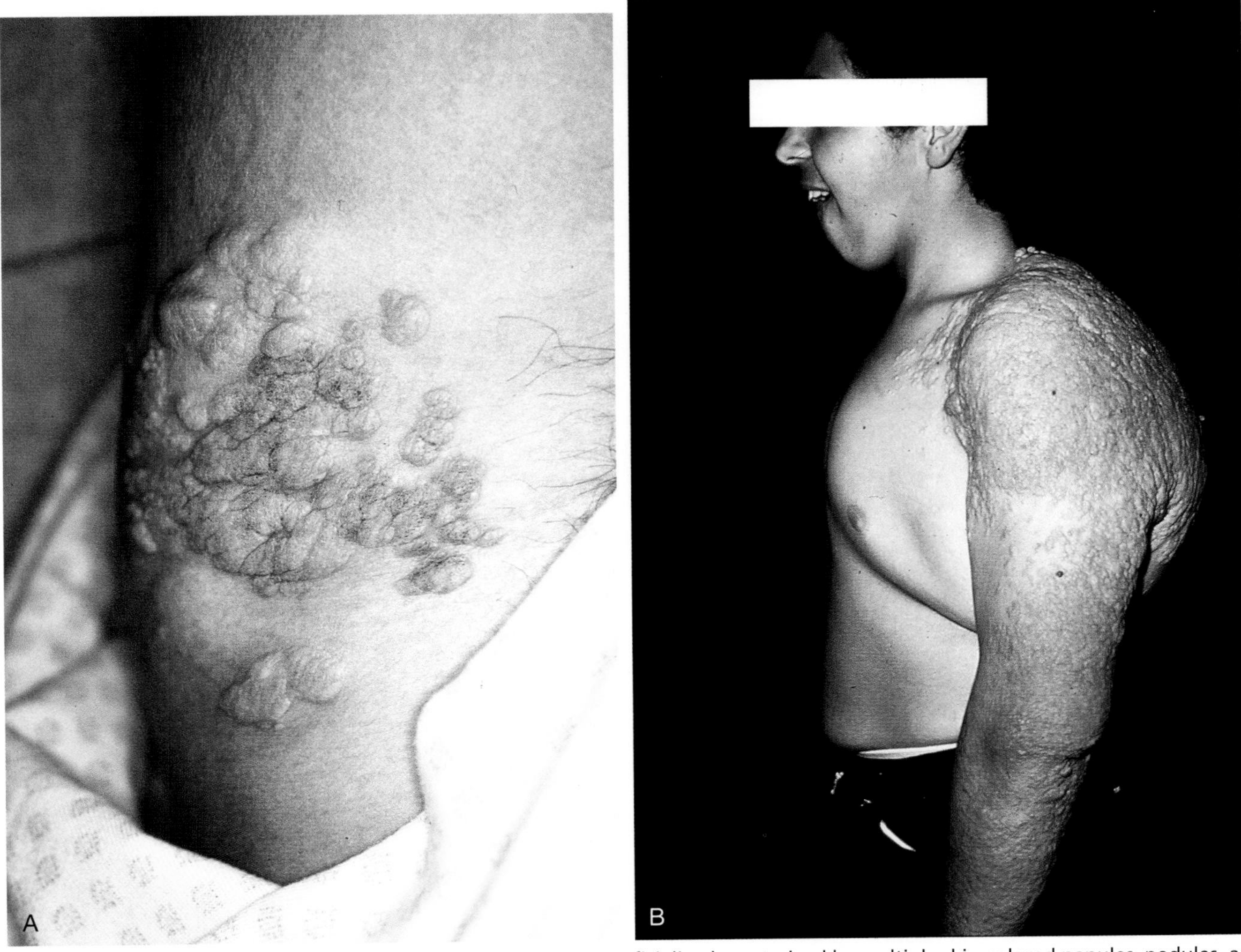

FIGURE 14-44. (A) Classic type of nevus lipomatosus cutaneous superficialis, characterized by multiple skin-colored papules, nodules, and plaques. (B) Unusual form of nevus lipomatosus cutaneous superficialis, with numerous lesions localized to the middle to upper back and proximal portion of the left arm.

with smooth muscle hamartomas and multiple anomalies has been described.[200]

HIBERNOMA

The term *hibernoma* refers to a benign lipomatous tumor in which the cells resemble brown fat, even though not all hibernomas occur at the few sites in which brown fat is encountered in humans. Such terms as *lipoma of immature adipose tissue*, *lipoma of embryonic fat*, and *fetal lipoma* have also been proposed by some authors because brown fat bears a close resemblance to early stages in the development of white fat.

Clinical Findings

Hibernomas occur chiefly in adults, with a peak incidence during the third decade of life; patients with hibernomas are on average considerably younger than those with lipoma. In the largest series published to date (170 cases derived from the files of the AFIP), there were 99 men and 71 women, whose ages ranged from 2 to 75 years (mean: 38 years).[201] Nine of these patients were in the pediatric age range. There are several other reports of hibernomas arising in infants, but it is possible that these are examples of lipoblastoma, perhaps with rare cells resembling brown fat.[202] Although traditionally believed to arise most commonly from the scapular and interscapular regions, in the AFIP series, the most common site was the soft tissues of the thigh, followed by the shoulder, back, neck, chest, arm, and abdominal cavity/retroperitoneum, in descending order of frequency. There are several reports of this tumor arising in the mediastinum,[203] breast,[204] and kidney.[205] Clinically, hibernomas are slowly growing painless tumors that typically arise in the subcutis, although about 10% of cases are intramuscular.

Pathologic Findings

Hibernomas are usually well-defined, soft, and mobile and are 5 to 15 cm (mean: 9.3 cm) in diameter, although tumors as

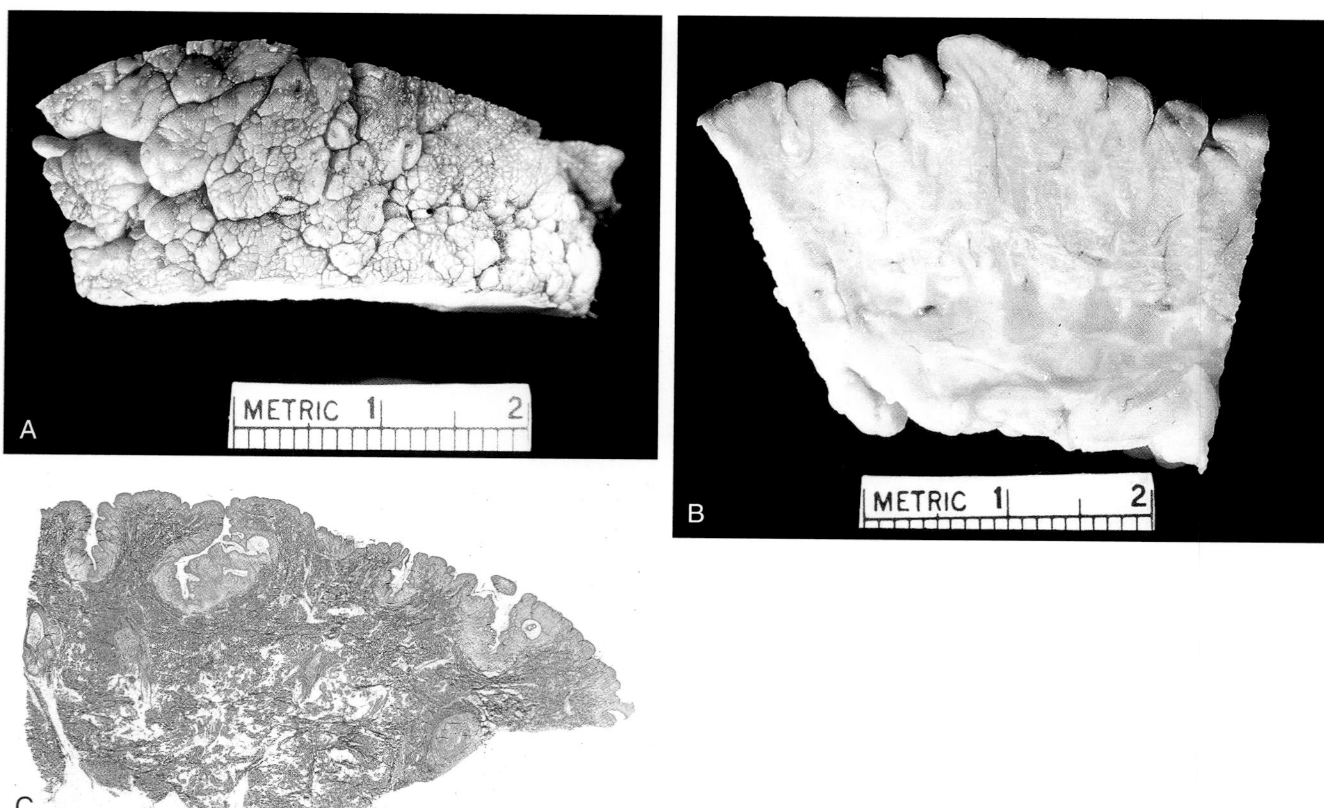

FIGURE 14-45. (A) Nevus lipomatosus cutaneous superficialis showing cerebriform wrinkled skin. (B) Cross-section of a nevus lipomatosus cutaneous superficialis showing the characteristic dermal accumulation of fat. (C) Low-power view of nevus lipomatosus cutaneous superficialis with characteristic infoldings of epidermis and accumulation of mature fat in the dermis.

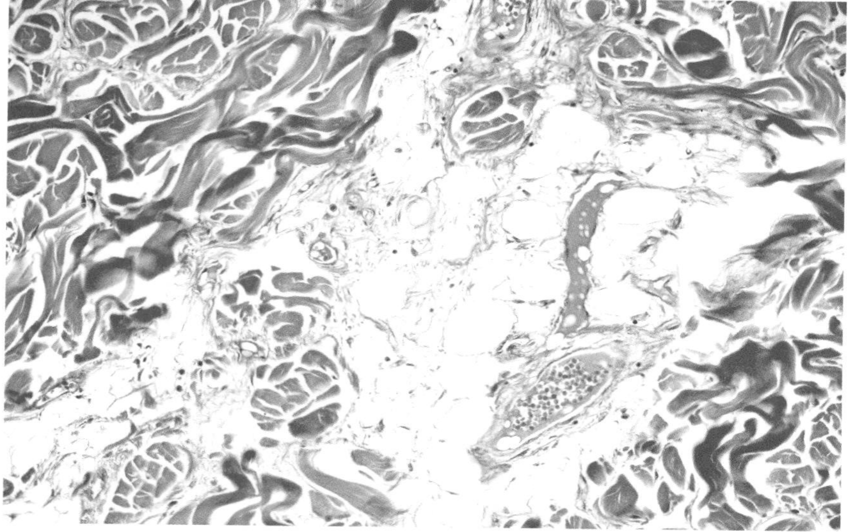

FIGURE 14-46. Nevus lipomatosus cutaneous superficialis with separation of dermal collagen by mature fat.

large as 24 cm have been reported.[201] Their color varies from tan to a deep red-brown (Fig. 14-47). CT scans and MRI clearly reveal a lipomatous tumor but are unreliable for distinguishing hibernoma from liposarcoma.[206] However, the morphologic findings in fine-needle aspiration specimens are quite reproducible and are helpful in excluding a preoperative diagnosis of liposarcoma.[207]

Microscopically, four morphologic variants are recognized. The most common (typical) displays a distinct lobular pattern and is composed of cells that show varying degrees of differentiation, ranging from uniform, round to ovoid, granular eosinophilic cells with a distinct cellular membrane to multivacuolated cells with multiple small lipid droplets and centrally placed nuclei (Figs. 14-48 to 14-51). There are also

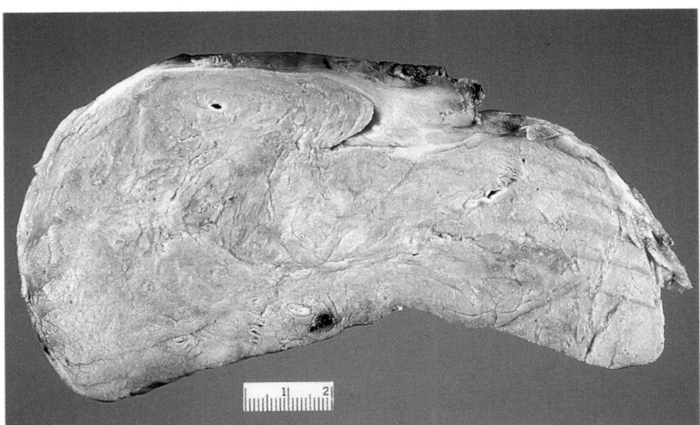

FIGURE 14-47. Gross appearance of a hibernoma of the retroperitoneum.

intermixed univacuolar cells with one or more large lipid droplets and peripherally placed nuclei resembling lipocytes. Far less commonly, hibernomas show diffuse myxoid change (myxoid variant) (Fig. 14-52). Very rarely, the cells take on a spindle cell morphology. The latter group tend to occur on the neck and scalp and can be easily confused with a spindle cell lipoma.[201,208] For all subtypes, the vascular supply is considerably more prominent in hibernomas than in lipomas. In fact, the distinct brown color of hibernoma is a result of the prominent vascularity and abundant mitochondria in the tumor.

Immunohistochemical Findings

Although immunohistochemistry is not necessary to render a diagnosis, these lesions usually stain strongly for S-100 protein. Rarely, the cells stain for CD34, although this seems

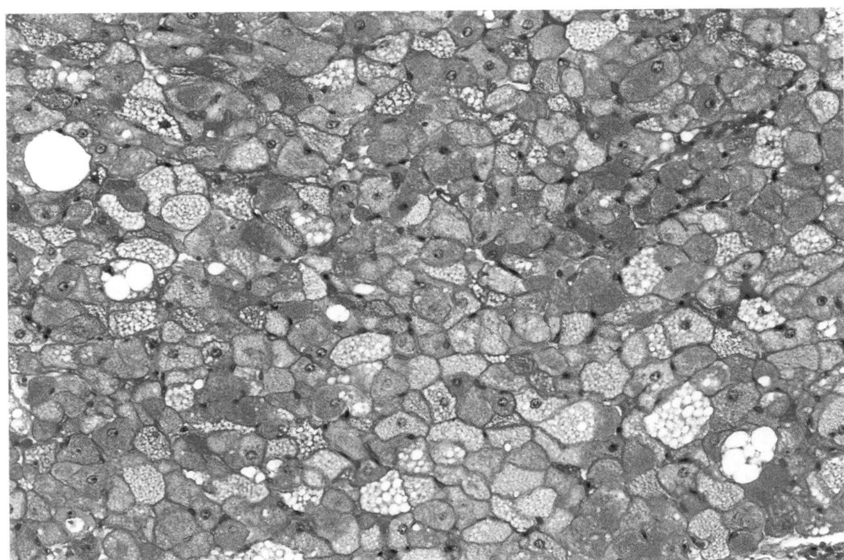

FIGURE 14-48. Hibernoma composed predominantly of vacuolated granular eosinophilic cells.

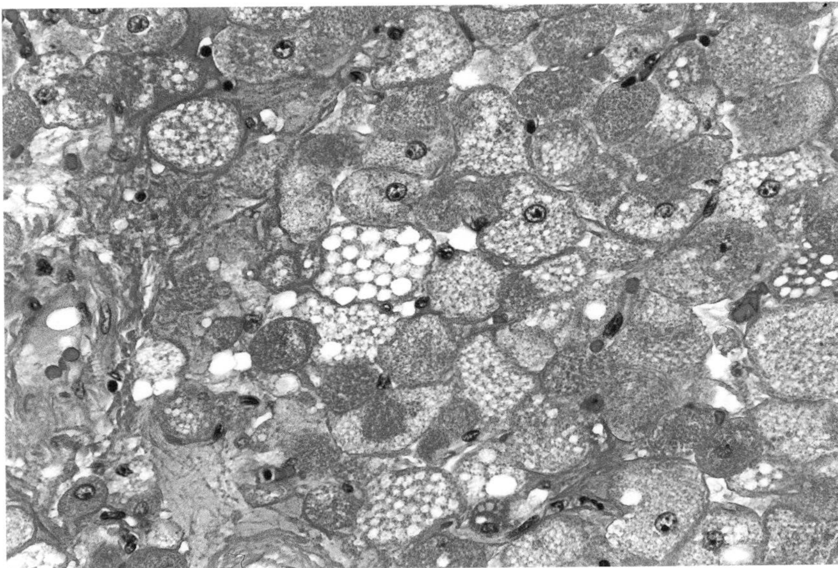

FIGURE 14-49. High-power view of granular and multivacuolated cells in a hibernoma.

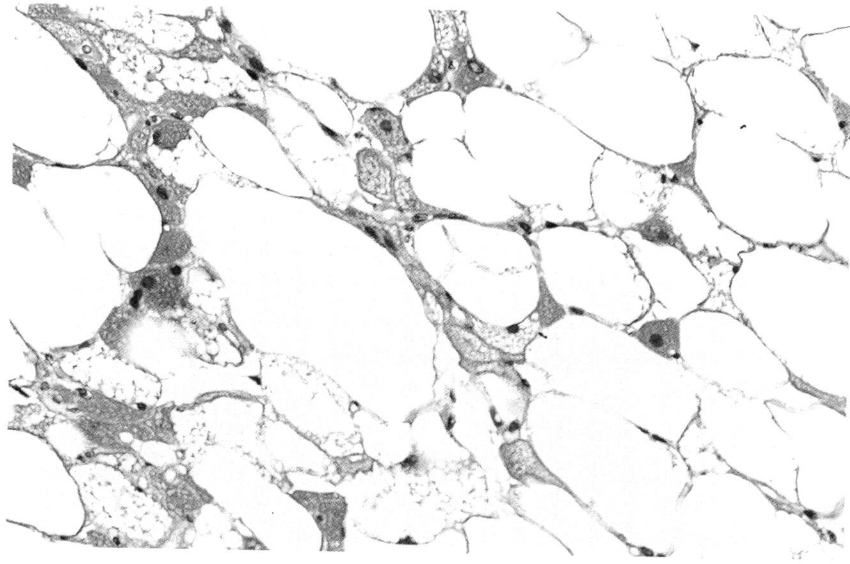

FIGURE 14-50. Hibernoma showing gradual transition between brown and white fat cells.

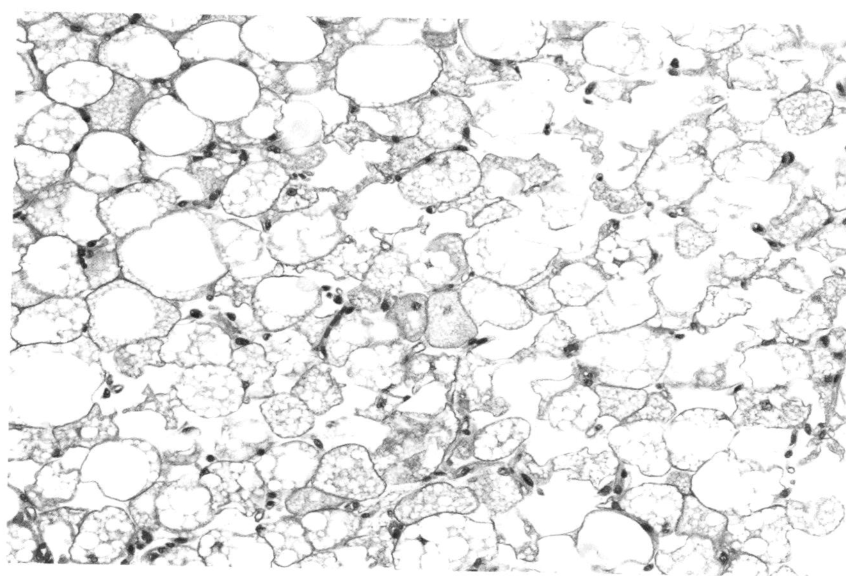

FIGURE 14-51. Hibernoma composed predominantly of fat cells with multiple cytoplasmic vacuoles.

limited to the spindle cell variant. Ultrastructural studies reveal multivacuolated and univacuolated cells packed with round to tubular mitochondria with parallel transverse cristae, a varying number of well-defined lipid droplets, and occasional lysosomes.[209]

Cytogenetic and Molecular Genetic Findings

Hibernomas have a characteristic cytogenetic aberration revealing structural rearrangements of 11q13-21, but there does not appear to be a consistent translocation partner.[210,211] Nord et al.[212] found this aberration to be consistently associated with concomitant deletions of nearby tumor suppressor genes *AIP* and *MEN1*, both of which were found to be underexpressed in hibernomas, suggesting a pathogenetic role for these tumor suppressor genes. Turaga[213] also reported a case of hibernoma with t(9;11)(q34;q13).

Differential Diagnosis

The likelihood of confusion with other tumors is minimal. *Adult rhabdomyoma* is composed of similar eosinophilic cells, but its cells are larger and contain considerable amounts of glycogen and, on careful search, crystals and cross-striations. *Granular cell tumors* bear a superficial resemblance to hibernoma but are more uniformly granular and lack typical adipocytes. S-100 protein staining is not helpful because both tumors are typically strongly positive for this antigen. The existence of malignant hibernoma is dubious. Possible cases have been encountered but interpreted microscopically as

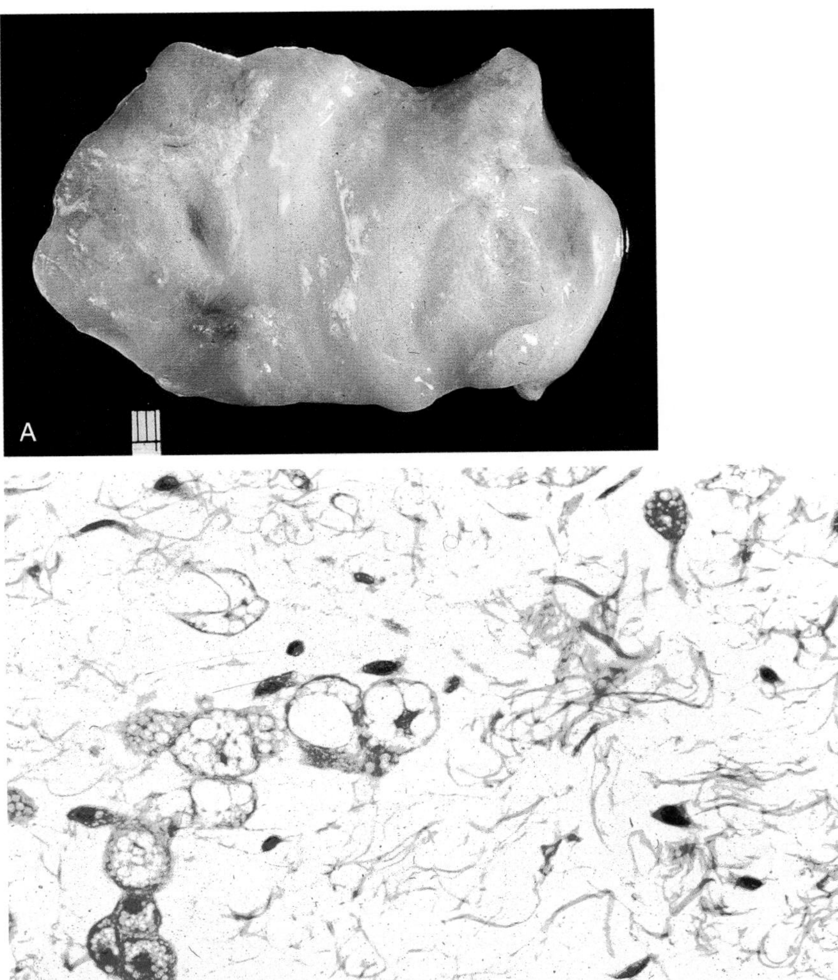

FIGURE 14-52. (A) Gross appearance of a hibernoma with extensive myxoid change. (B) Hibernoma with extensive myxoid change, with multivacuolated fat cells deposited in a mucoid matrix.

variants of round cell liposarcoma with multivacuolar eosinophilic lipoblasts; some of these cases have been confirmed by molecular analysis to harbor aberrations of *DDIT3* characteristic of myxoid/round cell liposarcoma.

Discussion

Hibernoma is a benign tumor. In the AFIP study, follow-up in 66 patients (mean follow-up period: 7.7 years) revealed no local recurrences or evidence of aggressive behavior, even though many of these tumors were incompletely excised.[201]

References

1. Poissonnet CM, Burdi AR, Bookstein FL. Growth and development of human adipose tissue during early gestation. Early Hum Dev 1983; 8(1):1–11.
2. Poissonnet CM, Burdi AR, Garn SM. The chronology of adipose tissue appearance and distribution in the human fetus. Early Hum Dev 1984; 10(1-2):1–11.
3. Ailhaud G, Massiera F, Weill P, et al. Temporal changes in dietary fats: role of n-6 polyunsaturated fatty acids in excessive adipose tissue development and relationship to obesity. Prog Lipid Res 2006;45(3):203–36.
4. Nnodim JO. Development of adipose tissues. Anat Rec 1987;219(4): 331–7.
5. Ravussin E, Galgani JE. The implication of brown adipose tissue for humans. Annu Rev Nutr 2011;31:33–47.
6. Ladanyi M. The emerging molecular genetics of sarcoma translocations. Diagn Mol Pathol 1995;4(3):162–73.
7. Adelmant G, Gilbert JD, Freytag SO. Human translocation liposarcoma-CCAAT/enhancer binding protein (C/EBP) homologous protein (TLS-CHOP) oncoprotein prevents adipocyte differentiation by directly interfering with C/EBPbeta function. J Biol Chem 1998;273(25): 15574–81.
8. Weiss SW, Langloss JM, Enzinger FM. Value of S-100 protein in the diagnosis of soft tissue tumors with particular reference to benign and malignant Schwann cell tumors. Lab Invest 1983;49(3):299–308.
9. Joyner CJ, Triffitt J, Puddle B, et al. Development of a monoclonal antibody to the aP2 protein to identify adipocyte precursors in tumours of adipose differentiation. Pathol Res Pract 1999;195(7): 461–6.
10. Rydholm A, Berg NO. Size, site and clinical incidence of lipoma. Factors in the differential diagnosis of lipoma and sarcoma. Acta Orthop Scand 1983;54(6):929–34.
11. Posadzy-Dziedzic M, Molini L, Bianchi S. Sonographic findings of parosteal lipoma of the radius causing posterior interosseous nerve compression with radiographic and magnetic resonance imaging correlation. J Ultrasound Med 2011;30(7):1033–6.
12. El-Monem MH, Gaafar AH, Magdy EA. Lipomas of the head and neck: presentation variability and diagnostic work-up. J Laryngol Otol 2006; 120(1):47–55.
13. Fletcher CD, Martin-Bates E. Intramuscular and intermuscular lipoma: neglected diagnoses. Histopathology 1988;12(3):275–87.
14. Macarenco RS, Erickson-Johnson M, Wang X, et al. Retroperitoneal lipomatous tumors without cytologic atypia: are they lipomas? A clinicopathologic and molecular study of 19 cases. Am J Surg Pathol 2009;33(10):1470–6.

15. Munk PL, Lee MJ, Janzen DL, et al. Lipoma and liposarcoma: evaluation using CT and MR imaging. AJR Am J Roentgenol 1997;169(2): 589–94.
16. Laskin WB, Fetsch JF, Michal M, et al. Sclerotic (fibroma-like) lipoma: a distinctive lipoma variant with a predilection for the distal extremities. Am J Dermatopathol 2006;28(4):308–16.
17. Chitnis M, Steyn T, Koeppen P, et al. Differentiation of a benign myxolipoma from a myxoid liposarcoma by tumour karyotyping–a diagnosis missed. Pediatr Surg Int 2002;18(1):83.
18. Martínez-Mata G, Rocío MF, Juan LE, et al. Angiomyxolipoma (vascular myxolipoma) of the oral cavity. Report of a case and review of the literature. Head Neck Pathol 2011;5(2):184–7.
19. Fritchie KJ, Renner JB, Rao KW, et al. Osteolipoma: radiological, pathological, and cytogenetic analysis of three cases. Skeletal Radiol 2011. Available at: http://www.ncbi.nlm.nih.gov/pubmed/21822651. Accessed August 13, 2011.
20. Simango S, Ramdial PK, Madaree A. Subpectoral post-traumatic lipoma. Br J Plast Surg 2000;53(7):627–9.
21. Ramdial PK, Madaree A, Singh B. Membranous fat necrosis in lipomas. Am J Surg Pathol 1997;21(7):841–6.
22. Nishio J. Contributions of cytogenetics and molecular cytogenetics to the diagnosis of adipocytic tumors. J Biomed Biotechnol 2011;2011: 524067.
23. Sandberg AA. Updates on the cytogenetics and molecular genetics of bone and soft tissue tumors: lipoma. Cancer Genet Cytogenet 2004;150(2):93–115.
24. Willén H, Akerman M, Dal Cin P, et al. Comparison of chromosomal patterns with clinical features in 165 lipomas: a report of the CHAMP study group. Cancer Genet Cytogenet 1998;102(1):46–9.
25. Wang X, Hulshizer RL, Erickson-Johnson MR, et al. Identification of novel HMGA2 fusion sequences in lipoma: evidence that deletion of let-7 miRNA consensus binding site 1 in the HMGA2 3' UTR is not critical for HMGA2 transcriptional upregulation. Genes Chromosomes Cancer 2009;48(8):673–8.
26. Schoenmakers EF, Wanschura S, Mols R, et al. Recurrent rearrangements in the high mobility group protein gene, HMGI-C, in benign mesenchymal tumours. Nat Genet 1995;10(4):436–44.
27. Petit MM, Mols R, Schoenmakers EF, et al. LPP, the preferred fusion partner gene of HMGIC in lipomas, is a novel member of the LIM protein gene family. Genomics 1996;36(1):118–29.
28. Kubo T, Matsui Y, Naka N, et al. Expression of HMGA2-LPP and LPP-HMGA2 fusion genes in lipoma: identification of a novel type of LPP-HMGA2 transcript in four cases. Anticancer Res 2009;29(6):2357–60.
29. von Ahsen I, Rogalla P, Bullerdiek J. Expression patterns of the LPP-HMGA2 fusion transcript in pulmonary chondroid hamartomas with t(3;12)(q27 approximately 28;q14 approximately 15). Cancer Genet Cytogenet 2005;163(1):68–70.
30. Kazmierczak B, Dal Cin P, Wanschura S, et al. HMGIY is the target of 6p21.3 rearrangements in various benign mesenchymal tumors. Genes Chromosomes Cancer 1998;23(4):279–85.
31. Tallini G, Dorfman H, Brys P, et al. Correlation between clinicopathological features and karyotype in 100 cartilaginous and chordoid tumours. A report from the Chromosomes and Morphology (CHAMP) Collaborative Study Group. J Pathol 2002;196(2):194–203.
32. Theumann N, Abdelmoumene A, Wintermark M, et al. Posttraumatic pseudolipoma: MRI appearances. Eur Radiol 2005;15(9):1876–80.
33. Veger HT, Ravensbergen NJ, Ottenhof A, et al. Familial multiple lipomatosis: a case report. Acta Chir Belg 2010;110(1):98–100.
34. Gámez J, Playán A, Andreu AL, et al. Familial multiple symmetric lipomatosis associated with the A8344G mutation of mitochondrial DNA. Neurology 1998;51(1):258–60.
35. Oktenli C, Gul D, Deveci MS, et al. Unusual features in a patient with neurofibromatosis type 1: multiple subcutaneous lipomas, a juvenile polyp in ascending colon, congenital intrahepatic portosystemic venous shunt, and horseshoe kidney. Am J Med Genet A 2004;127A(3): 298–301.
36. Wanner M, Celebi JT, Peacocke M. Identification of a PTEN mutation in a family with Cowden syndrome and Bannayan-Zonana syndrome. J Am Acad Dermatol 2001;44(2):183–7.
37. Pilarski R, Stephens JA, Noss R, et al. Predicting PTEN mutations: an evaluation of Cowden syndrome and Bannayan-Riley-Ruvalcaba syndrome clinical features. J Med Genet 2011;48(8):505–12.
38. Bogart MM, Arnold HE, Greer KE. Prune-belly syndrome in two children and review of the literature. Pediatr Dermatol 2006;23(4):342–5.
39. Gucev ZS, Tasic V, Jancevska A, et al. Congenital lipomatous overgrowth, vascular malformations, and epidermal nevi (CLOVE) syndrome: CNS malformations and seizures may be a component of this disorder. Am J Med Genet A 2008;146A(20):2688–90.
40. Abbasi NR, Brownell I, Fangman W. Familial multiple angiolipomatosis. Dermatol Online J 2007;13(1):3.
41. Nanassis K, Tsitsopoulos P, Marinopoulos D, et al. Lumbar spinal epidural angiolipoma. J Clin Neurosci 2008;15(4):460–3.
42. Levitt J, Lutfi Ali SA, Sapadin A. Multiple subcutaneous angiolipomas associated with new-onset diabetes mellitus. Int J Dermatol 2002; 41(11):783–5.
43. Kryvenko ON, Chitale DA, VanEgmond EM, et al. Angiolipoma of the female breast: clinicomorphological correlation of 52 cases. Int J Surg Pathol 2011;19(1):35–43.
44. Fletcher CD, Akerman M, Dal Cin P, et al. Correlation between clinicopathological features and karyotype in lipomatous tumors. A report of 178 cases from the Chromosomes and Morphology (CHAMP) Collaborative Study Group. Am J Pathol 1996;148(2):623–30.
45. Sciot R, Akerman M, Dal Cin P, et al. Cytogenetic analysis of subcutaneous angiolipoma: further evidence supporting its difference from ordinary pure lipomas: a report of the CHAMP Study Group. Am J Surg Pathol 1997;21(4):441–4.
46. Meis JM, Enzinger FM. Myolipoma of soft tissue. Am J Surg Pathol 1991;15(2):121–5.
47. Ulu EM, Kirbaş I, Töre HG, et al. Extraperitoneal pelvic myolipoma. Diagn Interv Radiol 2010;16(3):227–31.
48. Michal M. Retroperitoneal myolipoma. A tumour mimicking retroperitoneal angiomyolipoma and liposarcoma with myosarcomatous differentiation. Histopathology 1994;25(1):86–8.
49. Ben-Izhak O, Elmalach I, Kerner H, et al. Pericardial myolipoma: a tumour presenting as a mediastinal mass and containing oestrogen receptors. Histopathology 1996;29(2):184–6.
50. Meis JM, Enzinger FM. Chondroid lipoma. A unique tumor simulating liposarcoma and myxoid chondrosarcoma. Am J Surg Pathol 1993; 17(11):1103–12.
51. Chan JK, Lee KC, Saw D. Extraskeletal chondroma with lipoblast-like cells. Hum Pathol 1986;17(12):1285–7.
52. Darling MR, Daley TD. Intraoral chondroid lipoma: a case report and immunohistochemical investigation. Oral Surg Oral Med Oral Pathol Oral Radiol Endod 2005;99(3):331–3.
53. Gomez-Ortega JM, Rodilla IG, Basco López de Lerma JM. Chondroid lipoma. A newly described lesion that may be mistaken for malignancy. Oral Surg Oral Med Oral Pathol Oral Radiol Endod 1996;81(5):586–9.
54. Hyzy MD, Hogendoorn PC, Bloem JL, et al. Chondroid lipoma: findings on radiography and MRI (2006:7b). Eur Radiol 2006;16(10):2373–6.
55. Jiménez-Heffernan JA, González-Peramato P, Perna C. Diagnosis of chondroid lipoma by fine-needle aspiration biopsy. Arch Pathol Lab Med 2002;126(7):773; author reply 773–4.
56. Hoch B, Hermann G, Klein MJ, et al. Ossifying chondroid lipoma. Skeletal Radiol 2008;37(5):475–80.
57. Nielsen GP, O'Connell JX, Dickersin GR, et al. Chondroid lipoma, a tumor of white fat cells. A brief report of two cases with ultrastructural analysis. Am J Surg Pathol 1995;19(11):1272–6.
58. Kindblom LG, Meis-Kindblom JM. Chondroid lipoma: an ultrastructural and immunohistochemical analysis with further observations regarding its differentiation. Hum Pathol 1995;26(7):706–15.
59. Huang D, Sumegi J, Dal Cin P, et al. C11orf95-MKL2 is the resulting fusion oncogene of t(11;16)(q13;p13) in chondroid lipoma. Genes Chromosomes Cancer 2010;49(9):810–8.
60. Ballaux F, Debiec-Rychter M, De Wever I, et al. Chondroid lipoma is characterized by t(11;16)(q13;p12-13). Virchows Arch 2004;444(2): 208–10.
61. Enzinger FM, Harvey DA. Spindle cell lipoma. Cancer 1975;36(5): 1852–9.
62. Shmookler BM, Enzinger FM. Pleomorphic lipoma: a benign tumor simulating liposarcoma. A clinicopathologic analysis of 48 cases. Cancer 1981;47(1):126–33.
63. Evans HL, Soule EH, Winkelmann RK. Atypical lipoma, atypical intramuscular lipoma, and well differentiated retroperitoneal liposarcoma: a reappraisal of 30 cases formerly classified as well differentiated liposarcoma. Cancer 1979;43(2):574–84.
64. Azumi N, Curtis J, Kempson RL, et al. Atypical and malignant neoplasms showing lipomatous differentiation. A study of 111 cases. Am J Surg Pathol 1987;11(3):161–83.
65. Vecchio G, Amico P, Caltabiano R, et al. Spindle cell/pleomorphic lipoma of the oral cavity. J Craniofac Surg 2009;20(6):1992–4.
66. Harvell JD. Multiple spindle cell lipomas and dermatofibrosarcoma protuberans within a single patient: evidence for a common neoplastic

process of interstitial dendritic cells? J Am Acad Dermatol 2003;48(1): 82–5.
67. Fanburg-Smith JC, Devaney KO, Miettinen M, et al. Multiple spindle cell lipomas: a report of 7 familial and 11 nonfamilial cases. Am J Surg Pathol 1998;22(1):40–8.
68. Gurel D, Kargi A, Lebe B. Pedunculated cutaneous spindle cell/pleomorphic lipoma. J Cutan Pathol 2010;37(9):e57–9.
69. Reis-Filho JS, Milanezi F, Soares MF, et al. Intradermal spindle cell/pleomorphic lipoma of the vulva: case report and review of the literature. J Cutan Pathol 2002;29(1):59–62.
70. Mandal RV, Duncan LM, Austen WG Jr, et al. Infiltrating intramuscular spindle cell lipoma of the face. J Cutan Pathol 2009;36(Suppl. 1): 70–3.
71. Zelger BW, Zelger BG, Plörer A, et al. Dermal spindle cell lipoma: plexiform and nodular variants. Histopathology 1995;27(6):533–40.
72. Billings SD, Folpe AL. Diagnostically challenging spindle cell lipomas: a report of 34 "low-fat" and "fat-free" variants. Am J Dermatopathol 2007;29(5):437–42.
73. Sachdeva MP, Goldblum JR, Rubin BP, et al. Low-fat and fat-free pleomorphic lipomas: a diagnostic challenge. Am J Dermatopathol 2009; 31(5):423–6.
74. Fletcher CD, Martin-Bates E. Spindle cell lipoma: a clinicopathological study with some original observations. Histopathology 1987;11(8): 803–17.
75. Warkel RL, Rehme CG, Thompson WH. Vascular spindle cell lipoma. J Cutan Pathol 1982;9(2):113–8.
76. Hawley IC, Krausz T, Evans DJ, et al. Spindle cell lipoma–a pseudoangiomatous variant. Histopathology 1994;24(6):565–9.
77. Zamecnik M. Pseudoangiomatous spindle cell lipoma with "true" angiomatous features. Virchows Arch 2005;447(4):781–3.
78. Zamecnik M, Michal M. Angiomatous spindle cell lipoma: report of three cases with immunohistochemical and ultrastructural study and reappraisal of former "pseudoangiomatous" variant. Pathol Int 2007; 57(1):26–31.
79. Diaz-Cascajo C, Borghi S, Weyers W. Pleomorphic lipoma with pseudopapillary structures: a pleomorphic counterpart of pseudoangiomatous spindle cell lipoma. Histopathology 2000;36(5):475–6.
80. Suster S, Fisher C, Moran CA. Expression of bcl-2 oncoprotein in benign and malignant spindle cell tumors of soft tissue, skin, serosal surfaces, and gastrointestinal tract. Am J Surg Pathol 1998;22(7):863–72.
81. Magro G, Caltabiano R, Di Cataldo A, et al. CD10 is expressed by mammary myofibroblastoma and spindle cell lipoma of soft tissue: an additional evidence of their histogenetic linking. Virchows Arch 2007; 450(6):727–8.
82. Mandahl N, Höglund M, Mertens F, et al. Cytogenetic aberrations in 188 benign and borderline adipose tissue tumors. Genes Chromosomes Cancer 1994;9(3):207–15.
83. Dal Cin P, Sciot R, Polito P, et al. Lesions of 13q may occur independently of deletion of 16q in spindle cell/pleomorphic lipomas. Histopathology 1997;31(3):222–5.
84. Rubin BP, Dal Cin P. The genetics of lipomatous tumors. Semin Diagn Pathol 2001;18(4):286–93.
85. Flucke U, van Krieken JH, Mentzel T. Cellular angiofibroma: analysis of 25 cases emphasizing its relationship to spindle cell lipoma and mammary-type myofibroblastoma. Mod Pathol 2011;24(1):82–9.
86. Hameed M, Clarke K, Amer HZ, et al. Cellular angiofibroma is genetically similar to spindle cell lipoma: a case report. Cancer Genet Cytogenet 2007;177(2):131–4.
87. Maggiani F, Debiec-Rychter M, Vanbockrijck M, et al. Cellular angiofibroma: another mesenchymal tumour with 13q14 involvement, suggesting a link with spindle cell lipoma and (extra)-mammary myofibroblastoma. Histopathology 2007;51(3):410–2.
88. Maggiani F, Debiec-Rychter M, Verbeeck G, et al. Extramammary myofibroblastoma is genetically related to spindle cell lipoma. Virchows Arch 2006;449(2):244–7.
89. Vellios F, Baez J, Schumacker HB. Lipoblastomatosis: a tumor of fetal fat different from hibernoma; report of a case, with observations on the embryogenesis of human adipose tissue. Am J Pathol 1958;34(6): 1149–59.
90. Van Meurs DP. The transformation of an embryonic lipoma to a common lipoma. Br J Surg 1947;34(135):282–4.
91. Mentzel T, Calonje E, Fletcher CD. Lipoblastoma and lipoblastomatosis: a clinicopathological study of 14 cases. Histopathology 1993;23(6): 527–33.
92. Collins MH, Chatten J. Lipoblastoma/lipoblastomatosis: a clinicopathologic study of 25 tumors. Am J Surg Pathol 1997;21(10):1131–7.
93. Coffin CM, Lowichik A, Putnam A. Lipoblastoma (LPB): a clinicopathologic and immunohistochemical analysis of 59 cases. Am J Surg Pathol 2009;33(11):1705–12.
94. Jeong TJ, Oh YJ, Ahn JJ, et al. Lipoblastoma-like tumour of the lip in an adult woman. Acta Derm Venereol 2010;90(5):537–8.
95. Pham NS, Poirier B, Fuller SC, et al. Pediatric lipoblastoma in the head and neck: a systematic review of 48 reported cases. Int J Pediatr Otorhinolaryngol 2010;74(7):723–8.
96. Dillingh SJ, Merx TA, van Krieken HJ, et al. Rapid-growing tumor of the cheek mimicking a malignant tumor: lipoblastoma of infancy. J Pediatr Hematol Oncol 2011;33(2):113–5.
97. Salem R, Zohd M, Njim L, et al. Lipoblastoma: a rare lesion in the differential diagnosis of childhood mediastinal tumors. J Pediatr Surg 2011;46(5):e21–3.
98. Yu DC, Javid PJ, Chikwava KR, et al. Mesenteric lipoblastoma presenting as a segmental volvulus. J Pediatr Surg 2009;44(2):e25–8.
99. Koplin SA, Twohig MH, Lund DP, et al. Omental lipoblastoma. Pathol Res Pract 2008;204(4):277–81.
100. Kamal NM, Jouini R, Yahya S, et al. Benign intrascrotal lipoblastoma in a 4-month-old infant: a case report and review of literature. J Pediatr Surg 2011;46(7):e9–12.
101. Api O, Akil A, Uzun MG, et al. Fetal retroperitoneal lipoblastoma: ultrasonographic appearance of a rare embryonal soft tissue tumor. J Matern Fetal Neonatal Med 2010;23(9):1069–71.
102. Dutton JJ, Escaravage GK Jr, Fowler AM, et al. Lipoblastomatosis: case report and review of the literature. Ophthal Plast Reconstr Surg 2011. Available at: http://www.ncbi.nlm.nih.gov/pubmed/21743369. Accessed August 14, 2011.
103. Bourelle S, Viehweger E, Launay F, et al. Lipoblastoma and lipoblastomatosis. J Pediatr Orthop B 2006;15(5):356–61.
104. al-Qattan MM, Weinberg M, Clarke HM. Two rapidly growing fatty tumors of the upper limb in children: lipoblastoma and infiltrating lipoma. J Hand Surg Am 1995;20(1):20–3.
105. Chen CW, Chang WC, Lee HS, et al. MRI features of lipoblastoma: differentiating from other palpable lipomatous tumor in pediatric patients. Clin Imaging 2010;34(6):453–7.
106. Ahn KH, Boo YJ, Seol HJ, et al. Prenatally detected congenital perineal mass using 3D ultrasound which was diagnosed as lipoblastoma combined with anorectal malformation: case report. J Korean Med Sci 2010;25(7):1093–6.
107. Hill S, Rademaker M. A collection of rare anomalies: multiple digital glomuvenous malformations, epidermal naevus, temporal alopecia, heterochromia and abdominal lipoblastoma. Clin Exp Dermatol 2009; 34(8):e862–4.
108. Kok KY, Telisinghe PU. Lipoblastoma: clinical features, treatment, and outcome. World J Surg 2010;34(7):1517–22.
109. Chen Z, Coffin CM, Scott S, et al. Evidence by spectral karyotyping that 8q11.2 is nonrandomly involved in lipoblastoma. J Mol Diagn 2000; 2(2):73–7.
110. Gisselsson D, Hibbard MK, Dal Cin P, et al. PLAG1 alterations in lipoblastoma: involvement in varied mesenchymal cell types and evidence for alternative oncogenic mechanisms. Am J Pathol 2001;159(3):955–62.
111. Hibbard MK, Kozakewich HP, Dal Cin P, et al. PLAG1 fusion oncogenes in lipoblastoma. Cancer Res 2000;60(17):4869–72.
112. Morerio C, Nozza P, Tassano E, et al. Differential diagnosis of lipoma-like lipoblastoma. Pediatr Blood Cancer 2009;52(1):132–4.
113. Rossi M, Ravizza D, Fiori G, et al. Thoracic myelolipoma diagnosed by endoscopic ultrasonography and fine-needle aspiration cytology. Endoscopy 2007;39(Suppl. 1):E114–5.
114. Craig WD, Fanburg-Smith JC, Henry LR, et al. Fat-containing lesions of the retroperitoneum: radiologic-pathologic correlation. Radiographics 2009;29(1):261–90.
115. Gill KR, Hasan MK, Menke DM, et al. Presacral myelolipoma: diagnosis by EUS-FNA and Trucut biopsy. Gastrointest Endosc 2010;71(4):849; discussion 849–50.
116. Vaziri M, Sadeghipour A, Pazooki A, et al. Primary mediastinal myelolipoma. Ann Thorac Surg 2008;85(5):1805–6.
117. Radhi J. Hepatic myelolipoma. J Gastrointestin Liver Dis 2010;19(1): 106–7.
118. Sundaram M, Bauer T, von Hochstetter A, et al. Intraosseous myelolipoma. Skeletal Radiol 2007;36(12):1181–4.
119. Sukov WR, Remstein ED, Nascimento AG, et al. Sclerosing extramedullary hematopoietic tumor: emphasis on diagnosis by renal biopsy. Ann Diagn Pathol 2009;13(2):127–31.
120. Akamatsu H, Koseki M, Nakaba H, et al. Giant adrenal myelolipoma: report of a case. Surg Today 2004;34(3):283–5.

121. Goltz JP, Gattenlöhner S, Hahn D, et al. [Ruptured giant myelolipoma of the adrenal gland with acute retroperitoneal hemorrhage]. Rofo 2009;181(5):485–7.
122. Pereira JM, Sirlin CB, Pinto PS, et al. CT and MR imaging of extrahepatic fatty masses of the abdomen and pelvis: techniques, diagnosis, differential diagnosis, and pitfalls. Radiographics 2005;25(1):69–85.
123. Jhala NC, Jhala D, Eloubeidi MA, et al. Endoscopic ultrasound-guided fine-needle aspiration biopsy of the adrenal glands: analysis of 24 patients. Cancer 2004;102(5):308–14.
124. Yamada S, Tanimoto A, Wang KY, et al. Non-functional adrenocortical adenoma: a unique case of combination with myelolipoma and endothelial cysts. Pathol Res Pract 2011;207(3):192–6.
125. Sun X, Ayala A, Castro CY. Adrenocortical carcinoma with concomitant myelolipoma in a patient with hyperaldosteronism. Arch Pathol Lab Med 2005;129(6):e144–7.
126. Ukimura O, Inui E, Ochiai A, et al. Combined adrenal myelolipoma and pheochromocytoma. J Urol 1995;154(4):1470.
127. Courcoutsakis NA, Patronas NJ, Cassarino D, et al. Hypodense nodularity on computed tomography: novel imaging and pathology of micronodular adrenocortical hyperplasia associated with myelolipomatous changes. J Clin Endocrinol Metab 2004;89(8):3737–8.
128. Hagiwara H, Usui T, Kimura T, et al. Lack of ACTH and androgen receptor expression in a giant adrenal myelolipoma associated with 21-hydroxylase deficiency. Endocr Pathol 2008;19(2):122–7.
129. Cormio L, Ruutu M, Giardina C, et al. Combined adrenal adenoma and myelolipoma in a patient with Conn syndrome. Case report. Panminerva Med 1992;34(4):209–12.
130. Fowler MR, Williams RB, Alba JM, et al. Extra-adrenal myelolipomas compared with extramedullary hematopoietic tumors: a case of presacral myelolipoma. Am J Surg Pathol 1982;6(4):363–74.
131. Chang KC, Chen PI, Huang ZH, et al. Adrenal myelolipoma with translocation (3;21)(q25;p11). Cancer Genet Cytogenet 2002;134(1):77–80.
132. Bishop E, Eble JN, Cheng L, et al. Adrenal myelolipomas show nonrandom X-chromosome inactivation in hematopoietic elements and fat: support for a clonal origin of myelolipomas. Am J Surg Pathol 2006;30(7):838–43.
133. Kindblom LG, Angervall L, Stener B, et al. Intermuscular and intramuscular lipomas and hibernomas. A clinical, roentgenologic, histologic, and prognostic study of 46 cases. Cancer 1974;33(3):754–62.
134. Dionne GP, Seemayer TA. Infiltrating lipomas and angiolipomas revisited. Cancer 1974;33(3):732–8.
135. Bao L, Miles L. Translocation (1;4;12)(q25;q27;q15) in a childhood intramuscular lipoma. Cancer Genet Cytogenet 2005;158(1):95–7.
136. Pierron A, Fernandez C, Saada E, et al. HMGA2-NFIB fusion in a pediatric intramuscular lipoma: a novel case of NFIB alteration in a large deep-seated adipocytic tumor. Cancer Genet Cytogenet 2009;195(1):66–70.
137. Nishida J, Morita T, Ogose A, et al. Imaging characteristics of deep-seated lipomatous tumors: intramuscular lipoma, intermuscular lipoma, and lipoma-like liposarcoma. J Orthop Sci 2007;12(6):533–41.
138. Heim S, Mandahl N, Kristoffersson U, et al. Reciprocal translocation t(3;12)(q27;q13) in lipoma. Cancer Genet Cytogenet 1986;23(4):301–4.
139. Bryan RS, Dahlin DC, Sullivan CR. Lipoma of the tendon sheath. J Bone Joint Surg Am 1956;38-A(6):1275–80.
140. Pampliega T, Arenas AJ. An unusual trigger finger. Acta Orthop Belg 1997;63(2):132–3.
141. Chen CH, Wu T, Sun JS, et al. Unusual causes of carpal tunnel syndrome: space occupying lesions. J Hand Surg Eur Vol 2011. Available at: http://www.ncbi.nlm.nih.gov/pubmed/21825010. Accessed August 15, 2011.
142. Sheldon PJ, Forrester DM, Learch TJ. Imaging of intraarticular masses. Radiographics 2005;25(1):105–19.
143. Senocak E, Gurel K, Gurel S, et al. Lipoma arborescens of the suprapatellar bursa and extensor digitorum longus tendon sheath: report of 2 cases. J Ultrasound Med 2007;26(10):1427–33.
144. Chae EY, Chung HW, Shin MJ, et al. Lipoma arborescens of the glenohumeral joint causing bone erosion: MRI features with gadolinium enhancement. Skeletal Radiol 2009;38(8):815–8.
145. Wolf RS, Zoys GN, Saldivar VA, et al. Lipoma arborescens of the hip. Am J Orthop 2002;31(5):276–9.
146. Le Corroller T, Gaubert JY, Champsaur P, et al. Lipoma arborescens in the bicipitoradial bursa of the elbow: sonographic findings. J Ultrasound Med 2011;30(1):116–8.
147. Yacyshyn EA, Lambert RG. Lipoma arborescens: recurrent knee effusions with positive cyclic citrillunated peptide. J Rheumatol 2010;37(10):2188–9.
148. Coll JP, Ragsdale BD, Chow B, et al. Best cases from the AFIP: lipoma arborescens of the knees in a patient with rheumatoid arthritis. Radiographics 2011;31(2):333–7.
149. Silva L, Terroso G, Sampaio L, et al. Polyarticular lipoma arborescens—a clinical and aesthetical case. Rheumatol Int 2011. Available at: http://www.ncbi.nlm.nih.gov/pubmed/21526358. Accessed August 15, 2011.
150. Learch TJ, Braaton M. Lipoma arborescens: high-resolution ultrasonographic findings. J Ultrasound Med 2000;19(6):385–9.
151. Vilanova JC, Barceló J, Villalón M, et al. MR imaging of lipoma arborescens and the associated lesions. Skeletal Radiol 2003;32(9):504–9.
152. Kurihashi A, Yamaguchi T, Tamal K, et al. Lipoma arborescens with osteochondral metaplasia–a case mimicking synovial osteochondromatosis in a lateral knee bursa. Acta Orthop Scand 1997;68(3):304–6.
153. Hallel T, Lew S, Bansal M. Villous lipomatous proliferation of the synovial membrane (lipoma arborescens). J Bone Joint Surg Am 1988;70(2):264–70.
154. Kang HS, Wang KC, Kim KM, et al. Prognostic factors affecting urologic outcome after untethering surgery for lumbosacral lipoma. Childs Nerv Syst 2006;22(9):1111–21.
155. Al-Omari MH, Eloqayli HM, Qudseih HM, et al. Isolated lipoma of filum terminale in adults: MRI findings and clinical correlation. J Med Imaging Radiat Oncol 2011;55(3):286–90.
156. Lassman LP, James CC. Lumbosacral lipomas: critical survey of 26 cases submitted to laminectomy. J Neurol Neurosurg Psychiatr 1967;30(2):174–81.
157. Bekkali NL, Hagebeuk EE, Bongers ME, et al. Magnetic resonance imaging of the lumbosacral spine in children with chronic constipation or non-retentive fecal incontinence: a prospective study. J Pediatr 2010;156(3):461–5.
158. Park SH, Huh JS, Cho KH, et al. Teratoma in human tail lipoma. Pediatr Neurosurg 2005;41(3):158–61.
159. Samuels R, McGirt MJ, Attenello FJ, et al. Incidence of symptomatic retethering after surgical management of pediatric tethered cord syndrome with or without duraplasty. Childs Nerv Syst 2009;25(9):1085–9.
160. Cochrane DD, Finley C, Kestle J, et al. The patterns of late deterioration in patients with transitional lipomyelomeningocele. Eur J Pediatr Surg 2000;10(Suppl. 1):13–7.
161. Al-Jabri T, Garg S, Mani GV. Lipofibromatous hamartoma of the median nerve. J Orthop Surg Res 2010;5:71.
162. Bisceglia M, Vigilante E, Ben-Dor D. Neural lipofibromatous hamartoma: a report of two cases and review of the literature. Adv Anat Pathol 2007;14(1):46–52.
163. Silverman TA, Enzinger FM. Fibrolipomatous hamartoma of nerve. A clinicopathologic analysis of 26 cases. Am J Surg Pathol 1985;9(1):7–14.
164. Khan RA, Wahab S, Ahmad I, et al. Macrodystrophia lipomatosa: four case reports. Ital J Pediatr 2010;36:69.
165. Matsubara M, Tanikawa H, Mogami Y, et al. Carpal tunnel syndrome due to fibrolipomatous hamartoma of the median nerve in Klippel-Trénaunay syndrome. A case report. J Bone Joint Surg Am 2009;91(5):1223–7.
166. Jain TP, Srivastava DN, Mittal R, et al. Fibrolipomatous hamartoma of median nerve. Australas Radiol 2007;51 Spec No.:B98–100.
167. Woertler K. Tumors and tumor-like lesions of peripheral nerves. Semin Musculoskelet Radiol 2010;14(5):547–58.
168. Ogose A, Hotta T, Higuchi T, et al. Fibrolipomatous hamartoma in the foot: magnetic resonance imaging and surgical treatment: a report of two cases. J Bone Joint Surg Am 2002;84-A(3):432–6.
169. Greiss ME, Williams DH. Macrodystrophia lipomatosis in the foot. A case report and review of the literature. Arch Orthop Trauma Surg 1991;110(4):220–1.
170. El-Khatib HA. Unusual distribution of the lower body fatty tissue: classification, treatment, and differential diagnosis. Ann Plast Surg 2008;61(1):2–8.
171. Kim HK, Lee JY, Kim WS, et al. Atypical diffuse lipomatosis with multifocal abdominal involvement: a case report. J Plast Reconstr Aesthet Surg 2010;63(10):e742–4.
172. Komagata T, Takebayashi S, Hirasawa K, et al. Extensive lipomatosis of the small bowel and mesentery: CT and MRI findings. Radiat Med 2007;25(9):480–3.
173. Klein JA, Barr RJ. Diffuse lipomatosis and tuberous sclerosis. Arch Dermatol 1986;122(11):1298–302.

174. Gomes da Silva R, Detoffol Bragança R, Ribeiro Costa C, et al. Multiple symmetric lipomatosis. J Cutan Med Surg 2011;15(4):230–5.
175. Morelli F, De Benedetto A, Toto P, et al. Alcoholism as a trigger of multiple symmetric lipomatosis? J Eur Acad Dermatol Venereol 2003; 17(3):367–9.
176. Fernández-Vozmediano J, Armario-Hita J. Benign symmetric lipomatosis (Launois-Bensaude syndrome). Int J Dermatol 2005;44(3):236–7.
177. Gámez J, Playán A, Andreu AL, et al. Familial multiple symmetric lipomatosis associated with the A8344G mutation of mitochondrial DNA. Neurology 1998;51(1):258–60.
178. Stopar T, Jankovic VN, Casati A. Four different airway-management strategies in patient with Launois-Bensaude syndrome or Madelung's disease undergoing surgical excision of neck lipomatosis with a complicated postoperative course. J Clin Anesth 2005;17(4):300–3.
179. Ampollini L, Carbognani P. Images in clinical medicine. Madelung's disease. N Engl J Med 2011;364(5):465.
180. Nisoli E, Regianini L, Briscini L, et al. Multiple symmetric lipomatosis may be the consequence of defective noradrenergic modulation of proliferation and differentiation of brown fat cells. J Pathol 2002;198(3): 378–87.
181. Nielsen S, Levine J, Clay R, et al. Adipose tissue metabolism in benign symmetric lipomatosis. J Clin Endocrinol Metab 2001;86(6):2717–20.
182. Muñoz-Málaga A, Bautista J, Salazar JA, et al. Lipomatosis, proximal myopathy, and the mitochondrial 8344 mutation. A lipid storage myopathy? Muscle Nerve 2000;23(4):538–42.
183. Klopstock T, Naumann M, Seibel P, et al. Mitochondrial DNA mutations in multiple symmetric lipomatosis. Mol Cell Biochem 1997;174(1-2): 271–5.
184. Naumann M, Kiefer R, Toyka KV, et al. Mitochondrial dysfunction with myoclonus epilepsy and ragged-red fibers point mutation in nerve, muscle, and adipose tissue of a patient with multiple symmetric lipomatosis. Muscle Nerve 1997;20(7):833–9.
185. Di Candia M, Cormack GC. Rhytidectomy approach for recurrent Madelung disease. Aesthet Surg J 2011;31(6):643–7.
186. Enzi G, Busetto L, Ceschin E, et al. Multiple symmetric lipomatosis: clinical aspects and outcome in a long-term longitudinal study. Int J Obes Relat Metab Disord 2002;26(2):253–61.
187. Heyns CF. Pelvic lipomatosis: a review of its diagnosis and management. J Urol 1991;146(2):267–73.
188. Gajic O, Sprung J, Hall BA, et al. Fatal acute pulmonary embolism in a patient with pelvic lipomatosis after surgery performed after transatlantic airplane travel. Anesth Analg 2004;99(4):1032–4, table of contents.
189. Sharma S, Nabi G, Seth A, et al. Pelvic lipomatosis presenting as uraemic encephalopathy. Int J Clin Pract 2001;55(2):149–50.
190. Miglani U, Sinha T, Gupta SK, et al. Rare etiology of obstructive uropathy: pelvic lipomatosis. Urol Int 2010;84(2):239–41.
191. Sözen S, Gürocak S, Uzüm N, et al. The importance of re-evaluation in patients with cystitis glandularis associated with pelvic lipomatosis: a case report. Urol Oncol 2004;22(5):428–30.
192. Craig WD, Fanburg-Smith JC, Henry LR, et al. Fat-containing lesions of the retroperitoneum: radiologic-pathologic correlation. Radiographics 2009;29(1):261–90.
193. Siskind BN, Weiner FR, Frank M, et al. Steroid-induced mesenteric lipomatosis. Comput Radiol 1984;8(3):175–7.
194. Dhawan SS, Khouzam R. Atypical mediastinal lipomatosis. Heart Lung 2007;36(3):223–5.
195. Shukla LW, Katz JA, Wagner ML. Mediastinal lipomatosis: a complication of high dose steroid therapy in children. Pediatr Radiol 1988;19(1):57–8.
196. Viganò A, Zuccotti GV, Cerini C, et al. Lipodystrophy, insulin resistance, and adiponectin concentration in HIV-infected children and adolescents. Curr HIV Res 2011. Available at: http://www.ncbi.nlm.nih.gov/pubmed/21827385. Accessed August 16, 2011.
197. Lane JE, Clark E, Marzec T. Nevus lipomatosus cutaneus superficialis. Pediatr Dermatol 2003;20(4):313–4.
198. Park HJ, Park CJ, Yi JY, et al. Nevus lipomatosus superficialis on the face. Int J Dermatol 1997;36(6):435–7.
199. Sawada Y. Solitary nevus lipomatosus superficialis on the forehead. Ann Plast Surg 1986;16(4):356–8.
200. Nomura Y, Ota M, Tochimaru H. Self-healing congenital generalized skin creases: Michelin tire baby syndrome. J Am Acad Dermatol 2010;63(6):1110–1.
201. Furlong MA, Fanburg-Smith JC, Miettinen M. The morphologic spectrum of hibernoma: a clinicopathologic study of 170 cases. Am J Surg Pathol 2001;25(6):809–14.
202. Baskurt E, Padgett DM, Matsumoto JA. Multiple hibernomas in a 1-month-old female infant. AJNR Am J Neuroradiol 2004;25(8): 1443–5.
203. Barbetakis N, Asteriou C, Stefanidis A, et al. Mediastinal hibernoma presenting with hoarseness. Interact Cardiovasc Thorac Surg 2011;12(5): 845–6.
204. Padilla-Rodriguez AL. Pure hibernoma of the breast: insights about its origins. Ann Diagn Pathol 2011. Available at: http://www.ncbi.nlm.nih.gov/pubmed/21546293. Accessed July 26, 2011.
205. Delsignore A, Ranzoni S, Arancio M, et al. Kidney hibernoma: case report and literature review. Arch Ital Urol Androl 2010;82(3): 189–91.
206. Dursun M, Agayev A, Bakir B, et al. CT and MR characteristics of hibernoma: six cases. Clin Imaging 2008;32(1):42–7.
207. Thejasvi K, Niveditha SR, Suguna BV, et al. Cytomorphology of hibernoma: a report of 2 cases. Acta Cytol 2010;54(Suppl. 5):875–8.
208. Moretti VM, Brooks JS, Lackman RD. Spindle-cell hibernoma: a clinicopathologic comparison of this new variant. Orthopedics 2010;33(1): 52–5.
209. Manieri M, Murano I, Fianchini A, et al. Morphological and immunohistochemical features of brown adipocytes and preadipocytes in a case of human hibernoma. Nutr Metab Cardiovasc Dis 2010;20(8): 567–74.
210. Gisselsson D, Höglund M, Mertens F, et al. Hibernomas are characterized by homozygous deletions in the multiple endocrine neoplasia type I region. Metaphase fluorescence in situ hybridization reveals complex rearrangements not detected by conventional cytogenetics. Am J Pathol 1999;155(1):61–6.
211. Mertens F, Rydholm A, Brosjö O, et al. Hibernomas are characterized by rearrangements of chromosome bands 11q13-21. Int J Cancer 1994;58(4):503–5.
212. Nord KH, Magnusson L, Isaksson M, et al. Concomitant deletions of tumor suppressor genes MEN1 and AIP are essential for the pathogenesis of the brown fat tumor hibernoma. Proc Natl Acad Sci USA 2010;107(49):21122–7.
213. Turaga KK, Silva-Lopez E, Sanger WG, et al. A (9;11)(q34;q13) translocation in a hibernoma. Cancer Genet Cytogenet 2006;170(2):163–6.

Liposarcoma

CHAPTER CONTENTS

Liposarcoma, accounting for 15% to 25% of all sarcomas, is the most common sarcoma of adults. There are several subtypes that are histologically, biologically, cytogenetically, and, by molecular analyses, distinct from one another (Table 15-1). These subtypes range in behavior from nonmetastasizing neoplasms (e.g., atypical lipomatous neoplasm/well-differentiated liposarcoma [ALN/WDL]) to high-grade sarcomas with full metastatic potential (e.g., pleomorphic liposarcoma). So impressed were Enzinger and Winslow[1] by the diversity of this group of lesions that they wrote in their seminal work on liposarcoma in 1962, "Among mesenchymal tumors, liposarcomas are probably unsurpassed by their wide range in structure and behavior. In fact the variations are striking that it seems more apt [*sic*] to regard them as groups of closely related tumors rather than as a well defined entity." These words were truly prophetic. Molecular analysis has validated the distinctness of the subtypes. In no other group of sarcomas does the pathologist receive such a strong mandate to subclassify these lesions. Although histologic subtype remains the most reliable prognostic parameter in daily practice, recent evidence suggests that gene profiles may eventually factor into risk stratification of individual patients.[2]

Although the World Health Organization (WHO) divides liposarcomas into four subtypes (ALN/WDL, myxoid/round cell, dedifferentiated, pleomorphic),[3] it is useful to think of liposarcomas as three large groups from a conceptual point of view. ALN/WDL, also termed *atypical lipomatous neoplasm (ALN)* when it occurs in superficial soft tissue or in the muscles of the extremity because of its low-grade behavior, and dedifferentiated liposarcoma (DL) comprise one subgroup. Widely disparate in terms of biologic behavior, they are closely related from a pathogenetic point of view because a subset of ALN/WDL histologically progresses to dedifferentiated sarcomas. With dedifferentiation, the tumor acquires metastatic potential, a phenomenon accompanied by additional cytogenetic abnormalities. The second group is myxoid liposarcoma that ranges in appearance from pure myxoid tumors at one extreme to poorly differentiated round cell (poorly differentiated myxoid) tumors at the other. Pleomorphic liposarcomas are rare, poorly characterized tumors, many of which resemble undifferentiated pleomorphic sarcoma, except for the presence of pleomorphic lipoblasts. Finally, a small number of liposarcomas exhibit unusual features or combine patterns not accounted for in the previous classification (liposarcomas of mixed type). These are best individualized and diagnosed as liposarcomas of mixed or unclassifiable type, recognizing that the number of such lesions is dwindling because of the ability of molecular testing to assign them to a category.

Certain generalizations should be kept in mind when considering the diagnosis of liposarcoma. First, most liposarcomas occur in deep soft tissue, in contrast to lipomas, which occur in superficial soft tissue. This implies that subcutaneous ALN/WDL are rare and that the diagnosis should be made only after the more common mimics (e.g., spindle cell lipoma, pleomorphic lipoma, chondroid lipoma, cellular forms of angiolipoma) are excluded from the differential diagnosis. Second, there is little, if any, evidence that lipomas undergo malignant transformation to liposarcomas, an axiom that derives strong support from the marked difference in location of lipomas and liposarcomas. In reality, most lesions interpreted as malignant transformation of a lipoma are liposarcomas in which inadequate sampling led to an underdiagnosis of malignancy in the original material. Third, liposarcomas

TABLE 15-1 Comparison of Liposarcoma Subtypes

LIPOSARCOMA	AGE (YEARS)	LOCATION	CYTOGENETIC ABNORMALITY	BEHAVIOR
WDL	50-70	Extremity (75%); retroperitoneum	Giant marker + ring chromosome	Local recurrence high; no metastasis 5%-15% dedifferentiate
DL	50-70	Retroperitoneum (75%)	Giant marker + ring + additional abnormalities	High local recurrence; metastasis
MRCL	25-45	Extremity (75%)	t(12;16)	Recurrence + metastasis (determined by round cell component)

DL, dedifferentiated liposarcoma; MRCL, myxoid/round cell liposarcoma; WDL, well-differentiated liposarcoma.

rarely occur in children. Liposarcoma-like lesions in this age group usually represent lipoblastomas, a fetal form of lipoma. Last, liposarcomas, as a group, rarely develop as a postirradiation sarcoma.

There have been great strides in the understanding of liposarcomas during the last several years, largely as a result of cytogenetic studies. The reciprocal translocation between chromosomes 12 and 16, which characterizes most myxoid-round cell liposarcomas, results in the expression of a number of fusion transcripts, which appear to play a direct role in oncogenesis. The large group of ALN/WDL, on the other hand, has an entirely different abnormality in the form of giant and ring chromosomes, derived, at least in part, from chromosome 12, resulting in the amplification of a number of genes (e.g., *MDM2, CDK4*) that represent a recurring motif in a number of mesenchymal tumors.

CRITERIA AND IMPORTANCE OF LIPOBLASTS

Traditionally, great emphasis has been placed on the identification of lipoblasts for diagnosing liposarcoma. Although it is certainly an appropriate task for pathologists to search for these cells in some situations, their importance in other situations has been overemphasized. For example, sclerosing ALN/WDL usually have few lipoblasts. In these cases, the overall pattern and cellular components become more important determinants when making the diagnosis. On the other hand, imprecise criteria for the recognition of lipoblasts often lead to an erroneous diagnosis of liposarcoma.

Defined in the context of liposarcoma, the lipoblast is a neoplastic cell that, to some extent, recapitulates the differentiation cascade of normal fat. The earliest cells arise as pericapillary adventitial cells that closely resemble fibroblasts. These spindled cells, endowed with ample endoplasmic reticulum, slowly acquire fat droplets first at the poles of the cell and later throughout the cytoplasm. As fat accumulates in the cytoplasm, the cell loses its endoplasmic reticulum and assumes a round shape. Gradually, the nucleus becomes indented and pushed to one side of the cell. A similar range of changes can be identified in lipoblasts of some liposarcomas, notably the myxoid/round cell type (Fig. 15-1). In addition, pleomorphic cells with the features of lipoblasts can be identified in ALN/WDL and pleomorphic liposarcomas

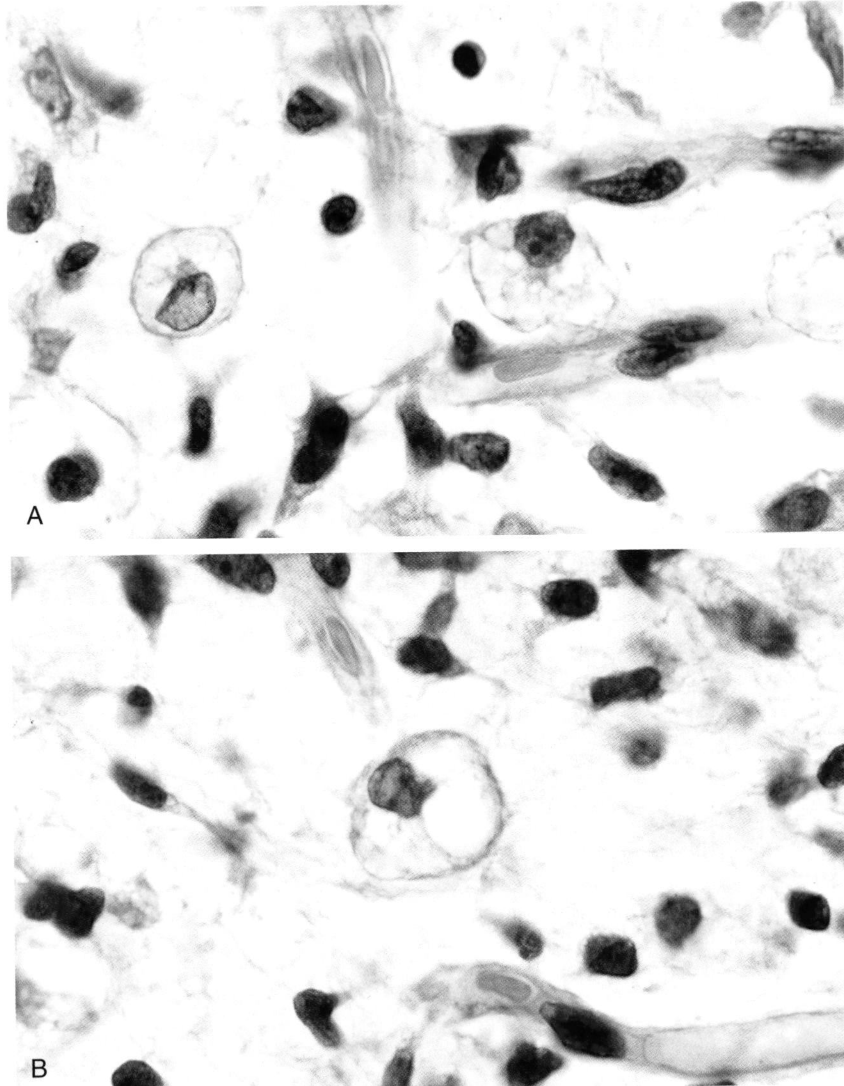

FIGURE 15-1. Developing lipoblasts from a myxoid liposarcoma, at an early stage of differentiation (A) with fine vacuoles, an intermediate stage (B, C), and a late stage (D) resembling mature white fat. *Continued*

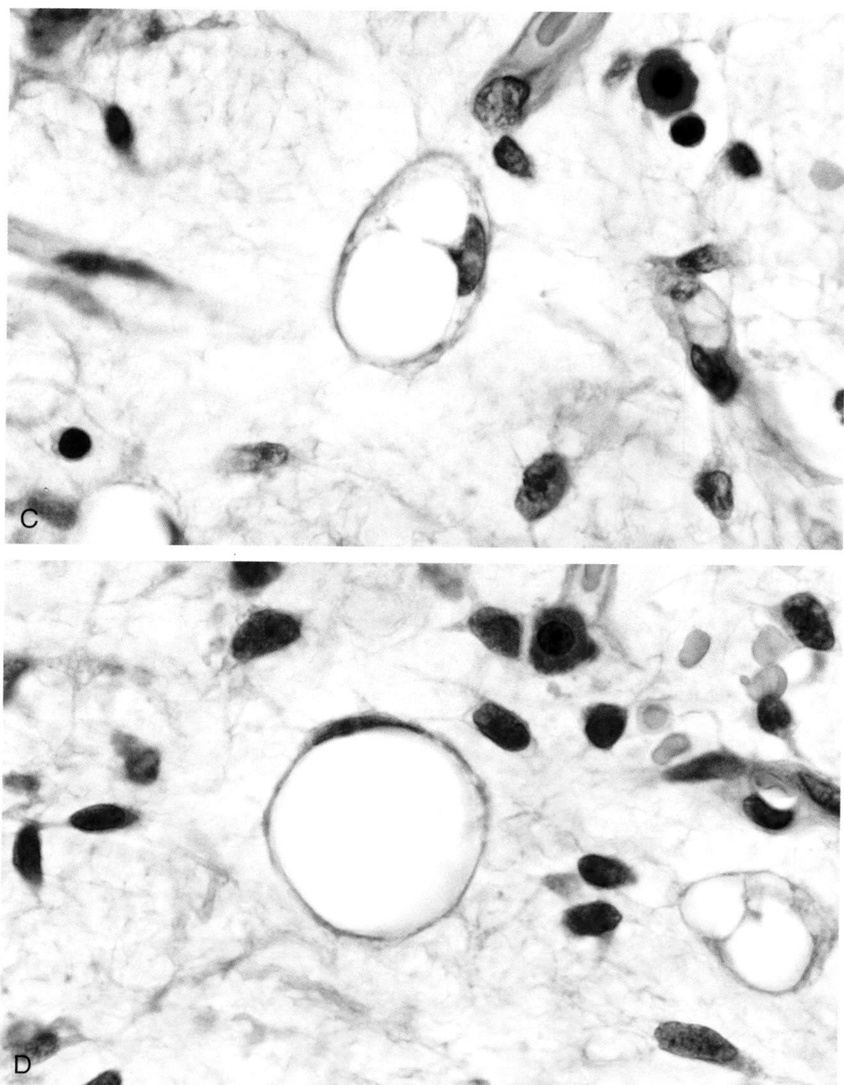

FIGURE 15-1, cont'd

(Fig. 15-2), but these cells have no equivalent in the differentiation sequence of normal fat. The task for the pathologist is to decide the point in the differentiation scheme at which the cell becomes sufficiently diagnostic to warrant the designation *lipoblast*.

Criteria that have proved useful for identifying *diagnostic* lipoblasts include the following: (1) a hyperchromatic indented or sharply scalloped nucleus; (2) lipid-rich (neutral fat) droplets in the cytoplasm; and (3) an appropriate histologic background. The importance of the last criterion cannot be overemphasized because lipoblast-like cells may be seen in a variety of conditions, and failure to take into consideration the overall appearance of a lesion can lead to an erroneous diagnosis of liposarcoma. For example, lipomas with fat necrosis (Fig. 15-3); fat with atrophic changes (Fig. 15-4); hibernomatous change in lipomas (Fig. 15-5); foreign body reaction to silicone (Fig. 15-6); nonspecific accumulation of intracytoplasmic stromal mucin (Fig. 15-7); fixation artifact (Fig. 15-8); and signet ring melanoma, carcinoma, and lymphoma (Fig. 15-9) all have cells that, to some extent, resemble lipoblasts. In each instance, other features indicate that the diagnosis of liposarcoma is not appropriate. Silicone reactions, for example, exhibit numerous multivacuolated histiocytes that fulfill some of the criteria of lipoblasts, yet the histologic background of foreign body giant cells and inflammation should alert the pathologist that the lesion is not a liposarcoma.

ATYPICAL LIPOMATOUS NEOPLASM (ALN)/ WELL-DIFFERENTIATED LIPOSARCOMA (WDL)

Clinical Findings

ALN/WDL liposarcoma, accounting for 30% to 40% of all liposarcomas,[4] is the most common form of liposarcoma encountered in late adult life. It reaches a peak incidence during the sixth and seventh decades of life. Men and women are equally affected, although at certain sites (e.g., groin) there

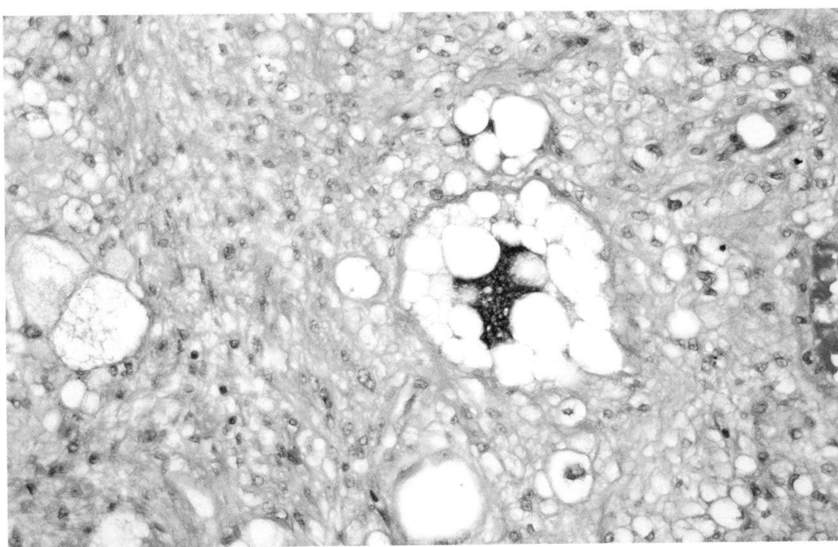

FIGURE 15-2. Pleomorphic lipoblast from a pleomorphic liposarcoma.

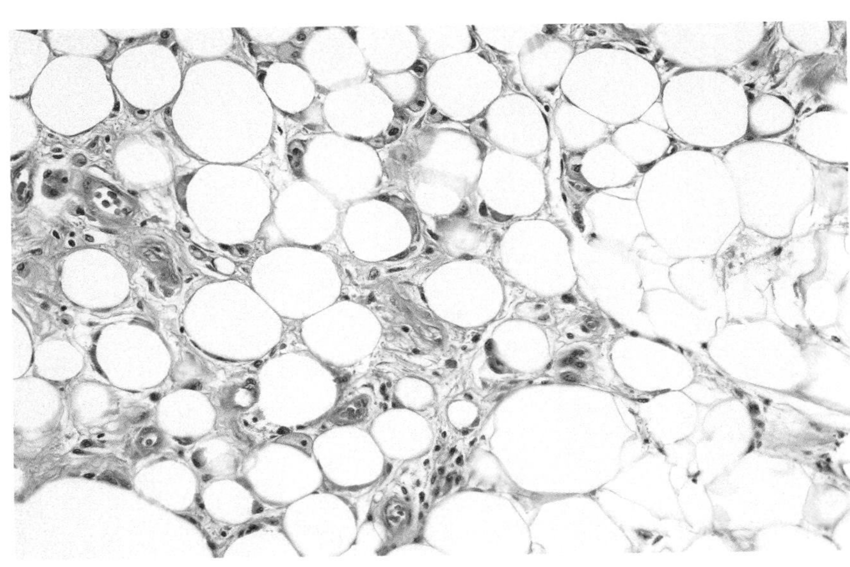

FIGURE 15-3. Fat necrosis in a lipoma. Scattered macrophages may be confused with atypical stromal cells of liposarcoma.

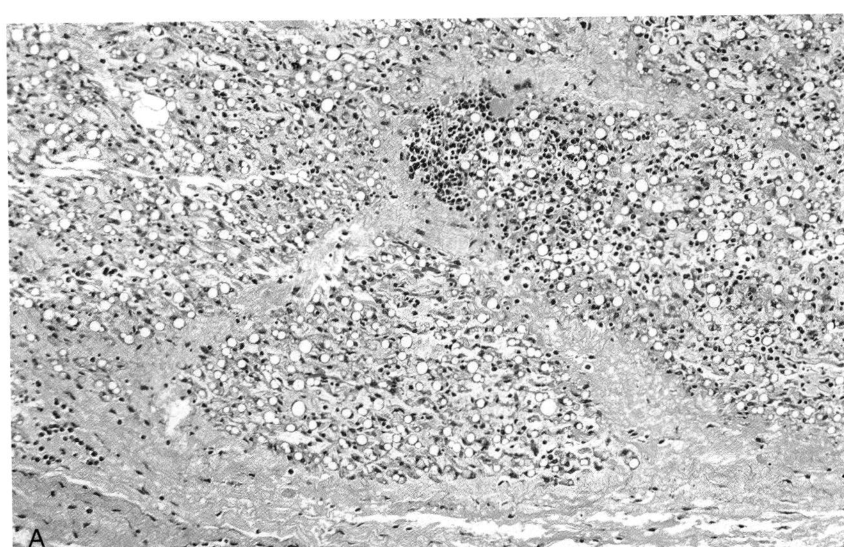

FIGURE 15-4. Atrophic fat occurring with malnutrition. Cells are arranged in lobules (A) and are uniformly small with lipofuscin pigment in the cytoplasm (B). *Continued*

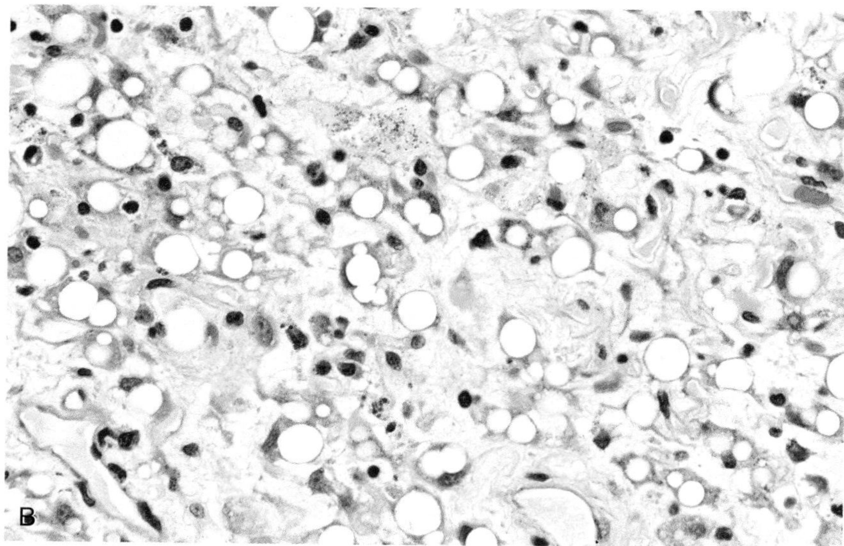

FIGURE 15-4, cont'd

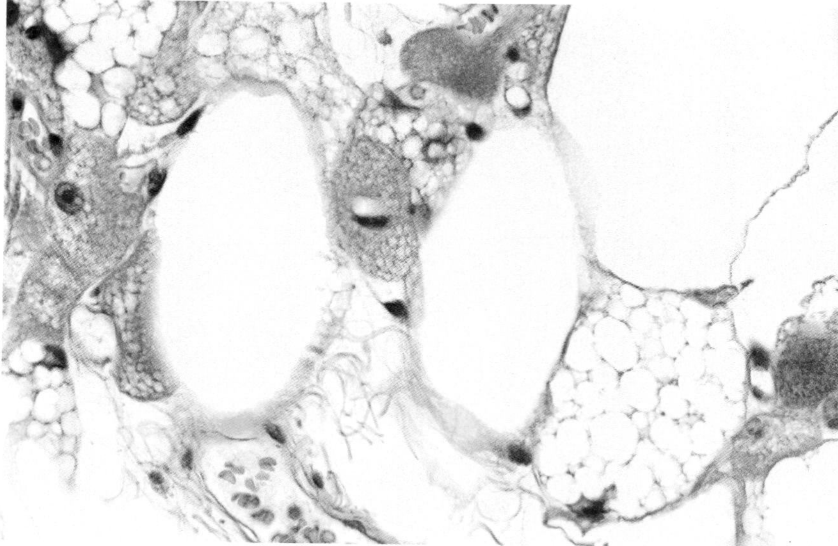

FIGURE 15-5. Finely vacuolated brown fat cells in a lipoma with hibernomatous changes mimicking lipoblasts.

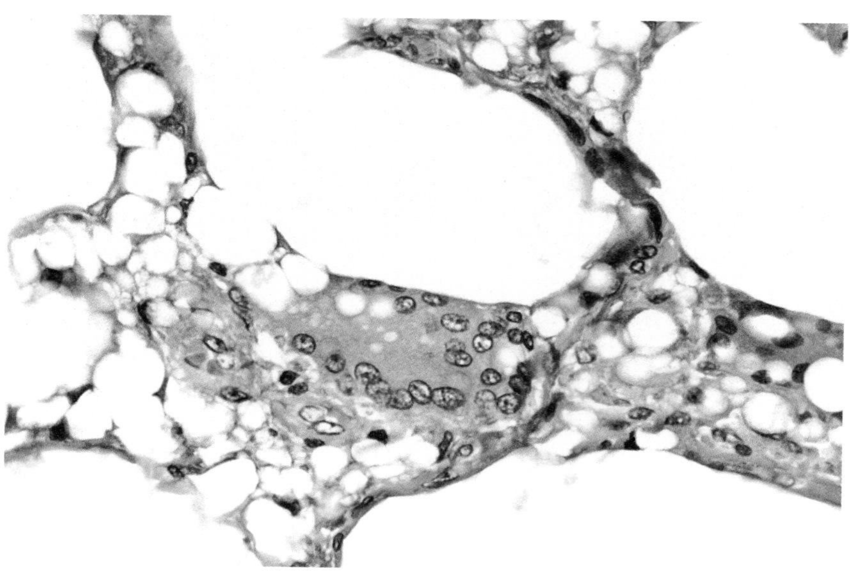

FIGURE 15-6. Silicone granuloma with multivacuolated histiocytes resembling lipoblasts.

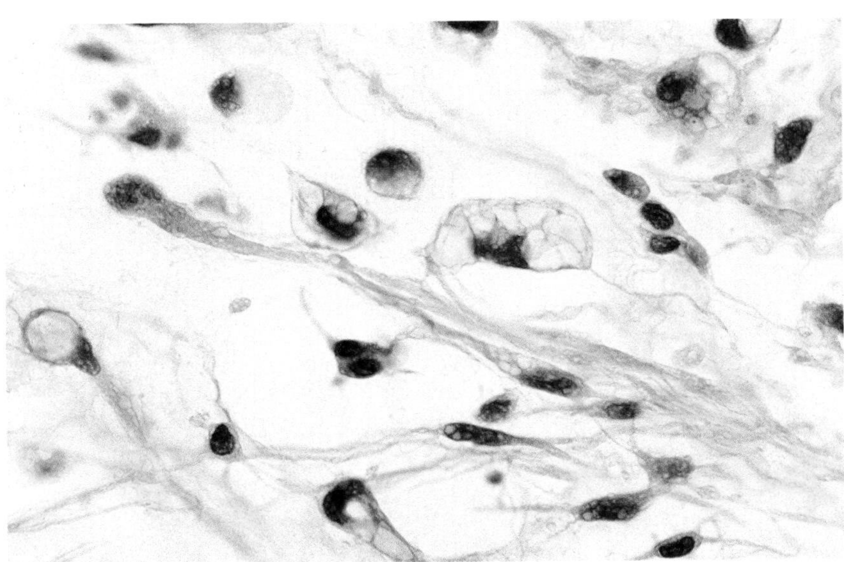

FIGURE 15-7. Cells of a myxoid undifferentiated pleomorphic sarcoma distended with hyaluronic acid. These cells are commonly misidentified as lipoblasts.

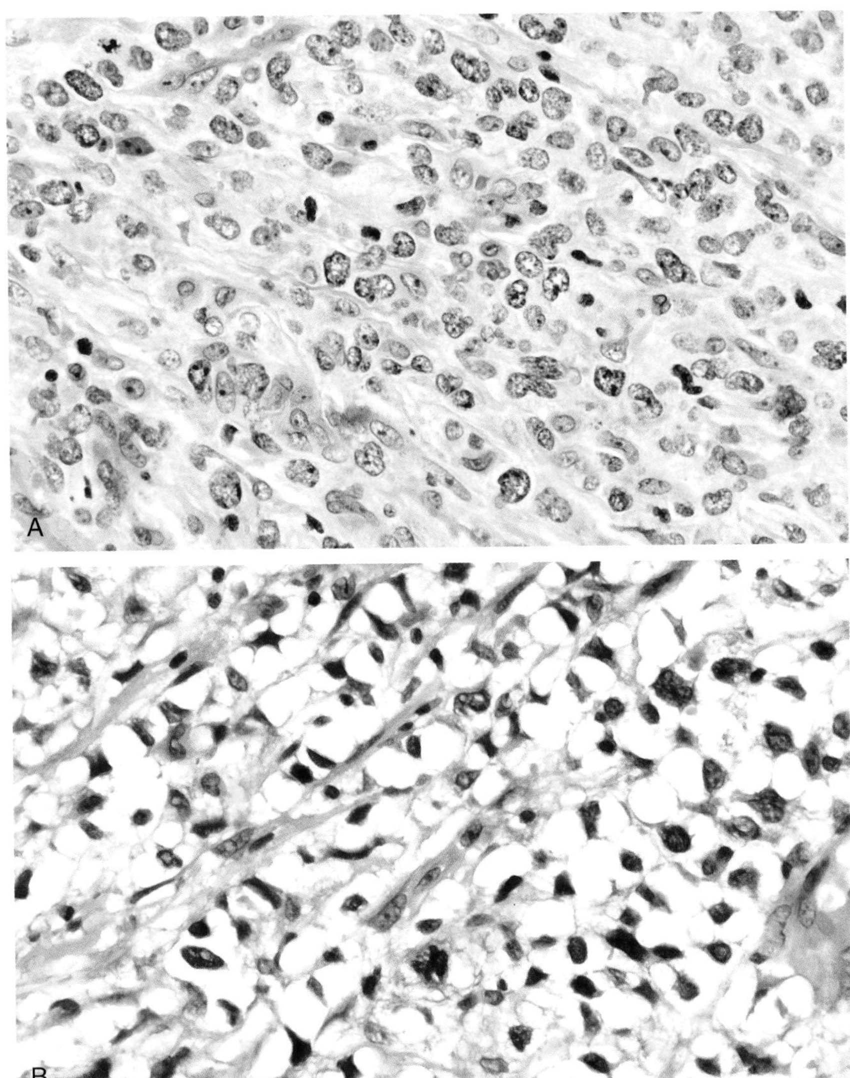

FIGURE 15-8. Large-cell lymphoma (A) with poorly fixed areas (B) in which the retraction artifact led to an erroneous diagnosis of liposarcoma.

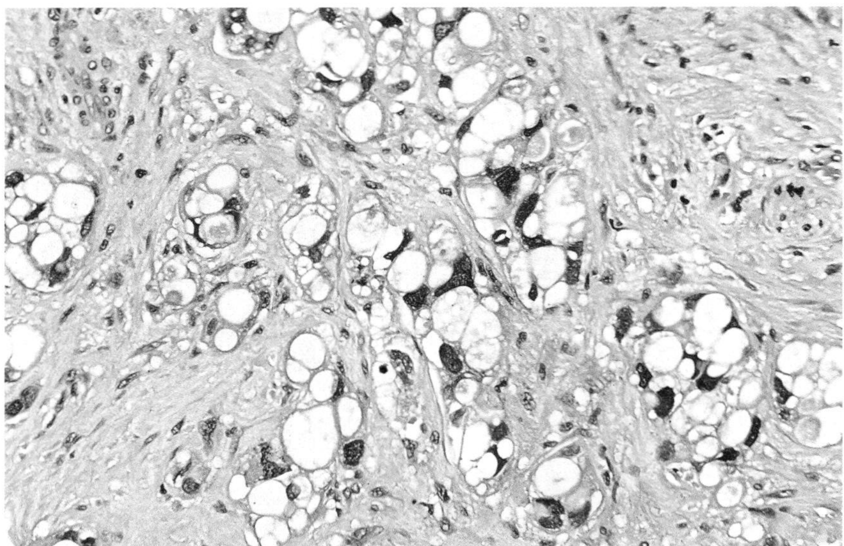

FIGURE 15-9. Adenocarcinoma arising in Barrett's mucosa showing a treatment effect with pseudolipoblasts.

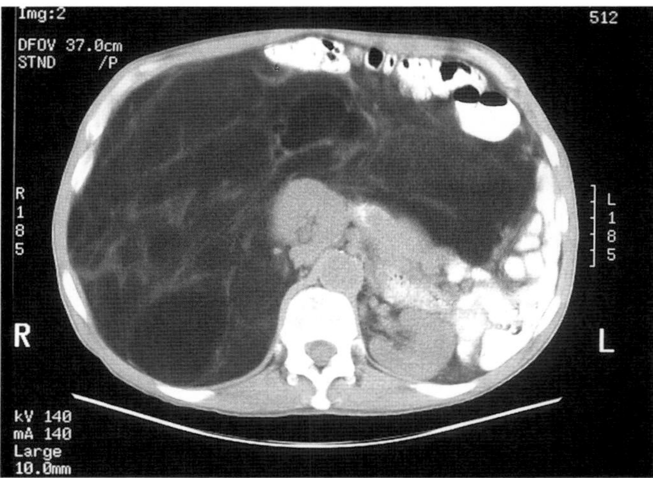

FIGURE 15-10. Computer tomography (CT) scan of ALN/WDL of the abdominal cavity and retroperitoneum. The mass, with a low attenuation value, replaces abdominal contents.

appears to be a predilection for men. In the collective experience of the Armed Forces Institute of Pathology (also known as AFIP) and the Mayo Clinic, 75% of cases developed in the deep muscles of the extremities and 20% in the retroperitoneum, with the remainder divided between the groin, spermatic cord, and miscellaneous sites.[5,6] Rarely do these tumors develop in the subcutis or in miscellaneous parenchymal sites.

Symptoms related to these tumors are dependent on the anatomic site. Those in the extremities develop as slowly growing masses that are present months or even several years before the patient seeks medical attention, whereas those in the retroperitoneum are associated with the usual symptoms of an intra-abdominal mass. In Computed tomography (CT), because ALN/WDL contain a significant component of mature fat, they present as fat density masses,[7-9] with mottled or streaky zones of higher density corresponding to the fibrous or sclerotic zones. They also tend to have less-well-defined borders than lipomas (Fig. 15-10).

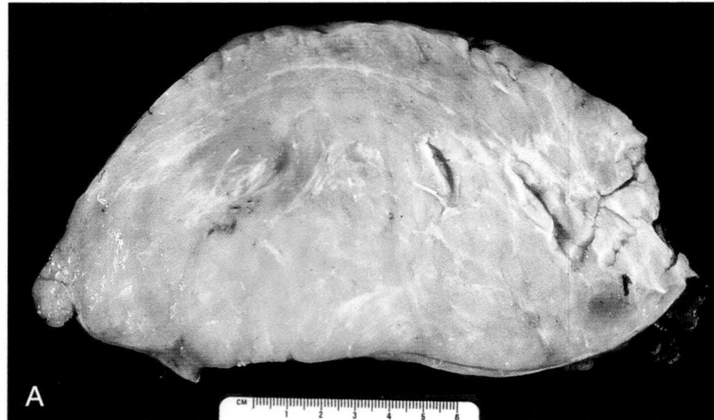

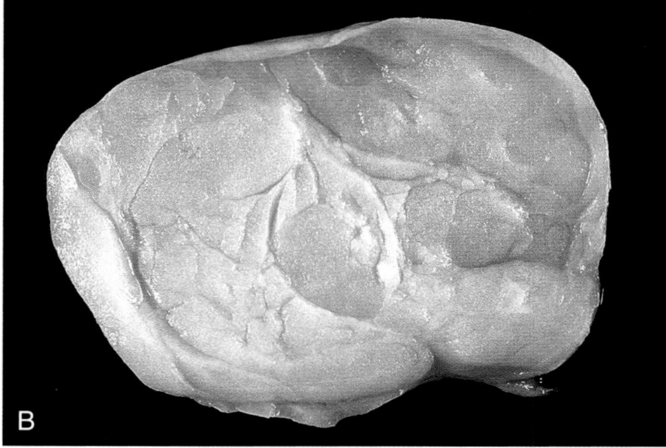

FIGURE 15-11. ALN/WDL closely resembling normal fat, except for fibrous bands (A). Others have a more gelatinous appearance (B).

Gross and Microscopic Features

Grossly, ALN/WDL are large multilobular lesions that range in color from deep yellow to ivory (Fig. 15-11). Many could be mistaken for a lipoma, except for their extremely large size

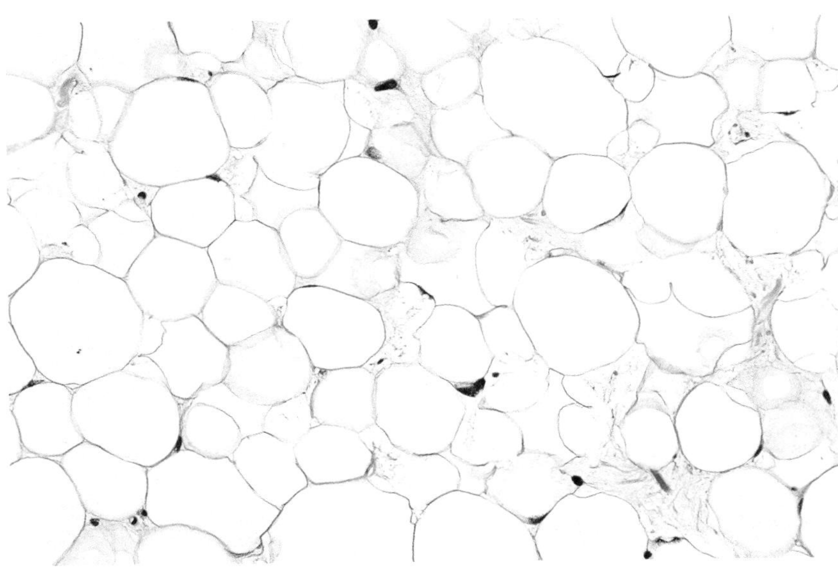

FIGURE 15-12. Well-differentiated (lipoma-like) liposarcoma showing only a rare atypical stromal cell amid a mature lipomatous backdrop.

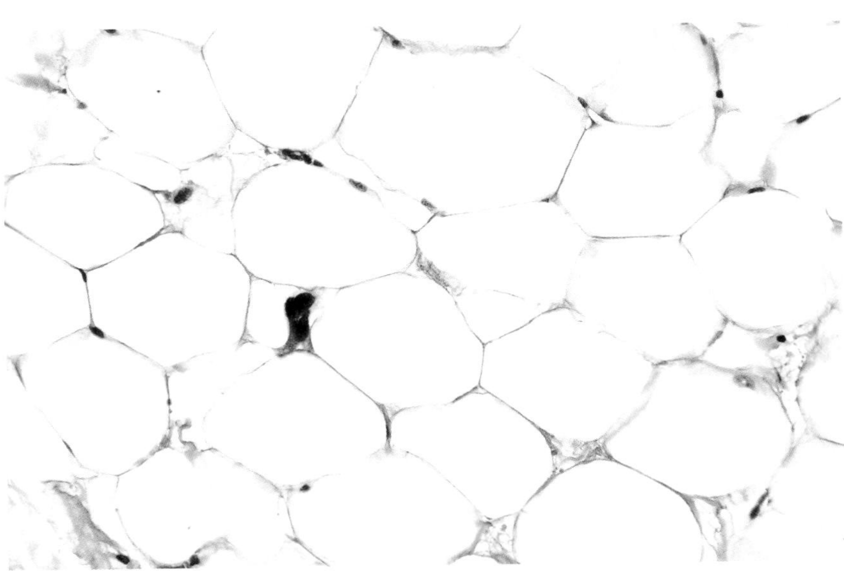

FIGURE 15-13. Atypical stromal cell in an ALN/WDL illustrating nuclear hyperchromatism.

and their tendency to have fibrous bands, gelatinous zones, or punctate hemorrhage.

ALN/WDL have traditionally been divided into three subtypes: (1) lipoma-like; (2) sclerosing; and (3) inflammatory. Because many ALN/WDL combine features of both lipoma-like and sclerosing subtypes, the distinction between these two types is often arbitrary and of limited practical importance. These lesions are rarely subclassified in daily practice, although the terms serve to draw attention to the range of appearances that these tumors may assume. In the typical lipoma-like ALN/WDL, the tumor consists predominantly of mature fat with a variable number of spindled cells with hyperchromatic nuclei and multivacuolated lipoblasts (Figs. 15-12 to 15-15). In some cases, these atypical spindled cells are numerous, whereas, in other cases, the cells are so rare as to require extensive sampling of the tissue. Sclerosing forms of ALN/WDL, prevailing in the groin and retroperitoneum, have dense fibrotic zones alternating with mature adipocytes (Figs. 15-16 to 15-19). In some cases, the fibrotic zones consist of trabeculae intersecting fat, and, in others, the fibrous areas consist of broad sheets (see Figs. 15-17 and 15-19). The fibrotic areas contain collagen fibrils of varying thickness in which are embedded scattered spindled and multipolar stromal cells with hyperchromatic nuclei. Similar cells may also be present between the mature adipocytes. Although lipoblasts may be present, they are usually rare. Therefore, the diagnosis for this pattern of liposarcoma is more dependent on the identification of stromal cells with a requisite degree of atypia than on the identification of diagnostic lipoblasts. The inflammatory form of ALN/WDL occurs almost exclusively in the retroperitoneum and consists of a dense lymphocytic or plasmacytic infiltrate superimposed on a lipoma-like or sclerosing form of ALN/WDL (Fig. 15-20).[10] Because of the intense inflammatory infiltrate, these tumors may be confused with lipogranulomatous inflammation.

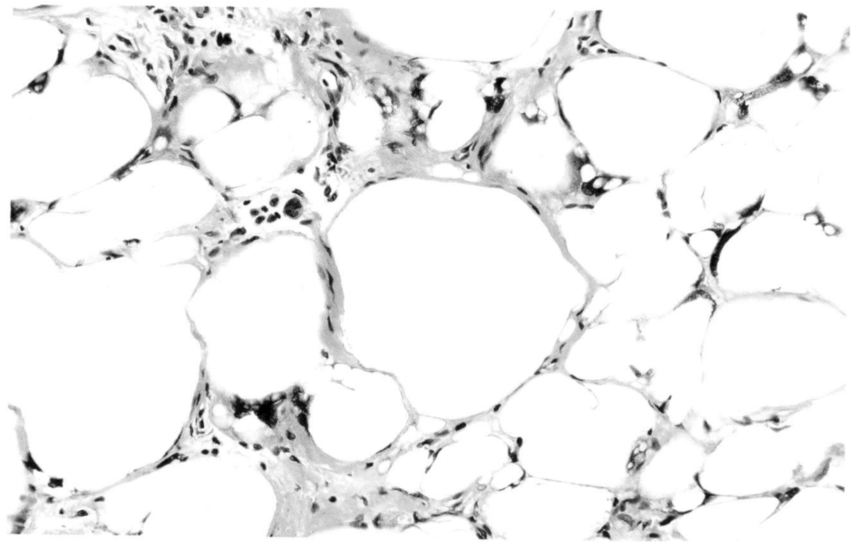

FIGURE 15-14. ALN/WDL with a larger number of atypical stromal cells and lipoblasts than in Figure 15-13.

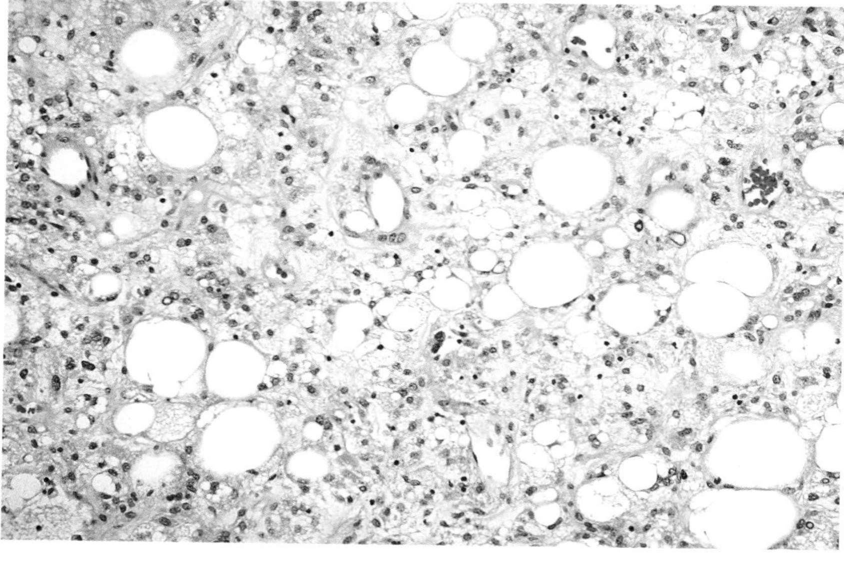

FIGURE 15-15. Well-differentiated (lipoma-like) liposarcoma with numerous lipoblasts.

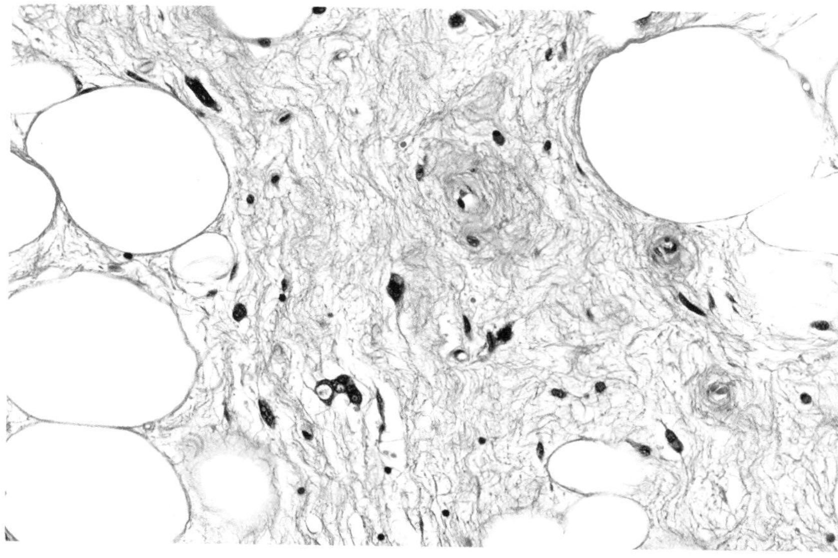

FIGURE 15-16. Sclerosing ALN/WDL.

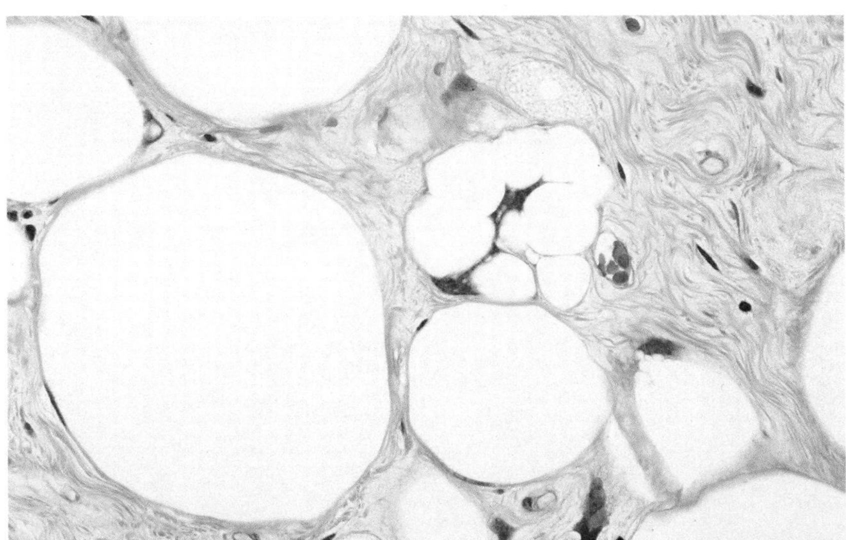

FIGURE 15-17. Well-differentiated (sclerosing) liposarcoma showing sheet-like areas of collagen and fat. Note the multivacuolated lipoblast in this lesion. These cells are typically rare.

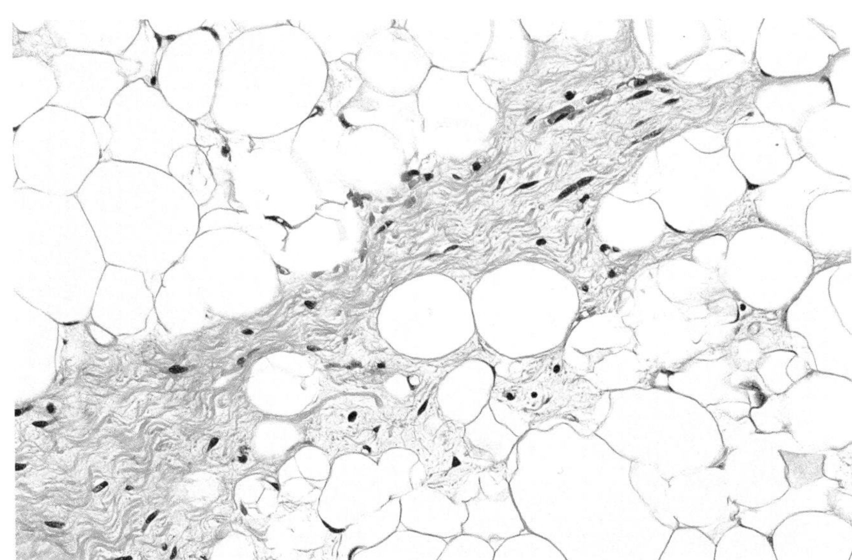

FIGURE 15-18. Well-differentiated (sclerosing) liposarcoma with fibrous bands containing atypical cells.

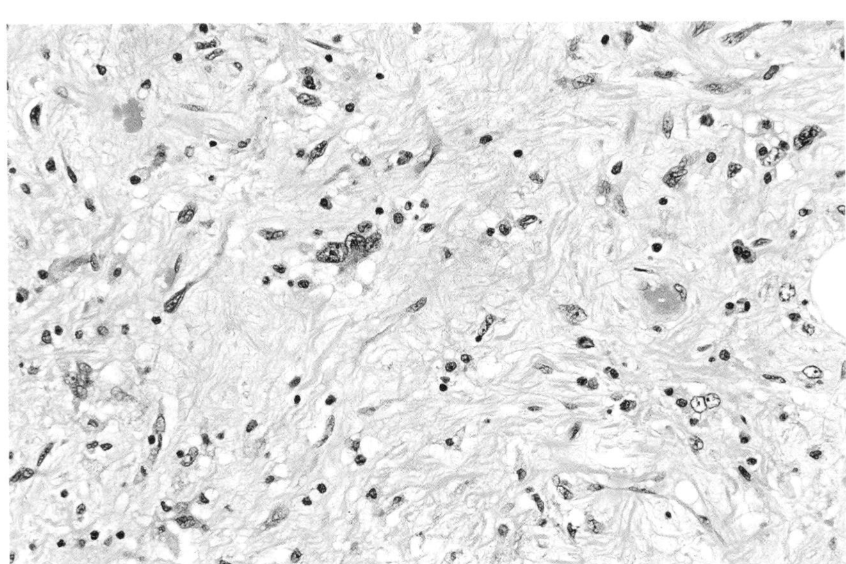

FIGURE 15-19. Nonlipogenic zone in a well-differentiated (sclerosing) liposarcoma. Note that the cellularity is far less than in nonlipogenic zones of dedifferentiated liposarcoma. Small-needle biopsies from these areas can lead to the erroneous conclusion that the tumor is not a liposarcoma.

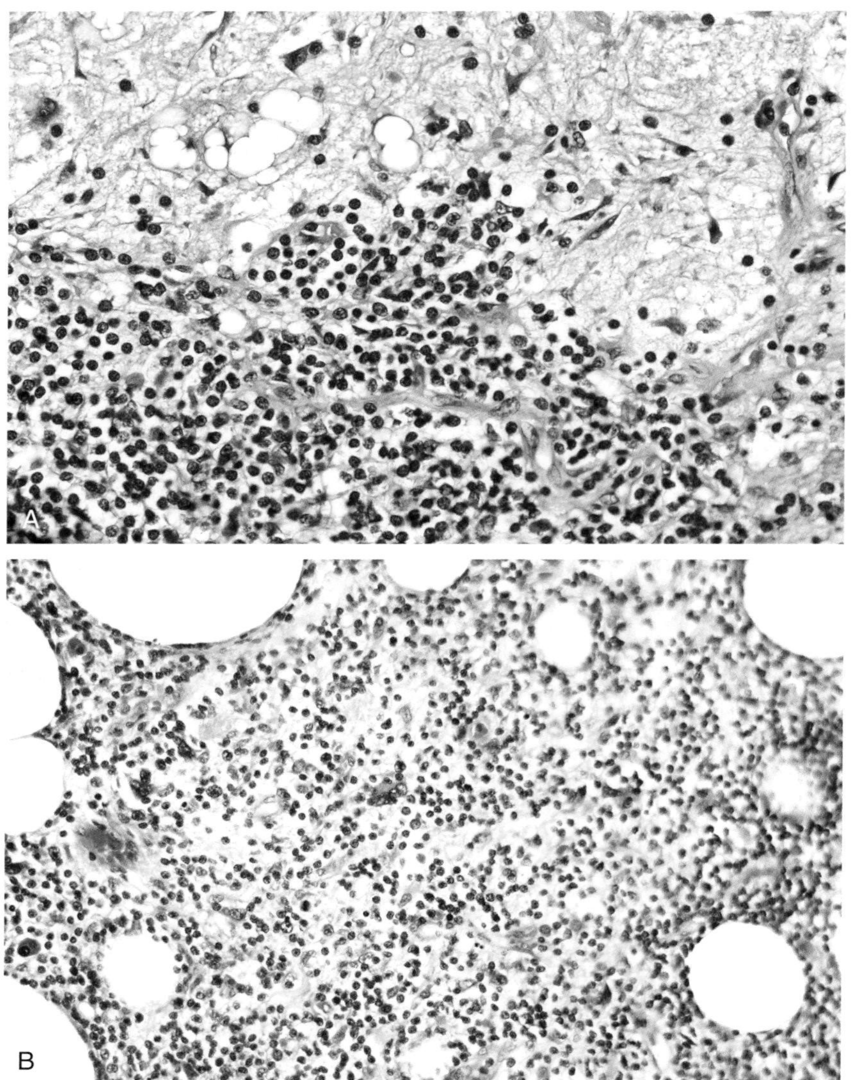

FIGURE 15-20. ALN/WDL of the inflammatory type with a dense lymphocytic infiltrate (A) and areas of lipoblastic differentiation (B).

ALN/WDL infrequently display areas of relatively mature smooth muscle (Figs. 15-21 and 15-22).[11-16] These so-called *lipoleiomyosarcomas* are dual-lineage sarcomas in which both the lipomatous and smooth muscle components are low grade. Biologically, they have a behavior identical to ALN/WDL, including the ability to dedifferentiate[15] and are recognized by areas of ALN/WDL blending with fascicles, nodules, or broad expanses of smooth muscle tissue having mild to moderate nuclear atypia and low levels of mitotic activity. In some cases, the smooth muscle appears to extend out from the walls of large vessels, which similarly contain atypical smooth muscle cells (see Fig. 15-22). The amount of smooth muscle varies considerably from case to case, with some tumors showing only occasional foci and others broad expanses. A less common association is ALN/WDL with low-grade osteosarcoma-like areas.[17] These tumors, occurring primarily in the retroperitoneum, consist of a lipomatous component, which usually predominates and blends with areas resembling parosteal or low-grade intramedullary osteosarcoma. These areas are characterized by relatively mature bone, with or without osteoblastic rimming, embedded in a low-grade fibroblastic backdrop. In a few cases, high-grade osteosarcoma coexists in the low-grade areas. In the few cases studied, MDM2 and CDK4 were demonstrated immunohistochemically in both the lipomatous and osteosarcomatous components.

Occasionally, ALN/WDL have a predominantly myxoid appearance, a phenomenon that has led to the conjecture that these tumors represent either a variant of myxoid liposarcoma or a mixed type of liposarcoma. Several studies have shown that these tumors lack the *DDIT3-FUS* fusion and, therefore, are unrelated to myxoid liposarcoma.[18,19]

Differential Diagnosis

Various neoplastic and non-neoplastic lesions enter the differential diagnosis of ALN/WDL (Box 15-1). For most of these conditions, none of the available histochemical or immunohistochemical stains is useful. Rather, careful sampling of the material and thin, well-stained hematoxylin and eosin

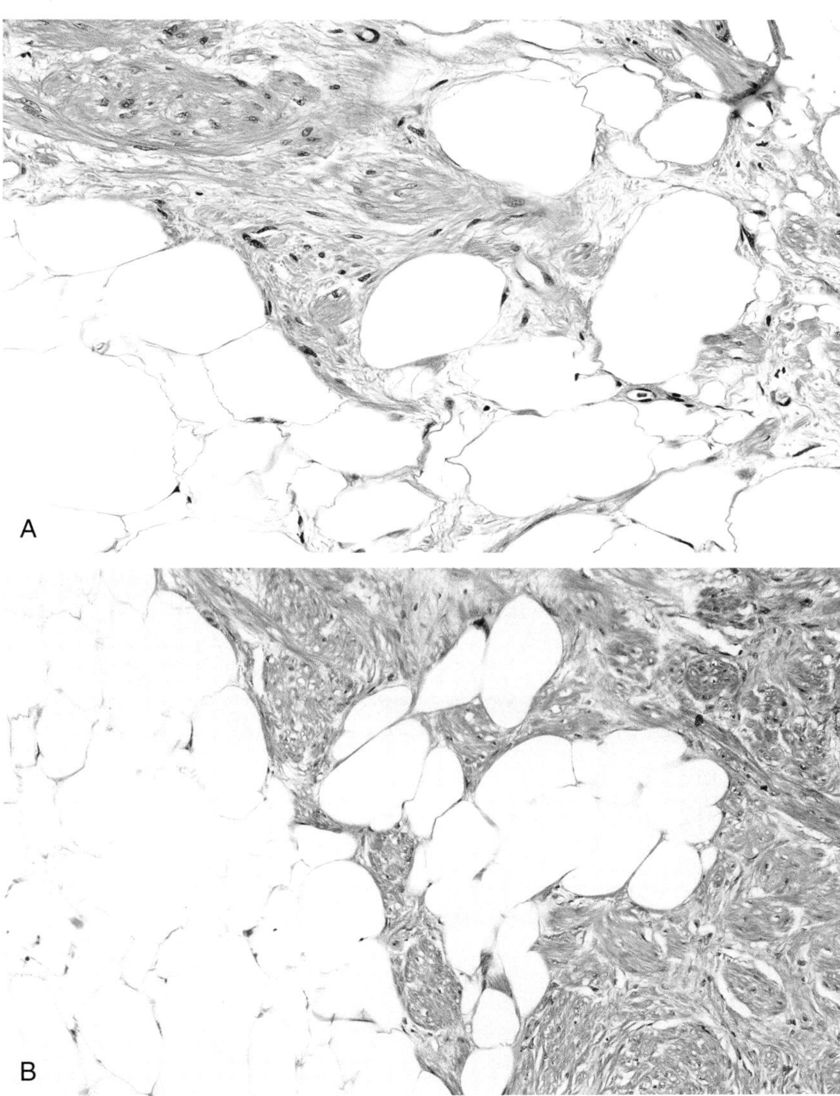

FIGURE 15-21. ALN/WDL with smooth muscle differentiation (lipoleiomyosarcoma) (A) and stained with Masson trichrome stain (B).

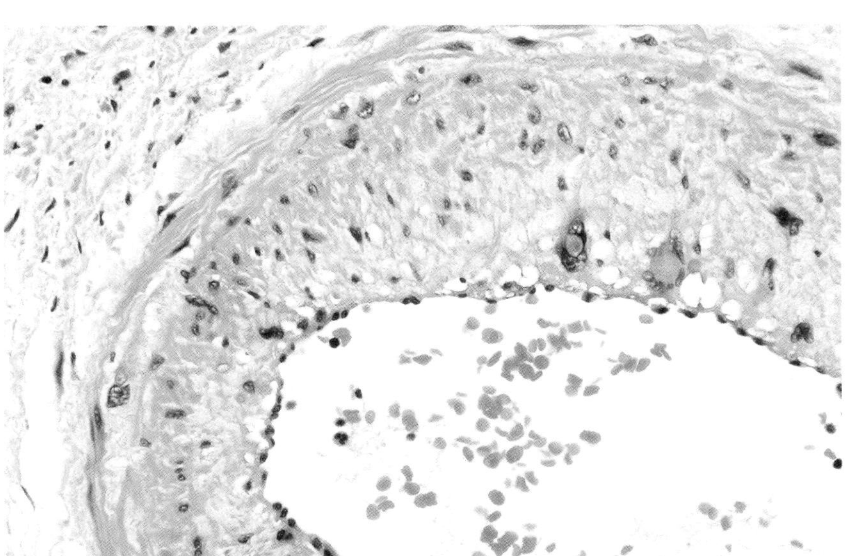

FIGURE 15-22. Lipoleiomyosarcoma showing atypia in a vessel wall.

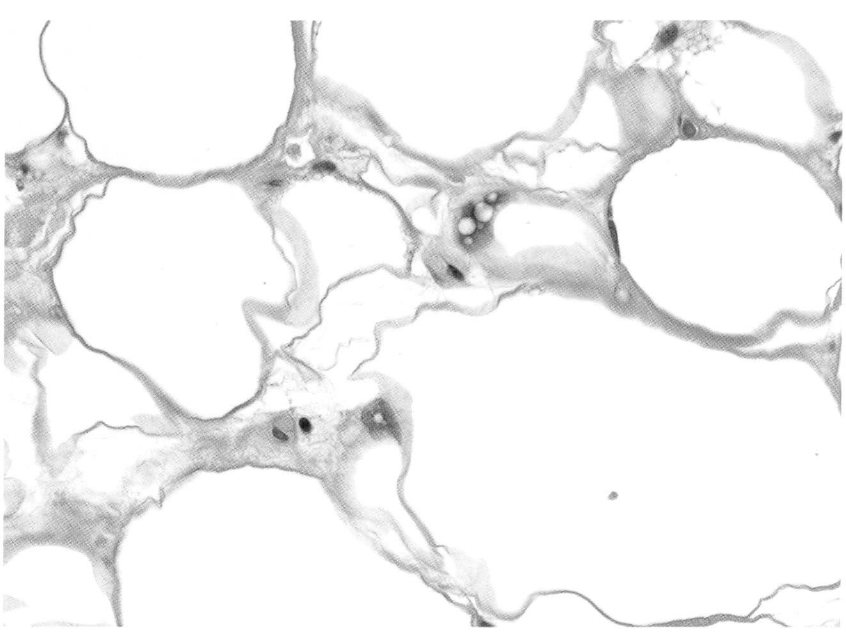

FIGURE 15-23. Nuclear vacuoles (*Lochkern*) in normal fat.

BOX 15-1 Lesions Simulating ALN/WDL

Lipoma with fat necrosis
Lipoma with *Lochkern*
Atrophy of fat
Silicone reaction
Diffuse lipomatosis
Spindle cell lipoma/pleomorphic lipoma
Myolipoma
Cellular angiolipoma
Angiomyolipoma
Lipomatous hemangiopericytoma/solitary fibrous tumor

sections comprise the mainstay of accurate diagnosis. Lipid stains, although obviously positive in ALN/WDL, also disclose lipid-positive deposits in the vast panorama of reactive lesions in fat and a variety of tumors.

Normal Fat with Lochkern. Normal white fat consists of spherical cells containing one large lipid vacuole that displaces the thin oval nucleus to one side. On routine sections, the nucleus of most fat cells is barely perceptible. From time to time, a section grazes an adipocyte nucleus so that it is viewed en face, displaying its characteristic central vacuole, termed *Lochkern* (German: "hole in the nucleus") (Fig. 15-23). *Lochkern* is viewed more frequently in thick sections and, therefore, are sometimes misinterpreted as evidence of lipoblastic differentiation and, therefore, a liposarcoma.

Fat necrosis. In areas of fat necrosis, finely granular or vacuolated macrophages are located in the vicinity of damaged fat characterized by diminished cell size, dropout of adipocytes, and chronic inflammation (see Fig. 15-3). Unlike lipoblasts, macrophages are of uniform size and have small, evenly dispersed vacuoles that do not indent the nucleus. The nucleus has a rounded shape with delicate staining. In thick sections, the nuclei of macrophages may overlap one another, giving the impression of hyperchromatism, which typifies the atypical stromal cells in ALN/WDL. It is important when making such distinctions to have suitably thin histologic sections.

Atrophy of fat. Starvation, malnutrition, and local trauma result in atrophy of fat. Atrophy is accompanied by a loss of intracellular lipid such that the cell shrinks dramatically and assumes an epithelioid shape (see Fig. 15-4). With loss of lipid, the nuclei become more prominent, and the cells superficially resemble lipoblasts. Important observations include cells that appear to be of uniform size and maintain their arrangement in lobules. With extreme atrophy, the cells may contain lipofuscin. Such changes are particularly noticeable in subcutaneous tissue and omentum.

Localized massive lymphedema. Massive forms of lymphedema restricted to a portion of the body may be confused clinically and histologically with ALN/WDL.[20] These lesions develop in morbidly obese individuals and appear to be the result of lymphedema secondary to chronic dependency of a fatty panniculus. Not surprisingly, these lesions develop in the proximal extremities and may be aggravated by underlying factors, such as lymphadenectomy. Grossly and microscopically, the lesions exhibit the changes of lymphedema, including thickening of overlying skin, dermal fibrosis, ectasia and proliferation of lymphatics with focal cysts, and expansion of connective tissue septa (Fig. 15-24). A misdiagnosis of liposarcoma is attributable to the expanded connective tissue septa that are believed to be part of a sclerosing liposarcoma. The septa contain mild to moderately atypical fibroblasts and delicate collagen fibrils separated by edema. In addition, there is often striking vascular proliferation at the interface between the expanded connective tissue septa and lobules of fat.

Silicone reaction. Injection of silicone for various therapeutic and cosmetic purposes results in sheets of massively distended multivacuolated histiocytes that are disarming replicas of lipoblasts (see Fig. 15-6). Lipoblasts of such quality and number are rarely encountered in true liposarcomas. Silicone reactions are also accompanied by a modest inflammatory and

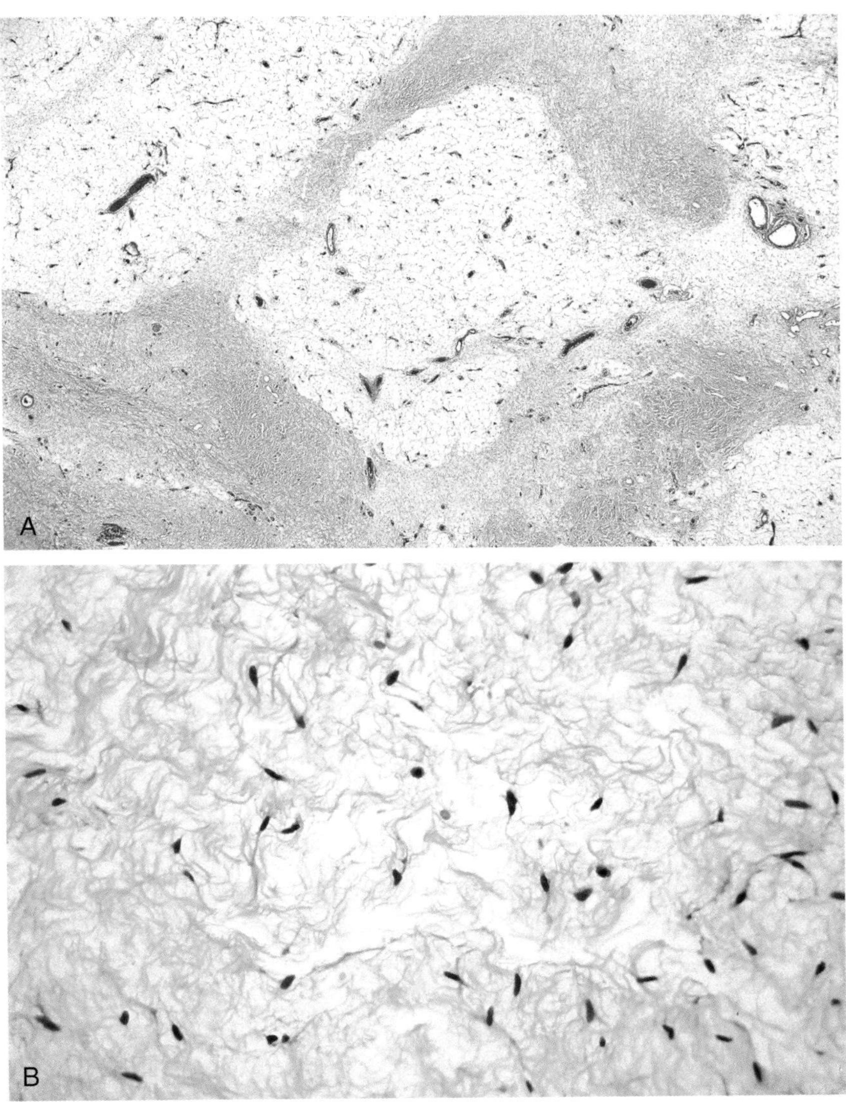

FIGURE 15-24. Changes of lymphedema that may mimic an ALN/WDL. Connective tissue septa are expanded (A), with mildly atypical fibroblasts in the septa (B).

giant cell reaction and a large cyst with eosinophilic borders. Most silicone reactions in clinical practice are encountered around silicone breast implants but, occasionally, are seen on the face and in the abdomen. Free silicone can also migrate under gravitational effect and, therefore, is found at sites distant from the original introduction site.

Intramuscular lipoma with atrophic muscle. Infrequently, atrophic skeletal muscle fibers are seen in intramuscular lipomas (Fig. 15-25). When these collections retain a clustered arrangement and have identifiable eosinophilic cytoplasm, this phenomenon is easily recognized. Isolated degenerating myofibers with barely perceptible cytoplasm understandably can be misidentified as atypical stromal cells of ALN/WDL. Positive identification can be accomplished with desmin immunostains.

Herniated orbital fat. Prolapse of subconjunctival intraconal fat is a rare cause of an intraorbital mass.[21] Herniated orbital fat, unlike normal orbital fat, contains floret-type giant cells, a feature that often leads to a mistaken diagnosis of liposarcoma (Fig. 15-26). This condition develops in adults in the region of the superotemporal quadrant of the orbit or the lateral canthus below the lacrimal gland. The lesion can be unilateral or bilateral.

Cytogenetic and Molecular Findings

ALN/WDL are characterized by giant marker and ring chromosomes,[4] sometimes as a sole finding or, occasionally, in association with other numerical or structural alterations.[3] The giant marker and ring chromosomes contain amplified sequences of 12q13-15, the site of several genes (e.g., *MDM2, GLI, SAS, CDK4,* and *HMGIC*). *MDM2*(12q13-14) and *HMGA2*(12q15), part of the same amplicon, are consistently amplified as a result of this abnormality. *CDK4*, located at 12q13, and *TSPAN31*, located at 12q13-q14, belong to a separate amplicon, which is co-amplified with *MDM2* and *HMGIC* in about 90% of cases. *GLI1* and *DDIT3*(12q13.1-q13.2) are infrequently amplified. Amplification of *MDM2* and *CDK4* results in downstream signaling, the net result of which is to inhibit apoptosis and increase cell proliferation. *MDM2* binds to p53, thereby decreasing apoptosis, whereas

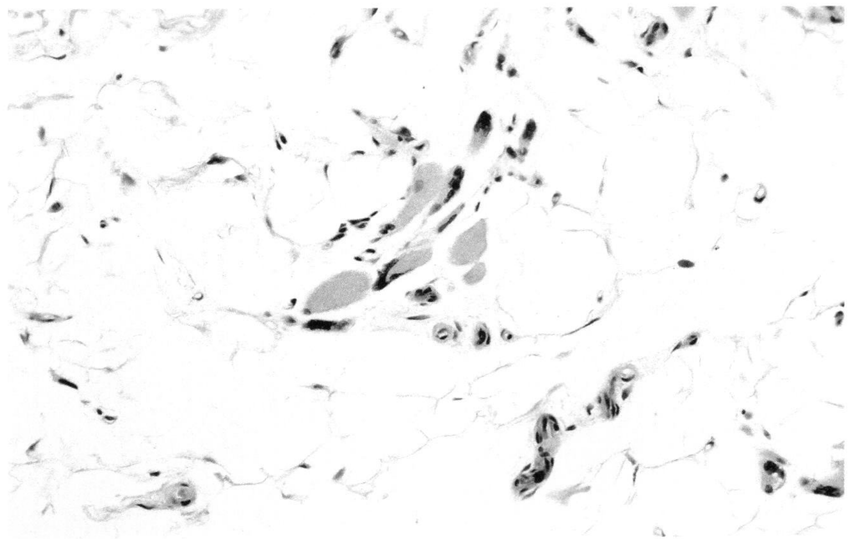

FIGURE 15-25. Atrophic muscle in an intramuscular lipoma. Degenerating myofibers are occasionally mistaken for atypical cells in liposarcomas.

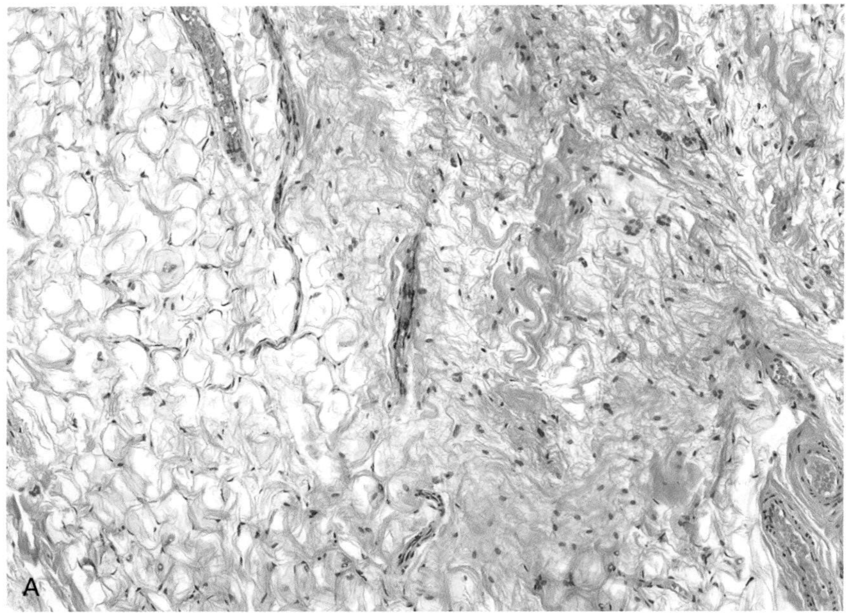

FIGURE 15-26. Herniated orbital fat at low power (A) and floret-type giant cells at high power (B).

CDK4 phosphorylates the *RB1* gene product preventing its interaction with E2F transcription factor allowing the cell cycle to escape the G1-S checkpoint.

The *MDM2*-p53 interaction can potentially be exploited for the purposes of targeted therapy. The nutlins are small molecule antagonists that inhibit the binding of MDM2 to p53, thereby restoring p53 activity and apoptosis. They have been shown to inhibit the growth of *MDM2*-amplified liposarcoma cell lines, but not in those without. Nutlins are currently in clinical trials.[22]

Immunohistochemical and Molecular Diagnosis of ALN/WDL and DL

Immunostaining for *CDK4* and *MDM2* is a reasonable first line tool for separating ALN/WDL from various benign lipomatous lesions.[23,24] Immunoreactivity can be detected within the majority of ALN/WDL and DL, although the percentage varies with the particular study. It is not generally present within deep lipomas. However, a small percentage of spindle cell–pleomorphic lipomas express *MDM2* and *CDK4*.[25,26] In addition, antibodies to CDK4 and MDM2 occasionally stain nuclei of histiocytes within areas of fat necrosis[4] making it imperative that the character of the immunopositive nuclei be evaluated. Nuclear MDM2 and CDK4 can also be detected by immunohistochemistry in a small subset of nonlipomatous sarcomas (e.g., malignant peripheral nerve sheath tumor).

In contrast, *MDM2* amplification evaluated by fluorescence in-situ hybridization (FISH) is a highly sensitive and specific means of diagnosing ALN/WDL[25,27,28] even in needle biopsy material.[29] It is significantly superior to immunostaining, which not only fails to identify all ANL/WDL but also is associated with a small, but definite, false-positive rate. Virtually all ALN/WDL display amplification of MDM2 in both biopsy

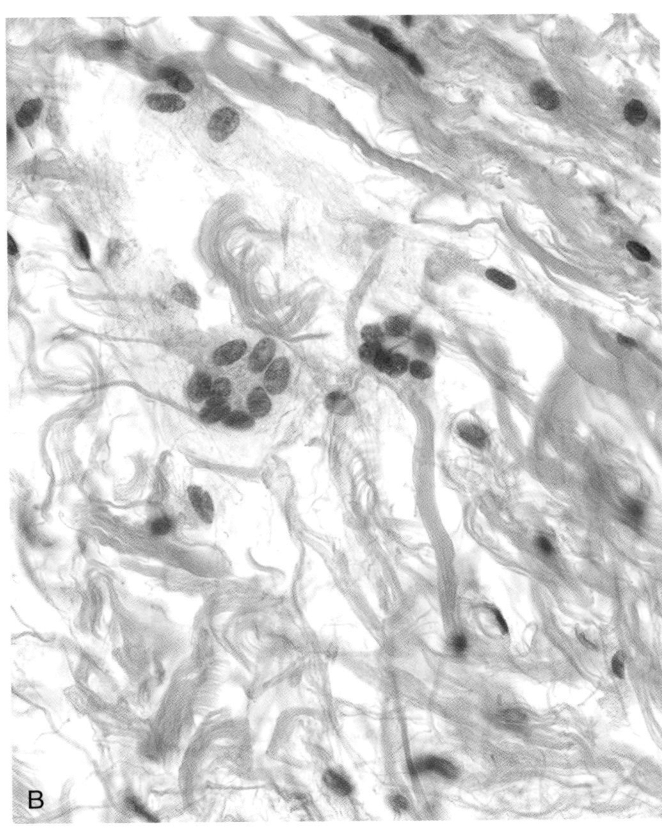

FIGURE 15-26, cont'd

and resection specimens. *MDM2* is not amplified in lipomas, although spindle cell/pleomorphic lipomas may display polysomy of the 12q locus. Because of the exquisite sensitivity and specificity of FISH in the diagnosis of ALN/WDL, it has been endorsed for evaluation of ambiguous, as opposed to obvious, lipomatous lesions. Most often these are tumors in which the degree of atypia falls short of a threshold level for the diagnosis of malignancy. Admittedly, this threshold is different from pathologist to pathologist, although the observation has been made that, as a group, pathologists tend to overestimate the degree of atypia in making the diagnosis of ALN/WDL. The situations in which molecular testing for MDM2 is highly recommended are lipomatous tumors with equivocal cytologic atypia, recurrent lipomas, deep lipomas without atypia that exceed 15 cm, and retroperitoneal or intra-abdominal lipomatous tumors lacking cytologic atypia (Box 15-2).[28] Using this approach, reasonable evidence has been mounted to establish the entity of retroperitoneal lipoma, a diagnosis formerly considered to be hearsay.[30] Nevertheless, although the existence of retroperitoneal lipomas has been established, they are exceedingly rare. The diagnosis should be made only after well-differentiated liposarcoma has been excluded.

BOX 15-2 Indications for MDM2 Gene Amplification Analysis in Lipomatous Tumors[28]

- Lipomatous tumors with equivocal cytologic atypia
- Recurrent lipomas
- Deep lipomas without atypia that exceed 15 cm
- Retroperitoneal or intra-abdominal lipomatous tumors lacking cytologic atypia

Clinical Behavior

ALN/WDL are nonmetastasizing lesions that are traditionally not graded. However, their rate of local recurrence and disease-related mortality is strongly influenced by location.[5,6,31,32] As depicted in Table 15-2, tumors in the extremities have significantly lower rates of local recurrence than those in the retroperitoneum. Extremity lesions recur in nearly one-half of cases, whereas, in the retroperitoneum, recurrence rates approach 100%.[6] One could legitimately argue that ALN/WDL of the retroperitoneum is basically an incurable lesion. About one-third of patients die as a direct result of their disease, but this figure increases with longer follow-up periods as a result of the indolent growth of these lesions. On the other hand, those rare ALN/WDL that occur in the subcutaneous tissues are not associated with tumor-related death[32] and are generally cured by limited excisions.

Because of the possibility of ALN/WDL being dismissed as little more than benign but locally aggressive lesions, a small percentage of these tumors over time dedifferentiate or progress histologically to a higher-grade lesion (DL).[5,6,33] Although this phenomenon occurs most frequently with retroperitoneal

TABLE 15-2 Behavior of 83 ALN/WDL

SITE	RECURRENCE (%)	DIED OF DISEASE (%)	DEDIFFERENTIATION (%)	YEARS OF FOLLOW-UP RANGE AND MEDIAN
Extremity	43	0	6	2-25 (9)
Retroperitoneum	91	33	17	1-35 (10)
Groin	79	14	28	2-25 (8)
Total	63	11	13	

From Weiss SW and Rao VK. ALN/WDL (atypical lipoma) of deep soft tissue of the extremities, retroperitoneum and miscellaneous sites: a follow-up study of 92 cases with analysis of the incidence of "dedifferentiation." Am J Surg Pathol 1992;16:1051–8.

liposarcomas, it also occurs with deep extremity lesions; it is rare in subcutaneous tumors. Therefore, it does not appear to be a site-specific phenomenon as was formerly believed but a time-dependent phenomenon encountered in those locations in which there is a high likelihood of clinical persistence of disease. With retroperitoneal tumors, for which complete excision is a veritable impossibility, there is a substantial risk of dedifferentiation (about 10% to 15%); it is somewhat lower for extremity lesions (5%). In ALN/WDL that have been followed longitudinally, dedifferentiation occurs after an average of 7 to 8 years but may be seen as long as 16 to 20 years after the original diagnosis. When dedifferentiation occurs, the lesions can usually be considered fully malignant sarcomas. An exception is the rare tumor in which dedifferentiation is restricted to an extremely small focus (see section, Minimal Dedifferentiation).

Because of site-dependent differences in the behavior of well-differentiated liposarcoma, *atypical lipoma* was a term originally introduced in 1979 by Evans et al.[31] At that time, these authors suggested retention of the term *ALN/WDL* for lesions in the retroperitoneum but later recommended that the term be abandoned altogether in favor of the term *atypical lipomatous tumor*. To avoid confusion, the WHO has endorsed the combined term *ALN/WDL* for all lesions previously diagnosed as atypical lipoma, ALN, or ALN/WDL. There is merit in retaining the term *WDL* for retroperitoneal, mediastinal, or body cavity lesions to emphasize the life-threatening nature of these tumors in these locations, to assure adequate therapy and follow-up care, and to acknowledge the risk of dedifferentiation over time. Implied in the foregoing discussion is the understanding that *ALN and ALN/WDL are synonyms, and the choice of one over the other is based on location, not a constellation of histologic differences*. Unfortunately, it has not been possible to predict, in the individual case, which ALN/WDL will dedifferentiate. Comparison of matched pairs of ALN/WDL with its respective dedifferentiated component discloses minor differences, which are discussed in the following section.

DEDIFFERENTIATED LIPOSARCOMA

Dedifferentiation or histologic progression to a higher-grade, less well-differentiated neoplasm was first described by Dahlin[34-36] as a late complication in the natural history of well-differentiated chondrosarcoma, but it is now known to occur in other low-grade mesenchymal tumors, including parosteal osteosarcoma, chordoma, and ALN/WDL. Traditionally, DL were defined as ALN/WDL juxtaposed to areas of high-grade nonlipogenic sarcoma, usually resembling either a fibrosarcoma or undifferentiated pleomorphic sarcoma (malignant fibrous histiocytoma). Dedifferentiation was believed to occur after a latent period of several years. These views have now been modified. Whereas most DL display high-grade dedifferentiation, a small number contain exclusively low-grade areas or a combination of low- and high-grade areas.[35,37,38] Although the concept of low grade dedifferentiation has been questioned by some[32] on the grounds that these tumors have a behavior more similar to ALN/WDL than classic DL, this is not borne out by the experience of most.[34,36,37]

Clinical Features

DL account for 18% of liposarcomas.[4] They develop in approximately the same age group as ALN/WDL and reach a peak during the early seventh decade.[35-37] The sexes are affected equally. Unlike ALN/WDL, location in the retroperitoneum is favored over deep soft tissues of the extremities by a margin of nearly 3 to 1. Fewer than 20% of DL occur collectively in the head, neck, trunk, and spermatic cord and rarely in the subcutis. Radiographically, they have areas characteristic of ALN/WDL but, in addition, have mass-like areas of nonfatty tissue. The latter has imaging characteristics similar to other sarcomas, with prolonged T1 and T2 relaxation by MRI and attenuation coefficients higher than those for normal fat on CT scans.[39]

Gross and Microscopic Features

The lesions present as large multinodular masses ranging in color from yellow to yellow-tan admixed with firm tan-gray areas that correspond to the dedifferentiated foci. Microscopically, the lesions consist of areas of ALN/WDL that display the range of changes described previously and a nonlipogenic (dedifferentiated) component. The interface between the two zones is typically abrupt (Fig. 15-27), although, in some cases, there is a gradual transition between the two (Fig. 15-28). Rarely, the two patterns co-mingle, giving the impression of mosaicism (Fig. 15-29).

In about 90% of cases, the dedifferentiated zones have the appearance of a high-grade fibrosarcoma or undifferentiated pleomorphic sarcoma (malignant fibrous histiocytoma) (Figs. 15-30 and 15-31). It has been proposed that dedifferentiated areas should have a mitotic count of at least 5 mitotic figures per 10 high-power fields.[32] This criterion has not been used because many high-grade non-lipomatous sarcomas do not meet this standard. Those areas resembling undifferentiated pleomorphic sarcoma (malignant fibrous

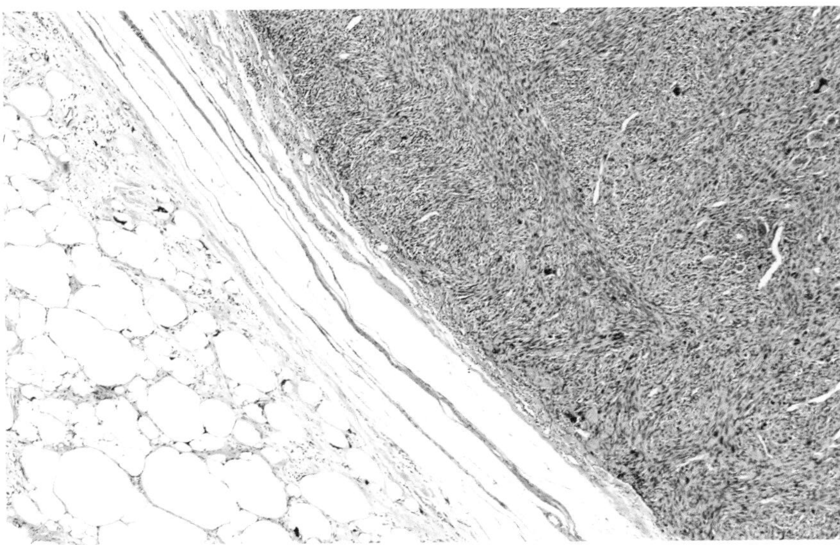

FIGURE 15-27. Dedifferentiated liposarcoma with sharp abutment of two zones.

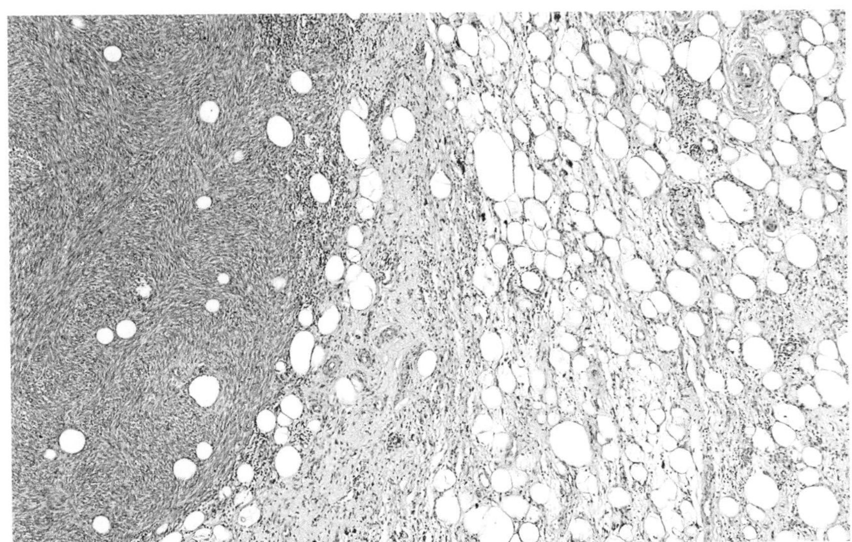

FIGURE 15-28. Dedifferentiated liposarcoma with an indistinct margin between well-differentiated and dedifferentiated zones.

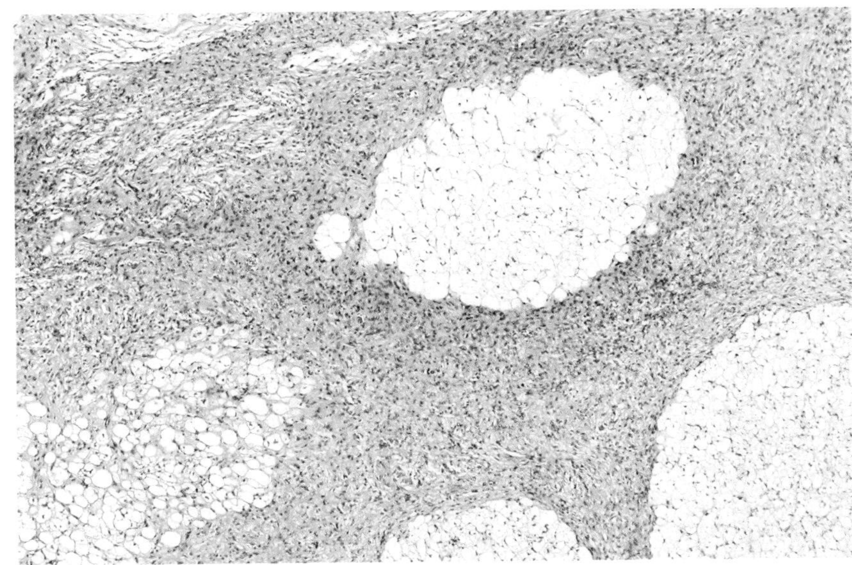

FIGURE 15-29. Mosaic pattern of a dedifferentiated liposarcoma.

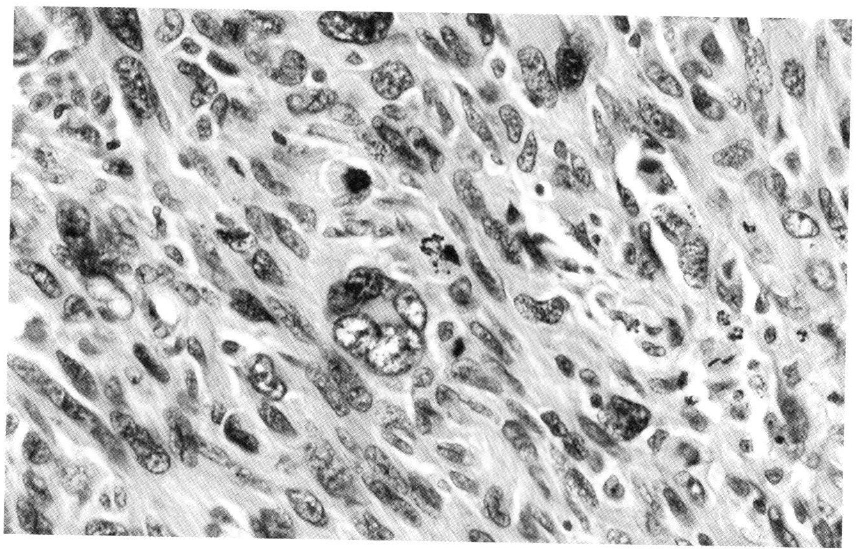

FIGURE 15-30. Dedifferentiated liposarcoma with areas resembling high-grade undifferentiated pleomorphic sarcoma (malignant fibrous histiocytoma).

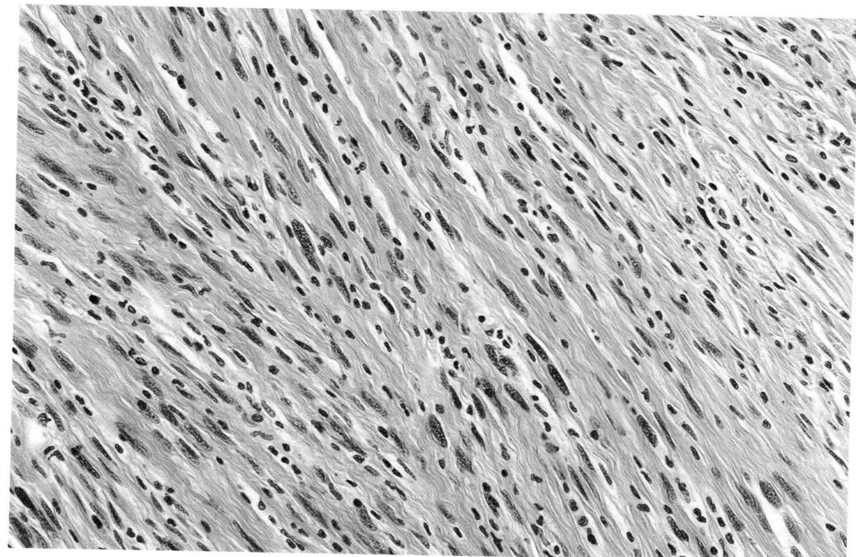

FIGURE 15-31. Dedifferentiated liposarcoma with areas having the appearance of a fibrosarcoma.

histiocytoma) display the full range of subtypes, from the common storiform-pleomorphic and myxoid types (high-grade myxofibrosarcoma) to the less common giant cell and inflammatory forms, including some with a dense lymphoid component.[40] Dedifferentiated areas resembling inflammatory undifferentiated pleomorphic sarcoma (malignant fibrous histiocytoma) have been associated with leukemoid blood reactions.[41] In fact, based on a combination of genomic profiling and *MDM2* and *CDK4* status, it has been suggested that most so-called inflammatory undifferentiated pleomorphic sarcoma (malignant fibrous histiocytoma) are, in fact, DL.[42,43] Some dedifferentiated areas depart from the foregoing description and resemble a low-grade fibrosarcoma or fibromatosis. Usually, these areas coexist with areas of high-grade dedifferentiation; however, in about 10% of cases, only low-grade areas are present (Fig. 15-32). A number of unusual patterns are seen in dedifferentiated zones (Figs. 15-33 and 15-34). They include undifferentiated large round cells in areas resembling a carcinoma or melanoma (see Fig. 15-34) and spindle cell areas containing whorled structures reminiscent of a meningioma or nerve sheath tumor (see Fig. 15-33).[35,44-46] The latter areas express actin and sometimes claudin-1, suggesting myofibroblastic or perineurial differentiation. Amianthoid fibers (Fig. 15-35) and divergent rhabdomyosarcomatous,[47] osteosarcomatous, or leiomyosarcomatous elements (Figs. 15-36 and 15-37) may also be seen.[35] Recently, two groups have independently identified ALN/WDL that coexisted with pleomorphic liposarcoma-like areas.[48,49] Because the pleomorphic liposarcoma displayed amplification of *MDM2*, they were considered dedifferentiated liposarcoma with homologous differentiation and are discussed in the following sections.

Differential Diagnosis

Sarcoma infiltrating fat. The most common problem in the differential diagnosis is distinguishing between a pleomorphic sarcoma infiltrating fat and a DL. There should be clear-cut evidence of ALN/WDL some distance from the

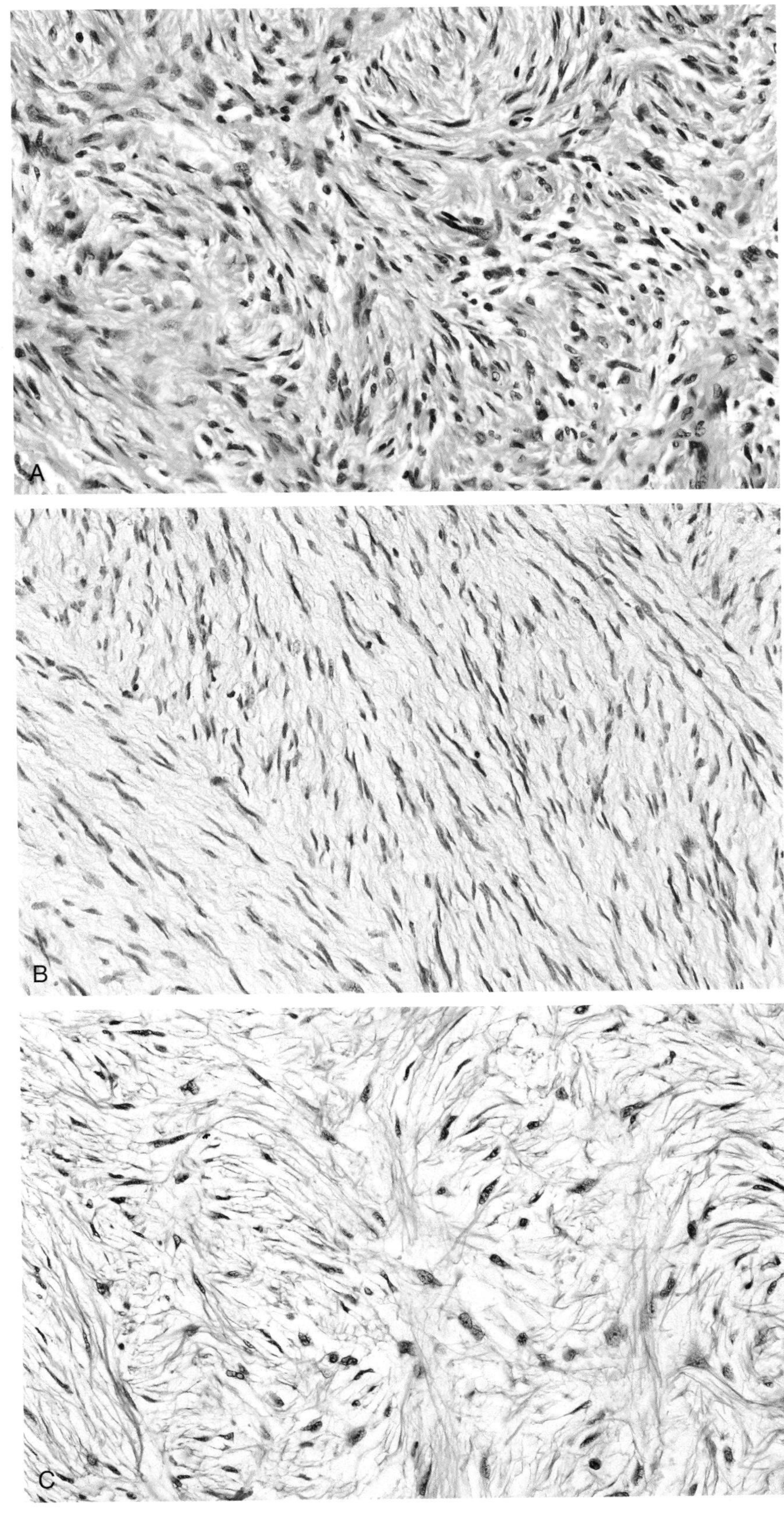

FIGURE 15-32. Dedifferentiated liposarcoma with low-grade dedifferentiation, ranging from grade II (A) to grade I (B, C).

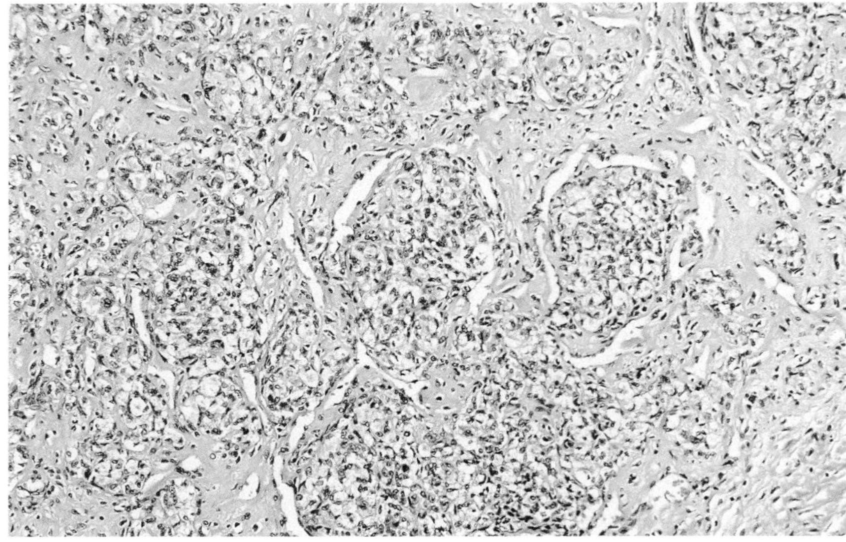

FIGURE 15-33. Dedifferentiated liposarcoma with areas of whorled structures.

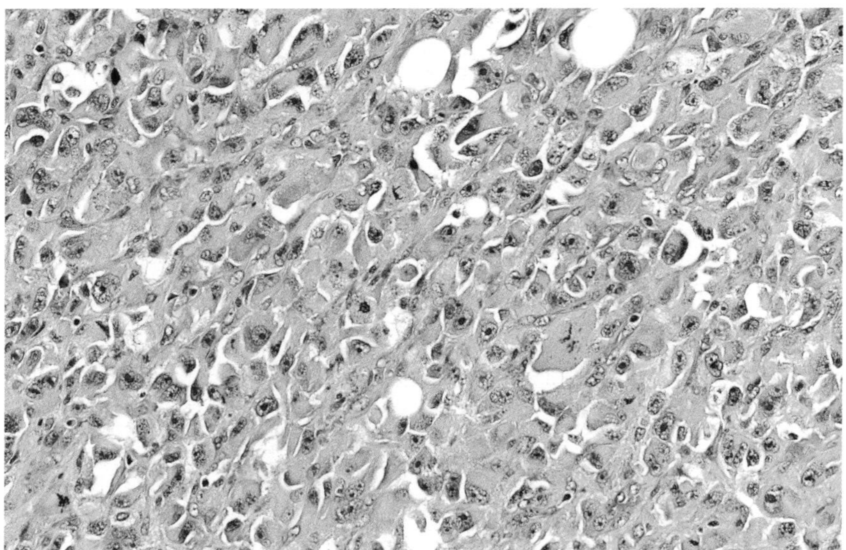

FIGURE 15-34. Dedifferentiated liposarcoma composed of undifferentiated large round cells.

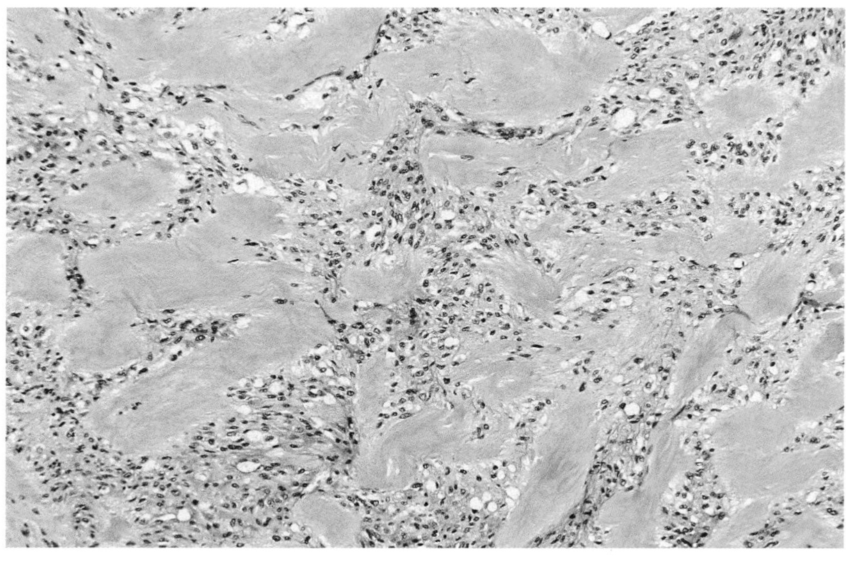

FIGURE 15-35. Dedifferentiated liposarcoma with amianthoid fibers.

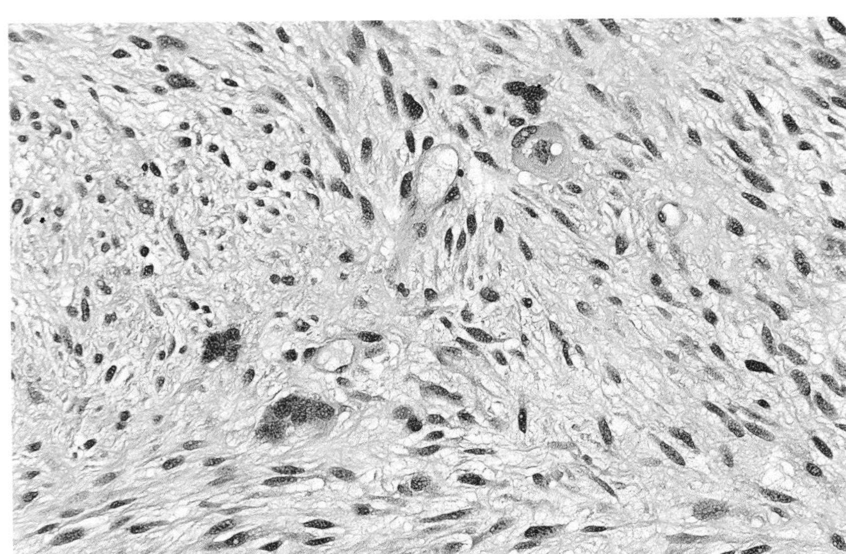

FIGURE 15-36. Dedifferentiated liposarcoma with rhabdomyosarcomatous differentiation in dedifferentiated areas.

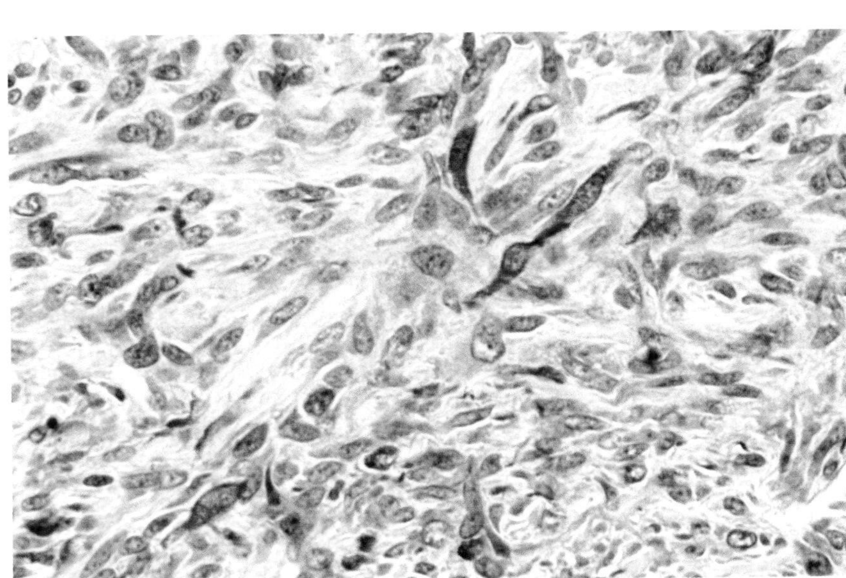

FIGURE 15-37. Dedifferentiated liposarcoma with rhabdomyosarcomatous differentiation in dedifferentiated areas. Desmin immunostain decorates rhabdomyoblasts.

dedifferentiated areas for the diagnosis of DL. Evaluating a high-grade sarcoma at its interface with normal fat results in an inappropriately low threshold for the diagnosis of DL.

Minimal dedifferentiation. A relatively rare problem is the significance of a microscopic focus of dedifferentiation in an otherwise typical ALN/WDL. The position that dedifferentiation ought to be macroscopically visible (greater than 1.0 cm) before the label "dedifferentiated liposarcoma" is applied has been adopted. Even so, it is likely that small foci of dedifferentiation (1 to 2 cm), which has been termed *minimal dedifferentiation*, are associated with a prolonged clinical course. For example, a patient with a 3-cm focus of dedifferentiation that evolved into a fully dedifferentiated tumor over a 25-year course was followed. Nonetheless, the previous case serves to illustrate that even tumors with minimal dedifferentiation can progress to full-fledged DL. Such cases should be individualized and signed out in a descriptive fashion, indicating the size of the dedifferentiated focus, until additional data are available.

Cytogenetic and Molecular Findings

The understanding of the molecular events that determine dedifferentiation is still evolving. Currently, there does not appear to be a consistent genetic aberration that separates ALN/WDL from DL in a statistically reproducible manner. In fact, the genetic similarity between matched pairs of a given ALN/WDL and its dedifferentiated component indicates that most of the abnormalities present in the lipomatous component of DL are present before phenotypic changes of dedifferentiation occur.[50] On the other hand, pure ALN/WDL without dedifferentiation have less complex abnormalities. These findings could offer the promise of identifying lesions that are at risk to dedifferentiate. At the same time, they do not negate the idea that dedifferentiation is a time-dependent phenomenon that occurs following a cumulative series of genetic events.

Generally, DL display more extensive chromosomal abnormalities than ALN/WDL. The 12q13-15 amplifications are more complex than those in ALN/WDL. Other amplifications, including 1q23, 12q24, and either 6q23 or 1p32, are encountered in about two-thirds of cases. The 6q23 amplicon is the seat of a candidate gene (MAP3K5) that inhibits lipogenic differentiation through c-JUN or PPaR-gamma-dependent pathways.[50]

Clinical Behavior

The behavior of DL appears to be similar to, but perhaps slightly better than, that of other pleomorphic high-grade sarcomas in adults. In the experience of Henricks et al.,[35] 41% of patients experience local recurrences, 17% metastasis, and 28% death from their tumors. An identical rate of metastasis was reported from the MD Anderson Cancer Center, Houston, Texas. Distant metastases occur most often to lung (76%) and liver (24%).[51] These figures reflect the accelerated tempo of the disease when dedifferentiation occurs. Whereas the metastatic rate might appear low compared to that of some high-grade sarcomas, two points should be emphasized. First, most patients die of the local effects of their tumor before distant metastasis becomes apparent, and, second, it is difficult to determine accurately which criteria differentiate between local (contiguous) intra-abdominal spread and local metastasis. For these reasons, the metastatic rate, determined with an average follow-up of 3 years, represents a conservative estimate of metastatic potential.[35]

Among the various prognostic factors, site appears to be the most significant. As with ALN/WDL, DLs located in the retroperitoneum have the worst prognosis. Although one might anticipate that the extent and grade of dedifferentiation would affect outcome, it does not appear to be true for the range of tumors commonly encountered in clinical practice.[35] What this seems to imply is that, when these tumors are clinically apparent, the amount of dedifferentiation is already so significant that quantitating and grading these zones do not provide any additional stratification that can identify good and poor prognosis subgroups. Furthermore, that patients with low-grade dedifferentiation may suffer the same untoward consequences as those with high-grade dedifferentiation indicates that the traditional definition of dedifferentiation (high-grade nonlipogenic sarcoma) should be expanded to include low-grade nonlipogenic sarcomas as well.

MYXOID LIPOSARCOMA

Myxoid liposarcoma embraces a continuum of lesions that includes, at one extreme, highly differentiated myxoid tumors with ample lipoblastic differentiation to poorly differentiated round cell tumors in which lipoblastic differentiation is inconspicuous, at best, and the latter end point sometimes referred to as *round cell liposarcoma*. Evidence supporting the idea that these two histologic extremes represent the same tumor category is derived from their similarity in terms of age, location, and cytogenetic abnormalities and by the identification of tumors with transitional or hybrid features.[52-54] Because of the range in observed behavior of this tumor, it is essential that some measure of biologic aggressiveness be given in either the form of a grade or an estimate of round cell areas (see the following sections).

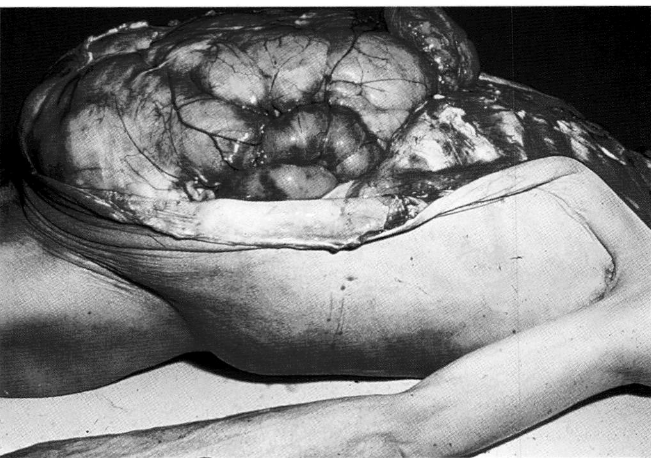

FIGURE 15-38. Myxoid liposarcoma massively replacing the abdominal contents.

Clinical Features

Myxoid liposarcomas account for about one-third to one-half of all liposarcomas. Unlike ALN/WDL and DL, this form occurs in a younger age group, with a peak incidence during the fifth decade. It develops preferentially in the lower extremity (75%), particularly the medial thigh and popliteal area, and less frequently in the retroperitoneum (Fig. 15-38). Radiographically, these lesions are quite varied. Typically, they appear as nonhomogeneous masses on CT scans. The attenuation values of highly myxoid lesions exceed those of normal fat but are less than those of the surrounding soft tissue. Less-differentiated round cell areas have attenuation values similar to those of other soft tissue sarcomas.[7]

Gross and Microscopic Features

Grossly, pure or predominantly myxoid liposarcomas are multinodular, gelatinous masses usually devoid of necrosis although, occasionally, hemorrhage is encountered (Fig. 15-39). Those tumors with discrete areas of round cell liposarcoma have corresponding opaque white nodules situated in the myxoid mass, whereas those that are predominantly round cell have a white fleshy appearance similar to that of other high-grade sarcomas.

Histologically, pure myxoid liposarcomas bear a marked similarity to developing fetal fat (Figs. 15-40 to 15-45). At low power, the lesion is a multinodular mass of low cellularity with enhanced cellularity at the periphery (see Fig. 15-41). Each nodule is composed of fusiform or round cells that lie suspended individually in a myxoid matrix composed of hyaluronic acid. The cells within pure myxoid liposarcomas characteristically are small without a discernible nuclear pattern and without much mitotic activity. Rarely, the nuclei are enlarged and hyperchromatic. (A distinctive pleomorphic variant of myxoid liposarcoma in children is described in the next sections.) A delicate plexiform capillary vascular network is present throughout these tumors and provides an important clue for distinguishing them from myxomas. The proliferating neoplastic cells recapitulate, albeit imperfectly,

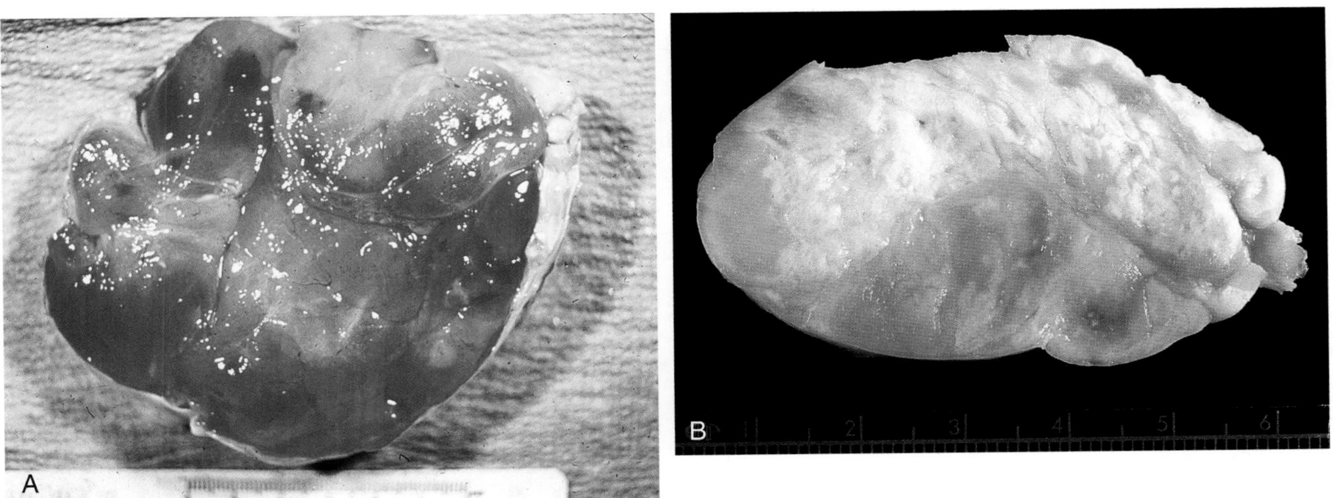

FIGURE 15-39. Gross specimen of a pure myxoid liposarcoma with a gelatinous cut surface (A) compared to a liposarcoma that contains myxoid (gelatinous) and round cell (opaque) areas (B).

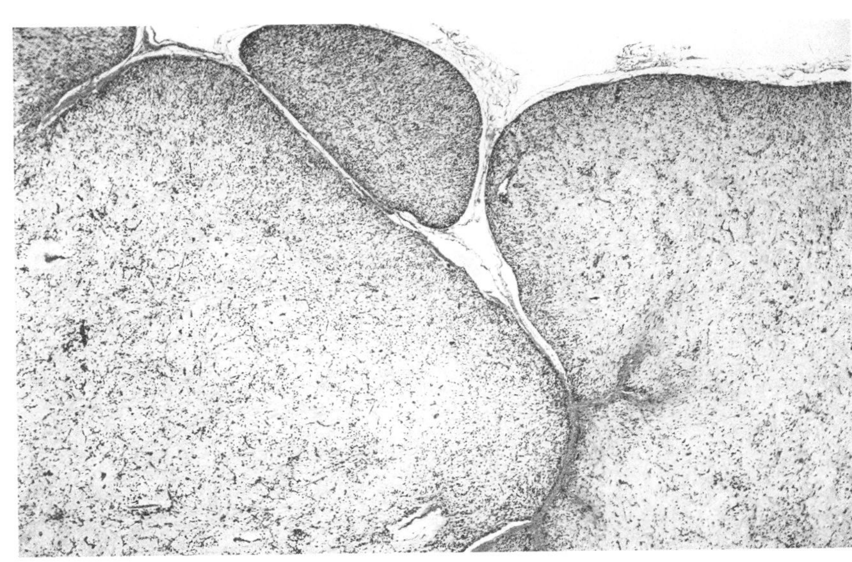

FIGURE 15-40. Multinodular appearance of a myxoid liposarcoma.

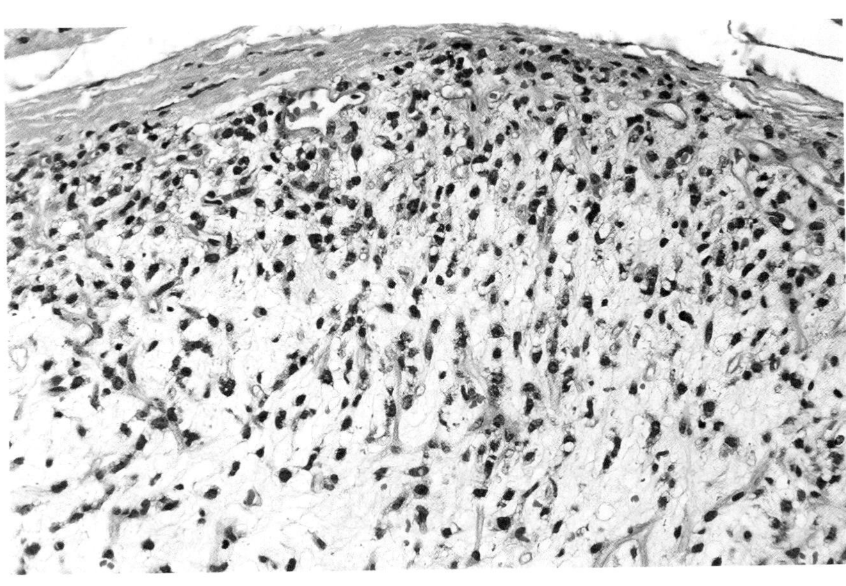

FIGURE 15-41. Enhanced cellularity at the periphery of nodules in a myxoid liposarcoma.

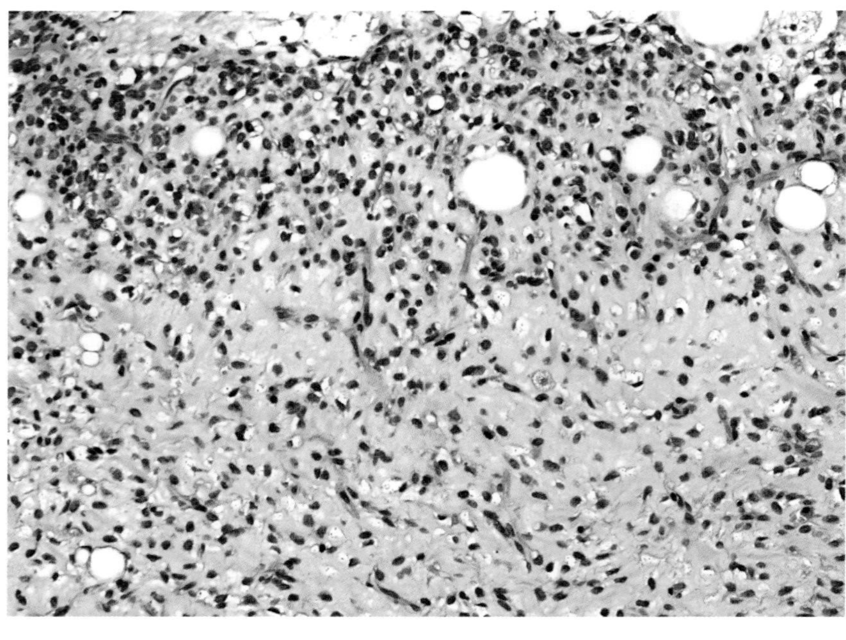

FIGURE 15-42. Myxoid liposarcoma with characteristic lipoblastic differentiation at the periphery.

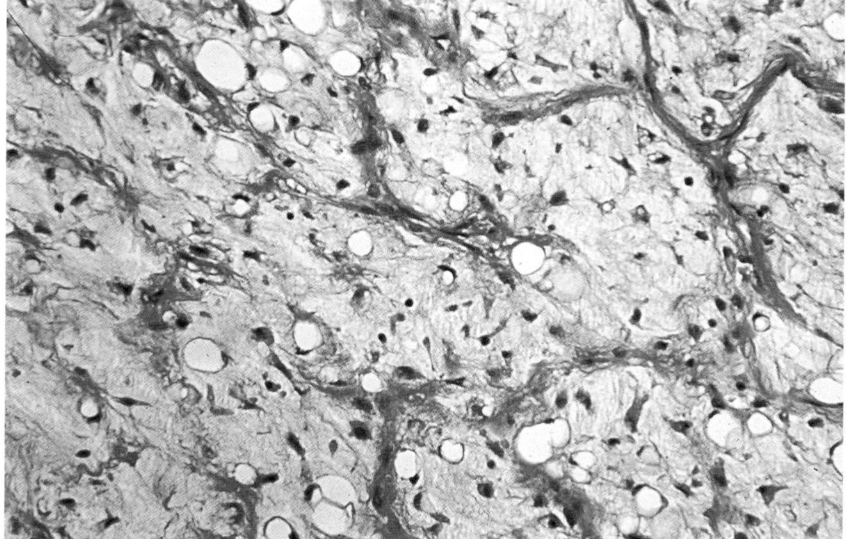

FIGURE 15-43. Typical appearance of a myxoid liposarcoma.

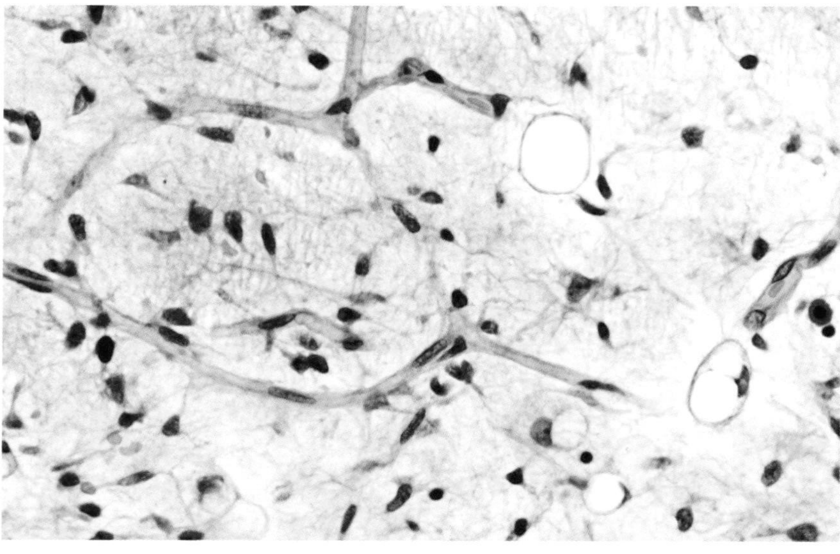

FIGURE 15-44. Myxoid liposarcoma with arborizing vasculature and lipoblasts at varying stages.

the sequence of adipocyte differentiation. Immature spindled cells lacking obvious lipogenesis may be seen next to multivacuolar and univacuolar lipoblasts. Although lipoblasts are usually easy to identify in these liposarcomas, they may be especially prominent at the periphery of the tumor nodules (see Fig. 15-42).

The hyaluronic acid-rich (Alcian blue-positive, hyaluronidase-sensitive)[55] stroma (Figs. 15-46 to 15-48) is present primarily in the extracellular space but may also be found in individual tumor cells. Frequently, the extracellular mucin forms large pools, creating a cribriform or lace-like pattern in the tumor and, infrequently, gross cysts (see Figs. 15-46 and 15-47). The cellular condensation at the rim of these pools produces a pseudoacinar pattern. In others, the weak staining of accumulated mucin and the flattened tumor cells mimic a lymphangioma. Interstitial hemorrhage is common and may be so prominent that the tumor is confused with a hemangioma. Focal cartilaginous,[56,57] leiomyomatous, or osseous differentiation occurs in myxoid liposarcomas. These elements do not appear to affect the prognosis. The significance of rhabdomyosarcomatous differentiation (Figs. 15-49 to 15-51), which has been encountered once by us and reported anecdotally in the literature, is uncertain.[58]

As myxoid liposarcomas lose their differentiation, they assume an increasingly round cell appearance, which is expressed in one of two ways. Amid a myxoid backdrop, one encounters a pure round cell nodule (Fig. 15-52) characterized by sheets of primitive round cells with a high nuclear/cytoplasmic ratio and a prominent nucleolus. The cells are so compact that they essentially lie back to back with no intervening myxoid stroma, and the capillary vascular pattern, though present, cannot be visualized easily. More commonly, however, the progression toward round cell areas is reflected in a more gradual fashion (Fig. 15-53). In these areas, the cellularity is clearly greater, and the cells are usually larger with a more rounded shape. At what point one applies the label "round cell" has been problematic. Round cell areas are

Text continued on p. 514

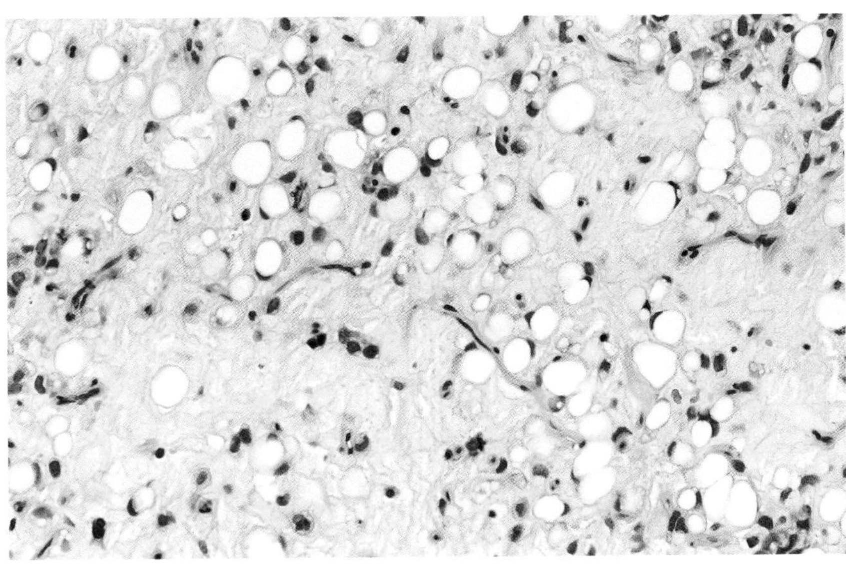

FIGURE 15-45. Myxoid liposarcoma with a larger number of mature lipoblasts than seen in Figure 15-44.

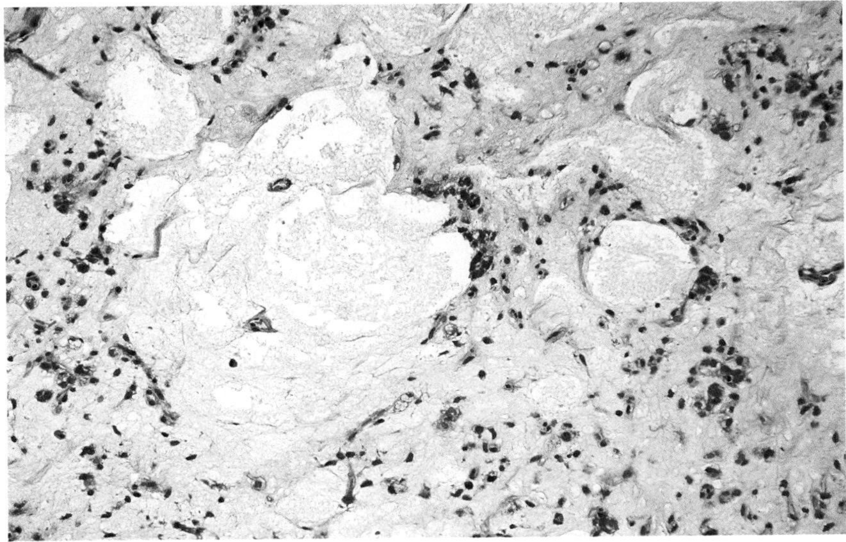

FIGURE 15-46. Small pools of stromal mucin in myxoid liposarcoma.

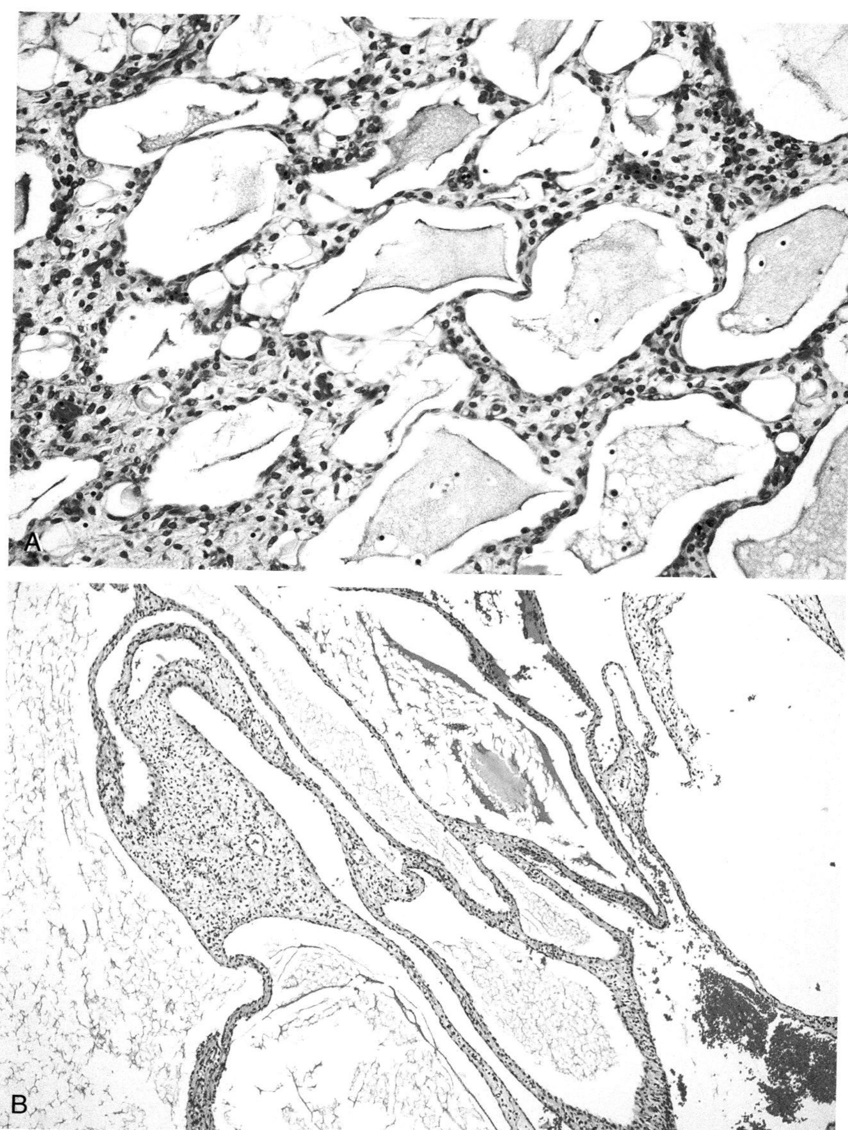

FIGURE 15-47. (A) Pools of stromal mucin in a myxoid liposarcoma forming a sieve pattern. (B) Pools of stromal mucin forming cysts.

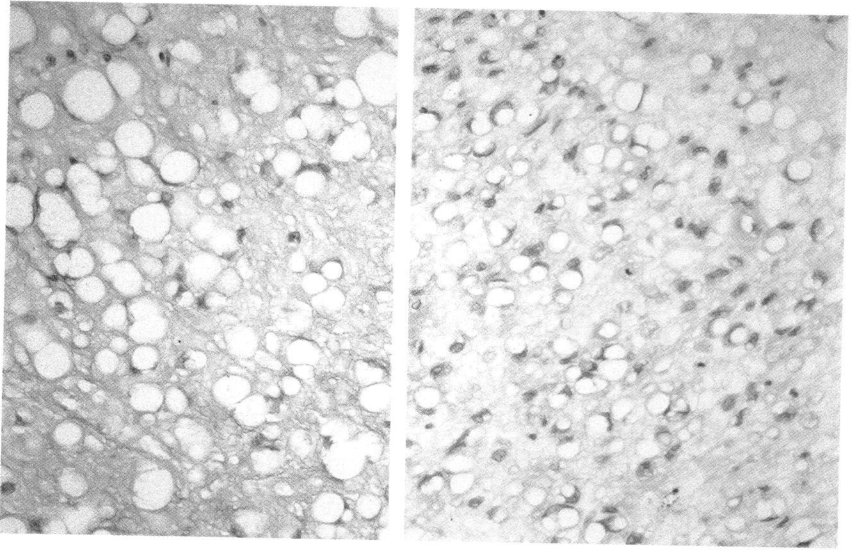

FIGURE 15-48. Alcian blue staining of myxoid liposarcoma before (left) and after (right) hyaluronidase digestion. Stromal mucin staining is abolished following enzyme treatment, indicating the presence of hyaluronic acid.

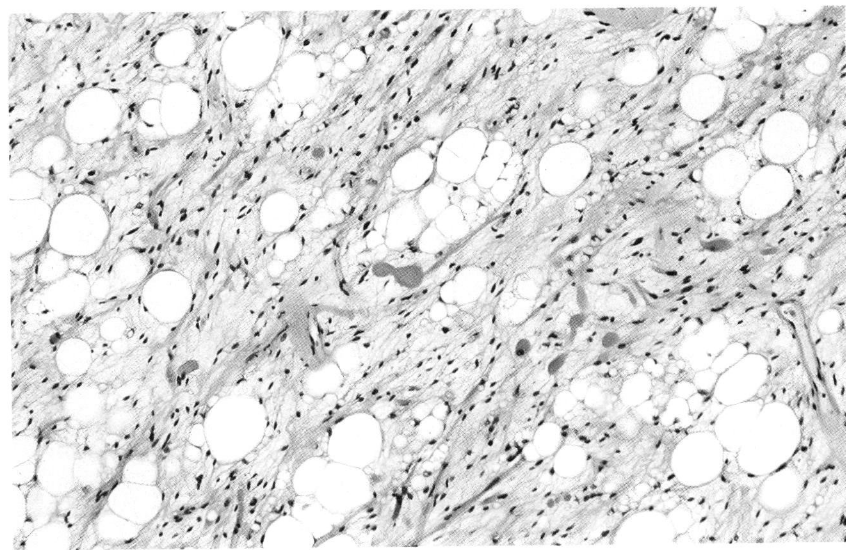

FIGURE 15-49. Unusual myxoid liposarcoma with rhabdomyoblastic differentiation.

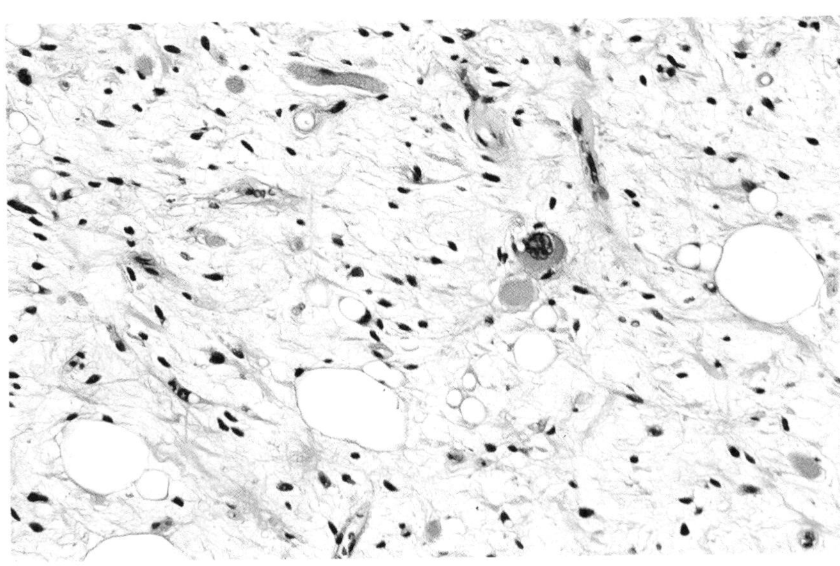

FIGURE 15-50. Rhabdomyoblasts in a myxoid liposarcoma.

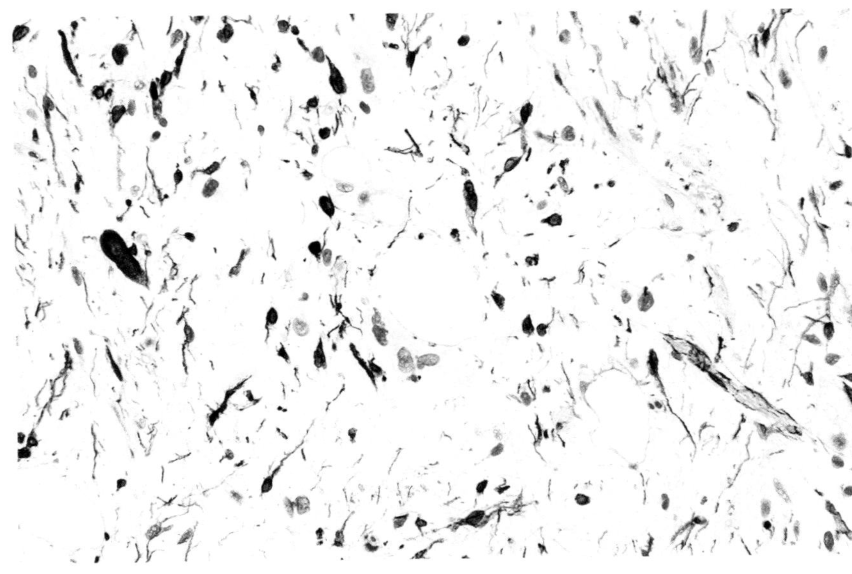

FIGURE 15-51. Desmin-positive rhabdomyoblasts in myxoid liposarcoma.

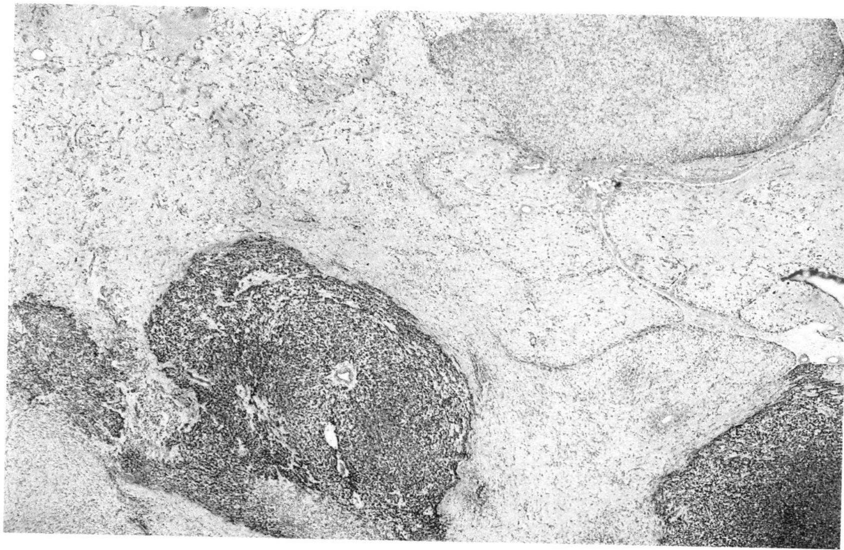

FIGURE 15-52. Myxoid liposarcoma with sharply demarcated nodules of round cell liposarcoma.

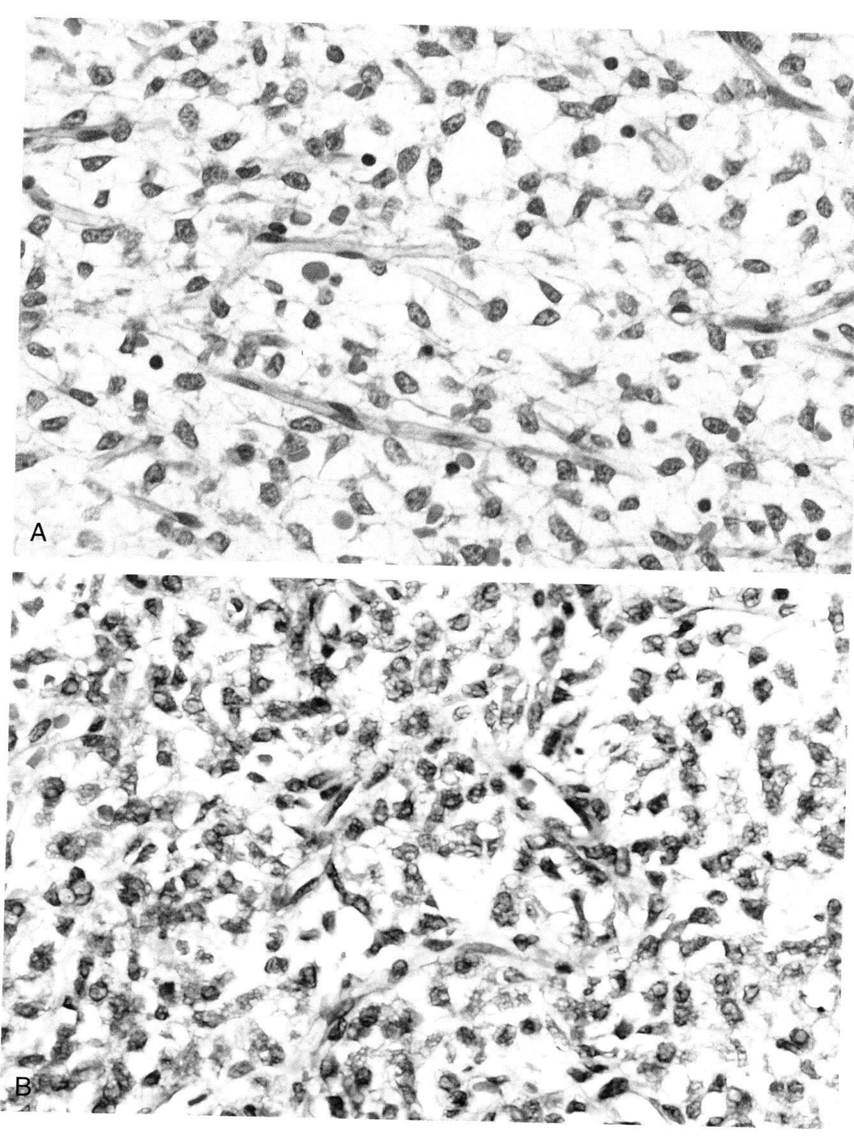

FIGURE 15-53. Myxoid/round cell liposarcoma with progressive transition, from somewhat cellular myxoid areas (A) to borderline areas (B) to round cell liposarcoma

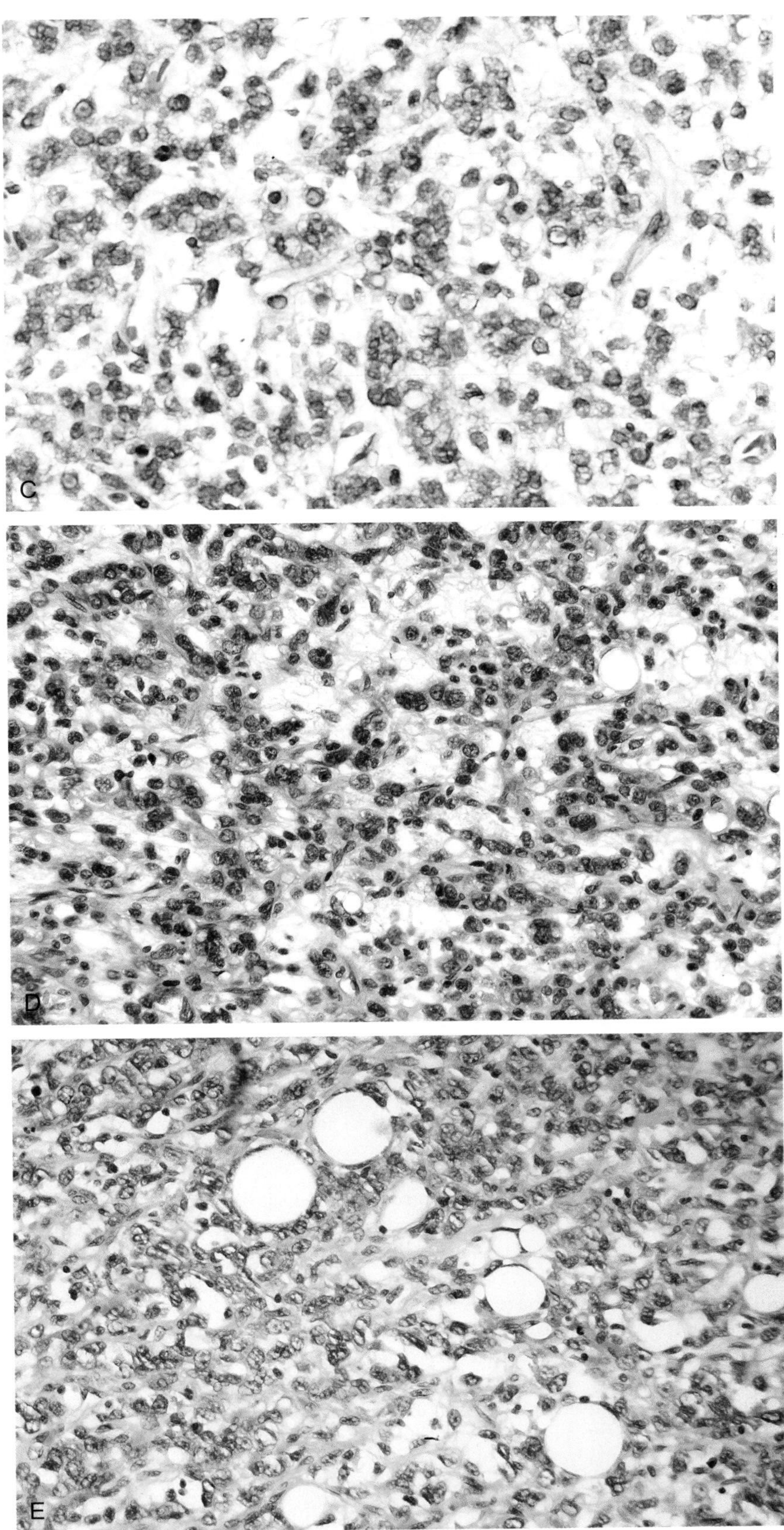

FIGURE 15-53, cont'd. (C, D) where cells have overlapping nuclei and some residual myxoid stroma. Round cell areas without myxoid stroma (E) may be impossible to diagnose as liposarcoma.

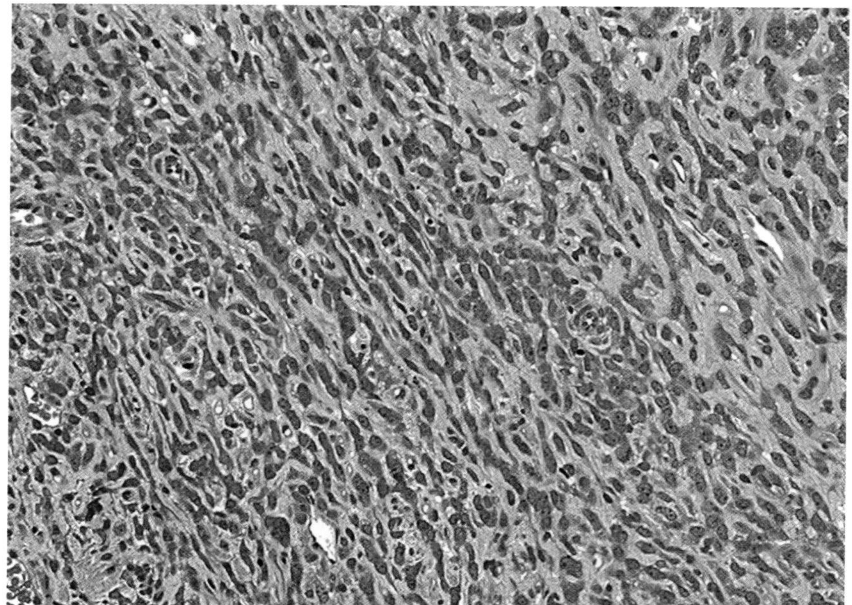

FIGURE 15-54. Cord-like pattern in a round cell liposarcoma.

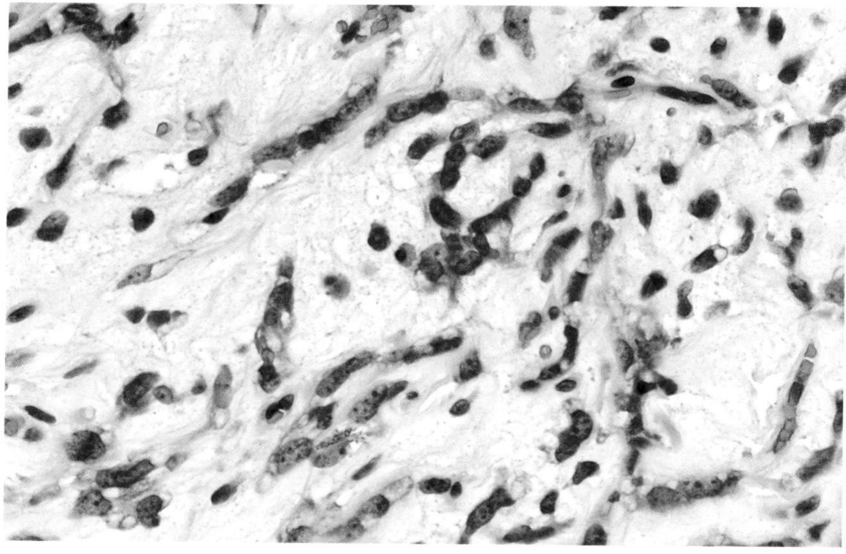

FIGURE 15-55. Cord-like pattern and stromal hyalinization in a round cell liposarcoma.

diagnosed when the cells acquire a rounded shape, sit back to back with overlapping nuclei, and obscure the vasculature.[59] The term *transitional* has been used for cellular areas of a myxoid liposarcoma that do not meet the criterion of a round cell. Transitional areas have not been correlated with an adverse outcome (see Fig. 15-53A).[60]

Occasionally, round cell areas are characterized by branching cords and rows of primitive small rounded cells (Figs. 15-54 and 15-55) or large cells with an eosinophilic granular or multivacuolar cytoplasm resembling malignant brown fat cells. Solidly cellular round cell areas, out of context, can be difficult to recognize as a liposarcoma, unless an occasional lipoblast is identified. In fact, in the absence of a lipoblast, one might entertain a diagnosis of another round cell sarcoma or a lymphoma. Finally, there have been a few exceptional myxoid/round cell liposarcomas that have displayed dedifferentiated areas similar to those seen in ALN/WDL.[61]

BOX 15-3 Lesions Simulating Myxoid Liposarcoma

Myxoma (intramuscular and cutaneous forms)
Angiomyxoma
Myxoid dermatofibrosarcoma protuberans
Myxoid chondrosarcoma
Myxoid undifferentiated pleomorphic sarcoma (low-grade myxofibrosarcoma)

Differential Diagnosis

The differential diagnosis of myxoid liposarcoma includes a wide range of lesions that appear myxoid (Box 15-3). The two most common myxoid sarcomas of adults that are commonly confused with myxoid liposarcoma are myxoid undifferentiated pleomorphic sarcoma (myxofibrosarcoma) and myxoid chondrosarcoma. The former is characterized by a significant degree of nuclear atypia and a coarser vasculature than is encountered in myxoid liposarcomas. It is tempting to interpret the pleomorphic vacuolated cells encountered in these tumors as lipoblasts and to draw the erroneous conclusion that the tumor is a liposarcoma (see Fig. 15-7). The vacuoles of these pseudolipoblasts are large, poorly defined, and filled with hyaluronic acid rather than lipid. Extraskeletal myxoid chondrosarcomas are composed of small, distinctly eosinophilic cells typically arranged in small clusters, cords, or pseudoacini, unlike the single cell arrangement in pure myxoid liposarcomas. The myxoid background in well-stained hematoxylin and eosin sections usually has a pale blue appearance in contrast to the clear appearance of the stroma in myxoid liposarcomas. Extremely myxoid forms of dermatofibrosarcoma protuberans occasionally closely mimic myxoid liposarcoma, but the superficial location of such lesions and the lack of lipoblastic differentiation are important observations that alert one to the correct diagnosis.

The diagnosis of myxoid liposarcoma with predominantly round cell areas fundamentally rests on finding unequivocal areas of myxoid liposarcoma or lipoblasts in the lesion. Fortunately, pure round cell liposarcomas are extraordinarily rare, and one can almost always find at least a few better differentiated diagnostic zones. Obviously, ancillary studies to exclude other round cell sarcomas such as rhabdomyosarcoma, poorly differentiated (round cell) synovial sarcoma, and Ewing sarcoma/primitive neuroectodermal tumors are important in selected cases (see Chapter 31).

Cytogenetic and Molecular Findings

Nearly all myxoid/round cell liposarcomas are characterized by a reciprocal translocation between chromosomes 12 and 16: t(12;16)(q13; p11).[53,56,62-64] This molecular event results in the fusion of the *DDIT3* (previously *CHOP)* gene on chromosome 12 with the *FUS* (*TLS*) gene on chromosome 16. Rarely, a translocation between chromosomes 12 and 22,[65,66] t(12;22)(q13; p11), or an insertion between chromosomes 12 and 16, (12;16)(q13; p11.2p13) occurs.[67] The normal *DDIT3* gene encodes a DNA transcription factor, whereas the *FUS* gene encodes an RNA binding protein with an affinity for steroid, thyroid hormone, and retinoid receptors.[68] The chimeric *FUS-DDIT3* gene gives rise to at least three fusion transcripts,[69-71] one of which (type II) has been identified in most myxoid/round cell liposarcomas. When introduced experimentally into preadipocyte cell lines, the transcript blocks adipogenesis and permits the evasion of cell cycle checkpoints.[70] *FUS-DDIT3* acts by way of several downstream targets, including PPARgamma2 and C/EBPalpha.[22] Targeted therapy for myxoid liposarcoma has been directed at nullifying the effect of the fusion protein. Trabectedin, a DNA minor groove-binding drug that interferes with the binding of the fusion protein to promoters, has had encouraging success in myxoid liposarcoma,[72,73] although there is some evidence that patients with certain fusion types respond better than others.

Various other molecular aberrations have been described in myxoid liposarcoma, indicating that targeted therapy could be aimed at several signaling points. For example, overexpression of several tyrosine kinase receptors (*RET, IGF1R, IGF1*) occurs in myxoid-round cell liposarcoma and is associated with a higher risk of metastasis after primary therapy. *P13K* mutations are also very frequent and associated with poor outcome.

A number of studies have focused on the integrity of the p53 pathway in this group of neoplasms.[74,75] Unlike ALN/WDL, in which only a small percentage demonstrates aberrations in this pathway, about 30% of myxoid/round cell liposarcomas have mutations in this gene, indicating differences among subsets of liposarcoma in terms of molecular oncogenic events.

Clinical Course

In the past, difficulty assessing the behavior of myxoid liposarcomas was the result of a lack of common criteria for making the diagnosis, the failure to distinguish the pure myxoid forms of the tumor from those having a significant round cell component, and the inability to compare outcome based on common therapeutic strategies.[76] There is general agreement now that the amount of round cell differentiation figures prominently into metastasis and outcome, the question centering on the appropriate threshold levels that one should use. Kilpatrick et al.[52] have used a three-tiered system (0 to 5%; 5% to 25%; greater than 25% round cell component), whereas Antonescu et al.[77] proposed a two-tiered system (less than or greater than 5% round cell component). Either way, tumors should be well sampled (using one section per centimeter tumor diameter) and the proportion of round cell component qualitatively estimated. This approach deals only with the percentage of round cell component, not the absolute amount. Therefore, it does not allow for disparities that might occur between a small liposarcoma containing a large proportion of round cells and a large liposarcoma containing a low proportion of round cells.

Despite the shortcomings, both a two- and three-tiered system correlate with survival and metastasis (Table 15-3). In the Mayo Clinic experience, 35% of patients with myxoid liposarcoma developed metastasis, and 31% died of their tumors. Using a multivariate analysis, age (less than 45 years), the percentage of round cell differentiation (less than or greater than 25%), and the presence of spontaneous necrosis were significantly associated with a poor prognosis (Table 15-4).[52] In the study by Antonescu et al.,[77] high histologic grade defined as greater than 5% round cell component, necrosis (greater than 5% of tumor mass), and overexpression of p53 immunostaining correlated significantly with reduced

TABLE 15-3 Myxoid/Round Cell Liposarcoma: Correlation of Round Cell Differentiation with Clinical Outcome

ROUND CELL POPULATION (%)	METASTASIS
0-5	11/48 (23%)
5-10	5/14 (35%)
>25%	14/24 (58%)

From Kilpatrick SE, Doyon J, Choong PF, et al. The clinicopathologic spectrum of myxoid and round cell liposarcoma: a study of 95 cases. Cancer 1996;77:1450–8.

TABLE 15-4 Myxoid/Round Cell Liposarcoma: Correlation of Clinical and Histologic Features with Survival

FEATURE	5-YEAR SURVIVAL (%)	10-YEAR SURVIVAL (%)
Age (Years)		
<45	88	80
>45	72	50
Necrosis		
Yes	25	0
No	90	70
Round Cell (%)		
<25	89	66
>25	79	40

From Kilpatrick SE, Doyon J, Choong PF, et al. The clinicopathologic spectrum of myxoid and round cell liposarcoma: a study of 95 cases. Cancer 1996;77:1450.

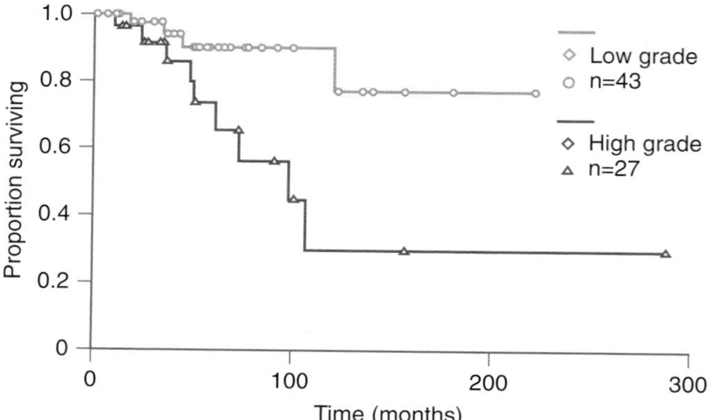

FIGURE 15-56. Disease-free survival in myxoid liposarcoma, based on amount of round cell component. Low-grade lesions have less than 5% round cell component, whereas high-grade lesions have greater than 5%. *(From Antonescu CR, Tschernyavsky SJ, Decuseara R, et al. Prognostic impact of P53 status, TLS-CHOP fusion transcript structure, and histological grade in myxoid liposarcoma: a molecular and clinicopathologic study of 82 cases. Clin Cancer Res 2001;7(12): 3977–87, with permission.)*

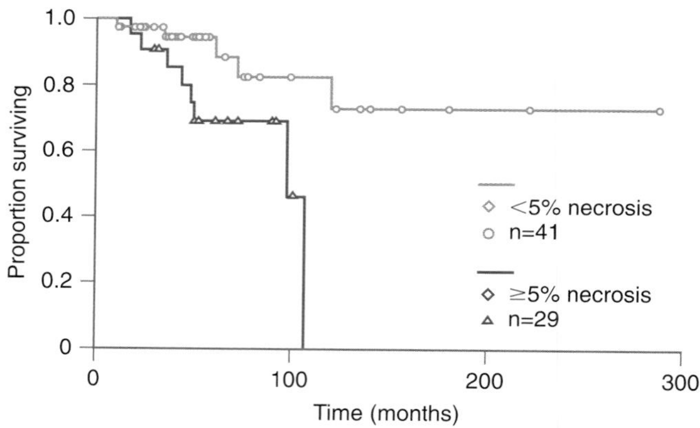

FIGURE 15-57. Disease-free survival in myxoid liposarcoma, based on amount of necrosis. *(From Antonescu CR, Tschernyavsky SJ, Decuseara R, et al. Prognostic impact of P53 status, TLS-CHOP fusion transcript structure, and histological grade in myxoid liposarcoma: a molecular and clinicopathologic study of 82 cases. Clin Cancer Res 2001;7(12): 3977–87, with permission.)*

metastasis-free survival (Figs. 15-56 and 15-57). Interestingly, there was no correlation between *FUS-DDIT3* fusion type and grade or disease-specific survival.[77]

Although myxoid/round cell liposarcoma metastasizes to usual sites, such as lung and bone, it displays a curious tendency, unlike all other liposarcomas, to metastasize to other soft tissue sites. Of the 16 metastatic myxoid liposarcomas reported by Evans,[78] 12 metastasized to soft tissue sites, 7 to lung, and 8 to bone.

PLEOMORPHIC LIPOSARCOMA

Pleomorphic liposarcoma is the least common and, consequently, the least well understood of the various liposarcomas. It represents less than 15% of all liposarcomas,[1,79-82] develops during late adult life, and is equally distributed between the retroperitoneum and deep somatic soft tissues of the extremities. About one-quarter develop in skin or subcutis.[83]

Pleomorphic liposarcomas display two related but clearly distinguishable histologic patterns that may coexist within the same tumor. Both share a disorderly growth pattern and an extreme degree of cellular pleomorphism, including bizarre giant cells, but they differ in their content of intracellular lipid material. The more common pattern resembles an undifferentiated pleomorphic sarcoma (malignant fibrous histiocytoma) but contains, in addition, giant lipoblasts with bizarre hyperchromatic, scalloped nuclei, many of which have a deeply acidophilic cytoplasm with eosinophilic hyaline droplets (Fig. 15-58). In the absence of these characteristic univacuolated or multivacuolated lipoblasts (that may require careful sampling to identify), these lesions are routinely diagnosed as undifferentiated pleomorphic sarcoma or rhabdomyosarcoma.

The second pattern in pleomorphic liposarcoma is less common. It consists mainly of sheets of large pleomorphic giant cells associated with smaller mononuclear forms (Figs. 15-59 to 15-61). Both cell types are highly vacuolated and lipid rich, and lipoblasts are easy to identify (in contrast to those in the first type of pleomorphic liposarcoma). Depending on the relative proportions of the two cell populations, this form of liposarcoma can be a highly anaplastic tumor or a small round clear-cell tumor resembling a carcinoma or melanoma. Tumors with a plethora of small round clear cells have been termed *epithelioid* variant of pleomorphic liposarcoma and are important because of their close mimicry to adrenal cortical carcinoma. Although these tumors can focally express keratin, actin, desmin, and S-100 protein,[83,84] they neither express inhibin nor manifest ultrastructural features of steroid-producing tumors (i.e., smooth endoplasmic reticulum).[85]

Pleomorphic liposarcomas are fully malignant high-grade sarcomas with local recurrence and metastatic rates of 30% to 40% and an overall 5-year survival of 55% to 65%.[83,84] In multivariate analyses, age, size, and central location were predictive of adverse outcome in pleomorphic liposarcoma. However, superficial lesions have an excellent prognosis. In a recent series of 33 cases of dermal and subcutaneous pleomorphic liposarcomas, local recurrence occurred in 10% and metastases in none.[86]

Given the rarity of these lesions, there are far fewer cytogenetic and molecular data pertaining to this form of

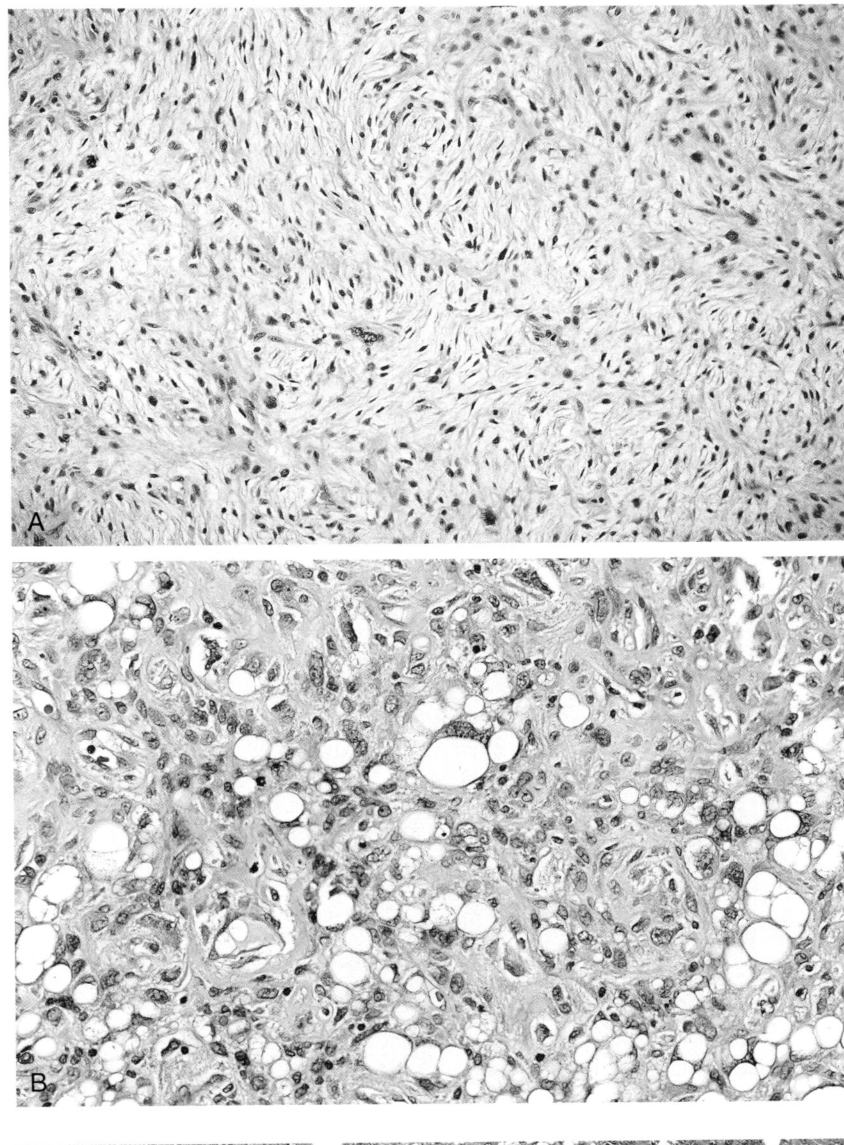

FIGURE 15-58. Pleomorphic liposarcoma with areas of undifferentiated pleomorphic sarcoma (malignant fibrous histiocytoma) (A) and areas containing pleomorphic lipoblasts (B).

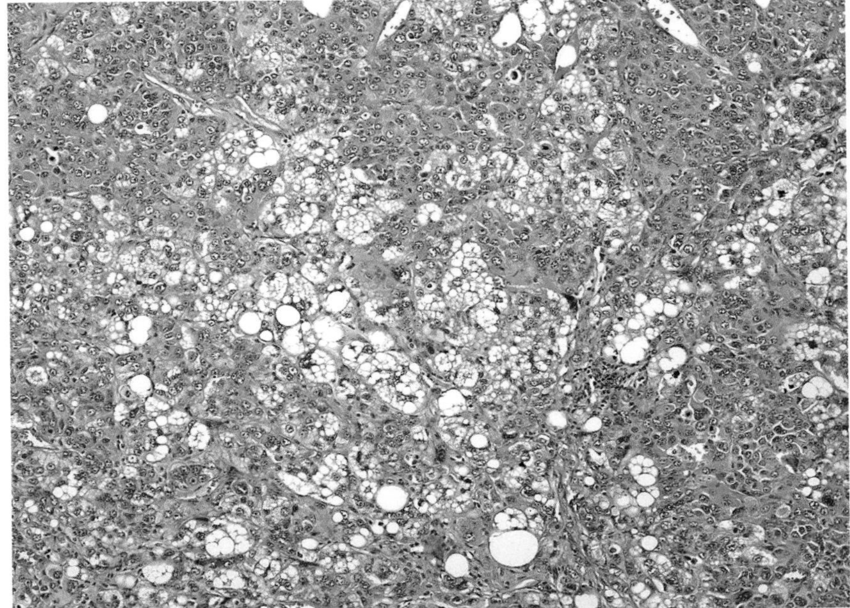

FIGURE 15-59. Pleomorphic liposarcoma showing sheets of epithelioid cells with scattered pleomorphic lipoblasts.

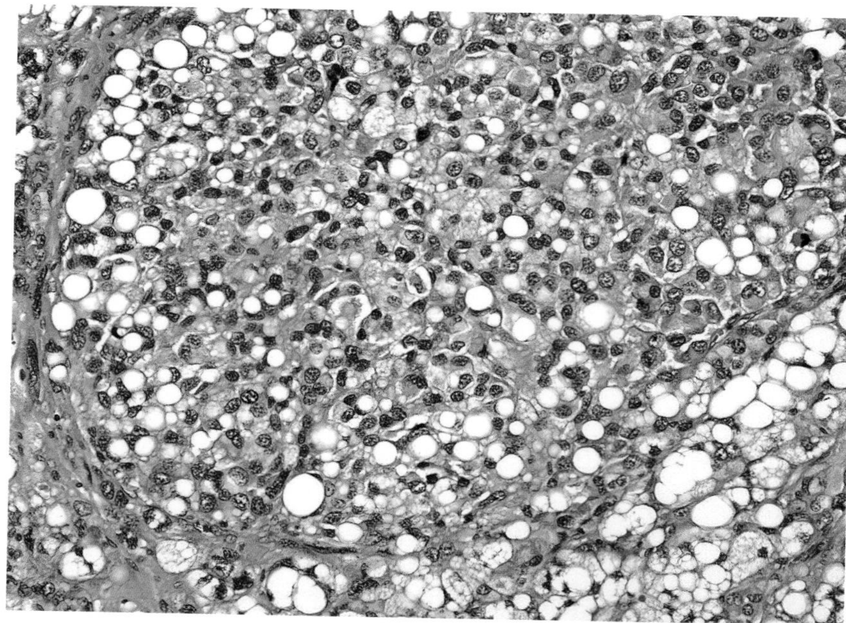

FIGURE 15-60. Pleomorphic liposarcoma showing sheets of vacuolated epithelioid lipoblasts.

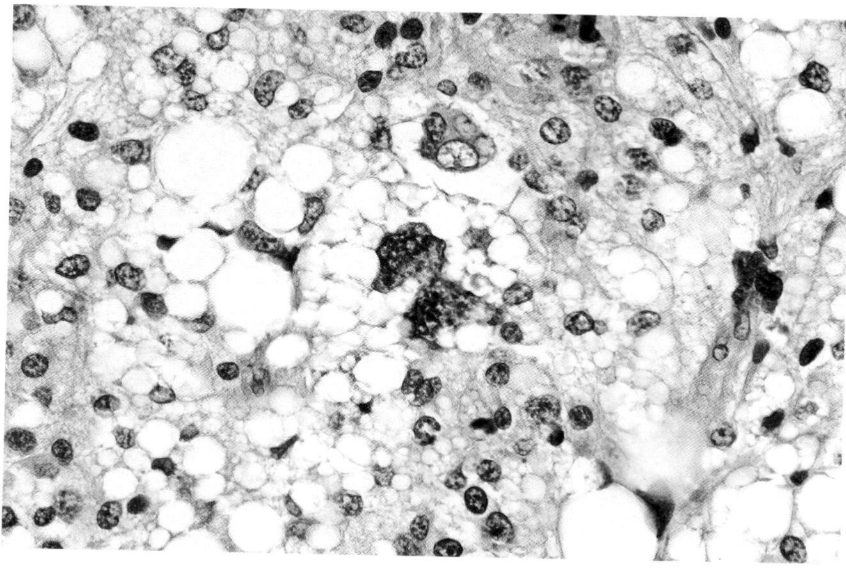

FIGURE 15-61. Pleomorphic liposarcoma showing pleomorphic lipoblasts.

liposarcoma. Cytogenetically, they exhibit complex structural genetic rearrangements that result in numerous gains and losses similar to other high-grade sarcomas. Dysregulation of several tumor suppressor pathways (e.g., *P53, Rb1, NF1*) commonly occurs in this subtype. Although possessing some histologic similarity to DL, they are, for the most part, molecularly distinct.[87,88] The only exceptions appear to be those pleomorphic liposarcomas that have occurred in association with ALN/DL[48,49] (see earlier section) as well as a small subset of cutaneous pleomorphic liposarcomas.[86]

SPINDLE CELL LIPOSARCOMA

A very rare and unusual form of lipomatous tumor consisting almost entirely of loosely arranged fibroblast-like spindle cells oriented along a single plane has been termed *spindle cell liposarcoma*.[89] Presumed to represent liposarcoma because of their similarity to a low-grade fibrosarcoma, the tumor cells' ability to metastasize has not yet been established. At low power, the tumor consists of nodules of slender fibroblast-like cells of low-nuclear grade arranged parallel to one amidst an arborizing vasculature. The cells have minimal atypia and mitotic activity (Figs. 15-62 to 15-63). At high power, it is possible to discern one or more minute fat vacuoles within the cytoplasm of many cells. In the more mature cells, the vacuoles coalesce to form a single vacuole that sits atop the slender indented nucleus like a scoop of ice cream on a cone. Where this lesion falls within the nosologic spectrum of liposarcoma has been debated. In no small part, this is related to authors having used different criteria in making the diagnosis, leading to the conclusion that these are variants of ALN/WDL or related to spindle cell lipoma.[90] Based on a recent series by Deyrup et al.,[91] spindle cell liposarcoma is a histologically

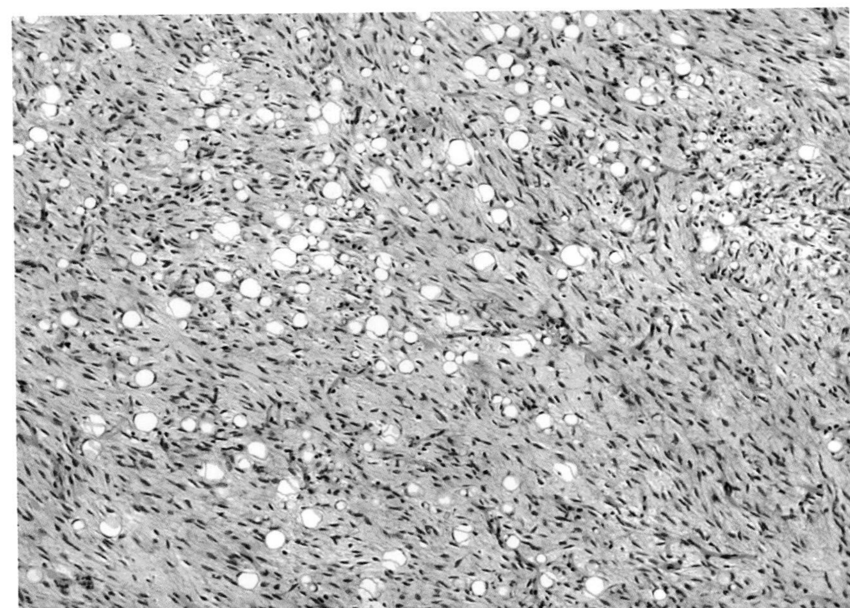

FIGURE 15-62. Spindle cell liposarcoma with prominent spindled tumor cells.

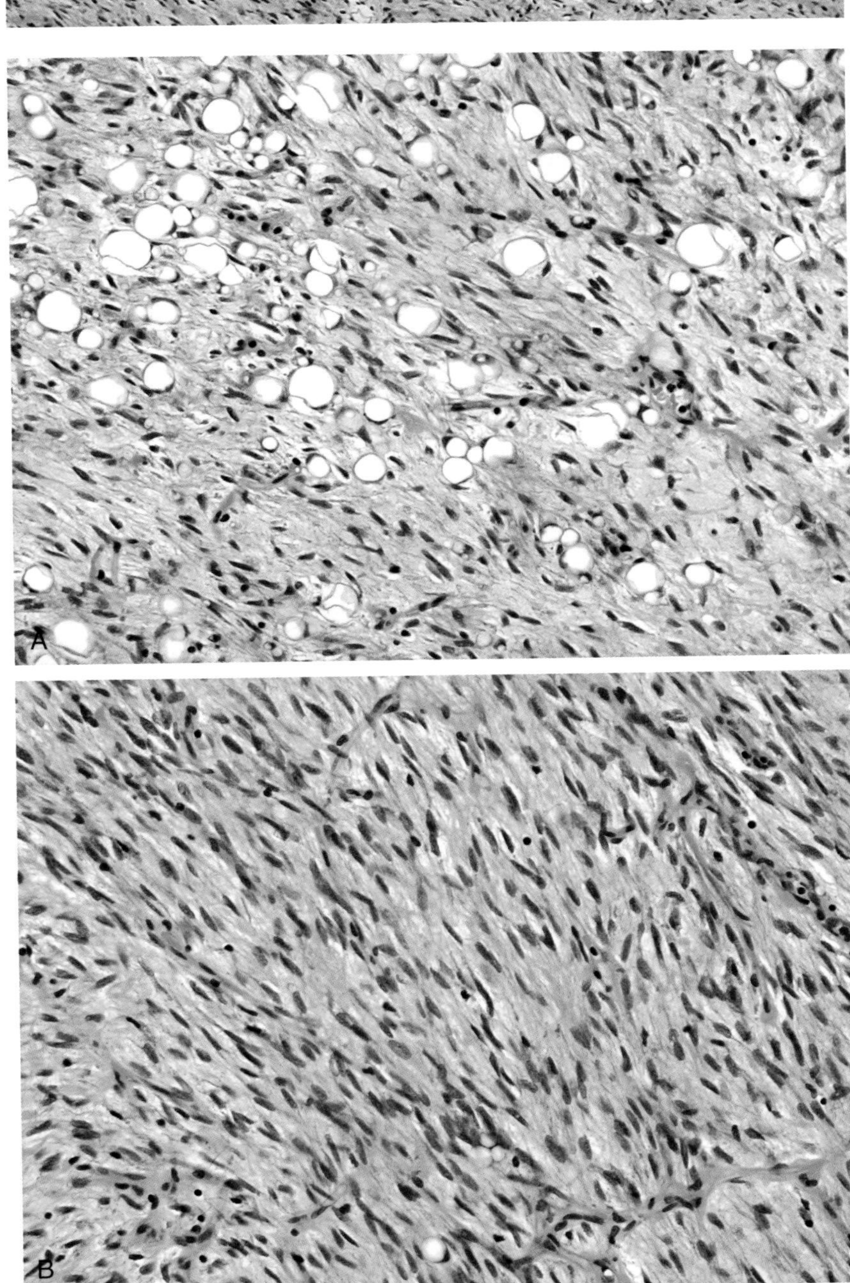

FIGURE 15-63. Spindle cell liposarcoma with scattered lipoblasts (A). The presence of lipoblasts and the variably sized spindle cells with hyperchromatic nuclei help distinguish this tumor from spindle cell lipoma. Area of spindle cell liposarcoma devoid of lipoblasts (B).

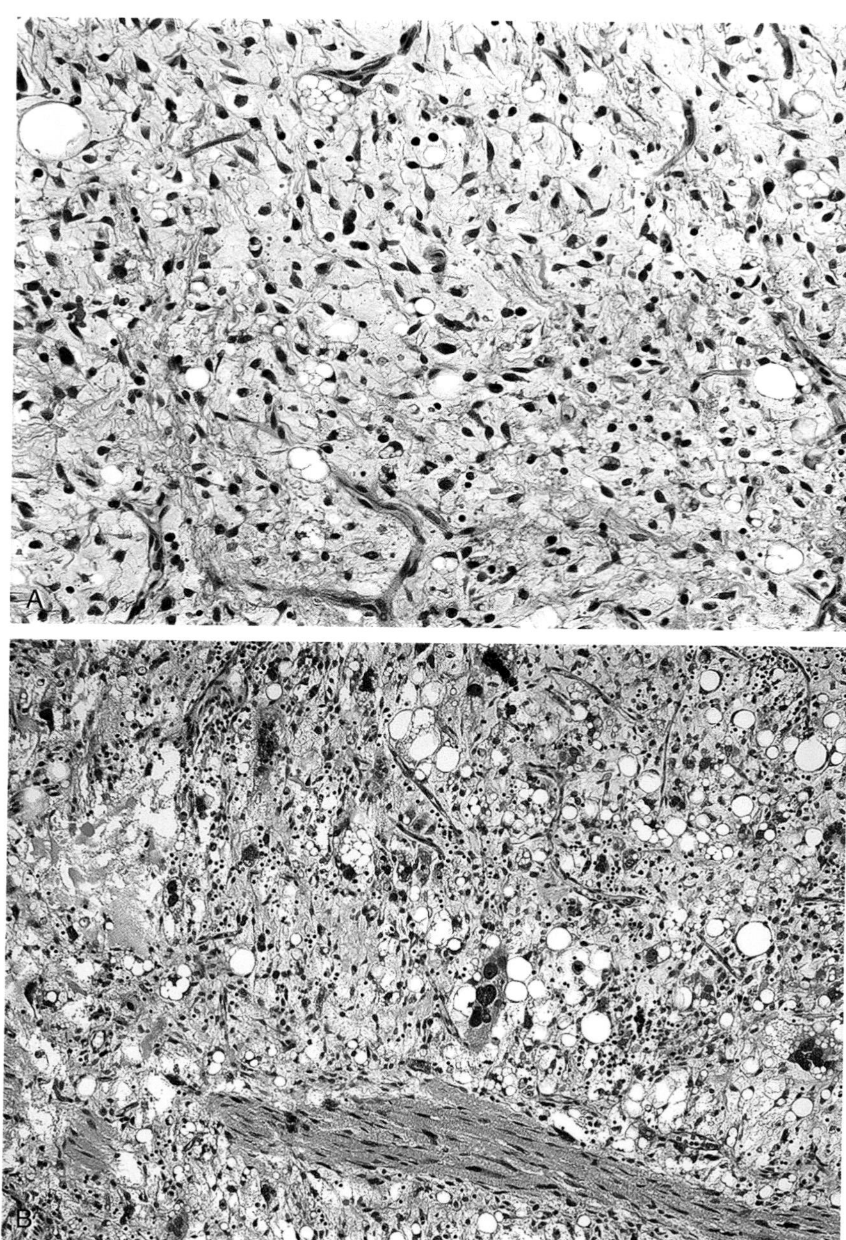

FIGURE 15-64. Pleomorphic myxoid liposarcoma occurring in a child showing area more closely resembling classic myxoid liposarcoma (A) and others with pleomorphic giant cells (B). *(From Alaggio R, Coffin CM, Weiss SW, et al. Liposarcomas in young patients: a study of 82 cases occurring in patients younger than 22 years of age. Am J Surg Pathol 2009;33(5):645–58, with permission.)*

distinctive lesion unrelated genetically to WDL, myxoid liposarcoma, and spindle cell lipoma. Although morphologically consistent with the diagnosis of a low-grade sarcoma, none of the 12 cases reported by Deyrup et al.[91] metastasized.

LIPOSARCOMA OF MIXED OR UNCLASSIFIABLE TYPE

Approximately 5% of liposarcomas do not fit easily into any of the foregoing categories, or they exhibit an unusual combination of patterns. The WHO has recommended that these maverick lesions be diagnosed as liposarcomas of mixed type. However, molecular tests have permitted some of these tumors to be classified within the current nosologic scheme. This implies that this category will become increasingly smaller over time. As an example of this, ALN/WDL with myxoid areas was identified as pure ALN/WDL rather than as a composite with myxoid liposarcoma. Quite recently, a distinct variant of liposarcoma has been described that combines features of ALN/WDL with pleomorphic liposarcoma.[49] These tumors occur primarily in the retroperitoneum of adults and consist of classic WDL associated with classic pleomorphic liposarcoma. The two components usually are present synchronously. Giant marker ring chromosomes and MDM2 amplification are present in the pleomorphic areas, leading to the conclusion they are variants of DL with homologous lipoblastic differentiation, rather than composite tumors. Like classic DL, they are high-grade sarcomas.

LIPOSARCOMA IN CHILDREN

Liposarcomas in infants and children are vanishingly uncommon.[92,93] Based on two recent studies of over 100 patients, the majority are classic myxoid liposarcomas, usually occurring on the extremity and having an excellent outcome with no proclivity to progress to round cell liposarcoma.[94,95] Two unusual histologic variants not generally encountered in adults were described in one study: a myxoid liposarcoma with spindled growth pattern (*spindle cell myxoid liposarcoma*) and a myxoid liposarcoma with pleomorphic areas (*pleomorphic myxoid liposarcoma*).[94] The former, consisting of conventional myxoid liposarcoma with low-grade spindled areas, had a behavior similar to classic myxoid liposarcoma. The latter, composed of conventional myxoid liposarcoma combined with pleomorphic areas and giant pleomorphic lipoblasts, occurred within the mediastinum and pursued an aggressive course (Fig. 15-64). The authors provisionally considered both to be variants of myxoid liposarcoma, albeit unique to the pediatric age group.

SO-CALLED MULTICENTRIC LIPOSARCOMA

The concept of multicentric liposarcoma was promulgated in the early literature because of the long interval between first and second liposarcomas in some patients. Recent molecular evidence using breakpoint analysis in a case of multifocal myxoid liposarcoma indicated clonality of all lesions consistent with metastasis.[96] Although difficult to exclude multifocality in rare multifocal cases, such as familial cancer syndromes, the plausible explanation for the overwhelming majority of multifocal liposarcomas is metastatic disease.

References

1. Enzinger FM, Winslow DJ. Liposarcoma. A study of 103 cases. Virchows Arch Pathol Anat Physiol Klin Med 1962;335:367–88.
2. Gobble RM, Qin LX, Brill ER, et al. Expression profiling of liposarcoma yields a multigene predictor of patient outcome and identifies genes that contribute to liposarcomagenesis. Cancer Res 2011;71(7):2697–705.
3. Fletcher CDM, Bridge JA, Hogendoorn P, et al, editors. WHO Classification of Tumours of Soft Tissue and Bone. 4th ed. Lyon: IARC WHO; 2013. p. 33–43.
4. Coindre JM, Pedeutour F, Aurias A. Well-differentiated and dedifferentiated liposarcomas. Virchows Archiv 2010;456(2):167–79.
5. Lucas DR, Nascimento AG, Sanjay BK, et al. Well-differentiated liposarcoma. The Mayo Clinic experience with 58 cases. Am J Clin Pathol 1994;102(5):677–83.
6. Weiss SW, Rao VK. Well-differentiated liposarcoma (atypical lipoma) of deep soft tissue of the extremities, retroperitoneum, and miscellaneous sites. A follow-up study of 92 cases with analysis of the incidence of "dedifferentiation". Am J Surg Pathol 1992;16(11):1051–8.
7. Arkun R, Memis A, Akalin T, et al. Liposarcoma of soft tissue: MRI findings with pathologic correlation. Skeletal Radiol 1997;26(3):167–72.
8. Ehara S, Rosenberg AE, Kattapuram SV. Atypical lipomas, liposarcomas, and other fat-containing sarcomas. CT analysis of fat element. Clin Imaging 1995;19(1):50–3.
9. Jelinek JS, Kransdorf MJ, Shmookler BM, et al. Liposarcoma of the extremities: MR and CT findings in the histologic subtypes. Radiology 1993;186(2):455–9.
10. Kraus MD, Guillou L, Fletcher CD. Well-differentiated inflammatory liposarcoma: an uncommon and easily overlooked variant of a common sarcoma. Am J Surg Pathol 1997;21(5):518–27.
11. Evans HL. Smooth muscle in atypical lipomatous tumors. A report of three cases. Am J Surg Pathol 1990;14(8):714–18.
12. Gomez-Roman JJ, Val-Bernal JF. Lipoleiomyosarcoma of the mediastinum. Pathology 1997;29(4):428–30.
13. Suster S, Wong TY, Moran CA. Sarcomas with combined features of liposarcoma and leiomyosarcoma. Study of two cases of an unusual soft-tissue tumor showing dual lineage differentiation. Am J Surg Pathol 1993;17(9):905–11.
14. Tallini G, Erlandson RA, Brennan MF, et al. Divergent myosarcomatous differentiation in retroperitoneal liposarcoma. Am J Surg Pathol 1993; 17(6):546–56.
15. Folpe AL, Weiss SW. Lipoleiomyosarcoma (well-differentiated liposarcoma with leiomyosarcomatous differentiation): a clinicopathologic study of nine cases including one with dedifferentiation. Am J Surg Pathol 2002;26(6):742–9.
16. Womack C, Turner AG, Fisher C. Paratesticular liposarcoma with smooth muscle differentiation mimicking angiomyolipoma. Histopathology 2000;36(3):221–3.
17. Yoshida A, Ushiku T, Motoi T, et al. Well-differentiated liposarcoma with low-grade osteosarcomatous component: an underrecognized variant. Am J Surg Pathol 2010;34(9):1361–6.
18. Antonescu CR, Elahi A, Humphrey M, et al. Specificity of TLS-CHOP rearrangement for classic myxoid/round cell liposarcoma: absence in predominantly myxoid well-differentiated liposarcomas. J Mol Diagn 2000;2(3):132–8.
19. Meis-Kindblom JM, Sjögren H, Kindblom LG, et al. Cytogenetic and molecular genetic analyses of liposarcoma and its soft tissue simulators: recognition of new variants and differential diagnosis. Virchows Arch 2001;439(2):141–51.
20. Farshid G, Weiss SW. Massive localized lymphedema in the morbidly obese simulating liposarcoma. Mod Pathol 1997;10:9A.
21. Schmack I, Patel RM, Folpe AL, et al. Subconjunctival herniated orbital fat: a benign adipocytic lesion that may mimic pleomorphic lipoma and atypical lipomatous tumor. Am J Surg Pathol 2007;31(2):193–8.
22. Hoffman A, Lazar AJ, Pollock RE, et al. New frontiers in the treatment of liposarcoma, a therapeutically resistant malignant cohort. Drug Resist Updat 2011;14(1):52–66.
23. Binh MB, Sastre-Garau X, Guillou L, et al. MDM2 and CDK4 immunostainings are useful adjuncts in diagnosing well-differentiated and dedifferentiated liposarcoma subtypes: a comparative analysis of 559 soft tissue neoplasms with genetic data. Am J Surg Pathol 2005;29(10): 1340–7.
24. Hostein I, Pelmus M, Aurias A, et al. Evaluation of MDM2 and CDK4 amplification by real-time PCR on paraffin wax-embedded material: a potential tool for the diagnosis of atypical lipomatous tumours/well-differentiated liposarcomas. J Pathol 2004;202(1):95–102.
25. Weaver J, Downs-Kelly E, Goldblum JR, et al. Fluorescence in situ hybridization for MDM2 gene amplification as a diagnostic tool in lipomatous neoplasms. Mod Pathol 2008;21(8):943–9.
26. Binh MB, Garau XS, Guillou L, et al. Reproducibility of MDM2 and CDK4 staining in soft tissue tumors. Am J Clin Pathol 2006;125(5): 693–7.
27. Sirvent N, Coindre JM, Maire G, et al. Detection of MDM2-CDK4 amplification by fluorescence in situ hybridization in 200 paraffin-embedded tumor samples: utility in diagnosing adipocytic lesions and comparison with immunohistochemistry and real-time PCR. Am J Surg Pathol 2007;31(10):1476–89.
28. Zhang H, Erickson-Johnson M, Wang X, et al. Molecular testing for lipomatous tumors: critical analysis and test recommendations based on the analysis of 405 extremity-based tumors. Am J Surg Pathol 2010; 34(9):1304–11.
29. Weaver J, Rao P, Goldblum JR, et al. Can MDM2 analytical tests performed on core needle biopsy be relied upon to diagnose well-differentiated liposarcoma? Mod Pathol 2010;23(10):1301–6.
30. Macarenco RS, Erickson-Johnson M, Wang X, et al. Retroperitoneal lipomatous tumors without cytologic atypia: are they lipomas? A clinicopathologic and molecular study of 19 cases. Am J Surg Pathol 2009; 33(10):1470–6.
31. Evans HL, Soule EH, Winkelmann RK. Atypical lipoma, atypical intramuscular lipoma, and well differentiated retroperitoneal liposarcoma: a reappraisal of 30 cases formerly classified as well differentiated liposarcoma. Cancer 1979;43(2):574–84.
32. Evans HL. Atypical lipomatous tumor, its variants, and its combined forms: a study of 61 cases, with a minimum follow-up of 10 years. Am J Surg Pathol 2007;31(1):1–14.
33. Brooks JJ, Connor AM. Atypical lipoma of the extremities and peripheral soft tissues with dedifferentiation: implications for management. Surg Pathol 1990;3:169.
34. Coindre JM, de Loynes B, Bui NB, et al. [Dedifferentiated liposarcoma. A clinico-pathologic study of 6 cases]. Ann Pathol 1992;12(1):20–8.

35. Henricks WH, Chu YC, Goldblum JR, et al. Dedifferentiated liposarcoma: a clinicopathological analysis of 155 cases with a proposal for an expanded definition of dedifferentiation. Am J Surg Pathol 1997;21(3):271–81.
36. McCormick D, Mentzel T, Beham A, et al. Dedifferentiated liposarcoma. Clinicopathologic analysis of 32 cases suggesting a better prognostic subgroup among pleomorphic sarcomas. Am J Surg Pathol 1994;18(12):1213–23.
37. Elgar F, Goldblum JR. Well-differentiated liposarcoma of the retroperitoneum: a clinicopathologic analysis of 20 cases, with particular attention to the extent of low-grade dedifferentiation. Mod Pathol 1997;10(2):113–20.
38. Huang HY, Brennan MF, Singer S, et al. Distant metastasis in retroperitoneal dedifferentiated liposarcoma is rare and rapidly fatal: a clinicopathological study with emphasis on the low-grade myxofibrosarcoma-like pattern as an early sign of dedifferentiation. Mod Pathol 2005;18(7):976–84.
39. Kransdorf MJ, Meis JM, Jelinek JS. Dedifferentiated liposarcoma of the extremities: imaging findings in four patients. AJR Am J Roentgenol 1993;161(1):127–30.
40. Kuhnen C, Mentzel T, Sciot R, et al. Dedifferentiated liposarcoma with extensive lymphoid component. Pathol Res Pract 2005;201(4):347–53.
41. Hisaoka M, Tsuji S, Hashimoto H, et al. Dedifferentiated liposarcoma with an inflammatory malignant fibrous histiocytoma-like component presenting a leukemoid reaction. Pathol Int 1997;47(9):642–6.
42. Coindre JM, Mariani O, Chibon F, et al. Most malignant fibrous histiocytomas developed in the retroperitoneum are dedifferentiated liposarcomas: a review of 25 cases initially diagnosed as malignant fibrous histiocytoma. Mod Pathol 2003;16(3):256–62.
43. Coindre JM, Hostein I, Maire G, et al. Inflammatory malignant fibrous histiocytomas and dedifferentiated liposarcomas: histological review, genomic profile, and MDM2 and CDK4 status favour a single entity. J Pathol 2004;203(3):822–30.
44. Fanburg-Smith JC, Miettinen M. Liposarcoma with meningothelial-like whorls: a study of 17 cases of a distinctive histological pattern associated with dedifferentiated liposarcoma. Histopathology 1998;33(5):414–24.
45. Nascimento AG, Kurtin PJ, Guillou L, et al. Dedifferentiated liposarcoma: a report of nine cases with a peculiar neurallike whorling pattern associated with metaplastic bone formation. Am J Surg Pathol 1998;22(8):945–55.
46. Thway K, Robertson D, Thway Y, et al. Dedifferentiated liposarcoma with meningothelial-like whorls, metaplastic bone formation, and CDK4, MDM2, and p16 expression: a morphologic and immunohistochemical study. Am J Surg Pathol 2011;35(3):356–63.
47. Salzano Jr RP, Tomkiewicz Z, Africano WA. Dedifferentiated liposarcoma with features of rhabdomyosarcoma. Conn Med 1991;55(4):200–2.
48. Mariño-Enriquez A, Fletcher CD, Dal Cin P, et al. Dedifferentiated liposarcoma with "homologous" lipoblastic (pleomorphic liposarcoma-like) differentiation: clinicopathologic and molecular analysis of a series suggesting revised diagnostic criteria. Am J Surg Pathol 2010;34(8):1122–31.
49. Boland JM, Weiss SW, Oliveira AM, et al. Liposarcomas with mixed well-differentiated and pleomorphic features: a clinicopathologic study of 12 cases. Am J Surg Pathol 2010;34(6):837–43.
50. Horvai AE, DeVries S, Roy R, et al. Similarity in genetic alterations between paired well-differentiated and dedifferentiated components of dedifferentiated liposarcoma. Mod Pathol 2009;22(11):1477–88.
51. Al-Zaid TJ, Ghadimi M, Peng T, et al. Metastasizing dedifferentiated liposarcoma: Clinical and Morphologic Analysis. Mod Pathol 2011: 24(1s);9A.
52. Kilpatrick SE, Doyon J, Choong PF, et al. The clinicopathologic spectrum of myxoid and round cell liposarcoma. A study of 95 cases. Cancer 1996;77(8):1450–8.
53. Orndal C, Mandahl N, Rydholm A, et al. Chromosomal evolution and tumor progression in a myxoid liposarcoma. Acta Orthop Scand 1990;61(2):99–105.
54. Tallini G, Akerman M, Dal Cin P, et al. Combined morphologic and karyotypic study of 28 myxoid liposarcomas. Implications for a revised morphologic typing, (a report from the CHAMP Group). Am J Surg Pathol 1996;20(9):1047–55.
55. Winslow DJ, Enzinger FM. Hyaluronidase-sensitive acid mucopolysaccharides in liposarcomas. Am J Pathol 1960;37:497–505.
56. Dijkhuizen T, Molenaar WM, Hoekstra HJ, et al. Cytogenetic analysis of a case of myxoid liposarcoma with cartilaginous differentiation. Cancer Genet Cytogenet 1996;92(2):141–3.
57. Siebert JD, Williams RP, Pulitzer DR. Myxoid liposarcoma with cartilaginous differentiation. Mod Pathol 1996;9(3):249–52.
58. Shanks JH, Banerjee SS, Eyden BP. Focal rhabdomyosarcomatous differentiation in primary liposarcoma. J Clin Pathol 1996;49(9):770–2.
59. Smith TA, Easley KA, Goldblum JR. Myxoid/round cell liposarcoma of the extremities. A clinicopathologic study of 29 cases with particular attention to extent of round cell liposarcoma. Am J Surg Pathol 1996; 20(2):171–80.
60. Fritchie KJ, Wang D, Goldblum J, et al. Myxoid liposarcoma: a clinicopathologic study of 27 cases of primary untreated disease with particular focus on so-called transitional and round cell areas. Mod Pathol 2011; 24(1s):14a.
61. Mentzel T, Fletcher CD. Dedifferentiated myxoid liposarcoma: a clinicopathological study suggesting a closer relationship between myxoid and well-differentiated liposarcoma. Histopathology 1997;30(5):457–63.
62. Gibas Z, Miettinen M, Limon J, et al. Cytogenetic and immunohistochemical profile of myxoid liposarcoma. Am J Clin Pathol 1995;103(1):20–6.
63. Knight JC, Renwick PJ, Dal Cin P, et al. Translocation t(12;16)(q13;p11) in myxoid liposarcoma and round cell liposarcoma: molecular and cytogenetic analysis. Cancer Res 1995;55(1):24–7.
64. Panagopoulos I, Höglund M, Mertens F, et al. Fusion of the EWS and CHOP genes in myxoid liposarcoma. Oncogene 1996;12(3):489–94.
65. Dal Cin P, Sciot R, Panagopoulos I, et al. Additional evidence of a variant translocation t(12;22) with EWS/CHOP fusion in myxoid liposarcoma: clinicopathological features. J Pathol 1997;182(4):437–41.
66. Panagopoulos I, Aman P, Mertens F, et al. Genomic PCR detects tumor cells in peripheral blood from patients with myxoid liposarcoma. Genes Chromosomes Cancer 1996;17(2):102–7.
67. Mrozek K, Szumigala J, Brooks JS, et al. Round cell liposarcoma with the insertion (12;16)(q13;p11.2p13). Am J Clin Pathol 1997;108(1):35–9.
68. Powers CA, Mathur M, Raaka BM, et al. TLS (translocated-in-liposarcoma) is a high-affinity interactor for steroid, thyroid hormone, and retinoid receptors. Mol Endocrinol 1998;12(1):4–18.
69. Kuroda M, Ishida T, Horiuchi H, et al. Chimeric TLS/FUS-CHOP gene expression and the heterogeneity of its junction in human myxoid and round cell liposarcoma. Am J Pathol 1995;147(5):1221–7.
70. Kuroda M, Ishida T, Takanashi M, et al. Oncogenic transformation and inhibition of adipocytic conversion of preadipocytes by TLS/FUS-CHOP type II chimeric protein. Am J Pathol 1997;151(3):735–44.
71. Yang X, Nagasaki K, Egawa S, et al. FUS/TLS-CHOP chimeric transcripts in liposarcoma tissues. Jpn J Clin Oncol 1995;25(6):234–9.
72. Forni C, Minuzzo M, Virdis E, et al. Trabectedin (ET-743) promotes differentiation in myxoid liposarcoma tumors. Mol Cancer Ther 2009;8(2):449–57.
73. Grosso F, Sanfilippo R, Virdis E, et al. Trabectedin in myxoid liposarcomas (MLS): a long-term analysis of a single-institution series. Ann Oncol 2009;20(8):1439–44.
74. Dei Tos AP, Piccinin S, Doglioni C, et al. Molecular aberrations of the G1-S checkpoint in myxoid and round cell liposarcoma. Am J Pathol 1997;151(6):1531–9.
75. Smith TA, Goldblum JR. Immunohistochemical analysis of p53 protein in myxoid/round-cell liposarcoma of the extremities. Appl Immunohistochem 1996;4(4):228–34.
76. Weiss SW. Lipomatous tumors. In: Weiss SW, Brooks JJ, editors. Soft tissue tumors. Baltimore: Williams & Wilkins; 1996.
77. Antonescu CR, Tschernyavsky SJ, Decuseara R, et al. Prognostic impact of P53 status, TLS-CHOP fusion transcript structure, and histological grade in myxoid liposarcoma: a molecular and clinicopathologic study of 82 cases. Clin Cancer Res 2001;7(12):3977–87.
78. Evans HL. Liposarcomas and atypical lipomatous tumors: a study of 66 cases followed for a minimum of 10 years. Surg Pathol 1988;1:41.
79. Hashimoto H, Enjoji M. Liposarcoma. A clinicopathologic subtyping of 52 cases. Acta Pathol Jpn 1982;32(6):933–48.
80. Kindblom LG, Angervall L, Svendsen P. Liposarcoma a clinicopathologic, radiographic and prognostic study. Acta Pathol Microbiol Scand Suppl 1975;(253):1–71.
81. Enterline HT, Culberson JD, Rochlin DB, et al. Liposarcoma. A clinical and pathological study of 53 cases. Cancer 1960;13:932–50.
82. Oliveira AM, Nascimento AG. Pleomorphic liposarcoma. Semin Diagn Pathol 2001;18(4):274–85.
83. Hornick JL, Bosenberg MW, Mentzel T, et al. Pleomorphic liposarcoma: clinicopathologic analysis of 57 cases. Am J Surg Pathol 2004;28(10):1257–67.
84. Gebhard S, Coindre JM, Michels JJ, et al. Pleomorphic liposarcoma: clinicopathologic, immunohistochemical, and follow-up analysis of 63 cases: a study from the French Federation of Cancer Centers Sarcoma Group. Am J Surg Pathol 2002;26(5):601–16.

85. Huang HY, Antonescu CR. Epithelioid variant of pleomorphic liposarcoma: a comparative immunohistochemical and ultrastructural analysis of six cases with emphasis on overlapping features with epithelial malignancies. Ultrastruct Pathol 2002;26(5):299–308.
86. Gardner JM, Dandekar M, Thomas D, et al. Cutaneous and subcutaneous pleomorphic liposarcoma: a clinicopathologic study of 29 cases with evalution of MDM2 gene amplification in 26. Am J Surg Pathol 2012; 36:1047–51.
87. Fritz B, Schubert F, Wrobel G, et al. Microarray-based copy number and expression profiling in dedifferentiated and pleomorphic liposarcoma. Cancer Res 2002;62(11):2993–8.
88. Rieker RJ, Joos S, Bartsch C, et al. Distinct chromosomal imbalances in pleomorphic and in high-grade dedifferentiated liposarcomas. Int J Cancer 2002;99(1):68–73.
89. Dei Tos AP, Mentzel T, Newman PL, et al. Spindle cell liposarcoma, a hitherto unrecognized variant of liposarcoma. Analysis of six cases. Am J Surg Pathol 1994;18(9):913–21.
90. Mentzel T, Palmedo G, Kuhnen C. Well-differentiated spindle cell liposarcoma ("atypical spindle cell lipomatous tumor") does not belong to the spectrum of atypical lipomatous tumor but has a close relationship to spindle cell lipoma: clinicopathologic, immunohistochemical, and molecular analysis of six cases. Mod Pathol 2010;23(5):729–36.
91. Deyrup A Chibon F, Guillou L, et al. Spindle cell liposarcoma: a distinct entity or histologic variant? Histologic and molecular analysis of 12 cases. Modern Pathology 2012;25(S2):11a.
92. Ferrari A, Casanova M, Spreafico F, et al. Childhood liposarcoma: a single-institutional twenty-year experience. Pediatr Hematol Oncol 1999;16(5):415–21.
93. Shmookler BM, Enzinger FM. Liposarcoma occurring in children. An analysis of 17 cases and review of the literature. Cancer 1983;52(3): 567–74.
94. Alaggio R, Coffin CM, Weiss SW, et al. Liposarcomas in young patients: a study of 82 cases occurring in patients younger than 22 years of age. Am J Surg Pathol 2009;33(5):645–58.
95. Huh WW, Yuen C, Munsell M, et al. Liposarcoma in children and young adults: a multi-institutional experience. Pediatr Blood Cancer 2011; 57(7):1142–6.
96. Antonescu CR, Elahi A, Healey JH, et al. Monoclonality of multifocal myxoid liposarcoma: confirmation by analysis of TLS-CHOP or EWS-CHOP rearrangements. Clin Cancer Res 2000;6(7):2788–93.

Benign Tumors of Smooth Muscle

CHAPTER CONTENTS

To a large extent, the distribution of benign smooth muscle tumors parallels the distribution of smooth muscle tissue in the body. The tumors tend to be relatively common in the genitourinary and gastrointestinal tracts, less frequent in the skin, and rare in deep soft tissue. In the experience of Farman,[1] based on 7748 leiomyomas, approximately 95% occurred in the female genital tract, and the remainder were scattered over various sites, including the skin (230 cases), gastrointestinal tract (67 cases), and bladder (5 cases). This study, based on surgical material, probably underestimates the large number of asymptomatic gastrointestinal and genitourinary lesions documented in autopsy material only. In general, soft tissue leiomyomas cause little morbidity; therefore, there are few studies in the literature concerning their presentation, diagnosis, and therapy. For purposes of classification, these tumors can be divided into several groups.

Cutaneous leiomyomas (leiomyoma cutis) comprise the most common group and are of two types. Those arising from the pilar arrector muscles of the skin are often multiple and associated with significant pain. Those arising from the network of muscle fibers that lie in the deep dermis of the scrotum (dartoic muscles), labia majora, and nipple are almost always solitary and are collectively referred to as *genital leiomyomas*. The second group of benign smooth muscle tumors includes the angiomyomas (vascular leiomyomas), which are distinctive, painful, subcutaneous tumors composed of a conglomerate of thick-walled vessels associated with smooth muscle tissue. They differ from cutaneous leiomyomas in their anatomic distribution, predominantly subcutaneous location, and predilection for women. The third group constitutes leiomyomas of deep soft tissue, lesions whose very existence has been questioned (see later section). Although recent studies provide reasonable evidence that soft tissue leiomyomas exist, they are, indeed, rare and should be diagnosed using the most stringent criteria only. Leiomyomatosis peritonealis disseminata can be conceptualized as a diffuse metaplastic response of the peritoneal surfaces in which multiple smooth muscle nodules form and may be confused with metastatic leiomyosarcoma because of its unusual growth pattern. Last, tumors of specialized genital stromal cell origin, including angiomyofibroblastoma, cellular angiofibroma, and aggressive angiomyxoma, are discussed in the chapter.

STRUCTURE AND FUNCTION OF SMOOTH MUSCLE CELLS

Smooth muscle cells are widely distributed throughout the body and contribute to the wall of the gastrointestinal, genitourinary, and respiratory tracts. They constitute the muscles of the skin, erectile muscles of the nipple and scrotum, and iris of the eye. Their characteristic arrangements in these organs determine the net effect of contraction. For instance, the circumferential arrangement in blood vessels results in a narrowing of the lumen during contraction, whereas contraction of the longitudinal and circumferential muscle layers in the gastrointestinal tract causes the propulsive peristaltic wave.

Smooth muscle cells are fusiform in shape and have centrally located cylindrical nuclei with round ends that develop deep indentations during contraction. The length of the muscle cell varies depending on the organ, achieving its greatest length in the gravid uterus, where it may measure as much as 0.5 mm. The cells are usually arranged in fascicles in which the nuclei are staggered so the tapered end of one cell lies in close association with the thick nuclear region of an adjacent cell. Typically, there are no connective tissue cells between individual muscle fibers, although a delicate basal lamina and small connective tissue fibers, presumably synthesized by the muscle cells,[2] can be seen as a thin periodic acid-Schiff-positive rim around individual cells in light microscopic preparations.

Ultrastructurally, the cells are characterized by clusters of mitochondria, rough endoplasmic reticulum, and free ribosomes, which occupy the zone immediately adjacent to the nucleus. The remainder of the cytoplasm (sarcoplasm) is filled with myofilaments oriented parallel to the long axis of the cell.[3-6] There are three types of filaments in the cell.[7-9] Thick myosin filaments (12 nm) are surrounded by seven to nine thin actin filaments (6 to 8 nm). Thick and thin filaments are aggregated into larger groups, or units, which correspond by light microscopy to linear myofibrils. In addition to the contractile proteins, intermediate filaments, measuring 10 nm and forming part of the cytoskeleton, are centered around the dense bodies or plaques, which are believed to be the smooth muscle analogue of the Z-band. The plasma membrane is dotted with tiny pinocytotic vesicles, and overlying the surface of the cell is a delicate basal lamina. Although the basal lamina separates individual cells, limited areas exist between cells in which the substance is lacking and in which the plasma membranes lie in close proximity, separated by a space of about 2 nm. This area, known as a *gap junction* or *nexus*, may allow the spread of electrical impulses between adjacent cells.

Smooth muscle cells display diversity in their content of contractile and intermediate filament proteins, depending on their location and function. It is useful to be aware of some of the regional variations when evaluating neoplasms. For example, the gamma isoform of muscle actin is present along with desmin in most smooth muscle cells, whereas, in vascular smooth muscle, the alpha isoform of muscle actin and vimentin predominates. Therefore, many smooth muscle tumors of vascular smooth origin may lack expression of desmin.

CUTANEOUS LEIOMYOMA (LEIOMYOMA CUTIS)

Superficial, or cutaneous, leiomyomas are of two types. Those arising from the pilar arrector muscles of the skin may be solitary or multifocal and are often associated with considerable pain and tenderness.[10-21] The other form, the genital leiomyoma, arises from the diffuse network of muscle in the deep dermis of the genital zones (e.g., scrotum, nipple, areola, vulva).[22-25] In the scrotum, leiomyomas arise from the dartoic muscles (dartoic leiomyoma) and, in the nipple, from the muscularis mamillae and areolae. This form is nearly always solitary and rarely causes significant pain.

Leiomyoma of Pilar Arrector Origin

Although formerly believed to be the more common form of cutaneous leiomyoma, leiomyomas of pilar arrector origin are probably far less common than previously thought and are probably outnumbered by those arising in genital sites. They may be solitary or multiple. Most develop during adolescence or early adult life, although occasional cases appear at birth or during early childhood. Some occur on a familial basis.[11,20] Recent evidence suggests that the majority of patients presenting with multiple cutaneous leiomyomas (MCL) have germline mutations of the fumarate hydratase gene, mapped to chromosome 1q43 and encoding an enzyme in the Krebs cycle.[26,27] This disease, known as MCL, also predisposes to early-onset uterine leiomyomas in women and to early-onset renal cell carcinoma of the collecting duct and papillary type in both men and women (hereditary leiomyomatosis and renal cell cancer, also referred to as *HLRCC*).[27] However, sporadic leiomyomas and leiomyosarcomas seemingly do not harbor somatic mutations of this gene very frequently.[28,29]

Typically, cutaneous leiomyomas develop as small brown-red to pearly discrete papules that, in the incipient stage, can be palpated more readily than they can be seen (Fig. 16-1). Eventually, they form nodules that coalesce into a fine linear pattern following a dermatome distribution. The extensor surfaces of the extremities are most often affected. The lesions often produce significant pain that can be triggered by exposure to cold. In one unusual case reported by Fisher and Helwig,[12] the patient claimed that strong emotions evoked pain in the lesions. It is not clear whether the pain produced by these tumors is the result of contraction of the muscle tissue or compression of nearby nerves by the tumors. Usually, the tumors grow slowly over a period of years, with new lesions forming as older lesions stabilize. The slowly progressive nature of the disease probably accounts for patients often seeking medical attention after a number of years.

Most pilar leiomyomas are 1 to 2 cm in diameter. They lie in the dermal connective tissue and are separated from the overlying atrophic epidermis by a grenz zone. The lesions are less well defined than are angiomyoma and blend in an irregular fashion with the surrounding dermal collagen and adjacent pilar muscle (Fig. 16-2). The central portions of the lesions are usually devoid of connective tissue and consist exclusively of packets or bundles of smooth muscle fibers. They usually intersect in an orderly fashion and often create the impression of hyperplasia or overgrowth of the pilar arrector muscle. The cells resemble normal smooth muscle cells, and myofibrils can

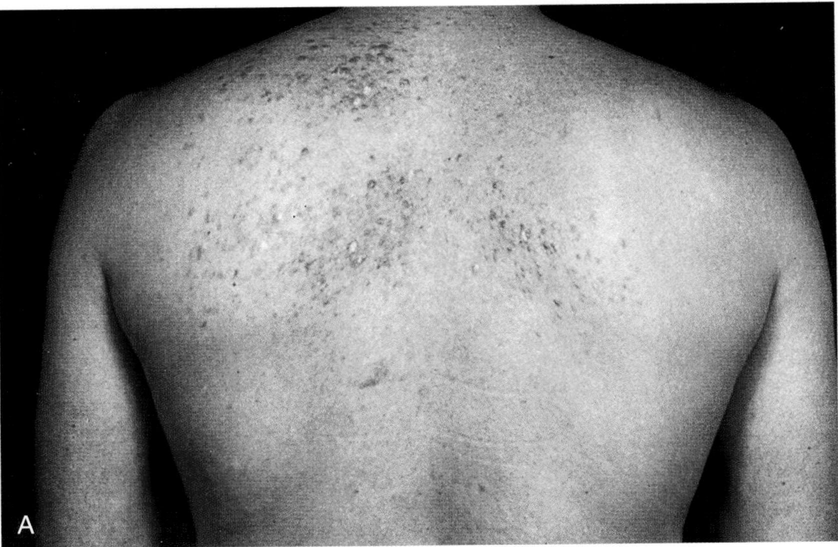

FIGURE 16-1. (A, B) Clinical appearance of multiple cutaneous leiomyomas. *Continued*

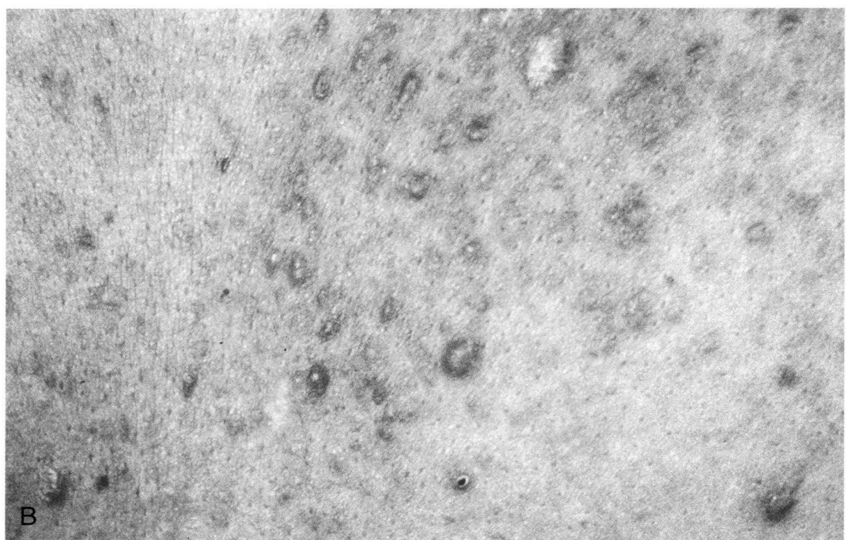

FIGURE 16-1, cont'd

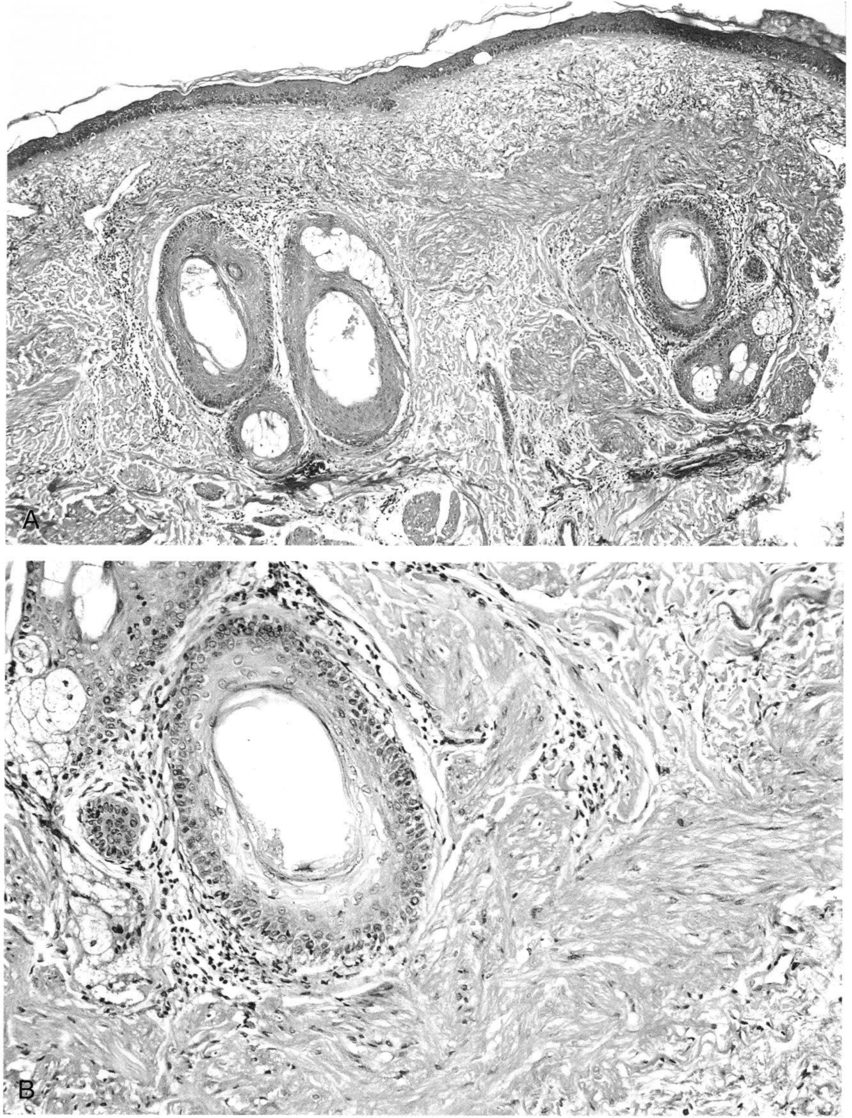

FIGURE 16-2. (A) Cutaneous leiomyoma of pilar arrector origin. (B) Smooth muscle bundles are closely associated with hair follicles and consist of well-differentiated, highly oriented cells.

be easily demonstrated with special stains, such as the Masson trichrome stain, in which they appear as red linear streaks traversing the cytoplasm in a longitudinal fashion. Muscle antigens, including actins, desmin and H-caldesmon are readily identified by immunohistochemistry (Fig. 16-3). Ultrastructurally, the cells have myofilaments, surface pinocytotic vesicles, and investing basal laminae.[17]

Diagnosis is rarely difficult in the typical case, particularly one with a characteristic history. Occasionally, solitary forms of the disease are mistaken for other benign tumors, such as cutaneous fibrous histiocytoma (dermatofibroma). The cells in fibrous histiocytoma are slender, less well ordered, and lack myofibrils. Secondary elements such as inflammatory cells, giant cells, and xanthoma cells, common to cutaneous fibrous histiocytomas, are lacking in cutaneous leiomyomas. Distinction of cutaneous leiomyomas from lesions reported as smooth muscle hamartomas of the skin is less clear-cut and may relate more to differences in clinical presentation than histologic features. Smooth muscle hamartomas are typically described as a single lesion measuring several centimeters in diameter and occurring in the lumbar region during childhood or early adult life.[19] Consisting of well-defined smooth muscle bundles in the dermis, these lesions are sometimes associated with hyperpigmentation and hypertrichosis (Becker nevus).[19] Because leiomyosarcomas also occur in the skin, care should be taken to ensure that neither atypia nor mitotic activity is encountered in a presumptive cutaneous leiomyoma. In this regard, it is not believed that atypia in dermal smooth muscle tumors is equivalent to atypia in uterine smooth muscle tumors, and that such lesions can be comfortably labeled "symplastic leiomyomas." Cutaneous smooth muscle tumors with significant atypia (even in the absence of mitotic activity) recur and progress over time, indicating that they should be considered leiomyosarcomas (see Chapter 17 for additional discussion).

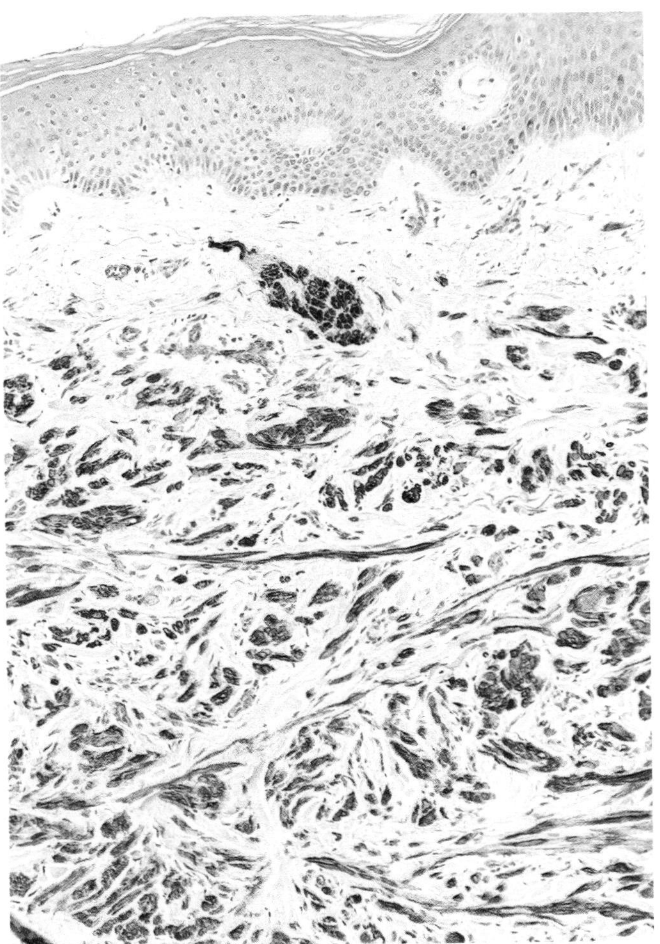

FIGURE 16-3. Actin immunostain of a cutaneous leiomyoma showing irregular packets and fascicles of spindle cells.

Cutaneous leiomyomas do not undergo malignant transformation; nonetheless, they may be difficult to treat. The lesions are often so numerous that total surgical excision is not possible. Laser therapy has been used with some success.

Genital Leiomyomas

Early studies based on referred consultations suggested that genital leiomyomas were far less common than those of pilar arrector origin.[12] Judging from more recent hospital-based series, genital leiomyomas may outnumber pilar ones by a margin of 2 to 1.[21] Affected sites include the areola of the nipple, scrotum, labium, penis, and vulva. The tumors are small, seldom exceeding 2 cm, and pain is not a prominent symptom. Histologically, genital leiomyomas, with the exception of the nipple lesions, differ from pilar leiomyomas in that they tend to be more circumscribed and more cellular, and they display a greater range of histologic appearances.[13] For example, Tavassoli and Norris,[25] in a review of 32 vulvar leiomyomas, noted myxoid change and an epithelioid phenotype of the cells, features not encountered in pilar leiomyomas.

ANGIOMYOMA (VASCULAR LEIOMYOMA)

Angiomyoma, a solitary form of leiomyoma that usually occurs in the subcutis, is composed of numerous thick-walled vessels. In the early literature, little attempt was made to distinguish these lesions from cutaneous leiomyomas, and the two were collectively termed *tuberculum dolorosum* because of their pain-producing properties.[30-36] Stout[30] later designated them vascular leiomyomas to contrast them with cutaneous leiomyoma, which has inconspicuous thin-walled vessels. These lesions account for about 5% of all benign soft tissue tumors[31] and one-fourth to one-half of all superficial leiomyomas. They occur more frequently in women,[32] except for those in the oral cavity where the reverse is true.[33] Unlike cutaneous leiomyomas, these tumors develop later in life, usually between the fourth and sixth decades, as solitary lesions.[31,32] They occur preferentially on the extremities, particularly the lower leg. In the series reported by Hachisuga et al.,[31] 375 of 562 occurred in the lower extremity, 125 on the upper extremity, 48 on the head, and 14 on the trunk. Most were less than 2 cm in diameter.

Affected patients complain most often of a small, slowly enlarging mass usually of several years' duration. Pain is a prominent feature in about half of the patients,[34] and, in some cases, it is exacerbated by pressure, change in temperature, pregnancy,[32] or menses.[34] The prevalence of pain has led some to suggest that these tumors are probably derived from arteriovenous anastomoses, similar to the glomus tumor.[35] However, they differ in appearance from the glomus tumor and are almost never encountered in a subungual location. The tumors are usually located in the subcutis and less often in the deep dermis, where they produce overlying elevations of the skin but without surface changes of the epidermis. Grossly, the tumors are circumscribed, glistening, white-gray nodules. Occasionally, they are blue or red, and rarely calcium flecks are visible grossly. The leiomyomas that visibly contract or writhe when touched or surgically manipulated are probably of this type.

Microscopically, the tumors have a characteristic appearance that varies little from case to case. The usual appearance is of a well-demarcated nodule of smooth muscle tissue punctuated with thick-walled vessels with partially patent lumens (Figs. 16-4 and 16-5). Typically, the inner layers of smooth muscle of the vessel are arranged in an orderly circumferential fashion, and the outer layers spin or swirl away from the vessel, merging with the less well-ordered peripheral muscle fibers. The morphological features of angiomyoma overlap to a degree with those of myopericytoma, and the distinction between these two entities may at times be quite subjective (see Perivascular Tumors, Chapter 25). Areas of myxoid change (Fig. 16-6), hyalinization, calcification, and fat may be seen. The vessels in these tumors are difficult to classify because they are not altogether typical of veins or arteries. Their thick walls and small lumens are reminiscent of arteries, but they consistently lack internal and external elastic laminae. In the experience of Hachisuga et al.,[31] a small number of angiomyomas are composed of predominantly cavernous-type vessels. Nerve fibers are usually difficult to demonstrate but undoubtedly are present, accounting for the exquisite sensitivity of these lesions to manipulation. Rarely, angiomyomas display degenerative nuclear atypia similar to that seen in symplastic leiomyomas.[36] Angiomyoma is a benign tumor, causing few problems apart from pain. Simple excision is adequate. None of the patients reported by Duhig and Ayer[32] developed recurrence following excision. In the series of Hachisuga et al.,[31] only two patients had a recurrence, although their follow-up data were incomplete.

LEIOMYOMA OF DEEP SOFT TISSUE

Unequivocal leiomyomas of deep soft tissue are exceptionally rare compared to their malignant counterpart, and, until recently, there has been no consensus as to how one separated soft tissue leiomyomas from leiomyosarcomas. In fact, the observation that some tumors that were initially labeled "leiomyoma" ultimately proved to be malignant enhanced the

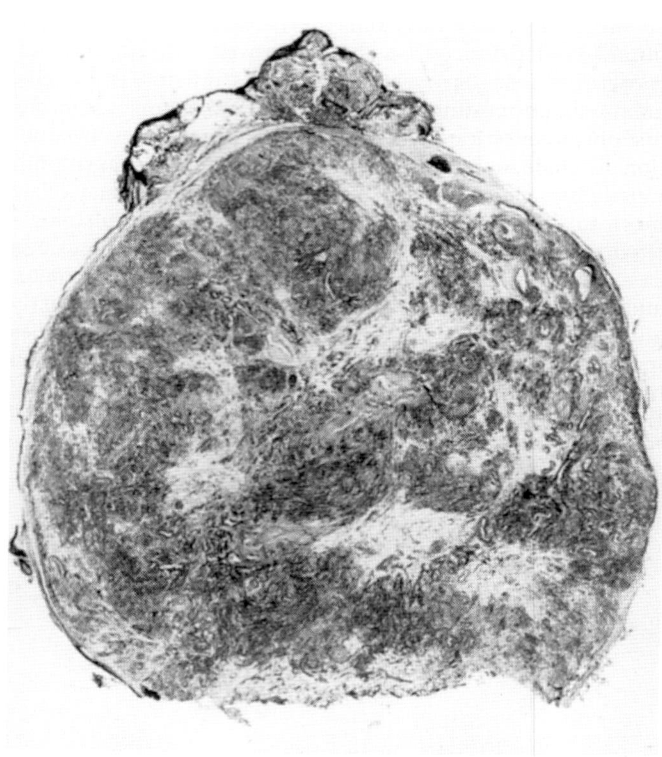

FIGURE 16-4. Angiomyoma of subcutaneous tissue. Congeries of thick-walled vessels constitute a major portion of the lesion and blend with surrounding smooth muscle tissue and focal myxoid stroma (Masson trichrome strain).

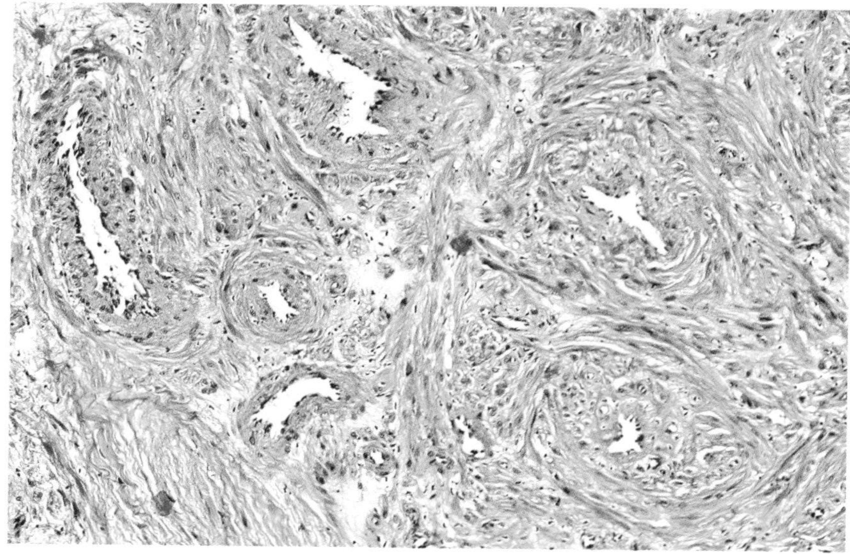

FIGURE 16-5. Thick-walled vessel of an angiomyoma. Inner layer of muscle is usually arranged circumferentially, and outer layer blends with less well-ordered smooth muscle tissue of tumors.

impression that it was nearly impossible to establish a minimum threshold for malignancy, leading inevitably to the conclusion that all smooth muscle tumors of deep soft tissue should be considered malignant.[37,38] Recent studies have presented convincing evidence that leiomyomas of deep soft tissue exist but are rare and should be diagnosed using strict criteria derived empirically from the evaluation of soft tissue smooth muscle tumors.[39-42] Soft tissue leiomyomas are of two distinct types (somatic and gynecologic) that differ in their clinical presentation and in the criteria of malignancy.

The less common somatic leiomyoma arises in the deep somatic soft tissue of the extremities and affects the sexes equally.[39] Measuring several centimeters at the time of presentation, about one-third also contain calcification (Fig. 16-7), probably a reflection of long duration and a feature that occasionally leads to a number of radiologic diagnoses, including "calcifying schwannoma," "synovial sarcoma," or "myositis ossificans." Histologically, these lesions are composed of fascicles of well-differentiated smooth muscle cells with abundant eosinophilic cytoplasm similar to vascular smooth muscle (Figs. 16-8 to 16-10). Rarely, somatic leiomyomas may have a predominantly clear cell appearance or display psammoma bodies (Figs. 16-11 and 16-12).

By definition, somatic leiomyomas should harbor no necrosis, at most mild atypia, and virtually no mitotic activity (less than 1 mitoses/50 high-power fields [HPF]). The number of somatic leiomyomas with extended follow-up information is still quite small but in the largest series reported by Billings et al.,[39] all 11 patients were alive and well from 5 to 97 months (median 67 months) after diagnosis.

The more common leiomyoma of gynecologic (or uterine) type occurs almost exclusively in women, usually in the perimenopausal period. They are situated predominantly in the pelvic retroperitoneum, although other peritoneal sites may be affected.[39,40] Benign-appearing inguinal smooth muscle tumors in women also appear to be of gynecologic (Mullerian) origin.[43] Although in the past, some of these lesions have undoubtedly been interpreted as autoamputated uterine leiomyomas, recent experience showing origin at sites clearly distinct from the uterus or in women without uterine fibroids suggests that they are more likely *de novo* soft tissue lesions.

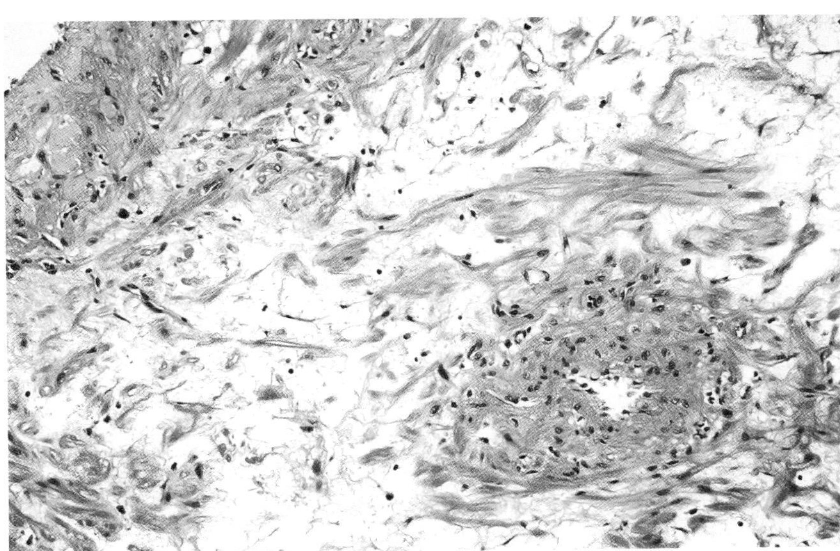

FIGURE 16-6. Focal myxoid change in an angiomyoma.

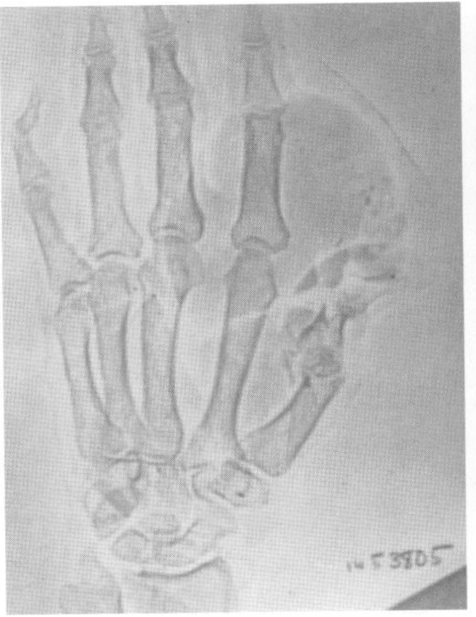

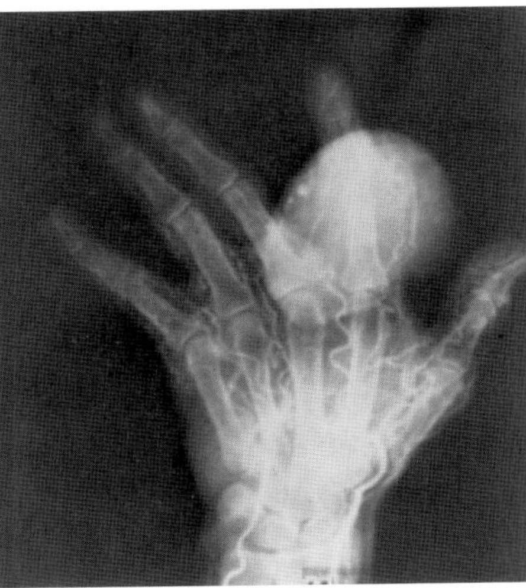

FIGURE 16-7. Radiograph showing calcification of a soft tissue leiomyoma.

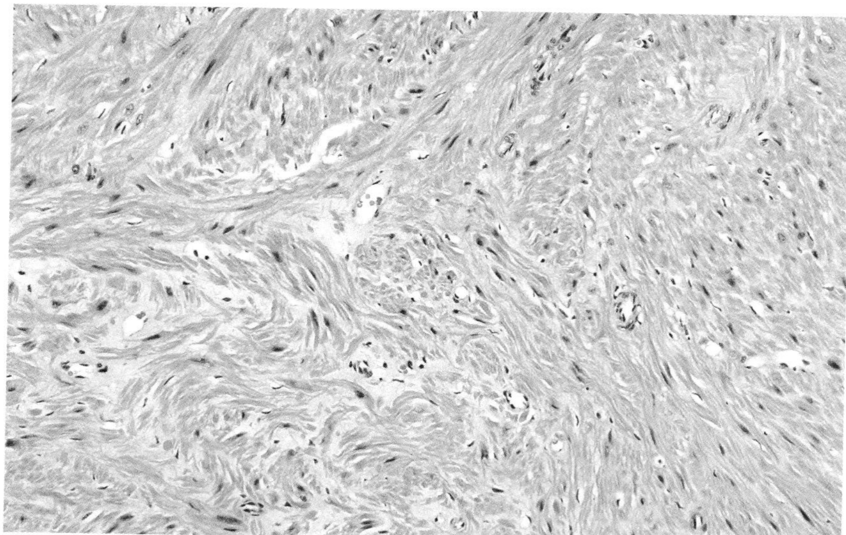

FIGURE 16-8. Somatic leiomyoma of deep soft tissue. Fascicles of smooth muscle tend to be less well oriented than in cutaneous leiomyomas.

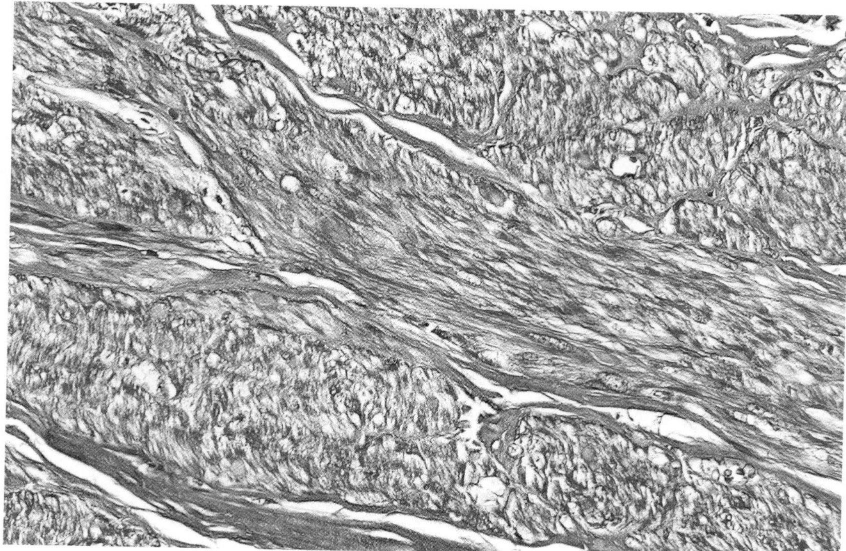

FIGURE 16-9. Masson trichrome stain of a deep leiomyoma. Cells are deeply fuchsinophilic with linear striations.

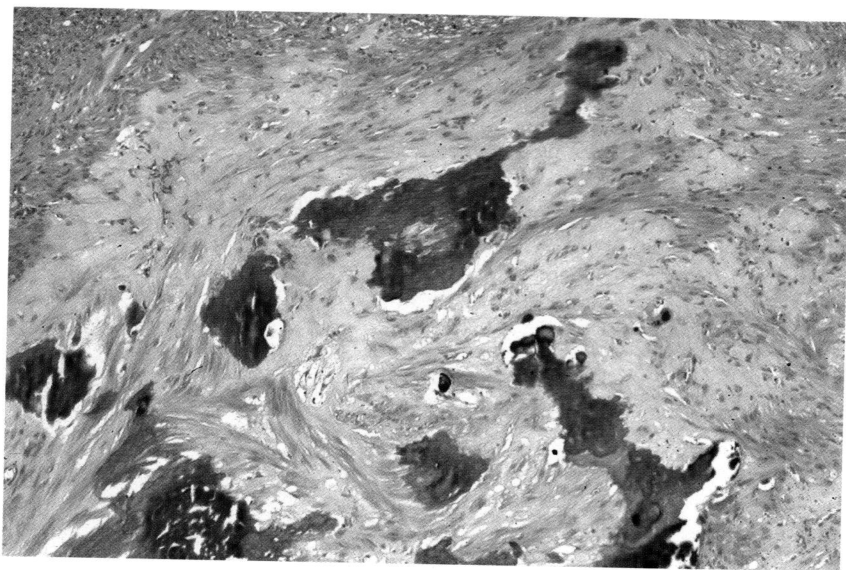

FIGURE 16-10. Somatic leiomyoma of soft tissue with calcification.

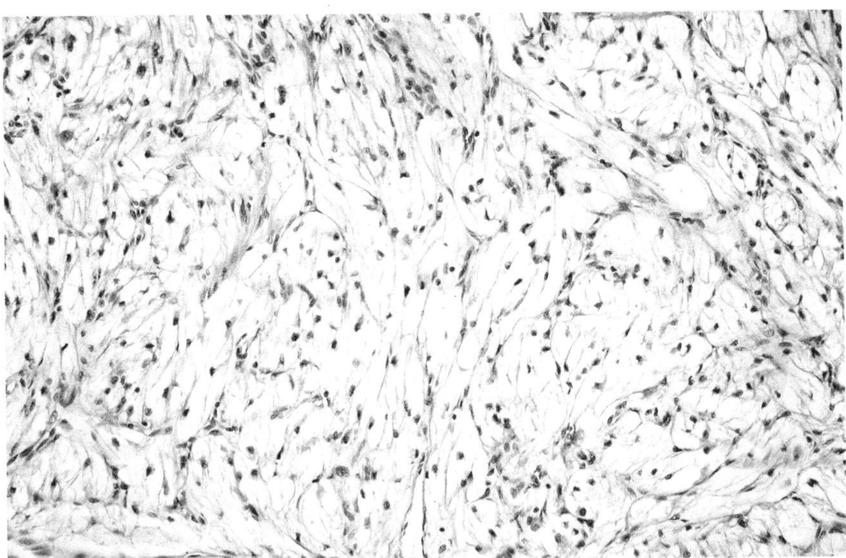

FIGURE 16-11. Clear-cell change of the cytoplasm in a somatic leiomyoma of soft tissue.

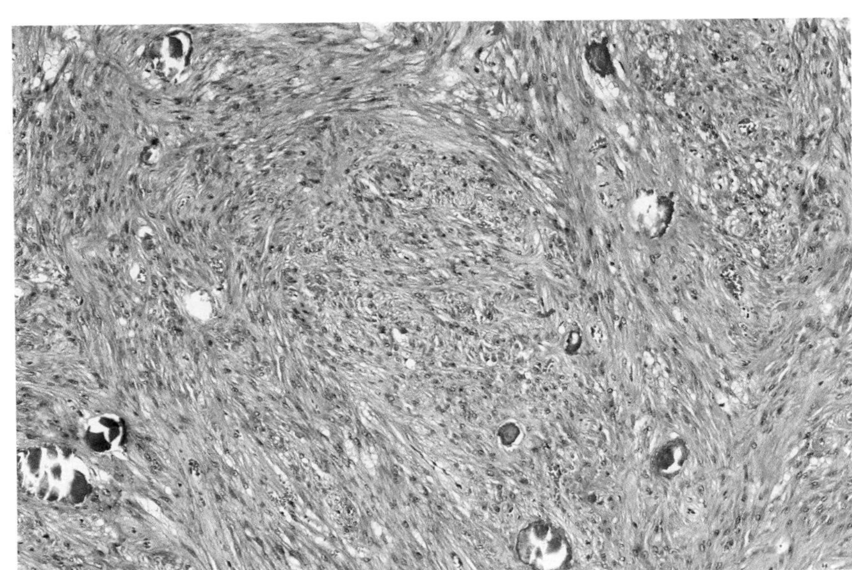

FIGURE 16-12. Somatic leiomyoma with psammomatous calcification.

Grossly and histologically, they bear an unmistakable similarity to uterine leiomyomas, thereby accounting for the term *leiomyoma of gynecologic type* (Figs. 16-13 to 16-17). Grossly, they are well circumscribed, gray-white lesions that range greatly in size from a few centimeters to more than 10 cm and consist of intersecting fascicles of slender-tapered smooth muscle cells with less cytoplasm than their somatic counterparts. The stroma contains vessels often with striking mural hyalinization (see Fig. 16-13). Other features of uterine leiomyomas are also encountered, such as hydropic (see Fig. 16-14) and myxoid change, hyaline necrosis, and an epithelioid or cord-like arrangement of the cells (see Fig. 16-16). Fatty change is quite common (see Fig. 16-17) and has led to the use of alternative terms (e.g., lipoleiomyoma, myolipoma).[44,45]

Unlike somatic leiomyomas, gynecologic leiomyomas typically display both nuclear estrogen and progesterone receptor protein (Fig. 16-18), suggesting that they arise from hormonally sensitive smooth muscle of the retroperitoneum. Not surprisingly, the criteria of malignancy for evaluating this group of lesions seem to approximate those used for uterine lesions (see later section). Although, by definition, neither necrosis nor more than mild atypia should be allowed in making this diagnosis, mitotic activity occurs frequently and does not seem to imply any adverse outcome. In two large studies, mitotic activity of 5/10 HPF was encountered in about one-quarter of cases with no observed adverse event. Although higher levels of mitotic activity may still be compatible with a benign diagnosis, the experience with such lesions is limited and they are best labeled as "uncertain malignant potential" until further data are accrued (Fig. 16-19). Given the similarity to uterine lesions, the question might also be raised as to whether there is a soft tissue analogue to a symplastic leiomyoma of the uterus (Fig. 16-20). Regrettably, there is no published information on this point. Until this time, it is recommended that such lesions be considered of uncertain

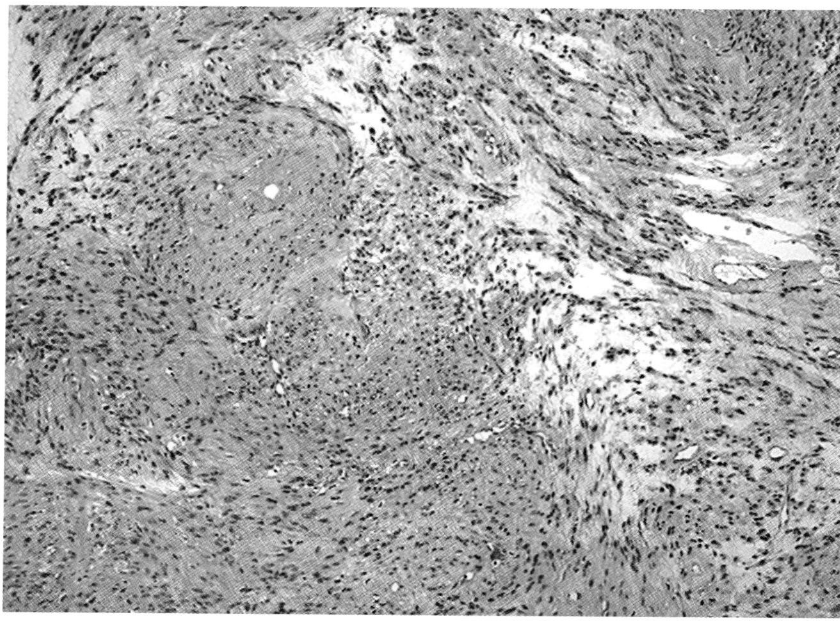

FIGURE 16-13. Gynecologic-type leiomyoma. Note prominent vessels and hyalinization.

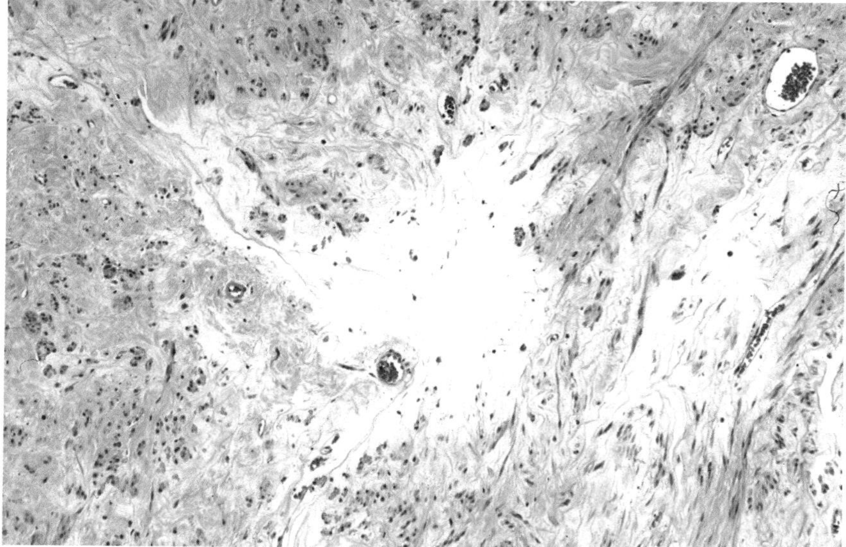

FIGURE 16-14. Gynecologic-type leiomyoma with hydropic change.

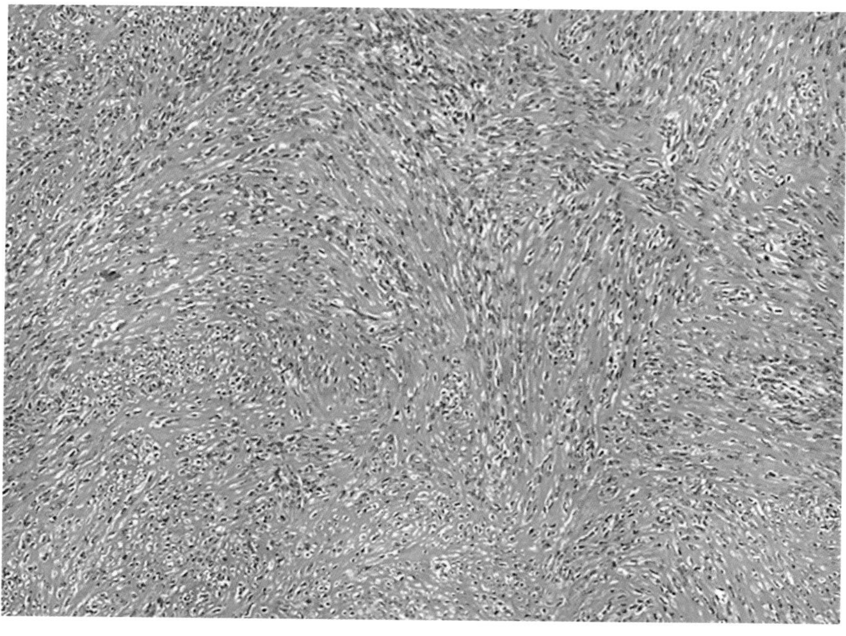

FIGURE 16-15. Prominent hyalinization within gynecologic-type leiomyoma.

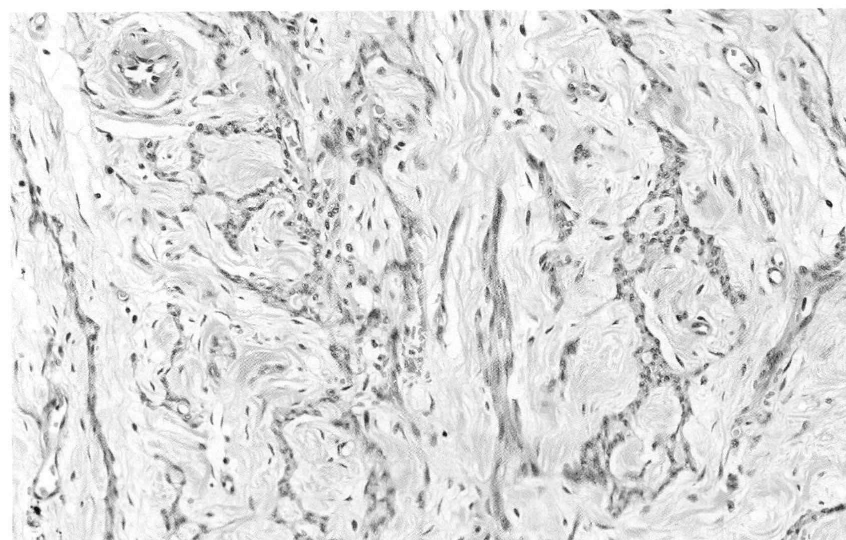

FIGURE 16-16. Gynecologic leiomyoma with cord-like arrangement of cells.

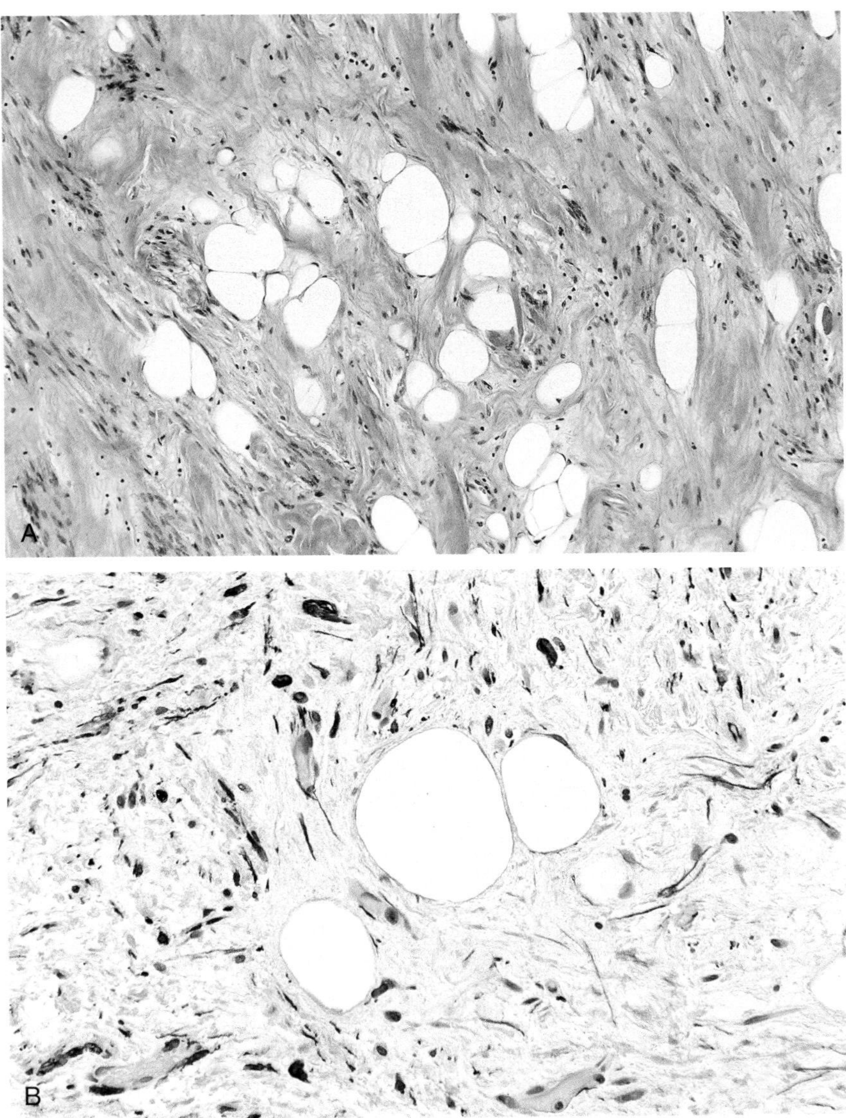

FIGURE 16-17. Leiomyoma with fat (myolipoma) (A). Desmin immunostain illustrates muscle cells between adipocytes (B).

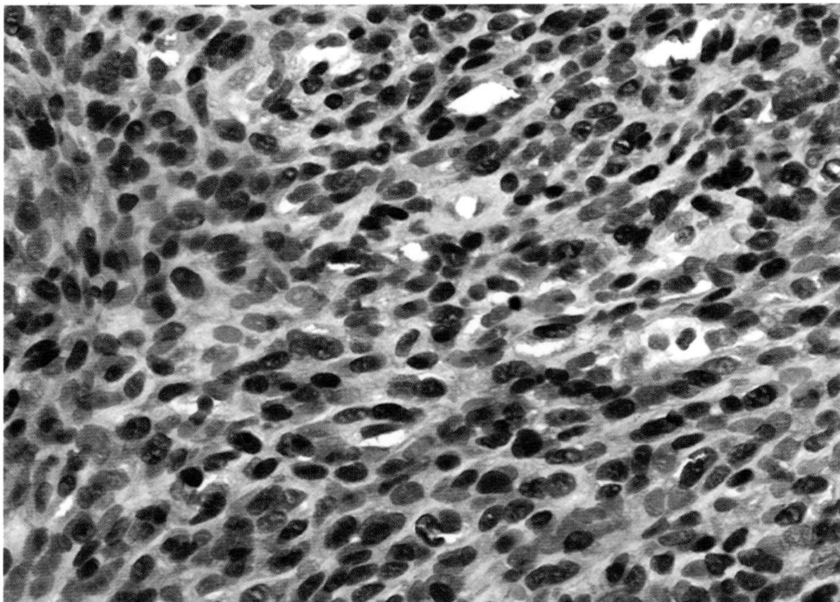

FIGURE 16-18. Estrogen receptor protein staining in gynecologic leiomyoma of retroperitoneum.

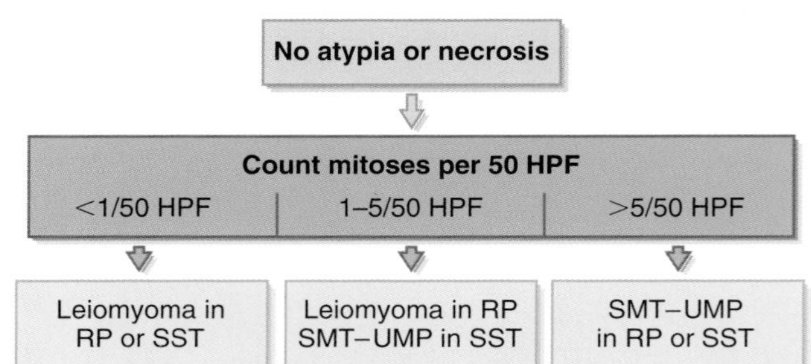

FIGURE 16-19. A schematic diagram showing the approach to an evaluation of differentiated smooth muscle tumors of soft tissue. (HPF, high-power field; RP, retroperitoneum; SST, somatic soft tissue; SMT, smooth muscle tumor; UMP, uncertain malignant potential.)

malignant potential. These criteria of benignancy have been validated in two recent large studies. Of the 54 patients reported collectively by Billings et al.[39] and Paal and Miettinen,[40] 20% experienced local recurrence, but no metastasis within an average follow-up period of 42 months in the former study and 142 months in the latter. Finally, even though hormone receptor proteins are characteristic of soft tissue leiomyomas of the gynecologic type, they may be expressed in leiomyosarcomas from women. Therefore, identification of positive receptor status in a deep smooth muscle tumor does not per se identify it as a leiomyoma; that feature should be assessed in the context of traditional histologic features.

LEIOMYOMATOSIS PERITONEALIS DISSEMINATA

Leiomyomatosis peritonealis disseminata is a rare condition in which multiple smooth muscle or smooth muscle-like nodules develop in a subperitoneal location throughout the abdominal cavity. The lesion occurs exclusively in women, usually during the childbearing years. Most cases reported in the United States have been in African-American women. More than half have occurred in pregnant women. Others have occurred in women taking oral contraceptives, and one patient had a functioning ovarian tumor.[46] These observations and that the lesion regresses following pregnancy[47] provide circumstantial evidence for the involvement of hormonal factors in its pathogenesis. The rarity of the condition suggests that other unknown factors must also be contributory. In most instances, leiomyomatosis is discovered incidentally at the time of surgery for other medical or obstetric conditions, although vague abdominal pain is often an accompanying symptom.

Grossly, the disease has an alarming appearance. The peritoneal surfaces, including the surfaces of the bowel, urinary bladder, and uterus, are studded with firm white-gray nodules of varying size (Fig. 16-21). The smallest nodules may be only a few millimeters in diameter whereas the largest are several centimeters. Although the diffuseness of the process initially suggests an intra-abdominal malignancy, the lesions lack hemorrhage and necrosis. Moreover, they do not violate the parenchyma of the affected organs, and they are not found in extra-abdominal sites, such as the lung or in lymph nodes. Leiomyomas of the uterus have been identified in some, but not all, cases of leiomyomatosis, indicating that the lesions do not represent localized spread of an intrauterine lesion.

Microscopic Findings

Although the term *leiomyomatosis* indicates the similarity to normal smooth muscle and to benign leiomyomas, reports in the literature coupled with cases reviewed at the Armed Forces Institute of Pathology, also known as AFIP,[48] suggest that there is a range of histologic changes perhaps not fully appreciated when the term was coined. In the classic case, the earliest nodules develop as microscopic foci of proliferating smooth

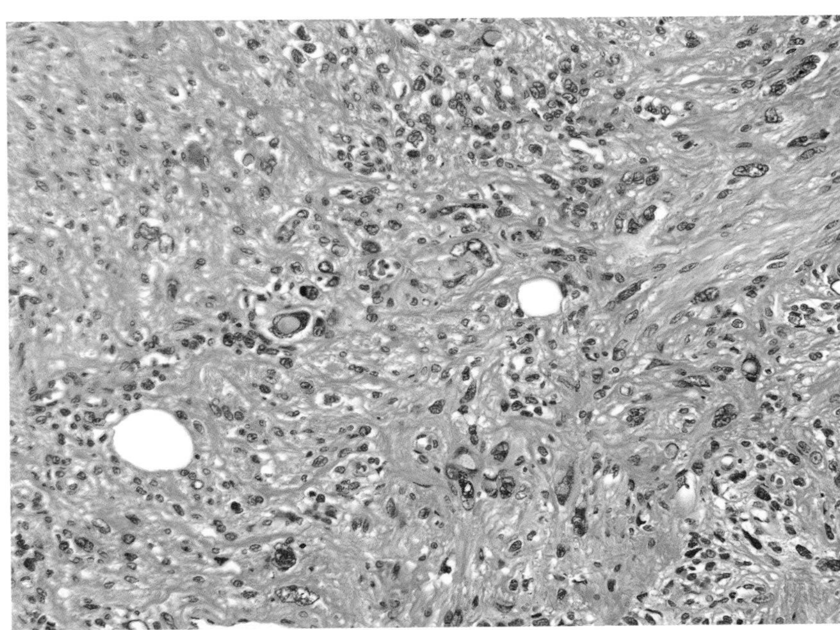

FIGURE 16-20. Localized area of atypia within an otherwise typical gynecologic-type leiomyoma. Whether these should be regarded as the equivalent to symplastic leiomyomas of uterus is uncertain.

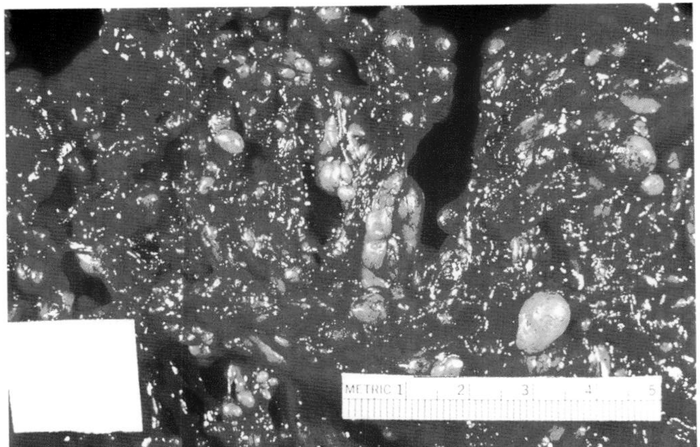

FIGURE 16-21. Gross appearance of leiomyomatosis peritonealis disseminata.

muscle immediately subjacent to the peritoneum (Figs. 16-22 to 16-25). With progressive growth, they may remain nodular or may, in addition, dissect through the underlying soft tissue in a more permeative fashion. The slender cells are arranged in close, compact fascicles oriented perpendicular to each other. The cells may show a minimal degree of nuclear pleomorphism that falls far short of that seen in leiomyosarcoma. Mitotic figures may be seen, but they are infrequent. In some cases, endometriosis has been present in the smooth muscle nodules.[49,50]

In a significant number of cases, the histologic appearance of these subperitoneal nodules is more fibroblastic or myofibroblastic. Cases of this type have been described by Parmley et al.,[51] Winn et al.,[52] and Pieslor et al.[53] The proliferating cell is usually large, has plump eosinophilic cytoplasm, and is usually not arranged in well-defined fascicles. Round decidual cells with an eosinophilic or foamy cytoplasm are usually scattered amid the spindled cells, and, at times, it is impossible to delimit these cells clearly from spindle cells by light microscopy. In these cases, the cells lack distinct longitudinal striations, as are seen in the foregoing type. Hyalinization of the nodules is seen in cases of regressing or regressed leiomyomatosis (see Fig. 16-25). The one case in the literature allegedly representing lipomatous differentiation in the cells is dubious, judging from the photomicrographs.[54] Glandular inclusions or sex cord-like structures may be seen infrequently in these lesions.[55,56]

Ultrastructural Findings

In view of the range of changes observed by light microscopy, it is not surprising that electron microscopy has produced conflicting reports regarding the histogenesis of this condition. In the studies of Nogales et al.,[57] Kuo et al.,[58] and Goldberg et al.,[59] most of the cells resembled mature smooth muscle cells and had an investiture of basal lamina, surface-oriented pinocytotic vesicles, and abundant longitudinally oriented myofilaments. In contrast, Parmley et al.[51] and Winn et al.[52] believed that the predominant cells were fibroblastic and, based on the close relation with the decidual cells, suggested that leiomyomatosis is a reparative fibrosis occurring in a preexisting decidual reaction (fibrosing deciduosis). Others have documented a variety of cell types, including fibroblasts, myofibroblasts, and smooth muscle cells[53] and suggested a close interrelation of all three.[48] The theory that leiomyomatosis represents metaplasia or differentiation of pluripotential cells of the serosa or subserosal tissue along several closely related cell lines is supported by the experimental work of Fujii et al.[60] Estrogen administered to guinea pigs induces peritoneal nodules similar to those of leiomyomatosis peritonealis. These nodules are composed of fibroblasts and myofibroblasts in animals receiving estrogen only, whereas smooth muscle differentiation and decidualization occur if estrogen plus progesterone are administered.

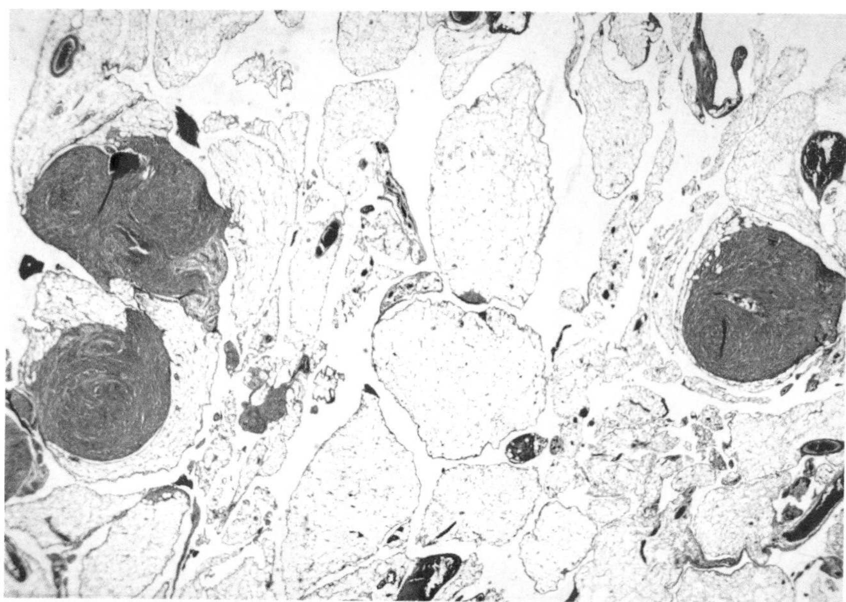

FIGURE 16-22. Leiomyomatosis peritonealis disseminata with numerous smooth muscle nodules of varying size arising underneath the peritoneal surface and involving underlying fat. Early nodules are present as microscopic foci.

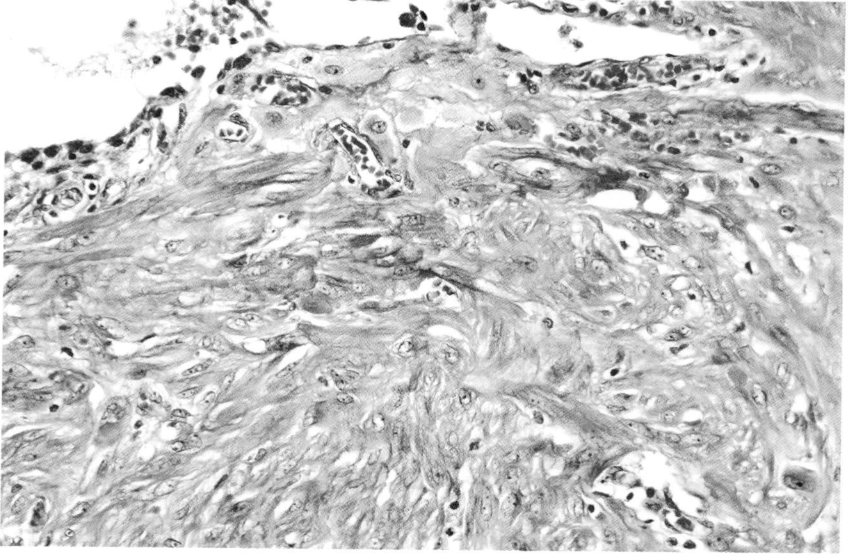

FIGURE 16-23. Subperitoneal nodule of leiomyomatosis peritonealis disseminata with decidualization.

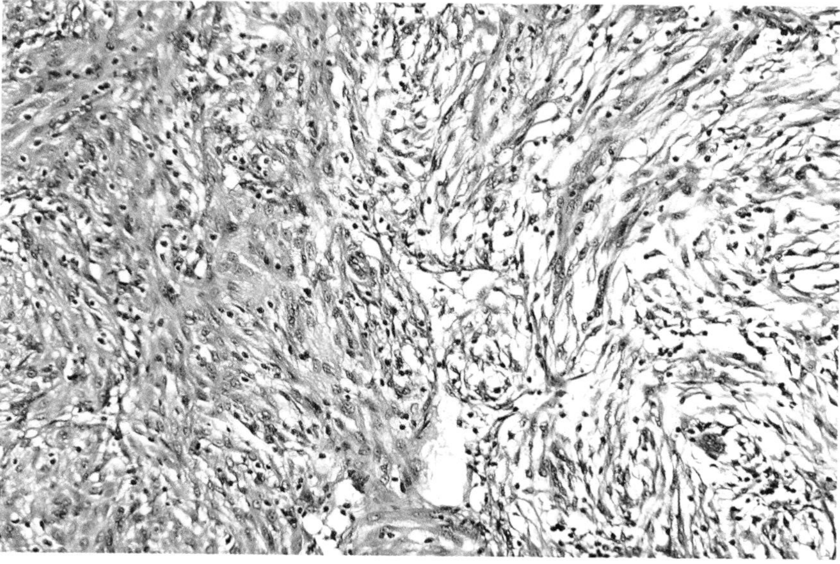

FIGURE 16-24. Leiomyomatosis peritonealis disseminata with a myofibroblastic appearance.

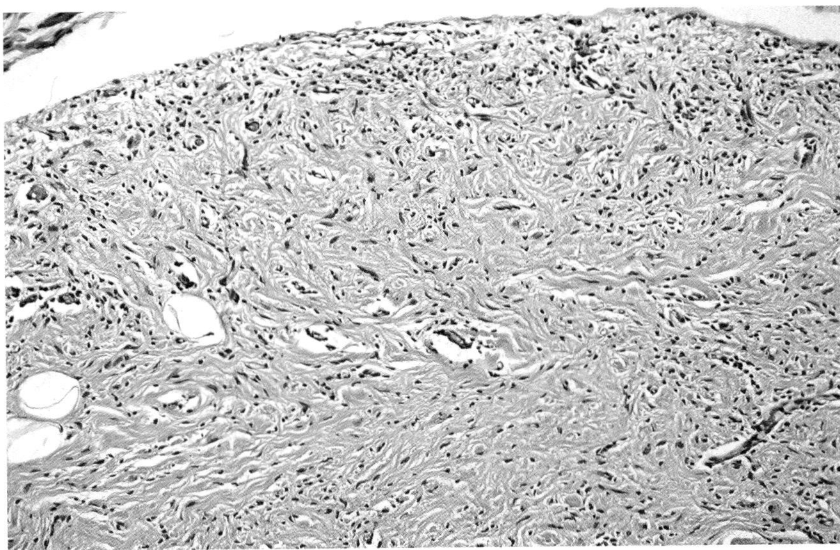

FIGURE 16-25. End-stage of leiomyomatosis peritonealis disseminata with extensive interstitial fibrosis.

Behavior and Treatment

In view of the benign nature of this condition, no particular therapy is warranted when the diagnosis has been firmly secured. In fact, there seems to be some evidence that the lesions regress following pregnancy or removal of the estrogenic source,[53] although with subsequent pregnancy, progression or recrudescence occurs.[50] The case reported by Aterman et al.[61] documented partial regression of lesions 5 months after the initial surgery without any intervening therapy and regression of another lesion within 12 weeks.[62] Gonadotropin-releasing hormone antagonists (e.g., leuprolide acetate) and megestrol acetate[63] have been used with some success to treat this disease.[64] There have been a few cases purporting to show malignant degeneration of the condition. The cases reported by Akkersdijk et al.[65] and Abulafia et al.[66] are scantily illustrated, and autopsies were not performed in either case. The case reported by Rubin et al.[67] is better documented.

In the past, leiomyomatosis peritonealis disseminata was regarded as a diffuse metaplastic process of the peritoneum. Quade et al.,[62] however, demonstrated clonality of multiple lesions in a given patient by assessing X-linked inactivation of the androgen receptor gene with the human androgen receptor assay (also known as HUMARA).[62] Although the authors believed that this indicated metastasis from a unicentric disease, they were careful to point out that their data were also consistent with multicentric clones selected for an X-linked gene.

BENIGN GENITAL STROMAL TUMORS

A number of benign mesenchymal tumors arising from or differentiating along the lines of specialized stroma of the female genital tract has been reported over the last two decades. This family of lesions includes angiomyofibroblastoma,[68] cellular angiofibroma,[69] angiomyofibroblastoma of male genital tract,[70] angiomyxoma, and superficial cervicovaginal myofibroblastoma.[71] They are closely related lesions as evidenced by their overlapping histologic and immunophenotypic features. Even among experts, distinction of these lesions may not be clear cut. For example, the lesion reported by Laskin et al.[70] as "angiomyofibroblastoma-like tumor of male genital tract" and regarded as a hybrid between classic angiomyofibroblastoma and spindle cell lipoma was described by Fletcher et al.[68] as "cellular angiofibroma." Although efforts are made to use the appropriate labels in typical cases, the term *benign genital stromal tumor* has been found to be very useful for hybrid or ambiguous cases, especially because these various distinctions have little clinical or biologic import.

Angiomyofibroblastoma

Angiomyofibroblastoma is a distinctive tumor that usually involves the vulva[68,69,72-75] but can involve the vagina and, rarely, the scrotum. These tumors develop as slowly growing, marginated masses in the subcutaneous tissues. Because of their preferential location on the vulva, they may be confused with a Bartholin cyst. The tumors contain prominent, sometimes ectatic vessels, surrounded by clusters of eosinophilic epithelioid cells, some of which blend or fan out from the muscular walls of the vessels. The prominence of the eosinophilic cytoplasm has lead to the term *plasmacytoid* for these distinctive cells that lie in small chains, cords, or singly in a matrix that varies from myxoid to hyaline (Figs. 16-26 and 16-27). In some cases, the cells spindle, and, in others, they separate from the stroma, creating pseudovascular spaces (Figs. 16-28 and 16-29). Lesions having a spindled appearance closely resemble cellular angiofibroma. Mature fat is occasionally encountered and, when prominent, has led to the proposed term *lipomatous variant of angiomyofibroblastoma*.[76] Immunohistochemically, the cells of angiomyofibroblastoma express vimentin, desmin, and hormone receptor proteins but usually not actin or CD34. Recently, fibroblast growth factor, vascular endothelial growth factor, and stem cell factor have been identified in the neoplastic cells.

The overwhelming majority of angiomyofibroblastomas are benign with recurrences occurring in those that are

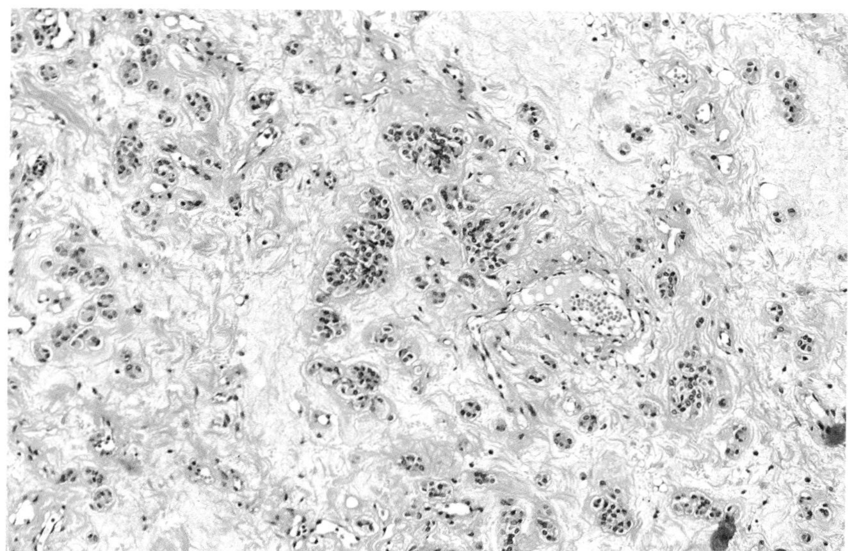

FIGURE 16-26. Angiomyofibroblastoma of the vulva.

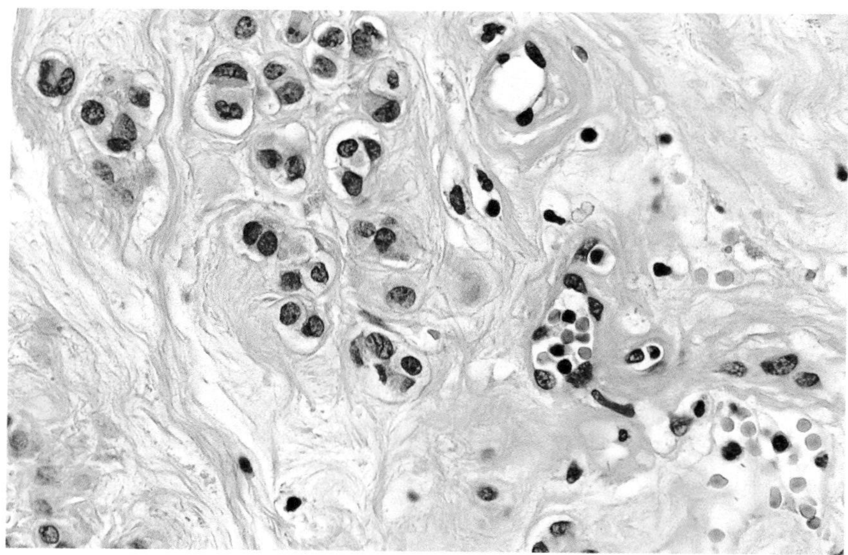

FIGURE 16-27. Epithelioid cells in an angiomyofibroblastoma.

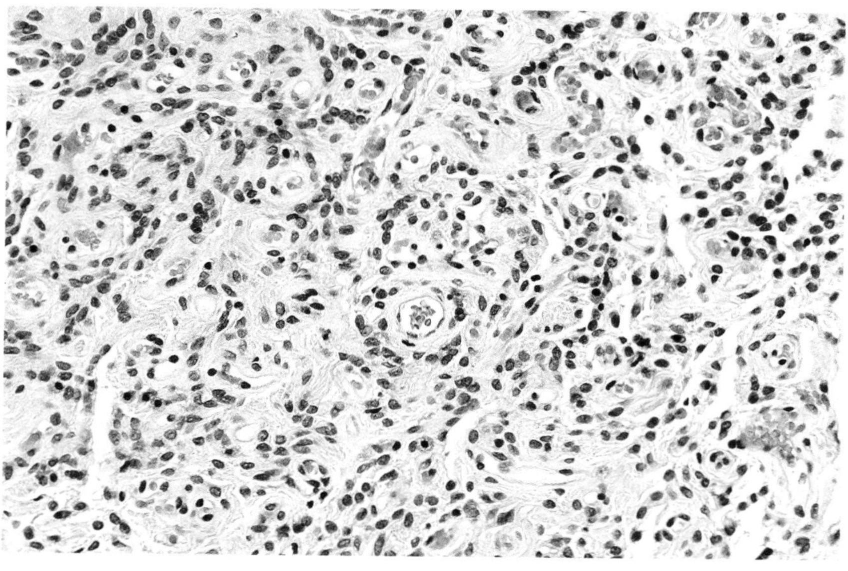

FIGURE 16-28. Angiomyofibroblastoma with more cellularity and spindling than is seen in Figure 16-38.

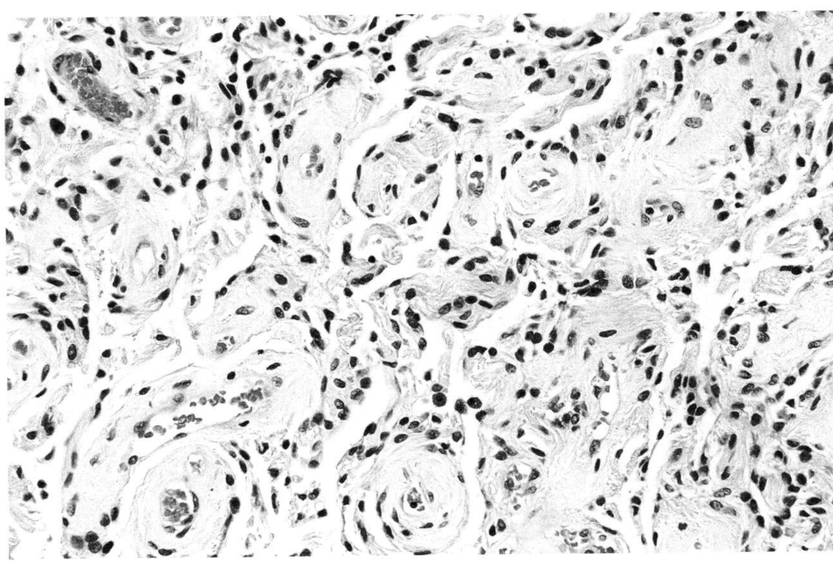

FIGURE 16-29. Pseudovascular spaces in an angiomyofibroblastoma.

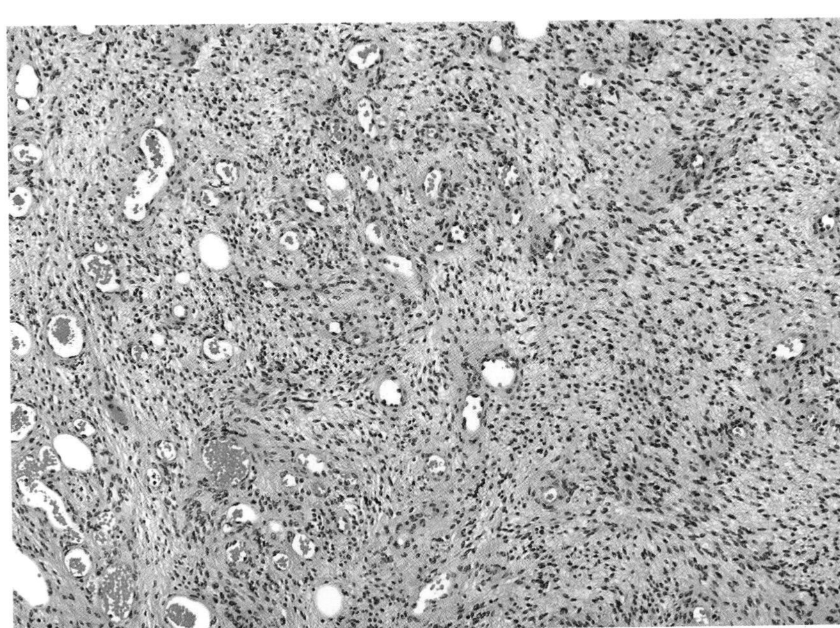

FIGURE 16-30. Cellular angiofibroma.

less marginated and, therefore, difficult to excise. Histologically malignant forms of angiomyofibroblastoma have been reported.[77,78] These tumors may either resemble an angiomyofibroblastoma, except that the cells possess marked atypia and mitotic activity, or they may assume a totally different appearance with areas resembling a leiomyosarcoma or undifferentiated sarcoma similar in nature to dedifferentiation in other mesenchymal tumors. None of these rare malignant tumors has metastasized to date, possibly as a result of their superficiality and ease of resection.

Cellular Angiofibroma (Angiomyofibroblastoma-Like Tumor of the Male Genital Tract)

Cellular angiofibroma was initially described in 1997 and later in a more extended form by Iwasa and Fletcher[79] in a series of 51 cases. As intimated previously, the lesion referred to as *angiomyofibroblastoma of the male genital tract*[79] is considered a similar, if not identical, tumor. Cellular angiofibroma occurs almost exclusively in the vulvovaginal region of women or in the inguinal–scrotal region of males. Unlike angiomyofibroblastoma, which is seen nearly exclusively in women, this lesion affects the sexes in roughly equal proportion and presents as a circumscribed dermal or subcutaneous tumor measuring a few centimeters in diameter. The lesions consist of two components, a cellular spindle cell component arranged randomly or in short fascicles, vague palisades, or swirls around a prominent vasculature (Figs. 16-30 and 16-31). The cells are either spindled or fusiform in shape with bland cytologic features and usually low mitotic activity (less than 1/10 HPF). The stroma contains evenly dispersed small-to-medium-sized vessels with mural hyalinization and delicate pale collagen interspersed with short, thicker ones. As in angiomyofibroblastoma, mature fat is seen in about one-quarter of

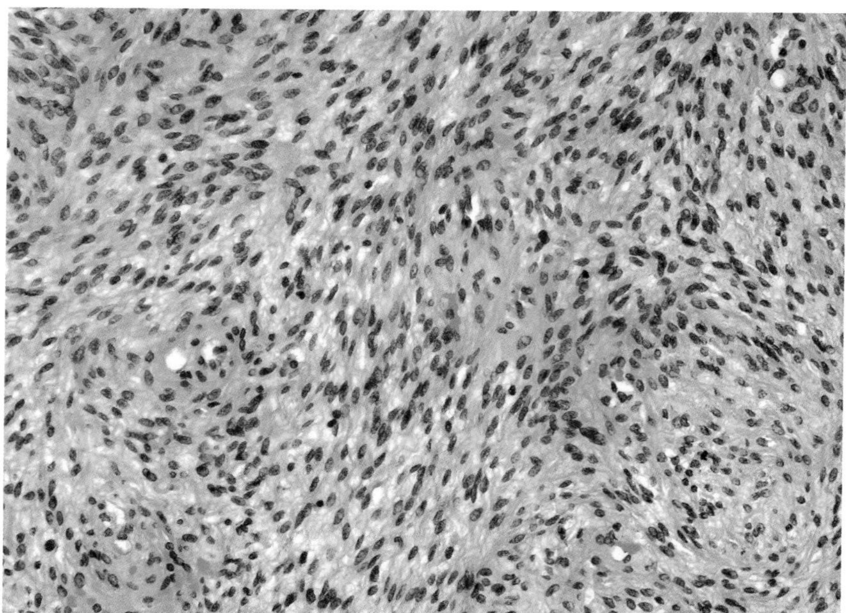

FIGURE 16-31. Cellular angiofibroma.

cases. The morphologic, immunophenotypic, and genetic features (e.g., abnormalities in 13q14, the *Rb* locus) of cellular angiofibroma overlap significantly with those of spindle cell lipoma and mammary-type myofibroblastoma. Also, it is likely that these represent different manifestations of a single entity.[80] As in angiomyofibroblastoma, a small number of cellular angiofibromas have been reported to show atypical or sarcomatous features, including foci resembling, undifferentiated pleomorphic sarcoma, and pleomorphic liposarcoma.[79,80] To date, the clinical behavior of these unusual tumors has been benign. Cellular angiofibromas are notable for strong and diffuse expression for CD34 (60%) with relatively less expression of smooth muscle actin (21%) and desmin (8%). Both estrogen and progesterone receptor proteins can be seen in a subset of cases but more often in tumors removed from women than men. Loss of Rb protein expression and monoallelic deletion of *Rb* gene are commonly seen.[81,82] Cellular angiofibromas are clinically benign tumors with a limited capacity for local recurrence.[79,81]

Aggressive Angiomyxoma

The term *aggressive angiomyxoma* was coined by Steeper and Rosai[83] in 1983 for a morphologically distinctive, slowly growing myxoid neoplasm that occurs chiefly in the genital, perineal, and pelvic regions of adult women. Despite its bland histologic features, it has a propensity to recur locally.

Clinical Findings

The neoplasm predominantly affects reproductive-age females with a peak incidence during the third decade of life. The female-to-male ratio is more than 6 to 1,[84] but this tumor has been increasingly recognized as arising in the inguinal region, along the spermatic cord, or in the scrotum or pelvic cavity of men.[85-89] In women, the vulvar region is the most common site of involvement and may be initially misdiagnosed clinically as a Bartholin cyst, periurethral cyst, or hernia.[69] Although slowly growing, these lesions aggressively infiltrate the perivaginal and perirectal soft tissues. The radiologic features of this tumor have been well described. MRI reveals a mass with high signal intensity on T2-weighted images with trans-levator extension and growth around perineal structures.[90]

Pathologic Findings

Grossly, aggressive angiomyxomas are soft, partly circumscribed, or polypoid; on a cross-section, they have a glistening, homogeneous, gelatinous appearance and range in size from a few centimeters to 20 cm or more. Steeper and Rosai[83] reported a pelvic/retroperitoneal tumor in a 34-year-old woman that measured 60 cm in greatest diameter. In the series by Fetsch et al.,[84] 23 of 27 tumors were 10 cm or larger. Most have a lobulated appearance. Although some areas of the tumor may be sharply marginated, others show adherence or infiltration into the surrounding soft tissues.

Microscopically, the tumor is composed of widely scattered spindled to stellate-shaped cells with ill-defined cytoplasm and variably sized, thin- or thick-walled vascular channels in a myxoid stroma that is rich in collagen fibers and, like other richly myxoid tumors, often contains foci of hemorrhage (Figs. 16-32 to 16-35). Although the cellularity is usually low and uniform throughout the tumor, some lesions have focal areas of increased cellularity, particularly around large vessels and at the periphery of the tumor.[69,84] The cells have small round to oval hyperchromatic nuclei with small centrally located nucleoli (Fig. 16-36). Mitotic figures are rare or absent and are not atypical. The stroma is characterized by prominent myxoid change with fine collagen fibrils, often with areas of erythrocyte extravasation. A characteristic feature is the presence of variably sized vessels that range from small thin-walled capillaries to large vessels with secondary changes, including perivascular hyalinization and medial hypertrophy (Fig. 16-37). Mast cells are often prominent, and some tumors have perivascular lymphoid aggregates. Small bundles of

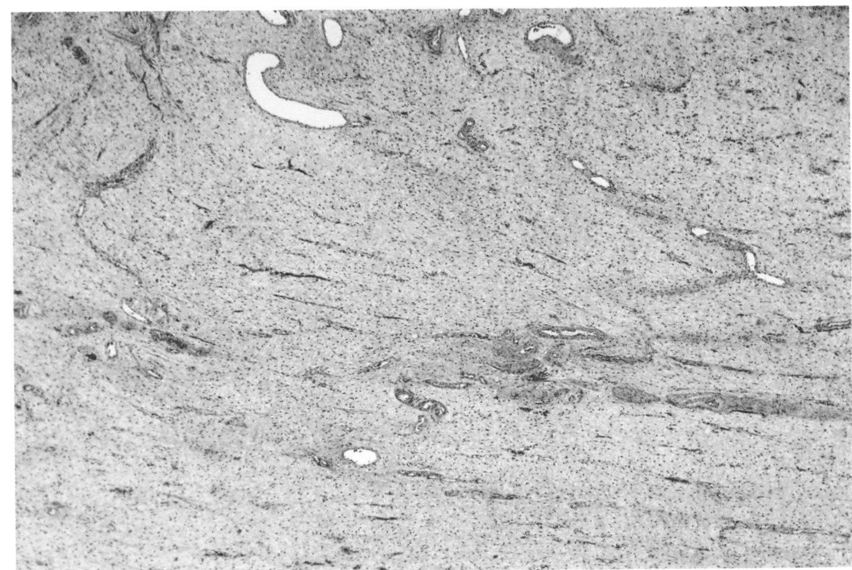

FIGURE 16-32. Aggressive angiomyxoma. The tumor is hypocellular and has prominent thin- and thick-walled vascular channels surrounded by a myxoid stroma.

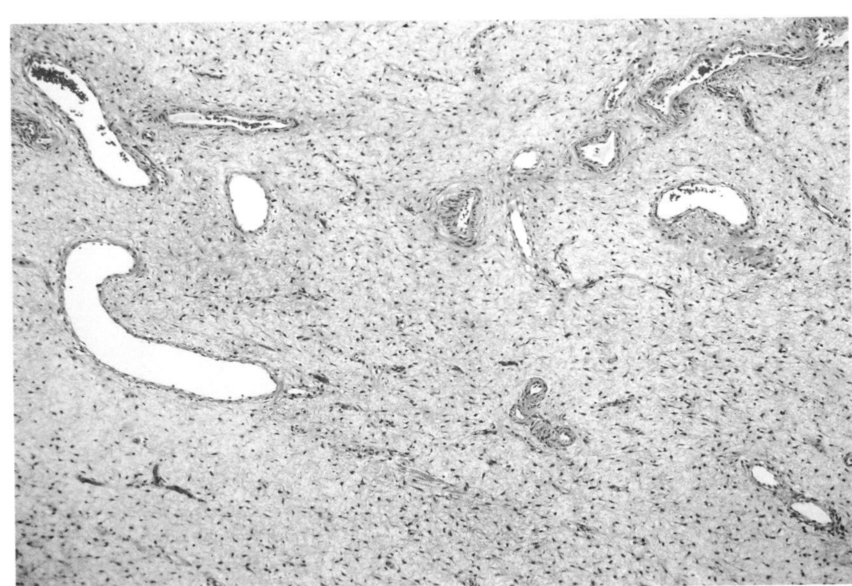

FIGURE 16-33. Aggressive angiomyxoma. Spindle-shaped cells are evenly distributed in a myxoid stroma. Prominent vessels are apparent.

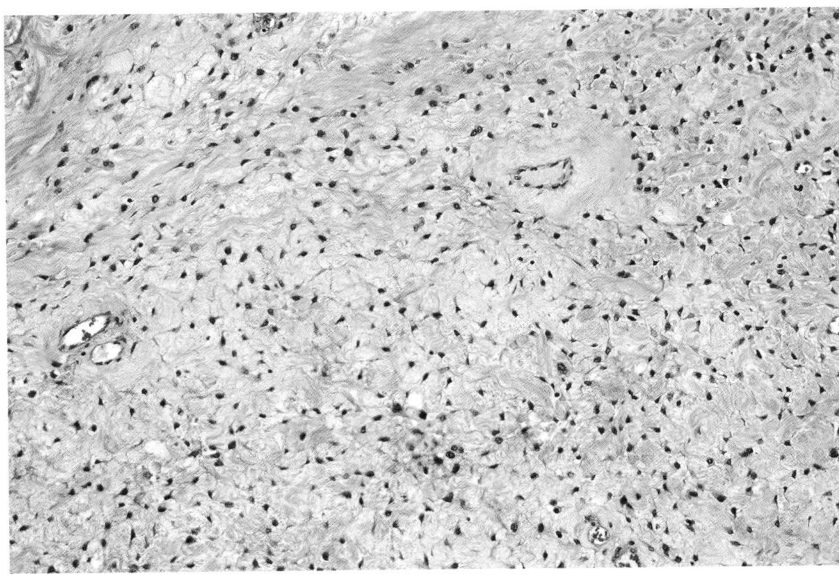

FIGURE 16-34. Aggressive angiomyxoma. Cytologically bland spindled and stellate-shaped cells are evenly distributed in a myxoid stroma.

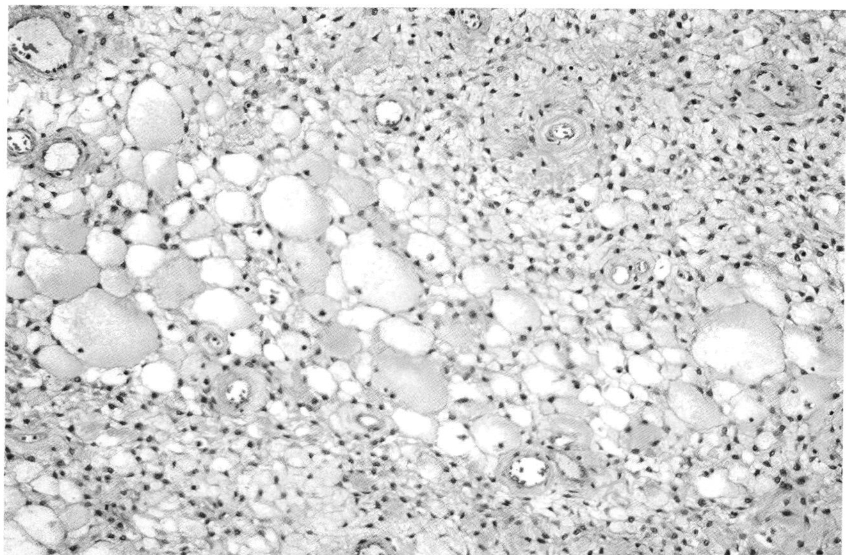

FIGURE 16-35. Microcystic change in an aggressive angiomyxoma.

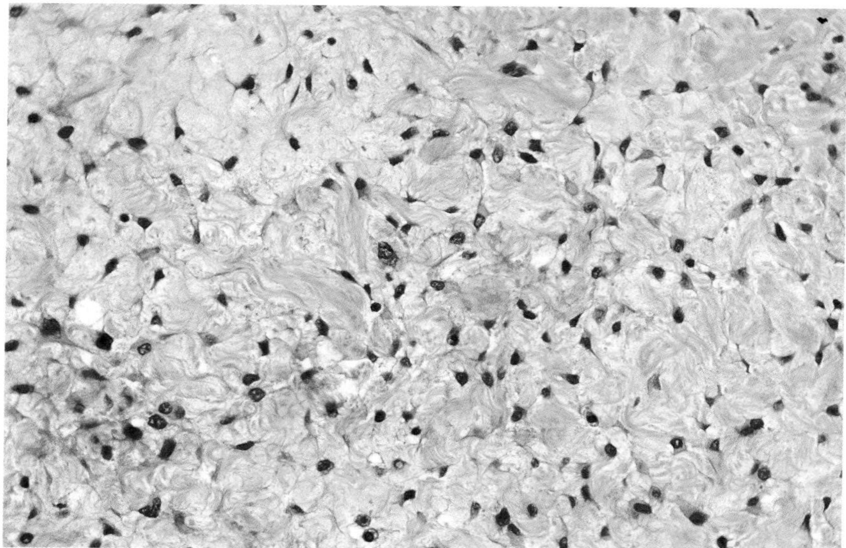

FIGURE 16-36. High-magnification view of bland spindled and stellate-shaped cells in an aggressive angiomyxoma.

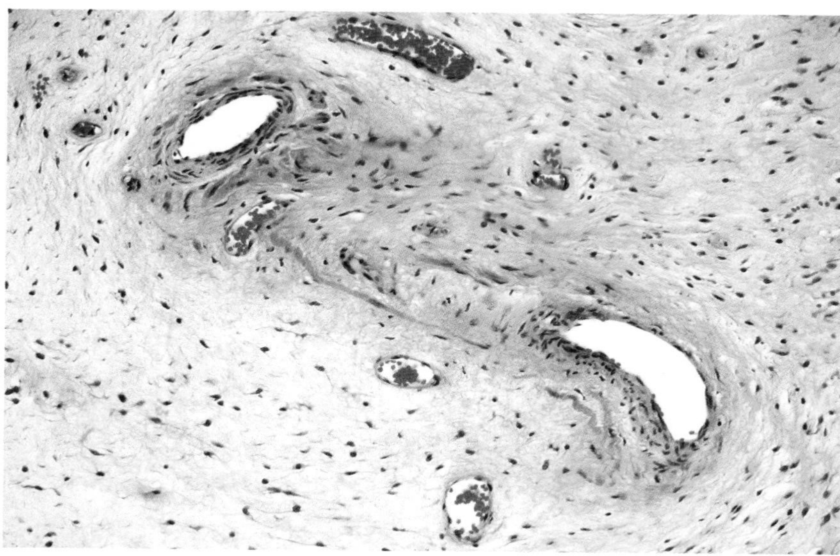

FIGURE 16-37. Characteristic thin- and thick-walled vascular channels in an aggressive angiomyxoma.

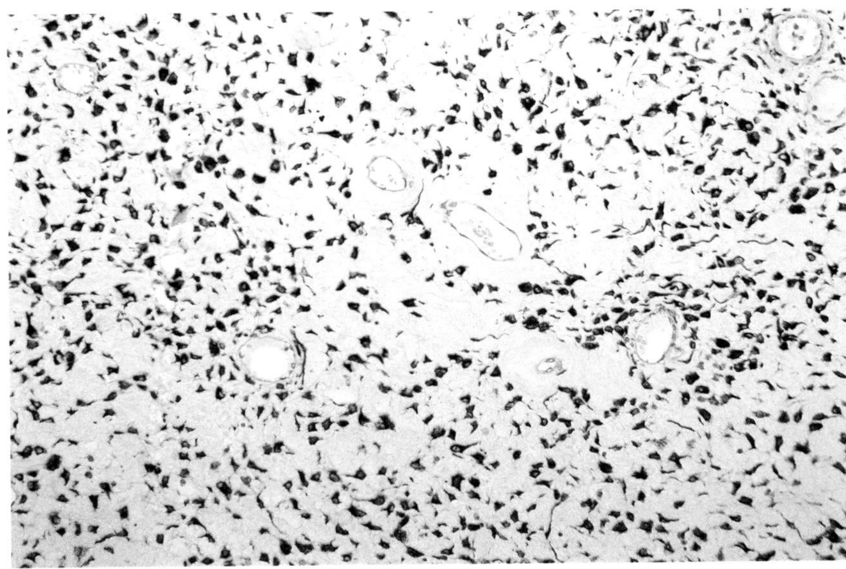

FIGURE 16-38. Diffuse desmin immunoreactivity in an aggressive angiomyxoma.

TABLE 16-1 Immunohistochemical Data in Series of Aggressive Angiomyxomas

MARKER	FETSCH ET AL.[84]	GRANTER ET AL.[69]	TOTAL (%)
Desmin	22/22	13/14	35/36 (97)
Smooth muscle actin	19/20	10/11	29/31 (94)
Muscle-specific actin	16/19	11/12	27/31 (87)
CD34	8/16	—	8/16 (50)
Estrogen receptor	13/14	—	13/14 (93)
Progesterone receptor	9/10	—	9/10 (90)
S-100 protein	0/20	0/14	0/34 (0)

spindle-shaped cells with eosinophilic cytoplasm may be present, frequently appearing to spin off from blood vessels.[69] These cells have more conventional features of smooth muscle cells, with cigar-shaped nuclei and perinuclear vacuoles.

Immunohistochemical and Ultrastructural Findings

Immunohistochemically, the cells of aggressive angiomyxoma show diffuse staining for vimentin. Although earlier reports of this entity noted an absence of desmin staining,[87] most recent studies have shown fairly consistent desmin immunoreactivity (Fig. 16-38; Table 16-1).[84,91] Immunostains for muscle-specific actin and smooth muscle actin are also positive in most cases, whereas S-100 protein and cytokeratins are not expressed by the neoplastic cells. A variable proportion of cells in some aggressive angiomyxomas also expresses CD34 and factor XIIIa.[92,93] The expression of both estrogen and progesterone receptors is a consistent finding in tumors from both genders, suggesting a hormonal role in the development or growth of these lesions.[94-96] Androgen receptors have been detected in tumors from males, but very few cases have been studied to determine whether this is a consistent finding or whether this is restricted to tumors in males.[85] As discussed in the following section, there may be some utility in staining for HMGA2, which is frequently overexpressed in this tumor.[97] Electron microscopic examination shows cells with fibroblastic, myofibroblastic, and smooth muscle differentiation.[98]

Genetic Findings

Relatively few examples of aggressive angiomyxoma have been studied cytogenetically. However, a consistent clonal aberration involving 12q13-15, the location of the *HMGA2* gene, has been identified.[99,100] Rearrangment of *HMGA2* has been demonstrated by fluorescence in-situ hybridization (FISH) in 33% of angiomyxomas and in rare genital leiomyomas, but not in angiomyofibroblastomas, cellular angiofibromas, and a variety of other stromal tumors of the female genital region.[101] In one case report by Nucci et al.,[100] an aggressive angiomyxoma harbored a t(8;12) resulting in deregulation of *HMGA2*. Micci et al.[102] reported a tumor with a t(11;12)(q23;q15) as the sole karyotypic aberration.

Clinical Behavior and Outcome

Aggressive angiomyxoma tends to locally recur in about 30% of patients (Fig. 16-39). Steeper and Rosai[83] reported five cases with more than 12-months follow-up, four of which recurred locally, one as late as 14 years after local excision. Begin et al.[87] described six cases with follow-up data, all of which recurred within 9 to 84 months after excision. A 36% rate of local recurrence was reported by both Fetsch et al.[84] and Granter et al.[69] More recent studies found a recurrence rate of less than 10% following aggressive surgical excision.[93,103] Neither size nor cellularity correlates with the risk of local recurrence. Because many of these tumors have infiltrative borders, complete excision is often difficult and likely accounts for the high rate of local recurrence (see Fig. 16-39). More recently, some patients have been successfully treated with adjuvant hormonal therapy, including gonadotropic-releasing hormone agonists.[104-106] There is a single believable report of aggressive angiomyxoma with lung metastases.[107]

Differential Diagnosis of Benign Genital Stromal Tumors

Angiomyofibroblastoma, cellular angiofibroma, and aggressive angiomyxoma have some overlapping clinical, morphologic, and immunophenotypic features (Table 16-2). In

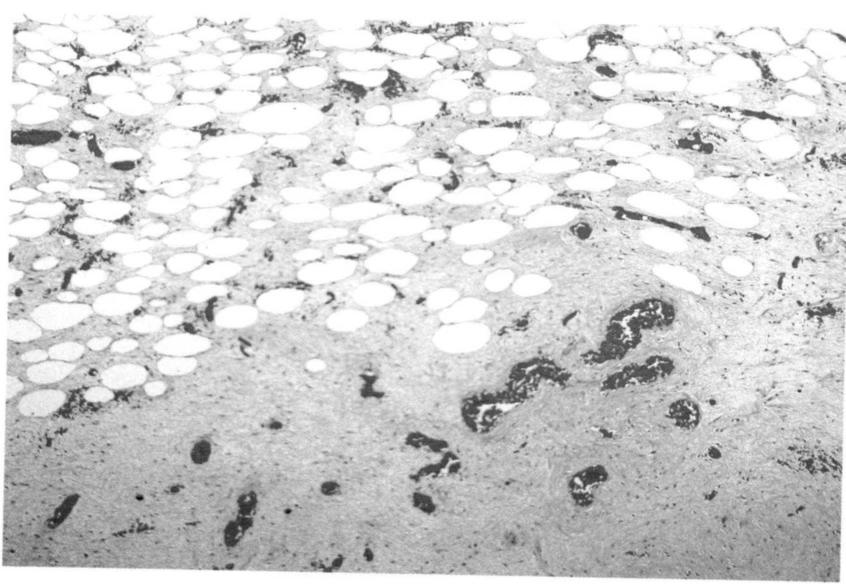

FIGURE 16-39. Infiltration of surrounding adipose tissue in an aggressive angiomyxoma. This pattern of infiltration likely accounts for the high rate of local recurrence of this tumor.

TABLE 16-2 Benign Genital Stromal Tumors

TUMOR	SEX PREDILECTION	DESMIN	ACTIN	CD34	ER/PR
Angiomyofibroblastoma	Females	+	+/–	Rare	+
Angiomyofibroblastoma-like tumor of male genital tract	Males	+	++	+++	+
Cellular angiofibroma	Females > males	Rare	+	+++	+
Angiomyxoma	Females	+	+	+	++

ER/PR, estrogen receptor, progesterone receptor.

TABLE 16-3 Differential Diagnostic Features of Aggressive Angiomyxoma and Angiomyofibroblastoma

FEATURE	AGGRESSIVE ANGIOMYXOMA	ANGIOMYOFIBROBLASTOMA
Gross appearance	Poorly circumscribed, infiltrative	Circumscribed
Size	Large (many >10 cm)	Most ≤3 cm
Cellularity	Uniform	Perivascular hypercellularity
Cell shape	Spindled	Epithelioid
Vasculature	Variably sized, thick-walled	Numerous, thin-walled, often perivascular hyalinization
Multinucleation	Absent	Present
Recurrence	50%	Rare

particular, the distinction of angiomyofibroblastoma and cellular angiofibroma, at times, may be somewhat subjective but is thankfully not of clinical significance. Thankfully, the more important distinction (between these two tumors and aggressive angiomyxoma) is less fraught with difficulty.

Both angiomyofibroblastoma and cellular angiofibroma present as circumscribed superficial nodules, with the latter having the greater propensity to occur in males and in sites outside of the gynecologic tract. The most distinctive feature of angiomyofibroblastoma is the characteristic nests or cords of distinctly epithelioid cells arranged around small vessels. In contrast, cellular angiofibroma is a uniformly cellular lesion showing a greater degree of spindling and lacking an epithelioid arrangement of cells around vessels. Strong expression of CD34 is more often seen in cellular angiofibroma. It is unclear whether there is a role for Rb immunohistochemistry or FISH in this differential diagnosis because angiomyofibroblastomas do not appear to have been studied for loss of Rb expression.

Aggressive angiomyxoma differs significantly from both angiomyofibroblastoma and cellular angiofibroma by virtue of its large size, deep location, prominent myxoid matrix, and infiltrative growth pattern (Table 16-3). In problematic cases, there may be some role for *HMGA2* FISH in this differential diagnosis, although careful clinical correlation and morphologic analysis should be sufficient in almost all instances. Other immunohistochemical markers are not of value here.

Aggressive angiomyxoma should also be distinguished from other myxoid neoplasms, in particular, superficial angiomyxoma (cutaneous myxoma), myxoid leiomyoma, pelvic fibromatosis with myxoid change, and myxofibrosarcoma. Superficial angiomyxoma is typically much smaller and more superficially located, and often shows a relatively well-circumscribed, lobular growth pattern. Stromal neutrophils may be seen, which is a valuable clue. Myxoid leiomyoma may reach a large size and involve the pelvic region but differs from aggressive angiomyxoma by its virtue of its less prominent vascular pattern and the presence of widely scattered smooth

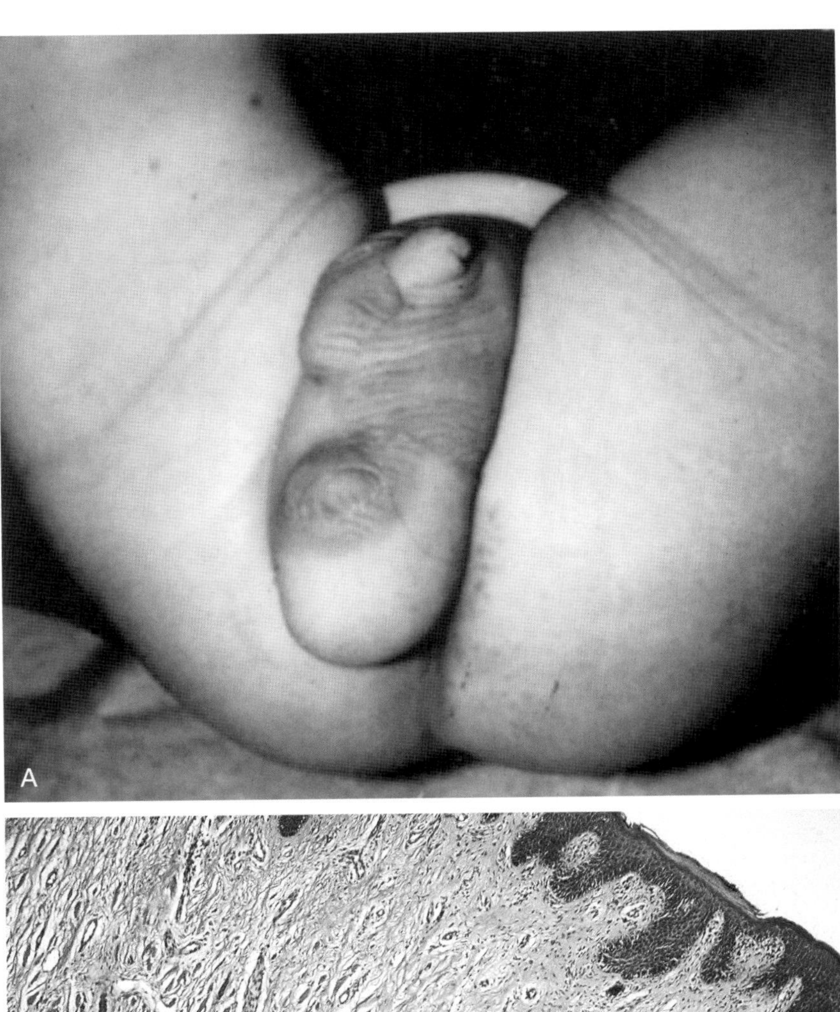

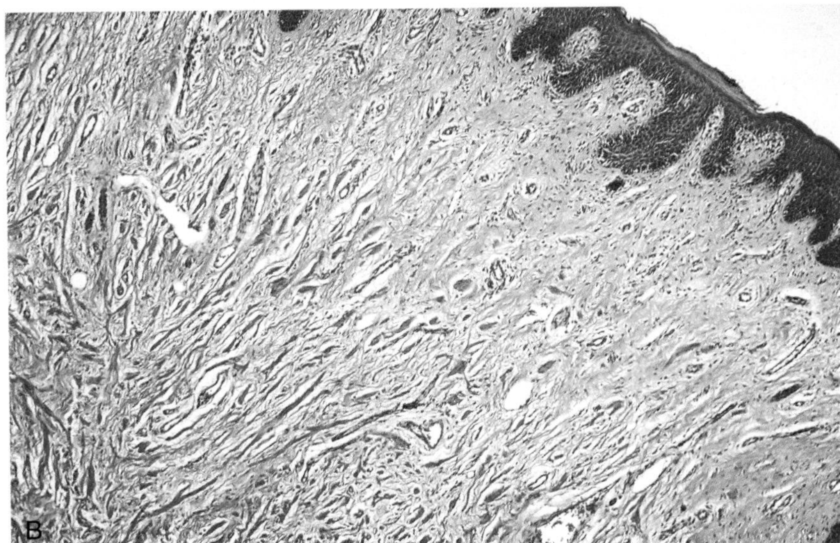

FIGURE 16-40. (A) Accessory scrotum in an infant. (B) Microscopic section shows well-differentiated smooth fibers oriented perpendicular to the skin surface.

muscle cells in a myxoid matrix. The cells of myxoid leiomyoma are larger and have more abundant eosinophilic cytoplasm than those of aggressive angiomyxoma, and tend to be arranged in small packets or loose fascicles. Pelvic fibromatoses tend to affect women in the third to fourth decades of life and may show prominent myxoid change and infiltrative growth, mimicking aggressive angiomyxoma. Careful inspection, however, will invariably reveal more typical zones of fibromatosis, with long, sweeping fascicles of uniform myofibroblastic cells arrayed about a thin-walled, dilated vasculature, often showing perivascular edema. Myxofibrosarcoma shows a much greater degree of cytologic atypia than does aggressive angiomyxoma, and shows a different vascular pattern with thick-walled arborizing vessels from which the neoplastic cells seem to emanate.

Finally, fibroepithelial stromal polyps of the vulvovaginal region have a wide spectrum of morphologic appearances and so they enter into the differential diagnosis of the various genital stromal tumors. Fibroepithelial stromal polyps usually arise in young to middle-aged women, most commonly in the vagina. Histologically, this lesion shows a distinctly polypoid growth pattern and lack a grenz zone with the overlying mucosa or skin. The absence of this grenz zone is in contrast to true genital stromal tumors and may be a valuable clue to

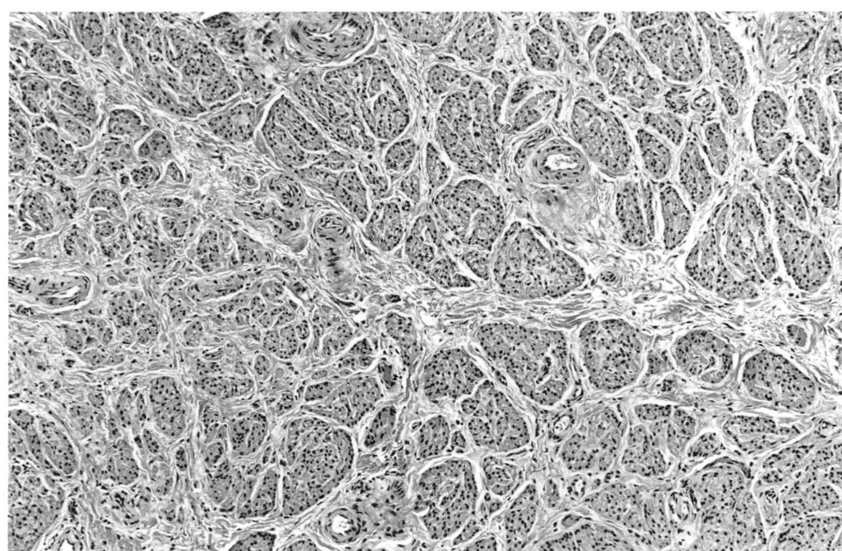

FIGURE 16-41. Round ligament removed at the time of inguinal herniorrhaphy. Cells are distinctly rounded with small centrally placed nuclei.

the correct diagnosis. Fibroepithelial stromal polyps show significant variability from case to case, with some being hypocellular and myxoid, and others showing marked hypercellularity and a pseudosarcomatous appearance.[97,108] Multinucleated stromal cells are characteristic and are usually found near the epithelial–stromal interface. There is a great deal of immunophenotypic overlap with the various genital stromal tumors because the stromal cells of fibroepithelial polyps may express desmin, actin, estrogen, and progesterone receptors.

MISCELLANEOUS LESIONS CONFUSED WITH LEIOMYOMAS

Although the diagnosis of leiomyoma is seldom difficult, occasionally, hamartomatous or choristomatous deposits of smooth muscle tissue suggest leiomyoma. Examples include accessory scrotal (Fig. 16-40) or areolar tissue. The clinical appearance and location of the lesions usually suggest the correct diagnosis. The round ligament, when removed incidentally during repair of an inguinal hernia, may also be misinterpreted as a leiomyoma. The round ligament is composed of distinctive, closely packed, polygonal muscle cells with small, dark, centrally placed nuclei (Fig. 16-41).

References

1. Farman AG. Benign smooth muscle tumors. S Afr Med J 1974;48:1214.
2. Ross R. The smooth muscle cell. II. Growth of smooth muscle in culture and formation of elastic fibers. J Cell Biol 1971;50(1):172–86.
3. Harman JW, O'Hegarty MT, Byrnes CK. The ultrastructure of human smooth muscle. I. Studies of cell surface and connections in normal and achalasia esophageal smooth muscle. Exp Mol Pathol 1962;1:204–28.
4. Hashimoto H, Komori A, Kosaka M, et al. Electron microscopic studies on smooth muscle of the human uterus. J Jpn Obstet Gynecol Soc 1960;7:115.
5. Morales AR, Fine G, Pardo V, et al. The ultrastructure of smooth muscle tumors with a consideration of the possible relationship of glomangiomas, hemangiopericytomas, and cardiac myxomas. Pathol Annu [Research Support, U.S. Gov't, Non-P.H.S. Review] 1975;10:65–92.
6. Rosenbluth J. Smooth muscle: an ultrastructural basis for the dynamic of its contraction. Science 1965;148:1337–9.
7. Schurch W, Skalli O, Seemayer TA, et al. Intermediate filament proteins and actin isoforms as markers for soft tissue tumor differentiation and origin: I. Smooth muscle tumors. Am J Pathol 1987;128(1):91–103.
8. Skalli O, Ropraz P, Trzeciak A, et al. A monoclonal antibody against alpha-smooth muscle actin: a new probe for smooth muscle differentiation. J Cell Biol 1986;103(6 Pt 2):2787–96.
9. Uehara Y, Campbell GR, Burnstock G. Cytoplasmic filaments in developing and adult vertebrate smooth muscle. J Cell Biol 1971;50(2):484–97.
10. Archer CB, Whittaker S, Greaves MW. Pharmacological modulation of cold-induced pain in cutaneous leiomyomata. Br J Dermatol 1988;118(2):255–60.
11. Auckland G. Hereditary multiple leiomyoma of the skin. Br J Dermatol 1967;79:63.
12. Fisher WC, Helwig EB. Leiomyomas of the skin. Arch Dermatol 1963;88:510–20.
13. Fox Jr SR. Leiomyomatosis cutis. N Engl J Med [Case Reports] 1960;263:1248–50.
14. Gagne EJ, Su WP. Congenital smooth muscle hamartoma of the skin. Pediatr Dermatol [Case Reports Review] 1993;10(2):142–5.
15. Jansen LH, Driessen FM. Leiomyoma cutis. Br J Dermatol [Case Reports] 1958;70(12):446–51.
16. Kloepfer HW, Krafchuk J, Derbes V, et al. Hereditary multiple leiomyoma of the skin. Am J Hum Genet 1958;10(1):48–52.
17. Mann PR. Leiomyoma cutis: an electron microscope study. Br J Dermatol 1970;82(5):463–9.
18. Montgomery H, Winkelmann RK. Smooth-muscle tumors of the skin. AMA Arch Derm [Case Reports] 1959;79(1):32–40; discussion 40–41.
19. Urbanek RW, Johnson WC. Smooth muscle hamartoma associated with Becker's nevus. Arch Dermatol [Case Reports] 1978;114(1):104–6.
20. Verma KC, Chawdhry SD, Rathi KS. Cutaneous leiomyomata in two brothers. Br J Dermatol 1974;90(3):351–3.
21. Yokoyama R, Hashimoto H, Daimaru Y, et al. Superficial leiomyomas. A clinicopathologic study of 34 cases. Acta Pathol Jpn 1987;37(9):1415–22.
22. Nascimento AG, Karas M, Rosen PP, et al. Leiomyoma of the nipple. Am J Surg Pathol 1979;3(2):151–4.
23. Newman PL, Fletcher CD. Smooth muscle tumours of the external genitalia: clinicopathological analysis of a series. Histopathology [Research Support, Non-U.S. Gov't] 1991;18(6):523–9.
24. Siegal GP, Gaffey TA. Solitary leiomyomas arising from the tunica dartos scroti. J Urol 1976;116(1):69–71.
25. Tavassoli FA, Norris HJ. Smooth muscle tumors of the vulva. Obstet Gynecol 1979;53(2):213–7.
26. Alam NA, Olpin S, Leigh IM. Fumarate hydratase mutations and predisposition to cutaneous leiomyomas, uterine leiomyomas and renal cancer. Br J Dermatol [Research Support, Non-U.S. Gov't Review] 2005;153(1):11–7.

27. Kiuru M, Launonen V. Hereditary leiomyomatosis and renal cell cancer (HLRCC). Curr Mol Med [Review] 2004;4(8):869–75.
28. Barker KT, Bevan S, Wang R, et al. Low frequency of somatic mutations in the FH/multiple cutaneous leiomyomatosis gene in sporadic leiomyosarcomas and uterine leiomyomas. Br J Cancer [Research Support, Non-U.S. Gov't] 2002;87(4):446–8.
29. Lehtonen R, Kiuru M, Vanharanta S, et al. Biallelic inactivation of fumarate hydratase (FH) occurs in nonsyndromic uterine leiomyomas but is rare in other tumors. Am J Pathol [Comparative Study Research Support, Non-U.S. Gov't] 2004;164(1):17–22.
30. Stout AP. Solitary cutaneous and subcutaneous leiomyoma. Am J Cancer 1937;24:435.
31. Hachisuga T, Hashimoto H, Enjoji M. Angioleiomyoma. A clinicopathologic reappraisal of 562 cases. Cancer [Research Support, Non-U.S. Gov't] 1984;54(1):126–30.
32. Duhig JT, Ayer JP. Vascular leiomyoma. A study of sixty one cases. Arch Pathol 1959;68:424–30.
33. Gutmann J, Cifuentes C, Balzarini MA, et al. Angiomyoma of the oral cavity. Oral Surg Oral Med Oral Pathol 1974;38(2):269–73.
34. Bardach H, H. E. Das Angioleiomyoma der Haut. Hautarzt 1975;26:638.
35. Ekestrom S. A comparison between glomus tumour and angioleiomyom. Acta Pathol Microbiol Scand 1950;27(1):86–93.
36. Carla TG, Filotico R, Filotico M. Bizarre angiomyomas of superficial soft tissues. Pathologica 1991;83(1084):237–42.
37. Kilpatrick SE, Mentzel T, Fletcher CD. Leiomyoma of deep soft tissue. Clinicopathologic analysis of a series. Am J Surg Pathol [Research Support, Non-U.S. Gov't] 1994;18(6):576–82.
38. Fletcher CD, Kilpatrick SE, Mentzel T. The difficulty in predicting behavior of smooth-muscle tumors in deep soft tissue. Am J Surg Pathol [Case Reports Comment Letter] 1995;19(1):116–7.
39. Billings SD, Folpe AL, Weiss SW. Do leiomyomas of deep soft tissue exist? An analysis of highly differentiated smooth muscle tumors of deep soft tissue supporting two distinct subtypes. Am J Surg Pathol 2001; 25(9):1134–42.
40. Paal E, Miettinen M. Retroperitoneal leiomyomas: a clinicopathologic and immunohistochemical study of 56 cases with a comparison to retroperitoneal leiomyosarcomas. Am J Surg Pathol [Comparative Study Research Support, Non-U.S. Gov't] 2001;25(11):1355–63.
41. Miettinen M, Fetsch JF. Evaluation of biological potential of smooth muscle tumours. Histopathology [Review] 2006;48(1):97–105.
42. Weiss SW. Smooth muscle tumors of soft tissue. Adv Anat Pathol 2002;9(6):351–9.
43. Patil DT, Laskin WB, Fetsch JF, et al. Inguinal smooth muscle tumors in women-a dichotomous group consisting of Mullerian-type leiomyomas and soft tissue leiomyosarcomas: an analysis of 55 cases. Am J Surg Pathol 2011;35(3):315–24.
44. Meis JM, Enzinger FM. Myolipoma of soft tissue. Am J Surg Pathol 1991;15(2):121–5.
45. Scurry JP, Carey MP, Targett CS, et al. Soft tissue lipoleiomyoma. Pathology 1991;23(4):360–2.
46. Willson JR, Peale AR. Multiple peritoneal leiomyomas associated with a granulosa-cell tumor of the ovary. Am J Obstet Gynecol 1952;64(1): 204–8.
47. Crosland DB. Leiomyomatosis peritonealis disseminata: a case report. Am J Obstet Gynecol 1973;117(2):179–81.
48. Tavassoli FA, Norris HJ. Peritoneal leiomyomatosis (leiomyomatosis peritonealis disseminata): a clinicopathologic study of 20 cases with ultrastructural observations. Int J Gynecol Pathol 1982;1(1):59–74.
49. Kaplan C, Benirschke K, Johnson KC. Leiomyomatosis peritonealis disseminata with endometrium. Obstet Gynecol [Case Reports] 1980; 55(1):119–22.
50. Lim OW, Segal A, Ziel HK. Leiomyomatosis peritonealis disseminata associated with pregnancy. Obstet Gynecol [Case Reports] 1980;55(1): 122–5.
51. Parmley TH, Woodruff JD, Winn K, et al. Histogenesis of leiomyomatosis peritonealis disseminata (disseminated fibrosing deciduosis). Obstet Gynecol [Case Reports] 1975;46(5):511–6.
52. Winn KJ, Woodruff JD, Parmley TH. Electron microscopic studies of leiomyomatosis peritonealis disseminata. Obstet Gynecol 1976;48: 225.
53. Pieslor PC, Orenstein JM, Hogan DL, et al. Ultrastructure of myofibroblasts and decidualized cells in leiomyomatosis peritonealis disseminata. Am J Clin Pathol [Case Reports] 1979;72(5):875–82.
54. Kitazawa S, Shiraishi N, Maeda S. Leiomyomatosis peritonealis disseminata with adipocytic differentiation. Acta Obstet Gynecol Scand [Case Reports] 1992;71(6):482–4.
55. Chen KT, Hendricks EJ, Freeburg B. Benign glandular inclusion of the peritoneum associated with leiomyomatosis peritonealis disseminata. Diagn Gynecol Obstet [Case Reports] 1982;4(1):41–4.
56. Ma KF, Chow LT. Sex cord-like pattern leiomyomatosis peritonealis disseminata: a hitherto undescribed feature. Histopathology [Case Reports] 1992;21(4):389–91.
57. Nogales Jr FF, Matilla A, Carrascal E. Leiomyomatosis peritonealis disseminata. An ultrastructural study. Am J Clin Pathol [Case Reports] 1978;69(4):452–7.
58. Kuo T, London SN, Dinh TV. Endometriosis occurring in leiomyomatosis peritonealis disseminata: ultrastructural study and histogenetic consideration. Am J Surg Pathol [Case Reports] 1980;4(2):197–204.
59. Goldberg MF, Hurt WG, Frable WJ. Leiomyomatosis peritonealis disseminata. Report of a case and review of the literature. Obstet Gynecol [Case Reports] 1977;49(Suppl. 1):S46–52.
60. Fujii S, Nakashima N, Okamura H, et al. Progesterone-induced smooth muscle-like cells in the subperitoneal nodules produced by estrogen. Experimental approach to leiomyomatosis peritonealis disseminata. Am J Obstet Gynecol 1981;139(2):164–72.
61. Aterman K, Fraser GM, Lea RH. Disseminated peritoneal leiomyomatosis. Virchows Arch A Pathol Anat Histol [Case Reports] 1977;374(1): 13–26.
62. Quade BJ, McLachlin CM, Soto-Wright V, et al. Disseminated peritoneal leiomyomatosis. Clonality analysis by X chromosome inactivation and cytogenetics of a clinically benign smooth muscle proliferation. Am J Pathol [Research Support, Non-U.S. Gov't Research Support, U.S. Gov't, P.H.S.] 1997;150(6):2153–66.
63. Hoynck van Papendrecht HP, Gratama S. Leiomyomatosis peritonealis disseminata. Eur J Obstet Gynecol Reprod Biol [Review] 1983;14(4): 251–9.
64. Parente JT, Levy J, Chinea F, et al. Adjuvant surgical and hormonal treatment of leiomyomatosis peritonealis disseminata. A case report. J Reprod Med [Case Reports] 1995;40(6):468–70.
65. Akkersdijk GJ, Flu PK, Giard RW, et al. Malignant leiomyomatosis peritonealis disseminata. Am J Obstet Gynecol [Case Reports] 1990; 163(2):591–3.
66. Abulafia O, Angel C, Sherer DM, et al. Computed tomography of leiomyomatosis peritonealis disseminata with malignant transformation. Am J Obstet Gynecol [Case Reports] 1993;169(1):52–4.
67. Rubin SC, Wheeler JE, Mikuta JJ. Malignant leiomyomatosis peritonealis disseminata. Obstet Gynecol [Case Reports] 1986;68(1):126–30.
68. Fletcher CD, Tsang WY, Fisher C, et al. Angiomyofibroblastoma of the vulva. A benign neoplasm distinct from aggressive angiomyxoma. Am J Surg Pathol [Research Support, Non-U.S. Gov't] 1992;16(4):373–82.
69. Granter SR, Nucci MR, Fletcher CD. Aggressive angiomyxoma: reappraisal of its relationship to angiomyofibroblastoma in a series of 16 cases. Histopathology 1997;30(1):3–10.
70. Laskin WB, Fetsch JF, Mostofi FK. Angiomyofibroblastomalike tumor of the male genital tract: analysis of 11 cases with comparison to female angiomyofibroblastoma and spindle cell lipoma. Am J Surg Pathol 1998;22(1):6–16.
71. McCluggage WG. A review and update of morphologically bland vulvovaginal mesenchymal lesions. Int J Gynecol Pathol [Review] 2005;24(1):26–38.
72. Horiguchi H, Matsui-Horiguchi M, Fujiwara M, et al. Angiomyofibroblastoma of the vulva: report of a case with immunohistochemical and molecular analysis. Int J Gynecol Pathol [Case Reports] 2003;22(3): 277–84.
73. Hiruki T, Thomas MJ, Clement PB. Vulvar angiomyofibroblastoma. Am J Surg Pathol [Comment Letter] 1993;17(4):423–4.
74. Hisaoka M, Kouho H, Aoki T, et al. Angiomyofibroblastoma of the vulva: a clinicopathologic study of seven cases. Pathol Int 1995;45(7):487–92.
75. Nielsen GP, Rosenberg AE, Young RH, et al. Angiomyofibroblastoma of the vulva and vagina. Mod Pathol 1996;9(3):284–91.
76. Cao D, Srodon M, Montgomery EA, et al. Lipomatous variant of angiomyofibroblastoma: report of two cases and review of the literature. Int J Gynecol Pathol [Case Reports] 2005;24(2):196–200.
77. Nielsen GP, Young RH, Dickersin GR, et al. Angiomyofibroblastoma of the vulva with sarcomatous transformation ("angiomyofibrosarcoma"). Am J Surg Pathol 1997;21(9):1104–8.
78. Folpe AL, Tworek JA, Weiss SW. Sarcomatous transformation in angiomyofibroblastomas: a clinicopathological and immunohistochemical study of eleven cases (abstract). Mod Pathol 2001;14:12A.
79. Iwasa Y, Fletcher CD. Cellular angiofibroma: clinicopathologic and immunohistochemical analysis of 51 cases. Am J Surg Pathol 2004;28(11): 1426–35.

80. Chen E, Fletcher CD. Cellular angiofibroma with atypia or sarcomatous transformation: clinicopathologic analysis of 13 cases. Am J Surg Pathol 2010;34(5):707–14.
81. Flucke U, van Krieken JH, Mentzel T. Cellular angiofibroma: analysis of 25 cases emphasizing its relationship to spindle cell lipoma and mammary-type myofibroblastoma. Mod Pathol 2011;24(1):82–9.
82. Maggiani F, Debiec-Rychter M, Vanbockrijck M, et al. Cellular angiofibroma: another mesenchymal tumour with 13q14 involvement, suggesting a link with spindle cell lipoma and (extra)-mammary myofibroblastoma. Histopathology 2007;51(3):410–2.
83. Steeper TA, Rosai J. Aggressive angiomyxoma of the female pelvis and perineum. Report of nine cases of a distinctive type of gynecologic soft-tissue neoplasm. Am J Surg Pathol 1983;7(5):463–75.
84. Fetsch JF, Laskin WB, Lefkowitz M, et al. Aggressive angiomyxoma: a clinicopathologic study of 29 female patients. Cancer 1996;78(1):79–90.
85. Chihara Y, Fujimoto K, Takada S, et al. Aggressive angiomyxoma in the scrotum expressing androgen and progesterone receptors. Int J Urol [Case Reports Review] 2003;10(12):672–5.
86. Carlinfante G, De Marco L, Mori M, et al. Aggressive angiomyxoma of the spermatic cord. Two unusual cases occurring in childhood. Pathol Res Pract [Review] 2001;197(2):139–44.
87. Begin LR, Clement PB, Kirk ME, et al. Aggressive angiomyxoma of pelvic soft parts: a clinicopathologic study of nine cases. Hum Pathol 1985;16(6):621–8.
88. Iezzoni JC, Fechner RE, Wong LS, et al. Aggressive angiomyxoma in males. A report of four cases. Am J Clin Pathol 1995;104(4):391–6.
89. Tsang WY, Chan JK, Lee KC, et al. Aggressive angiomyxoma. A report of four cases occurring in men. Am J Surg Pathol 1992;16(11):1059–65.
90. Jeyadevan NN, Sohaib SA, Thomas JM, et al. Imaging features of aggressive angiomyxoma. Clin Radiol [Case Reports] 2003;58(2):157–62.
91. Belge G, Caselitz J, Bonk U, et al. [Genetic studies of differential fatty tissue tumor diagnosis]. Pathologe [Case Reports] 1997;18(2):160–6.
92. Silverman JS, Albukerk J, Tamsen A. Comparison of angiomyofibroblastoma and aggressive angiomyxoma in both sexes: four cases composed of bimodal CD34 and factor XIIIa positive dendritic cell subsets. Pathol Res Pract [Case Reports Comparative Study] 1997;193(10):673–82.
93. van Roggen JF, van Unnik JA, Briaire-de Bruijn IH, et al. Aggressive angiomyxoma: a clinicopathological and immunohistochemical study of 11 cases with long-term follow-up. Virchows Arch [Case Reports] 2005;446(2):157–63.
94. Abu JI, Bamford WM, Malin G, et al. Aggressive angiomyxoma of the perineum. Int J Gynecol Cancer [Case Reports] 2005;15(6):1097–100.
95. McCluggage WG, Patterson A, Maxwell P. Aggressive angiomyxoma of pelvic parts exhibits oestrogen and progesterone receptor positivity. J Clin Pathol 2000;53(8):603–5.
96. McCluggage WG. Recent advances in immunohistochemistry in gynaecological pathology. Histopathology [Review] 2002;40(4):309–26.
97. Nucci MR, Fletcher CD. Vulvovaginal soft tissue tumours: update and review. Histopathology 2000;36(2):97–108.
98. Skalova A, Michal M, Husek K, et al. Aggressive angiomyxoma of the pelvioperineal region. Immunohistological and ultrastructural study of seven cases. Am J Dermatopathol 1993;15(5):446–51.
99. Kazmierczak B, Dal Cin P, Wanschura S, et al. Cloning and molecular characterization of part of a new gene fused to HMGIC in mesenchymal tumors. Am J Pathol 1998;152(2):431–5.
100. Nucci MR, Weremowicz S, Neskey DM, et al. Chromosomal translocation t(8;12) induces aberrant HMGIC expression in aggressive angiomyxoma of the vulva. Genes Chromosomes Cancer [Case Reports Research Support, U.S. Gov't, P.H.S.] 2001;32(2):172–6.
101. Medeiros F, Erickson-Johnson MR, Keeney GL, et al. Frequency and characterization of HMGA2 and HMGA1 rearrangements in mesenchymal tumors of the lower genital tract. Genes Chromosomes Cancer 2007;46(11):981–90.
102. Micci F, Panagopoulos I, Bjerkehagen B, et al. Deregulation of HMGA2 in an aggressive angiomyxoma with t(11;12)(q23;q15). Virchows Arch [Case Reports Research Support, Non-U.S. Gov't] 2006;448(6):838–42.
103. Amezcua CA, Begley SJ, Mata N, et al. Aggressive angiomyxoma of the female genital tract: a clinicopathologic and immunohistochemical study of 12 cases. Int J Gynecol Cancer 2005;15(1):140–5.
104. Shinohara N, Nonomura K, Ishikawa S, et al. Medical management of recurrent aggressive angiomyxoma with gonadotropin-releasing hormone agonist. Int J Urol [Case Reports] 2004;11(6):432–5.
105. Poirier M, Fraser R, Meterissian S. Case 1. Aggressive angiomyxoma of the pelvis: response to luteinizing hormone-releasing hormone agonist. J Clin Oncol [Case Reports] 2003;21(18):3535–6.
106. McCluggage WG, Jamieson T, Dobbs SP, et al. Aggressive angiomyxoma of the vulva: dramatic response to gonadotropin-releasing hormone agonist therapy. Gynecol Oncol [Case Reports] 2006;100(3):623–5.
107. Blandamura S, Cruz J, Faure Vergara L, et al. Aggressive angiomyxoma: a second case of metastasis with patient's death. Hum Pathol [Case Reports] 2003;34(10):1072–4.
108. Nucci MR, Young RH, Fletcher CD. Cellular pseudosarcomatous fibroepithelial stromal polyps of the lower female genital tract: an underrecognized lesion often misdiagnosed as sarcoma. Am J Surg Pathol 2000;24(2):231–40.

Leiomyosarcoma

CHAPTER CONTENTS

Leiomyosarcomas account for 5% to 10% of soft tissue sarcomas.[1-4] They are principally tumors of adults but are far outnumbered even in this age group by more common sarcomas, such as liposarcoma and undifferentiated pleomorphic sarcoma (malignant fibrous histiocytoma). Likewise, they are less common than leiomyosarcomas of uterine or gastrointestinal origin, and only some of the data gleaned from the collective experience with tumors in these two sites are directly applicable to the soft tissue counterpart. Few predisposing or etiologic factors are recognized for this disease. In general, these tumors are more common in women than men. About two-thirds of all retroperitoneal leiomyosarcomas[5,6] and more than three-quarters of all vena caval leiomyosarcomas occur in women.[7] The reasons for this are unclear, although growth and proliferation of smooth muscle tissue in women have been noted to coincide with pregnancy and estrogenic stimulation (see Chapter 16). Children rarely develop these tumors,[8,9] and there is conflicting evidence as to whether leiomyosarcomas in children have a better prognosis.[8,10,11] Many pediatric tumors reported as leiomyosarcoma appear to instead represent Epstein-Barr virus-related (also known as EBV) smooth muscle proliferations (see later section).

Leiomyosarcomas rarely occur following radiation[12-14] but may develop as a second malignancy in the setting of bilateral (hereditary) retinoblastoma.[15-17] Because these tumors may occur at sites distant from the previously irradiated site, their pathogenesis is directly attributable to the Rb1 mutation and not to irradiation. Deletions or mutations of the Rb1 locus can be identified in a small number of leiomyosarcomas that occur on a sporadic basis as well.[18,19] There is no evidence that leiomyomas undergo malignant transformation in more than extraordinarily rare instances. Well-differentiated areas resembling leiomyoma are often found in a leiomyosarcoma, but this by no means proves that malignant transformation occurred. In fact, the predilection of leiomyosarcomas for deep soft tissue, in contrast to the superficial location of leiomyomas, provides some evidence to the contrary. There is evidence that, as a group, leiomyosarcomas may have a poorer prognosis than other sarcomas when matched for other variables.[20-22]

It is useful to divide leiomyosarcomas into several site-related subgroups because of significant clinical and biologic differences. In fact, site alone is one of the most important prognostic factors in assessing outcome in this disease. Leiomyosarcomas of retroperitoneum and abdominal cavity are the most common subgroup and are associated with an aggressive clinical course. Leiomyosarcomas of somatic soft tissue are a second, but less common, subgroup associated with a better prognosis. There is increasing evidence that many, if not most, arise from small vessels, a relationship that may be important for defining the behavior and risk of metastasis. Although, technically, such lesions could be referred to as *vascular leiomyosarcomas*, this designation usually refers to a tumor arising from a major vessel so that clinical symptoms, radiographic findings, or both suggest the relationship preoperatively. Cutaneous leiomyosarcomas comprise a third subgroup that has an excellent prognosis because of its superficial location and limited clinical stage. The last subgroup comprises leiomyosarcomas of vascular origin. As implied previously in the chapter, this designation is used to refer to tumors arising from medium-size or large veins, in contrast to leiomyosarcomas in which the vascular origin is identified on the basis of microscopic examination. Defined in this fashion, these tumors are rare. Leiomyosarcomas may occur in an unusual soft tissue site, such as the head and neck and paratesticular region,[23,24] but these are decidedly uncommon.

RETROPERITONEAL/ABDOMINAL LEIOMYOSARCOMAS

About one-half to three-quarters of all soft tissue leiomyosarcomas arise in the retroperitoneum and a smaller number in the abdominal cavity or mediastinum. Two-thirds of affected patients are women. The peak incidence occurs in the seventh decade.[25] The presenting signs and symptoms are relatively nonspecific and include an abdominal mass or swelling, pain, weight loss, nausea, or vomiting (Fig. 17-1).

Gross and Microscopic Findings

Virtually all retroperitoneal tumors are more than 5 cm, and most are larger than 10 cm when first detected,[5,6,26] in striking contrast to the majority of somatic soft tissue leiomyosarcomas.[3] They commonly involve other structures, such as the kidney, pancreas, and vertebral column by direct extension. Grossly, some have a white-gray whorled appearance resembling a leiomyoma on a cut section (Fig. 17-2), whereas others are fleshy white-gray masses with foci of hemorrhage and necrosis, indistinguishable from other sarcomas.

Histologically, the typical cell of a leiomyosarcoma is elongated and has abundant cytoplasm that varies tinctorially from pink to deep red in routinely stained sections. The nucleus is usually centrally located and blunt-ended or cigar-shaped (Fig. 17-3). In some smooth muscle cells, a vacuole is seen at one end of the nucleus, causing a slight indentation, so the nucleus assumes a concave rather than a convex contour (see Fig. 17-3). In less well-differentiated tumors, the nucleus is larger and more hyperchromatic and often loses its central location. Multinucleated giant cells are common. Poorly differentiated leiomyosarcomas may consist of essentially undifferentiated-appearing pleomorphic spindled cells, resembling undifferentiated pleomorphic sarcoma, requiring a careful search for more typical areas. Likewise, depending on the degree of differentiation, the appearance of the cytoplasm varies. Differentiated cells have numerous well-oriented myofibrils that are demonstrable as deep red, longitudinally placed parallel lines running the length of the cell, as seen with a Masson trichrome stain (Fig. 17-4). In poorly differentiated cells, the longitudinal striations are less numerous, poorly oriented, and, therefore, more difficult to identify. In some tumors, the cytoplasm has a clotted appearance as a result of clumping of the myofilamentous material (Fig. 17-5). When this phenomenon occurs, it may be difficult to identify linear striations. Leiomyosarcomas are typically composed of slender or slightly plump cells arranged in fascicles of varying size (Figs. 17-6 to 17-9). In well-differentiated areas, the fascicles intersect at right angles so it is possible to see transverse and longitudinal sections side by side, similar to the pattern of a uterine myoma. However, in many areas, the pattern is not that orderly, and it more closely resembles the intertwining fascicular growth of an adult fibrosarcoma (Fig. 17-10). In occasional leiomyosarcomas, the nuclei align themselves to create palisades, similar to a schwannoma (Fig. 17-11). Hyalinization is a relatively

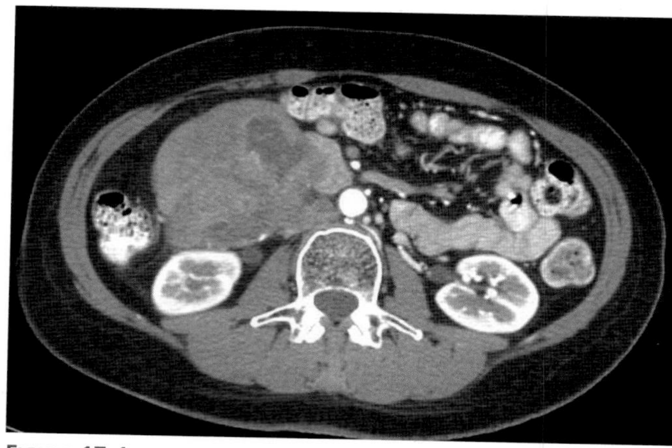

FIGURE 17-1. CT scan of retroperitoneal leiomyosarcoma, showing a large, heterogeneous mass displacing the internal organs. *(Courtesy of Dr. G. Petur Nielsen, Boston, MA, USA.)*

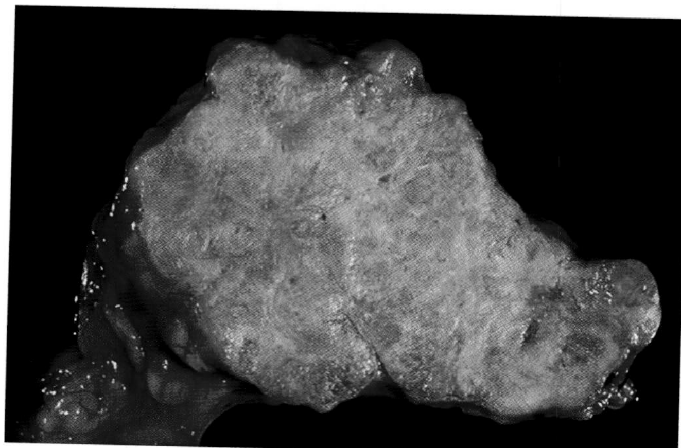

FIGURE 17-2. Retroperitoneal leiomyosarcoma characterized by fleshy white tissue with gelatinous change and necrosis. *(Courtesy of Dr. G. Petur Nielsen, Boston, MA, USA.)*

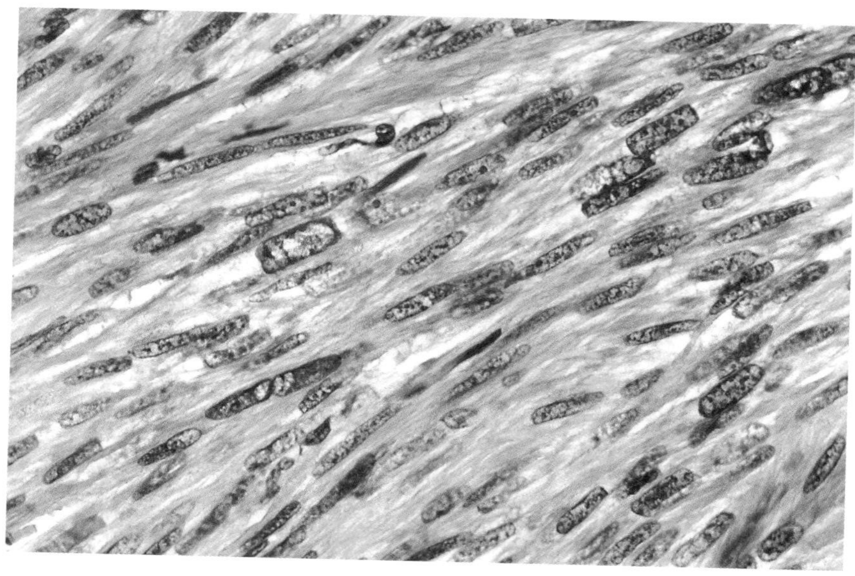

FIGURE 17-3. Cytologic features of leiomyosarcoma showing eosinophilic cytoplasm and blunt-ended nuclei. Occasional cells have perinuclear vacuoles.

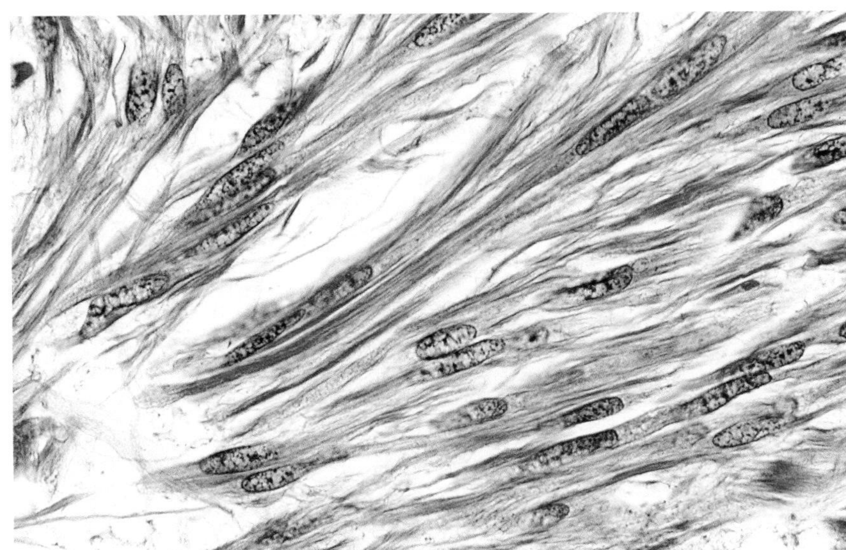

FIGURE 17-4. Masson trichrome stain illustrating longitudinal striations in a leiomyosarcoma. Striations appear as red, hair-like streaks in the cytoplasm.

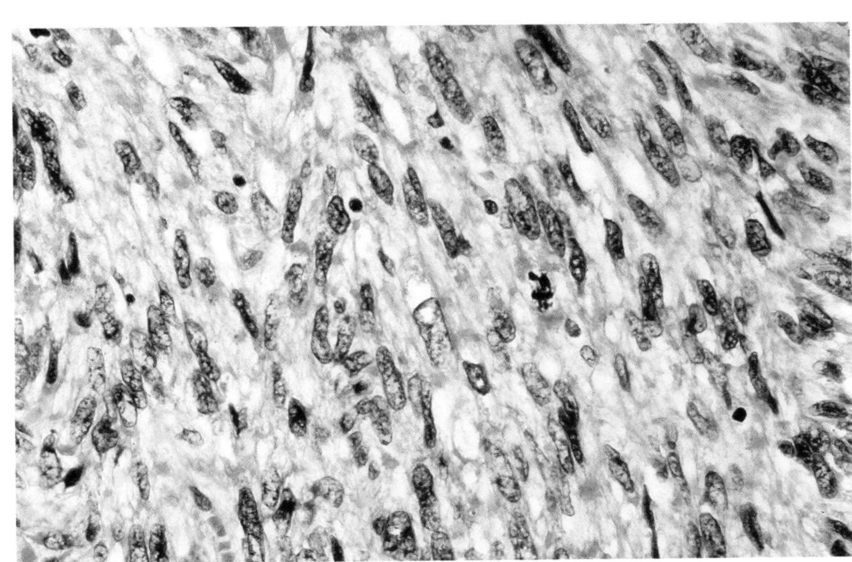

FIGURE 17-5. Leiomyosarcoma with clotted or clumped myofilamentous material in the cytoplasm.

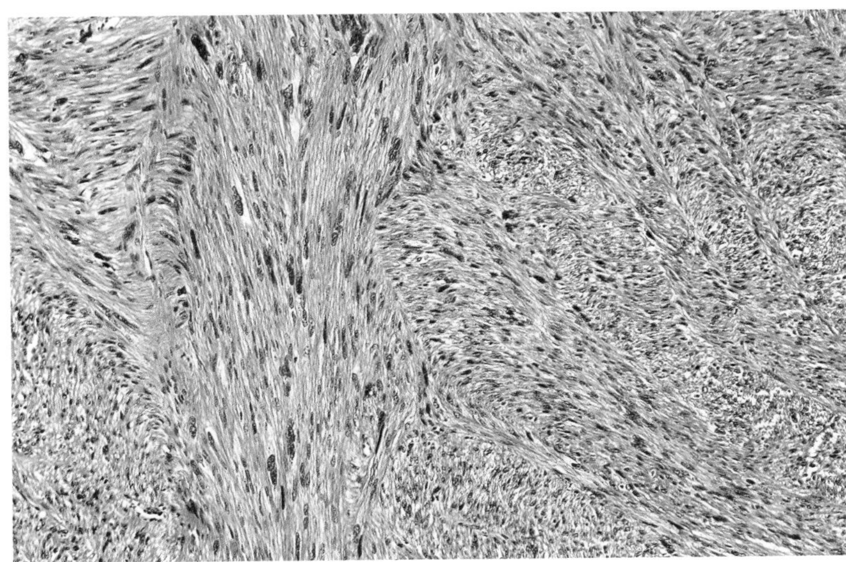

FIGURE 17-6. Moderately differentiated leiomyosarcoma composed of deeply eosinophilic fascicles intersecting at right angles.

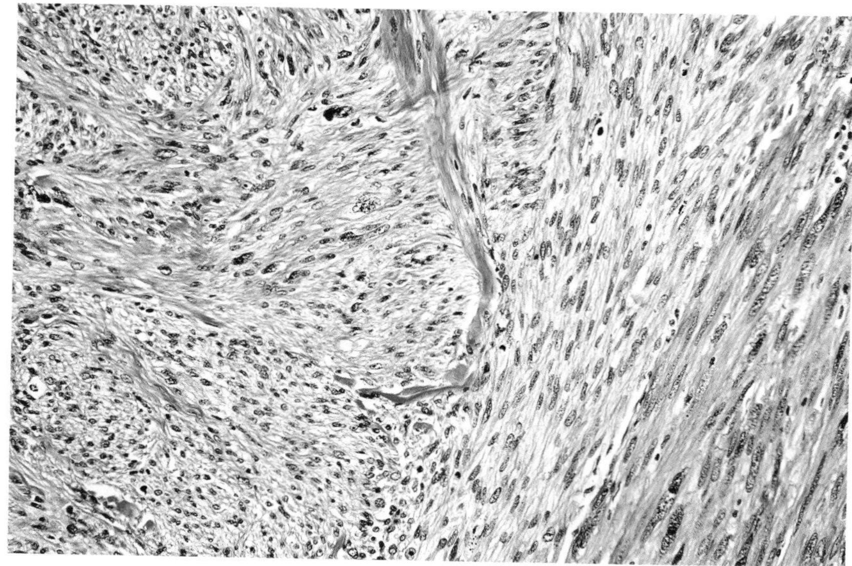

FIGURE 17-7. Moderately differentiated leiomyosarcoma composed of intersecting fascicles, some having a deeply eosinophilic hue and others a clear-cell appearance.

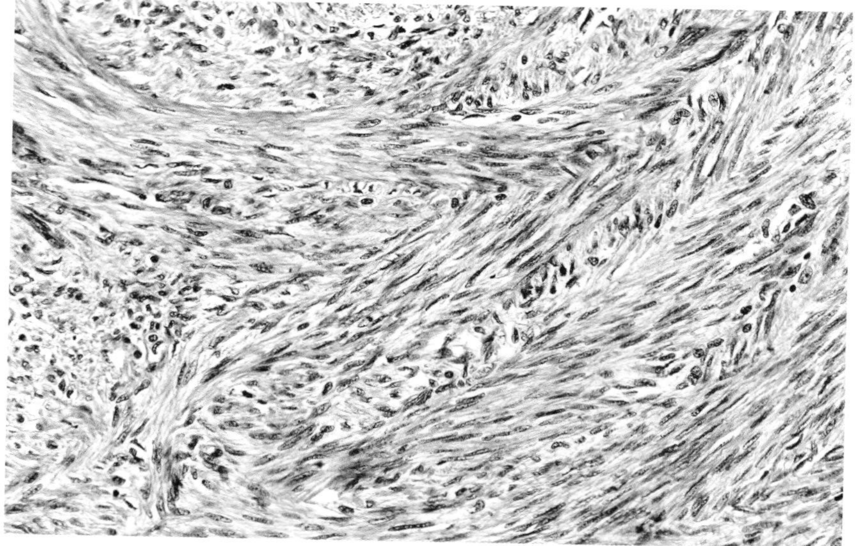

FIGURE 17-8. Well-differentiated leiomyosarcoma with a fascicular growth pattern.

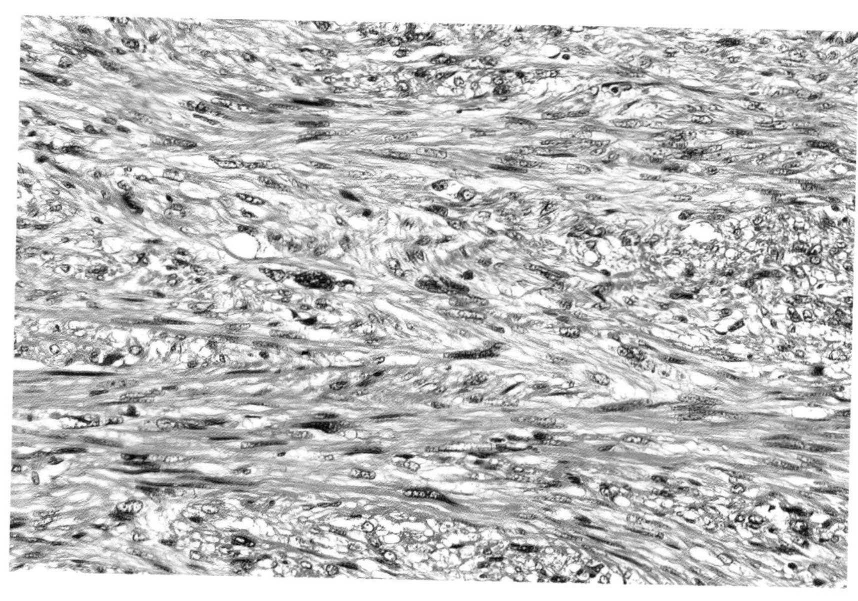

FIGURE 17-9. Moderately differentiated leiomyosarcoma with a fascicular growth pattern.

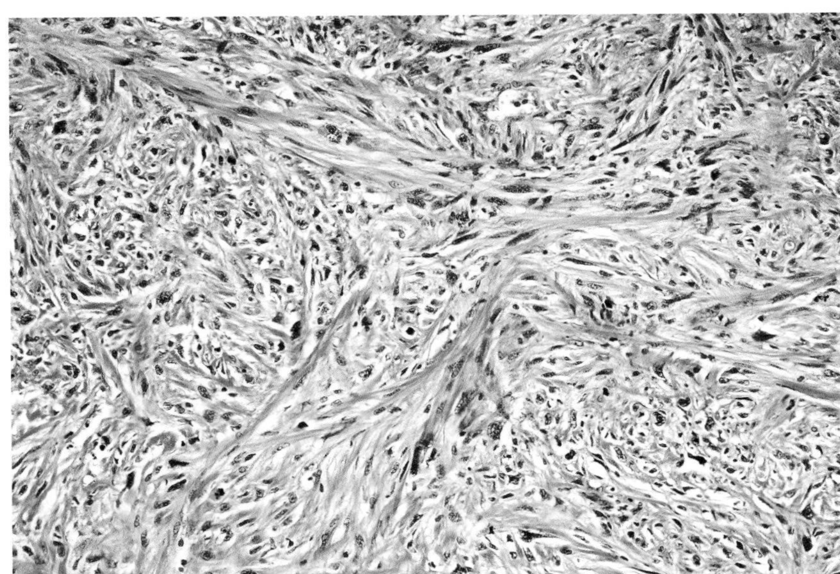

FIGURE 17-10. Leiomyosarcoma with a pattern of short intersecting fascicles.

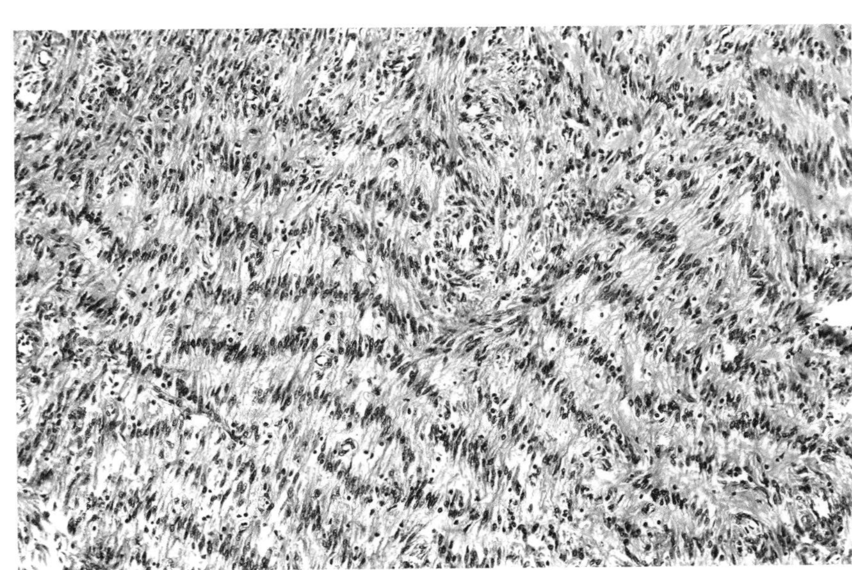

FIGURE 17-11. Leiomyosarcoma with nuclear palisading.

common, but usually focal, feature of many leiomyosarcomas (Fig. 17-12).[27] Extensively hyalinized leiomyosarcomas largely lack typical morphologic features, requiring ancillary immunohistochemical studies for a definitive diagnosis.

About 10% of retroperitoneal leiomyosarcomas are anaplastic tumors (Figs. 17-13 and 17-14), which, in the extreme case, resemble an undifferentiated pleomorphic sarcoma.[28] Some anaplastic leiomyosarcomas appear to arise in an abrupt fashion from preexisting well-differentiated tumors; such tumors have been referred to as *dedifferentiated leiomyosarcomas*, although this term is not universally accepted.[29,30] Anaplastic leiomyosarcomas contain numerous pleomorphic giant cells with deeply eosinophilic cytoplasm intimately admixed with a complement of more uniform-appearing spindle and round cells (Figs. 17-15 and 17-16). In contrast to undifferentiated pleomorphic sarcoma, these tumors have less interstitial collagen and few inflammatory cells. In addition, it is usually possible to document myogenic differentiation in the less pleomorphic areas. Necrosis, hemorrhage, and mitotic figures are frequent in these pleomorphic tumors. Osteoclastic giant cells may rarely be seen in leiomyosarcomas,[31-34] representing an unusual host response to the tumor. Some retroperitoneal leiomyosarcomas appear to represent dedifferentiated liposarcomas showing extensive heterologous differentiation.[35-38]

Histologic Variants of Leiomyosarcoma

So-called *inflammatory leiomyosarcoma* is a rare entity defined as a leiomyosarcoma containing xanthoma cells and a prominent inflammatory infiltrate (usually lymphocytes but, occasionally, neutrophils) (Fig. 17-17).[39] These tumors do not occur in any specific location and may be associated with constitutional or paraneoplastic symptoms such as anorexia, fever, night sweats, and diarrhea. Interestingly, whereas these tumors express desmin to a significant degree, they lack or only focally express other muscle markers, including muscle-specific actin, alpha smooth muscle actin, and caldesmon

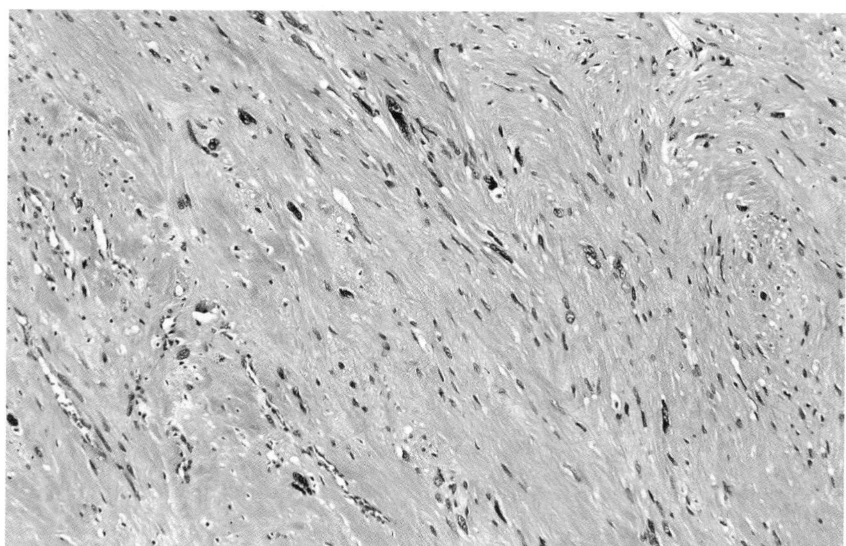

FIGURE 17-12. Hyalinization in a leiomyosarcoma.

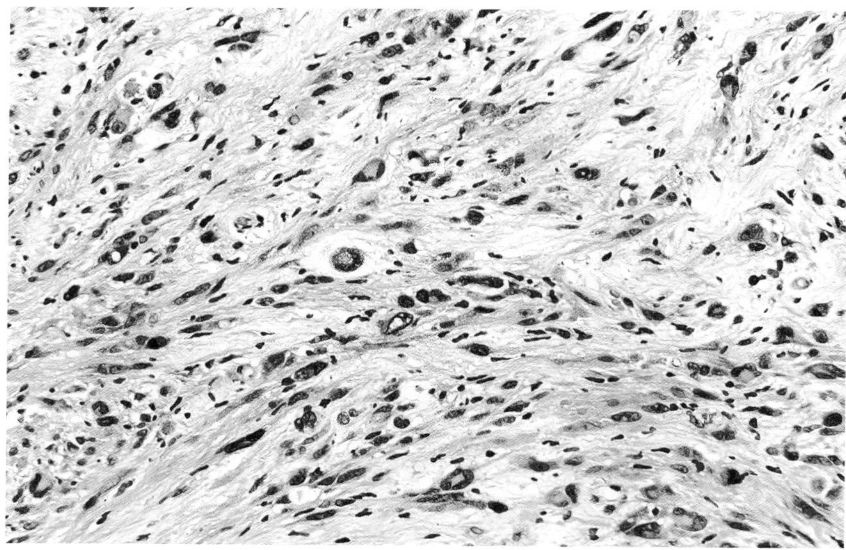

FIGURE 17-13. Pleomorphism in a leiomyosarcoma.

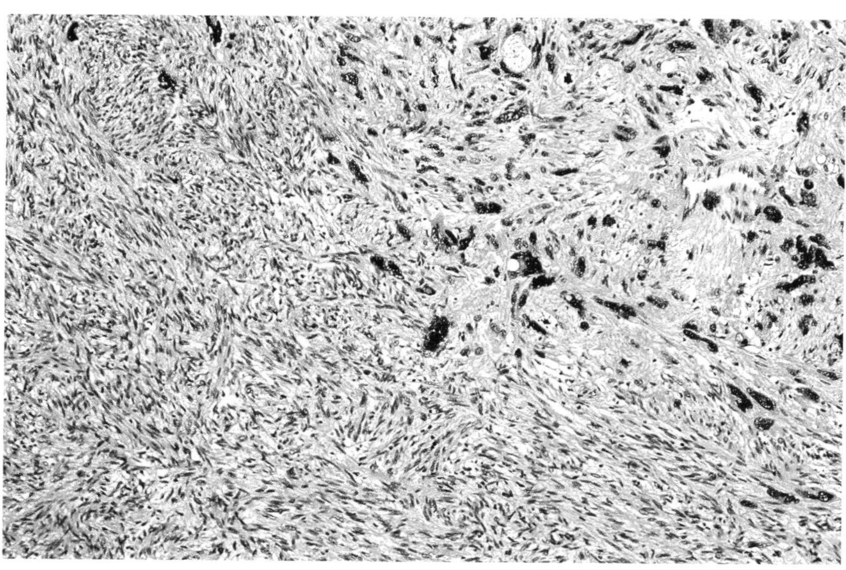

FIGURE 17-14. Leiomyosarcoma with pleomorphic areas resembling undifferentiated pleomorphic sarcoma (top right).

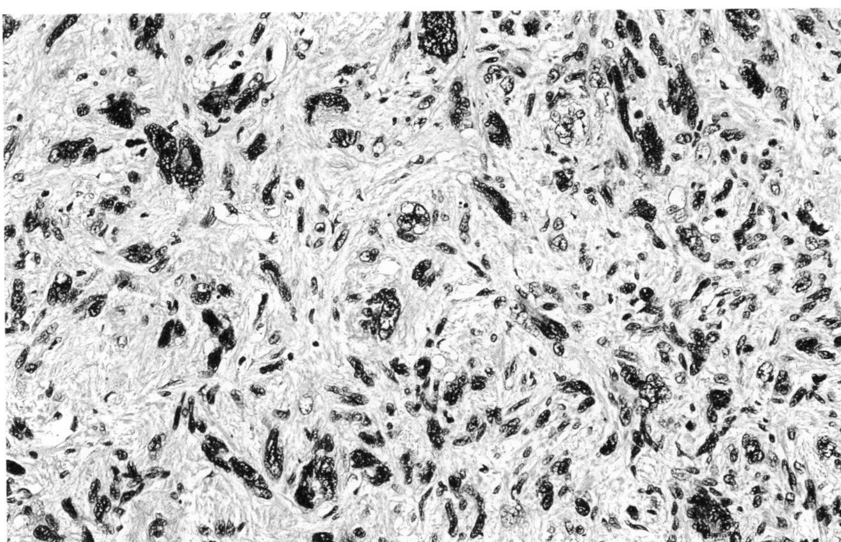

FIGURE 17-15. Pleomorphic area in leiomyosarcoma resembling undifferentiated pleomorphic sarcoma.

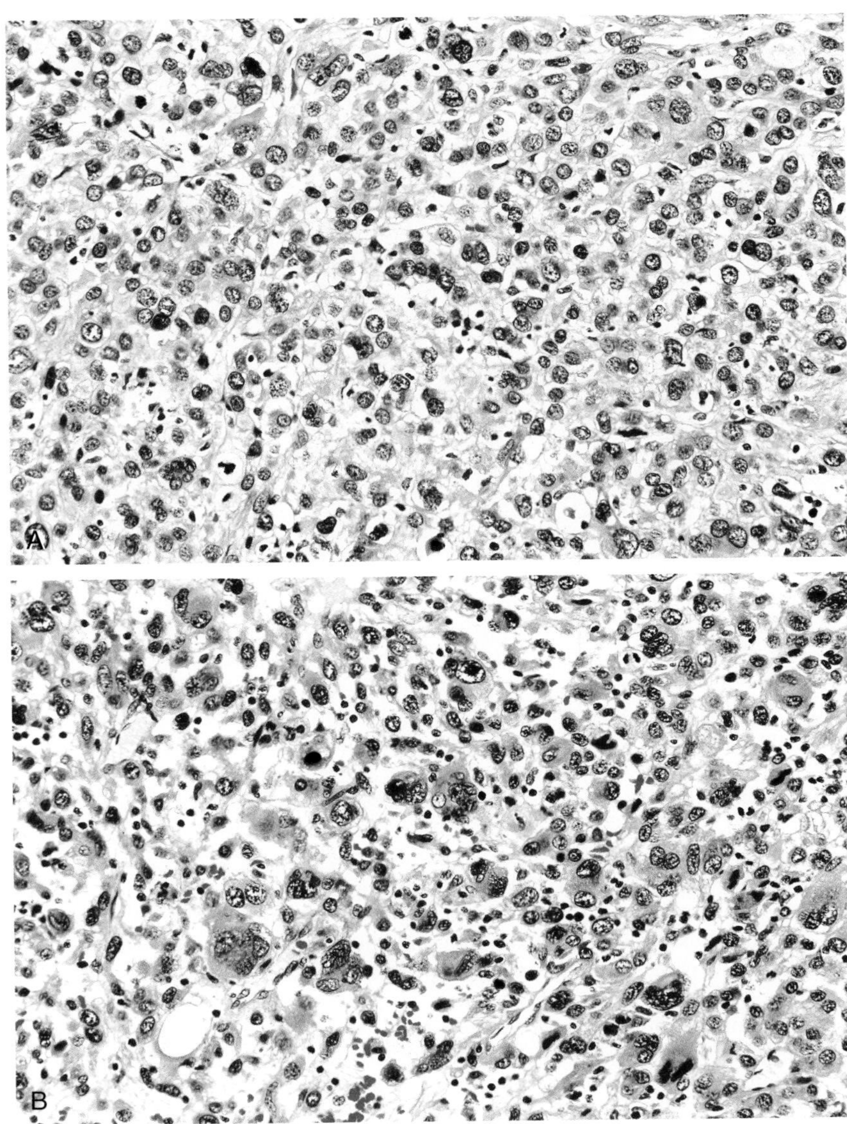

FIGURE 17-16. Leiomyosarcoma with round cell (A) and pleomorphic (B) areas.

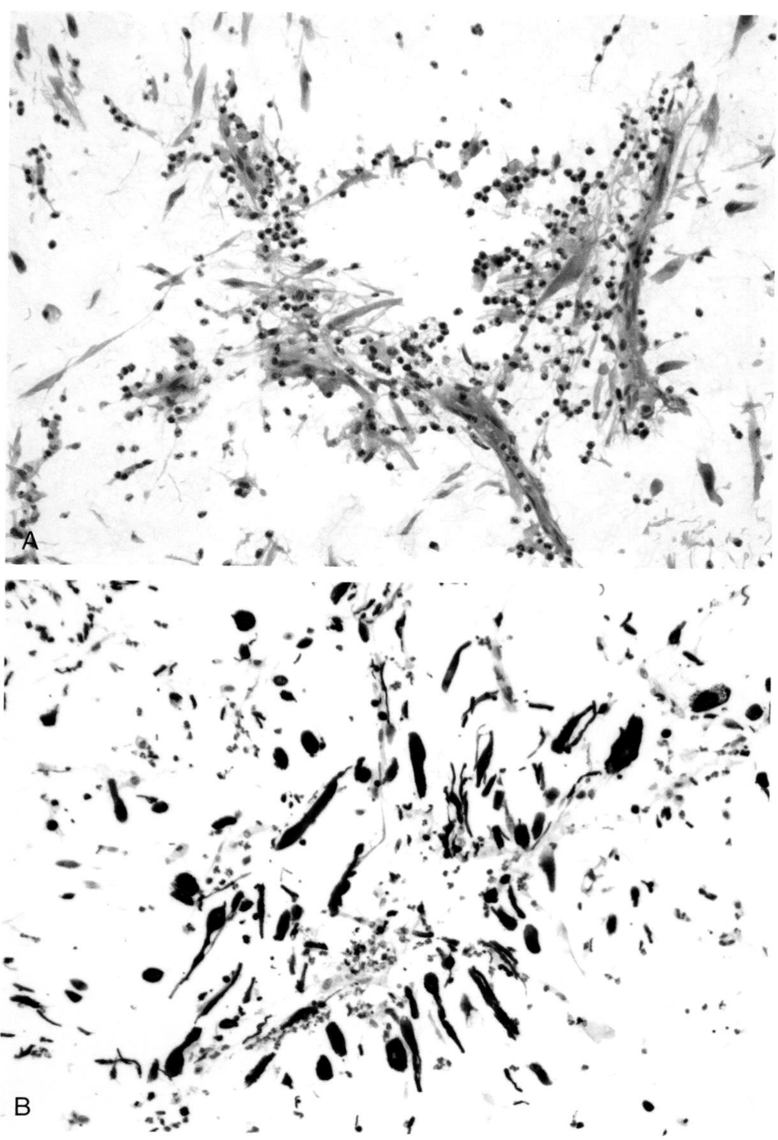

FIGURE 17-17. Inflammatory leiomyosarcoma consisting of small fascicles of cytologically atypical eosinophilic spindled cells in a myxoid background, with a prominent neutrophilic infiltrate (A). Diffuse desmin immunoreactivity in inflammatory leiomyosarcoma (B).

leading to the suggestion that these lesions may not be true smooth muscle tumors.[40] Most cases that have been analyzed have displayed a near-haploid karyotype. Although originally associated with an excellent prognosis, recent cases have been reported with metastases.

Myxoid change may occur in leiomyosarcomas. When extensive, these tumors appear grossly gelatinous and are referred to as *myxoid leiomyosarcoma*. Although most common in the uterus,[41,42] they develop in conventional soft tissue locations as well.[43] The spindled muscle cells are separated by pools of hyaluronic acid, and, in a cross-section, the fascicles resemble the cords of tumor seen in a myxoid chondrosarcoma (Figs. 17-18 and 17-19). Because these tumors are quite hypocellular relative to conventional leiomyosarcomas, mitotic rates estimated by counting high-power fields (HPF) are usually deceptively low, giving the false impression of a benign tumor. In general, myxoid leiomyosarcomas segregate toward the low-grade end of a grading spectrum. Of the 18 cases reported by Rubin and Fletcher,[43] 9 were considered grade 1, 8 grade 2, and only 1 grade 3. In their series, 5 of 13 patients experienced recurrences, often repeated, and 2 patients developed metastases. It is quite possible that spillage of the gelatinous matrix at the time of surgery contributes to the common phenomenon of local recurrence.

Rarely, leiomyosarcomas contain cells with granular eosinophilic cytoplasm[44] (granular cell leiomyosarcomas). This change corresponds to the presence of numerous granules that stain positively with periodic acid-Schiff (also known as PAS) and are resistant to diastase. Ultrastructurally, they are similar to the phagolysosomes seen in granular cell tumors.

Ultrastructural and Immunohistochemical Findings

Leiomyosarcomas are characterized by many of the same features as normal smooth muscle cells, but, in general, they are less developed. Differentiated leiomyosarcomas have deeply clefted nuclei and numerous well-oriented, thin (6 to 8 nm) myofilaments and dense bodies that occupy a large portion of

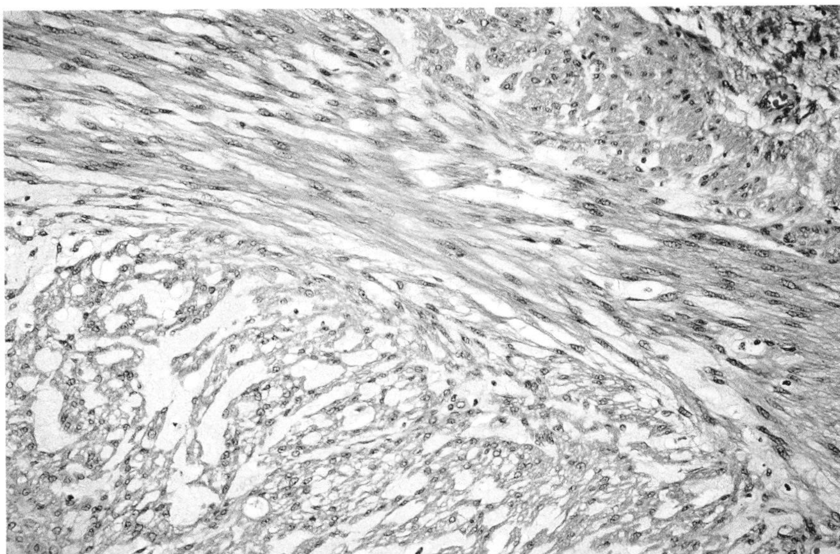

FIGURE 17-18. Myxoid leiomyosarcoma.

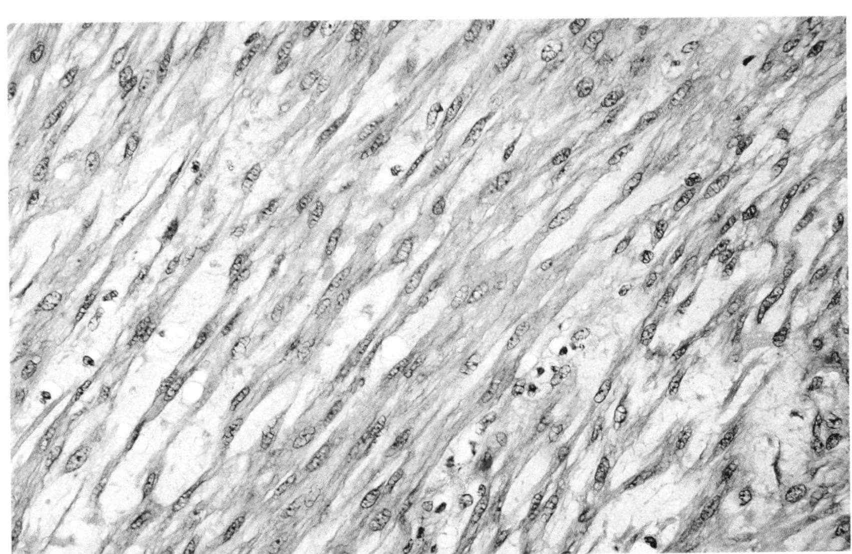

FIGURE 17-19. Myxoid leiomyosarcoma showing separation of spindle cells.

the cell (Fig. 17-20). Pinocytotic vesicles and intercellular connections are conspicuous, and basal lamina invests the entire cell membrane. The presence of these features is diagnostic of smooth muscle differentiation even without the benefit of light microscopic findings. On the other hand, poorly differentiated tumors show a loss of myofilaments, whereas rough endoplasmic reticulum and free ribosomes assume greater prominence.[45] Pinocytotic vesicles and intercellular attachments are sparse, and basal lamina may be incomplete or lacking altogether. All of these features must be evaluated *in toto* in these tumors and interpreted in conjunction with the light microscopic findings for diagnostic purposes. It should be emphasized that the mere presence of thin myofilaments with dense bodies does not identify a smooth muscle cell. Thin myofilaments are a nonspecific finding and can be seen in a variety of tumors where they typically occur underneath the cytoplasmic membrane.

Localization of muscle antigens by means of immunohistochemistry has largely replaced electron microscopy over the past decade. Although many leiomyosarcomas are easily diagnosed by light microscopic examination alone, poorly differentiated/anaplastic and extensively hyalinized tumors may require immunohistochemical confirmation of smooth muscle differentiation. It is important to keep in mind, however, that the distribution and intensity of muscle markers in highly pleomorphic areas of leiomyosarcoma are generally diminished compared to classic-appearing areas.[28]

Antibodies to smooth-muscle-specific (monoclonal antibody 1A4) and pan-muscle actins (monoclonal antibody HHF35)[46] are positive in most leiomyosarcomas.[9,28,47,48] Desmin, which is more variable, has been documented in one-half to nearly 100% of tumors,[28,48,49] depending on the series. Although there seems to be a general agreement that the presence of desmin diffusely throughout a tumor is usually indicative of myoid differentiation, the presence of actin or desmin focally should not necessarily be equated with myoid lineage because myofibroblasts in a variety of neoplastic and non-neoplastic conditions also display these phenotypes. The

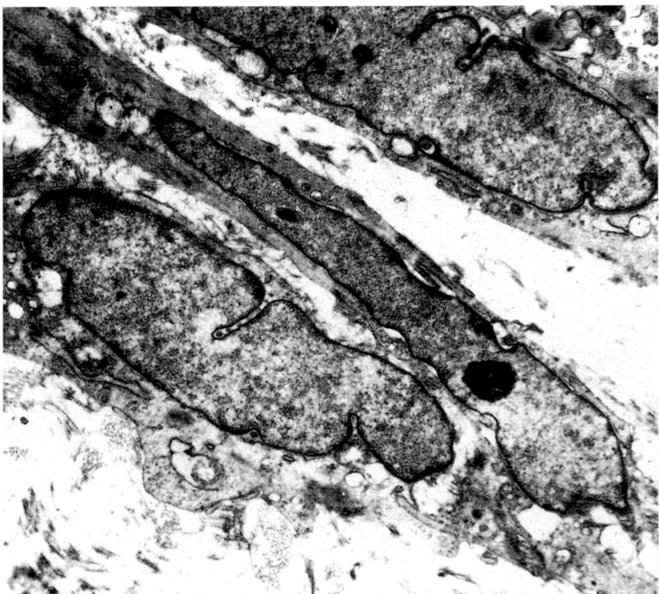

FIGURE 17-20. Electron micrograph of metastatic leiomyosarcoma. Cells are characterized by an elongated shape, deeply grooved nuclei, and numerous thin filaments with dense bodies.

pattern of smooth muscle actin expression may be helpful in discriminating true smooth muscle from myofibroblasts, with the former typically showing robust expression within the entire cell and the latter showing wispy expression confined to the periphery of the cytoplasm (tram-track pattern). Other markers of smooth muscle differentiation, including heavy caldesmon and smooth muscle myosin heavy chain, are less sensitive (approximately 40%) than are muscle actins and desmin for the diagnosis of leiomyosarcoma, although they are less often expressed in myofibroblasts.[50-52] These markers may, however, be expressed in myoepithelial cells, a potential pitfall in locations such as the skin and breast.[53] The immunophenotype of leiomyosarcomas may vary according to their origin. For example, tumors arising from vascular smooth muscle often show a desmin-negative/H-caldesmon-positive phenotype, and those arising in somatic soft tissue locations more often express desmin, and less often H-caldesmon.[54] Anomalous cytokeratin expression is relatively frequent in leiomyosarcomas, present in close to 40% of cases, and aberrant epithelial membrane antigen (also known as EMA) expression may also be seen.[55-59] Cytokeratin expression in leiomyosarcomas is limited to low-molecular weight types (keratins 8 and 18).[57] Leiomyosarcomas may also express CD34, S-100 protein, and estrogen and progesterone receptors.[23,48,60] Hormone receptor expression is not confined to leiomyosarcomas of gynecologic type in women and is not of value in the distinction of tumors of gynecologic and non-gynecologic origin.

Criteria of Malignancy

Criteria of malignancy in smooth muscle tumors were mentioned briefly in Chapter 16. In general, the finding of significant nuclear atypia even of a focal nature is a cause for concern in soft tissue smooth muscle tumors and should lead to an evaluation of mitotic activity. By definition, leiomyosarcomas possess some degree of nuclear atypia, but mitotic activity varies considerably. However, even very low levels of mitotic activity (less than 1/10 HPF) are accepted in the face of significant atypia as sufficient evidence of malignancy. In retroperitoneal lesions, coagulative necrosis is usually also present and can be quite impressive.

Differential Diagnosis

The differential diagnosis for leiomyosarcoma includes both non-pleomorphic spindle cell tumors, such as leiomyoma (of gynecologic and non-gynecologic types), cellular schwannoma, gastrointestinal stromal tumor, synovial sarcoma, malignant peripheral nerve sheath tumor, and inflammatory myofibroblastic tumor, as well as a variety of other pleomorphic sarcomas. Leiomyomas of gynecologic-type smooth muscle are common in the pelvis and retroperitoneum and pelvis and may achieve a large size at the time of diagnosis. As in the uterus, extrauterine gynecologic-type smooth muscle tumors may show mitotic activity but lack cytologic atypia and coagulative tumor cell necrosis (as distinct from infarct-type necrosis). Leiomyomas of gynecologic-type smooth muscle closely resemble uterine leiomyomas, with thick-walled blood vessels, trabecular and corded growth patterns, and occasionally fat. Leiomyomas of somatic soft tissue by definition are hypocellular, devoid of cytologic atypia, and essentially amitotic.[61] Cellular schwannomas are encapsulated, cellular, fascicular proliferations of well-differentiated, S-100 protein-positive, actin and (usually) desmin-negative Schwann cells, typically containing peripheral lymphoid aggregates, and intratumoral foamy macrophages. However, one should note that there have been exceptionally rare cases of cellular schwannoma exhibiting anomalous desmin immunoreactivity, apparently representing cross-reactivity with glial fibrillary acidic protein (also known as GFAP). Extraintestinal gastrointestinal stromal tumors show a lesser degree of cytoplasmic eosinophilia than is seen in true smooth muscle tumors and typically express both CD117 (c-Kit) and DOG1 (both positive in greater than 90% of gastrointestinal stromal tumors). Inflammatory myofibroblastic tumors usually arise in much younger patients than do true smooth muscle tumors and show a prominent mixed chronic inflammatory cell infiltrate, stromal hyalinization, and calcifications. Strong expression of ALK1 protein is seen in many inflammatory myofibroblastic tumors but not in smooth muscle tumors. Monophasic synovial sarcomas show alternating zones of hypocellularity and hypercellularity, carrot-shaped nuclei, wiry collagen, a staghorn vascular pattern, and numerous stromal mast cells. Expression of TLE1 and cytokeratins (focally), but not muscle markers, is typical of synovial sarcoma. Malignant peripheral nerve sheath tumors lack the diffuse cytoplasmic eosinophilia of leiomyosarcoma, have wavy or buckled nuclei, and show patchy expression of S-100 protein but not actins or desmin.

Genetic Findings

Karyotypic analyses of leiomyosarcomas typically show complex numeric and structural abnormalities, without consistent losses or gains.[62,63] Frequently lost chromosome regions include 3p21-23, 8p21-pter, 13q12-13, 13q32-qter, with areas of frequent gain, including the 1q21-31 region.[64] Comparative genomic hybridization studies have shown gain from chromosomes 1, 15, 17, 19, 20, 22, and X and loss from 1q, 2, 4q, 9p, 10, 11q, 13q, and 16.[65-67] Gain of material from chromosomes 6q and 8q may be seen in larger tumors. At the molecular genetic level, methylation-related inactivation of cancer-associated genes such as RASSF1A and p16INK4 has been associated with poor prognosis in patients with leiomyosarcomas.[68] The RB1 gene has been implicated in some cases of leiomyosarcoma, with frequent abnormalities in the Rb-cyclin D1 pathway.[69] P53 and MDM2 abnormalities seem to be less common than in other sarcoma subtypes, although alterations in these loci may be associated with a poor prognosis in leiomyosarcomas.[19] Specific gene expression signature patterns may offer the ability to further predict outcome.[70-72] Similarities between the gene expression patterns of leiomyosarcomas and undifferentiated pleomorphic sarcomas also suggest that some cases previously classified as the latter entity instead represent particularly poorly differentiated leiomyosarcomas.[73]

Clinical Behavior

Retroperitoneal leiomyosarcomas are aggressive lesions that cause death not only by distant metastasis but also by local extension. The survival figures differ among series and are obviously influenced by the criteria of malignancy, proportion of high-grade versus low-grade tumors, and length of the follow-up. Early studies reflected mortality rates of 80% to 90% within a 2 to 5 year follow-up period.[3,6,26] However, a recent multi-institutional study published by the National Federation of Centers in the Fight Against Cancer (FNCLCC) detailing experience with 165 retroperitoneal sarcomas of all types indicates that an improvement in complete resection rates in retroperitoneal sarcomas has reduced local recurrence to 50% and improved survival rates to 50%. Factors that influence outcome in (nonliposarcomatous) retroperitoneal sarcomas include size, grade, and whether extension to bone and nerve is present.[74] More recent studies have reported better outcome in retroperitoneal leiomyosarcomas treated with more aggressive surgical resection.[75,76]

LEIOMYOSARCOMAS OF SOMATIC SOFT TISSUE

Compared to retroperitoneal lesions, tumors arising from the soft tissues of the extremities and trunk are far less common and affect the sexes equally. Only 48 cases were identified by Gustafson et al.[1] in a 22-year review of a Swedish population in Lund, and Farshid et al.[4] have studied 42 cases largely based on referred consultations. The largest series to date from the Scandinavian Sarcoma Group Leiomyosarcoma Working Group includes 225 patients with leiomyosarcomas of nonvisceral soft tissue.[77] These tumors present as an enlarging mass, usually in the lower extremity. About half develop in the subcutis and the remainder in muscle. They have a circumscribed multinodular appearance and are significantly smaller (4 to 6 cm) than those in the retroperitoneum. When examined microscopically, at least one-third arise from a small vein causing expansion of the wall and protrusion into the lumen. Because many remain partially or completely confined by the adventitia, they give the impression of being discrete, encapsulated lesions, a feature that often leads to an inadvertent enucleation by the surgeon. Despite their vascular origin, few are associated with symptoms of vascular compromise as occurs with leiomyosarcomas arising from major vessels. The histologic features and criteria of malignancy in this group of leiomyosarcomas are similar to those in the retroperitoneum with some minor exceptions. Although, by definition, all display some degree of atypia, the range of mitotic activity can be quite wide with levels as low as less than 1/10 HPF. Necrosis is rarely encountered to the extent as that seen in retroperitoneal leiomyosarcomas.

As compared with retroperitoneal tumors, the behavior of somatic soft tissue leiomyosarcomas has been relatively poorly defined as a result of the smaller number of reported cases. In the most recent Scandinavian series, 84% of patients with localized disease at presentation remained free of locally recurrent disease at a median of 5.5 years of follow-up, with distant metastases in 34% and death from disease in 51% of patients, respectively.[77] Older series have shown local recurrence rates of 10% to 25% and metastatic rates from 44% to 45%, with a 5-year survival of 64%.[1,4] Most metastases develop in the lung and rarely in lymph nodes.

A number of variables affect the prognosis in this subgroup of leiomyosarcomas, but their relative importance differs, depending on the study. Gustafson et al.[1] found that age over 60 years and vascular invasion were independent risk factors for death from the tumor, whereas others have reported depth, tumor size, and stage as independent factors.[78,79] In the study of Farshid et al.,[4] factors that were predictive of metastasis at 36 months in a multivariate analysis were grade (FNCLCC system) and whether the tumor had been violated surgically (i.e., disruption). However, disruption also correlated with size and depth and, therefore, could represent a surrogate marker for both. On the other hand, this group of soft tissue sarcomas requires special scrutiny because their frequent origin from vessels may grant them greater accessibility to the bloodstream and hematogenous dissemination. This phenomenon was underscored by Berlin et al.,[80] who reported metastasis from all six extremity leiomyosarcomas that originated from veins. One patient with a small (3 cm) mass arising from the saphenous vein died 1 month after surgery with liver and lung metastases. Data from the Scandinavian group showed decreased metastasis-free survival to be associated with higher tumor grade, larger tumor size, and deeper tumor location, with higher tumor grade also significantly associated with decreased overall survival.[77]

CUTANEOUS LEIOMYOSARCOMAS

Although in the past the term *cutaneous leiomyosarcoma* referred to tumors arising in the dermis or subcutis, this designation should be restricted to lesions that arise from the dermis and only secondarily invade the subcutis. This is because leiomyosarcomas based exclusively in the subcutis arise in many instances from vessels and, therefore, have much in common with soft tissue leiomyosarcomas with respect to their origin, access to the bloodstream, and ultimate prognosis. Unfortunately, this definition has not been routinely used in the past, and so the distinction between these two potentially different diseases has been blurred.

Cutaneous leiomyosarcomas arise from the arrector pili muscle of the skin and its scrotal counterpart, dartoic smooth muscle. They may occur in patients of either sex and at any age but are most common in males between the fifth and seventh decades.[81-83] Cutaneous leiomyosarcomas typically present as solitary lesions on the scalp and hair-bearing extensor surfaces; the presence of multiple lesions should always raise the question of metastatic disease from a previously resected or occult leiomyosarcoma of retroperitoneal or deep soft tissue origin.[84] Cutaneous leiomyosarcomas are usually less than 2 cm at presentation and frequently cause changes in the overlying skin, such as discoloration and ulceration. Because of their rarity, these lesions seldom are correctly diagnosed preoperatively.

Gross and Microscopic Findings

Grossly, these leiomyosarcomas usually have a gray-white, whorled appearance and a varying degree of circumscription. Those in the dermis appear ill-defined by virtue of the intricate blending of tumor fascicles with the surrounding collagen and pilar arrector muscle. Those with extensions into the subcutis, in contrast, appear more circumscribed because they compress the surrounding tissue, creating a pseudocapsule. Most superficial leiomyosarcomas resemble retroperitoneal leiomyosarcomas in basic organization (Fig. 17-21).

Most are moderately well-differentiated tumors, differing principally by a lack of regressive or degenerative change. Hemorrhage, necrosis, hyalinization, and myxoid change are rarely encountered, which is probably a reflection of the smaller size of these lesions. Giant cells may be present, but, as in retroperitoneal tumors, it is uncommon to encounter a tumor that has a predominantly pleomorphic appearance. Mitotic figures, including atypical forms, are easily identified in these tumors. In the largest series, reported by Fields and Helwig,[14] 80% of these tumors had more than 2 mitoses/10 HPF. In general, those cutaneous smooth muscle tumors showing cytologic atypia and greater than 2 mitotic figures/10 HPF are diagnosed as leiomyosarcoma. Tumors showing cytologic atypia alone may be diagnosed as atypical pilar smooth muscle tumors but should be completely excised to prevent local recurrence and possible tumor progression. Muscle actin is present in virtually all tumors, although desmin is variably expressed and, when present, may be seen focally only.[85] A small number of cutaneous leiomyosarcomas contain cytokeratins.[85]

Clinical Behavior

The prognosis for cutaneous leiomyosarcoma is almost always excellent, with the overwhelming majority of tumors cured with a prompt wide surgical excision. This may, in part, reflect that the great majority of cutaneous leiomyosarcomas are small (less than 2 cm) and low-grade.[82] Cutaneous leiomyosarcomas that are confined to the dermis or show, at most, minimal involvement of the subcutaneous fat have a particularly good prognosis; it has been suggested that such tumors be labeled as *atypical pilar smooth muscle tumors* rather than *leiomyosarcoma*, although this suggestion has not been universally accepted.[83] These tumors are continued to be diagnosed as leiomyosarcoma, commenting on their excellent prognosis and recommending complete excision with histologically negative margins and careful follow-up with attention to local recurrence. Although it is difficult to quantify the metastatic risk for cutaneous leiomyosarcoma, it seems clear that the risk of metastasis increases with a greater degree of subcutaneous involvement, larger tumor size, high histologic grade, and previous local recurrence. In general, leiomyosarcomas confined to the dermis do not metastasize,[14,85,86] whereas those involving the subcutis metastasize in approximately 30% to 40% of cases.[14,85,86] The high rate of metastasis (50%) noted in the early report of Stout and Hill[87] reflects that most of their cases were subcutaneous lesions, and some even penetrated deep soft tissue, a phenomenon that substantially alters the outcome for the worse. Metastatic spread occurs hematogenously to the lung, although regional lymph nodes were

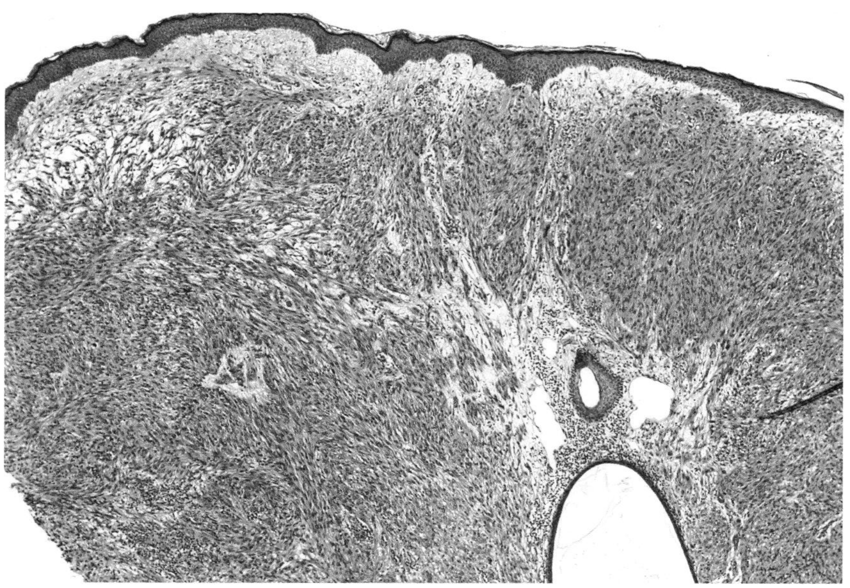

FIGURE 17-21. Superficial leiomyosarcoma arising from dermis.

involved in about 25% of Stout and Hill's[87] cases and have been noted in sporadic case reports.[87,88]

Because many of these lesions are potentially curable, every effort should be made to eradicate the tumor initially with a wide excision. Lesions allowed to recur run an increased risk of eventual metastasis because there is a distinct tendency for recurrent lesions to be larger and to involve deeper structures.[14] Mohs surgery has recently been used in the treatment of this disease[89,90] with a reported recurrence rate of 14%.[90]

LEIOMYOSARCOMAS OF VASCULAR ORIGIN

Leiomyosarcomas of vascular origin comprise a seemingly rare group of tumors illustrated because only a few hundred cases have been reported in the literature and only isolated instances are recorded in several large autopsy series. Hallock et al.[91] noted one case in 34,000 autopsies, Abell[92] reported two in 14,000 autopsies, and Dorfman and Fisher[93] found none in 30,000 autopsies. It should be emphasized that several features of this disease probably significantly affect its detection, diagnosis, and incidence. Lesions arising from major vessels, such as the vena cava, are likely to produce symptoms leading to their detection. Conversely, tumors arising from small vessels, vessels subserved by ancillary tributaries, or vessels in deep locations probably go unrecognized in a significant percentage of cases. It is difficult, therefore, to be certain what percentage of leiomyosarcomas of the retroperitoneum or other deep soft tissue sites may actually be of vascular origin. Hashimoto et al.[2] documented that, in their experience, at least one-fourth of leiomyosarcomas of peripheral soft tissue arose from or involved a vessel; this has been observed in at least one-third of cases.[4] Therefore, the recorded experience with vascular leiomyosarcomas is a biased one, which probably underestimates the true incidence and possibly also conveys a false impression concerning clinical behavior.

Clinical Findings

The distribution of vascular leiomyosarcomas parallels in a crudely inverse fashion the pressure in the vascular bed. Leiomyosarcomas are most common in large veins such as the vena cava, far less common in the pulmonary artery, and rare in systemic arteries. In an extensive review by Kevorkian and Cento,[7] of cases reported up to the early 1970s, a total of 33 cases arose in the inferior vena cava, and 35 collectively affected other medium-size or large veins; 10 occurred in the pulmonary artery alone, and 8 arose in systemic arteries. One report has indicated the unique occurrence of a leiomyosarcoma in a surgically created arteriovenous fistula.[94] The symptoms related to these tumors are diverse and are determined by the location of the tumor, rate of growth, and degree of collateral blood flow or drainage in an affected part.

Inferior Vena Cava Leiomyosarcoma

Inferior vena cava leiomyosarcomas occur during middle or late adult life, at an average age of about 50 years; 80% to 90% of patients are women.[95-97] The location of the tumor in the vessel is significant because it determines the symptoms and surgical resectability. Based on material submitted to the International Registry of Inferior Vena Cava Leiomyosarcomas, most tumors arise in the lower (44.2%) or middle (50.8%) portion, with only a small number (4.2%) arising from the upper third or suprahepatic region.[98] Patients with upper segment tumors develop Budd-Chiari syndrome, with hepatomegaly, jaundice, and massive ascites. Nausea, vomiting, and lower extremity edema may also be present. These tumors are surgically unresectable. Tumors of the middle segment involve the region between the renal veins and hepatic veins; they produce symptoms of right upper quadrant pain and tenderness, frequently mimicking biliary tract disease. Extension into the hepatic veins may cause some of the symptoms of the Budd-Chiari syndrome, whereas extension into the renal veins results in varying degrees of renal dysfunction, from mild elevation of blood urea nitrogen to nephrotic syndrome. Some of these lesions are surgically resectable. Lesions arising below the renal veins cause lower leg edema, but, unless they have spread extensively beyond the confines of the vessel, they are often amenable to surgical excision.

To date, the long-term outlook for this disease is poor. A large study comparing the effect of caval wall resection with a more extended segmental resection of the vessel demonstrated no significant difference in either a 5-year (55% versus 37%) or 10-year (42% versus 23%) survival. This seems to indicate that, at the time of clinical detection, the disease is relatively advanced and not curable by surgery in most instances. Very recently, improved outcome has been reported in a small series of Korean patients, with a multidisciplinary approach, including resection, prosthetic inferior vena cava grafting, chemotherapy, and radiotherapy.[99] Metastatic disease is seen most commonly in the lung, kidney, pleura, chest wall, liver, and bone.[100]

Leiomyosarcomas of Other Veins

Unlike vena cava lesions, those in other veins affect the sexes equally and most often arise in the veins of the lower extremity, including the saphenous, iliac, and femoral veins. They usually present as mass lesions of variable duration that occasionally produce lower leg edema. Pressure on nerves coursing close to the affected vessel may produce additional symptoms of numbness. Angiographically, the lesions are highly vascular and create compression of the accompanying artery. The compression appears to be the result of entrapment of the artery that resides in the same preformed fibrous sheath (conjunctiva vasorum) as the vein. Because an incisional biopsy of intravascular sarcomas can give rise to considerable seeding of tumor by hemorrhage, it has been suggested that thorough radiographic evaluation be followed by a needle biopsy in selected cases. The behavior of this group of leiomyosarcomas has been a controversial topic.[101] Although one series suggested that small intravascular leiomyosarcomas might have a relatively good prognosis,[101] all six patients reported by Berlin et al.[80] developed metastases, even those with relatively low mitotic rates. However, all but one of the tumors exceeded 4 cm in diameter.

Pulmonary Artery Leiomyosarcoma

Pulmonary artery leiomyosarcomas are the most common form of arterial leiomyosarcoma. They occur in adults and display no predilection for either sex. Their symptoms are referable to decreased pulmonary outflow and include chest pain, dyspnea, palpitations, dizziness, syncopal attacks, and eventual right heart failure. Until recently, the diagnosis was inevitably made at autopsy. Most of these tumors arise at the base of the heart and grow distally into the left and right main pulmonary arteries.

Gross and Microscopic Findings

In almost all reported cases, vascular leiomyosarcomas are described as polypoid or nodular masses that are firmly attached to the vessel at some point and have spread for a variable extent along its surface (Fig. 17-22). However, some reported cases describing extensive spread along the vena cava into the right heart may represent misdiagnosed intravenous leiomyomatosis (see Chapter 16).[102] In the case of thin-walled veins, extension to the adventitial surfaces and adjacent structures is a relatively early event, whereas, in arteries, the integrity of the internal elastic lamina is often preserved so that there is no spread outside of the vessel. Histologically, the tumors are similar to those in the retroperitoneum, although they usually do not exhibit as much hemorrhage or necrosis (Fig. 17-23). Mitoses are rather easy to identify in these tumors, and the histologic criteria of malignancy previously discussed are equally applicable to these lesions. True leiomyomas arising from vessels are rare, and this diagnosis should be made with extreme caution and only after the lesion has been sampled extensively.

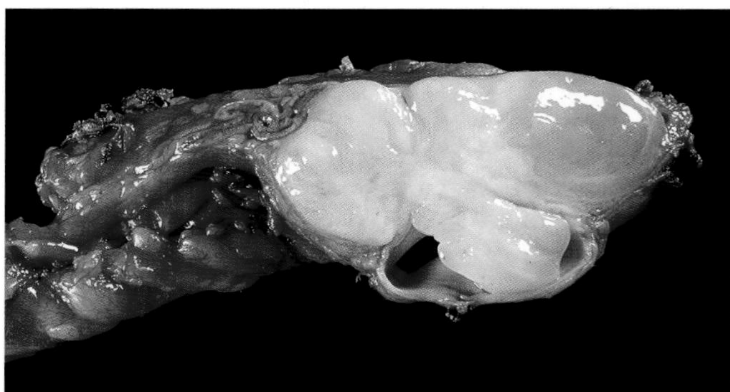

FIGURE 17-22. Leiomyosarcoma arising from the vena cava. Tumor partially occludes the lumen and involves the adjacent soft tissues, with displacement of the adrenal gland. *(Courtesy of Dr. G. Petur Nielsen, Boston, MA, USA.)*

Behavior and Treatment

The morbidity and mortality associated with these tumors are primarily a result of direct extension of the tumor along vessels, compromising the circulation. In only about half of the patients are metastases documented at the time of surgery or autopsy; they occur mainly in the liver or lung and less often in regional lymph nodes or intra-abdominal organs. Unfortunately, because only about half of the cases were diagnosed antemortem in the past, there is little information concerning the results of therapy. It may be anticipated that more sophisticated imaging techniques leading to an earlier diagnosis and therapy will improve survival rates, which so far have been poor. In 1973, Stuart and Baker[103] analyzed 10 such tumors in the vena cava that were treated surgically; they noted that all five patients who were followed longer than 1 year died. In a more recent series by Burke and Virmani,[100] only 7 of 13 inferior vena cava sarcomas developed metastases.

One of the greatest problems when treating this disease is that the location itself may preclude surgical resection. This is true of suprahepatic lesions, where ligation of the cava and partial hepatectomy have never been accomplished. Middle caval lesions may be resected with difficulty but require removal of one kidney and pelvic transplantation of the other if irradiation is contemplated.

MISCELLANEOUS SARCOMAS OF VASCULAR ORIGIN

Non-myogenic sarcomas arising from vessels are a veritable potpourri of lesions that are difficult to classify.[92,104-108] In contrast to the foregoing group, most of these peculiar hybrid

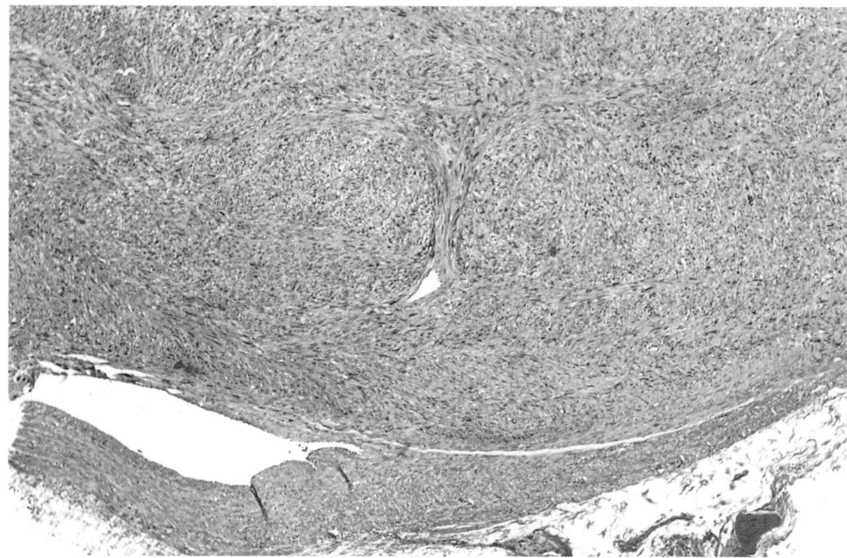

FIGURE 17-23. Leiomyosarcoma arising from a vein. Tumor protrudes into the vessel lumen.

lesions occur more often in the arterial system, particularly the pulmonary artery, where they tend to present during middle age with a constellation of symptoms associated with right ventricular outflow obstruction or pulmonary emboli.[100] Most of the tumors in this location probably arise from the base of the heart, although it is difficult to exclude an origin from the valve or even the heart itself. Aortic sarcomas tend to develop in older patients and involve the lower portion of the vessel. They are associated with myriad symptoms related to systemic embolization.[100] Arterial sarcomas grow in an intraluminal fashion similar to leiomyosarcomas, but there is a tendency for such lesions to creep along the vessel wall, splitting apart the layers of intima and media in their paths. This form of spreading was termed *intimal sarcomatosis* by Hedinger.[109] Histologically, a variety of terms have been applied to these tumors, including *pleomorphic sarcoma*, *intimal sarcoma*, *undifferentiated sarcoma*,[110] *fusocellular sarcoma*, *malignant mesenchymoma*,[111] *chondrosarcoma*,[106] and *osteosarcoma*.[98,112,113] The terms serve to emphasize that these tumors are, in general, highly pleomorphic tumors composed of haphazardly arranged giant cells and spindle cells.

The largest institutional review of arterial sarcomas was reported by the Armed Forces Institute of Pathology (also known as AFIP), which analyzed 11 and 16 cases from the aorta and pulmonary artery, respectively.[100] Histologically and for the most part, the sarcomas in both locations were pleomorphic, intima-based lesions. Of the 17 cases reported, 3 had the pattern of angiosarcoma and 3 osteosarcomas; the remainder were pleomorphic sarcomas that were difficult to classify. Other reports have documented the presence of cartilage or skeletal muscle differentiation in these tumors.[107,111]

Because these tumors occur in a different set of vessels, exhibit a strikingly different histologic appearance, and often remain confined to the superficial portions of the vessel suggests the possibility that they are intimal sarcomas, in contrast to the previous group, tumors that are more properly considered sarcomas of medial or adventitial origin. Because of their location, the diagnosis is rarely made antemortem, and death from local tumor extension, particularly to the lungs, is the rule.

EPSTEIN-BARR VIRUS-ASSOCIATED SMOOTH MUSCLE TUMORS

Smooth muscle tumors occur in immunocompromised patients with greater frequency than in the general population. Reported initially as a complication of renal transplantation and immunosuppression during the 1970s,[114,115] these smooth muscle tumors have been associated more recently with acquired immunodeficiency syndrome (AIDS)[116-124] and with cardiac and liver transplantation. However, it was not until 1995 that a causal link between these tumors and the Epstein-Barr virus (EBV) infection was established.[120,121] These tumors may be associated with either of the two EBV strains.

Most EBV smooth muscle tumors (EBVSMT) occur in children and, interestingly, develop in organs not traditionally considered preferred sites for leiomyosarcomas (soft tissue, liver, lung, spleen, dura). EBVSMT most often arise as a complication of kidney transplantation but typically do not involve the kidney itself, and they most often occur in the native or transplanted liver.[124] They typically represent late complications of transplantation and immunosuppression, with a median time to occurrence of 48 months.[124] About 50% of patients will have multiple lesions at the time of presentation, and small tumor seedlings can often be seen adjacent to small vessels, suggesting vascular smooth muscle as a site of infection (Fig. 17-24).

Although most reported tumors are scantily illustrated and have been variously diagnosed as leiomyoma, leiomyosarcoma, and smooth muscle tumor of uncertain malignant potential, all possess some level of mitotic activity. Histologically, these

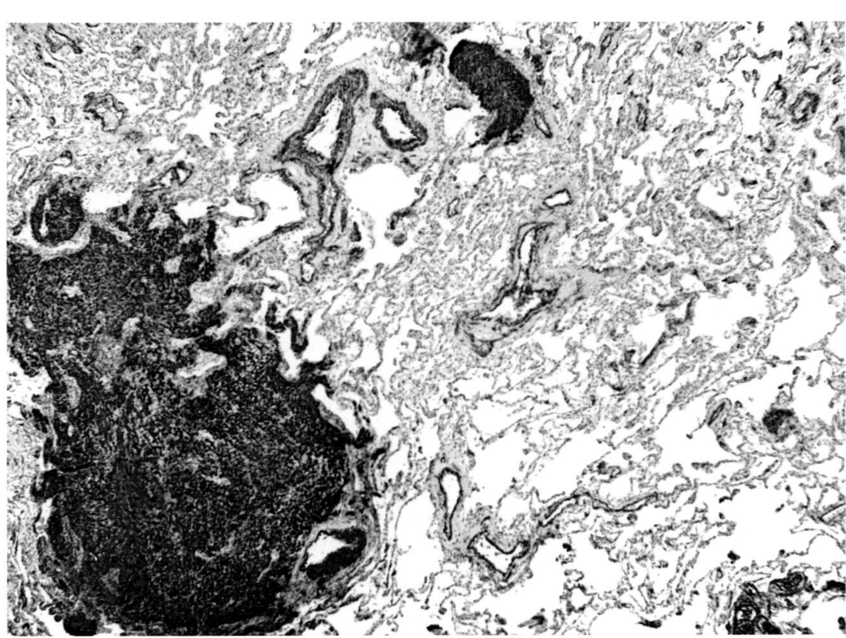

FIGURE 17-24. Actin immunostain of EBVSMT highlighting multifocal disease occurring within the lung.

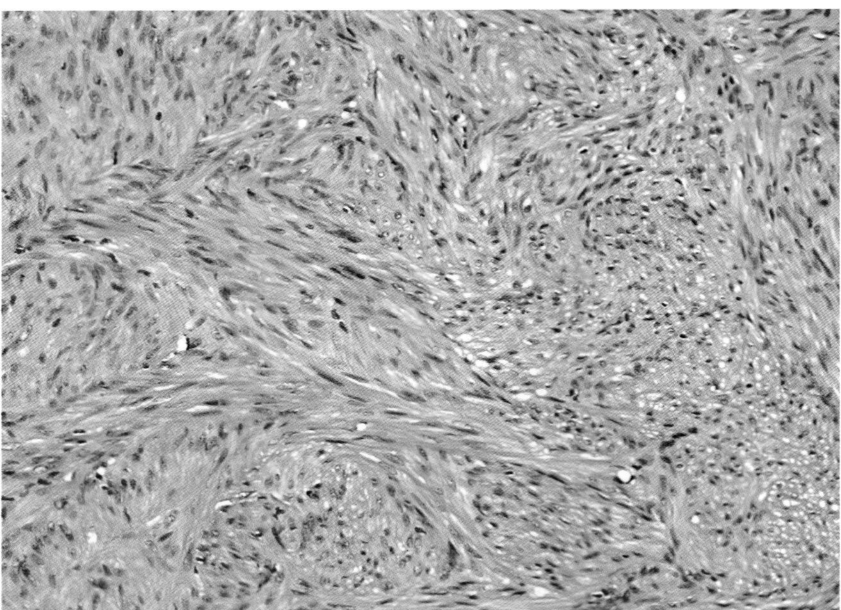

FIGURE 17-25. EBVSMT illustrating differentiated smooth muscle cells with some nuclear atypia.

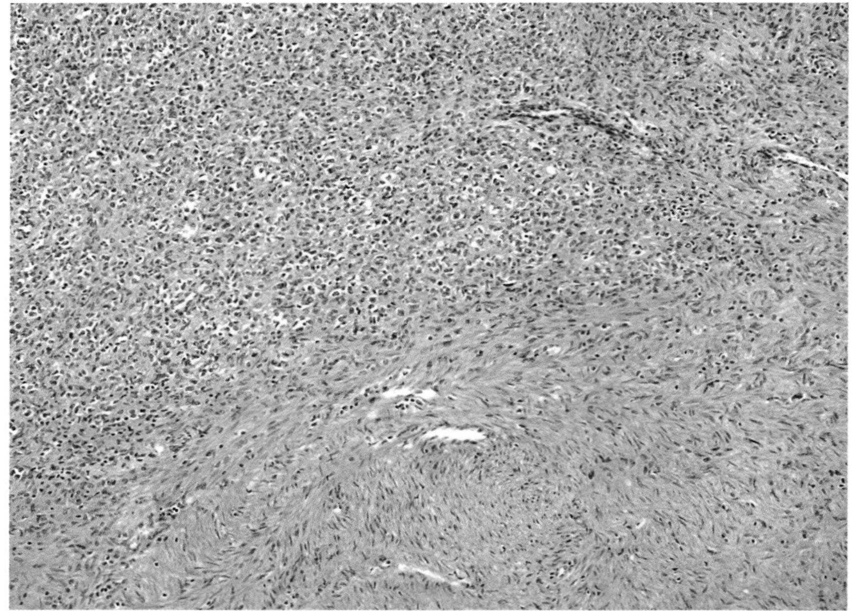

FIGURE 17-26. EBVSMT showing classic-appearing smooth muscle areas abutting round cell myoid areas (upper left).

lesions differ somewhat from classic leiomyosarcomas in several respects. Consisting of intersecting fascicles of differentiated smooth muscle cells, they never achieve the level of atypia noted in classic leiomyosarcomas, yet all display some level of mitotic activity (Fig. 17-25). In about one-half of cases, nodules of primitive rounded cells, representing an unusual altered smooth muscle cell can be identified (Figs. 17-26 and 17-27). Intralesional T lymphocytes are also a common feature (Fig. 17-28). Usually, the clinical setting in association with the foregoing features suggests the diagnosis of an EBVSMT, but the diagnosis can be confirmed by in-situ hybridization of Epstein-Barr virus early RNA (also known as EBER) (Fig. 17-29) if PCR-based methods for viral identification are not available.

Of 18 patients, over three-quarters were alive at the end of the follow-up period (mean 25 months) with most having persistent disease. Only one patient succumbed directly to a tumor. Surgery and reduced immunosuppression appear to be equally effective in the treatment of EBVSMT, with those tumors occurring in intracranial locations having a worse prognosis.[124] It is unclear whether the presence of multiple lesions indicates metastasis in the traditional sense (spread from a primary site) or instead multifocality as a result of multiple independent infection events. Based on a viral episomal analysis of lesions, it has been shown that multiple lesions are derived from separate viral clones and, therefore, likely to be multiple infection events.[125]

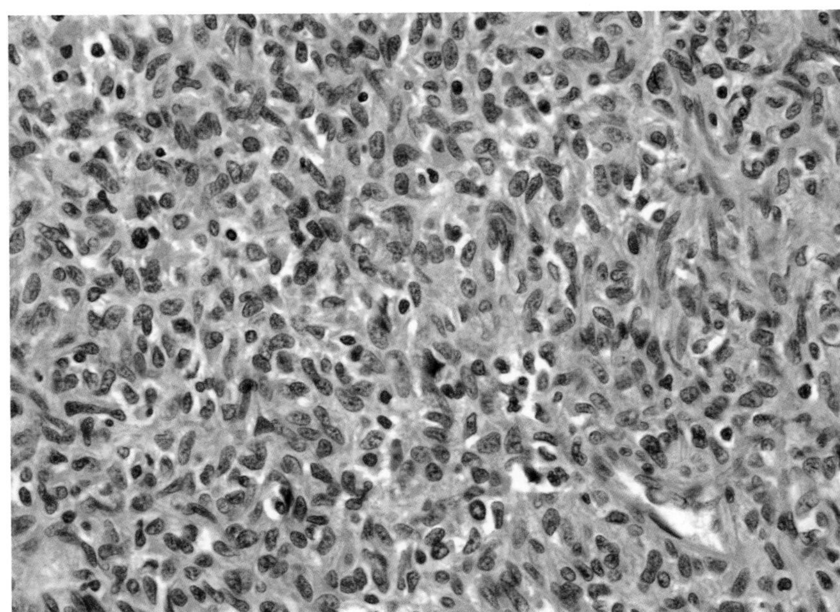

FIGURE 17-27. Round cell myoid areas within an EBVSMT.

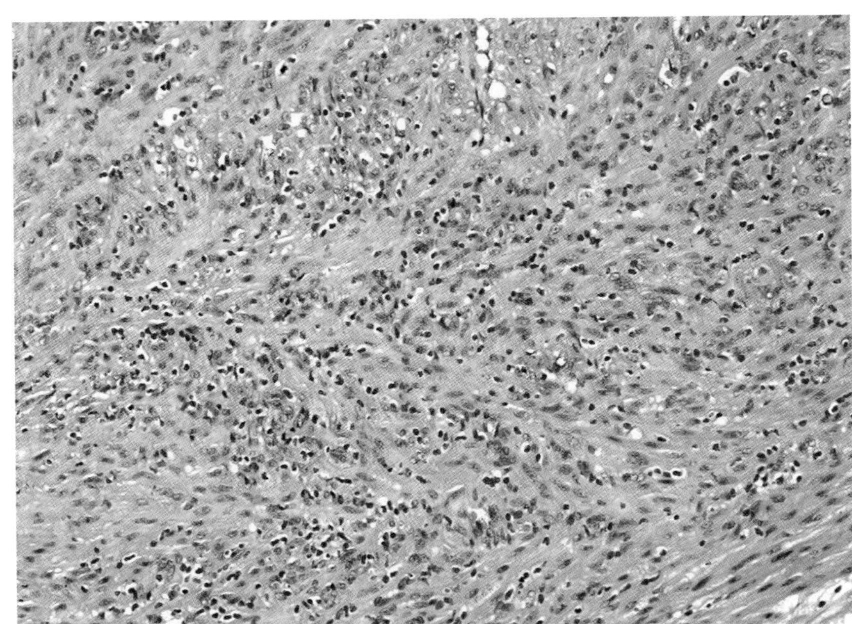

FIGURE 17-28. Intralesional lymphocytes in EBVSMT.

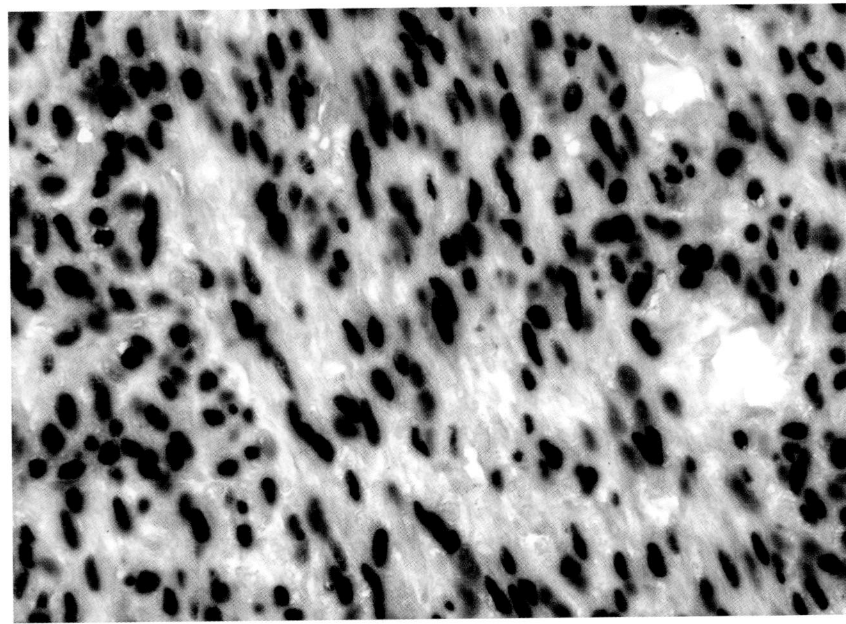

FIGURE 17-29. In-situ hybridization for EBER (Epstein-Barr virus early RNA) in an EBVSMT.

References

1. Gustafson P, Willen H, Baldetorp B, et al. Soft tissue leiomyosarcoma. A population-based epidemiologic and prognostic study of 48 patients, including cellular DNA content. Cancer 1992;70(1):114–9.
2. Hashimoto H, Daimaru Y, Tsuneyoshi M, et al. Leiomyosarcoma of the external soft tissues. A clinicopathologic, immunohistochemical, and electron microscopic study. Cancer 1986;57(10):2077–88.
3. Wile AG, Evans HL, Romsdahl MM. Leiomyosarcoma of soft tissue: a clinicopathologic study. Cancer 1981;48(4):1022–32.
4. Farshid G, Pradhan M, Goldblum J, et al. Leiomyosarcoma of somatic soft tissues: a tumor of vascular origin with multivariate analysis of outcome in 42 cases. Am J Surg Pathol 2002;26(1):14–24.
5. Hashimoto H, Tsuneyoshi M, Enjoji M. Malignant smooth muscle tumors of the retroperitoneum and mesentery: a clinicopathologic analysis of 44 cases. J Surg Oncol 1985;28(3):177–86.
6. Shmookler BM, Lauer DH. Retroperitoneal leiomyosarcoma. A clinicopathologic analysis of 36 cases. Am J Surg Pathol 1983;7(3):269–80.
7. Kevorkian J, Cento DP. Leiomyosarcoma of large arteries and veins. Surgery 1973;73(3):390–400.
8. Botting AJ, Soule EH, Brown Jr AL. Smooth muscle tumors in children. Cancer 1965;18:711–20.
9. Swanson PE, Wick MR, Dehner LP. Leiomyosarcoma of somatic soft tissues in childhood: an immunohistochemical analysis of six cases with ultrastructural correlation. Hum Pathol 1991;22(6):569–77.
10. de Saint Aubain Somerhausen N, Fletcher CD. Leiomyosarcoma of soft tissue in children: clinicopathologic analysis of 20 cases. Am J Surg Pathol 1999;23(7):755–63.
11. Lack EE. Leiomyosarcomas in childhood: a clinical and pathologic study of 10 cases. Pediatr Pathol 1986;6(2-3):181–97.
12. Laskin WB, Silverman TA, Enzinger FM. Postradiation soft tissue sarcomas. An analysis of 53 cases. Cancer 1988;62(11):2330–40.
13. Robinson E, Neugut AI, Wylie P. Clinical aspects of postirradiation sarcomas. J Natl Cancer Inst 1988;80(4):233–40.
14. Fields JP, Helwig EB. Leiomyosarcoma of the skin and subcutaneous tissue. Cancer 1981;47(1):156–69.
15. Font RL, Jurco S 3rd, Brechner RJ. Postradiation leiomyosarcoma of the orbit complicating bilateral retinoblastoma. Arch Ophthalmol 1983; 101(10):1557–61.
16. Francis JH, Kleinerman RA, Seddon JM, et al. Increased risk of secondary uterine leiomyosarcoma in hereditary retinoblastoma. Gynecol Oncol 2012;124(2):254–9.
17. Fitzpatrick SG, Woodworth BA, Monteiro C, et al. Nasal sinus leiomyosarcoma in a patient with history of non-hereditary unilateral treated retinoblastoma. Head Neck Pathol 2011;5(1):57–62.
18. Stratton MR, Williams S, Fisher C, et al. Structural alterations of the RB1 gene in human soft tissue tumours. Br J Cancer 1989;60(2):202–5.
19. Panelos J, Beltrami G, Scoccianti G, et al. Prognostic significance of the alterations of the G1-S checkpoint in localized leiomyosarcoma of the peripheral soft tissue. Ann Surg Oncol 2011;18(2):566–71.
20. Koea JB, Leung D, Lewis JJ, et al. Histopathologic type: an independent prognostic factor in primary soft tissue sarcoma of the extremity? Ann Surg Oncol 2003;10(4):432–40.
21. Deyrup AT, Haydon RC, Huo D, et al. Myoid differentiation and prognosis in adult pleomorphic sarcomas of the extremity: an analysis of 92 cases. Cancer 2003;98(4):805–13.
22. Coindre JM, Terrier P, Guillou L, et al. Predictive value of grade for metastasis development in the main histologic types of adult soft tissue sarcomas: a study of 1240 patients from the French Federation of Cancer Centers Sarcoma Group. Cancer 2001;91(10):1914–26.
23. Fisher C, Goldblum JR, Epstein JI, et al. Leiomyosarcoma of the paratesticular region: a clinicopathologic study. Am J Surg Pathol 2001;25(9):1143–9.
24. Montgomery E, Goldblum JR, Fisher C. Leiomyosarcoma of the head and neck: a clinicopathological study. Histopathology 2002;40(6): 518–25.
25. Weiss SW. Smooth muscle tumors of soft tissue. Adv Anat Pathol 2002;9(6):351–9.
26. Ranchod M, Kempson RL. Smooth muscle tumors of the gastrointestinal tract and retroperitoneum: a pathologic analysis of 100 cases. Cancer 1977;39(1):255–62.
27. Karroum JE, Zappi EG, Cockerell CJ. Sclerotic primary cutaneous leiomyosarcoma. Am J Dermatopathol 1995;17(3):292–6.
28. Oda Y, Miyajima K, Kawaguchi K, et al. Pleomorphic leiomyosarcoma: clinicopathologic and immunohistochemical study with special emphasis on its distinction from ordinary leiomyosarcoma and malignant fibrous histiocytoma. Am J Surg Pathol 2001;25(8):1030–8.
29. Chen E, O'Connell F, Fletcher CD. Dedifferentiated leiomyosarcoma: clinicopathological analysis of 18 cases. Histopathology 2011;59(6): 1135–43.
30. Nicolas MM, Tamboli P, Gomez JA, et al. Pleomorphic and dedifferentiated leiomyosarcoma: clinicopathologic and immunohistochemical study of 41 cases. Hum Pathol 2010;41(5):663–71.
31. Mentzel T, Calonje E, Fletcher CD. Leiomyosarcoma with prominent osteoclast-like giant cells. Am J Surg Pathol 1995;19:487.
32. Matthews TJ, Fisher C. Leiomyosarcoma of soft tissue and pulmonary metastasis, both with osteoclast-like giant cells. J Clin Pathol 1994; 47(4):370–1.
33. Mentzel T, Calonje E, Fletcher CD. Leiomyosarcoma with prominent osteoclast-like giant cells. Analysis of eight cases closely mimicking the so-called giant cell variant of malignant fibrous histiocytoma. Am J Surg Pathol 1994;18(3):258–65.
34. Wilkinson N, Fitzmaurice RJ, Turner PG, et al. Leiomyosarcoma with osteoclast-like giant cells. Histopathology 1992;20(5):446–9.
35. Evans HL, Khurana KK, Kemp BL, et al. Heterologous elements in the dedifferentiated component of dedifferentiated liposarcoma. Am J Surg Pathol [Case Reports] 1994;18(11):1150–7.
36. Folpe AL, Weiss SW. Lipoleiomyosarcoma (well-differentiated liposarcoma with leiomyosarcomatous differentiation): a clinicopathologic study of nine cases including one with dedifferentiation. Am J Surg Pathol 2002;26(6):742–9.
37. Suster S, Wong TY, Moran CA. Sarcomas with combined features of liposarcoma and leiomyosarcoma. Study of two cases of an unusual soft-tissue tumor showing dual lineage differentiation. Am J Surg Pathol 1993;17(9):905–11.
38. Tallini G, Erlandson RA, Brennan MF, et al. Divergent myosarcomatous differentiation in retroperitoneal liposarcoma. Am J Surg Pathol 1993;17(6):546–56.
39. Merchant W, Calonje E, Fletcher CD. Inflammatory leiomyosarcoma: a morphological subgroup within the heterogeneous family of so-called inflammatory malignant fibrous histiocytoma. Histopathology 1995; 27(6):525–32.
40. Chang A, Schuetze SM, Conrad EU 3rd, et al. So-called "inflammatory leiomyosarcoma'": a series of 3 cases providing additional insights into a rare entity. Int J Surg Pathol 2005;13(2):185–95.
41. King ME, Dickersin GR, Scully RE. Myxoid leiomyosarcoma of the uterus. A report of six cases. Am J Surg Pathol 1982;6(7):589–98.
42. Salm R, Evans DJ. Myxoid leiomyosarcoma. Histopathology 1985;9(2): 159–69.
43. Rubin BP, Fletcher CD. Myxoid leiomyosarcoma of soft tissue, an under-recognized variant. Am J Surg Pathol 2000;24(7):927–36.
44. Nistal M, Paniagua R, Picazo ML, et al. Granular changes in vascular leiomyosarcoma. Virchows Arch A Pathol Anat Histol 1980;386(2): 239–48.
45. Ferenczy A, Richart RM, Okagaki T. A comparative ultrastructural study of leiomyosarcoma, cellular leiomyoma, and leiomyoma of the uterus. Cancer 1971;28(4):1004–18.
46. Tsukada T, McNutt MA, Ross R, et al. HHF35, a muscle actin-specific monoclonal antibody. II. Reactivity in normal, reactive, and neoplastic human tissues. Am J Pathol 1987;127(2):389–402.
47. Rangdaeng S, Truong LD. Comparative immunohistochemical staining for desmin and muscle-specific actin. A study of 576 cases. Am J Clin Pathol 1991;96(1):32–45.
48. Swanson PE, Stanley MW, Scheithauer BW, et al. Primary cutaneous leiomyosarcoma. A histological and immunohistochemical study of 9 cases, with ultrastructural correlation. J Cutan Pathol 1988;15(3): 129–41.
49. Hisaoka M, Wei-Qi S, Jian W, et al. Specific but variable expression of h-caldesmon in leiomyosarcomas: an immunohistochemical reassessment of a novel myogenic marker. Appl Immunohistochem Mol Morphol 2001;9(4):302–8.
50. Watanabe K, Tajino T, Sekiguchi M, et al. h-Caldesmon as a specific marker for smooth muscle tumors. Comparison with other smooth muscle markers in bone tumors. Am J Clin Pathol 2000;113(5):663–8.
51. Watanabe K, Kusakabe T, Hoshi N, et al. h-Caldesmon in leiomyosarcoma and tumors with smooth muscle cell-like differentiation: its specific expression in the smooth muscle cell tumor. Hum Pathol 1999; 30(4):392–6.
52. Rush DS, Tan J, Baergen RN, et al. h-Caldesmon, a novel smooth muscle-specific antibody, distinguishes between cellular leiomyoma and endometrial stromal sarcoma. Am J Surg Pathol 2001;25(2):253–8.
53. Nan Ping W, Wan BC, Skelly M, et al. Antibodies to novel myoepithelium-associated proteins distinguish benign lesions and carcinoma in situ

from invasive carcinoma of the breast. Appl Immunohistochem 1997;5(3):141–51.
54. Matsuyama A, Hisaoka M, Hashimoto H. Vascular leiomyosarcoma: clinicopathology and immunohistochemistry with special reference to a unique smooth muscle phenotype. Pathol Int 2010;60(3):212–6.
55. Brown DC, Theaker JM, Banks PM, et al. Cytokeratin expression in smooth muscle and smooth muscle tumours. Histopathology 1987; 11(5):477–86.
56. Meredith RF, Wagman LD, Piper JA, et al. Beta-chain human chorionic gonadotropin-producing leiomyosarcoma of the small intestine. Cancer 1986;58(1):131–5.
57. Miettinen M. Immunoreactivity for cytokeratin and epithelial membrane antigen in leiomyosarcoma. Arch Pathol Lab Med 1988;112(6):637–40.
58. Miettinen M. Keratin subsets in spindle cell sarcomas. Keratins are widespread but synovial sarcoma contains a distinctive keratin polypeptide pattern and desmoplakins. Am J Pathol 1991;138(2):505–13.
59. Iwata J, Fletcher CD. Immunohistochemical detection of cytokeratin and epithelial membrane antigen in leiomyosarcoma: a systematic study of 100 cases. Pathol Int 2000;50(1):7–14.
60. Kelley TW, Borden EC, Goldblum JR. Estrogen and progesterone receptor expression in uterine and extrauterine leiomyosarcomas: an immunohistochemical study. Appl Immunohistochem Mol Morphol 2004; 12(4):338–41.
61. Billings SD, Folpe AL, Weiss SW. Do leiomyomas of deep soft tissue exist? an analysis of highly differentiated smooth muscle tumors of deep soft tissue supporting two distinct subtypes. Am J Surg Pathol 2001; 25(9):1134–42.
62. Mertens F, Fletcher CD, Dal Cin P, et al. Cytogenetic analysis of 46 pleomorphic soft tissue sarcomas and correlation with morphologic and clinical features: a report of the CHAMP Study Group. Chromosomes and MorPhology Genes Chromosomes Cancer [Multicenter Study Research Support, Non-U.S. Gov't] 1998;22(1):16–25.
63. Guillou L, Aurias A. Soft tissue sarcomas with complex genomic profiles. Virchows Arch 2010;456(2):201–17.
64. Yang J, Du X, Chen K, et al. Genetic aberrations in soft tissue leiomyosarcoma. Cancer Lett 2009;275(1):1–8.
65. Wang R, Lu YJ, Fisher C, et al. Characterization of chromosome aberrations associated with soft-tissue leiomyosarcomas by twenty-four-color karyotyping and comparative genomic hybridization analysis. Genes Chromosomes Cancer 2001;31(1):54–64.
66. Otano-Joos M, Mechtersheimer G, Ohl S, et al. Detection of chromosomal imbalances in leiomyosarcoma by comparative genomic hybridization and interphase cytogenetics. Cytogenet Cell Genet 2000;90(1-2):86–92.
67. Derre J, Lagace R, Nicolas A, et al. Leiomyosarcomas and most malignant fibrous histiocytomas share very similar comparative genomic hybridization imbalances: an analysis of a series of 27 leiomyosarcomas. Lab Invest 2001;81(2):211–5.
68. Kawaguchi K, Oda Y, Saito T, et al. Mechanisms of inactivation of the p16INK4a gene in leiomyosarcoma of soft tissue: decreased p16 expression correlates with promoter methylation and poor prognosis. J Pathol 2003;201(3):487–95.
69. Gibault L, Perot G, Chibon F, et al. New insights in sarcoma oncogenesis: a comprehensive analysis of a large series of 160 soft tissue sarcomas with complex genomics. J Pathol 2011;223(1):64–71.
70. Lee YF, John M, Falconer A, et al. A gene expression signature associated with metastatic outcome in human leiomyosarcomas. Cancer Res 2004;64(20):7201–4.
71. Ren B, Yu YP, Jing L, et al. Gene expression analysis of human soft tissue leiomyosarcomas. Hum Pathol 2003;34(6):549–58.
72. Beck AH, Lee CH, Witten DM, et al. Discovery of molecular subtypes in leiomyosarcoma through integrative molecular profiling. Oncogene 2010;29(6):845–54.
73. Mills AM, Beck AH, Montgomery KD, et al. Expression of subtype-specific group 1 leiomyosarcoma markers in a wide variety of sarcomas by gene expression analysis and immunohistochemistry. Am J Surg Pathol 2011;35(4):583–9.
74. Stoeckle E, Coindre JM, Bonvalot S, et al. Prognostic factors in retroperitoneal sarcoma: a multivariate analysis of a series of 165 patients of the French Cancer Center Federation Sarcoma Group. Cancer 2001; 92(2):359–68.
75. Nishimura J, Morii E, Takahashi T, et al. Abdominal soft tissue sarcoma: a multicenter retrospective study. Int J Clin Oncol 2010;15(4):399–405.
76. Schwarzbach MH, Hohenberger P. Current concepts in the management of retroperitoneal soft tissue sarcoma. Recent Results Cancer Res 2009;179:301–19.
77. Svarvar C, Bohling T, Berlin O, et al. Clinical course of nonvisceral soft tissue leiomyosarcoma in 225 patients from the Scandinavian Sarcoma Group. Cancer 2007;109(2):282–91.
78. Miyajima K, Oda Y, Oshiro Y, et al. Clinicopathologic prognostic factors in soft tissue leiomyosarcoma: a multivariate analysis. Histopathology 2002;40:353.
79. Mankin HJ, Casas-Ganem J, Kim JI, et al. Leiomyosarcoma of somatic soft tissues. Clin Orthop Relat Res 2004;(421):225–31.
80. Berlin O, Stener B, Kindblom LG, et al. Leiomyosarcomas of venous origin in the extremities. A correlated clinical, roentgenologic, and morphologic study with diagnostic and surgical implications. Cancer 1984;54(10):2147–59.
81. Orellana-Diaz O, Hernandez-Perez E. Leiomyoma cutis and leiomyosarcoma: a 10-year study and a short review. J Dermatol Surg Oncol 1983;9(4):283–7.
82. Kaddu S, Beham A, Cerroni L, et al. Cutaneous leiomyosarcoma. Am J Surg Pathol 1997;21(9):979–87.
83. Kraft S, Fletcher CD. Atypical intradermal smooth muscle neoplasms: clinicopathologic analysis of 84 cases and a reappraisal of cutaneous "leiomyosarcoma". Am J Surg Pathol 2011;35(4):599–607.
84. Vandergriff T, Krathen RA, Orengo I. Cutaneous metastasis of leiomyosarcoma. Dermatol Surg 2007;33(5):634–7.
85. Jensen ML, Myhre Jensen O, Michalski W, et al. Intradermal and subcutaneous leiomyosarcoma: a clinicopathological and immunohistochemical study of 451 cases. J Cutan Pathol 1996;23:458.
86. Dahl I, Angervall L. Cutaneous and subcutaneous leiomyosarcoma. A clinicopathologic study of 47 patients. Pathol Eur 1974;9(4):307–15.
87. Stout AP, Hill WT. Leiomyosarcoma of the superficial soft tissue. Cancer 1964;11:844.
88. Rising JA, Booth E. Primary leiomyosarcoma of the skin with lymphatic spread. Report of a case. Arch Pathol 1966;81(1):94–6.
89. Humphreys TR, Finkelstein DH, Lee JB. Superficial leiomyosarcoma treated with Mohs micrographic surgery. Dermatol Surg 2004;30(1): 108–12.
90. Huether M, Zitelli J, Brodland D. Mohs micrographic surgery for the treatment of spindle cell tumors of the skin. J Am Acad Dermatol 2001;44(4):656–9.
91. Hallock P, Watson CJ, Berman L. Primary tumor of inferior vena cava with clinical features suggestive of Chari's disease. Arch Intern Med 1940;66:50.
92. Abell MR. Leiomyosarcoma of the inferior vena cava; review of the literature and report of two cases. Am J Clin Pathol 1957;28(3):272–85.
93. Dorfman HD, Fisher ER. Leiomyosarcoma of the greater saphenous vein. Am J Clin Pathol 1963;39:73.
94. Weinreb W, Steinfeld A, Rodil J, et al. Leiomyosarcoma arising in an arteriovenous fistula. Cancer 1983;52(2):390–2.
95. Demers ML, Curley SA, Romsdahl MM. Inferior vena cava leiomyosarcoma. J Surg Oncol 1992;51(2):89–92; discussion 92–93.
96. Griffin AS, Sterchi JM. Primary leiomyosarcoma of the inferior vena cava: a case report and review of the literature. J Surg Oncol 1987;34(1):53–60.
97. Jurayj MN, Midell AI, Bederman S, et al. Primary leiomyosarcomas of the inferior vena cava. Report of a case and review of the literature. Cancer 1970;26(6):1349–53.
98. Mingoli A, Sapienza P, Cavallaro A, et al. The effect of extent of caval resection in the treatment of inferior vena cava leiomyosarcoma. Anticancer Res 1997;17(5/B):3877–81.
99. Kim JT, Kwon T, Cho Y, et al. Multidisciplinary treatment and long-term outcomes in six patients with leiomyosarcoma of the inferior vena cava. J Korean Surg Soc 2012;82(2):101–9.
100. Burke AP, Virmani R. Sarcomas of the great vessels. A clinicopathologic study. Cancer 1993;71(5):1761–73.
101. Leu HJ, Makek M. Intramural venous leiomyosarcomas. Cancer 1986;57(7):1395–400.
102. Jonasson O, Pritchard J, Long L. Intraluminal leiomyosarcoma of the inferior vena cava. Report of a case. Cancer 1966;19(9):1311–5.
103. Stuart FP, Baker WH. Palliative surgery for leiomyosarcoma of the inferior vena cava. Ann Surg 1973;177(2):237–9.
104. Haber LM, Truong L. Immunohistochemical demonstration of the endothelial nature of aortic intimal sarcoma. Am J Surg Pathol 1988; 12(10):798–802.
105. Hayata T, Sato E. Primary leiomyosarcoma arising in the trunk of pulmonary artery: a case report and review of literature. Acta Pathol Jpn 1977;27(1):137–44.
106. Hohbach C, Mall W. Chondrosarcoma of the pulmonary artery. Beitr Pathol 1977;160(3):298–307.

107. McGlennen RC, Manivel JC, Stanley SJ, et al. Pulmonary artery trunk sarcoma: a clinicopathologic, ultrastructural, and immunohistochemical study of four cases. Mod Pathol 1989;2(5):486–94.
108. Wright EP, Glick AD, Virmani R, et al. Aortic intimal sarcoma with embolic metastases. Am J Surg Pathol 1985;9(12):890–7.
109. Hedinger E. Ueber Intima Sarkomatose von Venen und Arterien in sarkomatoesen Strumen. Virchows Arch [Pathol Anat] 1901;164:199.
110. Shmookler BM, Marsh HB, Roberts WC. Primary sarcoma of the pulmonary trunk and/or right or left main pulmonary artery–a rare cause of obstruction to right ventricular outflow. Report on two patients and analysis of 35 previously described patients. Am J Med 1977;63(2):263–72.
111. Hagstrom L. Malignant mesenchymoma in pulmonary artery and right ventricle. Report of a case with unusual location and histological picture. Acta Pathol Microbiol Scand 1961;51:87–94.
112. McConnell TH. Bony and cartilaginous tumors of the heart and great vessels. Report of an osteosarcoma of the pulmonary artery. Cancer 1970;25(3):611–7.
113. Murthy MS, Meckstroth CV, Merkle BH, et al. Primary intimal sarcoma of pulmonary valve and trunk with osteogenic sarcomatous elements. Report of a case considered to be pulmonary embolus. Arch Pathol Lab Med 1976;100(12):649–51.
114. Shen SC, Yunis EJ. Leiomyosarcoma developing in a child during remission of leukemia. J Pediatr 1976;89(5):780–2.
115. Walker D, Gill TJ 3rd, Corson JM. Leiomyosarcoma in a renal allograft recipient treated with immunosuppressive drugs. JAMA 1971;215(13):2084–6.
116. Bluhm JM, Yi ES, Diaz G, et al. Multicentric endobronchial smooth muscle tumors associated with the Epstein-Barr virus in an adult patient with the acquired immunodeficiency syndrome: a case report. Cancer 1997;80(10):1910–3.
117. Boman F, Gultekin H, Dickman PS. Latent Epstein-Barr virus infection demonstrated in low-grade leiomyosarcomas of adults with acquired immunodeficiency syndrome, but not in adjacent Kaposi's lesion or smooth muscle tumors in immunocompetent patients. Arch Pathol Lab Med 1997;121(8):834–8.
118. Chadwick EG, Connor EJ, Hanson IC, et al. Tumors of smooth-muscle origin in HIV-infected children. JAMA 1990;263(23):3182–4.
119. Kingma DW, Shad A, Tsokos M, et al. Epstein-Barr virus (EBV)-associated smooth-muscle tumor arising in a post-transplant patient treated successfully for two PT-EBV-associated large-cell lymphomas. Case report. Am J Surg Pathol 1996;20(12):1511–9.
120. Lee ES, Locker J, Nalesnik M, et al. The association of Epstein-Barr virus with smooth-muscle tumors occurring after organ transplantation. N Engl J Med 1995;332(1):19–25.
121. McClain KL, Leach CT, Jenson HB, et al. Association of Epstein-Barr virus with leiomyosarcomas in children with AIDS. N Engl J Med 1995;332(1):12–8.
122. McLoughlin LC, Nord KS, Joshi VV, et al. Disseminated leiomyosarcoma in a child with acquired immune deficiency syndrome. Cancer 1991;67(10):2618–21.
123. Ross JS, Del Rosario A, Bui HX, et al. Primary hepatic leiomyosarcoma in a child with the acquired immunodeficiency syndrome. Hum Pathol 1992;23(1):69–72.
124. Jonigk D, Laenger F, Maegel L, et al. Molecular and clinicopathological analysis of Epstein-Barr virus-associated posttransplant smooth muscle tumors. Am J Transplant 2012;12(7):1908–17.
125. Deyrup AT, Lee VK, Hill CE, et al. Epstein-Barr virus-associated smooth muscle tumors are distinctive mesenchymal tumors reflecting multiple infection events: a clinicopathologic and molecular analysis of 29 tumors from 19 patients. Am J Surg Pathol 2006;30(1):75–82.

GIST and EGIST

BRIAN P. RUBIN

CHAPTER CONTENTS

Originally considered to be smooth muscle tumors (leiomyoblastomas), it is now known that gastrointestinal stromal tumors (GISTs) arise from interstitial cells of Cajal (ICC) or ICC precursor cells.[1] ICCs are pacemaker cells that are centered on the myenteric plexus along the entire length of the tubal gut (Fig. 18-1).[2] They function to set up a peristaltic wave that coordinates the movement of food through the digestion system. GISTs show many morphologic, immunohistochemical, and molecular features in common with ICC. The identification of *KIT* gene mutations in the majority of GIST has given GIST added importance because it has become a paradigm for targeted therapy of oncogenic proteins/oncogene addiction in solid tumors.[3] Indeed, many of the developments in GIST diagnostics within the last 10 years have been coupled with genetic findings of therapeutic importance.

EPIDEMIOLOGY AND CLINICAL FINDINGS FOR GASTROINTESTINAL STROMAL TUMORS

GISTs, at one time, were thought to be quite rare, but, because of an increased ability to reliably diagnose them, their incidence is now estimated at around 5000 new cases per year in the United States, which places them among the most common sarcomas.[1] Population-based studies estimate the annual incidence at 10 cases per million.[4] It should be emphasized that these GISTs are clinically significant GISTs of greater than 2 cm in size that require surgical evaluation and potentially systemic therapy. MicroGISTs, less than 1 cm in diameter, are quite common. Autopsy studies have identified microGISTs, known variably as *GIST tumorlets* or *GISTlets* in up to 22.5% of patients.[5] However, the vast majority of microGISTs do not progress to clinically important lesions that require medical attention.

GISTs arise over a wide age range, from children to the elderly with a peak median age of 64 years at the time of diagnosis.[6] They occur with an approximately equal sex predilection (47.3% female; 52.7% male), except in children, where there is a clear female predominance (see section on pediatric GIST). No etiologic factors related to GIST have been identified. However, although the vast majority of GISTs occur as sporadic tumors with somatic mutations, GISTs also occur rarely in various tumor syndromes (discussed separately later). They are found along the entire length of the digestive tract but are most common in the stomach (60%), jejunum and ileum (30%), duodenum (5%), and colon and rectum (less than 5%).[7] GISTs also rarely involve the esophagus, appendix, and gall bladder.[8-10]

A small number of GISTs do not have any apparent connection to the gastrointestinal (GI) tract. These GISTs, known as *extragastrointestinal* GISTs (EGISTs), involve the omentum, mesentery, retroperitoneum, and perineum.[10-12] The occasional finding of an omental or mesenteric GIST with a thin stalk attached to the stomach suggests that a subset of EGISTs are exophytic GISTs that arose within the GI tract but eventually lost their connection to it.[13] This is supported by molecular findings, which have shown that EGISTs in the omentum share molecular characteristics with gastric GISTs.[14]

Presenting symptoms include GI bleeding, anemia, abdominal fullness, or a mass.[15] GISTs can also present asymptomatically; because they arise from the wall of the gut, they do not become symptomatic until they erode/ulcerate the overlying mucosa or become large enough to cause mass-like symptoms.

GISTs have a characteristic pattern of metastasis. Unlike epithelial neoplasms of the gut, with one specific exception (succinate dehydrogenase [SDH] deficient GISTs—see later section), they do not metastasize to lymph nodes. They metastasize to the liver or disseminate throughout the peritoneal cavity as numerous metastatic nodules. It is unusual for GIST to metastasize outside of the abdomen, but dermal/subcutaneous, bone, brain, and lung metastases occur rarely.[16-18]

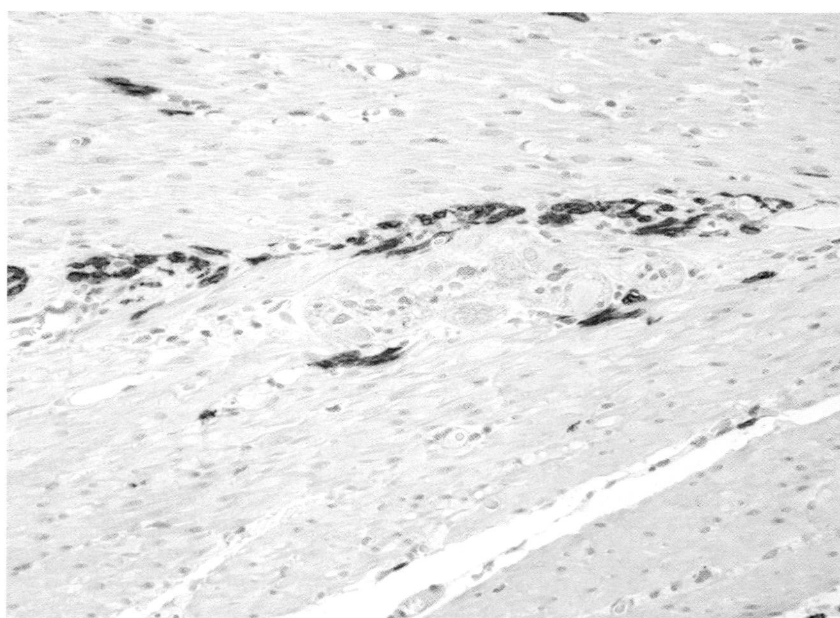

FIGURE 18-1. Interstitial cells of Cajal within the myenteric plexus of the small bowel (KIT immunohistochemical stain).

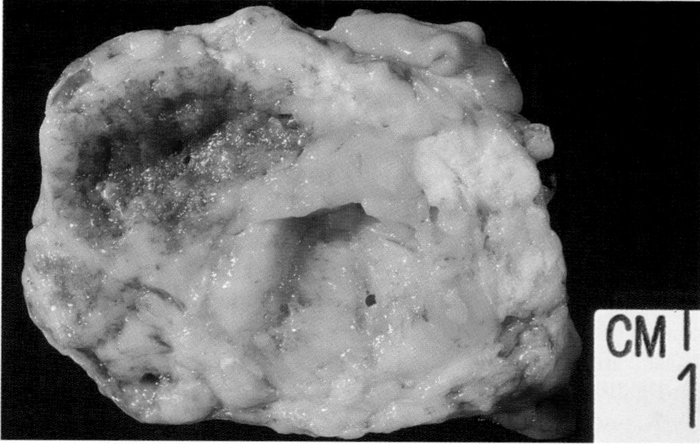

FIGURE 18-2. Gastric GIST with a typical fleshy appearance and central degeneration.

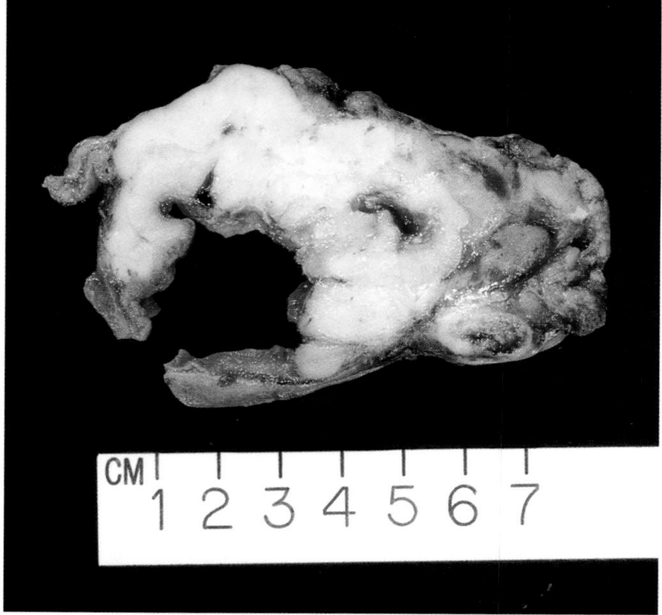

FIGURE 18-3. Aggressive GIST infiltrating through the wall of the small bowel.

MACROSCOPIC FINDINGS FOR GASTROINTESTINAL STROMAL TUMORS

GISTs range in size from 1 mm to very large tumors, occasionally measuring greater than 20 cm, with a median size of clinically significant GISTs of 6 cm in the stomach,[19] 4.5 cm in the duodenum,[20] and 7 cm in the jejunum/ileum.[21] It is important that, because GISTs arise from ICC or ICC precursors, they are centered on the wall of the gut (Figs. 18-2 and 18-3). This has important clinical ramifications because endoscopic biopsies may not be deep enough to obtain suitable tissue for a diagnosis. The use of endoscopic ultrasound and fine-needle aspiration overcomes this limitation by directing the biopsy needle directly into the lesion. GISTs frequently ulcerate the overlying mucosa.[22] On cross section, they are tan and fleshy with frequent cystification and hemorrhage. Necrosis can occur but is less common. GISTs usually grow as single tumor nodules but, occasionally, they are multifocal. Multifocality suggests an inherited disorder that predisposes to GIST or the presence of metastasis.

MICROSCOPIC FINDINGS FOR GASTROINTESTINAL STROMAL TUMORS

GISTs are centered on the muscularis propria and are usually circumscribed and tend to respect the muscularis mucosae (Fig. 18-4). When GISTs invade across the muscularis mucosae to involve the overlying mucosa, the lesional cells infiltrate amongst the glands. It is important to distinguish

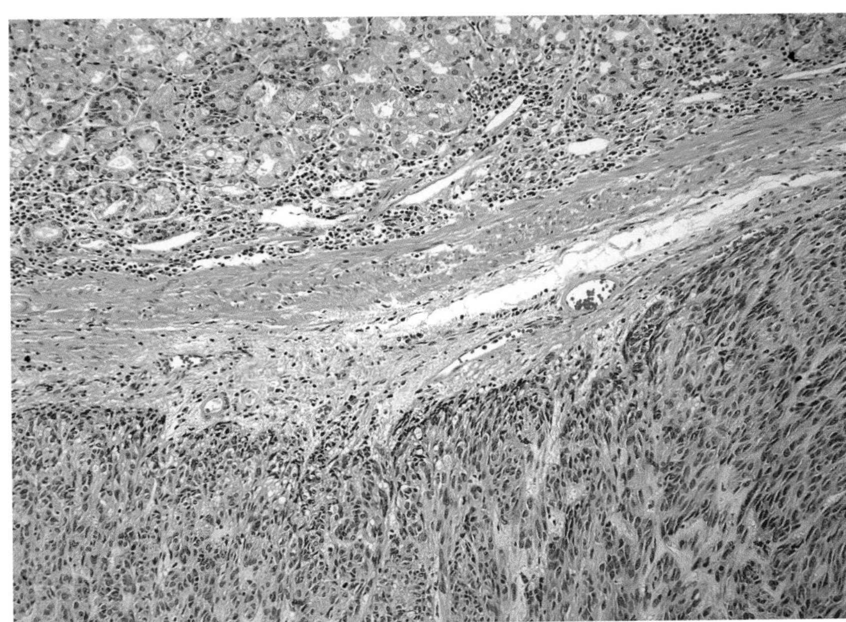

FIGURE 18-4. Typical spindle cell GIST with a smooth, non-infiltrative interface with the muscularis mucosae.

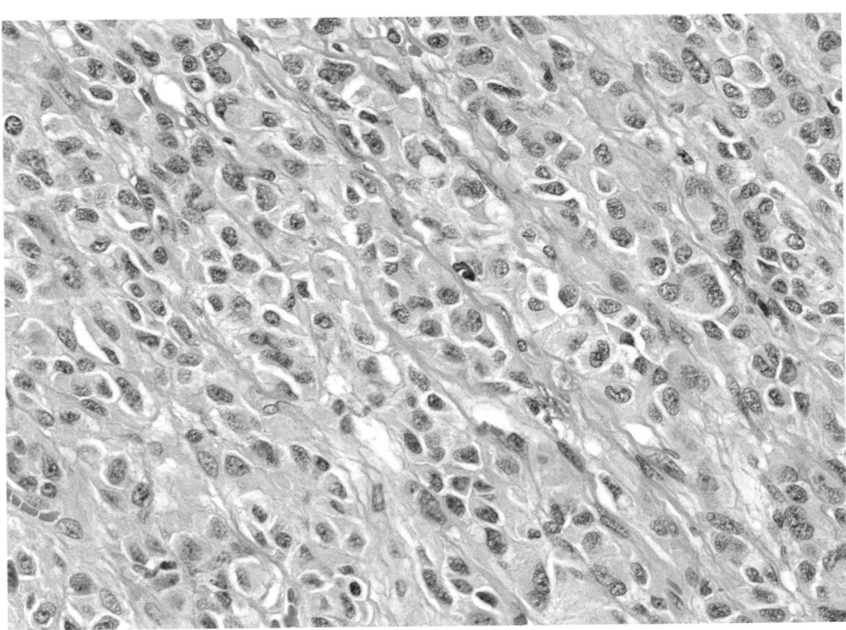

FIGURE 18-5. Epithelioid GIST with a nested growth pattern.

true invasion from simple erosion of the overlying mucosa because true invasion is associated with a worse prognosis and is almost always associated with aggressive clinical behavior. Lymphovascular invasion is very uncommon except in SDH-deficient GISTs; approximately 50% of SDH-deficient GISTs metastasize to lymph nodes.[23]

GISTs can have predominantly epithelioid (20%; Figs. 18-5 and 18-6) or spindle cell cytomorphology (70%; Figs. 18-7 to 18-9) or a combination of both epithelioid and spindle cell morphology (10%)[24, 25] and range from hypocellular to densely cellular lesions. The spindle cells have elongated nuclei with fine chromatin, inconspicuous nuclei, and a moderate amount of pale eosinophilic and fibrillary cytoplasm (Fig. 18-10). Spindle cell GISTs are always arranged in fascicles (see Figs. 18-7 to 18-9), whereas epithelioid GISTs can be arranged in a sheet-like or nested growth pattern (see Figs. 18-5 and 18-6). The stroma varies from hyalinized to, occasionally, myxoid. Coarse calcifications and stromal hyalinization (see Fig. 18-10) are typical of small, clinically insignificant micro-GISTs.[13] GISTs of all types are usually monomorphic with minimal cytologic pleomorphism. They also tend to have minimal mitotic activity. Atypical mitotic figures are rare and are usually a harbinger of high-grade or dedifferentiated GIST.

GISTs are well vascularized, and, in occasional examples, the blood vessels can be hyalinized, suggesting a schwannoma (Fig. 18-11). Gastric GISTs can have striking nuclear palisading, suggesting the diagnosis of schwannoma (Fig. 18-12). Ironically, gastric schwannomas are uniformly cellular and do

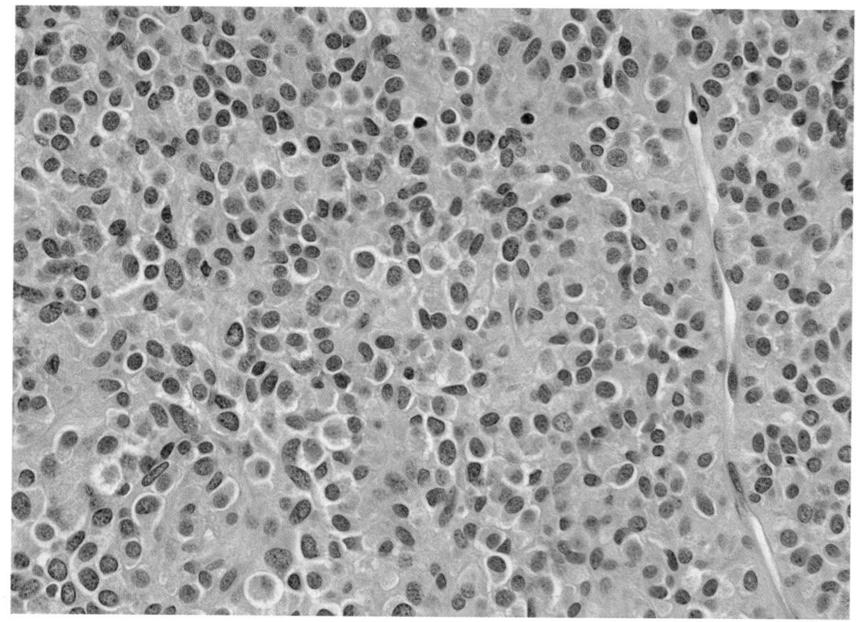

FIGURE 18-6. Epithelioid GIST with a diffuse growth pattern.

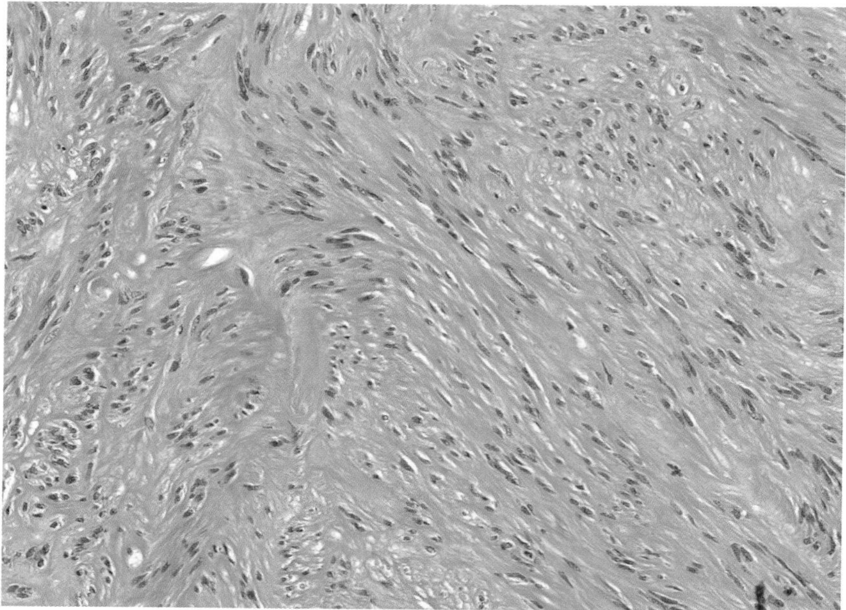

FIGURE 18-7. Hypocellular spindle cell GIST.

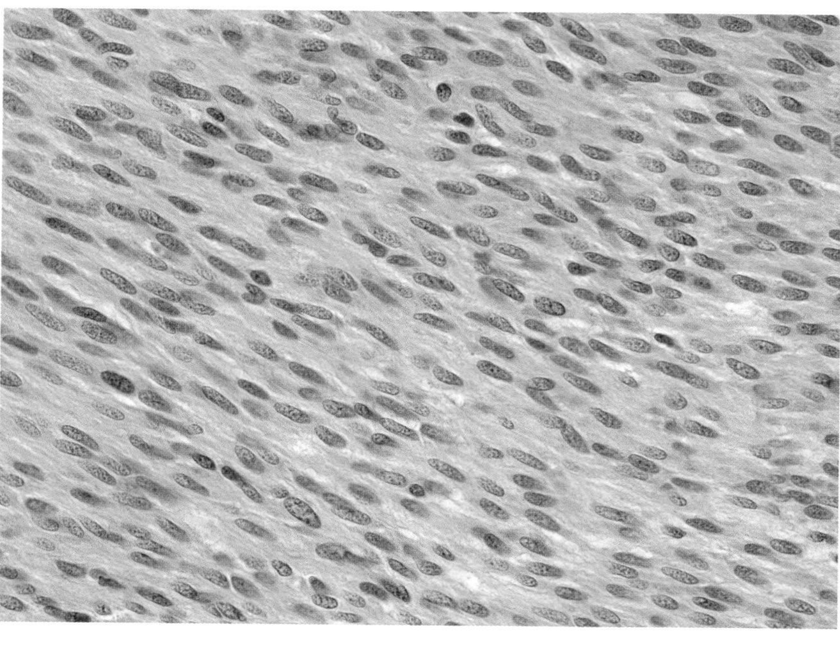

FIGURE 18-8. Moderately cellular spindle cell GIST.

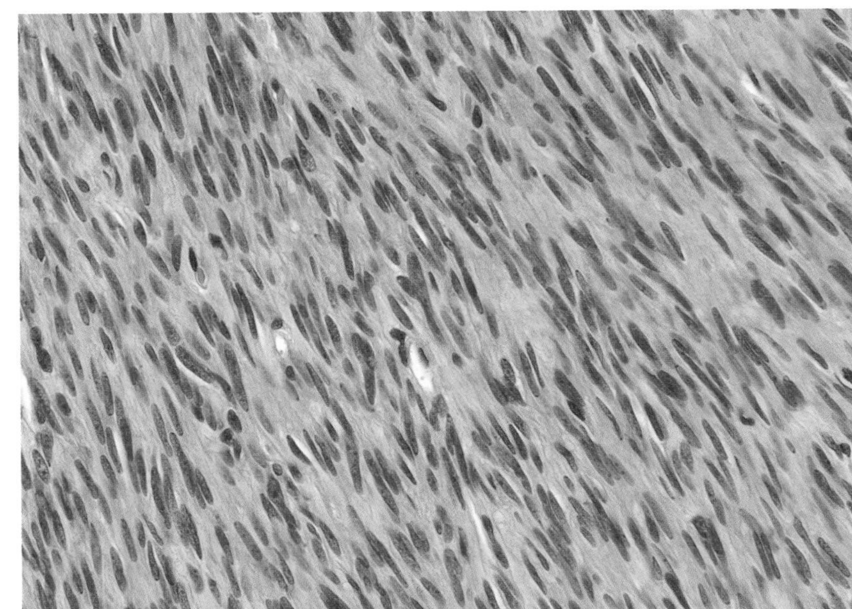

FIGURE 18-9. Hypercellular spindle cell GIST.

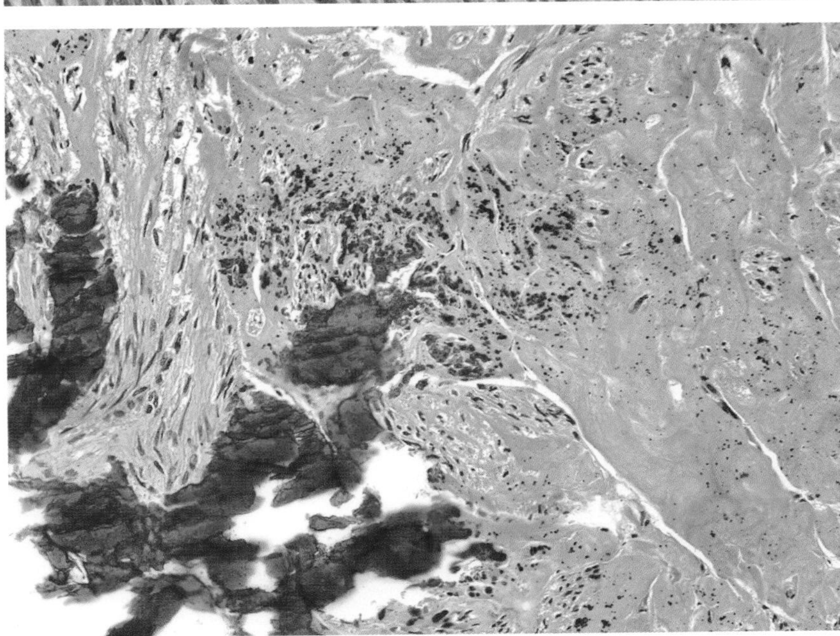

FIGURE 18-10. Hyalinized micro-GIST with coarse calcifications.

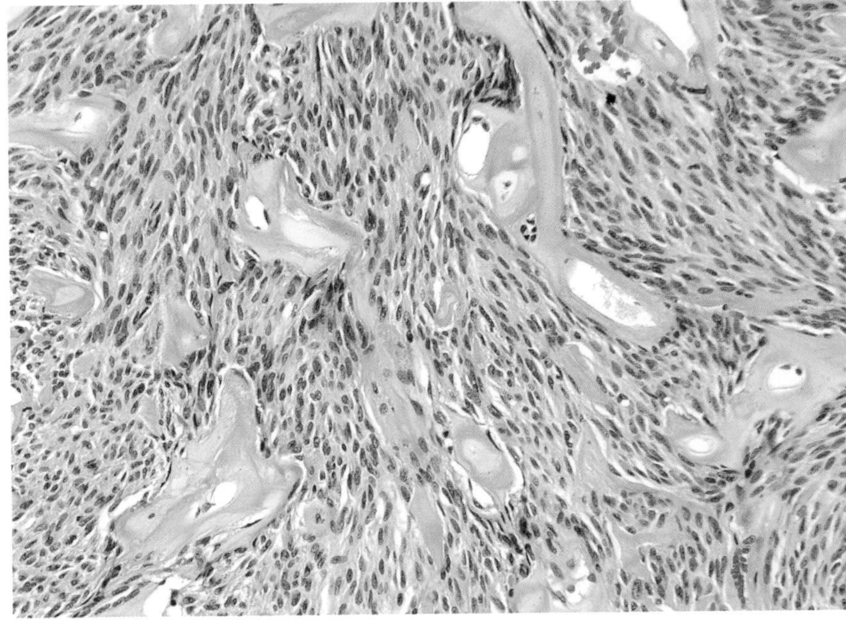

FIGURE 18-11. Spindle cell GIST with prominent hyalinized blood vessels mimicking a schwannoma.

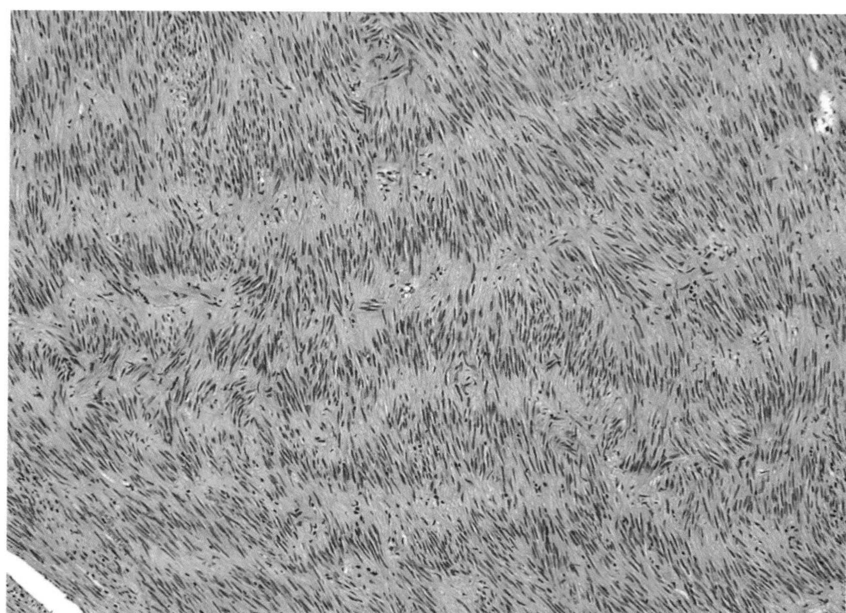

FIGURE 18-12. Gastric spindle cell GIST with nuclear palisading mimicking a schwannoma.

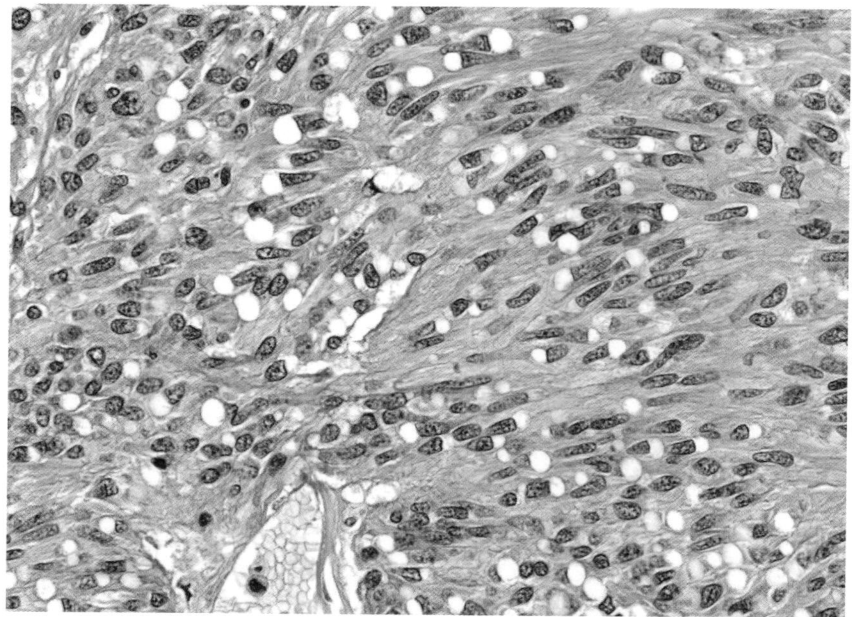

FIGURE 18-13. Gastric GIST with prominent cytoplasmic vacuolization.

not usually exhibit obvious nuclear palisading. Gastric GISTs can also have prominent cytoplasmic vacuolization (Fig. 18-13). Another interesting histologic feature frequently encountered in GIST is the presence of so-called skeinoid fibers, prominent deposits of collagen that are periodic-acid-Schiff-positive (Fig. 18-14),[26] which occur almost exclusively in small intestinal GISTs.

So-called dedifferentiated GISTs are characterized by the presence of morphologically typical GIST juxtaposed with high-grade sarcoma.[27] These lesions are very rare, but the available data demonstrate that the high-grade sarcomatous component loses KIT immunoreactivity, is more mitotically active, including atypical mitotic figures, and is clinically more aggressive than usual GIST (Figs. 18-15 and 18-16). Dedifferentiated GIST can be seen *de novo* and as a result of prolonged anti-KIT tyrosine kinase inhibitor therapy.

IMMUNOHISTOCHEMICAL FINDINGS FOR GASTROINTESTINAL STROMAL TUMORS

GISTs are diffusely and strongly positive for KIT (CD117) in approximately 95% of cases.[28,29] Immunoreactivity can be cytoplasmic (Fig. 18-17), membranous (Fig. 18-18), dot-like perinuclear (Fig. 18-19), or a combination of all of these patterns. There is no clinical significance to the different staining patterns. Because other GI neoplasms, such as leiomyoma and schwannoma, can mimic GIST, it is important to objectify the

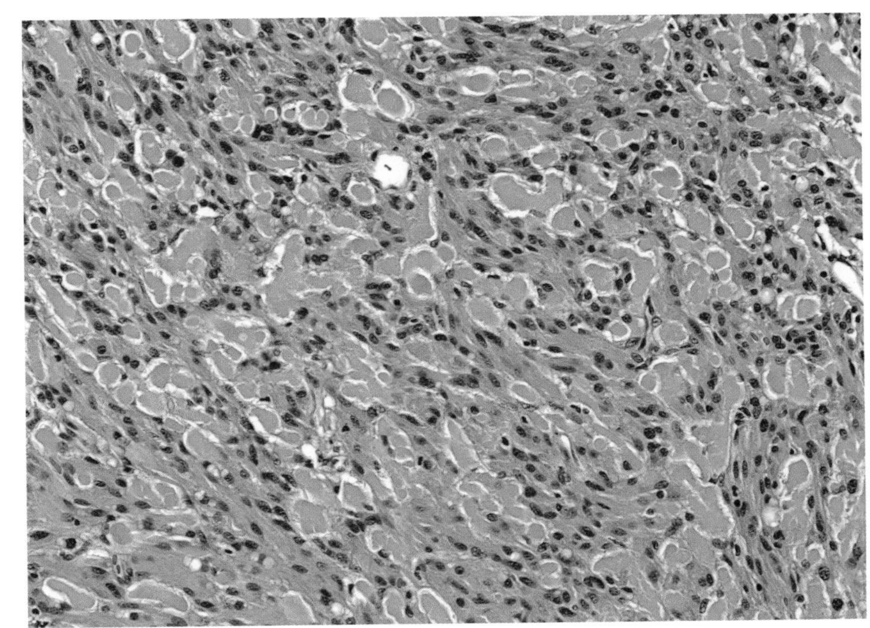

FIGURE 18-14. Skeinoid fibers in a jejunal GIST.

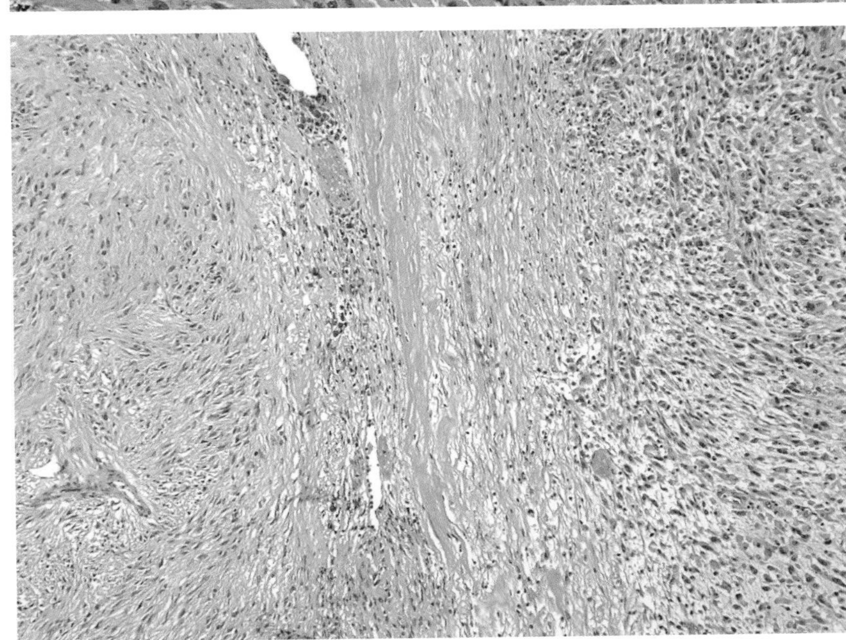

FIGURE 18-15. Dedifferentiated GIST (conventional component on left with an abrupt transition to a dedifferentiated component on right).

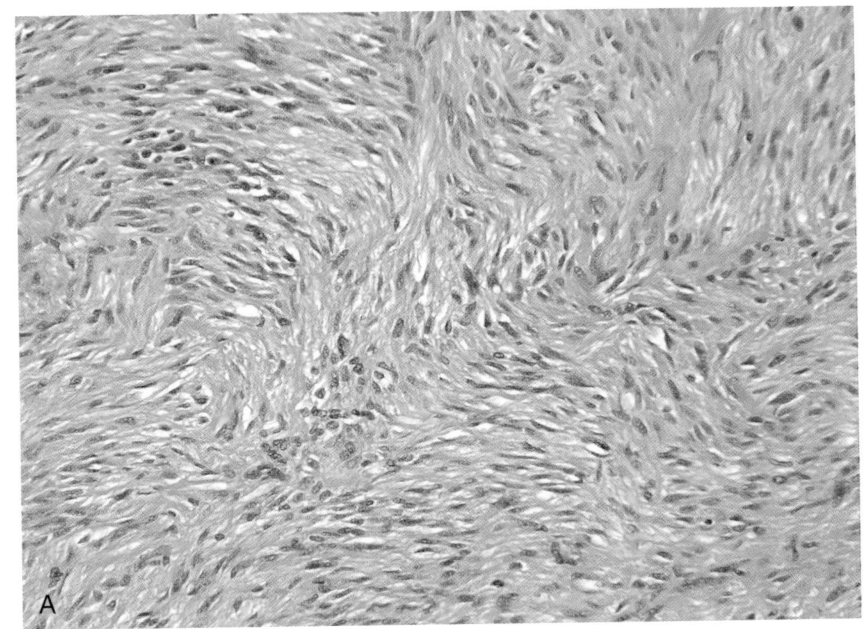

FIGURE 18-16. Conventional spindle cell component (A) and dedifferentiated component with rhabdoid morphology *Continued*

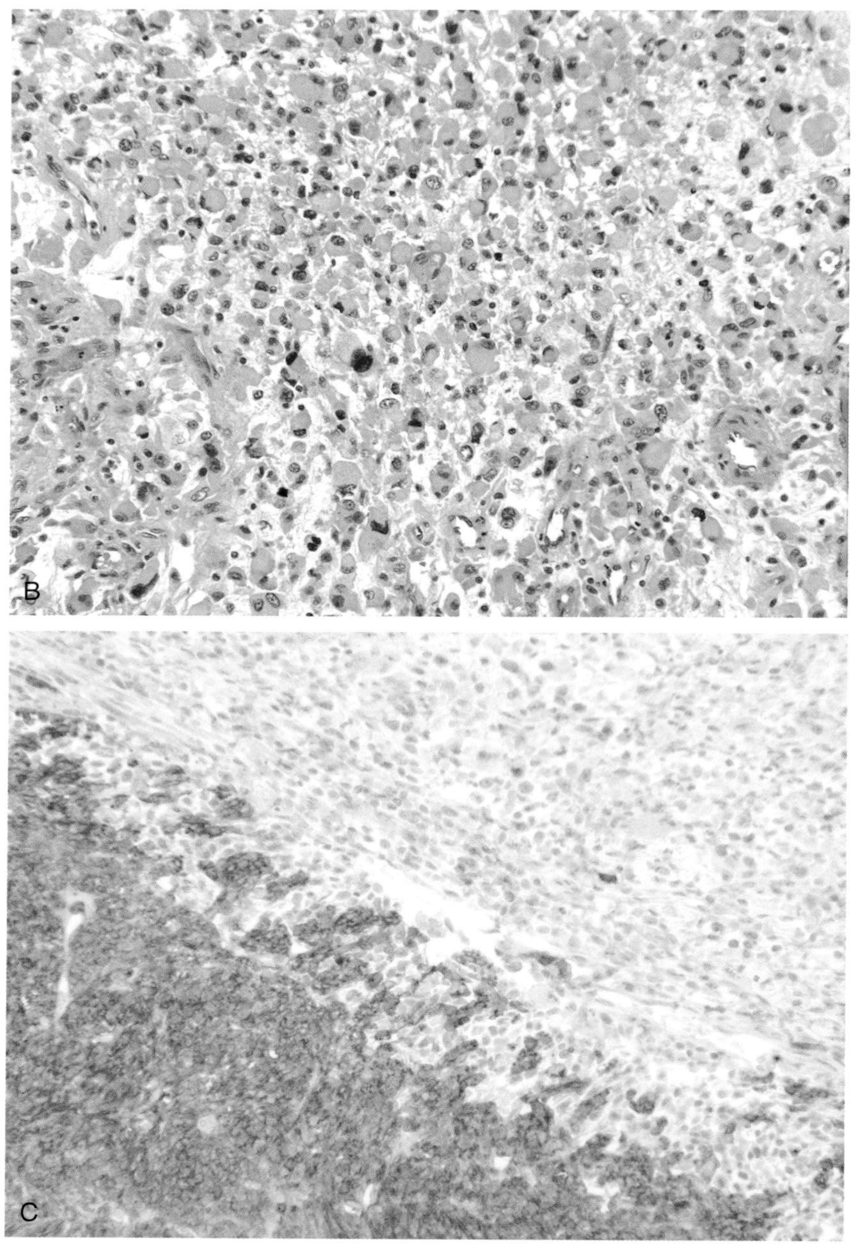

FIGURE 18-16, cont'd. (B) of dedifferentiated GIST. KIT immunohistochemical stain (C) shows abrupt loss of staining in the dedifferentiated component (upper right).

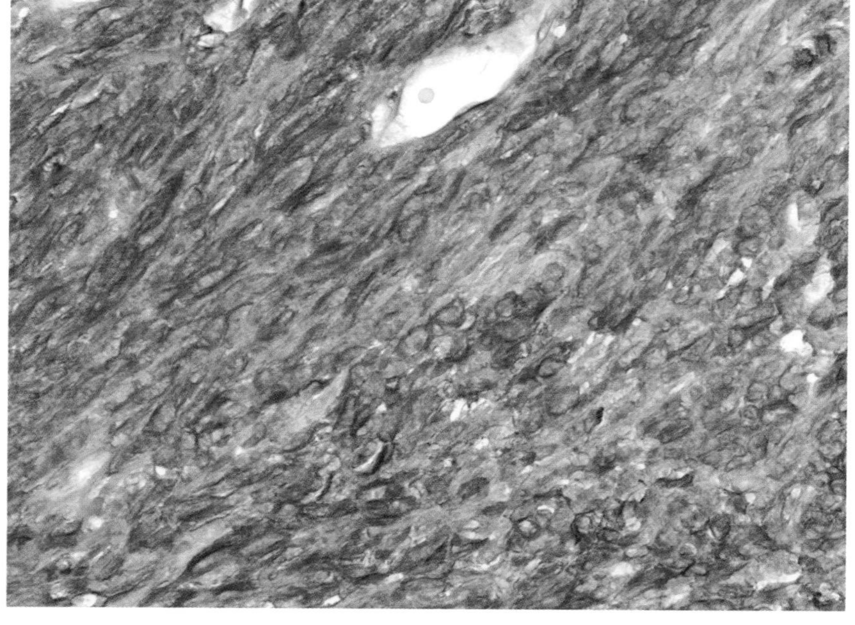

FIGURE 18-17. Cytoplasmic KIT immunoreactivity.

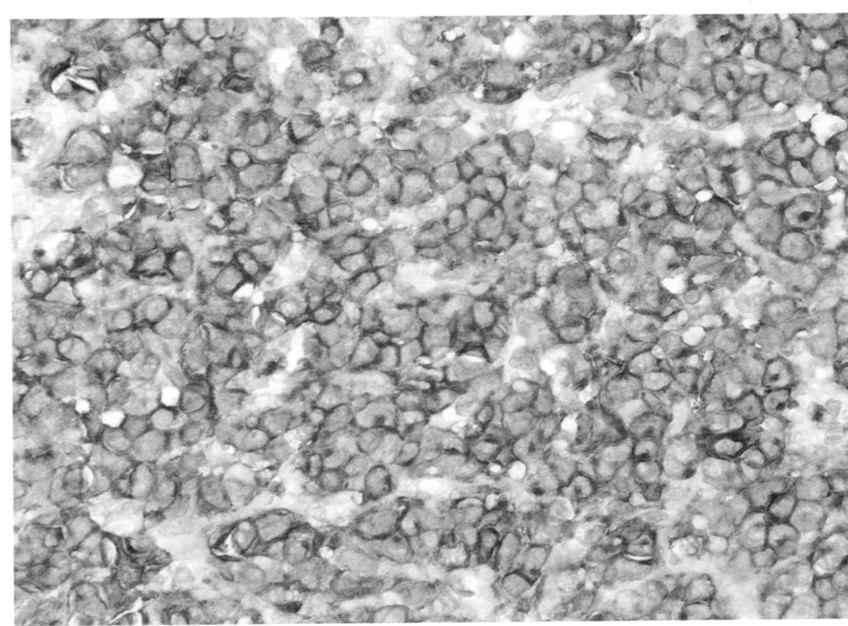

FIGURE 18-18. Membranous KIT immunoreactivity.

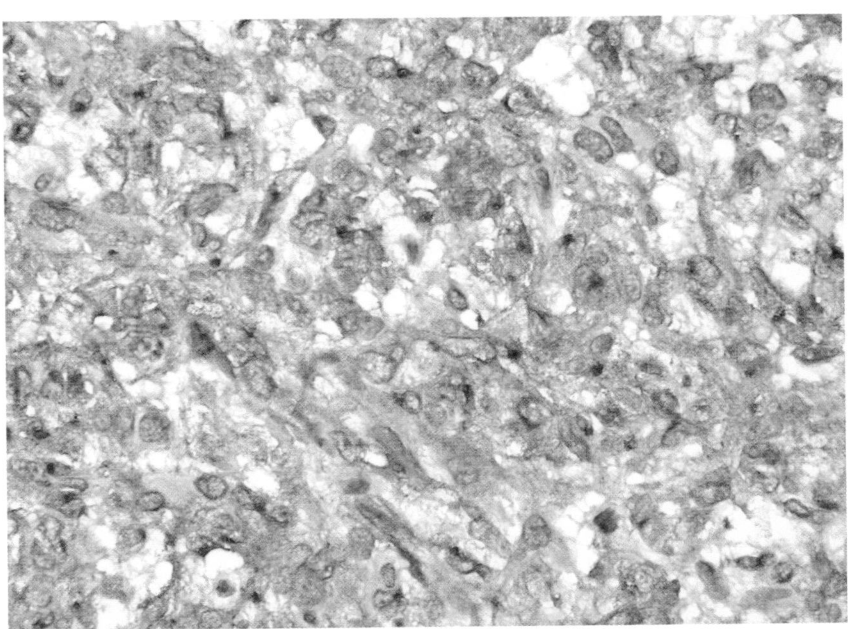

FIGURE 18-19. Dot-like KIT immunoreactivity.

histologic impression of GIST by confirmation with KIT immunohistochemistry. KIT immunoreactivity also has treatment implications because Food and Drug Administration (FDA)-approved treatment for GIST requires the presence of KIT immunoreactivity.

Approximately 5% of GISTs are negative for KIT by immunohistochemistry.[30] Most of these GISTs turn out to be *PDGFRA* mutant GISTs (Table 18-1; see later section).

DOG1 (discovered on GIST 1), also known as *ANO1*, is strongly expressed in ICC and is very sensitive and specific for the diagnosis of GIST.[31-34] DOG1 is strongly expressed in over 99% of GIST (Fig. 18-20). It is important to note that it is positive in most KIT-negative GISTs and, therefore, is useful in confirming the diagnosis of GIST in this subgroup (Fig. 18-21). For the time being, it is still necessary to confirm the diagnosis of GIST with KIT immunohistochemistry for treatment purposes. However, it is possible that DOG1 will eventually supplant KIT as the preeminent GIST immunohistochemical marker.

GISTs are also positive for CD34 (70%), but this immunohistochemical marker is no longer useful for the diagnosis of GIST.[1] Before the advent of KIT immunohistochemistry, CD34 was the go-to marker for diagnosing GIST. GISTs are also positive for smooth muscle actin in 30% to 40% of cases. In general, staining is more focal than that seen in leiomyomas and leiomyosarcomas. However, it is important to keep smooth muscle actin immunoreactivity in mind for the possible pitfall of misdiagnosing a GIST as a smooth muscle tumor. GISTs are occasionally positive for S-100 (5%), desmin (2%), and cytokeratins (2%), which is helpful in distinguishing GIST from schwannoma (KIT negative, diffusely S-100 positive), smooth muscle tumors (KIT negative, desmin positive), and metaplastic (sarcomatoid) carcinoma (KIT negative, keratin positive). S-100, desmin, and cytokeratins, when positive, are usually only focally positive in GIST. It is also important to remember that melanoma, which occasionally metastasizes to the bowel, is both S-100 and KIT-positive, although the degree of KIT immunoreactivity is typically less than that seen in

TABLE 18-1 Immunohistochemistry According to GIST Genotype

IMMUNOHISTOCHEMISTRY	GENOTYPE				
	KIT Mutation	*PDGFRA Mutation*	*BRAF Mutation*	*SDHB, C or D Mutation*	*SDHA Mutation*
KIT	+	–	+	+	+
DOG1	+	+	+	+	+
SDHB	+	+	+	–	–
SDHA	+	+	+	+	–

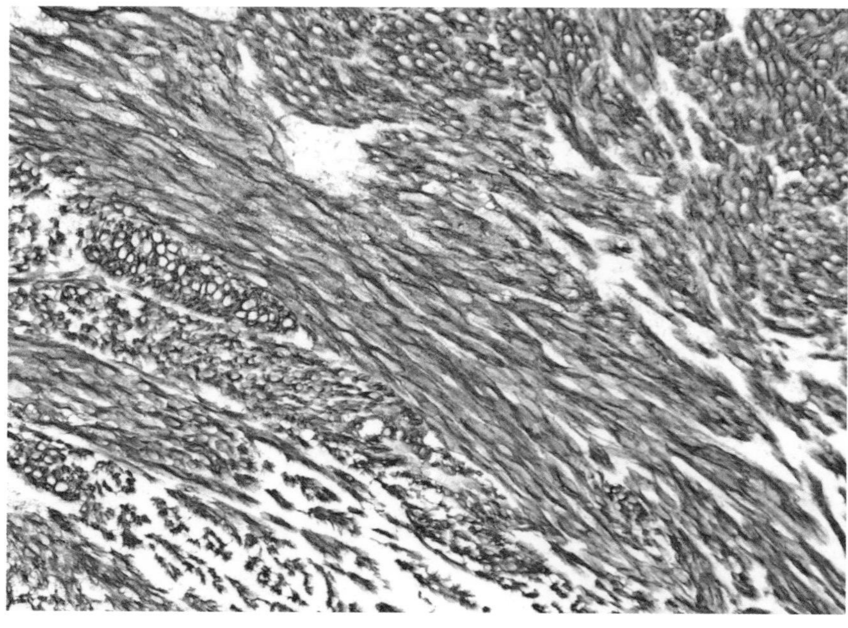

FIGURE 18-20. DOG1 immunohistochemistry in spindle cell GIST.

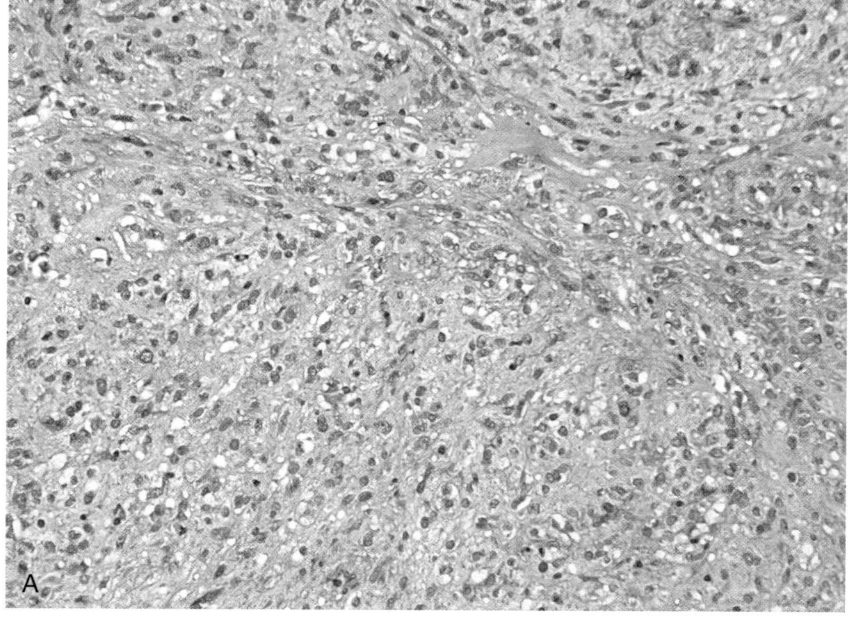

FIGURE 18-21. KIT (A) and DOG1

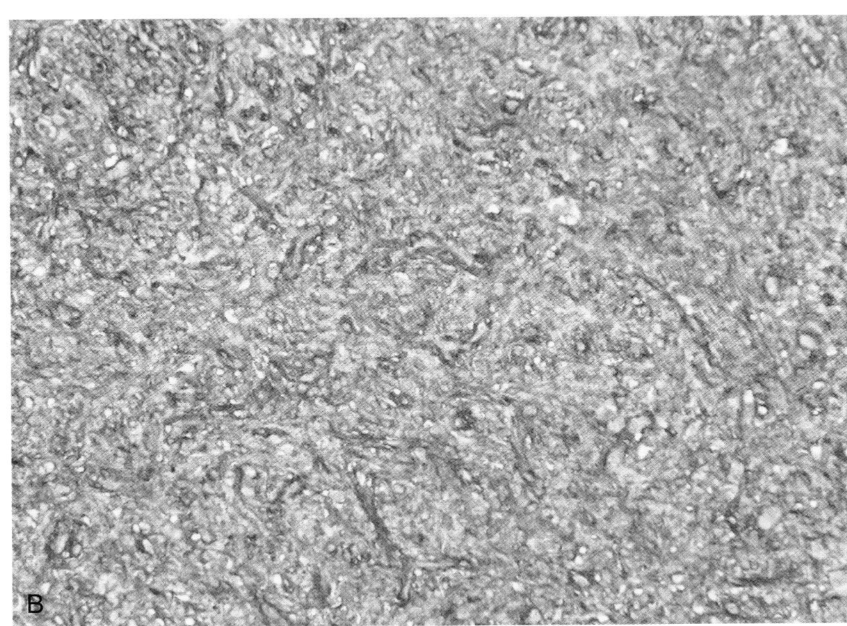

FIGURE 18-21, cont'd. (B) immunohistochemistry in KIT-negative GIST.

TABLE 18-2 Immunohistochemistry in Differential Diagnosis of GIST

DIAGNOSIS	KIT	DOG1	DESMIN	S-100
GIST	+++ (95%)	+++ (99%)	– (2%) Focal	– (5%) Focal
Leiomyoma	–	–	+++ (100%) Uniform	–
Leiomyosarcoma	–	–	++ (50%)	–
Schwannoma	–	–	–	+++ (100%) Uniform
Desmoid Fibromatosis	–	–	–	–

GIST. For the differential diagnosis of GIST, the most useful immunohistochemical panel is KIT, DOG1, S-100, and desmin (Table 18-2).

ULTRASTRUCTURAL FINDINGS FOR GASTROINTESTINAL AUTONOMIC NERVE TUMORS

Electron microscopic analysis of GIST reveals an organelle-poor undifferentiated phenotype or neural features, such as synaptic-type structures, perhaps as a result of their origin as ICC, which have neuron-like functions (Figs. 18-22 and 18-23).[35] The subset of GIST with poorly formed synaptic-like structures was previously known as *gastrointestinal autonomic nerve tumors (GANT)* or *plexosarcomas*.[36,37] Although GANT was formerly thought to be a distinct entity defined by unique electron microscopic features, more recent work has demonstrated that GANT is merely part of the spectrum of GIST, without distinct clinical or molecular features.[38] Because of its characteristic histologic, immunohistochemical, and genetic features, electron microscopy no longer plays an important role in the diagnosis of GIST.

GENETICS OF GASTROINTESTINAL STROMAL TUMORS

Approximately 70% to 80% of GISTs contain constitutively activating mutations in *KIT*, which encodes a receptor tyrosine kinase that is strongly expressed in ICC and is critical for ICC development and maintenance (Fig. 18-24).[3, 6, 39] *KIT* mutations are found in the smallest, sub-centimeter GISTs, suggesting that *KIT* mutation is the initiating tumorigenic event in most GISTs.[40, 41] This has been confirmed in mouse models where oncogenic KIT activation is all that is necessary to drive GIST tumorigenesis.[42-44] However, additional secondary changes are required to develop GISTs that are clinically aggressive.[45] *KIT* mutations are scattered along hotspots, including *KIT* exon 9, exon 11, exon 13, and exon 17 (see Fig. 18-24; Table 18-3).[46] Whereas most mutations are found throughout the length of the GI tract, *KIT* exon 9 mutant tumors arise predominantly in the small bowel.[47, 48] Approximately 67% of *KIT* mutations involve exon 11, 10% in exon 9, and 1% each in exons 13 and 17 (see Fig. 18-24 and Table 18-3). Other *KIT* mutations are rarely identified in exons 8, 12, 14, and 18. Mutations can be missense mutations, insertions, duplications, or deletions. Most *KIT* mutations are heterozygous. However, hemizygous and homozygous *KIT* mutations occur infrequently and are associated with aggressive clinical behavior.[46]

GISTs in the range of 7% to 15% have mutations in *PDGFRA*, which encodes a receptor tyrosine kinase that is related to *KIT* (see Fig. 18-24 and Table 18-3).[6, 39, 50] Both *KIT* and *PDGFRA* reside next to each other on chromosome 4q, suggesting that one of them was created through a gene duplication event from the other. *KIT* and *PDGFRA* mutations are mutually exclusive and, mechanistically, drive GIST tumorigenesis in exactly the same way. *PDGFRA* has one more exon than *KIT* so the numbering system is offset by one. *PDGFRA*

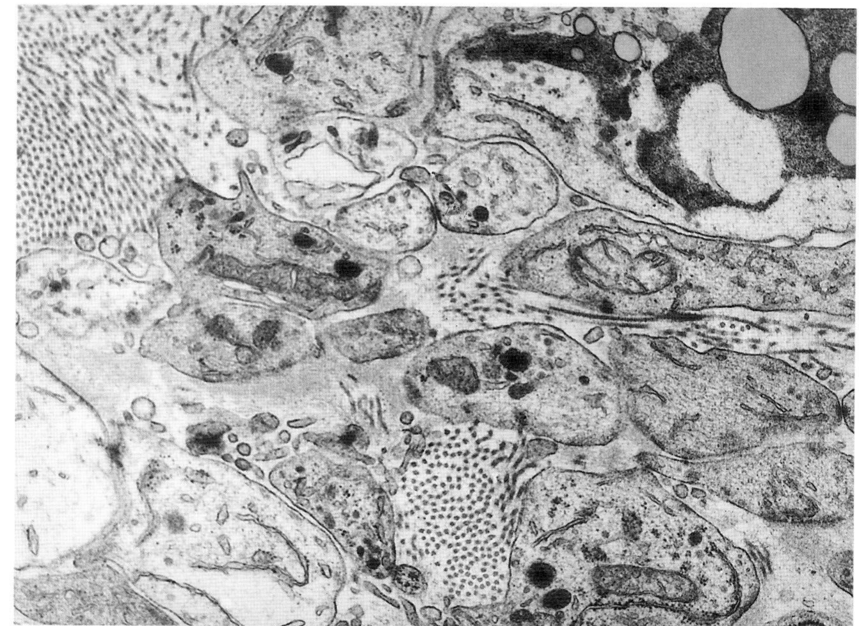

FIGURE 18-22. Electron micrograph of a GIST with neuronal and synapse-like structures containing dense-core neurosecretory granules and microtubules (X17700). *(Courtesy of Dr. Robert Erlandson.)*

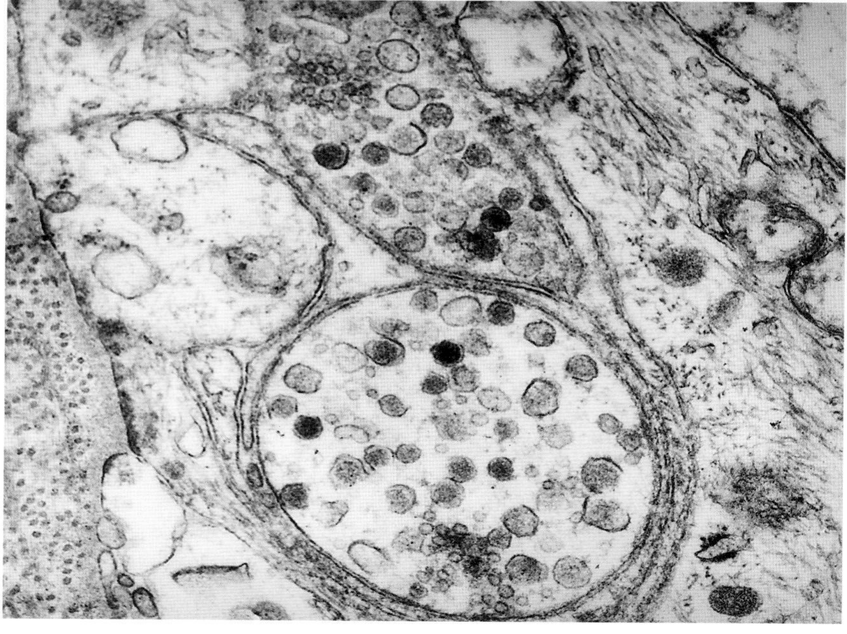

FIGURE 18-23. Electron micrograph of GIST illustrating details of the synapse-like structures. Note the neurosecretory granules and vesicles. A portion of a neurite is also present [X35700]). *(Courtesy of Dr. Robert Erlandson.)*

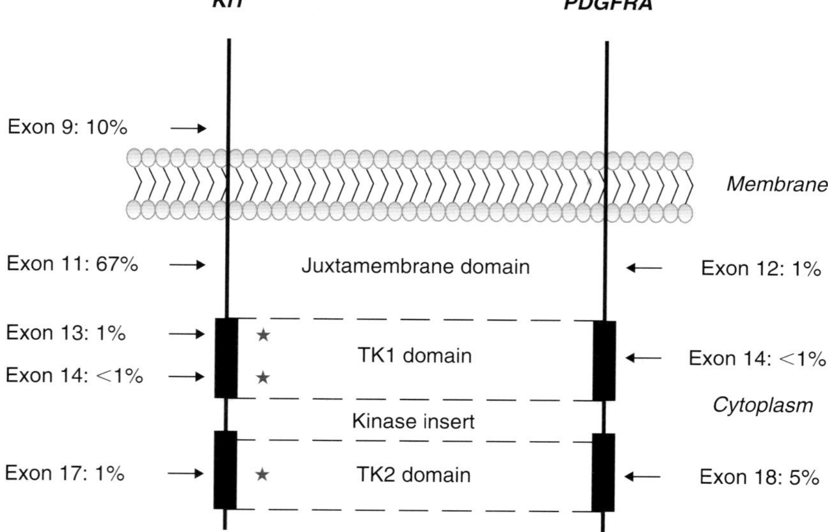

FIGURE 18-24. Schematic representation of KIT and PDGFRA with mutational hotspots.

TABLE 18-3 Genetics of Gastrointestinal Stromal Tumors

GENETIC TYPE	RELATIVE FREQUENCY	ANATOMIC DISTRIBUTION	GERMLINE EXAMPLES
KIT mutation (relative frequency 75% to 80%)			
Exon 8	Rare	Small bowel	One kindred
Exon 9 insertion AY502-503	10%	Small bowel and colon	None
Exon 11 (deletions, single nucleotide substitutions and insertions)	67%	All sites	Several kindreds
Exon 13 K642E	1%	All sites	Two kindreds
Exon 17 D820Y, N822K, and Y823D	1%	All sites	Five kindreds
PDGFRA mutation (relative frequency 5% to 8%)			
Exon 12 (such as V561D)	1%	All sites	Two kindreds
Exon 14 N659K	less than 1%	Stomach	None
Exon 18 D842V	5%	Stomach, mesentery, and omentum	None
Exon 18 (such as deletion of amino acids IMHD 842-846)	1%	All sites	One kindred
KIT and *PDGFRA* wild-type (relative frequency 12% to 15%)			
BRAF V600E	3%	Stomach and small bowel	None
SDHA, SDHB, SDHC, and *SDHD* mutations	3%	Stomach and small bowel	Carney-Stratakis
Sporadic pediatric GISTs	~1%	Stomach	Not heritable
GISTs as part of the Carney triad	~1%	Stomach	Not heritable
NF1-related	Rare	Small bowel	Numerous

GIST, gastrointestinal stromal tumor; NF1, neurofibromatosis type 1; PDGFRA, platelet-derived growth factor receptor a; SDH, succinate dehydrogenase.

Modified from Corless CL, Barnett CM, and Heinrich MC. Gastrointestinal stromal tumours: origin and molecular oncology. Nat Rev Cancer 2011;11:865–878.

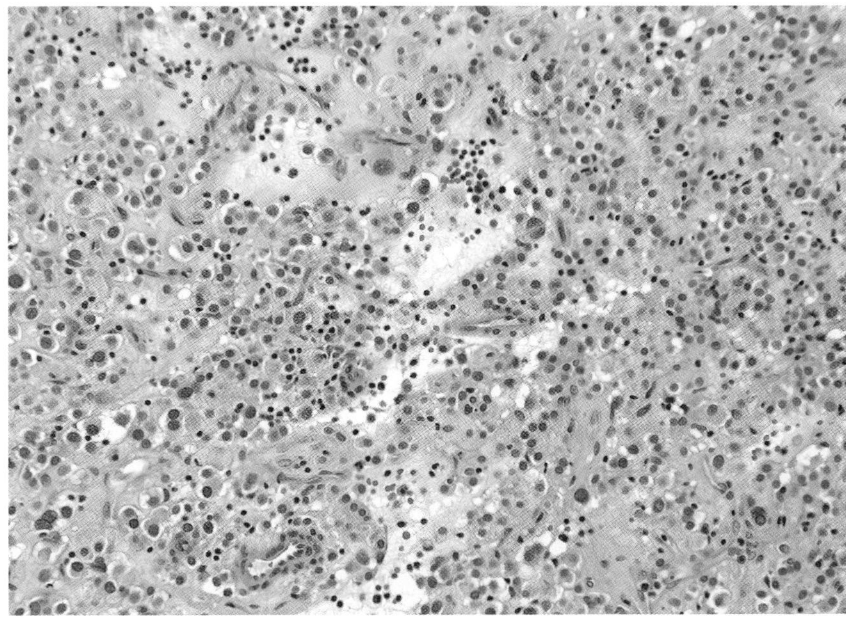

FIGURE 18-25. PDGFRA mutant GIST with epithelioid morphology with focal stromal edema.

mutations occur in exons 12 (less than 1%), 14 (less than 1%), and 18 (5% to 10%) (see Fig. 18-24 and Table 18-3). Exons 12, 14, and 18 of *PDGFRA* are homologous to exons 11, 13, and 17 of *KIT*. Most *PDGFRA* mutant GISTs arise in the stomach or omentum and have a specific morphology that is readily recognizable. *PDGFRA* mutant GISTs are negative or weakly positive for KIT immunohistochemistry (see Table 18-1), have epithelioid cytomorphology with prominent cell membranes, frequent binucleation, more pleomorphism than is usual in *KIT* mutant GIST, and focally myxoid stroma (Figs. 18-25 and 18-26).

Approximately 12% to 15% of GISTs lack *KIT* or *PDGFRA* mutations and have been collectively referred to as *wild-type* GISTs (see Table 18-3). Many of the molecular aberrations of these GISTs have now been characterized. BRAF V600E mutations have been identified in wild-type GISTs and account for approximately 3% of all GISTs.[51,52] *BRAF* mutant GISTs are positive for KIT by immunohistochemistry (see Table 18-1). BRAF V600E mutations are found in many different types of cancer, including melanoma and papillary thyroid cancer. BRAF V600E mutations are more common in small bowel (56%) than in gastric (22%) GISTs and have a tendency for aggressive behavior.

A subset of wild-type GISTs has loss-of-function mutations in SDH subunits A, B, C, or D (*SDHA, SDHB, SDHC,* and *SDHD*), which appear in SDH-deficient GISTs (see Tables 18-1 and 18-3; see later section).[53-56] Most *SDH* mutations are germline, but there is a single report of a somatic *SDHA* mutation.[56] *SDH* mutations are mutually exclusive with *KIT, PDGFRA,* and *BRAF* mutations.

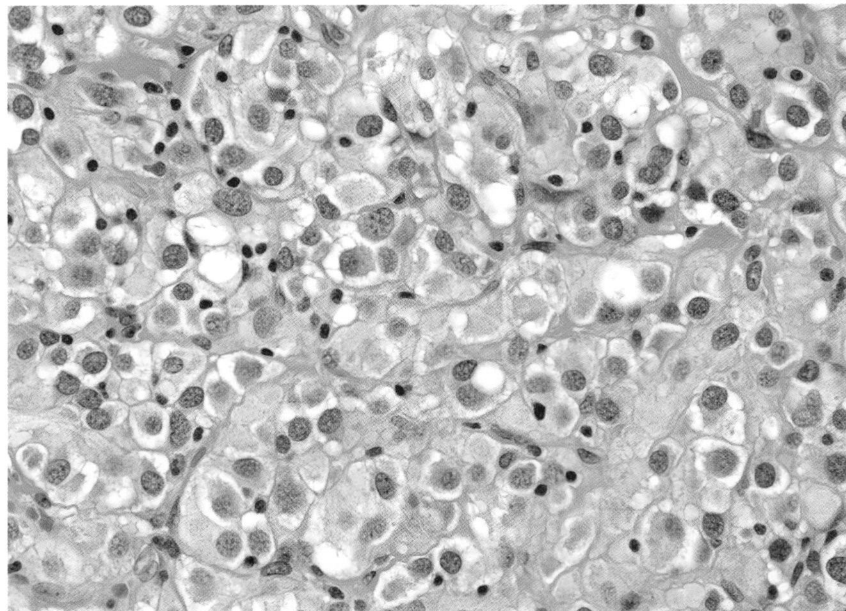

FIGURE 18-26. PDGFRA mutant GIST with epithelioid morphology, frequent binucleation, and prominent cell membranes.

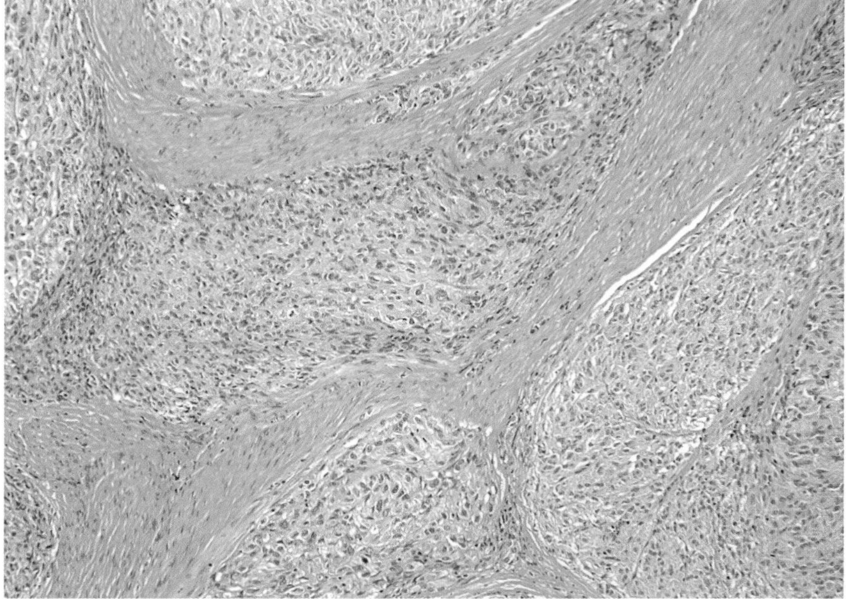

FIGURE 18-27. SDH-deficient GIST showing typical plexiform growth pattern with prominent fibrous bands.

KIT, PDGFRA, BRAF, and *SDH* mutations are undoubtedly the initiating events in GIST tumorigenesis, but other genetic events—secondary mutations—collaborate with these primary mutations.[45] Most of what is known about secondary mutations comes from comparative genomic hybridization and cytogenetic studies, which have implicated many gene regions in GIST tumorigenesis. Areas with frequent loss or gain of genetic information include deletions of 1p, 9p, 11p, 14q, 22q and gains of 8p and 17q. Unfortunately, most of the specific genes that are either amplified (oncogenes) or deleted (tumor suppressor) in these gene regions have not been identified. An exception is deletions within 9p that are associated with aggressive behavior and result in loss of the *CDKN2A* gene that encodes both p14(ARF) and p16(INK4A), two well-known tumor suppressors.[57]

SUCCINATE DEHYDROGENASE DEFICIENT GASTROINTESTINAL STROMAL TUMORS

The term *SDH-deficient GIST* has emerged to describe a recently identified subset of GIST, which comprises up to 42% of wild-type GISTs, 3% of all GISTs, and 7.5% of gastric GISTs.[58-60] These GISTs are characterized by a predilection for gastric location, are composed of epithelioid or mixed epithelioid and spindle cell morphology, have a distinctive multinodular/infiltrative growth pattern, frequently are multifocal, are diffusely and strongly positive for KIT by immunohistochemistry, and all demonstrate loss of SDHB expression by immunohistochemistry (see Table 18-1; Figs. 18-27 and 18-28). Approximately 27% of SDH-deficient GISTs also lack SDHA expression by immunohistochemistry.[55]

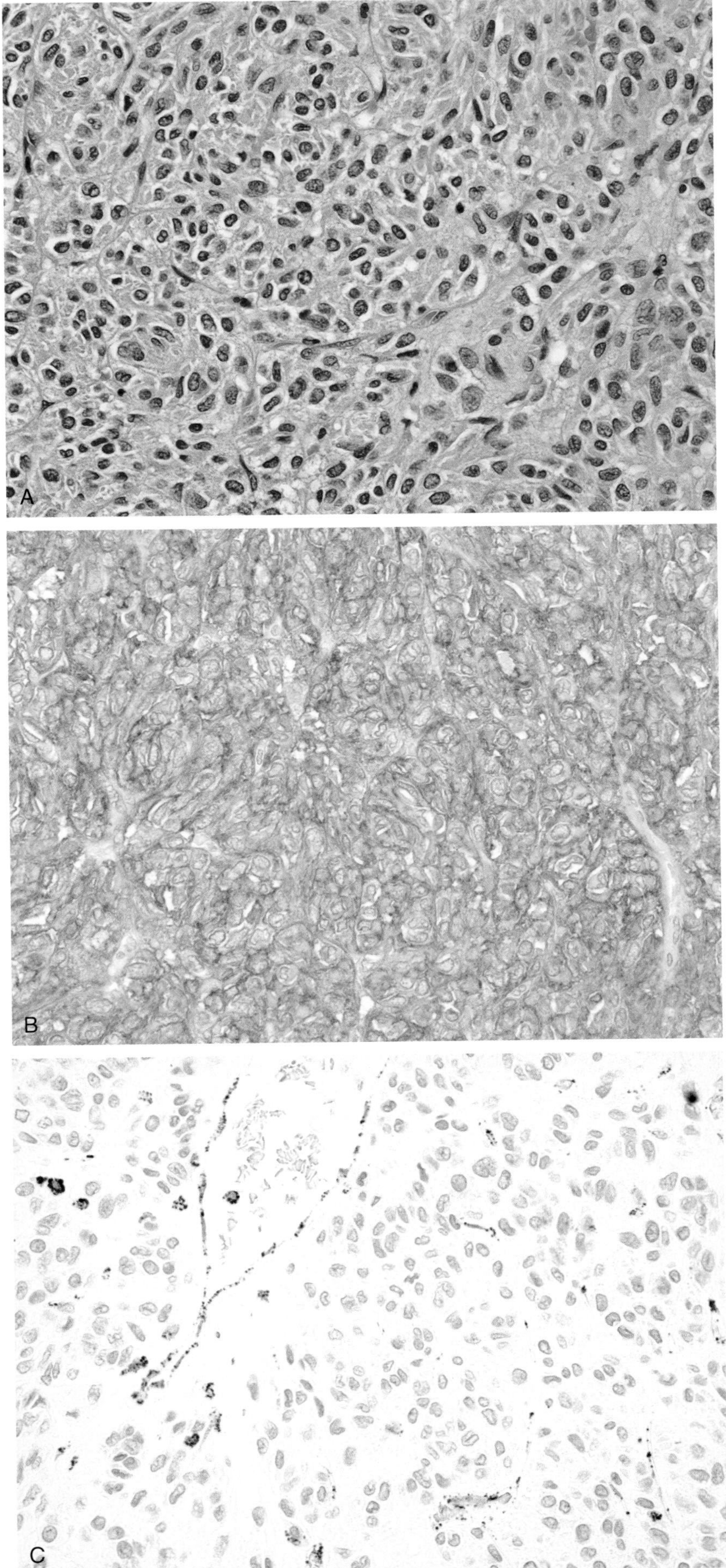

FIGURE 18-28. SDH-deficient GIST with epithelioid morphology (A). Corresponding KIT (B) and SDHB (C) immunohistochemical stains. Endothelial cells are positive internal controls in SDHB stain (C).

Germline mutations have been identified in SDH-deficient GISTs in the genes for four of the five protein subunits that comprise the SDH complex: *SDHA, SDHB, SDHC,* and *SDHD* (see Table 18-3).[53-56] A single somatic *SDHA* mutation has been identified.[56] Based on the limited data available, it is not possible to determine the overall frequency of these mutations at this time. However, *SDH* mutations have not been identified in the majority of SDH-deficient GISTs. Interestingly, loss of SDHA expression by immunohistochemistry accurately predicts the presence of inactivating mutations in *SDHA* (see Table 18-1).[55] Therefore, SDHA immunohistochemistry can be used as a surrogate for inactivating *SDHA* mutations.

SDH-deficient GISTs are also unusual with respect to clinical behavior. Unlike conventional GISTs, SDH-deficient GISTs have a propensity to metastasize to lymph nodes, which happens in approximately 50% of cases.[60] Even though they metastasize with high frequency, they appear to have relatively indolent metastases because patients can survive decades with metastatic disease. This has prompted the recommendation that standard criteria for risk stratification should not be used in SDH-deficient GISTs.

PEDIATRIC GASTROINTESTINAL STROMAL TUMORS

Pediatric GIST essentially describes all GISTs in patients 18 years of age or younger and occurs even in newborns.[61] GISTs in the pediatric population are rare, amounting to less than 1% of all GISTs (see Table 18-3); they have many characteristics that distinguish them from adult GISTs. Although *KIT* and *PDGFRA* mutations are found in 85% to 95% of adult GISTs, they occur in less than 15% of pediatric GISTs.

A subset of pediatric GIST patients, almost always male, has GISTs that are typical of adult patients with clinical, morphologic, and molecular findings (*KIT* or *PDGFRA* mutations) that are seen in adults. However, the majority of GISTs in the pediatric population occur in females, are multifocal gastric tumors, and have lymph node metastasis and epithelioid morphology. Also, despite frequent lymph node, liver, and peritoneal metastases, pediatric patients tend to have a much better prognosis than adult patients with GISTs. This is undoubtedly a result of the presence of a large number of germline *SDH* mutations in the pediatric GIST population. However, as a group, the majority of *SDH*-deficient GISTs occur in adults. Pediatric GISTs are also linked to the Carney triad and Carney-Stratakis syndrome (see later section).

GASTROINTESTINAL STROMAL TUMOR SYNDROMES

The majority of GISTs are sporadic without any known predisposing genetic factors. However, GIST also occurs in the setting of several syndromes, including familial GIST, neurofibromatosis type 1 (NF1), Carney triad, and Carney-Stratakis syndrome (see Table 18-3). NF1, Carney triad, and Carney-Stratakis syndrome GISTs are all examples of wild-type GISTs because they lack *KIT* or *PDGFRA* mutations.

Familial GIST is characterized by germline *KIT* or *PDGFRA* mutations that are inherited with an autosomal dominant pattern of inheritance (see Table 18-3).[46,62,63] Any family member that inherits a germline mutant *KIT* or *PDGFRA* allele will develop GISTs. Familial GISTs tend to be multifocal and can be accompanied by ICC hyperplasia. To date, germline *KIT* mutations have been identified in exons 8, 11, 13, and 17. Although most familial GIST kindreds harbor germline *KIT* mutations, germline *PDGFRA* mutations have also been identified in *PDGFRA* exons 12 and 18. In addition to GISTs, patients with germline *KIT* mutations may also have hyperpigmentation, urticaria pigmentosa, or dysphagia, depending on their genotype.[63] Patients with germline exon 18 *PDGFRA* mutations have large hands, in addition to multifocal GISTs. A single patient with a germline exon 12 *PDGFRA* mutation had multifocal gastric GISTs, multiple lipomas, and fibrous tumors of her intestine.[64]

NF1 is the most common tumor syndrome in humans and is characterized by the development of a variety of tumors, including, but not limited to, neurofibromas, malignant peripheral nerve sheath tumors, brainstem gliomas, and GISTs. Patients with NF1 have loss-of-function mutations within the *NF1* gene. Only a small number of patients with NF1 develop GISTs, estimated to be 7% of all NF1 patients in one study.[65] NF1 GISTs do not harbor *KIT* or *PDGFRA* mutations, suggesting that *NF1* mutations are the initiating tumorigenic event in these GISTs. However, the reason that only a small subset of NF1 patients develops GISTs is not clear. NF1 GISTs tend to occur in the small bowel, are multifocal, and may be clinically more indolent than *KIT* or a *PDGFRA* mutant GIST.[66] Resections of patients with NF1 GISTs frequently exhibit ICC hyperplasia (Fig. 18-29).

Carney triad was originally characterized by the presence of epithelioid gastric GIST, extra-adrenal paraganglioma, and pulmonary chondroma.[67,68] It affects mainly females and is sporadic (see Table 18-3). GISTs in Carney triad are part of the spectrum of SDH-deficient GISTs, clinically, histologically, and immunohistochemically.[69] However, Carney triad GISTs lack *SDHA, SDHB, SDHC,* and *SDHD* mutations.[70] As of the writing of this text, the genetic basis of Carney triad is unknown. As described in SDH-deficient GISTs, Carney-triad-associated GISTs have indolent clinical behavior, even in the presence of lymph node and liver metastasis.

Carney-Stratakis syndrome is characterized by the combination of epithelioid gastric GISTs and paragangliomas.[53] It is inherited with an autosomal dominant pattern of inheritance and affects both males and females. Carney-Stratakis syndrome GISTs are also SDH-deficient GISTs because they lack SDHB by immunohistochemistry, and patients with Carney-Stratakis syndrome have germline mutations in *SDHA, SDHB,* or *SDHD* (see Table 18-3). They have the clinical features as described for other cases of SDH-deficient GISTs.

BEHAVIOR OF GASTROINTESTINAL STROMAL TUMORS

As mentioned previously, SDH-deficient GISTs appear to have distinct clinical behavior from GISTs with *KIT, PDGFRA,* or *BRAF* mutations, which preclude them from being risk-stratified. Although there is some evidence that neurofibromatosis-1-associated GISTs may also be associated with more indolent behavior, the data are less clear, and,

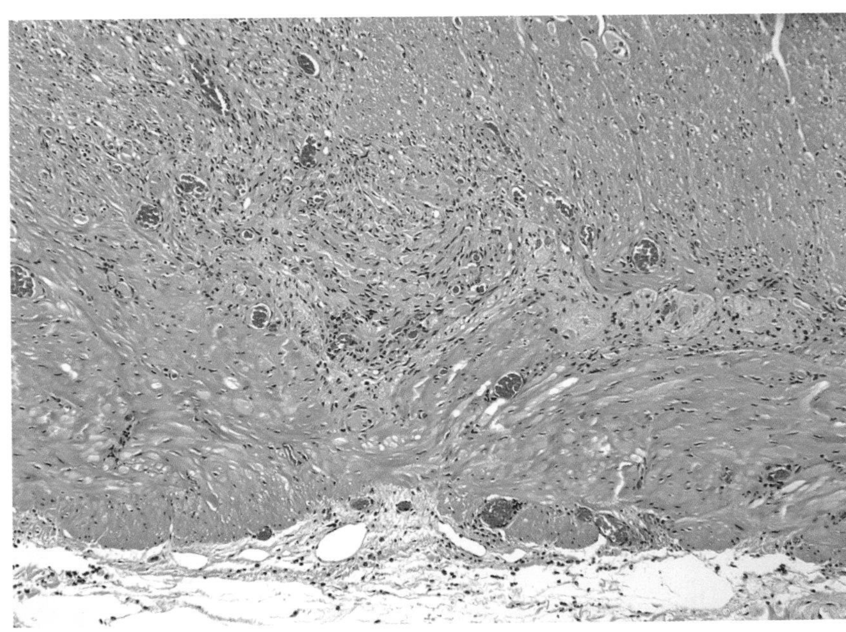

FIGURE 18-29. ICC hyperplasia arising from the myenteric plexus in a small bowel resection specimen from a patient with multifocal NF-1 GIST.

TABLE 18-4 NIH Consensus Criteria

RISK CATEGORY	TUMOR SIZE IN LARGEST DIMENSION	MITOTIC COUNT (PER 50 HPFs)
Very low	<2 cm	<5
Low	2-5 cm	<5
Intermediate	<5 cm	6-10
	5-10 cm	<5
High	>5 cm	>5
	>10 cm	Any mitotic rate
	Any size	>10

at this point, they should be risk-stratified as for conventional GISTs.

The most important risk factors for conventional GISTs are anatomic location, size, and mitotic rate.[71] Tumor rupture is also an important risk factor because GISTs that rupture have a far worse prognosis.[72] Finally, mucosal invasion is also associated with a poor prognosis. True mucosal invasion is rare and subjective, so it is not currently incorporated into the major risk-stratification schemes for GIST.

There is evidence that *KIT* mutation status is also of prognostic importance. *KIT* exon 9 mutations and *KIT* exon 11 codon 557-558 deletions have been linked to aggressive behavior.[73] GISTs with *PDGFRA* exon 18 mutations have been associated with a better prognosis.[74]

Several risk-stratification schemes have been proposed. The first scheme that was established, the National Institutes of Health (NIH) Consensus Criteria, used mitotic rate and size to determine risk for recurrence (Table 18-4).[25] After it was established, its utility was confirmed in independent sets of GISTs with long-term follow-up.[4,75] Based on several large studies, the Armed Forces Institute of Pathology (AFIP) modified the NIH Consensus criteria to add anatomic location (Table 18-5),[7] including the stomach, duodenum, jejunum/ileum, and rectum. Those GISTs that develop in other anatomic locations (such as EGISTs) are classified according to the criteria for jejunum/ileum. Mitotic rate is subdivided into those GISTs with less than or equal to 5 mitotic figures per 5 mm^2 and those with greater than 5 mitotic figures per 5 mm^2. Size is subdivided as less than or equal to 2 cm, greater than 2 cm and less than or equal to 5 cm, greater than 5 cm and less than or equal to 10 cm, and greater than 10 cm. The AFIP criteria are recommended by the College of American Pathologists (CAP) and included in their CAP GIST checklist.[76]

Joensuu[71] has proposed a simplification to the AFIP criteria that groups anatomic sites into either gastric or nongastric sites to reflect that gastric tumors have a better prognosis (Table 18-6). Furthermore, he subdivided mitotic rate into three categories instead of two: less than or equal to 5, 6-10, and greater than 10 mitotic figures per 50 high-power fields (HPF). The inclusion of the 6-10 mitotic figure category applies only to gastric GISTs that are less than or equal to 5 cm in greatest dimension and is meant to capture this group as intermediate risk. Finally, he added tumor rupture as automatic criteria for determining a GIST as high risk. The Joensuu[72] criteria were superior to other systems in identifying a single risk group (high risk) that were at risk for local recurrence/metastasis. This is critically important because the major use of risk stratification criteria, at this point, is for determining who should and should not receive adjuvant imatinib therapy after resection. The ability to definitively identify a single high-risk category is advantageous for this purpose.

The NIH, AFIP, and Joensuu criteria suffer from having to break size and mitotic rate down into discreet variables. This is obviously a problem when considering a GIST with five or six mitotic figures per 50 HPF because a difference of one mitotic figure can make a large difference in behavior prediction. Systems that are able to evaluate size and mitotic rate as continuous variables will more accurately reflect the continuum of biologic behavior. By pooling population-based studies, Joensuu et al.[77] were able to develop novel heat maps and contour maps that evaluated size and mitotic rates as continuous variables. Evaluation of these systems revealed

TABLE 18-5 AFIP Criteria

TUMOR PARAMETERS		RISK OF PROGRESSIVE DISEASE* (%), BASED ON SITE OF ORIGIN			
Mitotic Rate	Size	Gastric	Duodenum	Jejunum/Ileum	Rectum
≤5 per 50 HPF	≤2 cm	None (0%)	None (0%)	None (0%)	None (0%)
	>2, ≤5 cm	Very low (1.9%)	Low (8.3%)	Low (4.3%)	Low (8.5%)
	>5, ≤10 cm	Low (3.6%)	(Insuff. data)	Moderate (24%)	(Insuff. data)
	>10 cm	Moderate (10%)	High (34%)	High (52%)	High (57%)
>5 per 50 HPF	≤2 cm	None**	(Insuff. data)	High**	High (54%)
	>2, ≤5 cm	Moderate (16%)	High (50%)	High (73%)	High (52%)
	>5, ≤10 cm	High (55%)	(Insuff. data)	High (85%)	(Insuff. data)
	>10 cm	High (86%)	High (86%)	High (90%)	High (71%)

Modified from Miettinen M and Lasota J. Gastrointestinal stromal tumors: pathology and prognosis at different sites. Semin Diagn Pathol 2006; 23:70–83.
Data based on long-term follow-up of 1055 gastric, 629 small intestinal, 144 duodenal, and 111 rectal GISTs:
Miettinen M, Sobin LH, and Lasota J. Gastrointestinal stromal tumors of the stomach: a clinicopathologic, immunohistochemical, and molecular genetic study of 1765 cases with long-term follow-up. Am J Surg Pathol 2005 Jan;29(1):52–68; Miettinen M, Makhlouf H, Sobin LH, et al. Gastrointestinal stromal tumors of the jejunum and ileum: a clinicopathologic, immunohistochemical, and molecular genetic study of 906 cases before imatinib with long-term follow-up. Am J Surg Pathol 2006 Apr;30(4):477–489; Miettinen M and Lasota J. Gastrointestinal stromal tumors: pathology and prognosis at different sites. Semin Diagn Pathol 2006 May;23(2):70–83.

*Defined as metastasis or tumor-related death.
**Denotes small numbers of cases.

TABLE 18-6 Joensuu Criteria

RISK CATEGORY	TUMOR SIZE (CM)	MITOTIC INDEX (PER 50 HPFs)	PRIMARY TUMOR SITE
Very low risk	<2.0	≤5	Any
Low risk	2.1-5.0	≤5	Any
Intermediate risk	2.1-5.0	>5	Gastric
	<5.0	6-10	Any
	5.1-10.0	≤5	Gastric
High risk	Any	Any	Tumor rupture
	>10.0	Any	Any
	Any	>10	Any
	>5.0	>5	Any
	2.1-5.0	>5	Nongastric
	5.1-10.0	≤5	Nongastric

that they were more accurate in estimating the risk of recurrence after surgery than the conventional risk stratification systems mentioned previously.

In the event that a patient presents with metastasis, the GIST should be classified as malignant; it is not necessary to do a formal risk stratification in such lesions. Risk stratification is only for uninodular, primary GISTs that have not been treated. Neoadjuvant pre-treatment also invalidates risk stratification.

TREATMENT OF GASTROINTESTINAL STROMAL TUMORS

Treatment of primary GIST is surgical. However, approximately 40% of GISTs will recur or metastasize after complete resection of a primary disease. Treatment of recurrent metastatic GIST is based on targeting oncogenic KIT and PDGFRA mutant proteins. Imatinib mesylate (Gleevec, Novartis Pharmaceuticals) is a small molecule tyrosine kinase inhibitor that targets KIT and PDGFRA as well as other non-GIST relevant proteins, such as BCR-ABL kinase. Imatinib has been approved by the FDA for first-line use in the treatment of recurrent/metastatic GIST. Before the advent of imatinib, recurrent/metastatic GIST patients had a response rate to conventional chemotherapy of less than 5% and a median survival of 18 months.[78] With the use of imatinib, patients with unresectable GIST now have a median survival of 55 months.[79] Response to imatinib varies with *KIT* and *PDGFRA* mutation status. *KIT* exon 11 mutant GISTs respond the best to imatinib.[39] Increasing the imatinib dose from 400 mg/day to 800 mg/day improves the response of *KIT* exon 9 mutant GISTs.[80] The most common *PDGFRA* mutation that encodes PDGFRA D842V is unresponsive to imatinib. However, about one-third of *PDGFRA* and some wild-type GISTs respond to imatinib; therefore, the general procedure is to treat all recurrent or metastatic GIST patients with imatinib and escalate the dose from 400 to 800 mg per day if there is no response. The requirement to provide 800 mg/day of imatinib to *KIT* exon 9 mutant GISTs and the lack of efficacy in treating PDGFRA D842V mutant GISTs argues for determining the *KIT-PDGFRA* mutation status of each GIST before administration of imatinib, before initiating treatment of recurrent/metastatic GIST, or in the adjuvant setting.

Approximately 50% of GIST patients develop acquired resistance to imatinib within 2 years of the onset of therapy, and most will acquire imatinib resistance within 10 years.[81] Therapeutic resistance in these cases is a result of a second site intra-allelic *KIT* mutations within exons 13, 14, 17, or 18 that either inhibit binding to imatinib or render KIT insensitive to imatinib.[82] Resistance can be localized, often occurring as a single tumor nodule that is growing in the presence of other tumors that are under control or as generalized resistance with numerous sites of progression.

Sunitinib maleate (Sutent, Pfizer Pharmaceuticals) is another small molecule tyrosine kinase inhibitor that has been approved by the FDA for the treatment of patients who are intolerant of or resistant to imatinib. Sunitinib targets vascular endothelial growth factor receptors (VEGFR) 1-3, in addition to KIT and PDGFRA. In a placebo controlled trial of patients who were resistant to or intolerant of imatinib, the median time to tumor progression was 27.3 weeks in the treatment

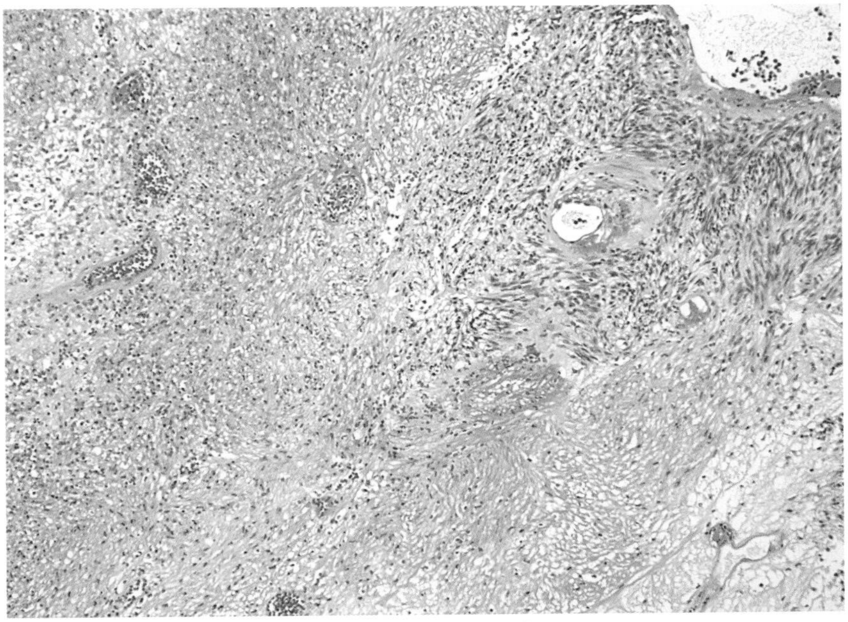

FIGURE 18-30. GIST treated with imatinib mesylate resulting in extensive necrosis with focal islands of viable appearing GIST cells surrounding blood vessels (upper right corner).

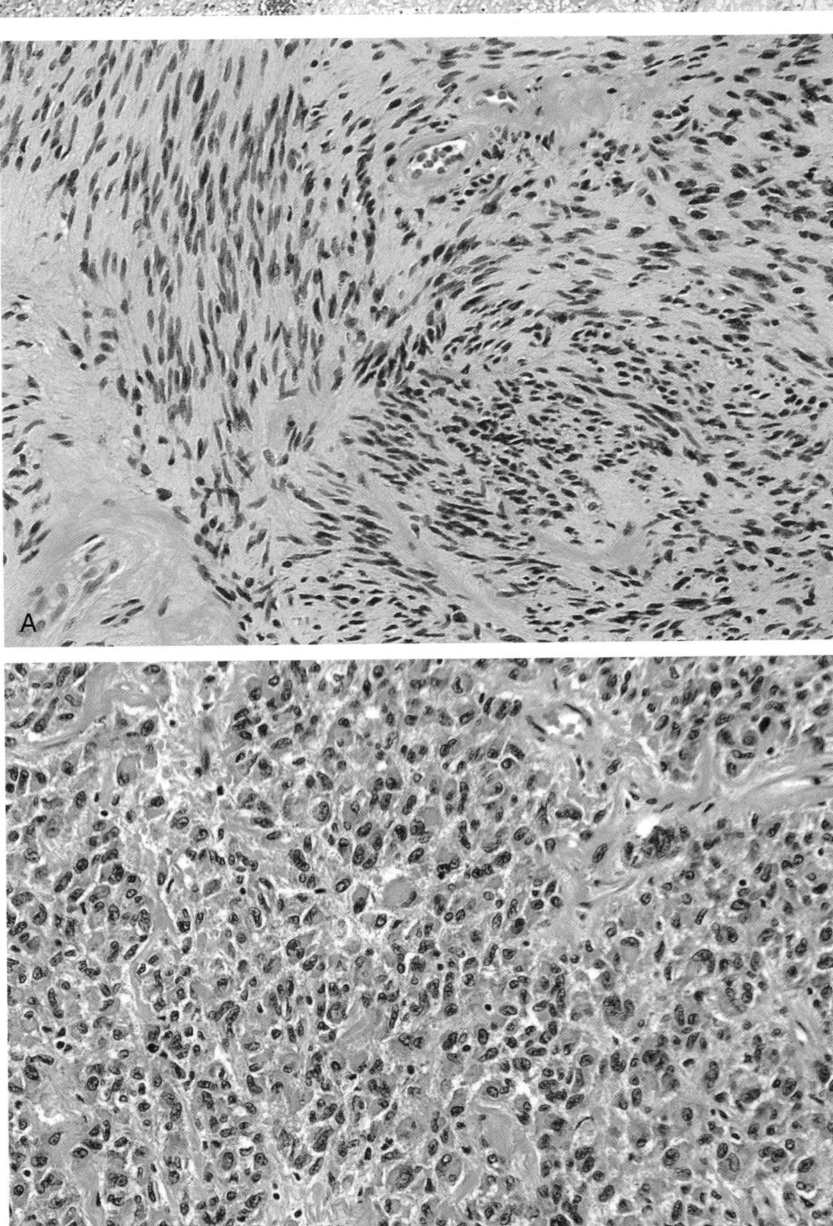

FIGURE 18-31. Spindle cell GIST (A) demonstrating a radical change to a more epithelioid and rhabdoid morphology (B) in an imatinib resistant nodule.

arm versus 6.4 weeks in the placebo arm.[83] The two most common *KIT* mutations that give rise to secondary resistance, KIT V654A and T670I, are sensitive to sunitinib.[84]

There are no currently FDA-approved treatments for patients who fail both primary therapy with imatinib and sunitinib. However, there are numerous other small-molecule tyrosine kinase inhibitors that are under various stages of development. Perhaps the most promising new therapy is regorafenib (Stivarga; Bayer), a multikinase inhibitor that targets KIT, PDGFR, VEGFR1-3, TIE2, RET, fibroblast growth factor receptor 1, RAF, and p38 mitogen-activated protein kinase. Of 33 patients that had received at least two cycles of regorafenib in a multicenter phase II trial in patients with advanced GIST who had failed at least imatinib and sunitinib, 4 patients achieved a partial response, and 22 had a stable disease at greater than or equal to 16 weeks.[85] The median progression free survival in this trial was 10 months.

The success of treatment of recurrent/metastatic unresectable GIST with imatinib suggested that adjuvant therapy with imatinib might delay the time to recurrence/metastasis. Most patients with localized, resectable GIST are cured by surgery and will not benefit from adjuvant therapy. However, about 40% of GIST patients will recur, and adjuvant therapy should be considered after resection in each patient with GIST. Adjuvant therapy has been examined in two large trials. Follow-up at 19.7 months of a large randomized placebo-controlled trial that examined recurrence-free survival (RFS) after 1 year of adjuvant imatinib demonstrated a 1 year RFS of 98% in the imatinib arm compared to an 83% RFS in the placebo arm.[86] A subsequent trial comparing 1 year to 3 years of adjuvant imatinib demonstrated an 87% RFS in the 3-year treatment group compared to 60% at 1 year of follow-up.[87] There was also a difference in overall survival in the 1-year and 3-year treatment groups. The overall survival was 92% versus 82% at 5 years of follow-up in the 3-year and 1-year treatment groups, respectively. Overall, the results of these two trials make an impressive argument for the use of adjuvant imatinib in patients with GIST, and, as a result, imatinib received FDA-approval for the adjuvant treatment of GIST.

HISTOLOGIC ASSESSMENT OF TREATED GASTROINTESTINAL STROMAL TUMORS

Because of the efficacy of imatinib, it is being used in the context of neoadjuvant therapy to shrink tumors and make them resectable.[88] Because of the use of neoadjuvant therapy, pathologists are occasionally asked to evaluate therapeutic response. Evaluation of morphologic changes in GISTs treated with imatinib reveals areas of hypocellularity, myxoid stroma, and necrosis (Fig. 18-30).[89] However, there are virtually always areas of viable cells. As a practical approach, the percentage of viable tumor cells after treatment should be reported.

Most GISTs that progress on tyrosine kinase inhibitor therapies retain their original morphology. However, rarely, they change morphology and can even lose KIT expression. Liegl et al.[90] described five cases of GIST that showed heterologous rhabdomyoblastic differentiation and a loss of KIT expression. Change from spindle cell morphology to epithelioid morphology with a loss of KIT expression has also been described (Fig. 18-31).[91]

References

1. Patil DT, Rubin BP. Gastrointestinal stromal tumor: advances in diagnosis and management. Arch Pathol Lab Med 2011;135(10):1298–310.
2. Sanders KM, Koh SD, Ward SM. Interstitial cells of Cajal as pacemakers in the gastrointestinal tract. Annu Rev Physiol 2006;68:307–43.
3. Hirota S, Isozaki K, Moriyama Y, et al. Gain-of-function mutations of c-kit in human gastrointestinal stromal tumors. Science 1998;279(5350):577–80.
4. Tryggvason G, Gíslason HG, Magnússon MK, et al. Gastrointestinal stromal tumors in Iceland, 1990-2003: the icelandic GIST study, a population-based incidence and pathologic risk stratification study. Int J Cancer 2005;117(2):289–93.
5. Agaimy A, Wünsch PH, Hofstaedter F, et al. Minute gastric sclerosing stromal tumors (GIST tumorlets) are common in adults and frequently show c-KIT mutations. Am J Surg Pathol 2007;31(1):113–20.
6. Emile JF, Brahimi S, Coindre JM, et al. Frequencies of KIT and PDGFRA mutations in the MolecGIST prospective population-based study differ from those of advanced GISTs. Med Oncol 2012;29(3):1765–72.
7. Miettinen M, Lasota J. Gastrointestinal stromal tumors: pathology and prognosis at different sites. Semin Diagn Pathol 2006;23(2):70–83.
8. Miettinen M, Sarlomo-Rikala M, Sobin LH, et al. Esophageal stromal tumors: a clinicopathologic, immunohistochemical, and molecular genetic study of 17 cases and comparison with esophageal leiomyomas and leiomyosarcomas. Am J Surg Pathol 2000;24(2):211–22.
9. Miettinen M, Sobin LH. Gastrointestinal stromal tumors in the appendix: a clinicopathologic and immunohistochemical study of four cases. Am J Surg Pathol 2001;25(11):1433–7.
10. Miettinen M, Sobin LH, Lasota J. Gastrointestinal stromal tumors presenting as omental masses–a clinicopathologic analysis of 95 cases. Am J Surg Pathol 2009;33(9):1267–75.
11. Reith JD, Goldblum JR, Lyles RH, et al. Extragastrointestinal (soft tissue) stromal tumors: an analysis of 48 cases with emphasis on histologic predictors of outcome. Mod Pathol 2000;13(5):577–85.
12. Lam MM, Corless CL, Goldblum JR, et al. Extragastrointestinal stromal tumors presenting as vulvovaginal/rectovaginal septal masses: a diagnostic pitfall. Int J Gynecol Pathol 2006;25(3):288–92.
13. Agaimy A, Wunsch PH. Gastrointestinal stromal tumours: a regular origin in the muscularis propria, but an extremely diverse gross presentation. A review of 200 cases to critically re-evaluate the concept of so-called extra-gastrointestinal stromal tumours. Langenbecks Arch Surg 2006; 391(4):322–9.
14. Yamamoto H, Kojima A, Nagata S, et al. KIT-negative gastrointestinal stromal tumor of the abdominal soft tissue: a clinicopathologic and genetic study of 10 cases. Am J Surg Pathol 2011;35(9):1287–95.
15. Demetri GD, von Mehren M, Antonescu CR, et al. NCCN Task Force report: update on the management of patients with gastrointestinal stromal tumors. J Natl Compr Canc Netw 2010;8(Suppl 2):S1–41; quiz S42-44.
16. Wang WL, Hornick JL, Mallipeddi R, et al. Cutaneous and subcutaneous metastases of gastrointestinal stromal tumors: a series of 5 cases with molecular analysis. Am J Dermatopathol 2009;31(3):297–300.
17. Jati A, Tatlı S, Morgan JA, et al. Imaging features of bone metastases in patients with gastrointestinal stromal tumors. Diagn Interv Radiol 2012;18(4):391–6.
18. Hamada S, Itami A, Watanabe G, et al. Intracranial metastasis from an esophageal gastrointestinal stromal tumor. Intern Med 2010;49(8):781–5.
19. Miettinen M, Sobin LH, Lasota J. Gastrointestinal stromal tumors of the stomach: a clinicopathologic, immunohistochemical, and molecular genetic study of 1765 cases with long-term follow-up. Am J Surg Pathol 2005;29(1):52–68.
20. Miettinen M, Kopczynski J, Makhlouf HR, et al. Gastrointestinal stromal tumors, intramural leiomyomas, and leiomyosarcomas in the duodenum: a clinicopathologic, immunohistochemical, and molecular genetic study of 167 cases. Am J Surg Pathol 2003;27(5):625–41.
21. Miettinen M, Makhlouf H, Sobin LH, et al. Gastrointestinal stromal tumors of the jejunum and ileum: a clinicopathologic, immunohistochemical, and molecular genetic study of 906 cases before imatinib with long-term follow-up. Am J Surg Pathol 2006;30(4):477–89.
22. Ito H, Inoue H, Ryozawa S, et al. Fine-needle aspiration biopsy and endoscopic ultrasound for pretreatment pathological diagnosis of gastric gastrointestinal stromal tumors. Gastroenterol Res Pract 2012;2012:139083.
23. Rege TA, Wagner AJ, Corless CL, et al. "Pediatric-type" gastrointestinal stromal tumors in adults: distinctive histology predicts genotype and clinical behavior. Am J Surg Pathol 2011;35(4):495–504.

24. Miettinen M, Lasota J. Gastrointestinal stromal tumors–definition, clinical, histological, immunohistochemical, and molecular genetic features and differential diagnosis. Virchows Arch 2001;438(1):1–12.
25. Fletcher CD, Berman JJ, Corless C, et al. Diagnosis of gastrointestinal stromal tumors: a consensus approach. Hum Pathol 2002;33(5):459–65.
26. Min KW. Small intestinal stromal tumors with skeinoid fibers. Clinicopathological, immunohistochemical, and ultrastructural investigations. Am J Surg Pathol 1992;16(2):145–55.
27. Antonescu C, Hornick JL, Nielsen GP. Dedifferentiation in gastrointestinal stromal tumor (GIST) to an anaplastic KIT-negative phenotype - a diagnostic pitfall. Mod Pathol 2007;20(Suppl. 2):11A.
28. Kindblom LG, Remotti HE, Aldenborg F, et al. Gastrointestinal pacemaker cell tumor (GIPACT): gastrointestinal stromal tumors show phenotypic characteristics of the interstitial cells of Cajal. Am J Pathol 1998;152(5):1259–69.
29. Sarlomo-Rikala M, Kovatich AJ, Barusevicius A, et al. CD117: a sensitive marker for gastrointestinal stromal tumors that is more specific than CD34. Mod Pathol 1998;11(8):728–34.
30. Medeiros F, Corless CL, Duensing A, et al. KIT-negative gastrointestinal stromal tumors: proof of concept and therapeutic implications. Am J Surg Pathol 2004;28(7):889–94.
31. Espinosa I, Lee CH, Kim MK, et al. A novel monoclonal antibody against DOG1 is a sensitive and specific marker for gastrointestinal stromal tumors. Am J Surg Pathol 2008;32(2):210–8.
32. Miettinen M, Wang ZF, Lasota J. DOG1 antibody in the differential diagnosis of gastrointestinal stromal tumors: a study of 1840 cases. Am J Surg Pathol 2009;33(9):1401–8.
33. Liegl B, Hornick JL, Corless CL, et al. Monoclonal antibody DOG1.1 shows higher sensitivity than KIT in the diagnosis of gastrointestinal stromal tumors, including unusual subtypes. Am J Surg Pathol 2009; 33(3):437–46.
34. Lopes LF, West RB, Bacchi LM, et al. DOG1 for the diagnosis of gastrointestinal stromal tumor (GIST): comparison between 2 different antibodies. Appl Immunohistochem Mol Morphol 2010;18(4):333–7.
35. Erlandson RA, Klimstra DS, Woodruff JM. Subclassification of gastrointestinal stromal tumors based on evaluation by electron microscopy and immunohistochemistry. Ultrastruct Pathol 1996;20(4):373–93.
36. Walker P, Dvorak AM. Gastrointestinal autonomic nerve (GAN) tumor. Ultrastructural evidence for a newly recognized entity. Arch Pathol Lab Med 1986;110(4):309–16.
37. Herrera GA, Pinto de Moraes H, Grizzle WE, et al. Malignant small bowel neoplasm of enteric plexus derivation (plexosarcoma). Light and electron microscopic study confirming the origin of the neoplasm. Dig Dis Sci 1984;29(3):275–84.
38. Lee JR, Joshi V, Griffin Jr JW, et al. Gastrointestinal autonomic nerve tumor: immunohistochemical and molecular identity with gastrointestinal stromal tumor. Am J Surg Pathol 2001;25(8):979–87.
39. Heinrich MC, Corless CL, Demetri GD, et al. Kinase mutations and imatinib response in patients with metastatic gastrointestinal stromal tumor. J Clin Oncol 2003;21(23):4342–9.
40. Corless CL, McGreevey L, Haley A, et al. KIT mutations are common in incidental gastrointestinal stromal tumors one centimeter or less in size. Am J Pathol 2002;160(5):1567–72.
41. Rossi S, Gasparotto D, Toffolatti L, et al. Molecular and clinicopathologic characterization of gastrointestinal stromal tumors (GISTs) of small size. Am J Surg Pathol 2010;34(10):1480–91.
42. Nakai N, Ishikawa T, Nishitani A, et al. A mouse model of a human multiple GIST family with KIT-Asp820Tyr mutation generated by a knock-in strategy. J Pathol 2008;214(3):302–11.
43. Sommer G, Agosti V, Ehlers I, et al. Gastrointestinal stromal tumors in a mouse model by targeted mutations of the Kit receptor tyrosine kinase. Proc Natl Acad Sci USA 2003;100:6706–11.
44. Rubin BP, Antonescu CR, Scott-Browne JP, et al. A knock-in mouse model of gastrointestinal stromal tumor harboring kit K641E. Cancer Res 2005;65(15):6631–9.
45. Wozniak A, Sciot R, Guillou L, et al. Array CGH analysis in primary gastrointestinal stromal tumors: cytogenetic profile correlates with anatomic site and tumor aggressiveness, irrespective of mutational status. Genes Chromosomes Cancer 2007;46(3):261–76.
46. Corless CL, Barnett CM, Heinrich MC. Gastrointestinal stromal tumours: origin and molecular oncology. Nat Rev Cancer 2011;11(12):865–78.
47. Antonescu CR, Sommer G, Sarran L, et al. Association of KIT exon 9 mutations with nongastric primary site and aggressive behavior: KIT mutation analysis and clinical correlates of 120 gastrointestinal stromal tumors. Clin Cancer Res 2003;9(9):3329–37.
48. Lux ML, Rubin BP, Biase TL, et al. KIT extracellular and kinase domain mutations in gastrointestinal stromal tumors. Am J Pathol 2000;156(3): 791–5.
49. Lasota J, Dansonka-Mieszkowska A, et al. A great majority of GISTs with PDGFRA mutations represent gastric tumors of low or no malignant potential. Lab Invest 2004;84(7):874–83.
50. Heinrich MC, Corless CL, Duensing A, et al. PDGFRA activating mutations in gastrointestinal stromal tumors. Science 2003;299(5607): 708–10.
51. Agaram NP, Wong GC, Guo T, et al. Novel V600E BRAF mutations in imatinib-naive and imatinib-resistant gastrointestinal stromal tumors. Genes Chromosomes Cancer 2008;47(10):853–9.
52. Hostein I, Faur N, Primois C, et al. BRAF mutation status in gastrointestinal stromal tumors. Am J Clin Pathol 2010;133(1):141–8.
53. Pasini B, McWhinney SR, Bei T, et al. Clinical and molecular genetics of patients with the Carney-Stratakis syndrome and germline mutations of the genes coding for the succinate dehydrogenase subunits SDHB, SDHC, and SDHD. Eur J Hum Genet 2008;16(1):79–88.
54. Janeway KA, Kim SY, Lodish M, et al. Defects in succinate dehydrogenase in gastrointestinal stromal tumors lacking KIT and PDGFRA mutations. Proc Natl Acad Sci U S A 2011;108(1):314–18.
55. Wagner AJ, Remillard SP, Zhang YX, et al. Loss of expression of SDHA predicts SDHA mutations in gastrointestinal stromal tumors. Mod Pathol 2013;26(2):289–94.
56. Italiano A, Chen CL, Sung YS, et al. SDHA loss of function mutations in a subset of young adult wild-type gastrointestinal stromal tumors. BMC Cancer 2012;12(1):408.
57. Schneider-Stock R, Boltze C, Lasota J, et al. High prognostic value of p16INK4 alterations in gastrointestinal stromal tumors. J Clin Oncol 2003;21(9):1688–97.
58. Gill AJ, Chou A, Vilain R, et al. Immunohistochemistry for SDHB divides gastrointestinal stromal tumors (GISTs) into 2 distinct types. Am J Surg Pathol 2010;34(5):636–44.
59. Miettinen M, Wang ZF, Sarlomo-Rikala M, et al. Succinate dehydrogenase-deficient GISTs: a clinicopathologic, immunohistochemical, and molecular genetic study of 66 gastric GISTs with predilection to young age. Am J Surg Pathol 2011;35(11):1712–21.
60. Doyle LA, Nelson D, Heinrich MC, et al. Loss of succinate dehydrogenase subunit B (SDHB) expression is limited to a distinctive subset of gastric wild-type gastrointestinal stromal tumours: a comprehensive genotype-phenotype correlation study. Histopathology 2012;61(5):801–9
61. Janeway KA, Pappo A. Treatment guidelines for gastrointestinal stromal tumors in children and young adults. J Pediatr Hematol Oncol 2012; 34(Suppl 2):S69–72.
62. Nishida T, Hirota S, Taniguchi M, et al. Familial gastrointestinal stromal tumours with germline mutation of the KIT gene. Nat Genet 1998; 19(4):323–4.
63. Postow MA, Robson ME. Inherited gastrointestinal stromal tumor syndromes: mutations, clinical features, and therapeutic implications. Clin Sarcoma Res 2012;2(1):16.
64. de Raedt T, Cools J, Debiec-Rychter M, et al. Intestinal neurofibromatosis is a subtype of familial GIST and results from a dominant activating mutation in PDGFRA. Gastroenterology 2006;131(6):1907–12.
65. Andersson J, Sihto H, Meis-Kindblom JM, et al. NF1-associated gastrointestinal stromal tumors have unique clinical, phenotypic, and genotypic characteristics. Am J Surg Pathol 2005;29(9):1170–6.
66. Miettinen M, Fetsch JF, Sobin LH, et al. Gastrointestinal stromal tumors in patients with neurofibromatosis 1: a clinicopathologic and molecular genetic study of 45 cases. Am J Surg Pathol 2006;30(1):90–6.
67. Carney JA. The triad of gastric epithelioid leiomyosarcoma, functioning extra-adrenal paraganglioma, and pulmonary chondroma. Cancer 1979; 43(1):374–82.
68. Zhang L, Smyrk TC, Young Jr WF, et al. Gastric stromal tumors in Carney triad are different clinically, pathologically, and behaviorally from sporadic gastric gastrointestinal stromal tumors: findings in 104 cases. Am J Surg Pathol 2010;34(1):53–64.
69. Gaal J, Stratakis CA, Carney JA, et al. SDHB immunohistochemistry: a useful tool in the diagnosis of Carney-Stratakis and Carney triad gastrointestinal stromal tumors. Mod Pathol 2011;24(1):147–51.
70. Matyakhina L, Bei TA, McWhinney SR, et al. Genetics of Carney triad: recurrent losses at chromosome 1 but lack of germline mutations in genes associated with paragangliomas and gastrointestinal stromal tumors. J Clin Endocrinol Metab 2007;92(8):2938–43.
71. Joensuu H. Risk stratification of patients diagnosed with gastrointestinal stromal tumor. Hum Pathol 2008;39(10):1411–19.

72. Rutkowski P, Bylina E, Wozniak A, et al. Validation of the Joensuu risk criteria for primary resectable gastrointestinal stromal tumour - the impact of tumour rupture on patient outcomes. Eur J Surg Oncol 2011;37(10):890–6.
73. Wardelmann E, Losen I, Hans V, et al. Deletion of Trp-557 and Lys-558 in the juxtamembrane domain of the c-kit protooncogene is associated with metastatic behavior of gastrointestinal stromal tumors. Int J Cancer 2003;106(6):887–95.
74. Wardelmann E, Büttner R, Merkelbach-Bruse S, et al. Mutation analysis of gastrointestinal stromal tumors: increasing significance for risk assessment and effective targeted therapy. Virchows Arch 2007;451(4):743–9.
75. Martin J, Poveda A, Llombart-Bosch A, et al. Deletions affecting codons 557-558 of the c-KIT gene indicate a poor prognosis in patients with completely resected gastrointestinal stromal tumors: a study by the Spanish Group for Sarcoma Research (GEIS). J Clin Oncol 2005;23(25):6190–8.
76. Rubin BP, Blanke CD, Demetri GD, et al. Protocol for the examination of specimens from patients with gastrointestinal stromal tumor. Arch Pathol Lab Med 2010;134(2):165–70.
77. Joensuu H, Vehtari A, Riihimäki J, et al. Risk of recurrence of gastrointestinal stromal tumour after surgery: an analysis of pooled population-based cohorts. Lancet Oncol 2012;13(3):265–74.
78. Dematteo RP, Heinrich MC, El-Rifai WM, et al. Clinical management of gastrointestinal stromal tumors: before and after STI-571. Hum Pathol 2002;33(5):466–77.
79. Blanke CD, Rankin C, Demetri GD, et al. Phase III randomized, intergroup trial assessing imatinib mesylate at two dose levels in patients with unresectable or metastatic gastrointestinal stromal tumors expressing the kit receptor tyrosine kinase: S0033. J Clin Oncol 2008;26(4):626–32.
80. Debiec-Rychter M, Sciot R, Le Cesne A, et al. KIT mutations and dose selection for imatinib in patients with advanced gastrointestinal stromal tumours. Eur J Cancer 2006;42(8):1093–103.
81. Gramza AW, Corless CL, Heinrich MC. Resistance to tyrosine kinase inhibitors in gastrointestinal stromal tumors. Clin Cancer Res 2009;15(24):7510–18.
82. Heinrich MC, Corless CL, Blanke CD, et al. Molecular correlates of imatinib resistance in gastrointestinal stromal tumors. J Clin Oncol 2006;24(29):4764–74.
83. Demetri GD, van Oosterom AT, Garrett CR, et al. Efficacy and safety of sunitinib in patients with advanced gastrointestinal stromal tumour after failure of imatinib: a randomised controlled trial. Lancet 2006;368(9544):1329–38.
84. Heinrich MC, Maki RG, Corless CL, et al. Primary and secondary kinase genotypes correlate with the biological and clinical activity of sunitinib in imatinib-resistant gastrointestinal stromal tumor. J Clin Oncol 2008;26(33):5352–9.
85. George S, Wang Q, Heinrich MC, et al. Efficacy and safety of regorafenib in patients with metastatic and/or unresectable GI stromal tumor after failure of imatinib and sunitinib: a multicenter phase II trial. J Clin Oncol 2012;30(19):2401–7.
86. Dematteo RP, Ballman KV, Antonescu CR, et al. Adjuvant imatinib mesylate after resection of localised, primary gastrointestinal stromal tumour: a randomised, double-blind, placebo-controlled trial. Lancet 2009;373(9669):1097–104.
87. Joensuu H, Eriksson M, Sundby Hall K, et al. One vs three years of adjuvant imatinib for operable gastrointestinal stromal tumor: a randomized trial. JAMA 2012;307(12):1265–72.
88. Wang D, Zhang Q, Blanke CD, et al. Phase II trial of neoadjuvant/adjuvant imatinib mesylate for advanced primary and metastatic/recurrent operable gastrointestinal stromal tumors: long-term follow-up results of Radiation Therapy Oncology Group 0132. Ann Surg Oncol 2012;19(4):1074–80.
89. Abdulkader I, Cameselle-Teijeiro J, Forteza J. Pathological changes related to Imatinib treatment in a patient with a metastatic gastrointestinal stromal tumour. Histopathology 2005;46(4):470–2.
90. Liegl B, Hornick JL, Antonescu CR, et al. Rhabdomyosarcomatous differentiation in gastrointestinal stromal tumors after tyrosine kinase inhibitor therapy: a novel form of tumor progression. Am J Surg Pathol 2009;33(2):218–26.
91. Vassos N, Agaimy A, Schlabrakowski A, et al. An unusual and potentially misleading phenotypic change in a primary gastrointestinal stromal tumour (GIST) under imatinib mesylate therapy. Virchows Arch 2011;458(3):363–9.

Rhabdomyoma

CHAPTER CONTENTS

STRIATED MUSCLE TISSUE: DEVELOPMENT AND STRUCTURE

Skeletal muscle is formed primarily within myotomes, which are arranged in segmental pairs along the spine and make their first appearance in the cephalic region during the third week of intrauterine life. In the region of the anterior head and neck, skeletal muscle may also develop from mesenchyme derived from the neural crest (mesectoderm).

At the earliest stage of muscle development, primitive mesenchymal cells differentiate along two lines: (1) as fibroblasts, which are loosely arranged spindle-shaped cells with the capacity to form collagen; and (2) as myoblasts, which are round or oval cells with single, centrally positioned nuclei and granular eosinophilic cytoplasm. Over the next few weeks, the individual myoblasts assume a more elongated bipolar shape with slender, symmetrically arranged processes and nonstriated longitudinal myofibrils that are laid down first in the peripheral portion of the cytoplasm; this phase is followed by successive alignment and fusion of the individual myoblasts into myotubes with multiple centrally placed nuclei (myotubular stage). During the 7th to 10th weeks of intrauterine development, as differentiation progresses, the myofibrils become thicker and more numerous by longitudinal division, and they develop increasingly distinct cross-striations. Finally, during the 11th to 15th weeks, the nucleus is moved from its initial central position toward the periphery of the muscle fiber. Muscles derived from the cervical and thoracic myotomes mature earlier than those arising more distally.

Ultrastructurally, the individual myofibrils are composed of two types of myofilaments: thin (actin) filaments measuring 50 to 70 nm in diameter and thick (myosin) filaments measuring 140 to 160 nm in diameter. The thin filaments are laid down first in a random fashion and later rearranged and form parallel bundles together with thick filaments and polyribosomes. In cross-section, the thin filaments are seen to surround the thick filaments in distinct, evenly spaced hexagonal patterns.

Mature striated muscle consists of parallel arrays of closely packed myofibrils embedded within sarcoplasm and enveloped by a thin sarcolemmal sheath. Each of the myofibrils shows distinct cross-banding, light and dark bands caused by the periodic arrangement and interdigitation of the thin and thick myofilaments. In this arrangement, isotropic (I) bands, anisotropic (A) bands, and H bands can be distinguished. The I band consists solely of thin (actin) filaments and is divided at its center by the Z line or disk, which is thought to serve as an attachment site for the sarcomeres, the repeating individual units of the muscle fiber. The adjacent A band is a zone of overlapping thin and thick (actin and myosin) filaments; it is separated by the H band, which consists of thick myofilaments only. The width of the individual bands and sarcomeres varies and depends on the state of muscle contraction (Fig. 19-1).

CLASSIFICATION OF RHABDOMYOMAS

Although, as a general rule, benign soft tissue neoplasms outnumber malignant neoplasms by a sizable margin, this does not hold true for neoplasms showing skeletal muscle differentiation; rhabdomyomas are considerably less common than rhabdomyosarcomas and account for no more than 2% of all striated muscle tumors.

There are two broad categories of rhabdomyomas: cardiac and extracardiac. Among the extracardiac rhabdomyomas, three clinically and morphologically different subtypes can be distinguished: (1) the *adult type*, a slowly growing lesion that is nearly always found in the head and neck area of elderly persons; (2) the *fetal type*, a rare tumor that also principally affects the head and neck region and occurs in both children and adults; and (3) the *genital type*, a polypoid mass found almost exclusively in the vagina and vulva of middle-aged women. A related lesion is the *rhabdomyomatous mesenchymal hamartoma*, a peculiar striated muscle proliferation that occurs chiefly in the periorbital and perioral region of infants and young children (Table 19-1).

CARDIAC RHABDOMYOMA

Cardiac rhabdomyoma occurs almost exclusively in the hearts of infants and young children, often as multiple intramural lesions in the right and left ventricles, although the interventricular septum and atria may be involved as well.[1,2] It often occurs in the setting of tuberous sclerosis and in association with other congenital abnormalities. In the study by Yinon et al.,[3] 33 of 40 fetal cardiac tumors were cardiac rhabdomyomas, and, of these, 88% proved to have tuberous sclerosis. Patients with a cardiac rhabdomyoma and a family history of tuberous sclerosis and those with multifocal lesions are far more likely to have tuberous sclerosis.[4] In studies that have examined patients with tuberous sclerosis by repeated echocardiograms, 47% to 67% of patients harbor one or more cardiac rhabdomyomas.[5,6]

Clinically, the lesion may be asymptomatic or may cause cardiac arrhythmia, tachycardia, ventricular outflow obstruction, Wolff-Parkinson-White syndrome, or even sudden death.[7,8] DeRosa et al.[7] found that clinical outcome is influenced by complications of outflow tract obstruction more than by dysrhythmic complications. The concurrence of cardiac and extracardiac rhabdomyomas in the same patient has not been observed, although rare examples of adult rhabdomyoma may occur in the heart.[9] These lesions tend to be more cellular, composed of smaller cells, and have fewer spider cells.

Extracardiac rhabdomyoma does not appear to be associated with the tuberous sclerosis complex.

Histologically, the lesions are composed predominantly of large polygonal spider cells with large cytoplasmic vacuoles secondary to loss of glycogen during processing (Figs. 19-2 and 19-3). The cells stain for muscle markers, including muscle-specific actin and desmin. Some authors have also reported HMB-45 immunoreactivity, supporting a relation with angiomyolipoma and lymphangioleiomyomatosis as components of the tuberous sclerosis complex. It has also been noted that the neoplastic cells lose expression of tuberin (protein coded for by the *TSC2* gene on chromosome 16) and hamartin (protein coded for by the *TSC1* gene on chromosome 9).[10,11]

Treatment of this lesion is reserved for those with life-threatening obstructive symptoms or arrhythmias refractory to medical therapy because these lesions have a tendency to regress spontaneously over time.[12,13] Interestingly, a recent report found complete regression of a cardiac rhabdomyoma following treatment with the mTOR inhibitor everolimus,[14] an observation that is not completely surprising given the apparent role of mTOR pathway abnormalities in the pathogenesis of tuberous sclerosis-associated cardiac rhabdomyomas.[15]

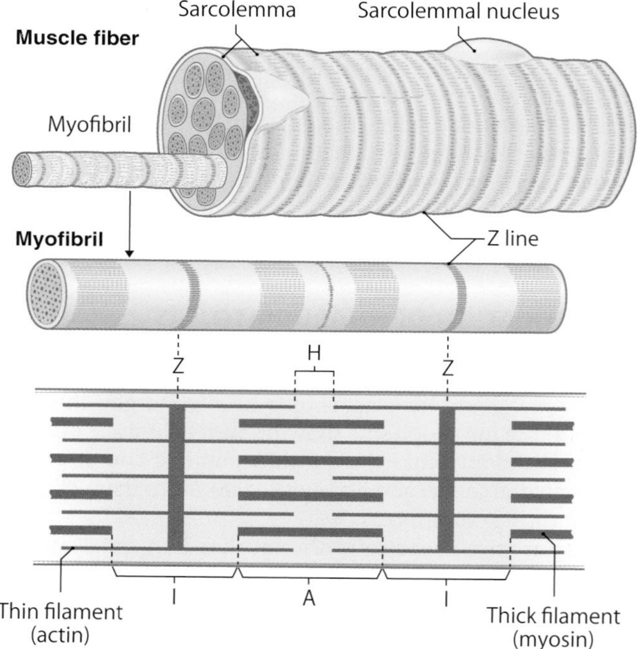

FIGURE 19-1. Muscle fiber, myofibril, and sliding actin and myosin filaments during the rest phase of muscle contraction.

ADULT RHABDOMYOMA

The adult type of rhabdomyoma is the most common subtype of extracardiac rhabdomyoma, but it is still quite rare. The

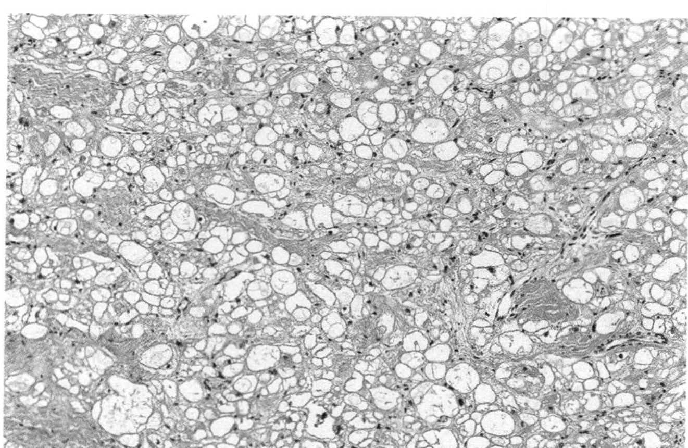

FIGURE 19-2. Cardiac rhabdomyoma. The lesion is composed predominantly of large polygonal spider cells with large cytoplasmic vacuoles.

TABLE 19-1 Clinical Features of Various Rhabdomyomas

PARAMETER	CARDIAC TYPE	ADULT TYPE	FETAL MYXOID TYPE	FETAL INTERMEDIATE TYPE	GENITAL TYPE	RMH
Peak age	Infants	>40 years	Infants	Children and adults	Young to middle-aged adults	Newborns
Gender (M/F)	1:1	3:1	3:1	3:1	Almost all female	Almost all male
Favored site(s)	Ventricles	Head and neck	Head and neck	Head and neck	Vagina, vulva	Chin
Associated conditions	Tuberous sclerosis	None	Nevoid BCC syndrome	Nevoid BCC syndrome	None	Congenital anomalies
Spontaneous regression	Yes	No	No	No	No	No

BCC, basal cell carcinoma; *RMH*, rhabdomyomatous mesenchymal hamartoma.

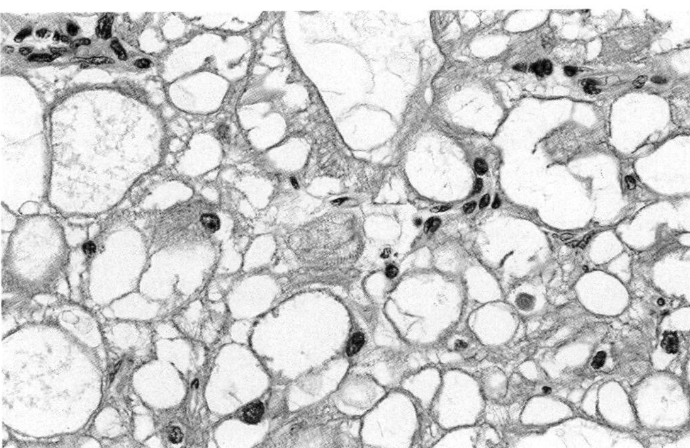

FIGURE 19-3. Cardiac rhabdomyoma with vacuolated spider cells. Cross-striations are rare but can be identified.

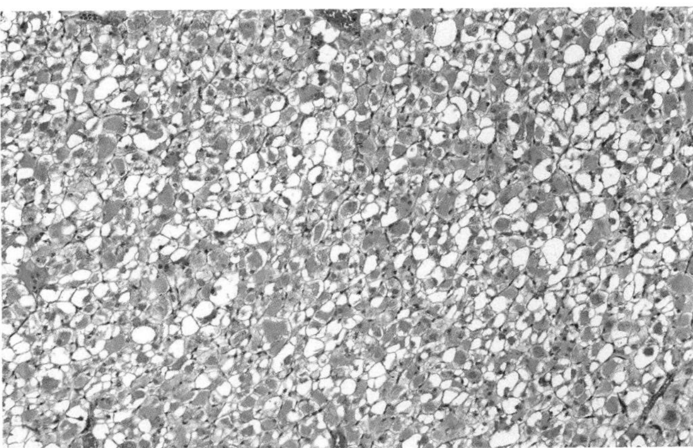

FIGURE 19-4. Low-power view of adult rhabdomyoma composed of an admixture of deeply eosinophilic polygonal cells and cells with vacuolated cytoplasm.

lesion usually presents as a solitary round or polypoid mass in the head and neck region of adults that causes neither tenderness nor pain; it may compress or displace the tongue or may protrude into and partially obstruct the pharynx or larynx. As a consequence, it may cause hoarseness or progressive difficulty with breathing or swallowing.[16] It is a slowly growing process, and several of the reported cases were present for many years before surgery. Most tumors occur in adults older than 40 years (median age 60 years); few cases arise in children.[17] Men are affected three to four times more commonly than women, but there is no predilection for any particular race. The principal site of involvement is the neck, where the tumor arises from the branchial musculature of the third and fourth branchial arches. It is found most frequently in the region of the pharynx, oral cavity, including the floor of the mouth or base of the tongue, and the larynx.[17,18] It may also involve the soft palate and the uvula, usually as an extension of a pharyngeal rhabdomyoma. Rare tumors have been described outside of the head and neck region in a myriad of locations.[19] Most adult rhabdomyomas are solitary, but about 20% are multifocal, mostly involving the general area of the neck.[20]

Pathologic Findings

As a rule, the tumor is well defined, rounded, or coarsely lobulated and ranges from 0.5 to 10.0 cm in greatest diameter (median 3.0 cm). Some are multinodular, and others form sessile or pedunculated polypoid submucosal masses. On cut section, it has a finely granular, gray-yellow to red-brown appearance.

Microscopically, this variant of rhabdomyoma is composed of tightly packed, large, round or polygonal cells 15 to 150 μm in diameter and separated from one another by thin, fibrous septa and narrow vascular channels. The cells have deeply acidophilic, finely granular cytoplasm, one or (rarely) two centrally or peripherally placed vesicular nuclei, and one or more prominent nucleoli (Figs. 19-4 and 19-5). Many of the cells are vacuolated because intracellular glycogen has been removed during processing; some of the vacuolated cells, in fact, contain merely a small central acidophilic cytoplasmic

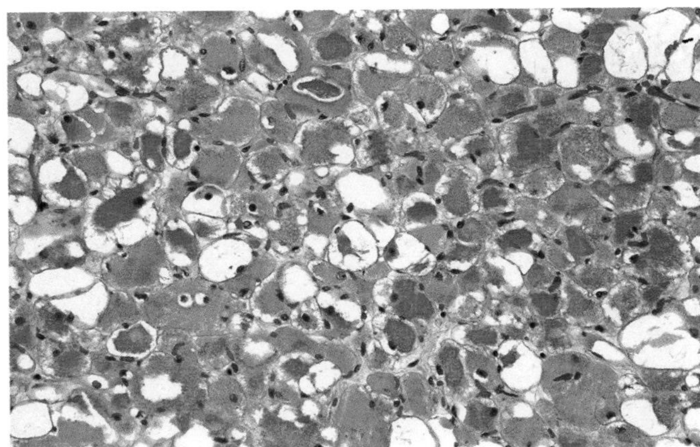

FIGURE 19-5. Adult rhabdomyoma composed of variously sized, deeply eosinophilic polygonal cells with small, peripherally placed nuclei and occasional intracellular vacuoles.

mass connected by thin strands of cytoplasm to a condensed rim of cytoplasm at the periphery (spider cells), but these cells are much more conspicuous in cardiac than in extracardiac rhabdomyomas. Mitotic figures are nearly always absent. Cross-striations can be discerned, in most cases, but sometimes they are detected only after a prolonged search; in many cases, additional features present are intracytoplasmic rod-like or jackstraw-like crystalline structures (Figs. 19-6 and 19-7). Both cross-striations and crystalline structures are identified much more readily with the phosphotungstic acid-hematoxylin (PTAH) stain than with hematoxylin-eosin.

Immunohistochemically, as one would expect, the cells stain strongly for desmin and muscle-specific actin (Fig. 19-8). By ultrastructure, the cytoplasm contains, in addition to a variable number of mitochondria with linear cristae and deposits of glycogen, thin and thick myofilaments showing a varying degree of differentiation and measuring 50 to 70 nm and 135 to 150 nm in diameter, respectively. Distinct Z lines are readily discernible within the I band, but sometimes A, H, M, and N bands are also apparent (Fig. 19-9). Crystalline intracytoplasmic inclusions may be seen and have been identified as hypertrophied Z bands.[21]

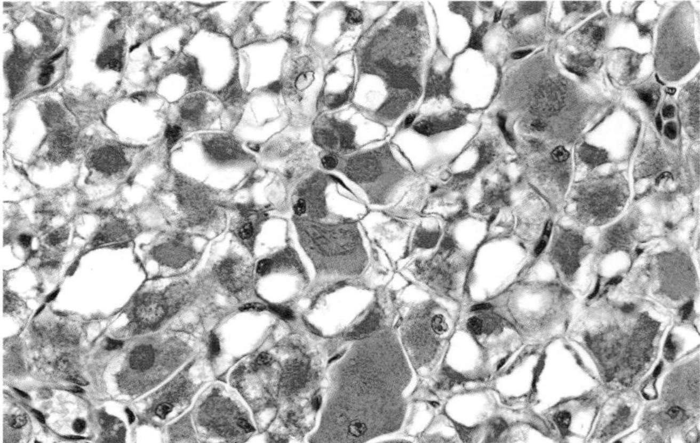

FIGURE 19-6. Adult rhabdomyoma with rare jackstraw-like crystalline structures within the cytoplasm of some of the eosinophilic polygonal cells.

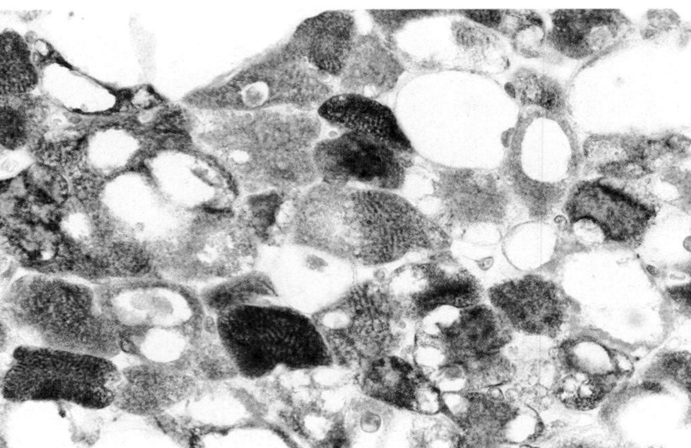

FIGURE 19-8. Adult rhabdomyoma showing immunoreactivity for desmin. Note accentuation of cross-striations.

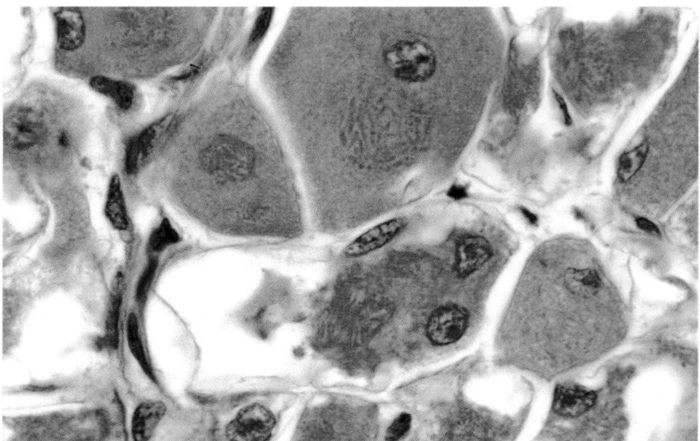

FIGURE 19-7. High-power view of adult rhabdomyoma with crystalline intracellular structures, probably representing Z-band material.

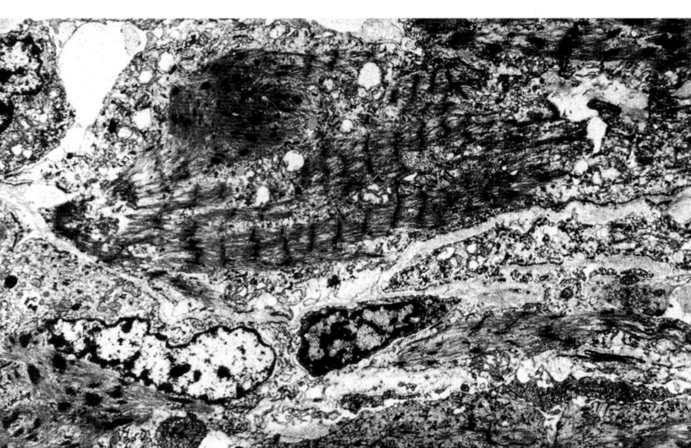

FIGURE 19-9. Electron micrograph of adult rhabdomyoma. Clearly discernible Z lines are present, along with bundles of actin and myosin filaments.

TABLE 19-2 Differential Diagnosis of Adult-Type Rhabdomyoma

PARAMETER	ADULT RHABDOMYOMA	GRANULAR CELL TUMOR	HIBERNOMA	PARAGANGLIOMA
Favored site	Head and neck	Skin, tongue	Interscapular	Extra-adrenal ganglia
Electron microscopy	Thin/thick filaments	Phagolysosomes	Mitochondria	Neurosecretory granules
S-100 protein	Rare, focal	Diffuse	Diffuse	Sustentacular cells
Muscle-specific actin	Diffuse	Negative	Negative	Negative
Chromogranin	Negative	Negative	Negative	Diffuse

Very few cytogenetic data are available pertaining to adult-type rhabdomyoma. Gibas and Miettinen,[22] in a cytogenetic study of a recurrent parapharyngeal rhabdomyoma in a 64-year-old man, found a reciprocal translocation of chromosomes 15 and 17 and abnormalities in the long arm of chromosome 10.

Differential Diagnosis

Despite its rarity, problems in diagnosis are unlikely for anyone familiar with the characteristic picture of the tumor (Table 19-2). *Granular cell tumor* can be confused with this lesion, but the cells tend to be less well defined and lack the characteristic vacuolation caused by intracellular glycogen; they are also devoid of cross-striations and usually are associated with more collagen. Moreover, the cells of granular cell tumors contain numerous periodic acid-Schiff (PAS)-positive, diastase-resistant granules that are related to the numerous intracytoplasmic phagolysosomes. Although S-100 protein is focally expressed in some cases of adult rhabdomyoma, its expression is more constant and diffuse in granular cell tumors.

Hibernoma also enters the differential diagnosis because of its frequent intracytoplasmic vacuoles and the presence of intracellular lipid. This tumor, however, is composed of small deeply eosinophilic granular cells that frequently contain distinct, variably sized lipid droplets in the cytoplasm. Clinically, hibernoma is most often found in the interscapular region of patients who are usually younger than 40 years of age. *Reticulohistiocytoma*, another lesion that must be included in the differential diagnosis, usually consists of an intimate mixture of deeply acidophilic histiocytes and fibroblasts intermingled with xanthoma cells, multinucleated giant cells, and chronic inflammatory elements. Typically, none of these cells contains glycogen, and the cells do not express myogenic antigens.

Crystal-storing histiocytosis associated with lymphoplasmacytic neoplasms may also simulate adult rhabdomyoma. In this lesion, however, the crystal-storing cells are histiocytes and stain positively for CD68 but are negative for skeletal muscle markers and S-100 protein.[23] Moreover, the associated lymphoplasmacytic infiltrate demonstrates monoclonality with immunostains for kappa and lambda chains (see Chapter 11).

Cardiac rhabdomyoma bears a close resemblance to adult rhabdomyoma, but its cells show a greater number of vacuolated spider cells and a more prominent population of giant cells. Cardiac rhabdomyoma is frequently encountered in association with tuberous sclerosis of the brain, sebaceous adenomas, and various other hamartomatous lesions of the kidney and other organs. Unlike adult rhabdomyoma, it has a propensity for spontaneous regression.

Rhabdomyosarcoma is composed of poorly differentiated and pleomorphic round or spindle-shaped cells associated with varying numbers of rhabdomyoblasts. Mitotic figures are common in rhabdomyosarcomas but are absent or rare in adult rhabdomyomas. *Oncocytoma* is an epithelial neoplasm of salivary gland origin composed of mitochondria-rich polyhedral cells with finely granular, eosinophilic cytoplasm. The cells stain for epithelial markers but do not express actin or desmin. *Paraganglioma* is a neuroendocrine neoplasm composed of cells arranged in an organoid pattern (Zellballen). As seen by immunohistochemistry, the cells express neuroendocrine markers, including neuron-specific enolase, synaptophysin, and chromogranin. S-100 protein outlines the sustentacular cells, and the cells lack myogenic antigens.

Prognosis and Therapy

The tumor is readily amenable to therapy but may recur locally if incompletely excised. In one series of 19 cases with follow-up information, the tumor recurred in 8 (42%) cases.[24] Examples of multiple and late recurrences have also been described.[24,25] Spontaneous regression, as is seen with some cardiac rhabdomyomas, has not been observed.

FETAL RHABDOMYOMA

Fetal rhabdomyoma is even rarer than adult-type rhabdomyoma, and only a small number of cases have been recorded in the medical literature. Awareness of the existence of this tumor, however, is of considerable importance because of its resemblance to embryonal rhabdomyosarcoma. The lesion has a variable histologic pattern, with a spectrum of skeletal muscle differentiation that ranges from immature, predominantly myxoid tumors, to those showing a high degree of cellular differentiation and hardly any myxoid matrix. The former have been described as *myxoid*[25] or *classic*[26] *fetal rhabdomyomas*; the latter are variously described as *intermediate*,[26] *cellular*,[25,27] or *juvenile*[28] *fetal rhabdomyomas*. Intermediate forms between these two types are not uncommon. There is also a third, still ill-defined morphologic variant of this tumor that is marked by prominent neural involvement showing some similarities to neuromuscular hamartoma.[29]

Clinical Features

The age incidence varies slightly according to the prevailing histologic type. Tumors of the *myxoid type* mainly affect boys during the first year of life (particularly in the postauricular region) or the vulvovaginal region of middle-aged women.[26,30] The *intermediate type* affects adults more often than children and occurs almost exclusively in the region of the head and neck, including the orbit, tongue, nasopharynx, and soft palate.[26] Rare cases of fetal rhabdomyoma have been described outside of the head and neck region, including the mediastinum, extremities, and skin.[31-33] For both types, males outnumber females by a ratio of approximately 3 to 1.

There are a number of reports in the literature of fetal rhabdomyoma associated with the nevoid basal cell carcinoma syndrome.[32,34,35] This syndrome is an autosomal dominant disorder characterized by multiple basal cell carcinomas that appear early during childhood, various skeletal abnormalities, and odontogenic keratocysts, among other findings. Mutations in the *PTCH* tumor suppressor gene have been implicated in the development of this syndrome.[36]

Pathologic Findings

On gross examination, the tumors are generally well circumscribed and most are between 2 and 6 cm in greatest diameter at the time of excision. Mucosal lesions tend to be smooth and polypoid or pedunculated. On sectioning, they are gray-white to pink, often with a mucoid, glistening surface. Unlike rhabdomyosarcoma, fetal rhabdomyoma is primarily a superficial tumor and is found more often in the subcutis or submucosa than in muscle. Most are solitary, but multicentric fetal rhabdomyomas have been reported in association with the nevoid basal cell carcinoma syndrome.[37]

Histologically, the *myxoid type* is chiefly composed of primitive oval or spindle-shaped cells with indistinct cytoplasm, interspersed immature skeletal muscle fibers reminiscent of fetal myotubes seen during the 7th to 10th weeks of intrauterine life, and a richly myxoid matrix (Figs. 19-10 and 19-11). The immature skeletal muscle cells have small uniform nuclei with delicate chromatin and inconspicuous nucleoli with bipolar or sometimes unipolar, finely tapered eosinophilic cytoplasmic processes. Cross-striations are rare and often difficult to discern; they are best seen with PTAH or Masson trichrome stains or with immunohistochemical stains for desmin or muscle-specific actin. The cells may be arranged in short bundles or isolated within the myxoid matrix. Sometimes, focal proliferation of abundant muscle fibers makes it difficult to draw a sharp line between tumor and normal muscle tissue. The primitive undifferentiated cells have oval nuclei with slight nuclear hyperchromasia and scanty, indistinct cytoplasm.

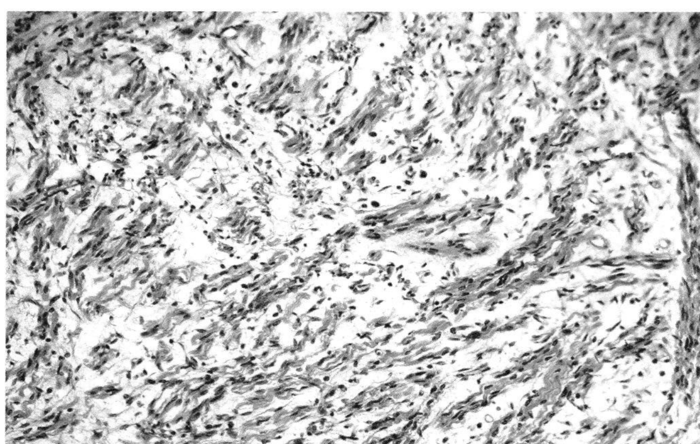

FIGURE 19-10. Fetal rhabdomyoma, myxoid type. The lesion is composed of an intimate mixture of primitive, round and spindle-shaped mesenchymal cells and differentiated myofibrils within a richly myxoid background.

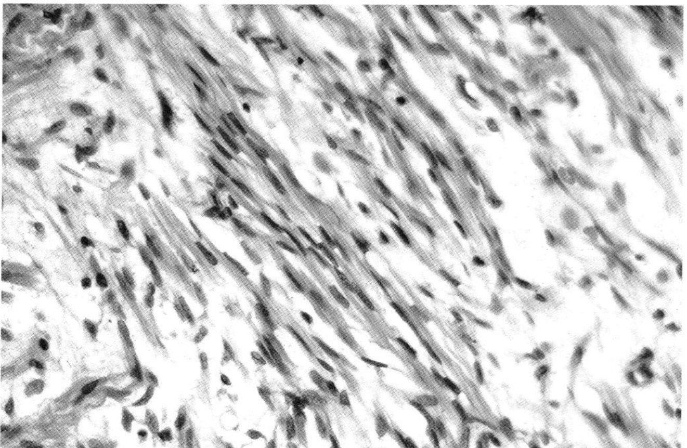

FIGURE 19-11. Fetal rhabdomyoma, myxoid type. Unlike embryonal rhabdomyosarcoma, the muscle cells vary little in size and shape, and there is no mitotic activity. The cells are deposited in an abundant myxoid matrix.

The *intermediate type* is characterized by the presence of numerous differentiated muscle fibers, less conspicuous or absent spindle-shaped mesenchymal cells, and little or no myxoid stroma (Fig. 19-12). In any given case, there may be a wide spectrum of skeletal muscle differentiation. The predominant cells are broad, strap-shaped muscle cells with abundant eosinophilic cytoplasm, centrally located vesicular nuclei, and frequent cross-striations reminiscent of the cells seen in adult rhabdomyomas; many of the cells contain glycogen and are often vacuolated. Others have prominent ganglion-like rhabdomyoblasts with large vesicular nuclei and prominent nucleoli. Mucosa-based lesions tend to have the widest spectrum of rhabdomyoblastic differentiation and the most mature-appearing cells. In some cases, there is mild cellular pleomorphism, but marked cellular atypia is not a feature of this tumor. Transitional forms between the myxoid and intermediate types do occur. In fact, age and duration may play a role in the maturation of some tumors, as suggested by the older mean age of patients with the intermediate (cellular) type and the reported long duration of some cases. In both types, mitotic figures are rare or absent. In addition to the myxoid and intermediate types, there are sporadic fetal rhabdomyoma-like tumors that are intimately associated with peripheral nerves reminiscent of neuromuscular choristoma (benign Triton tumor). By immunohistochemistry, similar to other rhabdomyoma subtypes, the muscle cells stain positively for desmin and muscle-specific actin. Ultrastructurally, the differentiated muscle cells consist of organized bundles of thick (myosin) and thin (actin) myofilaments with the characteristic banding in some of the more differentiated muscle cells.

Differential Diagnosis

Distinction from *embryonal* and *spindle cell rhabdomyosarcoma* is the principal issue (Table 19-3); unlike rhabdomyosarcoma, fetal rhabdomyoma tends to be fairly well circumscribed and is superficially located. Mitotic figures are rare, and the tumor lacks a significant degree of cellular pleomorphism and areas of necrosis; considerable cellularity, a mild degree of cellular pleomorphism, and occasional mitotic figures do not rule out this diagnosis.

Caution must also be exercised in the differential diagnosis because of the possible malignant transformation of fetal rhabdomyoma. One case was encountered in which the initial lesion, biopsied at 3 weeks of age, seemed to be characteristic of fetal rhabdomyoma, whereas the recurrent tumor, excised at 23 months, showed a much greater degree of cellularity and mitotic activity and was indistinguishable from embryonal rhabdomyosarcoma. Another possible case of cellular fetal rhabdomyoma with malignant transformation was reported by Kodet et al.[38] in the tongue of an 18-month-old infant. Of course, it is possible that these rare cases were actually examples of embryonal rhabdomyosarcoma all along.

Infantile fibromatosis may bear a close resemblance to fetal rhabdomyoma, especially if the tumor diffusely infiltrates muscle tissue and contains numerous residual muscle fibers that have been entrapped by the proliferating fibroblasts. Fetal rhabdomyoma, however, is better circumscribed than infantile fibromatosis, is situated in the subcutis rather than in muscle tissue, and lacks the fasciculated spindle cell pattern. In addition, interspersed fat cells, a frequent feature of diffuse infantile fibromatosis, are absent in fetal rhabdomyoma.

Prognosis and Therapy

Fetal rhabdomyoma, a benign lesion, is readily curable by local excision, with only rare reports of local recurrence.[26] It is a slowly growing process, and there are reports of lesions having been present for years with little change in size or histologic picture except for interstitial fibrosis. Whether it is a neoplasm or a hamartoma is unclear, but the ability to grow and recur strongly supports this being a benign neoplasm. There is no valid support for the contention that fetal rhabdomyoma is an early stage in the development of adult rhabdomyoma.

GENITAL RHABDOMYOMA

Although genital rhabdomyoma bears some resemblance to both adult and fetal rhabdomyomas, it has sufficiently

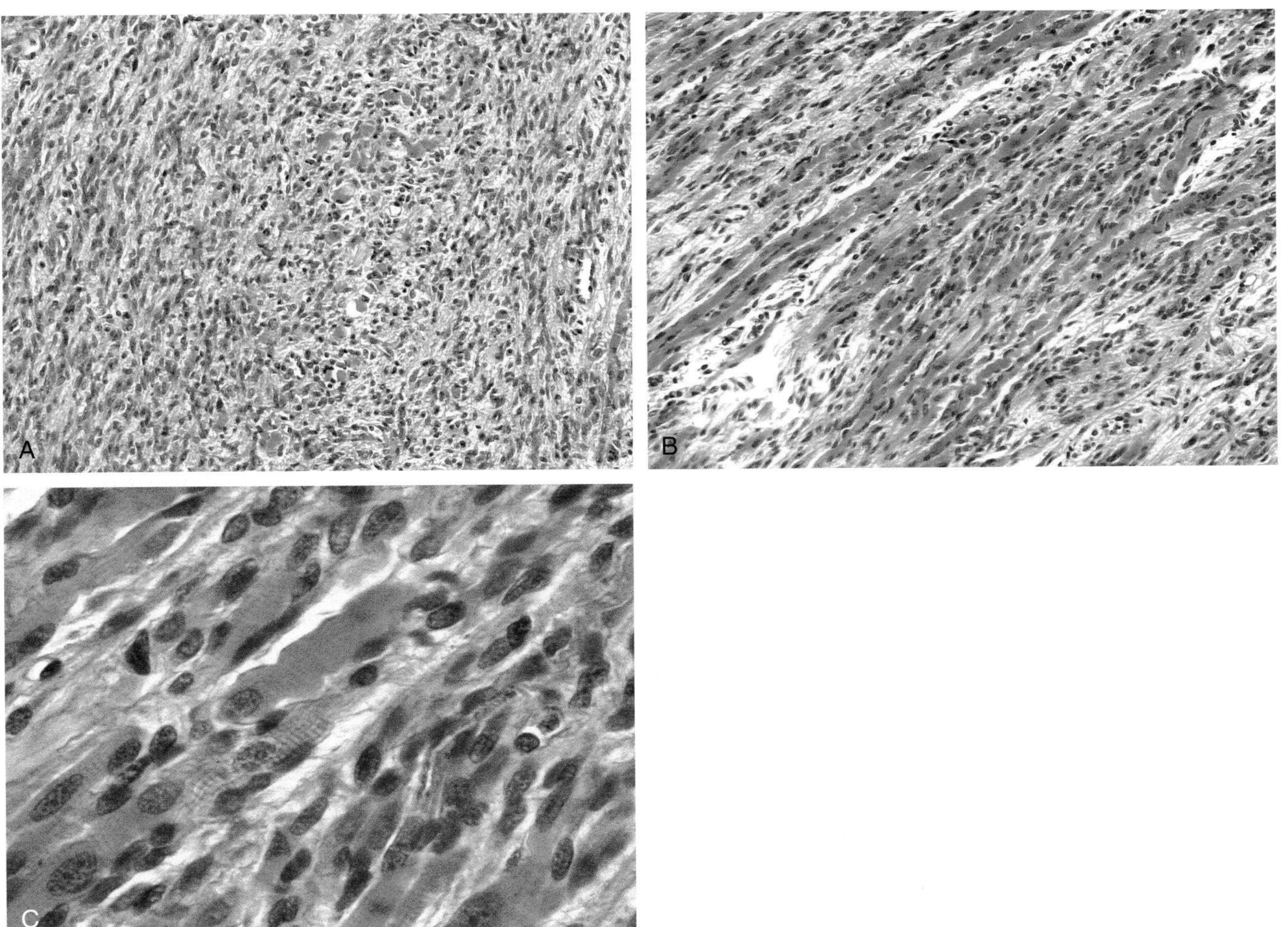

FIGURE 19-12. (A) Fetal rhabdomyoma, intermediate (cellular) type, consisting of intersecting bundles of differentiated eosinophilic myofibrils containing cross-striations. Myofibrils separated by small undifferentiated spindle cells. (B) Higher-magnification view of interspersed spindled cells with differentiated myofibrils. (C) High-magnification view of fetal rhabdomyoma, intermediate (cellular) type. *(Case courtesy of Dr. Cyril Fisher, Royal Marsden Hospital, London, England.)*

TABLE 19-3 Distinguishing Features of Fetal Rhabdomyoma and Embryonal Rhabdomyosarcoma

PARAMETER	FETAL RHABDOMYOMA	EMBRYONAL RHABDOMYOSARCOMA
Gross appearance	Well circumscribed	Infiltrative
Depth	Superficial	Deep
Mitotic figures	Absent or rare	Easily identified
Pleomorphism	Absent or slight	Moderate or marked
Necrosis	Absent	Often present

different clinical and microscopic characteristics to qualify as a separate entity. This is a very rare tumor, and only a small number of cases have been described, including some that were reported as fetal rhabdomyoma.[25] Almost all arise as a slowly growing polypoid mass or cyst in the vagina or vulva of young or middle-aged women,[39-41] although rare cases arise in the male genital region (epididymis).[42] Most are asymptomatic and are found on routine physical examination; some cause dyspareunia or vaginal bleeding secondary to mucosal erosion.

Microscopically, the tumor usually forms a polypoid or cauliflower-like mass covered by epithelium and rarely measures more than 3 cm in greatest diameter. It consists of scattered, more or less mature muscle fibers showing distinct cross-striations and a matrix containing varying amounts of collagen and mucoid material (Figs. 19-13 to 19-15). As with other rhabdomyomas, the cells are immunoreactive for desmin and muscle-specific actin. Electron microscopic examination of the lesion reveals a large nucleus with a prominent dense nucleolus and arrays of thick and thin myofilaments with Z lines and A and I bands.

The differential diagnosis includes benign *vaginal polyps* and *botryoid embryonal rhabdomyosarcoma (sarcoma botryoides)*. Benign vaginal polyps are characterized by atypical single or multinucleated stromal cells, but they lack classic strap cells with cross-striations. Botryoid embryonal rhabdomyosarcoma usually occurs in young children who present with a rapidly growing lesion that frequently ulcerates the overlying epithelium. In contrast, genital rhabdomyoma usually occurs in middle-aged women and is generally a

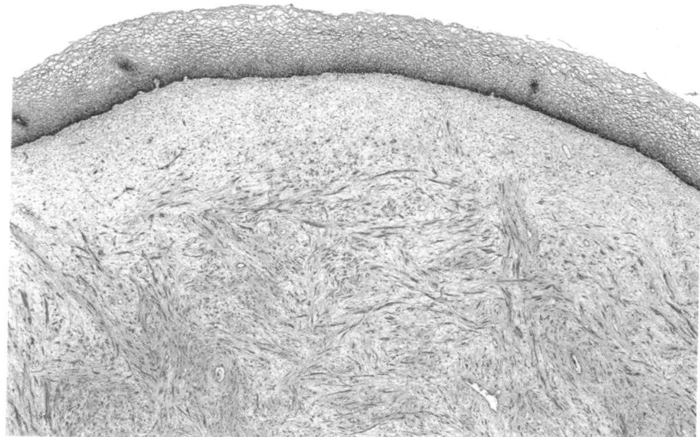

FIGURE 19-13. Genital (vaginal) rhabdomyoma. Submucosal proliferation of striated muscle cells separated by varying amounts of myxoid material and collagen.

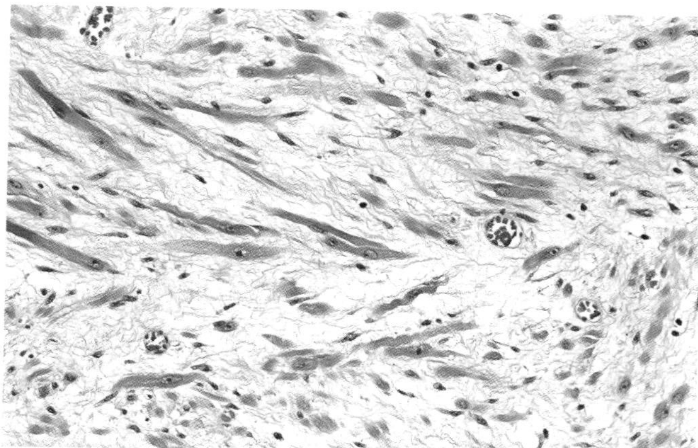

FIGURE 19-14. Genital rhabdomyoma composed of loosely arranged striated muscle cells and fibroblasts.

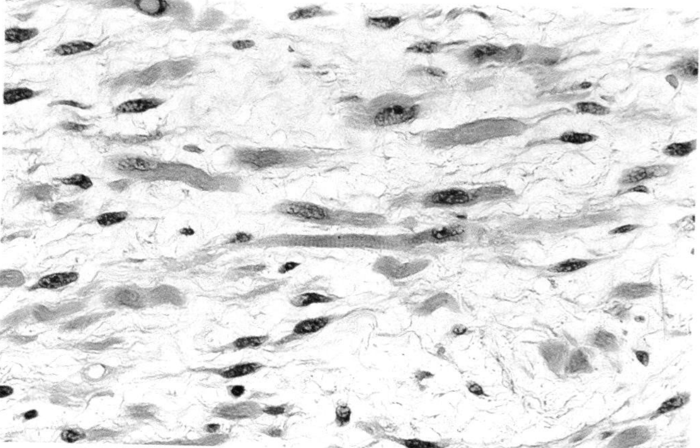

FIGURE 19-15. High-power view of genital rhabdomyoma showing rare striated muscle cells with cross-striations.

slowly growing tumor associated with an intact overlying epithelium. The subepithelial cambium layer characteristic of botryoid embryonal rhabdomyosarcoma is not found in genital rhabdomyomas. In addition, nuclear pleomorphism and mitotic figures are far more prominent in rhabdomyosarcomas than in rhabdomyomas (Table 19-4). The lesion, which pursues a benign course, is adequately treated by local excision.

TABLE 19-4 Distinguishing Features of Genital Rhabdomyoma and Botryoid Rhabdomyosarcoma

PARAMETER	GENITAL RHABDOMYOMA	BOTRYOID RHABDOMYOSARCOMA
Peak age	Young to middle-aged adults	Birth to 15 years
Gender (M/F)	Almost all females	1:1
Growth	Slowly growing	Rapidly growing
Epithelial ulceration	Absent	Often present
Cambium layer	Absent	Present
Mitotic figures	Absent or rare	Easily identified
Pleomorphism	Absent or slight	Moderate or marked

RHABDOMYOMATOUS MESENCHYMAL HAMARTOMA OF THE SKIN

Originally described in 1986 by Hendrick et al.[43] as *striated muscle hamartoma*, rhabdomyomatous mesenchymal hamartoma of skin, which occurs principally in the face and neck of newborns, is extremely rare. The lesion typically presents as a small dome-shaped papule or a polypoid pedunculated lesion in newborns. There are case reports of this lesion in adults, although it is not clear whether these lesions were present since childhood.[44] The lesions range in size from a few millimeters to 1 to 2 cm. The most common location appears to be the chin, followed by the periorbital, periauricular, and anterior mid-neck region.[45] Almost all lesions occur in males. Virtually all are solitary; Sahn et al.[46] described multiple pedunculated lesions arising in the periorbital and periauricular region in a newborn boy. Some patients have associated congenital anomalies.[47] For example, Takeyama et al.[48] described a case of rhabdomyomatous mesenchymal hamartoma associated with a nasofrontal meningocele and a dermoid cyst. One of the patients in the original report by Hendrick et al. had a cleft lip and cleft gum as well as circumferential amniotic bands around the head and distal left leg.[43]

Grossly, most lesions are polypoid and attached to the skin by a long stalk, with circumferential constriction of the distal attachment site. Other lesions are more globular in shape, occasionally with central umbilication. Histologically, single or small groups of mature-appearing skeletal muscle fibers are found within the subcutaneous tissue and dermis. The fibers frequently are deposited in a collagenous stroma admixed with mature adipose tissue and adnexal structures, often aligned perpendicular to the surface epithelium.[49] Blood vessels and nerves may also be found admixed among the mature skeletal muscle fibers. Rare cases show central calcification or ossification.

The differential diagnosis includes *nevus lipomatosis superficialis*, which shows mature adipose tissue within the dermis but lacks skeletal muscle elements. Similarly, *fibrous hamartoma of infancy* contains an admixture of mature adipose tissue, collagenous bundles, and more cellular areas deposited in a myxoid stroma but lacks the skeletal muscle fibers. *Neuromuscular choristoma (benign Triton tumor)*, a rare subcutaneous lesion found in association with peripheral nerves, is composed of mature skeletal muscle fibers and neural tissue. Finally, rhabdomyomatous mesenchymal hamartoma must be distinguished from the rare and much less differentiated *cutaneous embryonal rhabdomyosarcoma.*[50]

This congenital hamartomatous lesion is adequately treated by local excision, and recurrences have not been described. The identification of these lesions in female patients suggests that this entity is not an X-linked disorder, as previously suggested.[51]

MISCELLANEOUS LESIONS MIMICKING BENIGN STRIATED MUSCLE TUMORS

Various benign lesions of striated muscle may be confused with rhabdomyoma. Supernumerary muscles in the popliteal fossa and ankle region of young adults presenting as a tumor-like mass have been described.[52] Similar accessory muscles may occur in the hand, fingers, and other portions of the body. Likewise, unilateral or bilateral hypertrophy of the masseter muscle may be mistaken for a muscle tumor.[53] This condition occurs chiefly in young adults and is often accompanied by bony overgrowth or a spur at the angle of the mandible. Benign skeletal muscle differentiation is a rare phenomenon in uterine leiomyomas as well.[54]

References

1. Burke AP, Virmani R. Cardiac rhabdomyoma: a clinicopathologic study. Mod Pathol 1991;4(1):70–4.
2. Burke A, Virmani R. Pediatric heart tumors. Cardiovasc Pathol 2008;17(4):193–8.
3. Yinon Y, Chitayat D, Blaser S, et al. Fetal cardiac tumors: a single-center experience of 40 cases. Prenat Diagn 2010;30(10):941–9.
4. Gamzu R, Achiron R, Hegesh J, et al. Evaluating the risk of tuberous sclerosis in cases with prenatal diagnosis of cardiac rhabdomyoma. Prenat Diagn 2002;22(11):1044–7.
5. Harding CO, Pagon RA. Incidence of tuberous sclerosis in patients with cardiac rhabdomyoma. Am J Med Genet 1990;37(4):443–6.
6. Nir A, Tajik AJ, Freeman WK, et al. Tuberous sclerosis and cardiac rhabdomyoma. Am J Cardiol 1995;76(5):419–21.
7. De Rosa G, De Carolis MP, Pardeo M, et al. Neonatal emergencies associated with cardiac rhabdomyomas: an 8-year experience. Fetal Diagn Ther 2011;29(2):169–77.
8. Gupta A, Narula N, Mahajan R, et al. Sudden death of a young child due to cardiac rhabdomyoma. Pediatr Cardiol 2010;31(6):894–6.
9. Burke AP, Gatto-Weis C, Griego JE, et al. Adult cellular rhabdomyoma of the heart: a report of 3 cases. Hum Pathol 2002;33(11):1092–7.
10. Madueme P, Hinton R. Tuberous sclerosis and cardiac rhabdomyomas: a case report and review of the literature. Congenit Heart Dis 2011;6(2):183–7.
11. Vinaitheerthan M, Wei J, Mizuguchi M, et al. Tuberous sclerosis: immunohistochemistry expression of tuberin and hamartin in a 31-week gestational fetus. Fetal Pediatr Pathol 2004;23(4):241–9.
12. Fesslova V, Villa L, Rizzuti T, et al. Natural history and long-term outcome of cardiac rhabdomyomas detected prenatally. Prenat Diagn 2004;24(4):241–8.
13. Padalino MA, Vida VL, Boccuzzo G, et al. Surgery for primary cardiac tumors in children: early and late results in a multi-center European Congenital Heart Surgeons Association (ECHSA) Study. Circulation 2012;126(1):22–30.
14. Tiberio D, Franz DN, Phillips JR. Regression of a cardiac rhabdomyoma in a patient receiving everolimus. Pediatrics 2011;127(5):e1335–7.
15. Kotulska K, Larysz-Brysz M, Grajkowska W, et al. Cardiac rhabdomyomas in tuberous sclerosis complex show apoptosis regulation and mTOR pathway abnormalities. Pediatr Dev Pathol 2009;12(2):89–95.
16. Pichi B, Manciocco V, Marchesi P, et al. Rhabdomyoma of the parapharyngeal space presenting with dysphagia. Dysphagia 2008;23(2):202–4.
17. Solomon MP, Tolete-Velcek F. Lingual rhabdomyoma (adult variant) in a child. J Pediatr Surg 1979;14(1):91–4.
18. Zhang GZ, Zhang GQ, Xiu JM, et al. Intraoral multifocal and multinodular adult rhabdomyoma: report of a case. J Oral Maxillofac Surg 2012;70(10):2480–5.
19. Kuschill-Dziurda J, Mastalerz L, Grzanka P, et al. Rhabdomyoma as a tumor of the posterior mediastinum. Pol Arch Med Wewn 2009;119(9):599–602.
20. Koutsimpelas D, Weber A, Lippert BM, et al. Multifocal adult rhabdomyoma of the head and neck: a case report and literature review. Auris Nasus Larynx 2008;35(2):313–17.
21. Cornog Jr JL, Gonatas NK. Ultrastructure of rhabdomyoma. J Ultrastruct Res 1967;20(5):433–50.
22. Gibas Z, Miettinen M. Recurrent parapharyngeal rhabdomyoma. Evidence of neoplastic nature of the tumor from cytogenetic study. Am J Surg Pathol 1992;16(7):721–8.
23. Kapadia SB, Enzinger FM, Heffner DK, et al. Crystal-storing histiocytosis associated with lymphoplasmacytic neoplasms. Report of three cases mimicking adult rhabdomyoma. Am J Surg Pathol 1993;17(5):461–7.
24. Kapadia SB, Meis JM, Frisman DM, et al. Adult rhabdomyoma of the head and neck: a clinicopathologic and immunophenotypic study. Hum Pathol 1993;24(6):608–17.
25. Di Sant'Agnese PA, Knowles 2nd DM. Extracardiac rhabdomyoma: a clinicopathologic study and review of the literature. Cancer 1980;46(4):780–9.
26. Kapadia SB, Meis JM, Frisman DM, et al. Fetal rhabdomyoma of the head and neck: a clinicopathologic and immunophenotypic study of 24 cases. Hum Pathol 1993;24(7):754–65.
27. Elawabdeh N, Sobol S, Blount AC, et al. Unusual presentation of extracardiac fetal rhabdomyoma of the larynx in a pediatric patient with tuberous sclerosis. Fetal Pediatr Pathol 2013;31(1):43–7.
28. Crotty PL, Nakhleh RE, Dehner LP. Juvenilerhabdomyoma. An intermediate form of skeletal muscle tumor in children. Arch Pathol Lab Med 1993;117(1):43–7.
29. Vandewalle G, Brucher JM, Michotte A. Intracranial facial nerve rhabdomyoma. Case report. J Neurosurg 1995;83(5):919–22.
30. Dehner LP, Enzinger FM, Font RL. Fetal rhabdomyoma. An analysis of nine cases. Cancer 1972;30(1):160–6.
31. Premalata CS, Kumar RV, Saleem KM, et al. Fetal rhabdomyoma of the lower extremity. Pediatr Blood Cancer 2009;52(7):881–3.
32. Yang S, Zhao C, Zhang Y, et al. Mediastinal fetal rhabdomyoma in nevoid basal cell carcinoma syndrome: a case report and review of the literature. Virchows Arch 2011;459(2):235–8.
33. Walsh SN, Hurt MA. Cutaneous fetal rhabdomyoma: a case report and historical review of the literature. Am J Surg Pathol 2008;32(3):485–91.
34. DiSanto S, Abt AB, Boal DK, et al. Fetal rhabdomyoma and nevoid basal cell carcinoma syndrome. Pediatr Pathol 1992;12(3):441–7.
35. Watson J, Depasquale K, Ghaderi M, et al. Nevoid basal cell carcinoma syndrome and fetal rhabdomyoma: a case study. Ear Nose Throat J 2004;83(10):716–18.
36. Bree AF, Shah MR. Consensus statement from the first international colloquium on basal cell nevus syndrome (BCNS). Am J Med Genet A 2011;155A(9):2091–7.
37. Klijanienko J, Caillaud JM, Micheau C, et al. [Basal-cell nevomatosis associated with multifocal fetal rhabdomyoma. A case]. Presse Med 1988;17(42):2247–50.
38. Kodet R, Fajstavr J, Kabelka Z, et al. Is fetal cellular rhabdomyoma an entity or a differentiated rhabdomyosarcoma? A study of patients with rhabdomyoma of the tongue and sarcoma of the tongue enrolled in the intergroup rhabdomyosarcoma studies I, II, and III. Cancer 1991;67(11):2907–13.
39. López Varela C, López de la Riva M, La Cruz Pelea C. Vaginal rhabdomyomas. Int J Gynaecol Obstet 1994;47(2):169–70.
40. Willis J, Abdul-Karim FW, di Sant'Agnese PA. Extracardiac rhabdomyomas. Semin Diagn Pathol 1994;11(1):15–25.
41. Patrelli TS, Franchi L, Gizzo S, et al. [Rhabdomyoma of the vagina. Case report and short literature review]. Ann Pathol 2012;32(1):53–7.
42. Han Y, Qiu XS, Li QC, et al. Epididymis rhabdomyoma: a case report and literature review. Diagn Pathol 2012;7(1):47.
43. Hendrick SJ, Sanchez RL, Blackwell SJ, et al. Striated muscle hamartoma: description of two cases. Pediatr Dermatol 1986;3(2):153–7.
44. Brinster NK, Farmer ER. Rhabdomyomatous mesenchymal hamartoma presenting on a digit. J Cutan Pathol 2009;36(1):61–3.
45. Kim HS, Kim YJ, Kim JW, et al. Rhabdomyomatous mesenchymal hamartoma. J Eur Acad Dermatol Venereol 2007;21(4):564–5.
46. Sahn EE, Garen PD, Pai GS, et al. Multiple rhabdomyomatous mesenchymal hamartomas of skin. Am J Dermatopathol 1990;12(5):485–91.

47. Read RW, Burnstine M, Rowland JM, et al. Rhabdomyomatous mesenchymal hamartoma of the eyelid: report of a case and literature review. Ophthalmology 2001;108(4):798–804.
48. Takeyama J, Hayashi T, Sanada T, et al. Rhabdomyomatous mesenchymal hamartoma associated with nasofrontal meningocele and dermoid cyst. J Cutan Pathol 2005;32(4):310–13.
49. Williams NP, Shue AC. Rhabdomyomatous mesenchymal hamartoma: clinical overview and report of a case with spontaneous regression. West Indian Med J 2009;58(6):607–9.
50. Tari AS, Amoli FA, Rajabi MT, et al. Cutaneous embryonal rhabdomyosarcoma presenting as a nodule on cheek; a case report and review of literature. Orbit 2006;25(3):235–8.
51. Mills AE. Rhabdomyomatous mesenchymal hamartoma of skin. Am J Dermatopathol 1989;11(1):58–63.
52. Martinoli C, Perez MM, Padua L, et al. Muscle variants of the upper and lower limb (with anatomical correlation). Semin Musculoskelet Radiol 2010;14(2):106–21.
53. Eley KA, Shah KA, Watt-Smith SR. A slowly enlarging cheek mass. Oral Surg Oral Med Oral Pathol Oral Radiol Endod 2011;111(3):269–74.
54. Parker RL, Young RH, Clement PB. Skeletal muscle-like and rhabdoid cells in uterine leiomyomas. Int J Gynecol Pathol 2005;24(4):319–25.

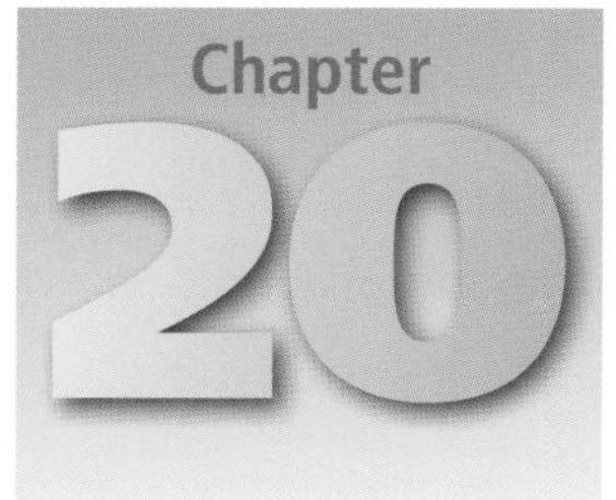

Rhabdomyosarcoma

CHAPTER CONTENTS

The concept of what constitutes rhabdomyosarcoma has changed over the years. During the 1930s and 1940s, the diagnosis of adult or pleomorphic rhabdomyosarcoma gained in popularity, and most of the rhabdomyosarcomas reported during this period were of this type.[1,2] These tumors occurred mainly in the muscles of the lower extremity and affected older patients. They displayed a striking degree of cellular pleomorphism, but cells with cross-striations were absent, in most instances. It became apparent that these tumors were other types of pleomorphic sarcoma. With the redefinition and acceptance of term *malignant fibrous histiocytoma*, most lesions that had formerly been labeled *pleomorphic rhabdomyosarcoma* were placed in the category of *malignant fibrous histiocytoma*, so that the very existence of pleomorphic rhabdomyosarcoma was questioned.

It also became gradually evident that many childhood sarcomas formerly diagnosed merely as round cell or spindle cell sarcomas were rhabdomyosarcomas of alveolar or embryonal type. Knowledge of these tumors was fostered by the introduction of newer, more effective modes of therapy. Before 1960, childhood rhabdomyosarcoma was known as an almost uniformly fatal neoplasm that recurred and metastasized in a high percentage of cases. During the last five decades, however, it has been shown that this tumor responds well to multimodality therapy—encompassing biopsy or conservative surgery, multiagent chemotherapy, and radiotherapy—and that many children treated by these modalities remain free of recurrent and metastatic disease. The numerous reports of the Intergroup Rhabdomyosarcoma Studies (IRS) (now recognized as the Soft Tissue Sarcoma Committee of the Children's Oncology Group) have greatly contributed to an understanding of childhood rhabdomyosarcomas and especially the effect of the various treatment modalities on the survival of patients with this tumor.[3-8]

As with other sarcomas, there is little to suggest that rhabdomyosarcoma arises from skeletal muscle cells. These tumors often arise at sites in which striated muscle tissue is normally absent (e.g., common bile duct, urinary bladder) or in areas in which striated muscle is scant (e.g., nasal cavity, middle ear, vagina).

Little is known about the underlying cause of the rhabdomyoblastic proliferations and the stimulus that induces their growth. Genetic factors are implicated by the rare occurrence of the disease in siblings,[9] the occasional presence of the tumor at birth,[10] and the association of the disease with other neoplasms in the same patient. Rhabdomyosarcoma has been described in conjunction with congenital retinoblastoma,[11] familial adenomatous polyposis,[12] multiple lentigines syndrome,[13] type 1 neurofibromatosis,[14] Costello syndrome,[15] Beckwith-Wiedemann syndrome,[16] and a variety of congenital anomalies.[17] There appears to be an increased risk of a familial cancer syndrome when embryonal rhabdomyosarcoma (or other soft tissue sarcoma) is diagnosed during the first 2 years of life, especially in a male child.[18] Savasan et al.[19] reported two children with alveolar rhabdomyosarcoma with constitutional balanced translocations and with peripheral blood lymphocytes harboring the same cytogenetic abnormality as that of the tumor cells. A recent report from the Children's Oncology Group found an association between first trimester x-ray exposure and embryonal rhabdomyosarcoma.[20]

INCIDENCE OF RHABDOMYOSARCOMA

Rhabdomyosarcoma is not only the most common soft tissue sarcoma in children under 15 years of age but also one of the most common soft tissue sarcomas of adolescents and young adults. It is estimated that rhabdomyosarcoma accounts for about 3% to 4% of all childhood cancers with an annual incidence of 4.5 cases per million per year.[18] It is rare in persons older than 45 years, and it has been estimated to account for between 2% and 5% of all adult sarcomas.[21]

HISTOLOGIC CLASSIFICATION OF RHABDOMYOSARCOMA

Arthur Purdy Stout[2] was the first to delineate rhabdomyosarcoma as a distinct entity, and Horn and Enterline[22] devised the first classification scheme in 1958, based on the clinical and

BOX 20-1 Modified Conventional (Horn and Enterline[22]) Classification Used by Intergroup Rhabdomyosarcoma Studies I and II

Embryonal
Botryoid
Alveolar
Pleomorphic
Sarcoma, not classified
Small round cell sarcoma, type indeterminate
Extraosseous Ewing sarcoma

BOX 20-2 International Society for Pediatric Oncology Classification for Rhabdomyosarcoma

- Embryonal sarcoma
- Embryonal rhabdomyosarcoma
  - Loose
    - Botryoid
    - Nonbotryoid
  - Dense
    - Well differentiated
    - Poorly differentiated
- Alveolar rhabdomyosarcoma
- Adult (pleomorphic) rhabdomyosarcoma
- Other specified soft tissue tumors
- Sarcoma, not otherwise specified

pathologic features of these tumors. This scheme, also known as the *conventional scheme*, recognized embryonal, botryoid, alveolar, and pleomorphic subtypes. Most patients in that series died of rhabdomyosarcoma, and the authors were unable to identify any prognostic differences among the four histologic subtypes. This scheme was adopted by the World Health Organization (also recognized as WHO) Classification of Soft Tissue Tumors and served as the basis for the numerous IRS studies to follow, with minor modifications (Box 20-1).[23]

Subsequently, Palmer et al.[24,25] devised a new classification scheme, based on tumor cytology rather than tumor architecture. This scheme, known as the *cytohistologic scheme*, identified two major unfavorable histologic subtypes: the monomorphous round cell type and the anaplastic type. This was the only classification that was not based on the Horn and Enterline scheme; rather, it was devised solely on nuclear morphology.

In 1989, the International Society of Pediatric Oncology (SIOP), including collaborators from 30 European countries, developed a classification scheme that emphasized the relation between clinical behavior and cellular differentiation in rhabdomyosarcoma subtypes with and without alveolar morphology (Box 20-2).[26] Based on a review of 513 rhabdomyosarcomas from the SIOP tumor registry, collaborators found that an alveolar architecture was not independently prognostically significant. Loose botryoid and dense well-differentiated rhabdomyosarcomas had a better prognosis

BOX 20-3 National Cancer Institute Classification of Rhabdomyosarcoma

- Embryonal rhabdomyosarcoma (favorable)
  - Conventional
  - Pleomorphic
  - Leiomyomatous
  - Aggressive histologic features
- Alveolar rhabdomyosarcoma (unfavorable)
  - Conventional
  - Solid alveolar
- Pleomorphic rhabdomyosarcoma
- Rhabdomyosarcoma (other)

than loose non-botryoid and dense poorly differentiated and alveolar rhabdomyosarcomas. This group also delineated embryonal sarcoma as a spindle cell tumor composed of peripheral mesenchymal cells with no evidence of myoblastic differentiation.

In 1992, collaborators at the Pediatric Branch of the National Cancer Institute (NCI) developed a modification of the conventional scheme, based on their review of 159 rhabdomyosarcomas (Box 20-3).[27] This scheme recognized the favorable prognosis of conventional embryonal rhabdomyosarcoma and three subtypes (pleomorphic, leiomyomatous, and those with aggressive histologic features) and the unfavorable prognosis of alveolar rhabdomyosarcoma. Most important, it also delineated the solid alveolar rhabdomyosarcoma, composed of round tumor cells identical to those in conventional alveolar rhabdomyosarcoma but lacking the characteristic alveolar architecture. These authors found that tumors with any degree of alveolar architecture or cytology had an unfavorable prognosis, regardless of extent.

From 1987 to 1991, the IRS committee conducted a comparative study of the various rhabdomyosarcoma classification systems to determine the reproducibility and prognostic significance of each of these systems.[28] Eight hundred representative rhabdomyosarcomas were reviewed by 16 pathologists and classified, using the conventional, SIOP, NCI, and cytohistologic classification systems; survival rates for all subtypes were compared. The highest degree of interobserver and intraobserver reproducibility was achieved using a modification of the conventional system, with fair-to-good observer agreement (Table 20-1). In addition, the histologic subtypes of the modified conventional system demonstrated a highly significant relation to survival. Based on the reproducibility and prognostic significance of this system, this group proposed a classification scheme, known as the International Classification of Rhabdomyosarcoma (ICR), which essentially was a modification of the conventional scheme with elements of the SIOP and NCI systems (Box 20-4).[29] The botryoid and spindle cell variants of embryonal rhabdomyosarcoma were found to have a superior prognosis, conventional embryonal rhabdomyosarcoma had an intermediate prognosis, and alveolar rhabdomyosarcoma and undifferentiated sarcoma had a poor prognosis. In addition, this classification scheme included those rhabdomyosarcoma subtypes in which the prognosis was yet to be determined (rhabdomyosarcoma with rhabdoid

TABLE 20-1 Interobserver and Intraobserver Variation in the Diagnosis of Rhabdomyosarcoma Subtypes

SYSTEM	INTEROBSERVER AVERAGE KAPPA (K)	INTRAOBSERVER AVERAGE KAPPA (K)
Modified conventional	0.451	0.605
SIOP	0.406	0.573
NCI	0.384	0.579
Cytohistologic	0.328	0.508
ICR	0.525	0.625

ICR, International Classification of Rhabdomyosarcoma; NCI, National Cancer Institute; SIOP, International Society for Pediatric Oncology.

Modified from Asmar L, Gehan EM, Newton WA Jr, et al. Agreement among and within groups of pathologists in the classification of rhabdomyosarcoma and related childhood sarcomas: report of an international study of four pathology classifications. Cancer 1994;74:2579.

TABLE 20-2 Anatomic Distribution of Rhabdomyosarcoma from Intergroup Rhabdomyosarcoma Group Studies (IRS-I, IRS-II, IRS-III), 1972-1991

ANATOMIC LOCATION	NO.	PERCENTAGE (%)
Head and neck	970	35
Parameningeal	437	16
Miscellaneous sites	276	10
Orbit	257	9
Genitourinary	650	24
Extremities	511	19
Other sites	616	22
Total	2747	100

Modified from Pappo AS, Shapiro DN, Crist WM, et al. Biology and therapy of pediatric rhabdomyosarcoma. J Clin Oncol 1995;13:2123.

BOX 20-4 International Classification of Rhabdomyosarcoma

- Superior prognosis
  - Botryoid rhabdomyosarcoma
  - Spindle cell rhabdomyosarcoma
- Intermediate prognosis
  - Embryonal rhabdomyosarcoma
- Poor prognosis
  - Alveolar rhabdomyosarcoma
  - Undifferentiated sarcoma
- Subtypes whose prognosis is not presently evaluable
  - Rhabdomyosarcoma with rhabdoid features

features). Similar to the NCI scheme, the ICR classified a tumor as the alveolar subtype if there was any alveolar architecture or cytology. Pleomorphic rhabdomyosarcoma was excluded given its extreme rarity in children. The classification has been modified to include the anaplastic variant of rhabdomyosarcoma.[30,31] Anaplasia is a histologic feature that may be found in any histologic subtype of rhabdomyosarcoma but is most common in embryonal rhabdomyosarcoma.

AGE AND GENDER DISTRIBUTION OF RHABDOMYOSARCOMA

Despite the striking diversity in location, clinical presentation, and histologic picture, rhabdomyosarcoma has a fairly uniform age distribution; it occurs predominantly in infants and children and somewhat less frequently in adolescents and young adults. In the series of Ragab et al.,[32] 5% of 1561 patients with rhabdomyosarcomas were younger than 1 year of age. About 2% of tumors are present at birth.[33] Each of the rhabdomyosarcoma subtypes occurs in a characteristic age group. For example, embryonal rhabdomyosarcomas and the botryoid and spindle cell subtypes affect mainly, but not exclusively, children between birth and 15 years of age. On the other hand, alveolar rhabdomyosarcoma tends to affect older patients, with peak ages of 10 to 25 years.

Rhabdomyosarcomas are uncommon in patients older than 40 years, but, when they occur, they are of the embryonal type; the spindle cell type also comprises a significant percentage of adult rhabdomyosarcomas,[34] but these differ somewhat from those described in childhood (see following text). There is some correlation between tumor location and age; for example, rhabdomyosarcomas of the urinary bladder, prostate, vagina, and middle ear tend to occur at a younger age (median: 4 years) than those in the paratesticular region (median: 14 years) or the extremities (median: 14 years).

Males are affected more commonly than females by a ratio of approximately 1.5 to 1.0, but the male predominance is less pronounced during adolescence and young adulthood and for rhabdomyosarcomas of the alveolar type.[18] African-Americans seem to be less commonly affected than Caucasians.

CLINICAL FEATURES OF RHABDOMYOSARCOMA

Although rhabdomyosarcomas may arise anywhere in the body, they occur predominantly in three regions: the head and neck, genitourinary tract and retroperitoneum, and upper and lower extremities. Each rhabdomyosarcoma histologic subtype may occur in virtually any location, but each subtype has a site predilection, as will be discussed in the specific sections.

The head and neck is the principal location of rhabdomyosarcoma; 970 (35%) of 2747 tumors from the IRS-I, IRS-II, and IRS-III studies occurred in this location (Table 20-2). In the head and neck, parameningeal tumors are the most common, accounting for 16% of all tumors in the IRS studies.[35] Parameningeal rhabdomyosarcomas are distinguished from the other rhabdomyosarcomas arising in the head and neck because of their potential intracranial extension and seeding—therefore, their less favorable clinical course.[36]

The orbit is the second most common head and neck site of rhabdomyosarcoma, accounting for 9% of cases from the IRS series. Most rhabdomyosarcomas in this location are of the embryonal subtype.[37] For example, 221 (90%) of 245 orbital tumors from the IRS-I through IRS-IV studies were of the embryonal subtype, although rare botryoid-type embryonal rhabdomyosarcomas and alveolar rhabdomyosarcomas also arise in the orbit.[38]

Rhabdomyosarcoma may also involve a variety of other sites in the head and neck, including the nasal cavity and nasopharynx, followed in frequency by the ear and ear canal, paranasal sinuses, soft tissues of the face and neck, and the oral cavity, including the tongue, lip, and palate.[39]

After the head and neck, the genitourinary tract is the second most common site for rhabdomyosarcoma.[40] In the IRS series, 650 (24%) of 2747 cases arose in this general region. Histologically, most tumors arising in this location are of the embryonal subtype. The tumors in this region most commonly arise in a paratesticular location and occur predominantly in adolescents. The spindle cell subtype of embryonal rhabdomyosarcoma has a propensity to arise in the paratesticular region.[41,42] They may also involve the spermatic cord and epididymis but usually are separate from the testis proper.

The retroperitoneum and pelvis are not uncommon sites of involvement. Approximately 45% of tumors in these sites are of the embryonal subtype, and up to 15% are alveolar rhabdomyosarcomas.[43,44] In general, effective therapy of rhabdomyosarcomas in the retroperitoneum and pelvic region is more difficult than that of paratesticular rhabdomyosarcomas.[45]

Approximately 5% of rhabdomyosarcomas arise in the urinary bladder or prostate. In fact, rhabdomyosarcoma is the most common bladder tumor in children under 10 years of age. Almost all pediatric tumors arising in this location are embryonal or botryoid rhabdomyosarcomas.[46] Those with a botryoid histology typically grow into the lumen of the urinary bladder as a grape-like, richly mucoid, multinodular or polypoid mass with a broad base that not infrequently causes an obstruction of the internal urethral orifice and prostatic urethra. This, in turn, results in incontinence and difficulty with urination. Interestingly, however, adult rhabdomyosarcomas of the urinary bladder are more often of the alveolar type, sometimes with anaplastic features, which can cause morphologic confusion with small cell carcinoma.[47] Rarely, rhabdomyosarcomas arise in other genitourinary sites, including the fallopian tube,[48] uterus,[49] cervix,[50] vagina,[51] labium and vulva,[52] and the perineum and perianal region.[53] Tumors in these locations are often (but not always) of the botryoid subtype. Rhabdomyosarcomas that arise in gynecologic organs in adults are morphologically similar to those arising in pediatric patients, but they seem to behave more aggressively.[48]

Unlike adult soft tissue sarcomas, rhabdomyosarcomas involve the extremities much less commonly; only 14.6% of cases from the Armed Forces Institute of Pathology (AFIP) series occurred in this location, with a similar incidence in the upper and lower extremities; alveolar rhabdomyosarcomas outnumbered embryonal rhabdomyosarcomas by a ratio of 4 to 3, similar to that found in the IRS-I and IRS-II studies.[6] Most pleomorphic rhabdomyosarcomas arise in the deep soft tissues of the extremities of adults.

Unusual rhabdomyosarcomas arise outside of the aforementioned sites. Tumors originating in the hepatobiliary tract usually arise from the submucosa of the common bile duct; most are botryoid type with typical myxoid grape-like gross and microscopic appearances.[54]

GROSS FINDINGS OF RHABDOMYOSARCOMA

There is little that is characterized grossly of this tumor. As with other rapidly growing sarcomas, the appearance of the tumor reflects the degree of cellularity, the relative amounts of collagenous or myxoid stroma, and the presence and extent of secondary changes such as hemorrhage, necrosis, and ulceration. In general, tumors growing into body cavities, such as those in the nasopharynx and urinary bladder, are fairly well circumscribed, multinodular, or distinctly polypoid with a glistening, gelatinous, gray-white surface that, on a cross-section, often shows patchy areas of hemorrhage or cyst formation. Deep-seated tumors involving or arising in the musculature are usually less well defined and nearly always infiltrate the surrounding tissues. They are firmer and rubbery and have a mottled gray-white to pink-tan, smooth or finely granular, often bulging surface. They rarely become large, averaging 3 to 4 cm in greatest diameter. There are often areas of focal necrosis and cystic degeneration.

RHABDOMYOSARCOMA SUBTYPES

Embryonal Rhabdomyosarcoma

Embryonal rhabdomyosarcoma (without other distinguishing features) accounts for approximately 60% of all rhabdomyosarcomas.[18] It mostly affects children younger than 10 years of age (mean age: near 7 years), but it also occurs in adolescents and young adults; it is uncommon in patients older than 40 years of age. The most common site of embryonal rhabdomyosarcoma is the head and neck, particularly the orbit and parameninges (Table 20-3). After the head and neck, this tumor is most commonly found in the genitourinary tract, followed by the deep soft tissues of the extremities and the pelvis and retroperitoneum.

Histologically, embryonal rhabdomyosarcoma bears a close resemblance to various stages in the embryogenesis of normal

TABLE 20-3 Distribution of Anatomic Sites of Rhabdomyosarcoma Subtypes for 1626 IRS-I and IRS-II Patients

SITE	EMBRYONAL	ALVEOLAR	BOTRYOID	PLEOMORPHIC	OTHER	TOTAL NO.
Head and neck	411 (71%)	76 (13%)	13 (2%)		77 (13%)	577
Genitourinary	246 (71%)	8 (2%)	70 (20%)	1 (<1%)	23 (7%)	348
Extremities	76 (24%)	156 (50%)		5 (2%)	74 (24%)	311
Trunk	27 (19%)	43 (30%)		3 (2%)	71 (49%)	144
Pelvis	45 (48%)	19 (20%)			29 (31%)	93
Retroperitoneum	44 (59%)	14 (19%)		1 (1%)	16 (21%)	75
Perineum/anus	13 (33%)	19 (48%)	1 (2%)	1 (2%)	6 (15%)	40
Other sites	15 (39%)	9 (24%)	4 (11%)		10 (26%)	38

Modified from Newton Jr WA, Soule EH, Hamoudi AB, et al. Histopathology of childhood sarcomas, Intergroup Rhabdomyosarcoma Studies I and II: clinicopathologic correlation. J Clin Oncol 1988;6:67.

skeletal muscle, but its pattern is much more variable, ranging from poorly differentiated tumors that are difficult to diagnose without immunohistochemical examination to well-differentiated neoplasms that resemble fetal muscle. Features common to most are the following: (1) varying degrees of cellularity with alternating densely packed, hypercellular areas and loosely textured myxoid areas (Figs. 20-1 to 20-4); (2) a mixture of poorly oriented, small, undifferentiated, hyperchromatic round or spindle-shaped cells (Fig. 20-5) and a varying number of differentiated cells with eosinophilic cytoplasm characteristic of rhabdomyoblasts; and (3) a matrix containing little collagen and varying amounts of myxoid material. Cross-striations are discernible in 50% to 60% of cases.

The least well-differentiated examples of this tumor correspond in appearance to developing muscle at 5 to 8 weeks' gestation. For the most part, they consist of small, round or spindle-shaped cells with darkly staining hyperchromatic nuclei and indistinct cytoplasm. The nuclei vary slightly in size and shape (more so than those of alveolar rhabdomyosarcoma), have one or two small nucleoli, and usually exhibit a high rate of mitotic activity. Differentiated rhabdomyoblasts are either absent entirely or are confined to a few small areas, making it mandatory to examine multiple sections from different portions of the tumor; adjunctive diagnostic procedures are required to confirm the diagnosis in virtually all cases.

Better-differentiated examples have, in addition to the primitive or undifferentiated cellular areas, larger round or

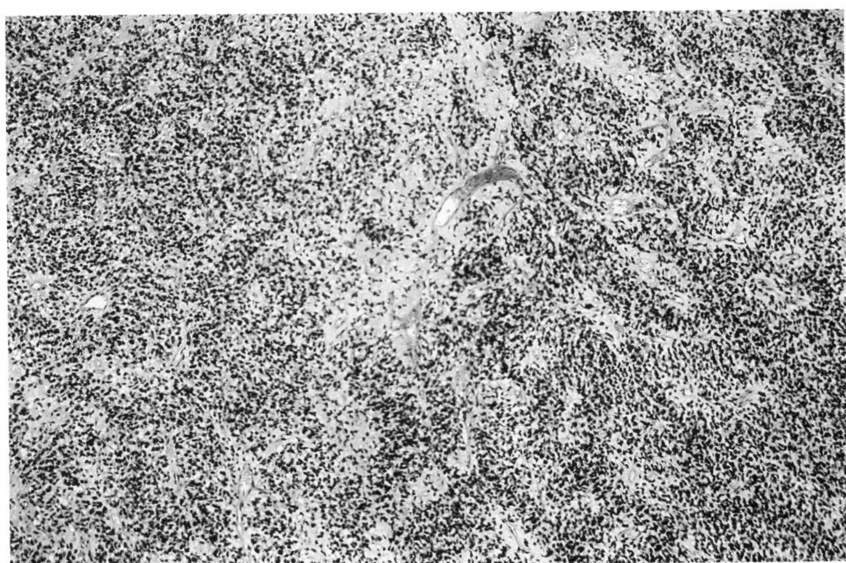

FIGURE 20-1. Low-power view of embryonal rhabdomyosarcoma with alternating cellular and myxoid areas, a characteristic feature of this tumor.

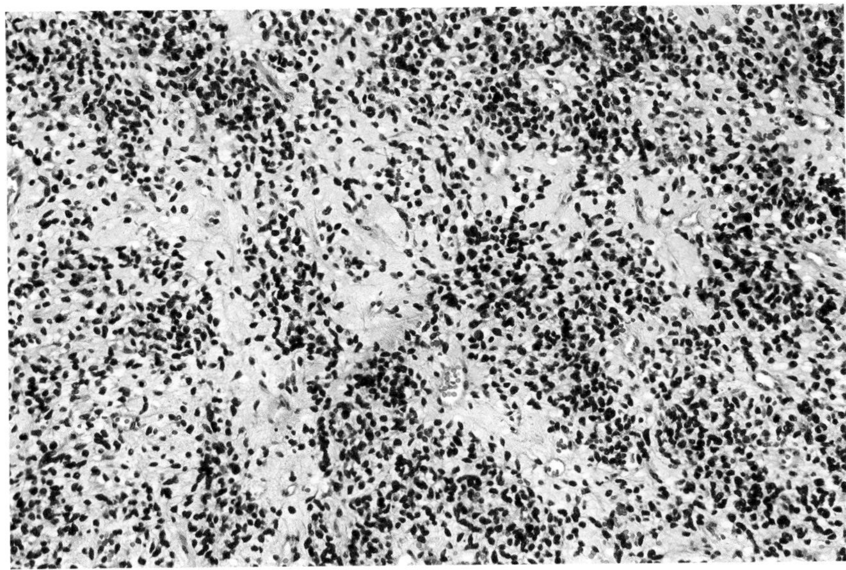

FIGURE 20-2. Alternating cellular and myxoid zones in an embryonal rhabdomyosarcoma.

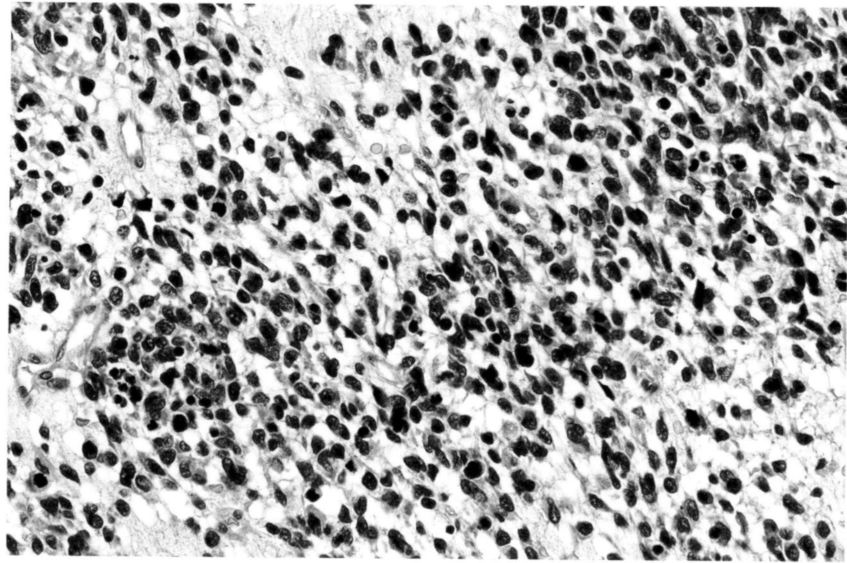

FIGURE 20-3. High-power view of an embryonal rhabdomyosarcoma composed predominantly of primitive ovoid cells.

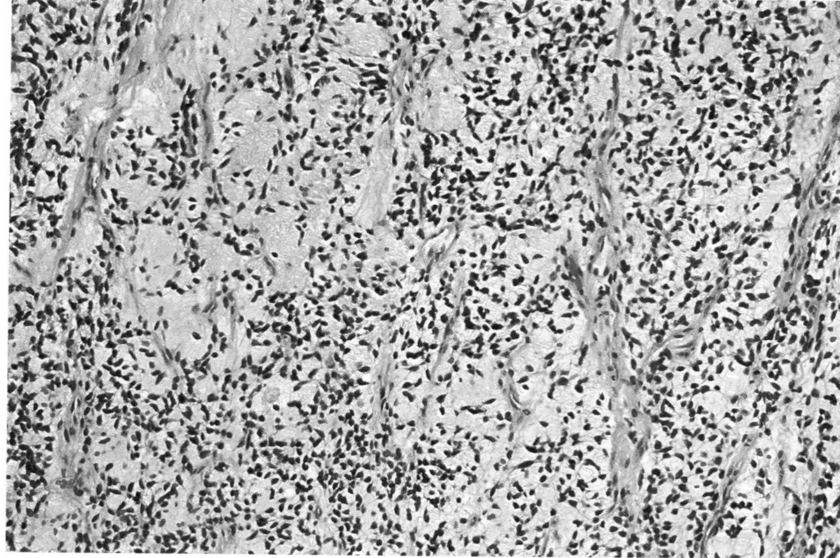

FIGURE 20-4. Primitive spindle-shaped cells deposited in an abundant myxoid stroma in an embryonal rhabdomyosarcoma.

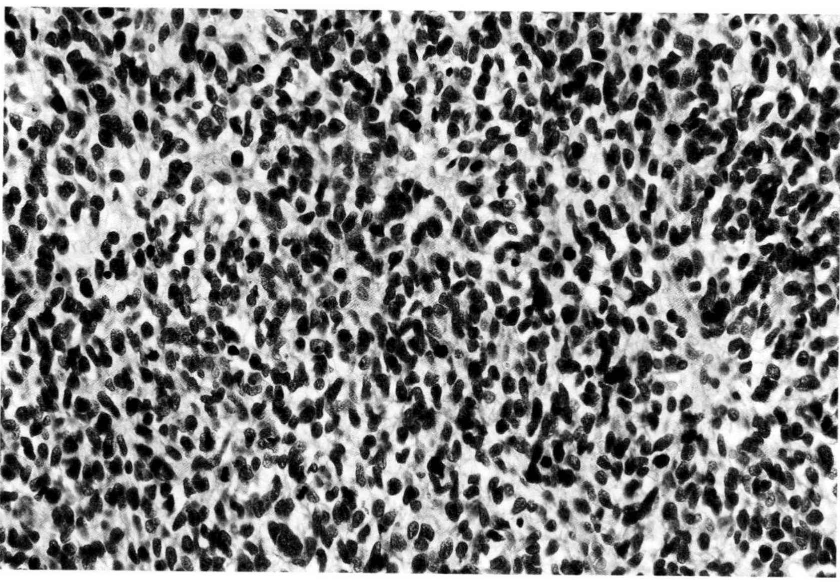

FIGURE 20-5. Embryonal rhabdomyosarcoma composed almost exclusively of primitive cells devoid of rhabdomyoblastic differentiation.

oval eosinophilic cells characteristic of rhabdomyoblasts (Figs. 20-6 to 20-8); the cytoplasm of these cells contains granular material or deeply eosinophilic masses of stringy or fibrillary material concentrically arranged near or around the nucleus. Cross-striations are rare in the round cells, and, if present, they are usually confined to narrow bundles of concentrically arranged myofibrils at the circumference of the rhabdomyoblast. Degenerated rhabdomyoblasts with a glassy or hyalinized deeply eosinophilic cytoplasm and pyknotic nuclei but without cross-striations are a frequent feature of this tumor.

Cross-striations are more readily discernible in embryonal rhabdomyosarcomas with a more prominent spindle cell component (Figs. 20-9 and 20-10), tumors that might be regarded as the morphologic equivalent of normal muscle at 9 to 15 weeks of intrauterine development; these neoplasms are composed mainly of a mixture of undifferentiated cells and differentiated fusiform or elongated cells that are readily identifiable as rhabdomyoblasts by light microscopy. The rhabdomyoblasts range from slender spindle-shaped cells with a small number of peripherally placed myofibrils to large eosinophilic cells with a strap, ribbon, tadpole, or racket shape and one or two centrally positioned nuclei and prominent nucleoli, with or without cross-striations. Cross-striations in neoplastic cells differ from those in residual or entrapped muscle cells by their more irregular distribution and because they often traverse only part of the tumor cell. Intracellular granules may be confused with cross-striations, but their granular nature is readily apparent after a careful examination of the cell under oil immersion. Sometimes, the strap-shaped cells are sharply angulated and form a diagnostically useful zigzag or broken straw pattern. Most of these tumors have only a moderate degree of cellular pleomorphism.

Embryonal rhabdomyosarcomas with a prominent degree of cellular pleomorphism (anaplasia) are rare and, in some

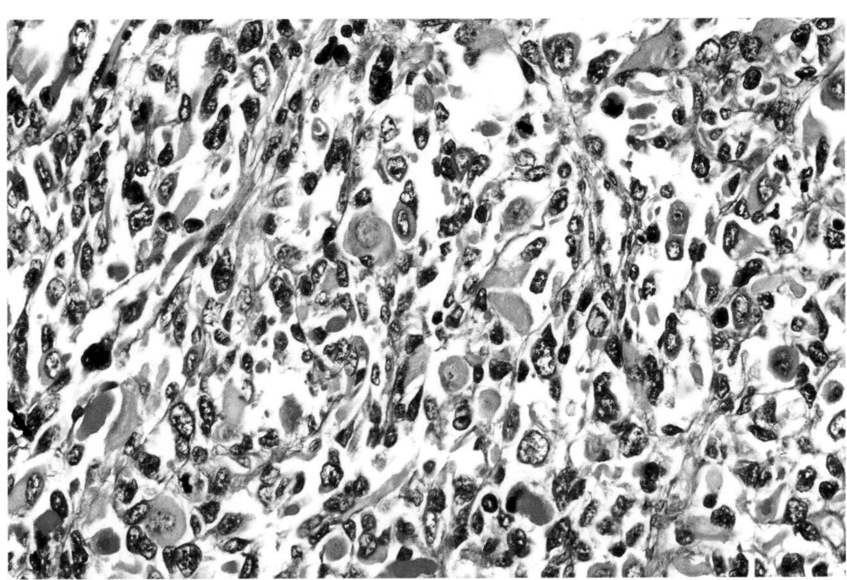

FIGURE 20-6. Embryonal rhabdomyosarcoma. Note the scattered cells with eosinophilic cytoplasm.

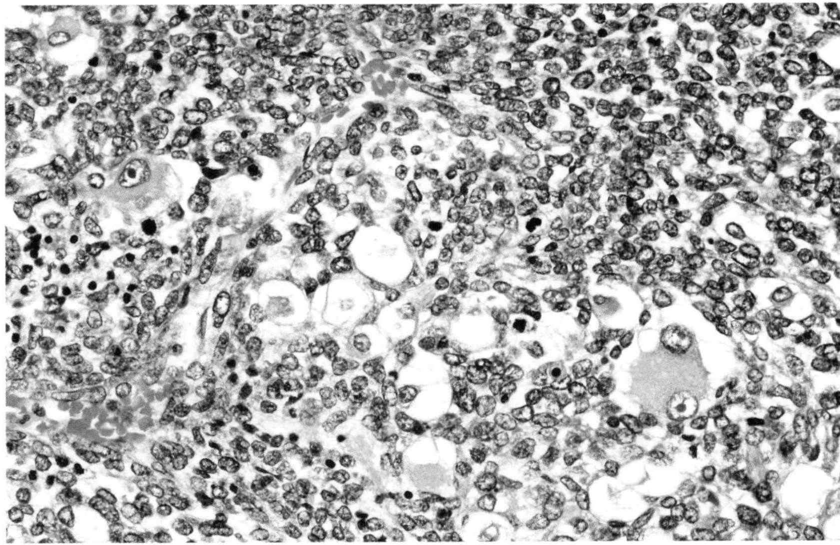

FIGURE 20-7. Embryonal rhabdomyosarcoma composed predominantly of primitive ovoid cells with scattered rhabdomyoblasts. The rhabdomyoblasts, in this case, have eccentric vesicular nuclei and abundant densely eosinophilic cytoplasm.

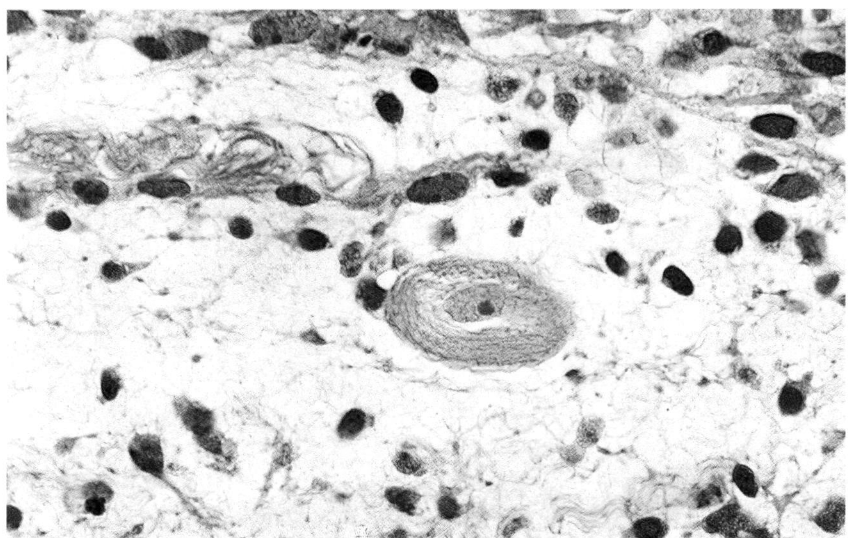

FIGURE 20-8. Characteristic rhabdomyoblast in an embryonal rhabdomyosarcoma. Deeply eosinophilic fibrillar material is concentrically arranged around the nucleus.

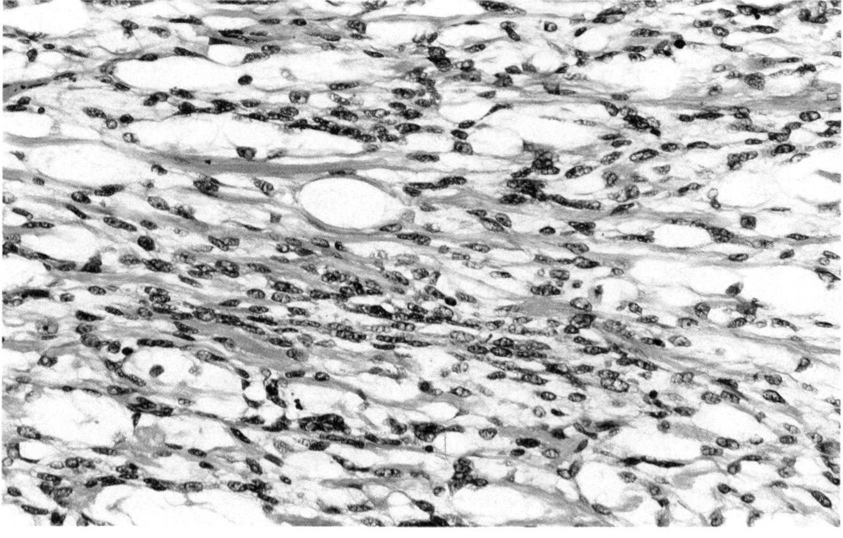

FIGURE 20-9. Embryonal rhabdomyosarcoma composed predominantly of atypical spindle-shaped cells with scattered elongated rhabdomyoblasts.

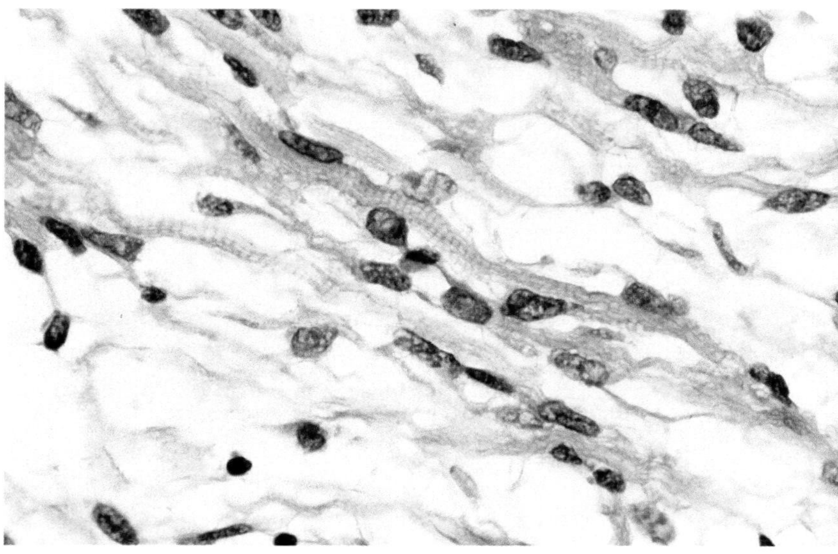

FIGURE 20-10. High-power view of elongated rhabdomyoblasts with distinct cross-striations in an embryonal rhabdomyosarcoma.

cases, difficult to distinguish from adult pleomorphic rhabdomyosarcomas (Fig. 20-11), except for the more frequent occurrence of cross-striations in childhood tumors and the identification of areas of more typical embryonal rhabdomyosarcoma. According to Kodet et al.,[55] survival in patients with diffuse anaplasia in embryonal rhabdomyosarcoma is similar to the unfavorable survival of patients with alveolar rhabdomyosarcoma.

There are also extremely well-differentiated embryonal rhabdomyosarcomas that consist almost entirely of well-differentiated rounded, spindle-shaped, or polygonal rhabdomyoblasts with abundant eosinophilic cytoplasm and frequent cross-striations. Some of these differentiated tumors are found in recurrent or metastatic neoplasms after prolonged therapy (Fig. 20-12), possibly as a result of the selective destruction of undifferentiated tumor cells.[56]

Glycogen is demonstrable in most rhabdomyosarcomas regardless of type; when the glycogen is removed during fixation, multivacuolated cells or spider cells result, which are large multivacuolated rhabdomyoblasts with narrow strands of cytoplasm connecting the center of the cell with its periphery. The centrally located nuclei and the irregular shape of the cytoplasmic vacuoles help distinguish these cells from the more rounded lipid-filled vacuoles of lipoblasts. In contrast to alveolar rhabdomyosarcoma, multinucleated giant cells are rare in embryonal rhabdomyosarcomas.

Occasionally, the embryonal rhabdomyosarcoma displays, in addition to its rhabdomyoblastic component, foci of immature cartilaginous (Fig. 20-13) or osseous tissue, or both. These tumors occur at any age and any location but seem to be more common in the genitourinary tract and the retroperitoneum.

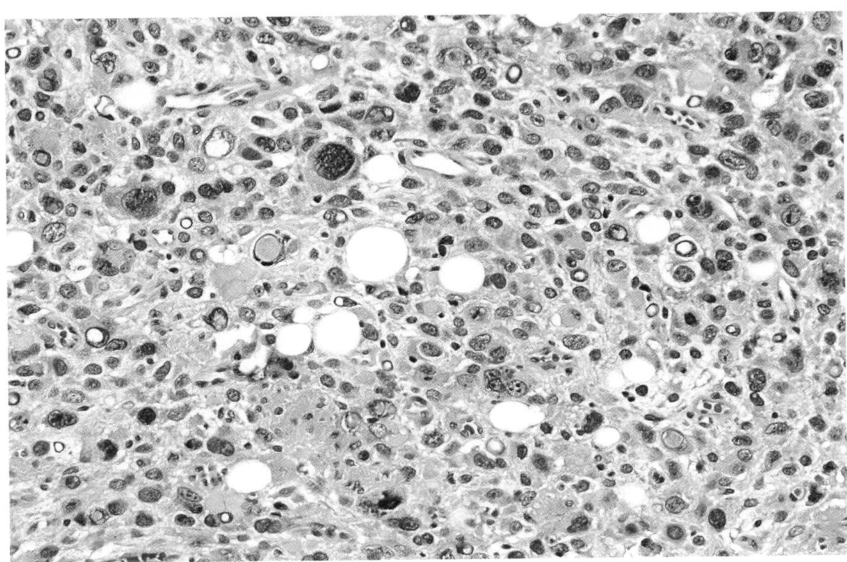

FIGURE 20-11. Embryonal rhabdomyosarcoma with anaplastic features arising in a 3-year-old child.

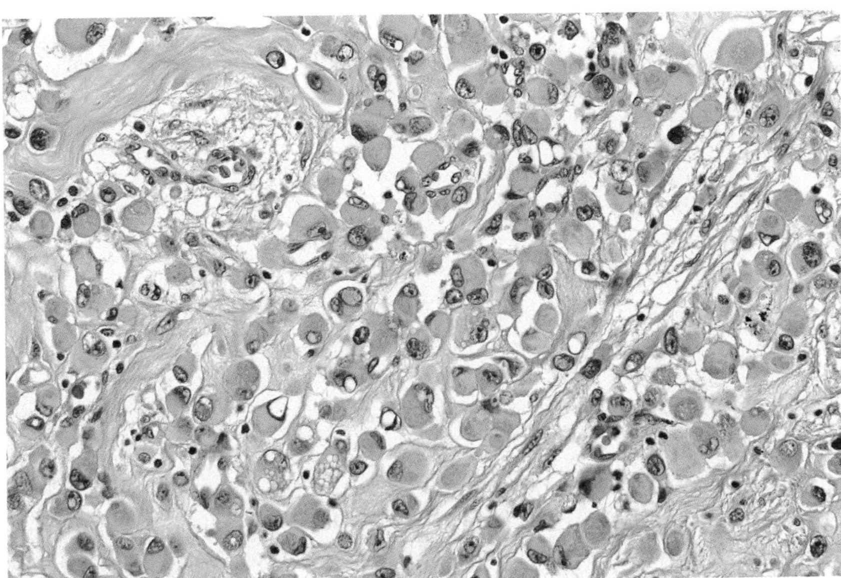

FIGURE 20-12. Embryonal rhabdomyosarcoma consisting almost entirely of differentiated rhabdomyoblasts, a feature occasionally encountered in recurrent tumors following therapy.

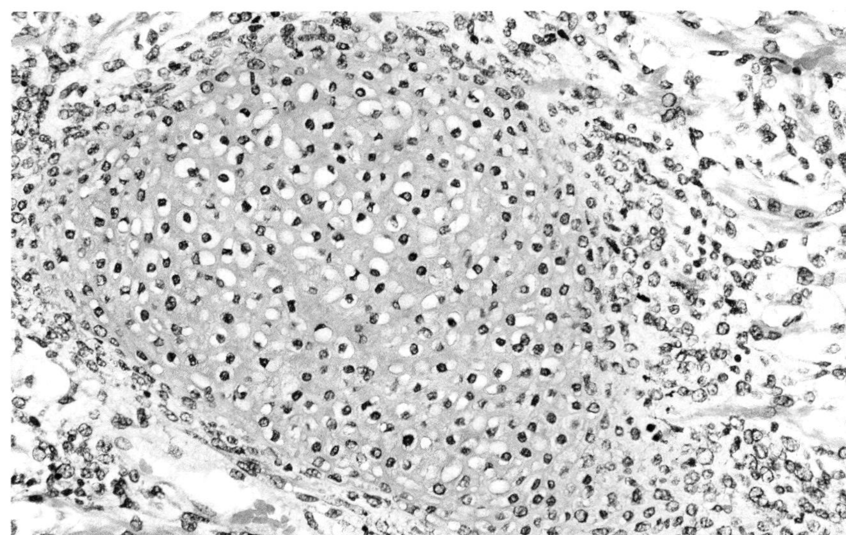

FIGURE 20-13. Embryonal rhabdomyosarcoma with foci of immature cartilage.

Cytogenetic and Molecular Genetic Findings

The cytogenetic abnormalities of embryonal and alveolar rhabdomyosarcomas are distinct. Embryonal rhabdomyosarcoma is characterized by a consistent loss of heterozygosity (LOH) for multiple closely linked loci at chromosome 11p15.5.[57,58] The LOH may result in activation of a tumor suppressor gene or genes, including *GOK*.[59] Rare cases of embryonal rhabdomyosarcoma have harbored translocations, including t(2;8)(q35;q13), which interestingly involved *PAX3*,[60] and t(4;22)(q35;q12), which involved *EWSR1*.[61] Others have reported trisomy 8 as a consistent finding in embryonal rhabdomyosarcomas.[62-64] More recently, a number of studies have implicated upregulation of genes involved in the hedgehog pathway, including *GLI1* and *Ptch1*.[65-68]

Spindle Cell Rhabdomyosarcoma

In 1992, Cavazzana et al.[42] reported 21 embryonal rhabdomyosarcomas composed predominantly (greater than 80%) of elongated spindle cells mimicking fetal myotubes at a late stage of cellular differentiation. In this study, there was a striking predilection for this tumor to arise in males, particularly in a paratesticular location. By immunohistochemistry and electron microscopy, the cells showed a high degree of skeletal muscle differentiation. The authors coined the term *spindle cell rhabdomyosarcoma* to distinguish this entity from the usual embryonal rhabdomyosarcoma because of its more favorable clinical course. Subsequent studies have confirmed the distinctive clinical and pathologic features of this rhabdomyosarcoma subtype.[41] Several studies have also described this variant of rhabdomyosarcoma in adults.[69,70] However, these adult-type spindle cell lesions have several distinctive features, including a predilection for the head and neck and extremities, a greater degree of cytologic atypia in the spindled cells, focal areas resembling pseudovascular sclerosing rhabdomyosarcoma, and a more aggressive clinical course than pediatric lesions.[69,70] So, in this instance, most of these cases are probably better classified as embryonal rhabdomyosarcoma because they deviate from the original description of spindle cell rhabdomyosarcoma. Whether this is a unique variant of rhabdomyosarcoma, part of a spectrum with sclerosing rhabdomyosarcoma (described later in the chapter) or simply the adult (more aggressive) variant of spindle cell rhabdomyosarcoma has yet to be fully elucidated.[71] Both variants are included under the rubric of spindle cell/sclerosing rhabdomyosarcoma in the new 2013 WHO classification.

TABLE 20-4 Anatomic Distribution of Spindle Cell Rhabdomyosarcomas[41,42]

ANATOMIC LOCATION	NO.	PERCENTAGE (%)
Paratesticular	30	38
Head and neck	21	27
Extremities	8	10
Genitourinary	8	10
Other	11	15
Total	78	100

Spindle cell rhabdomyosarcoma is a rare subtype of rhabdomyosarcoma, accounting for 21 (4.4%) of 471 rhabdomyosarcomas retrieved from the files of the German-Italian Cooperative Soft Tissue Sarcomas Study Group.[42] Of 800 randomly selected rhabdomyosarcomas from the IRS, this variant accounted for only 3% of all rhabdomyosarcomas.[72] Like other forms of embryonal rhabdomyosarcoma, the spindle cell type tends to arise in young patients (mean age: approximately 7 years), with a striking male predilection. The most common site of involvement is the paratesticular soft tissue (38%), followed by the head and neck (27%) (Table 20-4), but rare examples have also been described in a myriad of sites.

Histologically, the tumor is composed almost exclusively of elongated fusiform cells with cigar-shaped nuclei and prominent nucleoli (Figs. 20-14 to 20-16). The tumor cells have eosinophilic fibrillar cytoplasm with distinct cellular borders, closely resembling late-stage fetal myoblasts. Cytoplasmic cross-striations may be observed. The collagen-rich form is characterized by spindle cells separated by abundant collagen fibers arranged in a storiform or whorled growth pattern. The collagen-poor form is a more cellular proliferation of cells arranged in bundles, or fascicles, reminiscent of fibrosarcoma.

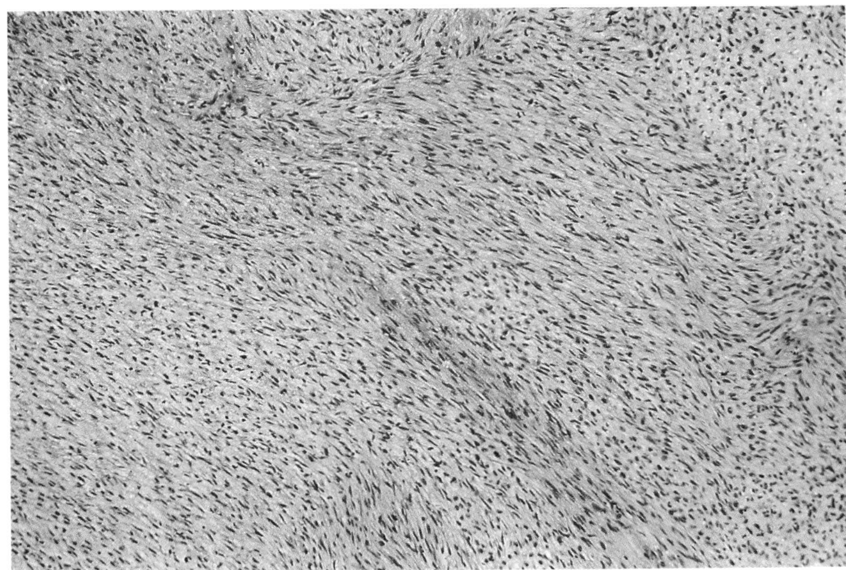

FIGURE 20-14. Low-power view of spindle cell type of embryonal rhabdomyosarcoma arising in the urinary bladder.

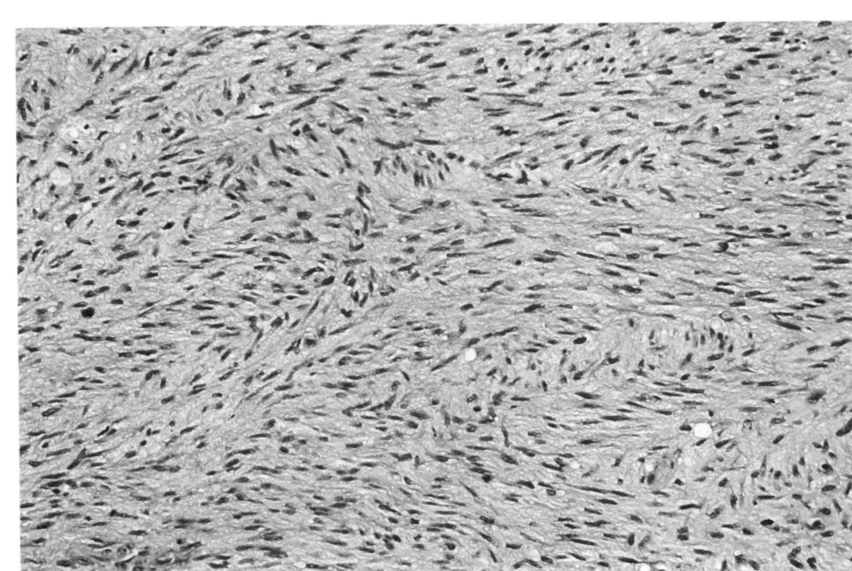

FIGURE 20-15. Spindle cell type of embryonal rhabdomyosarcoma composed of relatively uniform spindle-shaped cells deposited in a myxoid stroma. Cells are arranged in an irregular fascicular pattern reminiscent of leiomyosarcoma.

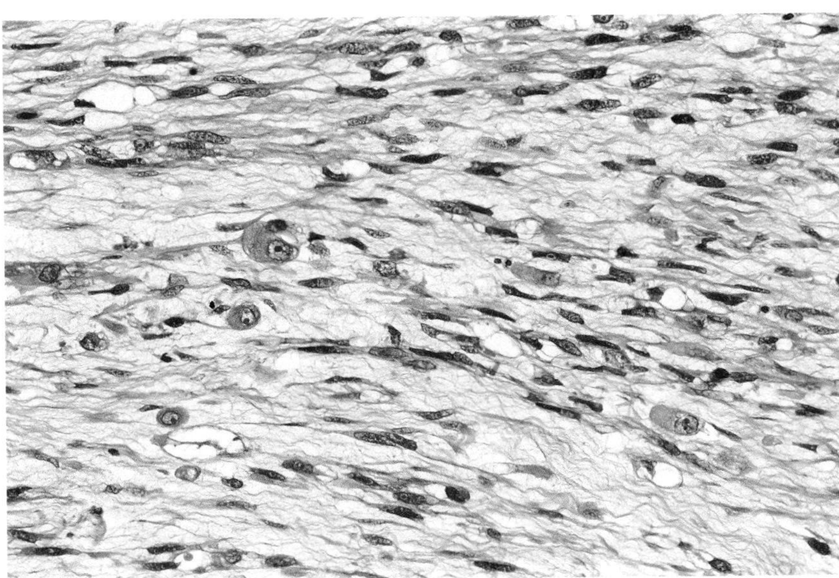

FIGURE 20-16. Scattered rhabdomyoblasts are apparent in this spindle cell type of embryonal rhabdomyosarcoma.

Immunohistochemically, the tumor cells consistently express myogenic antigens, including myogenin, muscle-specific actin and desmin. Interestingly, this rhabdomyosarcoma subtype more consistently expresses myogenic antigens that are generally expressed at a late stage of myogenesis (titin and troponin D), supporting a greater degree of differentiation of these spindle-shaped cells.[41,42] In the study by Mentzel et al.[71] of adult cases, some also expressed CD99 and WT1, which could lead to confusion with other mesenchymal neoplasms.

Few cases of spindle cell rhabdomyosarcoma have been evaluated by cytogenetics. Debiec-Rychter et al.[73] described one case arising in the cheek of an 18-year-old girl with a der (2)t(2;7), with apparent involvement of 2q36-37. Gil-Benso et al.[74] reported a case with structural rearrangements of chromosomes 8, 12, 21, and 22.

Embryonal Rhabdomyosarcoma, Botryoid Type

Botryoid rhabdomyosarcoma accounts for approximately 6% of all rhabdomyosarcomas.[29] The word *botryoid* is derived from the Greek word for *grapes*; this variant is characterized grossly by its polypoid (grape-like) growth and microscopically by its relative sparsity of cells and abundance of mucoid stroma, often resulting in a myxoma-like picture. Most botryoid rhabdomyosarcomas are found in mucosa-lined hollow organs, such as the nasal cavity, nasopharynx, bile duct, urinary bladder, and vagina (Fig. 20-17); tumors of this type may also be encountered in areas where the expanding neoplasm reaches the body surface, as in some rhabdomyosarcomas of the eyelid or the anal region.[75] Clearly, its unrestricted growth in body cavities or on body surfaces accounts for its characteristic edematous and grape-like appearance.

Although a grape-like configuration has traditionally been a defining feature of the botryoid variant, the ICR scheme does not require this characteristic gross appearance.[29] According to the ICR criteria, a cambium layer, characterized by a subepithelial condensation of tumor cells separated from an intact surface epithelium by a zone of loose stroma, must be present to recognize this variant (Figs. 20-18 to 20-20). The tumor cells should form a distinct zone that is several layers thick, although the thickness of this layer may vary in extent in different areas of the tumor. The cells range from primitive small cells to cells with clear-cut myoblastic differentiation (Fig. 20-21). Cells with stellate cytoplasmic processes are often prominent. The stroma is typically loosely cellular with a myxoid appearance, including a hypocellular zone that separates the surface epithelium from the underlying cambium layer. The surface epithelium may be hyperplastic or may undergo squamous changes, sometimes mimicking a carcinoma.

Immunohistochemically, there is usually strong staining for myogenic antigens, particularly in cells showing light microscopic evidence of myoblastic differentiation. By cytogenetics, Palazzo et al.[76] reported deletion of the short arm of chromosome 1 and trisomies of chromosomes 13 and 18. A second reported case showed a hyperdiploid clone with a

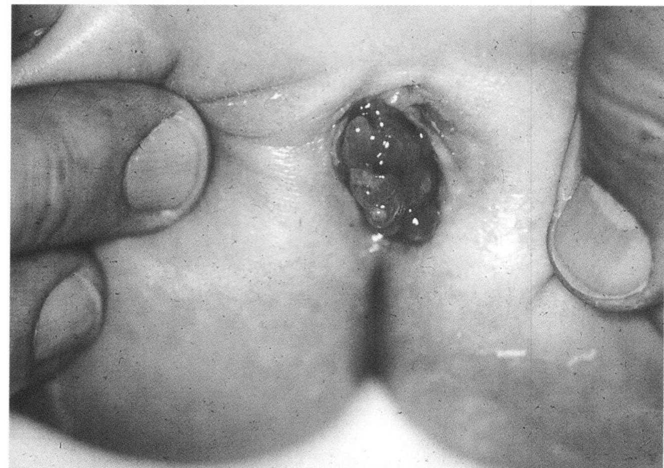

FIGURE 20-17. Botryoid-type embryonal rhabdomyosarcoma of the vagina.

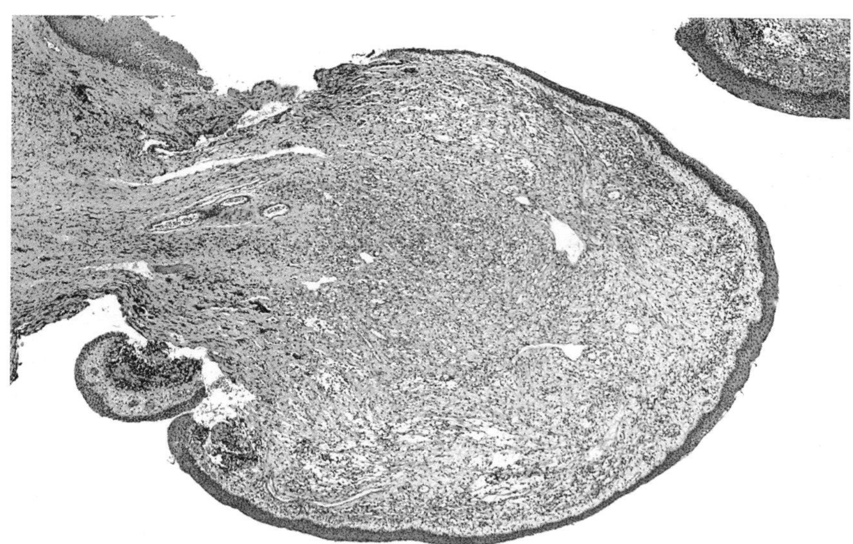

FIGURE 20-18. Polypoid fragment lined by squamous mucosa in a botryoid-type embryonal rhabdomyosarcoma of the vagina.

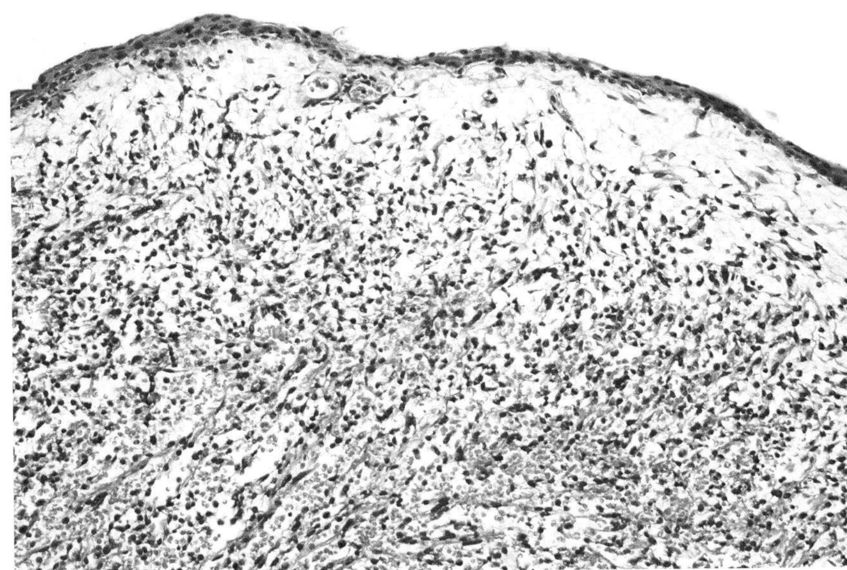

FIGURE 20-19. Botryoid-type embryonal rhabdomyosarcoma with the characteristic cambium layer, a submucosal zone of markedly increased cellularity.

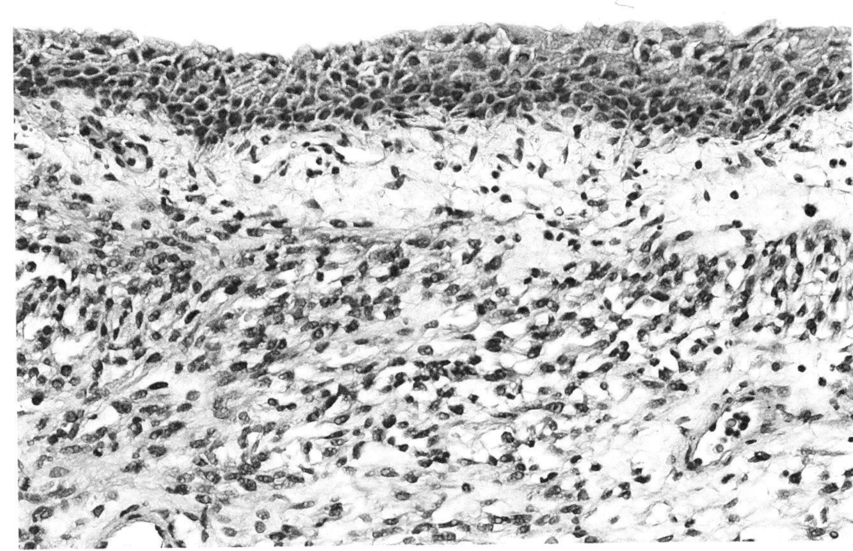

FIGURE 20-20. Primitive spindle-shaped and ovoid cells in the cambium layer of this botryoid-type embryonal rhabdomyosarcoma.

complex karyotype, including numerous chromosomal gains.[77] Manor et al.[78] recently described a case with trisomy 8.

Alveolar Rhabdomyosarcoma

Alveolar rhabdomyosarcoma is the second most common subtype, accounting for approximately 31% of all rhabdomyosarcomas.[29] This variant tends to arise at a slightly older age than embryonal, botryoid, and spindle cell rhabdomyosarcomas, with a peak incidence at 10 to 25 years of age. It has a predilection for the deep soft tissues of the extremities, although the tumor may arise in many other sites, including the head and neck,[79] bladder,[47] and gynecologic organs.[80,81]

Histologically, alveolar rhabdomyosarcoma is composed largely of ill-defined aggregates of poorly differentiated round or oval tumor cells that frequently show central loss of cellular cohesion and formation of irregular alveolar spaces (Figs. 20-22 to 20-24). The individual cellular aggregates are separated and surrounded by a framework of dense, frequently hyalinized fibrous septa that surround dilated vascular channels. Characteristically, the cells at the periphery of the alveolar spaces are well preserved and adhere in a single layer to the fibrous septa in a manner somewhat reminiscent of an adenocarcinoma or papillary carcinoma. The cells in the center of the alveolar spaces tend to be more loosely arranged, or freely floating (see Fig. 20-24); they are often poorly preserved and show evidence of degeneration and necrosis. In rare instances, viable cells are virtually absent, and the tumor

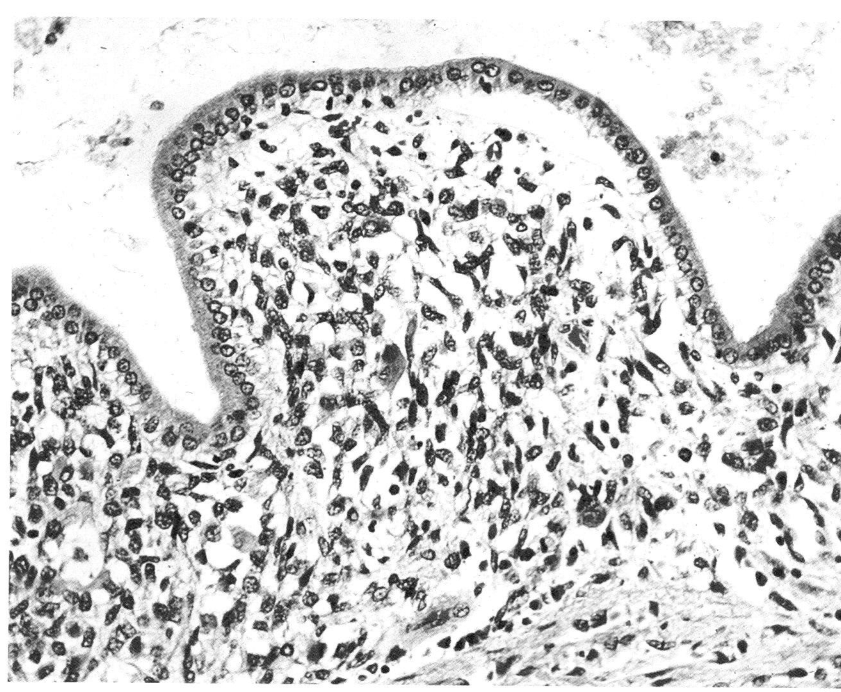

FIGURE 20-21. Embryonal rhabdomyosarcoma of the biliary tract with botryoid features. Scattered rhabdomyoblasts are apparent.

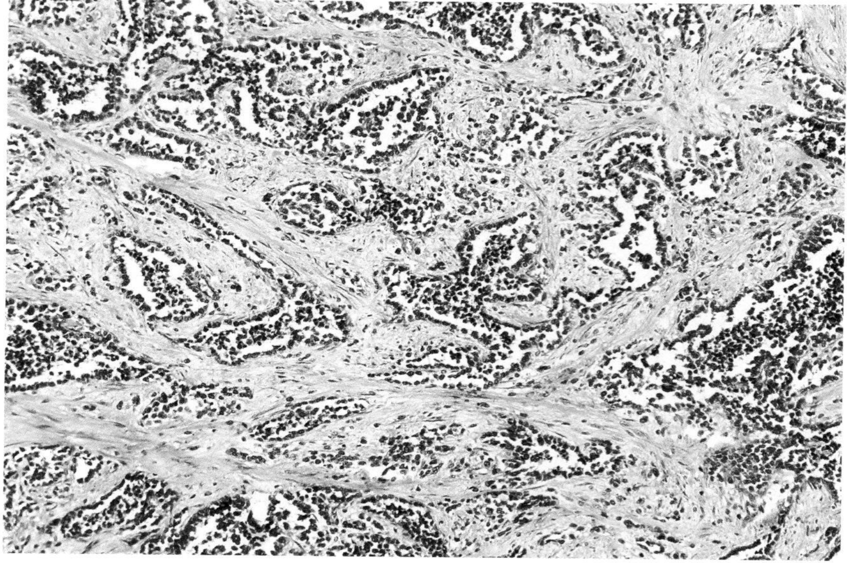

FIGURE 20-22. Alveolar rhabdomyosarcoma with the characteristic alveolar growth pattern.

consists merely of a coarse sieve-like or honeycomb-like meshwork of thick fibrous trabeculae surrounding small, loosely textured groups of severely degenerated cells with pyknotic nuclei and necrotic cellular debris.

There are also solid forms of this tumor that lack an alveolar pattern entirely and are composed of densely packed groups or masses of tumor cells resembling the round cell areas of embryonal rhabdomyosarcoma but with a more uniform cellular picture with little or no fibrosis (Figs. 20-25 and 20-26).[27] These solidly cellular areas are more commonly encountered at the periphery of the tumor and probably represent the most active and most cellular stage of growth. In most cases,

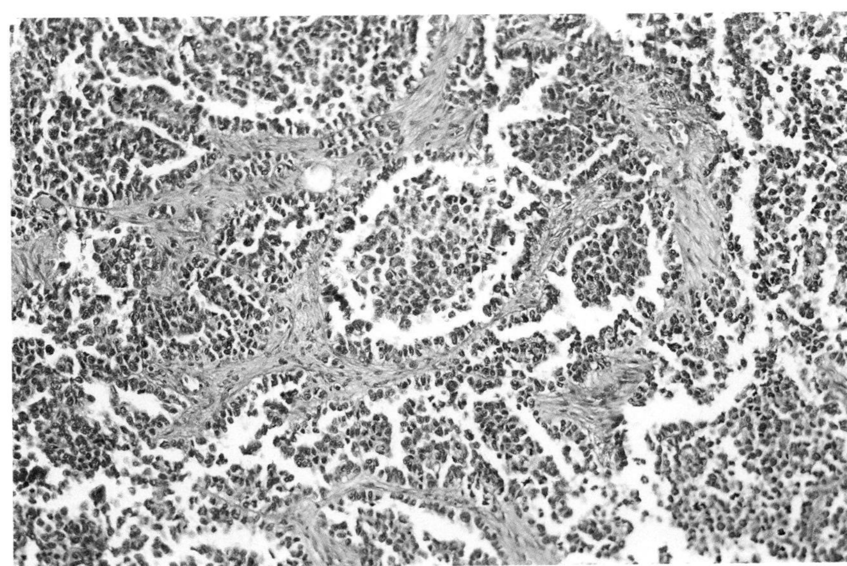

FIGURE 20-23. Alveolar rhabdomyosarcoma. A single layer of neoplastic cells adheres to dense fibrous septa with central loss of cellular cohesion.

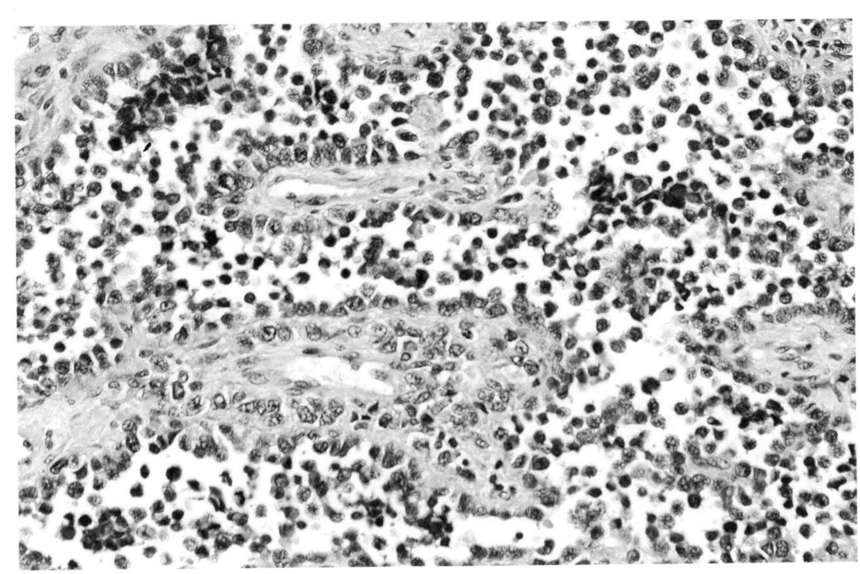

FIGURE 20-24. High-power view of alveolar rhabdomyosarcoma. Fibrovascular septa are lined by a single layer of round cells. There is loss of cellular cohesion and individual tumor cell necrosis between the fibrous septa.

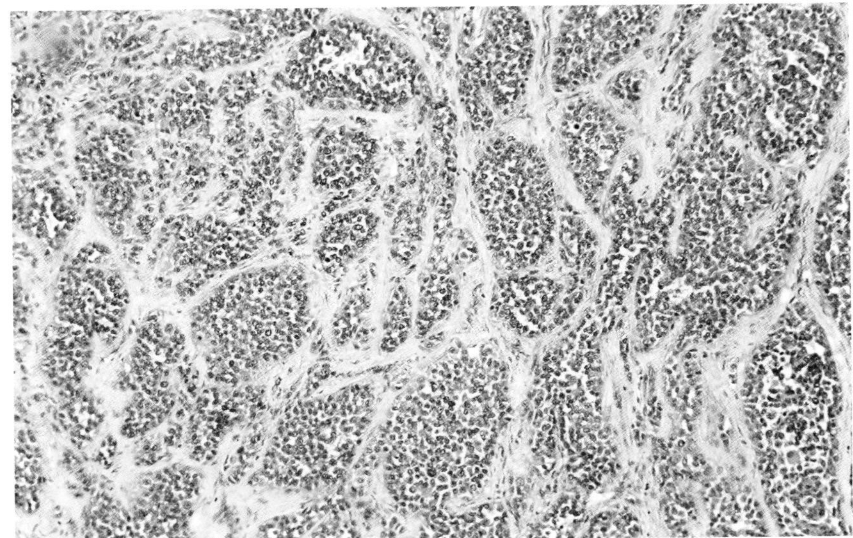

FIGURE 20-25. Low-power view of alveolar rhabdomyosarcoma with incipient loss of cellular cohesion in cellular nests.

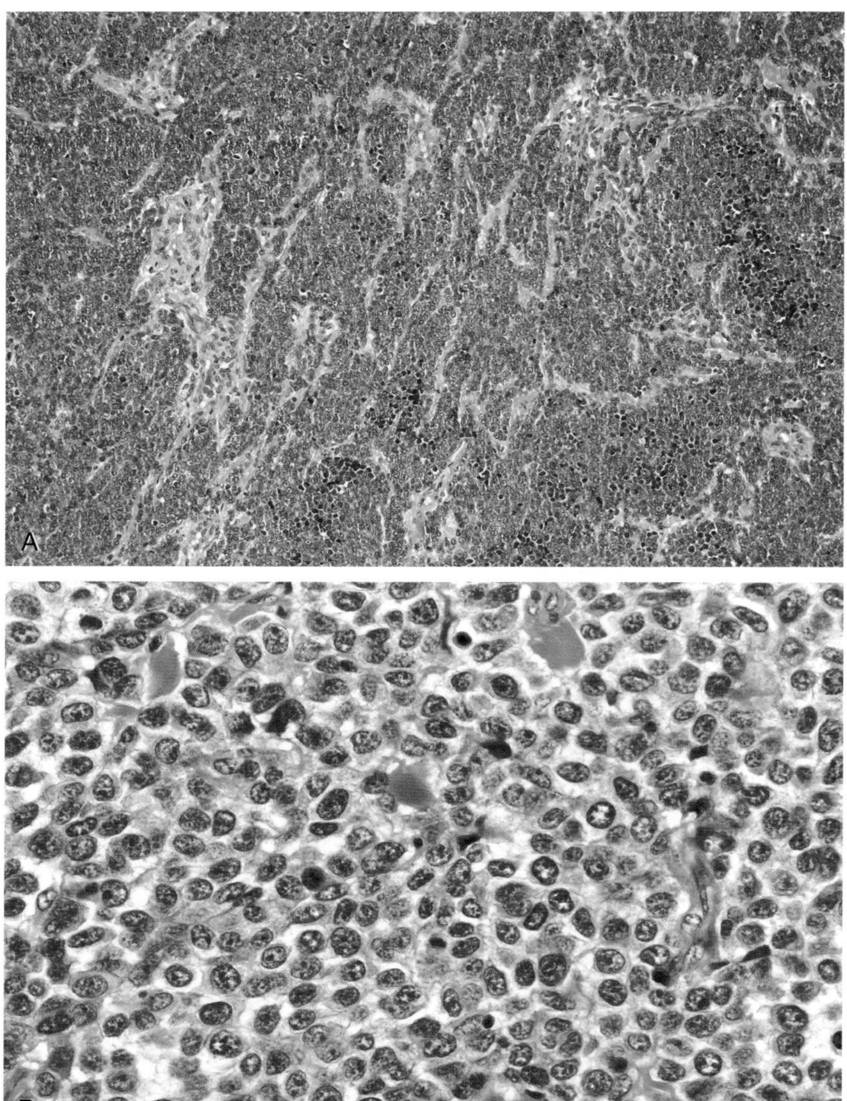

FIGURE 20-26. (A) Low-power view of a solid variant of alveolar rhabdomyosarcoma. Although the characteristic alveolar structures are not present, cellular nests are still separated by fibrovascular septa, characteristic of this tumor. (B) High-power view of a solid variant of alveolar rhabdomyosarcoma. The cytologic features are identical to those of the usual type of alveolar rhabdomyosarcoma. Cells are round with large nuclei and little cytoplasm.

examination of the solid tumor shows, in addition to the uniform cellular pattern, incipient alveolar features. Even in the solid areas, there is a regular arrangement of fibrous septa that surround the primitive round cells. There are also rare cases in which the cells have abundant pale-staining, glycogen-containing cytoplasm and vaguely resemble clear cell carcinoma or clear cell malignant melanoma (*clear cell rhabdomyosarcoma*).[82,83]

The individual cells in both alveolar and solid portions of the tumor have round or oval hyperchromatic nuclei with scant amounts of indistinct cytoplasm. Bulbous or club-shaped cells, sometimes with deeply eosinophilic cytoplasm, are often seen protruding from the fibrous walls into the lumen of the alveolar spaces. Mitotic figures are common. Neoplastic rhabdomyoblasts with pronounced stringy or granular eosinophilic cytoplasm are less common in alveolar than in embryonal rhabdomyosarcomas and are present in no more than 30% of cases. Most of the rhabdomyoblasts in the alveolar spaces have a round or oval configuration (Fig. 20-27); those located in or attached to the fibrous septa tend to be strap-shaped or spindle-shaped. If cross-striations are present, they are almost exclusively found in the spindle-shaped cells.

Multinucleated giant cells are a prominent and diagnostically important feature (Figs. 20-28 and 20-29). Usually, the giant cells have multiple, peripherally placed nuclei and pale-staining or weakly eosinophilic cytoplasm, without cross-striations. Transitional forms between rhabdomyoblasts and giant cells suggest that the latter are formed by cellular fusion. Collagen formation is usually confined to the intervening septa, but, occasionally, large portions of the tumor are obliterated by extensive fibroplasia. Some cases have areas that are indistinguishable from conventional embryonal rhabdomyosarcoma, but such cases should be classified as alveolar rhabdomyosarcomas for prognostic and therapeutic purposes.

Most alveolar rhabdomyosarcomas originate in muscle tissue, and entrapment of normal muscle fibers is common. These fibers are apt to be mistaken for neoplastic rhabdomyoblasts with cross-striations, a feature that sometimes results in the correct diagnosis for the wrong reason.

Metastatic alveolar rhabdomyosarcomas in lymph nodes, lung, and other viscera also display a distinct alveolar pattern (Fig. 20-30), making it unlikely that this pattern is merely the result of infiltrative growth along the fibrous framework of the involved musculature. Diffuse bone marrow metastases may be mistaken for leukemia.[84]

The immunoprofile of alveolar rhabdomyosarcoma is similar to that of other rhabdomyosarcomas. Because the differential diagnosis includes numerous other small round cell tumors, a large battery of immunostains is often required to exclude other entities, as discussed later in the chapter.

Alveolar rhabdomyosarcoma is characterized by distinctive cytogenetic abnormalities that allow its distinction from other rhabdomyosarcoma subtypes and other round cell neoplasms

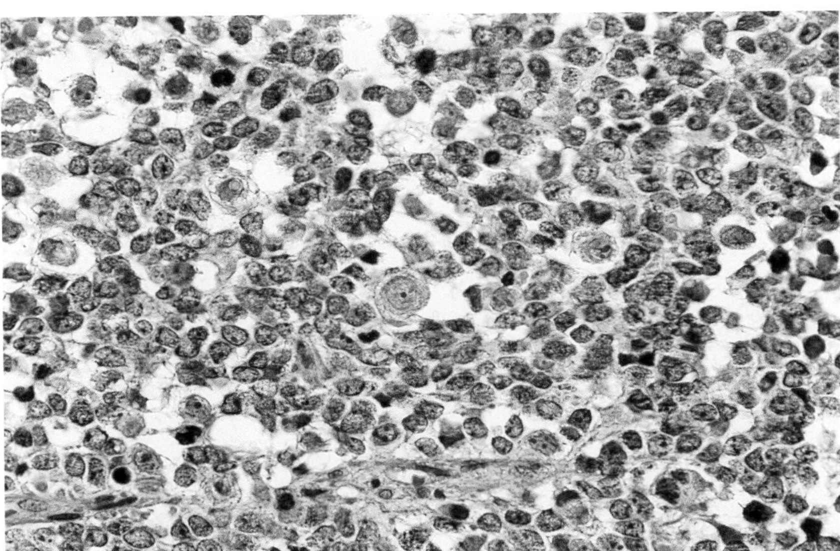

FIGURE 20-27. High-power view of an alveolar rhabdomyosarcoma with rare rhabdomyoblasts.

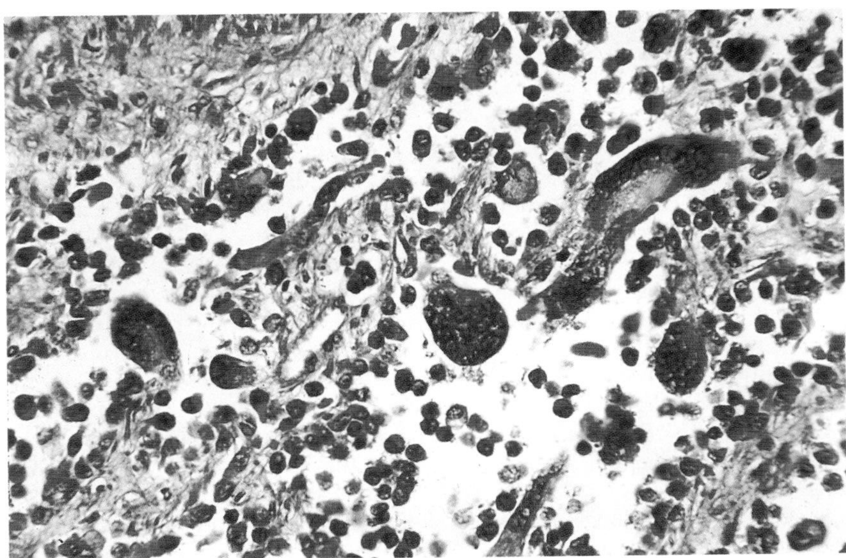

FIGURE 20-28. Multinucleated giant cells in an alveolar rhabdomyosarcoma.

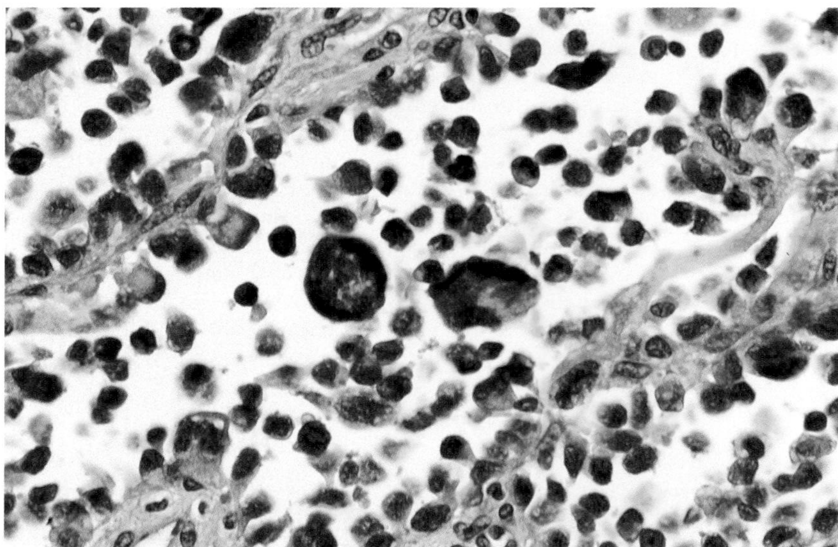

FIGURE 20-29. Alveolar rhabdomyosarcoma with multinucleated giant cells. These cells have peripherally placed wreath-like nuclei and are usually free-floating in alveolar structures.

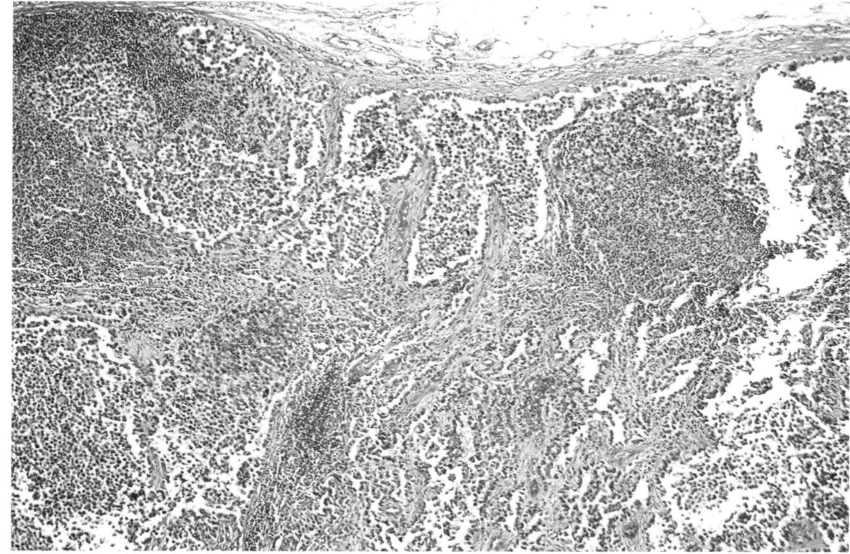

FIGURE 20-30. Metastatic alveolar rhabdomyosarcoma to a lymph node. The alveolar pattern is present in the metastasis as well.

in the differential diagnosis. Approximately 60% of cases have a t(2;13)(q35;q14) translocation, which results in the generation of two derivative chromosomes: a shortened chromosome 13 and an elongated chromosome 2.[85,86] The breakpoints occur within the *PAX3* gene on chromosome 2 and the *FOXO1A* gene (formerly known as *FKHR*) on chromosome 13, resulting in a *PAX3-FOXO1A* fusion gene on chromosome 13 and a *FOXO1A-PAX3* fusion gene on chromosome 2.[87] Both of these genes encode transcription factors that regulate the expression of specific target genes. The chimeric gene that results from this translocation encodes for a chimeric protein that acts as an aberrant transcription factor that excessively activates expression of genes with *PAX3* binding sites, including *MCYN*.[88,89] The *PAX3-FOXO1A* fusion appears to be more sensitive and specific than the *FOXO1A-PAX3* fusion in detecting this tumor.[90]

Approximately 20% of alveolar rhabdomyosarcomas are associated with a variant translocation, t(1;13)(p36;q14), which juxtaposes the *PAX7* gene on 1p36 with the *FOXO1A* gene on 13q14.[91-93] There is a high degree of homology between *PAX3* and *PAX7*, and it is likely that the fusion proteins that result from the translocations involving these genes aberrantly regulate a common set of target genes involved in the pathogenesis of alveolar rhabdomyosarcoma. In addition to cytogenetic examination, these molecular abnormalities can be detected by reverse transcriptase-polymerase chain reaction (also recognized as RT-PCR) or fluorescence in situ hybridization (FISH) using either frozen or paraffin-embedded tissues with a high degree of specificity.[94-99] Overall, about 80% of tumors diagnosed histologically as alveolar rhabdomyosarcoma are found to have the *PAX3-FOXO1A* or *PAX7-FOXO1A* fusions (Table 20-5).

TABLE 20-5 Frequency of PAX3-FOXO1A and PAX7-FOXO1A Fusion Transcripts in Alveolar and Embryonal Rhabdomyosarcomas

	ALVEOLAR		EMBRYONAL	
Study	PAX3-FOXO1A	PAX7-FOXO1A	PAX3-FOXO1A	PAX7-FOXO1A
Barr[99]	16/21 (76%)	2/21 (10%)	1/30 (3%)	1/30 (3%)
De Alava[97]	7/13 (54%)	2/13 (15%)	0/9 (0%)	0/9 (0%)
Downing[98]	20/23 (87%)		2/12 (17%)	
Arden[96]	8/13 (62%)	1/13 (8%)	0/11 (0%)	0/11 (0%)
Total	51/70 (73%)	5/47 (11%)	3/62 (5%)	1/50 (2%)

Therefore, approximately 20% of cases diagnosed histologically as alveolar subtype lack either of these fusions[85,100]; although some of these fusion-negative cases could be low expressors in which the fusion is actually present in rare cells only, or there are cryptic genomic fusions that cannot be detected by standard techniques. In addition, some cases of fusion-negative alveolar rhabdomyosarcoma are incorrectly classified, but it is clear that there are true fusion-negative tumors.[85,93] In a review of a large group of alveolar rhabdomyosarcomas blinded to fusion status, Parham et al.[93] found that histologic parameters were of limited utility in predicting fusion status. However, almost half of the fusion-negative cases had a totally solid architecture (versus none with a *PAX3-FOXO1A* and only rare *PAX7-FOXO1A* fusions). Nishio et al.[101] found some of these true fusion-negative cases to have a mixed histology with both alveolar and embryonal areas. Interestingly, gene expression array analyses have found distinct differences between fusion-positive and fusion-negative cases[57,102]; in fact, the fusion-negative cases show overlap with cases classified as embryonal rhabdomyosarcoma.[64]

Recently, several studies have implicated fibroblast growth factor receptor genes (*FGFR4* and *FGFR1*) in the pathogenesis of alveolar rhabdomyosarcoma.[65,103-106] Using array-comparative genomic hybridization, Williamson et al.[64] found amplification of *FGFR1* in 11% of fusion-negative alveolar rhabdomyosarcomas as well as 6% of embryonal rhabdomyosarcomas. Several other rare fusions have been reported, including a t(2;2)(p23;q53) resulting in a *PAX3-NCOA1* fusion and a t(2;8)(q35;q13) resulting in a *PAX3-NCOA2* fusion.[107]

Pleomorphic Rhabdomyosarcoma

Pleomorphic rhabdomyosarcoma is a rare variant of rhabdomyosarcoma that almost always arises in adults older than 45 years of age.[108-110] Given its extreme rarity in children,[111] this subtype was not included in the ICR. The concept of pleomorphic rhabdomyosarcoma has changed considerably since its inclusion in the Horn and Enterline[22] classification scheme reported in 1958. One-third of the 39 tumors in their study were designated as pleomorphic rhabdomyosarcomas, most of which arose in the deep soft tissues of the extremities of adults. Studies published in the 1960s described the clinical and pathologic features of pleomorphic rhabdomyosarcoma,[112] and this tumor was reported to account for between 9% and 14% of all soft tissue sarcomas.[1] However, with the emergence of the concept of malignant fibrous histiocytoma, many pleomorphic rhabdomyosarcomas were subsequently reclassified as storiform-pleomorphic variants of malignant fibrous histiocytoma,[113] and so pleomorphic rhabdomyosarcoma became regarded as rare or nonexistent.[113,114] Subsequently, with the advent of immunohistochemistry and refinement in recognizing tumors with skeletal muscle differentiation, studies confirmed the existence of pleomorphic rhabdomyosarcoma and delineated criteria by which this sarcoma could be distinguished from other pleomorphic sarcomas.[115,116]

Most of these tumors arise in adults with a peak incidence in the fifth decade of life, with a predilection for males. The tumor most commonly arises in the skeletal muscle of the extremities, particularly the thigh. Less commonly, these tumors arise in the abdomen/retroperitoneum, chest/abdominal wall, spermatic cord/testes, and upper extremities.[108] Rare examples have been reported in the uterus,[117] larynx,[118] and even the kidney.[119] Most present with a rapidly growing, painless mass of several months' duration.

The tumor is usually large (greater than 10 cm), and most are fleshy, well-circumscribed, intramuscular masses with focal hemorrhage and extensive necrosis. Histologically, pleomorphic rhabdomyosarcoma can be distinguished from embryonal and alveolar rhabdomyosarcoma by the association of loosely arranged, haphazardly oriented, large, round or pleomorphic cells with hyperchromatic nuclei and deeply eosinophilic cytoplasm (Figs. 20-31 and 20-32). As in embryonal rhabdomyosarcomas, there are racket-shaped and tadpole-shaped rhabdomyoblasts, but they are generally larger with more irregular outlines. Cells with cross-striations are commonly found in embryonal rhabdomyosarcomas with focal pleomorphic features[55] but are rare in adult pleomorphic rhabdomyosarcomas.[108] The tumor cells may be arranged in a haphazard pattern, but arrangement in a storiform pattern or a fascicular pattern reminiscent of leiomyosarcoma may be present (Fig. 20-33). The most helpful light microscopic feature suggesting this diagnosis is the presence of large bizarre tumor cells with deeply eosinophilic cytoplasm with some cell-to-cell molding (Fig. 20-34). Rare lesions have cells with a rhabdoid morphology characterized by the presence of a peripherally located vesicular nucleus, with a prominent nucleolus and an intracytoplasmic eosinophilic hyaline inclusion.[109] Other features include phagocytosis by tumor cells, the presence of intracytoplasmic glycogen, and a moderately dense lymphohistiocytic infiltrate. When primitive round cell areas are present, the diagnosis of pleomorphic rhabdomyosarcoma should be called into question, and a diagnosis of an alveolar variant should be strongly considered.

Ancillary techniques are required to confirm the diagnosis of pleomorphic rhabdomyosarcoma. Immunohistochemical detection of sarcomeric differentiation using antibodies to desmin (Fig. 20-35), muscle-specific actin, sarcomeric α-actin, MyoD1, and myogenin is essential in recognizing pleomorphic rhabdomyosarcoma and its distinction from other adult pleomorphic soft tissue sarcomas.[120-122] However, Furlong et al.[108] reported sensitivities of MyoD1 and myogenin of only 53% and 56%, respectively, in cases of pleomorphic rhabdomyosarcoma. This discrepancy may be related to differences in antibodies and antigen retrieval techniques.[123]

By cytogenetics, pleomorphic rhabdomyosarcoma does not have any characteristic aberration, and most have a highly complex karyotype.[124] In a study of 46 pleomorphic sarcomas

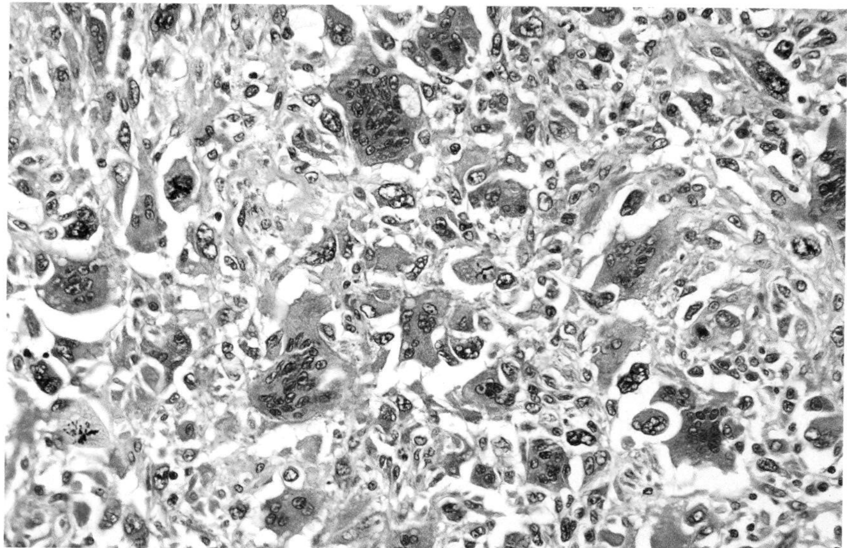

FIGURE 20-31. Pleomorphic rhabdomyosarcoma. This tumor was found in the deep soft tissues of the thigh in a 69-year-old man.

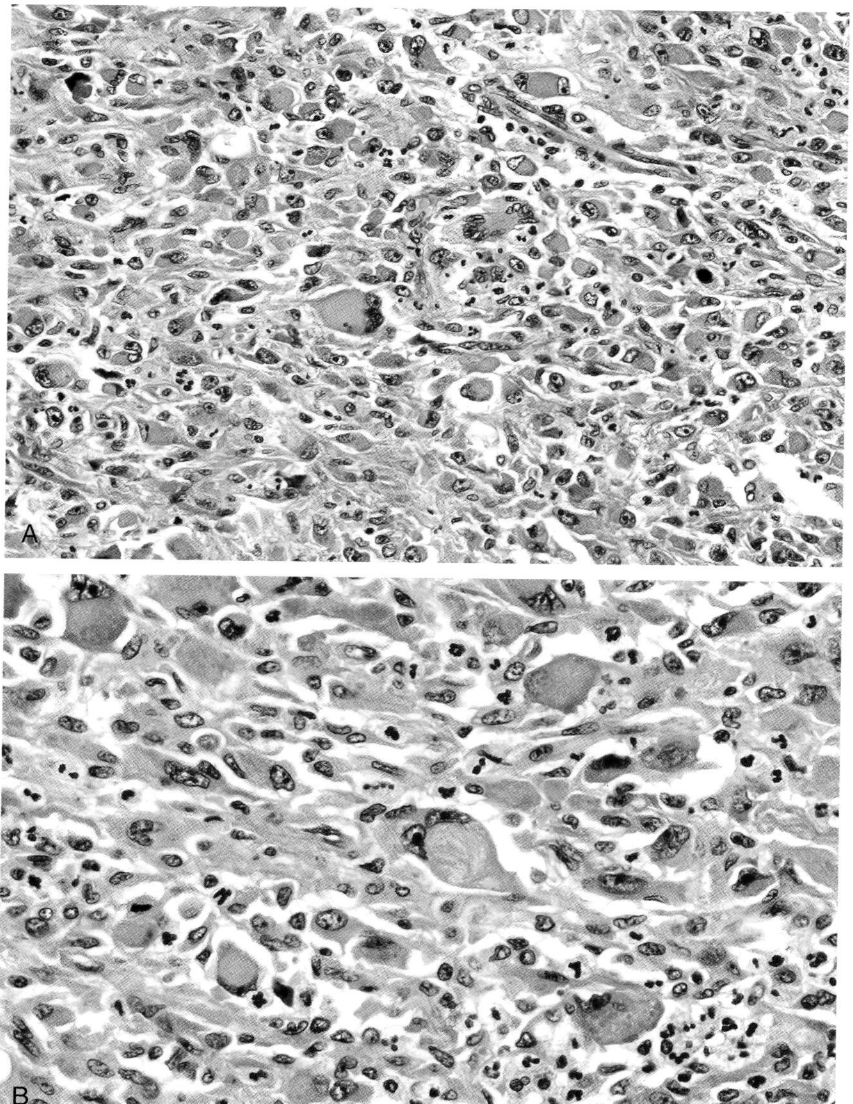

FIGURE 20-32. (A) Pleomorphic rhabdomyosarcoma composed predominantly of spindle-shaped cells with scattered large cells containing deeply eosinophilic cytoplasm. (B) Large cells with eosinophilic stringy cytoplasm in a pleomorphic rhabdomyosarcoma.

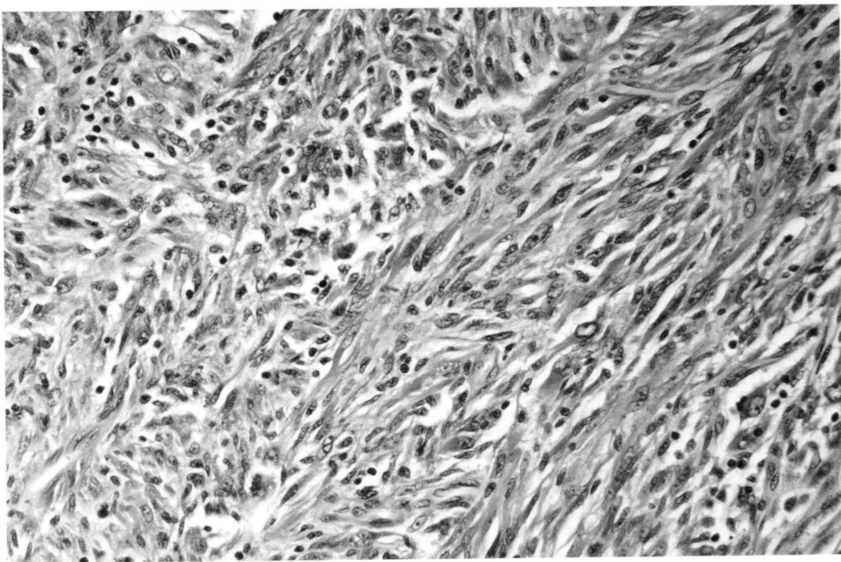

FIGURE 20-33. Pleomorphic rhabdomyosarcoma composed of spindle-shaped cells arranged in a fascicular pattern reminiscent of leiomyosarcoma.

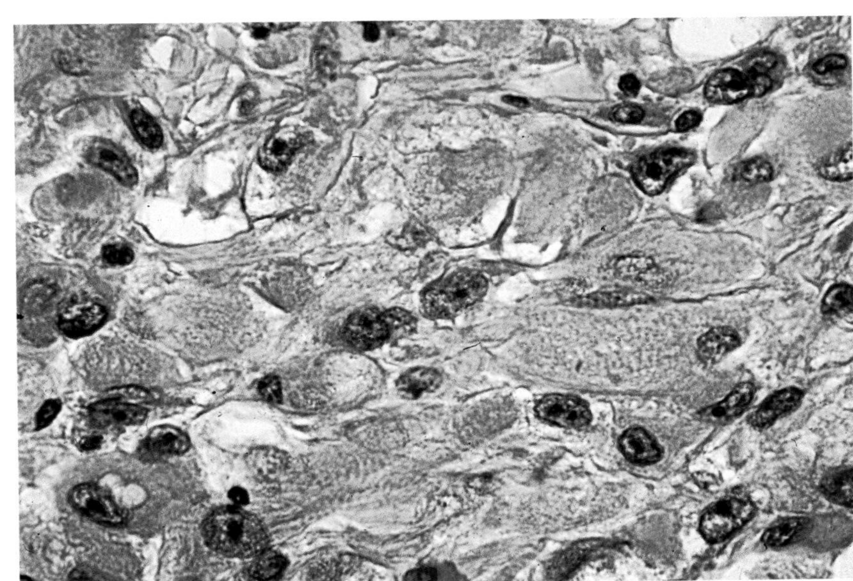

FIGURE 20-34. Unusual pleomorphic rhabdomyosarcoma. This focus was composed of numerous cells with eosinophilic fibrillar cytoplasm and cross-striations. Other portions of this tumor more closely resembled undifferentiated pleomorphic sarcoma.

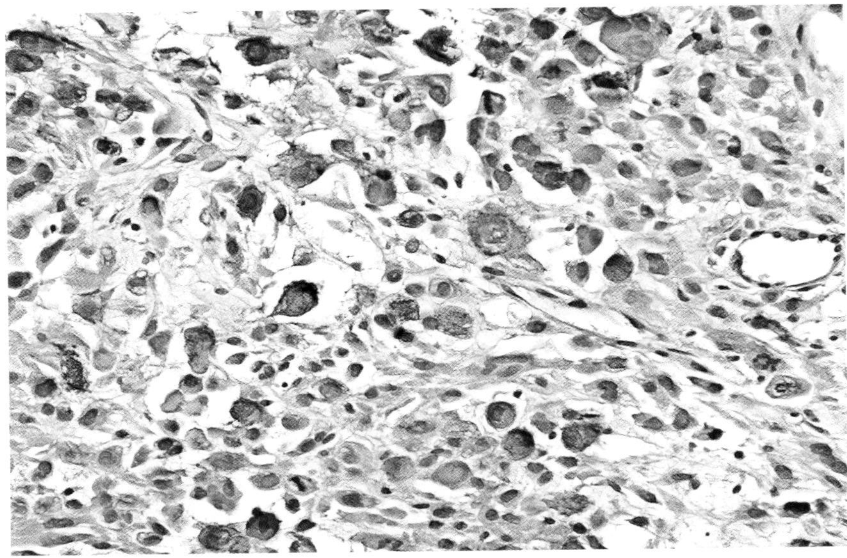

FIGURE 20-35. Desmin immunoreactivity in large eosinophilic cells in a pleomorphic rhabdomyosarcoma.

by Mertens et al.[125] from the CHAMP Study Group, karyotyping was not found to be useful in determining the line of differentiation in pleomorphic sarcomas.

The differential diagnosis includes a variety of other pleomorphic sarcomas and many other tumors that may simulate a pleomorphic sarcoma. First, pleomorphic rhabdomyosarcoma should be distinguished from the other rhabdomyosarcoma subtypes, all of which may have foci of pleomorphic cells. Adequate sampling of the latter usually reveals more typical areas of embryonal or alveolar rhabdomyosarcoma. Furthermore, pleomorphic rhabdomyosarcoma occurs in adults, whereas the other subtypes are seen mostly in children or adolescents. Pleomorphic rhabdomyosarcoma may be arranged in a fascicular growth pattern reminiscent of that seen in *pleomorphic leiomyosarcoma*. However, most cases of pleomorphic leiomyosarcoma have lower-grade areas that display a well-defined fascicular pattern composed of cells with typical smooth muscle features. Both tumors are immunoreactive for actin and desmin, but MyoD1 and myogenin are only present in pleomorphic rhabdomyosarcomas. These markers are also useful in distinguishing pleomorphic rhabdomyosarcoma from all other types of pleomorphic sarcoma, including undifferentiated pleomorphic sarcoma.

Like other pleomorphic sarcomas, pleomorphic rhabdomyosarcoma is a clinically aggressive neoplasm that frequently metastasizes early in its course.[110] In the series by Gaffney et al.,[109] seven of eight patients for whom follow-up information was available died of disease, including five patients within 8 months of diagnosis. The AFIP study reported that 70% of patients died of disease, with a mean survival of 20 months only.[108]

Sclerosing Rhabdomyosarcoma

In 2002, Folpe et al.[126] described four cases of an unusual hyalinizing, matrix-rich variant of rhabdomyosarcoma that could be easily confused with an osteosarcoma, chondrosarcoma, or angiosarcoma. All four of these tumors arose in adults whose ages ranged from 18 to 50 years, including three males and one female. These authors reported these lesions as sclerosing rhabdomyosarcomas, which they noted to be histologically similar, if not identical, to the two cases reported by Mentzel and Katenkamp[127] as sclerosing, pseudovascular rhabdomyosarcoma in adults. Subsequently, there have been several additional reports of sclerosing rhabdomyosarcoma that have contributed to an understanding of the clinical, histologic, and molecular genetic spectrum of this tumor.[120,128-130]

Clinically, sclerosing rhabdomyosarcoma does not appear to have a unique presentation because most patients present with a slowly enlarging mass. Although the four cases reported by Folpe et al.[126] arose in adults, subsequent reports have documented this tumor in children.[131,132] Chiles et al.[131] from the IRS reported 13 cases of sclerosing rhabdomyosarcoma in children and adolescents; these cases were identified from 1207 pediatric rhabdomyosarcomas. There are too few cases to determine whether there is a gender predilection.

Grossly, the tumor ranges in size from 3 cm to up to 8 cm. On gross examination, it is tan to yellow, rubbery in consistency, and typically infiltrates the surrounding soft tissues.

Histologically, sclerosing rhabdomyosarcoma has a characteristic constellation of features. The neoplastic cells are divided into lobules, small nests, microalveoli, and even single-file arrays by an abundantly hyalinized, eosinophilic to basophilic matrix that closely resembles primitive osteoid or chondroid material (Figs. 20-36 to 20-38). Overall, the tumors are usually of moderate cellularity and are composed of primitive-appearing nuclei with a small amount of eosinophilic cytoplasm, irregular nuclear contours, coarse nuclear chromatin, and small and, occasionally, multiple nucleoli. Wreath-like giant cells characteristic of alveolar rhabdomyosarcoma are not found. It is also unusual to identify rhabdomyoblasts, although strap cells may occasionally be seen. The

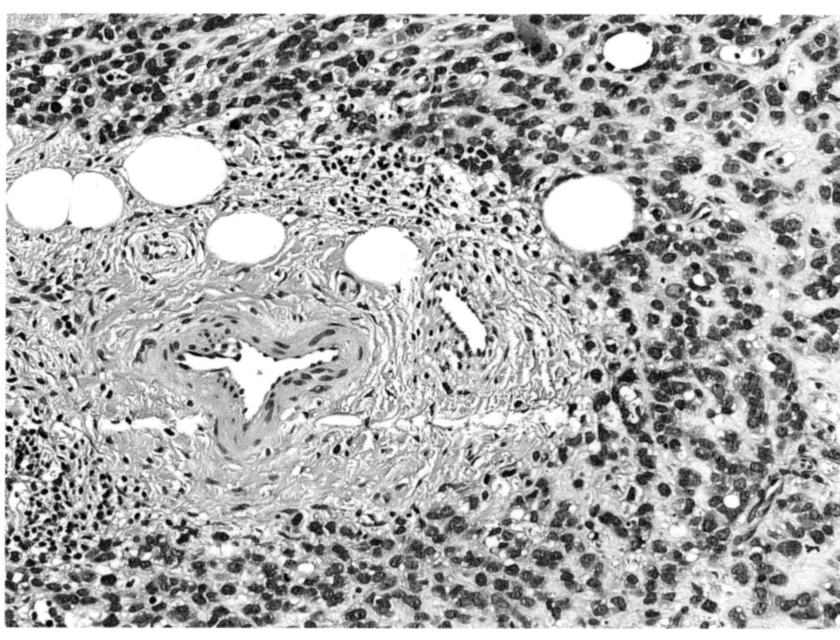

FIGURE 20-36. Sclerosing rhabdomyosarcoma composed of small nests and microalveoli of primitive round cells deposited in an abundantly hyalinized matrix.

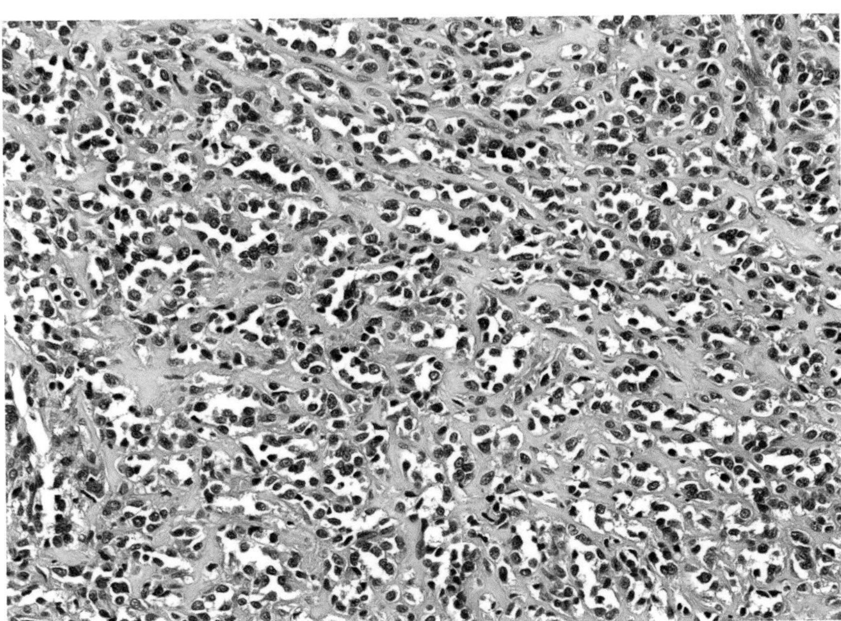

FIGURE 20-37. High-magnification view of sclerosing rhabdomyosarcoma composed of cords of primitive round cells arranged around a blood vessel and deposited in a densely hyalinized matrix.

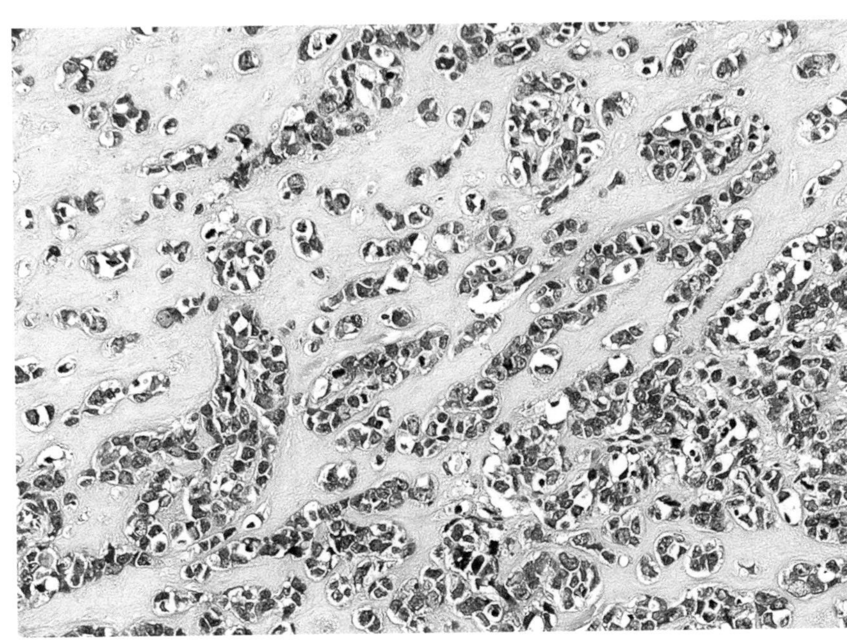

FIGURE 20-38. High-magnification view of sclerosing rhabdomyosarcoma.

mitotic rate is typically high. The hyalinized stroma is a dominant feature and often comprises up to 50% of the entire neoplasm. A number of cases have been described with pseudovascular features or with overlapping features of spindle cell rhabdomyosarcoma.[69,70,133,134]

The immunohistochemical features of this variant of rhabdomyosarcoma are somewhat unique. Folpe et al.[126] described focal and dot-like desmin staining in their four cases (Fig. 20-39), a pattern of desmin staining that is quite different from that seen in other variants of rhabdomyosarcoma. Although MyoD1 staining tends to be strong and diffuse (Fig. 20-40), myogenin staining is usually only focal and weak or completely negative.[135,136]

A small number of these lesions have been studied at the cytogenetic or molecular genetic level. At this point, there has generally been no evidence of *PAX* fusions as seen in alveolar rhabdomyosarcoma,[126,135] although Chiles et al.[131] did report a *PAX3-FOXO1A* fusion in one case. Kuhnen et al.[134] reported a unique case with pseudovascular features with loss of 10q22 and the Y chromosome and trisomy 18. Using whole genome genotyping by high-density single-nucleotide polymorphism (also known as SNP) analysis, Bouron-Dal Soglio et al.[137] found amplification of the 12q13-15 region with specific amplification of *MDM2* and *HMGA2*. Other reports indicate a complex, hyperdiploid karyotype with gains of a number of different chromosomes (2, 7 and 8, among

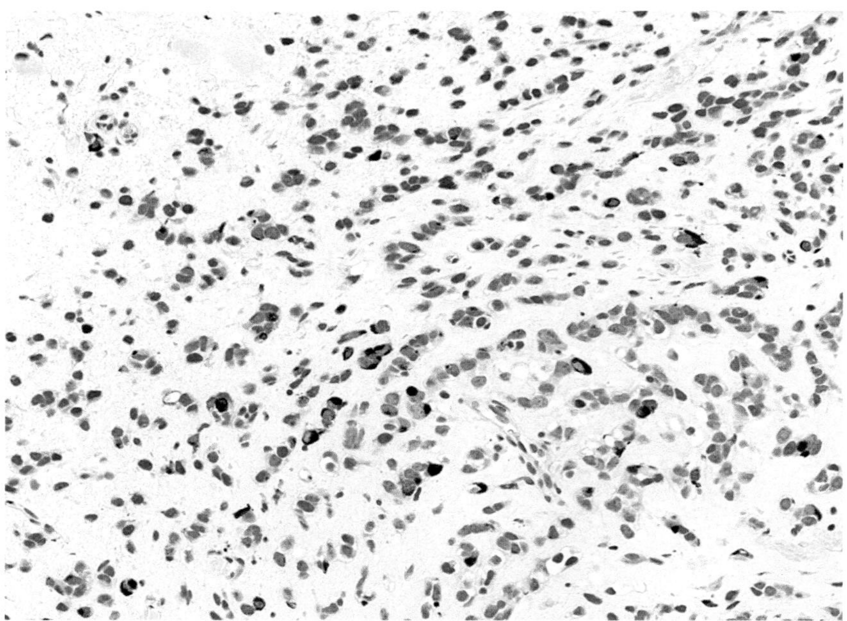

FIGURE 20-39. Peculiar pattern of desmin staining in sclerosing rhabdomyosarcoma.

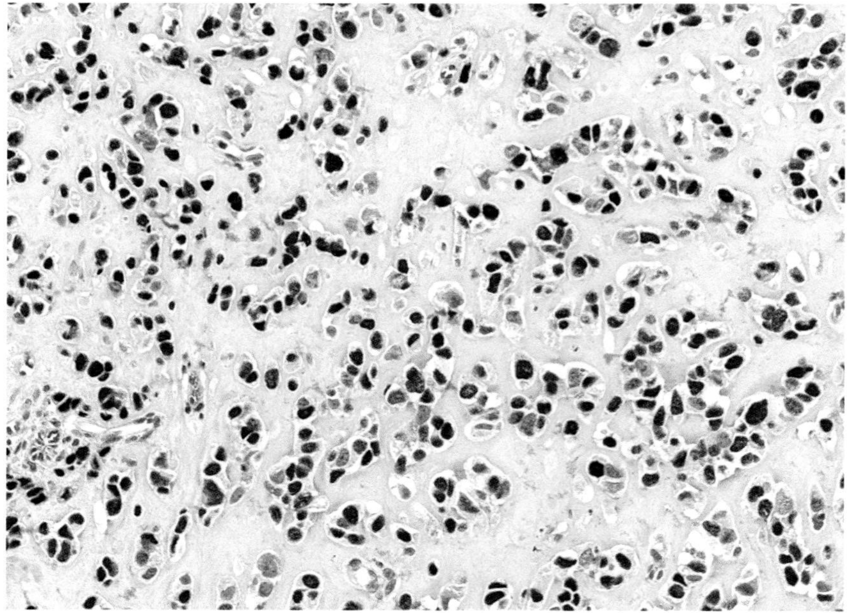

FIGURE 20-40. Strong nuclear staining for MyoD1 in sclerosing rhabdomyosarcoma.

others), similar to the complex karyotype of embryonal rhabdomyosarcoma.[131,132,138]

The exact relationship between sclerosing rhabdomyosarcoma and embryonal or alveolar rhabdomyosarcoma is uncertain. From a morphologic standpoint, sclerosing rhabdomyosarcoma does share some overlapping features with alveolar rhabdomyosarcoma. However, sclerosing rhabdomyosarcoma lacks well-formed alveoli and the wreath-like giant cells characteristic of alveolar rhabdomyosarcoma. An obvious difference is the more extensive hyalinized matrix as opposed to the fibrovascular septa of alveolar rhabdomyosarcoma. Immunohistochemically, alveolar rhabdomyosarcoma virtually always shows strong nuclear staining for myogenin.[139-142] In contrast, sclerosing rhabdomyosarcoma displays much stronger immunoreactivity for MyoD1 and only focal nuclear staining for myogenin.[143] As mentioned, only one case has ever been documented to harbor a *PAX* fusion.[131] A number of authors have suggested that sclerosing rhabdomyosarcoma is an unusual variant of embryonal rhabdomyosarcoma or possibly even a new subtype of rhabdomyosarcoma.

The differential diagnosis includes *sclerosing osteosarcoma*, although the latter can be distinguished from sclerosing rhabdomyosarcoma by virtue of matrix calcification, the frequent presence of osteoclasts, the typical coexistence of other patterns of osteosarcoma, and the epithelioid morphology of the osteoblasts. *Extraskeletal myxoid chondrosarcoma* is composed of cords and chains of eosinophilic cells deposited in a myxoid matrix and lacks the densely hyalinized matrix of sclerosing rhabdomyosarcoma. *Mesenchymal chondrosarcoma* shows an admixture of primitive round cells and nodules of well-differentiated cartilage, often with a prominent hemangiopericytoma-like vascular pattern. Cases of sclerosing rhabdomyosarcoma showing cords of cells embedded in a hyalinized stroma may also simulate *sclerosing epithelioid fibrosarcoma*. However, the latter usually shows at least focal areas of typical fibrosarcoma or low-grade fibromyxoid sarcoma. Immunohistochemical analysis is extremely useful in distinguishing sclerosing rhabdomyosarcoma from *angiosarcoma* because the latter typically shows strong membranous CD31 and nuclear ERG immunoreactivity and an absence of staining for MyoD1 and myogenin.

Epithelioid Rhabdomyosarcoma

In 2011, Jo et al.[144] described 16 cases of a distinct form of rhabdomyosarcoma composed of a sheet of uniformly sized epithelioid cells and abundant amphophilic to eosinophilic cytoplasm that arose in the deep soft tissues of elderly patients and pursued an aggressive clinical course (Fig. 20-41). Similar cases had been previously described by others and included in a larger series of unusual rhabdomyosarcoma.[145-148]

Clinically, the patients in the series by Jo et al.[144] ranged in age from 14 to 78 years with a median age of 70.5 years. Men outnumbered women by 2 to 1. Most of the cases arose in the deep soft tissues of the upper or lower extremities, head and neck, or trunk. Two patients presented with nodal metastases of unknown primary. The tumors ranged in size from 3 to 8.5 cm and had a nodular fleshy cut surface with necrosis and

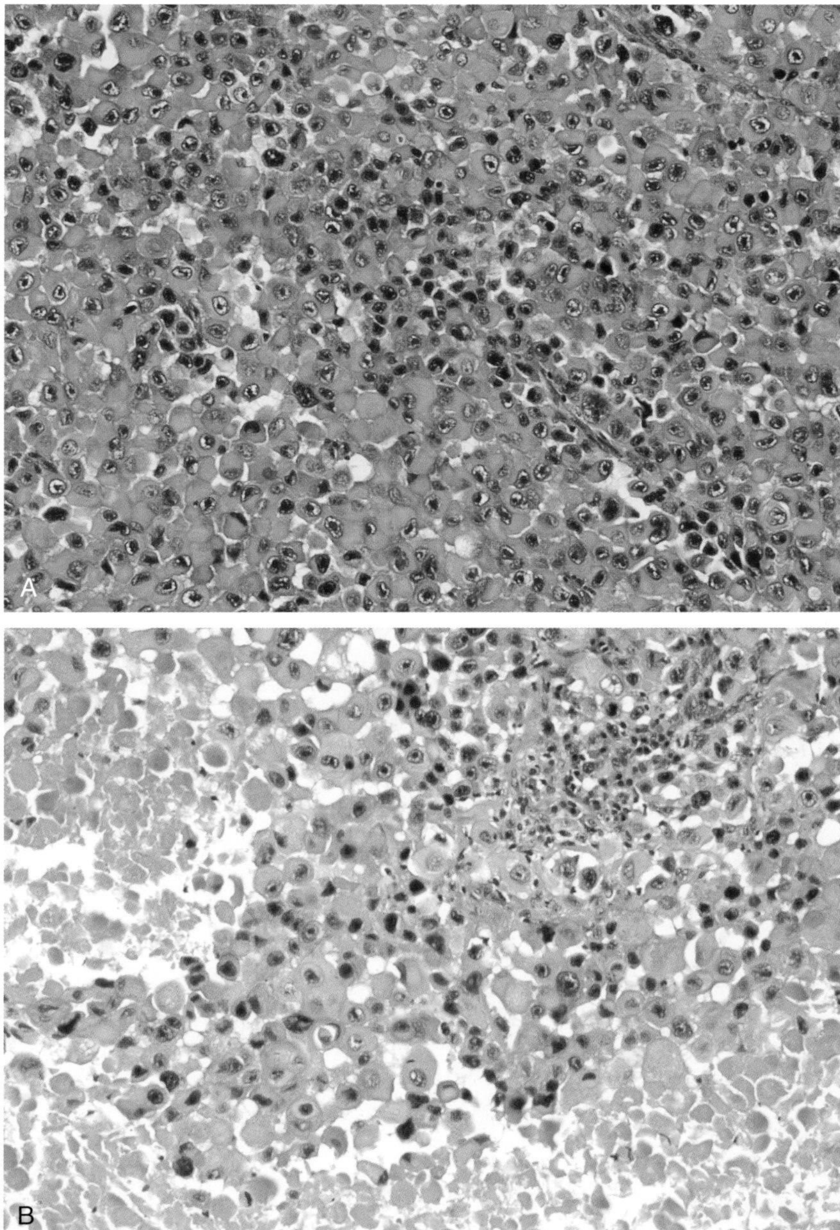

FIGURE 20-41. (A) Epithelioid rhabdomyosarcoma. Sheet-like proliferation of malignant epithelioid cells with prominent nucleoli and eosinophilic cytoplasm. (B) Necrotic focus surrounded by malignant epithelioid cells. *(Case courtesy of Dr. Hans Iwenofu, Ohio State University Medical Center, Columbus, OH.)*

infiltrative margins. Histologically, the neoplastic cells had large vesicular nuclei with prominent nucleoli and abundant cytoplasm that was usually densely eosinophilic, reminiscent of melanoma or poorly differentiated carcinoma (see Fig. 20-41; Fig. 20-42). The mitotic rates were consistently high (median: 23 per 10 high-power fields) with frequent atypical forms. Immunohistochemically, all showed evidence of myogenic differentiation with strong and diffuse desmin and consistent myogenin expression (Figs. 20-43 and 20-44), with an absence of S-100 protein and virtual absence of cytokeratin expression.

Most patients underwent surgical resection with chemotherapy and/or radiation therapy, although none were treated with rhabdomyosarcoma-specific protocols. Seven patients died of disease, all within 5 years of initial diagnosis; six patients developed regional lymph node metastases, and six patients developed distant metastases.

Too few cases of this subtype have been described to determine a relationship with other subtypes of rhabdomyosarcoma. None of the three cases tested by Jo et al.[144] had evidence of *FOXO1A* rearrangements by FISH. It is certainly likely that this variant has been underrecognized and misdiagnosed as

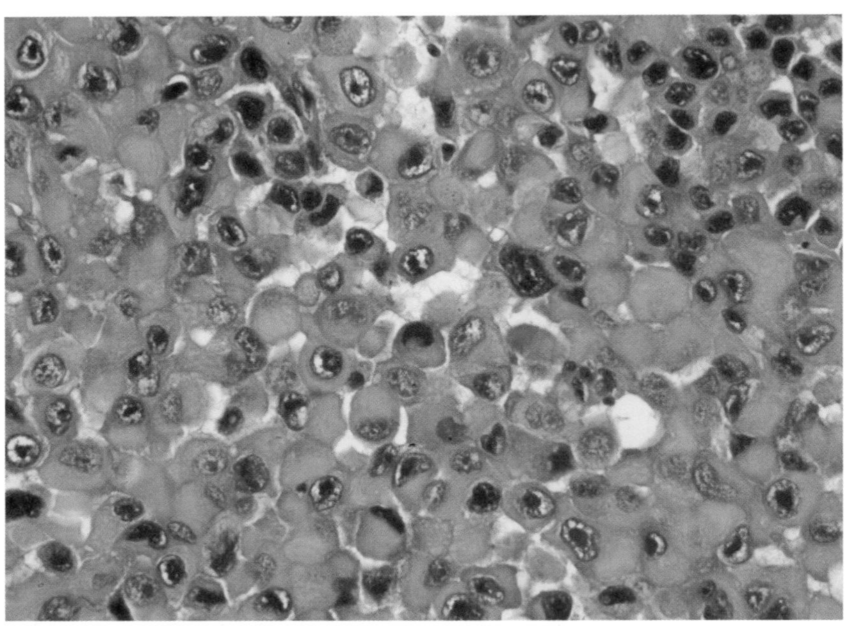

FIGURE 20-42. High-magnification view of neoplastic cells in epithelioid rhabdomyosarcoma. *(Case courtesy of Dr. Hans Iwenofu, Ohio State University Medical Center, Columbus, OH.)*

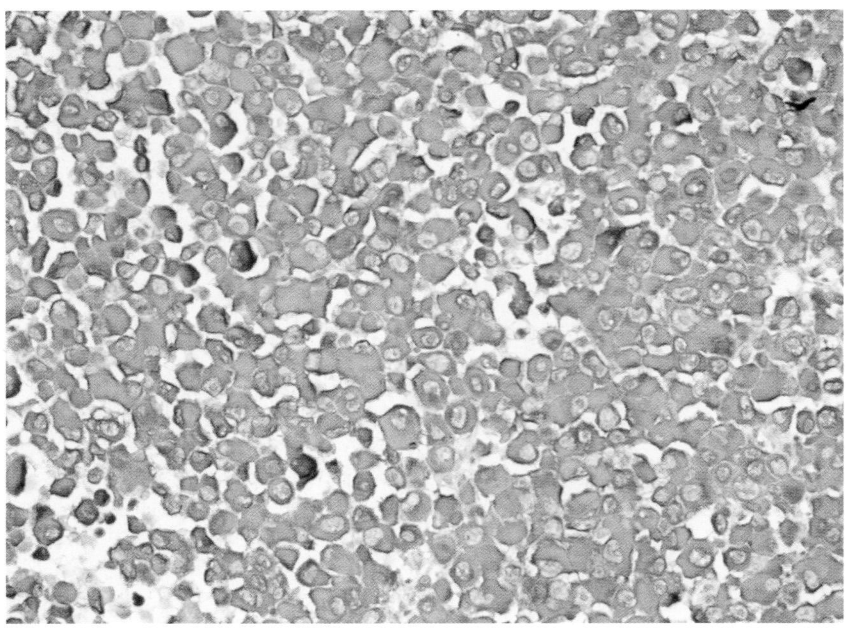

FIGURE 20-43. Strong and diffuse desmin staining in epithelioid rhabdomyosarcoma. *(Case courtesy of Dr. Hans Iwenofu, Ohio State University Medical Center, Columbus, OH.)*

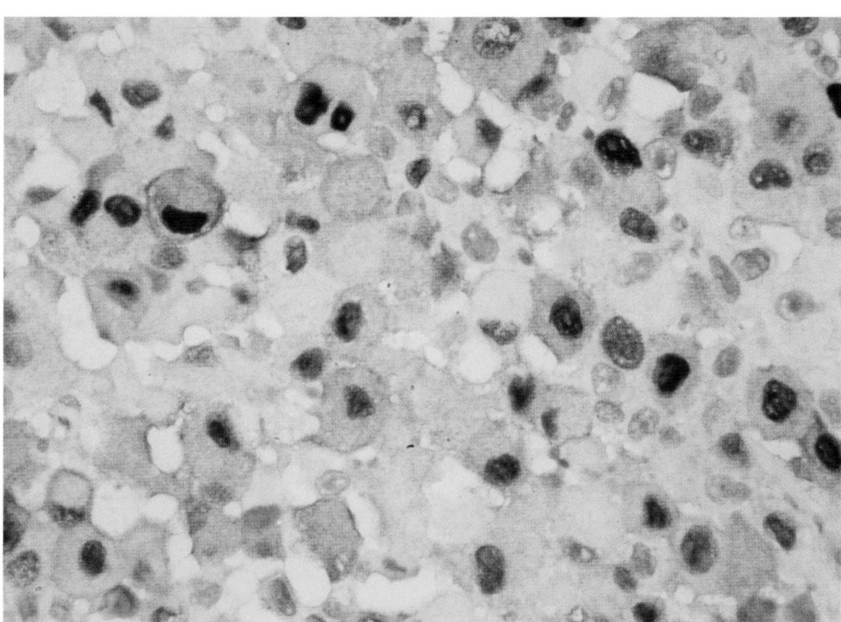

FIGURE 20-44. Nuclear myogenin staining in epithelioid rhabdomyosarcoma. *(Case courtesy of Dr. Hans Iwenofu, Ohio State University Medical Center, Columbus, OH.)*

some other type of pleomorphic sarcoma, melanoma, carcinoma, or undifferentiated malignant epithelioid neoplasm.

SPECIAL DIAGNOSTIC PROCEDURES FOR RHABDOMYOSARCOMA

Special Stains

Although many rhabdomyosarcomas can be diagnosed with routine sections, many poorly differentiated sarcomas masquerade as rhabdomyosarcomas (and vice versa), and ancillary diagnostic procedures are often essential for a reliable diagnosis. During the past three decades, conventional special stains, such as the periodic acid-Schiff (PAS) preparation or the Masson trichrome stain, have been essentially replaced by immunohistochemical procedures. Rhabdomyosarcomas contain considerable amounts of intracellular PAS-positive glycogen; in many tumors, the glycogen is irregularly distributed, and, as a rule, is much more conspicuous in well-differentiated than poorly differentiated tumor cells.

Immunohistochemical Findings

Many immunohistochemical markers have been applied to the diagnosis of rhabdomyosarcoma, but their diagnostic value, sensitivity, and specificity vary substantially. Of the various markers, antibodies against desmin (for the muscle type of intermediate filaments), muscle-specific actin (HHF35), and myoglobin have been the most widely used for diagnostic purposes.

Desmin is a reasonably sensitive marker of rhabdomyosarcoma (Fig. 20-45), although tumors composed predominantly of primitive cells may not stain for this antigen.[149] This marker is not useful for distinguishing rhabdomyosarcoma from leiomyosarcoma. Desmin is not entirely specific; it has been detected in a number of non-myogenic tumors, including rare tumors in the Ewing family of tumors, neuroblastoma, and malignant mesothelioma. Similarly, muscle-specific actin, although a sensitive marker of rhabdomyosarcoma, is expressed in the majority of leiomyosarcomas. This antigen is more resistant to formalin fixation than desmin but may also be negative in poorly differentiated rhabdomyosarcomas. Smooth muscle actin is an excellent marker of tumors with smooth muscle differentiation, but it may be found in up to 13% of rhabdomyosarcomas.[150]

Sarcomeric α-actin has also been reported to be a specific marker of rhabdomyosarcoma.[150] Monoclonal antibodies recognize both cardiac and skeletal α-actin; however, Schürch et al.[150] found that all variants of rhabdomyosarcoma express cardiac α-actin transcripts but not skeletal α-actin mRNA by Northern blot hybridization. Because cardiac α-actin is present in embryonic skeletal muscle, these authors suggested that rhabdomyosarcomas follow normal skeletal myogenesis but do not complete the final step of skeletal α-actin mRNA expression.

Myoglobin, although a specific marker of skeletal muscle tumors, is not particularly sensitive.[149] For example, Parham et al.[149] reported staining for myoglobin in only 17 (46%) of 37 formalin-fixed rhabdomyosarcomas. Furthermore, staining tends to be restricted to the more differentiated cells, and this antigen may also be detected in non-muscle cells as a result of diffusion.[151] This marker is not used in the evaluation of potential rhabdomyosarcomas.

Other somewhat less sensitive markers that have been used in the diagnosis of rhabdomyosarcoma include antibodies for fast, slow, and fetal myosin, creatine kinase (isoenzymes MM and BB), β-enolase, Z-protein, and titin.

Immunohistochemical expression of myoregulatory proteins has been found to be an excellent marker of all rhabdomyosarcoma subtypes, showing both high sensitivity and specificity (Table 20-6). MyoD1, which includes *myf-5* and *mrf-4-herculin/myf-6*, acts as a nodal point for the initiation of skeletal muscle differentiation by binding to enhancer sequences of muscle-specific genes.[152] These genes

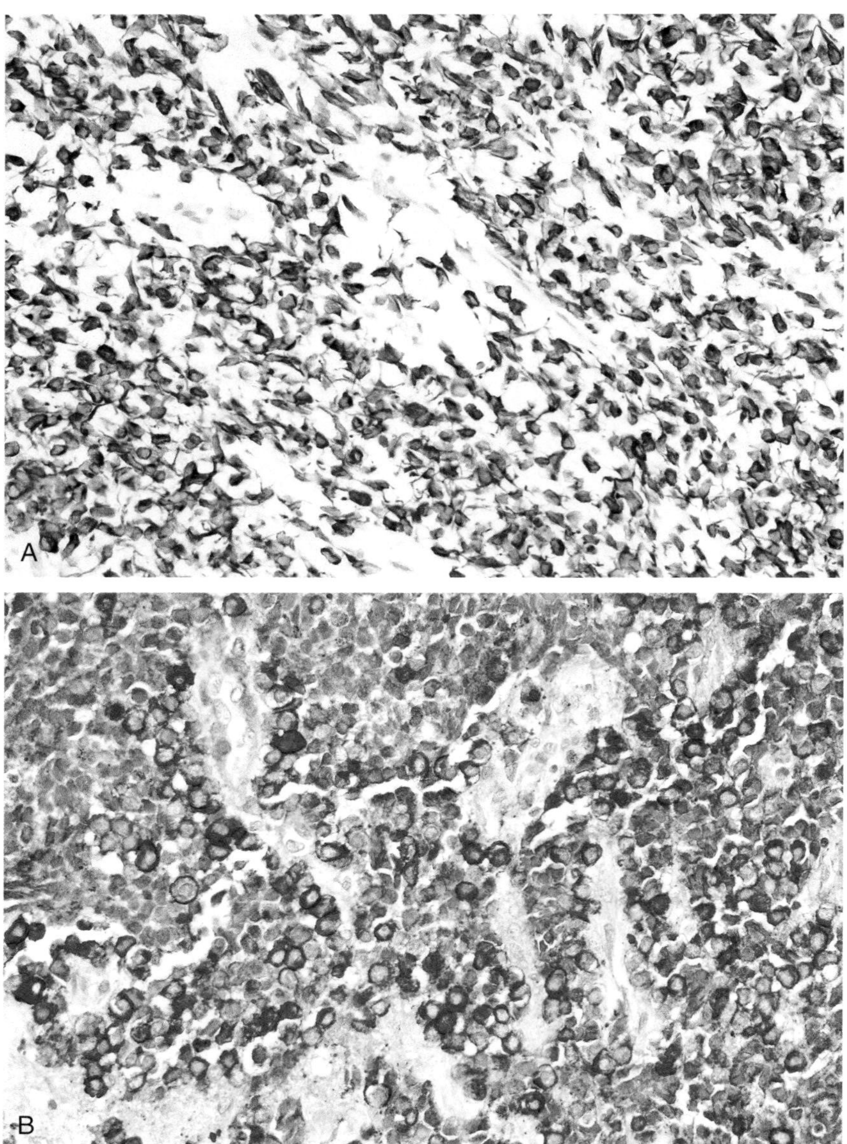

FIGURE 20-45. Diffuse, strong immunoreactivity for desmin in an embryonal rhabdomyosarcoma (A) and an alveolar rhabdomyosarcoma (B).

TABLE 20-6 Immunoreactivity for Myogenic Markers in Rhabdomyosarcoma and Other Pediatric Round Cell Tumors

TUMOR	MYOGENIN	MYOD1	ACTIN (HHF-35)	SARCOMERIC ACTIN	DESMIN	MYOGLOBIN
Rhabdomyosarcomas	30/33	30/33	30/33	21/33	33/33	8/28
Embryonal	22/25	23/25	22/25	18/25	25/25	6/20
Spindle cell	1/1	1/1	1/1	1/1	1/1	0/1
Alveolar	4/4	3/4	4/4	3/4	4/4	1/4
Pleomorphic	3/3	3/3	3/3	2/3	3/3	1/3
Ewing family of tumors	0/26	0/26	0/26	0/6	3/26	0/6
Neuroblastomas	0/12	0/12	0/12	0/12	0/12	0/12

Modified from Wang NP, Marx J, McNutt MA, et al. Expression of myogenic regulatory proteins (myogenin and MyoD1) in small blue round cell tumors of childhood. Am J Pathol 1995;147:1799.

are expressed at an early stage of skeletal muscle differentiation and are capable of converting multipotential murine fibroblasts into myoblasts.[153] Although originally detected using frozen tissues only, antigen retrieval techniques have allowed the detection of MyoD1 in formalin-fixed, paraffin-embedded tissues. Using formalin-fixed, paraffin-embedded tissues and antigen retrieval techniques, Wang et al.[120] detected nuclear expression of MyoD1 in 30 (91%) of 33 rhabdomyosarcomas, with no significant differences in sensitivity among the various histologic subtypes. Furthermore, none of the other round cell tumors tested demonstrated nuclear immunoreactivity for this antigen. These authors found a similar

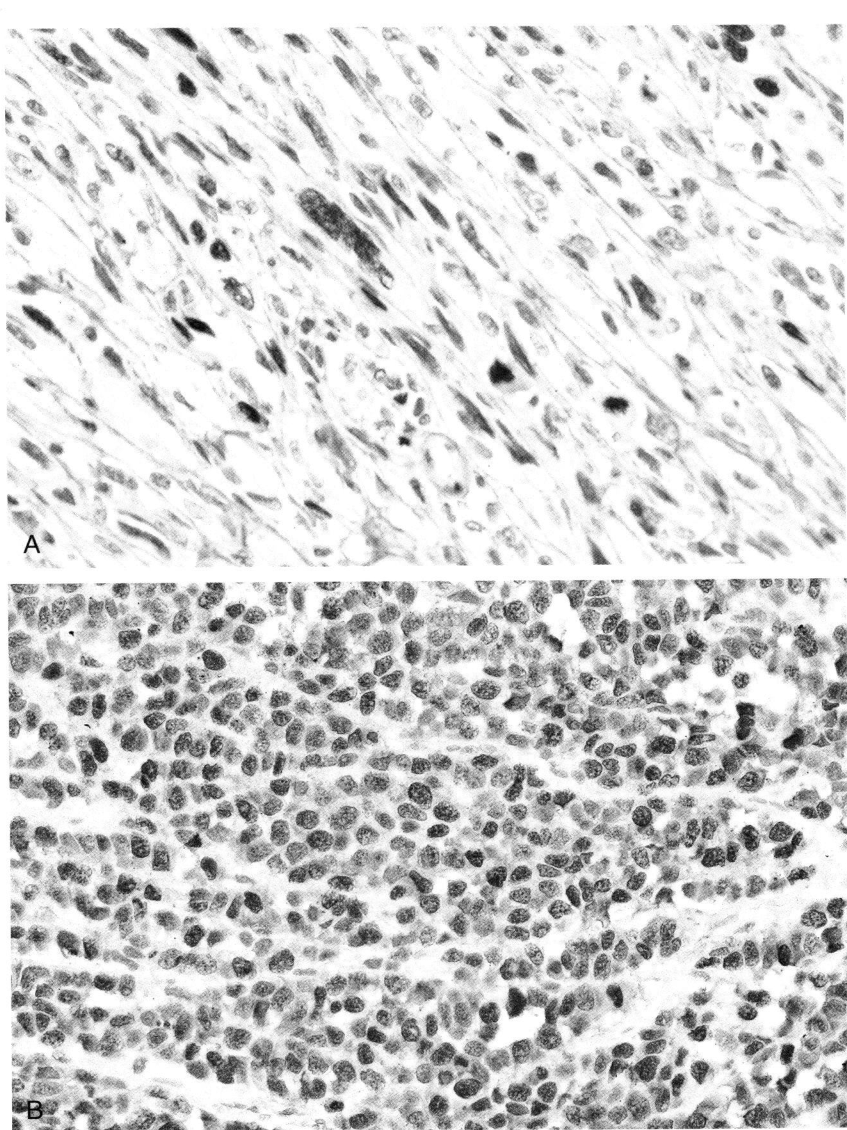

FIGURE 20-46. Nuclear staining for myogenin in an embryonal rhabdomyosarcoma (A) and an alveolar rhabdomyosarcoma (B).

percentage of lesions to stain with antibodies to myogenin. The antimyogenin antibody was found to have technical advantages over the anti-MyoD1 antibody in that there was an absence of non-specific cytoplasmic immunoreactivity, which was sometimes seen with the anti-MyoD1 antibody (Fig. 20-46). In this study, expression of both MyoD1 and myogenin was reciprocally related to the degree of cellular differentiation, with more primitive-appearing cells staining and decreased or absent immunoreactivity in large differentiated rhabdomyoblasts. In general, both myogenin and MyoD1 are expressed to a greater degree in alveolar rhabdomyosarcoma than embryonal subtypes.[142] In fact, a number of studies have found a much greater percentage of tumor cells to stain in alveolar versus embryonal cell types, with some suggesting that this pattern could be used to help distinguish these subtypes in difficult cases.[140] However, not all cases of alveolar rhabdomyosarcoma show diffuse, intense myogenin staining and, certainly, rare cases have been observed of embryonal rhabdomyosarcoma with this pattern of staining.[154] Recently, Heerema-McKenney et al.[155] found diffuse (greater than 80% of tumor cells) myogenin expression to be an independent marker of poor survival in pediatric rhabdomyosarcoma, regardless of histologic subtype, translocation status, tumor site, or stage.

PAX5 has recently been found to be a marker of alveolar rhabdomyosarcoma. As noted previously, the *PAX* gene family encodes for transcription factors critical to organogenesis, and translocations of this gene family are central to the pathogenesis of alveolar rhabdomyosarcoma. Sullivan et al.[156] found PAX5 immunoreactivity in 34 of 51 (67%) alveolar rhabdomyosarcomas, whereas none of the 55 embryonal rhabdomyosarcomas tested stained for this antigen. No other type of tumor stained, including neuroblastomas, lymphoblastic lymphomas, and the Ewing family of tumors. Of the cases with a known t(2;13) or t(1;13), all showed strong nuclear immunoreactivity for PAX5. In contrast, none of the fusion-negative cases stained for PAX5, although the number of cases tested was quite small. It is possible that this represents cross reactivity as opposed to true expression of this antigen.

Recent expression profiling studies have established newer markers of rhabdomyosarcoma that have also been associated with histologic subtype and fusion status. Wachtel et al.[157]

found coexpression of AP-2β and P-cadherin in fusion-positive alveolar rhabdomyosarcomas with a sensitivity and specificity of 64% and 98%, respectively. In contrast, coexpression of epidermal growth factor receptor (EGFR) and fibrillin-2 was found in embryonal rhabdomyosarcoma with a sensitivity and specificity of 60% and 90%, respectively. Coexpression of AP-2β and P-cadherin was associated with a significantly poorer outcome, whereas coexpression of EGFR and fibrillin-2 was associated with a significantly better outcome.

It should be noted that up to 50% of alveolar rhabdomyosarcomas stain for cytokeratins, including wide-spectrum cytokeratins and CAM5.2.[158] This certainly may contribute to difficulty in distinguishing this tumor from desmoplastic small round cell tumor and even the Ewing family of tumors, which themselves express cytokeratins in about 30% of cases.[159] Similarly, a number of different neuroendocrine markers may be expressed in alveolar rhabdomyosarcoma, including CD56 (almost ubiquitous), synaptophysin (up to 32%), and chromogranin A (up to 22%).[158] CD99 is expressed in some examples of alveolar rhabdomyosarcoma, leading to potential further confusion in its separation from the Ewing family of tumors.[160]

The ultrastructure of rhabdomyosarcoma bears a striking resemblance to that of embryonal muscle tissue in varying stages of development. The least differentiated cells contain only scattered or parallel bundles of thin (actin) myofilaments measuring 6 to 8 nm in diameter; this is a nonspecific finding that does not permit a reliable diagnosis of rhabdomyosarcoma; better-differentiated cells are characterized by distinct bundles of thick (myosin) filaments 12 to 15 nm in diameter, with attached ribosomes having an Indian-file arrangement (ribosome and myosin complex), a feature characteristic of rhabdomyoblastic differentiation. Further cellular maturation is marked by alternating thin (actin) and thick (myosin) filaments in a parallel arrangement, with a characteristic hexagonal pattern seen on cross sections and rod-like structures or disks composed of Z-band material. In many tumors, there are also well-differentiated rhabdomyoblasts with distinct sarcomeres, including the characteristic A and I banding and clearly discernible Z lines (Fig. 20-47).[161]

DIFFERENTIAL DIAGNOSIS OF RHABDOMYOSARCOMA

Poorly differentiated round and spindle cell sarcomas, especially in children or young adults, constitute the most common problem in differential diagnosis. Included in this group are neuroblastomas, Ewing family of tumors, poorly differentiated angiosarcomas, synovial sarcomas, malignant melanomas, melanotic neuroectodermal tumors of infancy, granulocytic sarcomas, and malignant lymphomas. Small cell carcinoma must also be considered when the tumor occurs in a patient older than 45 years. The differential diagnosis requires not only careful evaluation of clinical data, patient age, and tumor location, but also a painstaking examination of multiple sections for specific features such as rhabdomyoblasts, rosettes, biphasic cellular or vascular differentiation, and intracellular pigment, as well as immunohistochemical assessment with multiple markers and, possibly, cytogenetic/molecular testing.

Immunohistochemical analysis using a battery of stains is indispensable, including stains for muscle markers such as desmin, muscle-specific actin, and MyoD1 or myogenin. It must also be kept in mind that CD99, although a highly sensitive marker of the Ewing family of tumors, is sometimes detected in embryonal or alveolar rhabdomyosarcoma.[162]

Infantile rhabdomyofibrosarcoma is a rare tumor that resembles infantile fibrosarcoma but has ultrastructural and immunohistochemical evidence of rhabdomyoblastic differentiation. The spindle-shaped cells express desmin, smooth muscle actin, and sarcomeric actin; electron microscopy reveals fibroblastic and myofibroblastic features. The tumor shows cytogenetic alterations (monosomy 19 and monosomy

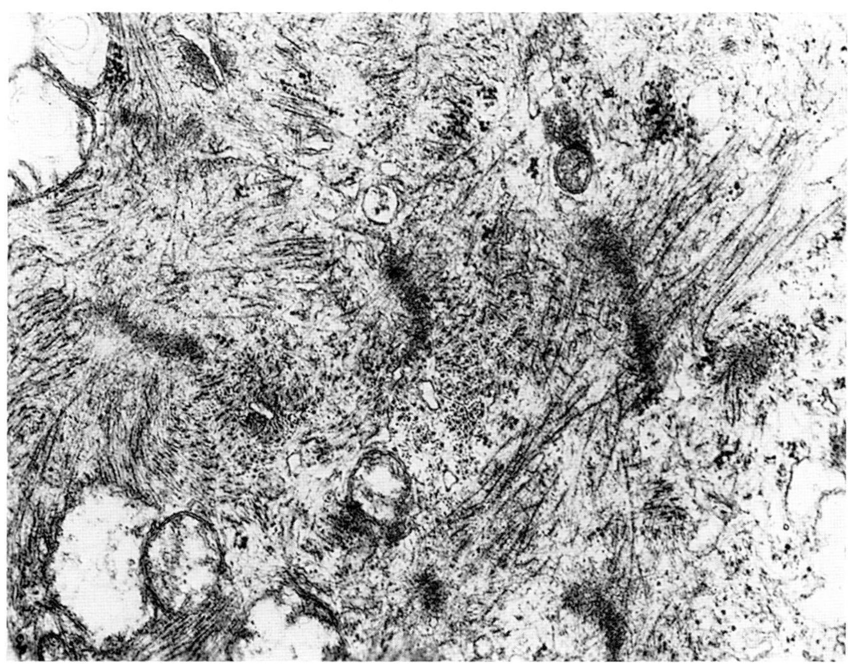

FIGURE 20-47. Ultrastructure of an embryonal rhabdomyosarcoma with a typical mixture of thick (myosin) and thin (actin) fibrils in longitudinal and cross section with distinct Z banding in several places.

22) distinct from those found in either infantile fibrosarcoma or embryonal or alveolar rhabdomyosarcoma.

Rhabdomyosarcoma with rhabdoid features is uncommon but well described.[145] These lesions have cells with cytoplasmic hyaline inclusions composed of intermediate filaments. A battery of immunostains, including stains for cytokeratins and myoregulatory proteins, is often necessary to distinguish this variant of rhabdomyosarcoma from other tumors with rhabdoid features, including *malignant extrarenal rhabdoid tumor*.

Problems in diagnosis may also be caused by benign reactive and neoplastic lesions such as polypoid cystitis, polyps and pseudosarcomatous myofibroblastic proliferations of the genitourinary tract, infectious granuloma, proliferative myositis, skeletal muscle regeneration, granular cell tumor, and fetal rhabdomyoma. Conversely, sparsely cellular botryoid-type rhabdomyosarcomas that were initially misinterpreted as *myxomas* have also been encountered. In these cases, consideration of age and location usually allows for the correct diagnosis because myxomas are virtually nonexistent in children and almost never occur in visceral organs.

Some tumors have *heterologous rhabdomyoblastic components*. Focal rhabdomyoblastic differentiation occurs in a variety of malignant neoplasms, including those with sarcomatous differentiation only, those with epithelial or germ cell elements, and tumors of neuroectodermal derivation (Box 20-5).[163] Identification of such elements may be obvious on light microscopic examination alone, but, in some cases, the use of immunohistochemistry is required to support rhabdomyoblastic differentiation. In addition, sarcomas with a propensity for undergoing dedifferentiation, including chondrosarcomas and liposarcomas, may have areas of divergent rhabdomyoblastic differentiation.[164]

Epithelial tumors may also exhibit rhabdomyoblastic differentiation, including malignant mixed mesodermal tumors of the uterus, cervix, or ovary, carcinosarcomas of the breast and stomach, pulmonary blastomas, nephroblastomas, and mixed-type hepatoblastomas. The rhabdomyoblastic component may even dominate the microscopic picture. Rhabdomyoblastic differentiation is also encountered in malignant or immature teratomas, but rarely as a major element. In most of these tumors, the rhabdomyoblastic component is accompanied by malignant epithelial and other mesenchymal elements such as cartilage and bone. Rare ovarian Sertoli-Leydig cell tumors contain heterologous rhabdomyoblastic foci.[165]

Last, rhabdomyoblastic elements may be found in various neuroectodermal neoplasms, including malignant peripheral nerve sheath tumor (so-called malignant Triton tumor), ganglioneuroma (ectomesenchymoma), medulloepithelioma, and medulloblastoma. Malignant peripheral nerve sheath tumors with rhabdomyoblastic differentiation chiefly occur in patients older than 30 years who have manifestations of neurofibromatosis.[166] Malignant ectomesenchymoma is primarily a tumor of children and is not known to be associated with neurofibromatosis; it consists of a mixture of rhabdomyoblastic elements, mature ganglion cells, and neuroma-like structures.[167] One case showed the initial tumor with features of an embryonal rhabdomyosarcoma, and the recurrent tumor was indistinguishable from a ganglioneuroma save for a few peripherally located groups of rhabdomyoblasts.

BOX 20-5 Tumors With Heterologous Rhabdomyoblastic Components

- Tumors with epithelial components
  - Carcinosarcoma (especially of breast, stomach, urinary bladder)
  - Malignant mixed Müllerian tumor (uterus, cervix, ovary)
  - Wilms tumor
  - Hepatoblastoma
  - Pulmonary blastoma
  - Thymoma
- Tumors with germ cell or sex cord elements
  - Germ cell tumors (seminoma, teratoma)
  - Sertoli-Leydig cell tumor
- Tumors with sarcomatous elements only
  - Malignant mesenchymoma
  - Dedifferentiated chondrosarcoma
  - Dedifferentiated liposarcoma
- Tumors of neuroectodermal derivation
  - Malignant peripheral nerve sheath tumor (malignant Triton tumor)
  - Ectomesenchymoma
  - Medulloepithelioma
  - Medulloblastoma
  - Congenital pigmented nevus (giant nevus)

Modified from Woodruff JM, Perino G. Non-germ-cell or teratomatous malignant tumors showing additional rhabdomyoblastic differentiation, with emphasis on the malignant Triton tumor. Semin Diagn Pathol 1994;11:69, with permission.

PROGNOSIS OF RHABDOMYOSARCOMA

During the past 50 years, the prognosis of rhabdomyosarcoma has improved dramatically. Before 1960, the prognosis was extremely poor, and there were few survivors even after radical, often destructive and disfiguring, surgical therapy. For example, an AFIP study in 1969 reported a 5-year mortality rate of 98%.[23]

Since the early 1960s, there has been marked improvement in the survival rates of patients with rhabdomyosarcoma because of a multidisciplinary therapeutic approach that consists of a biopsy or surgical removal of the neoplasm and multiagent chemotherapy with or without radiotherapy.[4] As a rule, treatment is carried out after a biopsy or resection and careful, comprehensive assessment of tumor stage or tumor group with radiography, computed tomographic (CT) scans, magnetic resonance imaging (MRI), bone scans and, if necessary, angiograms. Recommendations for therapy chiefly depend on the stage or clinical group of the disease and the site of the tumor following accurate microscopic diagnosis. Because rhabdomyosarcomas tend to metastasize to bone marrow, bilateral bone marrow aspiration/biopsy should be part of the staging process.

The IRS-II study, confined to patients younger than 21 years with a confirmed diagnosis of rhabdomyosarcoma, distinguished four clinical groups based on the amount of tumor remaining after initial surgery (Box 20-6). Because this approach is influenced by the variable practices of surgeons, the IRS Committee adopted a modification of the tumor-node-metastasis (TNM) system, which relies on a pretreatment assessment of tumor extent.[168] This system includes evaluation of the site of the primary tumor, the maximum diameter of the tumor, determination of tumor invasion into adjacent structures, status of regional lymph nodes, and the presence or absence of distant metastases. More recent studies of rhabdomyosarcoma rely on both the IRS clinical grouping system and the TNM stage to determine therapy. Both IRS clinical group and TNM stage have been found to have major prognostic significance (Box 20-7). Low-risk patients generally have localized embryonal histology tumors. Most of these patients have resected (group I or II) tumors, as well as group III tumors arising in favorable sites. Patients with embryonal tumors that are group III, stage 2 or 3, and all patients with nonmetastatic alveolar tumors are intermediate-risk. Patients with metastatic tumors (regardless of subtype) are treated with high-risk protocols. Based on data from the IRS-IV study, overall survival rates were 95%, 75%, and 27% for low-risk, intermediate-risk, and high-risk patients, respectively.[3] Similar results were reported from the European Cooperative Group studies using a four-tier risk system.[169,170] As a direct result of advances in risk stratification and therapy secondary to the collaborative group clinical trials, the 5-year failure-free survival rate for low-risk patients is as high as 90%[171]; the 4-year failure-free survival rate for intermediate risk patients is near 70%,[172] but there has been little progress made on improving survival for high-risk patients.[173]

Additional factors that influence the clinical course of the disease and necessitate more intensive therapy include the anatomic site and histologic subtype of the tumor. Tumors of the orbit have the best prognosis (92% 5-year survival) followed by tumors of the head and neck and nonbladder/prostate genitourinary tumors (about 80% 5-year survival).[3,174] A less favorable prognosis is found in patients whose tumors are located in a parameningeal location, bladder and prostate, and the extremities, with approximately 70% 5-year survivals for each. The poorest prognosis occurs in patients with tumors at other sites, including the retroperitoneum, biliary tract, and peritoneum. Late detection and large tumor size, difficulties encountered during surgical removal, extension into the meninges with or without spinal fluid spread, and lymph node metastasis are primarily responsible for the prognostic differences related to anatomic site.

Anatomic site is a major factor when determining the mode of therapy. For example, for rhabdomyosarcomas of the orbit, control is typically accomplished with biopsy, systemic chemotherapy, and irradiation alone.[8] Excellent results are achieved with rhabdomyosarcomas of the paratesticular region using radical orchiectomy with clear margins, radical retroperitoneal lymph node resection, and chemotherapy.[175] Tumors in parameningeal and paraspinal regions require extended irradiation and intrathecal chemotherapy to reduce local failure and spread of the disease.[176] Preoperative radiotherapy or chemotherapy for rhabdomyosarcomas of the

BOX 20-6 Clinical Staging of Patients with Rhabdomyosarcoma (Intergroup Rhabdomyosarcoma Studies Classification)

- Group I
  - Localized disease, completely resected (regional nodes not involved)
  - Confined to muscle or organ of origin
  - Contiguous involvement with infiltration outside of the muscle or organ of origin, as through fascial planes
- Group II
  - Grossly resected tumor with microscopic residual disease
  - No evidence of gross residual tumor; no evidence of regional node involvement
  - Regional disease, completely resected (regional nodes involved, extension of tumor into an adjacent organ, or both); all of tumor completely resected with no microscopic residual tumor
  - Regional disease with involved nodes, grossly resected, but with evidence of microscopic residual disease
- Group III
  - Incomplete resection or biopsy with gross residual disease
- Group IV
  - Distant metastatic disease present at onset (lung, liver, bones, bone marrow, brain, distant muscle, and nodes)

From Maurer HM, Beltangady M, Gehan EA, et al. The Intergroup Rhabdomyosarcoma Study I: a final report. Cancer 1988;61:209, with permission.

BOX 20-7 Favorable and Unfavorable Factors for Rhabdomyosarcomas

- Prognostically favorable factors
  - Age: infants and children
  - Orbital or genitourinary (nonbladder/prostate) location
  - Small size (<5 cm)
  - Botryoid or spindle cell type
  - Localized noninvasive tumor without regional lymph node involvement or distant metastasis
  - Complete initial resection
- Prognostically unfavorable factors
  - Age: adults
  - Location in head and neck (nonorbital), paraspinal region, abdomen, biliary tract, retroperitoneum, perineum, or extremities
  - Large size (>5 cm)
  - Alveolar (especially *PAX3/FOXO1A* fusion transcript-positive) or pleomorphic type
  - Diploid DNA content
  - Local tumor invasion, especially parameningeal or paraspinal region, sinuses, or skeleton
  - Local recurrence
  - Local recurrence during therapy
  - Regional lymph node involvement or distant metastasis
  - Incomplete initial excision or unresectability
  - Diffuse myogenin expression

urinary bladder and prostate usually allow less-extensive surgical therapy and better functional preservation.[46,177] Total excision of the tumor is part of the recommended therapy for rhabdomyosarcomas in the trunk and extremities.[178]

Histologic subtype has been found to be an important independent prognostic variable.[29] Newton et al.[29] found histologic subtype to be strongly predictive of survival by multivariate analysis, in addition to the known prognostic factors of primary site, clinical group, and tumor size. The latter study established that the botryoid and spindle cell subtypes of embryonal rhabdomyosarcoma have a superior prognosis (95% and 88% 5-year survivals, respectively); classic embryonal rhabdomyosarcoma has an intermediate prognosis (66% 5-year survival); and the alveolar subtype has a poor prognosis, with a 54% 5-year survival.

The degree of cellular differentiation (i.e., tumor cells resembling skeletal muscle cells) has been found by some to be of major prognostic significance. Wijnaendts et al.[179] found that a greater degree of cellular maturation was associated with prolonged survival, independent of histologic subtype. In addition, it has been repeatedly documented that tumor cells may undergo therapy-induced cytodifferentiation.[180] Botryoid and embryonal rhabdomyosarcoma subtypes are more likely to exhibit therapy-induced cytodifferentiation than other rhabdomyosarcoma subtypes.[180]

Age at diagnosis is also an independent predictor of outcome in patients with rhabdomyosarcoma.[181] Age has its greatest prognostic effect on patients with invasive but nonmetastatic tumors.[182]

The prognostic impact of the proliferative index of the tumor, including mitotic rate, Ki-67 index, and DNA ploidy analysis has been assessed in a number of different studies. However, conflicting results have been reported, and none of these factors have been clearly established as important prognostic parameters.[21,183-185] As mentioned previously, diffuse myogenin expression by immunohistochemistry was found to be an independent marker of poor survival in pediatric rhabdomyosarcomas, regardless of histologic subtype, translocation status, tumor site, or stage.[155]

The possible prognostic impact of various molecular alterations has been an area of intensive research in recent years. Accumulated intranuclear p53 protein has been detected by immunohistochemical techniques in a proportion of rhabdomyosarcomas.[186] Although some of these tumors harbor *p53* gene mutations, it appears that *MDM2* gene overexpression with subsequent *MDM2-p53* complex formation constitutes an alternative mechanism of inactivation of wild-type *p53* in some rhabdomyosarcomas.[187] The *MYCN* oncogene is amplified in some rhabdomyosarcomas, including both embryonal and alveolar subtypes, but seems to be significantly more common in the latter.[188] Barr et al.[188] found amplification of 2p24 and 12q13-14 in 13% and 12% of alveolar rhabdomyosarcomas, respectively; 2p24 amplification occurred preferentially in fusion-positive cases (either *PAX3-FOXO1A* or *PAX7-FOXO1A*), whereas 12q13-14 amplification occurred preferentially in *PAX3-FOXO1A* positive cases. *MYCN* was typically overexpressed in cases with 2p24 amplification, but this was not associated with clinical outcome. In contrast, multiple genes were overexpressed in cases with 12q13-14 amplification, which was associated with significantly worse overall and failure-free survival that was independent of gene fusion status.

Gene fusion subtype may also be important in determining prognosis in this group of patients. Several studies have found the *PAX7-FOXO1A* fusion to be associated with a better prognosis than the *PAX3-FOXO1A* fusion in patients with alveolar rhabdomyosarcoma.[100,189] For example, Sorensen et al.[100] evaluated 171 childhood rhabdomyosarcomas and found *PAX3-FOXO1A* and *PAX7-FOXO1A* fusions in 55% and 22% of alveolar rhabdomyosarcomas, respectively. Twenty-three percent of patients with alveolar tumors were fusion negative. Although fusion status was not correlated with outcome in patients with locoregional disease, there was a striking difference in outcome in patients presenting with metastatic disease, with estimated 4-year overall survivals of 75% and 8% for *PAX7-FOXO1A* and *PAX3-FOXO1A* fusions, respectively. Some studies suggest that the clinical behavior of fusion-negative alveolar rhabdomyosarcoma is comparable to that of embryonal rhabdomyosarcoma.[64]

Finally, expression profiling has started to identify signatures that are predictive of survival. For example, Davicioni et al.[57] assessed 120 rhabdomyosarcomas with a 22,000 probe set microarray and found the expression of a 34 gene set to be highly predictive of outcome, independent of patient age, stage, tumor size, or histology. This profile did correlate with a risk classification group (Children's Oncology Group) and certain biologic subsets of alveolar rhabdomyosarcomas.

RECURRENCE OF RHABDOMYOSARCOMA

Inadequately treated tumors grow in an infiltrative, destructive manner and recur in a high percentage of cases. Recurrence may herald metastasis, but by no means do all recurrent tumors metastasize. Bone does not constitute an effective barrier to growth of the tumor, and bone invasion is a frequent finding, particularly with rhabdomyosarcomas in the head and neck region and in the hands and feet. In the head and neck, the tumors tend to erode and destroy the bony walls of the orbit and sinuses, the temporal or mastoid bone, and the base of the skull; they may prove fatal because of extensive meningeal spread (parameningeal rhabdomyosarcomas) and spinal cord drop metastases.[190,191] Meningeal spread may also occur with rhabdomyosarcomas at other sites.

METASTASIS OF RHABDOMYOSARCOMA

Metastases develop during the course of the disease and are present at the time of diagnosis in about 20% of cases. Major metastatic sites include the lung, lymph nodes, and bone marrow followed by the heart, brain, meninges, pancreas, liver, and kidney. The lungs are involved in at least two-thirds of patients with metastases.[192] The incidence of lymph node metastasis largely depends on the location of the tumor. It is higher with rhabdomyosarcomas of the prostate, paratesticular region, and extremities than with those of the orbit and head and neck.[177] In fact, exploration and biopsy of ipsilateral retroperitoneal lymph nodes are recommended when assessing paratesticular rhabdomyosarcomas.[193] It is also useful to keep in mind that alveolar rhabdomyosarcoma is one of the few soft tissue tumors in which lymph node metastasis may antedate discovery of the primary mass. There is a surprisingly high incidence of cardiac metastasis.[194] Pratt et al.[195] found

8 of 23 fatal cases to have metastases to the heart. There are also reports of multiple skin metastases as the primary manifestation of the disease.[196]

Microscopically, the recurrent and metastatic lesions may be less well differentiated than the primary growth; but, unlike most other types of sarcoma, some recurrent or metastatic lesions for unknown reasons show a higher degree of differentiation. Several cases have been observed where a definitive diagnosis of rhabdomyosarcoma was possible only after rhabdomyoblasts with cross-striations were found in the pulmonary metastases. In addition, cytologic differentiation in rhabdomyosarcomas following polychemotherapy has been demonstrated, probably as a result of selective destruction of undifferentiated tumor cells.[56]

References

1. Pack GT, Eberjart WF. Rhabdomyosarcoma of skeletal muscle; report of 100 cases. Surgery 1952;32(6):1023–64.
2. Stout AP. Rhabdomyosarcoma of the skeletal muscles. Ann Surg 1946;123(3):447–72.
3. Crist WM, Anderson JR, Meza JL, et al. Intergroup rhabdomyosarcoma study-IV: results for patients with nonmetastatic disease. J Clin Oncol 2001;19(12):3091–102.
4. Crist W, Gehan EA, Ragab AH, et al. The Third Intergroup Rhabdomyosarcoma Study. J Clin Oncol 1995;13(3):610–30.
5. Maurer HM, Beltangady M, Gehan EA, et al. The Intergroup Rhabdomyosarcoma Study-I. A final report. Cancer 1988;61(2):209–20.
6. Newton Jr WA, Soule EH, Hamoudi AB, et al. Histopathology of childhood sarcomas, Intergroup Rhabdomyosarcoma Studies I and II: clinicopathologic correlation. J Clin Oncol 1988;6(1):67–75.
7. Maurer HM, Gehan EA, Beltangady M, et al. The Intergroup Rhabdomyosarcoma Study-II. Cancer 1993;71(5):1904–22.
8. Raney RB, Anderson JR, Barr FG, et al. Rhabdomyosarcoma and undifferentiated sarcoma in the first two decades of life: a selective review of intergroup rhabdomyosarcoma study group experience and rationale for Intergroup Rhabdomyosarcoma Study V. J Pediatr Hematol Oncol 2001;23(4):215–20.
9. Villella JA, Bogner PN, Jani-Sait SN, et al. Rhabdomyosarcoma of the cervix in sisters with review of the literature. Gynecol Oncol 2005; 99(3):742–8.
10. Megarbane H, Doz F, Manach Y, et al. Neonatal rhabdomyosarcoma misdiagnosed as a congenital hemangioma. Pediatr Dermatol 2011;28(3):299–301.
11. Turaka K, Shields CL, Meadows AT, et al. Second malignant neoplasms following chemoreduction with carboplatin, etoposide, and vincristine in 245 patients with intraocular retinoblastoma. Pediatr Blood Cancer 2012;59(1):121–5.
12. Armstrong SJ, Duncan AW, Mott MG. Rhabdomyosarcoma associated with familial adenomatous polyposis. Pediatr Radiol 1991;21(6): 445–6.
13. Heney D, Lockwood L, Allibone EB, et al. Nasopharyngeal rhabdomyosarcoma and multiple lentigines syndrome: a case report. Med Pediatr Oncol 1992;20(3):227–8.
14. Choi JS, Choi JS, Kim EJ. Primary pulmonary rhabdomyosarcoma in an adult with neurofibromatosis-1. Ann Thorac Surg 2009;88(4):1356–8.
15. Quezada E, Gripp KW. Costello syndrome and related disorders. Curr Opin Pediatr 2007;19(6):636–44.
16. Kuroiwa M, Sakamoto J, Shimada A, et al. Manifestation of alveolar rhabdomyosarcoma as primary cutaneous lesions in a neonate with Beckwith-Wiedemann syndrome. J Pediatr Surg 2009;44(3):e31–5.
17. Jongmans MC, Hoogerbrugge PM, Hilkens L, et al. Noonan syndrome, the SOS1 gene and embryonal rhabdomyosarcoma. Genes Chromosomes Cancer 2010;49(7):635–41.
18. Ognjanovic S, Linabery AM, Charbonneau B, et al. Trends in childhood rhabdomyosarcoma incidence and survival in the United States, 1975-2005. Cancer 2009;115(18):4218–26.
19. Savaşan S, Lorenzana A, Williams JA, et al. Constitutional balanced translocations in alveolar rhabdomyosarcoma. Cancer Genet Cytogenet 1998;105(1):50–4.
20. Grufferman S, Ruymann F, Ognjanovic S, et al. Prenatal X-ray exposure and rhabdomyosarcoma in children: a report from the children's oncology group. Cancer Epidemiol Biomarkers Prev 2009;18(4):1271–6.
21. Hawkins HK, Camacho-Velasquez JV. Rhabdomyosarcoma in children. Correlation of form and prognosis in one institution's experience. Am J Surg Pathol 1987;11(7):531–42.
22. Horn Jr RC, Enterline HT. Rhabdomyosarcoma: a clinicopathological study and classification of 39 cases. Cancer 1958;11(1):181–99.
23. Enzinger FM, Shiraki M. Alveolar rhabdomyosarcoma. An analysis of 110 cases. Cancer 1969;24(1):18–31.
24. Palmer N, Sachs N, Foukles M. Histopathology and prognosis in rhabdomyosarcoma. Proc Int Soc Pediatr Oncol 1981;1:113.
25. Palmer N, Sachs N, Foulkes M. Histopathology and prognosis in rhabdomyosarcoma (IRS-1). Proc Am Clin Oncol 1982;(1):170.
26. Caillaud JM, Gérard-Marchant R, Marsden HB, et al. Histopathological classification of childhood rhabdomyosarcoma: a report from the International Society of Pediatric Oncology pathology panel. Med Pediatr Oncol 1989;17(5):391–400.
27. Tsokos M, Webber BL, Parham DM, et al. Rhabdomyosarcoma. A new classification scheme related to prognosis. Arch Pathol Lab Med 1992;116(8):847–55.
28. Asmar L, Gehan EA, Newton WA, et al. Agreement among and within groups of pathologists in the classification of rhabdomyosarcoma and related childhood sarcomas. Report of an international study of four pathology classifications. Cancer 1994;74(9):2579–88.
29. Newton Jr WA, Gehan EA, Webber BL, et al. Classification of rhabdomyosarcomas and related sarcomas. Pathologic aspects and proposal for a new classification–an Intergroup Rhabdomyosarcoma Study. Cancer 1995;76(6):1073–85.
30. Qualman S, Lynch J, Bridge J, et al. Prevalence and clinical impact of anaplasia in childhood rhabdomyosarcoma: a report from the Soft Tissue Sarcoma Committee of the Children's Oncology Group. Cancer 2008;113(11):3242–7.
31. Qualman SJ, Bowen J, Parham DM, et al. Protocol for the examination of specimens from patients (children and young adults) with rhabdomyosarcoma. Arch Pathol Lab Med 2003;127(10):1290–7.
32. Ragab AH, Heyn R, Tefft M, et al. Infants younger than 1 year of age with rhabdomyosarcoma. Cancer 1986;58(12):2606–10.
33. Lobe TE, Wiener ES, Hays DM, et al. Neonatal rhabdomyosarcoma: the IRS experience. J Pediatr Surg 1994;29(8):1167–70.
34. Stock N, Chibon F, Binh MB, et al. Adult-type rhabdomyosarcoma: analysis of 57 cases with clinicopathologic description, identification of 3 morphologic patterns and prognosis. Am J Surg Pathol 2009;33 (12):1850–9.
35. Pappo AS, Shapiro DN, Crist WM, et al. Biology and therapy of pediatric rhabdomyosarcoma. J Clin Oncol 1995;13(8):2123–39.
36. Turner JH, Richmon JD. Head and neck rhabdomyosarcoma: a critical analysis of population-based incidence and survival data. Otolaryngol Head Neck Surg 2011;145(6):967–73.
37. Huh WW, Anderson JR, Rodeberg D, et al. Orbital sarcoma with metastases at diagnosis: a report from the Soft Tissue Sarcoma Committee of the Children's Oncology Group. Pediatr Blood Cancer 2010;54(7): 1045–7.
38. Kodet R, Newton Jr WA, Hamoudi AB, et al. Orbital rhabdomyosarcomas and related tumors in childhood: relationship of morphology to prognosis–an Intergroup Rhabdomyosarcoma study. Med Pediatr Oncol 1997;29(1):51–60.
39. Pappo AS, Meza JL, Donaldson SS, et al. Treatment of localized nonorbital, nonparameningeal head and neck rhabdomyosarcoma: lessons learned from intergroup rhabdomyosarcoma studies III and IV. J Clin Oncol 2003;21(4):638–45.
40. Breneman JC. Genitourinary rhabdomyosarcoma. Semin Radiat Oncol 1997;7(3):217–24.
41. Leuschner I, Newton Jr WA, Schmidt D, et al. Spindle cell variants of embryonal rhabdomyosarcoma in the paratesticular region. A report of the Intergroup Rhabdomyosarcoma Study. Am J Surg Pathol 1993; 17(3):221–30.
42. Cavazzana AO, Schmidt D, Ninfo V, et al. Spindle cell rhabdomyosarcoma. A prognostically favorable variant of rhabdomyosarcoma. Am J Surg Pathol 1992;16(3):229–35.
43. Huang CJ. Rhabdomyosarcoma involving the genitourinary organs, retroperitoneum, and pelvis. J Pediatr Surg 1986;21(2):101–7.
44. Cecchetto G, Bisogno G, Treuner J, et al. Role of surgery for nonmetastatic abdominal rhabdomyosarcomas: a report from the Italian and German Soft Tissue Cooperative Groups Studies. Cancer 2003;97(8): 1974–80.
45. Raney Jr RB, Crist W, Hays D, et al. Soft tissue sarcoma of the perineal region in childhood. A report from the Intergroup Rhabdomyosarcoma Studies I and II, 1972 through 1984. Cancer 1990;65(12):2787–92.

46. Seitz G, Dantonello TM, Int-Veen C, et al. Treatment efficiency, outcome and surgical treatment problems in patients suffering from localized embryonal bladder/prostate rhabdomyosarcoma: a report from the Cooperative Soft Tissue Sarcoma trial CWS-96. Pediatr Blood Cancer 2011;56(5):718–24.
47. Paner GP, McKenney JK, Epstein JI, et al. Rhabdomyosarcoma of the urinary bladder in adults: predilection for alveolar morphology with anaplasia and significant morphologic overlap with small cell carcinoma. Am J Surg Pathol 2008;32(7):1022–8.
48. Ferguson SE, Gerald W, Barakat RR, et al. Clinicopathologic features of rhabdomyosarcoma of gynecologic origin in adults. Am J Surg Pathol 2007;31(3):382–9.
49. da Silva BB, Dos Santos AR, Bosco Parentes-Vieira J, et al. Embryonal rhabdomyosarcoma of the uterus associated with uterine inversion in an adolescent: a case report and published work review. J Obstet Gynaecol Res 2008;34(4 Pt 2):735–8.
50. Adams BN, Brandt JS, Loukeris K, et al. Embryonal rhabdomyosarcoma of the cervix and appendiceal carcinoid tumor. Obstet Gynecol 2011;117(2 Pt 2):482–4.
51. Walterhouse DO, Meza JL, Breneman JC, et al. Local control and outcome in children with localized vaginal rhabdomyosarcoma: a report from the Soft Tissue Sarcoma committee of the Children's Oncology Group. Pediatr Blood Cancer 2011;57(1):76–83.
52. Puranik RB, Naik S, Kulkarni S, et al. Alveolar rhabdomyosarcoma of vulva. Indian J Pathol Microbiol 2010;53(1):167–8.
53. Okamura K, Yamamoto H, Ishimaru Y, et al. Clinical characteristics and surgical treatment of perianal and perineal rhabdomyosarcoma: analysis of Japanese patients and comparison with IRSG reports. Pediatr Surg Int 2006;22(2):129–34.
54. Kitagawa N, Aida N. Biliary rhabdomyosarcoma. Pediatr Radiol 2007; 37(10):1059.
55. Kodet R, Newton Jr WA, Hamoudi AB, et al. Childhood rhabdomyosarcoma with anaplastic (pleomorphic) features. A report of the Intergroup Rhabdomyosarcoma Study. Am J Surg Pathol 1993;17(5):443–53.
56. Coffin CM, Lowichik A, Zhou H. Treatment effects in pediatric soft tissue and bone tumors: practical considerations for the pathologist. Am J Clin Pathol 2005;123(1):75–90.
57. Davicioni E, Anderson MJ, Finckenstein FG, et al. Molecular classification of rhabdomyosarcoma–genotypic and phenotypic determinants of diagnosis: a report from the Children's Oncology Group. Am J Pathol 2009;174(2):550–64.
58. Xia SJ, Pressey JG, Barr FG. Molecular pathogenesis of rhabdomyosarcoma. Cancer Biol Ther 2002;1(2):97–104.
59. Sabbioni S, Barbanti-Brodano G, Croce CM, et al. GOK: a gene at 11p15 involved in rhabdomyosarcoma and rhabdoid tumor development. Cancer Res 1997;57(20):4493–7.
60. Meloni-Ehrig A, Smith B, Zgoda J, et al. Translocation (2;8)(q35;q13): a recurrent abnormality in congenital embryonal rhabdomyosarcoma. Cancer Genet Cytogenet 2009;191(1):43–5.
61. Sirvent N, Trassard M, Ebran N, et al. Fusion of EWSR1 with the DUX4 facioscapulohumeral muscular dystrophy region resulting from t(4;22)(q35;q12) in a case of embryonal rhabdomyosarcoma. Cancer Genet Cytogenet 2009;195(1):12–8.
62. Afify A, Mark HF. Trisomy 8 in embryonal rhabdomyosarcoma detected by fluorescence in situ hybridization. Cancer Genet Cytogenet 1999;108(2):127–32.
63. Muntean A, Bergsträsser E, Diepold M, et al. Karyotypic characterization of infant embryonal rhabdomyosarcoma. Cancer Genet Cytogenet 2008;180(2):145–8.
64. Williamson D, Missiaglia E, de Reyniès A, et al. Fusion gene-negative alveolar rhabdomyosarcoma is clinically and molecularly indistinguishable from embryonal rhabdomyosarcoma. J Clin Oncol 2010;28(13): 2151–8.
65. Paulson V, Chandler G, Rakheja D, et al. High-resolution array CGH identifies common mechanisms that drive embryonal rhabdomyosarcoma pathogenesis. Genes Chromosomes Cancer 2011;50(6):397–408.
66. Tostar U, Toftgård R, Zaphiropoulos PG, et al. Reduction of human embryonal rhabdomyosarcoma tumor growth by inhibition of the hedgehog signaling pathway. Genes Cancer 2010;1(9):941–51.
67. Pressey JG, Anderson JR, Crossman DK, et al. Hedgehog pathway activity in pediatric embryonal rhabdomyosarcoma and undifferentiated sarcoma: a report from the Children's Oncology Group. Pediatr Blood Cancer 2011;57(6):930–8.
68. Zibat A, Missiaglia E, Rosenberger A, et al. Activation of the hedgehog pathway confers a poor prognosis in embryonal and fusion gene-negative alveolar rhabdomyosarcoma. Oncogene 2010;29(48):6323–30.
69. Nascimento AF, Fletcher CD. Spindle cell rhabdomyosarcoma in adults. Am J Surg Pathol 2005;29(8):1106–13.
70. Mentzel T, Kuhnen C. Spindle cell rhabdomyosarcoma in adults: clinicopathological and immunohistochemical analysis of seven new cases. Virchows Arch 2006;449(5):554–60.
71. Mentzel T. [Spindle cell rhabdomyosarcoma in adults: a new entity in the spectrum of malignant mesenchymal tumors of soft tissues]. Pathologe 2010;31(2):91–6.
72. Qualman SJ, Coffin CM, Newton WA, et al. Intergroup Rhabdomyosarcoma Study: update for pathologists. Pediatr Dev Pathol 1998;1(6): 550–61.
73. Debiec-Rychter M, Hagemeijer A, Sciot R. Spindle-cell rhabdomyosarcoma with 2q36 approximately q37 involvement. Cancer Genet Cytogenet 2003;140(1):62–5.
74. Gil-Benso R, Carda-Batalla C, Navarro-Fos S, et al. Cytogenetic study of a spindle-cell rhabdomyosarcoma of the parotid gland. Cancer Genet Cytogenet 1999;109(2):150–3.
75. Lee MW, Chung WK, Choi JH, et al. A case of botryoid-type embryonal rhabdomyosarcoma. Clin Exp Dermatol 2009;34(8):e737–9.
76. Palazzo JP, Gibas Z, Dunton CJ, et al. Cytogenetic study of botryoid rhabdomyosarcoma of the uterine cervix. Virchows Arch A Pathol Anat Histopathol 1993;422(1):87–91.
77. Kadan-Lottick NS, Stork L, Ruyle SZ, et al. Cytogenetic abnormalities in a case of botryoid rhabdomyosarcoma. Med Pediatr Oncol 2000; 34(4):293–5.
78. Manor E, Bodner L, Kachko P, et al. Trisomy 8 as a sole aberration in embryonal rhabdomyosarcoma (sarcoma botryoides) of the vagina. Cancer Genet Cytogenet 2009;195(2):172–4.
79. Yasuda T, Perry KD, Nelson M, et al. Alveolar rhabdomyosarcoma of the head and neck region in older adults: genetic characterization and a review of the literature. Hum Pathol 2009;40(3):341–8.
80. Cakar B, Muslu U, Karaca B, et al. Alveolar rhabdomyosarcoma originating from the uterine cervix. Eur J Gynaecol Oncol 2011;32(2):196–8.
81. Fukunaga M. Pure alveolar rhabdomyosarcoma of the uterine corpus. Pathol Int 2011;61(6):377–81.
82. Jani P, Ye CC. Massive bone marrow involvement by clear cell variant of rhabdomyosarcoma with an unusual histological pattern and an unknown primary site. J Clin Pathol 2008;61(2):238–9.
83. Boman F, Champigneulle J, Schmitt C, et al. Clear cell rhabdomyosarcoma. Pediatr Pathol Lab Med 1996;16(6):951–9.
84. Krsková L, Mrhalová M, Hilská I, et al. Detection and clinical significance of bone marrow involvement in patients with rhabdomyosarcoma. Virchows Arch 2010;456(5):463–72.
85. Barr FG, Qualman SJ, Macris MH, et al. Genetic heterogeneity in the alveolar rhabdomyosarcoma subset without typical gene fusions. Cancer Res 2002;62(16):4704–10.
86. Mercado GE, Barr FG. Fusions involving PAX and FOX genes in the molecular pathogenesis of alveolar rhabdomyosarcoma: recent advances. Curr Mol Med 2007;7(1):47–61.
87. Barr FG. Gene fusions involving PAX and FOX family members in alveolar rhabdomyosarcoma. Oncogene 2001;20(40):5736–46.
88. Mercado GE, Xia SJ, Zhang C, et al. Identification of PAX3-FKHR-regulated genes differentially expressed between alveolar and embryonal rhabdomyosarcoma: focus on MYCN as a biologically relevant target. Genes Chromosomes Cancer 2008;47(6):510–20.
89. Xia SJ, Holder DD, Pawel BR, et al. High expression of the PAX3-FKHR oncoprotein is required to promote tumorigenesis of human myoblasts. Am J Pathol 2009;175(6):2600–8.
90. Frascella E, Toffolatti L, Rosolen A. Normal and rearranged PAX3 expression in human rhabdomyosarcoma. Cancer Genet Cytogenet 1998;102(2):104–9.
91. Biegel JA, Meek RS, Parmiter AH, et al. Chromosomal translocation t(1;13)(p36;q14) in a case of rhabdomyosarcoma. Genes Chromosomes Cancer 1991;3(6):483–4.
92. Stegmaier S, Poremba C, Schaefer KL, et al. Prognostic value of PAX-FKHR fusion status in alveolar rhabdomyosarcoma: a report from the cooperative soft tissue sarcoma study group (CWS). Pediatr Blood Cancer 2011;57(3):406–14.
93. Parham DM, Qualman SJ, Teot L, et al. Correlation between histology and PAX/FKHR fusion status in alveolar rhabdomyosarcoma: a report from the Children's Oncology Group. Am J Surg Pathol 2007;31 (6):895–901.
94. Barr FG, Smith LM, Lynch JC, et al. Examination of gene fusion status in archival samples of alveolar rhabdomyosarcoma entered on the Intergroup Rhabdomyosarcoma Study-III trial: a report from the Children's Oncology Group. J Mol Diagn 2006;8(2):202–8.

95. Downs-Kelly E, Shehata BM, López-Terrada D, et al. The utility of FOXO1 fluorescence in situ hybridization (FISH) in formalin-fixed paraffin-embedded specimens in the diagnosis of alveolar rhabdomyosarcoma. Diagn Mol Pathol 2009;18(3):138–43.
96. Arden KC, Anderson MJ, Finckenstein FG, et al. Detection of the t(2;13) chromosomal translocation in alveolar rhabdomyosarcoma using the reverse transcriptase-polymerase chain reaction. Genes Chromosomes Cancer 1996;16(4):254–60.
97. de Alava E, Ladanyi M, Rosai J, et al. Detection of chimeric transcripts in desmoplastic small round cell tumor and related developmental tumors by reverse transcriptase polymerase chain reaction. A specific diagnostic assay. Am J Pathol 1995;147(6):1584–91.
98. Downing JR, Khandekar A, Shurtleff SA, et al. Multiplex RT-PCR assay for the differential diagnosis of alveolar rhabdomyosarcoma and Ewing's sarcoma. Am J Pathol 1995;146(3):626–34.
99. Barr FG, Chatten J, D'Cruz CM, et al. Molecular assays for chromosomal translocations in the diagnosis of pediatric soft tissue sarcomas. JAMA 1995;273(7):553–7.
100. Sorensen PH, Lynch JC, Qualman SJ, et al. PAX3-FKHR and PAX7-FKHR gene fusions are prognostic indicators in alveolar rhabdomyosarcoma: a report from the children's oncology group. J Clin Oncol 2002;20(11):2672–9.
101. Nishio J, Althof PA, Bailey JM, et al. Use of a novel FISH assay on paraffin-embedded tissues as an adjunct to diagnosis of alveolar rhabdomyosarcoma. Lab Invest 2006;86(6):547–56.
102. Davicioni E, Anderson JR, Buckley JD, et al. Gene expression profiling for survival prediction in pediatric rhabdomyosarcomas: a report from the children's oncology group. J Clin Oncol 2010;28(7):1240–6.
103. Marshall AD, van der Ent MA, Grosveld GC. PAX3-FOXO1 and FGFR4 in alveolar rhabdomyosarcoma. Mol Carcinog 2012;51(10):807–15.
104. Cao L, Yu Y, Bilke S, et al. Genome-wide identification of PAX3-FKHR binding sites in rhabdomyosarcoma reveals candidate target genes important for development and cancer. Cancer Res 2010;70(16): 6497–508.
105. Taylor 6th JG, Cheuk AT, Tsang PS, et al. Identification of FGFR4-activating mutations in human rhabdomyosarcomas that promote metastasis in xenotransplanted models. J Clin Invest 2009;119(11): 3395–407.
106. Liu J, Guzman MA, Pezanowski D, et al. FOXO1-FGFR1 fusion and amplification in a solid variant of alveolar rhabdomyosarcoma. Mod Pathol 2011;24(10):1327–35.
107. Sumegi J, Nishio J, Nelson M, et al. A novel t(4;22)(q31;q12) produces an EWSR1-SMARCA5 fusion in extraskeletal Ewing sarcoma/primitive neuroectodermal tumor. Mod Pathol 2011;24(3):333–42.
108. Furlong MA, Mentzel T, Fanburg-Smith JC. Pleomorphic rhabdomyosarcoma in adults: a clinicopathologic study of 38 cases with emphasis on morphologic variants and recent skeletal muscle-specific markers. Mod Pathol 2001;14(6):595–603.
109. Gaffney EF, Dervan PA, Fletcher CD. Pleomorphic rhabdomyosarcoma in adulthood. Analysis of 11 cases with definition of diagnostic criteria. Am J Surg Pathol 1993;17(6):601–9.
110. Hollowood K, Fletcher CD. Rhabdomyosarcoma in adults. Semin Diagn Pathol 1994;11(1):47–57.
111. Furlong MA, Fanburg-Smith JC. Pleomorphic rhabdomyosarcoma in children: four cases in the pediatric age group. Ann Diagn Pathol 2001;5(4):199–206.
112. Patton RB, Horn Jr RC. Rhabdomyosarcoma: clinical and pathological features and comparison with human fetal and embryonal skeletal muscle. Surgery 1962;52:572–84.
113. Weiss SW. Malignant fibrous histiocytoma. A reaffirmation. Am J Surg Pathol 1982;6(8):773–84.
114. Seidal T. Rhabdomyosarcoma. Histopathology 1990;17(5):482–4.
115. Fletcher CD. Pleomorphic malignant fibrous histiocytoma: fact or fiction? A critical reappraisal based on 159 tumors diagnosed as pleomorphic sarcoma. Am J Surg Pathol 1992;16(3):213–28.
116. Schürch W, Bégin LR, Seemayer TA, et al. Pleomorphic soft tissue myogenic sarcomas of adulthood. A reappraisal in the mid-1990s. Am J Surg Pathol 1996;20(2):131–47.
117. Fadare O, Bonvicino A, et al. Pleomorphic rhabdomyosarcoma of the uterine corpus: a clinicopathologic study of 4 cases and a review of the literature. Int J Gynecol Pathol 2010;29(2):122–34.
118. Schrock A, Jakob M, Zhou H, et al. Laryngeal pleomorphic rhabdomyosarcoma. Auris Nasus Larynx 2007;34(4):553–6.
119. Dalfior D, Eccher A, Gobbo S, et al. Primary pleomorphic rhabdomyosarcoma of the kidney in an adult. Ann Diagn Pathol 2008;12(4): 301–3.
120. Wang NP, Marx J, McNutt MA, et al. Expression of myogenic regulatory proteins (myogenin and MyoD1) in small blue round cell tumors of childhood. Am J Pathol 1995;147(6):1799–810.
121. Wesche WA, Fletcher CD, Dias P, et al. Immunohistochemistry of MyoD1 in adult pleomorphic soft tissue sarcomas. Am J Surg Pathol 1995;19(3):261–9.
122. Tallini G, Parham DM, Dias P, et al. Myogenic regulatory protein expression in adult soft tissue sarcomas. A sensitive and specific marker of skeletal muscle differentiation. Am J Pathol 1994;144(4):693–701.
123. Folpe AL. MyoD1 and myogenin expression in human neoplasia: a review and update. Adv Anat Pathol 2002;9(3):198–203.
124. Li G, Ogose A, Kawashima H, et al. Cytogenetic and real-time quantitative reverse-transcriptase polymerase chain reaction analyses in pleomorphic rhabdomyosarcoma. Cancer Genet Cytogenet 2009;192(1): 1–9.
125. Mertens F, Fletcher CD, Dal Cin P, et al. Cytogenetic analysis of 46 pleomorphic soft tissue sarcomas and correlation with morphologic and clinical features: a report of the CHAMP Study Group. Chromosomes and MorPhology. Genes Chromosomes Cancer 1998;22(1):16–25.
126. Folpe AL, McKenney JK, Bridge JA, et al. Sclerosing rhabdomyosarcoma in adults: report of four cases of a hyalinizing, matrix-rich variant of rhabdomyosarcoma that may be confused with osteosarcoma, chondrosarcoma, or angiosarcoma. Am J Surg Pathol 2002;26(9):1175–83.
127. Mentzel T, Katenkamp D. Sclerosing, pseudovascular rhabdomyosarcoma in adults. Clinicopathological and immunohistochemical analysis of three cases. Virchows Arch 2000;436(4):305–11.
128. Chiles MC, Parham DM, Qualman SJ, et al. Sclerosing rhabdomyosarcomas in children and adolescents: a clinicopathologic review of 13 cases from the Intergroup Rhabdomyosarcoma Study Group and Children's Oncology Group. Pediatr Dev Pathol 2004;7(6):583–94.
129. Chiles MC, Parham DM, Qualman SJ, et al. Sclerosing rhabdomyosarcomas in children and adolescents: a clinicopathologic review of 13 cases from the Intergroup Rhabdomyosarcoma Study Group and Children's Oncology Group. Pediatr Dev Pathol 2005;8(1):141.
130. Zhu XW, Guo JP, Chen H, et al. [Deep sarcoma of the penis: a report of 2 cases and review of the literature]. Zhonghua Nan Ke Xue 2007; 13(10):915–7.
131. Chiles MC, Parham DM, Qualman SJ, et al. Sclerosing rhabdomyosarcomas in children and adolescents: a clinicopathologic review of 13 cases from the Intergroup Rhabdomyosarcoma Study Group and Children's Oncology Group. Pediatr Dev Pathol 2004;7(6):583–94.
132. Zambrano E, Pérez-Atayde AR, Ahrens W, et al. Pediatric sclerosing rhabdomyosarcoma. Int J Surg Pathol 2006;14(3):193–9.
133. Gavino AC, Spears MD, Peng Y. Sclerosing spindle cell rhabdomyosarcoma in an adult: report of a new case and review of the literature. Int J Surg Pathol 2010;18(5):394–7.
134. Kuhnen C, Herter P, Leuschner I, et al. Sclerosing pseudovascular rhabdomyosarcoma-immunohistochemical, ultrastructural, and genetic findings indicating a distinct subtype of rhabdomyosarcoma. Virchows Arch 2006;449(5):572–8.
135. Martorell M, Ortiz CM, Garcia JA. Testicular fusocellular rhabdomyosarcoma as a metastasis of elbow sclerosing rhabdomyosarcoma: A clinicopathologic, immunohistochemical and molecular study of one case. Diagn Pathol 2010;5:52.
136. Zhu L, Wang J. [Sclerosing rhabdomyosarcoma: a clinicopathologic study of four cases with review of literature]. Zhonghua Bing Li Xue Za Zhi 2007;36(9):587–91.
137. Bouron-Dal Soglio D, Rougemont AL, Absi R, et al. SNP genotyping of a sclerosing rhabdomyosarcoma: reveals highly aneuploid profile and a specific MDM2/HMGA2 amplification. Hum Pathol 2009;40(9): 1347–52.
138. Knipe TA, Chandra RK, Bugg MF. Sclerosing rhabdomyosarcoma: a rare variant with predilection for the head and neck. Laryngoscope 2005;115(1):48–50.
139. Kumar S, Perlman E, Harris CA, et al. Myogenin is a specific marker for rhabdomyosarcoma: an immunohistochemical study in paraffin-embedded tissues. Mod Pathol 2000;13(9):988–93.
140. Dias P, Chen B, Dilday B, et al. Strong immunostaining for myogenin in rhabdomyosarcoma is significantly associated with tumors of the alveolar subclass. Am J Pathol 2000;156(2):399–408.
141. Cessna MH, Zhou H, Perkins SL, et al. Are myogenin and MyoD1 expression specific for rhabdomyosarcoma? A study of 150 cases, with emphasis on spindle cell mimics. Am J Surg Pathol 2001;25(9):1150–7.
142. Morotti RA, Nicol KK, Parham DM, et al. An immunohistochemical algorithm to facilitate diagnosis and subtyping of rhabdomyosarcoma:

the Children's Oncology Group experience. Am J Surg Pathol 2006; 30(8):962–8.
143. Wang J, Tu X, Sheng W. Sclerosing rhabdomyosarcoma: a clinicopathologic and immunohistochemical study of five cases. Am J Clin Pathol 2008;129(3):410–5.
144. Jo VY, Mariño-Enríquez A, Fletcher CD. Epithelioid rhabdomyosarcoma: clinicopathologic analysis of 16 cases of a morphologically distinct variant of rhabdomyosarcoma. Am J Surg Pathol 2011;35(10): 1523–30.
145. Suárez-Vilela D, Izquierdo-Garcia FM, Alonso-Orcajo N. Epithelioid and rhabdoid rhabdomyosarcoma in an adult patient: a diagnostic pitfall. Virchows Arch 2004;445(3):323–5.
146. Bowe SN, Ozer E, Bridge JA, et al. Primary intranodal epithelioid rhabdomyosarcoma. Am J Clin Pathol 2011;136(4):587–92.
147. Fujiwaki R, Miura H, Endo A, et al. Primary rhabdomyosarcoma with an epithelioid appearance of the fallopian tube: an adult case. Eur J Obstet Gynecol Reprod Biol 2008;140(2):289–90.
148. Seidal T, Kindblom LG, Angervall L. Rhabdomyosarcoma in middle-aged and elderly individuals. APMIS 1989;97(3):236–48.
149. Parham DM, Webber B, Holt H, et al. Immunohistochemical study of childhood rhabdomyosarcomas and related neoplasms. Results of an Intergroup Rhabdomyosarcoma study project. Cancer 1991;67(12): 3072–80.
150. Schürch W, Bochaton-Piallat ML, Geinoz A, et al. All histological types of primary human rhabdomyosarcoma express alpha-cardiac and not alpha-skeletal actin messenger RNA. Am J Pathol 1994;144(4):836–46.
151. Eusebi V, Bondi A, Rosai J. Immunohistochemical localization of myoglobin in nonmuscular cells. Am J Surg Pathol 1984;8(1):51–5.
152. Davis RL, Cheng PF, Lassar AB, et al. The MyoD DNA binding domain contains a recognition code for muscle-specific gene activation. Cell 1990;60(5):733–46.
153. Miller JB. Myogenic programs of mouse muscle cell lines: expression of myosin heavy chain isoforms, MyoD1, and myogenin. J Cell Biol 1990; 111(3):1149–59.
154. Hostein I, Andraud-Fregeville M, Guillou L, et al. Rhabdomyosarcoma: value of myogenin expression analysis and molecular testing in diagnosing the alveolar subtype: an analysis of 109 paraffin-embedded specimens. Cancer 2004;101(12):2817–24.
155. Heerema-McKenney A, Wijnaendts LC, Pulliam JF, et al. Diffuse myogenin expression by immunohistochemistry is an independent marker of poor survival in pediatric rhabdomyosarcoma: a tissue microarray study of 71 primary tumors including correlation with molecular phenotype. Am J Surg Pathol 2008;32(10):1513–22.
156. Sullivan LM, Atkins KA, LeGallo RD. PAX immunoreactivity identifies alveolar rhabdomyosarcoma. Am J Surg Pathol 2009;33(5):775–80.
157. Wachtel M, Runge T, Leuschner I, et al. Subtype and prognostic classification of rhabdomyosarcoma by immunohistochemistry. J Clin Oncol 2006;24(5):816–22.
158. Bahrami A, Gown AM, Baird GS, et al. Aberrant expression of epithelial and neuroendocrine markers in alveolar rhabdomyosarcoma: a potentially serious diagnostic pitfall. Mod Pathol 2008;21(7):795–806.
159. Folpe AL, Goldblum JR, Rubin BP, et al. Morphologic and immunophenotypic diversity in Ewing family tumors: a study of 66 genetically confirmed cases. Am J Surg Pathol 2005;29(8):1025–33.
160. Folpe AL, Hill CE, Parham DM, et al. Immunohistochemical detection of FLI-1 protein expression: a study of 132 round cell tumors with emphasis on CD99-positive mimics of Ewing's sarcoma/primitive neuroectodermal tumor. Am J Surg Pathol 2000;24(12):1657–62.
161. Erlandson RA. The ultrastructural distinction between rhabdomyosarcoma and other undifferentiated "sarcomas." Ultrastruct Pathol 1987; 11(2-3):83–101.
162. Scotlandi K, Serra M, Manara MC, et al. Immunostaining of the p30/32MIC2 antigen and molecular detection of EWS rearrangements for the diagnosis of Ewing's sarcoma and peripheral neuroectodermal tumor. Hum Pathol 1996;27(4):408–16.
163. Woodruff JM, Perino G. Non-germ-cell or teratomatous malignant tumors showing additional rhabdomyoblastic differentiation, with emphasis on the malignant Triton tumor. Semin Diagn Pathol 1994; 11(1):69–81.
164. Binh MB, Guillou L, Hostein I, et al. Dedifferentiated liposarcomas with divergent myosarcomatous differentiation developed in the internal trunk: a study of 27 cases and comparison to conventional dedifferentiated liposarcomas and leiomyosarcomas. Am J Surg Pathol 2007; 31(10):1557–66.
165. Rekhi B, Karpate A, Deodhar KK, et al. Metastatic rhabdomyosarcomatous elements, mimicking a primary sarcoma, in the omentum, from a poorly differentiated ovarian Sertoli-Leydig cell tumor in a young girl: an unusual presentation with a literature review. Indian J Pathol Microbiol 2009;52(4):554–8.
166. Stasik CJ, Tawfik O. Malignant peripheral nerve sheath tumor with rhabdomyosarcomatous differentiation (malignant Triton tumor). Arch Pathol Lab Med 2006;130(12):1878–81.
167. Floris G, Debiec-Rychter M, Wozniak A, et al. Malignant ectomesenchymoma: genetic profile reflects rhabdomyosarcomatous differentiation. Diagn Mol Pathol 2007;16(4):243–8.
168. Lawrence Jr W, Anderson JR, Gehan EA, et al. Pretreatment TNM staging of childhood rhabdomyosarcoma: a report of the Intergroup Rhabdomyosarcoma Study Group. Children's Cancer Study Group. Pediatric Oncology Group. Cancer 1997;80(6):1165–70.
169. Stevens MC, Rey A, Bouvet N, et al. Treatment of nonmetastatic rhabdomyosarcoma in childhood and adolescence: third study of the International Society of Paediatric Oncology–SIOP Malignant Mesenchymal Tumor 89. J Clin Oncol 2005;23(12):2618–28.
170. Carli M, Colombatti R, Oberlin O, et al. European intergroup studies (MMT4-89 and MMT4-91) on childhood metastatic rhabdomyosarcoma: final results and analysis of prognostic factors. J Clin Oncol 2004;22(23):4787–94.
171. Meza JL, Anderson J, Pappo AS, et al. Analysis of prognostic factors in patients with nonmetastatic rhabdomyosarcoma treated on intergroup rhabdomyosarcoma studies III and IV: the Children's Oncology Group. J Clin Oncol 2006;24(24):3844–51.
172. Arndt CA, Stoner JA, Hawkins DS, et al. Vincristine, actinomycin, and cyclophosphamide compared with vincristine, actinomycin, and cyclophosphamide alternating with vincristine, topotecan, and cyclophosphamide for intermediate-risk rhabdomyosarcoma: children's oncology group study D9803. J Clin Oncol 2009;27(31):5182–8.
173. Huh WW, Skapek SX. Childhood rhabdomyosarcoma: new insight on biology and treatment. Curr Oncol Rep 2010;12(6):402–10.
174. Chisholm JC, Marandet J, Rey A, et al. Prognostic factors after relapse in nonmetastatic rhabdomyosarcoma: a nomogram to better define patients who can be salvaged with further therapy. J Clin Oncol 2011;29(10):1319–25.
175. Reeves HM, MacLennan GT. Paratesticular rhabdomyosarcoma. J Urol 2009;182(4):1578–9.
176. Lin C, Donaldson SS, Meza JL, et al. Effect of radiotherapy techniques (IMRT vs. 3D-CRT) on outcome in patients with intermediate-risk rhabdomyosarcoma enrolled in COG D9803—a report from the Children's Oncology Group. Int J Radiat Oncol Biol Phys 2012;82:1764–70.
177. Rodeberg DA, Anderson JR, Arndt CA, et al. Comparison of outcomes based on treatment algorithms for rhabdomyosarcoma of the bladder/prostate: combined results from the Children's Oncology Group, German Cooperative Soft Tissue Sarcoma Study, Italian Cooperative Group, and International Society of Pediatric Oncology Malignant Mesenchymal Tumors Committee. Int J Cancer 2011;128(5):1232–9.
178. Casanova M, Meazza C, Favini F, et al. Rhabdomyosarcoma of the extremities: a focus on tumors arising in the hand and foot. Pediatr Hematol Oncol 2009;26(5):321–31.
179. Wijnaendts LC, van der Linden JC, Van Unnik AJ, et al. Histopathological features and grading in rhabdomyosarcomas of childhood. Histopathology 1994;24(4):303–9.
180. Coffin CM, Rulon J, Smith L, et al. Pathologic features of rhabdomyosarcoma before and after treatment: a clinicopathologic and immunohistochemical analysis. Mod Pathol 1997;10(12):1175–87.
181. Perez EA, Kassira N, Cheung MC, et al. Rhabdomyosarcoma in children: a SEER population based study. J Surg Res 2011;170(2): e243–51.
182. La Quaglia MP, Heller G, Ghavimi F, et al. The effect of age at diagnosis on outcome in rhabdomyosarcoma. Cancer 1994;73(1):109–17.
183. Pappo AS, Crist WM, Kuttesch J, et al. Tumor-cell DNA content predicts outcome in children and adolescents with clinical group III embryonal rhabdomyosarcoma. The Intergroup Rhabdomyosarcoma Study Committee of the Children's Cancer Group and the Pediatric Oncology Group. J Clin Oncol 1993;11(10):1901–5.
184. Kilpatrick SE, Teot LA, Geisinger KR, et al. Relationship of DNA ploidy to histology and prognosis in rhabdomyosarcoma. Comparison of flow cytometry and image analysis. Cancer 1994;74(12):3227–33.
185. Staibano S, Franco R, Tranfa F, et al. Orbital rhabdomyosarcoma: relationship between DNA ploidy, p53, bcl-2, MDR-1 and Ki67 (MIB1) expression and clinical behavior. Anticancer Res 2004;24(1):249–57.
186. Ognjanovic S, Olivier M, Bergemann TL, et al. Sarcomas in TP53 germline mutation carriers: a review of the IARC TP53 database. Cancer 2012;118:1387–96.

187. Canner JA, Sobo M, Ball S, et al. MI-63: a novel small-molecule inhibitor targets MDM2 and induces apoptosis in embryonal and alveolar rhabdomyosarcoma cells with wild-type p53. Br J Cancer 2009;101(5):774–81.
188. Barr FG, Duan F, Smith LM, et al. Genomic and clinical analyses of 2p24 and 12q13-q14 amplification in alveolar rhabdomyosarcoma: a report from the Children's Oncology Group. Genes Chromosomes Cancer 2009;48(8):661–72.
189. Kelly KM, Womer RB, Sorensen PH, et al. Common and variant gene fusions predict distinct clinical phenotypes in rhabdomyosarcoma. J Clin Oncol 1997;15(5):1831–6.
190. Meazza C, Ferrari A, Casanova M, et al. Rhabdomyosarcoma of the head and neck region: experience at the pediatric unit of the Istituto Nazionale Tumori, Milan. J Otolaryngol 2006;35(1):53–9.
191. Raney B, Anderson J, Breneman J, et al. Results in patients with cranial parameningeal sarcoma and metastases (Stage 4) treated on Intergroup Rhabdomyosarcoma Study Group (IRSG) Protocols II-IV, 1978-1997: report from the Children's Oncology Group. Pediatr Blood Cancer 2008;51(1):17–22.
192. Dantonello TM, Winkler P, Boelling T, et al. Embryonal rhabdomyosarcoma with metastases confined to the lungs: report from the CWS Study Group. Pediatr Blood Cancer 2011;56(5):725–32.
193. Tomaszewski JJ, Sweeney DD, Kavoussi LR, et al. Laparoscopic retroperitoneal lymph node dissection for high-risk pediatric patients with paratesticular rhabdomyosarcoma. J Endourol 2010;24(1):31–4.
194. Thomas-de-Montpréville V, Nottin R, Dulmet E, et al. Heart tumors in children and adults: clinicopathological study of 59 patients from a surgical center. Cardiovasc Pathol 2007;16(1):22–8.
195. Pratt CB, Hustu HO, Kumar AP, et al. Treatment of childhood rhabdomyosarcoma at St. Jude Children's Research Hospital, 1962-78. Natl Cancer Inst Monogr 1981;56:93–101.
196. Piersigilli F, Danhaive O, Auriti C. Blueberry muffin baby due to alveolar rhabdomyosarcoma with cutaneous metastasis. Arch Dis Child Fetal Neonatal Ed 2010;95(6):F461.

Chapter 21 Benign Vascular Tumors and Malformations

CHAPTER CONTENTS

The term *hemangioma*, in the past, has been applied broadly to any benign, nonreactive vascular process with an increase in normal or abnormal-appearing vessels. Hemangiomas have been further subclassified pathologically, based on the predominant type of vessel. This was a simple and convenient approach for the pathologist who was often not apprised of the clinical or radiographic findings in a given case but conveyed a limited amount of biologic information to the clinicians. Advances in the understanding of the pathogenesis of this diverse group of lesions have led to a multidisciplinary consensus that benign vascular lesions be divided into two biologic groups: tumors and malformations. This dichotomy has important clinical implications.[1,2]

The International Society for the Study of Vascular Anomalies, based on earlier work,[2] has recommended that the term *hemangioma* be applied to lesions that arise as a result of cellular proliferation on the presumption that they are true neoplasms. Typically composed of capillary vessels, they grow in a disproportionately rapid fashion relative to the patient but may, depending on the type, involute. Vascular malformations, in contrast, are developmental abnormalities of the embryonic vasculature. They develop *in utero*, typically make their appearance at birth, grow proportionately with the patient, and display little proliferative activity. They are composed of any combination of arteries, veins, and capillaries. Some are associated with specific genetic defects (Table 21-1).

Despite these defining features, the histologic distinction between hemangiomas and vascular malformations is not always possible without clinical and imaging information. In fact, the growing number of vascular lesions linked to specific genetic defects suggests that these, too, may ultimately be incorporated into a comprehensive classification scheme. Dividing lesions into hemangiomas and vascular malformations has been attempted to the extent that is possible. Lesions for which the pathogenesis is uncertain are discussed at the end of the chapter.

HEMANGIOMAS

A hemangioma is one of the most common soft tissue tumors and is the most common tumor during infancy and childhood[1,3] (Table 21-2). Most hemangiomas are superficial lesions that have a predilection for the head and neck region, but they may also occur internally, such as in the liver. Hemangiomas are typically composed of capillary vessels arranged in lobules, which are subserved by a feeder vessel. This architectural organization has led to the term *lobular hemangioma* for some capillary hemangiomas. This term is descriptive and not useful for special forms of capillary hemangiomas occurring in the pediatric age group. Although some vascular tumors regress altogether (e.g., infantile hemangioma), most persist if untreated but have limited growth potential. Hemangiomas virtually never undergo malignant transformation, with the exception of those that have been irradiated. The concept of benign metastasizing hemangioma is no longer accepted. Most prove to be angiosarcomas with well-differentiated areas.

Capillary hemangiomas usually appear during the first few years of life, with the exception of the acquired adult form (e.g., cherry angiomas), and are located in the skin or subcutaneous tissue. Rare cases are familial; linkage analysis has localized the mutation to chromosome 5,[4] although the candidate gene has not been identified. However, sporadic hemangiomas also exhibit loss of heterozygosity in the region of 5q, which includes the *FLT4 (VEGFR3)*[5] gene. Typically elevated and red to purple in color, they are composed of a proliferation of capillary-sized vessels lined by flattened endothelium.

Cherry Angioma (Senile Angioma, Campbell de Morgan Spots)

Cherry angioma is a common acquired vascular lesion of adult life. Lesions present as ruby red papules with a pale halo and measure a few millimeters in diameter[6] and show a predilection for the trunk and extremity. These lesions may increase in number over time, and some have been noted to occur in crops in nursing homes, in association with infections, and with exposure to various chemicals. The lesions, located in the superficial corium, consist of lobules of capillaries lined by prominent endothelium. With age, the capillaries dilate resulting in elevation and mild atrophy of the skin (Fig. 21-1). Some lesions have a collarette similar to a pyogenic granuloma.

TABLE 21-1 Hereditary Vascular Malformations

MALFORMATION	LOCUS	LOCUS NAME	MUTATED GENE	TYPE OF MUTATION
Hereditary capillary malformation (CM)	5q13-15	CMC	?	
Cerebral cavernous (or capillary) malformation (CCM)	7q11-22	CCM1	*KRIT1*	Inactivating?
	7p13-35	CCM2	?	
	3q25.2-27	CCM3	?	
Hyperkeratotic cutaneous capillary venous malformation (HCCVM)	7q11-22	CCM1	*KRIT1*	Inactivating?
Arteriovenous malformation	5q13-15?	CMC1	?	
Hereditary hemorrhagic telangiectasia (HHT)	9q33-34	HHT1	*ENG*	Inactivating
	12q11-14	HHT2	*ALK1*	Inactivating?
Venous malformation (VM)	9p21	VMCM1	*TIE2 (TEK)*	Activating
Glomuvenous malformation	1p21-22	VMGLOM	*GLOMULIN*	Inactivating?
Primary congenital lymphedema (Milroy disease)	5q34-35	?	*FLT4 (VEGFR3)*	Inactivating?

Modified from Brouillard P, Vikkula M. Vascular malformations: localized defects in vascular morphogenesis. Clin Genet *2003;63(5):540–51.*

TABLE 21-2 Differential Diagnosis of Pediatric Vascular Tumors and Malformations

LESION	CLINICAL FEATURES	PATHOLOGIC FEATURES
Infantile hemangioma	Skin and/or subcutaneous lesion developing in early postnatal period. Rapidly grows and slowly involutes over 1 to 2 years.	Lobules of poorly canalized capillaries with mitotically active endothelium and prominent pericytes. Late lesions with canalized vessels and multilayered basement membrane. Endothelium is GLUT1 positive.
Congenital nonprogressive hemangioma	Fully formed at birth with little or no postnatal growth. Pursues non-involuting (NICH) or rapidly involuting course (RICH).	Lobules of capillaries with prominent draining veins separated by fibrotic stroma. Endothelium mitotically inactive and GLUT1 negative.
Kaposiform hemangioendothelioma	Congenital or acquired lesion of skin or deep tissues. Most common cause of Kasabach-Merritt phenomenon secondary to platelet trapping. Progressive growth and rare local metastasis.	Irregular cannon ball nodules infiltrating tissues composed of slit-like vessels circumscribing glomeruloid vessels containing fibrin thrombi. Endothelium express lymphatic markers (LYVE 1, PROX1) but not GLUT1.
Vascular malformation	Developmental abnormality of embryonic vasculature presenting at birth. In deep locations, lesions can present later. Grows proportionately with patient. No regression.	Variable mixture of large arteries, veins, venules, and capillaries some with arteriovenous shunting. Vessels are architecturally abnormal and mitotically inactive. Endothelium is mitotically inactive and GLUT1-negative.

Modified from North PE. Pediatric vascular tumors and malformations. Surg Pathol *2010;3:455–94.*

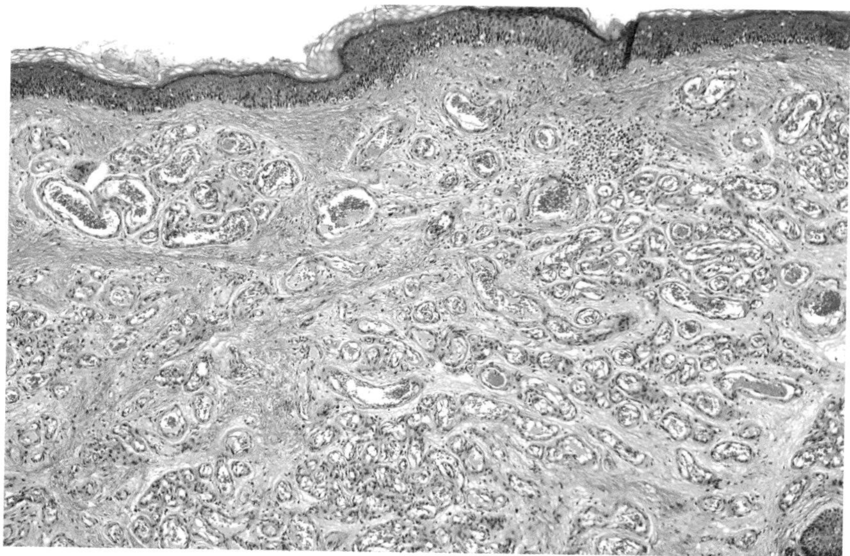

FIGURE 21-1. Adult form of capillary hemangioma consisting of small vessels lined by flattened mature endothelium.

Infantile Hemangioma

Infantile hemangioma, also known as *cellular hemangioma of infancy*, is a form of capillary hemangioma[4,7,8] that affects about 5% of children.[1] Females are affected more often than males by a ratio of 3 to 1. Although most cases are sporadic, some cases display familial segregation and have been linked to chromosome 5q31-33, suggesting that mutation at this locus predisposes to the tumor.[4,9] There is some evidence that sporadic cases are the result of somatic mutations.[5] A small subset of infantile hemangiomas has a segmental distribution and is associated with other abnormalities, including posterior fossa brain malformation, ***h***emangioma, ***a***rterial cerebrovascular abnormalities, ***c***ardiovascular anomalies, and ***e***ye anomalies (recognized as PHACE syndrome).[10]

During the early stage, the infantile hemangioma resembles a common birthmark and is a flat, red lesion that intensifies in color when the infant strains or cries. With time, it acquires an elevated, protruding appearance that distinguishes it from birthmarks and has earned it the fanciful designation of *strawberry nevus* (Fig. 21-2). Deeply situated lesions impart little color to the overlying skin and, consequently, may be misdiagnosed preoperatively. These tumors may be located on any body surface but are most common in the region of the head and neck, particularly the parotid, where they seemingly follow the distribution of cutaneous nerves and arteries.

The evolution of these lesions is characteristic. They appear within a few weeks after birth[7] and rapidly enlarge over a period of several months, achieving the largest size in about 6 to 12 months; they regress over a period of a few years. Regression is usually accompanied by fading of the lesion from scarlet to dull red-gray and by concomitant wrinkling of the once-taut skin. It has been estimated that by age 7 years, 75% to 90% have involuted, leaving a small pigmented scar. In the lesions that have ulcerated, the cosmetic defect may be more significant. The clinical phases of infantile hemangioma have distinctive physiologic differences elegantly detailed by Takahashi et al.,[8] as described in the following section.

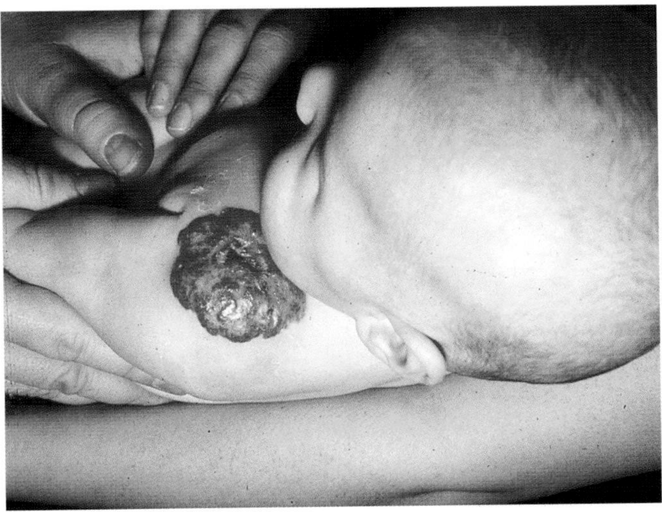

FIGURE 21-2. Clinical appearance of infantile hemangioma.

The tumors are multinodular masses fed by a single normally occurring arteriole (Fig. 21-3).[7] Because they are high flow lesions, draining vessels may be prominent. Histologically, the tumor varies with its age, although there is no sharp demarcation between proliferative and evolutional phase lesions. Early proliferative lesions are characterized by plump endothelial cells and pericytes with a clear cytoplasm, which form small capillaries with inconspicuous lumens (Figs. 21-4 to 21-6). The cellularity of the lesion is so striking as to obscure the fundamental vascular pattern. Mitotic figures are present in moderate numbers. Mast cells and factor XIIIa-positive interstitial cells are a consistent feature of these tumors. The former may be important in the production of angiogenic factors that regulate the growth of these tumors. As the lesions mature and blood flow through the lesion commences, the endothelium becomes flattened and resembles that seen in adult forms of capillary hemangioma (see Fig. 21-5). Maturation usually begins at the periphery of the tumors but ultimately involves all zones. Involution of the infantile hemangioma is accompanied by a disappearance of the capillaries, thickening of vascular basement membrane containing apoptotic dust, increased mast cells, and progressive interstitial fibrosis. Large arteries and veins may remain, however. In unusual cases, infarction of the tumor occurs, presumably as a result of thrombosis.

The clinical phases of infantile hemangiomas have been correlated with a distinctive immunophenotypic profile.[8] During the early proliferative phase (0 to 12 months), the tumors express proliferating cell nuclear antigen (PCNA), vascular endothelial growth factor (VEGF), and type IV collagenase, the former two localized to both endothelium and pericytes and the last to endothelium. All are associated with proliferation and growth of vessels. The adjacent epidermis potentially contributes to the production of angiogenic

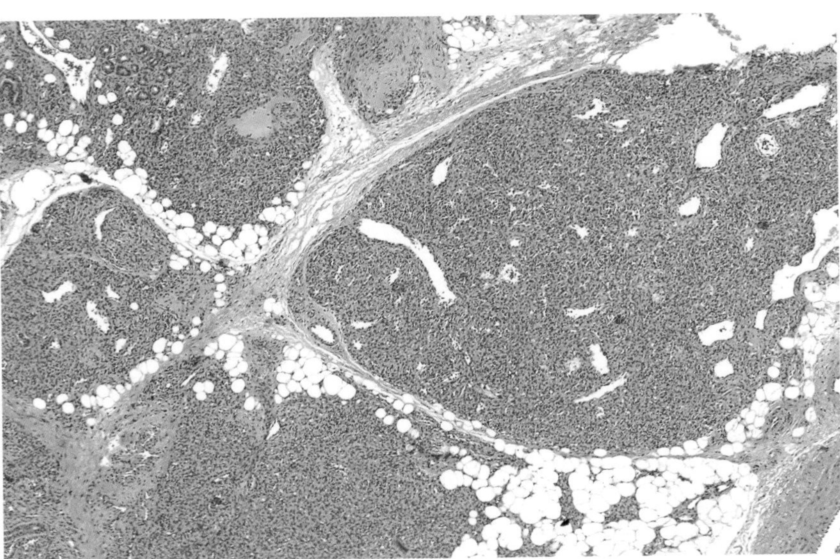

FIGURE 21-3. Low-power view of infantile hemangioma illustrating lobular growth. Lobules contain central feeding vessels.

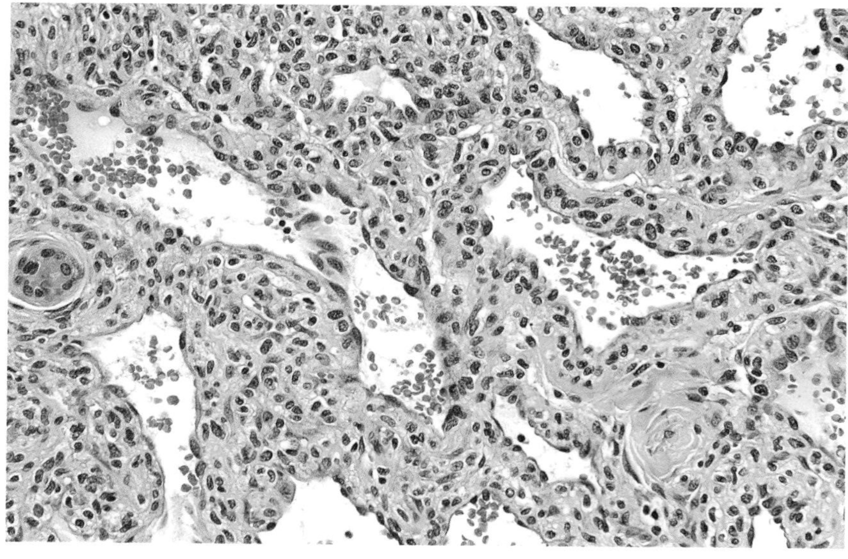

FIGURE 21-4. Infantile form of capillary hemangioma showing a combination of well-canalized and poorly canalized vessels.

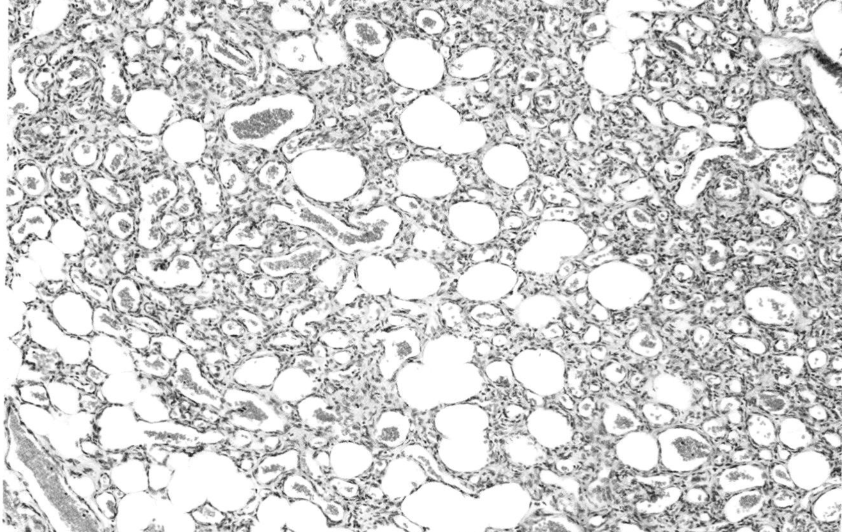

FIGURE 21-5. Infantile hemangioma showing canalization of most vessels.

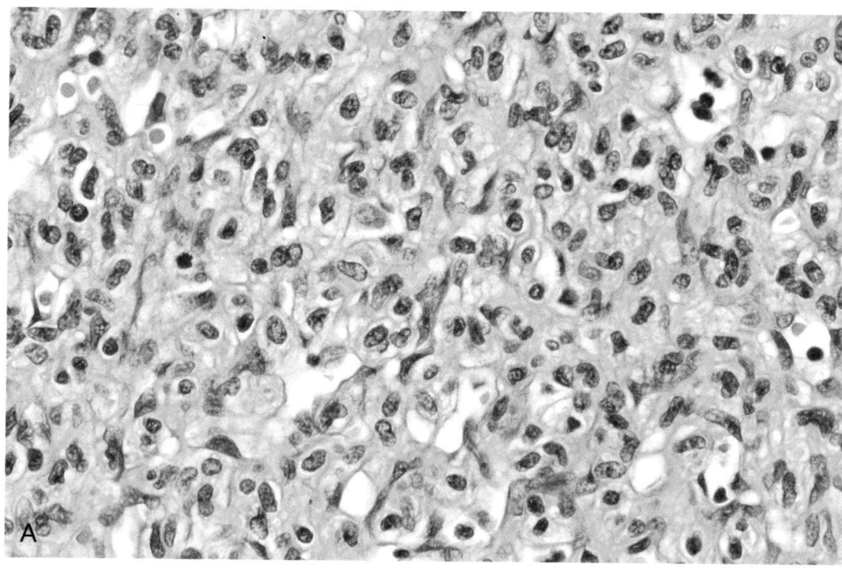

FIGURE 21-6. (A) High-power view of cellular areas of infantile hemangioma.

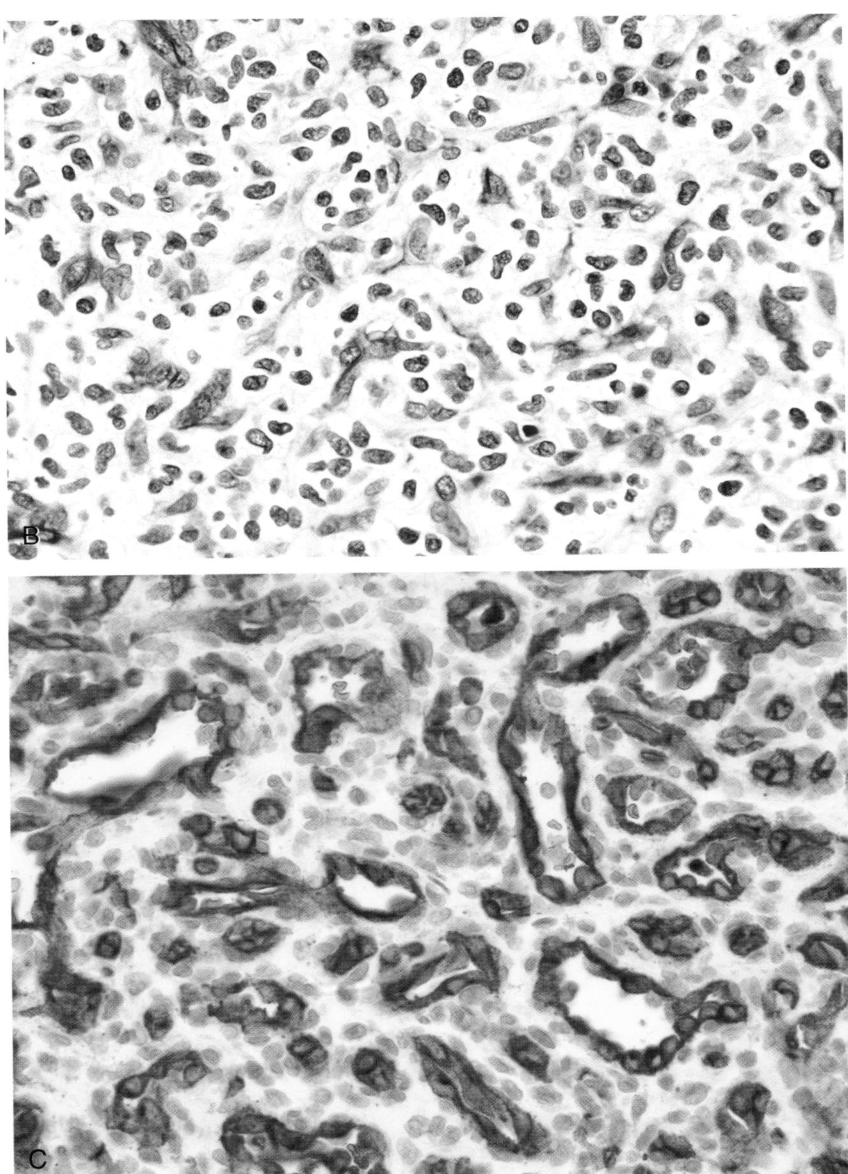

FIGURE 21-6, cont'd. (B) Immunostain for von Willebrand factor (vWF) illustrates a network of mature endothelial cells. Note the population of nonreactive cells representing a combination of immature endothelial cells and pericytes. (C) GLUT1 immunostaining within infantile hemangioma showing endothelial and erythrocyte staining.

factors. During the involution phase (1 to 5 years), these substances are dramatically reduced, whereas the tissue inhibitors of metalloproteinases (also known as TIMP), antiangiogenic factors, are markedly elevated. The traditional vascular markers, CD31, von Willebrand factor (vWF), and smooth muscle actin (a pericyte marker), are present during the proliferative and involution phases but are lost after the lesion is fully involuted. These findings contrast with congenital vascular lesions and malformations, which remain static throughout their natural history, and do not express PCNA, VEGF, and type IV collagenase. Infantile hemangiomas also express GLUT1, a glucose transport receptor.[1] The expression of this receptor is independent of proliferative activity and is not found in other forms of hemangioma, although it is present rarely in angiosarcomas. This protein is also expressed by human placenta and has led to the suggestion that these tumors arise from a vascular precursor cell in the placenta.[11]

Treatment of these lesions must be individualized and depends on factors such as the location and rate of growth. Most tumors can be masterfully neglected and allowed to regress spontaneously. Others require surgery, corticosteroids, pulsed dye laser, or off label use of propanolol.[1] Large, life-threatening lesions, impinging on critical structures (e.g., airway), have been treated with systemic glucocorticoids and interferon. The decision to use the latter requires prudence because of its association with spastic diplegia.

Congenital Nonprogressive Hemangioma

Congenital nonprogressive hemangioma is a recently recognized lesion, which, in the past, was grouped with infantile hemangioma but is clinically and morphologically distinct.[12-15] In contrast to infantile hemangioma, it presents at birth as a fully developed cutaneous lesion. It affects the sexes equally. Multiple lesions, some involving viscera, have been reported. Following birth, the lesions may remain static or rapidly involute. Static and involuting lesions are referred to as *non-involuting congenital hemangioma (NICH)* and *rapidly involuting congenital hemangioma (RICH)*, respectively. RICH typically regress at a much faster rate than infantile hemangiomas.

Despite the terms *NICH* and *RICH*, there is overlap between the two subtypes, indicating that they are part of a common spectrum. In fact, some use the term *congenital nonprogressive hemangioma* and modify it as appropriate when clinical history is available. Clinically, both RICH and NICH display a peripheral pallor. RICH, in addition, develops a central depression or ulcer as it regresses. Both are composed of capillary lobules separated by dense fibrous tissue containing atrophic adnexal structures (Fig. 21-7). The capillary vessels contain both plump endothelial cells and pericytes, which may closely resemble those of the proliferative phase of infantile hemangioma. But, in contrast, proliferative activity is low, and GLUT1 expression is absent. Draining and feeding vessels within these lesions can be quite prominent and give the superficial impression of a vascular malformation, particularly if involution has occurred.

Pyogenic Granuloma

The pyogenic granuloma is a polypoid form of capillary hemangioma occurring on the skin and mucosal surfaces.[16,17] Its pathogenesis is controversial, with some considering them neoplasms and others a reactive hyperplasia. Their lobular architecture has been used to justify their inclusion with other

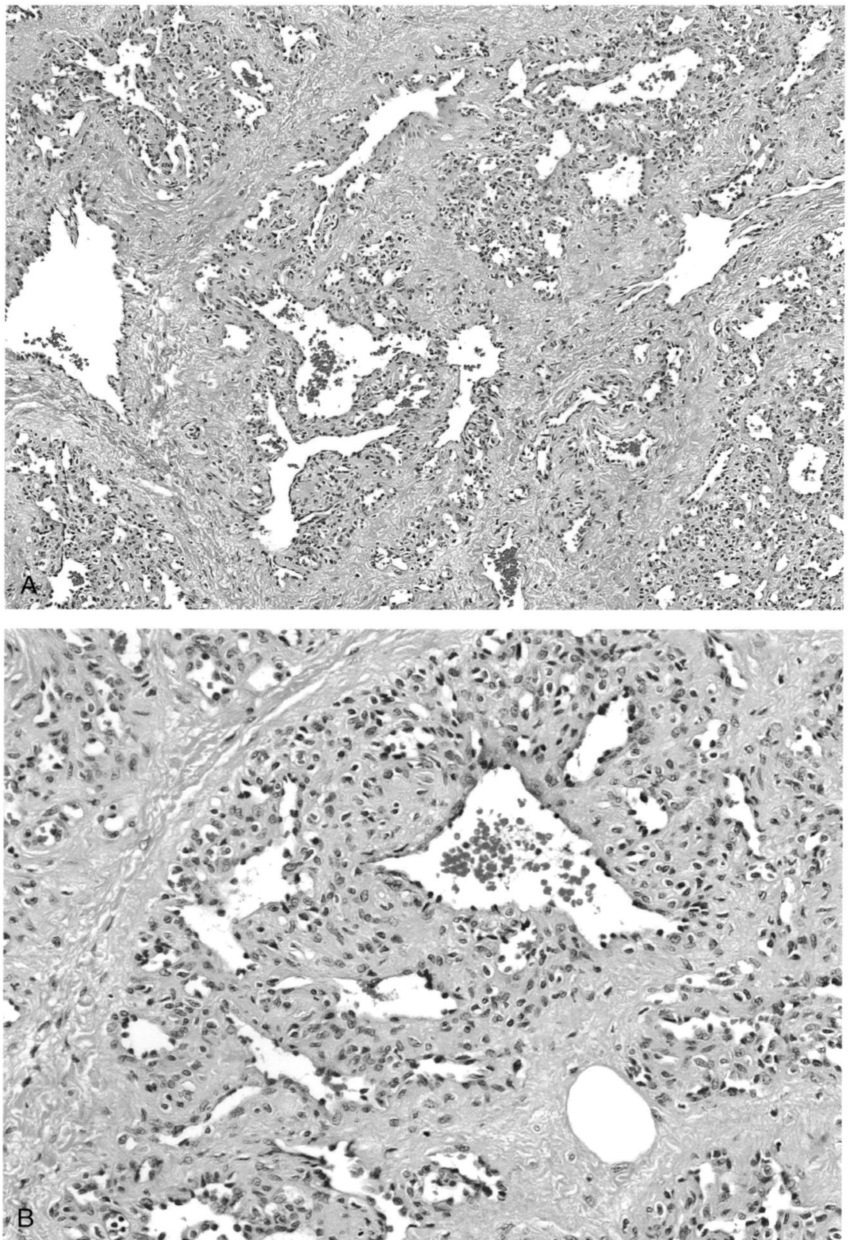

FIGURE 21-7. Congenital hemangioma. Non-involuting congenital non-progressive hemangioma (A, B).

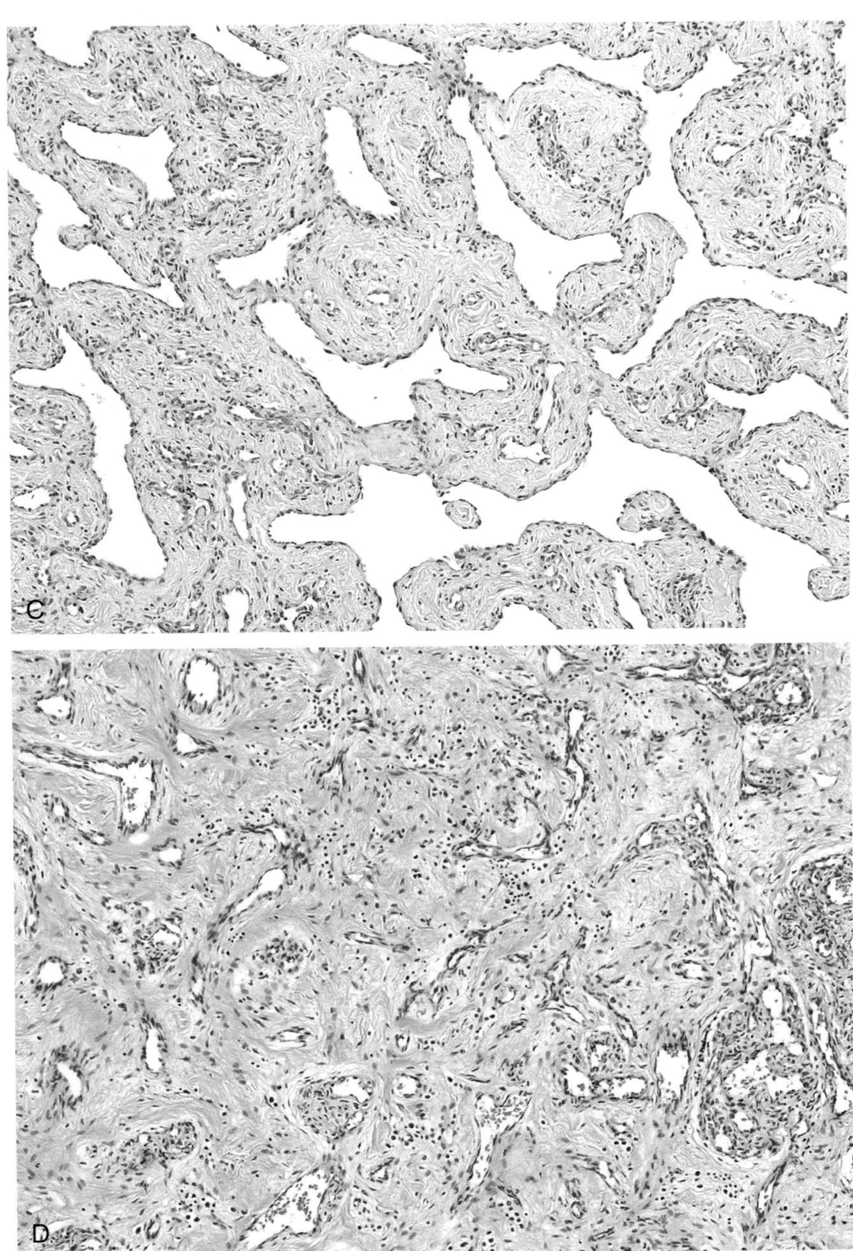

FIGURE 21-7, cont'd. Rapidly involuting congenital hemangioma (C, D). *(Case courtesy of Dr. Harry Kozekewich of Boston Children's Hospital.)*

capillary hemangiomas, but, conversely, their appearance following trauma, during pregnancy (see granuloma gravidarum), and during retinoid therapy mounts a compelling counterargument.

The pyogenic granuloma bears a striking resemblance to granulation tissue, and, in fact, most early pathologists considered them infectious. Poncet and Dor, credited with the first description, believed that these lesions were secondary to infection by *Botryomyces* organisms, whereas others implicated pyogenic bacteria, specifically staphylococci. Uncomplicated lesions, however, lack ulceration and inflammation and resemble other capillary (lobular) hemangiomas.

These tumors occur on either the skin or the mucosal surfaces, although the latter accounts for about 60% of all cases. In the extensive review of 289 cases by Kerr,[16] the gingiva, finger, lips, face, and tongue accounted for over 70% of cases. The genders are affected approximately equally, and the disease is evenly distributed over all decades. Approximately one-third develop following minor trauma and, in rare cases, in port-wine stains.[18] Multiple lesions may develop simultaneously, but this phenomenon almost always occurs in the cutaneous form rather than in the mucosal form of the disease. There have been a few reports of disseminated (eruptive) forms of pyogenic granuloma,[19] some following surgical removal of a solitary pyogenic granuloma. Disseminated pyogenic granulomas progress for a limited time and, ultimately, stabilize or regress. The mechanism for these initially alarming presentations is not clear, although some have suggested the release of angiogenic factors by the tumors. In the ordinary case, the tumors develop rapidly and achieve their maximal size of several millimeters to a few centimeters within a few weeks or months. The well-established lesion is a polypoid, friable, purple-red mass that bleeds easily and frequently ulcerates. Sessile forms of this tumor also occur, but they tend to be recurrent lesions.

The appearance of these lesions at low magnification immediately suggests the diagnosis. They are a distinctly exophytic growth connected to the skin by a stalk of varying diameter (Figs. 21-8 to 21-12) and, occasionally, are surrounded by a heaped-up collar of normal tissue. The adjacent epithelium is hyperkeratotic or acanthotic, but the epithelium overlying the lesion itself is flattened, atrophic, or ulcerated. The basic lesion is a lobular (capillary) hemangioma[20] set in a fibromyxoid matrix. Each lobule of the hemangioma is made up of a larger vessel, often with a muscular wall and surrounded by congeries of small capillaries. Most lesions, however, are altered by secondary inflammatory changes; as a result, they have been likened to granulation tissue. Both acute and chronic inflammatory cells are scattered throughout the lesion but, not unexpectedly, are most numerous at the surface. Secondary invading microorganisms are occasionally present in the superficial reaches of ulcerated lesions. Stromal edema may separate the capillary lumens and obscure the lobular arrangement of the tumor (see Fig. 21-11). Mitotic activity may be brisk in the endothelium and stromal fibroblasts when secondary changes, such as edema and inflammation, are present. In lesions that involute, a progressive stromal and perivascular fibrosis ensues. Rarely, the pyogenic granuloma displays epithelioid change of the endothelium (see the section on epithelioid hemangioma).

The clinical appearance of these lesions is quite characteristic and assists in the distinction between lesions such as well-differentiated angiosarcoma or an angiomatous form of Kaposi sarcoma. The pyogenic granuloma is a more or less circumscribed lesion, often with a lobular arrangement, in contrast to the rambling, poorly confined nature of malignant vascular neoplasms. The manner in which even well-differentiated angiosarcomas dissect through connective tissue and create irregular vascular spaces contrasts sharply with the pyogenic granuloma. Kaposi sarcoma also is not well circumscribed and contains at least focal cellular zones of spindled cells, which form the classic slit-like vascular spaces. However, these diagnostic areas are typically located in the central or deep areas of the tumor, whereas the well-differentiated angiomatous component is seen peripherally or superficially. In difficult cases, immunohistochemistry for

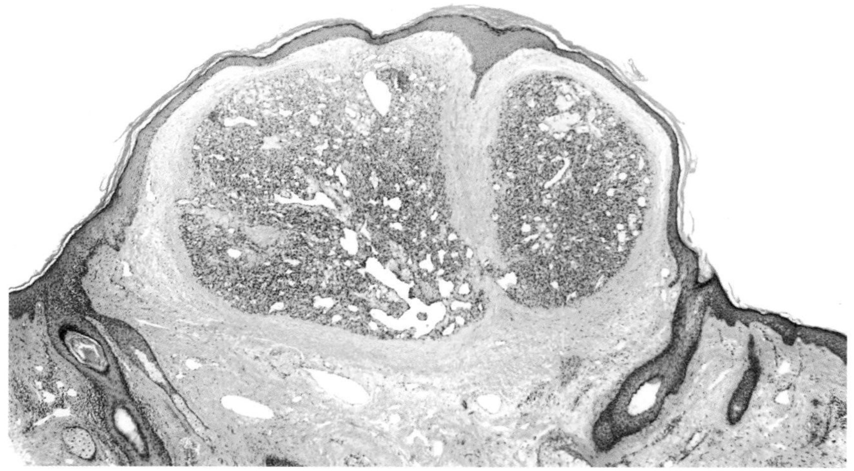

FIGURE 21-8. Pyogenic granuloma. Lesion is characterized by exophytic growth.

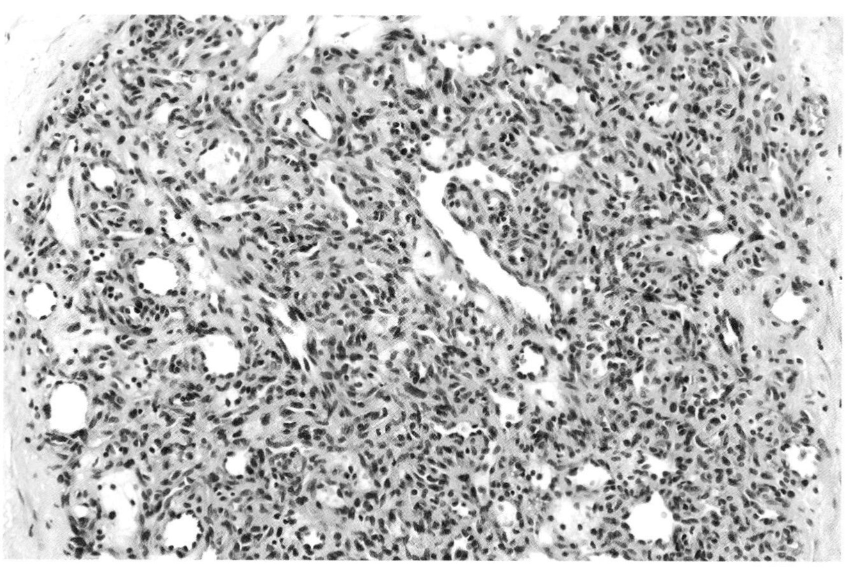

FIGURE 21-9. Lobular growth of vessels in a pyogenic granuloma.

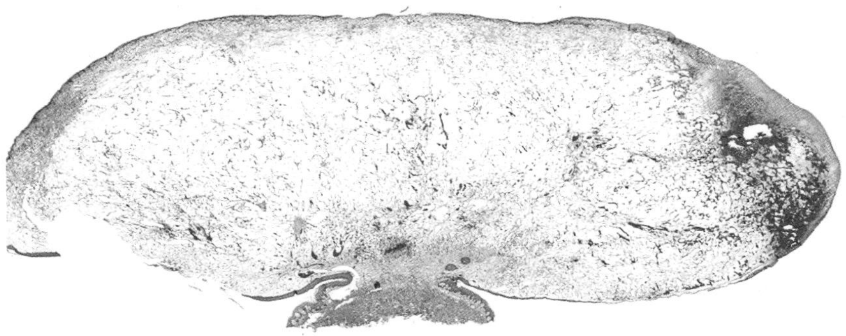

FIGURE 21-10. Pyogenic granuloma with ulceration of surface and marked stromal edema.

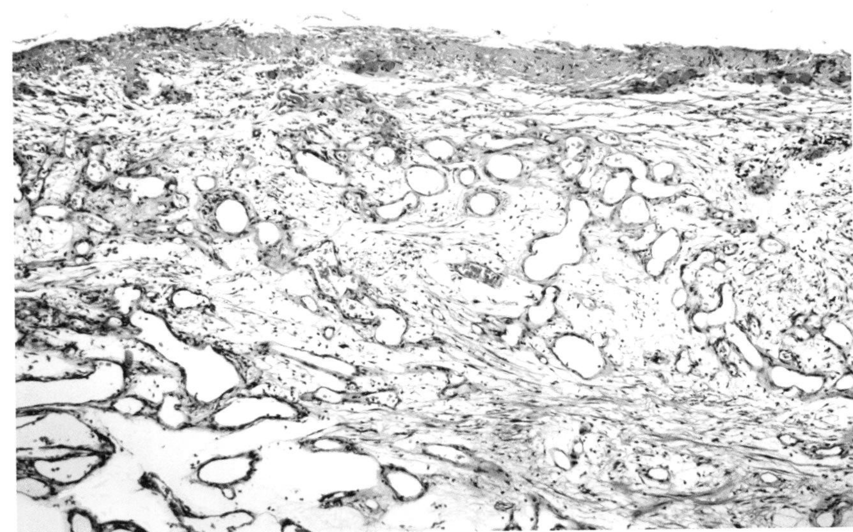

FIGURE 21-11. Stromal edema widely separating vessels of a pyogenic granuloma. (Same case as Fig. 22-10.)

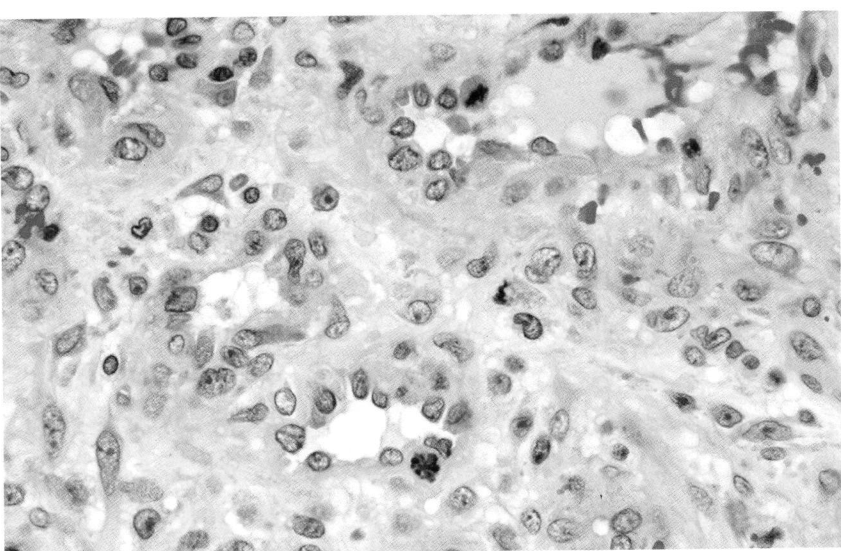

FIGURE 21-12. Mitotic activity in stromal and endothelial cells of a pyogenic granuloma.

HHV-8 LANA protein may be of value in the distinction of angiomatous forms of Kaposi sarcoma from pyogenic granuloma. Therefore, in some instances, a superficial biopsy of a vascular neoplasm may not be adequate to exclude malignancy.

Although the pyogenic granuloma is a benign lesion, 16% were noted to recur in one large series of tumors treated conservatively.[21] A significantly lower recurrence rate was noted in a series of 74 cases reported by Mills et al.[20] Recurrent disease may present as a solitary nodule or as multiple small satellite nodules around the site of the original lesion. The phenomenon of *satellitosis* in this disease was analyzed by Warner and Wilson-Jones,[22] who found that most of these lesions occurred on the trunk, particularly the scapular area, and most had been incompletely excised initially. In contrast to the original tumors, the satellites are usually not pedunculated but, rather, are sessile and have an intact surface epithelium. In these respects, they grossly resemble ordinary hemangiomas. Although the rapid development of numerous satellite lesions often causes considerable alarm on the part of the clinician, these lesions usually respond to reexcision and, in some instances, have even regressed spontaneously.

Pregnancy-Related Pyogenic Granuloma (Granuloma Gravidarum)

Granuloma gravidarum is a pyogenic granuloma that occurs on the gingival surface during pregnancy.[23] It is estimated that gingival changes occur in about 50% of pregnant women, but that only about 1% of this group develops localized tumors. Typically, these lesions develop abruptly during the first trimester and arise from the interdental area of the gum. They are grossly and histologically indistinguishable from the ordinary form of pyogenic granuloma. They usually regress dramatically following parturition, although many persist as small mucosal nodules capable of renewed growth at the time of subsequent pregnancies. This unusual tumor has provided some of the most compelling evidence that the pyogenic granuloma lacks the degree of autonomous growth that characterizes most vascular tumors of adulthood. In fact, hormone sensitivity manifested by granuloma gravidarum has led many to conclude that these are not neoplastic lesions.

Intravenous Pyogenic Granuloma

An intravenous counterpart of pyogenic granuloma was recognized by Cooper et al.[24] This tumor is most common on the neck and upper extremity. It presents as a red-brown intravascular polyp that can be easily mistaken for an organizing thrombus (Fig. 21-13). The tumor arises from the vein wall and protrudes deeply into the lumen but remains anchored to the wall by means of a narrow stalk containing the feeder vessels. The tumor is covered by a lining of endothelium, and the stroma often contains smooth muscle fibers, presumably remnants of the vein wall. Histologically, they are identical to uncomplicated pyogenic granulomas in that these tumors display no inflammatory or ulcerative change (Fig. 21-14). Like other pyogenic granulomas, they are benign and display no tendency to spread in the bloodstream.

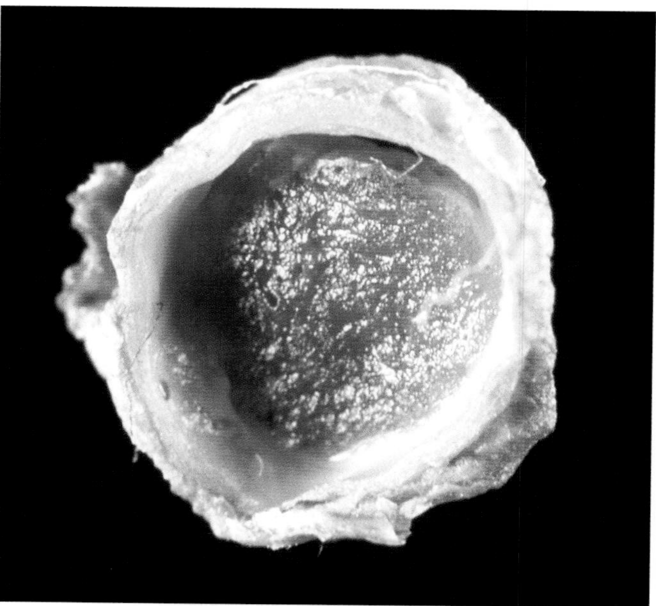

FIGURE 21-13. Gross specimen of the intravascular form of pyogenic granuloma.

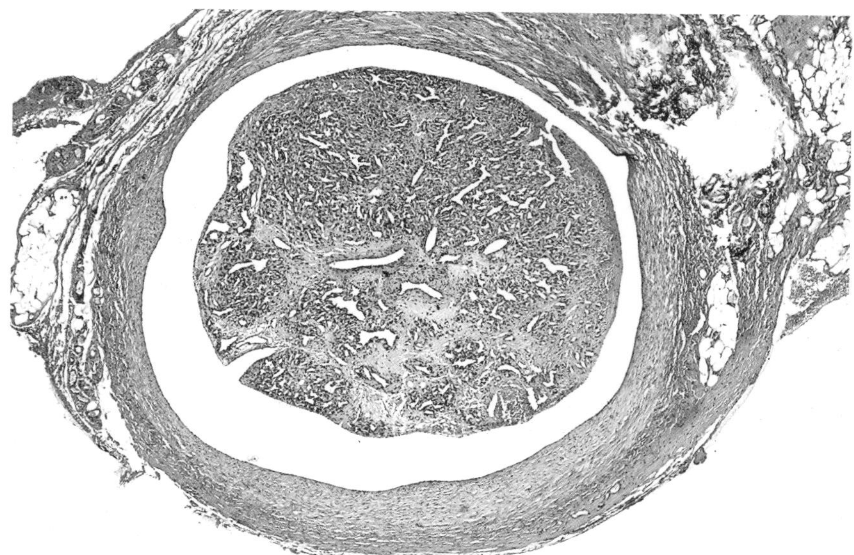

FIGURE 21-14. Intravascular pyogenic granuloma with preservation of the lobular arrangement of vessels.

Epithelioid Hemangioma (Angiolymphoid Hyperplasia with Eosinophilia)

Epithelioid hemangioma is an unusual but distinctive vascular tumor that was first described as *angiolymphoid hyperplasia with eosinophilia*,[25,26] and, subsequently, by others as *inflammatory angiomatous nodule, atypical or pseudopyogenic granuloma*, and *histiocytoid hemangioma*. However, the lesions reported in the Japanese literature as *Kimura disease*[27-30] represent a different entity.

Epithelioid hemangiomas typically occur during early to mid-adult life (ages 20 to 40 years) and affect women more often than men. Most are situated superficially in the head and neck, particularly the region around the ear. As a result, they can be detected relatively early as small, dull red, pruritic plaques. Crusting, excoriation, bleeding, and coalescence of lesions are common secondary features. About half of the patients develop multiple lesions, generally in the same area. Affected patients appear relatively well, although, occasionally, significant regional lymph node enlargement and eosinophilia of the peripheral blood accompany the lesions. These signs have suggested the possibility of an infectious agent, but, to date, none has been identified.

These tumors are circumscribed lesions of the subcutis or dermis (Figs. 21-15 and 21-16), but, occasionally, they involve deep soft tissue, vessels, or parenchymal organs.[31] Like other capillary hemangiomas, epithelioid hemangiomas consist of lobules of small capillary-sized vessels centered around a larger central vessel (Fig. 21-17). In most cases, the capillary vessels are well-formed, multicellular channels with perceptible lumina. However, in epithelioid hemangiomas that are large and deep, the canalization of the vessels may be poor and give the impression that the lesion consists of solid sheets of epithelioid to slightly spindled cells (Figs. 21-18 and 21-19). Solid forms of epithelioid hemangioma are problematic for pathologists and, occasionally, are diagnosed as epithelioid sarcoma or epithelioid angiosarcoma (see later text).

The hallmark of these lesions is the epithelioid endothelial cells (Figs. 21-20 to 21-23) that line a majority, but not necessarily all, of the vessels and protrude deeply into the lumen like tombstones. The epithelioid endothelial cells have rounded or lobated nuclei and abundant acidophilic cytoplasm containing occasional vacuoles that represent primitive vascular lumen formation. Although they have many of the ultrastructural features of normal endothelium, including micropinocytotic vesicles, antiluminal basal lamina, and Weibel-Palade bodies, there are also differences. Adjacent cells are often separated by rather large gaps and interdigitate only along their lateral basal borders by means of tight junctions. Organelles are more abundant in these cells and include increased numbers of mitochondria, smooth and rough endoplasmic reticulum, free ribosomes, and thin cytofilaments.

Epithelioid hemangiomas are typically associated with a prominent inflammatory component. Eosinophils are particularly characteristic of these tumors, but lymphocytes, mast cells, and plasma cells are also present. Lymphoid aggregates replete with germinal centers are occasionally present but are believed by some to be a feature of long-standing lesions or a peculiar host response.

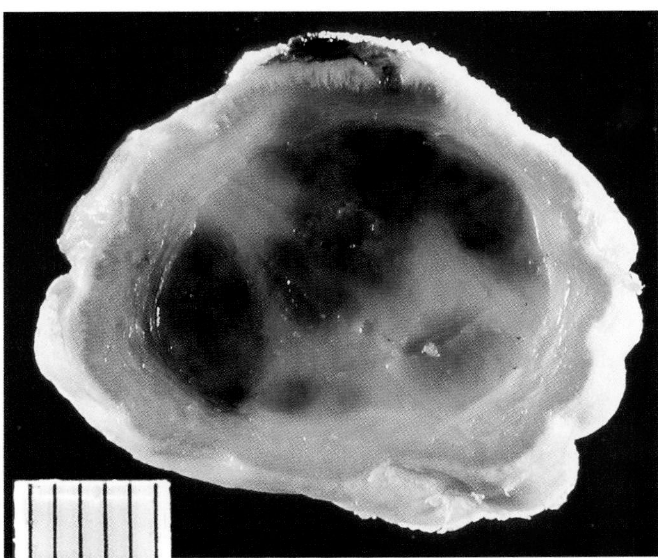

FIGURE 21-15. Gross appearance of a subcutaneous epithelioid hemangioma.

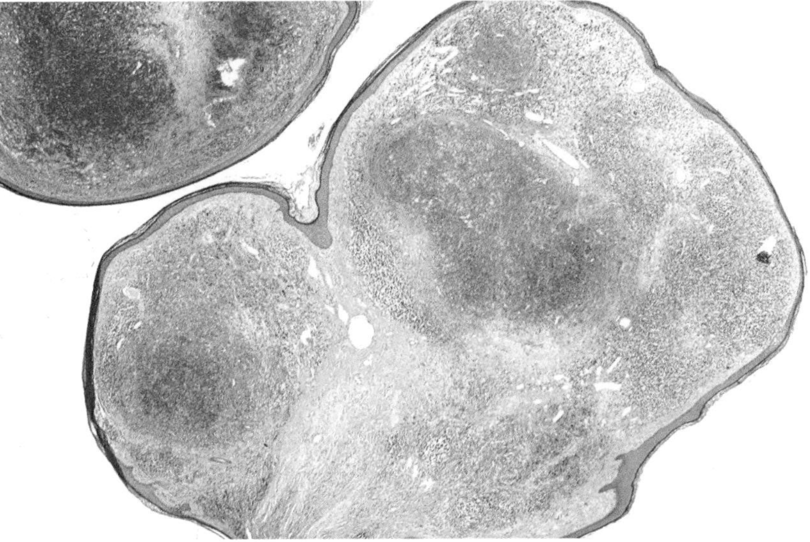

FIGURE 21-16. Low-power view of an epithelioid hemangioma with nodules of vessels surrounded by a prominent lymphoid cuff.

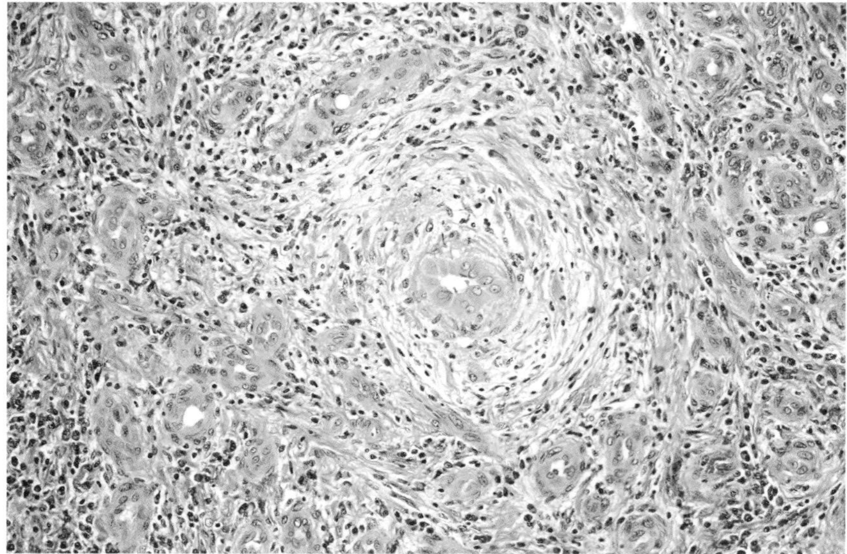

FIGURE 21-17. Epithelioid hemangioma with a central parent vessel surrounded by small vessels and dense inflammation.

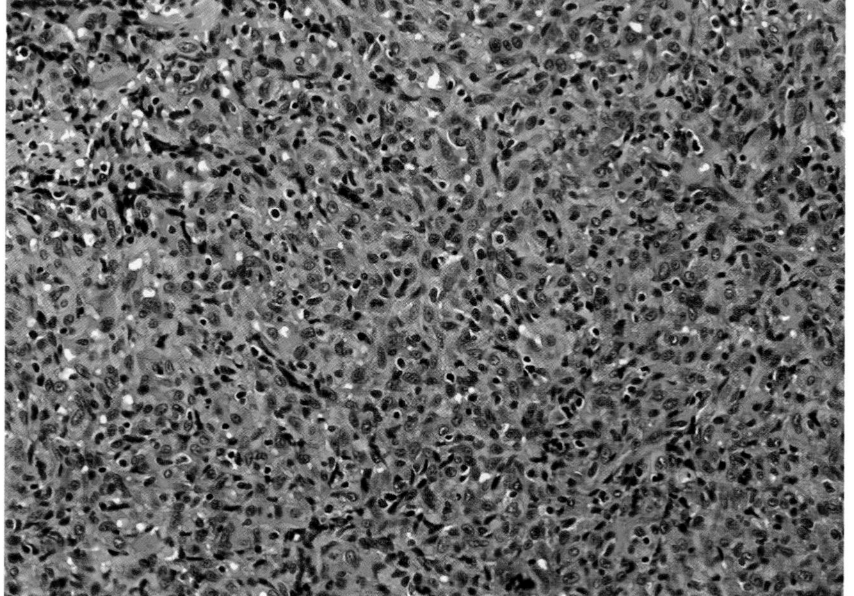

FIGURE 21-18. Solid form of epithelioid hemangioma in which luminal differentiation is subtle or inapparent.

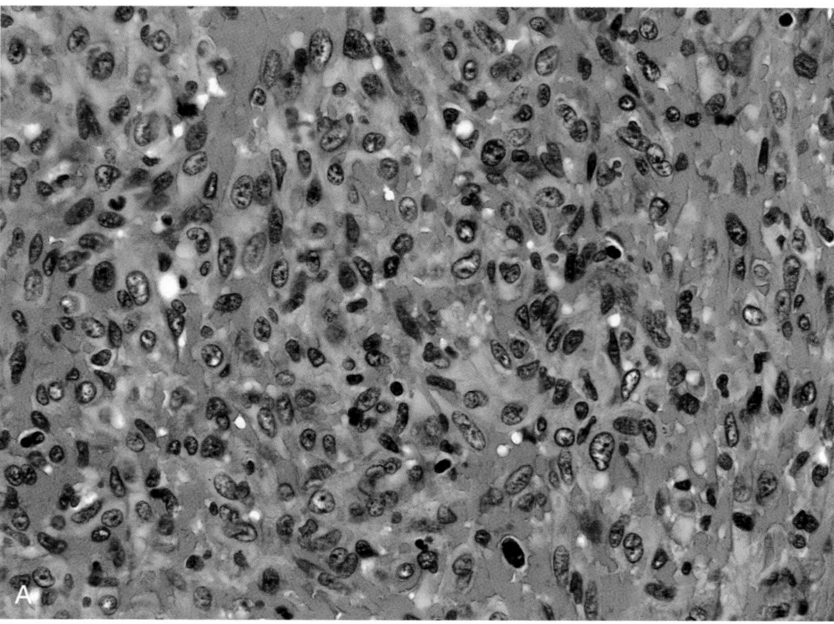

FIGURE 21-19. Solid form of epithelioid hemangioma showing epithelioid areas (A) and spindled areas (B).

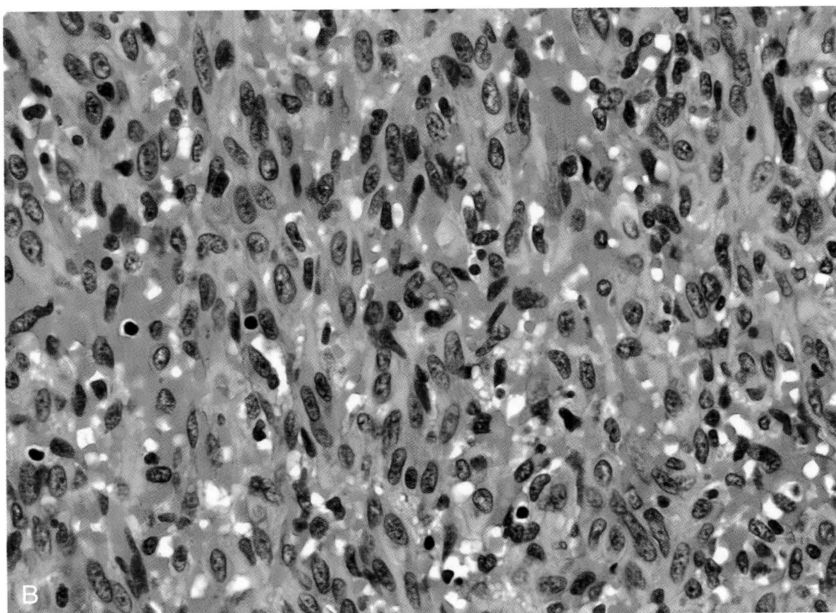

FIGURE 21-19, cont'd

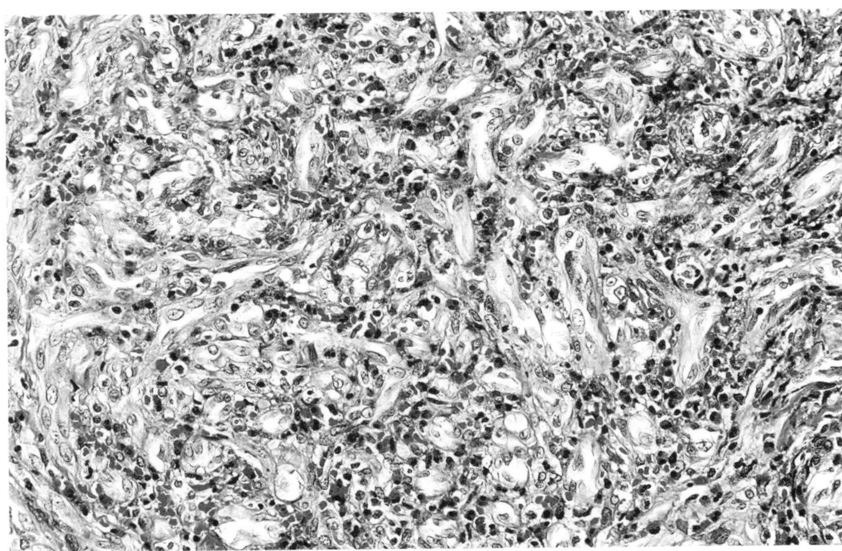

FIGURE 21-20. Epithelioid hemangioma. Vessels are lined by pale-staining cuboidal endothelial cells admixed with inflammatory elements, predominantly eosinophils.

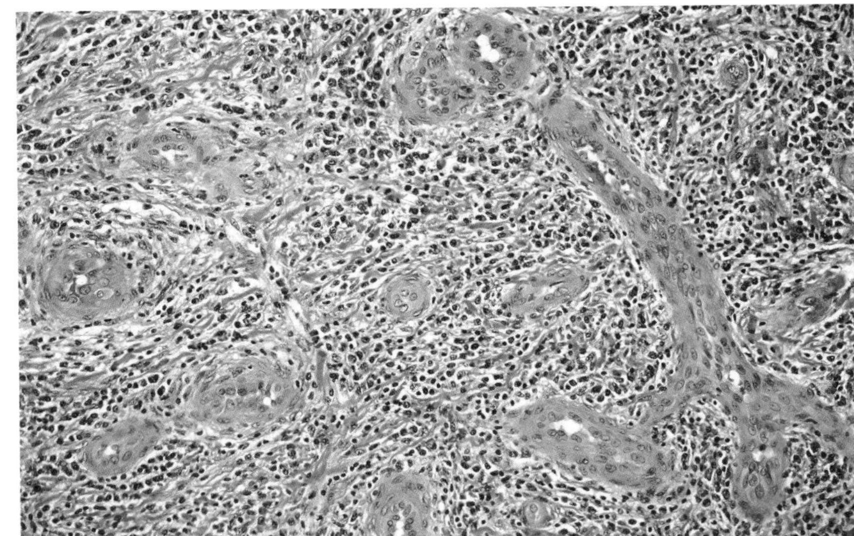

FIGURE 21-21. Epithelioid hemangioma in which some areas display more conventional-appearing endothelial cells interspersed with chronic inflammatory cells.

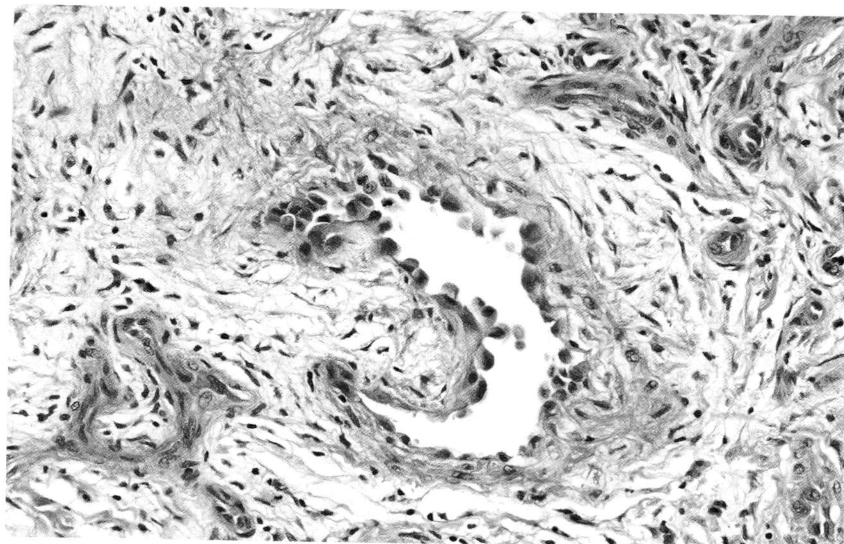

FIGURE 21-22. Tombstone-like appearance of cells in large vessels of epithelioid hemangioma.

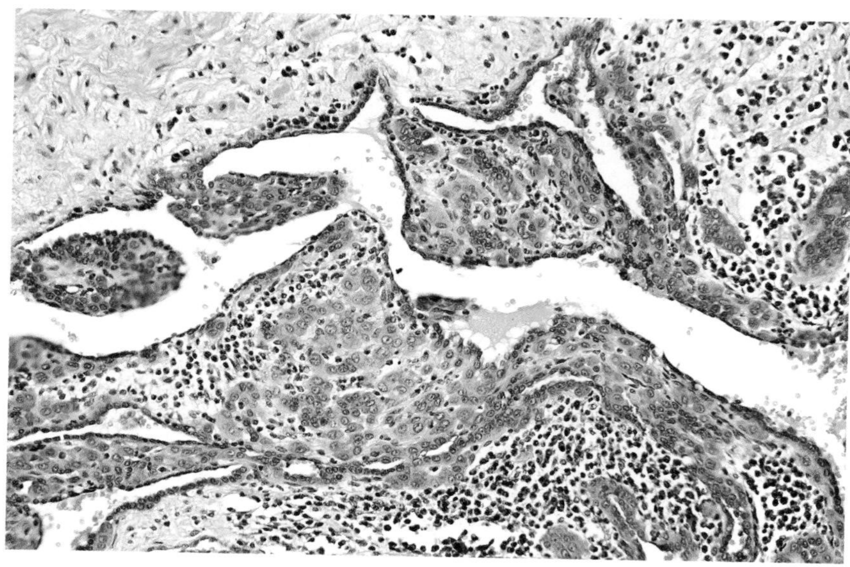

FIGURE 21-23. Epithelioid hemangioma involving the wall of a large vessel. This phenomenon should not be equated with malignancy.

Although about one-third of these lesions recur, virtually none has produced metastasis. One case reported by Reed and Terazakis[26] evidently gave rise to microscopic metastases in a regional lymph node, but this appears to be a unique event. Rare lesions have been noted to regress spontaneously, but, usually, surgical excision is required. About 80% of reported patients have responded at least partially to superficial radiotherapy, but cryotherapy and injection of intralesional steroids have not met with success.

Despite their benign behavior, controversy exists as to whether the lesions are reactive or neoplastic. The fact that 10% occur following trauma,[32] are symmetrically arranged around a vessel with mural damage,[33] and are associated with a prominent inflammatory response has led to the conclusion by some that they are reactive (Fig. 21-24). On the other hand, epithelioid hemangiomas can occur on a multifocal basis and are associated with local recurrences and, in extraordinary cases, by regional lymph node deposits. The most plausible reconciliation for these divergent observations is that the entity may be heterogeneous and that the various lesions embraced under this umbrella are linked by epithelioid change of the endothelium. In fact, the prevailing view is that epithelioid change is an altered functional state of endothelium that may be encountered in benign and malignant vascular tumors as well as in reactive vascular lesions.

The differential diagnosis of epithelioid hemangioma includes the full spectrum of epithelioid vascular lesions, most often epithelioid hemangioendothelioma, and, occasionally, other epithelioid tumors. In contrast to epithelioid hemangiomas, epithelioid hemangioendotheliomas are angiocentric tumors having a distinctive myxohyaline or chondroid background. The cells are arranged in short cords or chains rather than in multicellular vascular channels and rarely have a prominent inflammatory component. Those epithelioid hemangiomas that have solid or medullary zones may be mistaken for epithelioid angiosarcomas. The single most important observation in this regard is the nuclear grade of the cells. Epithelioid angiosarcomas are invariably high-grade lesions composed of large cells with prominent nuclei and nucleoli that sharply contrast with the nuclei of epithelioid hemangioma.

The *epithelioid angiomatous nodule* may be a variant of epithelioid hemangioma having a predominantly solid growth pattern.[34] Like epithelioid hemangioma, they present as dermal nodules, occasionally display multicellular vascular channel formation and inflammation, and pursue a benign course.

The lesion first described by Kim in the Chinese literature and later by Kimura et al.[27] in the Japanese literature as *Kimura disease* is a chronic inflammatory condition that appears to be endemic in the Asian population and occurs only infrequently in Westerners. Although formerly thought to be identical to epithelioid hemangioma (angiolymphoid hyperplasia), many data indicate that they are two entirely unrelated lesions bearing only a few superficial histologic similarities. Kimura disease is often confused with angiolymphoid hyperplasia (epithelioid hemangioma) largely because the term was inappropriately applied to classic examples of angiolymphoid hyperplasia. In fact, the two lesions are clinically and histologically quite different. Kimura disease presents as lymphadenopathy with or without an associated soft tissue mass. Peripheral eosinophilia is nearly always present. Increased serum immunoglobulin E (IgE), proteinuria, and nephrotic syndrome may also occur as part of the disease. Lesions are most frequent in the subcutis of the head and neck area, although lesions have been noted in the groin, extremities, and chest wall. There is a striking male predilection in this disease. The lesions are characterized by dense lymphoid aggregates containing prominent germinal centers (Fig. 21-25). Within the germinal centers, one occasionally

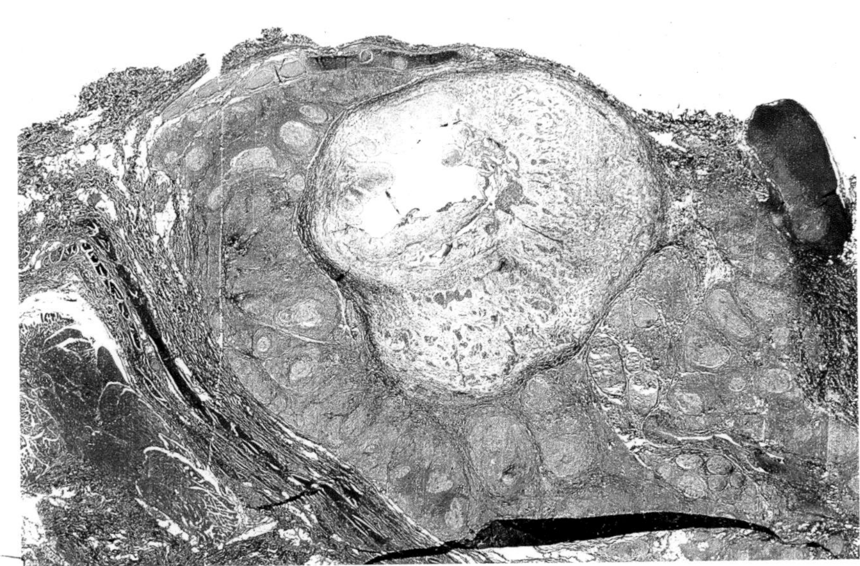

FIGURE 21-24. Changes of an epithelioid hemangioma arising from the wall of traumatized vessel. Note the prominent lymphocytic infiltrate around the lesions.

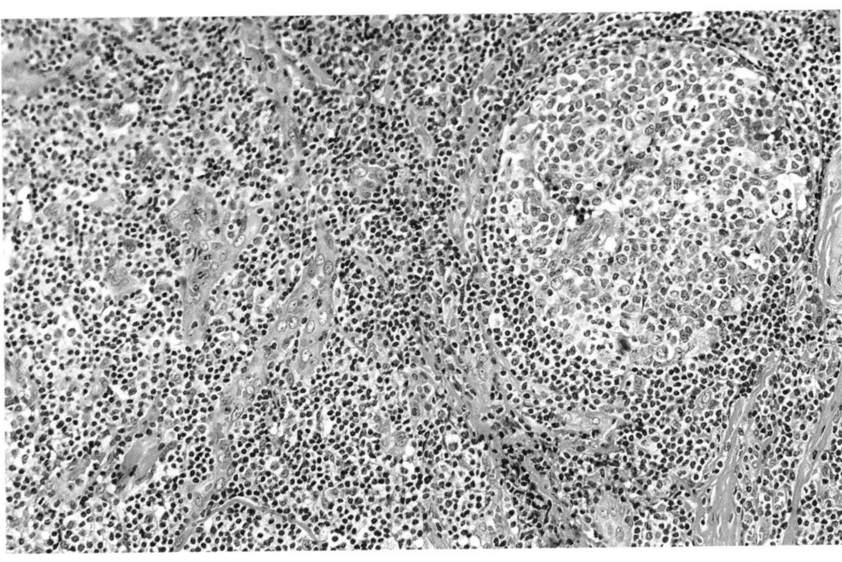

FIGURE 21-25. Kimura disease. Lesion differs from epithelioid hemangioma in that the lymphoid component overshadows the minor vascular component.

identifies nuclear debris, polykaryocytes, and a delicate eosinophilic matrix. Immunohistochemical procedures reveal that IgE-bearing cells, corresponding to the distribution of dendritic reticulum cells, populate the germinal center. Thin-walled vessels, with the characteristics of postcapillary venules, reside adjacent to the germinal centers, occasionally dipping into the centers. Dense infiltrates of eosinophils adjacent to the lymphoid aggregates occasionally form eosinophilic abscesses. During the late stages of the disease, a dense hyaline fibrosis supervenes. The adherence of the mass to the surrounding structures often triggers alarm on the part of the surgeon regarding the possibility of malignancy. In affected lymph nodes, there is exuberant follicular hyperplasia with preservation of the architecture. The changes in the germinal center are as described previously for soft tissue lesions.

The etiology of this condition is unknown, although the peripheral eosinophilia and elevated serum IgE suggest an immunologic reaction to an unknown stimulus. The lesions are benign, but recurrence may develop after surgical excision. There are no instances of malignancy supervening on these peculiar lymphoid proliferations.

Although Kimura disease and angiolymphoid hyperplasia have in common a lymphoid infiltrate with eosinophils, there are rather striking differences. The vascular proliferation in Kimura disease is relatively minor and is eclipsed by the inflammatory component. Moreover, the vessels in Kimura disease are not lined by epithelioid endothelium but by more attenuated endothelial cells.

VASCULAR MALFORMATIONS

Vascular malformations are developmental abnormalities of the embryonic vasculature that grow proportionately with the host.[2] Composed of combinations of arteries, veins, and capillaries, they may, in addition, manifest arteriovenous shunting. Unlike hemangiomas, they are static lesions that do not regress. Despite these differences, secondary factors can complicate or blur the distinction between the two. Vascular malformations with thrombosis and vascular ectasia can confer the impression of growth. Deeply situated malformations can present well after infancy or childhood, making the age at detection occasionally unreliable. Therefore, histologic diagnoses are ideally confirmed by clinical and imaging findings.

Vascular malformations are subclassified, based on the predominant vessel and the presence of arteriovenous shunting. Cavernous, venous, and arteriovenous hemangiomas are currently classified as malformations. Although malformations are often thought of as synonymous with anomalies of the blood vessels, malformations also involve the lymphatics (e.g., cystic and cavernous lymphangioma) (see Chapter 24) and glomuvenous system (e.g., glomulovenous hemangioma) (see Chapter 8).

Cutaneous Capillovenous Malformation

Anomalies of the cutaneous capillary network are heterogeneous and encompass malformations and telangiectasis, some of which are associated with specific genetic defects. Most are diagnosed clinically and, therefore, are rarely reflected in surgical pathology material.

Hereditary hemorrhagic telangiectasia (HHT) (Osler-Weber-Rendu disease) is characterized by vascular anomalies of capillaries and veins of the skin and mucosal membranes.[35] It is inherited as an autosomal dominant disease. Linkage analysis has identified two loci, *HHT1* on 9q33–34 and *HHT2* on 12q11–14. Premature stop codons of the endoglin (*ENG*) and activin receptor-like kinase 1 (*ALK-1*) genes, important for the TGF-beta receptor complex in vascular endothelial cells, suggest loss of function mutations.[36] The disease commences with the development of numerous small red papules on the skin and mucosa, particularly in the region of the face, lips, oral mucosa, and tongue. Similar lesions may be found in the gastrointestinal, genitourinary, and pulmonary systems. The lesions usually appear during childhood, increase with age, and, in the elderly, may have an appearance similar to that of the vascular spider. In contrast to the spider, the lesions are prone to bleeding, so the course of the disease is marked by repeated bouts of hemorrhage. Treatment must be supportive because treatment of ectasias by such modalities as electrocoagulation can result in the formation of satellite lesions.

The *port-wine stain* is a congenital, non-involuting lesion affecting less than 1% of newborns.[1] A small number of port-wine stains are inherited as an autosomal dominant trait. Preliminary data suggest locus heterogeneity for these lesions with one locus, CMC1, identified on 5q13–22.[37]

The lesion begins as a smooth red to purple macular lesion on the face or extremity. As the patient ages, the lesions become elevated and darker.[1,38] Biopsy of early lesions show dermis containing small vessels that are normal in number and appearance. More mature lesions consist of dilated vessels engorged with erythrocytes. Some have suggested that this change is the result of a loss of nerve tone secondary to denervation.[39] As the lesions evolve further, the vessels become thickened and fibrotic; some may, in addition, acquire a thickened muscle coat peripheral to the fibrosis. Protrusion of collections of vessels between adnexa occurs in very mature lesions and results in the cobblestone appearance of the skin.

Aside from the cosmetic problems it poses, the port-wine stain may indicate the presence of more extensive vascular malformation. Port-wine stains of the face that occur in the distribution of the trigeminal nerve may be associated with ipsilateral vascular malformations of the leptomeninges and, occasionally, of the retina (*Sturge-Weber syndrome*, *encephalotrigeminal angiomatosis*). Seizures, hemiplegia, and mental retardation, which characterize the full-blown syndrome, are the result of cerebral atrophy induced by the meningeal malformation. *Klippel-Trénaunay syndrome* includes a port-wine stain associated with varicosities and hypertrophy (gigantism) of an extremity. In most instances of this rare condition, the lower extremity is affected, and the extensive varicosities and edema appear to be the result of agenesis of the deep venous structures. In a small number of patients, there may be, in addition, a congenital arteriovenous fistula. It has been suggested that this subgroup be separately designated as *Parkes Weber syndrome* because the problems with management are different. In Parkes Weber syndrome, the major therapeutic thrust must be directed toward reducing or eliminating the arteriovenous fistula to prevent supervening congestive heart failure.

Venous Malformation (Venous Hemangioma)

Venous malformations encompass lesions previously labeled *venous hemangioma* and *cavernous hemangioma*. Some so-called intramuscular hemangiomas may be venous hemangiomas. Most are sporadic, although a subset is syndromic or linked to a specific genetic mutation. The *Blue rubber bleb nevus syndrome*, described by Bean[6] in 1958, is characterized by venous malformations of the skin and gastrointestinal tract. The term aptly describes the blue cutaneous lesions, which look and feel like rubber nipples. They compress easily with pressure, leaving a flaccid wrinkled appearance to the skin, and then regain their shape with cessation of pressure. Hyperhidrosis may occur over these lesions probably as a result of increased surface temperature. These internal lesions commonly bleed, so chronic anemia complicates the course of the disease.

Malformations have also been associated with mutations in the VMCM1 locus on chromosome 9, which results in ligand-independent autophosphorylation of the TIE-2 receptor with resultant downstream alterations.[40,41] This gene is responsible for endothelial growth and vascular wall remodeling. Venous hemangiomas have also been reported in Turner syndrome.

Venous malformations range from superficial varicosities to large, complex masses that infiltrate soft tissues[42] (Figs. 21-26 to 21-32). They are formed by congeries of venous vessels that are often not visualized on arteriography but require venography or direct injection to identify their presence and extent. Venous malformations consist principally of large veins with irregularly attenuated or disorganized walls (see Fig. 21-32). Because of slow flow, the vessels develop intraluminal thrombi, calcification, and phleboliths. Calcification may be of several types. Amorphous or curvilinear calcification is nonspecific, whereas phlebolith formation is a more frequent and more specific finding. Both are the result of dystrophic calcification in organizing thrombi.

Radiographically, the large deep lesions appear as localized or diffuse nonhomogeneous water density masses. Tortuous water density channels representing the afferent and efferent blood supplies are occasionally seen in adjacent fat.

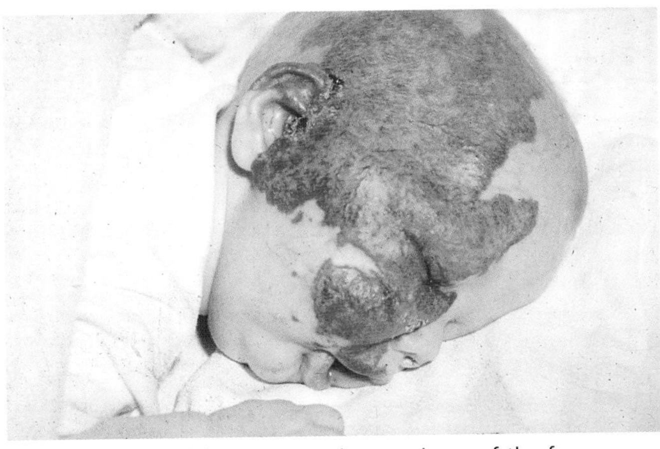

FIGURE 21-26. Cavernous hemangioma of the face.

Clinically, the color and surface appearances of these lesions relate to the location. Superficial lesions are blue, puffy masses with an irregular surface caused by dilatation of the vessels (see Fig. 21-26). Deep lesions may impart little or no color to the overlying skin.

Morphologically, venous malformations are poorly circumscribed lesions composed of collections of abnormal veins of varying sizes and proportions (see Figs. 21-30 to 21-32). Some vessels are large with irregularly attenuated thick muscle walls, whereas others are large but thin-walled. Lesions with a predominance of the former were those classically called *venous hemangioma*, whereas those with a predominance of the latter were usually diagnosed as *cavernous hemangioma*. Vessels may be grouped or haphazardly arranged in the stroma. The walls are occasionally thickened by an adventitial fibrosis, and inflammatory cells may be scattered. In some cases, a capillary or small venular component is present. Mature bone is occasionally present.

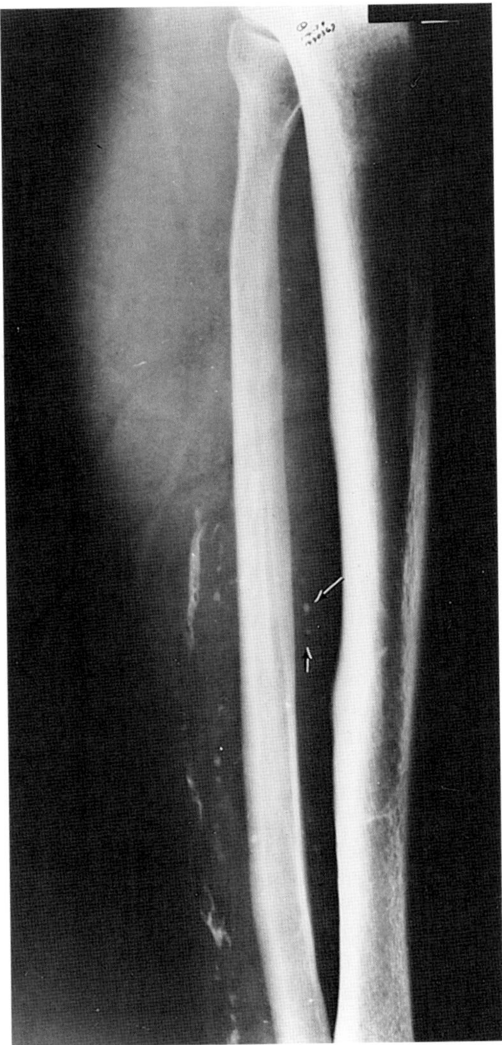

FIGURE 21-27. Venous malformation. Note the long curvilinear calcifications in addition to phleboliths (arrows). The latter are highly characteristic of cavernous hemangiomas. *(Courtesy of Dr. John Madewell, M.D. Anderson Cancer Hospital.)*

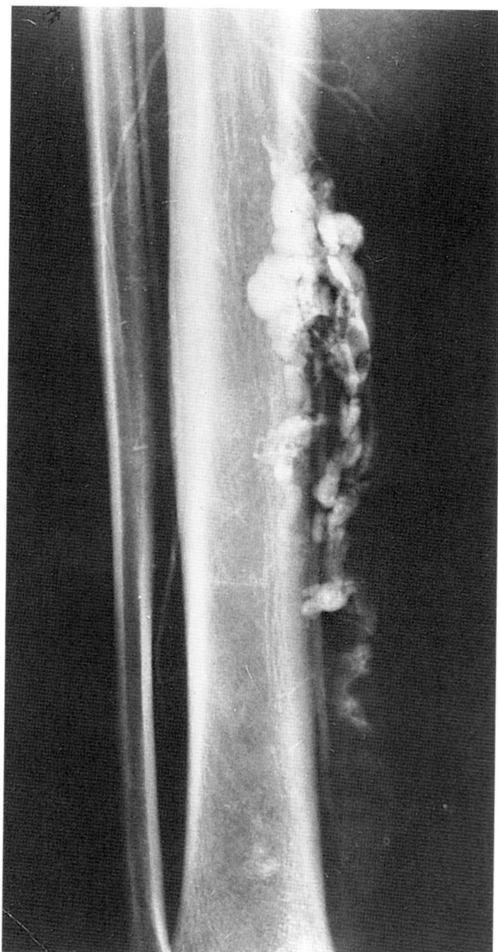

FIGURE 21-28. Venous malformation. Venous phase of the arteriogram portrays large saccular structures that correspond to tortuous, thick-walled muscular veins. *(Courtesy of Dr. John Madewell, M.D. Anderson Cancer Hospital)*

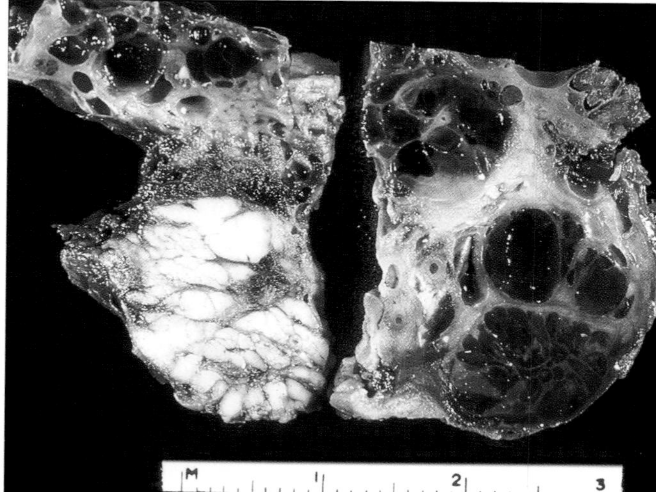

FIGURE 21-29. Gross specimen of venous malformation with large, thin-walled veins.

Arteriovenous Malformation (Arteriovenous Hemangioma)

Arteriovenous malformations, also known as *arteriovenous hemangioma*, are sporadic lesions occurring principally in the head, neck, and brain.[37,43,44] Some are associated with the following syndromes: capillary malformation-arteriovenous malformation, Parkes Weber, phosphatase and tensin homolog (also recognized as PTEN) hamartoma,[44a] and HHT (Osler-Weber-Rendu disease).[1] Typically, they present at birth or during childhood, remain quiescent until adolescence, and thereafter progress. Most cases of so-called *intramuscular hemangioma* or *angiomatosis* are most likely arteriovenous malformations, again underscoring the difficulty of accurately classifying vascular lesions without the benefit of clinical and imaging studies.

The presenting symptoms depend on the location, size, and amount of shunting in the lesion. Arteriovenous malformations involving the skin and superficial soft tissue may be associated with increased skin temperature, thrill, and pulsation, whereas those in deep soft tissue can result in arterial stealing and ischemia. The pathogenetic mechanism underlying this lesion is poorly understood but resides with aberrations of the capillary bed and the numerous small shunts.

Arteriovenous malformations are composed of a varying mixture of large arteries and veins, and small vessels within a fibrous or fibromyxoid background (Figs. 21-33 and 21-34). Consequently, the lesions vary in appearance, depending on the area sampled. Large tortuous arteries with fragmented elastic lamina are associated with thick-walled veins. In areas of shunting, the veins display hypertensive changes of intimal and mural thickening, whereas, in long-standing lesions, the vein walls become thinned and fibrotic. A variable small vessel component, consisting of capillaries, venules, or vessels of indeterminate type, is apparent in most arteriovenous malformations. When this component involves the overlying skin, the changes crudely simulate Kaposi sarcoma (see Chapter 23). These changes have been referred to as *kaposiform angiodermatitis* or *pseudo-Kaposi sarcoma*.[45] These changes consist of a proliferation of small capillary-sized vessels with thickened walls in association with fibroblasts and hemosiderin deposits (Fig. 21-35).

Some degree of small vessel proliferation is present in most arteriovenous malformations, but the reason for this is not well understood. Possibly, it is a compensatory mechanism secondary to shunting. It should be evident that the histologic variability and the myriad of small shunts not appreciated histologically make the diagnosis of these complex lesions extremely difficult without imaging studies.

The differential diagnosis of arteriovenous malformation ranges from capillary hemangioma to venous malformation, depending on the predominant vessel. However, the small vessels within arteriovenous malformations are mitotically quiescent and GLUT1-negative in contrast to those of infantile hemangiomas. Although arteriovenous fistulas have some of the features of arteriovenous malformation, they are acquired lesions composed of large vessels with only a few large dominant shunts.

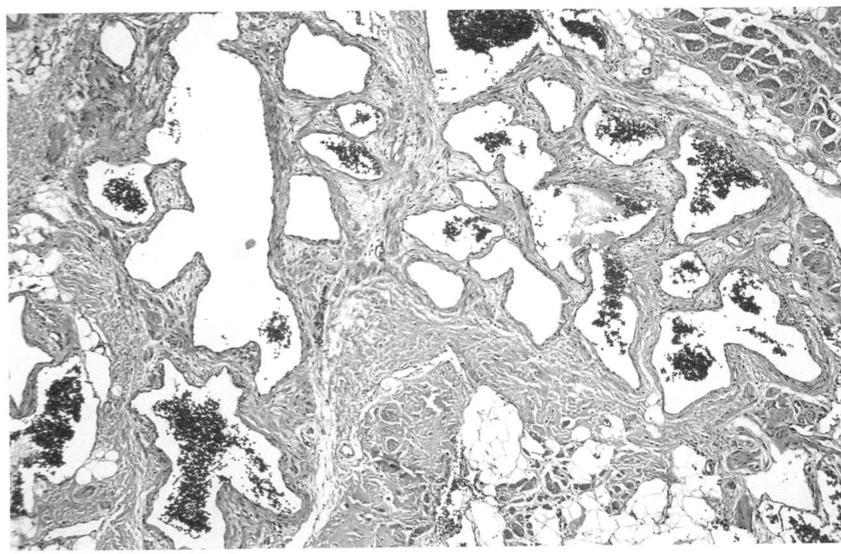

FIGURE 21-30. Venous malformation with thin-walled veins.

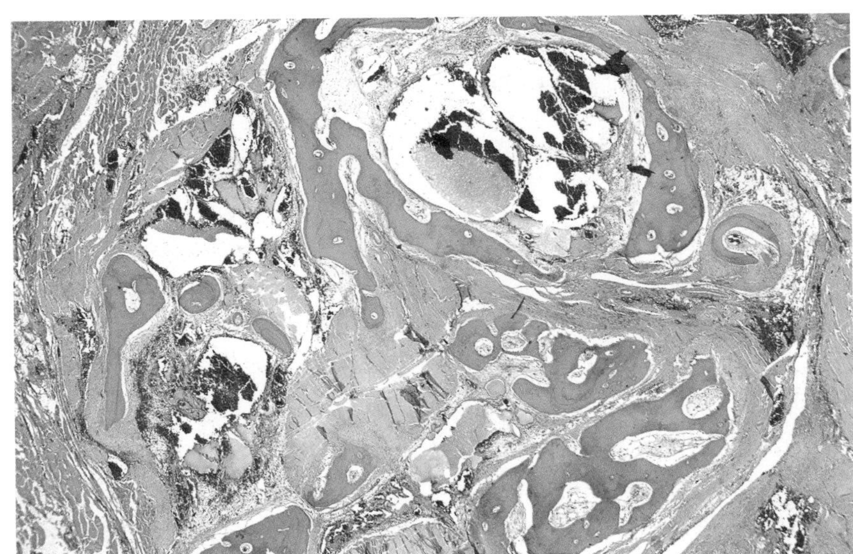

FIGURE 21-31. Venous malformation with bone.

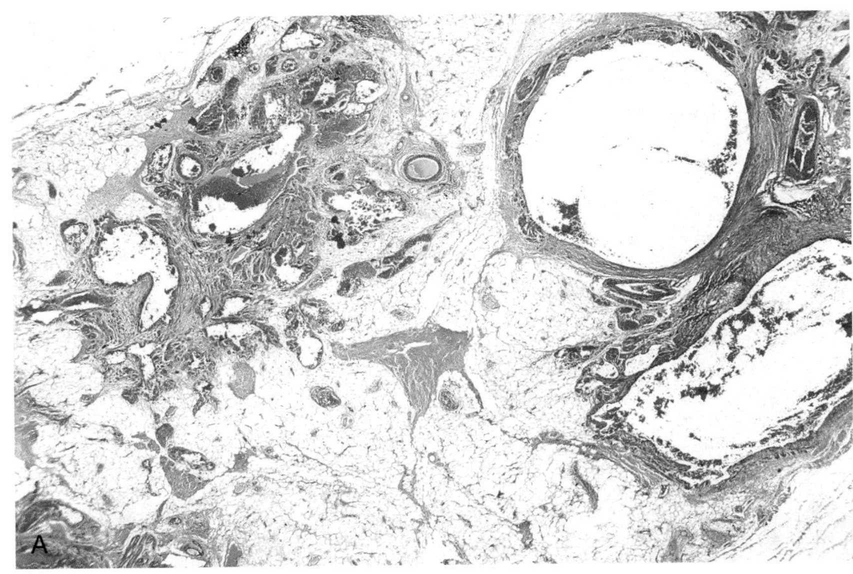

FIGURE 21-32. Large thick-walled veins of venous malformation (A, B). *Continued*

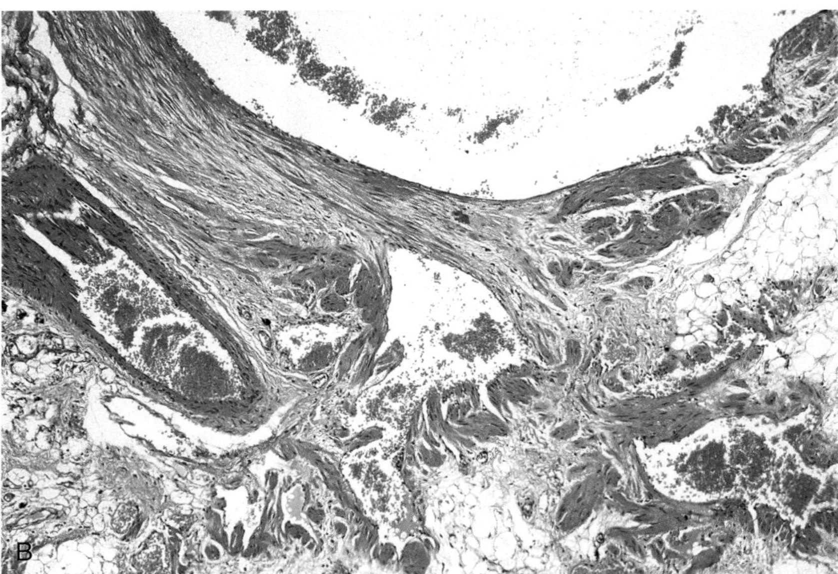

FIGURE 21-32, cont'd

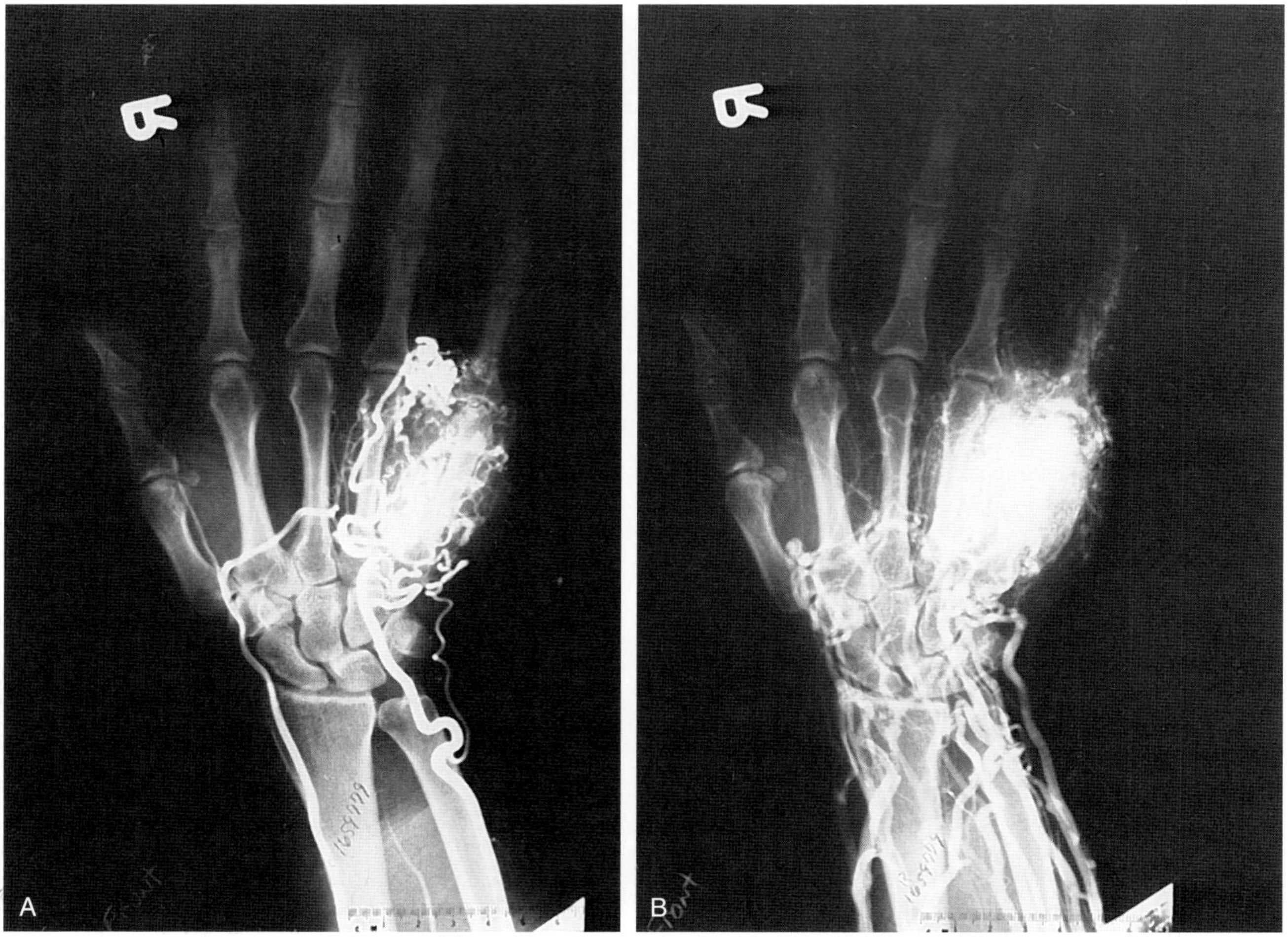

FIGURE 21-33. Arteriovenous malformation of hand. (A) Arteriogram shows filling of arterial vessels supplying tumor. (B) Opacification of tumor in the region of the fifth metacarpal and filling of draining veins while still in the arterial phase. *(Courtesy of Dr. John Madewell, M.D. Anderson Cancer Hospital.)*

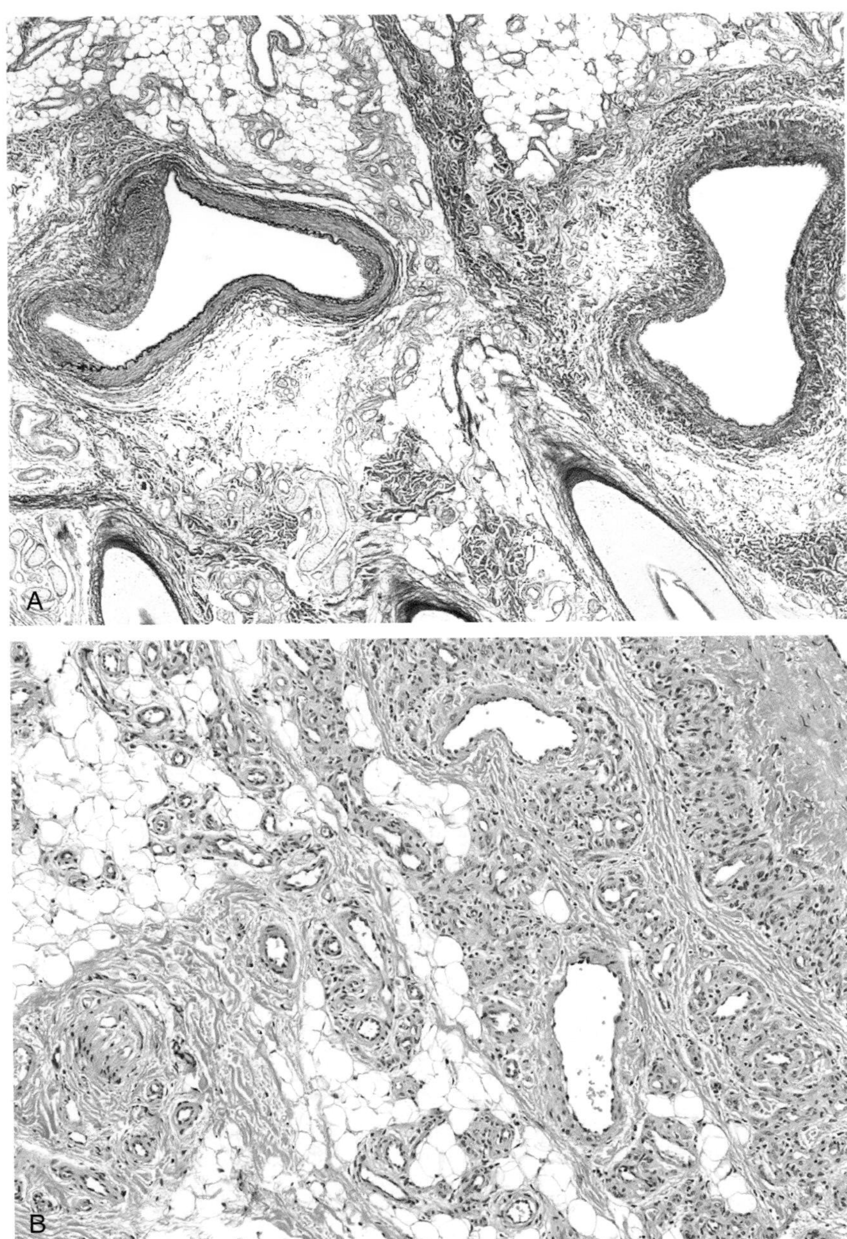

FIGURE 21-34. Arteriovenous malformation. (A) Elastic stain illustrates close juxtaposition of large artery and vein and an associated small vessel component. (B) Small vessel component in arteriovenous malformation. *(Courtesy of Dr. Harry Kosekevich, Boston Children's Hospital.)*

Intramuscular Hemangioma

Traditionally considered a vascular neoplasm, most intramuscular hemangiomas are probably arteriovenous malformations, although it is difficult to exclude the possibility that a subset is venous malformations or even true tumors. Unfortunately, based on published reports, it is not possible to make an accurate assessment. That 80% to 90% make their appearance before the age of 30 years[46] supports the idea that they are congenital malformations that slowly give rise to symptoms during late childhood or early adult life. Unlike cutaneous hemangioma, intramuscular hemangioma affects the genders in roughly equal numbers. Although any muscle can be affected, most intramuscular hemangiomas are located in the lower extremity, particularly the muscles of the thigh. There is some evidence that intramuscular hemangiomas of the capillary type have a greater predilection for the head and neck musculature.

Clinically, these lesions are more likely to pose diagnostic problems than are superficial hemangiomas. They present as enlarging soft tissue masses with few signs or symptoms to reveal their vascular nature. In particular, there is rarely any overlying discoloration of the skin, visible pulsation, or audible bruit. Radiography and arteriography are far more helpful for suggesting the diagnosis. Plain films may reveal phleboliths in addition to a soft tissue mass, and arteriography

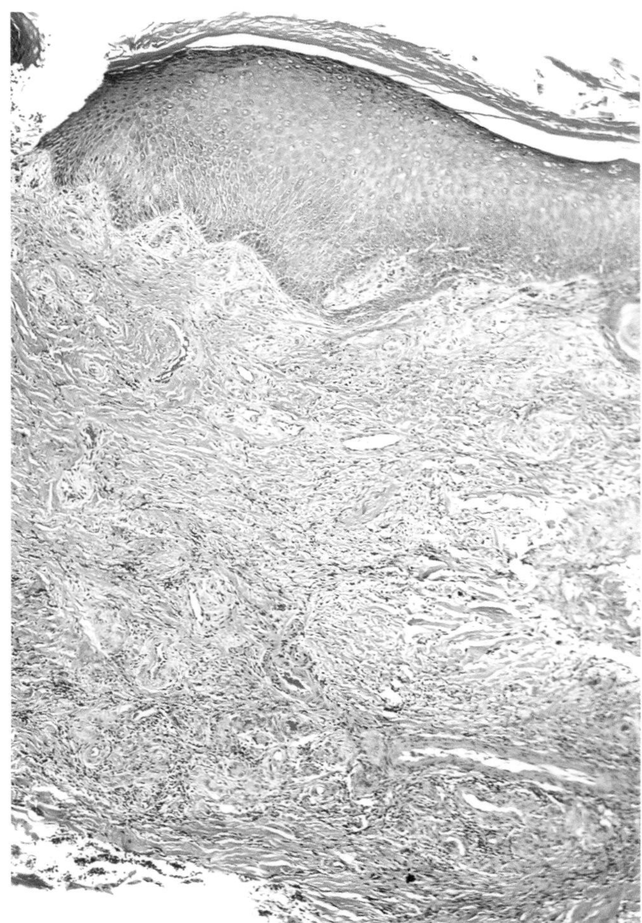

FIGURE 21-35. Kaposiform changes in skin overlying an arteriovenous fistula.

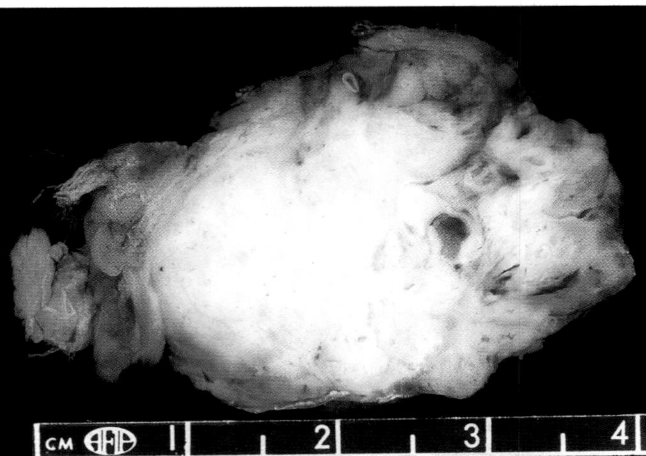

FIGURE 21-36. Gross appearance of an intramuscular hemangioma involving the medial thigh. Lesions often have a solid, nonhemorrhagic appearance.

may demonstrate a highly vascular lesion with early venous runoff. Moreover, the vessels are oriented parallel to one another in a striated pattern.[47] This pattern, created by the orderly entry and proliferation of vessels between fascicles of muscle, is considered a helpful feature in support of the benignancy of the lesion.[48] Pain is a frequent, but not invariable symptom, and is said to be more common with tumors involving long, narrow muscles where stretching of the muscle and nerve fibers by the tumor is more intense. Occasionally, function is impaired or anatomic deformity occurs. Although a history of trauma is given in about one-fifth of cases, there is no evidence that the lesions are caused by trauma.

Intramuscular hemangiomas vary in appearance, depending on whether they are of the capillary, cavernous, or mixed type. In many cases, it is not possible to sharply classify these types because they are all part of the same histologic spectrum.

Intramuscular hemangiomas of the capillary type are most common and are also likely to be confused with a malignant tumor. Grossly, they do not always appear vascular because they vary from tan to yellow or red (Fig. 21-36). They are composed of a myriad of small capillary-sized vessels with plump nuclei that extend between individual muscle fibers (Figs. 21-37 to 21-39). Well-developed lumen formation is apparent in most areas, although occasional tumors have a solidly cellular appearance similar to the early stage of the juvenile hemangioma. In occasional cases, mitotic activity, intraluminal papillary tufting, and a proliferation of capillary vessels in perineural sheaths are present. Although seemingly disturbing features, none of these features is indicative of malignancy.

In contrast, the large vessel form of intramuscular hemangioma is easily recognized as benign. They are blue-red masses composed of large vessels lined by bland, markedly attenuated endothelium, which seldom shows a significant degree of pleomorphism. The presence of adipose tissue in these tumors is common, and, at times, it may be so conspicuous as to suggest a diagnosis of lipoma. Tumors described in the early literature as *infiltrating angiolipomas of muscle* or *benign mesenchymoma* are examples of intramuscular hemangiomas with striking fatty overgrowth.

The most important consideration in the differential diagnosis of these lesions is the distinction from an angiosarcoma of skeletal muscle. Angiosarcomas of deep soft tissue, specifically skeletal muscle, are rare (see Chapter 23); therefore, a vascular lesion of skeletal muscle is far more likely to be benign than malignant. Moreover, intramuscular hemangiomas do not develop the freely anastomosing sinusoidal pattern, except in areas where organization of thrombus material occurs. The recurrence rate of hemangiomas varies from 18% to 50%, depending on adequacy of excision.[46,49] Treatment should be directed toward complete excision without resorting to radical surgery. Prior embolization of the tumor has been used as a means to facilitate surgical excision.[50]

ANGIOMATOSIS

Angiomatosis was a term formerly used to denote a clinically extensive hemangioma, which, by definition, either involved multiple tissue planes (e.g., subcutis, muscle, and bone) or was associated with extensive involvement of one type of tissue

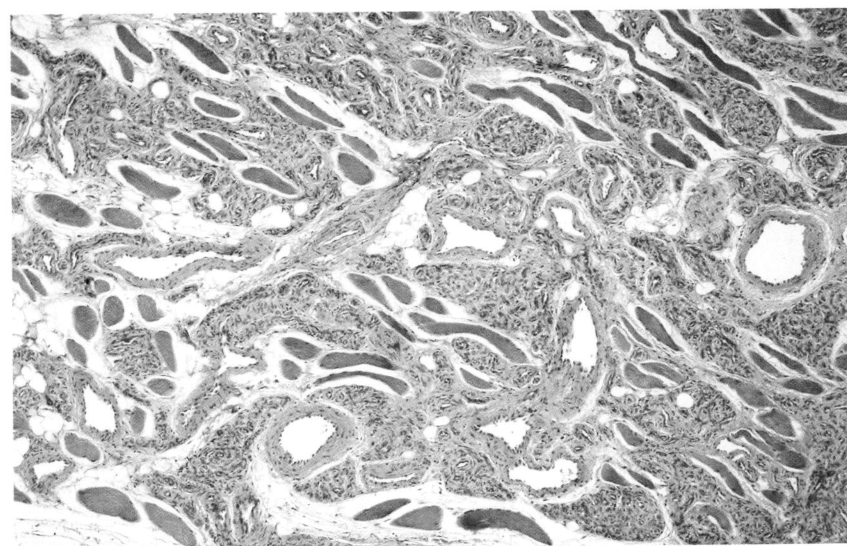

FIGURE 21-37. Intramuscular hemangioma with separation of muscle fibers by proliferating vessels. This pseudoinfiltrative pattern is often mistaken for evidence of malignancy.

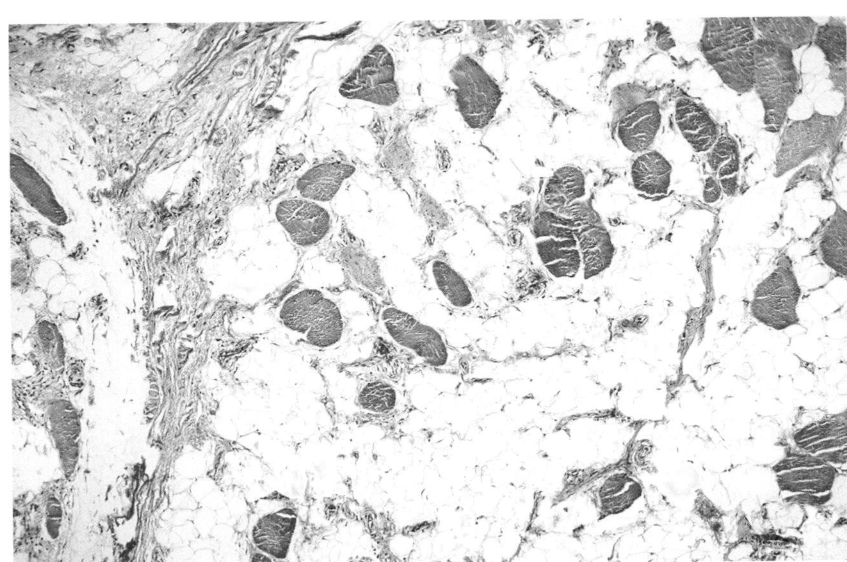

FIGURE 21-38. Intramuscular hemangioma with a significant admixture of fat. Such tumors have sometimes been classified as *angiolipomas of muscle.*

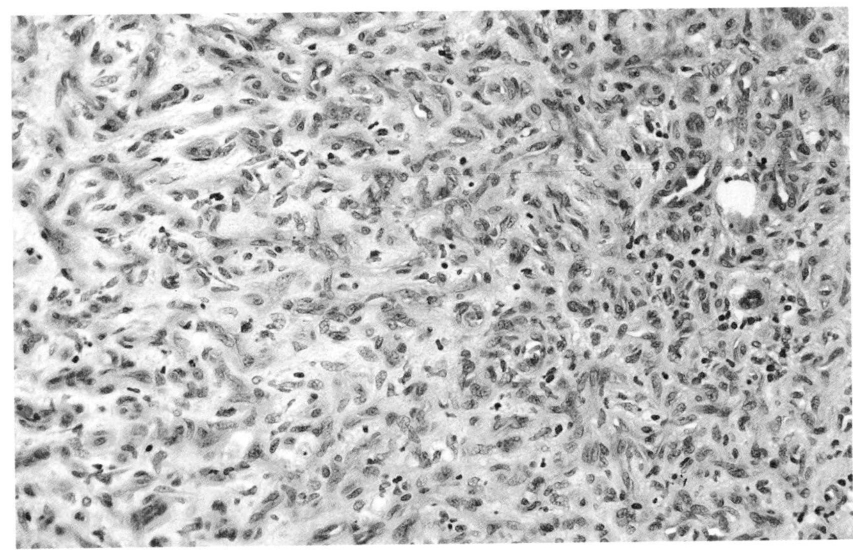

FIGURE 21-39. Small vessel (capillary) type of intramuscular hemangioma.

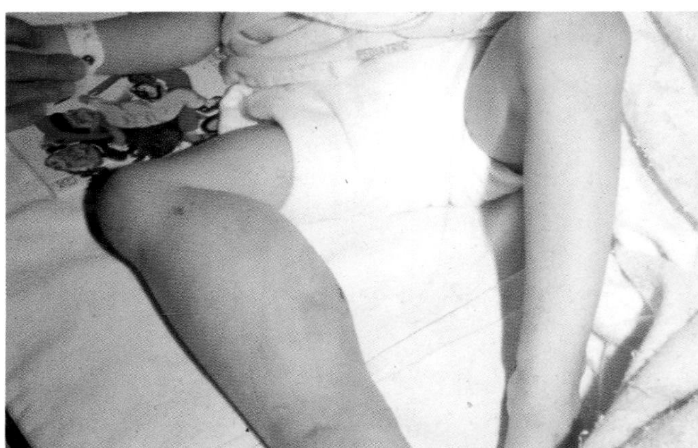

FIGURE 21-40. Child with angiomatosis affecting the entire lower leg.

(e.g., skeletal muscle)[51-53] (Fig. 21-40). Therefore, the label *angiomatosis* is based on combined clinical and histologic features. Like intramuscular hemangioma, the early onset of these lesions and their proportional growth provide compelling evidence that they, too, are malformations. Also, like intramuscular hemangioma, most are probably examples of arteriovenous malformation.

More than half of patients present within the first two decades of life, usually with symptoms of diffuse persistent swelling sometimes associated with pain and discoloration. Only rarely is hypertrophy, gigantism, or clinical evidence of arteriovenous shunting present. On computed tomography (CT) scans, the lesions appear as ill-defined nonhomogeneous masses that may resemble sarcoma, except for the presence of serpiginous dense areas that correspond to thick-walled, tortuous vessels (Fig. 21-41). Because of the presence of large amounts of fat, these tumors often appear as predominantly fatty tumors (Fig. 21-42).

Histologically, angiomatosis may assume one of two patterns. The first and more common pattern seen in most of the 50 cases reviewed consisted of a mélange of large venous, cavernous, and capillary-sized vessels scattered haphazardly throughout soft tissue (Figs. 21-43 to 21-45). The venous vessels are remarkable for their irregular, thick walls that have occasional attenuations and herniations (see Fig. 21-45). A rather characteristic feature of these veins is the presence of small vessels clustered just adjacent to or in the wall of a large vein (see Fig. 21-44). The second pattern, which occurs in a small number of cases, is virtually identical to that of a capillary hemangioma, except that the nodules of tumor diffusely infiltrate the surrounding soft tissue. The prominent amount of fat present in these lesions has led previous authors to use the term *infiltrating angiolipoma*.

In the study by Rao and Weiss,[52] nearly 90% of patients experienced recurrences, and 40% had more than one recurrence within a 5-year period. A somewhat lower recurrence rate was reported by Howat and Campbell.[51] Recurrence is related to incomplete excision as well as recruitment of collateral arterial flow into a low resistance vascular bed.[1] This behavior contrasts with the recurrence rate of intramuscular hemangiomas, which is usually less than 50%. Although there has been speculation that recurrence rates may be higher in young children affected with this condition, it appears not to be true. There is no evidence that such lesions ever progress to frank malignancy, so the goal of therapy is to treat the lesions as conservatively as possible, balancing the need for complete surgical extirpation with the morbidity of the procedure.

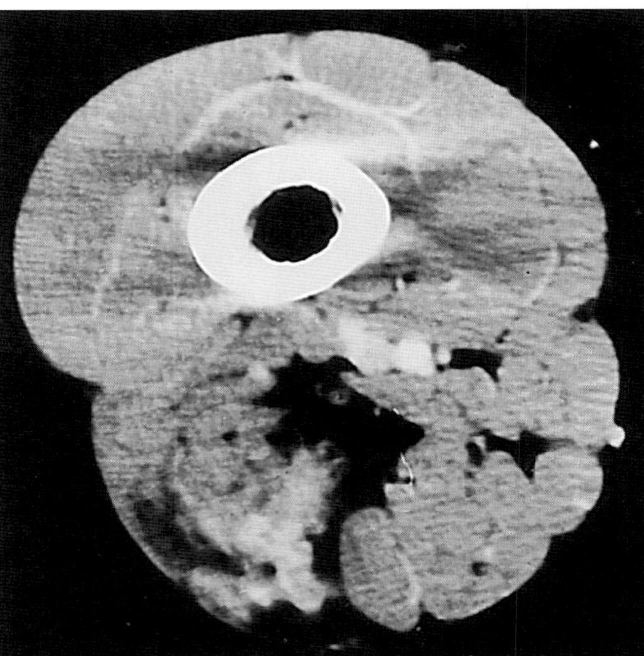

FIGURE 21-41. Computed tomography (CT) scan of angiomatosis illustrating diffuse nonhomogeneous regions in muscle. Serpiginous areas (arrow) represent tortuous vessels. *(From Rao VK, Weiss SW. Angiomatosis of soft tissue: an analysis of the histologic features and clinical outcome in 51 cases.* Am J Surg Pathol *1992;16(8):764–71.)*

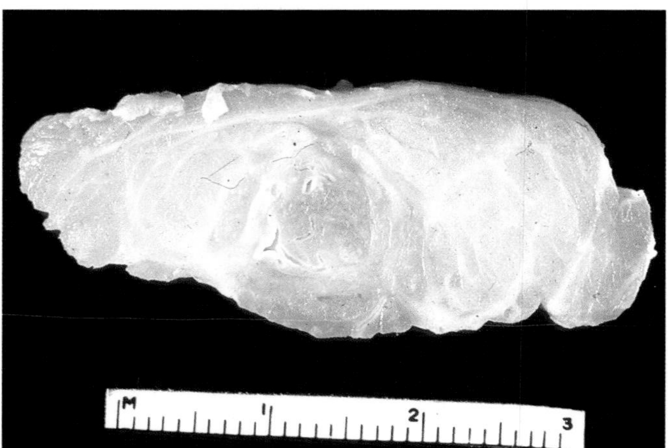

FIGURE 21-42. Cut section through a portion of angiomatosis. Pale appearance of muscle is typical and indicates replacement of fibers by vessels and fat.

MISCELLANEOUS HEMANGIOMAS AND MALFORMATIONS

Verrucous Hemangioma (Hyperkeratotic Vascular Stain)

Verrucous hemangioma is a variant of capillary or cavernous hemangioma that undergoes reactive hyperkeratosis of the

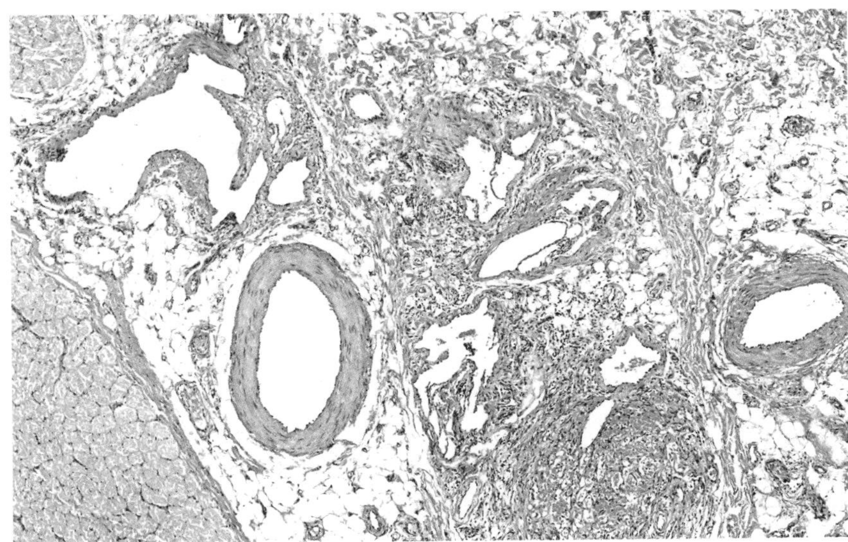

FIGURE 21-43. Angiomatosis with variously sized vessels involving muscle and fat.

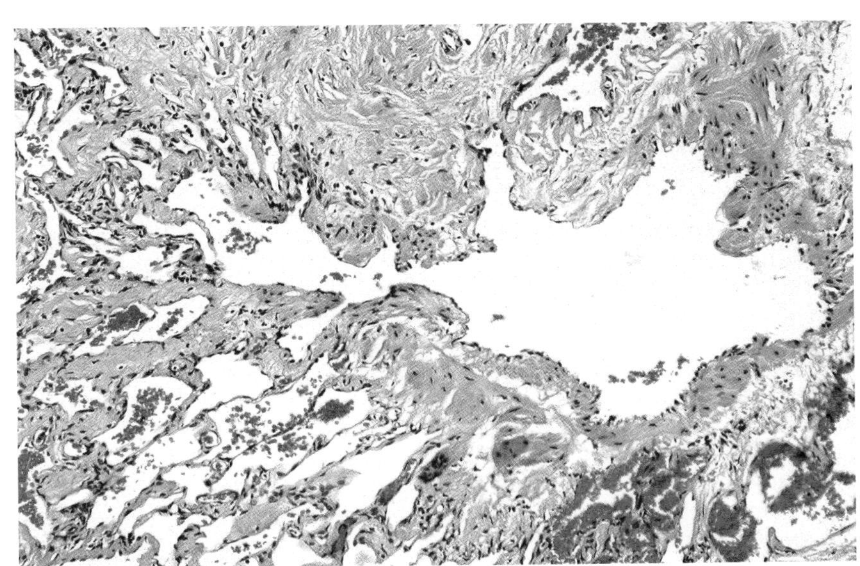

FIGURE 21-44. Angiomatosis with small vessels residing adjacent to and in the wall of a larger vessel.

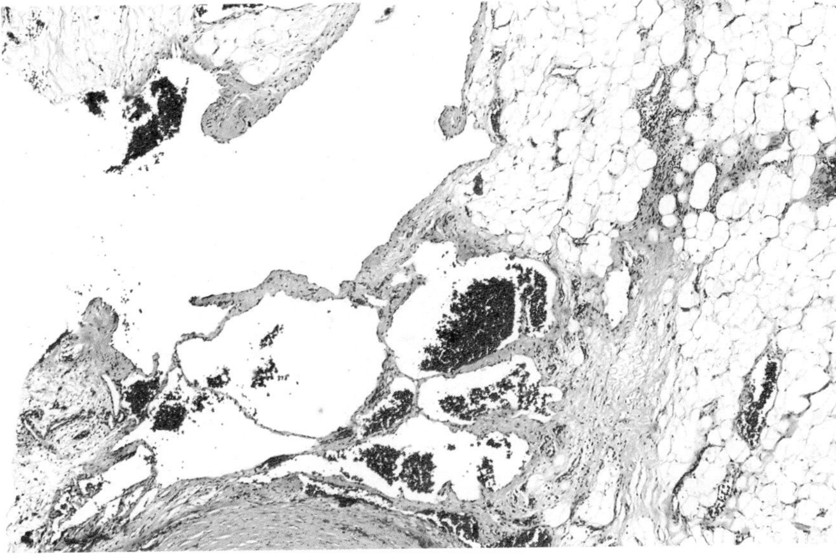

FIGURE 21-45. Venous vessel in angiomatosis illustrating irregular wall and herniations.

overlying skin and, consequently, may be confused with a wart or keratosis.[54-56] Some authors regard these as malformations (hyperkeratotic vascular stain).[57] Verrucous hemangiomas may occur as part of Cobb syndrome (cutaneous vascular lesion and spinal cord vascular malformation within a segment or two of involved dermatome).[57]

The lesions begin during childhood as unilateral lesions in the dermis of the lower extremity. Grossly and histologically, they resemble conventional hemangiomas during their early stage of development. With time, the overlying epidermis displays hyperkeratosis, acanthosis, and papillomatosis, features that obscure the vascular nature of the lesions. The vessels, a mixture of dilated capillaries and veins, involve superficial and deep dermis and sometimes extend into the subcutis. Because of their deep extension, complete excisions can be difficult, and recurrences and satellite lesions may develop. Angiokeratomas resemble these lesions clinically and histologically but are distinguished by a lack of a deep component.

Hobnail Hemangioma (Targetoid Hemosiderotic Hemangioma)

Hobnail hemangioma, described by Guillou et al.,[58] develops on the skin of the extremities in young adults as an angiomatous/pigmented or exophytic mass and has a distinctive biphasic appearance (Figs. 21-46 and 21-47). The superficial portion of the lesion consists of dilated vessels lined by hobnail endothelial cells (see Chapter 22) containing occasional intraluminal papillary tufts similar to the Dabska tumor. The deep portion consists of attenuated, slit-like capillaries that ramify in the dermis. Although the pattern is suggestive of an angiosarcoma, the vessels have an innocuous appearance. Hemorrhage, hemosiderin deposits, lymphocytes, and dermal sclerosis can accompany the lesions. The endothelial cells in hobnail hemangiomas are CD31, VEGFR3, and D2–40[59]-positive and CD34-negative, indicating a lymphatic phenotype similar to retiform hemangioendothelioma. The lesional vessels lack a pericytic cuff as would be expected for lymphatic vessels. Microshunts between small blood and lymphatic vessels have been imputed as the explanation for the frequent microaneurysms, hemorrhage, inflammatory changes, and scarring that are so typical of these lesions. The more than 50 cases that have been reported have had a benign clinical course.[58,59]

Hobnail hemangiomas correspond to some lesions originally termed *targetoid hemosiderotic hemangioma*.[60] However, *targetoid hemosiderotic hemangioma* is a clinical term referring to the presence of an ecchymotic halo surrounding a violaceous papule, and it is unclear whether these clinically defined lesions have a common pathologic appearance. The term *hobnail hemangioma* has, therefore, proven to be more useful to pathologists.

Sinusoidal Hemangioma

Sinusoidal hemangioma is a solitary-acquired hemangioma in adults, usually women. Considered originally to be a variant of cavernous hemangioma, it is well demarcated (Fig. 21-48) and composed of thin-walled cavernous vessels that ramify or interconnect in a sinusoidal pattern. In some tumors, this

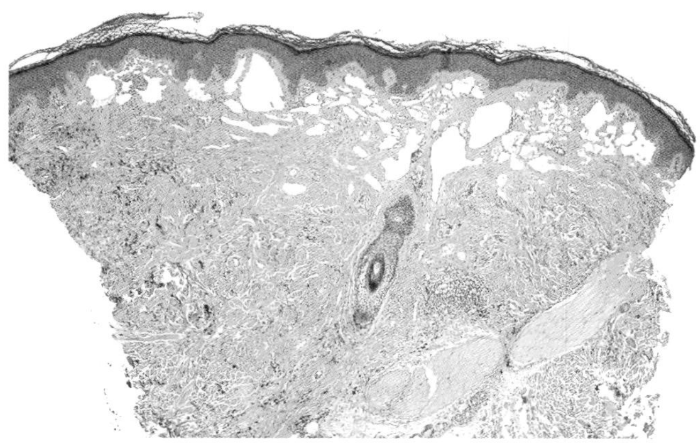

FIGURE 21-46. Hobnail hemangioma (targetoid hemosiderotic hemangioma).

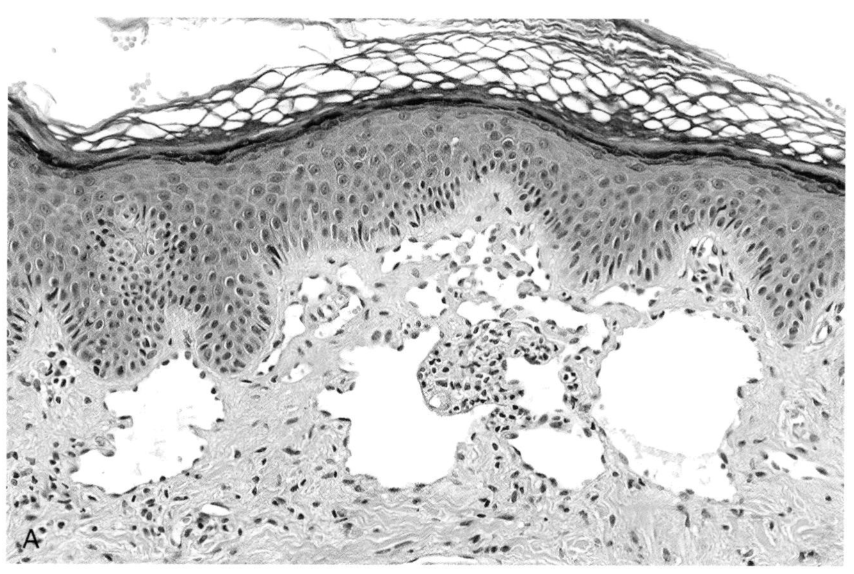

FIGURE 21-47. Hobnail hemangioma (targetoid hemosiderotic hemangioma) showing ectatic vessels at the surface (A) and in deeper regions illustrating the interface of ectatic vessels with attenuated slit-like vessels (B).

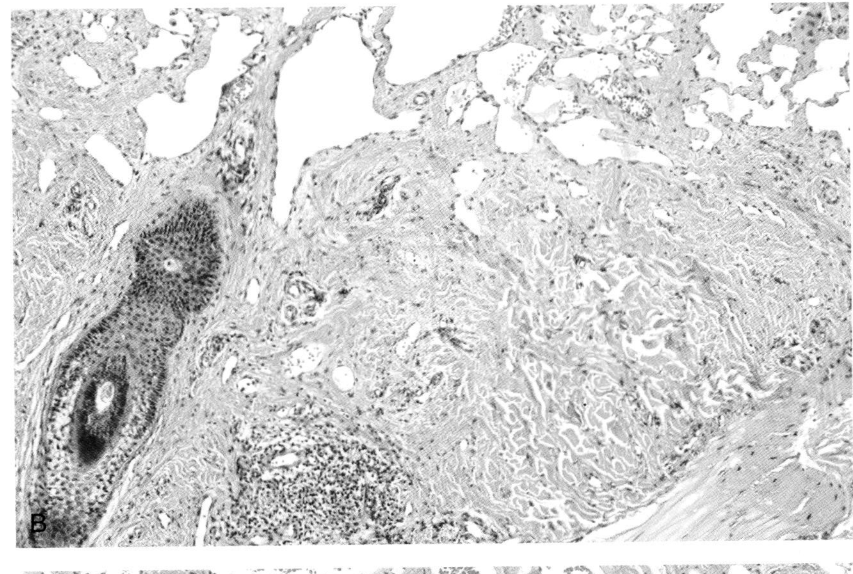

FIGURE 21-47, cont'd

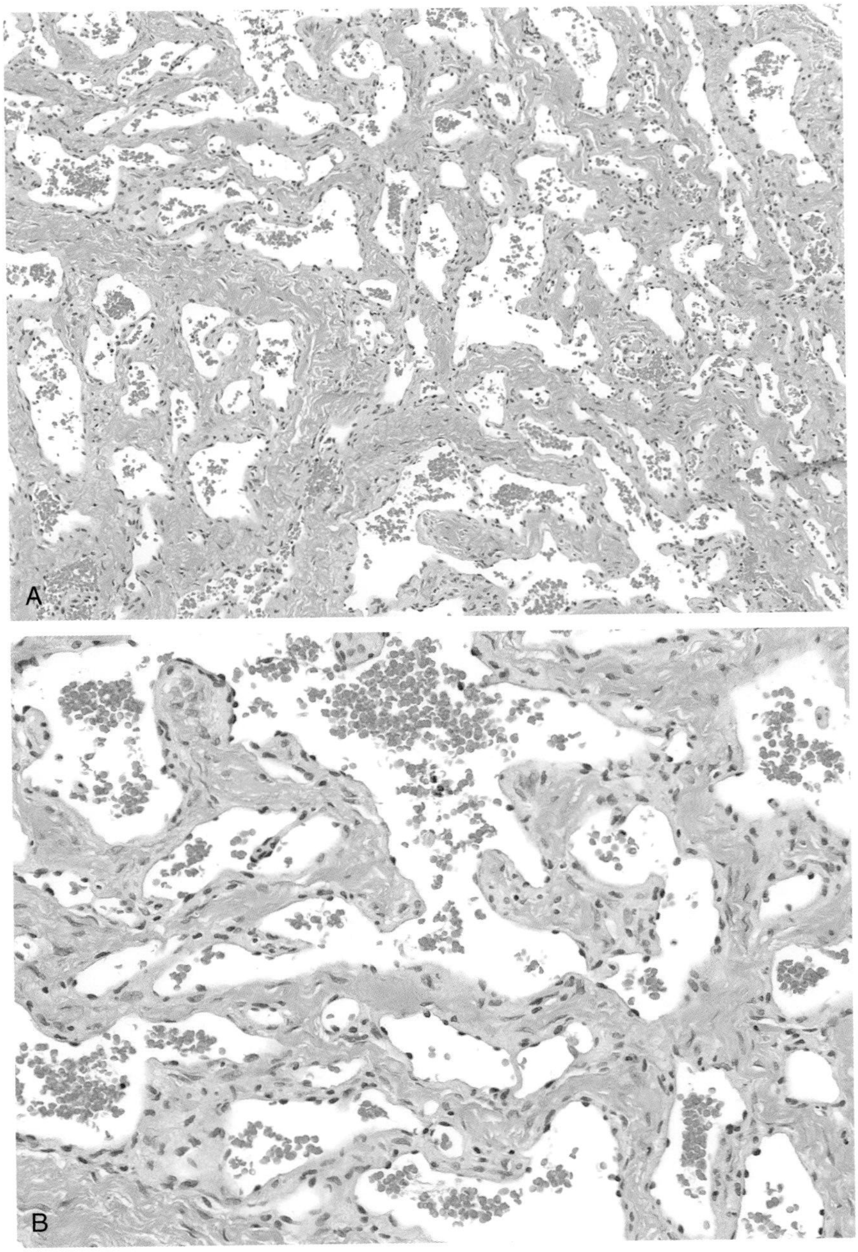

FIGURE 21-48. Sinusoidal hemangioma (A, B).

pattern may be the result of thrombosis and recanalization. Papillary infoldings of the endothelium are usually identified, and, in two cases reported by Calonje and Fletcher,[61] central infarction of the tumors occurred.

Anastomosing Hemangioma

Anastomosing hemangioma is a recently described variant of hemangioma that appears to have a predilection for the genitourinary tract, in particular, the kidney, as well as the retroperitoneum and paraspinal region.[62-64] Most are detected incidentally at the time of evaluation for other conditions, such as end-stage renal disease. Anastomosing hemangiomas are well marginated, mahogany lesions with a spongy consistency measuring a few centimeters in diameter. They are vaguely lobular with tightly packed capillary vessels arranged in an anastomosing or sinusoidal pattern (Fig. 21-49). Some have likened their appearance to red pulp of the spleen. The endothelial cells, which lack atypia and mitotic activity, occasionally have a hobnail appearance and contain hyaline globules. They are consistently CD34 and usually CD31-positive. Extramedullary hematopoiesis is occasionally present. Based on the small number of reported cases, the tumors are benign.

Acquired Tufted Angioma (Angioblastoma of Nakagawa)

Described by Wilson-Jones and Orkin[65] as *acquired tufted angioma*, and by Japanese authors as *angioblastoma of*

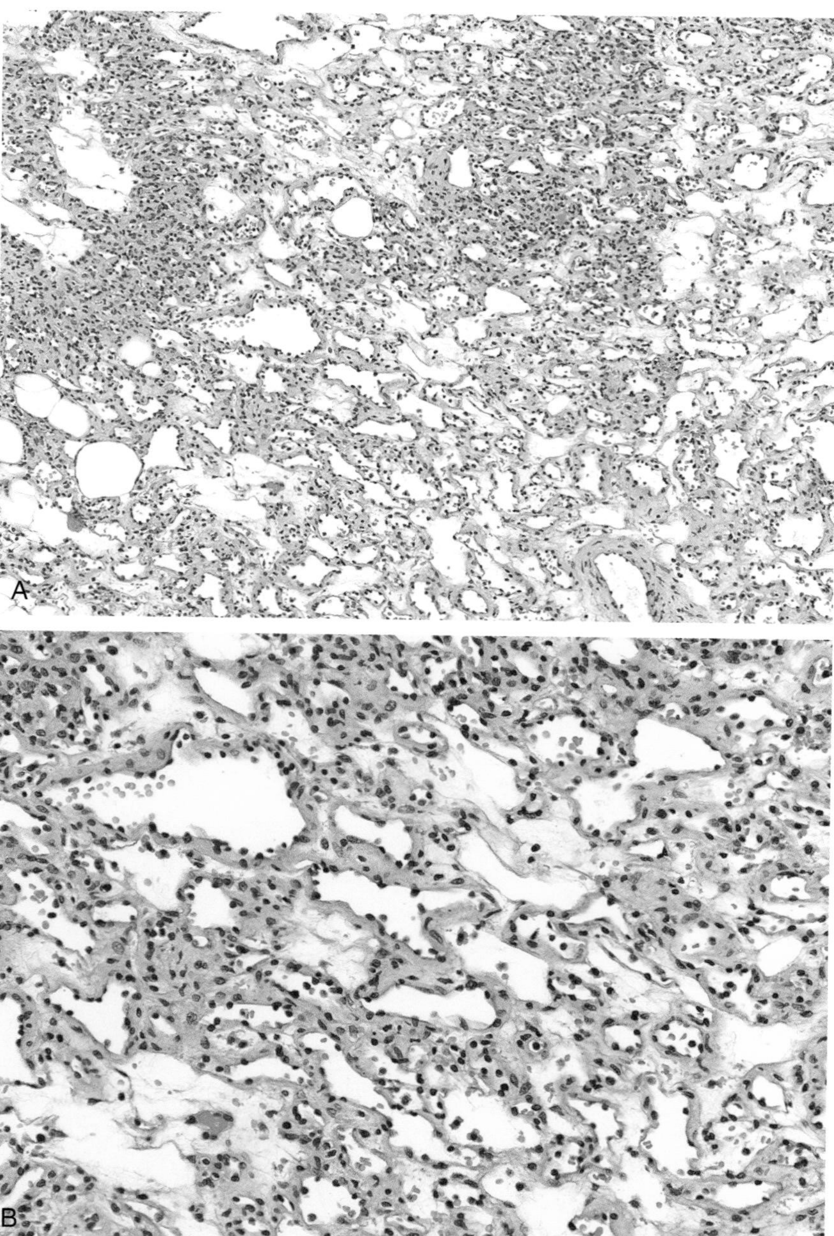

FIGURE 21-49. Anastomosing hemangioma (A) showing hobnail endothelium lining vessels (B).

Nakagawa,[66,67] this vascular lesion is considered to be identical to the kaposiform hemangioendothelioma. Evidence supporting this includes the following: both occur principally in children, are characterized by infiltrating nodules of tumor with focal glomeruloid structures, display a lymphatic component (see Chapter 22), and have a similar immunophenotype (Fig. 21-50). Several reports even comment that some lesions have features of both tumors or show transformation between the two. Many patients with acquired tufted angioma also develop Kasabach-Merritt phenomenon (KMP), but apparently less frequently than patients with kaposiform hemangioendothelioma. The relatively minor differences observed between the two lesions are best explained by the bias to label lesions occurring in an adult without manifestations of KMP as acquired tufted angioma and in children with KMP as kaposiform hemangioendothelioma. Although the term *kaposiform hemangioendothelioma* has been used for all lesions, there may be merit to retaining the term *acquired tufted angioma* for indolent cutaneous lesions in adults. Recently, a familial predisposition to acquired tufted hemangioma, suggesting an autosomal dominant pattern of inheritance linked to three possible candidate genes, *EDR*, *ENG* and *FLT4*,[68] has been reported. Similar observations have not yet been made in kaposiform hemangioendothelioma.

Spindle Cell Hemangioma

First described as *spindle cell hemangioendothelioma*,[69] the spindle cell hemangioma is an acral vascular lesion characterized by cavernous blood vessels and spindled areas reminiscent of Kaposi sarcoma. Although originally believed to be a tumor with limited metastatic potential, this benign, multifocal process is in all probability a vascular malformation.[70] The lesion occurs in young adults and affects the subcutis of the distal extremities, particularly the hand. The lesions produce so few symptoms that patients may delay seeking medical attention for several years. It is occasionally associated with Maffucci syndrome (Fig. 21-51).[70] In fact, it appears that many and maybe most lesions originally described as cavernous hemangiomas in Maffucci syndrome may well be spindle cell hemangiomas. In addition, spindle cell hemangiomas are also

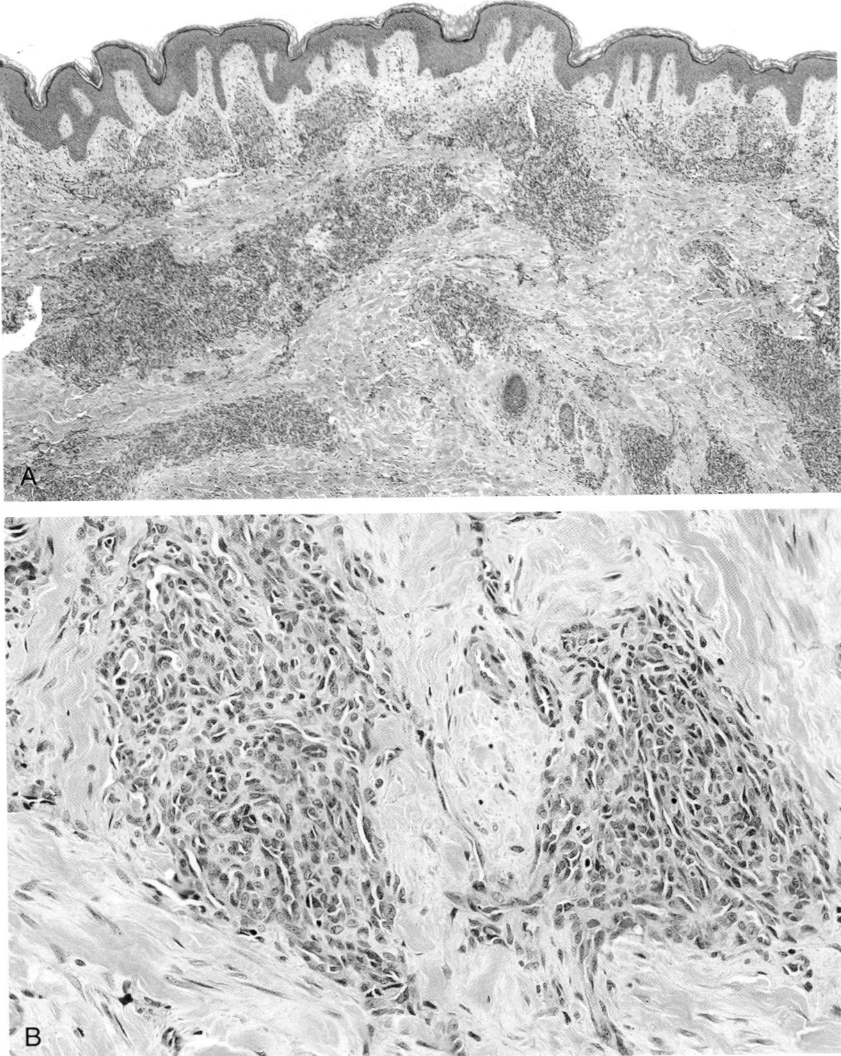

FIGURE 21-50. Acquired tufted hemangioma illustrating cannonball nests of tumor in the dermis (A). High-power view depicts irregular groups of capillary-sized vessels (B). *(Case courtesy of Dr. Philip Allen of Adelaide, Australia.)*

seen in Klippel-Trénaunay syndrome,[71] early-onset varicosities, congenital lymphedema, and rarely in association with epithelioid hemangioendothelioma. Most begin as a solitary nodule but have a remarkable tendency to give rise to multiple lesions in the same general area (Figs. 21-52 to 21-54). Approximately one-half of cases are intravascular; it appears that intravascular growth is the mechanism by which they give rise to multiple lesions in the same general area.

Histologically, the lesions are composed of thin-walled cavernous vessels lined by flattened endothelial cells and containing a mixture of erythrocytes and thrombi. Between the cavernous spaces are bland spindled areas reminiscent of Kaposi sarcoma (see Fig. 21-54; Figs. 21-55 and 21-56). Unlike Kaposi sarcoma, however, they contain distinctive round or epithelioid cells containing vacuoles or intracytoplasmic lumens similar to those in an epithelioid hemangioendothelioma (Fig. 21-57). In the extreme case, these clusters of vacuolated cells in the spindled stroma can be mistaken for entrapped fat (Fig. 21-58). The vWF can be identified in the endothelium lining of the cavernous spaces and in the epithelioid endothelium of the stroma. The spindled areas appear to be made up of collapsed vessels, pericytes, and fibroblastic cells, indicating that, architecturally, they are complex and have all of the elements of the vessel wall.

Abnormal vessels with irregularly attenuated muscle walls can be identified adjacent to many spindle cell hemangiomas. This feature and the association of these lesions with other vascular anomalies provide impressive evidence that spindle cell hemangioma is a superficial vascular malformation in which alterations in blood flow give rise to alternating areas of vascular expansion and collapse. That the cellular zones appear to have all of the elements of the vessel wall suggests that they are fundamentally similar to the cavernous areas but represent areas of vascular collapse.

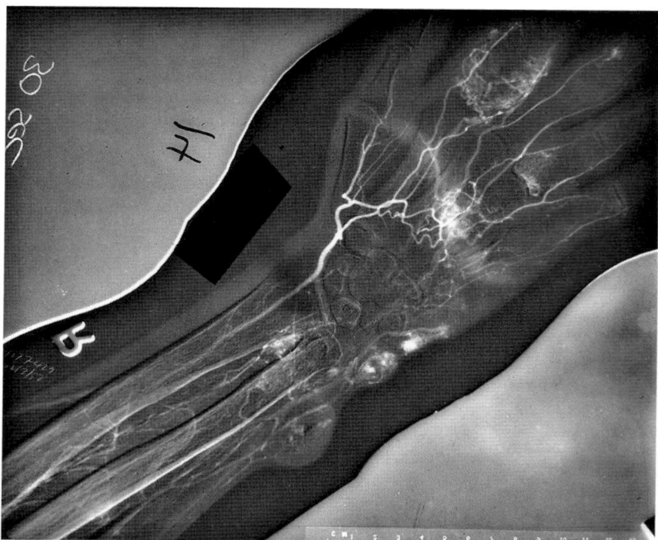

FIGURE 21-51. Radiograph of a patient with Maffucci syndrome and multiple spindle cell hemangiomas (some with phleboliths) on the lateral portion of the wrist and hand. Patient also has an enchondroma of the phalanx of the forefinger.

Synovial Hemangioma

Synovial hemangiomas arise from any synovium-lined surface and, therefore, may be found along the course of tendons or in a joint space.[72] In the former location, they present in the same fashion as a tenosynovial giant cell tumor, that is, as painless soft tissue swellings. The origin from synovium, in these cases, is only assumed because they may also involve superficial structures, and confinement by synovium is often not apparent. Therefore, the most characteristic form of synovial hemangioma is the intra-articular variety in which the

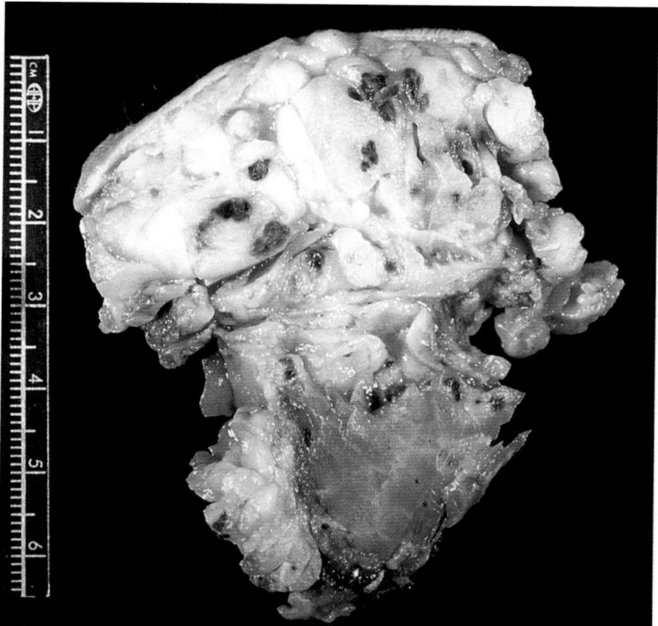

FIGURE 21-52. Gross specimen of a spindle cell hemangioma showing multiple lesions in the subcutis.

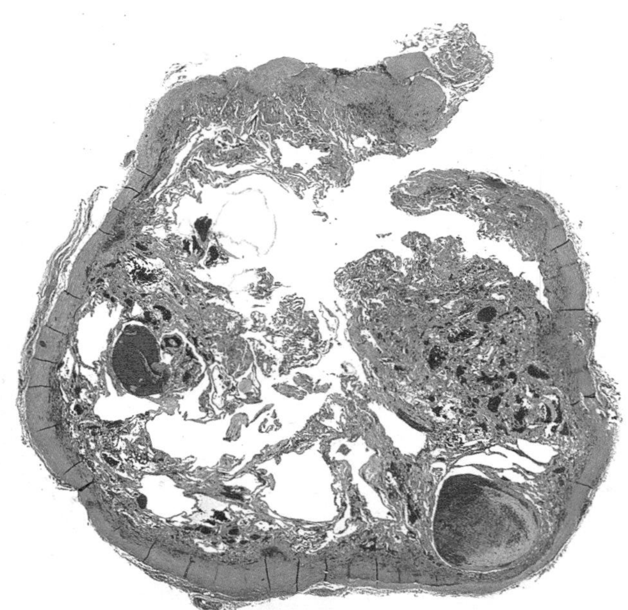

FIGURE 21-53. Subcutaneous spindle cell hemangioma with relative circumscription.

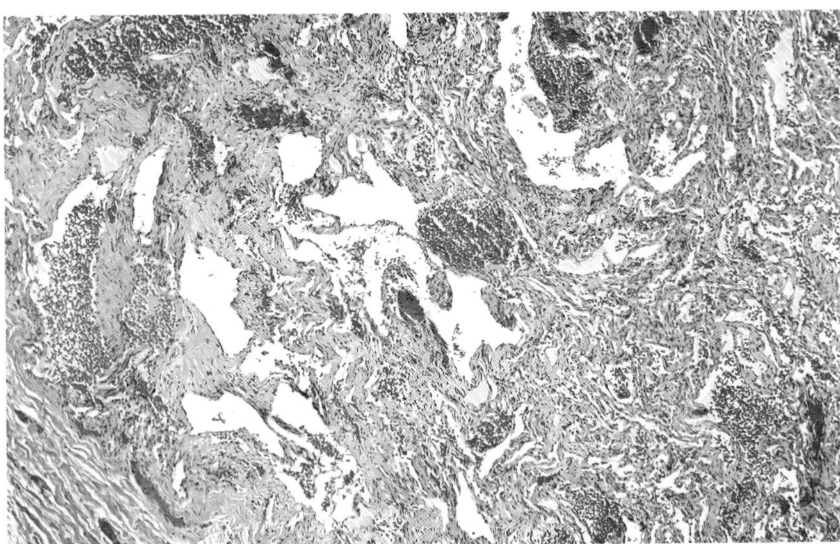

FIGURE 21-54. Spindle cell hemangioma with juxtaposition of the cellular and cavernous areas.

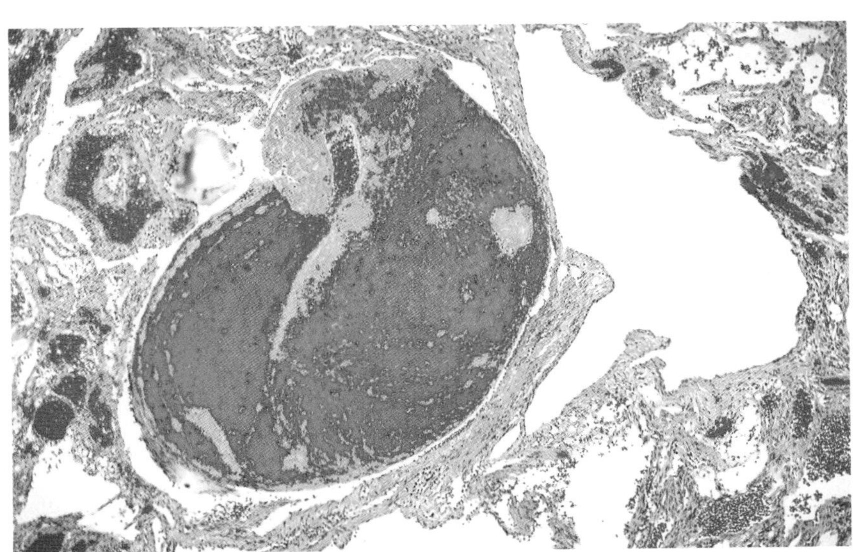

FIGURE 21-55. Spindle cell hemangioma with blood-filled cavernous spaces.

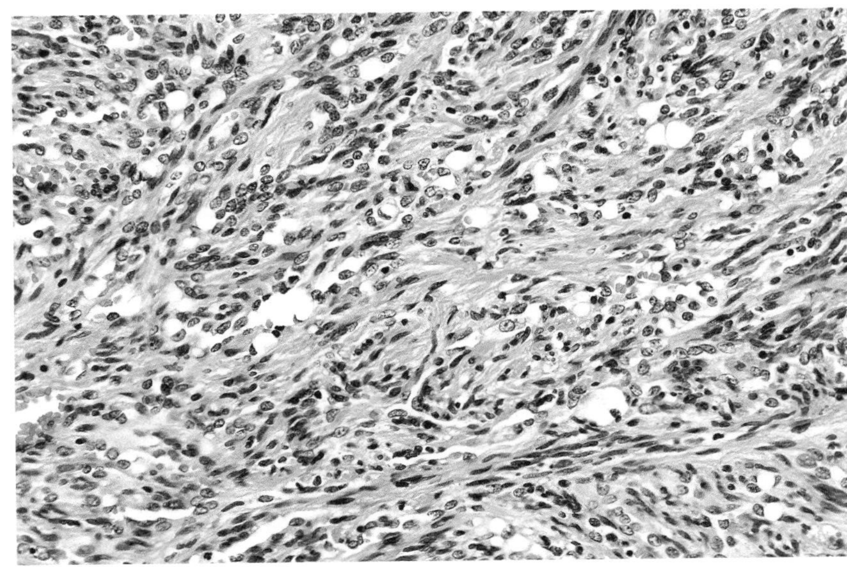

FIGURE 21-56. Spindle cell hemangioma with cellular (Kaposi sarcoma-like) areas.

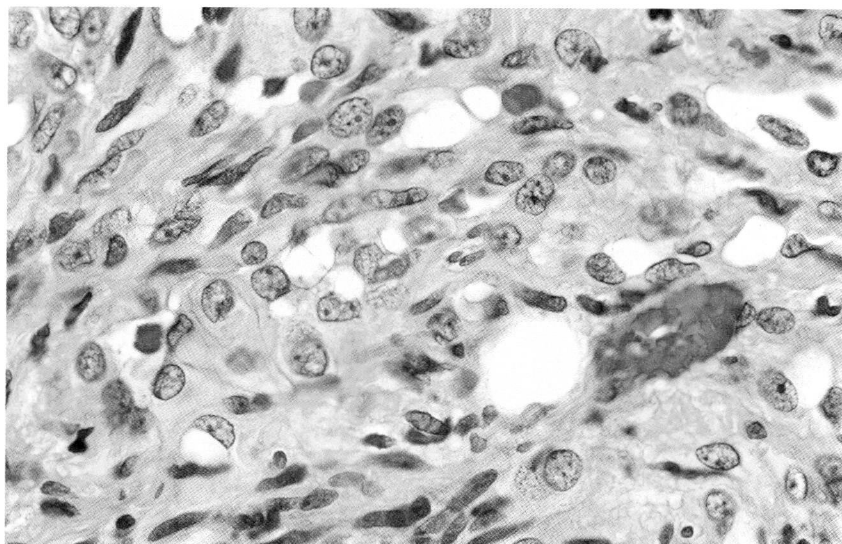

FIGURE 21-57. Spindle cell hemangioma with round epithelioid endothelial cells within cellular areas. Some show vacuolation.

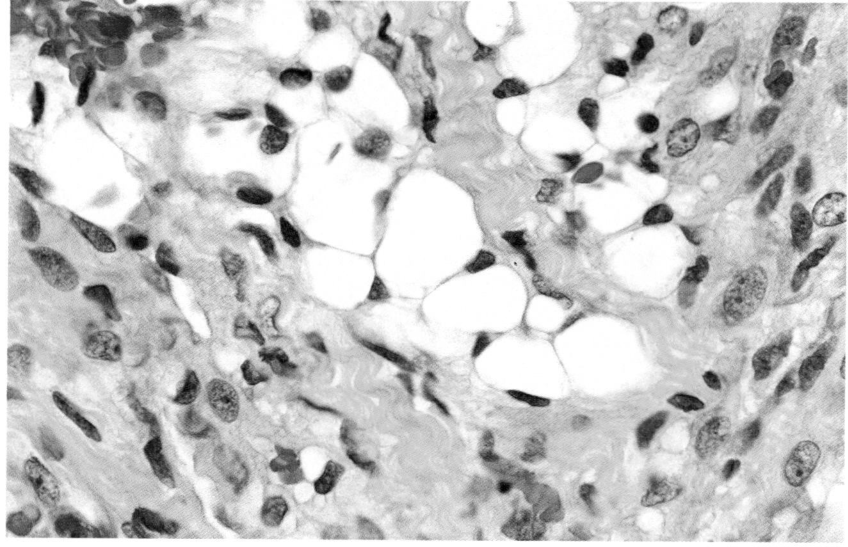

FIGURE 21-58. Spindle cell hemangioma with prominent vacuolation of endothelial cells. Such areas are frequently confused with fat.

tumor consists of a more or less discrete mass lined by a synovial membrane. These tumors almost invariably involve the knee joint and classically present as recurrent episodes of pain, swelling, and joint effusion. The symptoms usually begin during childhood and persist several years before the time of diagnosis. In most instances, a spongy compressible mass that decreases in size with elevation can be palpated over the joint. Plain films of the joint show nonspecific changes, including capsular thickening and vague soft tissue density and rarely erosion of bone or invasion of adjacent muscle. Arteriography is more diagnostic in that the pooling of blood over the mass suggests a vascular tumor. The tumor grows either as a discrete pedunculated lesion or as a diffuse process.

Histologically, the tumors are cavernous hemangiomas in which the vessels are separated by an edematous, myxoid, or focally hyalinized matrix, occasionally containing inflammatory cells and siderophages (Fig. 21-59). The synovium overlying the tumor is sometimes thrown into villous projections, and its cells contain moderate to marked amounts of hemosiderin pigment (see Fig. 21-59; Fig. 21-60). These synovial changes appear to be secondary phenomena but sometimes are so striking that they raise the possibility of primary synovitis. Proper evaluation depends on the recognition that the underlying vessels are far too numerous and large for the area in question.

It has been suggested that these lesions are not neoplasms but represent a reaction to trauma, although such a history is given in only a small number of cases. On the other hand, the young age of most afflicted patients again raises the question as to whether these lesions represent congenital malformations or tumors, especially because occasional patients have been noted to have hemangiomas elsewhere.

Treatment of local or pedunculated tumors is relatively easy, consisting of simple extirpation. Diffuse lesions are more difficult to eradicate surgically.

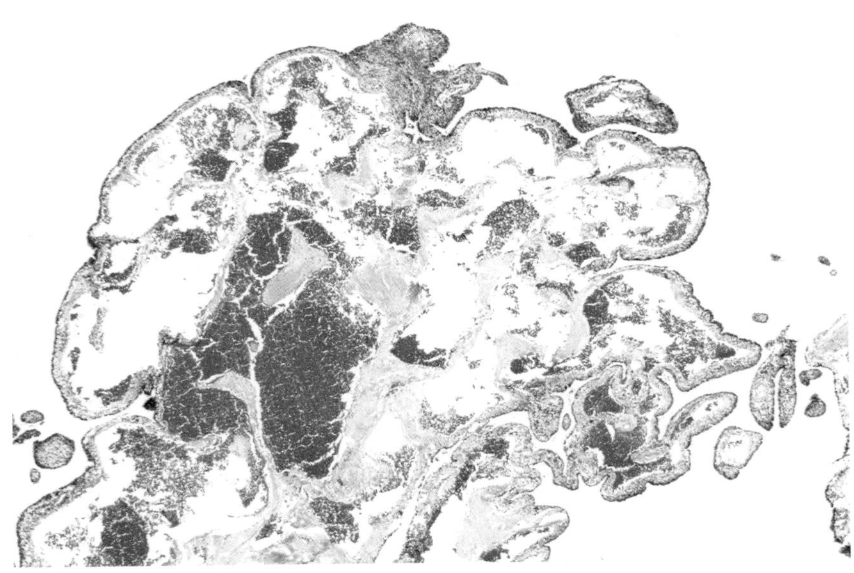

FIGURE 21-59. Synovial hemangioma depicting cavernous blood spaces located immediately subjacent to the synovial membrane.

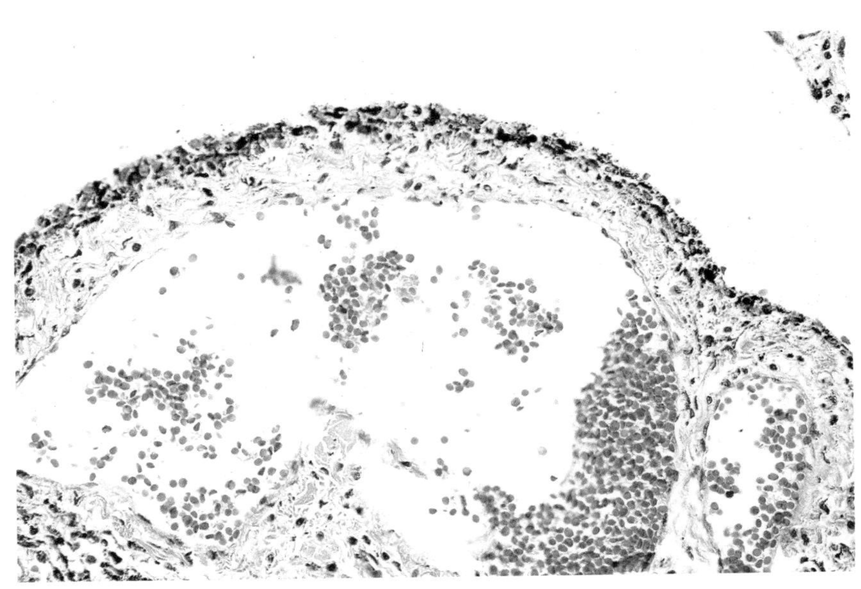

FIGURE 21-60. Synovial hemangioma. Pigmentation of synovial cells is a result of the presence of hemosiderin.

Hemangioma of Peripheral Nerves

Hemangiomas arising within the confines of the epineurium are rare. Pain is a common symptom and may be accompanied by numbness and muscle wasting in the affected region. In one case, symptoms of carpal tunnel syndrome were noted as a result of the location of the tumor in the median nerve. Involved nerves have included the trigeminal, ulnar, median, posterior tibial, and peroneal nerves. Histologically, most of the tumors have been cavernous hemangiomas with no histologic features suggesting malignancy.

Treatment of these benign tumors must be individualized. The benefits of total resection must be balanced against the morbidity of the procedure. Complete removal of an intraneural hemangioma has been accomplished by intrafascicular dissection, using dissecting microscopy. Such an approach offers complete removal with minimal morbidity.

REACTIVE VASCULAR PROLIFERATIONS

Papillary Endothelial Hyperplasia

Papillary endothelial hyperplasia is an exuberant, usually intravascular, endothelial proliferation that, in many respects, mimics an angiosarcoma.[73-75] It was first described by Masson, who designated it *vegetant intravascular hemangioendothelioma*. He regarded it as a true neoplasm that displays degenerative changes, including necrosis and thrombosis as it outgrows its blood supply, although now they are simply regarded as an exuberant form of organizing thrombus. Why only some thrombi display this form of organization is not clear.

Although this process may occur in virtually any vessel in the body, only those lesions that present as detectable masses are likely to come to the attention of the surgical pathologist. These lesions are most commonly located in veins on the head, neck, fingers, and trunk, where they appear as small, firm, superficial (deep dermis or subcutis) masses imparting a red to blue discoloration to the overlying skin (Fig. 21-61). Usually, a history of trauma is not elicited. Both the appearance and symptoms are nonspecific, so a biopsy is ultimately required to establish the identity of the lesion. In addition to its occurrence in a pure form in a dilated vessel, this lesion may be engrafted on a preexisting vascular lesion, such as a hemangioma, pyogenic granuloma, or vascular malformation. In these cases, the symptoms, appearance, and ultimate prognosis are related to the underlying lesion. In fact, most deeply situated papillary endothelial hyperplasias occur in intramuscular hemangiomas.

In its pure form, the lesion is a small (average 2 cm), purple-red, multicystic mass containing clotted blood and surrounded by a fibrous pseudocapsule containing residual smooth muscle or elastic tissue of the preexisting vessel wall (Fig. 21-62). In vessels of small caliber that are markedly dilated, little or no muscle is demonstrable in the pseudocapsule. Rarely, rupture of the vessel of origin permits spilling over of the process into surrounding soft tissue. In the early lesion, the ingrowth of endothelium along the contours of the thrombus partitions it into coarse papillae with fibrin cores (Fig. 21-63). In the well-established or typical lesion, myriad small delicate papillae project into the lumen and closely simulate the tufting growth of the angiosarcoma. These papillae are composed of a single layer of endothelium surrounding a collagenized core. The endothelial cells appear plump or swollen but lack significant pleomorphism and mitotic figures. During the late stage, clumping and fusing of the papillae give rise to an anastomosing network of vessels embedded in a loose mesh-like stroma of connective tissue (see Fig. 21-63D).

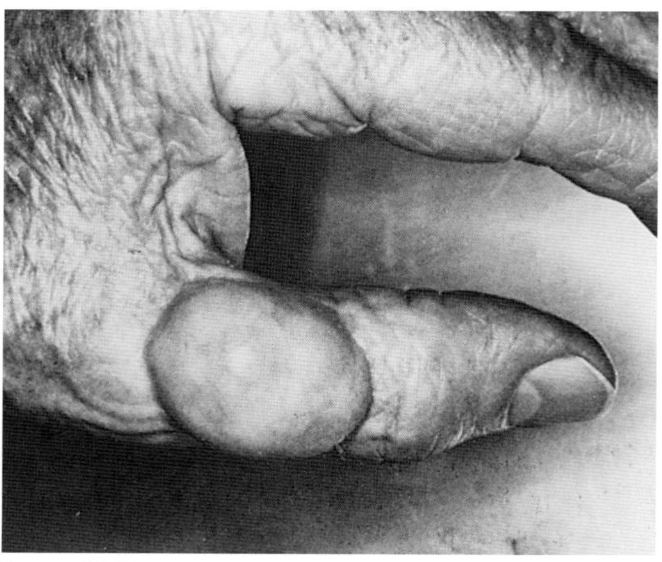

FIGURE 21-61. Papillary endothelial hyperplasia presenting as a localized nodule on the thumb.

Ultrastructurally, the cells lining the papillae appear to be differentiated endothelial cells with numerous micropinocytotic vesicles at the luminal aspect, tight junctions along the lateral boundaries, and occasional intracytoplasmic Weibel-Palade bodies. Basal lamina invests the antiluminal surface of the cells. In addition, pericytes and undifferentiated cells can be identified on the antiluminal aspects of the endothelial cells. The participation of several cell types is similar to the situation encountered in human granulation tissue and is further evidence of the reactive nature of this process.

The regularity with which this lesion is confused with an angiosarcoma is impressive. A helpful point in the differential diagnosis is its intravascular location because angiosarcomas are almost never confined to a vascular lumen. As mentioned earlier, passive extension of this process into soft tissue may occur following vessel rupture. However, even in these cases, the intravascular location of most of the lesion, coupled with the reactive changes in the vessel wall suggesting rupture, aid in the proper identification. On rare occasions, papillary endothelial hyperplasia occurs extravascularly as a result of organization of a hematoma, but this diagnosis should be made with caution. Apart from the usual intravascular location, papillary endothelial hyperplasia lacks the frank tissue necrosis, marked pleomorphism, and high mitotic rate that characterize many angiosarcomas.

The prognosis of this lesion is excellent. Essentially, all cases are cured by simple excision. Those that do recur are

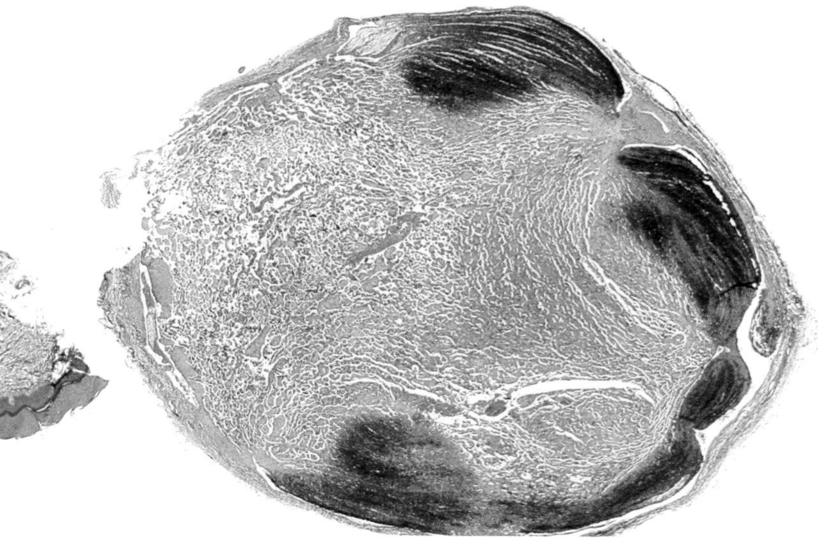

FIGURE 21-62. Organizing thrombus in a vessel showing early stages of papillary endothelial hyperplasia at the bottom of the picture.

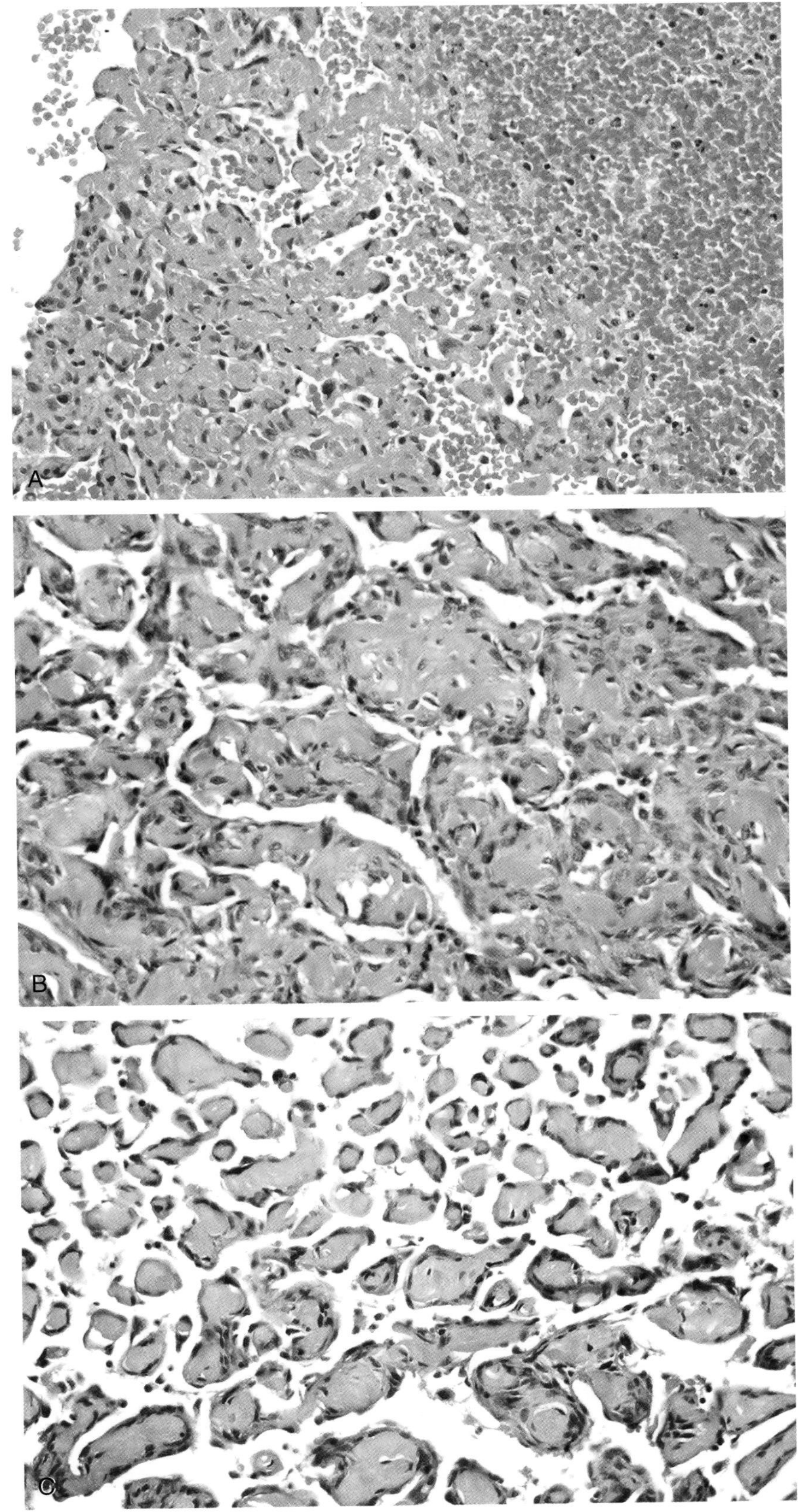

FIGURE 21-63. Stages of papillary endothelial hyperplasia. (A) Early stage is characterized by a thrombus with ingrowth of endothelial cells. Endothelium gradually subdivides the partially collagenized thrombus into coarse clumps (B), followed by papillae (C). *Continued*

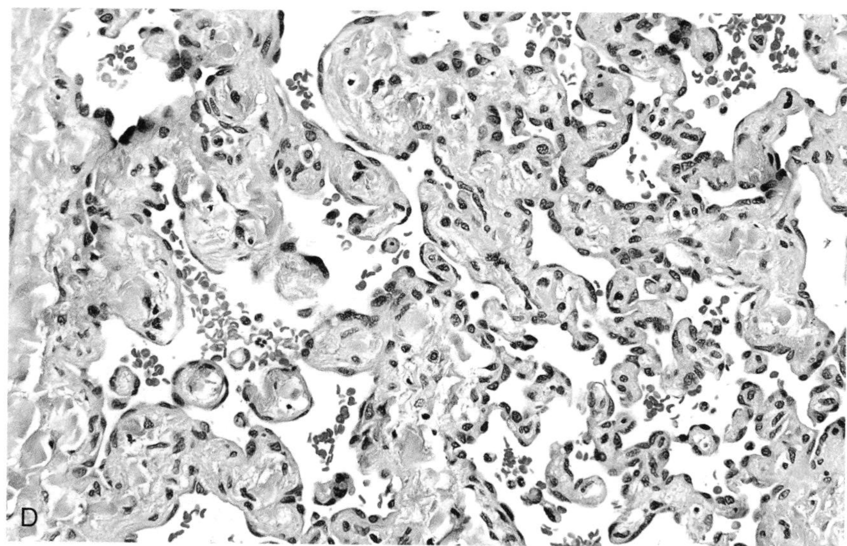

FIGURE 21-63, cont'd. (D) At the end stage, papillae fuse to form a loosely anastomotic secondary vascular pattern.

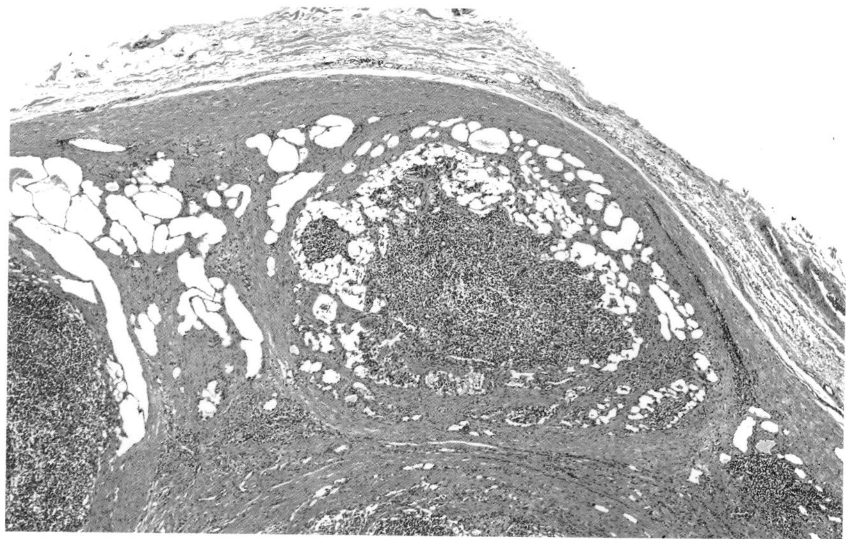

FIGURE 21-64. Vascular transformation in a lymph node (nodal angiomatosis). Vessels surround but preserve lymph follicles. Lymph node was removed as part of the regional lymph node dissection for carcinoma.

usually those that are superimposed on vascular tumors. The therapy in these cases should be dictated by the nature of the underlying lesions.

Vascular Transformation of Lymph Nodes

First described as *vascular transformation of lymph nodes* and later as *nodal angiomatosis*, this reactive change of lymph node occurs secondary to lymphatic or venous obstruction, or both, and has been observed particularly in axillary lymph nodes removed at the time of radical mastectomy for breast carcinoma.[76,77] The change may also occur in lymph nodes removed for a variety of other diagnostic or therapeutic reasons. Typically, the change involves the subcapsular space and sinuses in either a segmental or diffuse fashion. In the most readily recognized case, the small, ectatic, capillary-sized vessels are well formed (Figs. 21-64 and 21-65). Chan et al.[76] emphasized a greater range of changes in this condition than was previously appreciated. In extreme examples of vascular transformation, the vessels may be closely packed and slightly attenuated so that the resemblance to Kaposi sarcoma is more than fleeting. Usually, however, there is maturation of the vessels toward the periphery of the lymph node so that ectatic capillaries are present immediately subjacent to the capsule. Extravasation of erythrocytes occurs; in exceptional cases, hyaline droplets, similar to those in Kaposi sarcoma, are identified.

There are a number of features that serve to distinguish this lesion from Kaposi sarcoma, including the overall preservation of lymph node architecture, despite the expansion of the subcapsular and medullary sinuses, the peripheral maturation of the vessels, the lack of vessels arranged in distinct fascicles, and the presence of secondary sclerosis. However, the earliest stages of Kaposi sarcoma of lymph nodes, as seen in the patient with acquired immunodeficiency syndrome (AIDS), may prove exceptionally difficult and, at times, impossible to distinguish from vascular transformation of the lymph node. As noted previously, immunohistochemistry for HHV-8 LANA

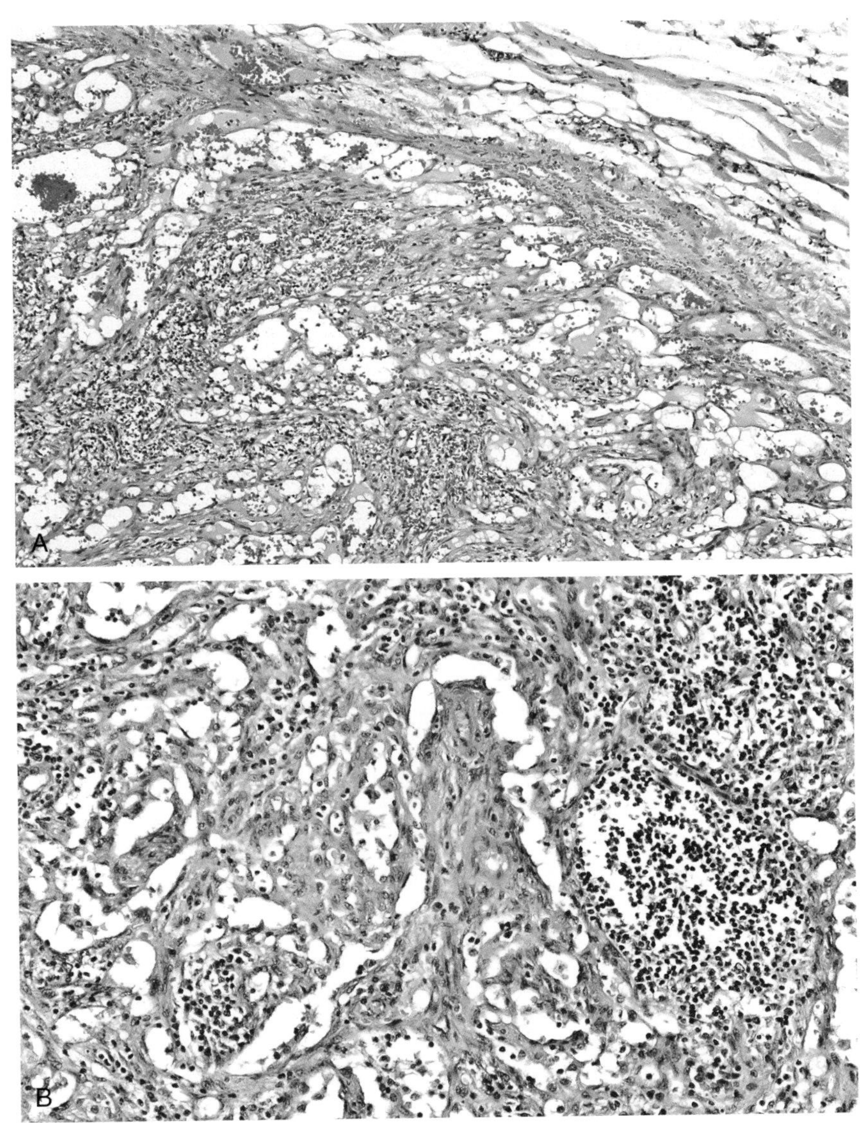

FIGURE 21-65. Vascular transformation of lymph node showing a subcapsular location (A) and prominent proliferation of vessels (B).

protein may be of considerable value in this differential diagnosis.

Glomeruloid Hemangioma

Glomeruloid hemangioma is a descriptive term coined by Chan et al.[78] for the reactive vascular proliferations that occur in *POEMS syndrome* (Takatsuki syndrome and Crowe-Fukase syndrome).[79,80] This syndrome is characterized by *p*olyneuropathy (peripheral neuropathy, papilledema), *o*rganomegaly (hepatosplenomegaly, lymphadenopathy), *e*ndocrinopathy (amenorrhea, gynecomastia, impotence, adrenal insufficiency, hypothyroidism, glucose intolerance), *M*-protein (plasmacytosis, paraproteinemia, bone lesions), and *s*kin lesions (hyperpigmentation, hypertrichosis, angiomas); in some instances, it overlaps with multicentric Castleman disease.[81]

The vascular lesions develop within the dermis underneath an intact, essentially normal epidermis. In the classic case, glomeruloid nests of capillaries lie in ectatic capillaries, creating a vessel-within-a-vessel appearance (Figs. 21-66 and 21-67). The intravascular capillaries are lined by normal-appearing endothelium and are filled with erythrocytes. A distinctive feature of the intravascular proliferation is the large round cells filled with eosinophilic globules corresponding to polytypic immunoglobulin (Fig. 21-68). Chan et al.[78] suggested that these cells, which reside principally outside of the basal lamina, are closely related to endothelial cells rather than pericytes or smooth muscle cells. Their unusual appearance is probably induced by the presence of cytoplasmic immunoglobulin, which is derived from serum. In some cases of POEMS syndrome, the vascular lesions are indistinguishable from an ordinary capillary hemangioma, and, in other cases, the lesions have features intermediate between a capillary hemangioma and the classic glomeruloid hemangioma, suggesting that they represent stages of the same process.

Bacillary (Epithelioid) Angiomatosis

Bacillary (epithelioid) angiomatosis is a pseudoneoplastic vascular proliferation, caused by *Bartonella* (formerly

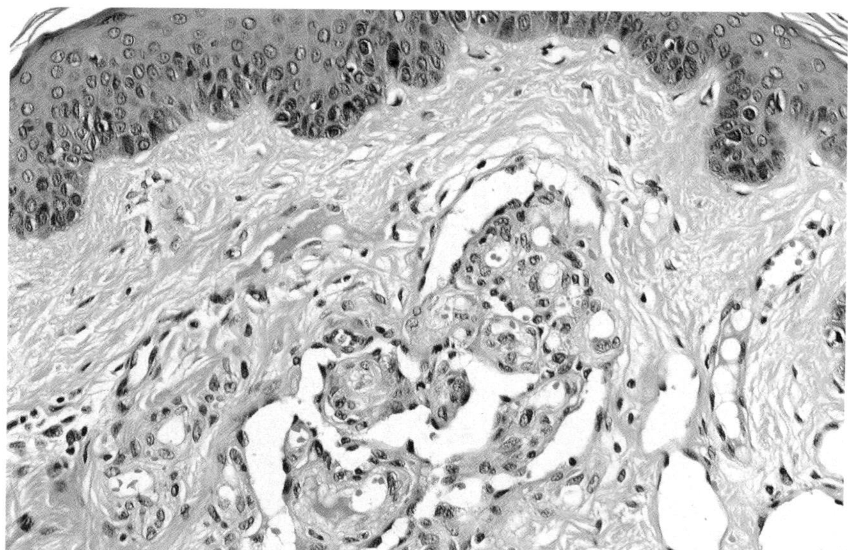

FIGURE 21-66. Glomeruloid hemangioma. *(Case courtesy of Dr. C.D.M. Fletcher, Brigham and Women's Hospital.)*

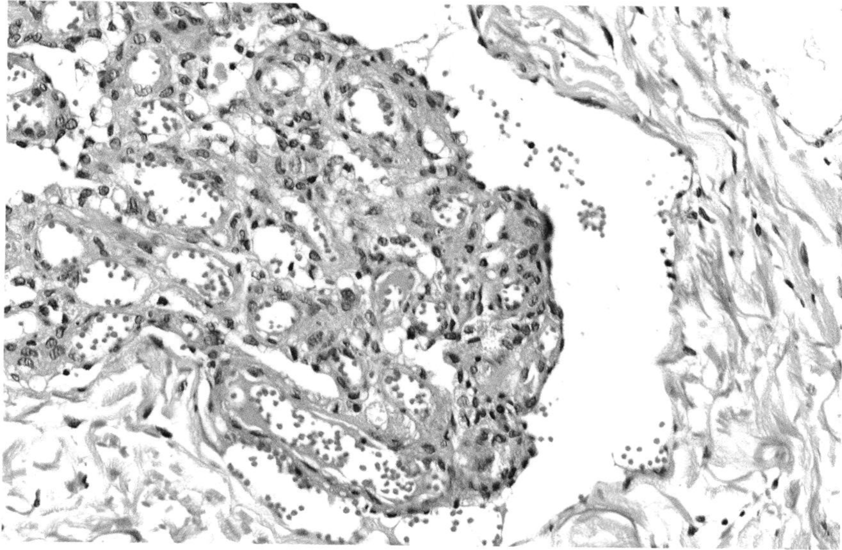

FIGURE 21-67. Glomeruloid hemangioma. *(Case courtesy of Dr. C.D.M. Fletcher, Brigham and Women's Hospital.)*

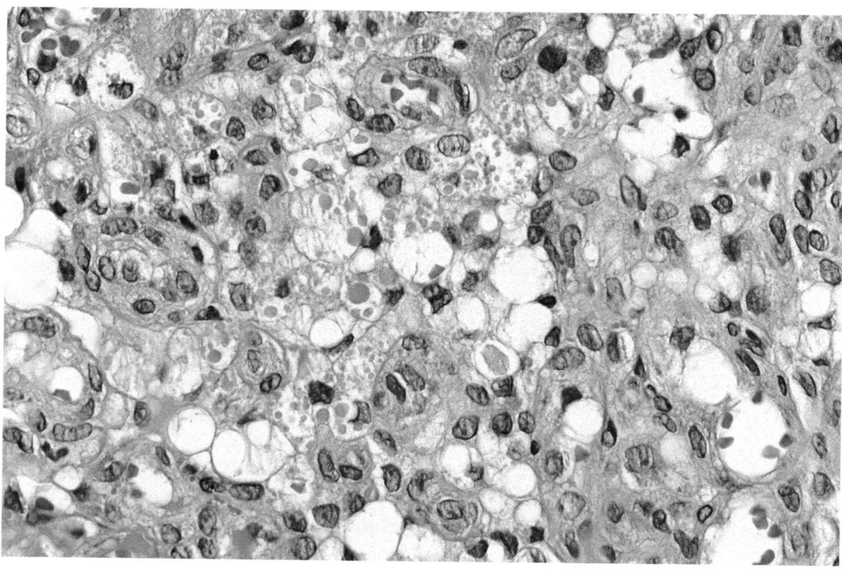

FIGURE 21-68. Hyaline droplets of immunoglobulin in a glomeruloid hemangioma. *(Case courtesy of Dr. C.D.M. Fletcher, Brigham and Women's Hospital.)*

Rochalimaea), which occurs almost exclusively in immunocompromised hosts. *Bartonella* is a family of small Gram-negative bacilli that includes a number of species pathogenic for humans: *B. henselae*, *B. quintana*, *B. bacilliformis*, and *B. elizabethae*. *Bartonella henselae* and *quintana* have been shown to be the causative agents for bacillary angiomatosis and bacillary peliosis, as well as for *Bartonella* bacterial endocarditis and classic cat-scratch disease.[82,83]

Most cases of bacillary angiomatosis occur in men in the setting of AIDS. Bacillary angiomatosis usually presents as multiple pink, elevated skin lesions that may resemble a pyogenic granuloma.[84,85] Usually, their pink color distinguishes them from the dusky violaceous lesions of Kaposi sarcoma. In some cases, there are also liver, spleen, lymph node, bone, and soft tissue lesions. In the classic case, bacillary angiomatosis consists of lobules of capillary-sized vessels lined by plump (epithelioid) endothelium with clear cytoplasm (Fig. 21-69). Mild atypia and occasional mitotic figures may be present in the endothelial cells. Although the strikingly clear cytoplasm of the endothelial cells bears some similarity to the endothelial changes in epithelioid hemangioma, there is a neutrophilic infiltrate in the interstitium along with collections of pink coagulum containing clusters of the organisms that are easily identified with the Warthin-Starry stain (Fig. 21-70). Unfortunately, some bacillary angiomatosis cases do not display the foregoing distinctive changes and may be virtually indistinguishable from granulation tissue.[83] Obviously, if the clinical setting suggests the diagnosis, one is obligated to rule out the diagnosis by means of special stains. On electron microscopy, the organisms appear as bacillary forms with a trilaminar cell wall. In the liver, the organisms induce peliotic changes. Large numbers of organisms can be identified around the peliotic zones in the liver. Treatment of bacillary angiomatosis is effectively accomplished with erythromycin.

Florid Vascular Proliferation of the Colon Secondary to Intussusception and Prolapse

A florid vascular proliferation occurring in adult patients with intussusception and prolapse has recently been reported by Bavikatty et al.[86] The lesion, consisting of a lobular

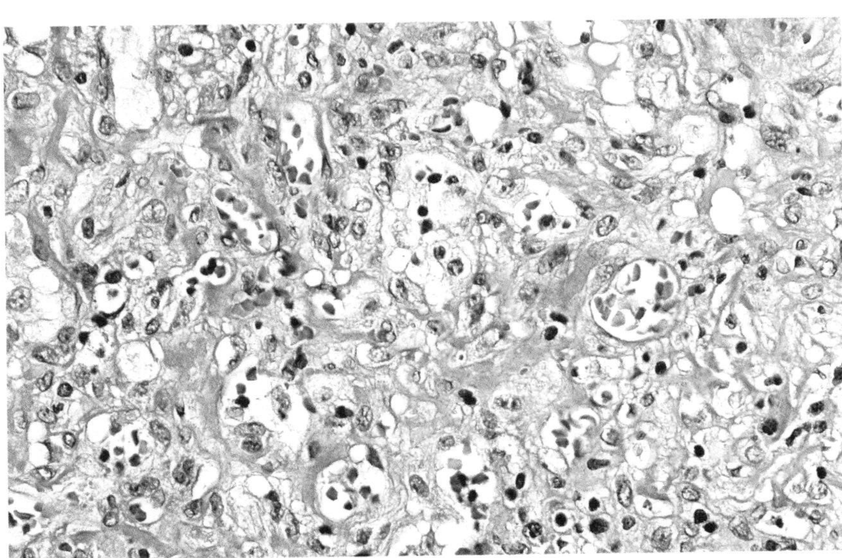

FIGURE 21-69. Bacillary angiomatosis showing endothelial cells with clear cytoplasm set in an inflammatory background.

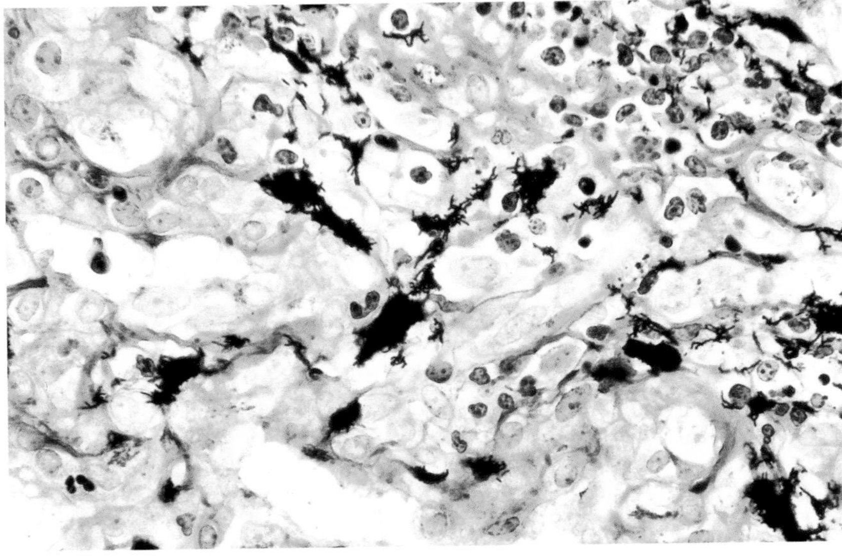

FIGURE 21-70. Warthin-Starry staining of bacillary angiomatosis showing numerous clumped rod-shaped organisms.

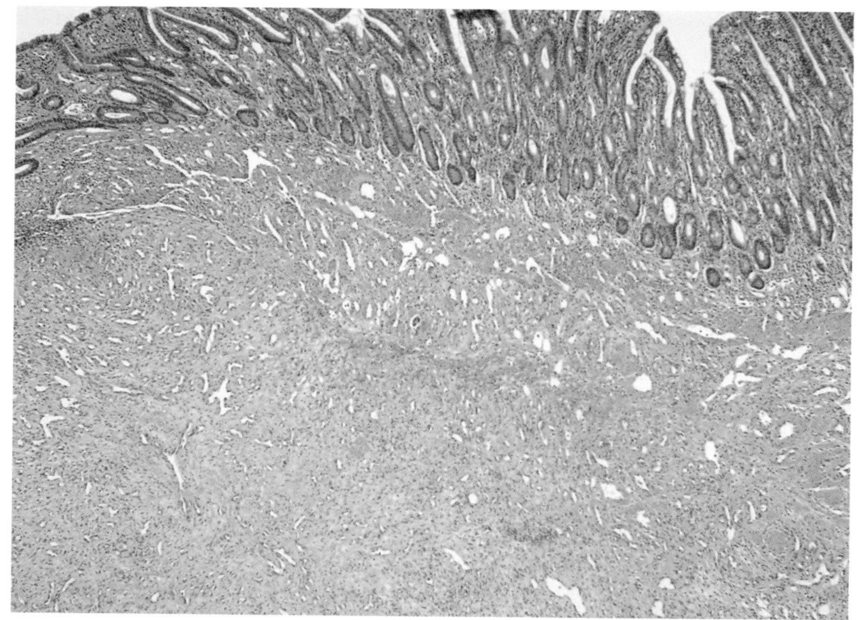

FIGURE 21-71. Florid vascular proliferation of the colon secondary to intussusception and colonic prolapse.

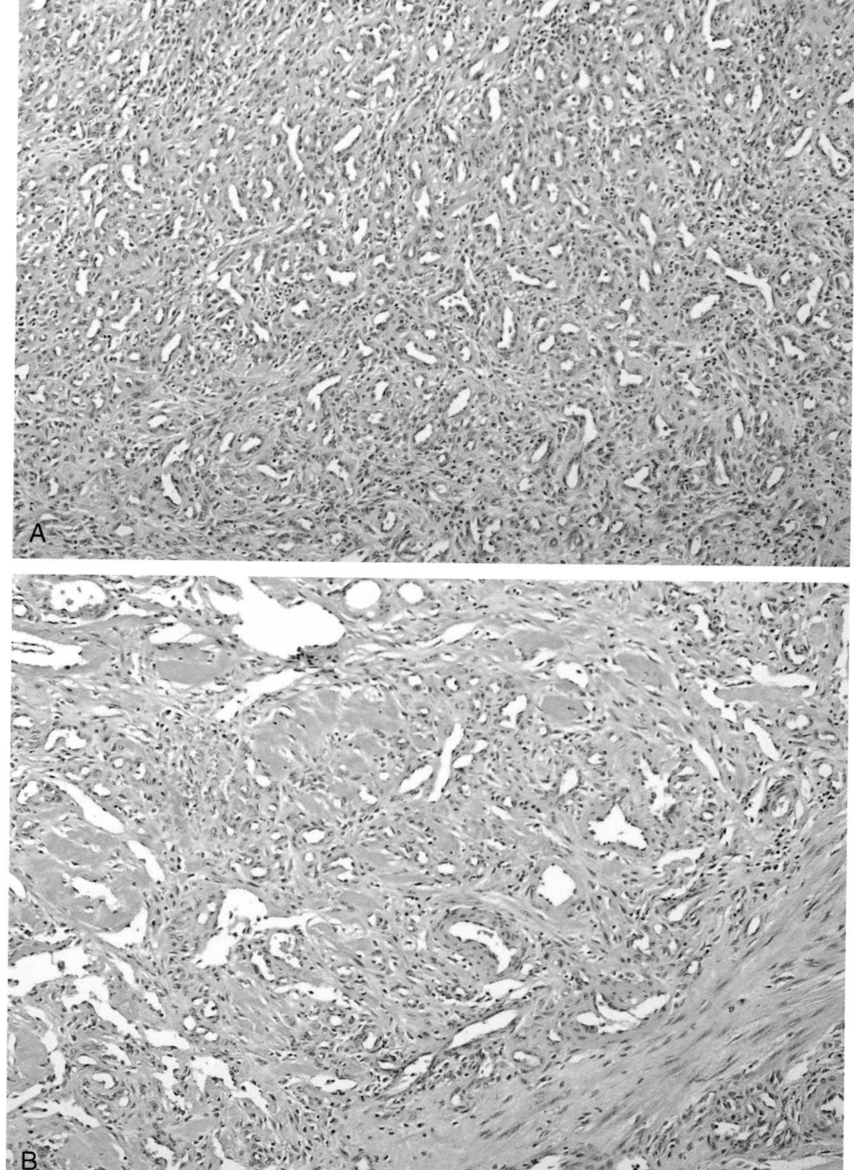

FIGURE 21-72. Florid vascular proliferation of the colon secondary to intussusception and colonic prolapse showing well-formed vessels (A) that involve muscularis propria (B).

proliferation of small capillary-sized vessels, extends from the submucosa through the entire bowel wall and is associated with mucosal ischemia and ulceration (Figs. 21-71 and 21-72). Although the vascular proliferation dissects muscle fibers, the vessels are well formed and display minimal nuclear atypia. In two of the five cases reported, an underlying vascular malformation was identified. The excellent follow-up in the reported cases underscores the reactive nature of these proliferations.

References

1. North PE. Pediatric vascular tumors and malformations. Surg Pathol 2010;3:455.
2. Mulliken JB, Glowacki J. Hemangioma and vascular malformations in infants and children: a classification based on endothelial characteristics. Plast Reconstr Surg 1982;69:412.
3. Lister WA. The natural history of strawberry nevi. Lancet 1938;1:1429.
4. Walter JW, Blei F, Anderson JL, et al. Genetic mapping of a novel familial form of infantile hemangioma. Am J Med Genet 1999;82:77.
5. Berg JN, Walter JW, Thisanagayam U, et al. Evidence for the loss of heterozygosity of 5q in sporadic hemangiomas: are somatic mutations involved in hemangioma formation. J Clin Pathol 2001;54:249.
6. Bean WB. Vascular spiders and related lesions of the skin. Springfield, IL: Charles C Thomas; 1958.
7. Walsh TS, Tompkins VN. Some observations on the strawberry nevus of infancy. Cancer 1956;9:869.
8. Takahashi K, Mulliken JB, Kozakewich HP, et al. Cellular markers that distinguish the phases of hemangioma during infancy and childhood. J Clin Invest 1994;93:2357.
9. Blei F, Walter J, Orlow SJ, et al. Familial segregation of hemangiomas and vascular malformations as an autosomal dominant trait. Arch Dermatol 1998;134:718.
10. Metry DW, Haggstrom AN, Drolet A, et al. A prospective study of PHACE syndrome in infantile hemangiomas: demographic features, clinical findings and complications. Am J Med Genet A 2006;140:975.
11. North PE, Waner M, Mizerack A, et al. A unique microvascular phenotype shared by juvenile hemangiomas and human placenta. Arch Dermatol 2001;137:559.
12. Boon LM, Enjolras O, Mulliken JB. Congenital hemangioma: evidence of accelerated involution. J Pediatr 1996;128:329.
13. North PE, Waner M, James CJ, et al. Congenital nonprogressive hemangioma: a distinct clinicopathological entity unlike infantile hemangioma. Arch Dermatol 2001;137:1607.
14. Enjolras O, Mulliken JB, Boon LM, et al. Noninvoluting congenital hemangioma: a rare cutaneous vascular anomaly. Plast Reconstr Surg 2001;107:1647.
15. Berenguer B, Mulliken JB, Enjolras O, et al. Rapidly involuting congenital hemangioma: clinical and histopathologic features. Pediatr Devel Pathol 2003;6:495.
16. Kerr DA. Granuloma pyogenicum. Oral Surg Oral Med Oral Pathol 1951;4:158.
17. Patrice SJ, Wiss K, Mulliken JB. Pyogenic granuloma (lobular capillary hemangioma): a clinicopathologic study of 178 cases. Pediatr Dermatol 1994;8:267.
18. Kim TH, Choi EH, Ahn SK, et al. Vascular tumors arising in port wine stains: two cases of pyogenic granuloma and a case of acquired tufted angiomas. J Dermatol 1999;26;813.
19. Wilson BB, Greer KE, Cooper PH. Eruptive disseminated lobular capillary hemangioma (pyogenic granuloma). J Am Acad Dermatol 1989;21:391.
20. Mills SE, Cooper PH, Fechner RE. Lobular capillary hemangioma: the underlying lesion of pyogenic granuloma. Am J Surg Pathol 1980;4:471.
21. Bhaskar SN, Jacoway JR. Pyogenic granuloma: clinical features, incidence, histology, and result of treatment: report of 242 cases. J Oral Surg 1966;24:391.
22. Warner J, Wilson-Jones E. Pyogenic granuloma recurring with multiple satellites: a report of 11 cases. Br J Dermatol 1968;80:218.
23. McDonald RH. Granuloma gravidarum. Am J Obstet Gynecol 1956;72:1132.
24. Cooper PH, McAllister HA, Helwig EB. Intravenous pyogenic granuloma: a study of 18 cases. Am J Surg Pathol 1979;3:221.
25. Wells GC, Whimster I. Subcutaneous angiolymphoid hyperplasia with eosinophilia. Br J Dermatol 1969;81:1.
26. Reed RJ, Terazakis N. Subcutaneous angioblastic lymphoid hyperplasia with eosinophilia (Kimura's disease). Cancer 1972;29:489.
27. Kimura T, Yoshimura S, Ishikawa E. Unusual granulation combined with hyperplastic change of lymphatic tissue. Trans Soc Pathol Jpn 1948;37:179.
28. Kung IT, Gibson JB, Bannatyne PM. Kimura's disease: a clinicopathological study of 21 cases and its distinction from angiolymphoid hyperplasia with eosinophilia. Pathology 1984;16:39.
29. Urabe A, Tsuneyoshi M, Enjoji M. Epithelioid hemangioma versus Kimura's disease: a comparative clinicopathologic study. Am J Surg Pathol 1987;11:758.
30. Chan JK, Hui PK, Ng CS, et al. Epithelioid hemangioma (angiolymphoid hyperplasia with eosinophilia) and Kimura's disease in Chinese. Histopathology 1989;15:557.
31. Fetsch JF, Sesterhenn IA, Miettinen M, et al. Epithelioid hemangioma of the penis: a clinicopathologic and immunohistochemical analysis of 19 cases, with special reference to exuberant examples often confused with epithelioid hemangioendothelioma and epithelioid angiosarcoma. Am J Surg Pathol 2004;28:523.
32. Moesner J, Pallesen R, Sorensen B. Angiolymphoid hyperplasia with eosinophilia (Kimura's disease): a case with dermal lesions in the knee and a popliteal arteriovenous fistula. Arch Dermatol 1981;117:650.
33. Fetsch JF, Weiss SW. Observations concerning the pathogenesis of epithelioid hemangioma (angiolymphoid hyperplasia). Mod Pathol 1991;4:449.
34. Brenn T, Fletcher CD. Cutaneous epithelioid angiomatous nodule: a distinct lesion in the morphologic spectrum of epithelioid vascular tumors. Am J Dermatopathol 2004;26:14.
35. Osler W. On a family form of recurring epistaxis associated with multiple telangiectases of the skin and mucous membranes. Bull Johns Hopkins Hosp 1901;12:333.
36. Brouillard P, Vikkula M. Vascular malformations: localized defects in vascular morphogenesis. Clin Genet 2003;63:340.
37. Eerola I, Boon LM, Mulliken JB, et al. Capillary malformation-arteriovenous malformation, a new clinical and genetic disorder caused by RASA1 mutations. Am J Hum Genet 2003;73:1240.
38. Finley JL, Noe JM, Arndt KA, et al. Port wine stains: morphologic variations and developmental lesions. Arch Dermatol 1984;120:1453.
39. Smoller B, Rosen S. Port-wine stains: a disease of altered neural modulation of blood vessels. Arch Dermatol 1986;122:177.
40. Gallione CJ, Pasyk KA, Boon LM, et al. A gene for familial venous malformations maps to chromosome 9p in a second large kindred. J Med Genet 1995;32:197.
41. Vikkula M, Boon LM, Carraway KL, et al. Vascular dysmorphogenesis caused by an activating mutation in the receptor tyrosine kinase TIE2. Cell 1996;87:1181.
42. Hein KD, Mulliken JB, Kozakewich HP, et al. Venous malformations of skeletal muscle. Plastic Reconstr Surg 2002;110:1625.
43. Tan WH, Baris HN, Burrows PE, et al. The spectrum of vascular anomalies in patients with PTEN mutations: implications for diagnosis and management. J Med Genet 2007;44:594.
44. Garzon MC, Huang JT, Enjolras I, et al. Vascular malformations. Part 1. J Am Acad Dermatol 2007;56:353.
44a. Kurek KC, Howard E, Tennant LB, et al. PTEN hamartoma of soft tissue: a distinctive lesions in PTEN syndromes. Am J Surg Pathol 2012;36(5):671–87.
45. Strutton G, Weedon D. Acro-angiodermatitis: a simulant of Kaposi's sarcoma. Am J Dermatopathol 1987;9:85.
46. Allen PW, Enzinger FM. Hemangiomas of skeletal muscle: an analysis of 89 cases. Cancer 1972;29:8.
47. Angervall L, Nielsen JM, Stener B, et al. Concomitant arteriovenous vascular malformation in skeletal muscle. Cancer 1979;44:232.
48. Angervall L, Nilsson L, Stener B, et al. Angiographic, microangiographic, and histologic study of vascular malformation in striated muscle. Acta Radiol 1968;7:65.
49. Beham A, Fletcher CD. Intramuscular angioma: a clinicopathologic analysis of 74 cases. Histopathology 1991;18:53.
50. Cohen AJ, Youkey JR, Clagett GP. Intramuscular hemangioma. JAMA 1983;249:2680.
51. Howat AJ, Campbell PE. Angiomatosis: a vascular malformation of infancy and childhood. Pathology 1987;19:377.
52. Rao VK, Weiss SW. Angiomatosis of soft tissue: an analysis of the histologic features and clinical outcome in 51 cases. Am J Surg Pathol 1992;16:764.
53. Devaney K, Vinh TN, Sweet DE. Skeletal-extraskeletal angiomatosis: a clinicopathological study of fourteen patients and nosological considerations. J Bone Joint Surg [Am] 1994;76:878.
54. Imperial R, Helwig EB. Verrucous hemangioma: a clinicopathologic study of 21 cases. Arch Dermatol 1967;96:247.

55. Chan JK, Tsang WY, Calonje E, et al. Verrucous hemangioma: a distinctive but neglected variant of cutaneous hemangioma. Int J Surg Pathol 1995;2:171.
56. Calduch L, Ortega C, Navarro V, et al. Verrucous hemangioma: report of two cases and review of the literature. Pediatr Dermatol 2000;17:213.
57. Clinton TS, Cooke LM, Graham BS. Cobb syndrome associated with a verrucous (angiokeratoma-like) vascular malformation. Cutis 2003;71:283.
58. Guillou L, Calonje E, Speight P, et al. Hobnail hemangioma: a pseudomalignant vascular lesion with a reappraisal of targetoid hemosiderotic hemangioma. Am J Surg Pathol 1999;23:97.
59. Mentzel TP, Partanen TA, Kutzner H. Hobnail hemangioma ("targetoid hemosiderotic hemangioma"): clinicopathologic and immunohistochemical analysis of 62 cases. J Cutan Pathol 1999;26:279.
60. Santa Cruz DJ, Aronberg J. Targetoid hemosiderotic hemangioma. J Am Acad Dermatol 1988;19:550.
61. Calonje E, Fletcher CD. Sinusoidal hemangioma: a distinctive benign vascular neoplasm within the group of cavernous hemangiomas. Am J Surg Pathol 1991;15:1130.
62. Montgomery EA, Epstein J. Anastomosing hemangioma of the genitourinary tract: a lesion mimicking angiosarcoma. Am J Surg Pathol 2009;33:1364.
63. Brown JG, Folpe AL, Rao P, et al. Primary vascular tumors and tumor-liked lesions of the kidney: a clinicopathologic analysis of 25 cases. Am J Surg Pathol 2010;34:942.
64. Kryvenko ON, Gupta NS, Meier FA, et al. Anastomosing hemangioma of the genitourinary system: eight cases in the kidney and ovary with immunohistochemical and ultrastructural analysis. Am J Clin Pathol 2011;136:450.
65. Wilson-Jones E, Orkin M. Tufted angioma (angioblastoma): a benign progressive angioma, not to be confused with Kaposi's sarcoma or low-grade angiosarcoma. J Am Acad Dermatol 1989;20:214.
66. Okada E, Tamura A, Ishikawa O, et al. Tufted angioma (angioblastoma): case report and review of 41 cases in the Japanese literature. Clin Exp Dermatol 2000;25:627.
67. Padilla RS, Orkin M, Rosai J. Acquired tufted angioma (progressive capillary hemangioma): a distinctive clinicopathologic entity related to lobular capillary hemangioma. Am J Dermatopathol 1987;9:292.
68. Tille JC, Morris MA, Brundler MA, et al. Familial predisposition to tufted angioma: identification of blood and lymphatic vascular components. Clin Genet 2003;63:393.
69. Weiss SW, Enzinger FM. Spindle cell hemangioendothelioma: a low grade angiosarcoma resembling a cavernous hemangioma and Kaposi's sarcoma. Am J Surg Pathol 1986;10:521.
70. Fletcher CD, Beham A, Schmid C. Spindle cell hemangioendothelioma: a clinicopathological and immunohistochemical study indicative of a non-neoplastic lesion. Histopathology 1991;18:291.
71. Perkins P, Weiss SW. Spindle cell hemangioendothelioma: an analysis of 78 cases with reassessment of its pathogenesis and biologic behavior. Am J Surg Pathol 1996;20:1196.
72. Harkins HN. Hemangioma of a tendon sheath: report of a case with a study of 24 cases from the literature. Arch Surg 1937;34:12.
73. Clearkin KP, Enzinger FM. Intravascular papillary endothelial hyperplasia. Arch Pathol Lab Med 1976;100:441.
74. Barr RJ, Graham JH, Sherwin LA. Intravascular papillary endothelial hyperplasia: a benign lesion mimicking angiosarcoma. Arch Dermatol 1978;114:723.
75. Hashimoto H, Daimaru Y, Enjoji M. Intravascular papillary endothelial hyperplasia: a clinicopathologic study of 91 cases. Am J Dermatopathol 1983;5:539.
76. Chan JK, Warnke RA, Dorfman R. Vascular transformation of sinuses in lymph nodes: a study of it morphological spectrum and distinction from Kaposi sarcoma. Am J Surg Pathol 1991;15:732.
77. Ostrowski ML, Siddiqui T, Barnes RE, et al. Vascular transformation of lymph node sinuses: a process displaying a spectrum of histologic features. Arch Pathol Lab Med 1990;114:656.
78. Chan JK, Fletcher CD, Hicklin GA, et al. Glomeruloid hemangioma: a distinctive cutaneous lesion of multicentric Castleman's disease associated with POEMS syndrome. Am J Surg Pathol 1990;14:1036.
79. Ishikawa AO, Nihei Y, Ishikawa H. The skin changes of POEMS syndrome. Br J Dermatol 1987;117:523.
80. Kanitakis J, Roger H, Soubrier M, et al. Cutaneous angiomas in POEMS syndrome: an ultrastructural and immunohistochemical study. Arch Dermatol 1988;124:695.
81. Yang SG, Cho KH, Bang YJ, et al. A case of glomeruloid hemangioma associated with multicentric Castleman's disease. Am J Dermatol 1998;20:266.
82. Spach DH, Koehler JF. Bartonella-associated infections. Infect Dis Clin North Am 1998;12:137.
83. Wong R, Tappero J, Cockerell CJ. Bacillary angiomatosis and other Bartonella species infections. Semin Cutan Med Surg 1997;16:186.
84. Cockerell CJ, Bergstresser PR, Myrie-Williams C, et al. Bacillary epithelioid angiomatosis occurring in an immunocompetent individual. Arch Dermatol 1990;126:787.
85. LeBoit PE, Berger TG, Egbert BM, et al. Bacillary angiomatosis: the histopathology and differential diagnosis of a pseudoneoplastic infection in patients with human immunodeficiency virus disease. Am J Surg Pathol 1989;13:909.
86. Bavikatty NR, Goldblum FR, Abdul-Karim FW, et al. Florid vascular proliferation of the colon related to intussusception and mucosal prolapse: potential diagnostic confusion with angiosarcoma. Mod Pathol 2001;14:1114.

Hemangioendothelioma: Vascular Tumors of Intermediate Malignancy

CHAPTER CONTENTS

VASCULAR TUMOR OF INTERMEDIATE MALIGNANCY

The term *hemangioendothelioma* is the designation for vascular tumors that have a biologic behavior intermediate between a hemangioma and a conventional angiosarcoma. Tumors included in this group have the ability to recur locally and some ability to metastasize but at a reduced level compared to angiosarcoma. The risk of metastasis varies from tumor to tumor within this group. For example, the epithelioid hemangioendothelioma, the most aggressive member of this family, produces distant metastasis and death in a minority of cases, whereas the retiform and Dabska-type hemangioendotheliomas, two closely related tumors, have been associated with regional lymph node metastasis only.

EPITHELIOID HEMANGIOENDOTHELIOMA

The epithelioid hemangioendothelioma, an angiocentric vascular tumor, can occur at almost any age but rarely occurs during childhood.[1,2] It affects the sexes about equally. To date, no predisposing factors have been identified. The tumor develops as a solitary, slightly painful mass in either superficial or deep soft tissue, although, in rare instances, it occurs multifocally in a localized region of the body (Fig. 22-1). At least half of cases are closely associated with or arise from a vessel, usually a vein (Fig. 22-2). In some cases, occlusion of the vessel accounts for more profound symptoms, such as edema or thrombophlebitis. Those tumors that arise from vessels usually have a variegated, white-red color and superficially resemble organizing thrombi, except that they are firmly attached to the surrounding soft tissue. Those that do not arise from vessels are white-gray and offer little hint of their vascular nature on gross inspection. Calcification is occasionally seen in large deeply situated tumors (see Fig. 22-1).

Microscopic Features

Lesions that arise from vessels have a characteristic appearance when seen at low power. They expand the vessel, usually preserving its architecture as they extend centrifugally from the lumen to the soft tissue (Figs. 22-3 and 22-4). The lumen is filled with a combination of tumor, necrotic debris, and dense collagen. Unlike the epithelioid hemangioma (see Chapter 21), in which vascular differentiation proceeds through the formation of multicellular, canalized vascular channels, vascular differentiation in these tumors is more primitive and is expressed primarily at the cellular level. The tumors are composed of short strands or solid nests of rounded to slightly spindled endothelial cells (Figs. 22-5 to 22-9). Large, distinct vascular channels are rarely seen, except in the more peripheral portions of the tumor (see Fig. 22-7). Instead, the tumor cells form small intracellular lumens, which are seen as clear spaces, or vacuoles, that distort (or blister) the cell (see Figs. 22-8 and 22-9). Frequently confused with the mucin vacuoles of adenocarcinoma, these miniature lumens occasionally contain erythrocytes. The stroma varies from highly myxoid to hyaline. The myxoid areas are light blue on hematoxylin-eosin staining, and conventional histochemical treatment with aldehyde fuchsin pH 1.0 may reveal sulfated acid mucopolysaccharides. This staining pattern should not be equated with cartilaginous differentiation; it simply reflects the tendency of some vascular tumors to produce sulfated acid mucins similar to the ground substance of vessel walls. Although occasional tumors contain eosinophils and lymphocytes, this feature is rarely as pronounced as it is in the epithelioid hemangioma.

A small subset of epithelioid hemangioendotheliomas has significant atypia, mitotic activity, or both (Figs. 22-10 to 22-12). It has been the practice to designate tumors with cytologic features of malignancy as *malignant epithelioid hemangioendothelioma*. These tumors typically also fulfill the criteria of high-risk lesions, as later described. Although risk stratification is seemingly redundant for malignant epithelioid hemangioendotheliomas, the value of the proposal lies in prognosticating for the remainder.

Differential Diagnosis

The differential diagnosis of this tumor includes metastatic carcinoma (or melanoma) and various sarcomas, which can assume an epithelioid appearance. In general, *carcinomas* and *melanomas* metastatic to soft tissue display far more nuclear atypia and mitotic activity than the epithelioid

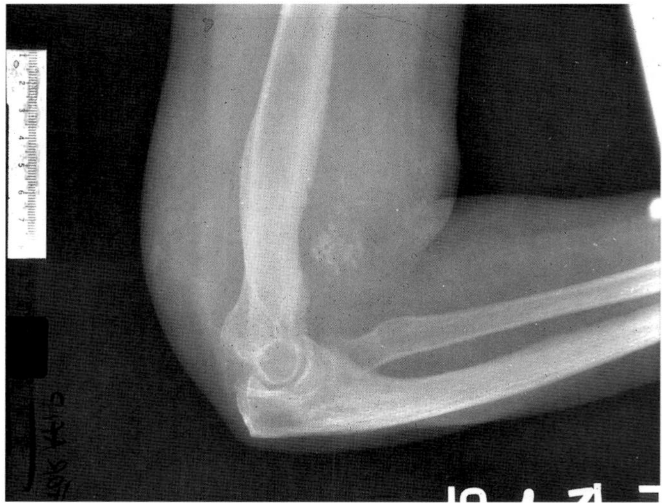

FIGURE 22-1. Plain film of arm showing an epithelioid hemangioendothelioma of the distal arm that has created erosion of bone. The mass is also partially calcified.

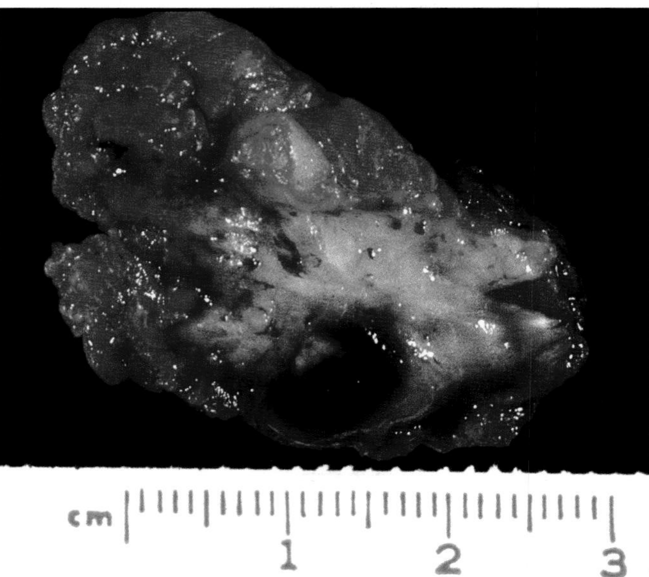

FIGURE 22-2. Gross specimen of epithelioid hemangioendothelioma. The tumor resembles an organizing thrombus in a small vein.

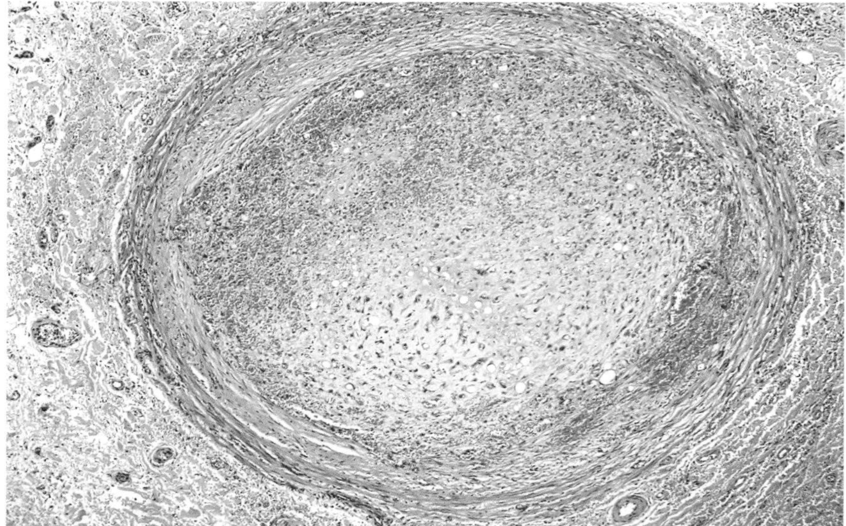

FIGURE 22-3. Epithelioid hemangioendothelioma illustrating origin from vessel.

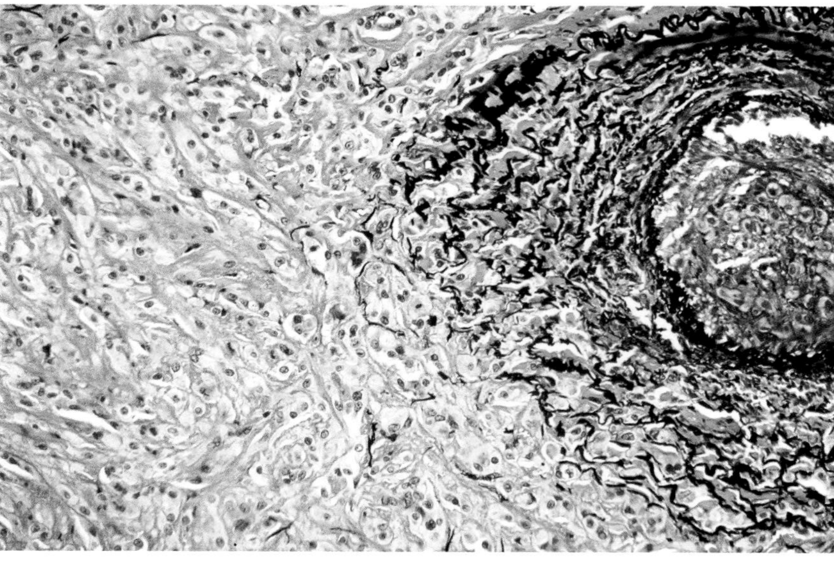

FIGURE 22-4. Epithelioid hemangioendothelioma arising in a small artery and extending centrifugally into soft tissue.

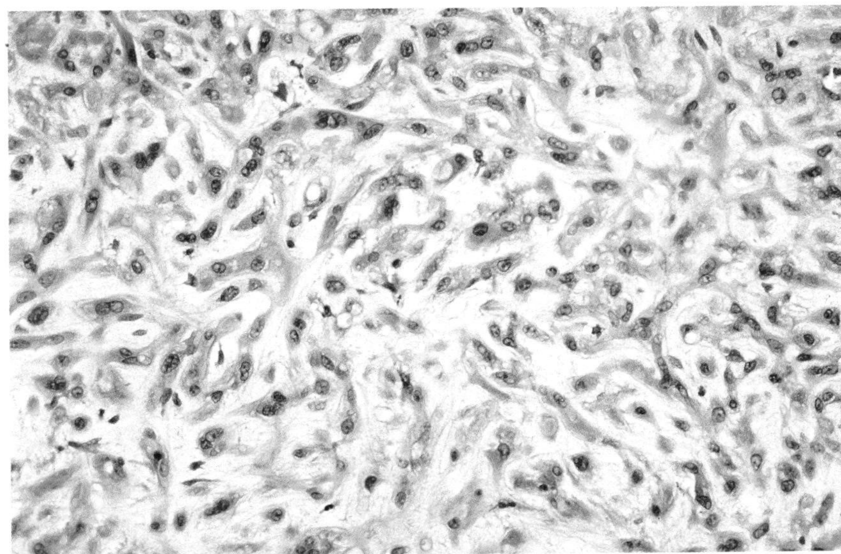

FIGURE 22-5. Epithelioid hemangioendothelioma composed of cords and chains of epithelioid endothelial cells in a myxoid background.

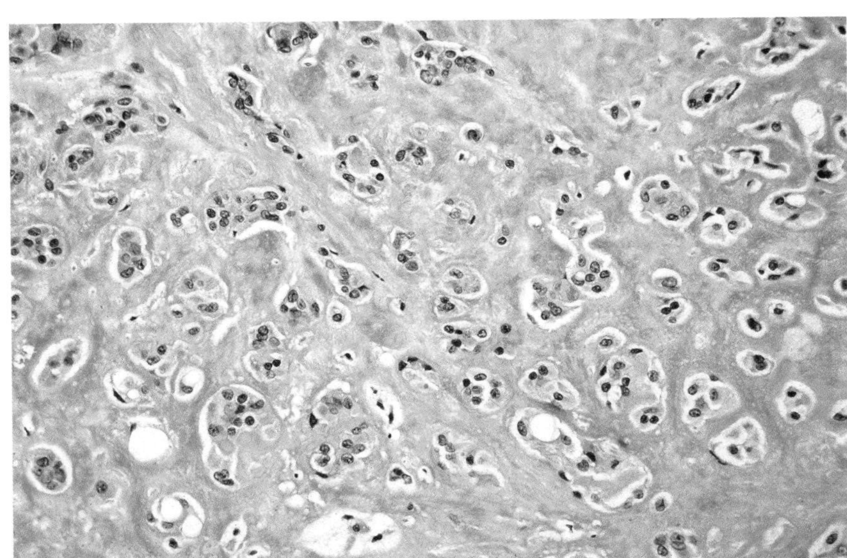

FIGURE 22-6. Epithelioid hemangioendothelioma with nests of cells in a hyalinized background.

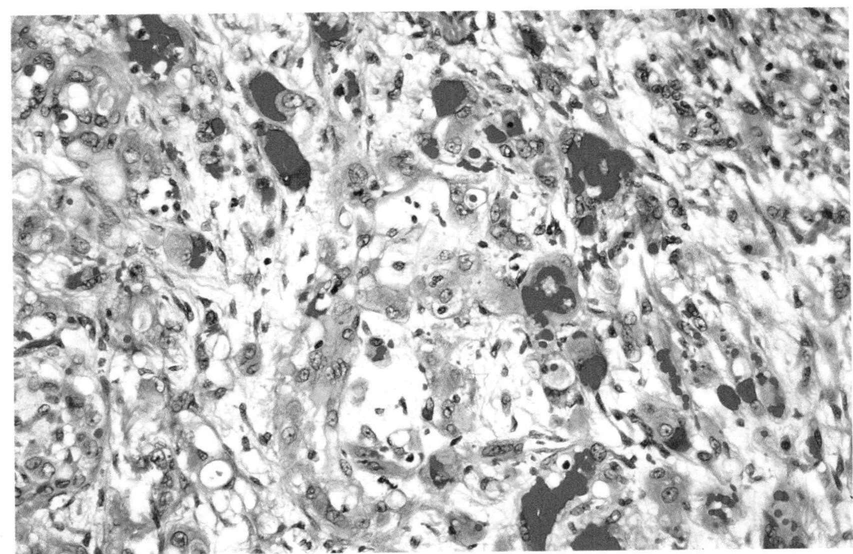

FIGURE 22-7. Peripheral areas of epithelioid hemangioendothelioma showing well-formed capillary-sized vessels.

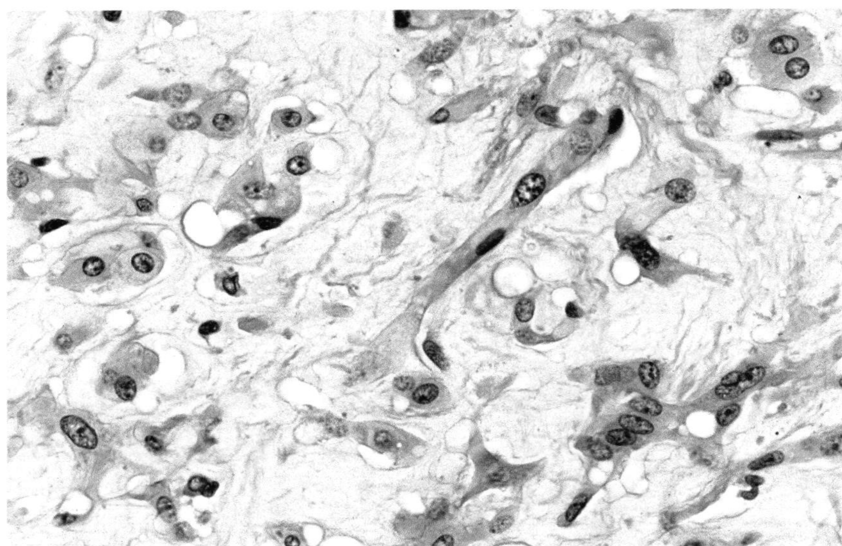

FIGURE 22-8. Cells of epithelioid hemangioendothelioma with characteristic intracytoplasmic vacuoles that blister the cell.

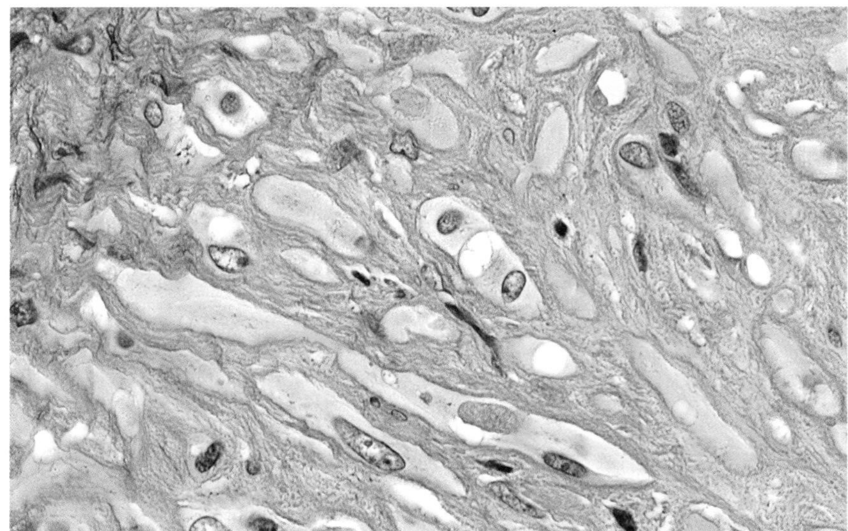

FIGURE 22-9. Epithelioid hemangioendothelioma with cytoplasmic vacuoles that blister the cell.

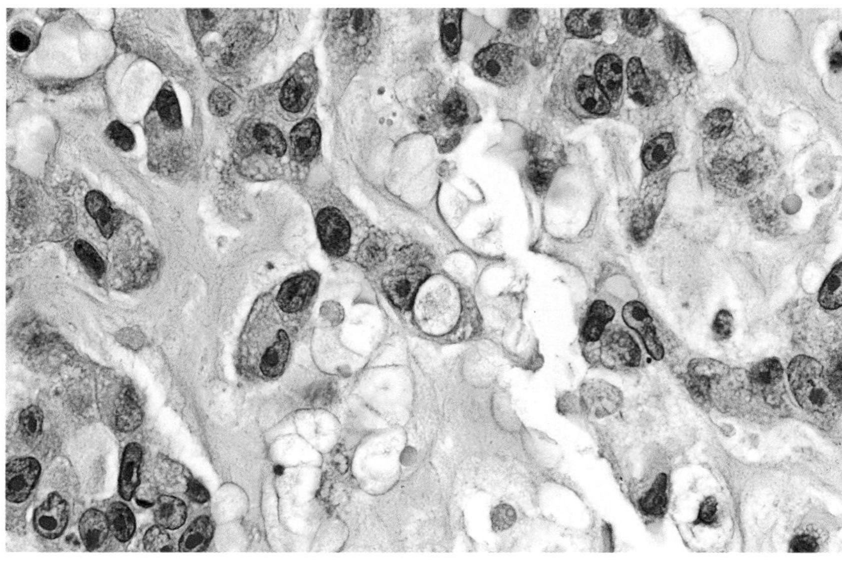

FIGURE 22-10. Malignant epithelioid hemangioendothelioma showing cells with marked atypia.

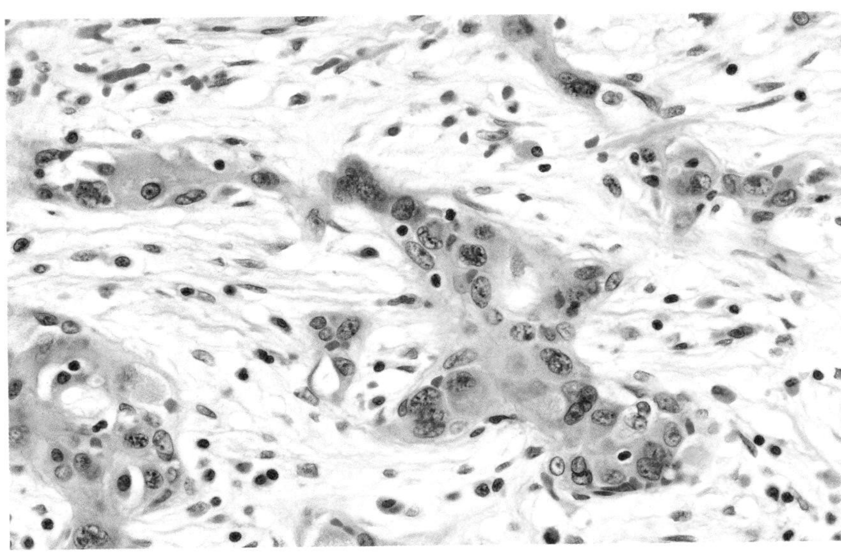

FIGURE 22-11. Malignant epithelioid hemangioendothelioma with cohesive nests of markedly atypical cells.

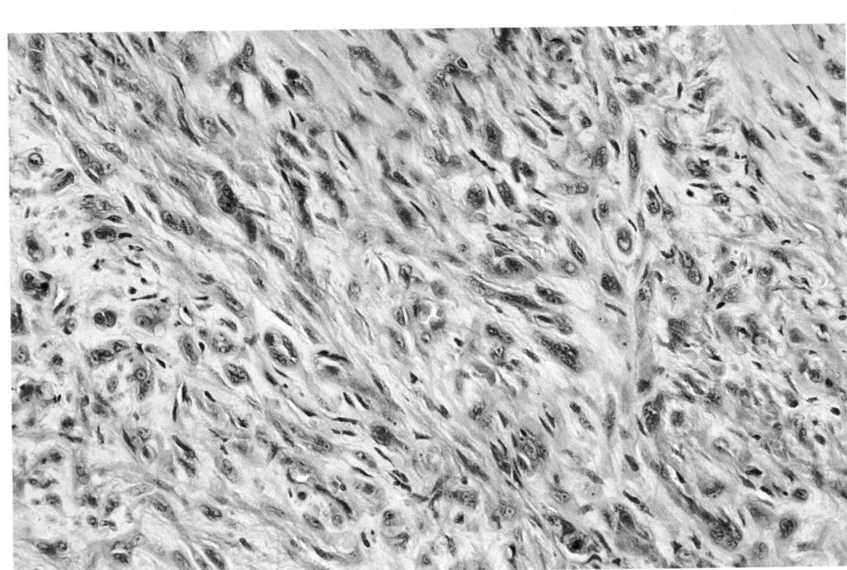

FIGURE 22-12. Marked spindling of cells in a malignant epithelioid hemangioendothelioma.

hemangioendothelioma and are rarely angiocentric. *Epithelioid angiosarcomas* are composed of solid sheets of highly atypical, mitotically active, epithelioid endothelial cells. Necrosis is common, and vascular differentiation is expressed primarily by the formation of irregular sinusoidal vascular channels.

Epithelioid sarcoma is perhaps the closest mimic of this tumor. Composed of nodules of rounded eosinophilic cells that surround cores of necrotic debris and collagen, epithelioid sarcoma develops primarily as a distal extremity lesion in young individuals. The polygonal cells usually blend and merge with the collagen in a close interplay between cell and stroma. In ambiguous cases, immunohistochemistry and electron microscopy may provide the most reliable clues for differentiation. With appropriate cocktails of monoclonal antibodies directed against a broad spectrum of cytokeratins, immunostaining is positive in virtually all carcinomas and epithelioid sarcomas. About one-fourth of epithelioid hemangioendotheliomas express cytokeratin,[3] but usually the staining is less intense and focal compared to epithelioid sarcoma. The cells of epithelioid hemangioendothelioma express CD31 and CD34 (Fig. 22-13), markers that are absent in epithelioid sarcoma and carcinoma, respectively. By electron microscopy, the cells have the characteristics of endothelium, including well-developed basal lamina, pinocytotic vesicles, and occasional Weibel-Palade bodies (Figs. 22-14 and 22-15).[1,4] They differ from normal endothelium principally by the superabundance of intermediate filaments that crowd the cytoplasm.

Behavior and Treatment

This tumor is capable of producing regional and distant metastasis but at a reduced frequency compared to soft tissue angiosarcomas. Deyrup et al.[5] reported a disease-specific survival of 81% at 5 years compared to a 1-year mortality of approximately 50% for soft tissue angiosarcomas. In this series of 49

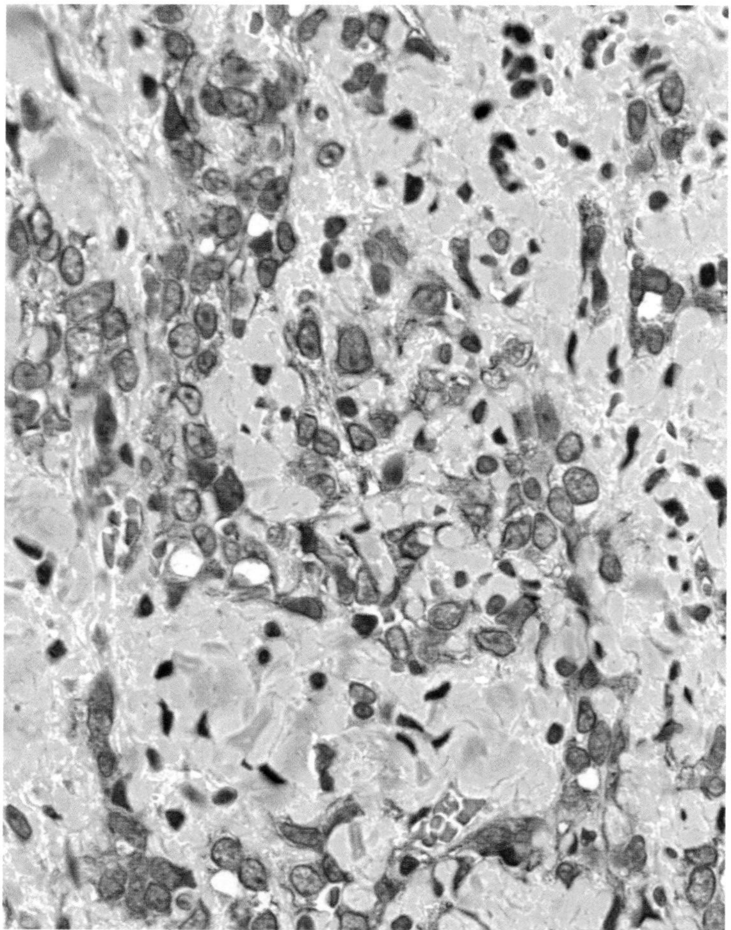

FIGURE 22-13. Membranous staining of epithelioid hemangioendothelioma for CD31.

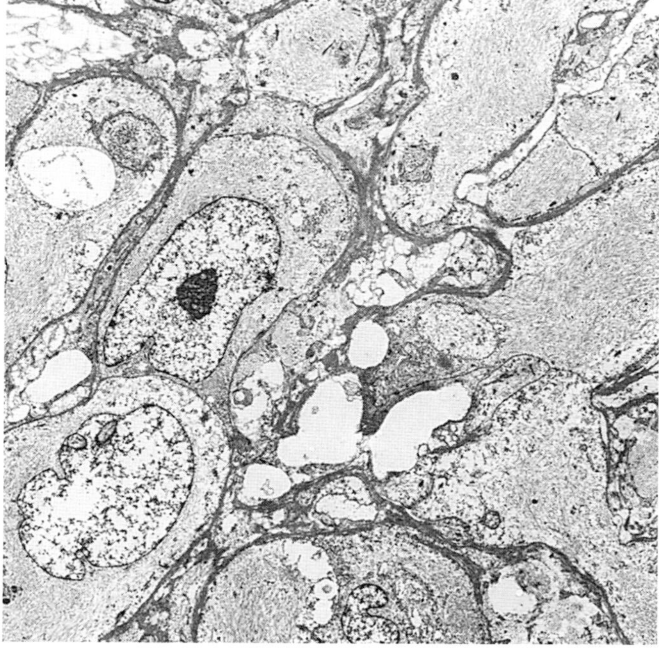

FIGURE 22-14. Electron micrograph of an epithelioid hemangioendothelioma showing complete investiture of cells with basal lamina, numerous intermediate filaments, and surface-oriented pinocytotic vesicles (X2200).

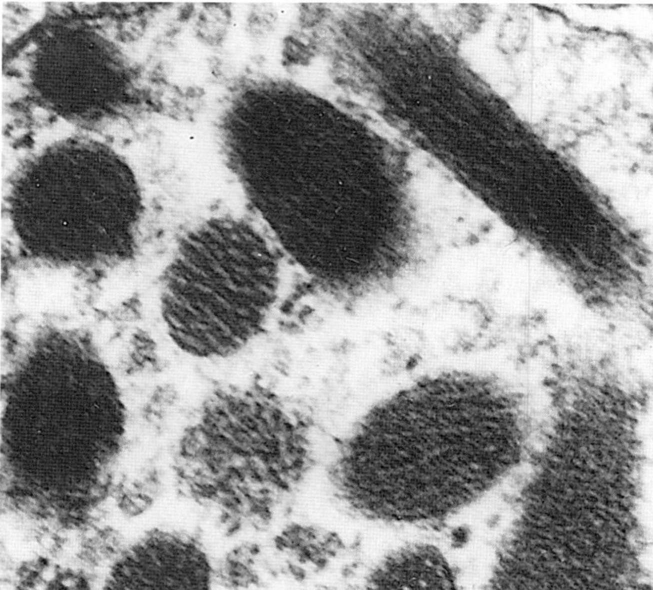

FIGURE 22-15. Weibel-Palade body in an epithelioid hemangioendothelioma. In a longitudinal section, the body has linear substructure; in a cross-section, a dot matrix pattern is seen (X75200).

patients with follow-up information (median 58 months), 31 (63%) were alive without disease, 5 (10%) were alive with disease, 9 (18%) died of disease, and 4 (8%) died of other causes. Lung and lymph nodes are the two most common metastatic sites (Table 22-1).[2] Similar data have been reported by others.[6]

Because the metastatic rate of epithelioid hemangioendotheliomas is significantly higher than that for other hemangioendotheliomas, the World Health Organization has recommended that epithelioid hemangioendotheliomas be grouped with angiosarcomas.[7] Because most epithelioid hemangioendotheliomas have innocuous histologic features and a better clinical course, there is continued value in separating them from angiosarcoma, a view reinforced by the finding of a unique disease-defining gene fusion (see later text). A risk stratification method has been proposed to identify lesions at high risk for tumor progression, with the idea that they can be targeted for more aggressive therapy.[5] Using size and mitotic activity, tumors can be divided into two groups: tumors larger than 3 cm and having greater than 3 mitoses/50 high-power fields (HPF) are high risk, and tumors lacking these features are low risk. Patients with high-risk tumors (19 cases) developed metastases in 32% of cases and had a specific survival of 59%. Low-risk patients (26 cases) developed metastases in 15% of cases, and all were alive within the follow-up period.

Armed with prior knowledge that a t(1;3)(p36.3;q25) was unique to epithelioid hemangioendothelioma, two groups have independently identified a novel gene fusion between *WWTR1* on chromosome 3 and *CAMTA1* on chromosome 1.[8,9] This is the first evidence that these genes participate in a disease process and that this fusion is specific to epithelioid hemangioendothelioma and to no other vascular lesion, in particular, epithelioid angiosarcoma. It is suggested that this fusion gene encodes a putative chimeric transcription factor capable of activating a novel transcriptional program by a yet unknown mechanism. In the normal state, *CAMTA1* is a highly conserved gene expressed almost exclusively in the brain in humans, whereas *WWTR1* is a transcriptional coactivator important in regulating organ size through cell proliferation and apoptosis.

TABLE 22-1 Behavior of Epithelioid Hemangioendotheliomas by Site

SITE	SOFT TISSUE[1,5,6]	BONE[15]	LIVER[19]
Cases with Follow up	104	26	60
Metastasis	22 (21%)	7 (27%)	16 (27%)
Mortality	13 (17%)*	8 (31%)	26 (43%)

*Based on 73 cases.

Epithelioid Hemangioendotheliomas in Other Sites

Epithelioid hemangioendotheliomas occur in sites other than soft tissue.[10-21] In epithelial organs, there is an even greater tendency to confuse them with carcinomas (Table 22-2). For example, in the lung, tumors were initially believed to be an unusual form of intravascular bronchioloalveolar carcinoma[10,11] (Fig. 22-16) and, in the liver, a sclerosing form of cholangiocarcinoma. Their vascular nature has been confirmed in numerous reports. Identical tumors have also been reported in bone.[15,16] They occur infrequently in the skin,[20,21]

TABLE 22-2 Comparison of Epithelioid Hemangioendotheliomas in Various Organs

ORGAN	AGE	GENDER	MULTIFOCAL	ANGIOCENTRICITY
Soft tissue	2nd to 9th decades	M = F	Rarely	One-half
Bone	2nd to 8th decades	M = F	>50%	
Lung	Median: 40 years	F > M	Common	Intravascular spread common
Liver	Median: 46 years	F > M	Common	Intravascular spread common

M, males; F, females.

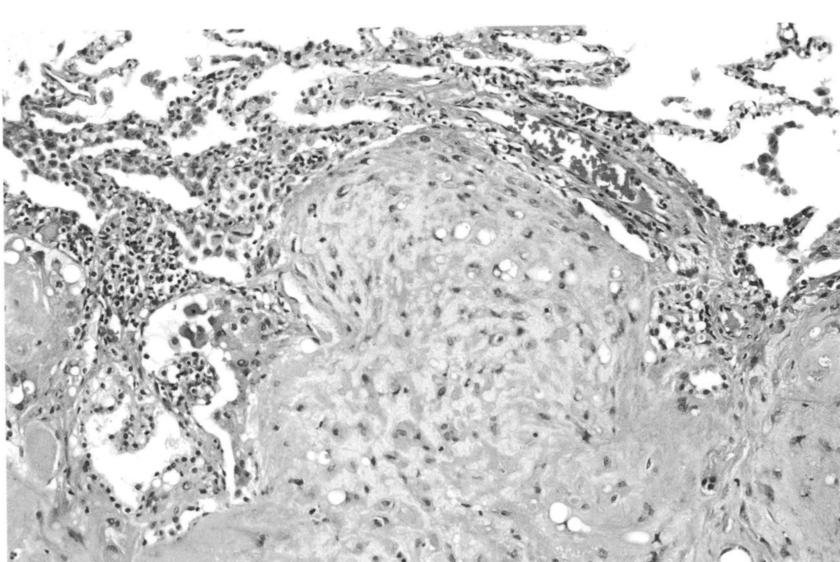

FIGURE 22-16. Epithelioid hemangioendothelioma of the lung (intravascular bronchioloalveolar tumor).

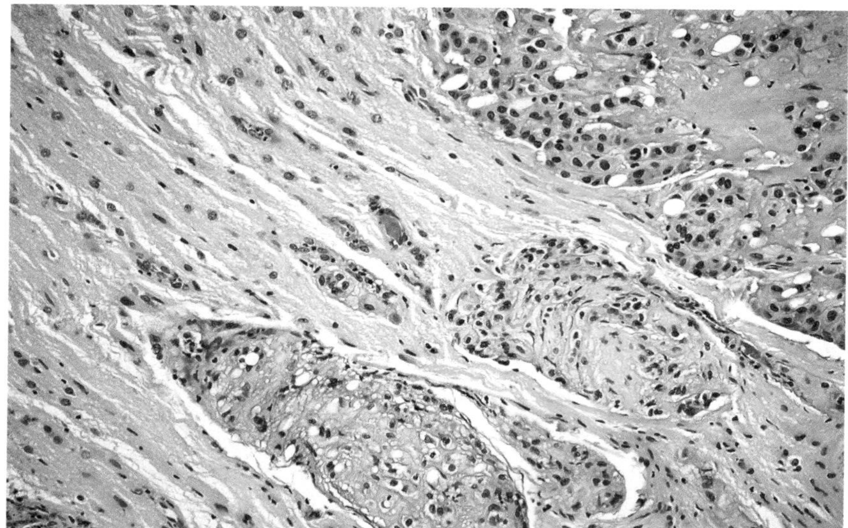

FIGURE 22-17. Epithelioid hemangioendothelioma of the meninges with brain involvement.

lymph nodes, brain and meninges[18] (Fig. 22-17), and peritoneum. Although the basic features of the tumor are similar in the various organs, the clinical presentation and disease-related signs and symptoms differ. In the liver and lung, the tumor occurs primarily in women and has a striking tendency to present in a multifocal fashion because of extensive growth along small vessels. The death rates from the disease in the lung and liver vary from 40% to 65%,[2,19] respectively, compared to a 13% death rate in soft tissues (see Table 22-1).[2] In a study by Marino et al.,[17] the projected 5-year survival rate of patients undergoing orthotopic liver transplantation was 76%, a figure that compares favorably to that for patients undergoing the procedure for nonmalignant disease.

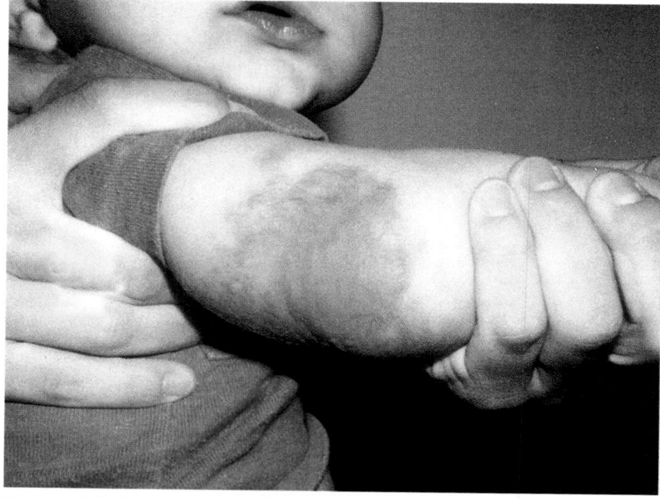

FIGURE 22-18. Kaposiform hemangioendothelioma with a violaceous plaque-like appearance on the arm of a child.

KAPOSIFORM HEMANGIOENDOTHELIOMA

The kaposiform hemangioendothelioma is a rare tumor that occurs nearly exclusively during the childhood and teenage years; one-half arise during the first year of life alone.[22,23] It has features common to both capillary hemangioma and Kaposi sarcoma and, for that reason, many terms were used in the past for these tumors, including *kaposi-like infantile hemangioendothelioma* and *hemangioma with Kaposi sarcoma-like features*. Although many were probably mistaken in the past for juvenile hemangiomas, there are compelling reasons for distinguishing between the two. The lesions occur in either superficial or deep soft tissue, although those in the latter sites, particularly the retroperitoneum, are associated with consumption coagulopathy and thrombocytopenia (Kasabach-Merritt phenomenon). Interestingly, it now appears that most cases of Kasabach-Merritt phenomenon (KMP) occur with kaposiform hemangioendotheliomas and not with hemangiomas of the usual type as was previously assumed.[24,25] A subset of cases is associated with lymphangiomatosis,[23] and one unique case supervened on congenital lymphedema.[26]

On the skin, they present as an ill-defined violaceous plaque (Fig. 22-18). In deep soft tissue, the tumor infiltrates as multiple coarse nodules that often evoke a striking desmoplasia. The tumor modulates between areas resembling a capillary hemangioma and Kaposi sarcoma (Figs. 22-19 to 22-26). The tumor is punctuated by glomeruloid structures, a signature feature of the tumor. They consist of small CD31-positive vessels invested with actin-positive pericytes and represent a specialized zone of platelet and red cell sequestration and destruction as evidenced by the presence of red blood cell fragments, hyaline droplets, finely granular hemosiderin and CD61-positive fibrin microthrombi (see Fig. 22-23C). When carefully studied, most kaposiform hemangioendotheliomas have an impressive lymphatic component consisting of thin-walled vessels surrounding the vascular tumor nodules or, in the extreme case, by a discrete lymphangioma (Fig. 22-25).

Immunohistochemically, these tumors have a profile indicating the participation of both blood-vascular and lymphatic components.[27-29] With the advent of new lymphatic markers, it has been possible to immunologically dissect the components of these tumors. Lymphatic markers (PROX1, LYVE1, and podoplanin) are highly expressed in the kaposi-like

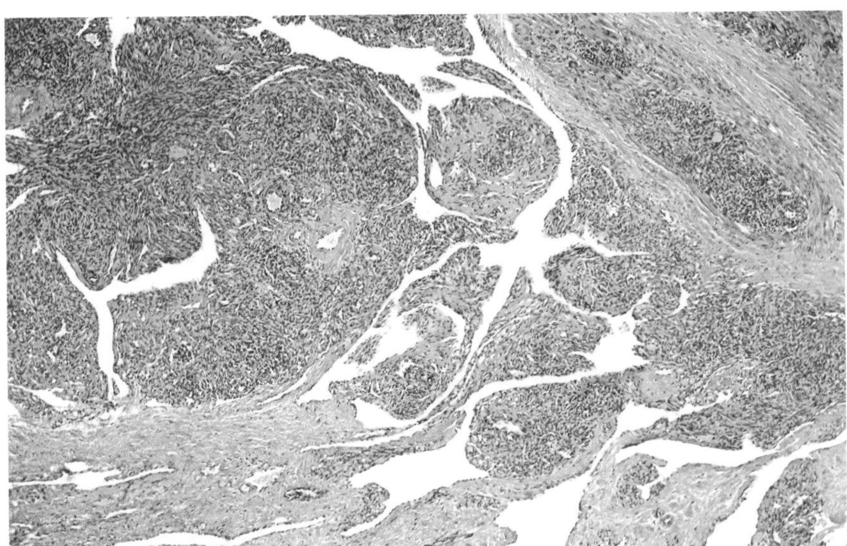

FIGURE 22-19. Kaposiform hemangioendothelioma with irregular nodules of tumor coursing through soft tissue.

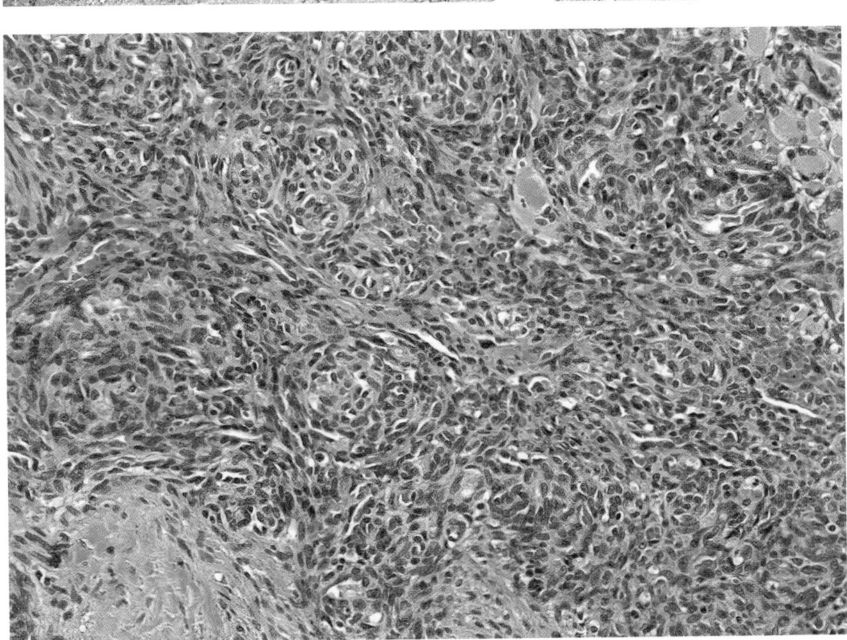

FIGURE 22-20. Kaposiform hemangioendothelioma with spindled zones merging with glomeruloid nests of rounded or epithelioid endothelial cells.

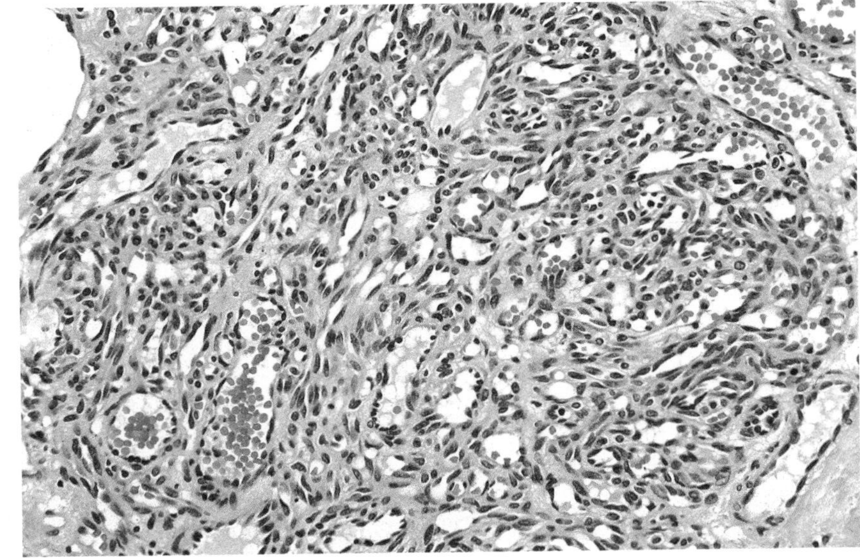

FIGURE 22-21. Capillary hemangioma-like areas in a kaposiform hemangioendothelioma.

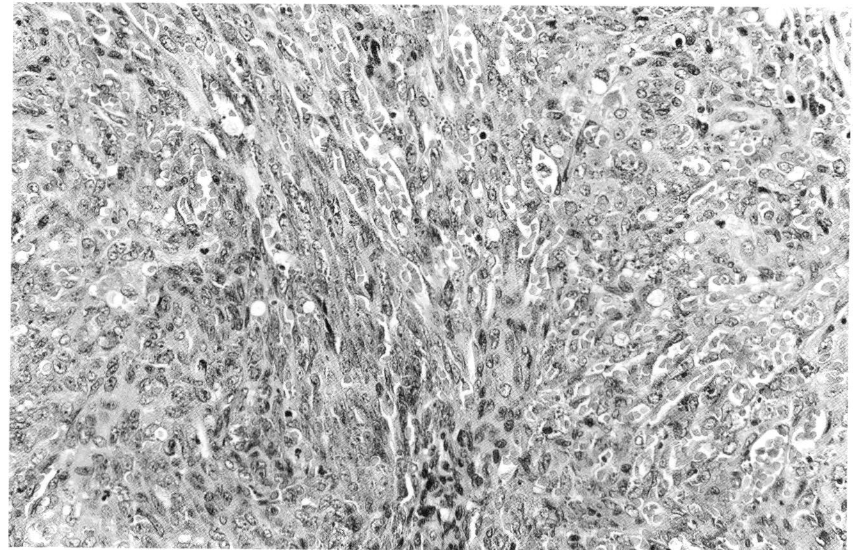

FIGURE 22-22. Kaposi-sarcoma-like areas in a kaposiform hemangioendothelioma.

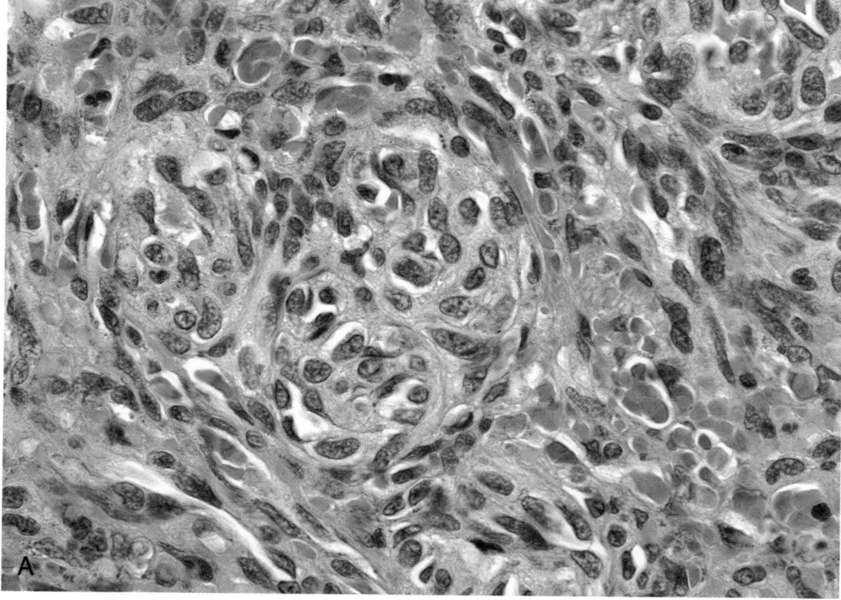

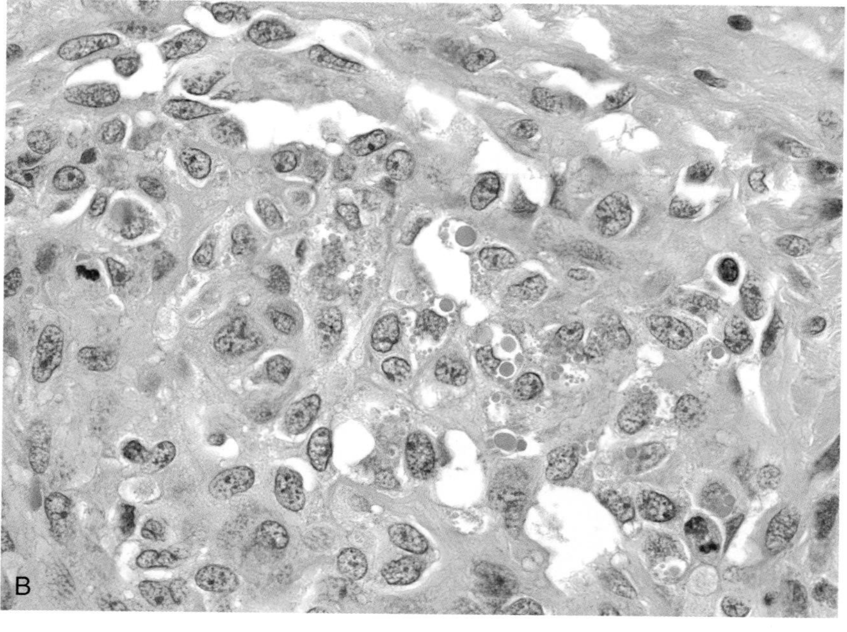

FIGURE 22-23. High-power view of glomeruloid-like areas in a kaposiform hemangioendothelioma illustrating (A) hyaline globules, (B) hemosiderin, and

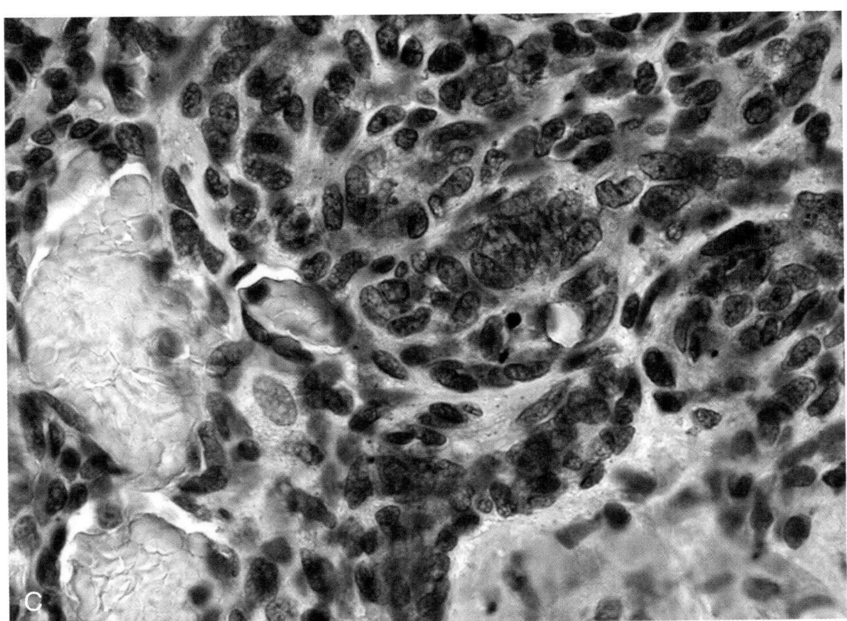

FIGURE 22-23, cont'd. (C) fibrin thrombi immunostained with CD61.

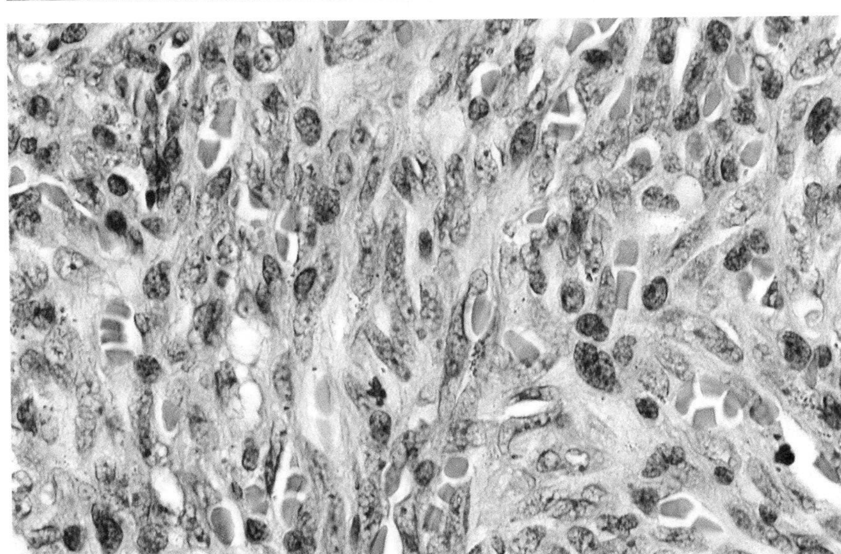

FIGURE 22-24. High-power view of Kaposi-sarcoma-like areas in a kaposiform hemangioendothelioma.

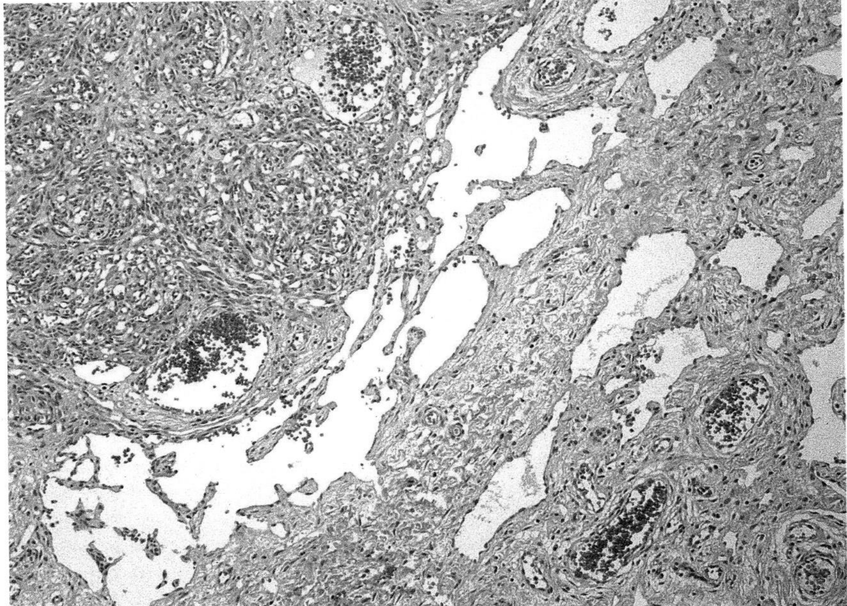

FIGURE 22-25. Kaposiform hemangioendothelioma associated with lymphangiomatosis.

areas, whereas the glomeruloid structures lack these antigens and, instead, express CD31 and CD34 only.[29] The large lymphatic-type vessels adjacent to the tumors are variably PROX1-positive. GLUT1, a member of a family of facilitative glucose transporter proteins, which is strongly expressed in infantile hemangioma, is absent in kaposiform hemangioendothelioma and provides yet another contrasting point between these two tumors.

In contrast to infantile hemangiomas, these lesions show no tendency to regress, and the eventual outcome is strongly influenced by site, clinical extent, and the development of consumption coagulopathy. A majority of patients can be cured following surgical excision of the tumor. Medical intervention is required when surgery is not possible or when KMP is present. Treatment of KMP has proven to be the most challenging issue in the disease and may require a multimodality approach using steroids, cytotoxic agents, interferon, and other agents.[30-33] Unfortunately, there is evidence that kaposiform hemangioendothelioma may be less responsive to interferon than the common infantile hemangioma. Death occurs in about 10% of patients either from the local effects of disease or from complications of KMP. Regional lymph node metastases are rare (Fig. 22-27) and, to date, no distant metastases have been reported. However, because fewer than 100 cases have been reported, it is not inconceivable that the potential for distant metastasis exists but at a very low, and as yet undetectable, rate.

It is still not clear as to the reason that this tumor, above all others, should be so closely associated with KMP. It does not appear to be strictly related to size because far larger vascular tumors, and even metastatic angiosarcomas, are rarely associated with KMP. More likely, it is related to unique attributes of vascular architecture or endothelium. Interestingly, the introduction of PROX1 into a mouse model of kaposiform hemangioendothelioma confers upon the tumor a more aggressive course.[34]

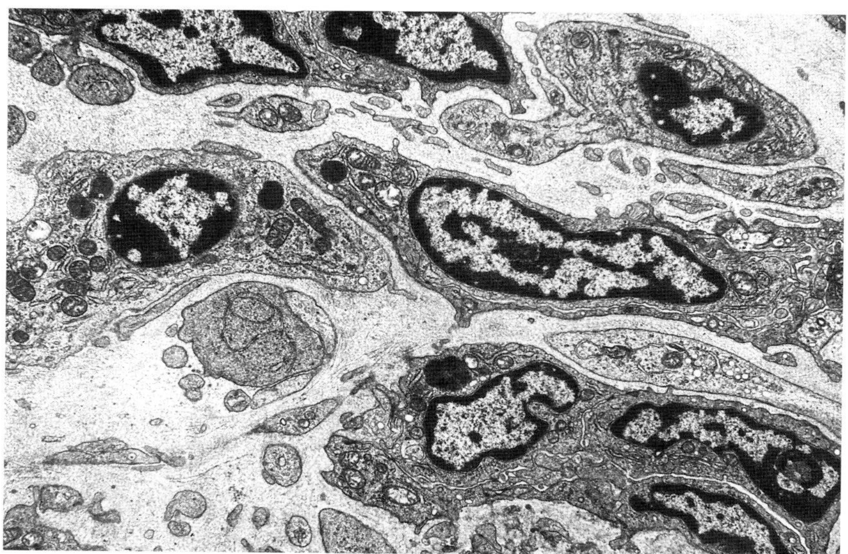

FIGURE 22-26. Electron micrograph of a kaposiform hemangioendothelioma illustrating primitive endothelial cells.

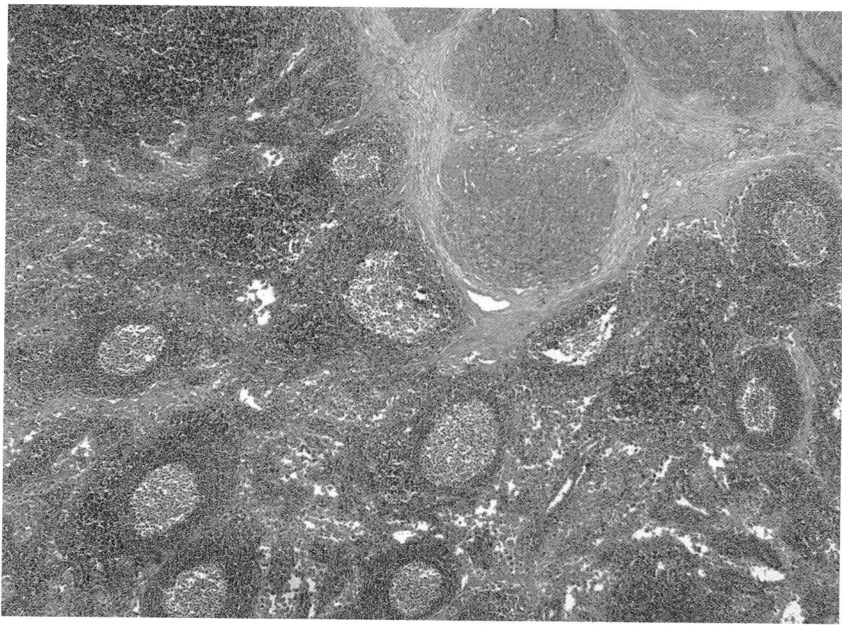

FIGURE 22-27. Kaposiform hemangioendothelioma metastatic to lymph node.

The two most important differential considerations in this disease are infantile hemangioma and Kaposi sarcoma. Infantile hemangiomas are composed of distinct nodules of small capillary-sized vessels. Although canalization can be imperfect during the early phase of growth, infantile hemangiomas do not display spindling of the cells, and they do not contain the signature glomeruloid structures of kaposiform hemangioendothelioma. Kaposi sarcoma is an exceptionally rare tumor during childhood, with the exception of lymphadenopathic forms described in Africa. It is characterized by uniform spindling of the cells and often a peripheral inflammatory infiltrate. Although portions of kaposiform hemangioendothelioma may be indistinguishable from Kaposi sarcoma, the former shows much greater variation from area to area. Kaposi sarcoma-associated herpesvirus (HHV8) has not been associated with kaposiform hemangioendothelioma, and, therefore, staining for this antigen can readily distinguish between the tumors. Acquired tufted hemangioma, a skin lesion reported initially in adults, bears an unmistakable histologic and immunohistochemical similarity to kaposiform hemangioendothelioma. The lesions are identical, differing in the manner of presentation only (see Chapter 21).

HOBNAIL (DABSKA-RETIFORM) HEMANGIOENDOTHELIOMA

Hobnail hemangioendothelioma is a term used for two closely related tumors, the retiform hemangioendothelioma and Dabska-type hemangioendothelioma, both of which are characterized by a hobnail or cuboidal endothelial cell (Fig. 22-28). This cell is characterized by a high nuclear/cytoplasmic ratio and an apically placed, occasionally grooved nucleus that produces a surface bulge, accounting for the term *hobnail* or *matchstick*. Hobnail endothelial cells vary in size and shape, from small lymphocytoid cells to larger cuboidal cells and, in the extreme case, tall columnar cells that appear to be of lymphatic lineage.[27,35] The two tumors have similar biologic behavior but display minor clinical and pathologic differences (Table 22-3). For purposes of clarity, the classic features of each are presented, but tumors with overlapping features occur, and patients falling outside of the normal age range for each tumor may be encountered.

Dabska-type hemangioendotheliomas were first described in 1969 in a small series of six patients.[36,37] All occurred in the skin or subcutis of infants and young children and were characterized by a distinctive small cuboidal or hobnail endothelial cell lining vascular spaces and forming intravascular glomeruloid papillations. Termed *endovascular papillary angioendothelioma* and more recently *papillary endolymphatic angioendothelioma*, these rare tumors have never lent themselves to extensive studies. It has even been intimated that these lesions might not represent a distinct entity. More recently, another low-grade angiosarcoma, also characterized by hobnail endothelial cells but occurring in adults and forming long retiform vessels largely without intravascular papillations, has been described as *retiform hemangioendothelioma*.[38]

Clinical Features

Hobnail hemangioendotheliomas may be seen in a broad age range, although lesions with classic features of the Dabska tumor typically occur in children, whereas retiform ones more commonly occur in adults (mean: fourth decade) (see Table 22-3). Both, however, develop as ill-defined or plaque-like

TABLE 22-3 Comparison of Dabska and Retiform Hemangioendotheliomas

PARAMETER	DABSKA	RETIFORM
Age	Children (25% adult)	Adults (15% child)
Location	Distal extremities (50%)	Distal extremities (50%)
Local recurrence	≈40%	≈60%
Lymph node metastasis	<10%	<10%
Distant metastasis	One case	None
Associations	Vascular/lymphatic malformation of tumor	Lymphedema, radiation

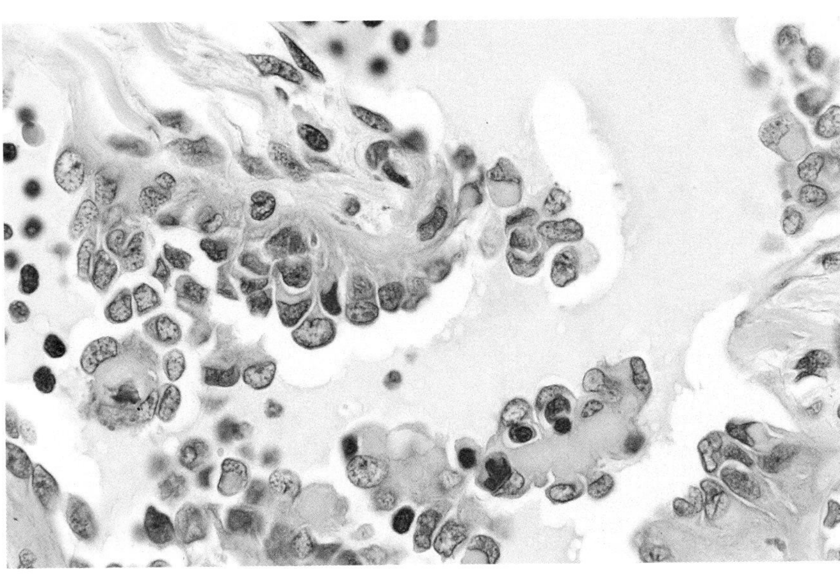

FIGURE 22-28. Hobnail, or matchstick, endothelium, which characterizes the retiform and Dabska forms of hemangioendothelioma.

lesions of the skin and subcutaneous tissue sometimes associated with overlying violaceous discoloration. About one-half of cases occur in the distal portion of the extremity, but other sites may be affected. Rare cases of the Dabska type have been recorded in the spleen and in deep locations.[39,40]

Microscopic Features

The Dabska-type hemangioendothelioma is characterized by well-formed vessels lined by cuboidal endothelium and featuring intraluminal growth of papillary endothelial structures (Figs. 22-29 to 22-33; Table 22-4). The vessels are often flanked by dense hyaline zones containing lymphocytes (see Figs. 22-30 and 22-33). The papillations are lined by a hobnail endothelial cell with central hyaline cores (see Fig. 22-31) composed of accumulated basement membrane material presumably synthesized by the tumor cells.[41] These structures have been compared to renal glomeruli. Intracytoplasmic vacuolation of the endothelium may be observed, a phenomenon seen in epithelioid vascular tumors. In some cases, there is a close intermingling of endothelial cells with the intravascular lymphocytes, an observation that has led some to suggest that the tumor cells express some of the properties of the high endothelial cell of the postcapillary venule.[42] Although the intravascular papillations are admittedly the most spectacular part of the tumor, there is usually an underlying lesion, which may range from a lymphangioma to a more complex tumor with areas of hemangioma and lymphangioma (see Fig. 22-29). Two cases in the literature have documented Dabska tumors arising in preexisting benign vascular tumors/malformations.[39,43]

The typical retiform hemangioendothelioma, on the other hand, consists of numerous elongated vessels, resembling the shape of the rete testis, that replace the dermis and extend into the subcutis (see Table 22-4). These vessels are lined by a single layer of hobnail endothelial cells (Figs. 22-34 and 22-35). In the vicinity of the epidermal junction, the vessels may become ectatic so that the retiform pattern is lost. The vessels, often surrounded by hyaline sclerosis and lymphocytes, intercommunicate with one another; however, dissection of the collagen planes by small groups of endothelial cells, as is seen

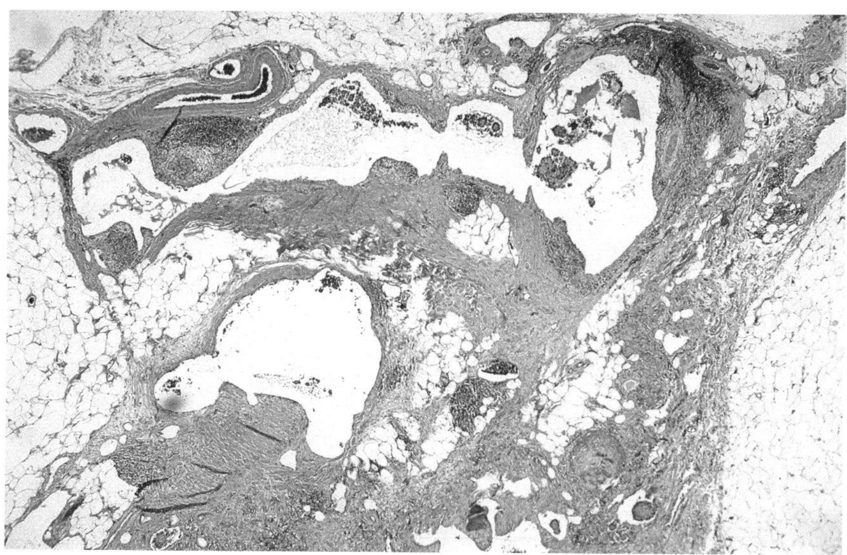

FIGURE 22-29. Dabska-type hobnail hemangioendothelioma with a lymphangiomatous background with intraluminal papillary growth.

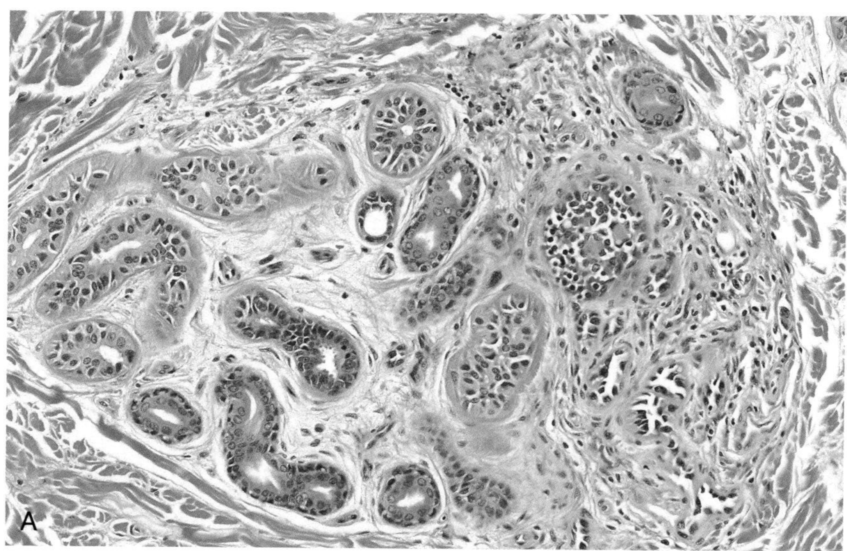

FIGURE 22-30. Dabska-type hemangioendothelioma with vessels lined by cuboidal-columnar endothelium (A)

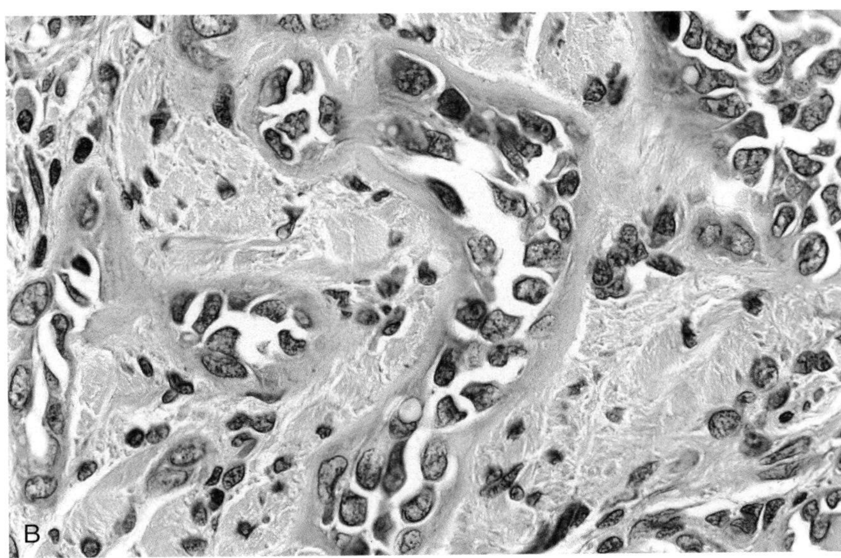

FIGURE 22-30, cont'd. and surrounded by hyaline material (B).

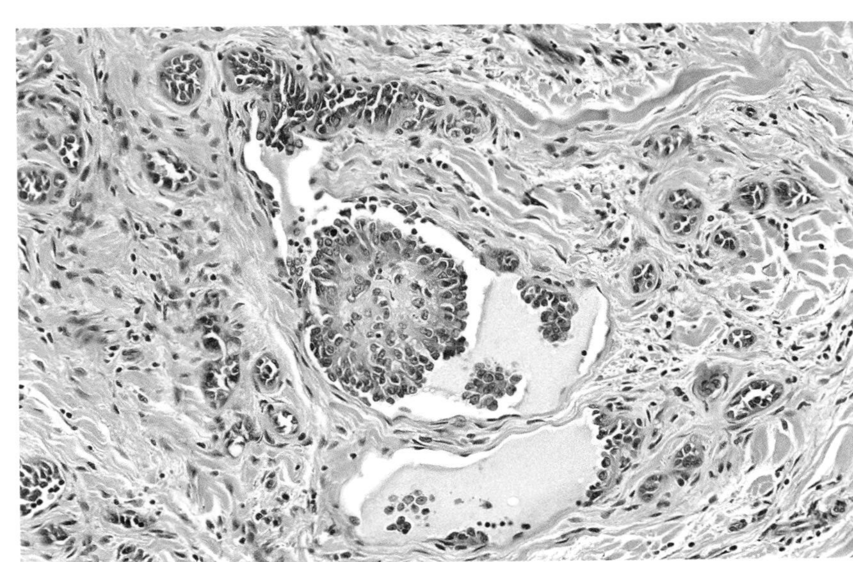

FIGURE 22-31. Intravascular papillations in a Dabska-type hemangioendothelioma.

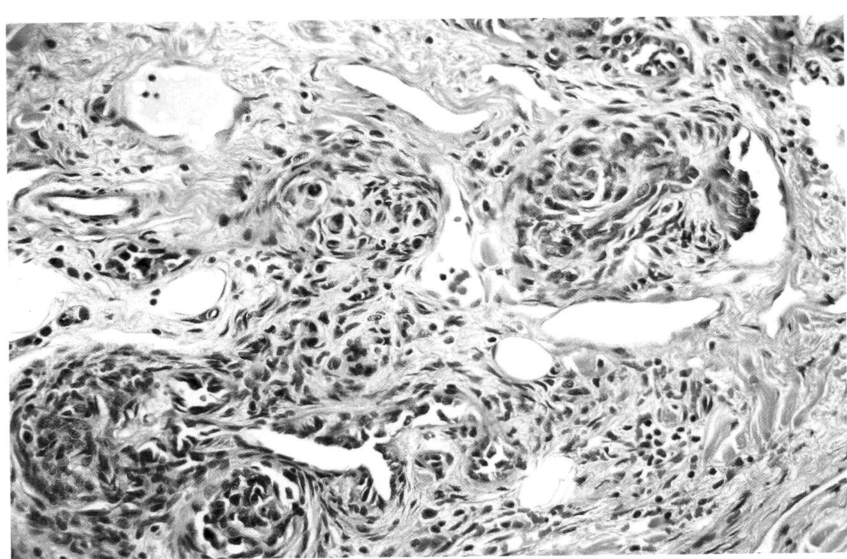

FIGURE 22-32. Solid areas of intravascular growth in a Dabska-type hemangioendothelioma.

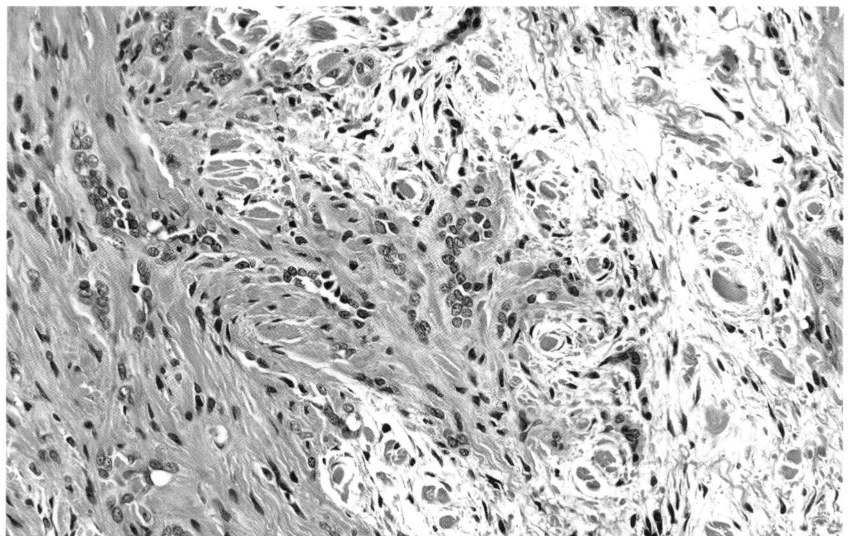

FIGURE 22-33. Dense hyaline sclerosis around vessels in a Dabska-type hemangioendothelioma.

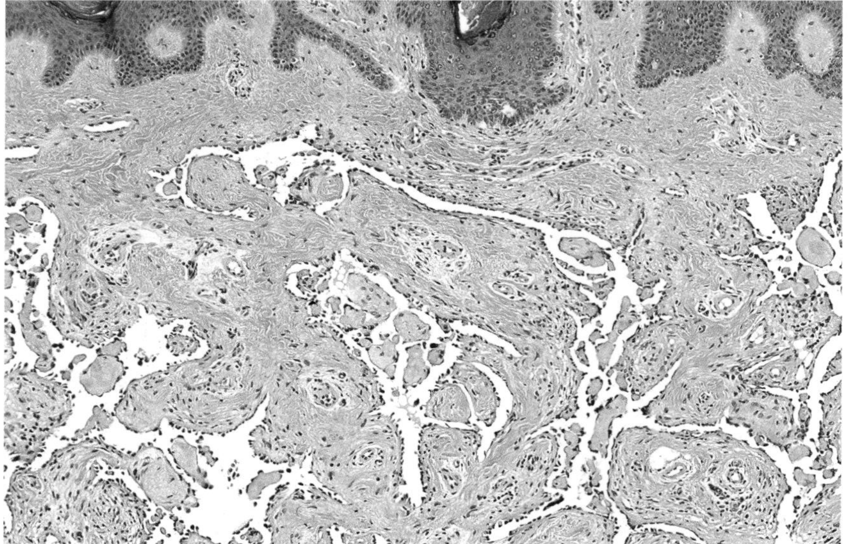

FIGURE 22-34. Retiform hemangioendothelioma involving the dermis.

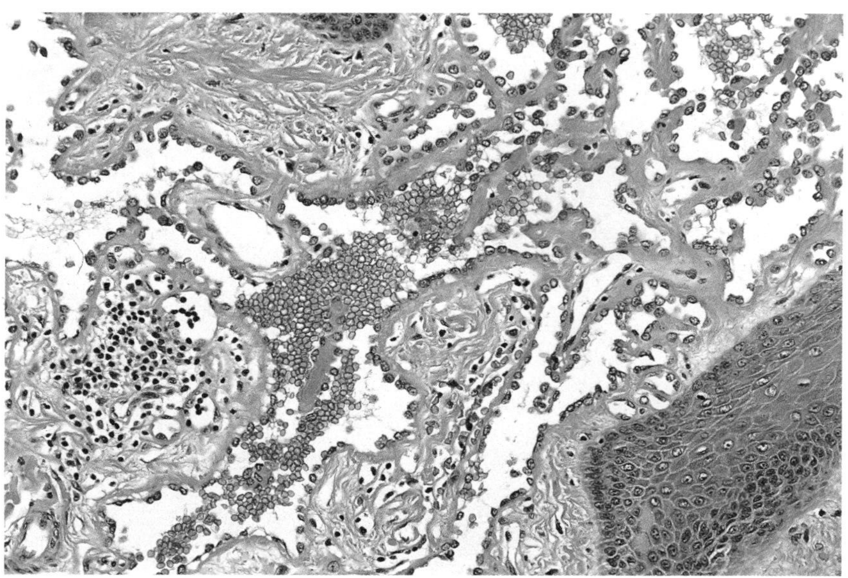

FIGURE 22-35. Retiform hemangioendothelioma with elongated vessels lined by cuboidal endothelium.

in a conventional angiosarcoma, does not occur. Intraluminal papillary tufts of endothelial cells similar to the Dabska-type hemangioendothelioma can be identified but are usually infrequent (Fig. 22-36).

Although the foregoing descriptions seemingly depict two different lesions, one occasionally encounters hybrid tumors that defy precise classification. These tumors may be made up of vessels lined by hobnail endothelium but not arranged in a retiform pattern and with only rare intraluminal papillations and no underlying vascular malformation. The tumors underscore the need to create a designation that embraces all of the lesions under discussion.

TABLE 22-4 Histiologic Comparison of Dabska and Retiform Hemangioendotheliomas

FEATURE	DABSKA	RETIFORM
Hobnail endothelium	+++	+++
Lymphocytes	+++	+++
Perivascular hyalinization	+++	+++
Intravascular papillary tufts	+++	+
Retiform vessels	—	+++
Lymphangioma areas	++	—

Immunohistochemical Findings

The immunohistochemistry of the Dabska and retiform lesions is remarkably similar. The neoplastic endothelial cells usually express von Willebrand factor, CD31, and CD34, although staining of the first two is usually significantly less intense than that of the last. In addition, these lesions strongly express lymphatic markers (Fig. 22-37).[27,35] For this reason, Fanburg-Smith et al.[35] suggested that the Dabska-type hemangioendothelioma be termed *papillary intralymphatic angioendothelioma*. The lymphocytic infiltrate usually shows a mixture of B ($CD20^+$) and T ($CD3^+$) cells, although the intraluminal ones are predominantly T cells.[38]

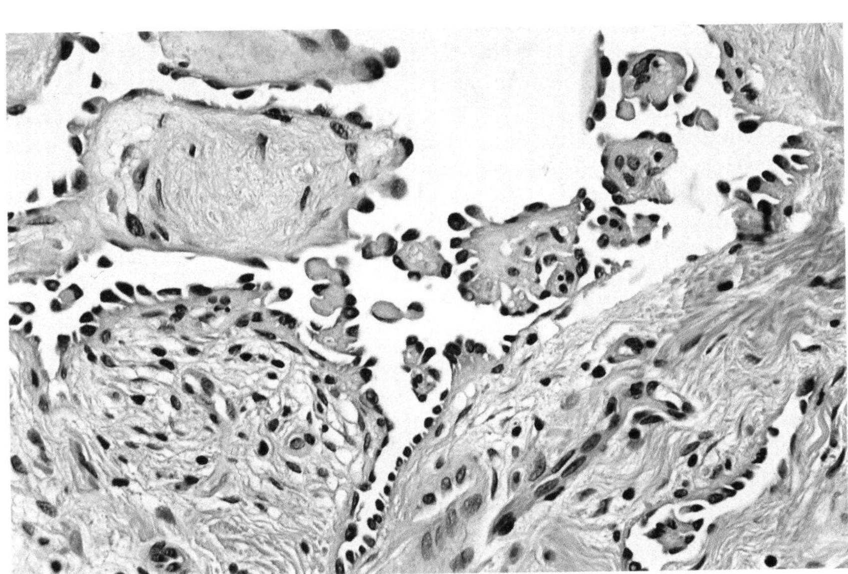

FIGURE 22-36. Retiform hemangioendothelioma with small intravascular papillations similar to a Dabska-type hemangioendothelioma.

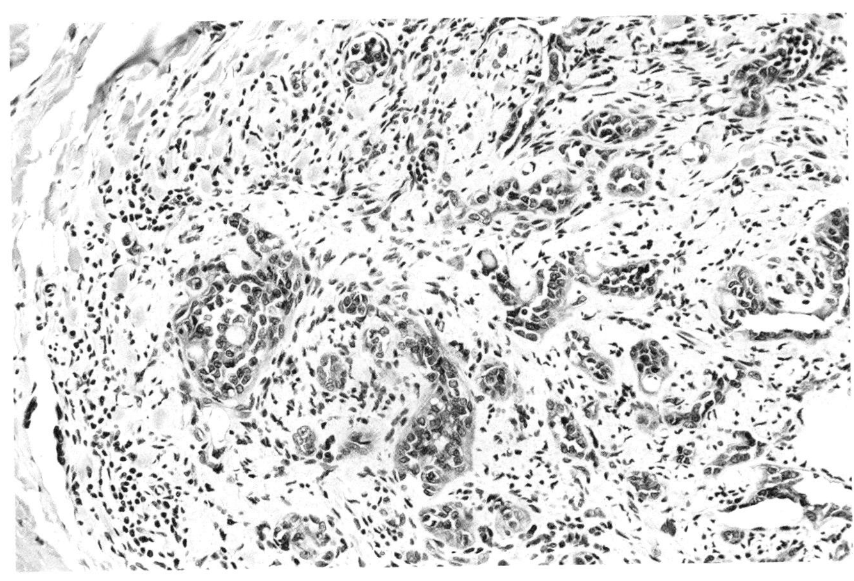

FIGURE 22-37. VEGFR-3 immunostaining in a Dabska-type hemangioendothelioma suggesting lymphatic differentiation.

Discussion

Hobnail hemangioendotheliomas, regardless of whether they are of the Dabska or retiform type, appear to be low-grade lesions with a capacity to extend to regional lymph nodes. Of the six patients reported by Dabska, two developed regional lymph node metastasis, and one eventually died of metastasis (as cited by Argani and Athanasian[39]). In the experience of Calonje et al.,[38] nearly 60% of patients developed local recurrence, and 1 of 14 patients developed a lymph node metastasis. In another study with 10 cases, including both Dabska and retiform types, 4 developed local recurrences, and 1 patient, with a tumor of an exclusively retiform pattern, developed a regional lymph node metastasis. In the series of Dabska-type hemangioendotheliomas reported by Fanburg-Smith et al.,[35] none of eight patients developed recurrence or metastasis during a median follow-up of 9 years.

It should be emphasized that these data are based on tumors that fulfill a strict definition. Specifically, hobnail hemangioendotheliomas are composed of (hobnail) endothelium of low nuclear grade with an overall architectural pattern, as described previously. Intravascular tufts of atypical endothelium occur in angiosarcomas, but these lesions do not qualify as Dabska-type hemangioendotheliomas. There are also rare angiosarcomas characterized by high-grade hobnail cells growing in solid sheets or as permeative vessels. These, too, should be designated angiosarcomas, rather than hobnail hemangioendotheliomas.

EPITHELIOID SARCOMA-LIKE HEMANGIOENDOTHELIOMA

The epithelioid sarcoma-like hemangioendothelioma is a rare vascular tumor described by Billings et al.[44] in 2003 and named for its resemblance to epithelioid sarcoma, the most common referring diagnosis. More recently, a large series of cases was reported under the rubric of *pseudomyogenic hemangioendothelioma.*[45] The lesions typically present as superficial or deep nodules of the extremities similar to epithelioid sarcoma. Over half of patients present with multiple nodules, and males are affected more often than females (Figs. 22-38 to 22-41). Measuring up to a few centimeters in diameter, these tumors consist of nodules of glassy, eosinophilic epithelioid cells that show frequent transitions to spindled and multipolar cells with little cellular cohesion. The atypia within the lesions varies from mild to moderate, but mitotic activity is usually low (less than 5/50 HPF). The diagnosis of a vascular tumor is seldom suspected because these lesions do not recreate multicellular vascular channels or manifest the cytoplasmic vacuolization typical of epithelioid vascular tumors, in general (see section on epithelioid hemangioendothelioma). Expression of vascular markers is variable. FLI-1 is consistently expressed; CD31 is expressed in 50% to 100%, depending on the study; and CD34 is absent. Cytokeratin and INI1 are consistently expressed; In addition, a balanced t(7;19)(q22;q13) has been identified as the sole abnormality in one case of epithelioid sarcoma-like hemangioendothelioma and an unbalanced der(7)t(7;19) in another.[46] Collectively, these findings reinforce the view that this lesion is distinct from both epithelioid sarcoma and epithelioid hemangioendothelioma. Additional contrasting features are given in Table 22-5.

The disease course is marked by the development of multiple tumor nodules in the same location, which could arguably be considered local recurrence or regional metastasis. Based on the combined reported experience with 38 patients,[44,45] 1 has developed regional lymph node metastasis and another developed distant metastasis 16 years after primary excision.

COMPOSITE HEMANGIOENDOTHELIOMA

The composite hemangioendothelioma is a locally aggressive but rarely metastasizing tumor composed of a mixture of benign, intermediate, and malignant vascular components.[47]

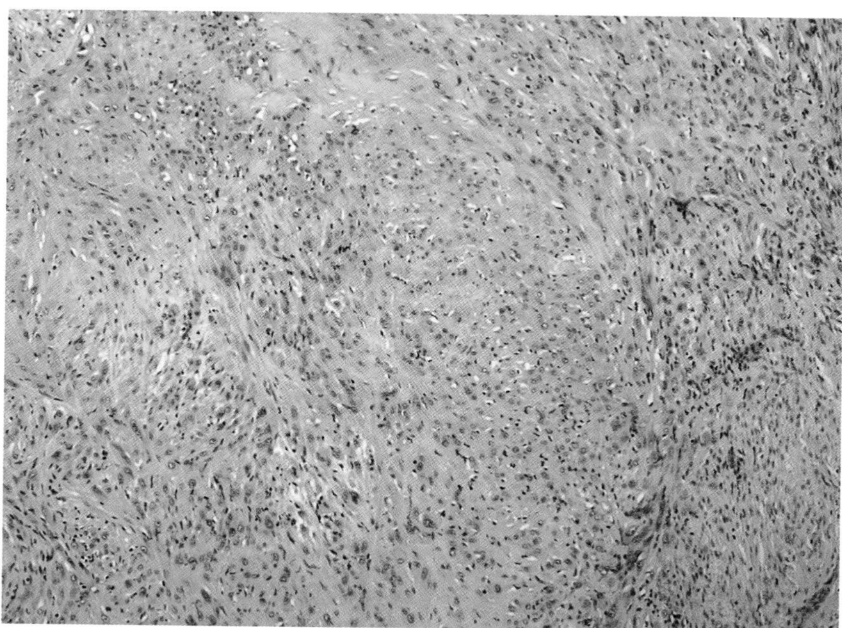

FIGURE 22-38. Low-power view of epithelioid sarcoma-like hemangioendothelioma.

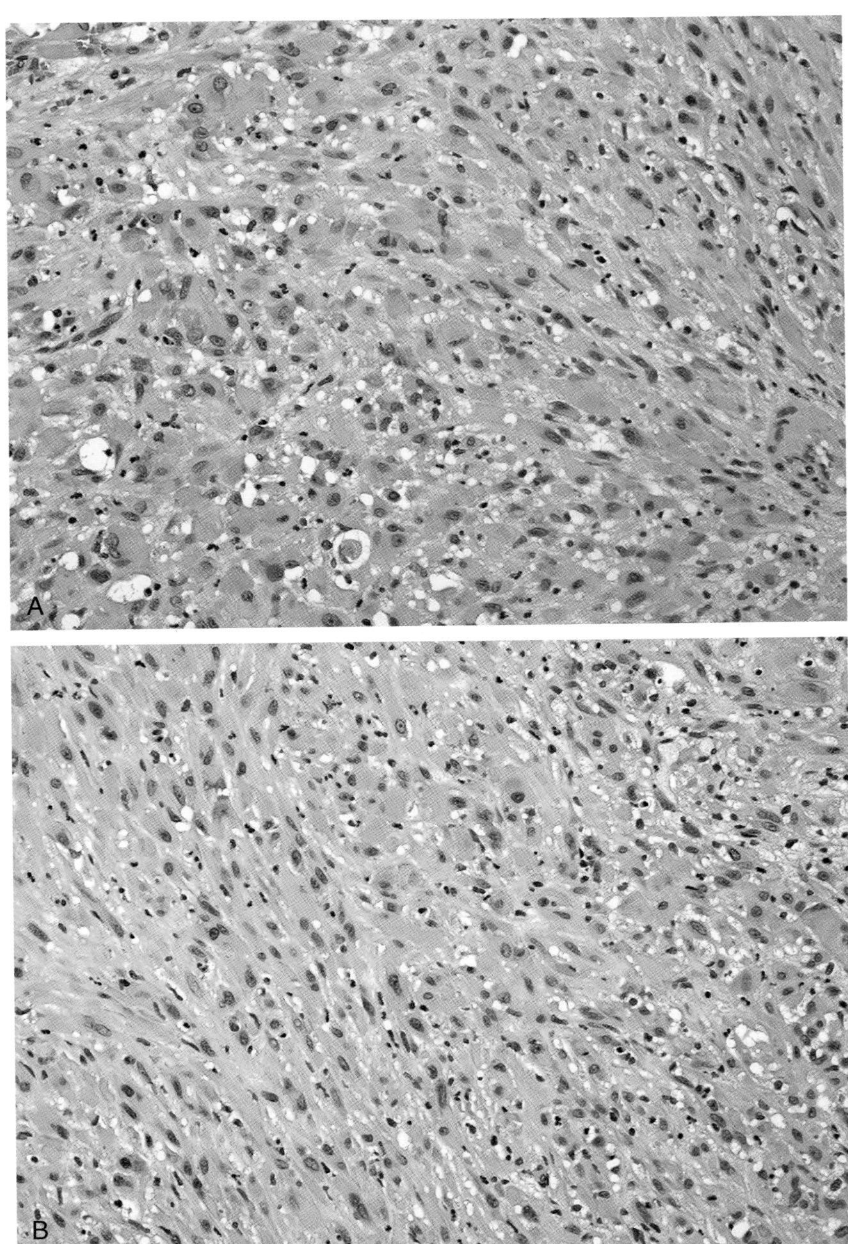

FIGURE 22-39. Epithelioid endothelial cells within an epithelioid sarcoma-like hemangioendothelioma (A). Transition between epithelioid and spindled endothelial cells within an epithelioid sarcoma-like hemangioendothelioma (B).

Because of the variation in the type and amount of these various components, no two tumors look exactly alike. This has led to an ongoing debate as to whether composite hemangioendothelioma should be considered a distinct entity. The problem is compounded by published reports either poorly illustrating or inaccurately diagnosing the various lesional components,[48,49] leaving few legitimate cases for analyses. True *composite* tumors are exceptionally rare and, therefore, this term is used rarely. The wisdom of labeling a lesion *composite hemangioendothelioma* is also questioned when areas of unequivocal angiosarcoma are present, as has been suggested.

Of the fewer than 20 cases of composite hemangioendothelioma, most occur as long-standing masses of the superficial tissues of the extremity of adults. Some are congenital. The majority are associated with an underlying vascular lesion such as lymphedema, angiomatosis, arteriovenous malformation, cavernous hemangioma, and, in one case, Maffucci syndrome.[50] Tumors vary one from another histologically, but the most consistent combination of elements is epithelioid hemangioendothelioma and hobnail (retiform) hemangioendothelioma.[50] Although angiosarcoma has been reported as a component of some cases, illustrations suggest that these may represent areas of hobnail hemangioendothelioma growing in a more racemose vascular pattern.

The behavior of these lesions is incompletely defined. Based on the comprehensive analysis by Fukunaga et al.,[50] about one-half of cases recur undoubtedly because of their propensity for infiltrative growth, but only rare cases have metastasized to lymph node and soft tissue.

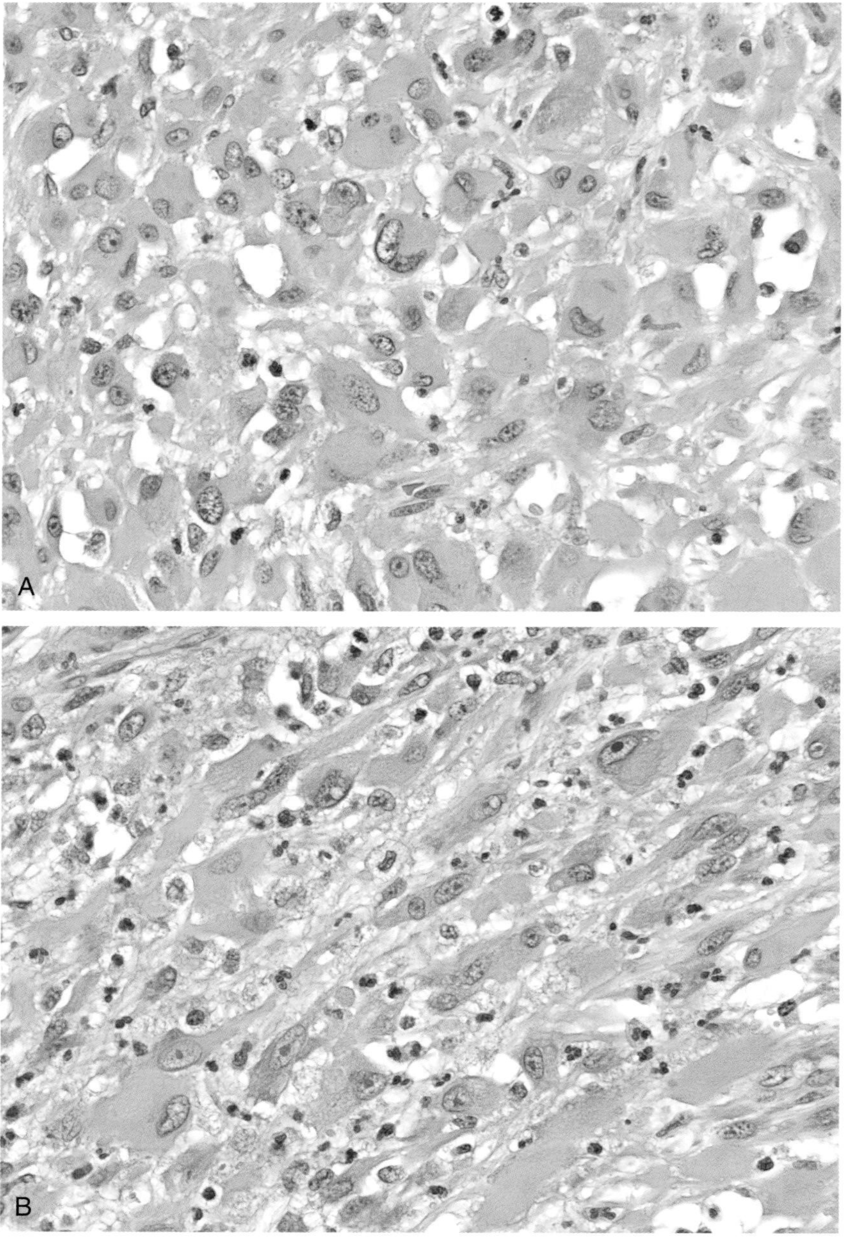

FIGURE 22-40. High-power view of epithelioid sarcoma-like hemangioendothelioma showing epithelioid (A) and spindled (B) endothelial cells.

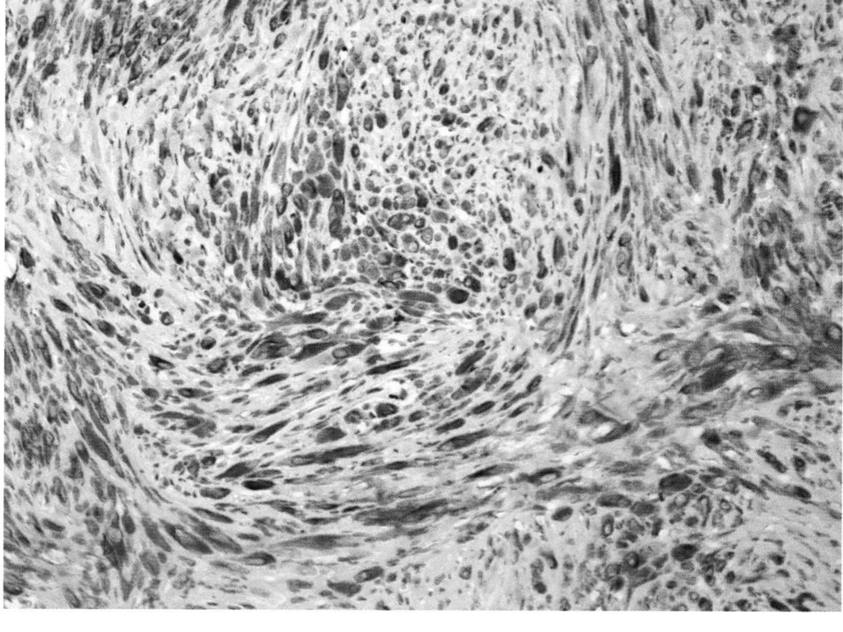

FIGURE 22-41. Diffuse keratin immunoreactivity within epithelioid sarcoma-like hemangioendothelioma.

TABLE 22-5 Comparison of Epithelioid Sarcoma-Like Hemangioendothelioma and Its Mimics

	EHE	ES-LIKE HE	ES
Cord-like growth pattern	+++	–	–
Coarse nodules often with central necrosis	+ (in malignant forms)	–	+++
Intracytoplasmic vacuoles	Common	Rare	Rare
Myxochondroid background	+++	–	–
Origin from vessel	More than 50%	No	No
Keratin	+/++	+++	+++
CD31	+++	+++	–
CD34	+++	None so far	60%
Molecular genetics	t(7;16) fusion *WWTR1-CAMTA1*	t(7;19)(q22;q13) der (7)t(7;19)	*INI1* mutation

EHE, epithelioid hemangioendothelioma; ES-like HE, epithelioid sarcoma-like hemangioendothelioma; ES, epithelioid sarcoma.

References

1. Weiss SW, Enzinger FM. Epithelioid hemangioendothelioma: a vascular tumor often mistaken for a carcinoma. Cancer 1982;50:970.
2. Weiss SW, Ishak KG, Dail DH, et al. Epithelioid hemangioendothelioma and related lesions. Semin Diagn Pathol 1986;3:259.
3. Gray MH, Rosenberg AE, Dickersin GR, et al. Cytokeratin expression in epithelioid vascular neoplasms. Hum Pathol 1990;21:212.
4. Vasquez M, Ordonez NG, English GW, et al. Epithelioid hemangioendothelioma of soft tissue: report of a case with ultrastructural observations. Ultrastruct Pathol 1998;22:73.
5. Deyrup AT, Tighiouart M, Montag AG, et al. Epithelioid hemangioendothelioma of soft tissue: a proposal for risk stratification based on 49 cases. Am J Surg Pathol 2008;32:924.
6. Mentzel T, Beham A, Calonje E, et al. Epithelioid hemangioendothelioma of skin and soft tissues: clinicopathologic and immunohistochemical study of 30 cases. Am J Surg Pathol 1997;21:363.
7. Fletcher CDM, Bridge JA, Hogendoorn FCW, et al, editors. WHO Classification of Tumors of Soft Tissue and Bone. International Agency for Research on Cancer. Lyon, 2013.
8. Errani C, Zhang L, Sung YS, et al. A novel WWTR1-CAMTA1 gene fusion is a consistent abnormality in epithelioid hemangioendothelioma of different anatomic sites. Genes Chromosomes Cancer 2011;50:644.
9. Tanas M, Sboner A, Oliveira A, et al. Identification of a disease-defining gene fusion in epithelioid hemangioendothelioma. Sci Transl Med 2011;3:98ra82.
10. Bhagavan BS, Dorfman HD, Murthy MS, et al. Intravascular bronchioloalveolar tumor (IVBAT): a low-grade sclerosing epithelioid angiosarcoma of lung. Am J Surg Pathol 1982;6:41.
11. Dail DH, Liebow AA, Gmelich JT, et al. Intravascular, bronchiolar, and alveolar tumor of the lung (IVBAT): an analysis of twenty cases of a peculiar sclerosing endothelial tumor. Cancer 1983;51:451.
12. Dean PJ, Haggitt RC, O'Hara CJ. Malignant epithelioid hemangioendothelioma of the liver in young women: relationship to oral contraceptive use. Am J Surg Pathol 1985;9:695.
13. Ishak KG, Sesterhenn IA, Goodman ZD, et al. Epithelioid hemangioendothelioma of the liver: a clinicopathologic and follow-up study of 32 cases. Hum Pathol 1984;15:839.
14. Kelleher MB, Iwatsuki S, Sheahan DG. Epithelioid hemangioendothelioma of the liver: clinicopathological correlation of 10 cases treated with orthotropic liver transplantation. Am J Surg Pathol 1989;13:999.
15. Kleer CG, Unni KK, McLeod RA. Epithelioid hemangioendothelioma of bone. Am J Surg Pathol 1996;20:1301.
16. Tsuneyoshi M, Dorfman HD, Bauer TW. Epithelioid hemangioendothelioma of bone: a clinicopathologic, ultrastructural, and immunohistochemical study. Am J Surg Pathol 1986;10:754.
17. Marino I, Todo S, Tzakis AG, et al. Treatment of hepatic epithelioid hemangioendothelioma with liver transplantation. Cancer 1988;62:2079.
18. Nora FE, Scheithauer BW. Primary epithelioid hemangioendothelioma of the brain. Am J Surg Pathol 1996;20:707.
19. Makhlouf HR, Ishak KG, Goodman ZD. Epithelioid hemangioendothelioma of the liver: a clinicopathologic study of 137 cases. Cancer 1999; 85:562.
20. Quante M, Patel NK, Hill S, et al. Epithelioid hemangioendothelioma presenting in the skin: a clinicopathologic study of eight cases. Am J Dermatopathol 1998;20:541.
21. Kato N, Tamura A, Okushiba M. Multiple cutaneous epithelioid hemangioendotheliomas: a case with spindle cells. J Dermatol 1998;25: 453.
22. Zukerberg LR, Nickoloff BJ, Weiss SW. Kaposiform hemangioendothelioma of infancy and childhood: an aggressive neoplasm associated with Kasabach-Merritt syndrome and lymphangiomatosis. Am J Surg Pathol 1993;17:321.
23. Lyons LL, North PE, Mac-Moune Lai F, et al. Kaposiform hemangioendothelioma: a study of 33 cases emphasizing its pathologic, immunophenotypic, and biologic uniqueness from juvenile hemangiomas. Am J Surg Pathol 2004;28:559.
24. Enjolras O, Wassef M, Mazoyer E, et al. Infants with Kasabach-Merritt syndrome do not have "true" hemangiomas. J Pediatr 1997;130:631.
25. Sarkar M, Mulliken JB, Kozakewich HP, et al. Thrombocytopenic coagulopathy (Kasabach-Merritt phenomenon) is associated with kaposiform hemangioendothelioma and not with common infantile hemangioma. Plast Reconstruct Surg 1997;100:1377.
26. Mendez R, Capdevila A, Tellado MG. Kaposiform hemangioendothelioma associated with Milroy's disease (primary hereditary lymphedema). J Pediatr Surg 2003;38:E9.
27. Folpe AL, Veikkola T, Valtola R, et al. Vascular endothelial growth factor receptor-3 (VEGFR-3): a marker of vascular tumors with presumed lymphatic differentiation, including Kaposi's sarcoma, kaposiform and Dabska-type hemangioendotheliomas, and a subset of angiosarcomas. Mod Pathol 2000;13:180.
28. Debelenko LV, Perez-Atade AR, Mulliken JB, et al. D2-40 immunohistochemical analysis of pediatric vascular tumors reveals positivity in kaposiform hemangioendothelioma. Mod Pathol 2005;18:1454.
29. Huu AR, Jokinen CH, Rubin BP, et al. Expression of PROX1, lymphatic endothelial nuclear transcription factor in kaposiform hemangioendothelioma and tufted angioma. Am J Surg Pathol 2010;34:1563.
30. Deb G, Jenkner A, DeSio L, et al. Spindle cell (kaposiform) hemangioendothelioma with Kasabach-Merritt syndrome in an infant: successful treatment with alpha-2A interferon. Med Pediatr Oncol 1997;28:358.
31. Haisley-Royster C, Enjoiras O, Frieden IJ. Kasabach-Merritt phenomenon: a retrospective study of treatment with vincristine. J Pediatr Hemato Oncol 2002;24:459.
32. Hermans DJ, van Beynum IM, van der Vijver RJ, et al. Kaposiform hemangioendothelioma with Kasabach Merritt syndrome: a new indication for propranolol treatment. J Pediatr Hematol 2011;23:e171.
33. Blatt J, Stavas J, Moats-Staats B, et al. Treatment of childhood kaposiform hemangioendothelioma with sirolimus. Pediatr Blood Cancer 2010;55: 1396.
34. Dadras SS, Skrzypek A, Nguyen L, et al. Prox-1 promotes invasion of kaposiform hemangioendotheliomas. J Invest Dermatol 2008;128:2798.
35. Fanburg-Smith JC, Michal M, Partanen TA, et al. Papillary intralymphatic angioendothelioma (PILA): a report of twelve cases of a distinctive vascular tumor with phenotypic feature of lymphatic vessels. Am J Surg Pathol 1999;23:1004.
36. Dabska M. Malignant endovascular papillary angioendothelioma of the skin in childhood. Cancer 1969;24:503.
37. Schartz RA, Dabski C, Dabska M. The Dabska tumor: a thirty year retrospect. Dermatology 2001;201:1.
38. Calonje E, Fletcher CD, Wilson-Jones E, et al. Retiform hemangioendothelioma: a distinctive form of low-grade angiosarcoma delineated in a series of 15 cases. Am J Surg Pathol 1994;18:115.

39. Argani P, Athanasian E. Malignant endovascular papillary angioendothelioma (Dabska tumor) arising within a deep intramuscular hemangioma. Arch Pathol Lab Med 1997;121:992.
40. Katz JA, Mahoney DH, Shukla LW, et al. Endovascular papillary angioendothelioma in the spleen. Pediatr Pathol 1988;8:185.
41. Patterson K, Chandra RS. Malignant endovascular papillary angioendothelioma: a cutaneous borderline tumor. Arch Pathol Lab Med 1985;109: 671.
42. Manivel JC, Wick MR, Swanson PE, et al. Endovascular papillary angioendothelioma of childhood: a vascular lesion possibly characterized by "high" endothelial cell differentiation. Hum Pathol 1986;17:1240.
43. Quecedo E, Martinez-Escribano JA, Febrer I, et al. Dabska tumor developing within a preexisting vascular malformation. Am J Dermatopathol 1996;18:303.
44. Billings SD, Folpe AL, Weiss SW. Epithelioid sarcoma-like hemangioendothelioma. Am J Surg Pathol 2003;27:4857.
45. Hornick JL, Fletcher CD. Pseudomyogenic hemangioendothelioma: a distinctive often multicentric tumor with indolent behavior. Am J Surg Pathol 2011;35:190.
46. Trombetta D, Magnusson L, von Steyem FV, et al. Translocation t(7;19)(q22;q13)—a recurrent chromosome aberration in pseudomyogenic hemangioendothelioma? Cancer Genet 2011;204:211.
47. Nayler SJ, Rubin BP, Calonje E, et al. Composite hemangioendothelioma: a complex, low-grade vascular lesion mimicking angiosarcoma. Am J Surg Pathol 2000;24(3):352.
48. Cakir E, Demirag G, Gulhan E et al. Mediastinal composite hemangioendothelioma: a rare tumor in an unusual location. Tumori 2009;95(1):98.
49. Requena I, Luis Diaz J, Manzarbeitia F, et al. Cutaneous composite hemangioendothelioma with satellitosis and lymph node metastases. J Cutan Pathol 2008;35(2):225.
50. Fukunaga M, Suzuki K, Saegusa N, et al. Composite hemangioendothelioma: report of 5 cases including one with associate Maffucci syndrome. Am J Surg Pathol 2007;31(10):1567.

Malignant Vascular Tumors

CHAPTER CONTENTS

ANGIOSARCOMA

Angiosarcomas are malignant tumors that recapitulate many of the functional and morphologic features of normal endothelium. They vary from highly differentiated tumors resembling a hemangioma to anaplastic ones difficult to distinguish from a poorly differentiated carcinoma or sarcoma. Angiosarcomas are no longer subdivided into lymphangiosarcomas and hemangiosarcomas because this distinction cannot be reliably made by conventional methods. In fact, there is evidence that some angiosarcomas have a mixed phenotype.[1] *Hemangioendothelioma*, a term formerly used as a synonym for *angiosarcoma*, particularly in sites such as the bone, is used for vascular tumors of borderline malignancy only (see Chapter 22).

Incidence

Angiosarcomas are collectively one of the rarest soft tissue neoplasms. They account for a vanishingly small proportion of all vascular tumors, and they comprise less than 1% of all sarcomas. Although they may occur at any location in the body, they rarely arise from major vessels and have a decided predilection for skin and superficial soft tissue, a phenomenon that contrasts sharply with the deep location of most soft tissue sarcomas. These tumors infrequently occur during childhood, but, when they do, they seem to occur in an epidemiologic pattern different from that of adults.[2,3] For example, there is a greater tendency for them to develop in internal organs or with various disease states (e.g., Klippel-Trénaunay syndrome). Over the past two decades, the distribution pattern of angiosarcomas has changed. Cutaneous angiosarcomas, formerly constituting about one-third of all angiosarcomas, now account for about one-half. This increase probably reflects the increasing frequency of cutaneous postirradiation sarcomas. About 10% of angiosarcomas are located in deep soft tissue, and the remainder is located in parenchymal organs such as the breast, bone, heart, and spleen. (Table 23-1).[4]

TABLE 23-1 Anatomic Distribution of Angiosarcomas

LOCATION	NO. OF CASES (N = 222)	PERCENTAGE (%)
Skin	110	49.6
Breast (parenchyma)	32	14.4
Soft tissue	25	11.2
Heart	15	6.7
Bone	9	4.1
Other	31	14

Data from Lahat G, Dhuka AR, Hallevi H, et al. Angiosarcoma: clinical and molecular insights. Ann Surg 2010;251(6):1098.

Because there are pathogenetic and behavioral differences among angiosarcomas, it is useful to conceptualize them not as one disease but as several interrelated ones linked by the common presence of the malignant endothelial cell. Angiosarcomas are divided into several clinical groups: (1) primary cutaneous angiosarcoma (unassociated with lymphedema or radiation); (2) lymphedema-associated angiosarcoma; (3) postirradiation angiosarcoma; (4) angiosarcoma of deep soft tissue; and (5) angiosarcoma of parenchymal organs such as bone, liver, spleen, heart, and breast. Angiosarcomas also develop adjacent to foreign material, in the vicinity of arteriovenous fistulas in renal transplant patients, within other tumors, or in association with rare genetic syndromes. Although eclipsed in number by the other forms of angiosarcoma, these unusual associations suggest more than a fortuitous occurrence.

Etiologic Factors

Chronic lymphedema and radiation are the most widely recognized predisposing factors for angiosarcomas of skin and soft tissue. Typically, lymphedema-associated angiosarcomas occur in women who have undergone (modified) radical mastectomy for breast carcinoma and have suffered chronic severe lymphedema for years. But virtually all forms of lymphedema have been associated with this complication.

Several theories have been advanced to explain the association of lymphedema and angiosarcoma. Some have suggested that the growth and proliferation of obstructed lymphatics eventually fail to respond to normal control mechanisms. Others have subscribed to the idea that carcinogens in lymphatic fluid induce the neoplastic change or that the lymphedematous extremity represents an immunologically privileged site[5] that is unable to perform immunologic surveillance of normally occurring mutant cell populations.

Radiation has been clearly associated with angiosarcoma, independent of lymphedema. Definitionally, such tumors must (1) be biopsy proven, (2) arise in the radiation field, (3) occur after a latency of several years, and (4) arise in an area without lymphedema. Previously, postirradiation angiosarcomas followed radiotherapy for carcinoma of the cervix, ovary, endometrium, and Hodgkin lymphoma after an interval of more than 10 years. In the past two decades, this epidemiologic prolife has been changing because of the common practice of administering radiation to women following lumpectomy for breast cancer. The interval in these patients is far shorter than the foregoing group.

A number of angiosarcomas have developed at the site of defunctionalized arteriovenous fistulas[6-8] in renal transplant patients and have been attributed to immunosuppression. However, this does not explain those cases that have occurred in the absence of immunosuppression or the invariable presence of angiosarcoma in the immediate vicinity of the fistula. Some have proposed that immunosuppression provides the ideal context in which deviant patterns of blood flow upregulate growth factors and adhesion molecules to promote endothelial proliferation and migration.[9] Angiosarcomas also have been reported adjacent to foreign material introduced into the body iatrogenically or accidentally. In an extensive review of the literature by Jennings et al.,[10] nine angiosarcomas associated with foreign material were identified. Common to all was a long latent period between the time of introduction of the foreign material and the development of the tumor. Although one case occurred within 3 years, the remainder appeared more than a decade later. A variety of solid materials were implicated, including shrapnel, steel, plastic and synthetic (usually Dacron) vascular graft material, surgical sponges, and bone wax.[10] The authors suggest that an exuberant host response in the form of a fibrous tissue capsule around the foreign material may represent an important intermediate step in the development of the sarcoma. An angiosarcoma occurring in a long-standing gouty tophus suggests that urate deposits may function as the equivalent of foreign material.[11]

Angiosarcomas supervening on other tumors such as port-wine stains, hemangiomas, lymphangiomas,[12,13] benign and malignant nerve sheath tumors,[14-18] malignant germ cell tumors,[19] and leiomyomas[20] have been well documented but are extraordinarily rare. In addition, angiosarcomas may develop in association with other diseases such as neurofibromatosis,[16] bilateral retinoblastoma (Rb1 deletion),[21] Klippel-Trénaunay syndrome,[12] xeroderma pigmentosum,[22] and Aicardi syndrome.[23] The latter is an X-linked disorder associated with multiple congenital abnormalities, including agenesis of the corpus callosum.

Unfortunately, there is little information concerning the possible role of environmental carcinogens in the pathogenesis of soft tissue angiosarcomas. That these factors exist is suggested by the relatively strong evidence linking various substances to the induction of hepatic angiosarcomas. About one-fourth of hepatic angiosarcomas occur in patients who have received thorium dioxide (Thorotrast) for cerebral angiography, in vineyard workers exposed to AsO_3-containing insecticides, or in industrial workers exposed to vinyl chloride during the production of synthetic rubber. A few cases have been recorded in patients receiving long-term androgenic anabolic steroids. Mutations of the K-*ras-2* gene have been detected in both sporadic and Thorotrast-induced hepatic angiosarcomas.[24]

Molecular-Genetic Findings

Angiosarcomas constitute a tight genomic group that differs from other sarcomas by overexpression of genes implicated in the stages of angiogenesis. These include genes for vascular-specific receptor tyrosine kinases: *TIE1, KDR (VEGFR2), SNRK, TEK,* and *FLT1 (VEGFR1)*.[25] Angiosarcomas can be further separated into two genomic subgroups: radiation-induced lesions characterized by overexpression of *LYN* and *PRKCθ* and nonradiation-induced lesions characterized by overexpression of *FLT1* and *AKT3*. A small subset of angiosarcoma also harbors activating mutations of *KDR*, suggesting that small molecule receptor inhibitors (e.g., sunitinib) could be effective therapeutic agents.

High-level *MYC* amplification has recently been demonstrated in postirradiation and lymphedema-associated angiosarcoma. *MYC* amplification has been identified in 50% to 100% of postirradiation and lymphedema-associated angiosarcomas but not in other forms.[26-28] Furthermore, amplification status is independent of grade, location, and histologic features.

Clinical Subtypes

Primary Cutaneous Angiosarcoma

Primary cutaneous angiosarcoma (i.e., those unassociated with radiation or lymphedema) is the most common clinical form accounting for one-half of all cases.[3] It usually occurs after the seventh decade. Males and females are equally affected. Nearly 90% occur in the Caucasian population. About half develop on the head, neck, and face, particularly the area of the scalp and upper forehead. Although sun exposure is often imputed causally, this has not been proven. Clinically, the appearance of these lesions is variable. Most begin as ill-defined bruise-like areas with indurated borders. Advanced lesions are elevated, nodular, and occasionally ulcerated (Fig. 23-1). It is difficult to determine clinically the extent of these lesions. This fact, coupled with

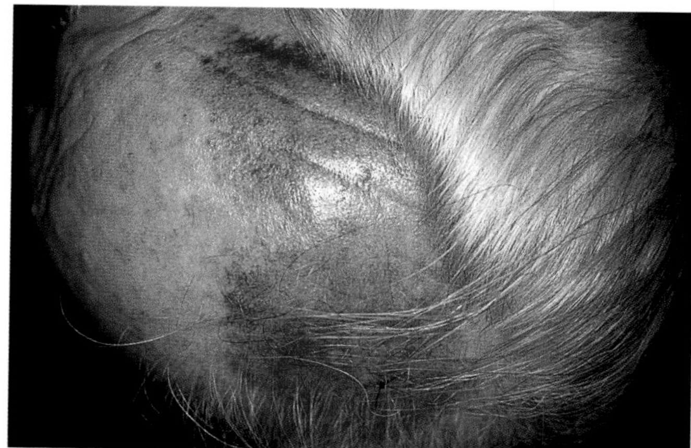

FIGURE 23-1. Angiosarcoma of the scalp in an elderly man. *(Case courtesy of Dr. Vernon Sondak, University of Michigan Hospitals.)*

multifocality in about half of the cases, seriously complicates therapy and probably results in suboptimal initial therapy in a large number of cases. Preoperative mapping of angiosarcoma using grid-pattern biopsies or Mohs surgery has resulted in better delineation of tumor extent and treatment planning.[29]

Grossly, the tumors consist of ill-defined hemorrhagic areas (Fig. 23-2) that flatten or ulcerate the overlying skin. Rarely, the epidermis displays verrucous hyperplasia. On a cut section, the tumors have a microcystic or sponge-like quality as a result of the presence of blood-filled spaces. The tumors extensively involve the dermis and extend well beyond their apparent gross confines. In poorly differentiated, rapidly growing tumors, deep structures, such as the subcutis and fascia, are invaded. The periphery of the tumors contains a fringe of dilated lymphatic vessels surrounded by chronic inflammatory cells and usually small capillaries in which piling up and tufting of the endothelium suggest incipient malignant change.

Most cutaneous angiosarcomas are moderately differentiated lesions that form distinct vascular channels, albeit of irregular size and shape (Figs. 23-3 to 23-8). These tumors, at first, may suggest poorly confined hemangiomas because of the numerous channels and the flattened, innocuous appearance of the cells. Yet, in contrast to true hemangiomas, the vascular channels seem to create their own tissue planes, dissecting through the dermal collagen (see Fig. 23-6) and fascia or splitting apart groups of subcutaneous fat cells. Moreover, there is a tendency for the channels to communicate with each other to form an anastomosing network of sinusoids (see Figs. 23-4 and 23-5). Although the cells resemble normal

Text continued on p. 710

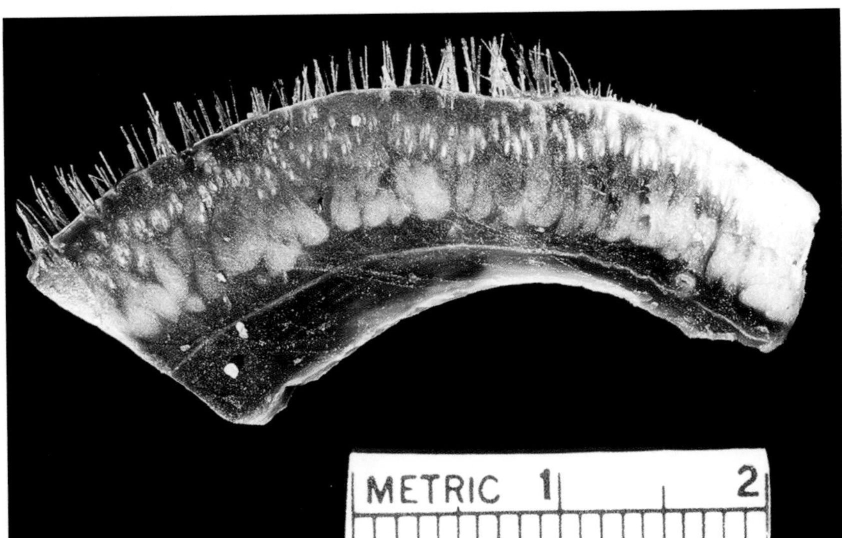

FIGURE 23-2. Angiosarcoma of the scalp. Hemorrhagic appearance frequently suggests a diagnosis of dissecting hemorrhage or hematoma.

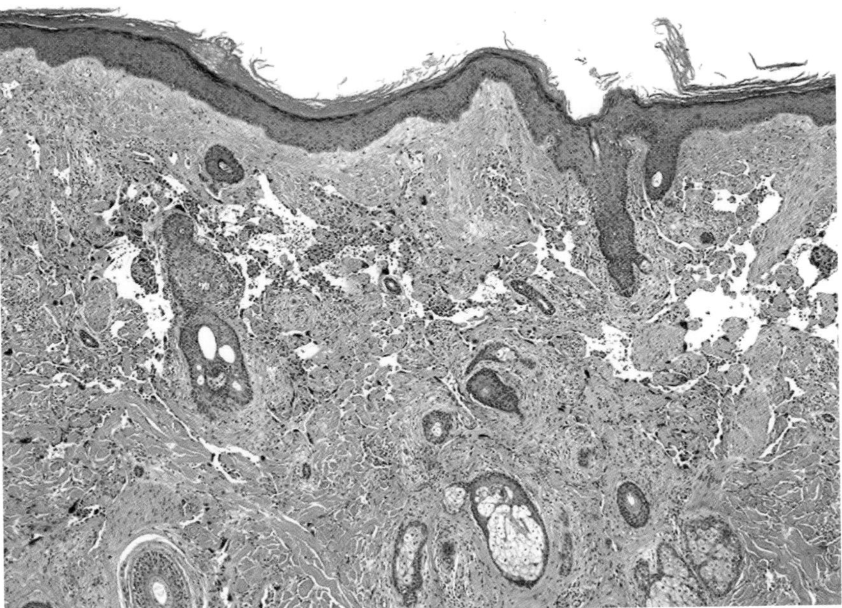

FIGURE 23-3. Cutaneous angiosarcoma composed of irregular vascular channels infiltrating the dermis.

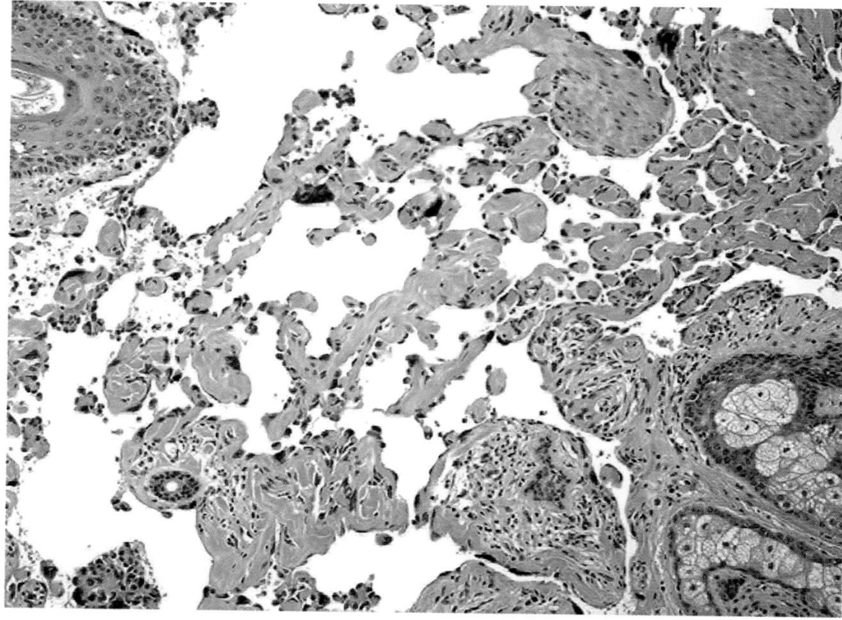

FIGURE 23-4. Cutaneous angiosarcoma showing a sinusoidal pattern of vessels.

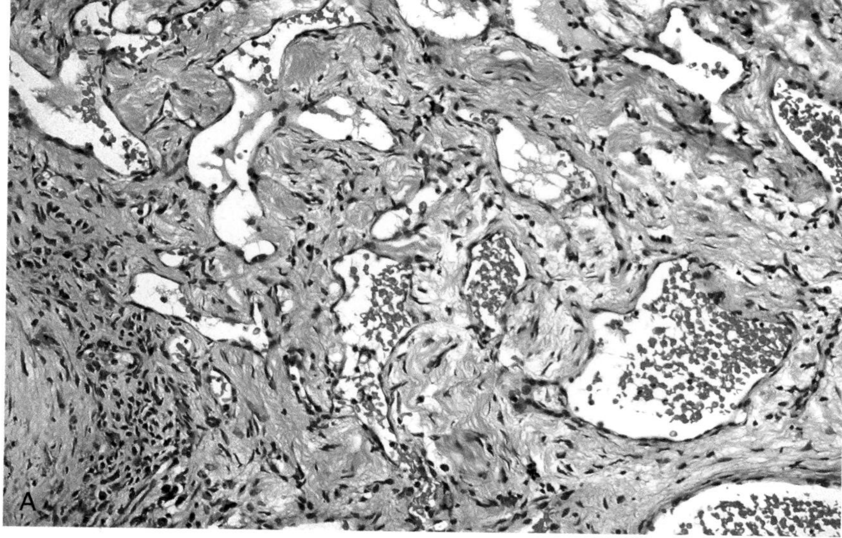

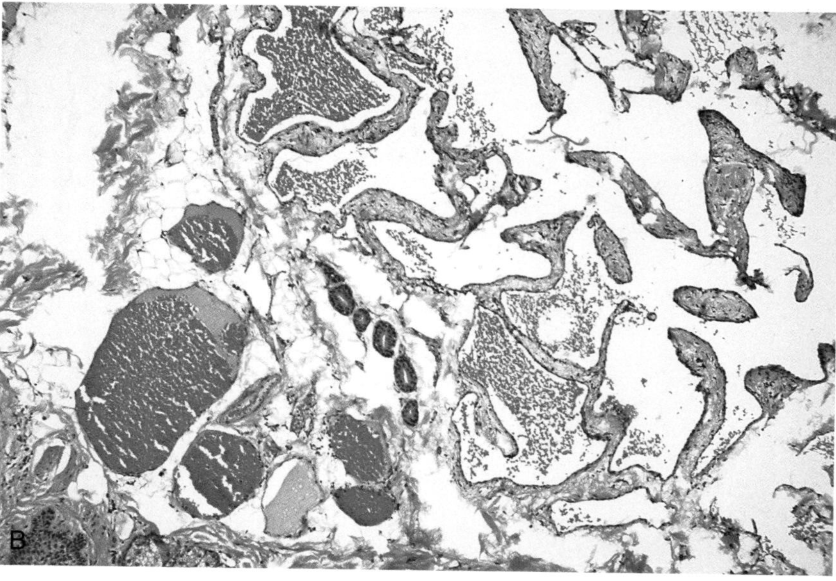

FIGURE 23-5. Varying patterns in cutaneous angiosarcomas. (A) Irregular ectatic vessels dissecting the dermis. (B) Large cavernous vascular spaces resembling a cavernous hemangioma.

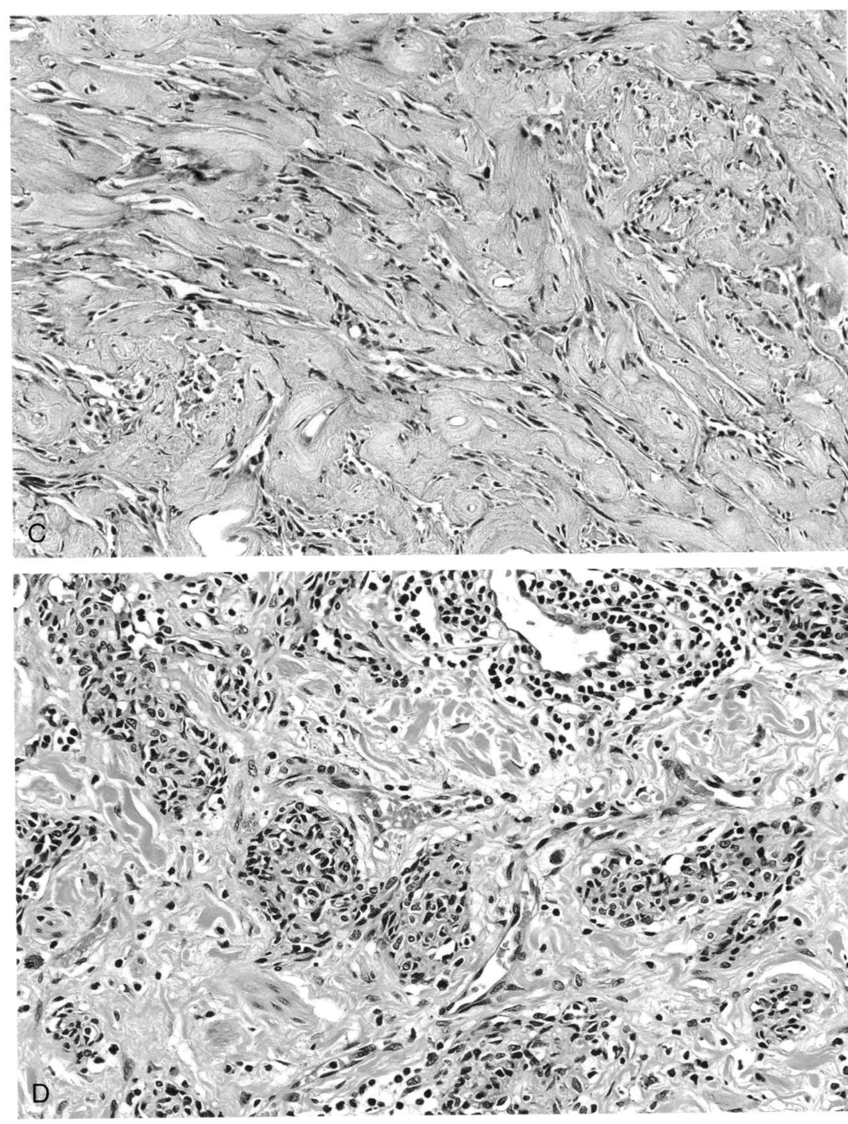

FIGURE 23-5, cont'd. (C) Slit-like vessels dissecting collagen. (D) Small clusters of slit-like vessels surrounded by chronic inflammatory cells.

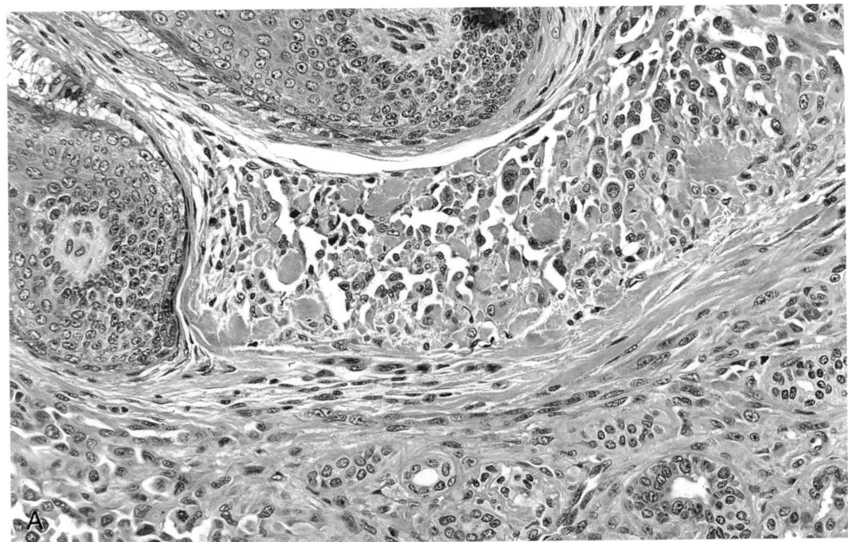

FIGURE 23-6. Infiltrative growth of an angiosarcoma around a hair shaft (A), within fat (B), and between collagen bundles (C).

Continued

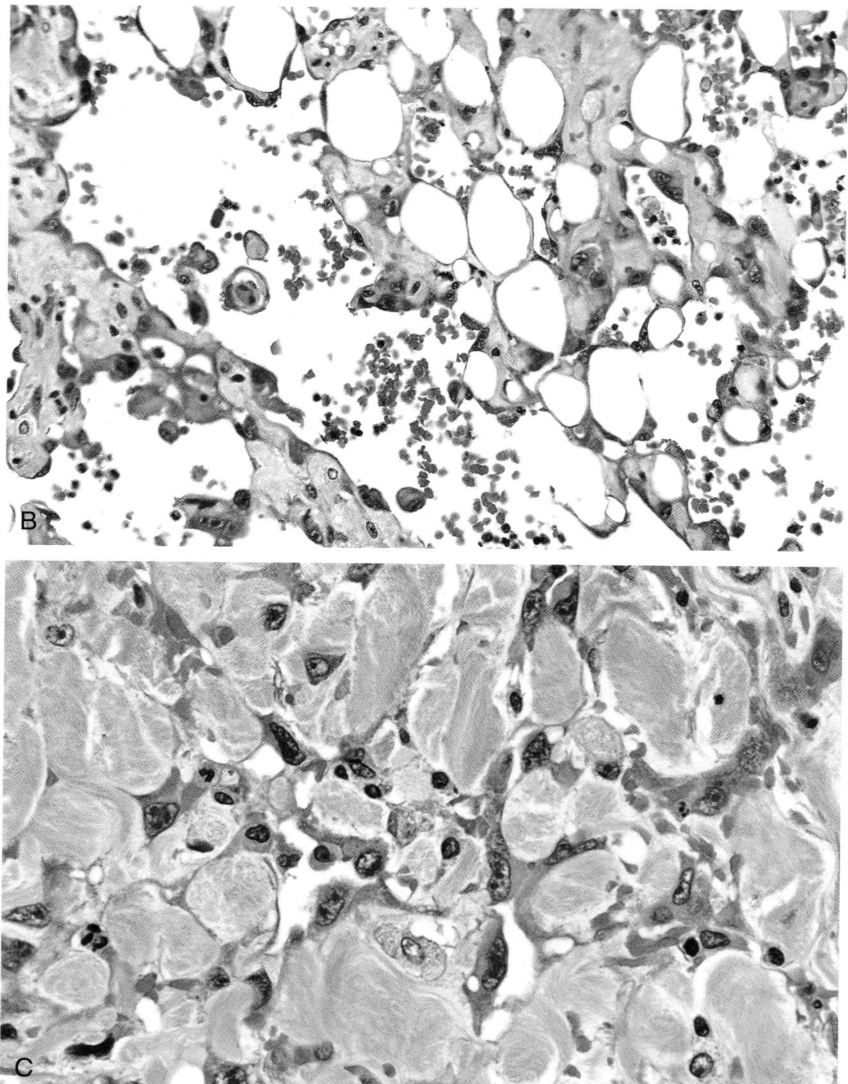

FIGURE 23-6, cont'd

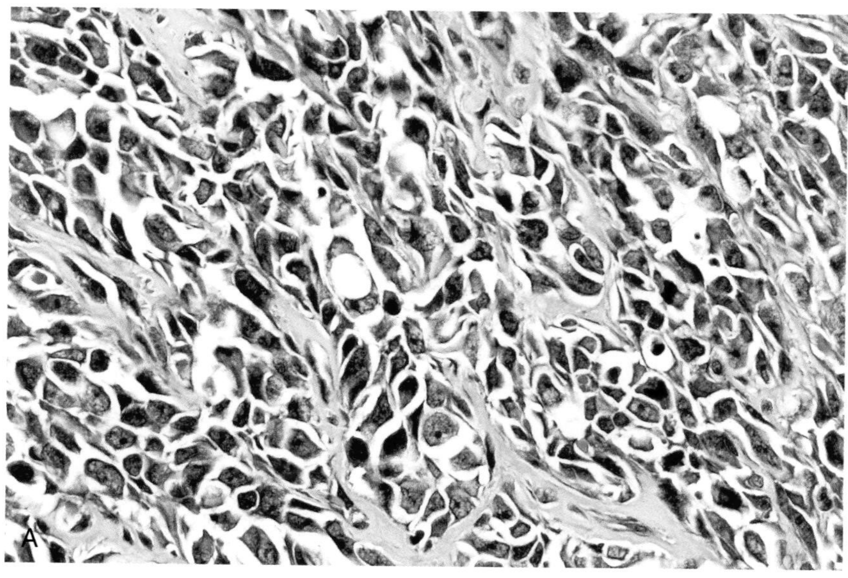

FIGURE 23-7. Variety of patterns in a high-grade angiosarcoma, including a solid or medullary focus (A) and marked spindling of the cells (B, C). Highly pleomorphic tumor with rudimentary lumen formation (D).

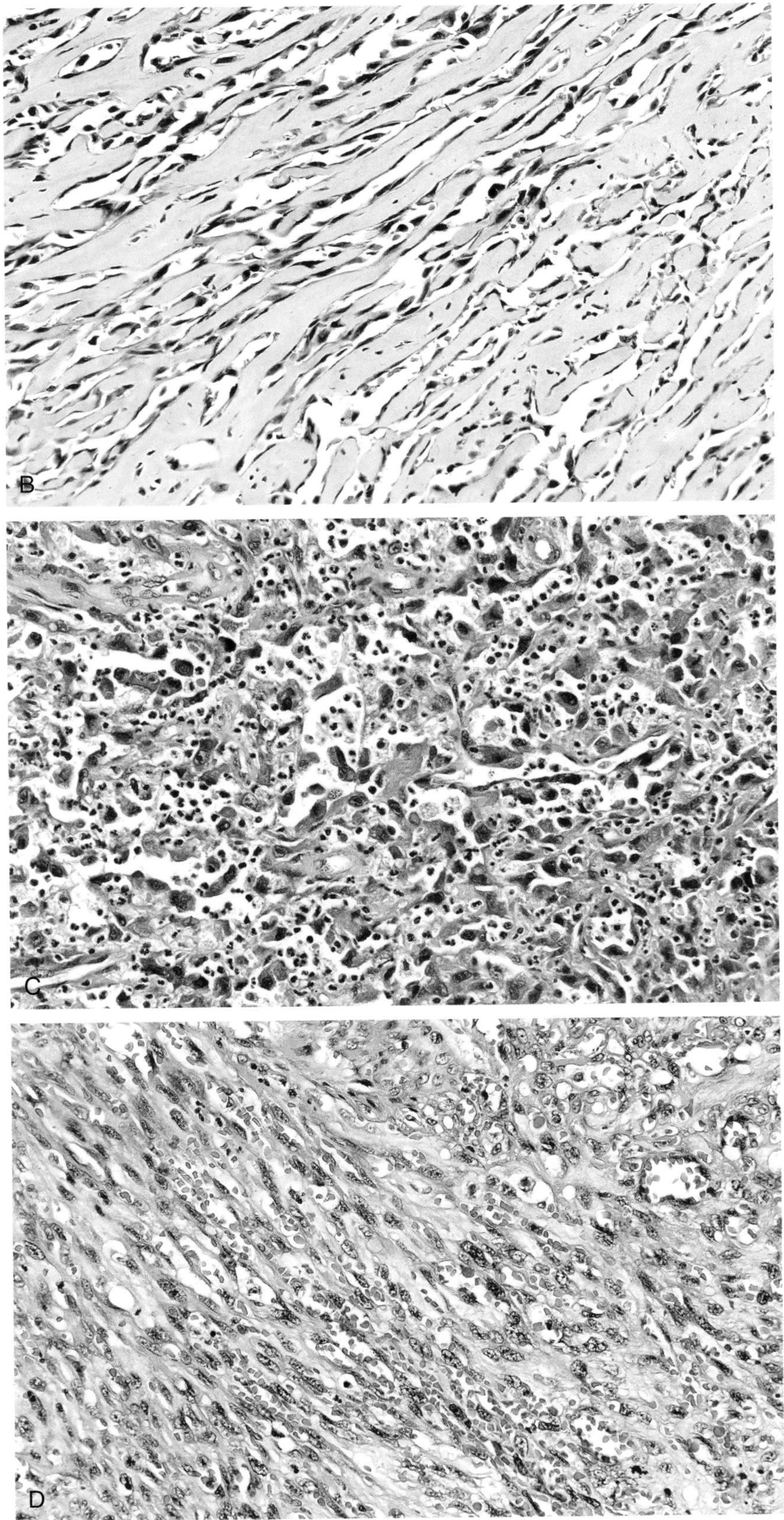

FIGURE 23-7, cont'd

endothelium to some extent, they usually have larger, hyperchromatic nuclei and often pile up along the lumens, creating the papillations so typical of angiosarcomas (but which may also be seen in reactive vascular proliferations, such as papillary endothelial hyperplasia).

A small number of cutaneous angiosarcomas are high-grade tumors that are difficult to distinguish from carcinomas or high-grade fibrosarcomas (see Fig. 23-7). These tumors may have occasional well-differentiated areas, as described earlier, that facilitate diagnosis. Others are composed exclusively of

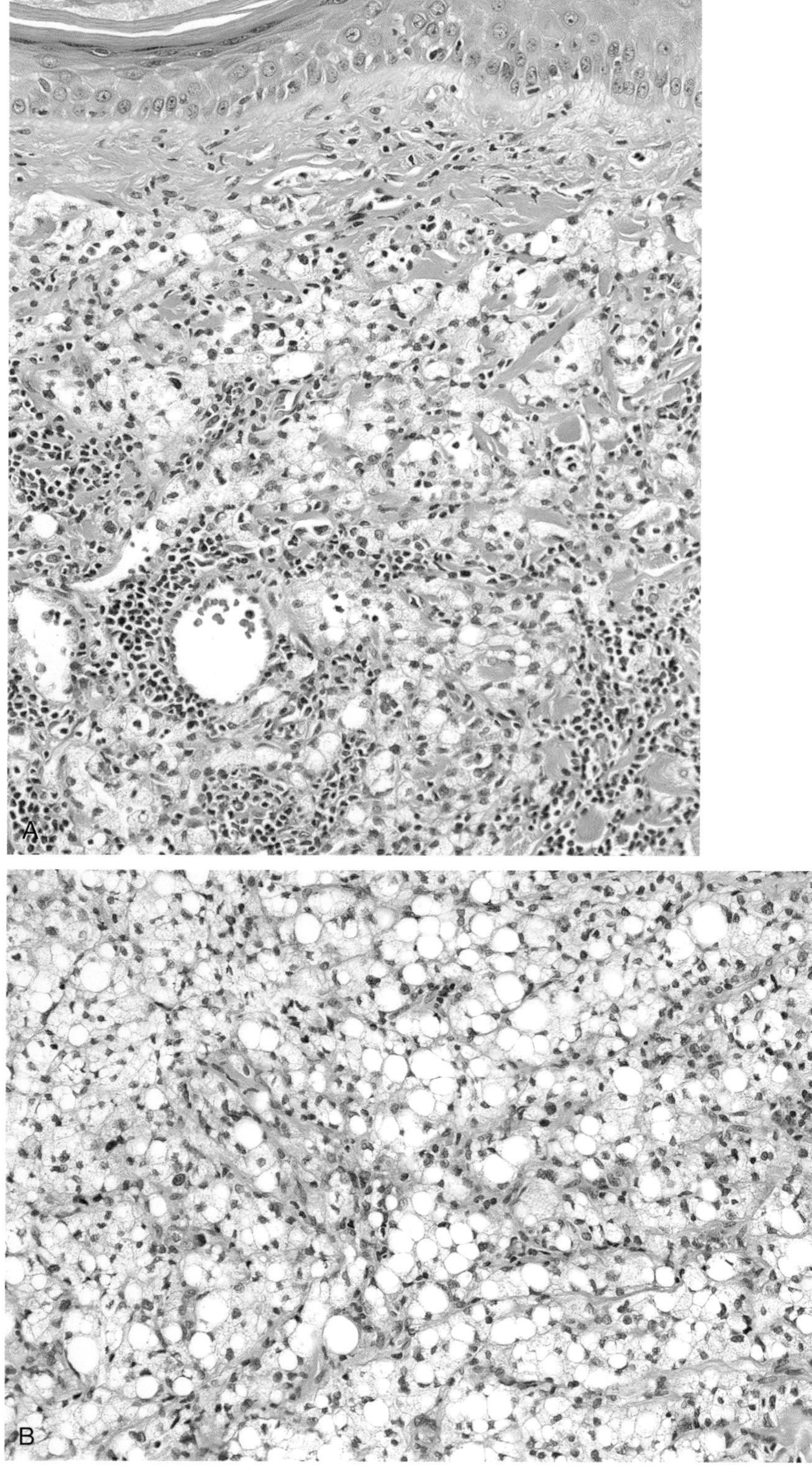

FIGURE 23-8. Foamy cell variant of angiosarcoma (A) illustrating finely vacuolated endothelial cells (B) expressing CD31 (C).

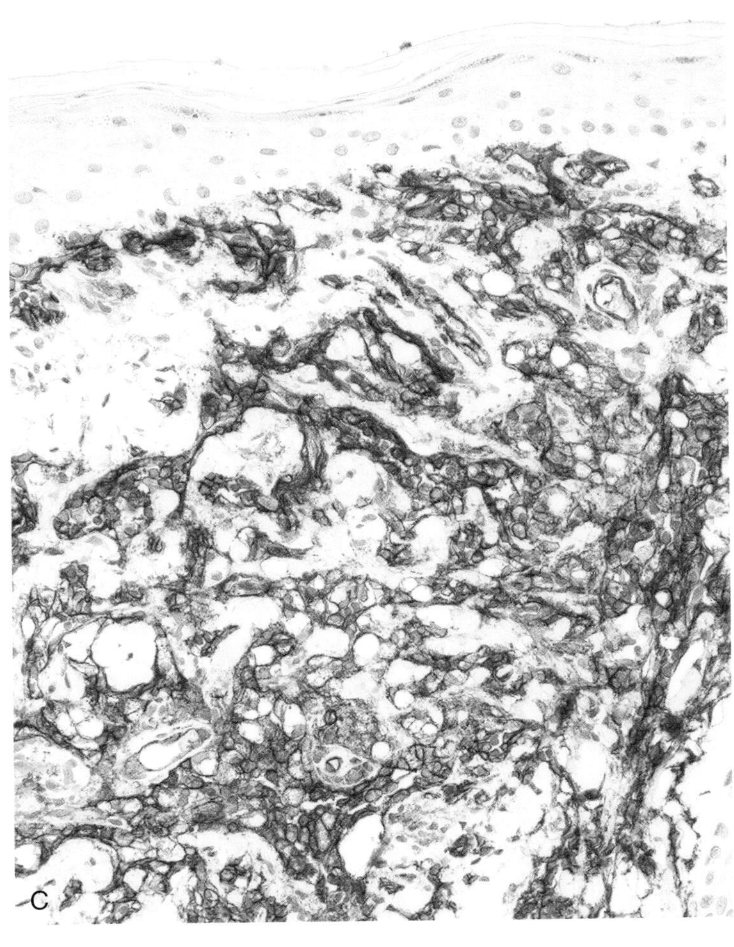

FIGURE 23-8, cont'd

poorly differentiated areas. The cells in the poorly differentiated tumors may be pleomorphic and mitotically active. Rarely, angiosarcomas have a uniformly low-grade appearance consisting of innocuous vessels infiltrating soft tissue and containing intraluminal papillations. The diagnosis, in these cases, is based more on the pattern of growth than on the degree of cytologic atypia and mitotic activity. A rare form of angiosarcoma is the so-called *foamy cell variant*.[30] Composed of sheets of cytologically bland, finely vacuolated endothelial cells, these lesions are easily mistaken for a xanthomatous reaction (see Fig. 23-8). Those with more atypia may bring to mind a signet ring carcinoma.

Ultrastructural Findings

Given the superiority of immunohistochemistry in assessing endothelial differentiation, ultrastructural analysis is rarely (if ever) used diagnostically. Electron microscopy achieves greatest success in those angiosarcomas that are well differentiated and display many of the features of normal endothelium, including a partial investiture of basal lamina along the antiluminal borders (Fig. 23-9), tight junctions between cells, pinocytotic vesicles, and occasional cytofilaments. Weibel-Palade bodies, an organelle specific to endothelium, are rarely seen, however. Endothelial differentiation is difficult to document in poorly differentiated lesions; sometimes the topographic relationship of the neoplastic cells to one another and to erythrocytes can be used to infer endothelial differentiation.

Immunohistochemical Findings

Immunohistochemical confirmation of the diagnosis of angiosarcoma, even those that are poorly differentiated, can usually be accomplished using a panel of vascular markers (see Chapter 7). Using both CD34 and CD31, nearly all angiosarcomas, even poorly differentiated ones, can be identified. There are a few caveats, however. Although CD34 is expressed by many angiosarcomas and Kaposi sarcoma, it is also seen in some soft tissue tumors (e.g., epithelioid sarcoma) that may enter into the differential diagnosis of angiosarcoma. CD31 (platelet-endothelial cell adhesion molecule), on the other hand, seems to be the more sensitive and more specific antigen for endothelial differentiation (Fig. 23-10). In the context of soft tissue neoplasia, virtually all benign and malignant vascular tumors express this membrane protein, whereas nonvascular tumors do not. Because histiocytes are CD31-positive in a granular membranous pattern, it is important to accurately assess the characteristics of positive cells. The prudent approach is to use immunohistochemical studies to rule out other diagnoses that may legitimately enter the differential diagnosis coupled with a panel of vascular markers (e.g., CD31, CD34) that, if positive, support the diagnosis of angiosarcoma.

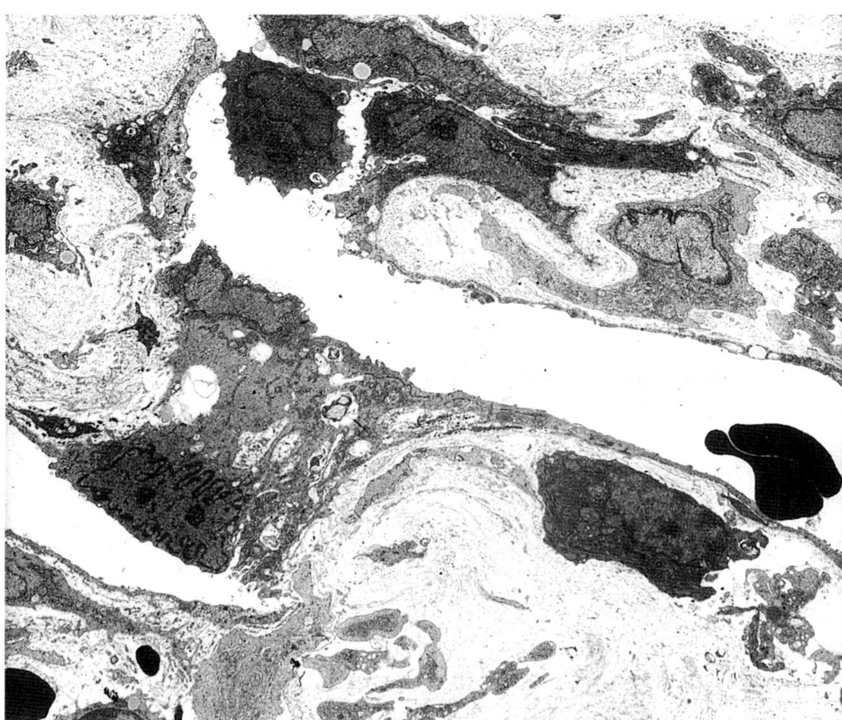

FIGURE 23-9. Electron micrograph of an angiosarcoma. An irregularly shaped blood vessel is lined by neoplastic endothelial cells with segments of basal lamina. Several perithelial cells and their processes are present outside of the vessel wall. *(Courtesy of Dr. Jerome B. Taxy.)*

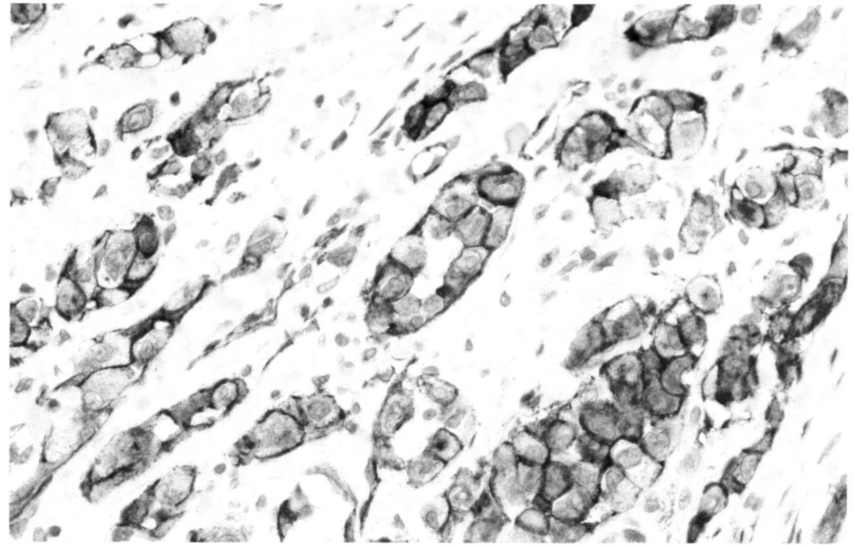

FIGURE 23-10. Immunostain for CD31 shows intense staining of most angiosarcoma cells.

Newer antibodies to FLI1 and ERG proteins are highly sensitive and relatively highly specific markers of angiosarcoma.[31-33] FLI1, a nuclear transcription factor, has been shown to identify more than 95% of vascular tumors, regardless of type and level of malignancy.[31] But it is also expressed by some adenocarcinomas and melanomas,[32] making it important that one not prejudge a malignant tumor as an angiosarcoma without considering these as well. ERG, an ETS family transcription factor, is expressed in normal endothelial cells. Nuclear ERG expression has recently been shown to be an exquisitely sensitive endothelial marker of vascular differentiation. In a study of over 200 vascular tumors, Miettinen et al.[33] have shown that virtually all benign and malignant vascular tumors express the protein, including lymphatic lesions as well. Because ERG expression is highly retained in angiosarcomas, it indicates that the marker is independent of the level of malignancy. In contrast, it is absent in a wide variety of benign and malignant mesenchymal tumors.

Claudin-5, a tight junction protein expressed in endothelial and some epithelial cells, is a new and promising marker for angiosarcoma. Miettinen et al[34] have found that virtually all angiosarcomas and Kaposi sarcoma express claudin-5 compared to approximately 5% of nonvascular mesenchymal tumors. Among those that were positive were biphasic synovial sarcoma. However, the full range of expression of claudin-5 among mesenchymal tumors has not been completely defined. Actin immunostains can be used to judge the presence of pericytes investing the endothelium in histologically ambiguous vascular lesions. Angiosarcomas typically lack pericytes. However, care must be exercised not to misinterpret stromal myofibroblasts as pericytes.

Clinical Behavior

The overall 5-year survival of patients with cutaneous angiosarcomas varies from 30% to 50%.[4,35,36] Most patient deaths are the result of metastases to lung, liver, and lymph node.[36,37] Outcome is influenced by a number of factors, including age, size, and margin status.[4,35,36,38] Younger patients have a decidedly better prognosis than older ones. In a retrospective analysis of patients entered into the Surveillance, Epidemiology, and End Results Program, patients less than 50 years of age had a 10-year relative survival rate of 71.7% compared to 36.8% for those older than 50 years.[39] A similar trend has been reported by others.[35,36]

Size, too, is a parameter most consistently linked to outcome. Although, in the past, most angiosarcomas were large (greater than 5 cm) at the time of presentation,[37] this demographic has changed. Approximately one-half of angiosarcomas are less than 5 cm at the time of presentation.[4,36] Tumors less than 5 cm in diameter (T1) have a significantly better prognosis than those that are larger (T2).[35,37,40-42] Mark et al.[40] reported a 5-year survival of 32% for lesions less than 5 cm compared to 13% for those greater than 5 cm, and Pawlik et al.[35] noted a mortality of less than 10% in patients with lesions less than 5 cm and 75% in those with lesions greater than 5 cm. It should be noted that pathologic size correlates better with outcome than clinical size because the latter commonly underestimates the size.

Negative margin status is highly correlated with improved survival,[4,38] although it is both difficult to achieve negative margins in angiosarcoma and to assess them at the time of a frozen section. At one institution, as many as two-thirds of margins interpreted as negative at the time of a frozen section were judged to be positive on a permanent section.[35] For this reason, Pawlik et al. recommend that reconstruction surgery be postponed until the results of permanent sections are available.[35]

Although conventional histologic grading is not widely applied to angiosarcomas, Deyrup et al.[36] have recently proposed a risk stratification scheme, based on a combination of necrosis and epithelioid morphology. Patients whose tumors had both necrosis and epithelioid morphology (high-risk histologic group) had a 24% 3-year survival. In contrast, patients whose tumors lacked both (low-risk histologic group) had a 77% 3-year survival. The importance of necrosis[43] and epithelioid appearance[4] in prognosis have been validated by others. Recently, a purely epithelioid form of cutaneous angiosarcoma with predilection for the extremities and aggressive course has been described.[44,45]

Angiosarcoma Associated with Lymphedema

In 1949, Stewart and Treves[46] reported six patients who developed vascular sarcomas (so-called *lymphangiosarcoma*) following radical mastectomy and axillary lymph node dissection for breast carcinoma. Although some of the patients had also undergone radiotherapy, the common denominator in each of the cases appeared to be the presence of chronic lymphedema, which usually supervened shortly after mastectomy. Since this original description, many cases of vascular sarcomas complicating chronic lymphedema have been recorded. Not unexpectedly, most have occurred in women following mastectomy, although tumors have been documented on the abdominal wall following lymph node dissection for carcinoma of the penis and the arm or leg affected by congenital, idiopathic, traumatic and filarial lymphedema. Recently, angiosarcomas have also been reported in obesity-associated lymphedema (localized massive lymphedema).[47] This has led to the conjecture that the obesity epidemic may well increase the incidence of angiosarcoma.

Clinical Findings

About 90% of all angiosarcomas associated with chronic lymphedema occur after surgery for breast carcinoma, although the frequency of this complication has been estimated as less than 1% of all women who survive 5 years after mastectomy. These patients are typically women in their seventh decade who have developed a significant degree of lymphedema, usually within a year of mastectomy. The tumors develop within 10 years of the original surgery, although the interval may be as short as 4 years or as long as 27 years. In rare instances, the tumor has been reported in post-mastectomy patients who have experienced little or no lymphedema. Whether some patients truly have no lymphedema is questionable because minor degrees of lymphedema in obese patients can go undetected clinically.

When these tumors occur in congenital or idiopathic lymphedema, the affected patients are usually younger, the lymphedema is of longer duration, and any extremity may be affected. Most patients are in their fourth or fifth decade and have experienced lymphedema for two decades or longer.

Regardless of the clinical setting, the onset of cancer is heralded by the development of one or more polymorphic lesions superimposed on the brawny, nonpitting edema of the affected extremity. Deeply situated lesions in the subcutis may impart only a mottled purple-red hue to the overlying skin, whereas superficial lesions can be palpated as distinct nodules that coalesce to form large polypoid growths (Fig. 23-11).

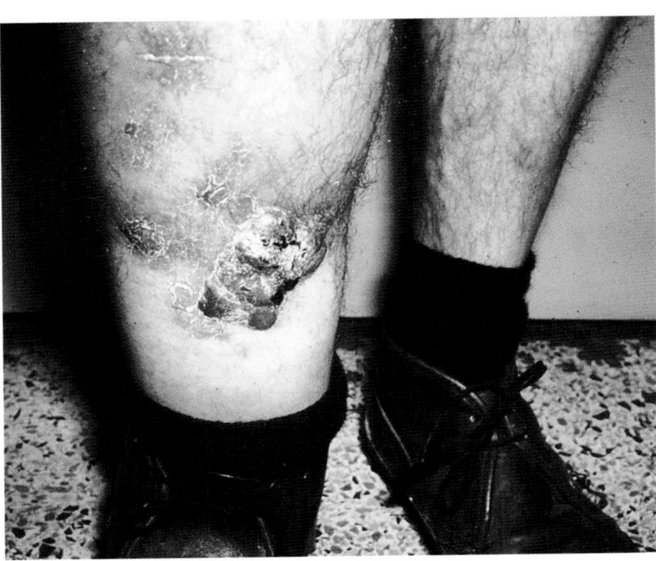

FIGURE 23-11. Angiosarcoma in a lymphedematous extremity.

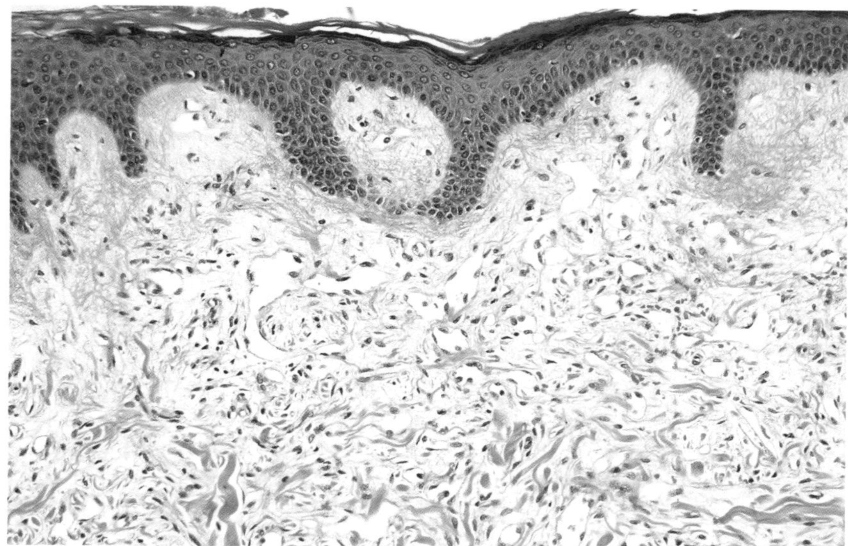

FIGURE 23-12. Diffuse proliferation of dermal lymphatic vessels (lymphangiomatosis) containing atypical endothelium. Lesion occurred in a patient a few years after mastectomy for breast carcinoma. Minimal lymphedema was present. Such changes have been considered premalignant and may herald the onset of frank angiosarcoma (lymphangiosarcoma).

Ulceration, accompanied by a serosanguineous discharge, characterizes late lesions. Repeated healing and breakdown give rise to lesions of various stages that spread distally to the hands and feet or proximally to the chest wall or trunk, in advanced cases.

Microscopic Findings

The hallmark of the lesion is the presence of small capillary-sized vessels composed of obviously malignant cells that infiltrate soft tissue and skin. The lumens may be empty, filled with clear fluid, or engorged with erythrocytes, a finding that has made it difficult to classify these tumors as to blood vessel or lymphatic origin and has led to the suggestion that two lines of differentiation may be present. Lymphocytes are occasionally found around the neoplastic vessels, but, because this feature is also seen in other angiosarcomas, it does not provide sufficient evidence of lymphatic differentiation.

Perhaps the only feature that sets this tumor apart from the conventional angiosarcomas discussed in the chapter and provides some support for lymphatic differentiation is its association with areas of so-called *lymphangiomatosis*.[48] These changes appear to represent premalignant changes of small vessels, presumably lymphatics. The vessels become dilated and form a diffuse ramifying network throughout the soft tissue (Fig. 23-12). They are lined by plump endothelial cells with hyperchromatic nuclei. These areas may merge imperceptibly with areas of frank angiosarcoma or may exist alone in patients who have not yet developed discrete clinical lesions.

Therapy for this premalignant lesion is problematic. These patients probably are at risk of developing angiosarcoma and deserve scrupulous follow-up care. It seems best to recommend therapy for patients with clinical lesions only.

Angiosarcoma of the Breast

Angiosarcomas of the breast are those that originate in the mammary parenchyma as opposed to those overlying the skin.[49-53] They may, however, extend secondarily into the skin. This has led to a blurring of the distinction between angiosarcomas arising in breast parenchyma from those arising in the skin of the breast following radiation. Extracting the behavior of parenchymal breast angiosarcoma from published reports is also problematic. Some studies fail to make the distinction between the two types or, if they do, they combine data from both groups for the purposes of reporting.

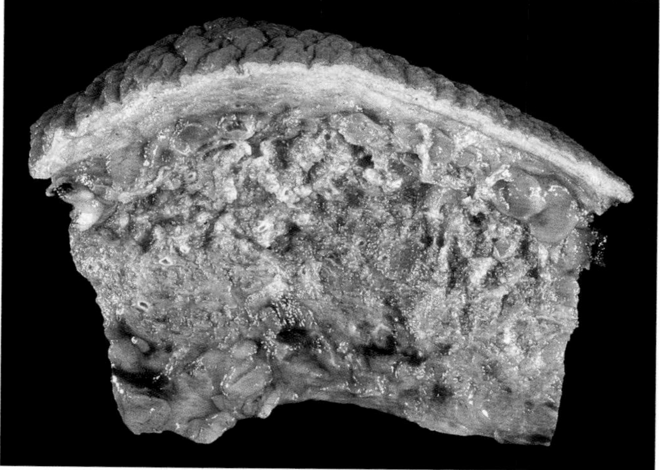

FIGURE 23-13. Angiosarcoma of the breast with a sponge-like quality.

True parenchymal angiosarcomas account for approximately 1 in 1700 to 2000 primary malignant tumors of the breast. Unlike other angiosarcomas, this type occurs exclusively in women, usually during the third or fourth decade, although occasional cases have been reported in menopausal or pregnant women.[49]

The typical presentation is an intramammary mass averaging about 5 to 7 cm associated with variable discoloration of the overlying skin (Fig. 23-13). About 80% of women have localized disease at presentation.[50] Rarely, metastases in the regional lymph nodes or contralateral breast are present.[53] Despite the size, classic features of carcinoma, such as nipple retraction, are absent. Located deep in the substance of the breast, they often invade the skin but seldom extend into the pectoral fascia. The tumors are ill-defined, hemorrhagic, spongy masses surrounded by a rim of engorged vessels. The tumors share similar histologic features to other angiosarcomas. It has been recommended that breast angiosarcomas be graded.[54] Grade I lesions are composed of well-formed, anastomosing vascular channels that permeate fat and breast. The vessels are lined by a single layer attenuated endothelium with minimal atypia. Grade II lesions are more cellular. Vessels are lined by cells with distinct nuclear atypia and multilayering. However, solid areas are not present. Grade III lesions are composed of sheets of cells of high nuclear grade interrupted by intralesional blood lakes. The three grades are represented roughly equally within this group of angiosarcomas.[53] Whether grading actually predicts outcome is controversial. In a large series by Rosen,[54] survival probability amongst the three grades at 1 year was similar, but at 5 and 10 years, grade III lesions fared worse. A more recent review by Nascimento et al.[53] did not define statistically significant differences among the three grades. The approach has been to provide a grade and indicate that its significance is uncertain.

Whether this form of angiosarcoma has a similar or different behavior from cutaneous angiosarcomas of the breast is also debated. Some maintain that they have a comparable course,[50] whereas others maintain a higher risk of mortality.[52] In one of the largest series of 59 patients, the 5-year overall survival was 61%, and the 5-year disease-free survival was 44%.[52] Both were significantly associated with tumor size but not with various other factors, including age or administration of chemotherapy. However, grade was not assessed and evaluated.

Differential Diagnosis

The differential diagnosis of this lesion lies principally in distinguishing it from *benign hemangioma* or *angiolipoma*, two *nonpalpable* breast lesions that are increasingly detected and removed as a result of more sophisticated imaging techniques. Angiosarcomas of the breast are ill-defined lesions that grow infiltratively within fat and breast lobules. It is the pattern of destructive growth that distinguishes them from benign lesions when the degree of atypia is minimal. Hemangiomas and angiolipomas of the breast are usually sharply demarcated from normal breast tissue. The vessels of a hemangioma are regular in shape, and those of angiolipoma have fibrin microthrombi.

Angiosarcoma of Soft Tissue

Angiosarcomas arising from and essentially restricted to deep soft tissue account for about 10% of all angiosarcomas (see Table 23-1). Unlike their cutaneous counterpart, they occur at any age and are evenly distributed throughout all decades.[12] About one-third develop in association with other conditions such as inherited diseases (neurofibromatosis, Klippel-Trénaunay syndrome, Maffucci syndrome), synthetic vascular grafts, and other neoplasms. Like the more common adult soft tissue sarcomas, they develop on the extremities or in the abdominal cavity where they present as a large, hemorrhagic mass (Fig. 23-14). It is not unusual for these tumors to be confused with a chronic hematoma, even after biopsy of the tumor, especially if the biopsy material is limited or nonrepresentative. In the very young, the large size of this tumor may result in hematologic abnormalities, such as thrombocytopenia, high-output cardiac failure from arteriovenous shunting, or even death as a result of massive exsanguination.[2] Unlike angiosarcomas of the skin, deep angiosarcomas more commonly have an epithelioid appearance (Figs. 23-15 and 23-16).[12,13] These so-called *epithelioid angiosarcomas* consist of sheets of high-grade rounded endothelial cells with prominent nuclei, some of which contain intracytoplasmic lumens. Because many express cytokeratin, it is essential that CD31 stains be performed in parallel.

Based on the largest series so far, soft tissue angiosarcomas are aggressive neoplasms.[12] Altogether, 53% of patients were dead of the disease within 1 year; another 31% had no evidence of disease at 46 months. Overall, 20% of patients experienced local recurrences and 49% distant metastasis, most often to the lung followed by lymph node, bone, and soft tissue. The features statistically associated with poor outcome included older age, retroperitoneal location, large size, and high Ki67 values (greater than 10%). In a smaller series of epithelioid angiosarcomas, four of six patients died of the disease.[13]

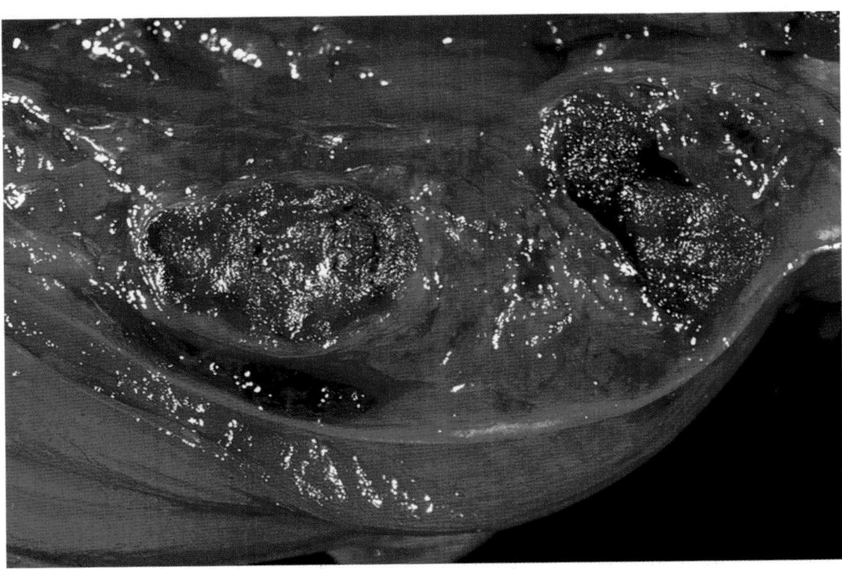

FIGURE 23-14. Angiosarcoma in deep soft tissue with prominent hemorrhage.

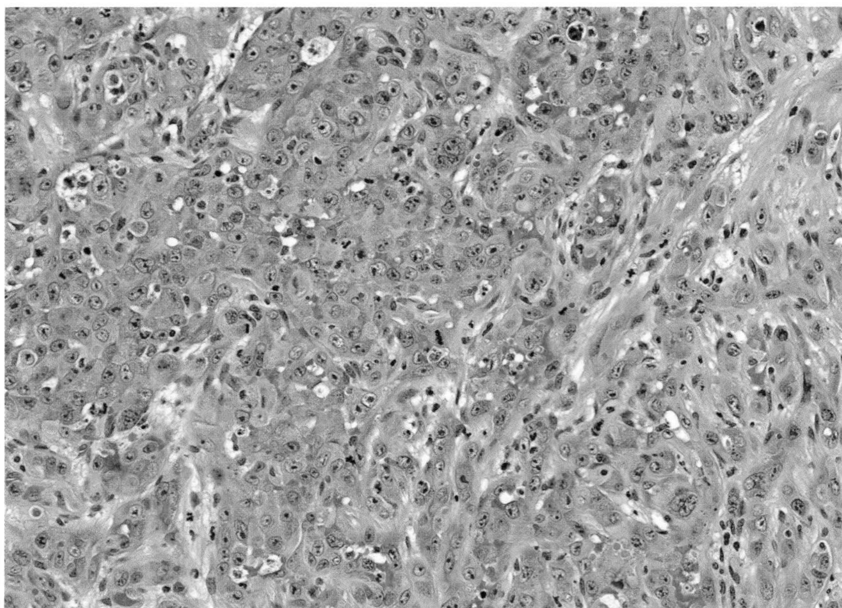

FIGURE 23-15. Epithelioid angiosarcoma of deep soft tissue.

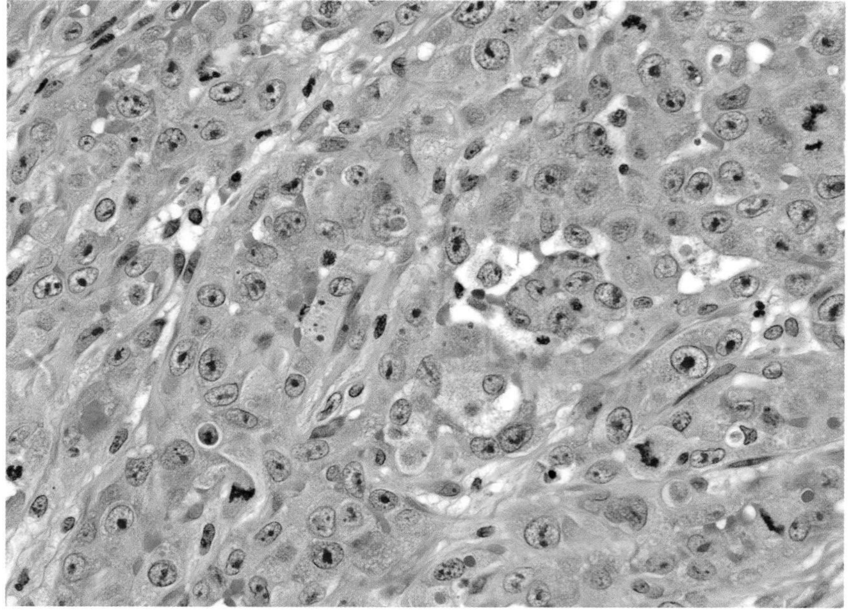

FIGURE 23-16. Epithelioid angiosarcoma of deep soft tissue composed of epithelioid endothelial cells with prominent nucleoli.

Radiation-Induced Angiosarcoma

About one-quarter of angiosarcomas occur following radiation. In previous decades, these angiosarcomas commonly presented in the abdominal wall or cavity following irradiation for carcinoma of the cervix, ovary, or uterus, with a small number of cases occurring after irradiation for various other malignant or benign conditions. This demographic profile has changed in recent years. Currently, about one-half of postirradiation angiosarcomas develop on the skin of the breast in women who have had breast-sparing surgery and whole breast irradiation.[4] The incidence of this complication has been estimated at 0.05 to 0.14% of all patients.[55,56]

Most develop within 5 years following high doses of radiation (median 50 Gy), but a significant subset occurs with a latency as short as 3 years.[57] The onset of these lesions is heralded by ecchymoses or thickening of the skin with one or more elevated lesions that develop in the background of little or no lymphedema but with changes of radiation damage in the epidermis (Fig. 23-17). Typically multifocal, they vary greatly in size (0.4 to 20 cm) but on an average are significantly larger than the atypical vascular lesion described later in the chapter. Histologically, they involve dermis and rarely extend into the underlying breast parenchyma. Their features are similar to other cutaneous angiosarcomas. Approximately 50% of patients experience recurrences and 40% metastases, which occur most commonly in the lung, contralateral breast, and bone. To date, histologic features have not been especially helpful in predicting outcome. Although there have been a few

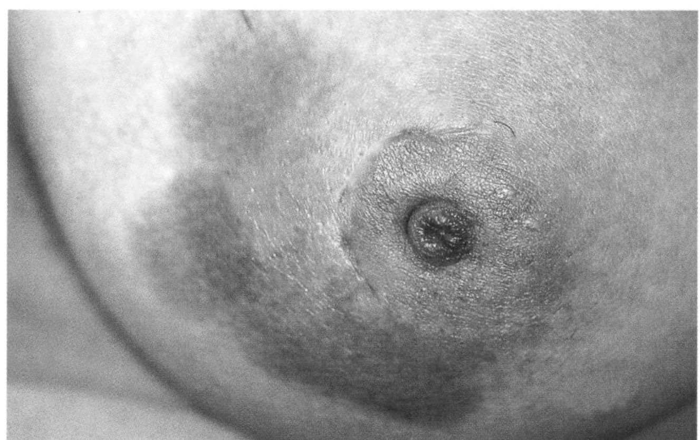

FIGURE 23-17. Cutaneous angiosarcoma of the breast after breast-conserving surgery and irradiation for carcinoma.

reports suggesting that tumors with low-grade features have a good prognosis, there have been too few cases of this type for statistical analysis.[57]

This form of postirradiation angiosarcoma differs from others by the relatively short interval between radiation and the development of a tumor. The reason for this shorter latency is not well understood, but the large volume of skin encompassed in the radiation field has been suggested as one explanation.[57]

Prognostic Factors and Clinical Behavior

Although angiosarcomas are considered several interrelated clinical diseases, most large studies combine them to analyze outcome.[4,43] This approach has the advantage of providing cohort sizes amenable to statistical analysis, but it also runs the risk of obscuring differences that may exist among the various clinical subtypes. Nevertheless, the themes that emerge from such studies underscore that clinical factors are more relevant in determining prognosis than histologic features. That is not to say that histologic features play no role in the assessment of outcome, but that the features commonly used in grading systems do not lend themselves well to angiosarcomas. As noted previously, the use of risk stratification schemes using angiosarcoma-specific histologic criteria may prove useful in the future.[36]

Collectively, patients with angiosarcomas have a 5-year survival that averages between 30% and 40%.[4,38] Many prognostic factors have been studied in this disease, including patient age, location, size, depth, extent, and margin status (Table 23-2). The importance accorded to each varies from study to study. There is a general agreement, however, that older patients have a worse prognosis than their younger counterparts, as has been noted previously for cutaneous angiosarcomas.[4,35,39] Tumor size, which has been most extensively studied in cutaneous lesions,[38-40] is strongly linked to outcome in all angiosarcomas.[4] Clinical extent, resectability, and margin status are important determinants of outcome, based on several studies and are detailed in Table 23-3. Studies also reaffirm the belief that angiosarcomas of deep soft tissue, body cavities, or body organs fare worse than cutaneous lesions.[38]

TABLE 23-2 Prognostic Factors in Angiosarcoma: All Sites

	FAVORABLE PROGNOSTIC FACTOR	UNFAVORABLE PROGNOSTIC FACTOR
Age[35,39]	<50 yr	>50 yr
Location[39]	Trunk[39]	Head/neck
Focality	Unifocal[35]	Multifocal
Clinical extent[37,39]	Local	Regional/distant
Size[4,39-41]	<5 cm[4,39]	>5 cm
Depth[38]	Superficial	Deep soft tissue-body cavity
Margin status[4]	Negative	Positive
Histology	Nonepithelioid	Epithelioid[4,36]
	No necrosis	Necrosis[36,43]

TABLE 23-3 Relationship Between Prognostic Factors and Outcome in Angiosarcoma

ALL SITES	MEDIAN SURVIVAL
Excision[4]	
Complete	66 mo
Incomplete	19 mo
Margins[38]	
Negative	4.9 yr
Positive	2.0 yr
Size[38]	
<5 cm	3.6 yr
>5 cm	2.3 yr
Location[38]	
Superficial	3.6 yr
Deep soft tissue	2.3 yr

Treatment for localized regional disease consists of complete surgical excision with negative margins. Because of the risk of local recurrence and the difficulty of achieving negative margins, adjuvant radiotherapy is typically combined with surgery.[35,58-60] There is no conclusive evidence to support the use of adjuvant chemotherapy for localized disease after surgery and radiation.[55,56]

Cytotoxic chemotherapy, which includes the use of anthracyclines, ifosfamide, and taxanes, is the primary treatment for metastatic angiosarcoma. Taxanes have become increasingly popular over the past decade because of their antiangiogenic activity. There is some evidence that head and neck angiosarcomas are more responsive to taxanes than those in other sites.[60] At the vanguard of therapeutic research is the use of tyrosine kinase inhibitors, such as sorafenib, to target the VEGFR signaling pathways.[60]

ATYPICAL VASCULAR LESION

Atypical vascular lesion (AVL) is a term that refers to a continuum of cutaneous lesions that develop following radiation and have some, but not all, of the features of angiosarcoma[61-65] (Figs. 23-18 to 23-23). The term was first used by Fineberg and Rosen[66] to refer to small, sharply circumscribed intradermal vascular lesions that resembled a lymphangiectasia or

Text continued on p. 722

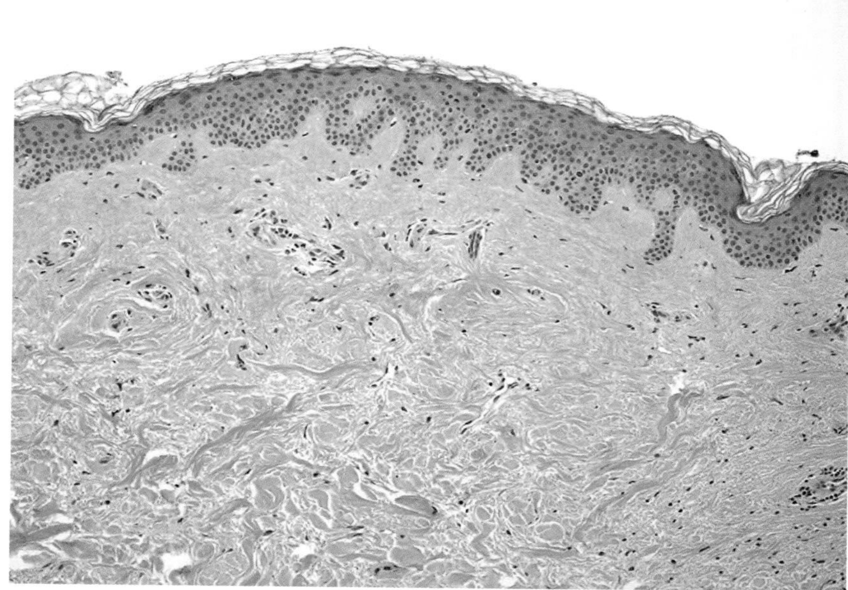

FIGURE 23-18. Radiation changes in the epidermis in a patient who had angiosarcoma following a lumpectomy and radiation. Note the homogenized, eosinophilic appearance of superficial dermis.

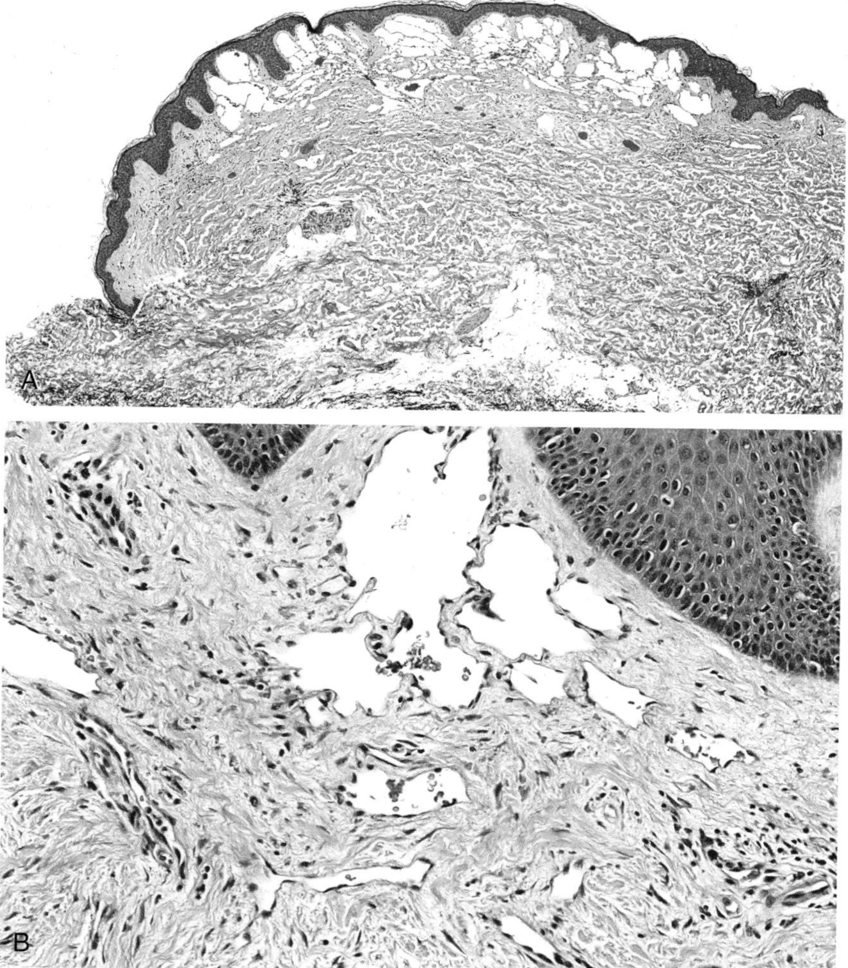

FIGURE 23-19. Atypical vascular lesion of the breast, lymphatic type, after breast-conserving surgery and irradiation for carcinoma. This lesion is a circumscribed dermal nodule (A) with minimal endothelial atypia but some anastomotic growth (B). Lesions of this type, so far, have proved to be benign.

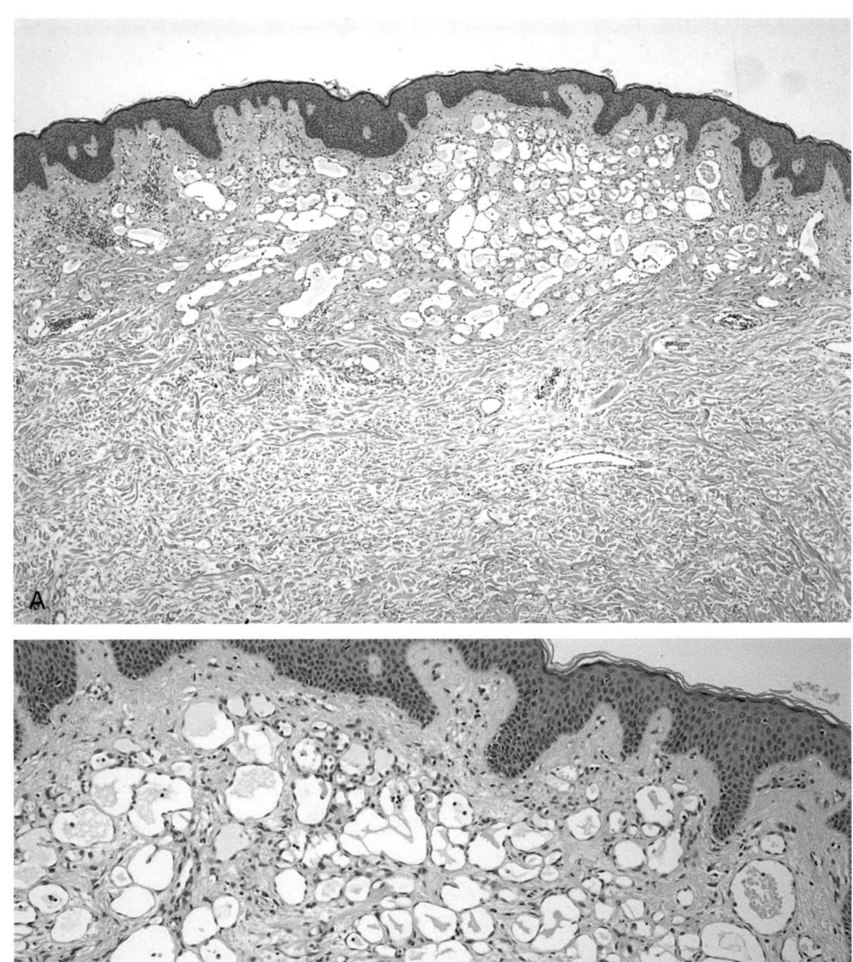

FIGURE 23-20. Atypical vascular lesion of the breast, lymphatic type, showing more irregular vascular proliferation in the dermis (A) consisting of anastomosing vessels (B).

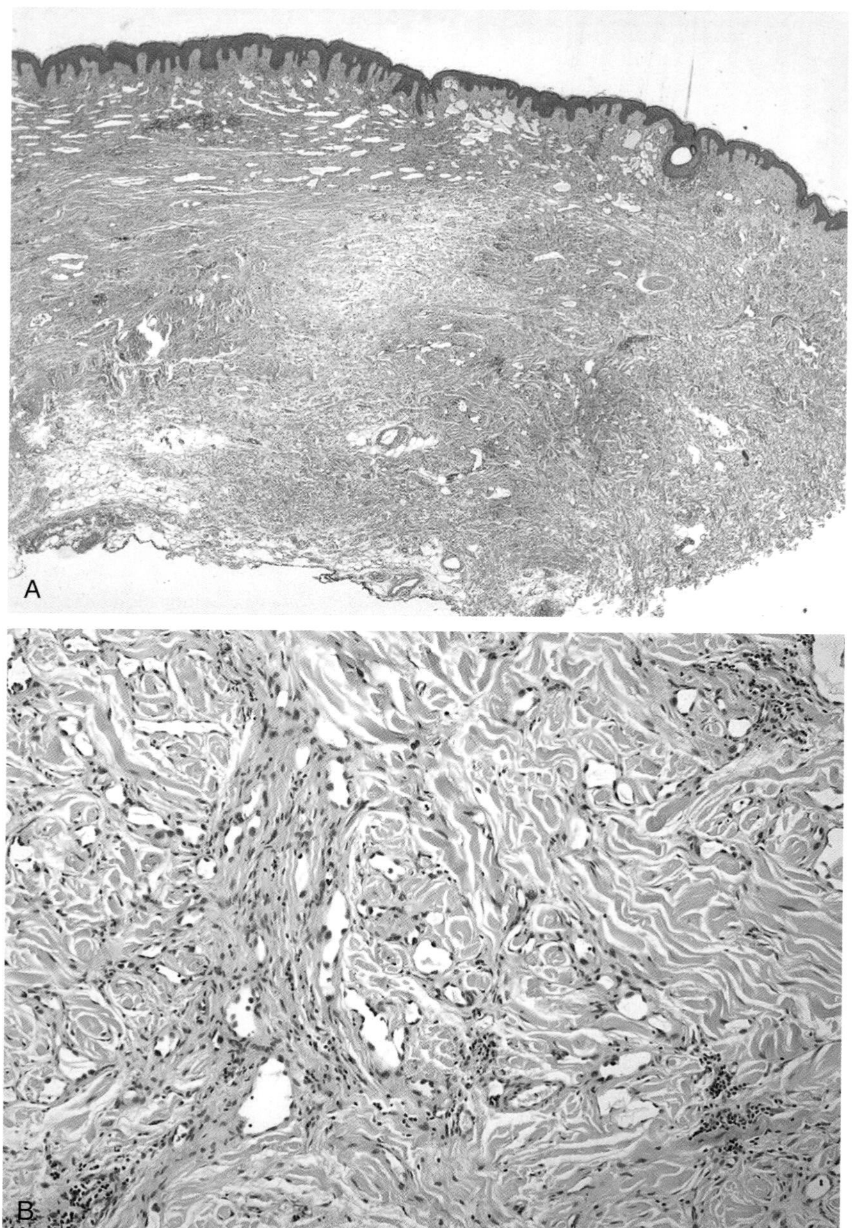

FIGURE 23-21. Atypical vascular lesion of breast, lymphatic type, with involvement of deep dermis (A) and more permeative growth of vessels (B).

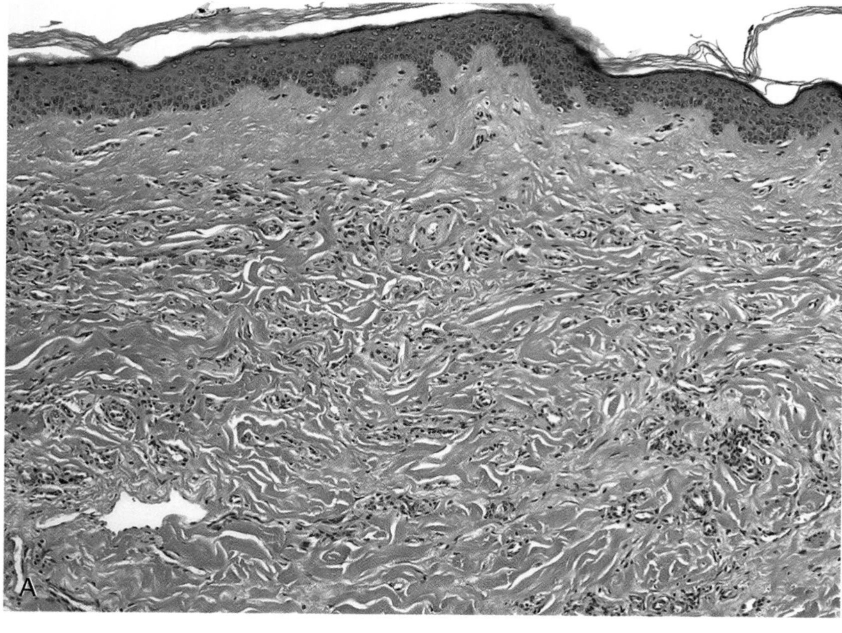

FIGURE 23-22. Atypical vascular lesion of breast, vascular type, showing proliferation of small capillary type vessels within the dermis (A, B).

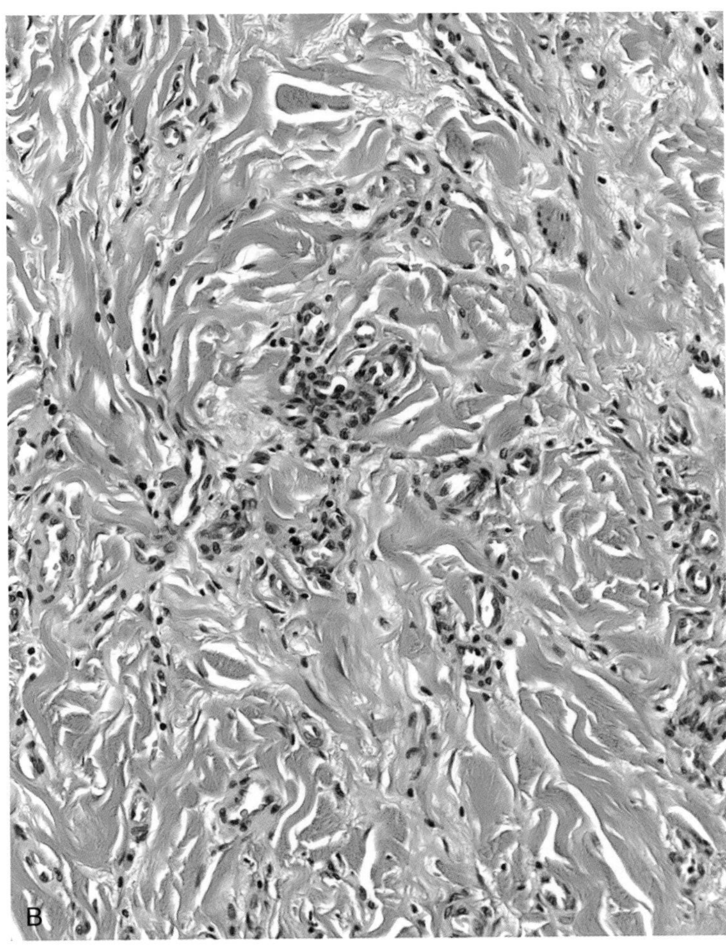

FIGURE 23-22, cont'd

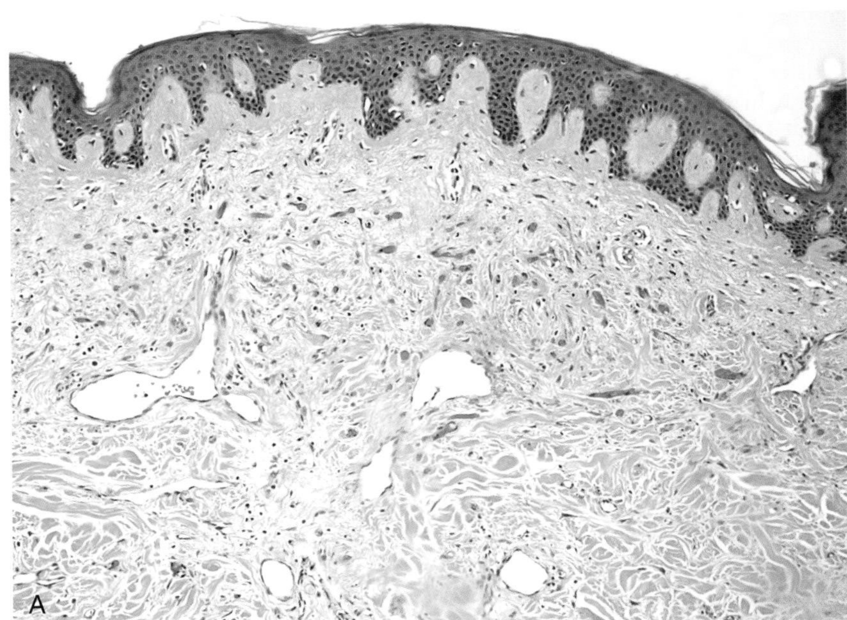

FIGURE 23-23. Atypical vascular lesion of breast, vascular type, showing more pronounced proliferation of small capillary-type vessels (A, B).

Continued

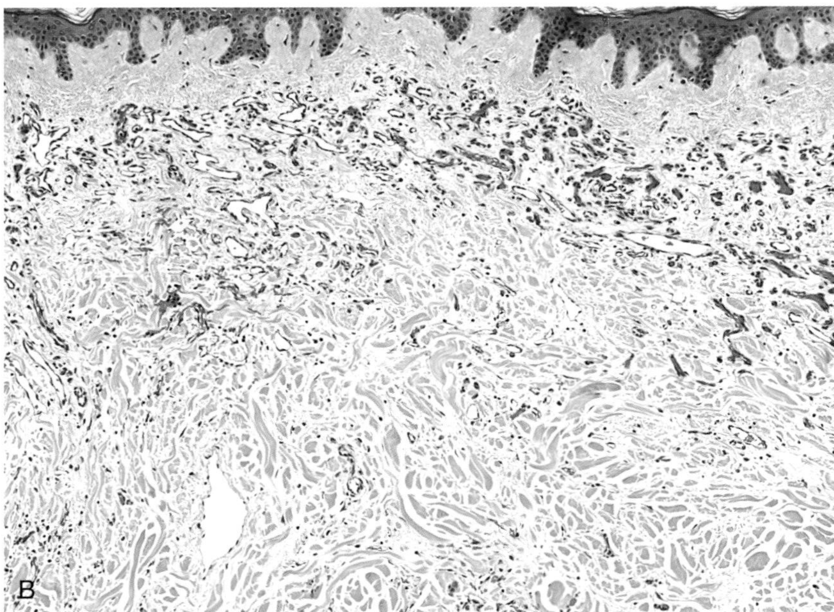

FIGURE 23-23, cont'd

lymphangioma and pursued a benign course. It is now evident that the spectrum of histologic changes that occur in this clinical setting is more diverse than originally appreciated and that some lesions, although not diagnostic of angiosarcoma, are, nonetheless, quite worrisome and, therefore, deserve careful scrutiny (Table 23-4).

Clinically, AVLs are small, pink-brown cutaneous papules (less than 1 cm) that are frequently multifocal and usually develop within 3 years of radiation. Histologically, AVLs embrace a histologic spectrum that ranges from banal appearing lesions resembling a lymphangioma circumscriptum to capillary vascular proliferations with nuclear atypia. This has led to the proposal that AVLs be divided into two types: a lymphatic type (LT) and a capillary vascular type (VT). The more common LT consists of ectatic lymphatic vessels usually confined to the superficial dermis and often referred to as *benign lymphangiomatous papules*. The vessels are lined by flattened or slightly protuberant (hobnail) lymphatic endothelium, which expresses CD31, podoplanin (D2-40), and, variably, CD34. Although the nuclei may appear hyperchromatic, they are not enlarged or irregular in shape (see Figs. 23-19 to 23-21). In a minority of LT-AVLs, the vessels infiltrate and intercommunicate more extensively within the dermis (see Figs. 23-20 and 23-21). Such lesions are reminiscent of progressive lymphangiomas. VT-AVLs resemble capillary hemangiomas and consist of blood-filled, pericyte-invested capillary vessels involving the superficial and/or deep dermis. Extravasated erythrocytes and hemosiderin may be present in the dermis (see Figs. 23-22 and 23-23). A small number of VT-AVLs display nuclear atypia.

Recently, it has been suggested that *MYC* amplification status be used to discriminate between AVLs and postirradiation angiosarcomas[67] because all AVLs studied to date have had no amplification. This can be carried out by either immunohistochemistry or fluorescence in situ hybridization (also known as FISH) because both yield comparable results.[67] The approach has been to evaluate *MYC* amplification status in histologically ambiguous situations, recognizing that the majority of typical AVLs do not require such refined studies.

The understanding of the behavior of these lesions is still evolving. Approximately 10% to 20% of patients with AVLs will develop additional lesions.[64,65] The critical question, of course, is whether these lesions carry an increased risk for angiosarcoma. Opinions on this point are divided. One view maintains that the two are unrelated, based on the observation that the vast majority of patients with AVLs have a favorable clinical course following excision of one or more lesions. This is borne out by a recent large study from the French Sarcoma Group.[68] That radiation-association angiosarcomas display *MYC* amplification and AVLs do not has buttressed this view.[27,28, 65] On the other hand, others maintain that the two are related and represent a histologic continuum.[63-65] This view is supported by the rare instances in which sequential biopsies of patients with AVLs document histologic progression of the

TABLE 23-4 Comparison of Atypical Vascular Lesion and Postirradiation Angiosarcoma

	ATYPICAL VASCULAR LESION	ANGIOSARCOMA
Size	Usually <1 cm	Typically >1 cm Average about 4.0 cm
Multifocality	Common	Common
Circumscription	++	–
Subcutaneous extension	Rare	Common
Anastomotic vessels	++	+++
Cytologic atypia and prominent nucleoli	–	+++
Multilayered endothelium	–	+++
Blood lakes	–	++

Data from Brenn T, Fletcher CD. Radiation-associated cutaneous atypical vascular lesions and angiosarcoma: clinicopathologic analysis of 42 cases. Am J Surg Pathol 2005;29:983.

lesion to angiosarcoma[63-65] as well as by TP53 mutational analysis defining common mutations in both.[69] Recently, Patton et al.[65] have proposed that the risk for angiosarcoma varies, depending on the type of AVL. They suggest that the LT-AVLs, which represent the overwhelming majority of lesions reported in the literature, probably carry very little risk, whereas the VT-AVLs have a higher, but as yet not defined, risk. VT-AVLs displaying nuclear atypia are at greatest risk for angiosarcoma and may be a direct precursor lesion. They recommend a diagnostic biopsy for the ordinary LT-AVL, complete excision with excellent follow-up care for VT-AVLs, and more extensive surgery for those having atypia.

KAPOSI SARCOMA

In 1872, Kaposi[70] described five cases of an unusual tumor that principally affected the skin of the lower extremities of elderly men in a multifocal, often symmetric fashion. Termed *idiopathic multiple pigmented sarcoma of the skin*, by Kaposi, this form of the disease later became known as *sporadic* or *classic* Kaposi sarcoma. Other forms were subsequently recognized and included an endemic form prevalent in sub-Saharan Africa, a rapidly progressive or epidemic form associated with AIDS, and an iatrogenic form following organ transplantation. Despite these apparent differences, epidemiologic data strongly pointed to an infectious etiology for all. A seminal study by Chang et al.[71] identified DNA fragments within Kaposi sarcoma tissue that shared a sequence identity to Epstein-Barr virus (also known as EBV) and herpesvirus saimiri (also known as HVS). The agent, subsequently classified as a gamma 2 herpesvirus, is known as Kaposi sarcoma-associated herpesvirus (KSHV) or human herpesvirus 8 (HHV8). This virus is also responsible for primary effusion lymphoma and multifocal Castleman disease. KSHV, unlike other herpesvirus infection, does not occur ubiquitously but has distinct pockets of prevalence. It is most common in sub-Saharan Africa (greater than 50%), moderately prevalent in the Mediterranean (20% to 30%), and less common in Europe and the United States (less than 10%).

KSHV is now considered the causative agent for all forms of Kaposi sarcoma, based on a number of key observations[72,73]: (1) the incidence of Kaposi sarcoma mirrors the prevalence of KSHV in all populations studied; (2) KSHV seroconversion is a predictor of Kaposi sarcoma and occurs before clinically evident lesions in all forms of the disease; (3) KSHV can be identified in Kaposi sarcoma cells and is capable of transforming endothelial cells[74]; (4) Kaposi sarcoma is never observed in the absence of KSHV; and (5) the genome of KSHV contains homologues of cellular genes (e.g., v-*cyclin*) that can stimulate cell growth and angiogenesis. The marked variation in the incidence of Kaposi sarcoma in various risk groups implies that KSHV *per se* is not sufficient for the development of Kaposi sarcoma. In the course of the infection, the virus preempts various host genes.

Transmission of KSHV occurs principally through saliva.[75] Once introduced, the virus is capable of infecting a number of cell types, including B lymphocytes and endothelium, where it establishes a latent infection. Reactivation of latent virus, believed to be pivotal in the development of Kaposi sarcoma, results in the expression of a number of viral genes that dysregulate the immune response and signaling pathways. These genes, which bear homology to cellular genes of humans, include cyclins, inhibitors of apoptosis, and cytokines and receptors. Tumor growth is further enhanced by HIV coinfection. HIV-1 induces various inflammatory cytokines and growth factors (e.g., fibroblast growth factor) that enhance tumor growth, and the HIV-1 Tat protein, secreted extracellularly, stimulates Kaposi sarcoma cells to produce metalloproteinase that promotes tumor invasion and angiogenesis. Finally, Kaposi sarcoma cells themselves produce a number of cytokines (e.g., VEGF), which, through their own receptors, autoregulate growth.[76]

Clinical Findings

Classic Kaposi Sarcoma

The chronic or classic form of Kaposi sarcoma occurs primarily in men (90%) during late adult life (peak incidence, sixth and seventh decades). The disease is prevalent in certain parts of the world, including Poland, Russia, Italy, and the central equatorial region of Africa. In the last region, it accounts for up to 9% of all reported cancers.[77] It is rare in the United States and accounts for only 0.02% of all cancers. This form is statistically and significantly associated with a second malignant tumor or altered immune state.

The disease commences with the development of multiple cutaneous lesions, usually on the distal portion of the lower extremity. Less commonly, the lesions occur on the upper extremity and rarely in a visceral organ in the absence of cutaneous manifestations. The initial lesion is a blue-red nodule often accompanied by edema of the extremity. The latter sign has been interpreted by some as indicating deep soft tissue or lymphatic involvement by the tumor. The lesions slowly increase in size and number, spreading proximally and coalescing into plaques or polypoid growths that may resemble pyogenic granuloma. Occasional lesions even ulcerate. In some patients, the early lesions regress, whereas others evolve so that many stages of the disease are present at the same time. The course of the disease is characteristically indolent and prolonged.

Endemic (African) Kaposi Sarcoma

Before the development of the AIDS pandemic, African Kaposi sarcoma was a disease primarily encountered in young males and very young children who presented with bulky lymph node disease. Its prevalence, furthermore, coincided with that of podoconiosis, a form of lymphedema associated with barefoot exposure to soil containing silica, a substance thought to result in localized immune suppression.[72] With the advent of AIDS, it has become increasingly difficult to delineate a pure (non-AIDS) endemic form of Kaposi sarcoma. Kaposi sarcoma in this region is more frequent in women and children than in anywhere else in the world and occurs in several forms, one of which resembles classic Kaposi sarcoma and the others of which resemble the progressive Kaposi sarcoma of AIDS. One of the latter forms, in particular, occurs in very young children (less than 3 years), who present with localized or generalized lymphadenopathy and occasionally ocular and salivary gland disease. Skin lesions are usually minimal. The fulminant course of the disease is attributed to a tendency for internal involvement.

Iatrogenic (Transplantation-Associated) Kaposi Sarcoma

The development of Kaposi sarcoma in transplant patients is well established, although the incidence varies, depending on the patient population, again suggesting the importance of cofactors. It occurs almost exclusively in renal transplant recipients and not recipients of solid organ or bone marrow transplants. Renal transplant recipients who are seropositive for KSHV before the transplant or who receive cyclophosphamide as part of their immunosuppressive regime are also more likely to develop Kaposi sarcoma than others. The disease develops several months to a few years after the transplant (average 16 months), and the extent of the disease can be correlated directly with the loss of cellular immunity. Interestingly, renal transplant patients on cyclosporine-based immunosuppression have a regression of Kaposi sarcoma when their regimen is changed to rapamycin, a drug now thought to have direct antitumor activity.[75]

AIDS-Related Kaposi Sarcoma

Caused by HIV-1, AIDS produces profound immunodeficiency and susceptibility to opportunistic infections and various tumors. AIDS originated in Africa, where its epidemic proportions have been attributed to heterosexual transmission and to transmission through contaminated medical equipment (e.g., syringes). In the United States, most cases occur in the male homosexual population, although other risk groups, including intravenous drug users and hemophiliacs receiving factor VIII-enriched blood fractions, are also well recognized. During the zenith of the AIDS epidemic, approximately 30% of patients with AIDS developed Kaposi sarcoma, but this incidence has been markedly reduced with the advent of antiretroviral therapy (ART). Kaposi sarcoma, however, does not equally affect the known risk groups. At one time, as many as 40% of homosexual patients with AIDS developed Kaposi sarcoma compared to less than 5% in the other recognized risk groups. It has only rarely occurred in transfusion recipients. The typical presentation is a young adult male who presents with multiple small, flat, pink patches (Fig. 23-24), which later acquire the classic blue-violet papular appearance (Fig. 23-25). They occur in almost any location but have a predilection for lines of cleavage, mucosal surfaces, and internal organs.

Microscopic Findings

There is no fundamental difference in the appearance of Kaposi sarcoma among the various clinical groups. The early lesions of Kaposi sarcoma are now seen most commonly in the AIDS patient, and the subtlety of changes, in many cases, presents an ongoing challenge to the surgical pathologist.

The earliest (*patch*) stage of Kaposi sarcoma is a flat lesion characterized by a proliferation of miniature vessels surrounding larger ectatic vessels. A slightly more advanced patch lesion displays, in addition, a loosely ramifying network of jagged vessels in the upper dermis (Figs. 23-26 and 23-27). In some respects, this stage resembles a well-differentiated angiosarcoma, except that the cells are so unimpressive that they resemble normal capillary or lymphatic endothelium. There is also a sparse infiltrate of lymphocytes and plasma cells surrounding the patch lesion. The histologic changes seen in patch lesions have also been noted in clinically normal areas of skin in patients who have Kaposi sarcoma elsewhere. This observation underscores the diffuseness of the disease process.

The more advanced (*plaque*) stage of the disease produces a slight elevation of the skin; it is, at this point, that the vascular proliferation usually involves most of the dermis and may extend to the subcutis. A discernible but relatively bland spindle cell component, initially centered around the proliferating vascular channels, appears at this stage. In time, the spindle cell foci coalesce and produce the classic nodular lesions of Kaposi sarcoma. Diagnosis of the well-established case is seldom difficult. Graceful arcs of spindle cells intersect one another as in a well-differentiated fibrosarcoma (Figs. 23-28 to 23-32); but, unlike fibrosarcoma, slit-like spaces containing erythrocytes separate the spindle cells and vascular channels (see Fig. 23-29). In a cross-section, these arcs of spindle cells are equally diagnostic by virtue of the sieve-like or honeycomb pattern they create. Inflammatory cells (lymphocytes and plasma cells), hemosiderin deposits, and dilated vessels are commonly seen at the periphery of nodular lesions (see Fig. 23-28). A characteristic, but not specific, feature of the well-established lesion is the presence of the hyaline globule. These periodic acid-Schiff-positive, diastase-resistant spherules may be located both intracellularly and extracellularly (see Fig. 23-32). Some of the hyaline globules are effete

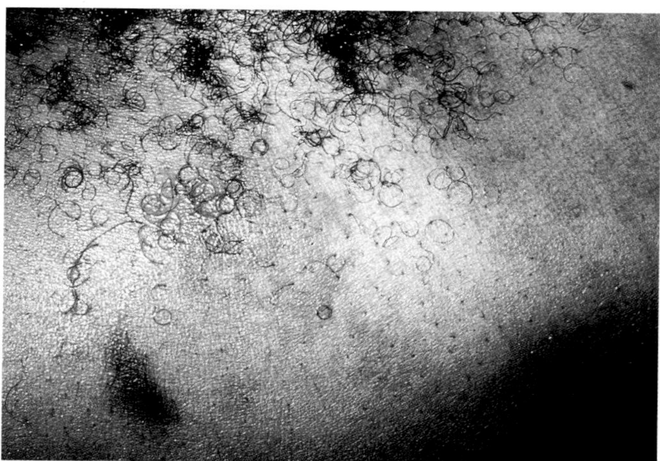

FIGURE 23-24. Early patch stage of Kaposi sarcoma, as seen in a patient with AIDS. Lesion is flat and mottled. *(Courtesy of Dr. Abe Macher.)*

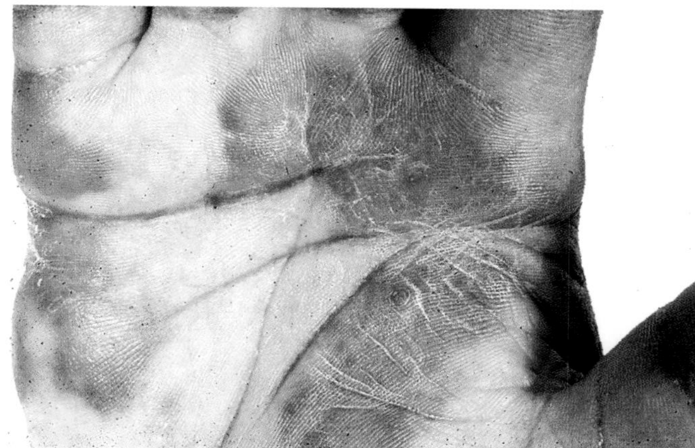

FIGURE 23-25. Advanced stage of Kaposi sarcoma in an AIDS patient with a combination of patch, plaque, and nodular lesions. *(Courtesy of Dr. Abe Macher.)*

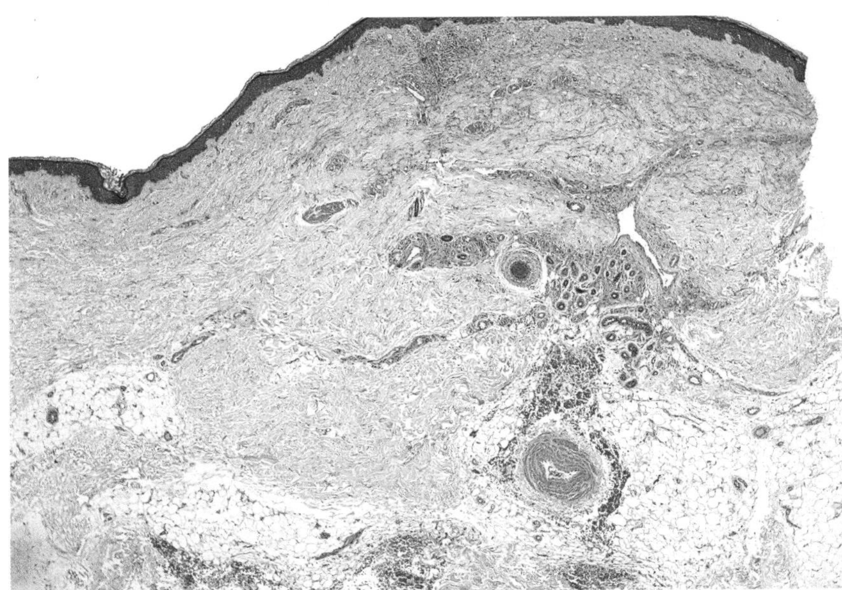

FIGURE 23-26. Early lesion of Kaposi sarcoma in an AIDS patient. Lesions are flat or slightly elevated.

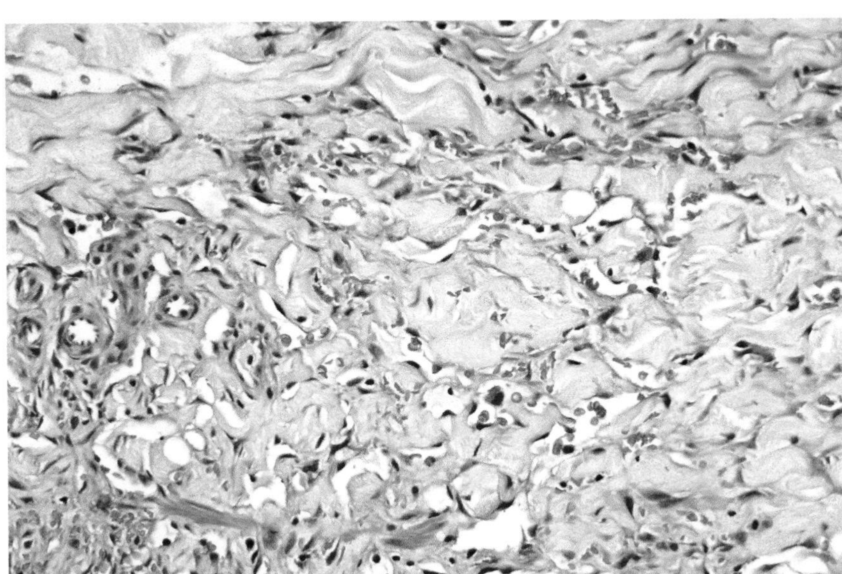

FIGURE 23-27. Early lesion of Kaposi sarcoma illustrating irregular proliferation of miniature vessels in the dermis somewhat reminiscent of the pattern of an angiosarcoma.

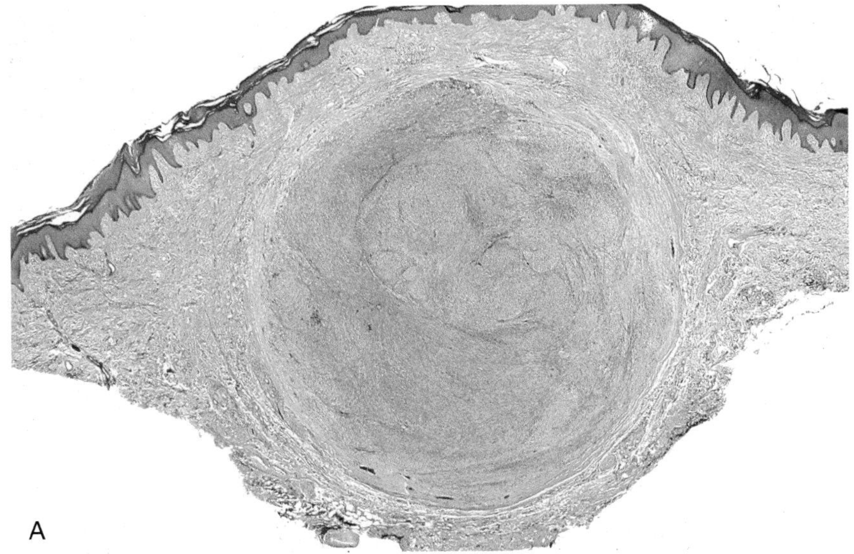

A

FIGURE 23-28. (A) Well established lesion of Kaposi sarcoma. *Continued*

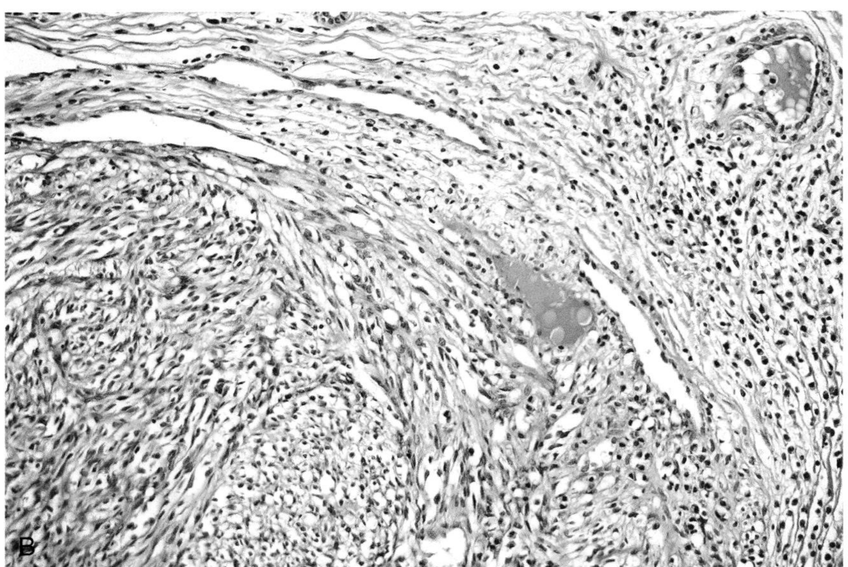

FIGURE 23-28, cont'd. (B) Tumor nodule is circumscribed by lymphocytes and ectatic or crescentic vessels.

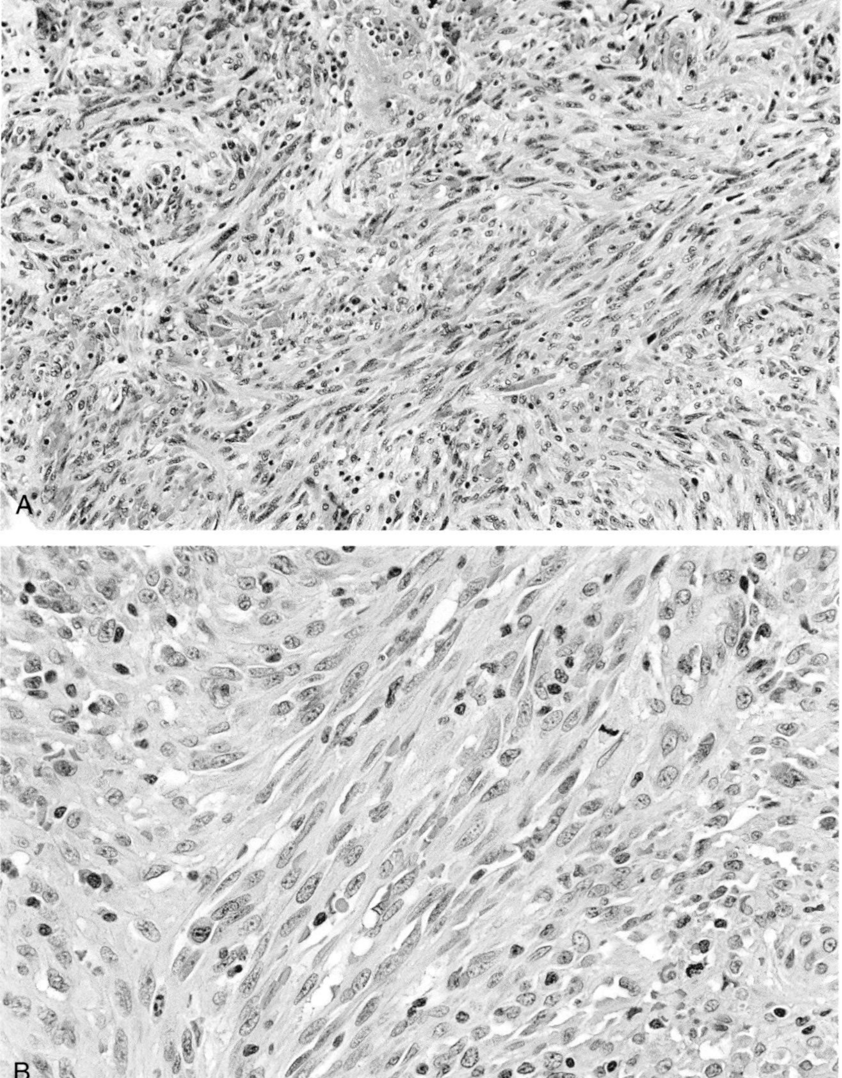

FIGURE 23-29. (A) Kaposi sarcoma illustrating monomorphic spindle cells arranged in ill-defined fascicles. (B) Cells are separated by slit-like vessels containing erythrocytes.

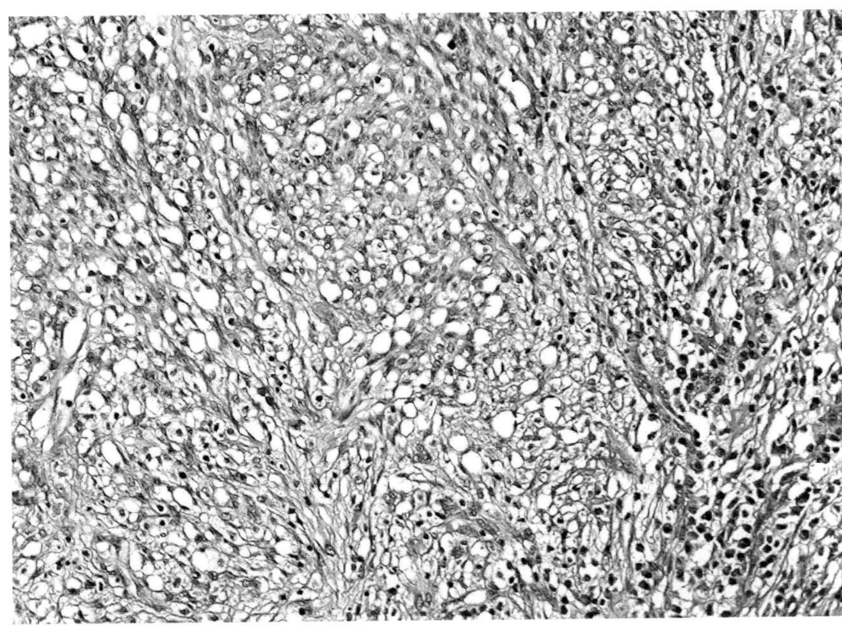

FIGURE 23-30. Transverse section through a fascicle of Kaposi sarcoma illustrating the sieve-like pattern.

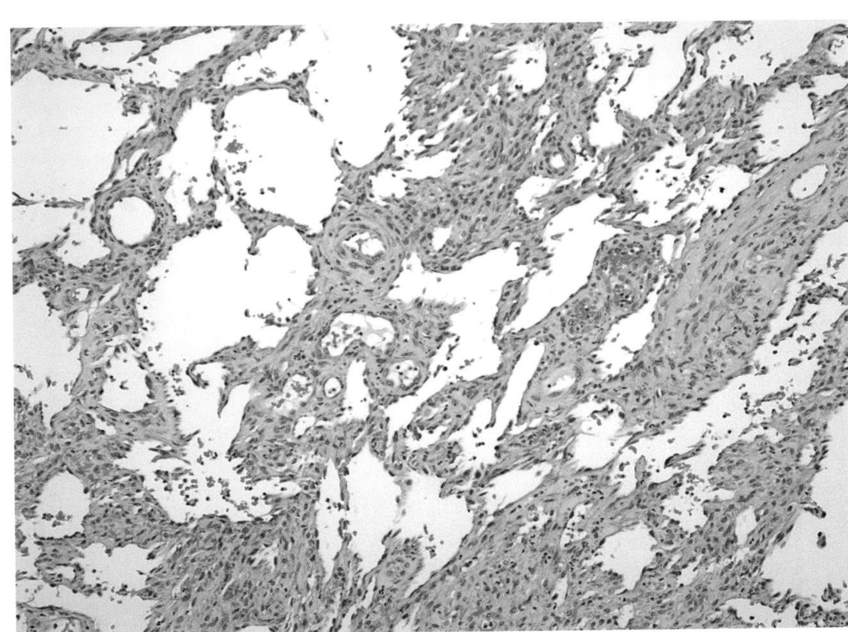

FIGURE 23-31. Kaposi sarcoma with lymphangioma-like areas.

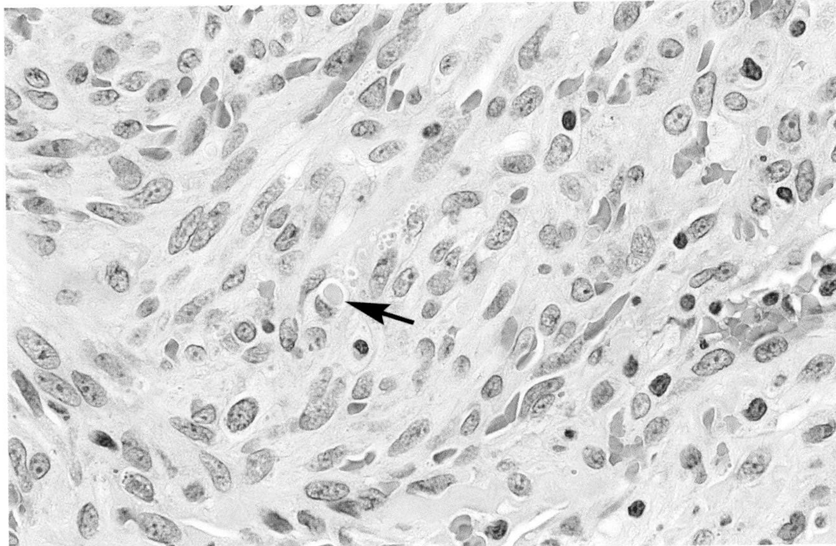

FIGURE 23-32. High-power view of Kaposi sarcoma with hyaline globules (H&E).

erythrocytes, an idea that derives support from the finding of erythrocytes in phagolysosomes by ultrastructural analysis and by certain common histochemical features (positive for toluidine blue and endogenous peroxidase).

Although the typical lesions of Kaposi sarcoma are devoid of pleomorphism and a significant number of mitotic figures, histologically aggressive forms of Kaposi sarcoma can be seen. They may result from progressive histologic dedifferentiation in otherwise typical cases. Poorly differentiated tumors may also arise *ab initio* and seem to be more common in cases of Kaposi sarcoma originating in Africa. In these tumors, the cells not only appear more pleomorphic, but also there may be a brisk level of mitotic activity. Kaposi sarcoma, particularly in the setting of AIDS, may show transitional areas that appear more akin to angiosarcoma. These areas may contain large ectatic vascular spaces similar to a hemangioma or lymphangioma and, in addition, have papillary tufts lined by atypical endothelial cells (see Fig. 23-31). These tumors have been termed *lymphangioma-like Kaposi sarcoma*.[78]

Just as the early changes of Kaposi sarcoma in the skin present a diagnostic challenge, so do early changes of this tumor in other organs (Fig. 23-33). A particularly common problem is the evaluation of lymph nodes in the AIDS patient. The earliest changes in lymph nodes may be represented by a mild angiectasia and proliferation of vessels in the subcapsular sinus. The interfollicular sinuses are gradually involved and expanded. The earliest stages may closely resemble the reactive lymph node condition, known variously as nodal angiomatosis and vascular transformation of the subcapsular sinus, which occurs as a result of lymph node obstruction. Others have noted the similarity of these lymph nodes to Castleman disease, when the proliferating vessels are centered around the follicles. Fortunately, immunostaining is extremely helpful as even subliminal lymph node lesions express HHV8 (see later text). Well-advanced cases of Kaposi sarcoma involving lymph nodes do not present a problem because they exhibit partial or complete lymph node effacement by a monotonous spindle cell proliferation. Because patients with AIDS are prone to develop mycobacterial pseudotumors of the lymph node, special stains may be needed to distinguish these changes from Kaposi sarcoma of the node.

Immunohistochemical Findings

Identification of KSHV as the causative agent of Kaposi sarcoma has made possible the targeting of viral antigens as markers for the diagnosis of Kaposi sarcoma. Latency-associated nuclear antigen (LANA-1), encoded by the open reading frame 73 of KSHV, is responsible for anchoring viral DNA to host heterochromatin and is constitutively expressed in infected tissues. Commercially available antibodies to this protein have high sensitivity and specificity for identifying Kaposi sarcoma. Over 90% of Kaposi sarcoma of all types display strong nuclear immunoreactivity for this protein in both the endothelium and spindled components (Fig. 23-34B),[79-81] whereas other vascular tumors, even those from HIV-infected patients, are negative for this antigen. Although usually not needed to diagnose classic examples of Kaposi sarcoma, LANA-1 antibodies have proved to be useful for diagnosing the early or subtle lesions of Kaposi sarcoma or for discriminating spindled cell angiosarcomas from Kaposi sarcoma.

CD31, a panendothelial marker, is expressed by both the spindled and endothelial components of Kaposi lesions (Fig. 23-34A). In addition, VEGFR-3 and podoplanin (D2-40), generally considered markers of lymphatic endothelium, are strongly expressed by these tumors.[82-85] Although usually cited as evidence that Kaposi sarcoma is a lymphatic lesion, KSHV infection is known to alter the pattern of endothelial marker expression. When vascular endothelial cells are infected with KSHV, they upregulate markers of lymphatic lineage; conversely, following infection, lymphatic endothelial cells shift in the direction of vascular transcriptional profile. The ability of the virus to reprogram target cells explains the unusual pattern of marker expression Kaposi sarcoma and why lineage assignment is problematic.[86]

Ultrastructural Observations

Electron microscopy has traditionally supported the idea of endothelial differentiation in these tumors. In the early lesions, slender endothelial cells with oval nuclei and small nucleoli

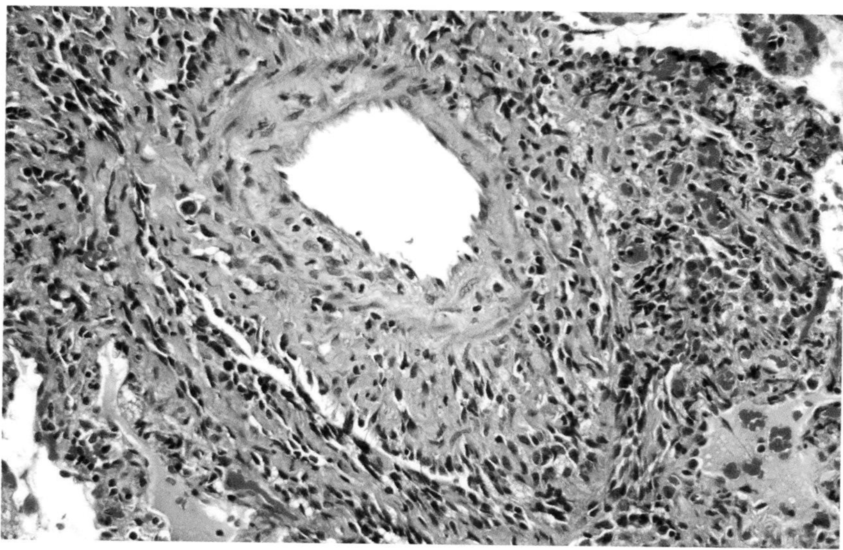

FIGURE 23-33. Kaposi sarcoma involving lung. Note the permeation of the septa and perivascular connective tissue.

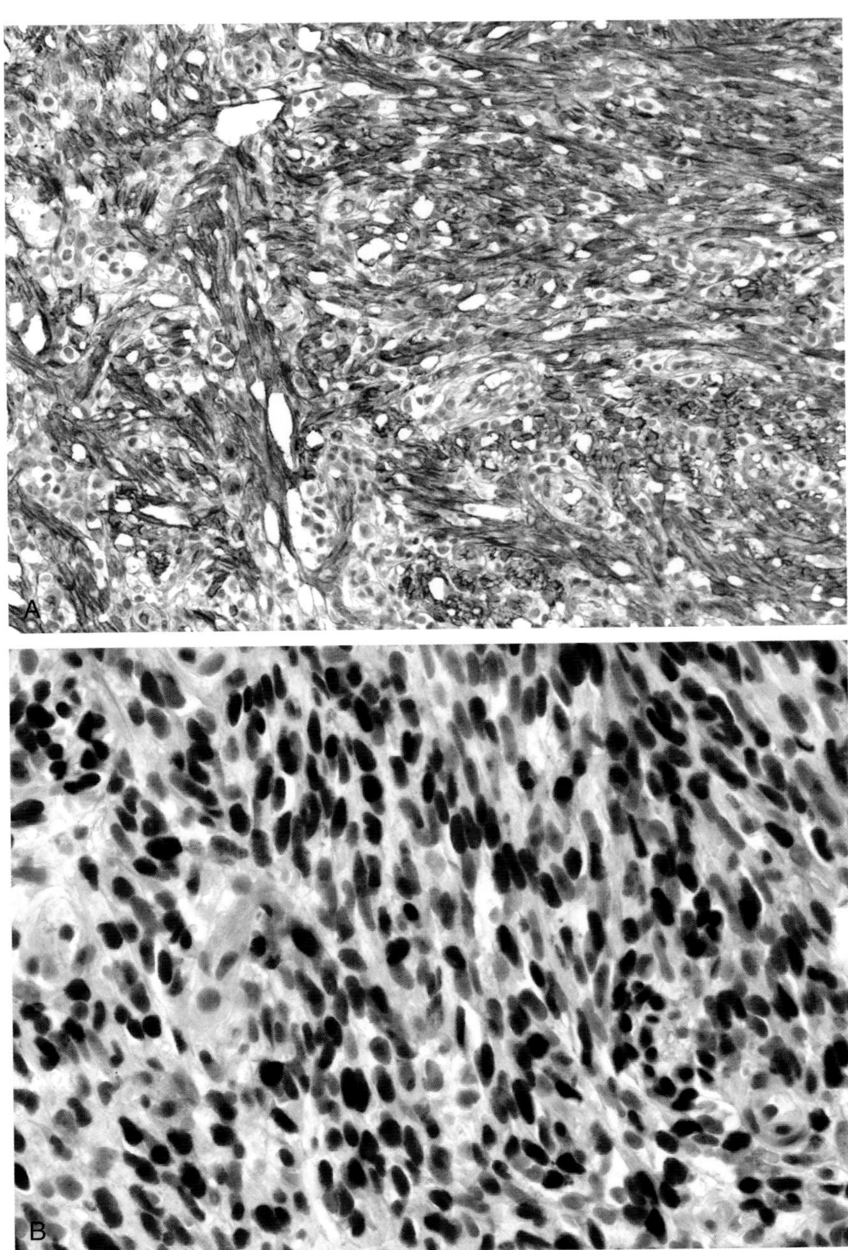

FIGURE 23-34. CD31 immunostaining of Kaposi sarcoma illustrating immunoreactivity of majority of spindled cells (A). Immunostaining for LANA-1 of KSHV decorates most nuclei within lesional cells of Kaposi sarcoma (B).

line slit-like lumens (Fig. 23-35). Few intercellular junctions are noted, and focally gaps may be present between the cells. Fragmented basal lamina encircles the abluminal surface of the cells, and few, if any, pericytes are observed.[87] The latter observations are more consistent with lymphatic differentiation. Advanced lesions not unexpectedly contain cells that have been variously described as *perithelial* or *fibroblastic*, although immunohistochemical observations indicate that they are actually modified endothelial cells. Ultrastructurally, the spindled perithelial cells have lysosomes and ferritin and appear to be actively phagocytic.

Differential Diagnosis

In the past, recognition of the early changes of Kaposi sarcoma, especially in the AIDS patient, remained one of the most difficult diagnostic problems but has been greatly simplified using immunostains for HHV8. The irregular infiltrative pattern of the endothelial cells in early lesions is more helpful for the diagnosis than the degree of cytologic atypia, although the changes may be virtually indistinguishable from those in a well-differentiated angiosarcoma. The well-advanced case may be confused with a fibrosarcoma. Features that distinguish a highly cellular form of Kaposi sarcoma from a fibrosarcoma include the presence of ectatic vessels and inflammatory cells at the periphery of the lesions, the more curvilinear fascicles, and the presence of hyaline globules.

HHV8 immunostaining has also proved to be valuable in discriminating Kaposi sarcoma from various mimics, although histologic features should never be ignored. Arteriovenous malformations occasionally give rise to cutaneous lesions that clinically duplicate the picture of Kaposi sarcoma. These lesions have been termed *pseudo-Kaposi sarcoma.*

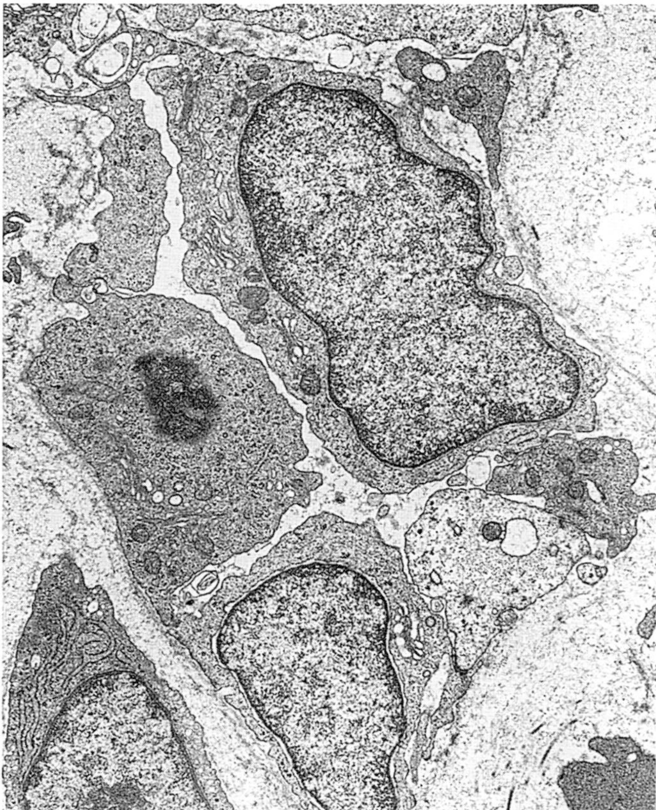

FIGURE 23-35. Electron micrograph of Kaposi sarcoma. Cells exhibit endothelial characteristics and are surrounded by fragmented basal lamina. Pericytes are absent or greatly reduced (x9000). *(From McNutt NS, Fletcher V, Conant MA. Early lesions of Kaposi sarcoma in homosexual men: an ultrastructural comparison with other vascular proliferations in the skin. Am J Pathol 1983;111:62, with permission.)*

TABLE 23-5 Revised AIDS Clinical Trials Group Staging Classification for Kaposi Sarcoma

	GOOD RISK (0; ALL OF THE FOLLOWING)	POOR RISK (1; ANY OF THE FOLLOWING)
Tumor (T)	Confined to skin and/or lymph nodes.	Tumor associated edema or ulceration; extensive oral KS; gastrointestinal KS; KS in other non-nodal visceral locations.
Immune system (I; not included if HIV sensitive to HAART)*	CD4 cells >150 μL.	CD4 cells <150 μL.
Systemic illness (S)	No history of opportunistic infection or thrush; no "B" symptoms (unexplained fever, night sweats, >10% involuntary weight loss, or diarrhea) persistent more than 2 weeks; performance status >70 (Karnofsky).	History of opportunistic infections and/or thrush; "B" symptoms present; performance status <70; other HIV-related illness (e.g., lymphoma).

Data from Krown SE, Testa MA, Huang J. AIDS-related Kaposi sarcoma: prospective validation of the AIDS Clinical Trials Group staging classification. AIDS Clinical Trials Group Oncology Committee. J Clin Oncol 1997;15:3085; Nasti G, Talamini R, Antinori A, et al. AIDS-related Kaposi sarcoma: evaluation of potential new prognostic factors and assessment of the AIDS Clinical Trial Group staging system in the HAART era—the Italian Cooperative Group on AIDS and Tumors and the Italian Cohort of Patients naïve from antiretrovirals. J Clin Oncol 2003;21:2876.

KS, Kaposi sarcoma; *HAART,* highly active antiretroviral therapy.
*CD4 cutoff of 200 μL previously proposed has been revised to 150 μL.

Histologically, these lesions consist of a proliferation of small capillary-sized vessels occasionally surrounded by extravasated erythrocytes and hemosiderin. Frank spindling and formation of slit-like lumens are not seen. Arteriographic studies documenting the presence of an underlying arteriovenous malformation and the clinical findings of a bruit in the area of the lesions provide additional contrasting points.

The spindle cell hemangioma (see Chapter 21) is frequently confused with Kaposi sarcoma. The presence of cavernous vessels and epithelioid endothelial cells (which are not seen in Kaposi sarcoma) are important histologic features for distinguishing the two tumors.

Behavior and Treatment

The behavior of Kaposi sarcoma is dependent on a number of interrelated factors, such as the form of the disease, clinical stage, immunocompetence of the host, and presence or absence of opportunistic infections.

In the classic or chronic form of the disease, which occurs in more immunocompetent individuals who present with limited cutaneous disease, the disease-related mortality rate is 10% to 20%. Even in patients in this group who die of their disease, the duration of the disease is 8 to 10 years, although an additional 25% of patients die of a second malignancy. Local therapy consisting of cryotherapy, intralesional injections, and radiation therapy is usually sufficient for limited mucocutaneous disease. Surgery is used principally to provide diagnostic biopsy material before therapy.

Before the advent of ART, the mortality among AIDS-associated Kaposi sarcoma patients approached 90%. Effective ART now not only prevents the development of Kaposi sarcoma lesions but also is responsible for substantial disease regression in AIDS patients.[75] It is now recommended that patients with AIDS-associated Kaposi sarcoma receive ART and that those with advanced symptomatic disease receive chemotherapy as well. To accurately evaluate the efficacy of various drug combinations, the AIDS Clinical Trials Group Oncology Committee has devised specific definitions of *clinical response* along with a staging system unique for AIDS-related Kaposi sarcoma.[88,89] This staging system replaces traditional ones and encompasses a number of parameters, including extent of tumor (T), status of the immune system (I), and severity of the illness (S) (Table 23-5). Good risk is designated with subscript 0 following the criteria and poor risk with 1. In the pre-ART era, poor risk in any category denoted poor risk overall. With the advent of ART, the CD4 level does not seem to provide additional prognostic information. Therefore, two risk groups are currently recognized: good (T0S0, T1S0, T0S1) and poor (T1S1).

References

1. Breiteneder-Geleff S, Soleiman A, Kowalski H. Angiosarcomas express mixed endothelial phenotypes of blood and lymphatic capillaries: podoplanin as a specific marker for lymphatic endothelium. Am J Pathol 1999;154:385.
2. Deyrup AT, Miettinen M, North PE, et al. Angiosarcomas arising in the viscera and soft tissue of children and young adults: a clinicopathologic study of 15 cases. Am J Surg Pathol 2009;33:264.
3. Deyrup AT, Miettinen M, North PE, et al. Pediatric cutaneous angiosarcomas: a clinicopathologic study of 10 cases. Am J Surg Pathol 2011;35:70.
4. Lahat G, Dhuka AR, Hallevi H, et al. Angiosarcoma: clinical and molecular insights. Ann Surg 2010;251:1098.
5. Schreiber H, Barry FM, Russell WC, et al. Stewart-Treves syndrome: a lethal complication of postmastectomy lymphedema and regional immune deficiency. Arch Surg 1979;114:82.
6. Bessis D, Sotto A, Roubert P, et al. Endothelin-secreting angiosarcoma occurring at the site of an arteriovenous fistula for haemodialysis in a renal transplant recipient. Br J Dermatol 1998;138:361.
7. Wehrli BM, Janzen DL, Shokeir O, et al. Epithelioid angiosarcoma arising in a surgically constructed arteriovenous fistula: a rare complication of chronic immunosuppression in the setting of renal transplantation. Am J Surg Pathol 1998;22:1154.
8. Chanyaputhipong J, Hock DL, Sebastian MG. Disseminated angiosarcoma of the dialysis fistula in 2 patients without kidney transplants. Am J Kidney Dis 2011;57:917.
9. Qureshi YA, Strauss DC, Thway K, et al. Angiosarcoma developing in a nonfunctioning arteriovenous fistula post-renal transplant. J Surg Oncol 2010;101:520.
10. Jennings TA, Peterson L, Axiotis CA, et al. Angiosarcoma associated with foreign body material: a report of three cases. Cancer 1988;62:2436.
11. Folpe AL, Johnston CA, Weiss SW. Cutaneous angiosarcoma arising in a gouty tophus: report of a unique case and a review of foreign material-associated angiosarcoma. Am J Dermatopathol 2000;22:418.
12. Meis-Kindblom JM, Kindblom LG. Angiosarcoma of soft tissue: a study of 80 cases. Am J Surg Pathol 1998;22:683.
13. Fletcher CD, Beham A, Bekir S, et al. Epithelioid angiosarcoma of deep soft tissue: a distinctive tumor readily mistaken for an epithelial neoplasm. Am J Surg Pathol 1991;15:915.
14. Brown RW, Tornos C, Evans HL. Angiosarcoma arising from malignant schwannoma in a patient with neurofibromatosis. Cancer 1992;70:1141.
15. Chaudhuri B, Ronan SG, Manaligod JR. Angiosarcoma arising in a plexiform neurofibroma. Cancer 1980;46:605.
16. Meis JM, Kindblom LG, Enzinger FM. Angiosarcoma arising in von Recklinghausen's disease (NF1): report of five additional cases. Mod Pathol 1994;7:8A.
17. Morphopoulos GD, Banerjee SS, Ali HH, et al. Malignant peripheral nerve sheath tumour with vascular differentiation: a report of four cases. Histopathology 1996;28:401.
18. Trassard M, LeDoussal V, Bui BN, et al. Angiosarcoma arising in a solitary schwannoma (neurilemoma) of the sciatic nerve. Am J Surg Pathol 1996;20:1412.
19. Ulbright TM, Clark SA, Einhorn LH. Angiosarcoma associated with germ cell tumors. Hum Pathol 1985;16:268.
20. Tallini G, Price FV, Carcangiu ML. Epithelioid angiosarcoma arising in uterine leiomyomas. Am J Clin Pathol 1993;100:514.
21. Dunkel IJ, Gerald WL, Rosenfield NS, et al. Outcome of patients with history of bilateral retinoblastoma treated for a second malignancy: the Memorial Sloan Kettering experience. Med Pediatr Oncol 1998;30:59.
22. Leake J, Sheehan MP, Rampling D, et al. Angiosarcoma complicating xeroderma pigmentosum. Histopathology 1992;21:179.
23. Tso CY, Sommer A, Hamoudi AB. Aicardi syndrome, metastatic angiosarcoma of the leg, and scalp lipoma. Am J Med Genet 1993;45:594.
24. Przygodski RM, Finkelstein SD, Keohayong P, et al. Sporadic and Thorotrast-induced angiosarcoma of the liver manifest frequent and multiple point mutations in K-ras-2. Lab Invest 1997;76:153.
25. Antonescu CR, Yoshida A, Guo T, et al. KDR activating mutations in human angiosarcomas are sensitive to specific kinase inhibitors. Cancer Res 2009;69:7175.
26. Manner J, Radiwimmer B, Hohenberger P, et al. MYC high level gene amplification is a distinctive feature of angiosarcomas after irradiation or chronic lymphedema. Am J Pathol 2010;176:34.
27. Guo T, Zhang L, Chang NE, et al. Consistent MYC and FLT4 gene amplification in radiation-induced angiosarcoma but not in other radiation-associated atypical vascular lesions. Genes Chromosomes Cancer 2011; 50:25.
28. Mentzel T, Schildhaus HU, Palmedo G, et al. Postradiation cutaneous angiosarcoma after treatment of breast carcinoma is characterized by MYC amplification in contrast to atypical vascular lesions after radiotherapy and control cases: clinicopathologic immunohistochemical and molecular analysis of 66 cases. Mod Pathol 2012;25(1):75.
29. Bullen R, Larson PO, Landeck AE, et al. Angiosarcoma of the head and neck managed by a combination of multiple biopsies to determine tumor margin and radiation therapy: report of three cases and review of the literature. Dermatol Surg 1998;24:1105.
30. Tatsas AD, Keedy VL, Florell SR, et al. Foam cell angiosarcoma: a rare and deceptively bland variant of cutaneous angiosarcoma. J Cutan Pathol 2010;37:901.
31. Folpe AL, Chand EM, Goldblum J, et al. Expression of Fli-1, a nuclear transcription factor, distinguishes vascular neoplasm from potential mimics. Am J Surg Pathol 2001;25:1061.
32. Rossi S, Orvieto E, Furlanetto A, et al. Utility of the immunohistochemical detection of Fli-1 expression in round cell and vascular neoplasm using a monoclonal antibody. Mod Pathol 2004;17:547.
33. Miettinen M, Wang AG, Paetau A, et al. ERG transcription factor as an immunohistochemical marker for vascular endothelial tumors and prostatic carcinoma. Am J Surg Pathol 2011;35:432.
34. Miettinen M, Sarlomo-Rikala M, Wang ZF. Claudin-5 as an immunohistochemical marker for angiosarcoma and hemangioendothelioma. Am J Surg Pathol 2011;35:1848.
35. Pawlik TM, Paulino AF, McGinn CJ, et al. Cutaneous angiosarcoma of the scalp: a multidisciplinary approach. Cancer 2003;98:1716.
36. Deyrup AT, McKenney JK, Tighiouari M, et al. Sporadic cutaneous angiosarcomas: a proposal for risk stratification based on 69 cases. Am J Surg Pathol 2008;32:72.
37. Holden CA, Spittle MF, Jones EW. Angiosarcoma of the face and scalp: prognosis and treatment. Cancer 1987;59:1046.
38. Fury MG, Antonescu CR, Van Zee KF, et al. A 14-year retrospective review of angiosarcomas: clinical characteristics, prognostic factors, and treatment outcomes with surgery and chemotherapy. Cancer J 2005; 11:241.
39. Albores-Saavedra J, Schwartz AM, Henson DE, et al. Cutaneous angiosarcoma. Analysis of 434 cases from the Surveillance, Epidemiology and End Results Program 1973-2007. Ann Diagn Pathol 2011;15:93.
40. Mark RJ, Poen JC, Tran LM, et al. Angiosarcoma: a report of 67 patients and a review of the literature. Cancer 1996;77:2400.
41. Maddox JC, Evans HL. Angiosarcoma of skin and soft tissue: a study of 44 cases. Cancer 1981;48:1907.
42. Morgan MB, Swann M, Somach S, et al. Cutaneous angiosarcoma: a case series with prognostic correlation. J Am Acad Dermatol 2004;50:867.
43. Fayette J, Martin E, Piperno-Neumann S, et al. Angiosarcomas, a heterogeneous group of sarcomas with specific behavior depending on primary site: a retrospective study of 161 cases. Ann Oncol 2007;2030.
44. Bacchi CE, Silva TR, Zambrano E, et al. Epithelioid angiosarcoma of the skin: a study of 18 cases with emphasis on its clinicopathologic spectrum and unusual morphologic features. Am J Surg Pathol 2010;34:1334.
45. Suchak R, Thway K, Zelger B, et al. Primary cutaneous epithelioid angiosarcoma: a clinicopathologic study of 13 cases of a rare neoplasm occurring outside the setting of conventional angiosarcomas and with predilection for the limbs. Am J Surg Pathol 2011;35:60.
46. Stewart FW, Treves N. Lymphangiosarcoma in postmastectomy lymphedema. Cancer 1949;1:64.
47. Shon W, Ida CM, Boland-Froemming JM, et al. Cutaneous angiosarcoma arising in massive localized lymphedema of the morbidly obese: a report of five cases and review of the literature. J Cutan Pathol 2011;38:560.
48. Woodward AH, Ivins JC, Soule EH. Lymphangiosarcoma. Cancer 1981;48:1674.
49. Steingaszner LC, Enzinger FM, Taylor HB. Hemangiosarcoma of the breast. Cancer 1965;18:352.
50. Hodgson NC, Bowen-Wells C, Moffat F, et al. Angiosarcoma of the breast: a review of 70 cases. Am J Clin Oncol 2007;30:570.
51. Luini A, Gatti G, Diaz J, et al. Angiosarcoma of the breast: the experience of the European Institute of Oncology and review of the literature. Breast Cancer Res Treat 2002;105:81.
52. Sher T, Hennessy BT, Valero V, et al. Primary angiosarcomas of the breast. Cancer 2007;110:173.
53. Nascimento AF, Raut CP, Fletcher CD. Primary angiosarcoma of the breast: clinicopathologic analysis of 49 cases, suggesting that grade is not prognostic. Am J Surg Pathol 2008;32:1896.
54. Rosen PP, Kimmel M, Ernsberger D. Mammary angiosarcoma. The prognostic significance of tumor differentiation. Cancer 1988;62:2145.

55. Marchal C, Weber B, de Lafontan B. Nine breast angiosarcomas after conservative treatment for breast carcinoma: a survey from French comprehensive cancer centers. Int J Radiat Oncol Biol Phys 1999;44:113.
56. Fodor J, Orosz Z, Szabo E, et al. Angiosarcoma after conservation treatment for breast carcinoma: our experience and a review of the literature. J Am Acad Dermatol 2006;54:499.
57. Billings SD, McKenney JK, Folpe AL, et al. Cutaneous angiosarcoma following breast-conserving surgery and radiation: an analysis of 27 cases. Am J Surg Pathol 2004;28:781.
58. Mendenhall WM, Mendenhall CM, Werning JW, et al. Cutaneous angiosarcoma. Am J Clin Oncol 2006;29:524.
59. Abraham JA, Hornicek FJ, Kaufman AM, et al. Treatment and outcome of 82 patients with angiosarcoma. Ann Surg Oncol 2007;14:1953.
60. Young RJ, Brown NJ, Reed MW, et al. Angiosarcoma. Lancet Oncology 2010;11:983.
61. Sener SF, Milos S, Feldman JL, et al. The spectrum of vascular lesions in the mammary skin including angiosarcoma after breast conservation treatment for breast cancer. J Am Coll Surg 2001;193:22.
62. Requena L, Kutzner H, Mentzel T, et al. Benign vascular proliferations in irradiated skin. Am J Surg Pathol 2002;26:328.
63. Brenn T, Fletcher CD. Radiation-associated cutaneous atypical vascular lesions and angiosarcoma: clinicopathologic analysis of 42 cases. Am J Surg Pathol 2005;29:983.
64. Brenn T, Fletcher CD. Postradiation vascular proliferations: an increasing problem. Histopathology 2006;48:106.
65. Patton KT, Deyrup AT, Weiss SW. Atypical vascular lesions after surgery and radiation of the breast: a clinicopathologic study of 32 cases analyzing histologic heterogeneity and association with angiosarcoma. Am J Surg Pathol 2008;32:943.
66. Fineberg S, Rosen PP. Cutaneous angiosarcoma and atypical vascular lesions of the skin and breast after radiation therapy for breast carcinoma. Am J Clin Pathol 1994;102:7.
67. Fernandez AP, Sun Y, Tubbs RR, et al. FISH for MYC amplification and anti-MYC immunohistochemistry: useful diagnostic tools in the assessment of secondary angiosarcoma and atypical vascular proliferations. J Cutan Pathol 2012;39:234.
68. Gengler C, Coindre JM, Leroux A, et al. Vascular proliferation of the skin after radiation therapy for breast cancer: clinicopathologic analysis of a series in favor of a benign process: a study from the French Sarcoma Group. Cancer 2007;109:1584.
69. Santi R, Cetica V, Franchi A, et al. Tumour suppressor gene TP53 mutations in atypical vascular lesion of breast skin following radiotherapy. Histopathology 2011;58:455.
70. Kaposi M. Idiopathisches multiples Pigmentsarkom der Haut. Arch Dermatol Syph 1872;4:265.
71. Chang Y, Cesarman E, Pessin MS, et al. Identification of herpesvirus-like DNA sequences in AIDS-associated Kaposi sarcoma. Science 1994;266:1865.
72. Dourmishev L, Dourmishev AL, Paleri D, et al. Molecular genetics of Kaposi sarcoma-associated herpesvirus (human herpesvirus 8) epidemiology and pathogenesis. Microbiol Mol Biol Rev 2003;67:175.
73. Pantanwitz L, Dezube BJ. Advances in the pathobiology and treatment of Kaposi sarcoma. Curr Opin Oncol 2004;16:443.
74. Flore O, Rafii S, Ely S, et al. Transformation of primary human endothelial cells by Kaposi sarcoma-associated herpes virus. Nature 1998;394:588.
75. Uldrick TS, Whitby D. Update on KSHV epidemiology, Kaposi Sarcoma pathogenesis, and treatment of Kaposi sarcoma. Cancer Lett 2011;305:150.
76. Masood R, Cai J, Zheng T, et al. Vascular endothelial growth factor/vascular permeability factor is an autocrine growth factor for AIDS-Kaposi sarcoma. Proc Natl Acad Sci USA 1997;94:979.
77. Bluefarb SM. Kaposi sarcoma. Springfield, IL: Charles C Thomas; 1966.
78. Cossu S, Satta R, Cottoni F, et al. Lymphangioma-like variant of Kaposi sarcoma: clinicopathologic study of seven cases with review of the literature. Am J Dermatopathol 1997;19:16.
79. Cheuk WW, Wong KO, Wong SC, et al. Immunostaining for human herpesvirus 8 latent nuclear antigen-1 helps distinguish Kaposi sarcoma from its mimickers. Am J Clin Pathol 2004;121:335.
80. Patel RM, Goldblum JR, His ED. Immunohistochemical detection of human herpesvirus-8 latent nuclear antigen-1 is useful in the diagnosis of Kaposi sarcoma. Mod Pathol 2004;17:456.
81. Hammock L, Reisenauer A, Wang W, et al. Latency associated nuclear antigen expression and human herpesvirus 8 polymerase chain reaction in the evaluation of Kaposi sarcoma and other vascular tumors in HIV positive patients. Mod Pathol 2005;18:463.
82. Weninger W, Partanen TA, Breiteneder-Geleff S, et al. Expression of vascular endothelial growth factor receptor-3 and podoplanin suggests a lymphatic endothelial cell origin of Kaposi sarcoma tumor cells. Lab Invest 1999;79:243.
83. Folpe AL, Veikkola T, Valtola R, et al. Vascular endothelial growth factor receptor-3 (VEGFR-3): a marker of vascular tumors with presumed lymphatic differentiation, including Kaposi sarcoma, kaposiform and Dabska-type hemangioendotheliomas, and a subset of angiosarcomas. Mod Pathol 2000;13:180.
84. Kahn HJ, Bailey D, Marks A. Monoclonal antibody D2-40, a new marker of lymphatic endothelium, reacts with Kaposi sarcoma and a subset of angiosarcomas. Mod Pathol 2002;15:434.
85. Fukunaga M. Expression of D2-40 in lymphatic endothelium of normal tissues and in vascular tumors. Histopathology 2005;46:396.
86. Ganem D. KSHV and the pathogenesis of Kaposi sarcoma: listening to the human biology and medicine. J Clin Invest 2010;120:939.
87. McNutt NS, Fletcher V, Conant MA. Early lesions of Kaposi sarcoma in homosexual men: an ultrastructural comparison with other vascular proliferations in the skin. Am J Pathol 1983;111:62.
88. Krown SE, Testa MA, Huang J. AIDS-related Kaposi sarcoma: prospective validation of the AIDS Clinical Trials Group staging classification. AIDS Clinical Trials Group Oncology Committee. J Clin Oncol 1997;15:3085.
89. Nasti G, Talamini R, Antinori A, et al. AIDS-related Kaposi sarcoma: evaluation of potential new prognostic factors and assessment of the AIDS Clinical Trial Group staging system in the HAART era—the Italian Cooperative Group on AIDS and Tumors and the Italian Cohort of Patients naïve from antiretrovirals. J Clin Oncol 2003;21:2876.

Tumors and Malformations of Lymphatic Vessels

CHAPTER CONTENTS

The lymphatics are an extensive unidirectional system of blunt-ending vessels that regulate normal tissue pressure by retrieving excess fluid from the interstitium, transporting it to regional lymph nodes, and returning it to the venous system by way of the thoracic duct. The lymphatic system makes its appearance during the sixth week of human embryonic development as an outgrowth from the venous system. On a molecular level, lymphangiogenesis is heralded by the polarized expression of the homeobox transcription factor *PROX1* in a subpopulation of endothelial cells located within the cardinal vein.[1,2] This event is accompanied by a budding of the endothelium from primitive veins and by the induction of lymphatic specific genes, *LYVE1* and *VEGFR3* (FLT4). Expression of *PROX1* appears to be a master event in lymphangiogenesis, for in its absence there is agenesis of the entire lymphatic system. *VEGFR3*, in turn, is largely responsible for the migration and formation of primary lymphatic sacs, which, through budding growth, give rise to the lymphatic vasculature. When lymphatic sacs are formed, the lymphatic and blood vasculature develop independently and only remain connected at certain specific points to allow return of the lymph fluid. The molecular events underlying late lymphangiogenesis are less well understood. One gene, *FOXC2*, which is mutated in inherited lymphedema, appears highly associated with the morphogenesis of lymphatic valves, and deficiencies in angiopoietin 2 are associated with defects in both patterning and function of the lymphatic system.

Small lymphatics closely resemble capillaries but can be distinguished ultrastructurally and immunohistochemically. Unlike the vascular endothelial cell, the lymphatic endothelial cell is invested by neither a basement membrane nor pericytes, with the exception of large collecting lymphatic channels. These observations are borne out by immunohistochemistry. Whereas antibodies to type IV collagen and laminin demonstrate a linear pattern of immunoreactivity around vascular capillary endothelium, this pattern is lacking around lymphatic capillary endothelium.[3] Although lymphatic endothelial cells occasionally manifest tight junctions (zonula adherens) and macula adherens, and desmosomes are present, there are many areas of simple overlapping of cells with no junctions.[4,5] This arrangement creates a swinging-door effect so that fluid can passively enter the lymphatic space during periods of increased interstitial pressure. Pinocytotic vesicles, thin cytofilaments, modest numbers of mitochondria, and endoplasmic reticulum, similar to those in capillaries, are also present in lymphatic cells.

Further differences between vascular and lymphatic capillary endothelium can be demonstrated by means of immunohistochemistry, using antibodies targeted against lineage-specific proteins, basal lamina, and pericytes. Lymphatic endothelium typically expresses PROX1, LYVE1, VEGFR3, but usually lacks CD34 and does not possess an investiture of actin-positive pericytes. The reverse phenotype is observed in blood vascular endothelium.[3,6,7]

LYMPHATIC MALFORMATIONS (LYMPHANGIOMA, CYSTIC HYGROMA)

Regarded as an abnormality of morphogenesis rather than as a neoplasm, lymphangiomas are now referred to as *lymphatic malformations* (Fig. 24-1). They are subclassified as *microcystic*, *macrocystic* (cysts greater than 0.5 cm), or *combined*.[8,9] Diffuse lymphatic malformations involving multiple organs are still often referred to as *lymphangiomatosis*.

The pathogenetic mechanisms underlying lymphatic malformations are poorly understood but likely vary, depending

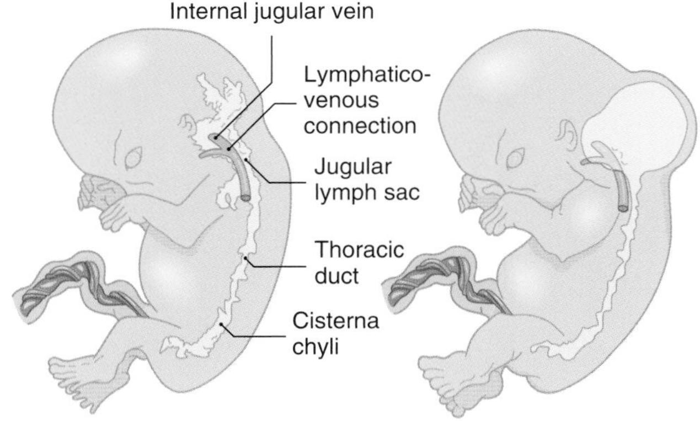

FIGURE 24-1. Proposed mechanism for formation of a lymphatic malformation. Lymphatic system in a normal fetus (left) with a patent connection between the jugular lymph sac and the internal jugular vein and a lymphatic malformation from a failed lymphaticovenous connection (right). *(Modified from Chervenak FA, Issacson G, Blakemore KJ. Fetal cystic hygroma: cause and natural history. N Engl J Med 1983;309:822.)*

on the type of malformation. Type I hereditary lymphedema, a malformation of small lymphatic vessels that presents shortly after birth, is the result of a germline mutation of *VEGFR3*.[10] Type II hereditary lymphedema, a malformation presenting later in life and associated with distichiasis (double eyelashes), is caused by mutations in the *FOXC2* transcription factor gene.[11] Lymphatic abnormalities also occur in association with mutations in *SOX18* transcription factor gene and the *NEMO* (IKBKG) gene. But the vast majority of lymphatic malformations are sporadic. Given an understanding of the molecular basis of normal lymphangiogenesis, it is not unreasonable to assume that, in the future, many will be traced to somatic mutations in genes controlling normal lymphangiogenesis.

Clinical Findings

Relative to vascular malformations, lymphatic ones are rare. Bill and Sumner[12] estimated that they accounted for 5 of 3000 admissions at Children's Orthopedic Hospital. The gender incidence is roughly equal.[12,13] Half of all lymphatic malformations are present at birth and as many as 90% are evident by the end of the second year of life.[12,14-17] Those that present during adult life are superficial cutaneous malformations (lymphangioma circumscriptum).[18-20]

Lymphatic malformations affect almost any part of the body served by the lymphatic system but show a predilection for the head, neck, and axilla (Figs. 24-2 and 24-3), sites that account for one-half to three-fourths of all lymphatic malformations (Table 24-1). They also occur sporadically in various organs, including lung, gastrointestinal tract, spleen, liver, and bone. In the last three locations, they occasionally signify the presence of diffuse or multifocal disease (see section on lymphangiomatosis). Lymphatic malformations also occur in association with hemangiomas in Maffucci syndrome.

The most common presentation of a lymphatic malformation is that of a soft fluctuant mass that enlarges, remains static, or waxes and wanes during the period of clinical observation. The overlying skin may appear normal or slightly blue. In some cases, rapid enlargement is the result of an upper respiratory tract infection, which causes obstruction in the lymphatics draining the lesion.

Lymphatic malformations also produce site-specific signs and symptoms. For example, malformations of the major lymphatic ducts produce chylous pleural or pericardial effusions; those in the soft tissues of the extremities produce overgrowth and gigantism whereas those in the bone produce osteolysis, so-called *disappearing bone disease* (Gorham disease).

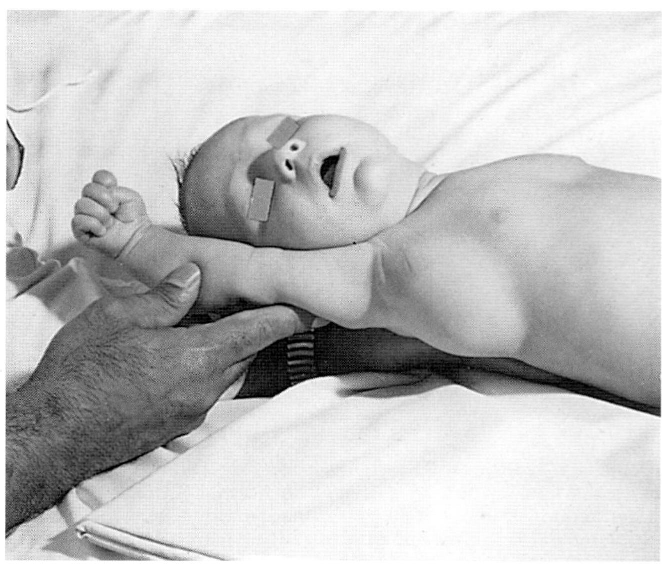

FIGURE 24-2. Lymphatic malformation (cystic hygroma) of the axilla.

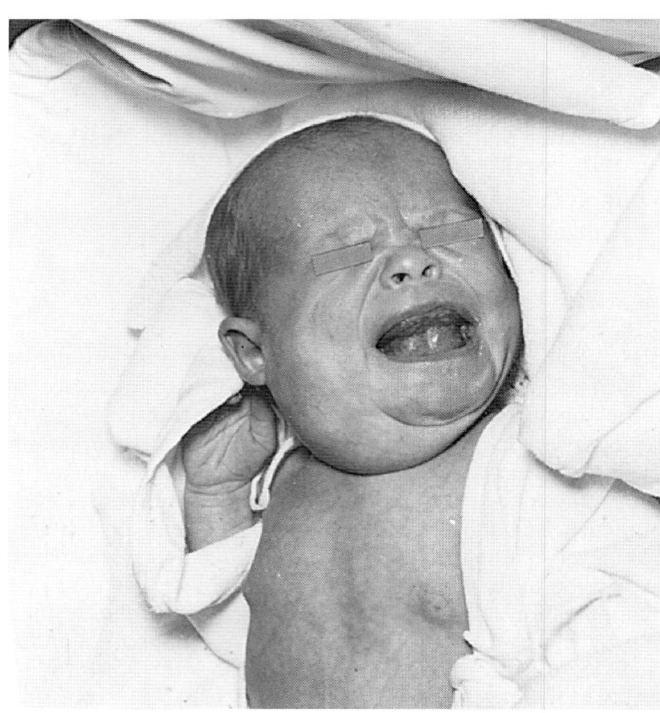

FIGURE 24-3. Lymphatic malformation (cystic hygroma) of the neck.

TABLE 24-1 Anatomic Location of Lymphatic Malformations (61 Patients)*

ANATOMIC LOCATION	NO.
Head	35
Tongue	8
Cheek	7
Floor of the mouth	7
Parotid	5
Other	8
Neck	25
Trunk and extremities	43
Axilla	15
Pectoral	10
Arm	6
Scapula	5
Other	7
Internal	6
Mediastinum	5
Abdomen	1

Modified from Bill AH, Sumner DS. A unified concept of lymphangioma and cystic hygroma. Surg Gynecol Obstet 1965;120:79.

*There are more than 61 tumors because large tumors were tabulated under several locations.

Lymphatic malformations can be effectively imaged by MRI or, in the case of macrocystic lymphatic malformations, by ultrasonography. *In utero* imaging of lymphatic malformations is especially important because they are associated with hydrops fetalis and Turner syndrome and a high death rate (Figs. 24-4 and 24-5).[21,22] Chervenak et al.[22] found that 11 of 15 intrauterine macrocystic lymphatic malformations (cystic hygromas) were associated with the cytogenetic abnormalities of Turner syndrome (45,X/O or 46,XO/46,XX). Of the 15 fetuses, 13 had severe hydrops, and none of the 15 ultimately survived. The authors suggested that severe aberrations of the lymphatic system in this condition are incompatible with life; milder forms are compatible with survival but give rise to webbing of the neck and edema of the hands and feet, which characterize the Turner syndrome infantile phenotype (Fig. 24-6). Other syndromes may also be associated with fetal macrocystic lymphatic malformations, including Noonan syndrome, familial pterygium colli, fetal alcohol syndrome, and several chromosomal aneuploidies.[23] Because aneuploidic conditions may recur during subsequent pregnancies, cytogenetic analysis of fetuses born with a macrocystic lymphatic malformation is indicated.

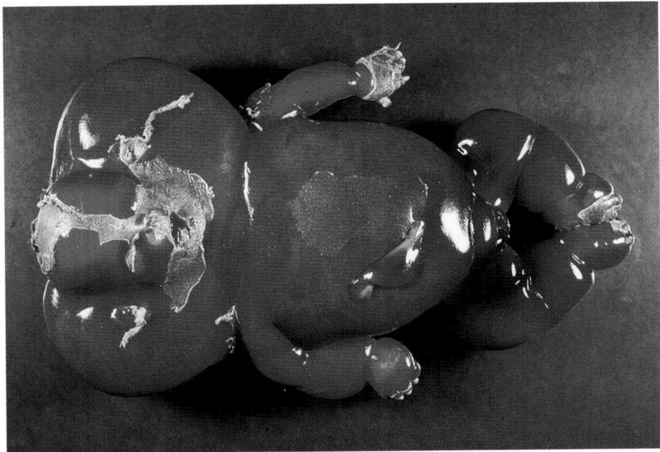

FIGURE 24-4. Abortus with Turner syndrome (XX/XO). A large macrocystic lymphatic malformation (cystic hygroma) had been detected in utero by ultrasonography.

Lymphatic Malformations of the Head and Neck

Lymphatic malformations are most common in the neck, where they typically lie in the supraclavicular fossa of the posterior cervical triangle or extend toward the crest of the shoulder. Less frequently, they are located in the anterior cervical triangle just below the angle of the jaw. Tumors in this location may present with airway or feeding problems.[24] Lymphatic malformations are the most common cause of enlargement of the tongue. About 10% of lymphatic malformations of the neck extend into the mediastinum and require careful imaging to define the surgical approach. Grossly, the lesions are unicystic or multicystic masses that involve the superficial soft tissue and tend to bulge outward rather than extend inward (see Fig. 24-3). Consequently, they usually do not compromise vital structures, such as the trachea and esophagus, unless they are large. In contrast, malformations involving the soft tissues of the lips, cheek, tongue, and mouth frequently involve deep soft tissue structures and cause functional impairment, depending on their size.

Intra-Abdominal Lymphatic Malformations

Intra-abdominal lymphatic malformations are rare (Fig. 24-7). Galifer et al.[25] tabulated only 139 cases from the English literature. Although 60% are present in patients under the age of 5 years, a significant percentage does not manifest until adult life.[16] The most common location is the mesentery, followed by the omentum, mesocolon, and retroperitoneum. In addition to a palpable mass, patients with lesions in the first three locations often develop symptoms of an acute abdomen because of intestinal obstruction, volvulus, and infarction. In fact, a provisional diagnosis of acute appendicitis is frequently

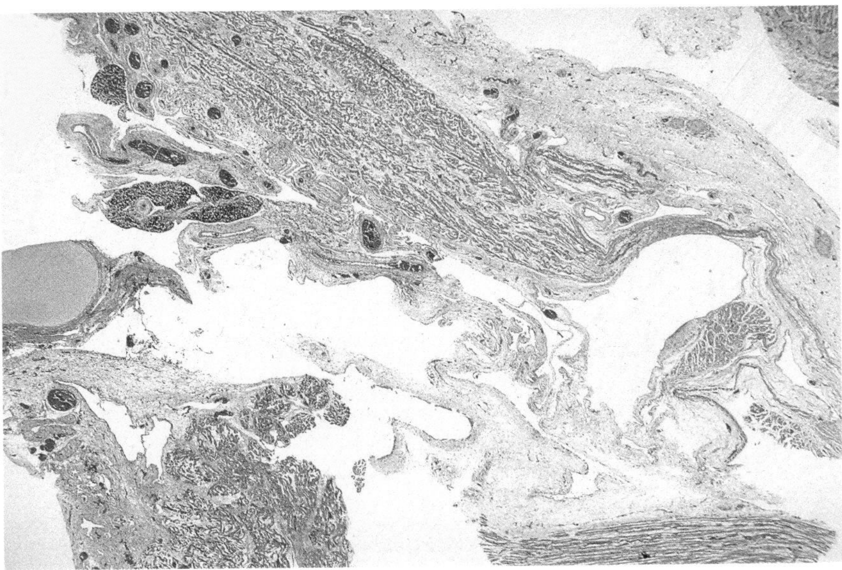

FIGURE 24-5. Macrocystic lymphatic malformation (cystic hygroma) from a fetus with Turner syndrome.

entertained because of the common occurrence of right lower quadrant pain. In contrast, retroperitoneal tumors produce few acute symptoms but, ultimately, are diagnosed by virtue of a large palpable mass causing displacement of one or more organs. Most arise in the lumbar area and cause displacement of the kidney, usually without urinary tract obstruction. Those arising in the superior portion of the retroperitoneum shift the pancreas and duodenum anteriorly.

In the past, an abdominal lymphatic malformation was seldom diagnosed preoperatively. The diagnosis can usually be suspected with a combination of radiologic studies.[26] Ultrasonography is useful for localizing and determining the cystic nature of the tumors. As seen by arteriography, the lesions are poorly vascularized, and, in a few reported cases, connections between lower extremity lymphatics and the tumors can be demonstrated with lymphangiography. On CT scans, the tumors appear as multiple, homogeneous, nonenhancing areas with variable attenuation values, depending on whether the fluid is chylous or serous.

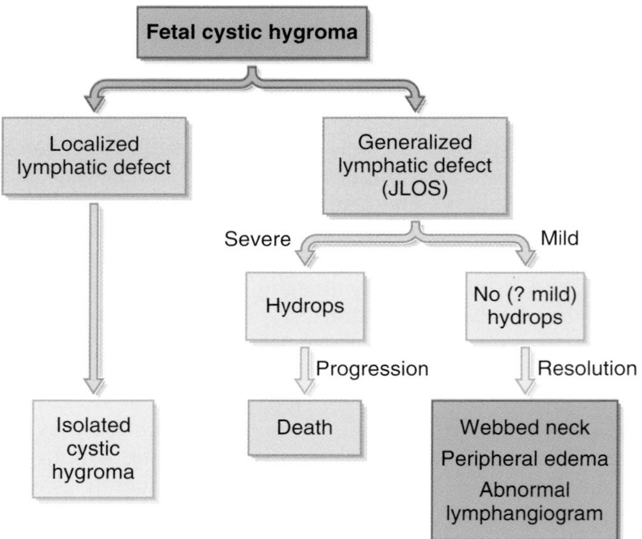

FIGURE 24-6. Natural history of a fetal nuchal lymphatic malformation. Generalized lymphatic defect results from the jugular lymphatic obstruction sequence (also known as JLOS). Depending on the severity of the obstruction, varying degrees of hydrops are noted. *(Modified from Chervenak FA, Issacson G, Blakemore KJ. Fetal cystic hygroma: cause and natural history. N Engl J Med 1983;309:822.)*

Cutaneous Lymphatic Malformations

Cutaneous lymphatic malformations can be divided into superficial and deep forms. The latter form is histologically and clinically identical to the usual lymphatic malformation described previously and histologically later (Fig. 24-8). The superficial intradermal form, sometimes referred to as *lymphangioma circumscriptum*,[19] has rather characteristic features. These lesions develop as multiple small vesicles or wart-like nodules that cover localized areas of skin (Fig. 24-9), although, in some cases, large areas of the body are affected. Histologically, dilated irregular lymphatic channels fill the papillary dermis and protrude into the epidermis, giving the impression of being intraepidermal. The overlying epidermis is acanthotic and thrown into papillae. Generally, the lesions

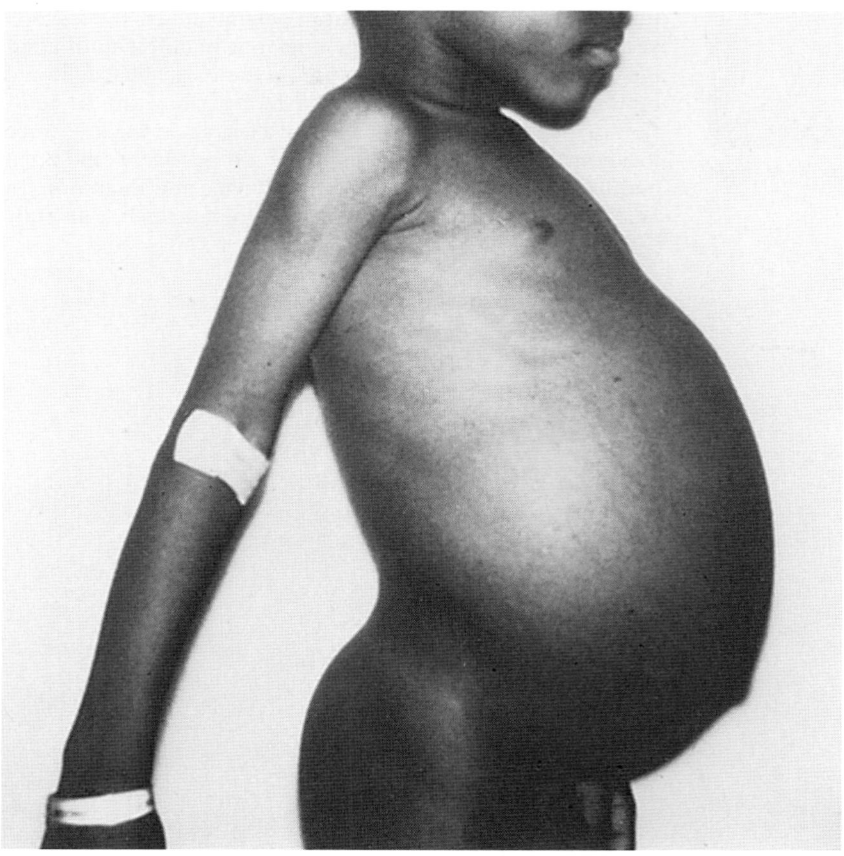

FIGURE 24-7. Large intra-abdominal lymphatic malformation.

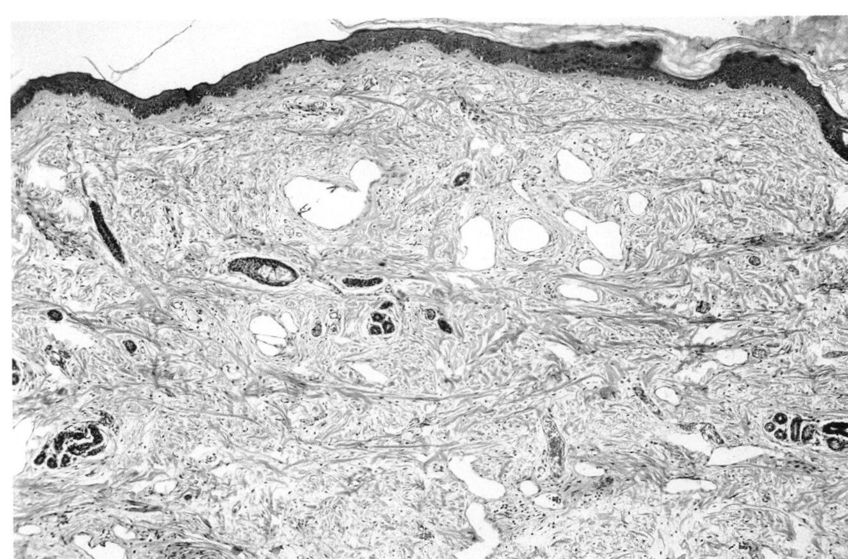

FIGURE 24-8. Cutaneous lymphatic malformation of the deep type. Dilated lymphatic channels extend over large areas of skin and involve superficial and deep dermis.

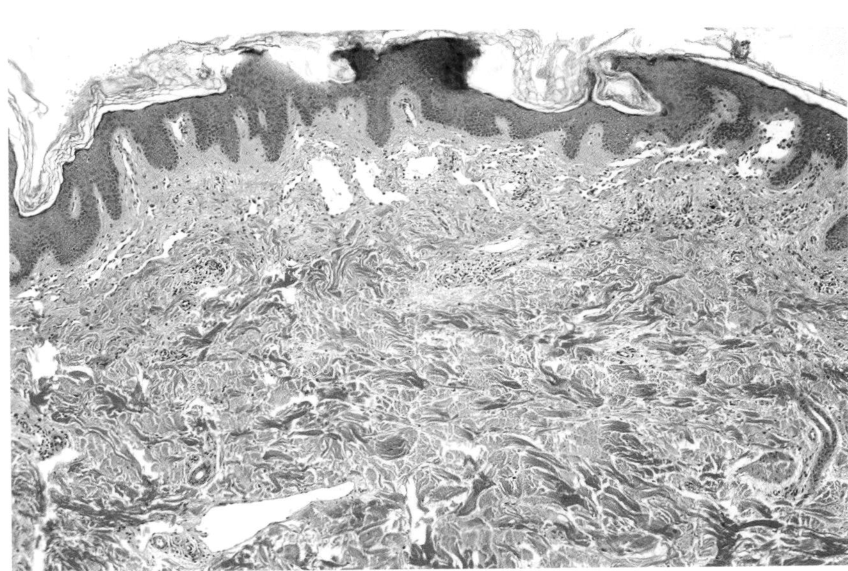

FIGURE 24-9. Cutaneous lymphatic malformation of superficial type (lymphangioma circumscriptum). Lymphatic vessels are localized and restricted to superficial dermis.

are asymptomatic unless they become irritated. They may arise *de novo* or secondary to surgery.

(Acquired) progressive lymphangioma is a term used for a cutaneous slowly progressive lymphatic proliferation that occurs primarily in adults (Figs. 24-10 to 24-12).[27] In most patients, the lesions present as a bruise-like area or pigmented patch that evolves over several years and achieves a size of several centimeters. Some have been reported to be well over 10 cm. Clinically, the lesion consists of ectatic lymph vessels in the subpapillary region of the dermis that create the papular or vesicular appearance. The vessels ramify in the dermis and occasionally extend into the subcutis. The vessels, filled with clear fluid, are lined by attenuated endothelial cells that do not exhibit atypia, mitotic activity, or solid areas of growth. Lymphoid aggregates accompany the lymphatic channels. Follow-up of a limited number of cases of acquired progressive lymphangioma reflects a benign clinical course with no evidence of metastasis.[27] The label *(acquired) progressive lymphangioma* has also been applied to atypical vascular lesions that occur following radiation (see Chapter 23). Given the differences in presentation and management, this practice should be discouraged.

Gross and Microscopic Findings

Lymphatic malformations vary from well-circumscribed lesions made up of one or more large interconnecting cysts to ill-defined, sponge-like compressible lesions (Figs. 24-13 to 24-21) composed of microscopic cysts. Lymphatic malformations composed of large lymphatic channels greater than 0.5 cm are referred to as *macrocystic lymphatic malformations* and those with smaller cysts, *microcystic*. Often lesions have features of both.

Regardless of the size of the lymphatic spaces, both lesions are lined by attenuated or hobnailed endothelium resembling that in normal lymphatics. Small lymphatic spaces have only an inconspicuous adventitial coat surrounding them, whereas

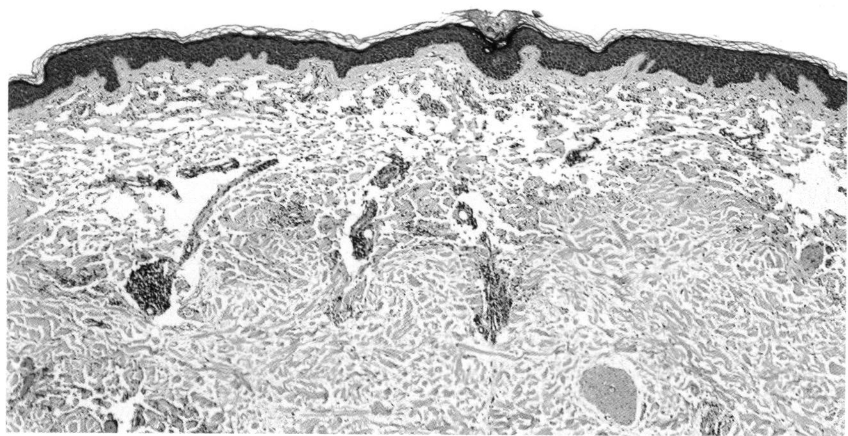

FIGURE 24-10. Acquired progressive lymphangioma with superficial proliferation of lymphatic vessels.

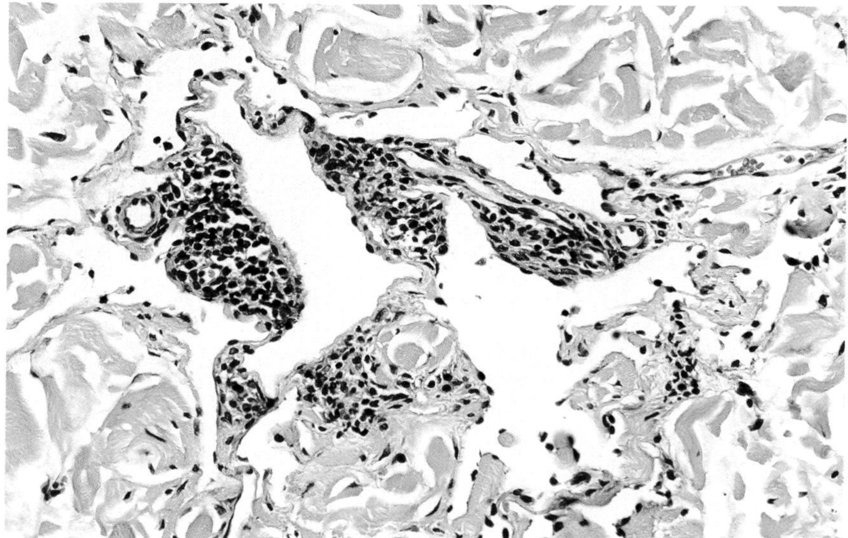

FIGURE 24-11. Acquired progressive lymphangioma with dissection of dermis by well-differentiated lymphatic vessels.

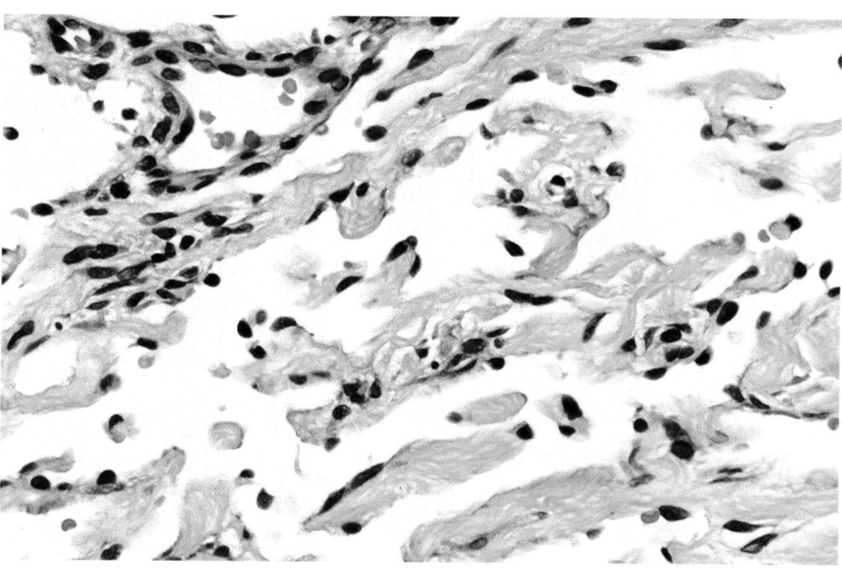

FIGURE 24-12. Acquired progressive lymphangioma with a single layer of endothelial cells without atypia.

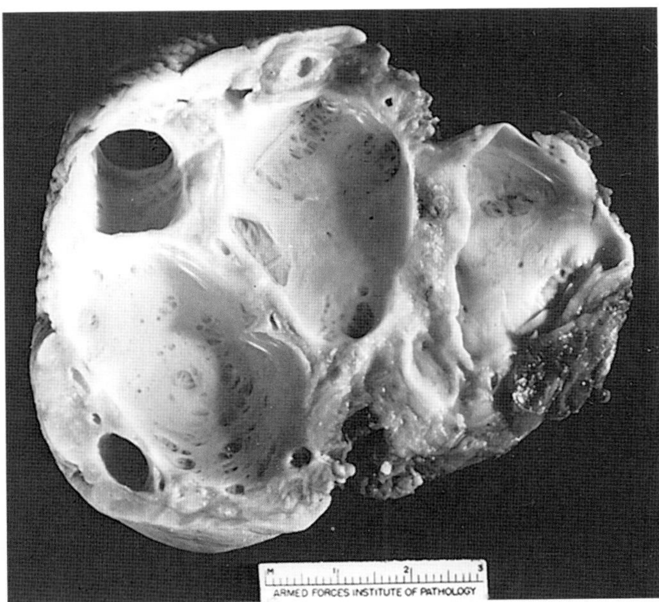

FIGURE 24-13. Cut section of a macrocystic lymphatic malformation with thick-walled cysts of various sizes.

large lymphatic spaces have, in addition, poorly developed fascicles of smooth muscle (see Figs. 24-16 and 24-17). The spaces are empty, filled with proteinaceous fluid and lymphocytes, or contain extravasated blood secondary to hemorrhage. The stroma is composed of a delicate meshwork of collagen punctuated by small lymphoid aggregates (see Fig. 24-15). With repeated bouts of infection, the stroma of a lymphatic malformation becomes inflamed, edematous (see Fig. 24-21), and, ultimately, fibrotic.

In most cases, there is little difficulty establishing the correct diagnosis, although lymphatic malformations with secondary hemorrhage can resemble a cavernous hemangioma, and those with a significant amount of smooth muscle within the wall of the lymphatic spaces resemble a venous malformation. Histologic features that favor the diagnosis of lymphatic malformation over a vascular malformation are lymphoid aggregates in the stroma and more irregular lumens with widely spaced nuclei. Immunohistochemistry for lymphatic lineage markers is ultimately the most reliable method for distinguishing the two (see Fig. 24-18).[6,28] PROX1 and VEGFR3 antibodies have been shown to have greater sensitivity than podoplanin (D2-40) in making this distinction.[29]

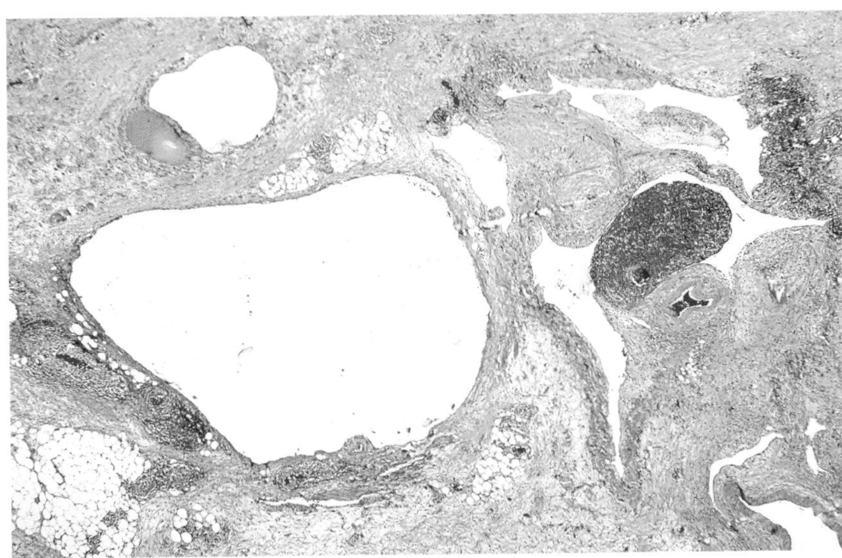

FIGURE 24-14. Low-power view of lymphatic malformation.

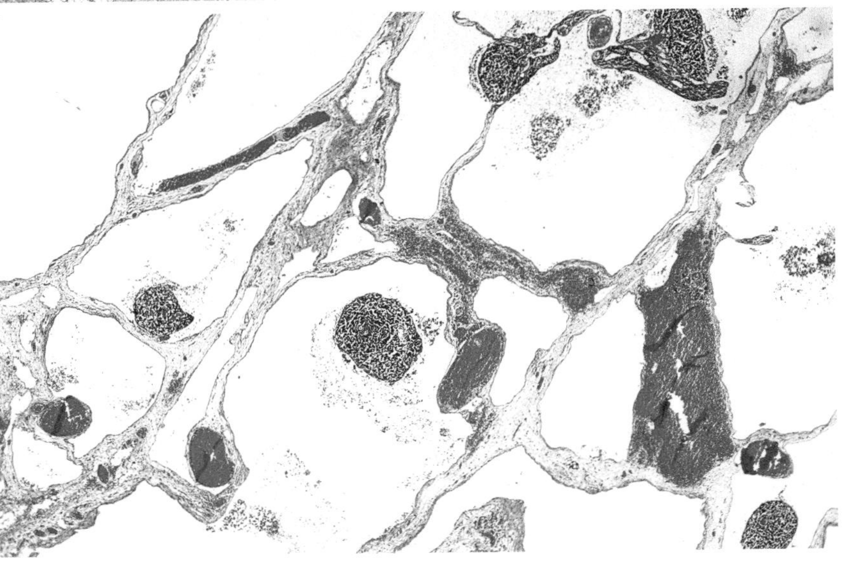

FIGURE 24-15. Lymphatic malformation containing dense lymphoid aggregates.

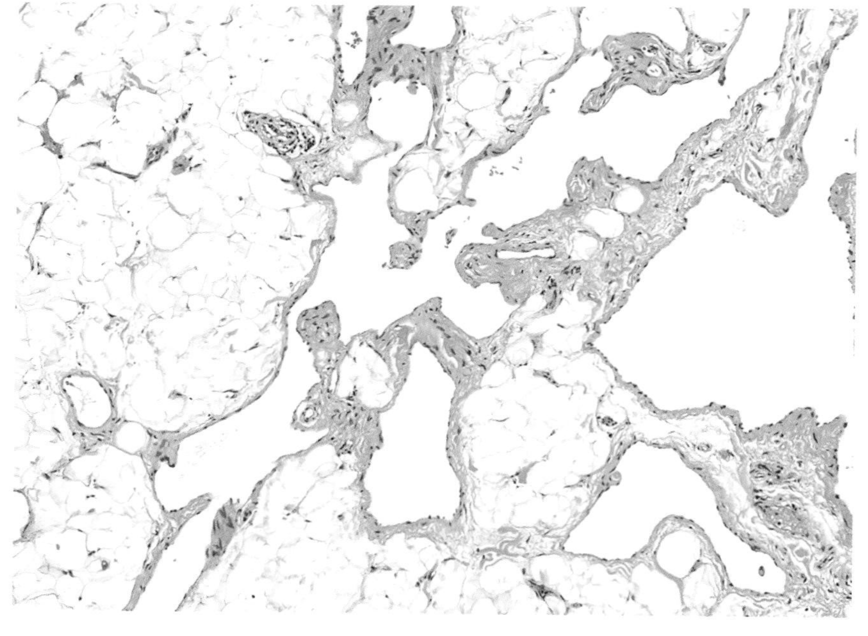

FIGURE 24-16. Microcystic lymphatic malformation illustrating irregular vascular channels, some containing slips of smooth muscle.

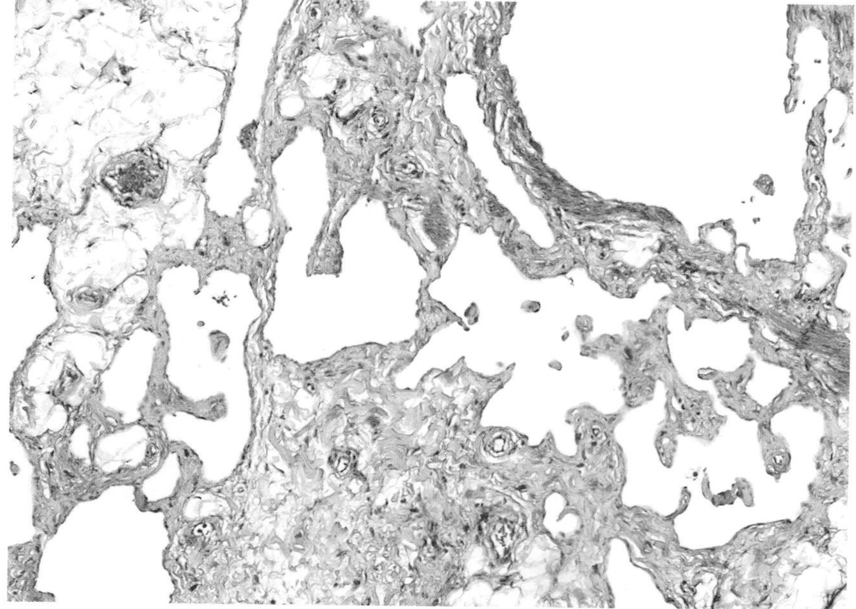

FIGURE 24-17. Masson trichrome stain of microcystic lymphatic malformation illustrating scattered collection of smooth muscle in walls of larger vascular channels (same case as Figure 24-16).

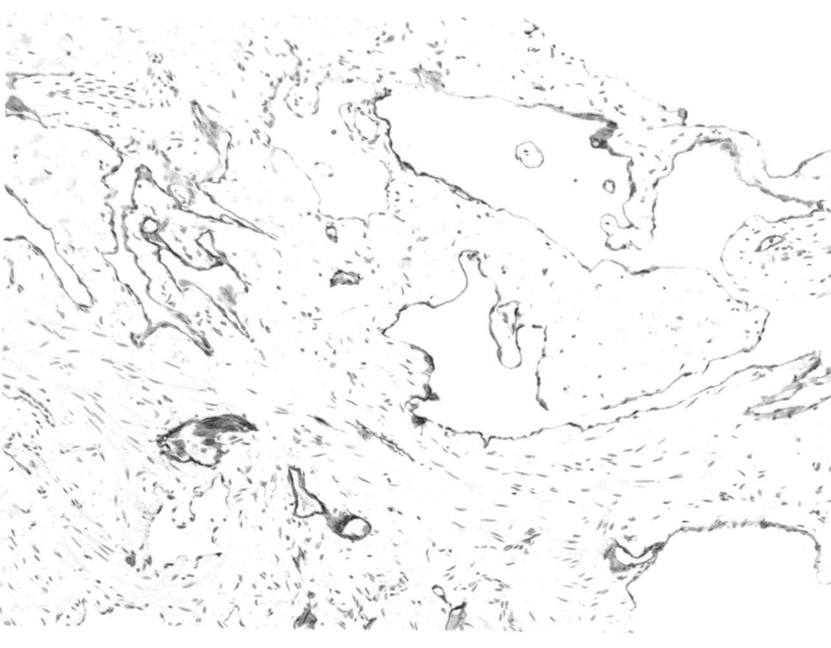

FIGURE 24-18. D2-40 (podoplanin) immunostaining of microcystic lymphatic malformation illustrating staining of virtually all vascular (lymphatic) channels.

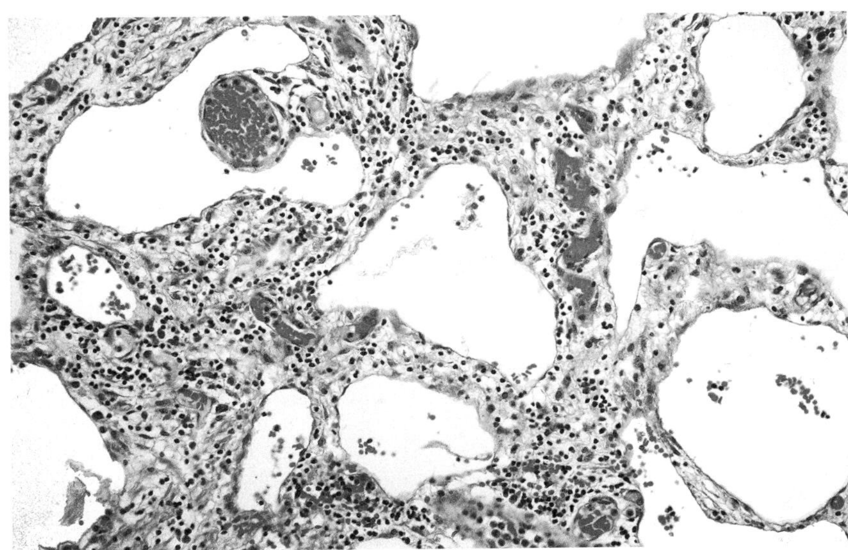

FIGURE 24-19. Lymphatic malformation with engorged vascular spaces.

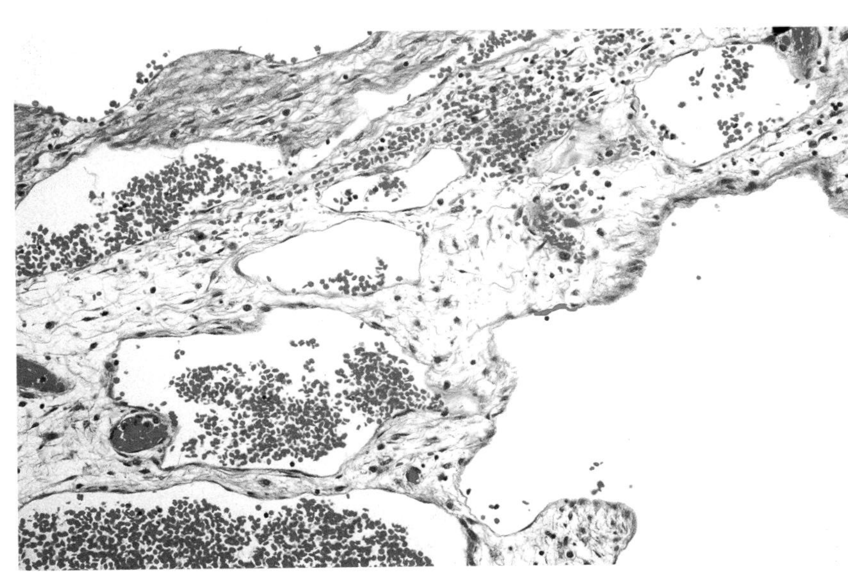

FIGURE 24-20. Lymphatic malformation with stromal hemorrhage.

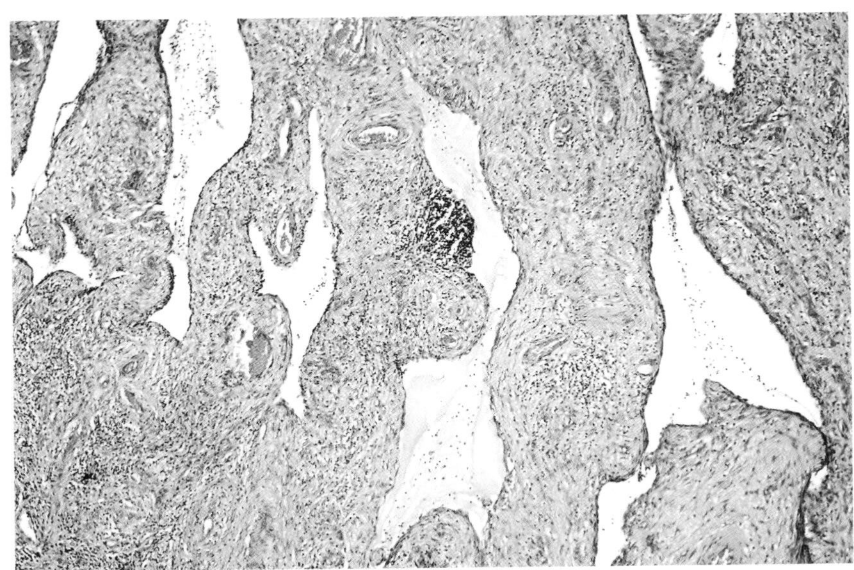

FIGURE 24-21. Inflamed intra-abdominal lymphatic malformation.

It is important to distinguish an intra-abdominal lymphatic malformation from a multicystic mesothelioma or microcystic adenoma of the pancreas. The cystic mesothelioma presents as a multicystic mass affecting a large area of peritoneum and requires repeated surgery for control. Cystic mesotheliomas are composed of pseudoglandular structures that show greater variation in size than the vascular spaces of the lymphatic malformation. Moreover, there is a transition from normal or reactive mesothelium to the glandular spaces of the mesothelioma. Out of context, however, the cells may look surprisingly similar. The cells of mesotheliomas have numerous microvilli, whereas those of lymphatic malformations are smoothly contoured and resemble normal lymphatic endothelium. In ambiguous situations, immunohistochemical procedures are an easy and reliable means to make this distinction. Multicystic mesothelioma, like other mesothelial tumors, expresses cytokeratin and epithelial membrane antigen. Microcystic adenomas of the pancreas are composed of cystic spaces lined by cuboidal or low columnar, keratin-positive epithelium. The glandular spaces are regular in shape and rest on a stroma containing a rich network of small blood capillaries.

Behavior and Treatment

Although the lymphatic malformation is a benign lesion, it can cause significant morbidity because of its large size, location, or proclivity to become secondarily infected. Only rare cases are known to have regressed spontaneously. Therefore, the mainstay of therapy is surgery, an approach that has been refined through better imaging and staging procedures. Lymphatic malformations producing life-threatening symptoms require immediate surgical treatment. For those with minimal symptoms, treatment can be delayed beyond infancy and include a combination of surgery and sclerotherapy with OK-432, a lyophilized mixture of group A *Streptococcus pyogenes*.[30] Approximately one-third of all lymphatic malformations respond to sclerotherapy with this agent. Factors that predict good response include head and neck location, size less than 5 cm, and macrocystic architecture.[31,32] Surgery achieves its best results when lesions are circumscribed and amenable to complete excision and is less successful for infiltrating microcystic or combined microcystic-macrocystic lesions.

LYMPHANGIOMATOSIS

Lymphatic malformations affecting soft tissue or parenchymal organs in a diffuse or multifocal fashion are termed *lymphangiomatosis*. This rare disease can be conceptualized as the lymphatic counterpart of angiomatosis (see Chapter 21).

Like angiomatosis, this disease principally affects children and rarely manifests after age 20. Diagnosis of this condition at birth is uncommon because it seems that a latent period is required for these lesions to achieve sufficient size to become symptomatic. There is no gender predilection. The presenting symptoms are varied and depend on the site and extent of involvement. More than three-fourths of patients have multiple bone lesions. These well-delimited osteolytic lesions with a variable degree of sclerosis (Figs. 24-22 to 24-24) are usually asymptomatic, discovered incidentally, and frequently diagnosed as fibrous dysplasia or bone changes associated with hyperparathyroidism. Acute symptoms more often relate to the presence of lymphatic malformations in soft tissue, mediastinum, liver, spleen, or lung. The prognosis is determined by the extent of the disease.[33] Patients with liver, spleen, lung, and thoracic duct involvement usually have a poor prognosis[33] because the lesions tend to be diffuse and are not amenable to surgical excision. On the other hand, patients with soft tissue involvement with or without skeletal involvement enjoy an excellent prognosis[34] because, in most cases, the bone lesions eventually stabilize and the soft tissue lesions respond to limited surgical resection. In contrast, patients with lesions in the vertebrae may develop cord compression and, ultimately, die of their disease.

Lymphangiomatosis affecting principally soft tissue and bone presents with fluctuant brawny swelling of an extremity that corresponds on the lymphangiogram to numerous interconnecting lymphatic channels (Fig. 24-25). The skin is thickened, and the soft tissue has a brown sponge-like quality because of the extensive replacement by proliferating lymphatic channels (Fig. 24-26). The proliferating vessels are lined by a single layer of flattened endothelium that ramifies in the soft tissue in a pattern analogous to a well-differentiated angiosarcoma. Stromal hemosiderin deposits in the absence of active hemorrhage can be seen. Atypical features, such as endothelial tufting, atypia, and mitotic activity of the lymphatic endothelium, are not present. In these respects, lymphangiomatosis is similar histologically to the deep portions of acquired progressive lymphangioma. The diagnosis of lymphangiomatosis may be difficult to establish when only bone biopsy is undertaken. To the unsuspecting pathologist, the bland dilated lymph channels devoid of cells may appear so innocuous as to be overlooked altogether, and more emphasis may be placed on the surrounding bone resorption and atrophy.

The differential diagnosis of lymphangiomatosis includes angiomatosis, acquired progressive lymphangioma, and, most

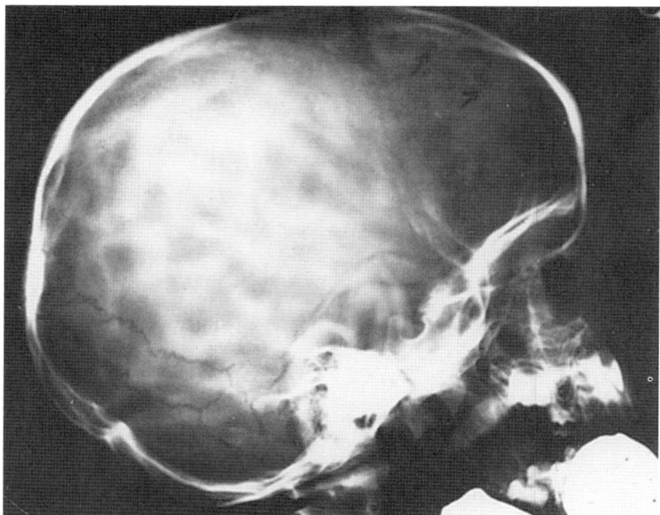

FIGURE 24-22. Male child with lymphangiomatosis affecting multiple bones and soft tissue sites. Multiple osteolytic lesions are present in the skull.

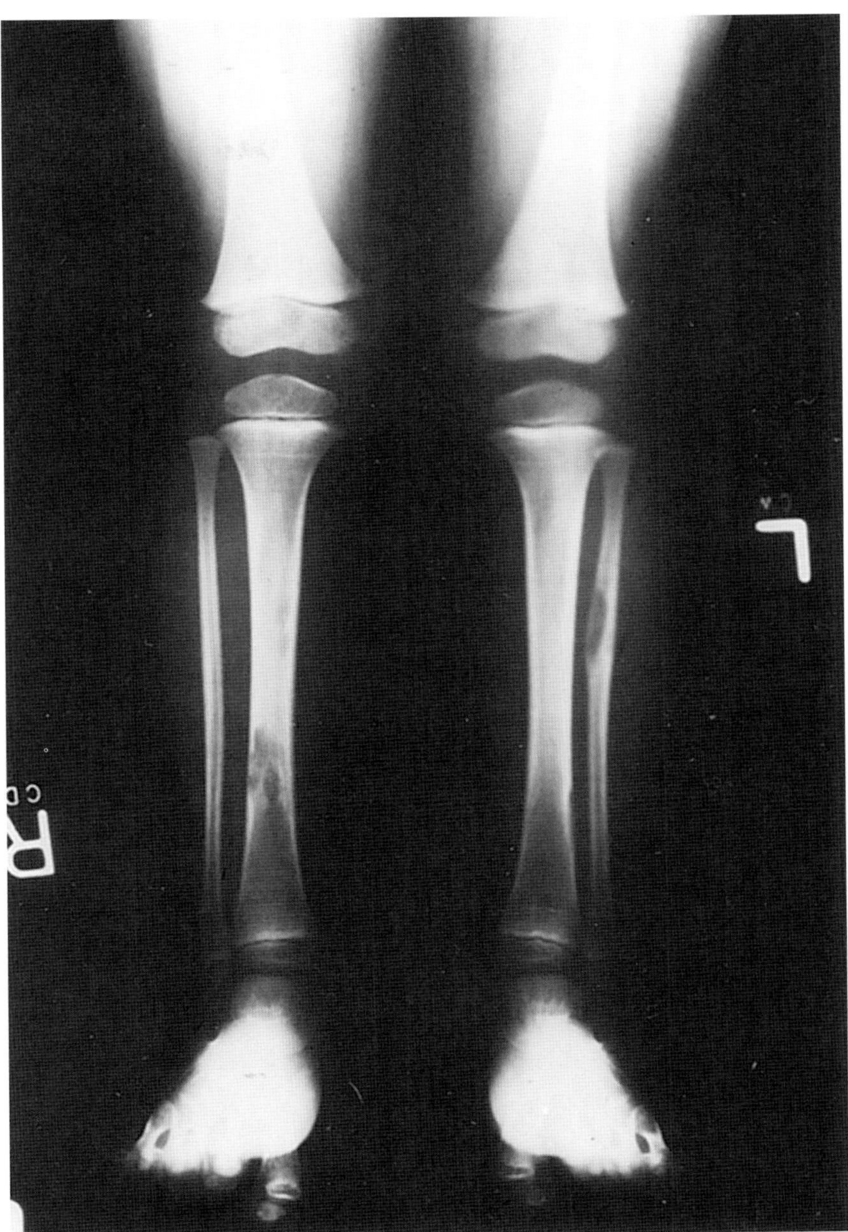

FIGURE 24-23. Lymphangiomatosis (same case as in Figure 24-22) with multiple, bilateral osteolytic lesions in long bones.

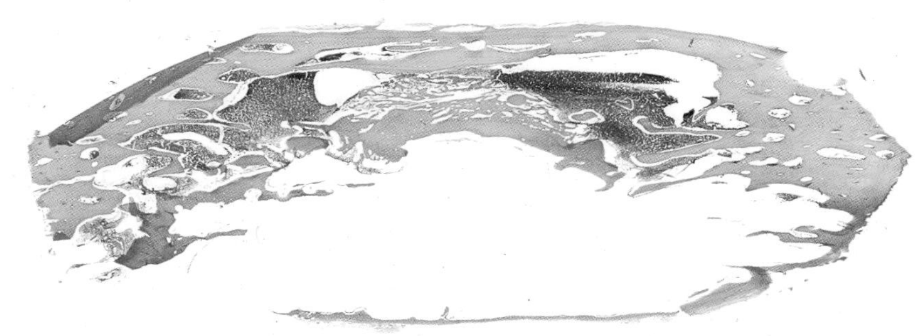

FIGURE 24-24. Section of lymphatic malformation removed from the rib of a patient with lymphangiomatosis. Note the delicate lining of lymphatic cells around the defect (same case as in Figure 24-22).

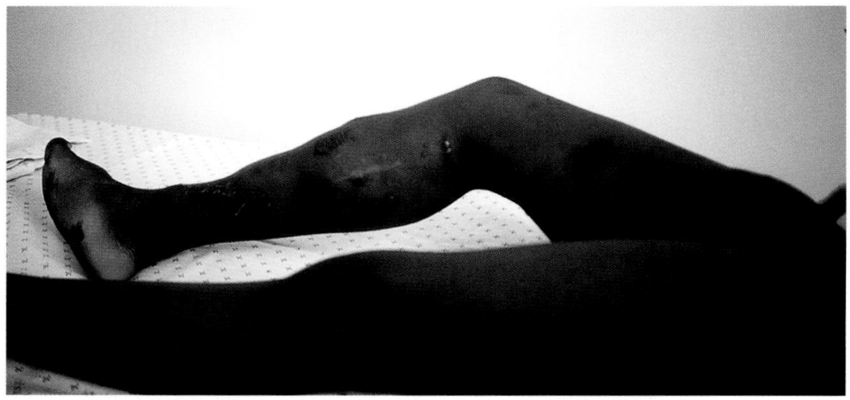

FIGURE 24-25. Lymphangiomatosis affecting one lower extremity.

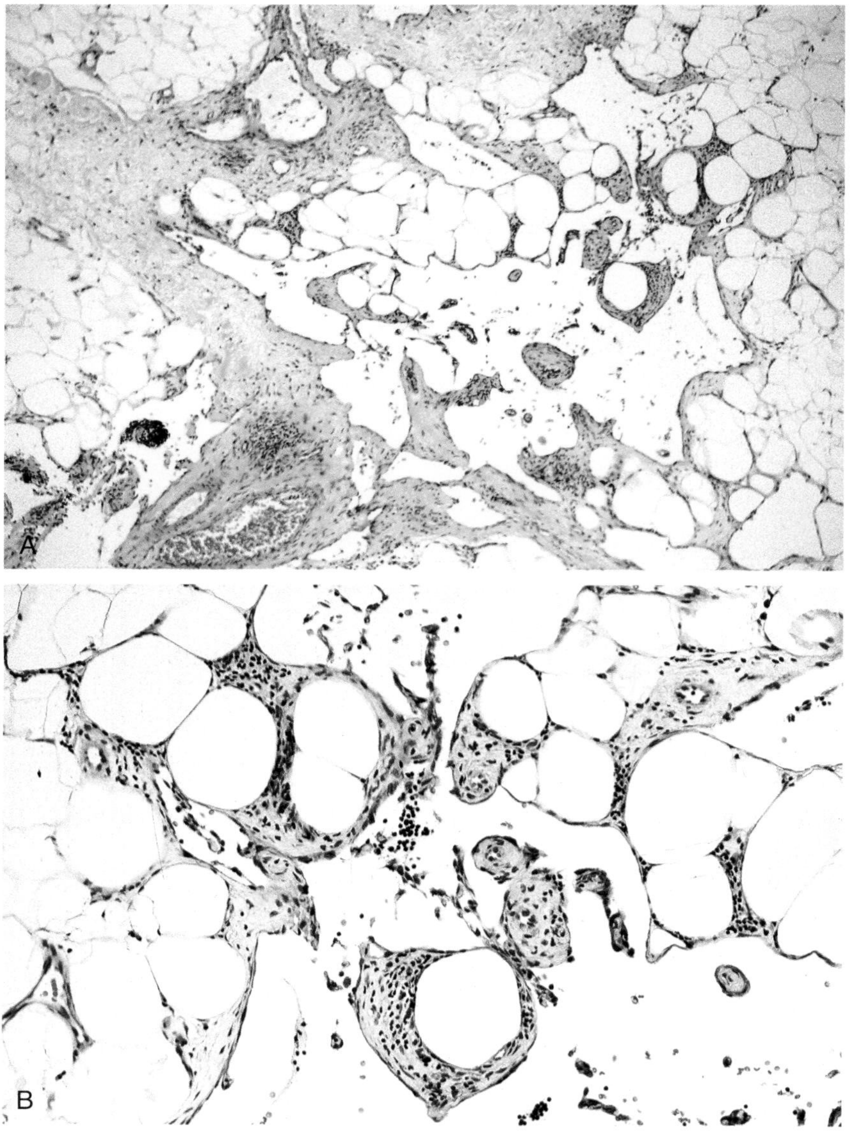

FIGURE 24-26. Persistently recurring lymphangiomatosis of the leg. Lymphatic channels diffusely involve soft tissue (A) and are composed of cells with little atypia (B).

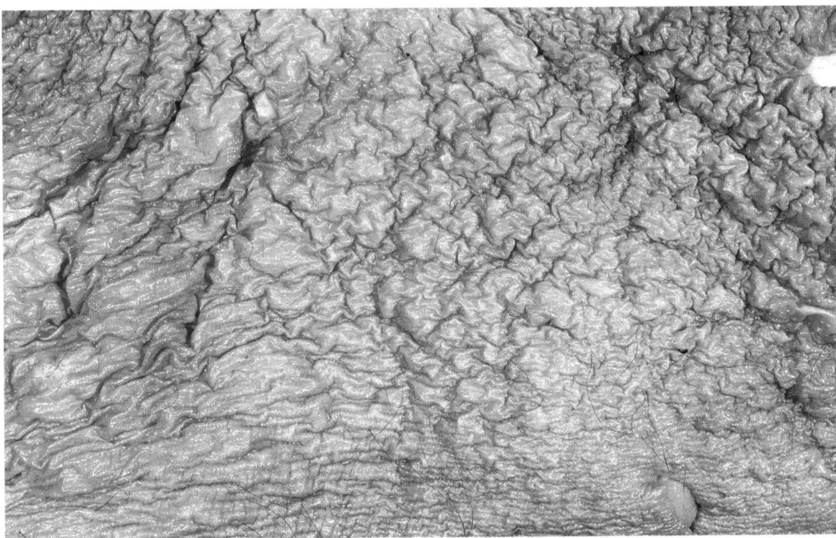

FIGURE 24-27. Localized massive lymphedema showing thickened pebble-like skin.

important, angiosarcoma. Although the infiltrative appearance at low power immediately suggests angiosarcoma, one is always struck by the apparent discordance between the infiltrative pattern, which suggests an aggressive process, and the relatively innocuous appearance of the lymphatic endothelium. Features, such as endothelial redundancy and nuclear atypia, which are the hallmark of virtually all angiosarcomas, are absent in lymphangiomatosis. Angiomatosis is typically composed of vessels of varying size and complexity (see Chapter 21). Although some have a prominent capillary vascular component, the capillary vessels do not dissect and ramify throughout the soft tissue to the extent seen in lymphangiomatosis. The distinction between acquired progressive lymphangioma and lymphangiomatosis is more problematic. Portions of acquired progressive lymphangioma are virtually indistinguishable from lymphangiomatosis. Therefore, one could conceptualize the acquired progressive lymphangioma, in some cases, as a limited or superficial form of lymphangiomatosis. Therefore, the distinction between the two is best made, based on presentation and clinical extent.

LOCALIZED MASSIVE LYMPHEDEMA

Localized areas of massive lymphedema develop in morbidly obese individuals and frequently simulate a well-differentiated liposarcoma.[35,36] The pathogenetic mechanism of this pseudoneoplastic condition is a functional lymphatic obstruction as a result of the weight of large dependent folds of fat. In some cases, the condition is probably exacerbated by previous surgery that has interrupted lymphatics and contributes to obstruction. Patients with this condition usually weigh in excess of 300 pounds and develop lesions preferentially in the medial portion of the extremities or abdominal wall. Clinically, the lesions are pendulous masses with a thickened hyperkeratotic or peau d'orange-like appearance of skin (Fig. 24-27). Radiologically, the mass corresponds to expanded subcutaneous tissue with soft tissue streaking but without a discrete mass lesion. On a cut section, one is impressed by the amount of fibrous tissue traversing the fat and by

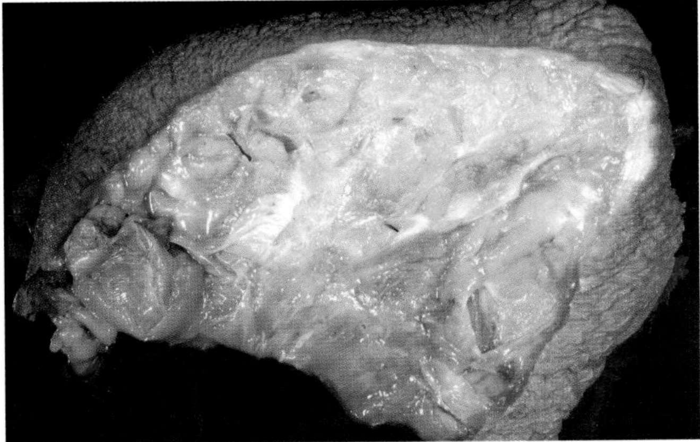

FIGURE 24-28. Localized massive lymphedema with multiple cysts of the subcutis and exaggerated fibrous trabeculae.

the presence of cysts of various sizes that weep serous fluid (Fig. 24-28).

Histologically, the changes are those of chronic lymphedema. The overlying skin is thickened and, occasionally, hyperkeratotic (Fig. 24-29), whereas the underlying dermis is hyalinized and contains numerous small lymphatic channels surrounded by clusters of lymphocytes (Fig. 24-30). In the subcutis, the interlobular septa are markedly expanded by edema fluid and mildly atypical fibroblasts that eclipse the fat lobule (Figs. 24-31 and 24-32). At the interface of the septa and the residual fat, one occasionally finds a fringe of reactive capillary-sized vessels.

Although these lesions represent a reactive condition involving the lymphatic system, they are commonly confused with liposarcoma (see Chapter 15) because the expanded interlobular septa are misinterpreted as the fibrous bands of a sclerosing well-differentiated liposarcoma. The salient observations when making this distinction are the overall preservation of the architecture of normal subcutaneous fat and the lack of significant atypia in the fibrous bands separating the fat. Because the underlying cause of the condition is morbid

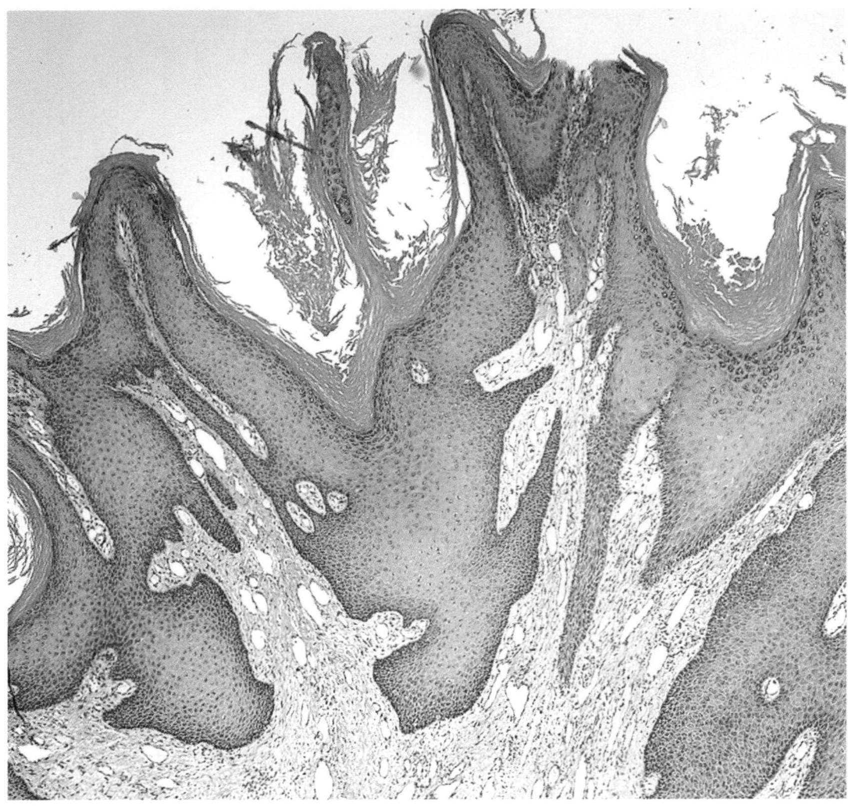

FIGURE 24-29. Thickened hyperkeratotic skin in localized massive lymphedema.

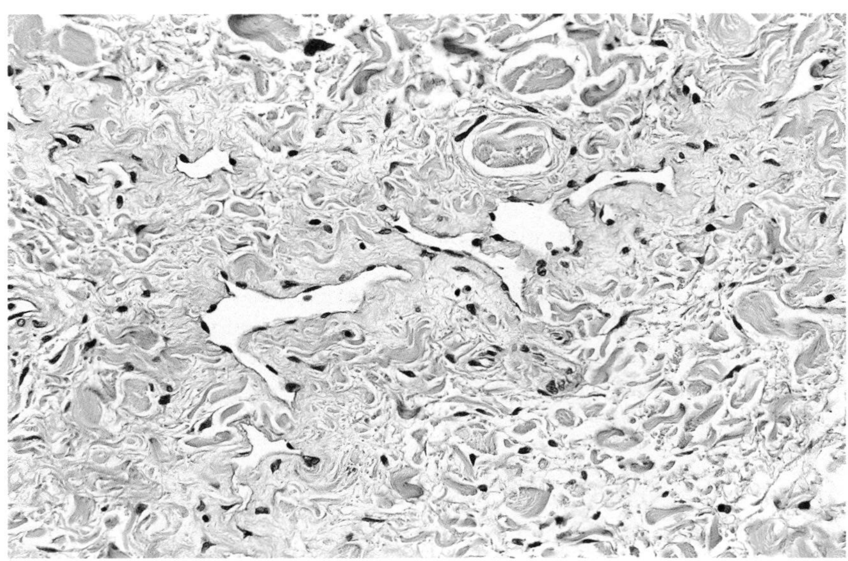

FIGURE 24-30. Irregular lymphatic channels in sclerotic dermis in localized massive lymphedema.

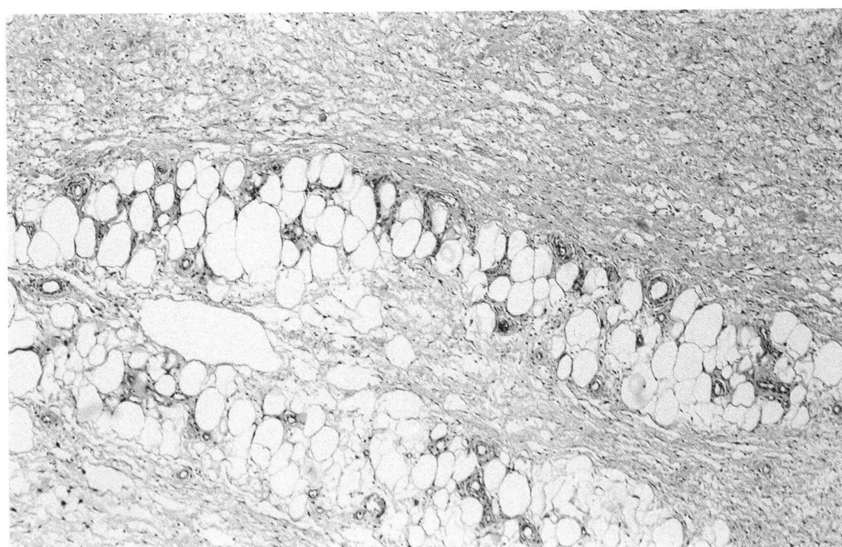

FIGURE 24-31. Widened fibrous trabeculae in the subcutis in massive localized lymphedema. Note fringe at the capillaries of interface of fat and fibrous trabeculae.

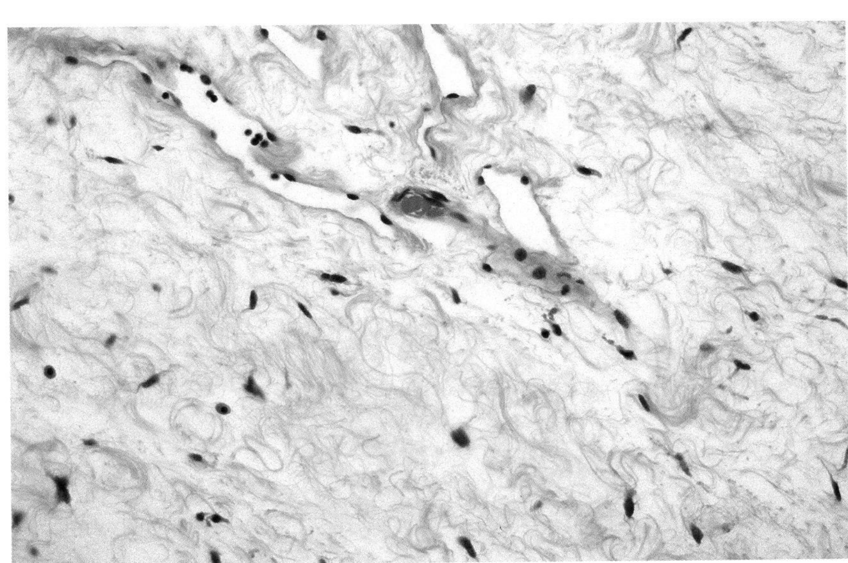

FIGURE 24-32. Mildly atypical fibroblasts in fibrous trabeculae within massive localized lymphedema.

obesity, persistence or even recurrence of these lesions is to be expected following surgery. None has behaved in an aggressive manner. Quite recently, several cases of cutaneous angiosarcoma arising in long-standing localized massive lymphedema have been reported. The authors warn of the increased risk of angiosarcoma given the preponderance of obesity in Western society.[37]

References

1. Tammela T, Petrova TV, Alitalo K. Molecular lymphangiogenesis: new players. Trends Cell Biol 2005;15(8):434–41. Epub 2005/07/12.
2. Hong YK, Detmar M. Prox1, master regulator of the lymphatic vasculature phenotype. Cell Tissue Res 2003;314(1):85–92. Epub 2003/07/29.
3. Barsky SH, Baker A, Siegal GP, et al. Use of anti-basement membrane antibodies to distinguish blood vessel capillaries from lymphatic capillaries. Am J Surg Pathol 1983;7(7):667–77. Epub 1983/10/01.
4. Fraley EE, Weiss L. An electron microscopic study of the lymphatic vessels in the penile skin of the rat. Am J Anat 1961;109:85–101. Epub 1961/07/01.
5. Leak LV, Burke JF. Fine structure of the lymphatic capillary and the adjoining connective tissue area. Am J Anat 1966;118(3):785–809. Epub 1966/05/01.
6. Fukunaga M. Expression of D2-40 in lymphatic endothelium of normal tissues and in vascular tumours. Histopathology 2005;46(4):396–402. Epub 2005/04/07.
7. Folpe AL, Veikkola T, Valtola R, et al. Vascular endothelial growth factor receptor-3 (VEGFR-3): a marker of vascular tumors with presumed lymphatic differentiation, including Kaposi's sarcoma, kaposiform and Dabska-type hemangioendotheliomas, and a subset of angiosarcomas. Mod Pathol 2000;13(2):180–5. Epub 2000/03/04.
8. Mulliken JB, Fishman SJ, Burrows PE. Vascular anomalies. Curr Probl Surg 2000;37(8):517–84.
9. North PE. Pediatric vascular tumors and malformations. Surg Pathol 2010;3:455–94.
10. Ferrell RE, Levinson KL, Esman JH, et al. Hereditary lymphedema: evidence for linkage and genetic heterogeneity. Hum Mol Genet 1998;7(13):2073–8.
11. Fang J, Dagenais SL, Erickson RP, et al. Mutations in FOXC2 (MFH-1), a forkhead family transcription factor, are responsible for the hereditary lymphedema-distichiasis syndrome. Am J Hum Genet 2000;67(6):1382–8.

12. Bill Jr AH, Sumner DS. A unified concept of lymphangioma and cystic hygroma. Surg Gynecol Obstet 1965;120:79–86. Epub 1965/01/01.
13. Kindblom LG, Angervall L. Tumors of lymph vessels. Contemp Issues Surg Pathol 1991;18:163.
14. Alqahtani A, Nguyen LT, Flageole H, et al. 25 years' experience with lymphangiomas in children. J Pediatr Surg 1999;34(7):1164–8. Epub 1999/08/12.
15. Castanon M, Margarit J, Carrasco R, et al. Long-term follow-up of nineteen cystic lymphangiomas treated with fibrin sealant. J Pediatr Surg 1999;34(8):1276–9. Epub 1999/08/31.
16. Chung JH, Suh YL, Park IA, et al. A pathologic study of abdominal lymphangiomas. J Korean Med Sci 1999;14(3):257–62. Epub 1999/07/13.
17. Fonkalsrud EW. Congenital malformations of the lymphatic system. Semin Pediatr Surg 1994;3(2):62–9. Epub 1994/05/01.
18. Fisher I, Orkin M. Acquired lymphangioma (lymphangiectasis). Report of a case. Arch Dermatol 1970;101(2):230–4. Epub 1970/02/01.
19. Peachey RD, Lim CC, Whimster IW. Lymphangioma of skin. A review of 65 cases. Br J Dermatol 1970;83(5):519–27. Epub 1970/11/01.
20. Whimster IW. The pathology of lymphangioma circumscriptum. Br J Dermatol 1974;91(10):35–6.
21. Byrne J, Blanc WA, Warburton D, et al. The significance of cystic hygroma in fetuses. Hum Pathol 1984;15(1):61–7. Epub 1984/01/01.
22. Chervenak FA, Isaacson G, Blakemore KJ, et al. Fetal cystic hygroma. Cause and natural history. N Engl J Med 1983;309(14):822–5. Epub 1983/10/06.
23. Fryns JP, Kleczkowska A, Vandenberghe K, et al. Cystic hygroma and hydrops fetalis in dup(11p) syndrome. Am J Med Genet 1985;22(2):287–9. Epub 1985/10/01.
24. Emery PJ, Bailey CM, Evans JN. Cystic hygroma of the head and neck. A review of 37 cases. J Laryngol Otol 1984;98(6):613–9. Epub 1984/06/01.
25. Galifer RB, Pous JG, Juskiewenski S, et al. Intro-abdominal cystic lymphangiomas in childhood. Prog Pediatr Surg 1978;11:173–238. Epub 1978/01/01.
26. Koshy A, Tandon RK, Kapur BM, et al. Retroperitoneal lymphangioma. A case report with review of the literature. Am J Gastroenterol 1978;69(4):485–90. Epub 1978/04/01.
27. Guillou L, Fletcher CD. Benign lymphangioendothelioma (acquired progressive lymphangioma): a lesion not to be confused with well-differentiated angiosarcoma and patch stage Kaposi's sarcoma. Am J Surg Pathol 2000;24(8):1047–57.
28. Galambos C, Nodit L. Identification of lymphatic endothelium in pediatric vascular tumors and malformations. Pediatr Dev Pathol 2005;8(2):181–9. Epub 2005/02/19.
29. Castro E, Galambos C. Prox-1 and VEGFR3 antibodies are superior to D2-40 in identifying endothelial cells of lymphatic malformations—a proposal of a new immunohistochemical panel to differentiate lymphatic from other vascular malformations. Pediatr Dev Pathol 2009;12(3):187–94.
30. Perkins JA, Manning SC, Tempero RM, et al. Lymphatic malformations: review of current treatment. Otolaryngol Head Neck Surg 2010;142(6):795–803.
31. Banieghbal B, Davies MR. Guidelines for the successful treatment of lymphangioma with OK-432. Eur J Pediatr Surg 2003;13(2):103–7. Epub 2003/05/31.
32. Hall N, Ade-Ajayi N, Brewis C, et al. Is intralesional injection of OK-432 effective in the treatment of lymphangioma in children? Surgery 2003;133(3):238–42. Epub 2003/03/28.
33. Ramani P, Shah A. Lymphangiomatosis. Histologic and immunohistochemical analysis of four cases. Am J Surg Pathol 1993;17(4):329–35. Epub 1993/04/01.
34. Gomez CS, Calonje E, Ferrar DW, et al. Lymphangiomatosis of the limbs. Clinicopathologic analysis of a series with a good prognosis. Am J Surg Pathol 1995;19(2):125–33. Epub 1995/02/01.
35. Farshid G, Weiss SW. Massive localized lymphedema in the morbidly obese: a histologically distinct reactive lesion simulating liposarcoma. Am J Surg Pathol 1998;22(10):1277–83. Epub 1998/10/20.
36. Manduch M, Oliveira AM, Nascimento AG, et al. Massive localised lymphoedema: a clinicopathological study of 22 cases and review of the literature. J Clin Pathol 2009;62(9):808–11.
37. Shon W, Ida CM, Boland-Froemming JM, et al. Cutaneous angiosarcoma arising in massive localized lymphedema of the morbidly obese: a report of five cases and review of the literature. J Cutan Pathol 2011;38(7):560–4.

Perivascular Tumors

CHAPTER CONTENTS

Perivascular tumors recapitulate the appearance of the modified myoid cells that support or invest blood vessels (i.e., glomus cell and pericyte). Sometimes referred to as *perivascular myoid tumors*, they include glomus tumor and its variants, myopericytoma, and hemangiopericytoma-like tumor of the nasal passages (HTNP). So-called *hemangiopericytoma*, although a distinctive lesion histologically, does not display true pericytic differentiation but shares many histologic, immunophenotypic and cytogenetic features with a solitary fibrous tumor. Because there is a consensus that hemangiopericytoma and a solitary fibrous tumor are part of the same spectrum of lesions and of uncertain lineage, they are covered in Chapter 32.

CLASSIC (SPORADIC) GLOMUS TUMOR

The glomus tumor is a distinctive neoplasm that resembles the normal glomus body. It was originally considered a form of angiosarcoma until Masson[1] published his classic paper on the subject in 1924. His work was based on observations of three patients who had experienced strikingly similar symptoms. Each suffered paroxysms of lancinating pain in the upper extremity that abated abruptly after removal of the tumor. Masson compared the tumors to the normal glomus body and suggested that the lesion represented hyperplasia or overgrowth of this structure.

The normal glomus body is a specialized form of arteriovenous anastomosis that regulates heat. It is located in the stratum reticularis of the dermis and is most frequently encountered in the subungual region, the lateral areas of the digits, and the palm.[2] Glomus bodies are also identified in the precoccygeal soft tissue as one or more grouped structures (glomus coccygeum) varying in diameter from less than 1 to 4 mm. According to Popoff,[2] the structure does not develop until several months after birth and gradually undergoes atrophy during late adult life. Although it may be damaged in certain disease states, there is evidence that it may regenerate, probably as a result of differentiation of perivascular cells. The glomus body is made up of an afferent arteriole derived from the small arterioles supplying the dermis and branching into two or four preglomic arterioles (Figs. 25-1 to 25-3). These arterioles are endowed with the usual complement of muscle cells and an internal elastic lamina, but they blend gradually into a thick-walled segment with an irregular lumen known as the *Sucquet-Hoyer canal*. This region is the arteriovenous anastomosis proper. It is lined by plump cuboidal endothelial cells, which, in turn, are surrounded by longitudinal and circular muscle fibers but no elastic tissue. Scattered throughout the muscle fibers are the rounded, epithelioid glomus cells. These canals drain into a series of thin-walled collecting veins. The entire glomic complex is encompassed by lamellated collagenous tissue containing small nerves and vessels.

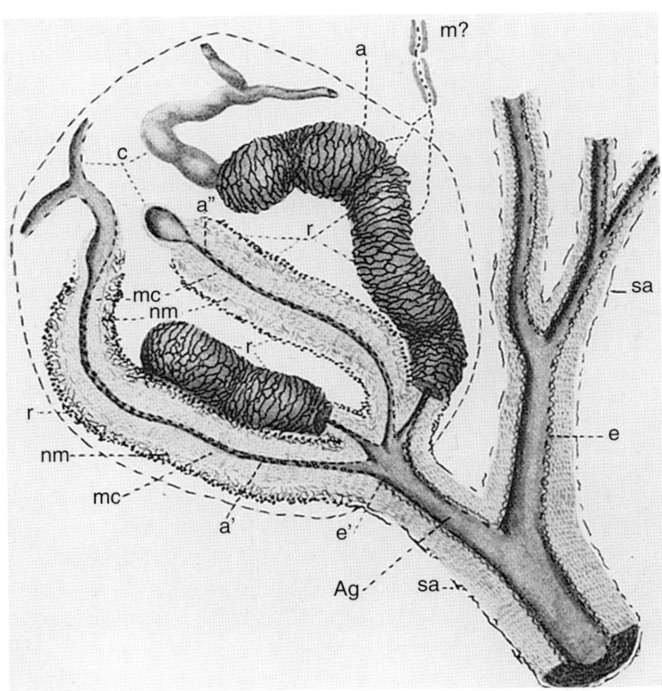

FIGURE 25-1. Normal glomus body according to Masson.[1] Afferent arteriole (Ag) gives rise to four preglomic arterioles, which blend with an irregular, thick-walled segment known as the Sucquet-Hoyer canal containing the arteriovenous anastomosis. It terminates in the collecting veins (c). *(From Masson P. Le glomus neuromyoarterial des regions tactiles et ses tumeurs. Lyon Chir 1924;21:257.)*

Clinical Findings

Glomus tumors are uncommon, with an estimated incidence of 1.6% among the 500 consecutive soft tissue tumors reported from the Mayo Clinic.[3] The tumor is about equally common in both genders, although there is a striking female predominance (3 to 1) among patients with subungual lesions.[4,5] Multiple subungual glomus tumors have been reported in neurofibromatosis 1.[6,7] Most glomus tumors are diagnosed during adult life (20 to 40 years of age), although symptoms have often been present for several years before the diagnosis. The lesions develop as small blue-red nodules that are usually located in the deep dermis or subcutis of the upper or lower extremity. The single most common site is the subungual region of the finger, but other common sites include the palm, wrist, forearm, and foot (Table 25-1). Glomus tumors probably also occur in the subcutaneous tissue near the tip of the spine, where they presumably arise from the glomus coccygeum (Fig. 25-4). However, many incidental glomus tumors arising in the region of the coccyx may well represent the normal glomus coccygeum[8,9] because this structure can reach several millimeters in diameter in the absence of clinical symptoms, suggesting a neoplasm.[10] Rare glomus tumors have been reported in almost every location, including the gastrointestinal tract,[11,12] penis,[13-15] bladder,[16] mediastinum,[17] nerve,[18] bone,[19] and lung.[20] Classic glomus tumors are typically solitary. The symptoms produced by glomus tumors are characteristic and often well out of proportion to the size of the neoplasm. Paroxysms of pain radiating away from the lesion are the most common complaint. These episodes can be elicited by changes in temperature, particularly exposure to cold, and tactile stimulation of even a minor degree. In some patients, the pain is accompanied by additional signs of hypesthesia, muscle atrophy, or osteoporosis of the affected part. In unusual instances, disturbances of autonomic function (e.g., Horner syndrome) have been reported.[1] Although the mechanism of pain production has not been fully elucidated, identification of nerve fibers containing immunoreactive substance P (pain-associated vasoactive peptide) in glomus tumors suggests pain mediation through a release of this substance.[21]

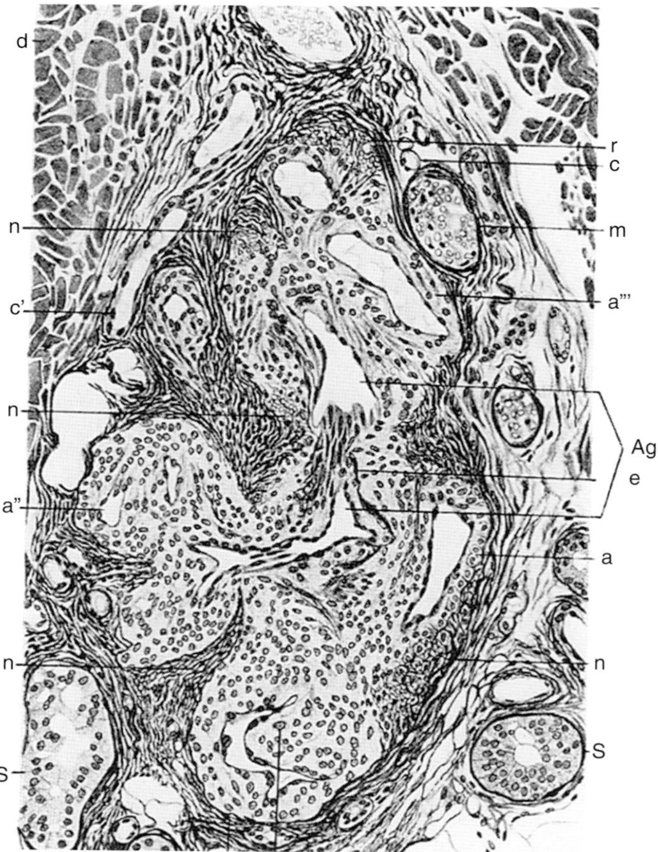

FIGURE 25-2. Histologic cross section through a glomus body according to Masson.[1] Glomic arterioles of Sucquet-Hoyer canal (a, a", a'") contain glomus cells in their walls. Collecting veins are located at the periphery (c). Small nerves and collagen fibers encircle the glomus body. *(From Masson P. Le glomus neuromyoarterial des regions tactiles et ses tumeurs. Lyon Chir 1924; 21:257.)*

Gross Findings

Grossly, the lesions are small blue-red nodules (usually less than 1 cm) that are immediately apparent during a clinical

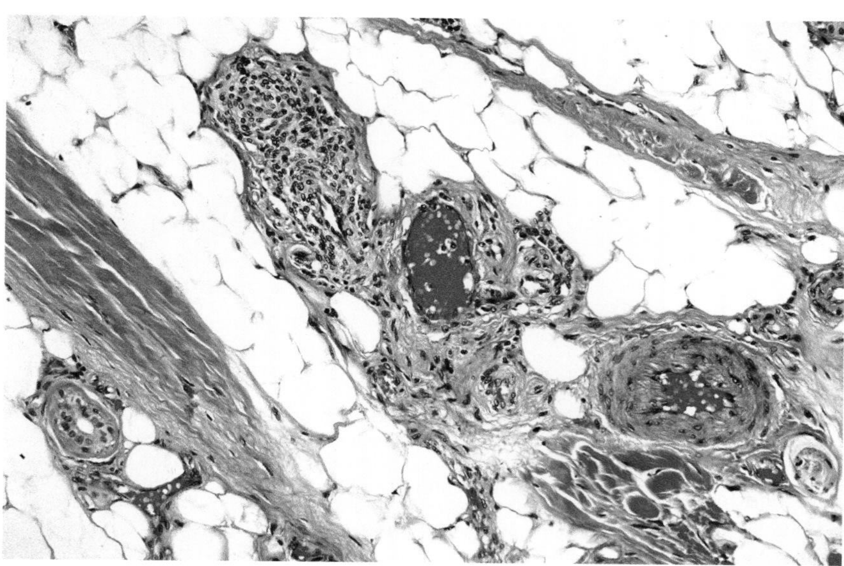

FIGURE 25-3. Normal glomus body from the foot.

TABLE 25-1 Anatomic Distribution of Glomus Tumors According to Histologic Subtype: AFIP, 506 Cases

	GLOMUS TUMOR		GLOMANGIOMA		GLOMANGIOMYOMA	
Anatomic Location	No. of Cases	%	No. of Cases	%	No. of Cases	%
Upper extremities	176	34	45	9	16	3
Finger	81	—	9	—	3	—
Lower extremities	98	19	29	6	14	3
Head and neck	29	6	6	1	5	1
Trunk	24	5	8	2	0	0
Other	45	9	4	1	7	1
Total	372	73	92	19	42	8

AFIP, Armed Forces Institute of Pathology.

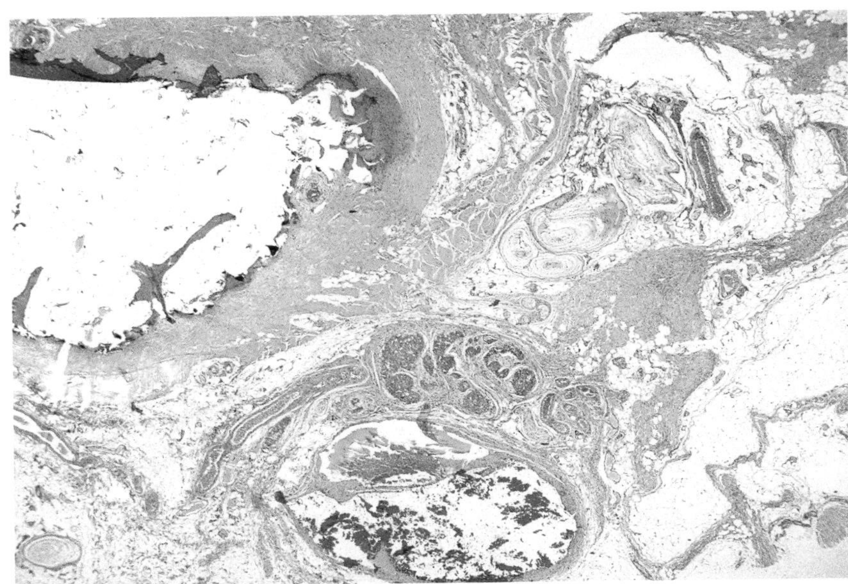

FIGURE 25-4. Glomus coccygeum located at the ventral tip of the coccyx.

examination. Subungual lesions may be more difficult to detect, and care should be taken to look for ridging of the nail or discoloration of the nail bed. Radiographs are helpful when they demonstrate a small scalloped osteolytic defect with a sclerotic border in the terminal phalanx because this finding is highly characteristic of a glomus tumor and epidermal inclusion cyst (Fig. 25-5). The more recent use of high-resolution magnetic resonance imaging (MRI) offers the promise of detecting extremely small soft tissue-based lesions.[22]

Classic glomus tumors are most common in the upper extremity and have a marked predilection for the finger, particularly the subungual region. The common form of glomus tumor accounts for about three-fourths of all cases in the material (see Table 25-1). It is a well-circumscribed lesion consisting of tight convolutes of capillary-sized vessels surrounded by collars of glomus cells set in a hyalinized or myxoid stroma (Fig. 25-6). Rarely, it appears as a poorly circumscribed, diffuse lesion. Depending on the size of the nests of glomus cells, the tumor may have a vascular appearance reminiscent of a hemangiopericytoma or paraganglioma or a cellular appearance suggestive of an epithelial tumor (Fig. 25-7).[23] The glomus cell is distinctive, and its appearance is one of the most reliable means of distinguishing this tumor from others with similar growth patterns. The cell has a rounded, regular shape with a sharply punched-out rounded nucleus set off from the amphophilic or eosinophilic cytoplasm (Fig. 25-8). The outlines of the cells are not fully appreciated on routine hematoxylin-eosin-stained sections but can be accentuated with a periodic acid-Schiff (PAS) or toluidine blue stain. In these preparations, a chicken-wire network of matrix material is present between the cells.

Only rarely do glomus cells deviate from the foregoing description, but, when they do, alterations in either the nucleus or the cytoplasm may be seen. Large hyperchromatic nuclei, probably representing a degenerative change, may replace the typical round, regular nuclei. If this change is present as an isolated finding in an otherwise typical glomus tumor, it should not be equated with malignancy. Such tumors are referred to as *symplastic glomus tumors* (see later text). A less common phenomenon is the acquisition of abundant granular, eosinophilic cytoplasm such that portions of the tumor appear oncocytic (Fig. 25-9).[24,25] Intravascular growth and signet-ring changes in the cells have been noted in a multifocal gastric glomus tumor.[11]

Although the cells are regarded as variants of smooth muscle cells, the cytoplasm is usually devoid of glycogen, and there is only minimal fuchsinophilia observed on staining with the Masson trichrome stain, two features that contrast with the staining reactions of conventional smooth muscle cells. Peripherally, the tumors have an ill-defined rim of collagen containing small nerves and vessels. This rim seldom serves as a complete or totally confining capsule because isolated nests of glomus cells can be identified outside of its boundaries and occasionally in the walls of small vessels surrounding the main tumor mass (Fig. 25-10). Vascular invasion is rarely seen in benign glomus tumors and does not appear to be predictive in and of itself of malignancy.

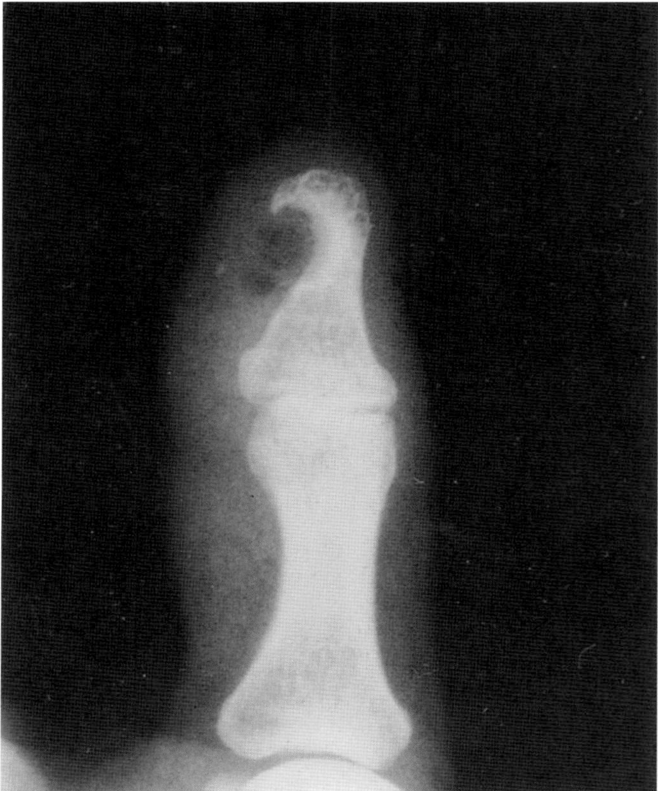

FIGURE 25-5. Postoperative radiograph showing a defect in the distal phalanx created by a subungual glomus tumor.

Because glomus tumors are quite distinctive by virtue of their characteristic cells, location, and symptoms, errors in diagnosis are infrequent. Nonetheless, highly cellular glomus tumors are occasionally mistaken for adnexal tumors or, less frequently, intradermal nevi. In the former instance, it is important to note the intimate relation of glomus cells around small vessels at the periphery of the tumor (see Fig. 25-10) and the total lack of ductular differentiation or epithelial mucin production. Immunohistochemistry can reliably discriminate glomus tumors from solid forms of hidradenoma (the adnexal tumor most closely resembling a glomus tumor).[26] Virtually all hidradenomas express keratins, whereas glomus tumors do not. In addition, hidradenomas frequently also express carcinoembryonic and epithelial membrane antigens, which are not encountered in glomus tumors. Likewise, S-100 protein is a reliable marker for distinguishing melanocytic nevi from glomus tumors.[27] Although electron microscopy can serve as a diagnostic adjunct, it is seldom needed, given the reliability of immunohistochemistry, in most cases.

Ultrastructural and Immunohistochemical Findings

The glomus cell is rounded or polygonal in shape and measures 8 to 12 μm with a rounded nucleus with occasional clefts and prominent nucleoli (Fig. 25-11). The cells are closely spaced and often interdigitate with each other along their short, knobby processes. Their surfaces are invested by a thick, often continuous, basal lamina. The cytoplasm contains modest numbers of mitochondria and endoplasmic reticulum but is most notable for the bundles of thin (8 nm) actin-like filaments that fill the cytoplasm. The bundles are well oriented, have typical dense bodies, and, occasionally, terminate in dense attachment plaques on the cytoplasmic membrane.[28] In the glomus tumors with oncocytic features,

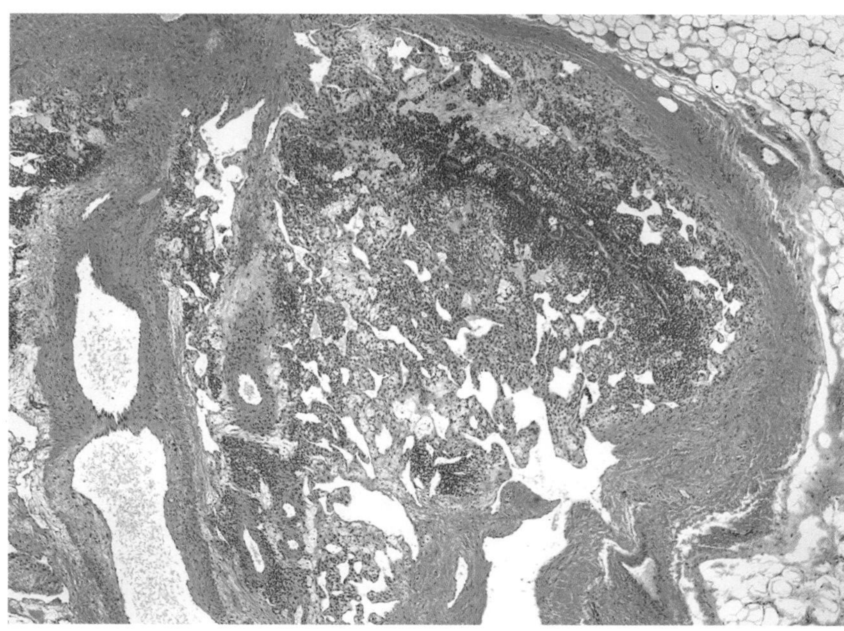

FIGURE 25-6. Typical glomus tumor, consisting of a well-circumscribed proliferation of uniform round cells, surrounding numerous blood vessels of varying caliber.

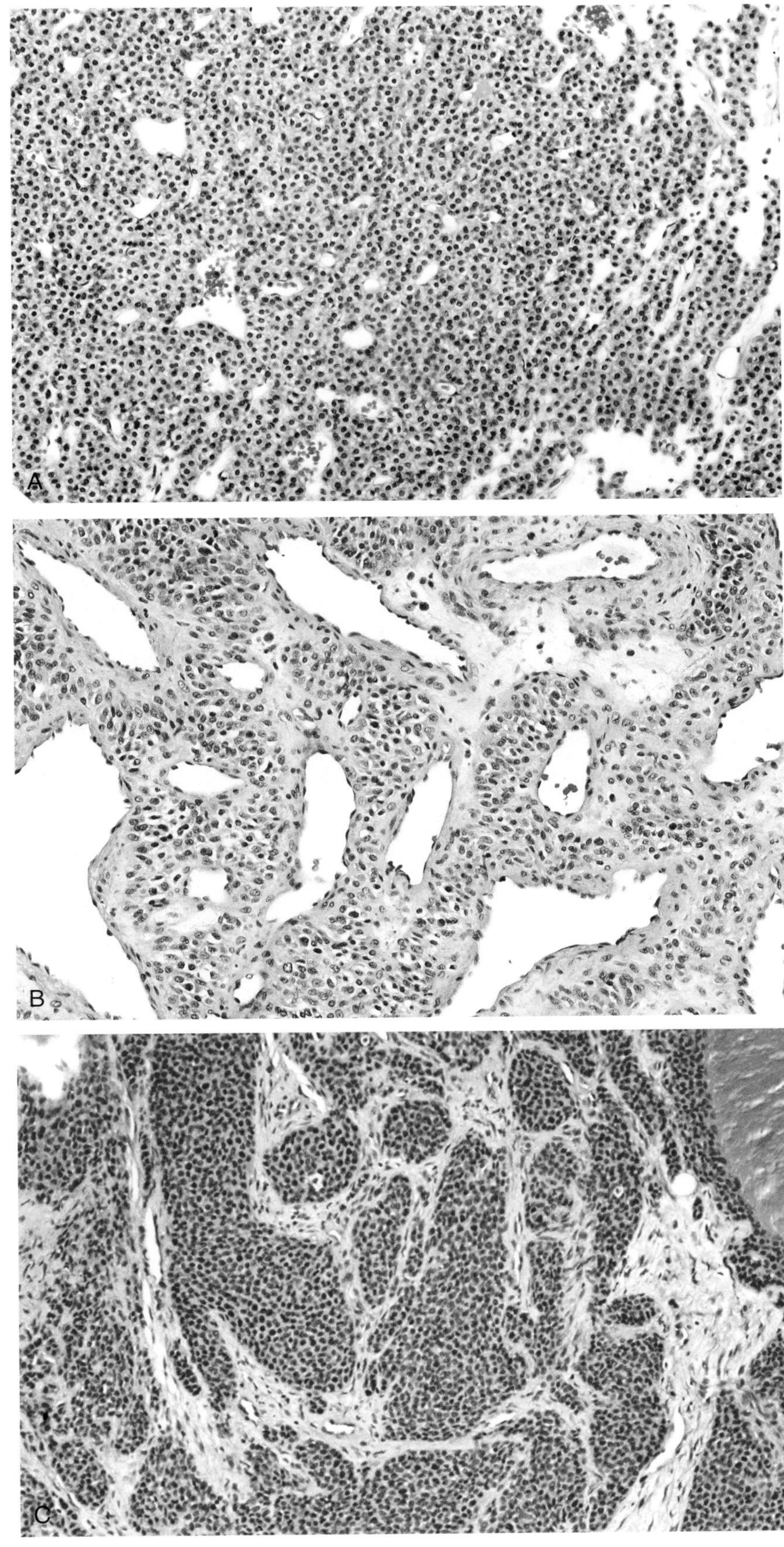

FIGURE 25-7. Variable patterns in glomus tumors. Most tumors are composed of solid sheets of cells interrupted by vessels of varying size (A, B). Some areas have an organoid or epithelioid pattern of growth (C).

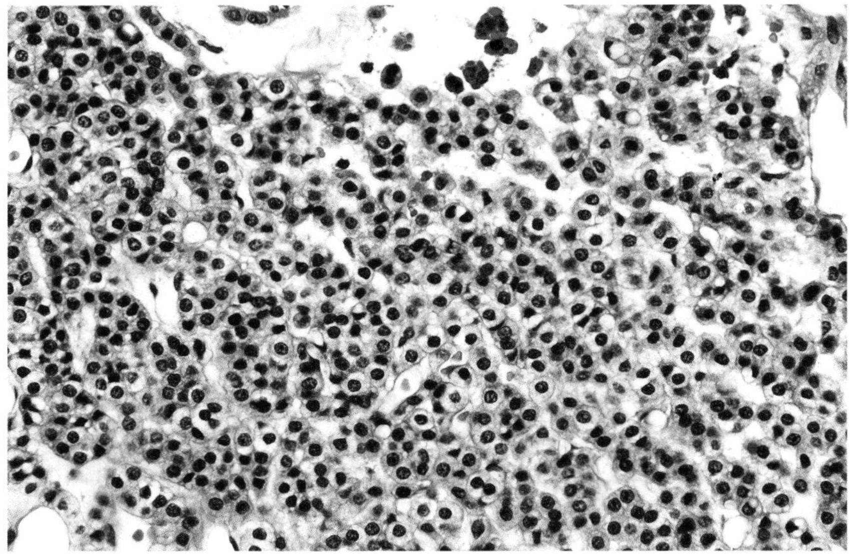

FIGURE 25-8. Glomus tumor with round cells exhibiting punched-out nuclei, pale cytoplasm, and a lacework of basement membrane material around the cells.

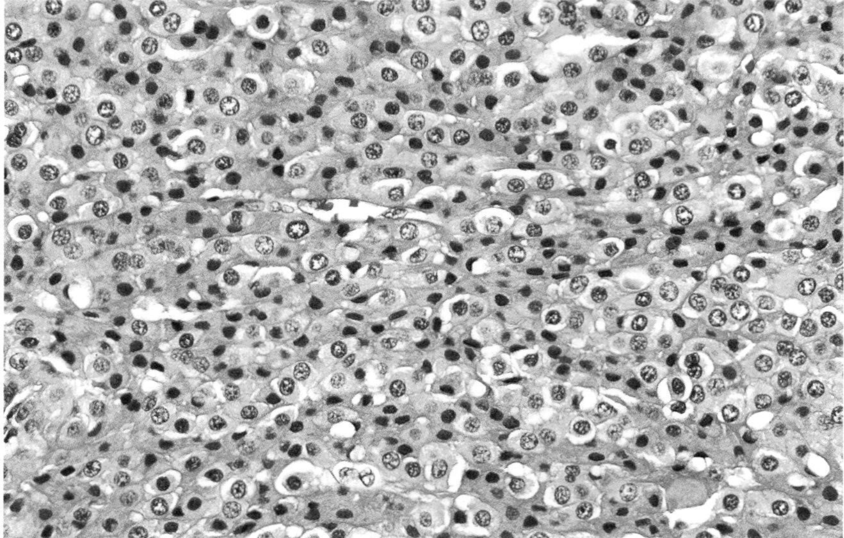

FIGURE 25-9. Oncocytic change in a glomus tumor.

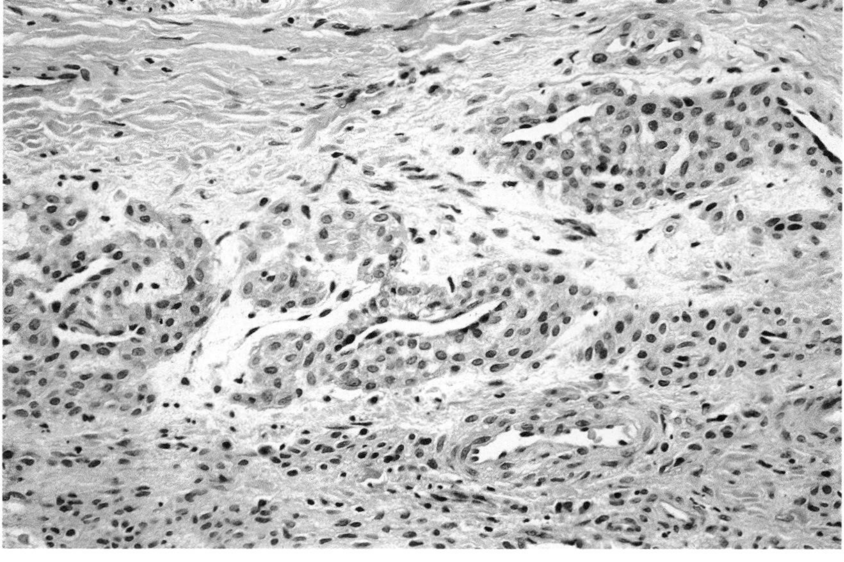

FIGURE 25-10. Proliferation of glomus cells in vessels at the periphery of a glomus tumor. This feature may be helpful for distinguishing solid glomus tumors from adnexal tumors.

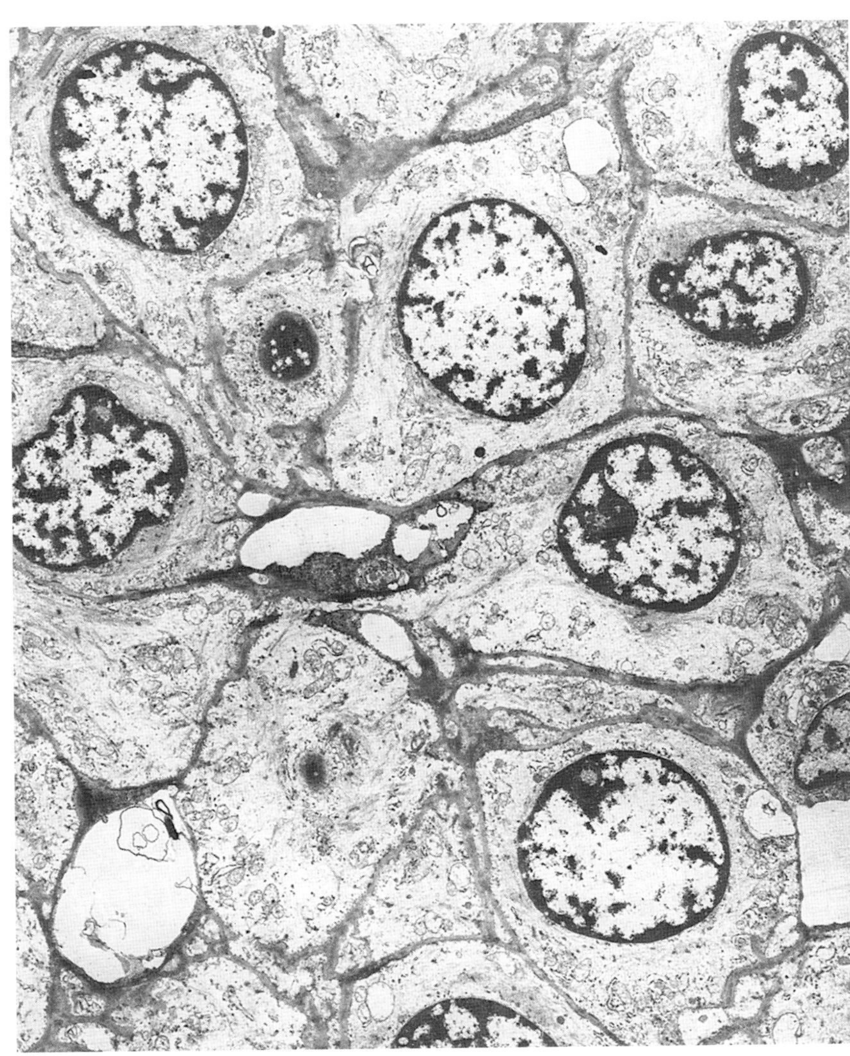

FIGURE 25-11. Electron micrograph of a glomus tumor. Cells are invested by dense basal lamina, have pinocytic vesicles along their surfaces, and contain cytoplasmic myofilaments with dense bodies (Magnification reduced from x5000). *(Courtesy of the Department of Pathology, Veterans Administration Hospital, Hines, IL.)*

not surprisingly, the cytoplasm is filled with numerous mitochondria, making it more difficult to identify microfilaments.[25] Originally, glomus cells were thought to be pericytes on the basis of certain morphologic similarities noted in tissue culture. However, as a result of determining the foregoing ultrastructural features, the glomus tumor is generally considered more closely related to the smooth muscle cell. Certainly, the quantity of myofilaments present in these cells exceeds those normally encountered in the pericyte, and the cell processes are less well developed than those of the latter cell.

Vimentin and muscle actin isoforms can be identified in nearly all glomus tumors (Fig. 25-12A).[2,29-33] However, desmin is highly variable.[32,33] Heavy-caldesmon may be present.[34] Corresponding to the ultrastructural features of the neoplasm, laminin and type IV collagen, two constituents of basal lamina, outline the cells or small groups of cells (Fig. 25-12B).[11]

Behavior and Treatment

Most glomus tumors are benign and can be treated adequately by simple excision. Only 10% recur following conservative excision.[35] Infrequent local recurrences probably represent persistence of tumor following inadequate excision or, infrequently, a benign glomus tumor growing in a diffuse or infiltrative fashion (see later text).[36,37]

GLOMUVENOUS MALFORMATION (GLOMANGIOMA, FAMILIAL GLOMANGIOMA)

Glomuvenous malformations, formerly called *glomangioma* and considered variants of classic glomus tumor, comprise only about one-fifth of glomus lesions.[38] Recent genetic studies have demonstrated that they arise secondary to truncating mutations of the glomulin gene located at 1p21-22 and are likely malformations.[39] Although glomulin is a normal component of vascular smooth muscle during embryogenesis, it is not yet understood how its functional absence relates to the development of these malformations. Based on an analysis of several families with predominantly inherited lesions, four principal germline mutations have been identified. Random post-zygotic mutations may explain both the variation in the number and distribution of lesions in familial cases and the occurrence of nonfamilial cases.

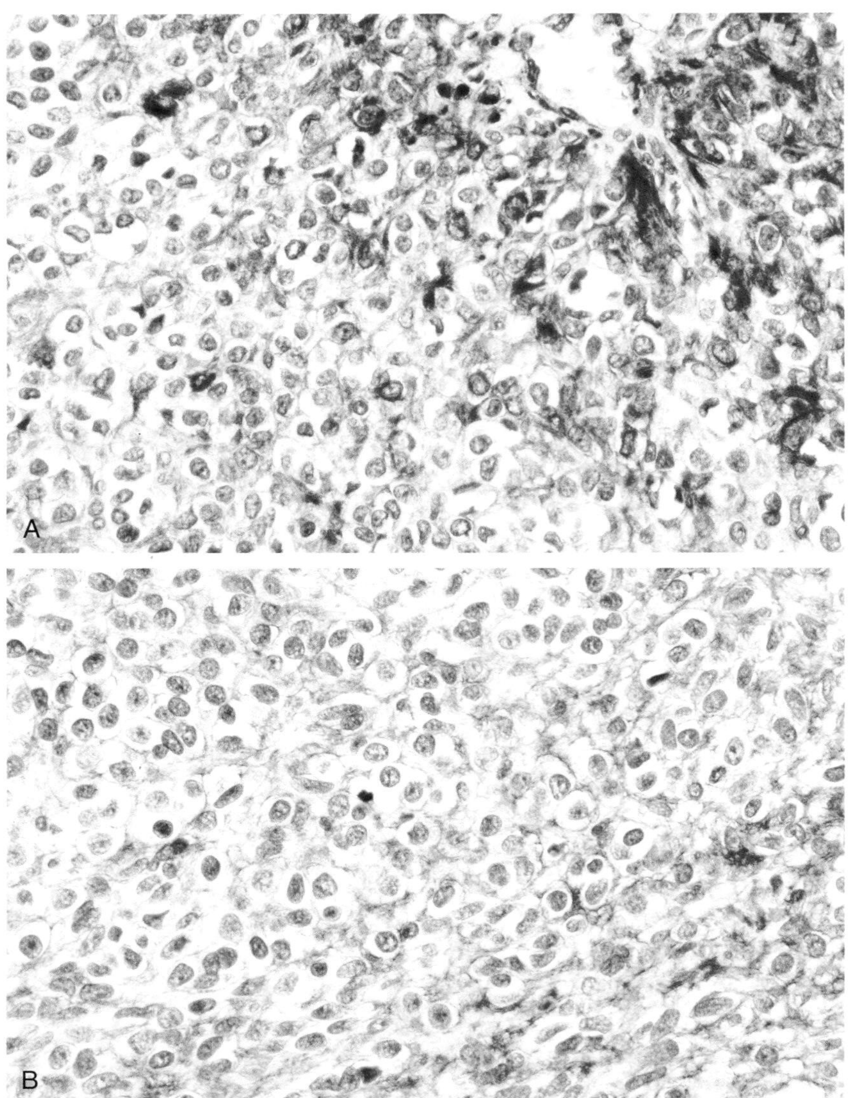

FIGURE 25-12. (A) Immunostains for actin reveal strong cytoplasmic positivity in glomus cells. (B) Immunostains for type IV collagen in a glomus tumor show intricate chicken-wire pattern between cells.

Unlike classic glomus tumor, glomuvenous malformations occur more often during childhood, are rarely subungual, and are less likely to be painful or symptomatic. Most predominate on the hand and forearm. Histologically, they are usually poorly circumscribed, occasionally plaque-like lesions that resemble cavernous hemangiomas,[40] in contrast to the classic glomus tumor, which is usually better circumscribed and more cellular. Grossly and microscopically, they resemble cavernous hemangiomas (Figs. 25-13 to 25-15). They are composed of gaping veins with small clusters of glomus cells in their walls. Secondary thrombosis and phlebolith formation may occur in these lesions as they would in an ordinary hemangioma.

GLOMANGIOMYOMA

Glomangiomyoma are glomus lesions that display focal or partial smooth muscle differentiation. In actuality, most probably represent variations in either a classic glomus tumor or glomuvenous malformation. Those glomangiomyomas with the architectural pattern of classic glomus tumor show transitions between glomus cells and cells with partial smooth muscle features, as evidenced by their fusiform shape and cytoplasmic eosinophilia. Usually, these transitional areas comprise only a small portion of the lesions. In glomangiomyomas with the architectural features of a glomuvenous malformation, the glomus cells intermingle with the mature smooth muscle of the large vessels. Many cases reported in the pediatric literature as glomangiomyoma are examples of this form and, therefore, glomuvenous malformations (Figs. 25-16 and 25-17).[41,42] The term *glomangiopericytoma* has been used recently for glomus tumors with prominent thin and thick-walled vessels and slight spindling of the glomus cells (Fig. 25-18).

GLOMANGIOMATOSIS (DIFFUSE GLOMUS TUMOR)

Glomus tumors can present as diffusely infiltrating lesions similar to some vascular tumors and malformations. They are

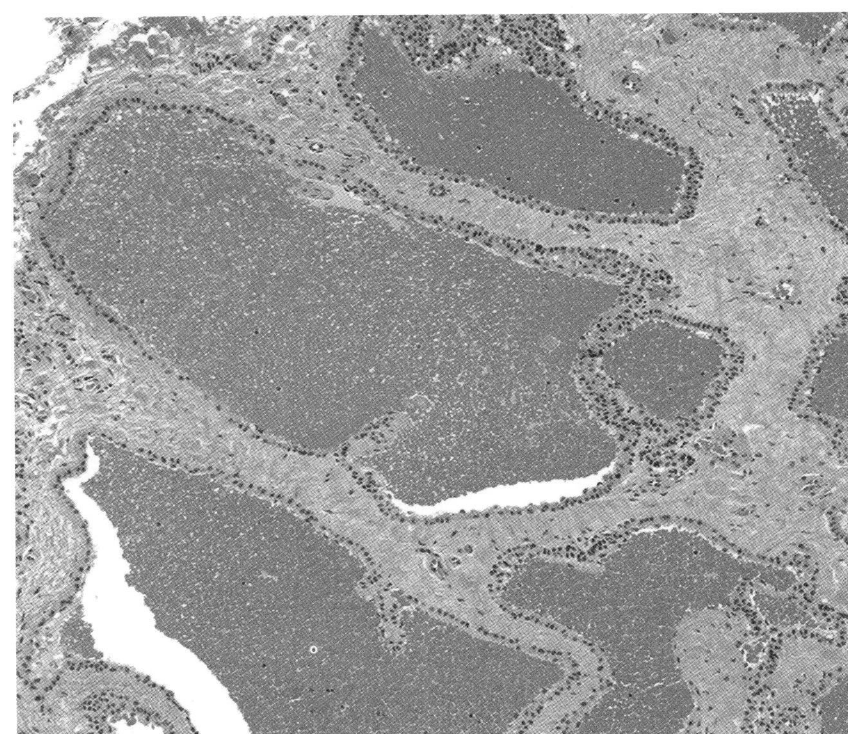

FIGURE 25-13. Glomuvenous malformation (glomangioma) with dilated veins surrounded by a cuff of glomus cells.

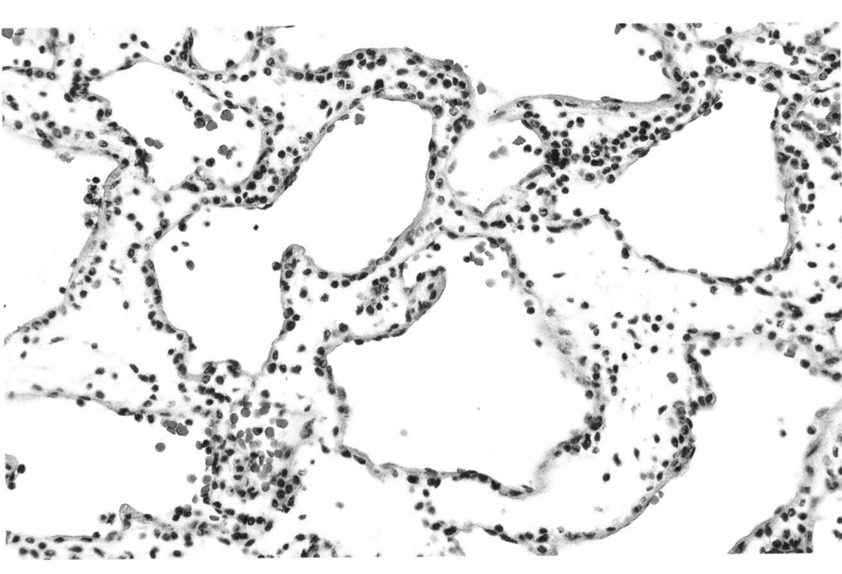

FIGURE 25-14. Glomuvenous malformation (glomangioma) with cuffs of cells around dilated vessels.

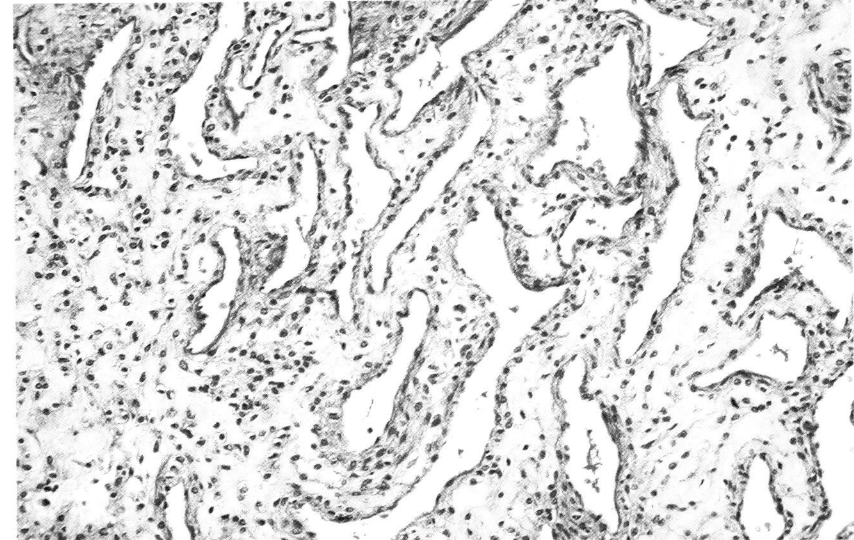

FIGURE 25-15. Glomangioma with marked hyalinization (Masson trichrome stain).

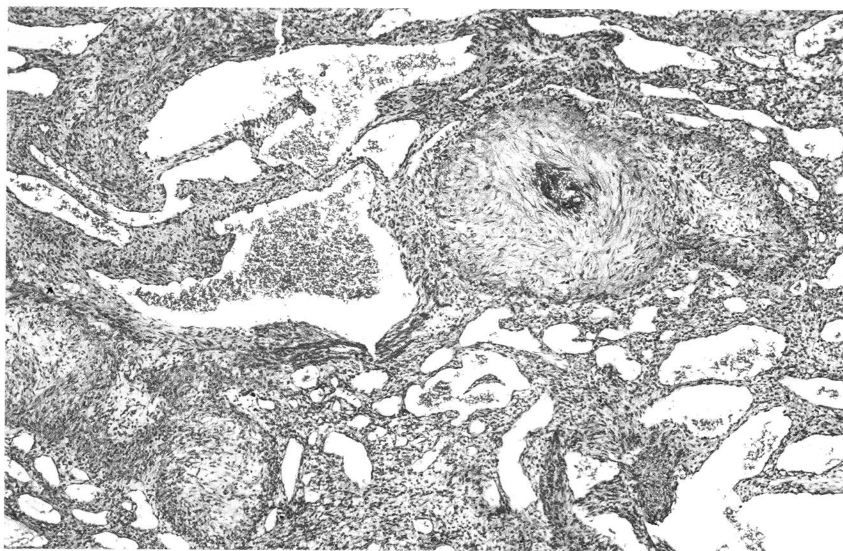

FIGURE 25-16. Glomangiomyoma. Note the blending of muscle in the vessels with tumor (Masson trichrome stain).

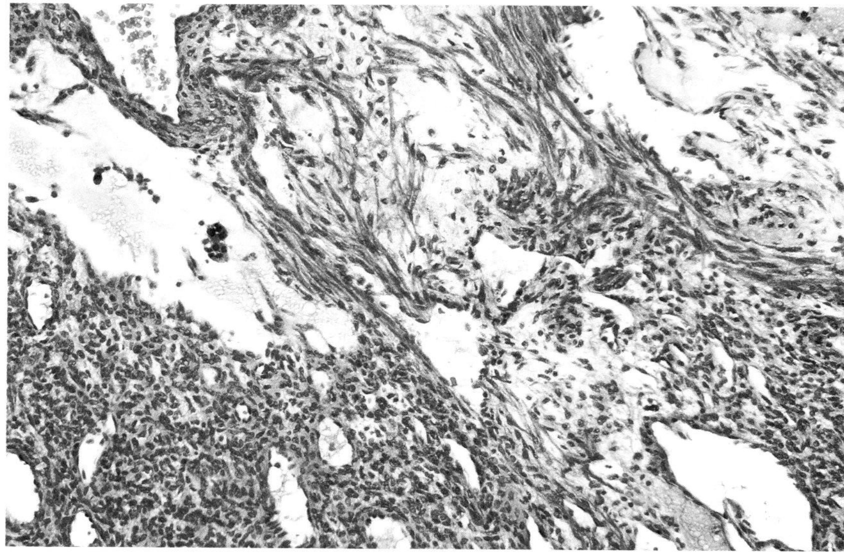

FIGURE 25-17. Glomangiomyoma. Glomus cells undergo transition to smooth muscle cells (Masson trichrome stain).

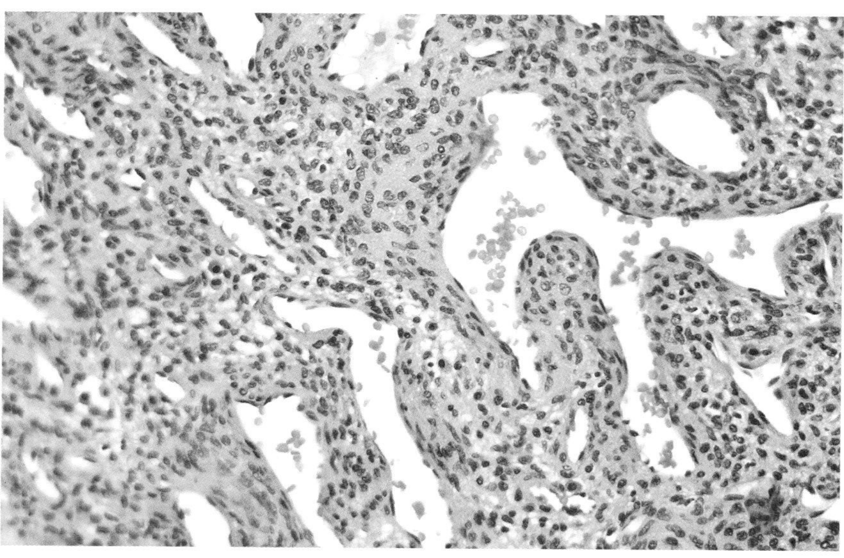

FIGURE 25-18. Glomus tumor that recurred with predominantly pericytic features: a so-called *glomangiopericytoma*.

referred to as *glomangiomatosis* and conceptualized as the glomoid counterpart of angiomatosis. Glomangiomatosis is rare, accounting for only 5% of glomus tumors with unusual or atypical features and a vanishingly smaller percentage of all glomus tumors. This form of glomus tumor may be more prevalent among patients who present during childhood.[43] Others have been reported in the literature.[37,44-50] Typically, these lesions are extensive, deep, and often pain-producing. Like angiomatosis, they consist of well-formed vessels of varying size that grow in a diffuse or infiltrative fashion (Fig. 25-19). Mature fat sometimes accompanies the vessels. Clusters of glomus cells invest the vessels, particularly small vessels. There is no evidence that these lesions are malignant or undergo malignant transformation, but, like angiomatosis, they may be difficult to eradicate. In fact, one remarkable case is known in which microscopic residua of glomangiomatosis were associated with persistence of pain and required wide excision to alleviate symptoms. In general, the extent of excision is gauged by the symptomatic and cosmetic needs of the patient.

ATYPICAL AND MALIGNANT GLOMUS TUMORS

Over the years, the malignancy of glomus tumors has been more of a concept than a reality. Although several histologically malignant glomus tumors have been reported, biologic confirmation of malignancy in these cases was lacking,[17,36,51-56] probably because many were superficial and therefore cured by therapy. A second compounding factor was that the rare malignant glomus tumors that produced metastases lacked a benign glomus component, and so the accuracy of the diagnosis was questioned. The tumor reported by Lumley and Stansfeld,[44] which produced metastases, is an example of this phenomenon. Two other reports, one by Brathwaite and Poppiti[57] and a second by Watanabe et al.,[58] detailed two patients with malignant glomus tumors clearly arising in the setting of a benign glomus tumor. The first case, a mitotically active glomus tumor of the nose in a patient with multiple glomus tumors, produced disseminated disease documented at autopsy. The second case was a glomangiomyoma that produced pulmonary metastases in 2 years.

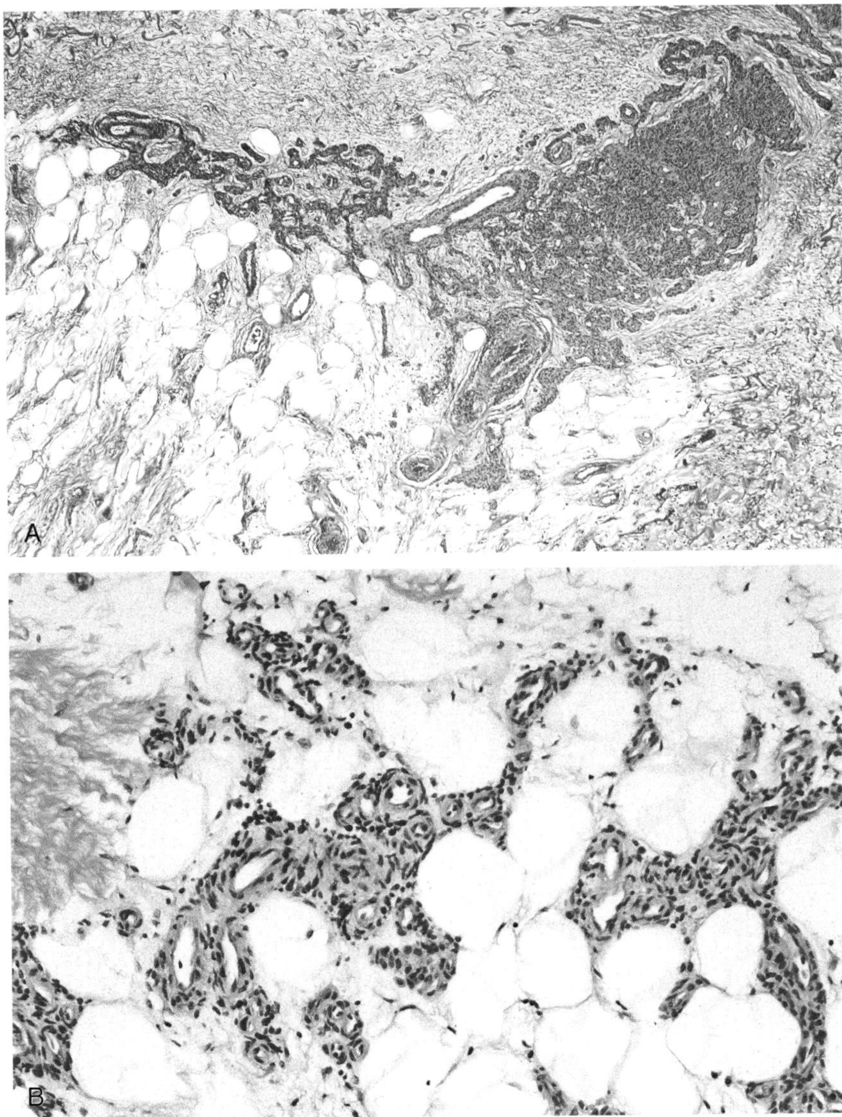

FIGURE 25-19. Diffuse glomus tumor (glomangiomatosis) with infiltrative growth of vessels (A), which are encircled by glomus cells (B).

A malignant glomus tumor can be diagnosed in the absence of a benign glomus component, provided that ancillary immunohistochemical data are available. In fact, only about one-half of malignant glomus tumors have a discernible benign component. Box 25-1 details the classification of glomus tumors with unusual features such as large size, nuclear atypia, and mitotic activity.

Malignant Glomus Tumor

Malignant glomus tumors are defined as those that (1) have marked nuclear atypia and elevated mitotic rates (greater than 5 mitoses/50 high-power fields [HPF]) or (2) display atypical mitotic figures.[50] Although large (greater than 2 cm) and deeply located glomus tumors are considered to be malignant, evidence has shown that most of these cases behave in a clinically benign fashion. Therefore, these lesions are better considered glomus tumors of uncertain malignant potential (see later text). A compressed rim of benign glomus tumor surrounding the malignant areas is seen in about one-half of cases (Fig. 25-20). The malignant areas can assume one of two patterns (Figs. 25-21 and 25-22). In the first, the tumor retains its architectural similarity to a benign glomus tumor and consists of sheets of round cells with a high nuclear/cytoplasmic ratio, high nuclear grade, and typical or atypical mitotic figures. At first glance, these lesions resemble a round cell sarcoma such as Ewing sarcoma (see Fig. 25-22). In the second pattern, the malignant areas differ cytoarchitecturally from a glomus tumor and are composed of spindle or fusiform cells arranged in short fascicles reminiscent of a fibrosarcoma or leiomyosarcoma (see Fig. 25-21). In the absence of a benign glomus component, the diagnosis of a malignant glomus tumor nearly always requires ancillary immunohistochemistry. Identification of cytoplasmic actin and the lattice-work of type IV collagen, at least focally, are highly suggestive of the diagnosis. Of the 21 glomus tumors meeting the criteria of malignancy detailed previously, 38% developed metastases, providing support for the validity of the criteria.[50] The validity of these criteria is also supported in more recent reports of histologically and clinical malignant glomus tumors.[15,16,59-73]

BOX 25-1 Classification of Glomus Tumors with Atypical Features

- Malignant glomus tumor
  - Marked atypia + mitotic activity (>5/50 HPF) or
  - Atypical mitotic figures
- Glomus tumor of uncertain malignant potential
  - Superficial location + high mitotic activity (>5/50 HPF) or
  - Large size (>2 cm) and/or deep location
- Symplastic glomus tumor
  - Lacks criteria for malignant glomus tumor and
  - Marked nuclear atypia only
- Glomangiomatosis
  - Lacks criteria for malignant glomus tumor or glomus tumor of uncertain malignant potential and
  - Diffuse growth resembling angiomatosis with prominent glomus component

Modified from Folpe AL, Fanburg-Smith JC, Miettinen M, et al. Atypical and malignant glomus tumors: analysis of 53 cases with a proposal for the reclassification of glomus tumors. *Am J Surg Pathol* 2001;25:1.

Glomus Tumor of Uncertain Malignant Potential

Some glomus tumors fail to meet the minimum criteria of malignancy but display features that are clearly beyond the realm of an ordinary glomus tumor. These lesions are designated as *glomus tumor of uncertain malignant potential.* Most lesions falling into this category are superficial tumors with high mitotic activity and no significant nuclear atypia, or are large or deep but otherwise devoid of atypical features (see Box 25-1). As noted previously, it is no longer believed that this second group of tumors should be classified as malignant.

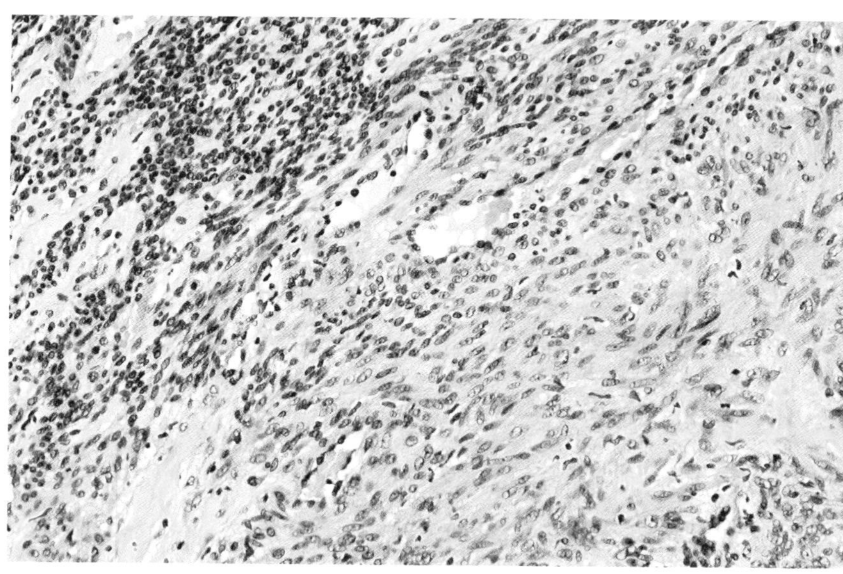

FIGURE 25-20. Malignant glomus tumor. There is a compressed rim of benign glomus tumor (upper left) next to a histologically malignant glomus tumor with a spindled pattern.

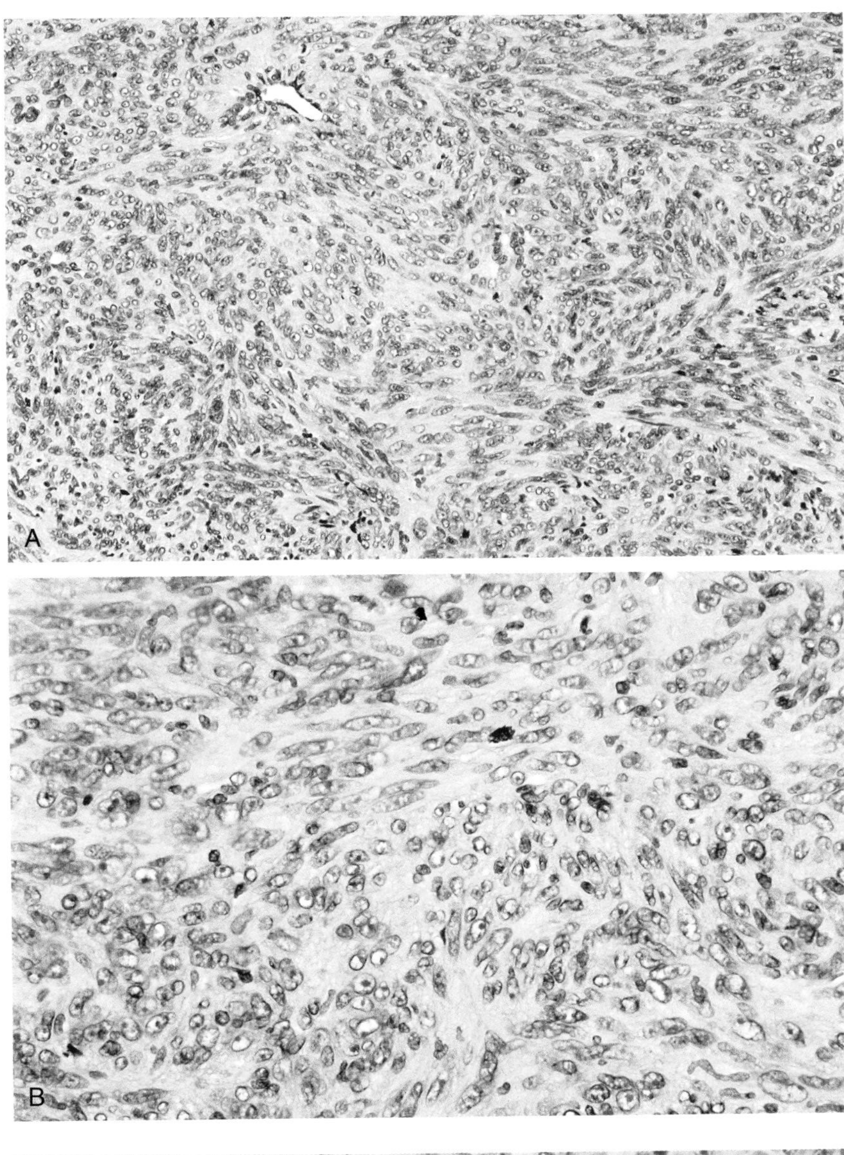

FIGURE 25-21. Malignant glomus tumor with a predominantly spindled pattern (A). Cells have myoid features with marked atypia and mitotic activity (B). Same case as in Figure 25-20.

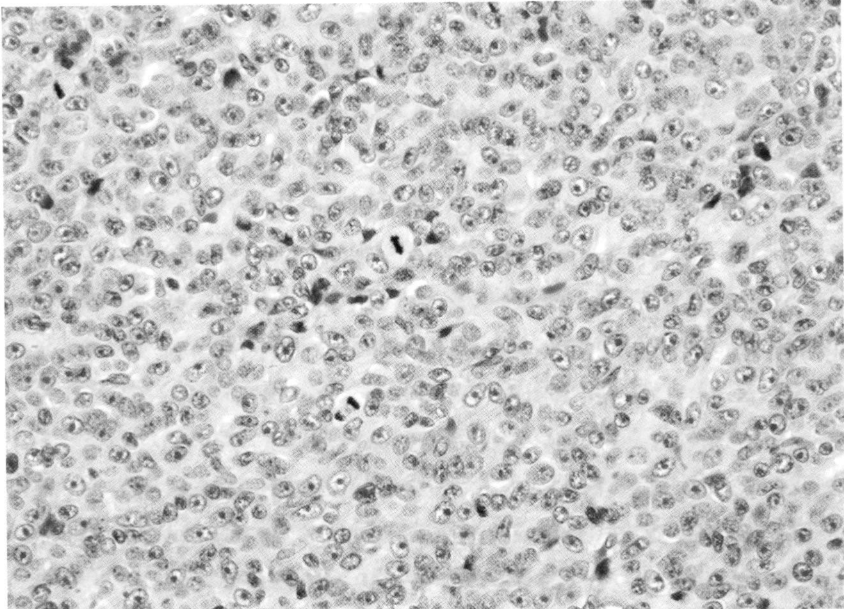

FIGURE 25-22. Malignant glomus tumor with the features of a predominantly round cell sarcoma. Such tumors may be confused with Ewing sarcoma or lymphoma.

The behavior of these tumors appears unpredictable, with most following a benign clinical course, but a minority eventually resulting in distant metastases, typically to the lungs. To date, the follow-up of other glomus tumors of uncertain malignant potential has been good, but the number of cases is small and the follow-up relatively short. Affixing the label *uncertain malignant potential* guarantees adequate follow-up for this problematic group of lesions.

Symplastic Glomus Tumor

Glomus tumors that have marked nuclear atypia as their sole unusual feature can be labeled *symplastic glomus tumors* (Fig. 25-23). The marked nuclear atypia that characterizes tumors in this group appears to be a degenerative phenomenon that can be likened to symplastic change in uterine leiomyomas. To date, symplastic glomus tumors have a benign course, similar to ordinary glomus tumors.[50,74-76]

MYOPERICYTOMA

Myopericytoma is a benign perivascular myoid tumor that has some overlapping features with glomus tumor and myofibroma.[77-79] It develops as a solitary, painless, slowly growing mass in the subcutaneous tissues of the lower extremity. Usually well marginated and measuring only a few centimeters in diameter, it is composed of oval to short fusiform cells that demonstrate a striking multilayered concentric growth around the vessels that may appear small and rounded or elongated and ectatic (Fig. 25-24). Architecturally, the close

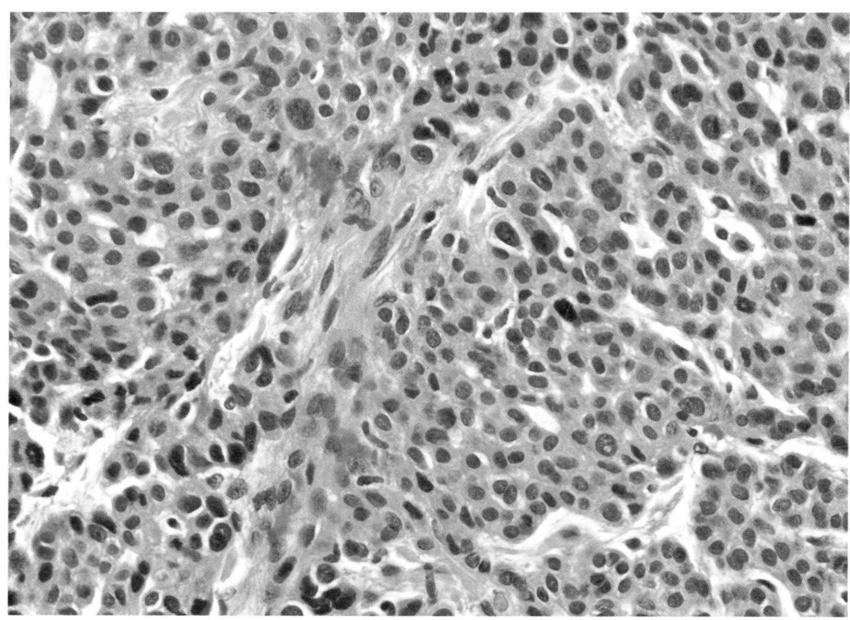

FIGURE 25-23. Glomus tumor with degenerative atypia (*symplastic glomus tumor*).

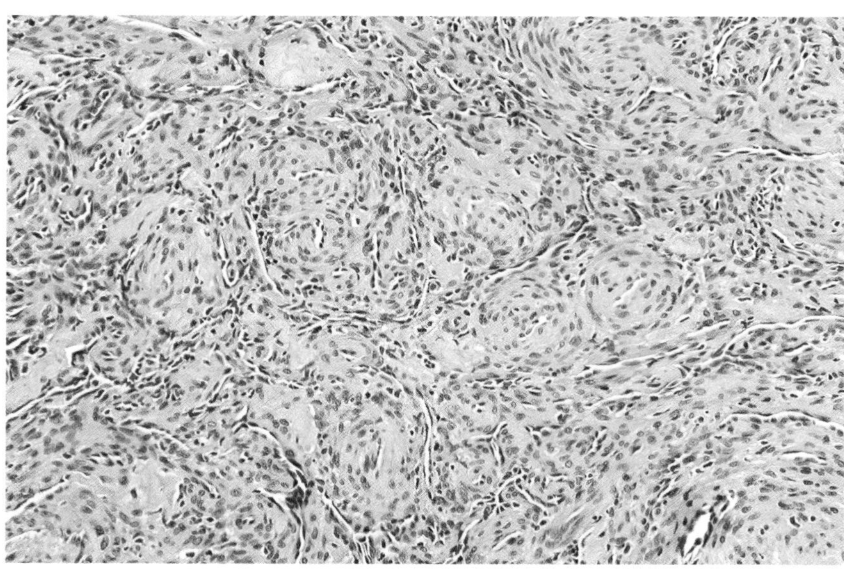

FIGURE 25-24. Myopericytoma. Muscle from the walls of small-caliber vessels spin off into the stroma of the lesion, giving it an appearance intermediate between a hemangiopericytoma and an angiomyoma.

and intricate arrangement of myoid cells to vessels in this tumor brings to mind the arrangement of angiomyoma, except that the cells of myopericytoma do not display a mature muscle phenotype. A small subset of myopericytomas may occur in an intravascular location. By immunohistochemistry, the cells of myopericytomas have a distinct myoid phenotype and express smooth muscle actin, h-caldesmon, and, less frequently, desmin and CD34.

Myopericytomas are almost always benign. Most do not recur following excision; those that do are likely poorly marginated. Rare examples of malignant myopericytoma have been reported[78,79] and are recognized by deeply infiltrative growth, marked atypia, and increased proliferative activity. Very recently, myopericytoma-like tumors, sometimes multiple, have been reported as arising in the setting of Epstein-Barr virus infection.[80-82] These lesions likely represent morphologic variants of Epstein-Barr virus-associated smooth muscle tumors (see Chapter 17).

HEMANGIOPERICYTOMA-LIKE TUMOR OF NASAL PASSAGES

First described by Compagno and Hyams[83] in 1976, the hemangiopericytoma-like tumor of the nasal passages (HTNP) is a distinctive tumor characterized by spindled myoid cells that are arranged around a prominent vasculature (Figs. 25-25 and 25-26). Both features have led to the suggestion that this lesion has little in common with the classic hemangiopericytoma of soft tissue but is more closely related to other perivascular myoid lesions, specifically the glomus tumor.[83a-86] It has been suggested that these lesions are better classified as *glomangiopericytoma*,[87] although the morphology of these distinctive tumors is somewhat different than that of glomangiopericytoma of soft tissue, as originally described by Granter et al.[77]

The HTNP appears unique to the nasal cavity and passages and seems to have no counterpart in soft tissue proper.

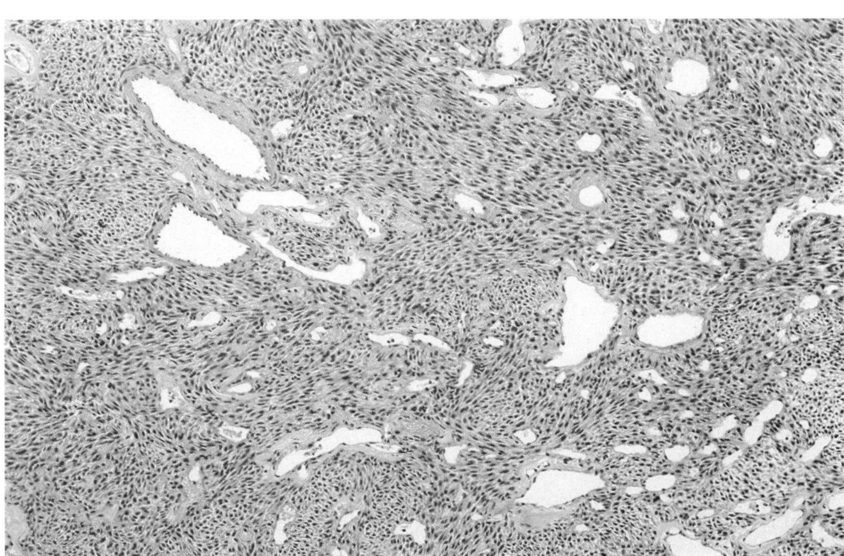

FIGURE 25-25. Hemangiopericytoma-like tumor of the nasal passage. The rounded to spindled myoid cells are arranged around an intricate vasculature.

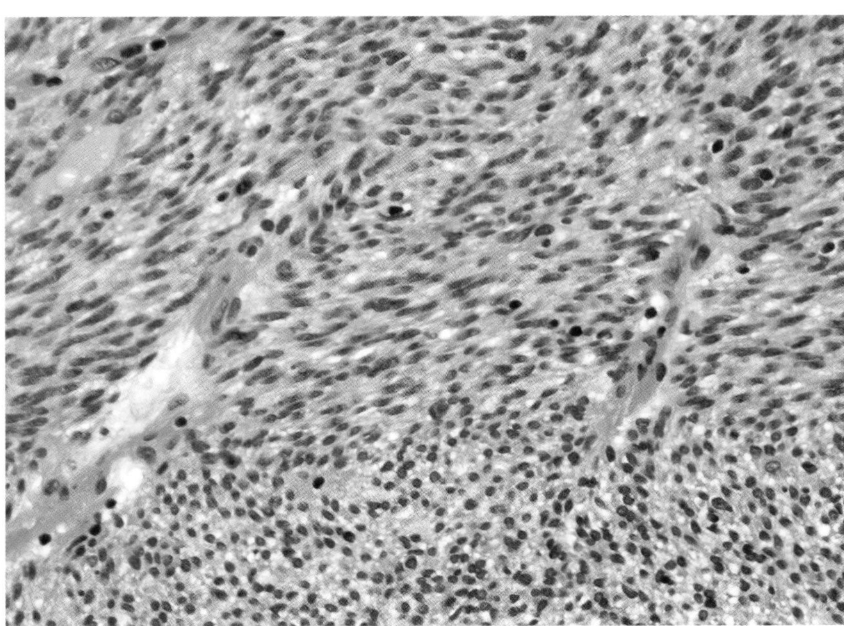

FIGURE 25-26. Higher power view of hemangiopericytoma-like tumor of the nasal passage, showing uniform spindled cells with minimal cytologic atypia surrounding small blood vessels.

Patients typically present with nasal obstruction or epistaxis. The majority are polypoid lesions that involve the nasal cavity or paranasal sinuses and grow as diffuse submucosal masses encircling minor salivary glands. Spindled to oval cells are arranged in short fascicular, storiform, whorled, or mixed patterns. The thin-walled vessels are occasionally staghorn shaped and hyalinized. Atypia is generally absent, and mitotic activity is low (1/10 HPF). Mast cells and eosinophils are noted, in most cases.

The cells within HTNP have a distinctly myoid phenotype, despite that they do not resemble mature smooth muscle cells. The vast majority express smooth muscle actin and muscle-specific actin, but not desmin. Only a minority of cases express CD34, the classic marker of the solitary fibrous tumor (hemangiopericytoma) family of lesions. Most behave in a benign manner.[84] In the largest experience reported to date, the 5- and 10-year disease-free survival was 74.2% and 64.4%, respectively. Patients at greatest risk to die of their disease are those with a long history of symptoms or those whose tumors display marked atypia or bone invasion.

References

1. Masson P. Le glomus neuromyoarterial des regions tactiles et ses tumeurs. Lyon Chir 1924;21:257.
2. Popoff N. The digital vascular system with reference to the state of the glomus in inflammation, arteriosclerotic gangrene, thromboangiitis obliterans, and supernumerary digits in man. Arch Pathol 1934;18: 295.
3. Shugart RR, Soule EH, Johnson EW. Glomus tumor. Surg Gynecol Obstet 1963;117:334.
4. Takata H, Ikuta Y, Ishida O, et al. Treatment of subungual glomus tumour. Hand Surg 2001;6(1):25–7.
5. Van Geertruyden J, Lorea P, Goldschmidt D, et al. Glomus tumours of the hand. A retrospective study of 51 cases. J Hand Surg [Br] 1996;21(2):257–60.
6. Okada O, Demitsu T, Manabe M, et al. A case of multiple subungual glomus tumors associated with neurofibromatosis type 1. J Dermatol 1999;26(8):535–7.
7. Sawada S, Honda M, Kamide R, et al. Three cases of subungual glomus tumors with von Recklinghausen neurofibromatosis. J Am Acad Dermatol 1995;32(2 Pt 1):277–8.
8. Albrecht S, Zbieranowski I. Incidental glomus coccygeum. When a normal structure looks like a tumor. Am J Surg Pathol 1990;14(10): 922–4.
9. Duncan L, Halverson J, DeSchryver-Kecskemeti K. Glomus tumor of the coccyx. A curable cause of coccygodynia. Arch Pathol Lab Med [Case Reports] 1991;115(1):78–80.
10. Gatalica Z, Wang L, Lucio ET, et al. Glomus coccygeum in surgical pathology specimens: small troublemaker. Arch Pathol Lab Med 1999;123(10): 905–8.
11. Haque S, Modlin IM, West AB. Multiple glomus tumors of the stomach with intravascular spread. Am J Surg Pathol 1992;16(3):291–9.
12. Miettinen M, Paal E, Lasota J, et al. Gastrointestinal glomus tumors: a clinicopathologic, immunohistochemical, and molecular genetic study of 32 cases. Am J Surg Pathol 2002;26(3):301–11.
13. Kiyosawa T, Umebayashi Y, Nakayama Y, et al. Hereditary multiple glomus tumors involving the glans penis. A case report and review of the literature. Dermatol Surg 1995;21(10):895–9.
14. Saito T. Glomus tumor of the penis. Int J Urol 2000;7(3):115–7.
15. Masson-Lecomte A, Rocher L, Ferlicot S, et al. High-flow priapism due to a malignant glomus tumor (glomangiosarcoma) of the corpus cavernosum. J Sex Med 2011;8(12):3518–22.
16. Shim HS, Choi YD, Cho NH. Malignant glomus tumor of the urinary bladder. Arch Pathol Lab Med 2005;129(7):940–2.
17. Hirose T, Hasegawa T, Seki K, et al. Atypical glomus tumor in the mediastinum: a case report with immunohistochemical and ultrastructural studies. Ultrastruct Pathol 1996;20(5):451–6.
18. Calonje E, Fletcher CD. Cutaneous intraneural glomus tumor [see comments]. Am J Dermatopathol 1995;17(4):395–8.
19. Rozmaryn LM, Sadler AH, Dorfman HD. Intraosseous glomus tumor in the ulna. A case report. Clin Orthop Relat Res 1987;(220):126–9.
20. Gaertner EM, Steinberg DM, Huber M, et al. Pulmonary and mediastinal glomus tumors–report of five cases including a pulmonary glomangiosarcoma: a clinicopathologic study with literature review. Am J Surg Pathol 2000;24(8):1105–14.
21. Kishimoto S, Nagatani H, Miyashita A, et al. Immunohistochemical demonstration of substance P-containing nerve fibres in glomus tumours. Br J Dermatol 1985;113(2):213–8.
22. Idy-Peretti I, Cermakova E, Dion E, et al. Subungual glomus tumor: diagnosis based on high-resolution MR images. AJR Am J Roentgenol [Case Reports Letter] 1992;159(6):1351.
23. Pulitzer DR, Martin PC, Reed RJ. Epithelioid glomus tumor. Hum Pathol 1995;26(9):1022–7.
24. Shin DH, Park SS, Lee JH, et al. Oncocytic glomus tumor of the trachea. Chest [Case Reports] 1990;98(4):1021–3.
25. Slater DN, Cotton DW, Azzopardi JG. Oncocytic glomus tumour: a new variant. Histopathology 1987;11(5):523–31.
26. Haupt HM, Stern JB, Berlin SJ. Immunohistochemistry in the differential diagnosis of nodular hidradenoma and glomus tumor. Am J Dermatopathol 1992;14(4):310–4.
27. Kaye VM, Dehner LP. Cutaneous glomus tumor. A comparative immunohistochemical study with pseudoangiomatous intradermal melanocytic nevi. Am J Dermatopathol [Comparative Study] 1991;13(1):2–6.
28. Venkatachalam MA, Greally JG. Fine structure of glomus tumor: similarity of glomus cells to smooth muscle. Cancer 1969;23(5):1176–84.
29. Brooks JJ, Miettinen M, Virtanen I. Desmin immunoreactivity in glomus tumors. Am J Clin Pathol [Letter] 1987;87(2):292.
30. Dervan PA, Tobbia IN, Casey M, et al. Glomus tumours: an immunohistochemical profile of 11 cases. Histopathology 1989;14(5):483–91.
31. Nuovo M. Glomus tumors: clinicopathologic and immunohistochemical analysis of forty cases. Surg Pathol 1990;3:31.
32. Porter PL, Bigler SA, McNutt M, et al. The immunophenotype of hemangiopericytomas and glomus tumors, with special reference to muscle protein expression: an immunohistochemical study and review of the literature. Mod Pathol 1991;4(1):46–52.
33. Schurch W, Skalli O, Lagace R, et al. Intermediate filament proteins and actin isoforms as markers for soft-tissue tumor differentiation and origin. III. Hemangiopericytomas and glomus tumors. Am J Pathol 1990;136(4): 771–86.
34. Watanabe K, Kusakabe T, Hoshi N, et al. Suzuki T. h-Caldesmon in leiomyosarcoma and tumors with smooth muscle cell-like differentiation: its specific expression in the smooth muscle cell tumor. Hum Pathol 1999; 30(4):392–6.
35. Tsuneyoshi M, Enjoji M. Glomus tumor: a clinicopathologic and electron microscopic study. Cancer [Research Support, Non-U.S. Gov't] 1982; 50(8):1601–7.
36. Gould EW, Manivel JC, Albores-Saavedra J, et al. Locally infiltrative glomus tumors and glomangiosarcomas. A clinical, ultrastructural, and immunohistochemical study. Cancer 1990;65(2):310–8.
37. Rao VK, Weiss SW. Angiomatosis of soft tissue. An analysis of the histologic features and clinical outcome in 51 cases. Am J Surg Pathol 1992; 16(8):764–71.
38. Boon LM, Mulliken JB, Enjolras O, et al. Glomuvenous malformation (glomangioma) and venous malformation: distinct clinicopathologic and genetic entities. Arch Dermatol 2004;140(8):971–6.
39. Brouillard P, Boon LM, Mulliken JB, et al. Mutations in a novel factor, glomulin, are responsible for glomuvenous malformations ("glomangiomas"). Am J Hum Genet 2002;70(4):866–74.
40. Eyster Jr WH, Montgomery H. Multiple glomus tumors. AMA Arch Dermatol Syphilol 1950;62(6):893–906.
41. Yang JS, Ko JW, Suh KS, et al. Congenital multiple plaque-like glomangiomyoma. Am J Dermatopathol [Case Reports] 1999;21(5):454–7.
42. Calduch L, Monteagudo C, Martinez-Ruiz E, et al. Familial generalized multiple glomangiomyoma: report of a new family, with immunohistochemical and ultrastructural studies and review of the literature. Pediatr Dermatol [Case Reports Review] 2002;19(5):402–8.
43. Stout A. Tumors of the neuromyoarterial glomus. Am J Cancer 1935;24:255.
44. Lumley JS, Stansfeld AG. Infiltrating glomus tumour of lower limb. Br Med J 1972;1(798):484–5.
45. Negri G, Schulte M, Mohr W. Glomus tumor with diffuse infiltration of the quadriceps muscle: a case report. Hum Pathol [Case Reports] 1997;28(6):750–2.
46. Skelton HG, Smith KJ. Infiltrative glomus tumor arising from a benign glomus tumor: a distinctive immunohistochemical pattern in the infiltrative component. Am J Dermatopathol [Case Reports] 1999;21(6): 562–6.

47. Zhou P, Zhang H, Bu H, et al. Paravertebral glomangiomatosis. Case report. J Neurosurg 2009;111(2):272–7.
48. Park EA, Hong SH, Choi JY, et al. Glomangiomatosis: magnetic resonance imaging findings in three cases. Skeletal Radiol 2005;34(2):108–11.
49. Jalali M, Netscher DT, Connelly JH. Glomangiomatosis. Ann Diagn Pathol 2002;6(5):326–8.
50. Folpe AL, Fanburg-Smith JC, Miettinen M, et al. Atypical and malignant glomus tumors: analysis of 52 cases, with a proposal for the reclassification of glomus tumors. Am J Surg Pathol 2001;25(1):1–12.
51. Aiba M, Hirayama A, Kuramochi S. Glomangiosarcoma in a glomus tumor. An immunohistochemical and ultrastructural study. Cancer 1988;61(7):1467–71.
52. Hegyi L, Cormack GC, Grant JW. Histochemical investigation into the molecular mechanisms of malignant transformation in a benign glomus tumour. J Clin Pathol [Case Reports] 1998;51(11):872–4.
53. Hiruta N, Kameda N, Tokudome T, et al. Malignant glomus tumor: a case report and review of the literature. Am J Surg Pathol 1997;21(9): 1096–103.
54. Lopez-Rios F, Rodriguez-Peralto JL, Castano E, et al. Glomangiosarcoma of the lower limb: a case report with a literature review. J Cutan Pathol [Case Reports Review] 1997;24(9):571–4.
55. Noer H, Krogdahl A. Glomangiosarcoma of the lower extremity. Histopathology 1991;18(4):365–6.
56. Wetherington RW, Lyle WG, Sangueza OP. Malignant glomus tumor of the thumb: a case report. J Hand Surg Am 1997;22(6):1098–102.
57. Brathwaite CD, Poppiti Jr RJ. Malignant glomus tumor. A case report of widespread metastases in a patient with multiple glomus body hamartomas. Am J Surg Pathol 1996;20(2):233–8.
58. Watanabe K, Sugino T, Saito A, et al. Glomangiosarcoma of the hip: report of a highly aggressive tumour with widespread distant metastases. Br J Dermatol 1998;139(6):1097–101.
59. Lancerotto L, Salmaso R, Sartore L, et al. Malignant glomus tumor of the leg developed in the context of a superficial typical glomus tumor. Int J Surg Pathol 2012;20(4):420–4.
60. Uchiyama M, Kato T, Kunitani K, et al. [Multiple glomus tumors in chest wall and buttocks]. Kyobu Geka 2011;64(2):116–9.
61. Terada T, Fujimoto J, Shirakashi Y, et al. Malignant glomus tumor of the palm: a case report. J Cutan Pathol 2011;38(4):381–4.
62. Lamba G, Rafiyath SM, Kaur H, et al. Malignant glomus tumor of kidney: the first reported case and review of literature. Hum Pathol 2011;42(8):1200–3.
63. Cecchi R, Pavesi M, Apicella P. Malignant glomus tumor of the trunk treated with Mohs micrographic surgery. J Dtsch Dermatol Ges 2011;9(5):391–2.
64. Zhang Q, Wang S, Divakaran J, et al. Malignant glomus tumour of the lung. Pathology 2010;42(6):594–6.
65. Song SE, Lee CH, Kim KA, et al. Malignant glomus tumor of the stomach with multiorgan metastases: report of a case. Surg Today 2010;40(7): 662–7.
66. Oh SD, Stephenson D, Schnall S, et al. Malignant glomus tumor of the hand. Appl Immunohistochem Mol Morphol 2009;17(3):264–9.
67. Hayashi M, Kitagawa Y, Kim Y, et al. Malignant glomus tumor arising among multiple glomus tumors. J Orthop Sci 2008;13(5):472–5.
68. Cibull TL, Gleason BC, O'Malley DP, et al. Malignant cutaneous glomus tumor presenting as a rapidly growing leg mass in a pregnant woman. J Cutan Pathol 2008;35(8):765–9.
69. Vasenwala SM, Iraqi AA, Ahmad S, et al. Malignant glomus tumour–a case report. Indian J Pathol Microbiol 2006;49(1):40–1.
70. Perez de la Fuente T, Vega C, Gutierrez Palacios A, et al. Glomangiosarcoma of the hypothenar eminence: a case report. Chir Main 2005; 24(3-4):199–202.
71. Khoury T, Balos L, McGrath B, et al. Malignant glomus tumor: a case report and review of literature, focusing on its clinicopathologic features and immunohistochemical profile. Am J Dermatopathol 2005;27(5): 428–31.
72. Park JH, Oh SH, Yang MH, et al. Glomangiosarcoma of the hand: a case report and review of the literature. J Dermatol 2003;30(11):827–33.
73. De Chiara A, Apice G, Mori S, et al. Malignant glomus tumour: a case report and review of the literature. Sarcoma 2003;7(2):87–91.
74. Kamarashev J, French LE, Dummer R, et al. Symplastic glomus tumor—a rare but distinct benign histological variant with analogy to other "ancient" benign skin neoplasms. J Cutan Pathol 2009;36(10):1099–102.
75. Chong Y, Eom M, Min HJ, et al. Symplastic glomus tumor: a case report. Am J Dermatopathol 2009;31(1):71–3.
76. Arsenovic N, Ramaiya A, Moreira R. Symplastic glomangioma: information review and addition of a new case. Int J Surg Pathol 2011;19(4): 499–501.
77. Granter SR, Badizadegan K, Fletcher CD. Myofibromatosis in adults, glomangiopericytoma, and myopericytoma: a spectrum of tumors showing perivascular myoid differentiation. Am J Surg Pathol 1998;22(5): 513–25.
78. McMenamin ME, Fletcher CD. Malignant myopericytoma: expanding the spectrum of tumours with myopericytic differentiation. Histopathology [Case Reports] 2002;41(5):450–60.
79. Mentzel T, Dei Tos AP, Sapi Z, et al. Myopericytoma of skin and soft tissues: clinicopathologic and immunohistochemical study of 54 cases. Am J Surg Pathol 2006;30(1):104–13.
80. Calderaro J, Polivka M, Gallien S, et al. Multifocal Epstein Barr virus (EBV)-associated myopericytoma in a patient with AIDS. Neuropathol Appl Neurobiol 2008;34(1):115–7.
81. Lau PP, Wong OK, Lui PC, et al. Myopericytoma in patients with AIDS: a new class of Epstein-Barr virus-associated tumor. Am J Surg Pathol 2009;33(11):1666–72.
82. Ramdial PK, Sing Y, Deonarain J, et al. Periampullary Epstein-Barr virus-associated myopericytoma. Hum Pathol 2011;42(9):1348–54.
83. Compagno J, Hyams VJ. Hemangiopericytoma-like intranasal tumors. A clinicopathologic study of 23 cases. Am J Clin Pathol 1976;66(4): 672–83.
83a. Fletcher C. Hemangiopericytoma-a dying breed? Reappraisal of an entity and its variant: a hypothesis. Curr Diagn Pathol 1994;1:19.
84. Thompson LD, Miettinen M, Wenig BM. Sinonasal-type hemangiopericytoma: a clinicopathologic and immunophenotypic analysis of 104 cases showing perivascular myoid differentiation. Am J Surg Pathol 2003;27(6): 737–49.
85. Tse LL, Chan JK. Sinonasal haemangiopericytoma-like tumour: a sinonasal glomus tumour or a haemangiopericytoma? Histopathology 2002; 40(6):510–7.
86. Kuo FY, Lin HC, Eng HL, et al. Sinonasal hemangiopericytoma-like tumor with true pericytic myoid differentiation: a clinicopathologic and immunohistochemical study of five cases. Head Neck 2005;27(2): 124–9.
87. Thompson LD. Sinonasal tract glomangiopericytoma (hemangiopericytoma). Ear Nose Throat J 2004;83(12):807.

Benign Tumors and Tumor-Like Lesions of Synovial Tissue

CHAPTER CONTENTS

The synovial membrane forms the lining of joints, tendons, and bursae. In addition, its cells synthesize hyaluronate, a major component of synovial fluid, and facilitate the exchange of substances between blood and synovial fluid. The synovial membrane varies considerably in appearance, depending on local mechanical factors and the nature of the underlying tissue. For instance, the synovial surface of joints subjected to high pressure is flat and acellular, whereas joints under less stress have a redundant surface lined by cells that resemble cuboidal or columnar epithelium.[1] Unlike epithelial lining cells, the synovial cells do not rest on a basal lamina but blend with the underlying stromal elements, occasionally forming an incomplete layer at the surface only.[2] Therefore, joint fluid and blood vessels come in close contact with each other, a relationship that probably enhances solute exchange between the two compartments.

Electron microscopically, the synovial membrane is composed of two cell types. Type A cells are found beneath the surface and are characterized by filopodia that extend upward and form a ramifying network of overlapping processes devoid of junctional attachments. Under appropriate conditions, these cells engage in phagocytosis. The surface synoviocytes are termed *type B cells*. These cells have ovoid nuclei and long cytoplasmic processes that circumferentially surround the nucleus. Although seemingly different, these cells probably represent functional modulations of the same cell because transitional forms are often seen.[1,3] Both cells are embedded in a collagen-rich extracellular matrix with pools of amorphous ground substance. Immunohistochemically, both synoviocyte types stain for CD68, but they do not express actins, desmin, CD34, CD45, S-100 protein, or cytokeratins.

A number of benign tumors and tumor-like lesions arise from the synovium, such as chondroma of the tendon sheath, fibroma of the tendon sheath, synovial chondromatosis, and synovial hemangioma; yet only the giant cell tumor is considered prototypical. This tumor is the most common benign tumor of the tendon sheath and synovium and is the only one that generally recapitulates the appearance of the normal synovial cell.

The most significant contribution to the understanding of giant cell tumor of tendon sheath was made by Jaffe et al.,[4] who regarded the synovium of the tendon sheath, bursa, and joint as an anatomic unit that could give rise to a common family of lesions, including the giant cell tumor of tendon sheath (nodular tenosynovitis), localized and diffuse forms of pigmented villonodular synovitis, and rare cases of extra-articular pigmented villonodular synovitis arising from bursae (diffuse type giant cell tumor of tendon sheath). These authors maintained that the differences in clinical extent and growth were influenced by the anatomic location. Lesions of the joints tended to expand inward and grow along the joint surface as the path of least resistance. Tumors of the tendon sheath, of necessity, grew outward, molded and confined by the shearing forces of the tendon. At present, there has been no improvement of the elegant unifying concept of Jaffe et al.[4] On the other hand, their hypothesis that these lesions are reactive in nature is incorrect; the preponderance of evidence indicates that they are neoplastic.

Although a number of terms have been applied in the literature, the term *tenosynovial giant cell tumor* is preferred, and the tumors are divided into localized and diffuse forms, depending on their growth characteristics.[5] The localized type primarily affects the digits and arises from the synovium of tendon sheaths or interphalangeal joints. The diffuse form occurs in areas adjacent to large weight-bearing joints such as the knee and ankle and, in many instances, represents an extra-articular extension of pigmented villonodular synovitis. A small number of diffuse giant cell tumors have no intra-articular component and probably take origin from bursae associated with large joints. Pigmented villonodular synovitis restricted to the joint proper is not specifically discussed in the chapter.

GIANT CELL TUMOR OF TENDON SHEATH, LOCALIZED TYPE (TENOSYNOVIAL GIANT CELL TUMOR, LOCALIZED TYPE)

The localized form of giant cell tumor of tendon sheath is characterized by a discrete proliferation of rounded synovial-like cells accompanied by a variable number of multinucleated giant cells, inflammatory cells, siderophages, and xanthoma cells.

Clinical Findings

Giant cell tumor of tendon sheath may occur at any age but is most common in patients 30 to 50 years of age. Women are affected about twice as often as men.[6,7] The tumors occur predominantly on the hand, where they represent the most common neoplasm of that region (Figs. 26-1 and 26-2). Less common sites include the feet, ankles, and knees.[8,9] In the study by Ushijima et al.,[7] 183 of 208 tumors occurred in the digits, most commonly one of the fingers (158 cases); only 25 tumors were found in the larger joints, including the ankle/foot (10 cases), knee (8 cases), wrist (6 cases), and elbow (1 case). Finger lesions are typically located adjacent to the interphalangeal joint, although other sites may also be affected.

The tumors develop gradually over a long period of time and often remain the same size for several years. On physical examination, they are fixed to deep structures but are usually not attached to skin unless the lesion occurs in the distal portion of the fingers where skin is closely related to tendon. Serum cholesterol levels are invariably normal. Antecedent trauma occurs in a variable number of patients, but its association with the lesions is likely fortuitous. Radiographic studies usually demonstrate a circumscribed soft tissue mass and, occasionally, degenerative changes of the adjacent joint.[10] In only a small portion of patients (perhaps 10%), however, there is cortical erosion of bone,[11] and bony invasion is exceedingly uncommon.

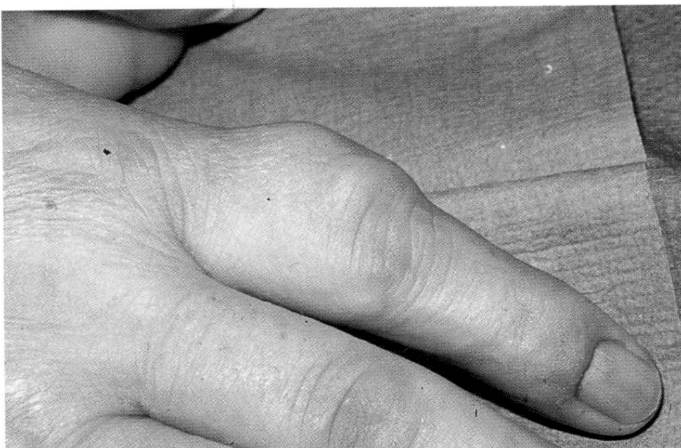

FIGURE 26-1. Localized giant cell tumor involving the proximal portion of the finger.

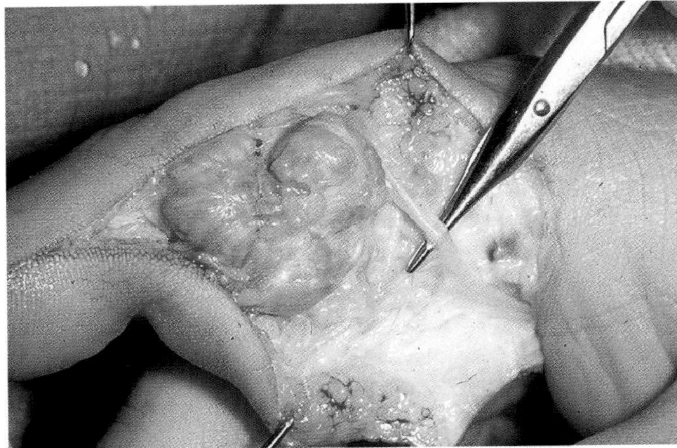

FIGURE 26-2. Localized giant cell tumor. Lobulated mass is present adjacent to the tendon (same case as in Figure 26-1).

Gross Findings

Giant cell tumor of tendon sheath is a circumscribed lobulated mass that has occasional shallow grooves along its deep surfaces, created by the underlying tendons (Figs. 26-3 and 26-4). They are usually relatively small, ranging from 0.5 to between 3.0 and 4.0 cm in diameter. Those on the feet are often larger and more irregular in shape than those on the hands. On a cut section, the tumors have a mottled appearance: a pink-gray background flecked with yellow or brown, depending on the amount of lipid and hemosiderin. Tumors arising in the large joints are usually of greater size and more irregular in shape than tumors in the digits.

Microscopic Findings

The earliest lesion is a villous structure that projects into the synovial space of the tendon sheath. Limited space prevents continued growth into the cavity so, ultimately, the tumor grows outward in a cauliflower fashion and compresses synovium-lined clefts into its substance. At the stage at which most lesions are surgically excised, they are exophytic masses attached to the tendon sheath and have smooth but lobulated contours. They are partially invested by a dense collagenous capsule that penetrates the tumor, dividing it into vague nodules. The capsule is not totally confining because isolated nests of tumor can be identified outside of its bounds, especially at the deep margin where the tumor blends with the synovial membrane.

The histologic appearance of this tumor varies, depending on the proportion of mononuclear cells, giant cells, xanthoma

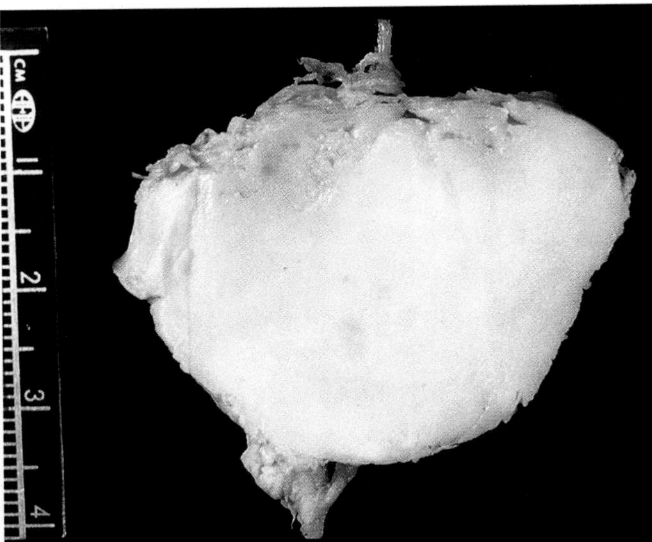

FIGURE 26-3. Gross appearance of giant cell tumor of the tendon sheath, localized type.

cells, hemosiderin, and the degree of collagenization (Figs. 26-5 to 26-7). Most tumors are moderately cellular and are composed of sheets of round or polygonal cells that blend with hypocellular collagenized zones in which the cells appear slightly spindled. Cleft-like spaces are occasionally present, particularly in lesions arising near large joints. Some probably represent synovium-lined spaces, whereas others are artifactual spaces caused by shrinkage and loss of cellular cohesion. Multinucleated giant cells are scattered throughout the lesions. In the typical case, they are relatively numerous but become sparse in highly cellular lesions, particularly recurrent ones (Fig. 26-8). These cells, which form by fusion of the more prevalent mononuclear cells, have a variable number of nuclei, ranging from as few as 3 to 4 to as many as 50 to 60. Xanthoma cells are also frequent, tend to be located geographically in these tumors, and often contain fine hemosiderin granules and/or cholesterol clefts (Fig. 26-9). Cartilaginous and osseous metaplasia is a rare focal finding.

The diagnosis of giant cell tumor of tendon sheath is rarely difficult, but the evaluation of certain atypical features can be problematic. For instance, the presence of mitotic figures occasionally leads to a mistaken diagnosis of a malignant neoplasm. Rao and Vigorita[12] documented three or more mitotic figures per 10 high-power fields (HPF) in more than 10% of their cases. Although it may indicate an actively growing lesion that is likely to recur, no evidence suggests that these lesions are at increased risk to metastasize (Figs. 26-10 and 26-11). In about 1% to 5% of cases, tumor thrombi are observed in small veins draining these lesions (Fig. 26-12). Likewise, this feature does not correlate with the ability to produce metastasis, based on follow-up information in the cases of the authors of this edition. In fact, because of the extreme rarity of metastasizing forms of giant cell tumor of tendon sheath, it is justifiable to adopt a conservative approach when interpreting these atypical features.

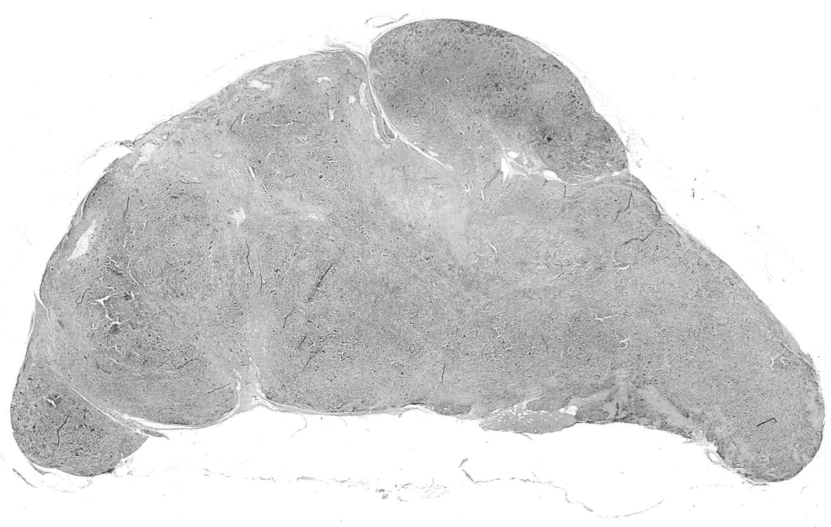

FIGURE 26-4. Localized giant cell tumor illustrating a late-stage lesion. Deep synovial clefts are obliterated and replaced by fibrous bands that impart a vague lobular pattern to the tumor. Concave surface at the bottom is created by underlying tendon.

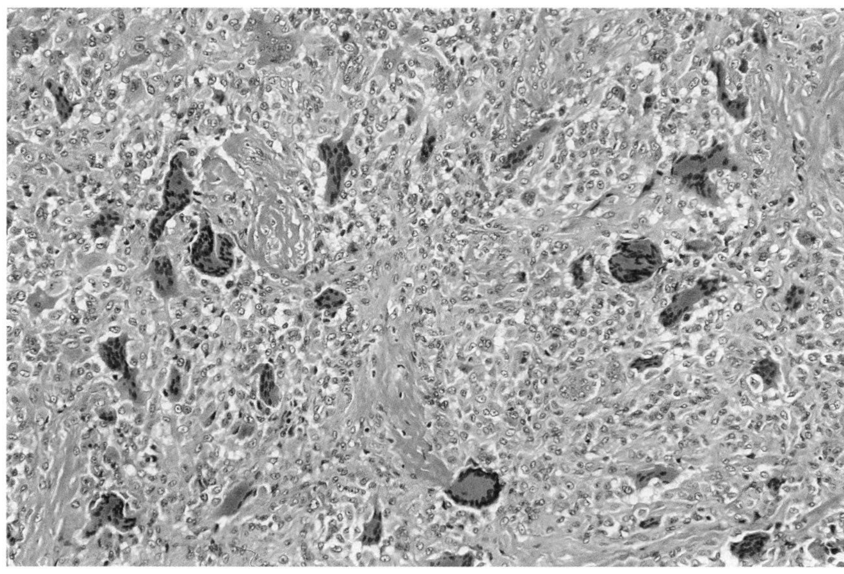

FIGURE 26-5. Localized form of giant cell tumor with a regular distribution of multinucleated giant cells admixed with round cells and collagen.

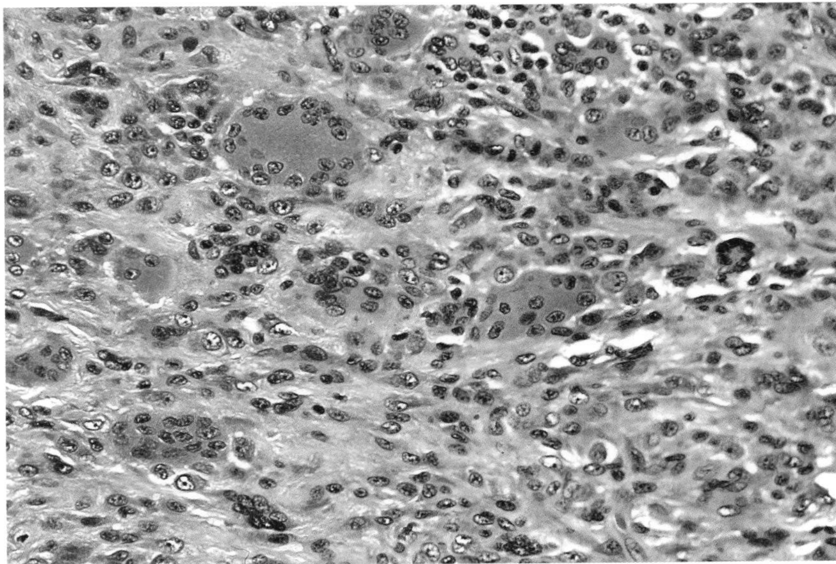

FIGURE 26-6. Giant cell-rich area of a localized form of giant cell tumor.

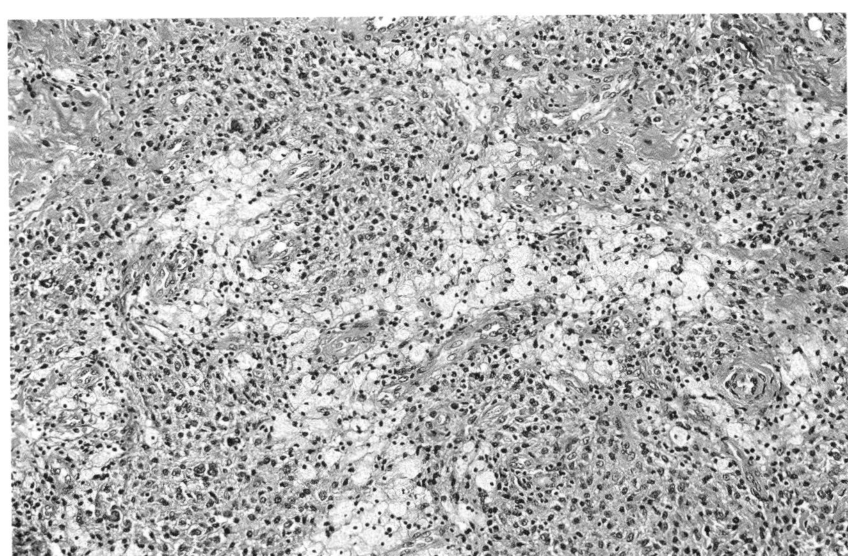

FIGURE 26-7. Localized form of giant cell tumor showing focal collections of xanthoma cells intermixed with round cells.

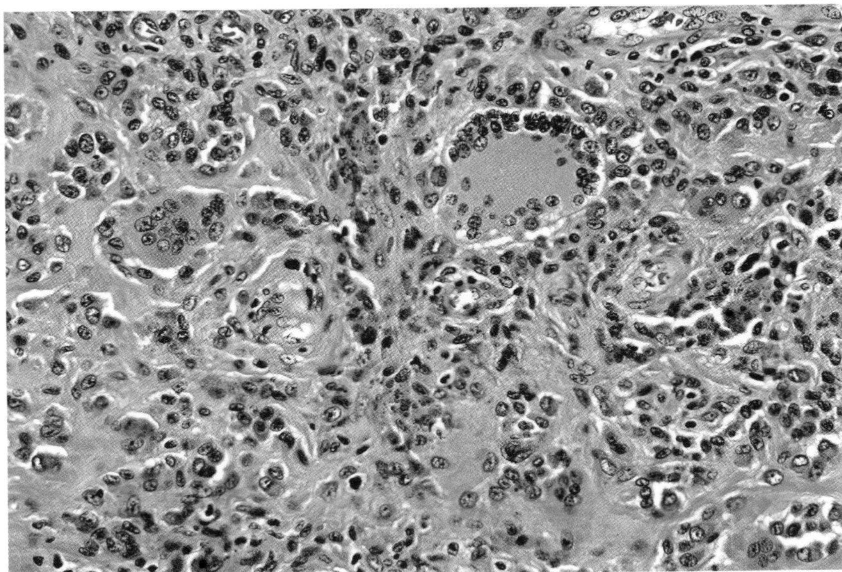

FIGURE 26-8. Rare giant cells admixed with round cells and areas of hemosiderin deposition in a giant cell-poor localized form of giant cell tumor.

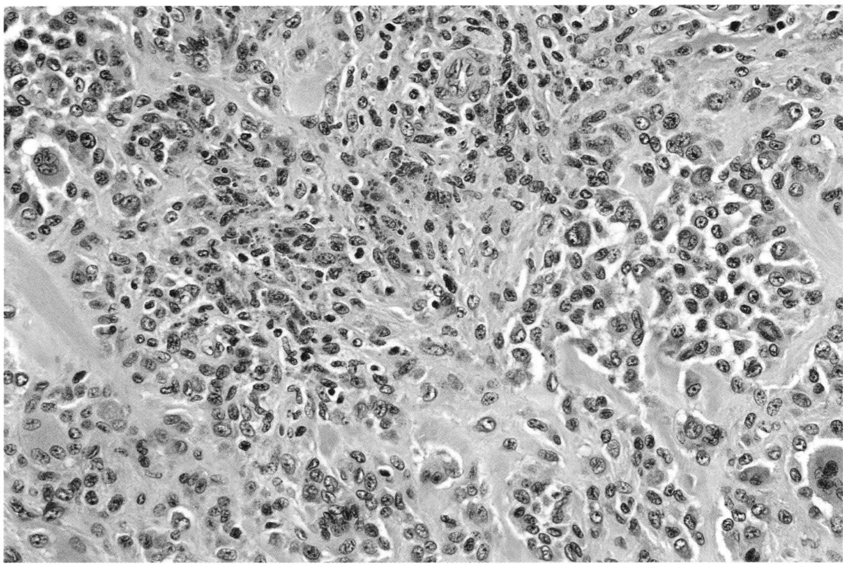

FIGURE 26-9. Abundant hemosiderin deposition in a localized giant cell tumor.

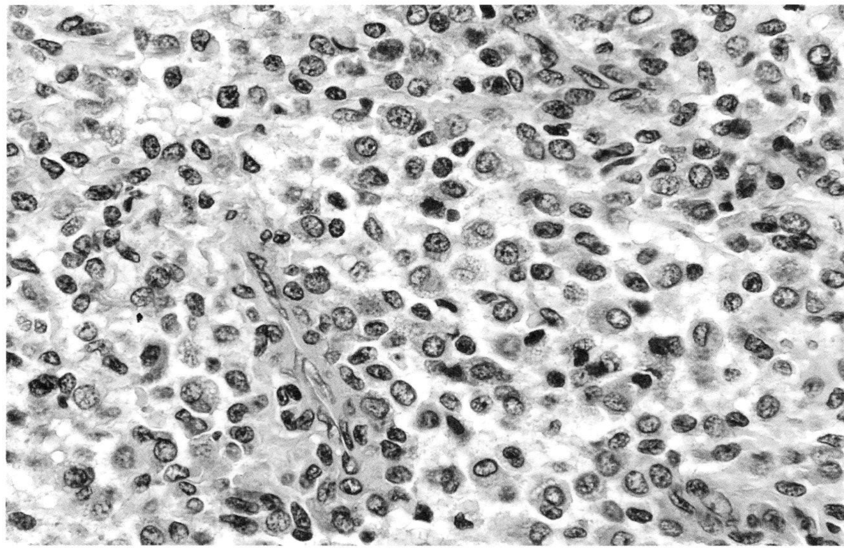

FIGURE 26-10. High-power view of round cells in a giant cell tumor with a paucity of giant cells. Some of the cells contain intracytoplasmic hemosiderin.

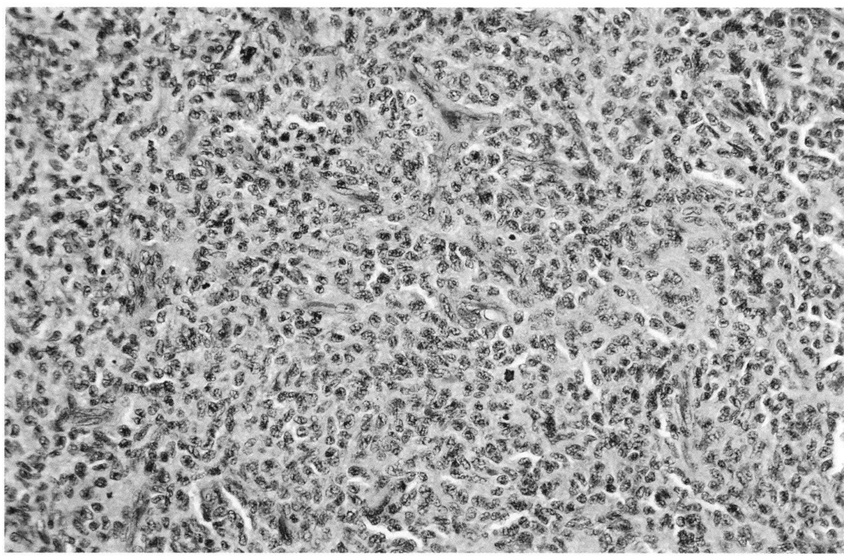

FIGURE 26-11. Cellular example of a localized form of giant cell tumor with a paucity of giant cells. Rare mitotic figures can be seen.

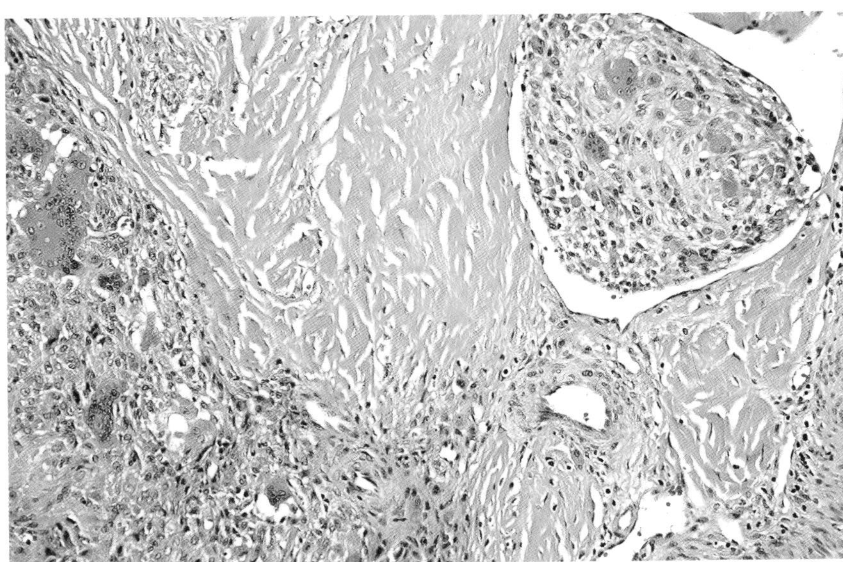

FIGURE 26-12. Focus of tumor in a vein in a localized giant cell tumor. This feature does not necessarily indicate malignancy.

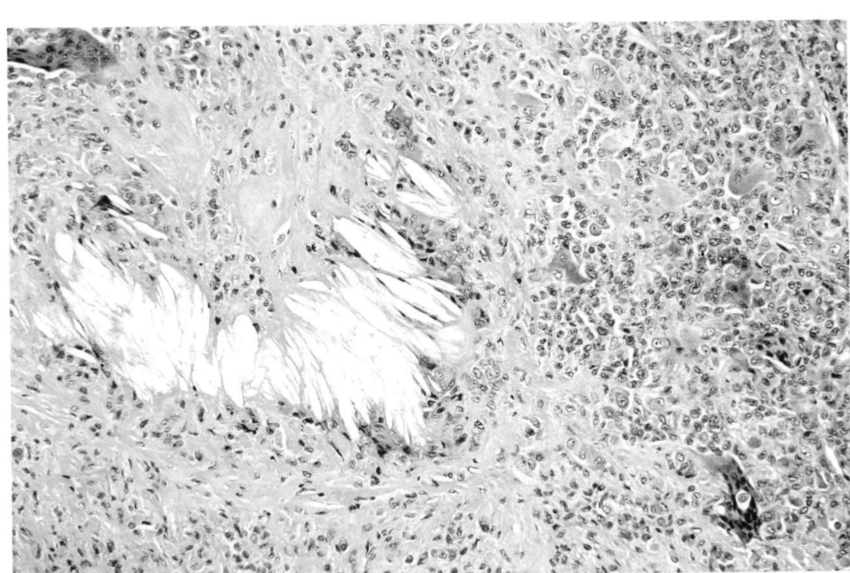

FIGURE 26-13. Cholesterol clefts in a localized giant cell tumor.

Differential Diagnosis

Occasionally, other benign lesions located in the vicinity of the tendon sheath are confused with giant cell tumors, including foreign body granulomas, necrobiotic granulomas, tendinous xanthomas, and fibromas of the tendon sheath. *Granulomatous lesions*, however, are less localized and have a greater complement of inflammatory cells. *Necrobiotic granulomas* are characterized by cores of degenerating collagen rimmed by histiocytes and a prominent zone of proliferating capillaries. Giant cells are usually scarce or nonexistent. The distinction of giant cell tumor of tendon sheath with a prominent xanthomatous component (Fig. 26-13) and *tendinous xanthoma* formerly represented a problem in differential diagnosis. As a result of the recognition and early treatment of hyperlipidemia, it is seldom a practical problem for the surgical pathologist today. In contrast to giant cell tumors, tendinous xanthomas that arise in the setting of hyperlipidemia are often multiple and occur in the tendon proper. Histologically, they consist almost exclusively of xanthoma cells, with only a few multinucleated giant cells and chronic inflammatory cells. *Fibromas of the tendon sheath* bear some similarity to hyalinized forms of giant cell tumor (Fig. 26-14), and some believe that the former represents an end-stage of the latter.[13] In general, the cells of fibroma of the tendon sheath appear fibroblastic and are deposited in a more uniformly hyalinized stroma, although some lesions have areas reminiscent of giant cell tumors. Occasionally, *epithelioid sarcomas* with numerous giant cells mimic a giant cell tumor. The relatively monomorphic population of cells with dense cytoplasmic eosinophilia and strong and diffuse expression of keratin distinguish it from giant cell tumor. Clefted areas of a giant cell tumor may also suggest the glandular component of a *biphasic synovial sarcoma*, but the cells lining the spaces are identical to those found in the solid portion of the tumor and lack epithelial features, as determined by immunohistochemistry.

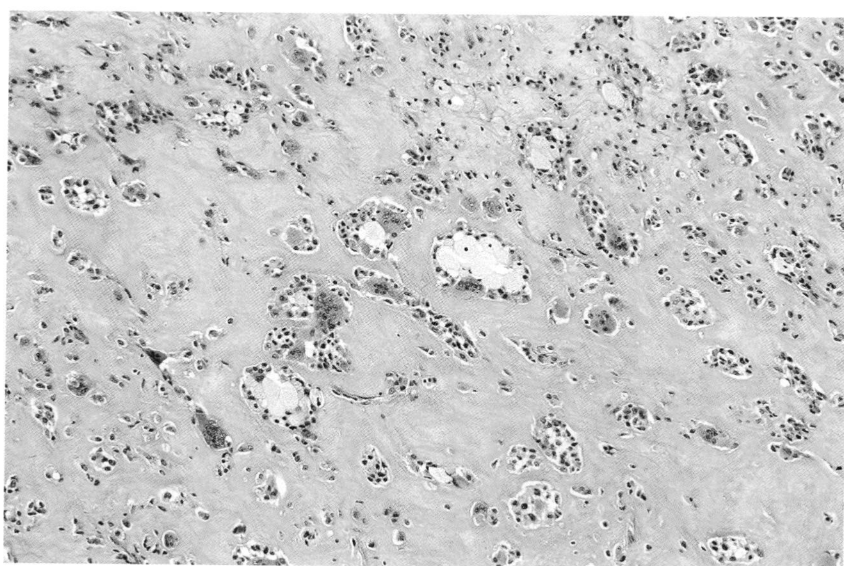

FIGURE 26-14. Localized giant cell tumor with extensive hyalinization bearing some resemblance to a fibroma of the tendon sheath.

TABLE 26-1 Immunohistochemical Features of Cell Types in Tenosynovial Giant Cell Tumor

	LARGE MONONUCLEAR CELLS	HISTIOCYTOID CELLS	MULTINUCLEATED GIANT CELLS	NORMAL SYNOVIOCYTES
Clusterin	Strong, diffuse +	—	—	+
Desmin	Usually +, focal	—	—	Focal +
CD163	—	Strong, diffuse +	—	—
CD21	—	—	—	—
CD35	—	—	—	—

Modified from Boland JM, Folpe AL, Hornick JL, et al. Clusterin is expressed in normal synoviocytes and in tenosynovial giant cell tumors of localized and diffuse types: diagnostic and histogenetic implications. Am J Surg Pathol 2009;33(8):1225–1229.

Immunohistochemical Findings

Immunohistochemical findings are variable within the different cell populations of this tumor. The small histiocytoid cells with pale cytoplasm stain for CD45, CD68, and CD163, consistent with histiocytic differentiation.[14-16] These cells do not express CD21 or CD35. The large mononuclear cells do not stain for CD163, CD21, or CD35, but they do express clusterin, a follicular dendritic cell-associated glycoprotein.[17] In a recent study by Boland et al.,[18] all cases of localized (11 cases) and diffuse (29 cases) giant cell tumors showed strong and diffuse cytoplasmic clusterin staining in these large mononuclear cells, whereas the smaller histiocytoid cells and the multinucleated giant cells were negative for this marker (Table 26-1). As noted previously,[14] the majority of cases (71%) also showed desmin expression in these same large mononuclear cells, which also highlighted their dendritic processes.[18] Desmin was not expressed in the small histiocytoid cells or multinucleated giant cells. Interestingly, normal synoviocytes also stained for both clusterin and, to a lesser degree, desmin, suggesting that this tumor shows synoviocytic as opposed to histiocytic differentiation.[18]

Cytogenetic and Molecular Genetic Findings

A number of studies have found clonal cytogenetic abnormalities in giant cell tumor of tendon sheath. Gains of chromosomes 5 and 7 are common, as are rearrangements of 1p11-13.[19-23] Aberrations of the *CSF1* gene, located at 1p13-21, have been implicated as central to the pathogenesis of this tumor.[24] This gene encodes for macrophages colony stimulating factor, a protein involved in macrophage function, differentiation, and proliferation.[25] A fascinating scenario has emerged whereby *CSF1* rearrangements in the large mononuclear cells create a landscape of reactive inflammatory cells that have been recruited by CSF1 secreted by the tumor cells.[24,26] In fact, the CSF1 receptor is expressed by the majority of mononuclear and multinucleated giant cells.[24] *COL6A3*, located on chromosome 2q37, seems to be the most frequent translocation partner for *CSF1*.[24] However, alternative mechanisms of CSF1 overexpression also seem to occur because some tumors show high expression of mRNA and protein without detectable *CSF1* rearrangements.[26] Others have also found that rearrangements of 1p11-13 are frequent in both localized and diffuse forms of giant cell tumor of tendon sheath. Although the most common translocation partner is 2q35-37, others include 5q22-31, 11q11-12, and 8q21-22.

Discussion

Giant cell tumor of tendon sheath is a benign lesion that nonetheless has a capacity for local recurrence in about 10% to 20% of cases.[6,7,27] In a study by Williams et al.,[27] of 213 cases of giant cell tumor of tendon sheath involving the hand, 27

(13%) cases locally recurred with a mean follow-up period of 51 months. Cases located on the extensor tendon more commonly recurred than those in other locations. Recurrences are nondestructive and are easily controlled by re-excision. Local excision with a small cuff of normal tissue is usually considered adequate therapy, even for lesions with increased cellularity and mitotic activity. Most are cured by this approach, and more extended surgery can always be planned at a later time for persistently recurring lesions. Interestingly, imatinib mesylate has been found to be effective in the treatment of locally advanced and metastatic examples of giant cell tumor of tendon sheath and pigmented villonodular synovitis.[28]

GIANT CELL TUMOR OF TENDON SHEATH, DIFFUSE TYPE (TENOSYNOVIAL GIANT CELL TUMOR, DIFFUSE TYPE; EXTRA-ARTICULAR PIGMENTED VILLONODULAR SYNOVITIS)

The diffuse tenosynovial giant cell tumor can be regarded as the soft tissue counterpart of pigmented villonodular synovitis of the joint space. In most instances, the lesion represents extra-articular extension of a primary intra-articular process, a contention supported by the similarity in age, location, clinical presentation, and symptoms of the two processes. Far less commonly, this disease resides completely outside of a joint, in which case its origin must be ascribed to the synovium of the bursa or tendon sheath.[16,22,29] In their original description of villonodular synovitis, Jaffe et al.[4] described four extra-articular cases, including two arising from the popliteal bursa, one from the bursa anserina, and one from the ankle bursa. Only one of 34 cases of pigmented villonodular synovitis reported by Atmore et al.[30] was located extra-articularly. In many instances, it is difficult to define the origin of the tumor. Therefore, the term *tenosynovial giant cell tumor of the diffuse type* is used when there is a poorly confined soft tissue mass with or without involvement of the adjacent joint.

Compared with the localized giant cell tumor, this form is far less common and exhibits certain clinical differences. There is a tendency for these lesions to occur in young persons. In the largest study to date of 50 cases, Somerhausen and Fletcher[16] reported an age range of 4 to 76 years, with a median age of 41 years. Females are affected slightly more often than males. Typically, symptoms are of relatively long duration, often several years, and include pain and tenderness in the affected extremity. The additional presence of joint effusion, hemarthrosis, limitation of joint motion, and locking signify articular involvement. Its anatomic distribution parallels that of pigmented villonodular synovitis and includes the knee followed by the ankle and foot. Uncommon locations are the finger, elbow, toe, and temporomandibular and sacroiliac areas. Radiographically, a soft tissue mass is usually evident and may be accompanied by osteoporosis, widening of the joint space, and cortical erosion of the adjacent bone (Fig. 26-15).

At surgery, the lesions are large, firm or sponge-like, multinodular masses. Color varies from white to yellow or brown, although usually staining with hemosiderin is less evident than in their articular counterparts, and they usually do not have grossly discernible villous patterns (Figs. 26-16 and 26-17).

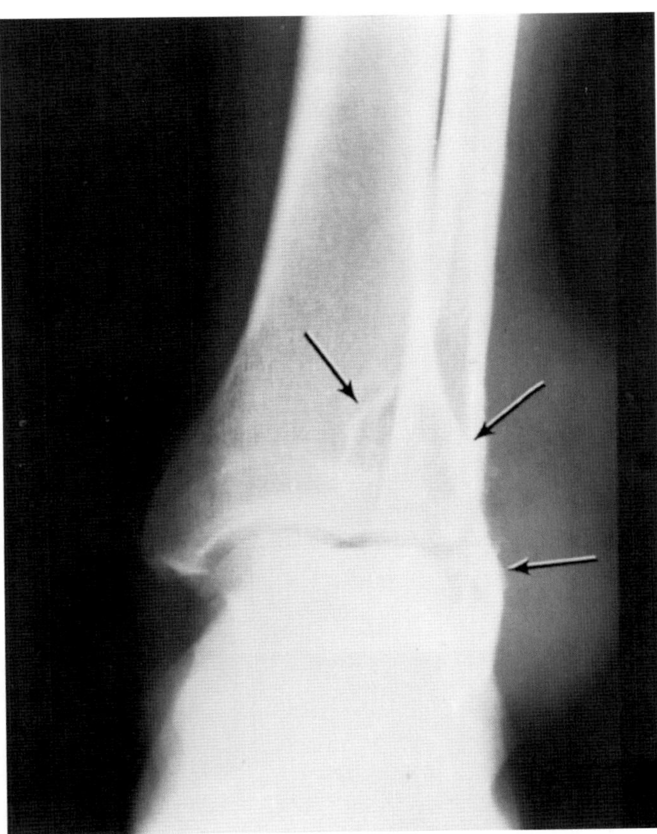

FIGURE 26-15. Radiograph of a diffuse form of giant cell tumor. Large soft tissue mass is present in the ankle region and has caused secondary destruction of the distal tibia and fibula *(arrows)*. Minimal changes in the joint space suggest that the tumor arose in an extra-articular location.

In contrast to localized giant cell tumors, this form is not surrounded by a mature collagenous capsule but instead grows in expansive sheets (Figs. 26-18 and 26-19) interrupted by cleft-like or pseudoglandular spaces (Fig. 26-20). Many of the spaces represent residual synovial membrane, whereas others are probably artifactual. The predominant cell is round or polygonal (Fig. 26-21) with clear or deeply brown cytoplasm when laden with hemosiderin. Gradual transition between these cells, spindle cells, and xanthoma cells is common; and, in some tumors, the diagnosis of xanthoma is suggested. Multinucleated giant cells and chronic inflammatory cells are intermingled so the net effect is that of a highly polymorphic population of cells. In general, giant cells are less numerous than in localized tumors. In cellular areas, the collagenous stroma is delicate and inconspicuous, whereas, in hypocellular areas, the stroma may be quite hyalinized.

These lesions usually present greater diagnostic problems than their localized counterparts. The pronounced cellularity, coupled with the clinical findings of an extensive, destructive mass is likely to lead to a diagnosis of malignancy. Particular problems arise in the early lesions, which are characterized by a monomorphic population of round cells with a high nuclear to cytoplasmic ratio and a brisk mitotic rate (Figs. 26-22, 26-23). Focal necrosis may be present if torsion of a pedunculated tumor nodule has occurred. In such cases, attention should be paid to the synovium-based location

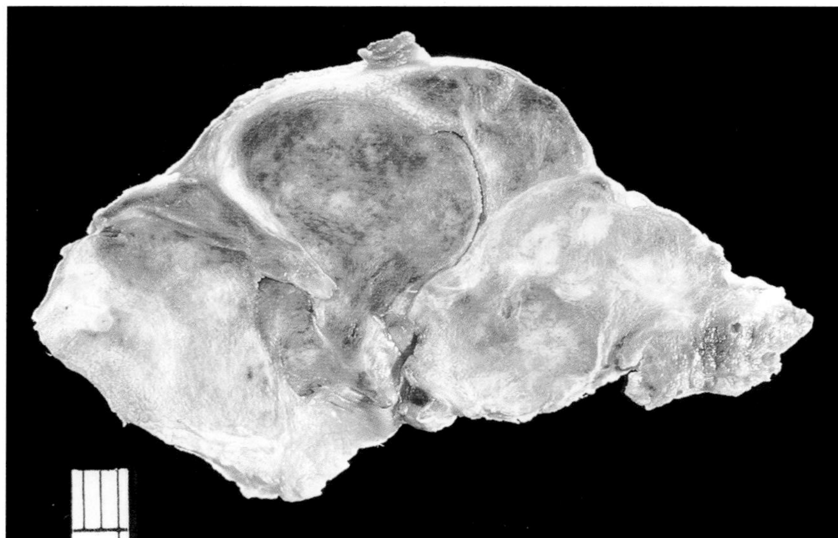

FIGURE 26-16. Diffuse form of giant cell tumor. The lesion has a multinodular appearance with variegated color. Shaggy villous projections, typical of pigmented villonodular synovitis, are not seen.

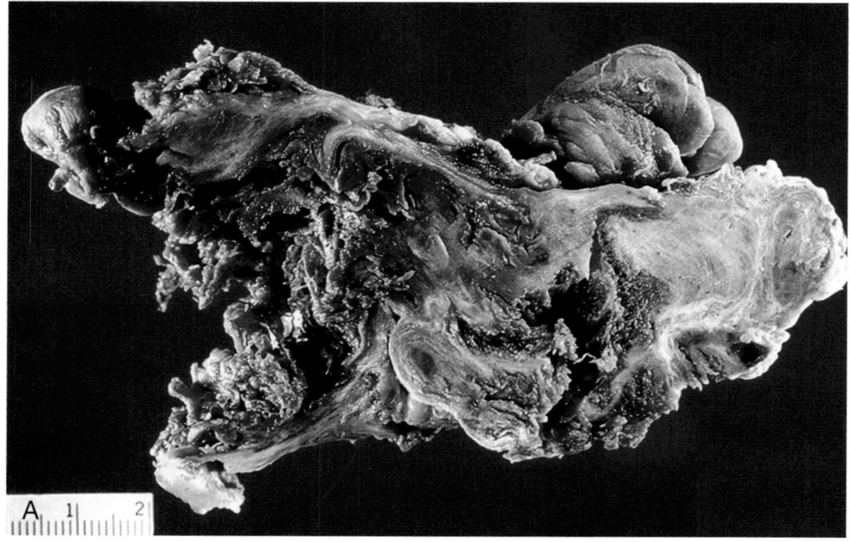

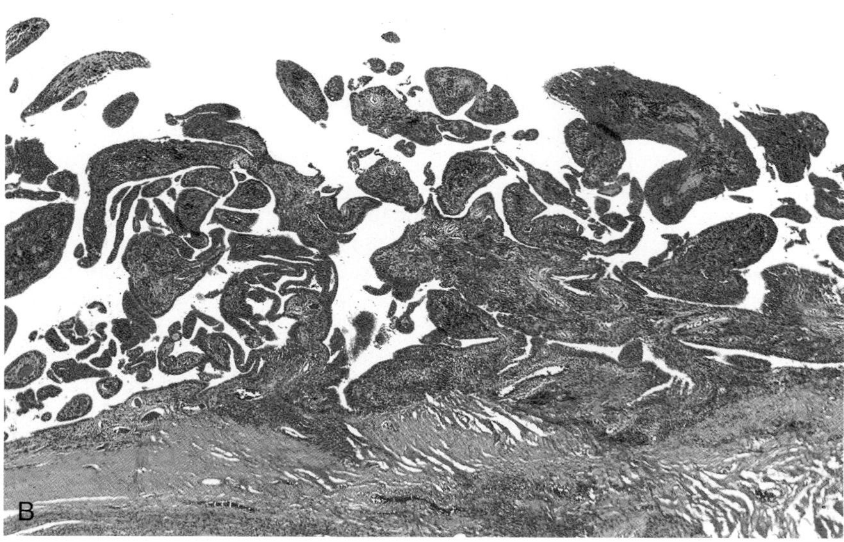

FIGURE 26-17. Intra-articular form of diffuse giant cell tumor (pigmented villonodular synovitis). Note the shaggy villous appearance in the gross (A) and microscopic (B) specimens.

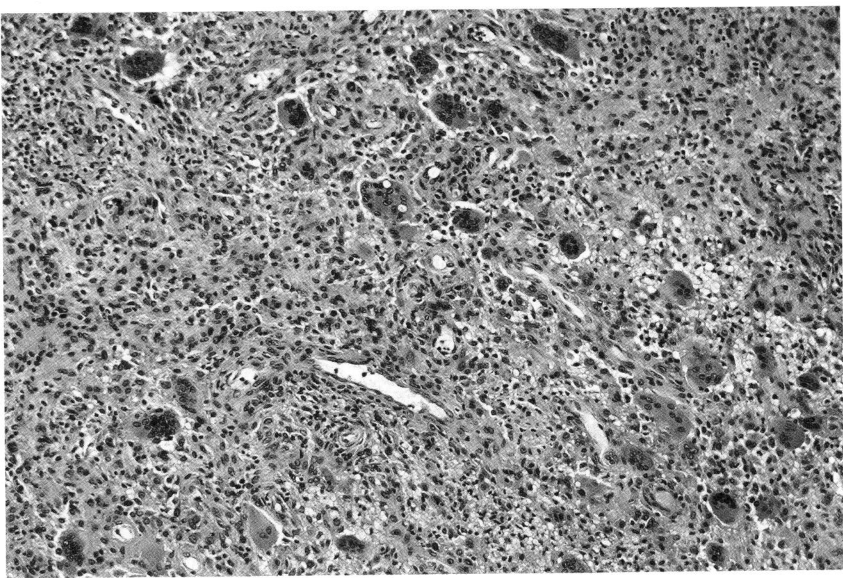

FIGURE 26-18. Diffuse form of giant cell tumor characterized by sheets of rounded synovial-like cells admixed with multinucleated giant cells and xanthoma cells with hemosiderin.

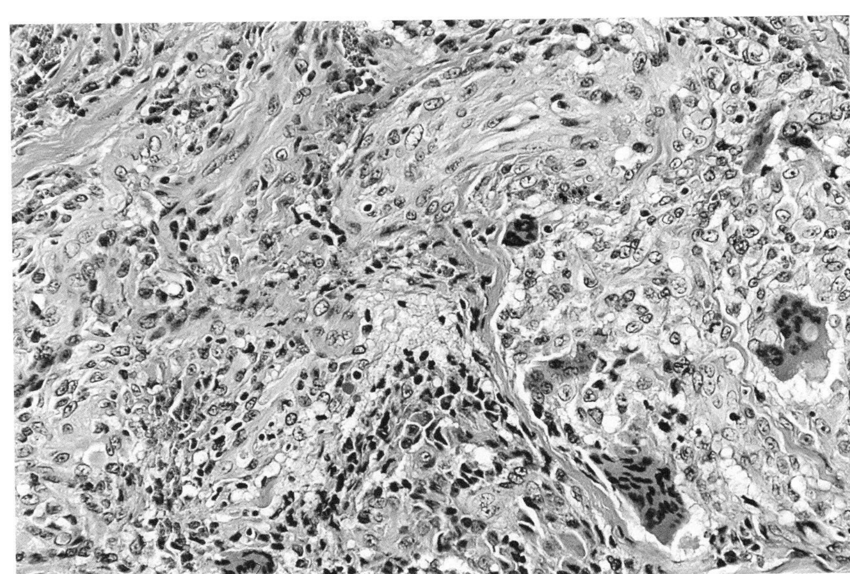

FIGURE 26-19. High-power view of diffuse type of giant cell tumor.

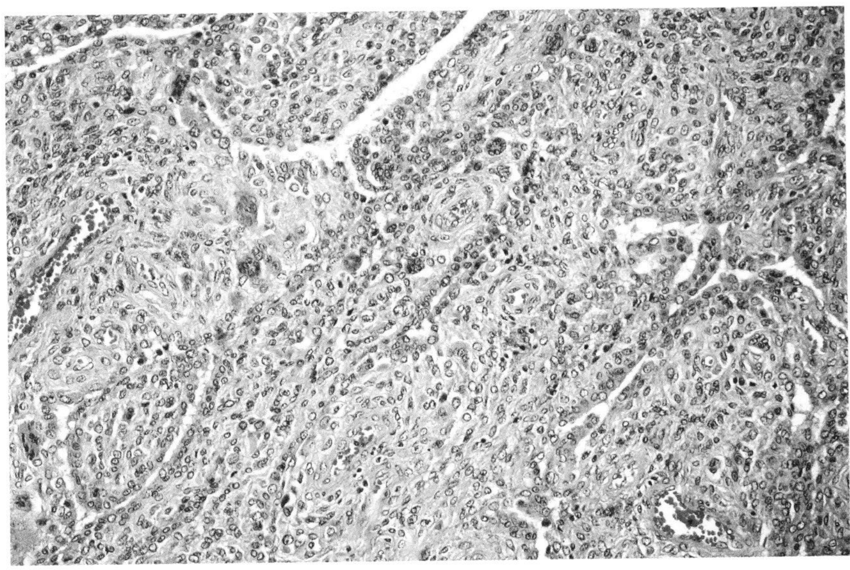

FIGURE 26-20. Pseudoglandular spaces in a diffuse giant cell tumor.

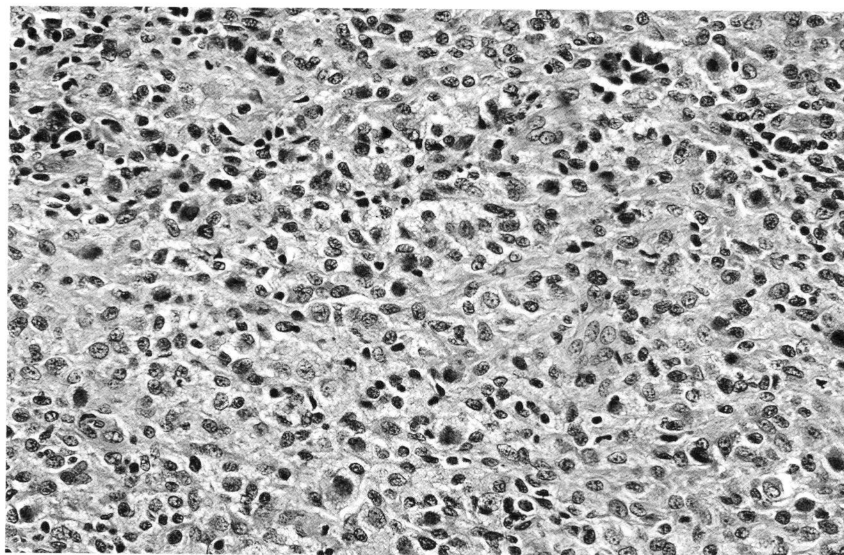

FIGURE 26-21. High-power view of monotonous round cells in a diffuse type of giant cell tumor.

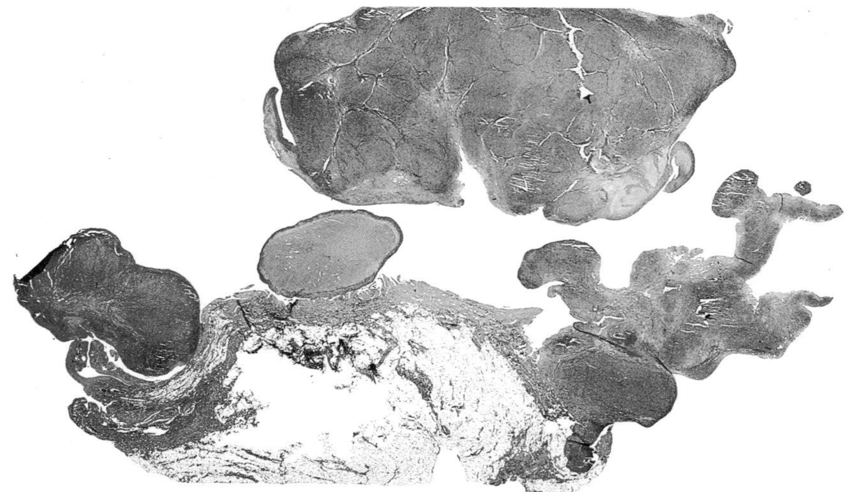

FIGURE 26-22. Early stage of a diffuse intra-articular giant cell tumor. Note necrosis of one of the nodules due to torsion of the tumor on its stalk.

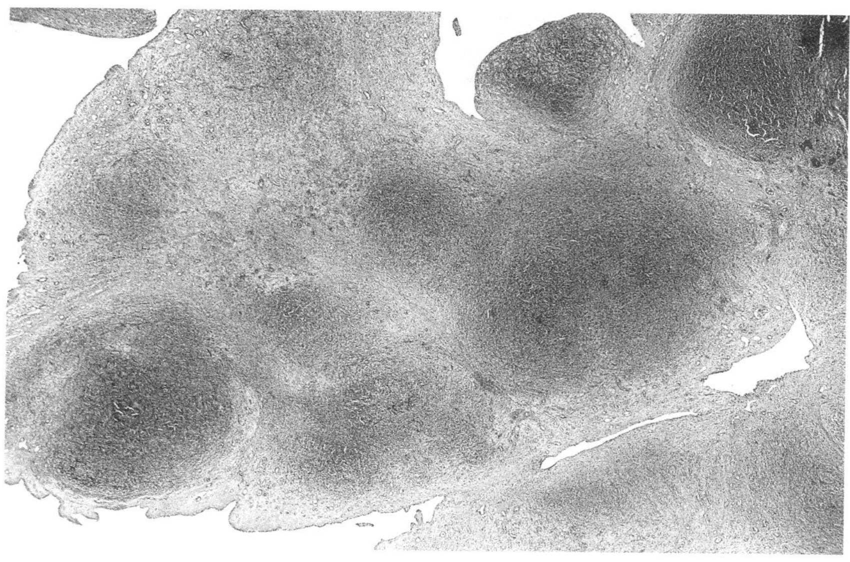

FIGURE 26-23. Early stage of a diffuse giant cell tumor (same case as Figure 26-22). The lesion has a distinctly nodular appearance.

and to the apparent maturation of these tumor nodules at their periphery where the cells acquire a more prominent, slightly xanthomatous-appearing cytoplasm. Additional sections occasionally disclose focal giant cells, and iron staining may identify modest amounts of hemosiderin not discernible in routine sections. In more advanced lesions consisting of the classic polymorphic cellular population, other problems in differential diagnosis occur. For example, the pseudoglandular spaces are often misinterpreted as glandular spaces of a synovial sarcoma or the alveolar spaces of a rhabdomyosarcoma. The giant cell tumor shows great variation in type and arrangement of cells. Its geographic pattern of xanthomatous regions alternating with cellular hyalinized regions contrasts with the more uniform spindled appearance of most synovial sarcomas and the primitive round cells of alveolar rhabdomyosarcomas. The immunohistochemical features of the diffuse type of giant cell tumor are identical to those found in the localized form. Similarly, this tumor has identical cytogenetic and molecular genetic aberrations as the localized form, including *CSF1* aberrations.

Behavior and Treatment

Although much has been reported concerning the behavior and treatment of pigmented villonodular synovitis, there are few data concerning extra-articular forms of the disease. Follow-up information in the cases of the authors of this edition indicates that 40% to 50% of patients develop local recurrence. In the series by Somerhausen and Fletcher,[16] follow-up information available in 24 patients revealed recurrences in 8 (33%), with a median follow-up of 55 months. All recurrences occurred between 4 and 6 months after initial excision, and five patients had multiple recurrences. Six cases had atypical histologic features, including increased mitotic activity, necrosis, cytologic atypia, and spindling of mononuclear cells, but these features did not predict local recurrence. In addition, four cases harbored areas of overt sarcomatous transformation, and one of these patients developed pulmonary metastases and died after 35 months, confirming the existence of rare malignant variants (discussed further in the chapter). Also reviewed is one recurrent diffuse giant cell tumor arising from the foot that metastasized to the lung after several years (Fig. 26-24).

From a practical point of view, these lesions should be regarded as locally aggressive but (usually) nonmetastasizing lesions. Therapy should be based on a desire to remove the tumor as completely as possible without producing severe disability for the patient. Although wide excision or amputation is the best choice for local control of the disease, it implies significant morbidity, especially for lesions located adjacent to major joints. Therefore, less radical excision is justified in these cases. Although radiotherapy has been endorsed for treatment of surgically unresectable villonodular synovitis,[31] there is no significant experience concerning its use for the extra-articular form of the disease. For those cases arising in the knee, arthroscopic synovectomy appears to offer short-term relief of symptoms, but most of these patients ultimately develop local recurrences.[32]

MALIGNANT GIANT CELL TUMOR OF THE TENDON SHEATH/PIGMENTED VILLONODULAR SYNOVITIS

Malignant giant cell tumors of the tendon sheath/pigmented villonodular synovitis comprise a rare group of tumors, the existence of which has been doubted by some and the diagnosis of which is difficult. The belief that the giant cell tumor is an inflammatory condition has led to the conclusion by some that malignant forms of this disease do not exist. Others have accepted any sarcoma that contains giant cells arising in the vicinity of a tendon as a malignant giant cell tumor of the tendon sheath.[33] Consequently, malignant giant cell tumors of the tendon sheath, as reported in the literature, constitute a variety of lesions, including clear cell sarcoma, fibrosarcoma, epithelioid sarcoma, and undifferentiated pleomorphic sarcoma. Still others have implied that diffuse forms of the giant cell tumor, which behave in a locally aggressive fashion, should be considered malignant, although the morphologic appearance may remain unaltered during the course of the disease. The designation of malignant giant cell tumor

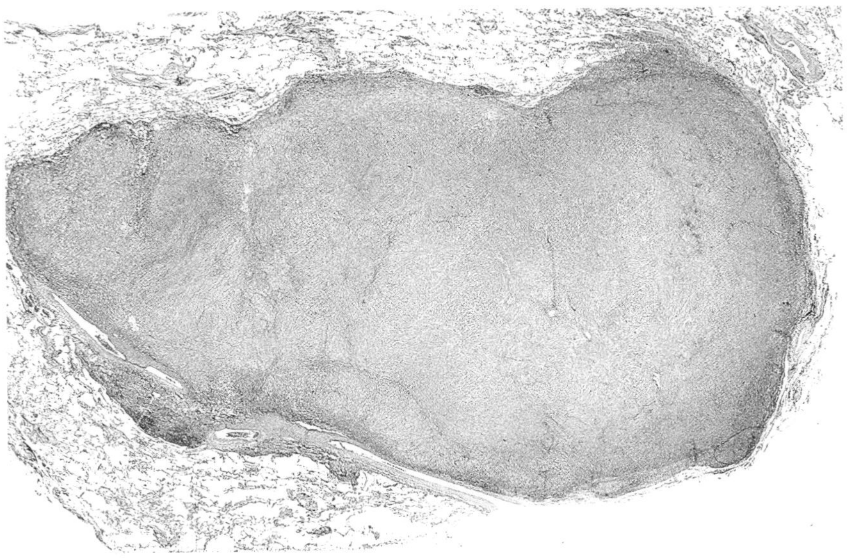

FIGURE 26-24. Pulmonary metastasis from a diffuse form of giant cell tumor of the foot.

of the tendon sheath/pigmented villonodular synovitis is reserved for lesions in which a typical-appearing benign giant cell tumor or pigmented villonodular synovitis coexists with frankly malignant areas, or when the original lesion is typical of a benign giant cell tumor or pigmented villonodular synovitis and the recurrence appears histologically malignant (Fig. 26-25). Defined in this fashion, true malignant giant cell tumors of the tendon sheath/pigmented villonodular synovitis comprise an extremely rare group of tumors and are far outnumbered by benign lesions or even tumors with atypical features.

Castens and Howell[34] were the first to report a malignant giant cell tumor. The patient's original lesion was described as a giant cell tumor of the tendon sheath with atypical features that arose in the dorsum of the right foot. Following local excision, the lesion recurred repeatedly over many years and ultimately gave rise to numerous local metastases on the same extremity. There are several other documented cases of giant cell tumors of tendon sheath/pigmented villonodular synovitis that appeared histologically malignant following recurrence, some of which metastasized[16,29,35,36] and others of which did not.[37]

In 1997, Bertoni et al.[38] described three cases of typical pigmented villonodular synovitis that had histologic features of malignancy in recurrent lesions. No pathologic features were useful for predicting malignant transformation. In addition, they reported five cases of malignant pigmented villonodular synovitis that were primary (i.e., did not arise in

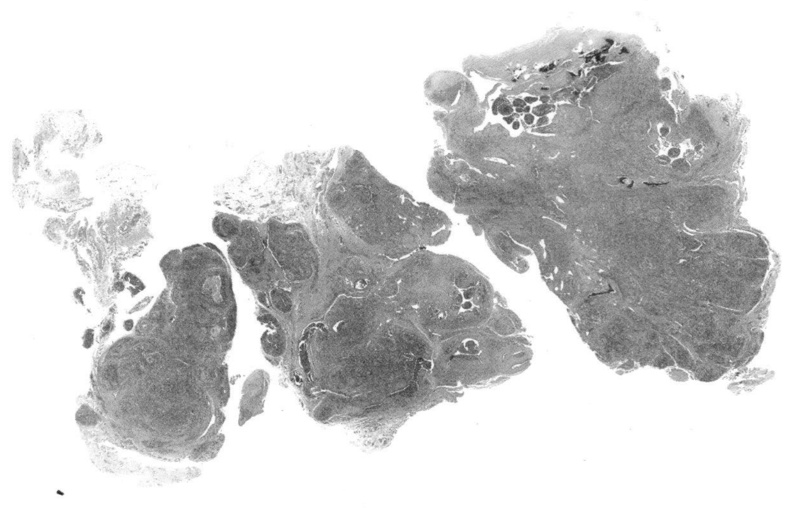

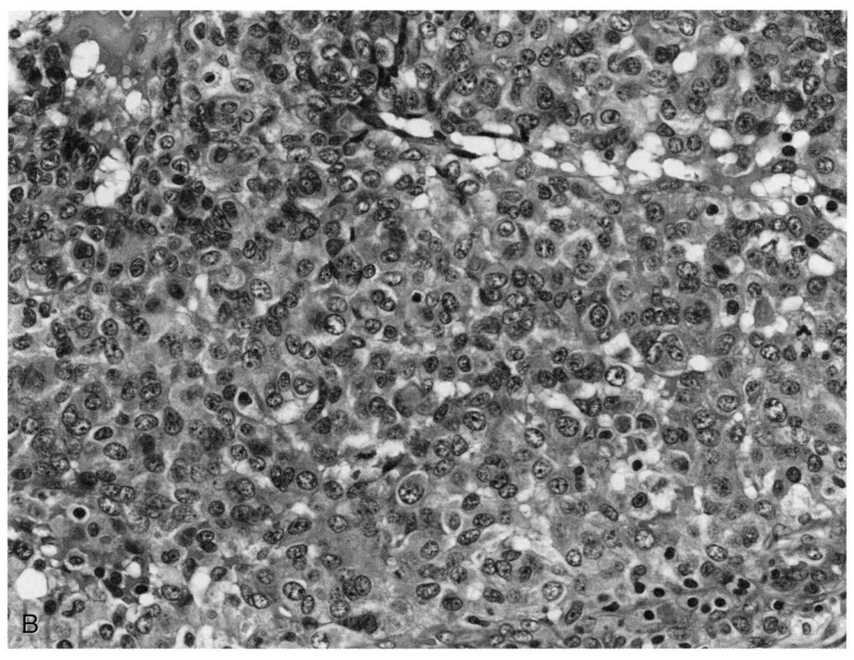

FIGURE 26-25. Low-power (A) and high-power (B) views of a malignant giant cell tumor of the tendon sheath. This tumor is characterized by sheets of large round cells devoid of intervening stroma.

previously documented pigmented villonodular synovitis) but had histologic features similar to those found in the cases of secondary malignant pigmented villonodular synovitis.

Histologically, the cases of primary malignant pigmented villonodular synovitis were characterized by nodules or sheets of oval to round cells with larger hyperchromatic nuclei and more prominent nucleoli than are found in typical cases of pigmented villonodular synovitis. Mitotic figures, including atypical mitoses, were seen, as was more extensive necrosis than is usually seen in pigmented villonodular synovitis. Furthermore, the zoning phenomenon seen in pigmented villonodular synovitis, in which the cells at the periphery of the nodules have smaller nuclei and more cytoplasm, was not found in the malignant cases (Table 26-2). In this series, four patients died with pulmonary or nodal metastases or secondary to local extension into the pelvis or cranium; four patients were alive after wide aggressive surgical procedures. A similar case of primary malignant pigmented villonodular synovitis was reported by Nielsen and Kiaer.[39]

Recently, Li et al.[40] reported an additional 7 cases of malignant diffuse-type giant cell tumors and summarized the literature of the 30 cases (including 7 of their own) published to date (Table 26-3). According to their review, 17 cases were primary malignant giant cell tumors and 13 arose from a prior histologically benign lesion. Histologically, the most common pattern of malignancy was the giant cell tumor-like pattern described by Bertoni,[38] with solid sheets or multiple discrete nodules of enlarged ovoid cells with prominent nucleoli and little intervening stroma. Less commonly, areas resembling fibrosarcoma, myxofibrosarcoma, and malignant fibrous histiocytoma-like areas were seen. Immunohistochemically, these tumors had similar staining patterns to their benign counterparts, including scattered desmin-positive cells with dendritic processes. Ki-67 labeling indices were higher in malignant cases when compared to their benign counterparts, but there was some overlap among individual cases.

Clinically, approximately 50% of cases reported in the literature have metastasized, most commonly to regional lymph nodes, a feature that is unusual for sarcomas. These tumors arise predominantly in proximity to large joint spaces of limbs, similar to their benign counterparts. Huang et al.[41] found significantly greater expression of cyclin A and p63 in malignant tumors, without overlap of labeling indices. Deletions of 15q were found only in a malignant diffuse giant cell tumor (15q22-24), suggesting a candidate tumor suppressor gene at this locus. Wide excision or amputation of true malignant forms of tenosynovial giant cell tumor/pigmented villonodular synovitis is indicated.

TABLE 26-2 Clinical Features of Malignant Giant Cell Tumor of the Tendon Sheath/Pigmented Villonodular Synovitis and Pigmented Villonodular Synovitis

PARAMETER	PVNS	MPVNS
Age	50% <40 years	12-79 years (peak: 6th decade)
Gender	Females >males	Females >males
Local recurrence (%)	25-50	60-70
Metastasis (%)		60-70
Died of tumor	None	40-50

Modified from Bertoni F, Unni KK, Beabout JW, Sim FH. Malignant giant cell tumor of the tendon sheaths and joints (malignant pigmented villonodular synovitis). Am J Surg Pathol 1997;21(2):153-163.

PVNS, pigmented villonodular synovitis; *MPVNS,* malignant pigmented villonodular synovitis.

TABLE 26-3 Clinicopathologic Features in Benign and Malignant Diffuse Tenosynovial Giant Cell Tumors

	MALIGNANT D-TGCT	BENIGN D-TGCT
Age (years)	61.0±12.8	39.5±15.6*
Gender	3 males/3 females	9 males/15 females
Tumor size (cm)	9.4±4.1	6.5±2.7*
Necrosis	7/7 (100%)	1/24 (4%)
Atypical mitotic figures	6/7 (85.7%)	2/24 (8.3%)*
Mitotic counts/10 HPF	17.9±20.7	2.1±3.1

Modified from Li CF, Wang JW, Huang WW, et al. Malignant diffuse-type tenosynovial giant cell tumors: a series of 7 cases comparing with 24 benign lesions with review of the literature. Am J Surg Pathol 2008;32(4): 587–599.

*Statistically significant.
D-TGCT, diffuse tenosynovial giant cell tumor.

MISCELLANEOUS CONDITIONS RESEMBLING DIFFUSE GIANT CELL TUMOR

Occasionally, reactive synovial lesions mimic the appearance of a diffuse giant cell tumor, particularly lesions of the intra-articular type (pigmented villonodular synovitis). Perhaps the most common condition that produces this picture is intra-articular hemorrhage (hemosiderotic synovitis). Long known to be associated with synovitis in hemophiliacs, intra-articular hemorrhage can give rise to hyperplastic changes of the synovium, consisting of villous change and large deposits of hemosiderin.[15,42] However, only in the early stages of chronic hemarthrosis are the lesions reminiscent of pigmented villonodular synovitis. During the late stage, the synovium is flattened and the subjacent tissue markedly fibrotic. A second condition that can histologically resemble pigmented villonodular synovitis is the synovitis associated with failed orthopedic prosthetic devices.[43,44] Collectively termed *detritic synovitis*, these lesions are characterized by villous hyperplasia of the synovium (Fig. 26-26A). The subsynovial space is infiltrated with histiocytes, multinucleated giant cells, and a variable number of chronic inflammatory cells. The prosthetic material can be detected under polarized light as weakly birefringent intracellular or extracellular spicules (Fig. 26-26B). Finally, synovial tissue was reviewed from a patient with α-mannosidase deficiency who developed bilateral destructive synovitis of the ankle region.[45] The hyperplastic villous-appearing synovium was infiltrated with clear-appearing histiocytes containing periodic acid-Schiff (PAS)-positive, diastase-resistant material representing partially degraded oligosaccharides in lysosomes (Figs. 26-27 to 26-30). A similar case was reported by Hale et al.[46] in which this deficiency was associated with bilateral patellar dislocation. Although definitive diagnosis requires an adequate clinical history with confirmatory biochemical data, the presence of a systemic disease was suspected because of the bilaterally symmetric distribution of the lesions, a distribution seldom encountered in pigmented villonodular synovitis.

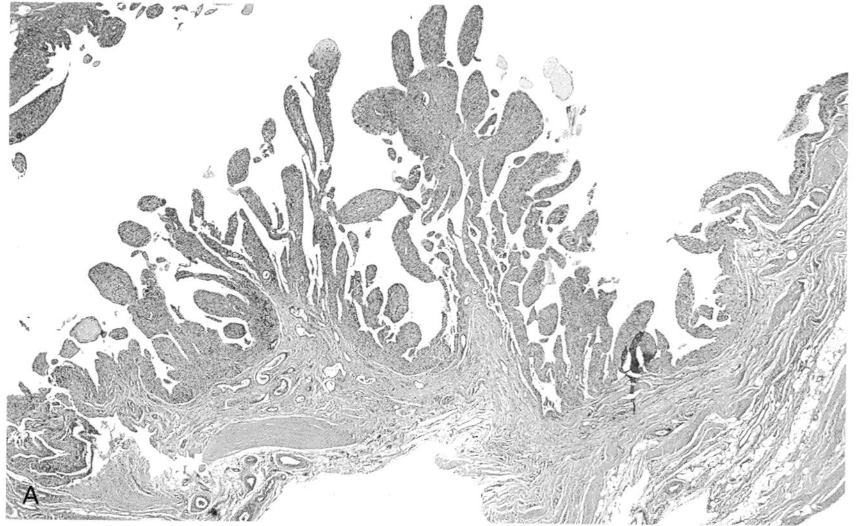

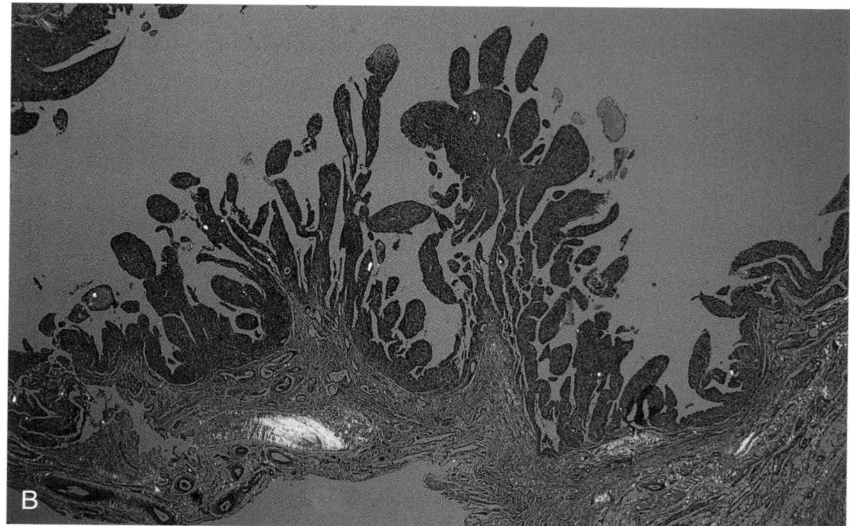

FIGURE 26-26. (A) Detritic synovitis showing villous configuration of the synovium. (B) Graft material is visible as birefringent particles in this partially polarized view.

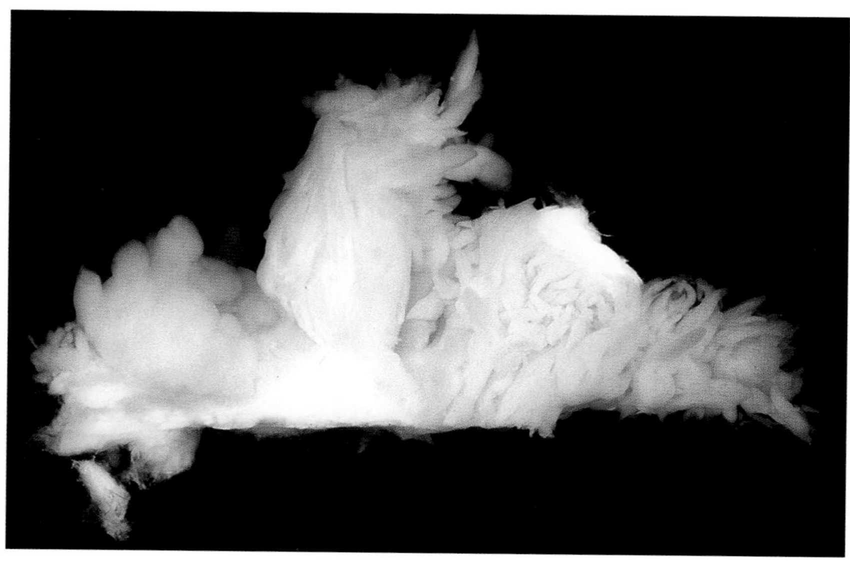

FIGURE 26-27. Gross appearance of synovium in a patient with α-mannosidase deficiency. Note that the synovium has delicate villous fronds.

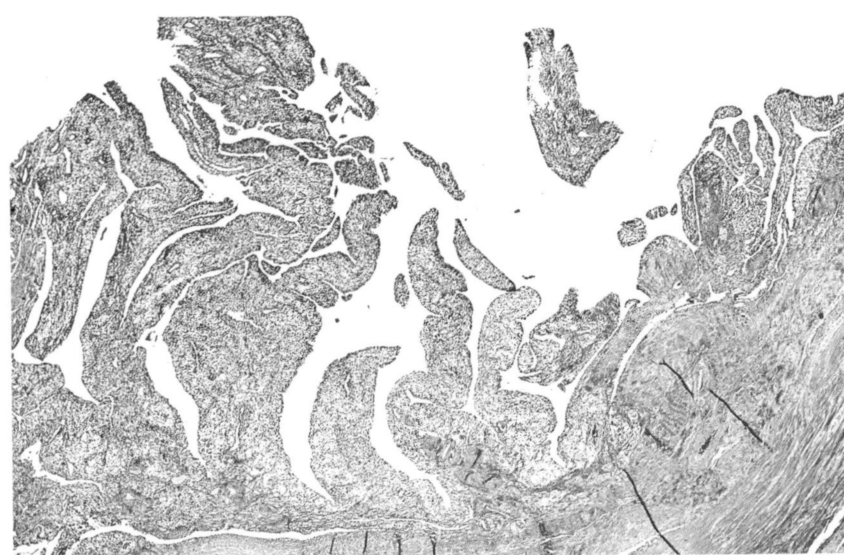

FIGURE 26-28. Synovitis due to α-mannosidase deficiency. At low power, the lesion superficially resembles pigmented villonodular synovitis.

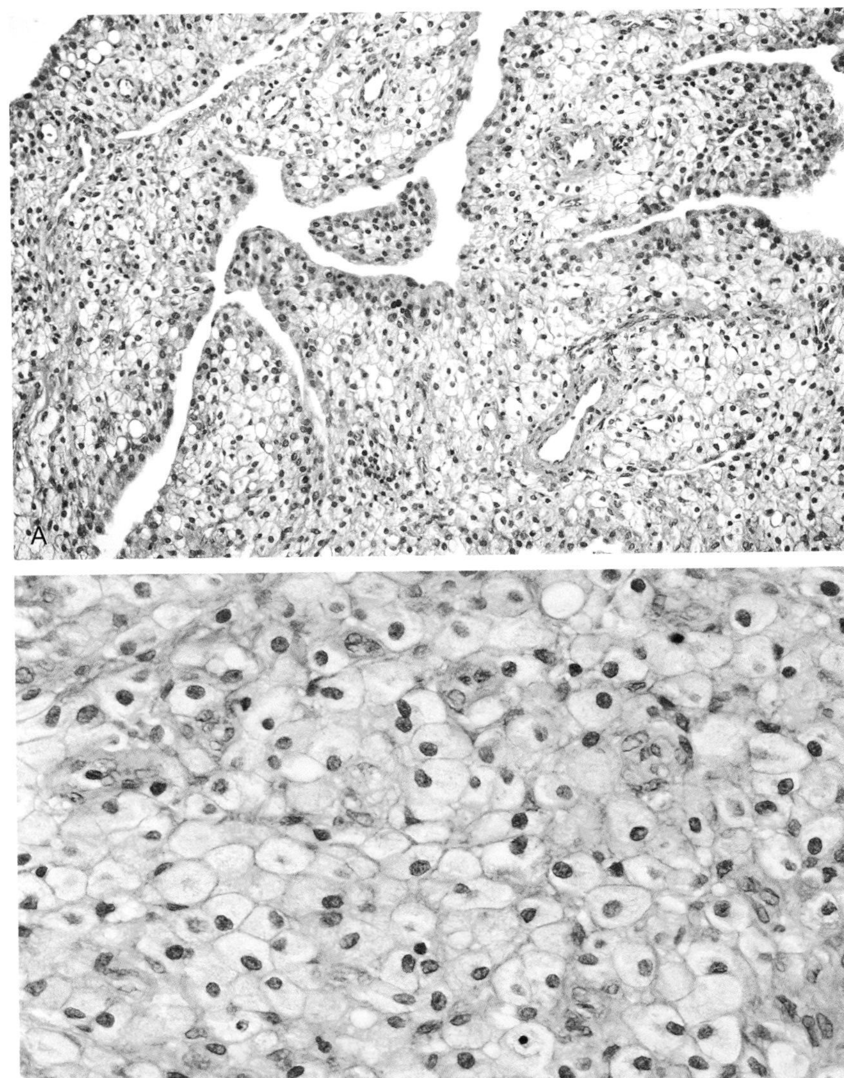

FIGURE 26-29. (A) Synovitis due to α-mannosidase deficiency composed of synovial-lined papillary projections with centrally located vacuolated cells. (B) At high power, the infiltrate consists of clear-appearing histiocytes containing PAS-positive, diastase-resistant bodies representing partially degraded oligosaccharides. *(From Weiss SW, Kelly WD. Bilateral destructive synovitis associated with alpha-mannosidase deficiency. Am J Surg Pathol 1983;7:487.)*

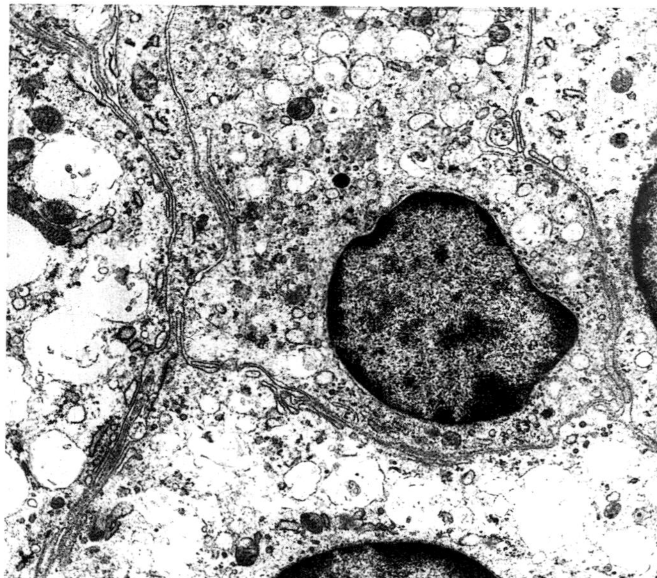

FIGURE 26-30. Electron micrograph of histiocytes from the synovium of a patient with α-mannosidase deficiency. Oligosaccharide is represented by granuloamorphous material in lysosomes. *(From Weiss SW, Kelly WD. Bilateral destructive synovitis associated with α-mannosidase deficiency. Am J Surg Pathol 1983;7:487.)*

References

1. O'Connell JX. Pathology of the synovium. Am J Clin Pathol 2000;114(5):773–84.
2. Cohen MJ, Kaplan L. Histology and ultrastructure of the human flexor tendon sheath. J Hand Surg Am 1987;12(1):25–9.
3. Steinberg PJ, Hodde KC. The morphology of synovial lining of various structures in several species as observed with scanning electron microscopy. Scanning Microsc 1990;4(4):987–1019; discussion 1019-20.
4. Jaffe HL, Lichtenstein L, Sutro CJ. Pigmented villonodular synovitis, bursitis and tenosynovitis: a discussion of the synovial and bursal equivalents of the tenosynovial lesions commonly denoted as xanthoma, xanthogranulomas, giant cell tumor or myeloma of the tendon sheath, with some consideration of the tendon sheath lesion itself. Arch Pathol 1941;31:731.
5. Rubin BP. Tenosynovial giant cell tumor and pigmented villonodular synovitis: a proposal for unification of these clinically distinct but histologically and genetically identical lesions. Skeletal Radiol 2007;36(4):267–8.
6. Monaghan H, Salter DM, Al-Nafussi A. Giant cell tumour of tendon sheath (localised nodular tenosynovitis): clinicopathological features of 71 cases. J Clin Pathol 2001;54(5):404–7.
7. Ushijima M, Hashimoto H, Tsuneyoshi M, et al. Giant cell tumor of the tendon sheath (nodular tenosynovitis). A study of 207 cases to compare the large joint group with the common digit group. Cancer 1986;57(4):875–84.
8. Findling J, Lascola NK, Groner TW. Giant cell tumor of the flexor hallucis longus tendon sheath: a case study. J Am Podiatr Med Assoc 2011;101(2):187–9.
9. Chechik O, Amar E, Khashan M, et al. Giant cell tumors in the patellar tendon area. J Knee Surg 2010;23(2):115–9.
10. Wan JM, Magarelli N, Peh WC, et al. Imaging of giant cell tumour of the tendon sheath. Radiol Med 2010;115(1):141–51.
11. Kitagawa Y, Ito H, Amano Y, et al. MR imaging for preoperative diagnosis and assessment of local tumor extent on localized giant cell tumor of tendon sheath. Skeletal Radiol 2003;32(11):633–8.
12. Rao AS, Vigorita VJ. Pigmented villonodular synovitis (giant-cell tumor of the tendon sheath and synovial membrane). A review of eighty-one cases. J Bone Joint Surg Am 1984;66(1):76–94.
13. Satti MB. Tendon sheath tumours: a pathological study of the relationship between giant cell tumour and fibroma of tendon sheath. Histopathology 1992;20(3):213–20.
14. Folpe AL, Weiss SW, Fletcher CD, et al. Tenosynovial giant cell tumors: evidence for a desmin-positive dendritic cell subpopulation. Mod Pathol 1998;11(10):939–44.
15. O'Connell JX, Fanburg JC, Rosenberg AE. Giant cell tumor of tendon sheath and pigmented villonodular synovitis: immunophenotype suggests a synovial cell origin. Hum Pathol 1995;26(7):771–5.
16. Somerhausen NS, Fletcher CD. Diffuse-type giant cell tumor: clinicopathologic and immunohistochemical analysis of 50 cases with extraarticular disease. Am J Surg Pathol 2000;24(4):479–92.
17. Grogg KL, Macon WR, Kurtin PJ, et al. A survey of clusterin and fascin expression in sarcomas and spindle cell neoplasms: strong clusterin immunostaining is highly specific for follicular dendritic cell tumor. Mod Pathol 2005;18(2):260–6.
18. Boland JM, Folpe AL, Hornick JL, et al. Clusterin is expressed in normal synoviocytes and in tenosynovial giant cell tumors of localized and diffuse types: diagnostic and histogenetic implications. Am J Surg Pathol 2009;33(8):1225–9.
19. Nilsson M, Höglund M, Panagopoulos I, et al. Molecular cytogenetic mapping of recurrent chromosomal breakpoints in tenosynovial giant cell tumors. Virchows Arch 2002;441(5):475–80.
20. Ohjimi Y, Iwasaki H, Ishiguro M, et al. Short arm of chromosome 1 aberration recurrently found in pigmented villonodular synovitis. Cancer Genet Cytogenet 1996;90(1):80–5.
21. Ray RA, Morton CC, Lipinski KK, et al. Cytogenetic evidence of clonality in a case of pigmented villonodular synovitis. Cancer 1991;67(1):121–5.
22. Rowlands CG, Roland B, Hwang WS, et al. Diffuse-variant tenosynovial giant cell tumor: a rare and aggressive lesion. Hum Pathol 1994;25(4):423–5.
23. Sciot R, Rosai J, Dal Cin P, et al. Analysis of 35 cases of localized and diffuse tenosynovial giant cell tumor: a report from the Chromosomes and Morphology (CHAMP) study group. Mod Pathol 1999;12(6):576–9.
24. West RB, Rubin BP, Miller MA, et al. A landscape effect in tenosynovial giant-cell tumor from activation of CSF1 expression by a translocation in a minority of tumor cells. Proc Natl Acad Sci USA 2006;103(3):690–5.
25. Morris SW, Valentine MB, Shapiro DN, et al. Reassignment of the human CSF1 gene to chromosome 1p13-p21. Blood 1991;78(8):2013–20.
26. Cupp JS, Miller MA, Montgomery KD, et al. Translocation and expression of CSF1 in pigmented villonodular synovitis, tenosynovial giant cell tumor, rheumatoid arthritis and other reactive synovitides. Am J Surg Pathol 2007;31(6):970–6.
27. Williams J, Hodari A, Janevski P, et al. Recurrence of giant cell tumors in the hand: a prospective study. J Hand Surg Am 2010;35(3):451–6.
28. Cassier PA, Gelderblom H, Stacchiotti S, et al. Efficacy of imatinib mesylate for the treatment of locally advanced and/or metastatic tenosynovial giant cell tumor/pigmented villonodular synovitis. Cancer 2011. Available at: http://www.ncbi.nlm.nih.gov/pubmed/21823110. Accessed January 25, 2012.
29. Abdul-Karim FW, el-Naggar AK, Joyce MJ, et al. Diffuse and localized tenosynovial giant cell tumor and pigmented villonodular synovitis: a clinicopathologic and flow cytometric DNA analysis. Hum Pathol 1992;23(7):729–35.
30. Atmore WG, Dahlin DC, Ghormley RK. Pigmented villonodular synovitis; a clinical and pathologic study. Minn Med 1956;39(4):196–202.
31. Ofluoglu O. Pigmented villonodular synovitis. Orthop Clin North Am 2006;37(1):23–33.
32. Chin KR, Brick GW. Extraarticular pigmented villonodular synovitis: a cause for failed knee arthroscopy. Clin Orthop Relat Res 2002;(404):330–8.
33. Myers BW, Masi AT. Pigmented villonodular synovitis and tenosynovitis: a clinical epidemiologic study of 166 cases and literature review. Medicine (Baltimore) 1980;59(3):223–38.
34. Castens HP, Howell RS. Malignant giant cell tumor of tendon sheath. Virchows Arch A Pathol Anat Histol 1979;382(2):237–43.
35. Kalil RK, Unni KK. Malignancy in pigmented villonodular synovitis. Skeletal Radiol 1998;27(7):392–5.
36. Layfield LJ, Meloni-Ehrig A, Liu K, et al. Malignant giant cell tumor of synovium (malignant pigmented villonodular synovitis). Arch Pathol Lab Med 2000;124(11):1636–41.
37. Ushijima M, Hashimoto H, Tsuneyoshi M, et al. Malignant giant cell tumor of tendon sheath. Report of a case. Acta Pathol Jpn 1985;35(3):699–709.
38. Bertoni F, Unni KK, Beabout JW, et al. Malignant giant cell tumor of the tendon sheaths and joints (malignant pigmented villonodular synovitis). Am J Surg Pathol 1997;21(2):153–63.

39. Nielsen AL, Kiaer T. Malignant giant cell tumor of synovium and locally destructive pigmented villonodular synovitis: ultrastructural and immunohistochemical study and review of the literature. Hum Pathol 1989; 20(8):765–71.
40. Li CF, Wang JW, Huang WW, et al. Malignant diffuse-type tenosynovial giant cell tumors: a series of 7 cases comparing with 24 benign lesions with review of the literature. Am J Surg Pathol 2008;32(4):587–99.
41. Huang HY, West RB, Tzeng CC, et al. Immunohistochemical and biogenetic features of diffuse-type tenosynovial giant cell tumors: the potential roles of cyclin A, P53, and deletion of 15q in sarcomatous transformation. Clin Cancer Res 2008;14(19):6023–32.
42. Mahendra G, Kliskey K, Athanasou NA. Immunophenotypic distinction between pigmented villonodular synovitis and haemosiderotic synovitis. J Clin Pathol 2010;63(1):75–8.
43. Hameed MR, Erlandson R, Rosen PP. Capsular synovial-like hyperplasia around mammary implants similar to detritic synovitis. A morphologic and immunohistochemical study of 15 cases. Am J Surg Pathol 1995; 19(4):433–8.
44. Slobodin G, Lurie M, Rozenbaum M, et al. Osteolysis with detritic synovitis: appearance in a patient with connective tissue disease. Arthritis Rheum 2005;53(1):126–8.
45. Weiss SW, Kelly WD. Bilateral destructive synovitis associated with alpha mannosidase deficiency. Am J Surg Pathol 1983;7(5):487–94.
46. Hale SS, Bales JG, Rosenzweig S, et al. Bilateral patellar dislocation associated with alpha-mannosidase deficiency. J Pediatr Orthop B 2006;15(3): 215–9.

Benign Tumors of Peripheral Nerves

CHAPTER CONTENTS

Benign peripheral nerve sheath tumors differ from other soft tissue tumors in several important respects. Most soft tissue tumors arise from mesodermally derived tissue and display a range of features consonant with that lineage. Nerve sheath tumors arise from tissues considered to be of neuroectodermal or neural crest origin and display a range of features that mirrors the various elements of the nerve (e.g., Schwann cell, perineurial cell). Whereas most soft tissue tumors only seem to be encapsulated by virtue of the compression of surrounding tissues against their advancing border, benign nerve sheath tumors arising in a nerve are completely surrounded by epineurium or perineurium and, therefore, have a true capsule, a feature that facilitates their enucleation. Finally, benign nerve sheath tumors represent the most important group of benign soft tissue lesions in which malignant transformation is an acknowledged phenomenon. Sarcomas develop in neurofibromas in a subset of patients with neurofibromatosis 1, thereby providing an excellent model in which to study the molecular pathway of malignant transformation.

This chapter discusses the two principal benign nerve sheath tumors, schwannoma and neurofibroma, their associated syndromes, and the more recently recognized perineurioma. The schwannoma recapitulates in a more or less consistent fashion the appearance of the differentiated Schwann cell, whereas the neurofibroma displays a spectrum of cell types ranging from the Schwann cell to the fibroblast. Schwannomas and neurofibromas are distinctive lesions that can be reproducibly distinguished from one another, in most instances, by their pattern of growth, cellular composition, associated syndromes, and cytogenetic alterations (Table 27-1). The perineurioma mirrors the barrier (perineurial) cell of the nerve sheath recognized by certain characteristic ultrastructural and immunophenotypic features.

NORMAL ANATOMY

The peripheral nervous system consists of nervous tissue outside of the brain and spinal cord and includes somatic and autonomic nerves, end-organ receptors, and supporting structures. It develops when axons lying close to one another grow

TABLE 27-1 Comparison of Schwannoma and Neurofibroma

PARAMETER	SCHWANNOMA	NEUROFIBROMA
Age	20-50 years	20-40 years; younger in NF1
Common locations	Head-neck; flexor portion of extremities; less often retroperitoneum and mediastinum	Cutaneous nerves; deep locations in NF1
Encapsulation	Usually	Usually not
Growth patterns	Encapsulated tumor with Antoni A and B areas; plexiform type uncommon	Localized, diffuse and plexiform patterns
Associated syndromes	Most lesions sporadic; some NF2 and schwannomatosis, rarely NF1	Most lesions sporadic; some NF1
S-100 protein immunostaining	Strong and uniform	Variable staining of cells
Malignant transformation	Exceptionally rare	Rare in sporadic cases but occurs in 2%-3% of NF1 patients

out from the neural tube and are gradually invested with Schwann cells. Schwann cells arise from the neural crest, a group of cells that arise from and lie lateral to the neural tube and underneath the ectoderm of the developing embryo. The major peripheral nerve trunks form by fusion and division of segmental spinal nerves and contain mixtures of sensory, motor, and autonomic elements.

In the fully developed nerve, a layer of connective tissue or epineurium surrounds the entire nerve trunk (Fig. 27-1). This structure varies in size, depending on the location of the nerve, and it is composed of a mixture of collagen and elastic fibers along with mast cells. Several nerve fascicles lie within the confines of the epineurium, and each, in turn, is surrounded by a well-defined sheath known as the *perineurium*. The outer portion of the perineurium consists of layers of connective tissue, and the inner portion is represented by a multilayered, concentrically arranged sheath of flattened cells. The perineurium, which is continuous with the pia-arachnoid of the central nervous system, represents the principal diffusion barrier for the peripheral nerve. Unlike the Schwann cell, the perineurial cell is a mesodermal derivative sharing an immunophenotype with the cells of the pia-arachnoid (S-100 protein negative; epithelial membrane antigen [EMA], GLUT1, and claudin 1 positive).[1] Ultrastructurally, perineurial cells form close junctions with each other and have basal lamina along the endoneurial and perineurial aspects of the cell, features not encountered in the ordinary fibroblast and Schwann cell.

Despite the undoubted importance of the investing connective tissue, the critical supporting element is the Schwann cell. It provides mechanical protection for the axon, produces and maintains the myelin sheath, and serves as a tube to guide regenerating nerve fibers. Ultrastructurally, the Schwann cell is easily identified by its intimate relation to its axons and by a continuous basal lamina that coats the surface of the cell facing the endoneurium. In routine preparations, it is difficult to distinguish the axon from the myelin sheath. This distinction, however, is easily accomplished with special stains. Silver stains selectively stain the axon (Fig. 27-2), whereas stains such as Luxol fast blue stains myelin. The variation in diameter

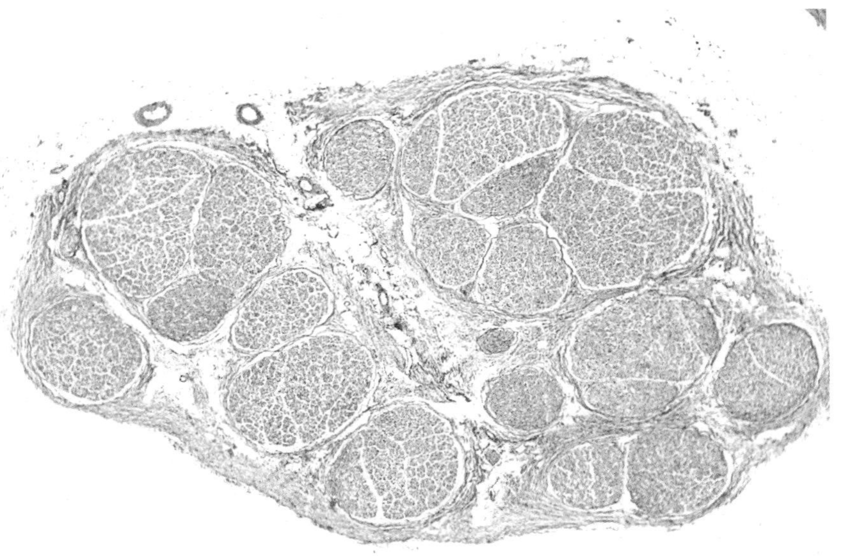

FIGURE 27-1. Normal sciatic nerve in cross section. The entire nerve is surrounded by epineurium, and smaller nerve fascicles are encompassed by perineurium.

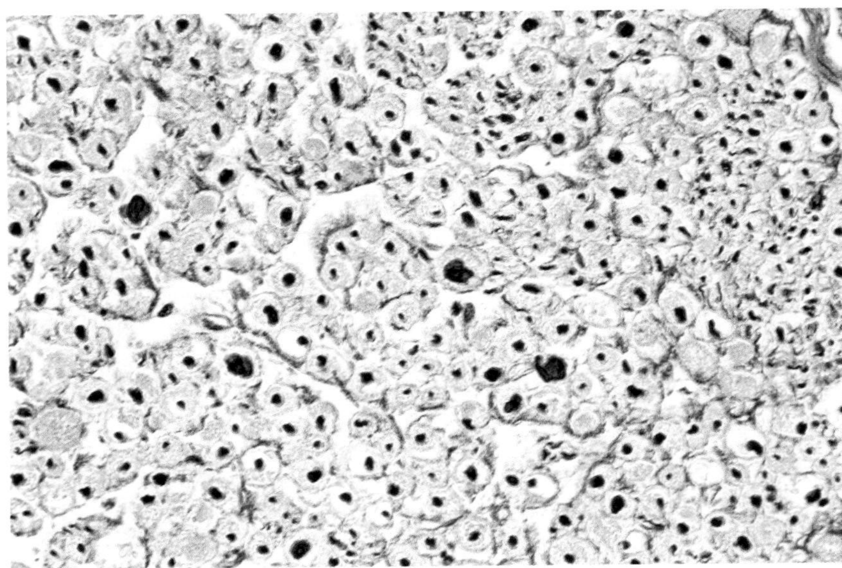

FIGURE 27-2. Normal peripheral nerve cut in cross section and stained with Bodian (silver) stain. Individual axons stain positively; surrounding myelin sheath does not stain. The thickness of axons and the myelin sheath varies and determines the conduction speed.

of axon and myelin sheath can be appreciated with these stains. In general, moderate or heavily myelinated fibers correspond to sensory and motor fibers with fast conduction speeds, whereas lightly myelinated or unmyelinated fibers correspond to autonomic fibers with slower conduction speeds. Ultrastructurally, the cytoplasm of the axon is characterized by numerous cytoplasmic filaments, slender mitochondria, and a longitudinally oriented endoplasmic reticulum. Nissl substance, a feature of the nerve cell body, is not present in the axoplasm. In addition, small vesicles are observed occasionally; they may represent packets of neurotransmitter substance en route to the nerve terminal.

TRAUMATIC (AMPUTATION) NEUROMA

Traumatic neuroma is an exuberant, but non-neoplastic, proliferation of a nerve occurring in response to injury or surgery. Under ideal circumstances, the ends of a severed nerve reestablish continuity by an orderly growth of axons from proximal to distal stump through tubes of proliferating Schwann cells. However, if close apposition of the ends of a nerve is not maintained or if there is no distal stump, a disorganized proliferation of the proximal nerve gives rise to a neuroma. Symptomatic neuromas are usually the result of surgery, notably amputation. Occasionally, other surgical procedures, such as cholecystectomy, have been incriminated in their pathogenesis. A rare form of traumatic neuroma is seen in rudimentary (supernumerary) digits that undergo autoamputation *in utero.* These lesions appear as raised nodules on the ulnar surface of the proximal fifth finger and contain a disordered proliferation of nerves similar to a conventional traumatic neuroma (Fig. 27-3).[2]

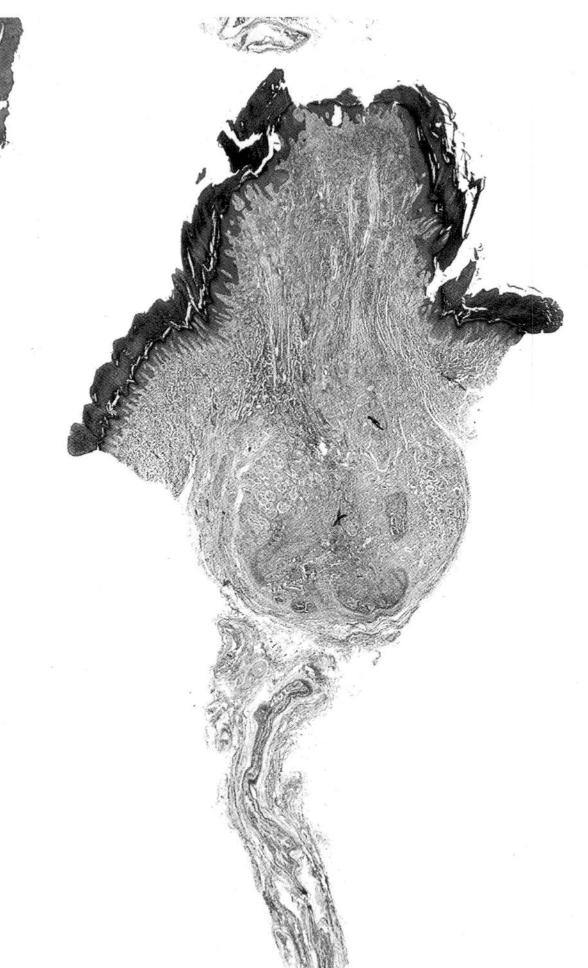

FIGURE 27-3. Rudimentary digit that underwent autoamputation in utero and showed areas of traumatic neuroma.

Clinically, the neuroma presents as a firm nodule that is occasionally tender or painful. Strangulation of the proliferating nerve by scar tissue, local trauma, and infection have been invoked as possible explanations of the pain. Grossly, the lesions are circumscribed, white-gray nodules seldom exceeding 5 cm in diameter; they are located in continuity with the proximal end of the injured or transected nerve. They consist of a haphazard proliferation of nerve fascicles, including axons with their investitures of myelin, Schwann cells, and fibroblasts. The fascicles are usually less well-myelinated than the parent nerve and are embedded in a background of collagen (Fig. 27-4).

Traumatic neuromas are sometimes confused with palisaded encapsulated neuromas and neurofibromas. Participation of all elements of the nerve fascicles and identification of a damaged nerve distinguish a traumatic neuroma from neurofibroma. In areas where the fascicles are small and the matrix is poorly collagenized and highly myxoid, the similarity to neurofibroma may be striking (Fig. 27-5) and, therefore, may require identification of more subtle clues such as the characteristic collagen bundles of neurofibroma. Palisaded encapsulated neuromas arise exclusively in the skin, predominantly in women; they consist of a more circumscribed, orderly arrangement of nerve fascicles.

Treatment of traumatic neuromas is, in part, prophylactic. After traumatic nerve injury, an attempt should be made to reappose the ends of the severed nerve so that regeneration of the proximal end proceeds down the distal trunk in an orderly fashion. Once a neuroma has formed, removal is indicated when it becomes symptomatic or when it must be distinguished from recurrent tumor in a patient who has had cancer-related surgery. Simple excision of the lesion and re-embedding the proximal nerve stump in an area away from the old scar constitute the conventional therapy.

MUCOSAL NEUROMA

Germline activating mutations of the RET proto-oncogene are responsible for several familial syndromes, one of which is multiple endocrine neoplasia 2B (MEN-2b) (thyroid carcinoma, pheochromocytoma, and mucosal neuromas).[3] Patients with this disease develop characteristic neuromas of the mucosal surfaces of the lips, mouth, eyelids, and intestines. Because mucosal neuromas may represent an early manifestation of this life-threatening syndrome, recognition of these lesions is of more than academic interest. The lesions manifest during the first few decades of life and present as multiple nodules of varying size, which may result in diffuse enlargement of the affected area.

Focally, the lesions are notable for the irregular, tortuous bundles of nerve with a prominent perineurium that lie

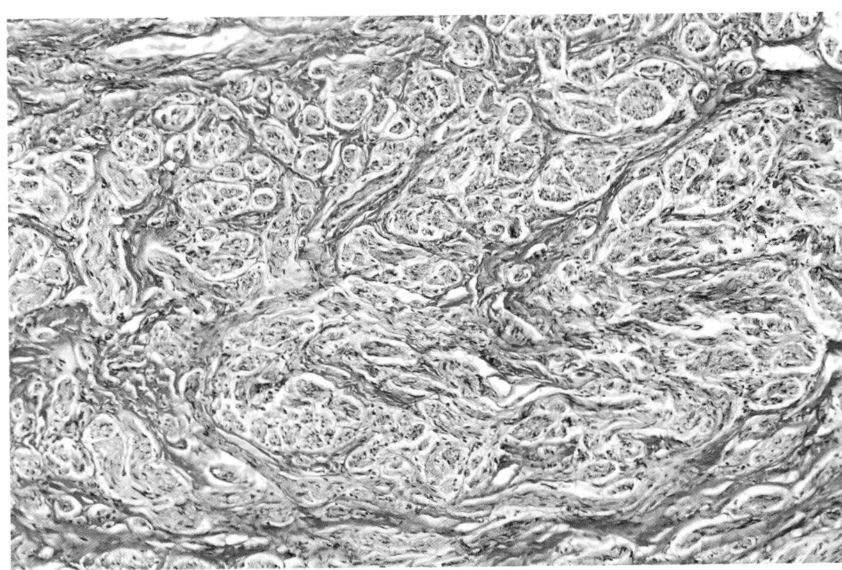

FIGURE 27-4. Traumatic neuroma composed of small proliferating fascicles of nerve enveloped in collagen.

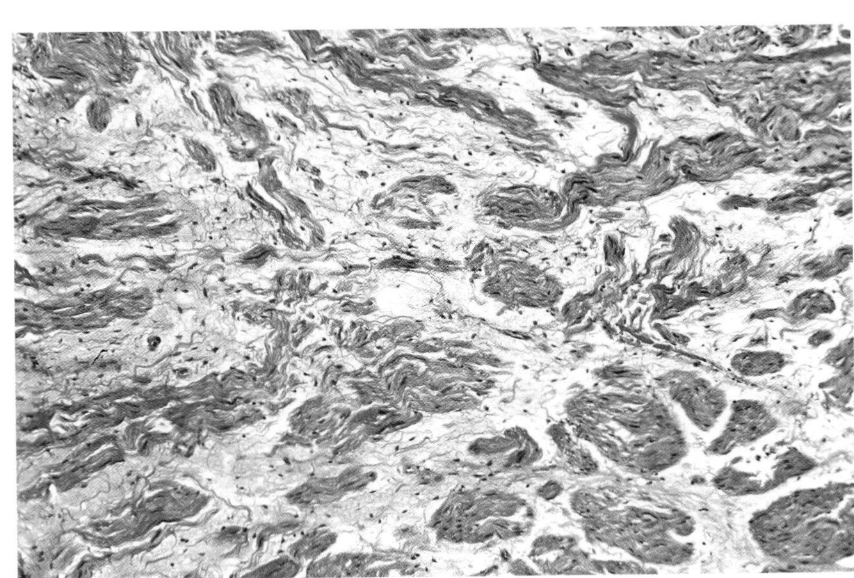

FIGURE 27-5. Myxoid areas in a traumatic neuroma resembling a neurofibroma.

scattered throughout the submucosa of the oral cavity (Fig. 27-6). The nerves and perineurium may be distinguished by a prominent degree of myxoid change. In the gastrointestinal tract, both submucosal and myenteric plexus appear hyperplastic, with an increase in all elements of the plexus, including Schwann cells, neurons, and ganglion cells (Fig. 27-7).[4]

PACINIAN NEUROMA

Pacinian neuroma refers to localized hyperplasia or hypertrophy of the pacinian corpuscles, which occurs following trauma and commonly produces pain.[5-9] Typically, it develops on the digits, where it produces a localized mass. Pacinian neuromas range in appearance from small nodules attached to the nerve by a slender stalk to one or more contiguous subepineural nodules (Fig. 27-8). Histologically, it consists of mature pacinian corpuscles that are increased in size or number (or both) and are often associated with degenerative changes and fibrosis of the adjacent nerve. The principal problem in the differential diagnosis is the distinction of these lesions from a normal pacinian body, which can achieve a size sufficient to be visualized macroscopically. For example, normal pacinian bodies can be identified in the abdominal cavity, where they are occasionally misinterpreted as tumor implants.[5] In pacinian neuromas, the structures usually are larger than 1.5 mm in diameter. In general, a pacinian neuroma is diagnosed when the histologic features described previously are associated with a discrete pain-producing mass. Pacinian neuromas should not be confused with *pacinian neurofibromas*, a term loosely used to describe a heterogeneous group of lesions that probably includes neurofibroma, congenital nevi, perineurioma, and neurothekeoma.

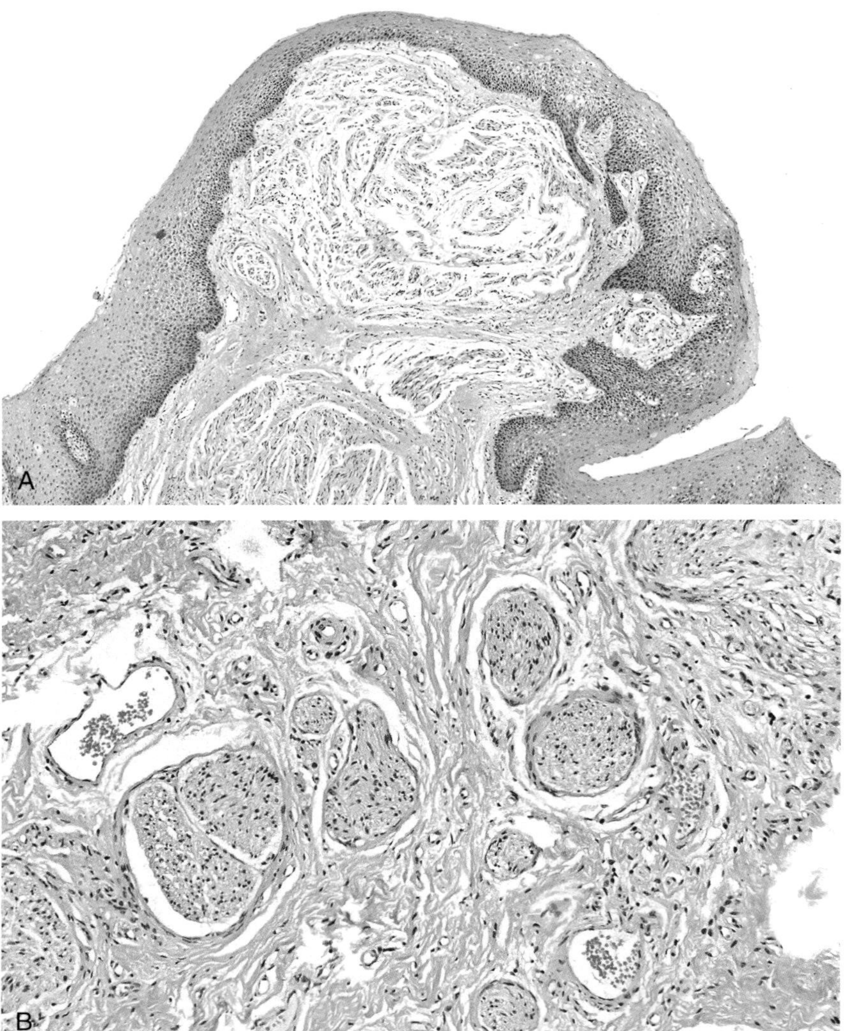

FIGURE 27-6. Mucosal neuroma from a patient with multiple endocrine neoplasia type 2b (A). Irregular, convoluted nerves with prominent perineurium and focal myxoid change lie in submucosal tissue (B).

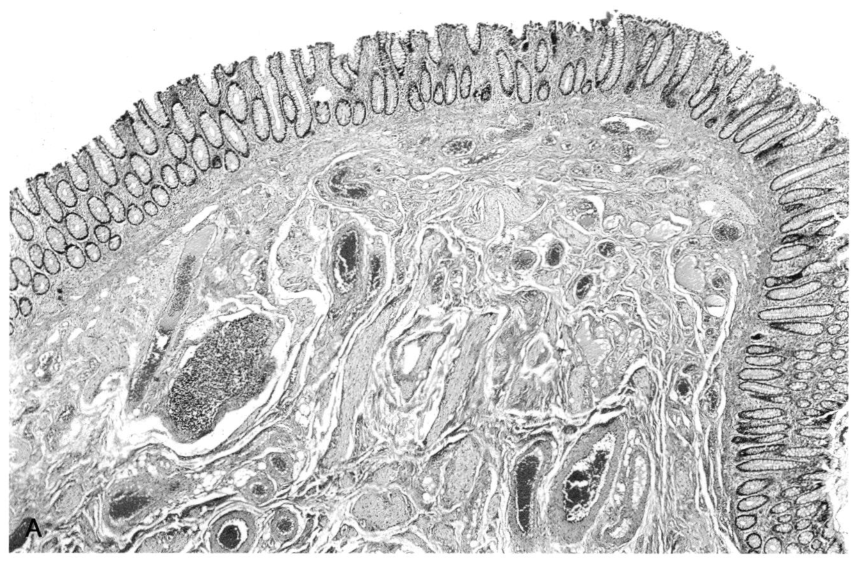

FIGURE 27-7. Ganglioneuromatosis of the gastrointestinal tract in a patient with MEN-2b (A).

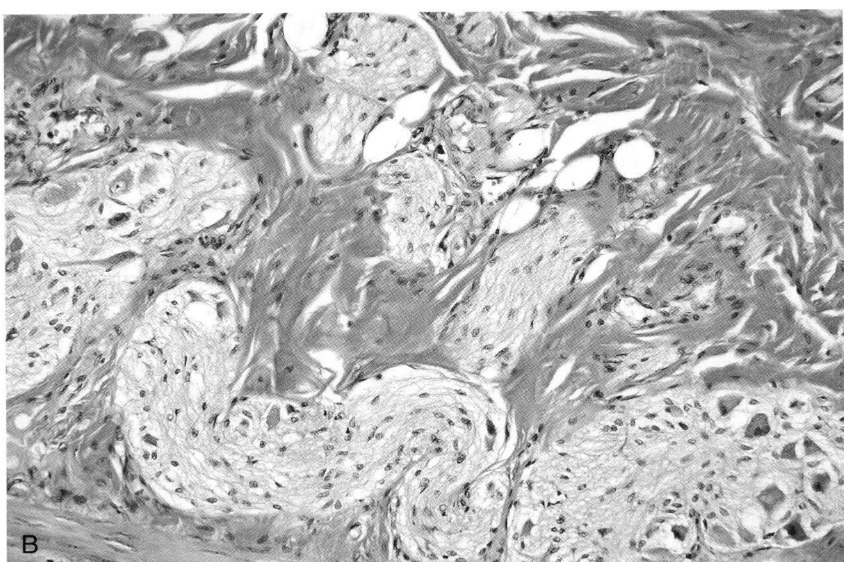

FIGURE 27-7, cont'd. Autonomic nerves in the muscle wall are increased in size and number (B).

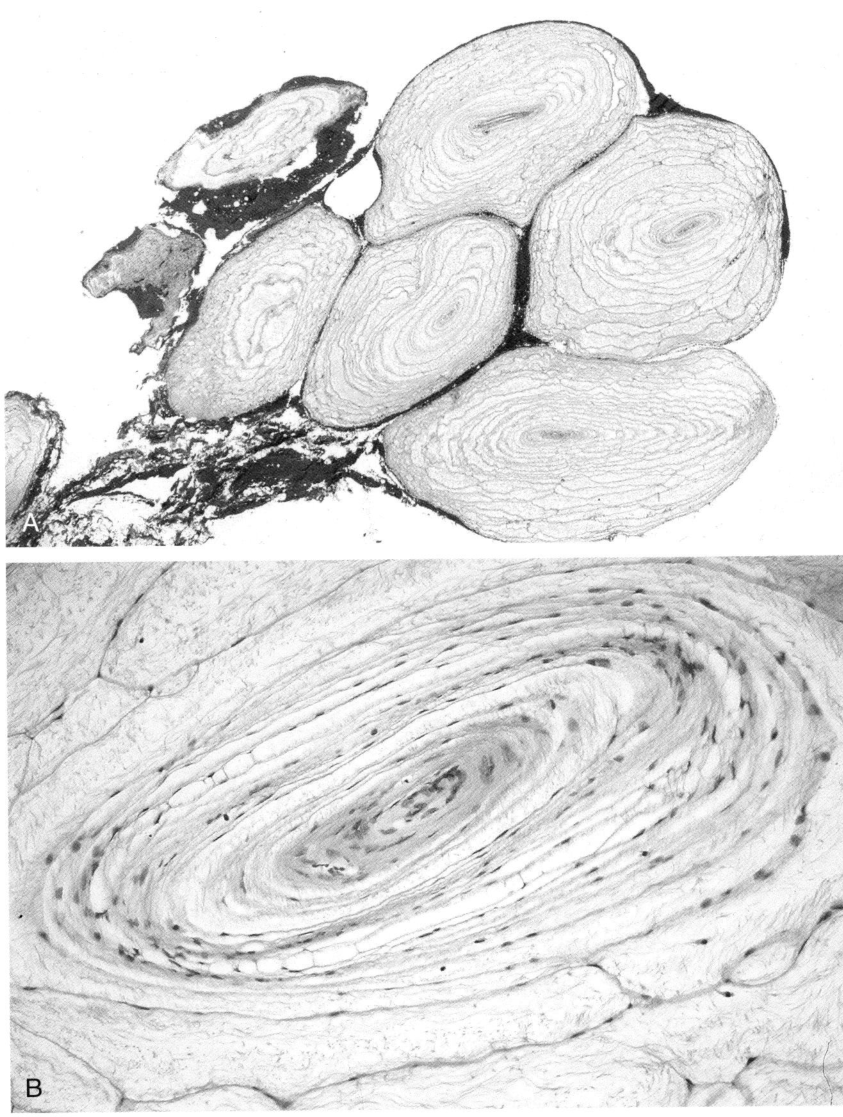

FIGURE 27-8. Pacinian neuroma (A). High-power view (B).

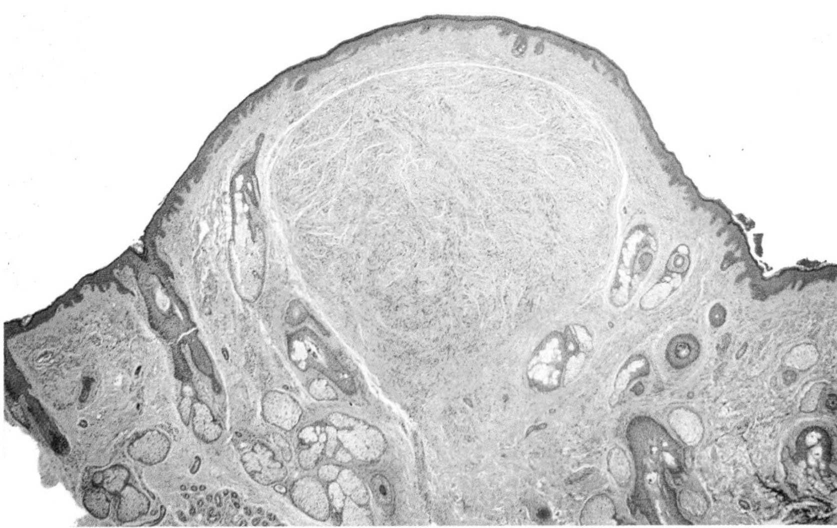

FIGURE 27-9. Palisaded encapsulated neuroma.

PALISADED ENCAPSULATED NEUROMA

The palisaded encapsulated neuroma can be conceptualized as a hyperplastic expansion of Schwann cells and axons of a cutaneous peripheral nerve. Although slow to gain acceptance because of some similarity to the schwannoma, it has distinct clinical features.[10-13] The palisaded encapsulated neuroma develops as a small asymptomatic nodule in the area of the face of adult patients. Rare cases on the distal extremities have been reported.[14] Males and females are involved equally. Affected patients do not display manifestations of neurofibromatosis 1 or MEN-2b.

Histologically, it is composed of one or more circumscribed or encapsulated nodules that occupy the deep dermis and subcutaneous tissues (Fig. 27-9). In some cases, the nodules form club-like extensions into the subcutaneous tissue [15] or may even have a plexiform architecture. They consist of a solid proliferation of Schwann cells and lack the variety of stromal changes (e.g., myxoid change, hyalinization) that may be encountered in schwannomas and neurofibromas (Fig. 27-10). Although, superficially, these neuromas may resemble schwannomas, particularly if minor degrees of nuclear palisading are noted, they differ by the presence of axons, best demonstrated with silver stains, that traverse the lesion in close association with the Schwann cells. Schwannomas may contain axons, but they are typically located peripherally immediately underneath the capsule. In most instances, simple excision of these lesions has proved curative. In contrast to a traumatic neuroma, these lesions are encapsulated, more uniform appearing, and unassociated with a damaged nerve.

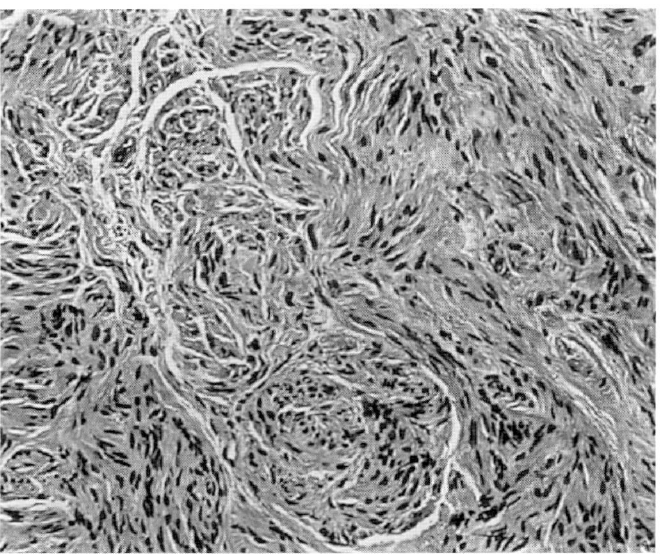

FIGURE 27-10. Palisaded encapsulated neuroma with irregular bundles of nerves containing both nerve and nerve sheath cells.

MORTON NEUROMA (MORTON METATARSALGIA)

Morton interdigital neuroma is not a true tumor but, rather, a fibrosing process of the plantar digital nerve that results in paroxysmal pain in the sole of the foot, usually between the heads of the third and fourth metatarsals and less often between the second and third.[16,17] The pain typically commences with exercise, is alleviated by rest, and may radiate into the toes or leg. In some cases, a small area of point tenderness can be defined, although generally no mass can be palpated. Many theories have been advanced to explain this condition and have included chronic trauma, ischemia, and bursitis. Evidence favors the idea that Morton neuroma is a nerve entrapment syndrome caused by impingement on the plantar digital nerve by the deep transverse intermetatarsal ligament or by the adjacent metatarsal heads. Because women are affected more often than men, the wearing of ill-fitting high-heeled shoes has been incriminated in the pathogenesis of this condition. Lesions histologically similar to Morton neuroma are sometimes seen in relation to nerves in the hand, where they are undoubtedly related to chronic occupational or recreational injury.

At surgery, the characteristic lesion is a firm fusiform enlargement of the plantar digital nerve at its bifurcation point. In advanced cases, the nerve may be firmly attached to the adjacent bursa and soft tissue. Although grossly the lesion resembles a traumatic neuroma or neurofibroma, it is different histologically. Proliferative changes characterize traumatic neuromas, whereas degenerative changes are the hallmark of Morton neuroma. Edema, fibrosis, and demyelinization occur within the nerve (Fig. 27-11A). Hyalinization of endoneurial vessels is also present in some cases (Fig. 27-11B). Elastic fibers are diminished in the center of the lesions but are increased at its periphery, where they have a bilaminar appearance similar to the elastic fibers in an elastofibroma.[18] As the lesion progresses, the fibrosis becomes marked and envelops the epineurium and perineurium in a concentric fashion and may even extend into the surrounding tissue. Although conservative treatment such as wearing of orthopedic footwear and steroid injections are first-line measures, the most successful therapy is removal of the affected nerve segment.

GANGLIONEUROMA

Ganglioneuroma is a differentiated ganglionic tumor that contains no immature neuroblastic elements. They are rare compared to other benign neural tumors such as schwannoma or neurofibroma but outnumber neuroblastomas of the sympathetic axis by a margin of 3 to 1. Most ganglioneuromas are diagnosed in patients older than 10 years and are most often located in the posterior mediastinum followed by the retroperitoneum (Table 27-2). The difference in distribution of neuroblastomas and ganglioneuromas supports the idea that most ganglioneuromas develop *de novo* rather than by way of maturation in a neuroblastoma.

Ganglioneuromas may also be found at other sites, including the skin, retropharynx or parapharynx, the paratesticular region, and gastrointestinal tract. In the gastrointestinal tract, polypoid ganglioneuromas have been reported in association with several inherited diseases, including Cowden syndrome,[19] tuberous sclerosis,[20] and juvenile polyposis.[21,22]

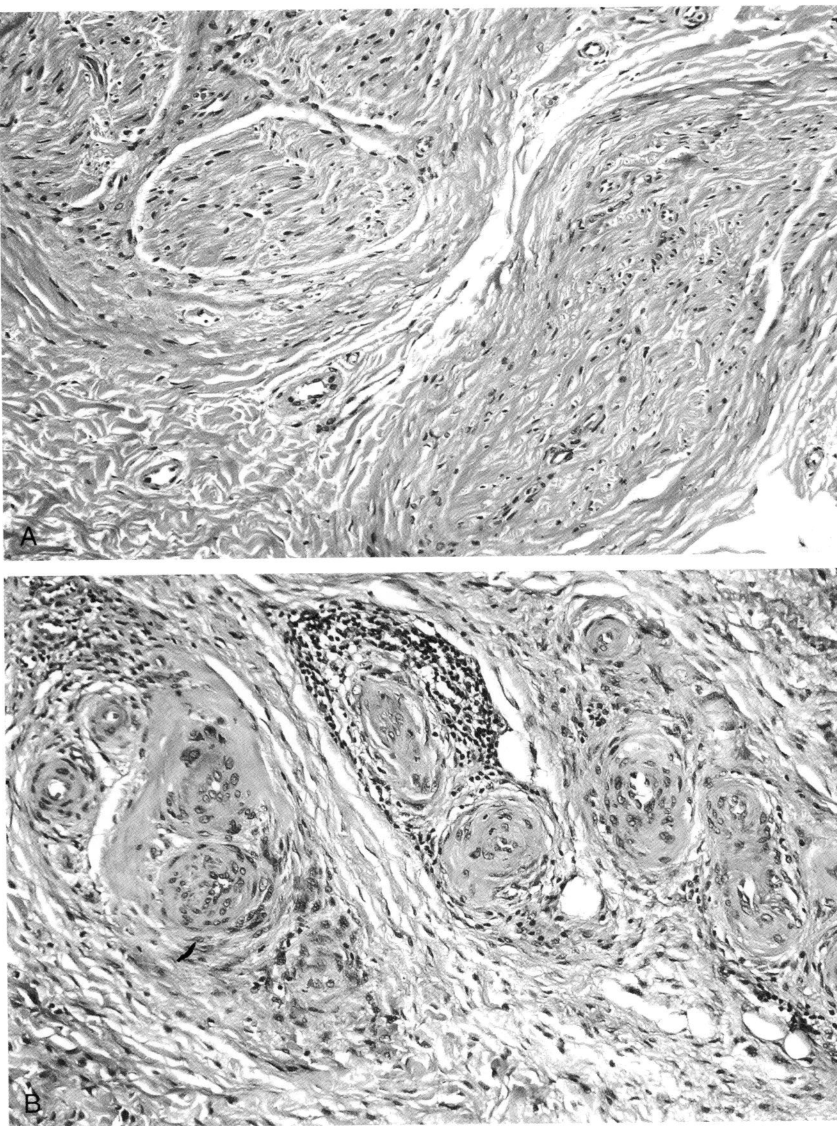

FIGURE 27-11. Morton neuroma. Dense perineural (A) and perivascular (B) fibrosis characterize the lesion.

Ganglioneuromatous polyposis has been described in patients with type 1 neurofibromatosis[23] and multiple endocrine neoplasia type 2b (MEN-2b).[24]

Clinically, ganglioneuromas present as large masses in the retroperitoneum or mediastinum. Most patients have normal levels of urinary catecholamine metabolites, although there is an increased incidence of elevated values in patients with extremely large tumors. However, extreme elevations should prompt careful evaluation for occult neuroblastomatous foci. On radiographic examination, about one-third of cases have intralesional calcification. Clinically, patients may present with sweating, hypertension, virilization, and diarrhea.[25] Diarrheal symptoms in patients with these tumors may be related to the presence of vasoactive intestinal peptide, which can be localized to the cytoplasm of the ganglion cells by means of immunoperoxidase techniques.[26]

Grossly, the ganglioneuroma is a well-circumscribed tumor with a fibrous capsule. On a cut section, it is gray to yellow and sometimes displays a trabecular or whorled pattern similar to that of leiomyoma. Histologically, it has a uniform appearance throughout. The background consists of bundles of longitudinal and transversely oriented Schwann cells that crisscross each other in an irregular fashion (Figs. 27-12 and 27-13). Rarely, fat is present in the stroma.[27] Scattered throughout the schwannian backdrop are relatively mature ganglion cells (Figs. 27-14 to 27-17). Although they may occur in an isolated fashion, usually they are found in small clusters or nests. In general, they are not fully mature and lack satellite cells and Nissl bodies. Typically, their voluminous cytoplasm is bright pink and contains one to three nuclei, which may exhibit a mild to moderate degree of atypia. Pigment is sometimes present in the ganglion cells and is believed to represent catecholamine products that undergo auto-oxidation to a melanin-like substance (neuromelanin).[28] Although the pigment has tinctorial properties of dermal melanin (Fontana-positive), ultrastructurally, it does not have the regular subunit structure but consists instead of large lysosomal structures with myelin figures.[28] There are a number of reports in the literature of composite tumors composed of ganglioneuroma and paraganglioma/pheochromocytoma,[29,30] some of which have arisen in patients with type 1 neurofibromatosis[31] or MEN-2.[32]

Biologically, ganglioneuromas are benign tumors. However, it should be pointed out that rarely an apparent metastatic focus of ganglioneuroma is encountered in a lymph node adjacent to the main tumor mass or at a more distant site (Fig. 27-18).[33] It is assumed that these lesions represent neuroblastomas in which the metastasis and the primary tumor matured. Rare ganglioneuromas undergo malignant transformation,[34,35] including *de novo* ganglioneuromas as well as those derived from maturation in a neuroblastoma. Most commonly, the malignant component resembles a malignant peripheral nerve sheath tumor (MPNST) (Fig. 27-19).

TABLE 27-2 Age and Anatomic Distributions of Ganglioneuroma: 1970–1980 (88 Cases)

PARAMETER	NO. OF CASES
Age (years)	
0-4	5
5-9	9
10-19	23
20-29	22
30-39	12
40-49	4
50-59	6
60-69	4
>69	3
Location	
Mediastinal	27
Retroperitoneal	19
Adrenal	5
Pelvic	2
Cervical	1
Parapharyngeal	34

Data from the Armed Forces Institute of Pathology (AFIP).

NERVE SHEATH GANGLION

Rarely, ganglia occur in intraneural locations.[36-38] These lesions present as tender masses with pain or numbness in the

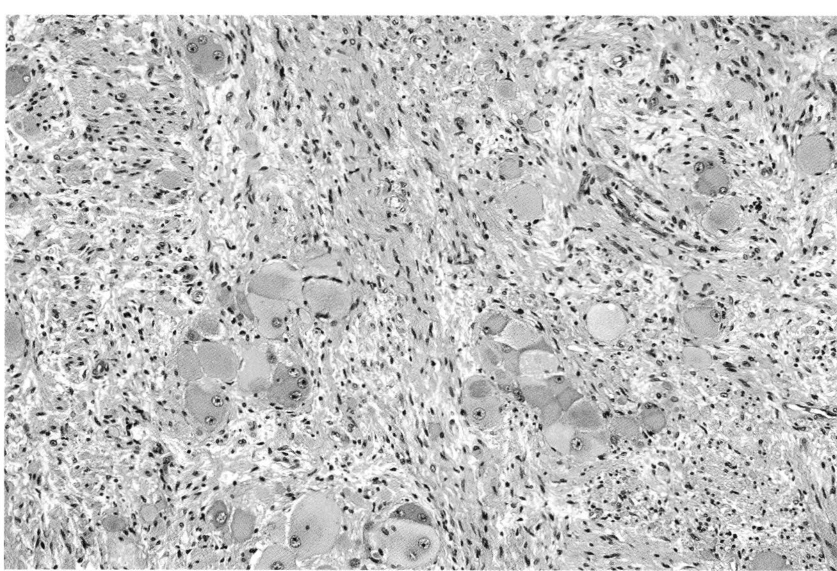

FIGURE 27-12. Ganglioneuroma composed of clusters of ganglion cells deposited in a neuromatous stroma.

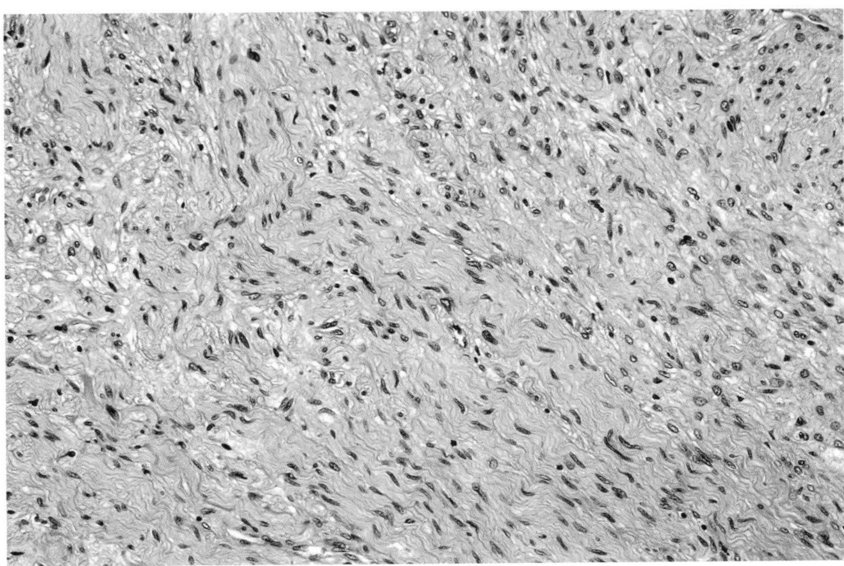

FIGURE 27-13. Neuromatous stroma devoid of ganglion cells in a ganglioneuroma.

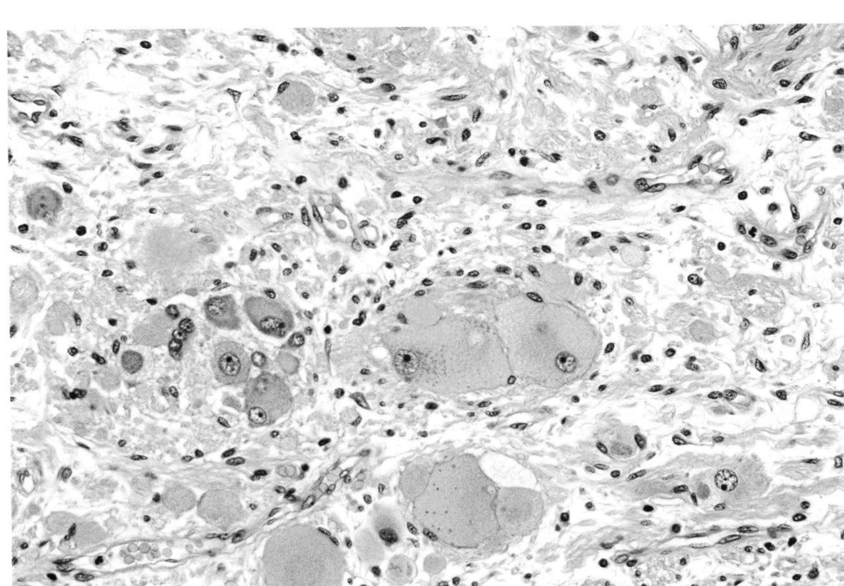

FIGURE 27-14. Ganglioneuroma with clusters of variably sized ganglion cells.

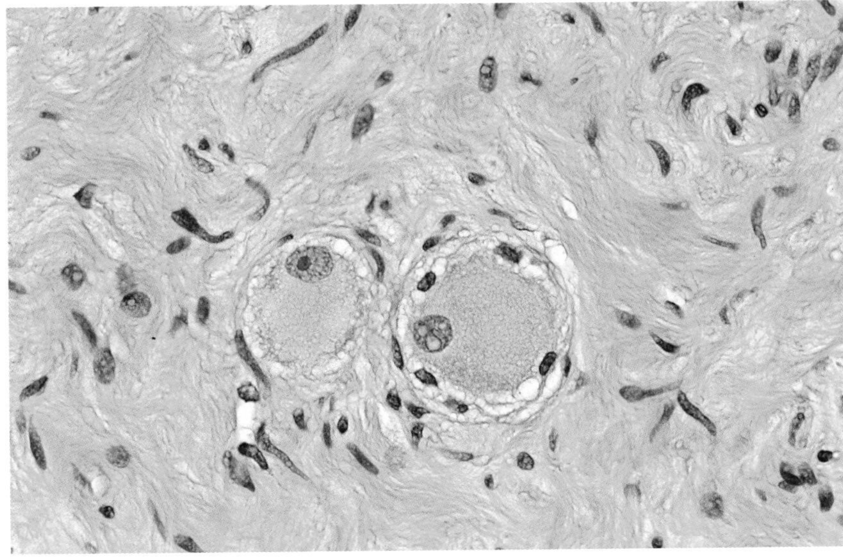

FIGURE 27-15. Mature ganglion cells with satellite cells in a ganglioneuroma.

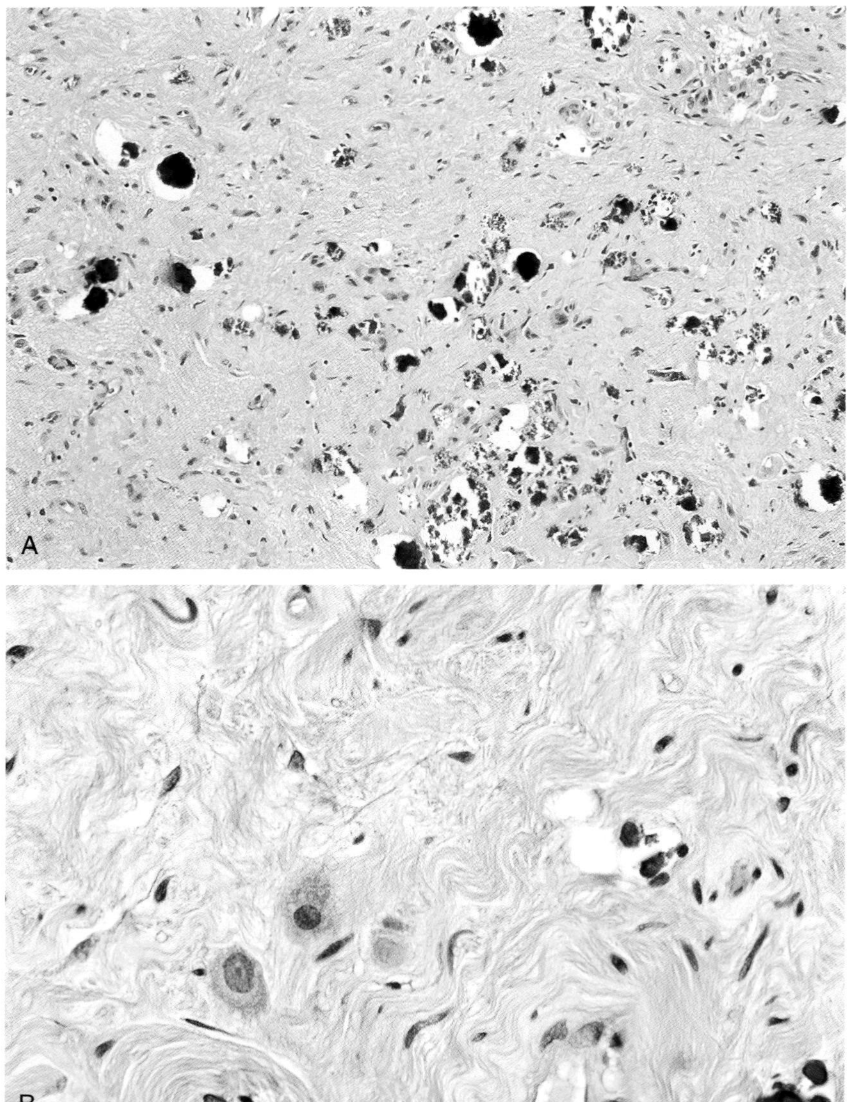

FIGURE 27-16. Ganglion cells from a ganglioneuroma having less Nissl substance and fewer satellite cells than their normal counterparts. Focal calcification is seen.

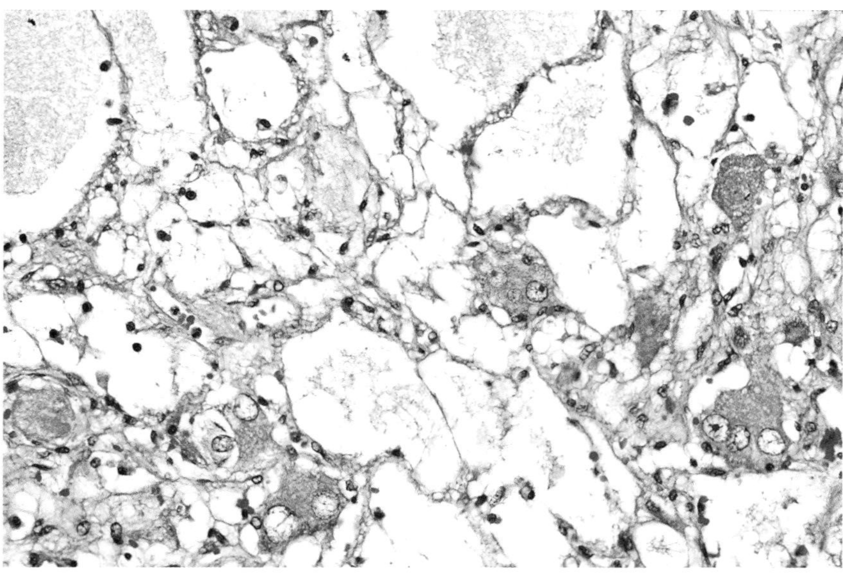

FIGURE 27-17. Cystic change in a ganglioneuroma obscuring the basic architecture of this lesion. Obvious ganglion cells can still be identified.

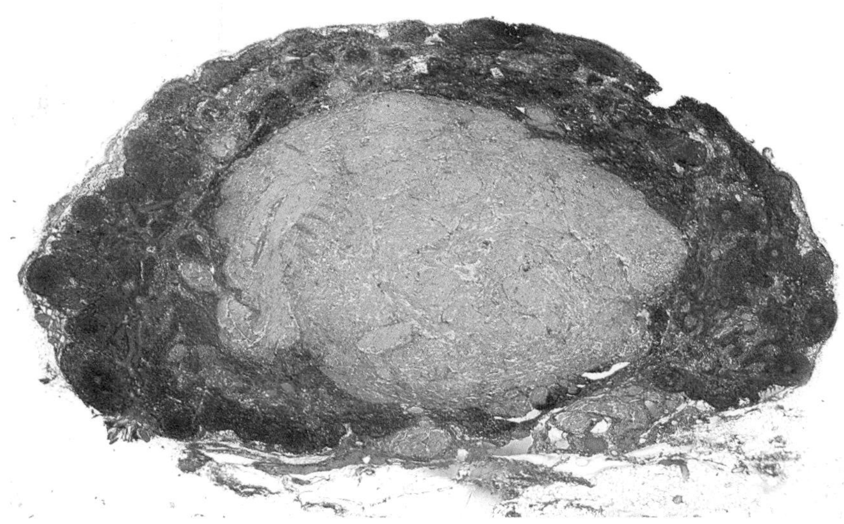

FIGURE 27-18. Apparent metastatic focus of a ganglioneuroma in a lymph node probably representing maturation of a neuroblastoma.

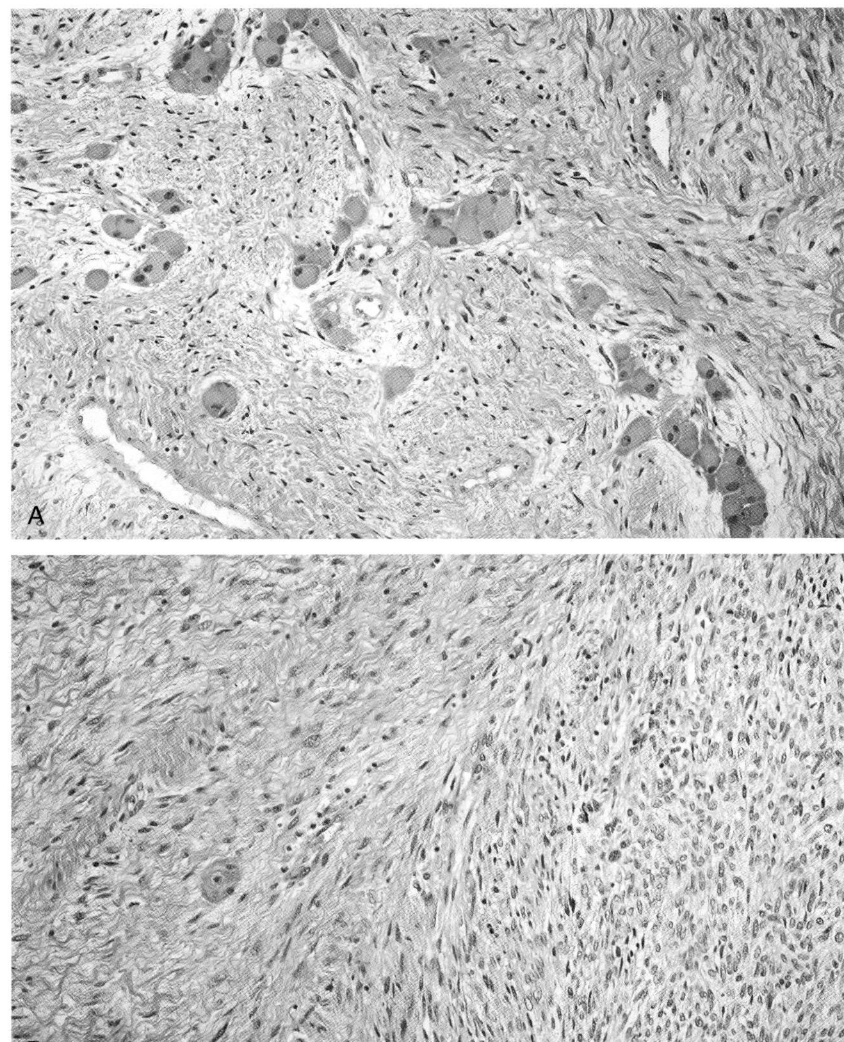

FIGURE 27-19. Rare example of malignant transformation of a ganglioneuroma to a malignant peripheral nerve sheath tumor. (A) Ganglioneuromatous portion of the tumor. (B) Interface between a ganglioneuroma and a malignant peripheral nerve sheath tumor.

distribution of the affected nerve. Most of these lesions are located in the external popliteal nerve[36] at the head of the fibula, which suggests that a particular type of injury or irritation leads to their development. The nerve exhibits localized swelling that corresponds to myxoid change with secondary cyst formation. In some cases, however, the unlined cysts dominate the histologic picture and cause marked displacement of the nerve fascicles toward one side of the sheath (Fig. 27-20). This lesion, like its soft tissue counterpart, represents a degenerative process rather than a neoplasm. The myxoid zones in these lesions, unfortunately, have led to some confusion with the so-called nerve sheath myxoma, a true neoplasm probably of Schwann cell origin, which is quite distinct from nerve sheath ganglion. Therapy of a nerve sheath ganglion consists of local excision, although decompression is acceptable if the integrity of the nerve is threatened.

NEUROMUSCULAR HAMARTOMA (NEUROMUSCULAR CHORISTOMA, BENIGN TRITON TUMOR)

Tumors composed of skeletal muscle and neural elements are collectively referred to as *Triton tumors* in accord with an early hypothesis concerning their histogenesis (see Chapter 28).[39] The best recognized of these mosaic tumors is the MPNST with rhabdomyoblastic differentiation (malignant Triton tumor), although combinations such as rhabdomyosarcoma with ganglion cells (ectomesenchymoma) also occur. Benign lesions composed of neural and skeletal muscle differentiation are rare and are represented principally by the neuromuscular hamartoma or choristoma and the neurofibroma with a rhabdomyomatous component. *Benign Triton tumor* is often used loosely to refer to neuromuscular hamartomas, although it is technically incorrect if these are hamartomas or choristomas that occur when primitive mesenchyme of developing limb buds is included in the nerve sheath. Karyotypic analysis in one case was normal, supporting a hamartomatous process.

Of the fewer than 50 cases from the literature, the majority occurred in young children as solitary masses involving large nerve trunks, particularly the brachial and sciatic.[40] Tumors arising from the cranial nerves also occur but usually present during adult life.[41] The case described by O'Connell and Rosenberg[42] presented as multiple lesions outside of the nerve. Because of their strategic locations, neurologic symptoms are prominent.[40] MRI may be helpful in diagnosis because the signal characteristics are similar to skeletal muscle. Grossly, the lesions simulate a benign nerve sheath tumor. The tumors are multinodular masses subdivided by fibrous bands into smaller nodules or fascicles. Each fascicle is composed of highly differentiated skeletal muscle fibers that vary in size but are often larger than normal. Intimately associated with the skeletal muscle and sharing the same perimysial sheath are both small myelinated and nonmyelinated nerves (Fig. 27-21). Immunohistochemical stains for neural and muscle markers highlight the close juxtaposition of both components. Smooth muscle is rarely present.[43] At times, the fibrous component surrounding the lesions is so dense and cellular that it suggests the diagnosis of fibromatosis replacing muscle and nerve. Follow-up information in the cases of the authors of this edition and those in the literature supports their benignity. Even incomplete excision has resulted in amelioration of symptoms and progressive decrease in size. Therefore, after a correct diagnosis, treatment should be conservative and aimed at maintaining the integrity of the nerve.

NEUROFIBROMA

Neurofibromas may assume one of three growth patterns: localized, diffuse, or plexiform. The localized form is seen most commonly as a superficial, solitary tumor in normal individuals. Diffuse and plexiform neurofibromas have a close association with neurofibromatosis 1 (NF1), the latter being nearly pathognomonic of the disease and are later discussed in that context.

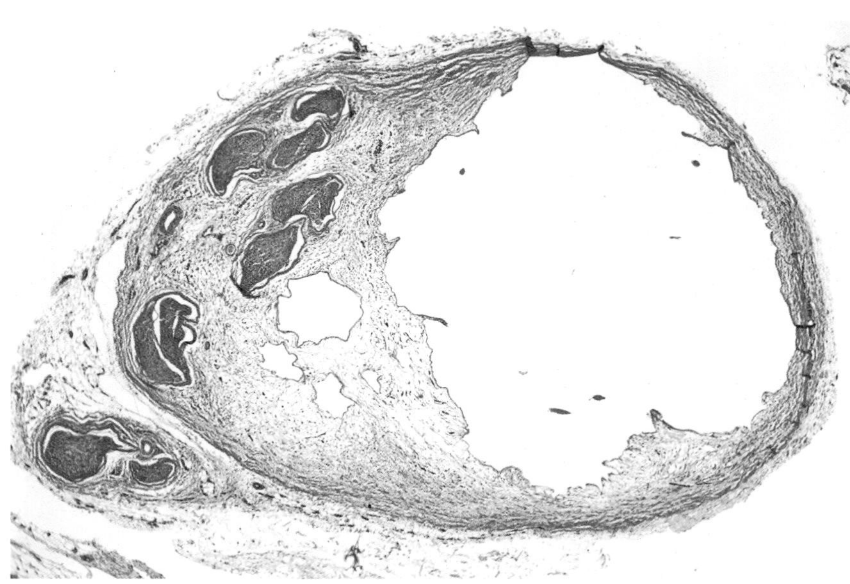

FIGURE 27-20. Ganglion of nerve sheath. Connective tissue of the nerve undergoes myxoid change and cystification.

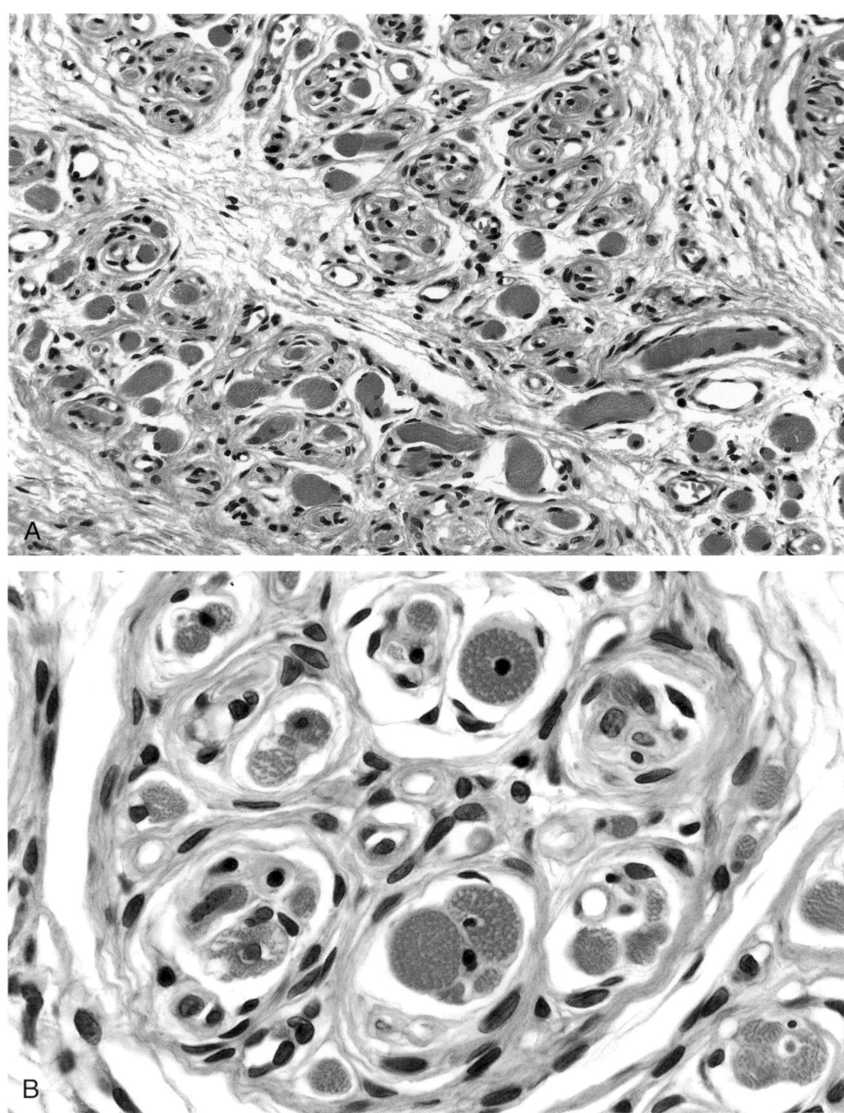

FIGURE 27-21. Neuromuscular hamartoma composed of short bundles of mature nerve and muscle (A). High-power view of neuromuscular hamartoma (B).

Localized (Sporadic) Neurofibroma

Localized neurofibromas occur most often as sporadic lesions in patients who do not have NF1. Their exact incidence is unknown because of the difficulty in excluding the diagnosis of NF1 in some persons such as the young, in whom the initial presentation of the disease may be a solitary neurofibroma, or patients who have no affected family members. Despite these problems, it appears that sporadic neurofibromas outnumber those occurring in NF1 by a considerable margin.

Clinical Findings

Localized sporadic neurofibromas, like their inherited counterparts, affect the genders equally. Most develop in persons between the ages of 20 and 30 years. Because most are superficial lesions of the dermis or subcutis, they are found evenly distributed over the body surface. They grow slowly as painless nodules that produce few symptoms. Grossly, they are glistening tan-white tumors that lack the secondary degenerative changes common to schwannomas. If they arise in major nerves, they expand the structure in a fusiform fashion, and normal nerves can be seen entering and exiting from the mass (Fig. 27-22). If this lesion remains confined by the epineurium, it has a true capsule. More commonly, these tumors arise in small nerves and readily extend into soft tissue. These tumors appear circumscribed but not encapsulated.

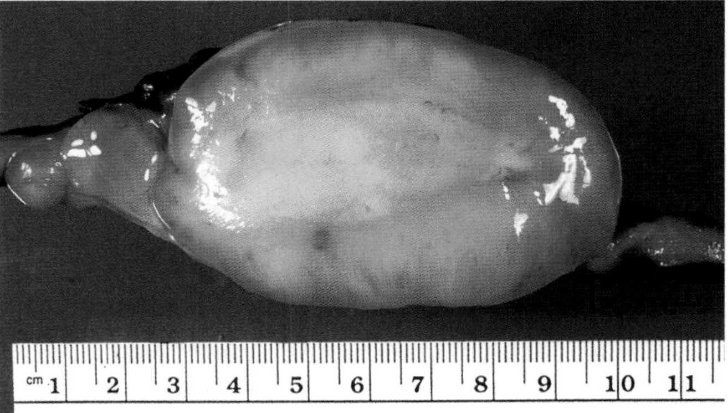

FIGURE 27-22. Gross specimen of neurofibroma arising as fusiform expansion of nerve. *(Case courtesy of Dr. Steve Bonsib.)*

Microscopic Findings

Histologically, the neurofibroma varies, depending on its content of cells, stromal mucin, and collagen (Figs. 27-23 to 27-27). In its most characteristic form, the neurofibroma contains interlacing bundles of elongated cells with wavy, darkly stained nuclei. The cells are intimately associated with wire-like strands of collagen that have been likened to shredded carrots. Small to moderate amounts of mucoid material separate the cells and collagen. The stroma of the tumor is dotted with mast cells, lymphocytes, and, rarely, xanthoma cells. Less frequently, the neurofibroma is highly cellular and consists of Schwann cells set in a uniform collagen matrix devoid of mucosubstances (see Fig. 27-24). The cells may be arranged in short fascicles, whorls, or even a storiform pattern. In certain respects, these cellular neurofibromas resemble Antoni A areas of a schwannoma. Unlike schwannoma, they are not encapsulated and lack a clear partition into two zones. Moreover, small neurites can usually be demonstrated throughout these tumors. Least commonly, these tumors are highly myxoid and, therefore, often confused with myxomas; this form of neurofibroma usually occurs on the extremities. These hypocellular neoplasms contain pools of acid mucopolysaccharide with widely spaced Schwann cells. In contrast to the cells of myxoma, neurofibroma cells usually have a greater degree of orientation. The vascularity is also more prominent, and, with careful searching, features of specific differentiation (e.g., pseudomeissnerian bodies) may be found. Rare variations in neurofibromas are epithelioid change of the Schwann cells (see Fig. 27-27) and skeletal muscle. Extraordinarily rare cases contain benign glands or rosettes. S-100 protein can be identified in these tumors but stains only a subset of cells, in keeping with the observation that neurofibromas contain a mixed population of cells (see Fig. 27-26).

Although solitary neurofibromas are not associated with the same incidence of malignant change as their inherited counterparts, the exact risk is unknown. It is probably extraordinarily small. Simple excision of these tumors is considered adequate therapy.

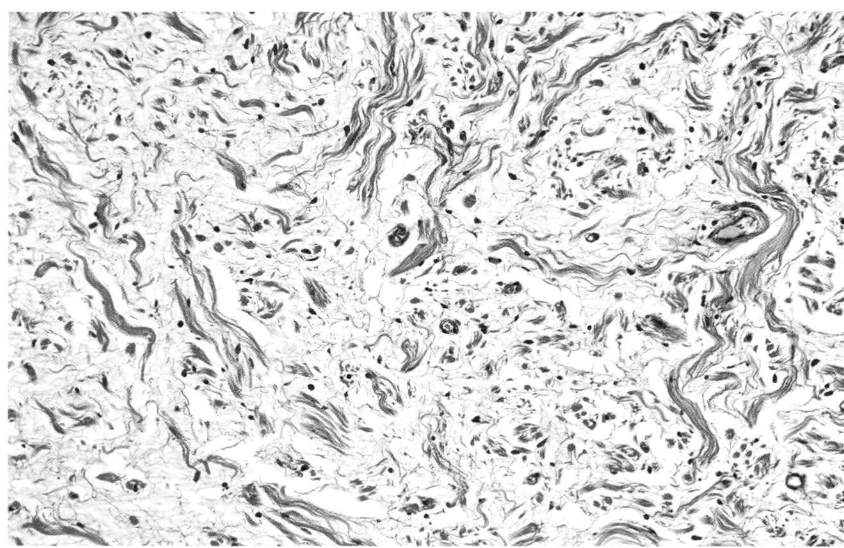

FIGURE 27-23. Neurofibroma with a myxoid matrix containing neoplastic cells and ropey collagen bundles.

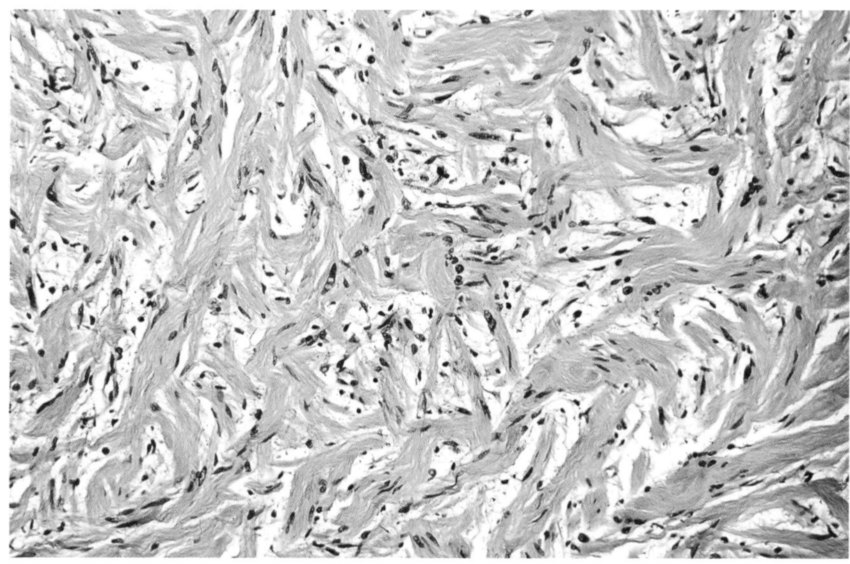

FIGURE 27-24. Neurofibroma with dense collagen bundles.

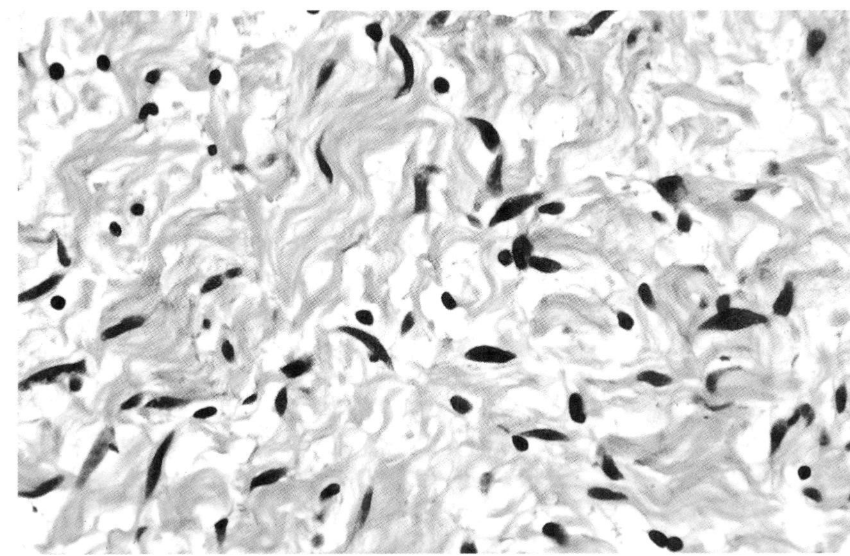

FIGURE 27-25. Neurofibroma with Schwann cells of an irregular shape, mononuclear cells, and occasional mast cells.

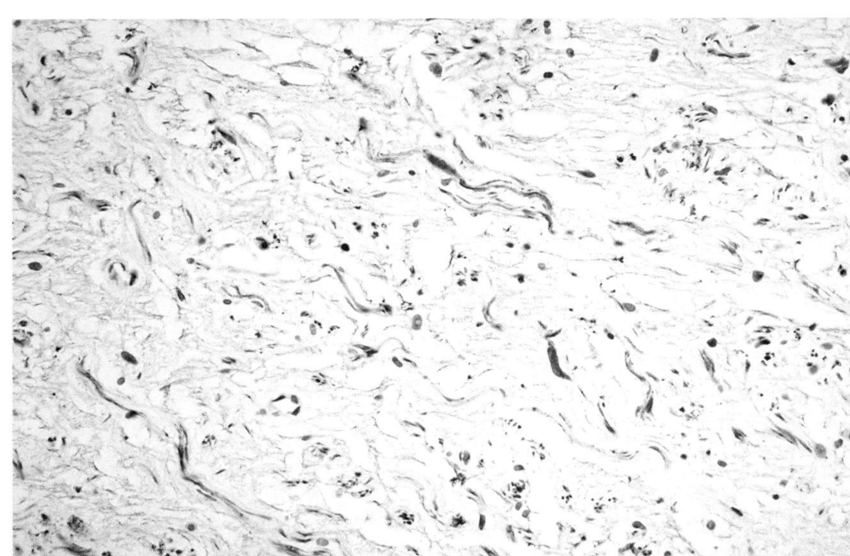

FIGURE 27-26. S-100 protein immunostain of a neurofibroma illustrating that not all cells in the lesion express the antigen.

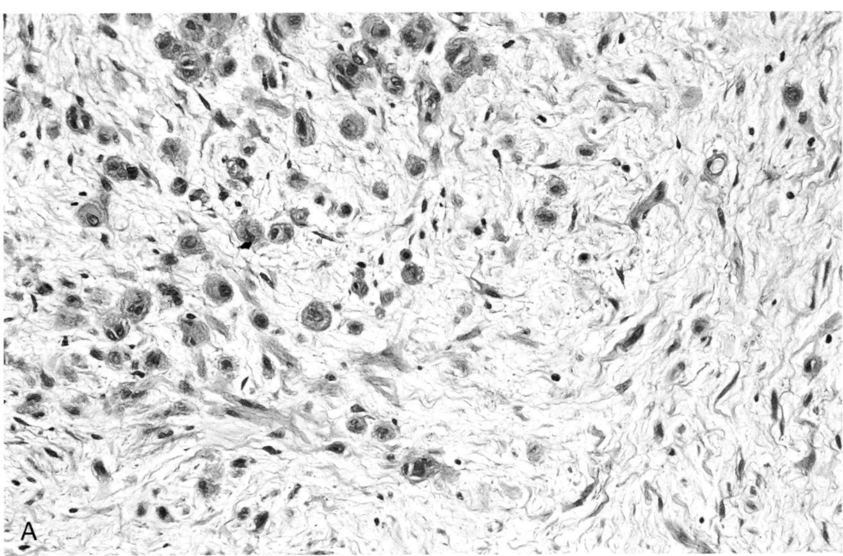

FIGURE 27-27. Epithelioid neurofibroma arising in a nerve in a patient with neurofibromatosis 1 (NF1). (A) shows transition between epithelioid areas and those with appearance of conventional neurofibroma. *Continued*

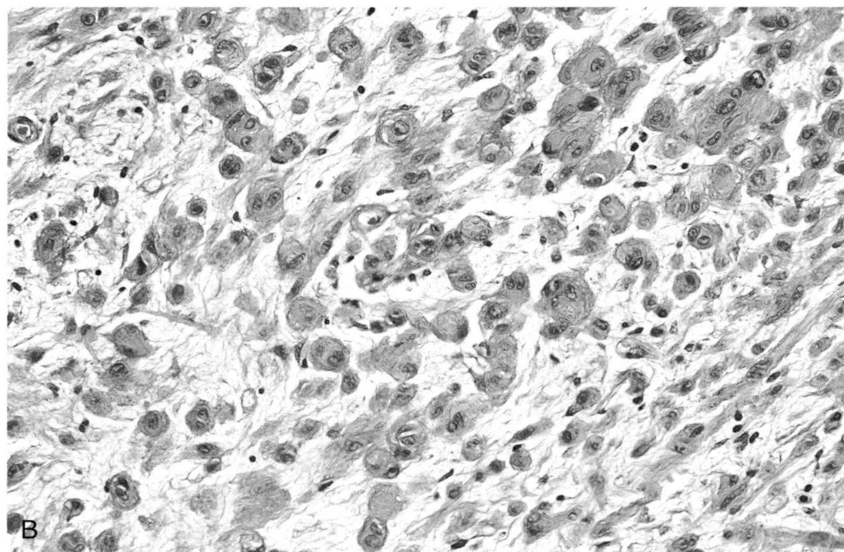

FIGURE 27-27, cont'd. High-power view of epithelioid areas (B).

NEUROFIBROMATOSIS 1 (NF1)

Neurofibromatosis, also named *von Recklinghausen disease* for the man who described the disease in 1882, was formerly considered a single disease but is now known to be at least two clinically and genetically distinct diseases. The more common disease, formerly known as the peripheral form of neurofibromatosis, is designated *neurofibromatosis 1 (NF1)*, whereas the less common disease, formerly known as the central form, is designated *neurofibromatosis 2 (NF2) (bilateral vestibular schwannoma)*.

A common genetic disease, NF1 affects 1 in every 3500 individuals.[44,45] It is inherited as an autosomal dominant trait with a high rate of penetrance. Because only half of the patients with this disease have affected family members, the disease in the remaining patients represents new mutations. The mutation rate, estimated at 10^{-4} per gamete per generation, is among the highest for a dominantly inherited trait. About 80% of new mutations are of paternal origin.

NF1 is caused by deletions, insertions, stop mutations, amino acid substitutions, and splicing mutations in the *NF1* gene, a tumor suppressor gene located in the pericentromeric region of chromosome 17.[46,47] Spanning a distance of 300 kb and containing at least 60 exons, it is one of the largest human genes, an observation that likely explains its high mutation rate. It encodes an approximately 2800 amino acid protein known as *neurofibromin*, several isoforms of which are differentially expressed in tissues such as brain, neurons, and peripheral nerve. A small portion of neurofibromin possesses sequence homology to the RAS GTPase activating protein (RAS-GAP) family of proteins that inactivate RAS. Loss of *NF1* gene expression, therefore, results in increased RAS activity, cell proliferation, and tumorigenesis.[48] Neurofibromin has other functions as well. For example, neurofibromin positively regulates c-AMP which, in turn, modulates astrocytic growth and differentiation in the brain.[49] Understanding these additional signaling pathways will likely begin to explain the protean manifestations of the disease.

BOX 27-1 Diagnostic Criteria for Neurofibromatosis 1

Neurofibromatosis 1 is diagnosed in an individual with two or more of the following signs or factors:

- Six or more café au lait macules: >5 mm in greatest diameter in prepubertal individuals; >15 mm in greatest diameter in postpubertal individuals
- Two or more neurofibromas of any type or one plexiform neurofibroma
- Freckling in the axillary or inguinal region
- Optic glioma
- Two or more Lisch nodules (iris hamartomas)
- A distinctive osseous lesion such as sphenoid dysplasia or thinning of long bone cortex with or without pseudoarthrosis
- First-degree relative (parent, sibling, offspring) with neurofibromatosis 1 by the above criteria

From National Institutes of Health.[167]

Clinical Findings

Although, in principal, diagnosis of NF1 should be possible through genetic testing, the large size of the gene and the myriad of mutations have precluded this. Instead, a protein truncation assay to screen for stop mutations has been devised. Unfortunately, it detects only two-thirds of cases and does not predict severity of the disease.[47] For these reasons, the diagnosis of NF1 is still dependent on identification of the cardinal signs of the disease, two or more of which must be present (Box 27-1) to establish the diagnosis. The severity of the disease varies widely from patient to patient and from family to family. Because of the complexity of the disease and size of the gene, it has been difficult to perform precise genotypic–phenotypic correlations. Only in patients with extremely severe forms of the disease who harbor large deletions have such correlations been possible. It is, therefore, likely that genetic modifiers outside of the NF1 locus play a role in disease symptoms.[45] Complete gene deletions are associated with severe symptoms of NF1, a large number of neurofibromas and significantly higher lifetime risk for MPNST,[47] whereas mutations at the 3' end of the gene correlate with familial spinal neurofibromatosis. Segmental forms of neurofibromatosis may be explained by somatic mosaicism.

In the typical patient, NF1 becomes evident within the first few years of life when café au lait spots develop. These pigmented macular lesions resemble freckles, especially during the early stage when they are small. Typically, they become much larger and darker with age and occur mainly on unexposed surfaces of the body (Fig. 27-28). One of the most characteristic locations for these spots is the axilla (axillary freckle sign). Pathologically, they are characterized by an increase in melanin pigment in the basal layer of the epidermis. In adults, only lesions larger than 1.5 cm are considered café au lait spots for purposes of diagnosis.[50] Because the number of café au lait spots increases with age and more than 90% of patients with neurofibromatosis have these lesions, their number serves as a useful guideline when making the diagnosis. Not only do these lesions herald the onset of the disease, but also in older patients they often give some indication as to the form and severity of the disease.[50] For instance, patients with few café au lait spots tend to have either (1) late onset of palpable neurofibromas, (2) localization of neurofibromas to one segment of the body, or (3) NF2.

Neurofibromas, the hallmark of the disease, make their appearance during childhood or adolescence after the café au lait spots. The time course varies greatly: some tumors emerge at birth, and others appear during late adult life (Fig. 27-29). They may be found in virtually any location and, in rare instances, may be restricted to one area of the body (segmental neurofibromatosis). Unusual symptoms have been related to the presence of these tumors in various organs such as the gastrointestinal tract. The tumors are usually slowly growing lesions. Acceleration of their growth rate has been noted during pregnancy and at puberty. A sudden increase in the size of one lesion should always raise the question of malignant change.

In addition to peripheral neurofibromas, patients with NF1 also develop central nervous system tumors, including optic nerve glioma, astrocytoma, and a variety of heterotopias. Vestibular schwannoma, the hallmark of NF2, is virtually never encountered in NF1. Unusual bright objects are detected by T2-weighted MRI in the brain in over 60% of patients with NF1 and are thought to provide some indication of the degree of cognitive dysfunction in the disease.[49]

Pigmented hamartomas of the iris (Lisch nodules)[51] may also be found. These asymptomatic lesions are not present in normal individuals or in those with NF2 (Figs. 27-30 and 27-31). Although they cannot be correlated with other specific manifestations of NF1, they are helpful for establishing the diagnosis.

Skeletal abnormalities occur in almost 40% of patients with this disease.[50,52] They include erosive defects secondary to impingement by soft tissue tumors and primary defects, such as scalloping of the vertebra, congenital bowing of long bones with pseudoarthrosis, unilateral orbital malformations, and cystic osteolytic lesions. In the past, the intraosseous cystic

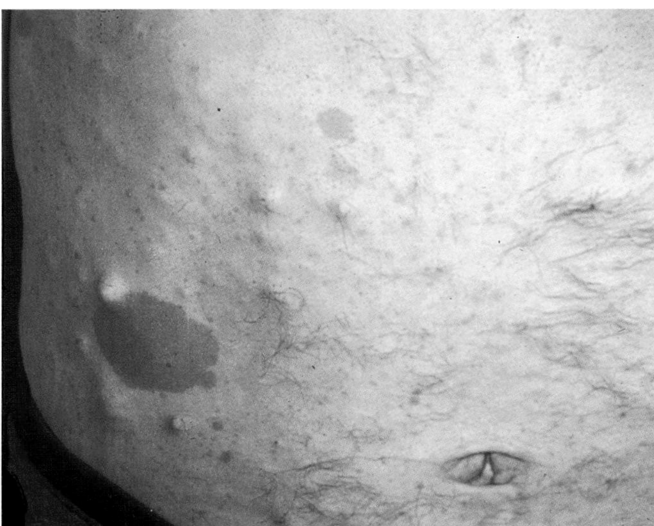

FIGURE 27-28. Café au lait spot. These pigmented lesions usually herald the onset of NF1. They are usually multiple, occur on unexposed surfaces, and typically are several centimeters in diameter.

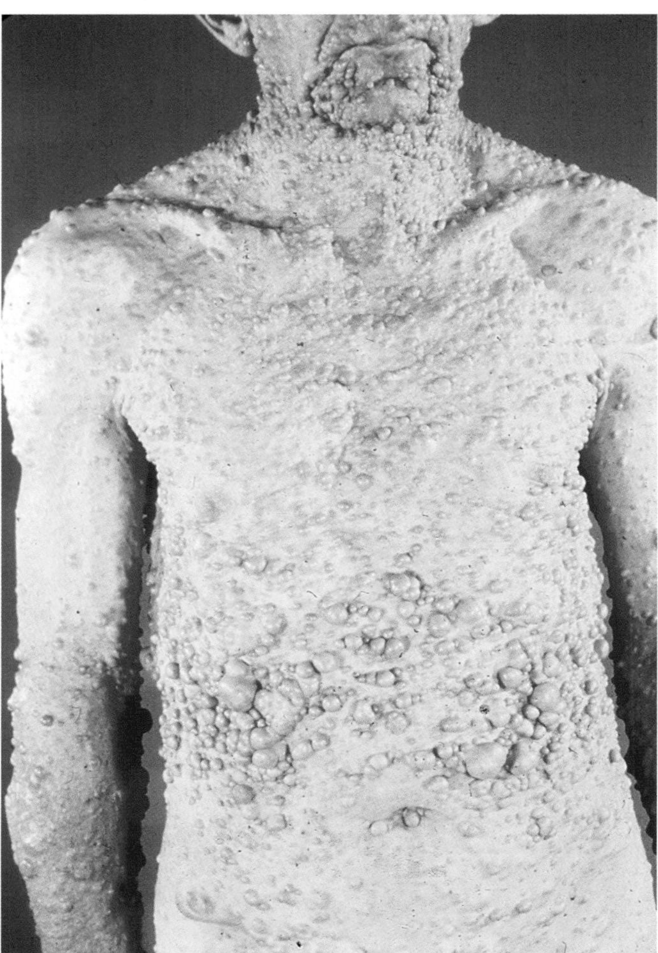

FIGURE 27-29. Male patient with neurofibromatosis of long duration.

lesions were believed to be skeletal neurofibromas, but most of these lesions have the histologic appearance of nonossifying fibroma or fibrous cortical defect characterized by fascicles of fibroblasts arranged in short intersecting fascicles (sometimes in a storiform pattern) and punctuated with occasional giant cells.

Vascular abnormalities, specifically vascular stenoses, secondary to proliferation of intimal cells, are a significant cause of premature death due to renovascular hypertension or stroke. Gynecomastia-like changes (pseudogynecomastia) consisting of stromal hyalinization with nerve fibers and fibroblasts, some of which are multinucleated, have been reported in young males with the disease. In addition to these well-recognized signs and symptoms, NF1 is associated with diverse symptoms not clearly referable to the presence of tumors. They include disorders of growth, sexual maturation, and cognition[50] and abnormalities of the lung. Patients with NF1 are also prone to develop non-neural tumors, notably pheochromocytoma, myelogenous leukemia, and multifocal gastrointestinal stromal tumors.

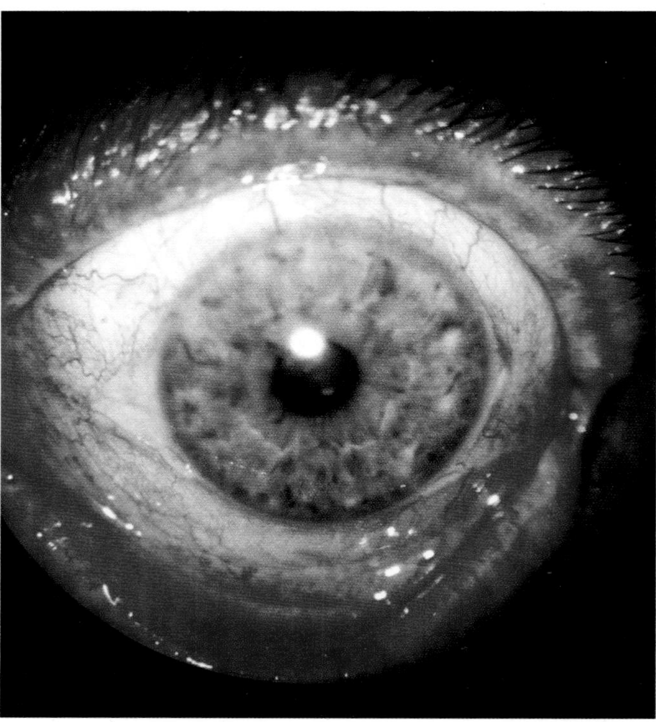

FIGURE 27-30. Lisch nodule in a patient with NF1. Pigmented areas are seen as brown areas in the iris.

Variants of NF1

In addition to classic NF1, there appear to be variant forms in which the features are atypical or incomplete. They include (1) *segmental NF* manifesting as neurofibromas in a segmental distribution caused by somatic mosaicism of NF1 mutations, (2) *gastrointestinal NF*, (3) *familial spinal NF*, and (4) *familial café au lait spots.*

Pathologic Findings

Several types of neurofibroma occur with this disease. They are distinguished on the basis of their gross and microscopic appearances.

Localized Neurofibroma

Localized neurofibroma is the most common type encountered, but it is histologically the least characteristic because identical lesions also occur on a sporadic basis. These tumors are typically located in the dermis and subcutis but may be located in deep soft tissue as well. The tumors are larger than solitary neurofibromas. Large pendulous tumors of the skin were referred to as *fibroma molluscum* in the early literature.

Histologically, these tumors are no different from solitary neurofibromas and embrace a spectrum from highly cellular to highly myxoid tumors. When malignant transformation occurs, it is usually in deeply situated lesions and is discussed later.

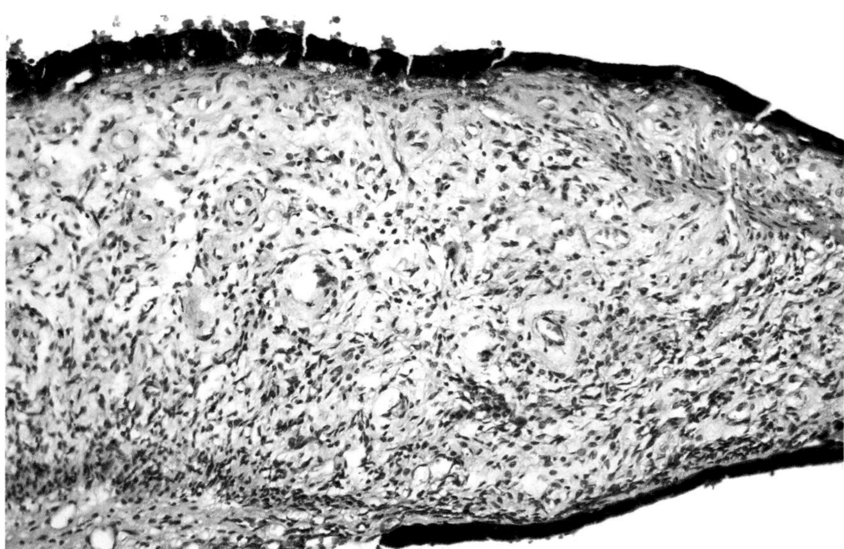

FIGURE 27-31. Lisch nodule showing collections of pigment in the iris.

Plexiform Neurofibroma

Plexiform neurofibroma is pathognomonic of this disease, provided that the definition of a plexiform neurofibroma is stringent (Figs. 27-32 to 27-35). Plexiform neurofibromas always develop during early childhood, often before the cutaneous neurofibromas have fully developed. Those plexiform neurofibromas involving an entire extremity give rise to the condition known as *elephantiasis neuromatosa*, in which the extremity is enlarged (Fig. 27-36). The overlying skin is loose, redundant, and hyperpigmented, and the

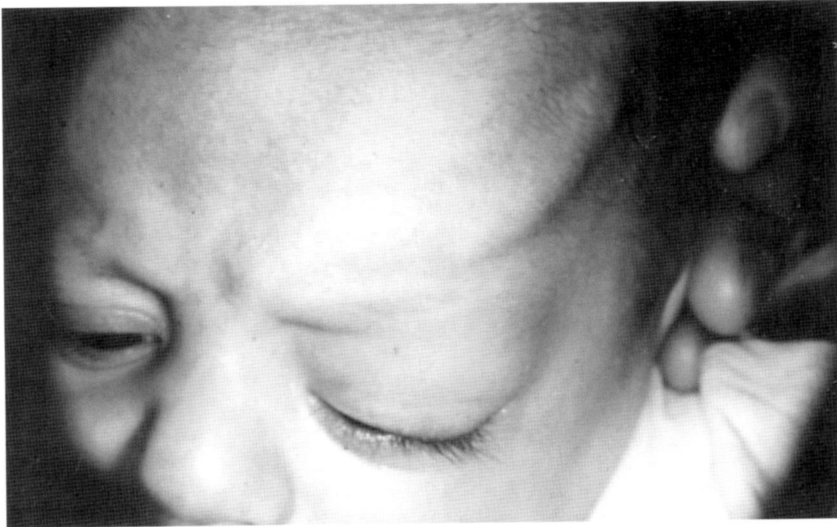

FIGURE 27-32. Plexiform neurofibroma in the subcutis of the scalp and involving the upper eyelid. Note the irregular, tortuous contour of the tumor. Lesions of this type are virtually pathognomonic of NF1.

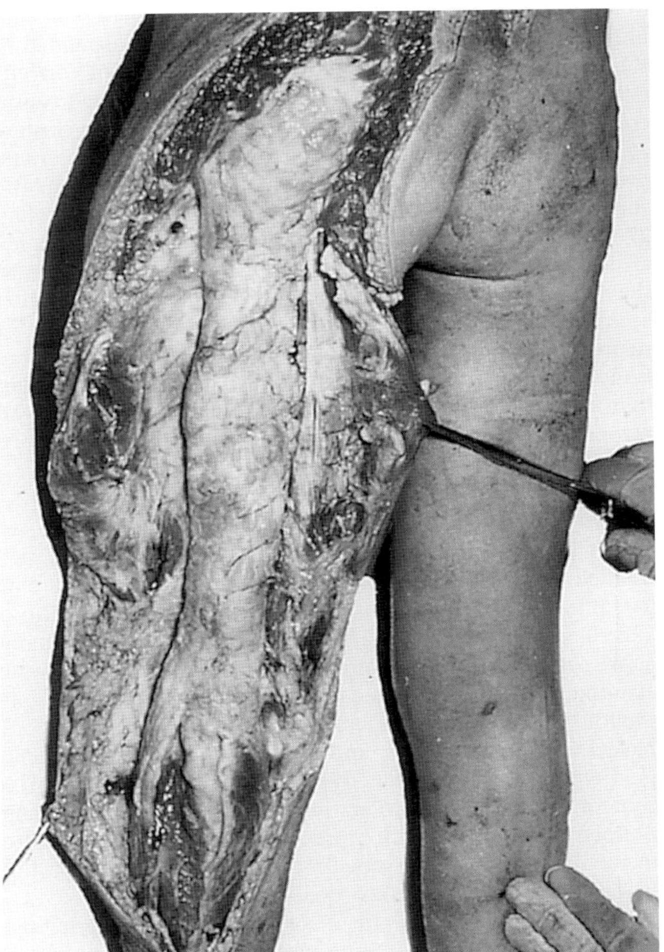

FIGURE 27-33. Plexiform neurofibroma of the lower extremity in a patient with NF1.

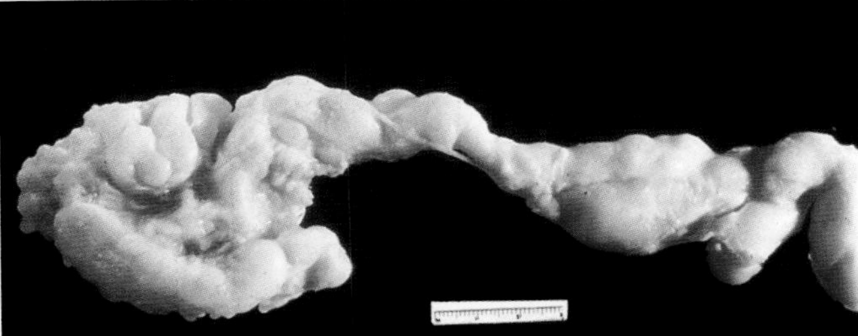

FIGURE 27-34. Gross appearance of a plexiform neurofibroma. The nerve is converted to a thick convoluted mass, which has been likened to a bag of worms.

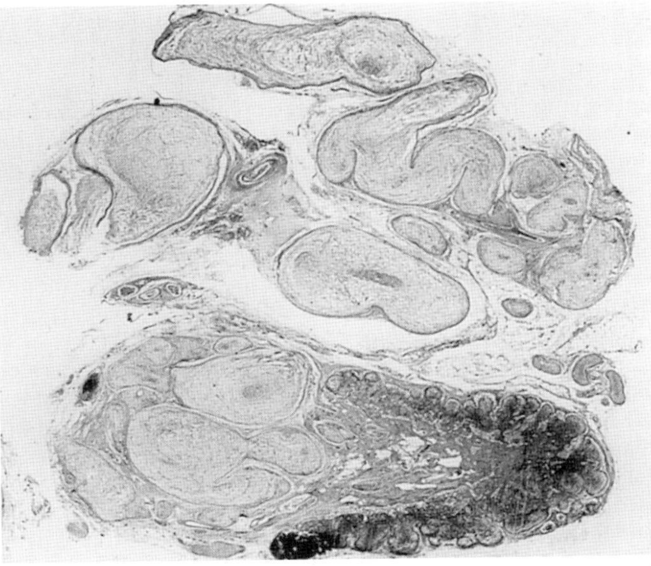

FIGURE 27-35. Plexiform neurofibroma involving nerve and extending into the hilum of a lymph node. Apparent lymph node involvement does not indicate malignancy but simply reflects the diffuseness of the process (x5).

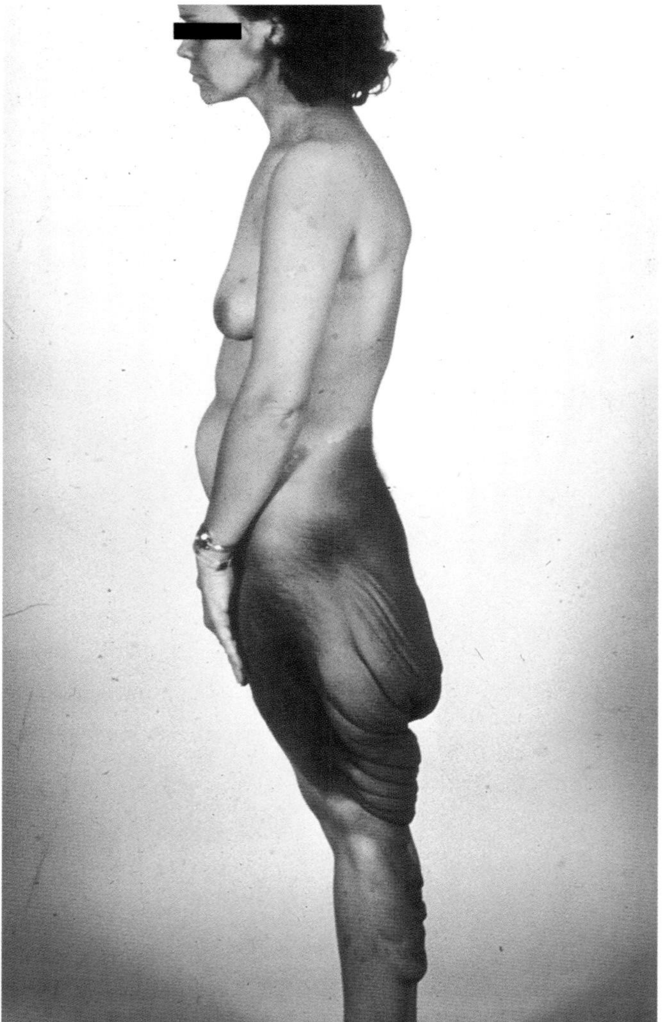

FIGURE 27-36. Patient with NF1 and a large neurofibroma of leg resulting in elephantiasis neuromatosa.

underlying bone may be hypertrophied, a phenomenon probably related to the increased vascular supply to the limb. Macroscopically, plexiform neurofibromas are large lesions that affect large segments of a nerve, distorting it and contorting it into a "bag of worms" (see Fig. 27-34). Smaller lesions, which simply have a plexiform pattern when viewed microscopically rather than macroscopically, should not be interpreted as plexiform neurofibromas for purposes of establishing the diagnosis of NF1.

Microscopically, the lesion consists of a tortuous mass of expanded nerve branches, which are seen cut in various planes of section (Figs. 27-37 to 27-39). In the early stages, the nerves may simply have an increase in the endoneurial matrix material, resulting in a wide separation of the small nerve fascicles (see Fig. 27-38). With continued growth, the cells spill out of the nerves into soft tissue, creating a diffuse backdrop of neurofibromatous tissue (see Fig. 27-39) so that NF1 lesions can have both plexiform and diffuse areas. Plexiform neurofibromas, like localized neurofibromas, may display nuclear atypia. Because these lesions are at greatest risk to undergo malignant transformation, care should be paid to lesions displaying heightened cellularity and atypia. The sequence of histologic changes and the inherent problems are discussed later.

Electron microscopy of these lesions has documented the participation of several cell types. The predominant cell is the Schwann cell, which is surrounded by basal lamina (Fig. 27-40). These cells may invest small axons, spiral around themselves, or lie singly in the matrix. A significant number of fibroblasts are also present, which are distinguished from Schwann cells by their prominent endoplasmic reticulum and their lack of basal lamina.

Diffuse Neurofibroma

Diffuse neurofibroma is an uncommon but distinctive form that occurs principally in children and young adults. A subset of patients with this lesion also has neurofibromatosis.

Clinically, this tumor is most common in the head and neck region and presents as a plaque-like elevation of the skin. On a cut section, the entire subcutis between superficial fascia and dermis is thickened by firm, grayish tissue (Fig. 27-41). As its name implies, this form of neurofibroma is ill-defined and spreads extensively along connective tissue septa and between fat cells. Despite its infiltrative growth, it does not destroy but, rather, envelops the normal structures that it encompasses in much the same fashion as dermatofibrosarcoma protuberans (Fig. 27-42). It differs from the conventional neurofibroma in that it has a uniform matrix of fine fibrillary collagen. The Schwann cells, which lie suspended in the matrix, are usually less elongated than those of conventional neurofibromas and have short fusiform or even round contours (Figs. 27-43 and 27-44). The tumor contains clusters of pseudomeissnerian body-like structures, a characteristic feature of this lesion that serves to distinguish it from the superficial aspect of dermatofibrosarcoma protuberans (Fig. 27-45). Some diffuse neurofibromas consist of a rather complex arrangement of several mesenchymal elements in addition to the neurofibromatous tissue (Fig. 27-46). These tumors, which seem to be more common in neurofibromatosis, consist of neurofibromatous tissue admixed with mature fat or large ectatic vessels. The latter structures, at times, are so striking that they eclipse the neural component and can result in the erroneous impression of exuberant granulation tissue. Rarely, nuclear palisading is present in diffuse neurofibromas.

Pigmented Neurofibroma

About 1% of all neurofibromas contain melanin-bearing pigmented cells.[53,54] Most occur in patients with NF1 and are of the diffuse type, although some have features of both diffuse and plexiform types (Fig. 27-47). The pigment is not usually appreciated on gross examination and requires histologic examination. The pigmented cells, which are dendritic or epithelioid in shape, are dispersed throughout the tumors but have a tendency to cluster and localize toward the superficial portions of the lesion (Fig. 27-48). They express both S-100 protein and melanin markers in contrast to the surrounding nonpigmented cells, which express S-100 protein only. Because of the diffuse pattern of growth, these lesions may recur, but metastasis has not been recorded.

These lesions should be distinguished from pigmented forms of dermatofibrosarcoma protuberans (Bednar tumor), a tumor that in the past was sometimes referred to as a

Text continued on p. 809

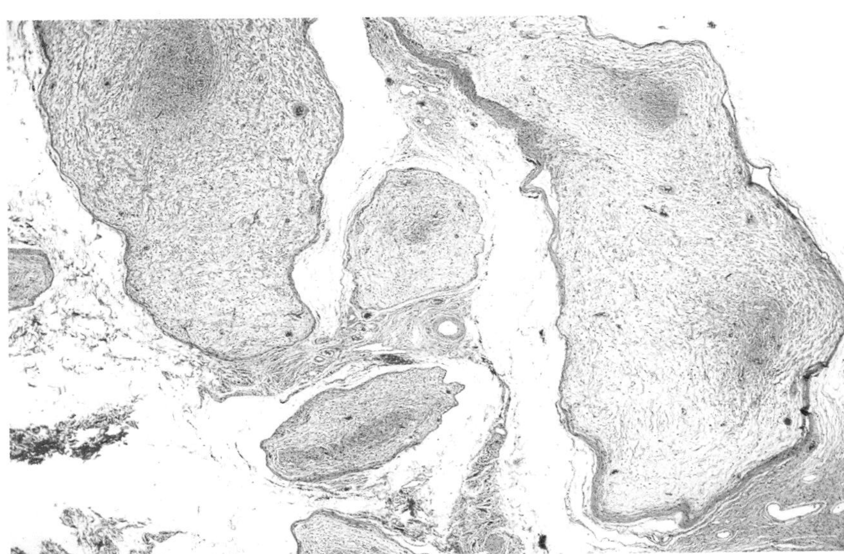

FIGURE 27-37. Plexiform neurofibroma with tortuous enlargement of the nerves.

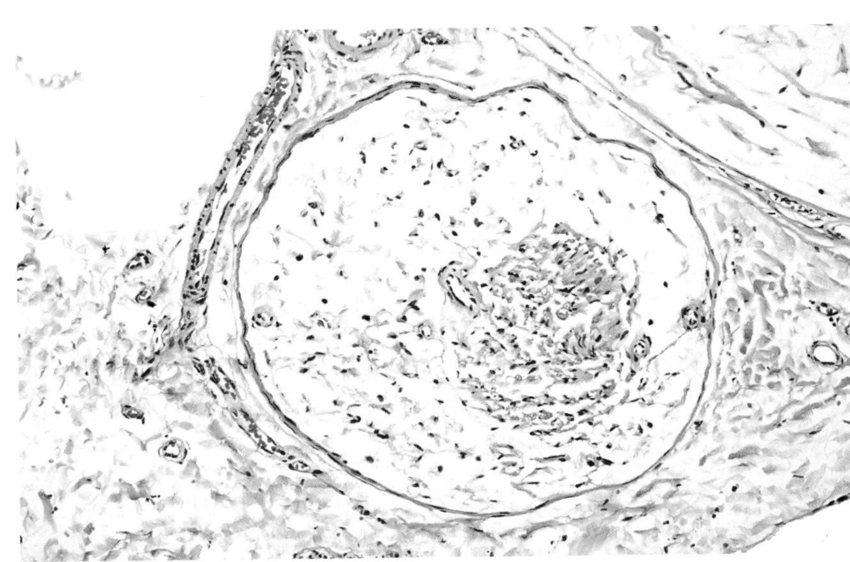

FIGURE 27-38. Plexiform neurofibroma with expansion of the endoneurium by myxoid ground substance.

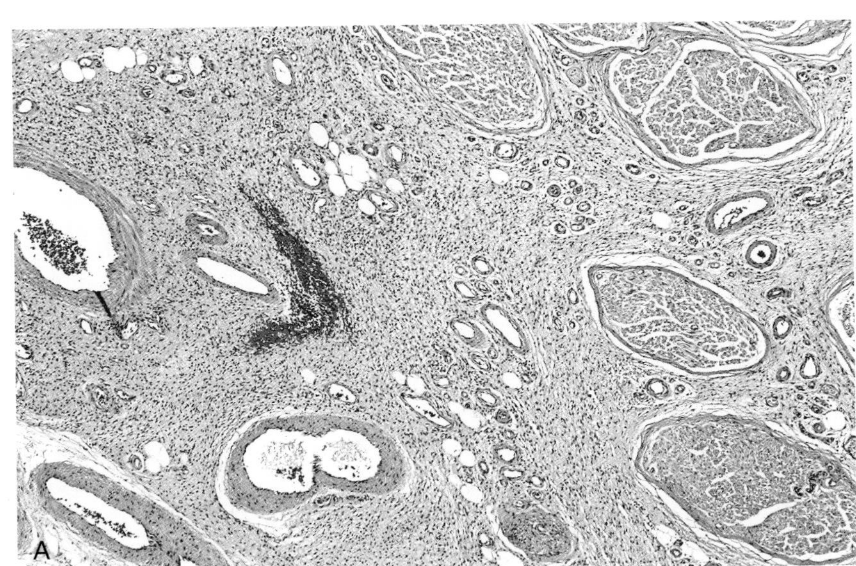

FIGURE 27-39. (A, B) Portion of a plexiform neurofibroma illustrating the lesion spilling out into soft tissue. These areas may resemble areas of diffuse neurofibroma. *Continued*

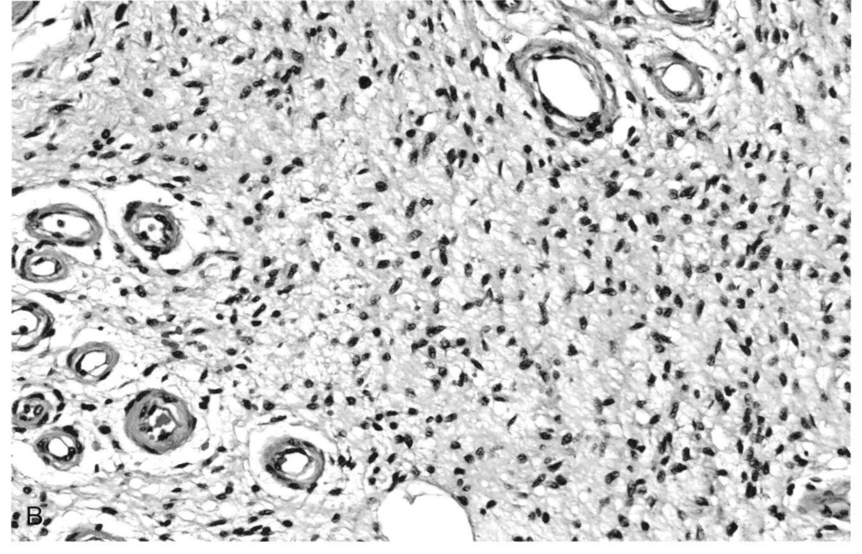

Figure 27-39, cont'd

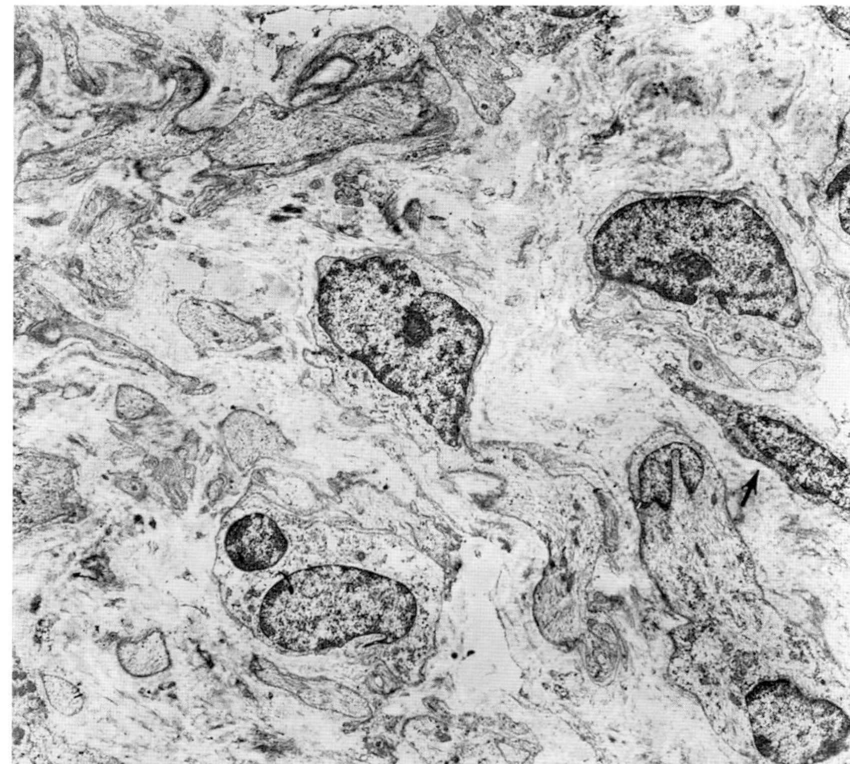

Figure 27-40. Electron micrograph of a neurofibroma with predominantly Schwann cells and occasional fibroblasts (arrow) (x5775).

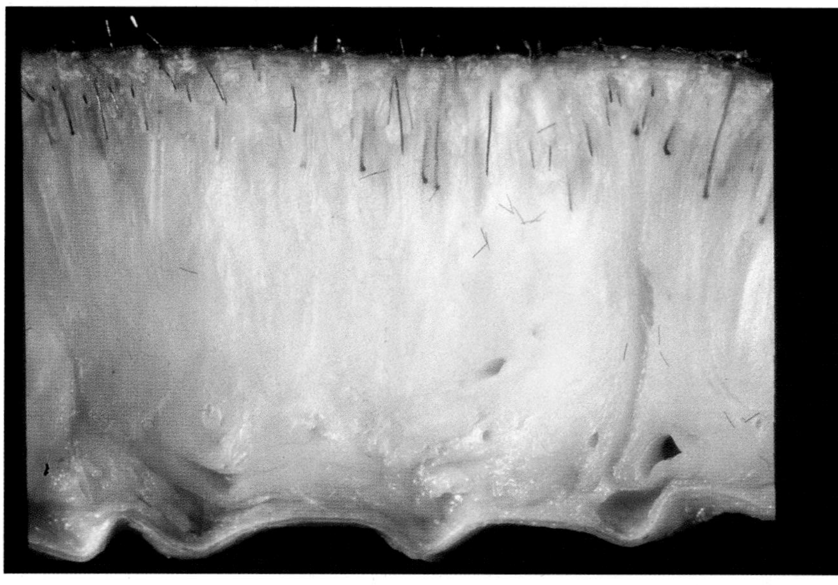

Figure 27-41. Diffuse neurofibroma presenting as an ill-defined expansion of the subcutaneous region of the scalp.

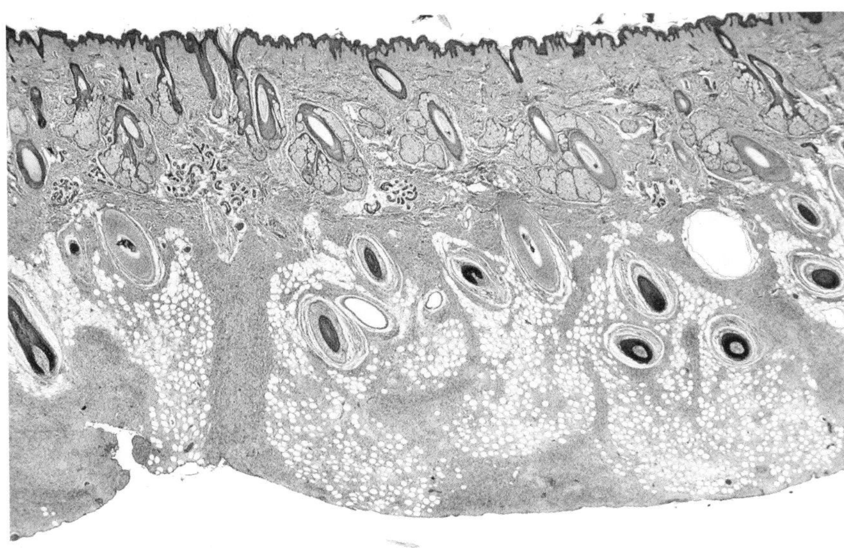

FIGURE 27-42. Diffuse neurofibroma with extensive permeation of subcutaneous tissue similar to a dermatofibrosarcoma protuberans.

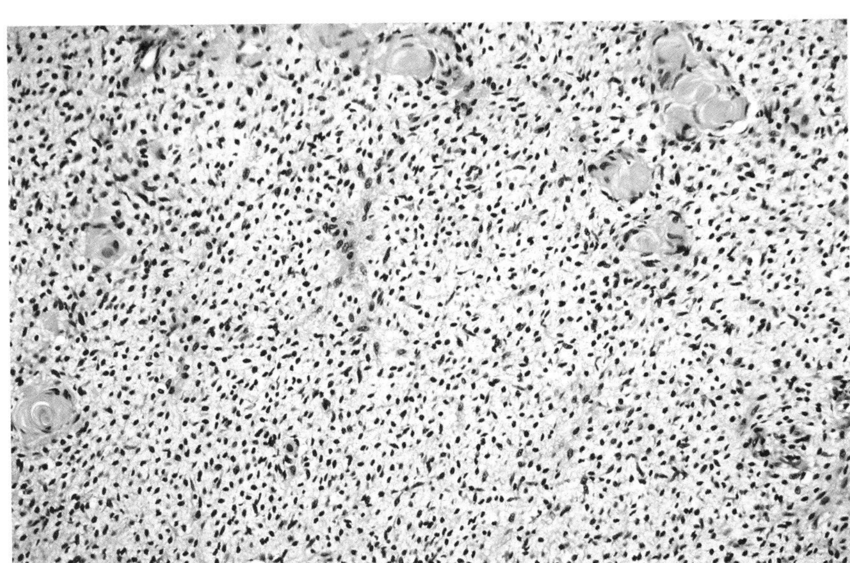

FIGURE 27-43. Diffuse neurofibroma showing the fine fibrillary collagenous background punctuated with pseudomeissnerian bodies.

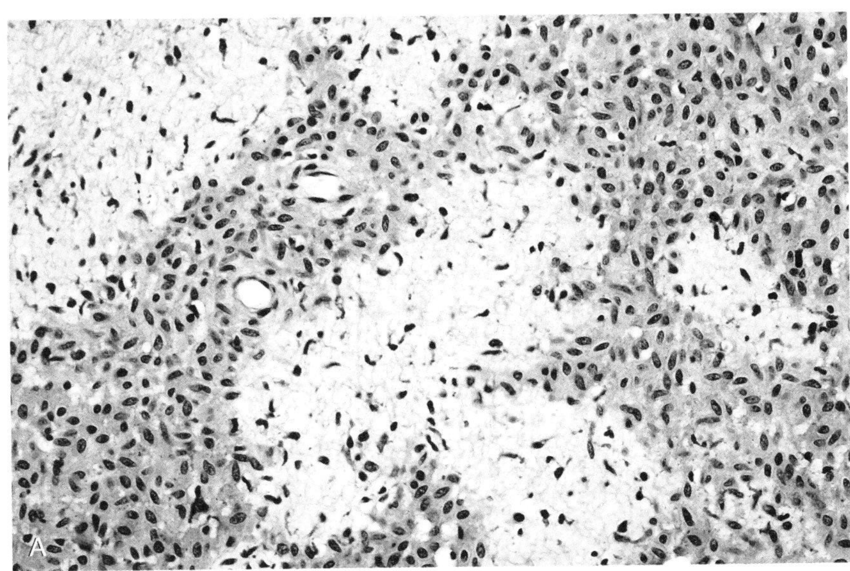

FIGURE 27-44 Diffuse neurofibroma with characteristic short fusiform or rounded Schwann cells. Shown at medium (A) and high power (B).

Continued

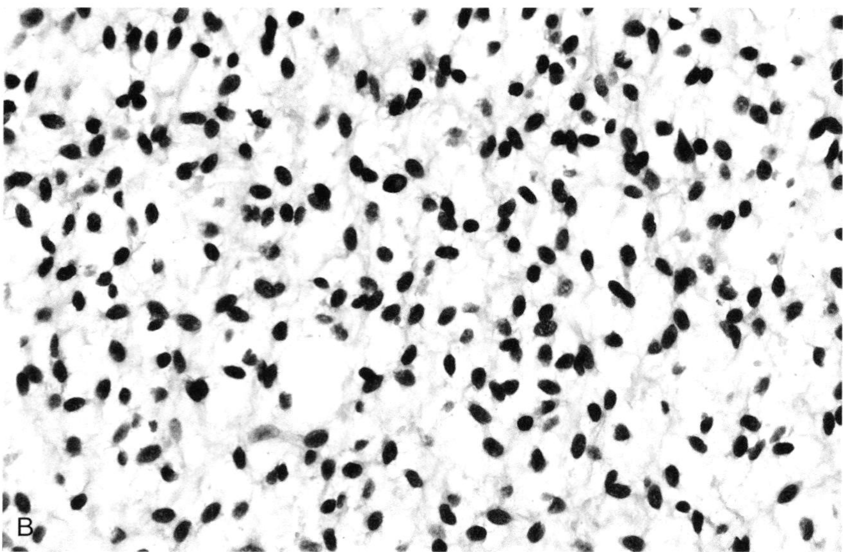

FIGURE 27-44, cont'd

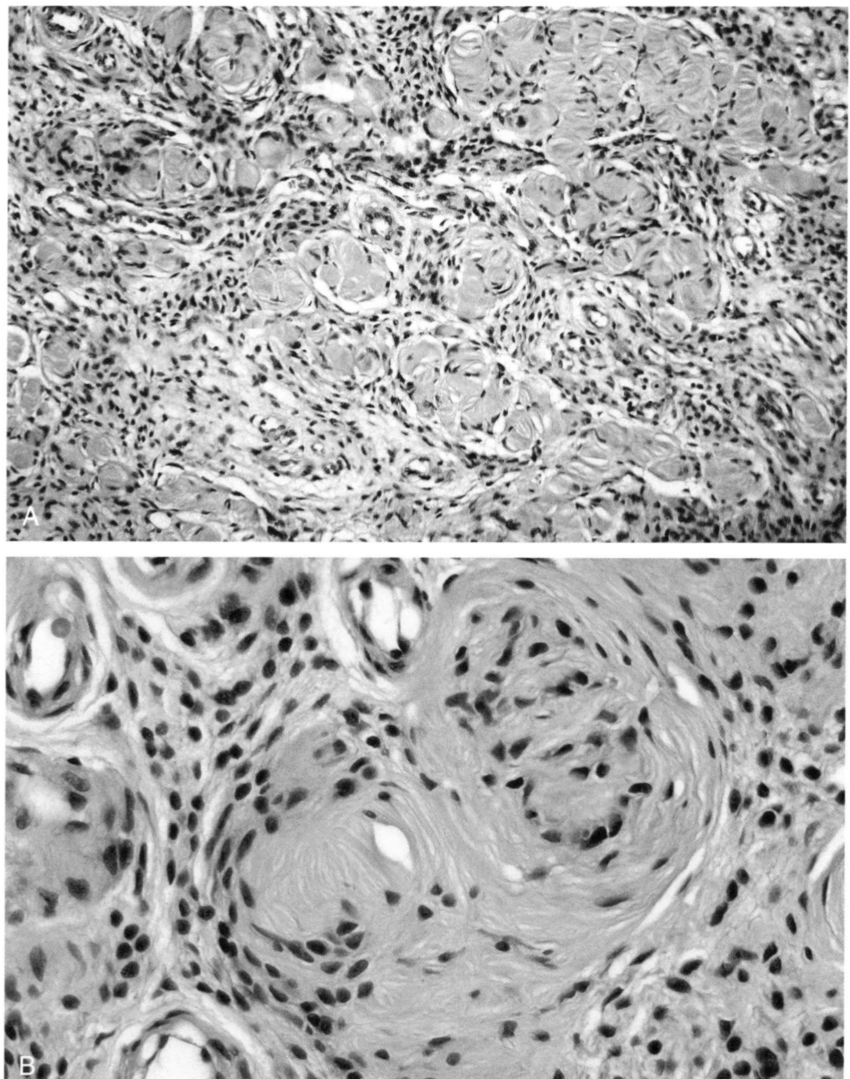

FIGURE 27-45. Pseudomeissnerian bodies in a diffuse neurofibroma at medium (A) and high (B) power.

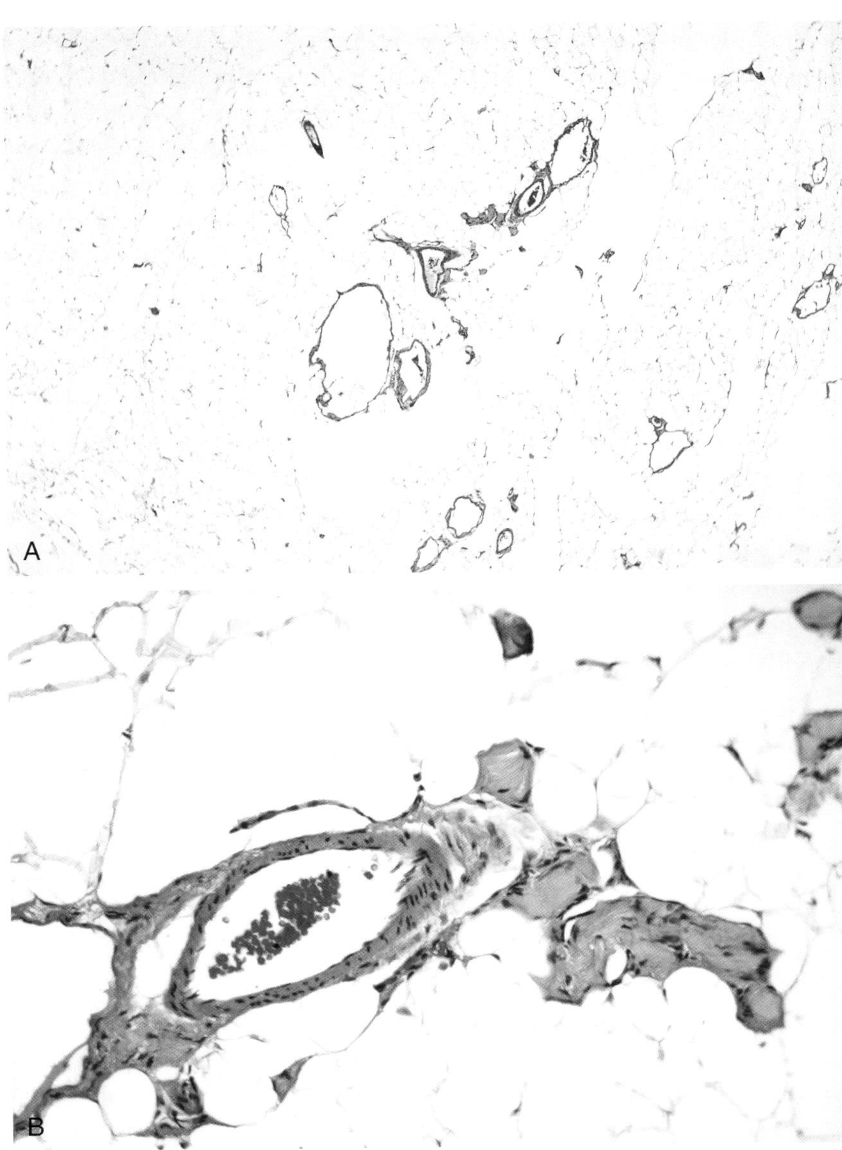

FIGURE 27-46. (A) Diffuse neurofibroma with extensive fatty overgrowth. (B) Pseudomeissnerian bodies in the fat identify the neural nature of the lesion.

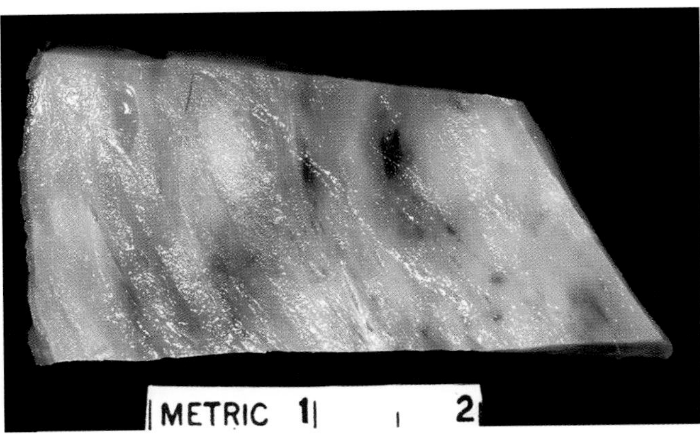

FIGURE 27-47. Pigmented neurofibroma developing in a neurofibroma of the diffuse type.

storiform pigmented neurofibroma. The uniform fibroblastic cells, repetitive storiform pattern, and lack of S-100 protein immunoreactivity usually make this distinction apparent. The distinction between congenital pigmented nevi with neuroid features and pigmented neurofibroma is less clear-cut. The lack of a junctional or superficial nevoid component supports the diagnosis of a pigmented neurofibroma over that of a congenital neuroid nevus.

Malignant Change in Neurofibromas

In a subset of NF1 patients, an MPNST emerges from a preexisting neurofibroma, typically a deep-seated plexiform lesion (Figs. 27-49 and 27-50). The histologic demarcation between a neurofibroma with atypical histologic features and a low-grade MPNST is difficult because, in effect, these lesions represent a histologic continuum (Figs. 27-51 to 27-54). Furthermore, in neurofibromas that have undergone malignant

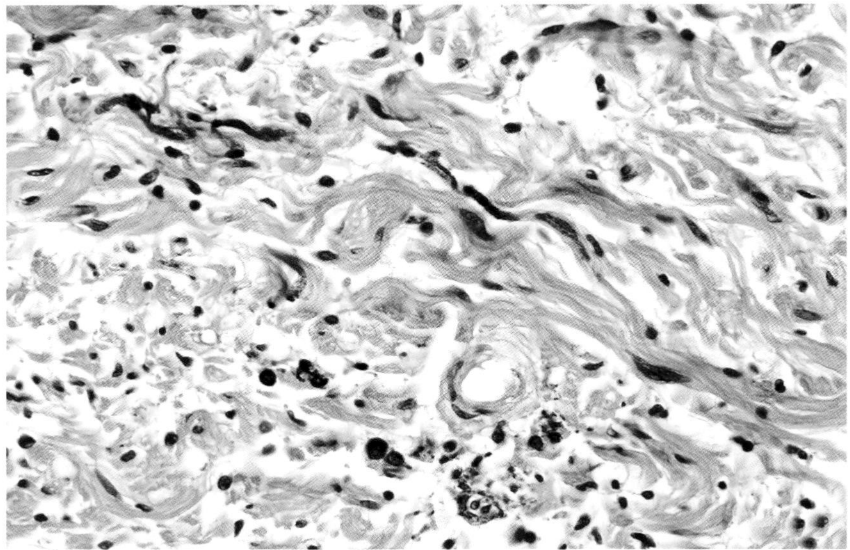

FIGURE 27-48. Pigmented neurofibroma. Melanin pigment is present in irregularly shaped Schwann cells.

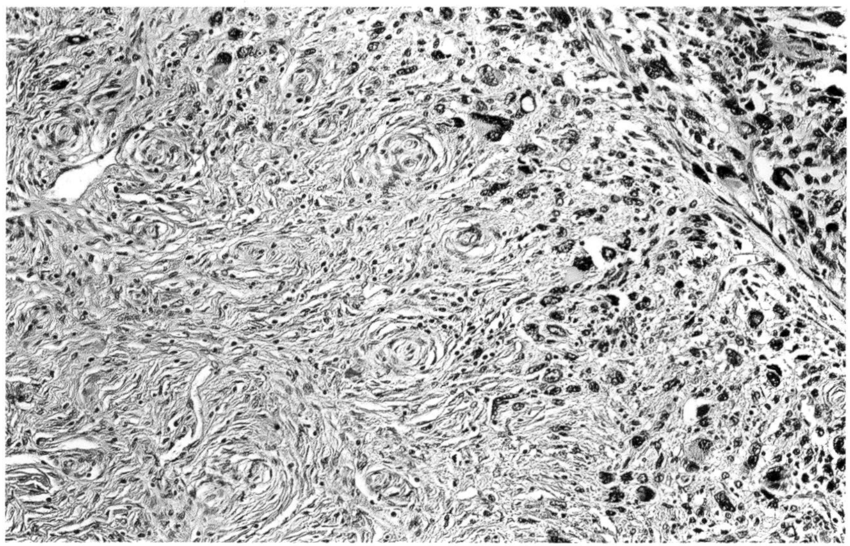

FIGURE 27-49. Neurofibroma with malignant transformation (right).

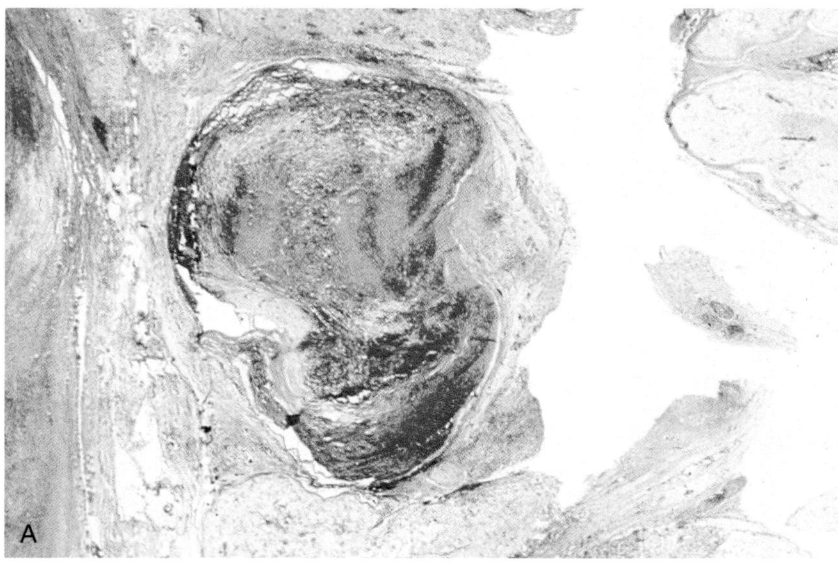

FIGURE 27-50. (A) Plexiform neurofibroma with an area of angiosarcoma (hemorrhagic zone). The tumor was an epithelioid angiosarcoma.

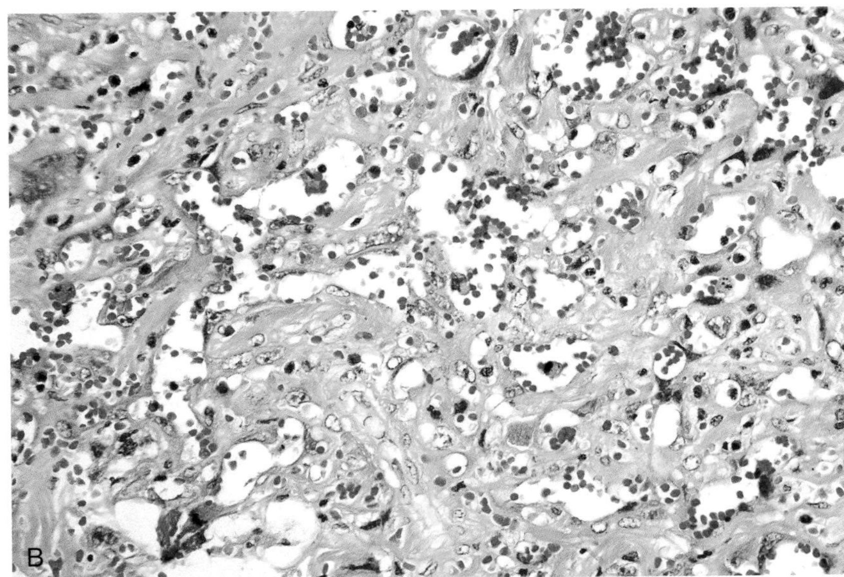

FIGURE 27-50, cont'd (B) This pattern of malignant transformation is rare and is discussed in Chapter 28.

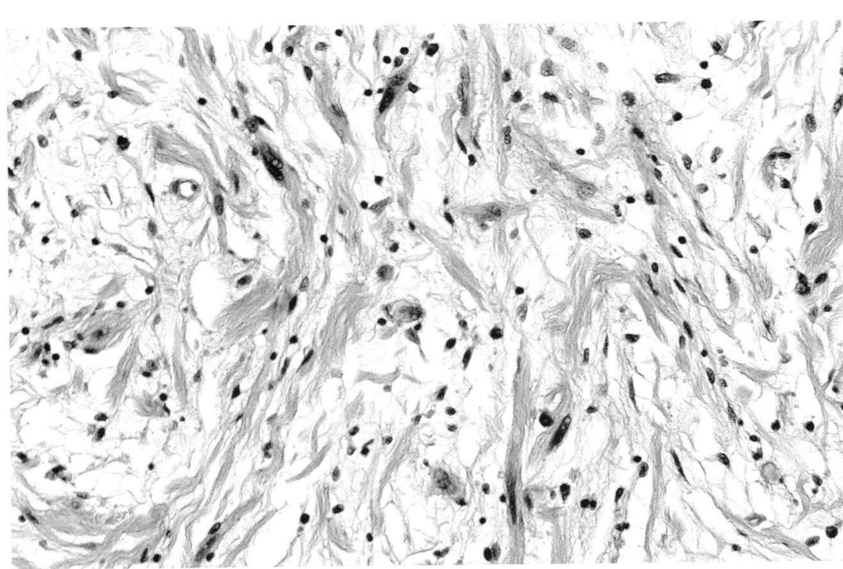

FIGURE 27-51. Neurofibroma with nuclear atypia of occasional cells without increased cellularity or mitotic activity.

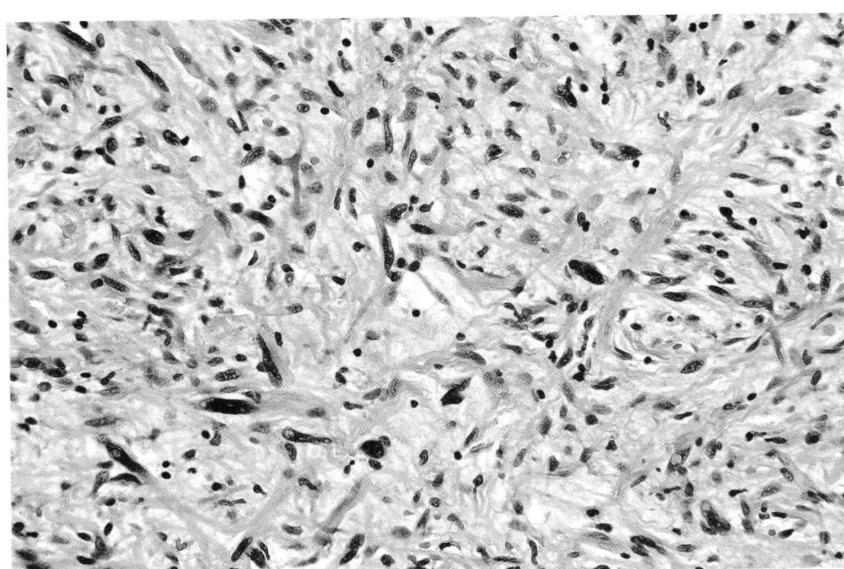

FIGURE 27-52. Neurofibroma with moderate cellularity and nuclear atypia. The designation neurofibroma with atypical features is used for changes of this type. This change was adjacent to areas of frank sarcoma.

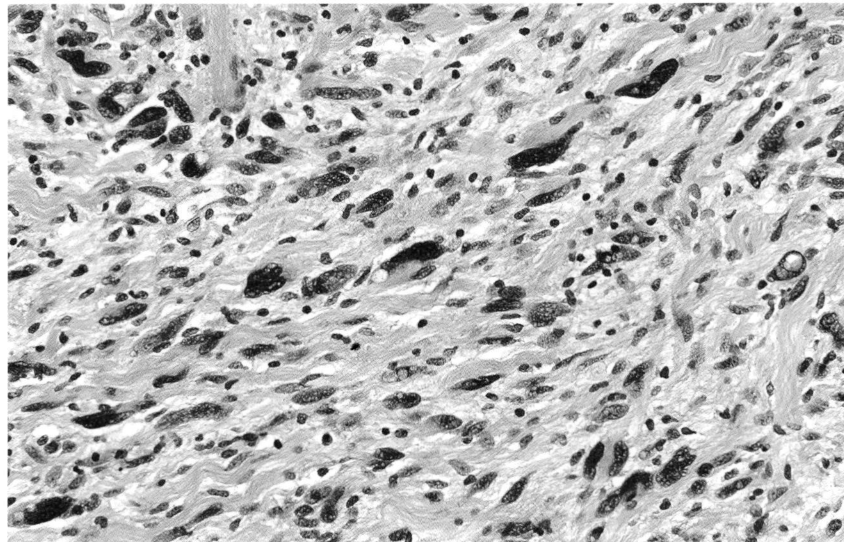

FIGURE 27-53. Low-grade malignant peripheral nerve sheath tumor arising in a neurofibroma. This neurofibromatous lesion is characterized by marked cellularity so that cells are nearly back-to-back. The nuclear atypia is marked and generalized.

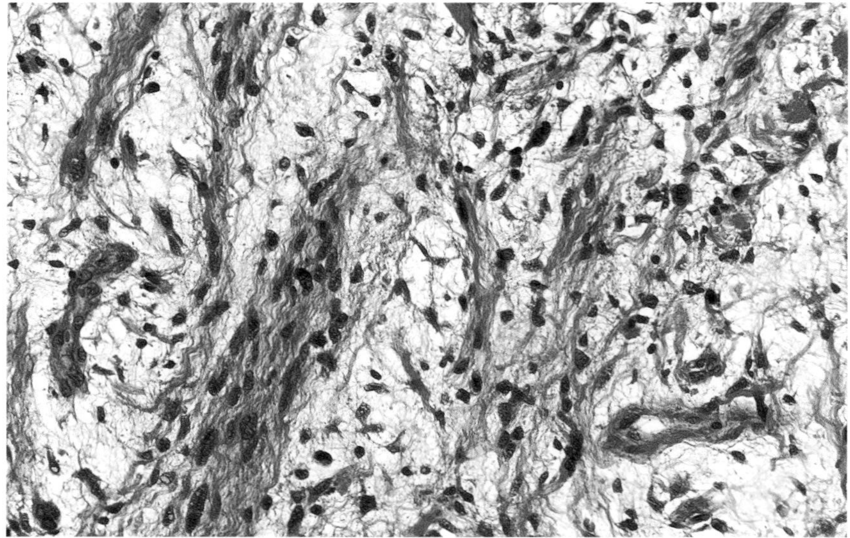

FIGURE 27-54. Low-grade malignant peripheral nerve sheath tumor arising in a neurofibroma. There is generalized marked atypia and increased cellularity so that the cells appear arranged in small fascicles. Low levels of mitotic activity were identified in the lesion.

transformation, it is commonplace to have neurofibroma with a range of atypical features adjacent to areas of frank MPNST. To date, there has been no large study correlating the number and degree of atypical features in neurofibromas with either outcome or with molecular alterations. Because the progression to MPNST is associated with additional mutational events (see later section), immunohistochemistry to detect loss of tumor suppressor gene proteins may prove to be helpful in the future. Immunohistochemistry for p16 can be demonstrated in neurofibromas but is lacking in MPNST. However, there is not yet sufficient information to recommend its routine use in diagnosis, which remains principally a light microscopic diagnosis.

A small study with short-term follow-up by Lin et al.[55] suggested that cellularity, atypia, and low levels of mitotic activity were still associated with good outcome. Similar findings were reported by others.[56] Some believe the presence of mitotic figures in an otherwise innocuous neurofibroma is insufficient for a diagnosis of malignancy,[57] but it should be pointed out that mitotic activity and cellularity seem to covary; it is unusual to encounter a mitotically active neurofibroma without some increase in cellularity. The following paragraphs represent a general approach to this problem. In the final analysis, although labels are convenient, borderline neurofibromatous lesions require careful sampling, dialogue with the clinician, and potentially complete removal, depending on the clinical setting.

Neurofibroma is used for conventional neurofibromas, including those with nuclear atypia only (see Fig. 27-51). The latter, as an isolated focal or diffuse change, is common in neurofibromas and does not correlate with malignancy. Although some use the term *atypical neurofibroma* for these lesions, it is preferred not to use a term that could be misconstrued as reflecting concern about malignancy.

Neurofibroma with atypical features is the term used for neurofibromas that have any combination of atypical features (cellularity, atypia, mitotic activity) that fall short of the minimum criteria for a diagnosis of low-grade MPNST (see

Fig. 27-52). This category excludes lesions characterized by nuclear atypia only, as described previously.

Low-grade MPNST arising in neurofibroma is diagnosed when there is generalized nuclear atypia, diffuse cellularity, and usually low levels of mitotic activity (see Figs. 27-53 and 27-54). Nuclear atypia consists of nuclear enlargement and hyperchromatism. Some require that nuclear enlargement should be at least three times the size of a normal Schwann cell nucleus.[57] If mitotic activity is not present, a low-grade MPNST is diagnosed if the cellularity and atypia are marked and the haphazard architectural pattern gives way to one that is fascicular.

Discussion

Unlike solitary neurofibromas, those encountered in neurofibromatosis cause significant morbidity. The large number of lesions usually makes surgical therapy impossible. Therefore, surgery has traditionally been reserved for lesions that are large, painful, or located in strategic areas where continued expansion would compromise organ function. Even after attempted complete excision of these lesions, clinical recurrences occasionally develop, a phenomenon related to the ill-defined nature of the tumors. Targeted therapies, therefore, may prove to be extremely important. Treatment of plexiform neurofibromas with cis-retinoic acid, a maturational agent, and interferon-alpha, an antiangiogenic factor, have shown growth stabilization in a majority of patients.[58] Some patients have also responded to thalidomide, known to have antiangiogenic properties.[59]

A problem of greater importance is that of malignant transformation. The exact incidence is difficult to determine and has been estimated at 2% to 29% of patients with the disease[44,50,60] but seems dependent on the severity of the disease among the population studied. A large follow-up study of a nationwide cohort of 212 Danish patients with neurofibromatosis found 9 sarcomas and 16 gliomas but noted the tumors occurred in the proband group (84 patients), who, by definition, required hospitalization and were probably more severely affected by the disorder.[61] The authors suggest that the natural history of neurofibromatosis may be more accurately reflected by the largest group of patients, relatives of the probands (128 patients) who did not require hospitalization and whose prognosis may have been better than previously thought. Both groups, however, had decreased survival rate after 40 years when compared with the general population. A more recent study by Evans et al.[62] documented an 8% to 13% lifetime risk for MPNST, and de Raedt et al.[63] identified an association between large genomic deletions and malignancy in NF1 patients. The latter suggests that certain mutations may be more closely linked to the risk for malignant transformation.[64] In general, patients with NF1 and MPNST have had the disease for many years and present with rapid enlargement or pain in a preexisting neurofibroma.[65] Both symptoms, especially the former, should always lead to biopsy. Unfortunately, the prognosis is poor for patients developing an MPNST in this setting (see Chapter 28).

With the identification of the NF1 gene in 1990, it has become possible to examine the molecular events underlying tumorigenesis in this disease. Because conventional mice knockout models in which *NF1* is completely inactivated ($NF1^{-/-}$) prove lethal in utero, conditional mice knockout models in which Schwann cell-specific *NF1* is inactivated have been used.[49,66] In this system, Zhu et al.[67] have shown that Schwann cell-specific knockout mice ($NF1^{-/-}$) develop Schwann cell hyperplasias but rarely neurofibromas, whereas Schwann cell-specific knockout mice having one mutant and one wild type allele ($NF1^{+/-}$) readily develop plexiform neurofibromas containing $NF1^{+/-}$ mast cells. These observations have led to the hypothesis that neurofibromin-deficient Schwann cells ($NF1^{-/-}$) require other haploinsufficient ($NF1^{+/-}$) (e.g., mast cells, fibroblasts) cells in the microenvironment for tumorigenesis.[67,68] Progression of neurofibromas to MPNST requires additional mutational events involving mitogenic and cell cycle regulatory pathways. Mutations in *p53*, *INK4* ($p16^{INK4a}$ and $p14^{ARF}$ genes),[69-72] $p27^{kip1}$,[70] and amplification of *EGFR* have been reported in MPNSTs and suggest a synergistic effect with *NF*.

SCHWANNOMA

Schwannoma is an encapsulated nerve sheath tumor consisting of two components: a highly ordered cellular component (Antoni A area) and a loose myxoid component (Antoni B area). The presence of encapsulation and the two types of Antoni areas plus uniformly intense immunostaining for S-100 protein distinguish schwannoma from neurofibroma.

Clinical Findings

Schwannomas occur at all ages but are most common in persons between the ages of 20 and 50 years. They affect the genders in roughly equal numbers. The tumors have a predilection for the head, neck, and flexor surfaces of the upper and lower extremities. Consequently, the spinal roots and the cervical, sympathetic, vagus, peroneal, and ulnar nerves are most commonly affected. Deeply situated tumors predominate in the posterior mediastinum and the retroperitoneum. Schwannomas are usually solitary sporadic lesions. In a population-based study of schwannomas, about 90% were sporadic, 3% occurred in patients with NF2, 2% in those with schwannomatosis, and 5% in association with multiple meningiomas in patients with or without NF2.[73] Rarely, schwannomas occur as part of NF1. About 60% of sporadic and NF2-associated schwannomas have inactivating mutations of the *NF2* gene. These events are small frameshift mutations that occur throughout the coding sequence and predict a truncated product. Usually these mutations are accompanied by inactivation of the remaining wild type allele on 22q. In about one-third of tumors, there is a loss of 22q without detectable mutations, and the remaining tumors seem to have no detectable *NF2* alteration. Nevertheless, all schwannomas, whether sporadic or syndromic, lack the protein product, merlin.[74] This suggests that schwannomas with apparent intact *NF2* gene either have undetectable mutations or epigenetic modification of the gene.[75]

Schwannoma is a slowly growing tumor that is usually present several years before diagnosis. When it involves small nerves, it is freely movable except for a single point of attachment. In large nerves, the tumor is movable except along the long axis of the nerve where the attachment restricts mobility.

Pain and neurologic symptoms are uncommon unless the tumor becomes large. In some instances, the patient is vaguely aware that the tumor waxes and wanes in size,[76] a phenomenon that might be related to fluctuations in the amount of cystic change in the lesion. Of particular significance is the posterior mediastinal schwannoma, which often originates from or extends into the vertebral canal. Such lesions, termed *dumbbell tumors*, pose difficult management problems because patients may develop profound neurologic difficulties.

Gross Findings

Because these tumors arise in nerve sheaths, they are surrounded by a true capsule consisting of the epineurium. Depending on the size of the involved nerve, the appearance of the tumor varies. Tumors of small nerves may resemble neurofibromas by virtue of their fusiform shape, and they often eclipse or obliterate the nerve of origin. In large nerves, the tumors present as eccentric masses over which the nerve fibers are splayed.

On a cut section, these tumors have a pink, white, or yellow appearance and usually measure less than 5 cm (Figs. 27-55 and 27-56). Tumors in the retroperitoneum and mediastinum

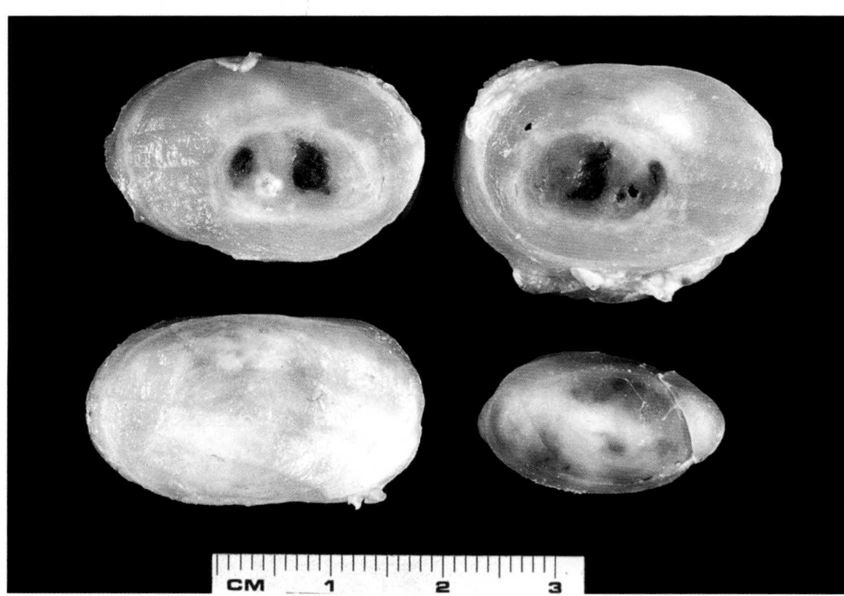

FIGURE 27-55. Multiple transverse sections through a schwannoma. Tumors are well circumscribed and commonly display foci of hemorrhage and cyst formation.

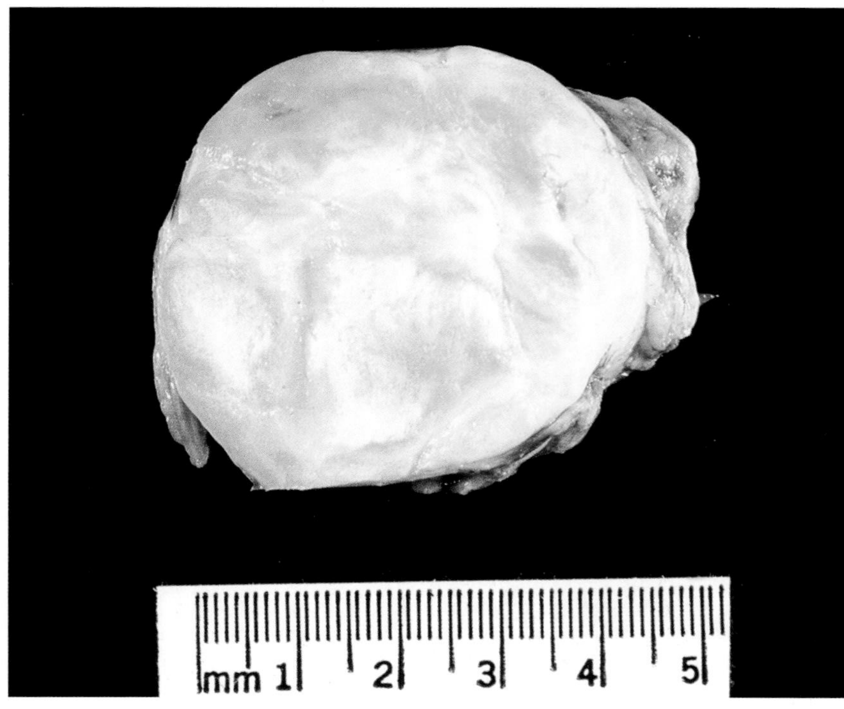

FIGURE 27-56. Mottled yellow-white appearance of a presacral schwannoma.

are considerably larger. As a result, these tumors are more likely to manifest secondary degenerative changes such as cystification and calcification (see later discussion of the ancient schwannoma).

Microscopic Findings

Most schwannomas are uninodular masses surrounded by a fibrous capsule consisting of epineurium and residual nerve fibers (Fig. 27-57). Neurites are generally not demonstrable in the substance of the tumor. In rare cases, the schwannoma arises intradermally or, as mentioned previously, manifests as a plexiform or multinodular growth similar to a plexiform neurofibroma.

The hallmark of a schwannoma is the pattern of alternating Antoni A and B areas (Figs. 27-58 to 27-59). The relative amounts of these two components vary, and they may blend imperceptibly or change abruptly. Antoni A areas are composed of compact spindle cells that usually have twisted nuclei, indistinct cytoplasmic borders, and, occasionally, clear intranuclear vacuoles. They are arranged in short bundles or interlacing fascicles (see Figs. 27-59 to 27-61). In highly differentiated Antoni A areas, there may be nuclear palisading, whorling of the cells (similar to meningioma), and Verocay bodies, formed by two compact rows of well-aligned nuclei separated by fibrillary cell processes (see Fig. 27-59). Mitotic figures are occasionally present but can usually be dismissed if the lesion otherwise has all the hallmarks of schwannoma. Antoni B areas are far less orderly and less cellular. The spindle or oval cells are arranged haphazardly in the loosely textured matrix, which is punctuated by microcystic change, inflammatory cells, and delicate collagen fibers (see Figs. 27-62 to 27-65). The large, irregularly spaced vessels, which are characteristic of schwannomas, become most conspicuous in the

Text continued on p. 820

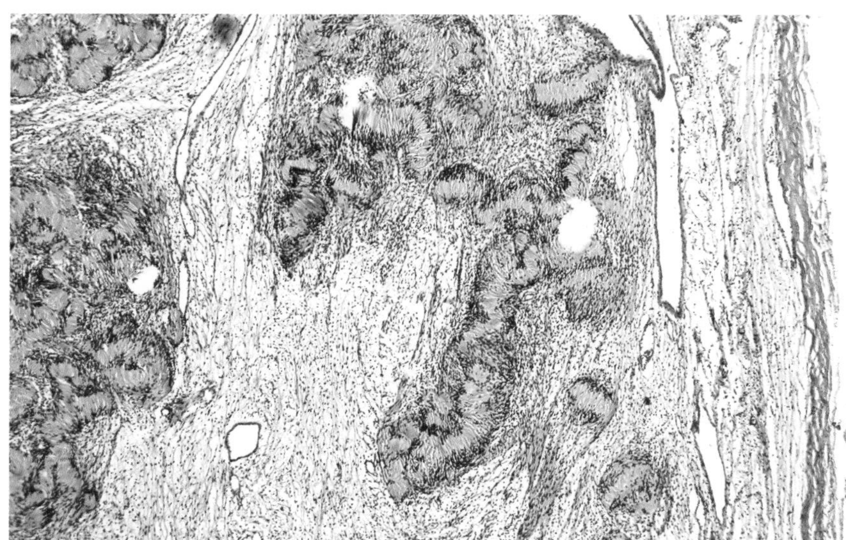

FIGURE 27-57. Schwannoma with a discrete, confining capsule.

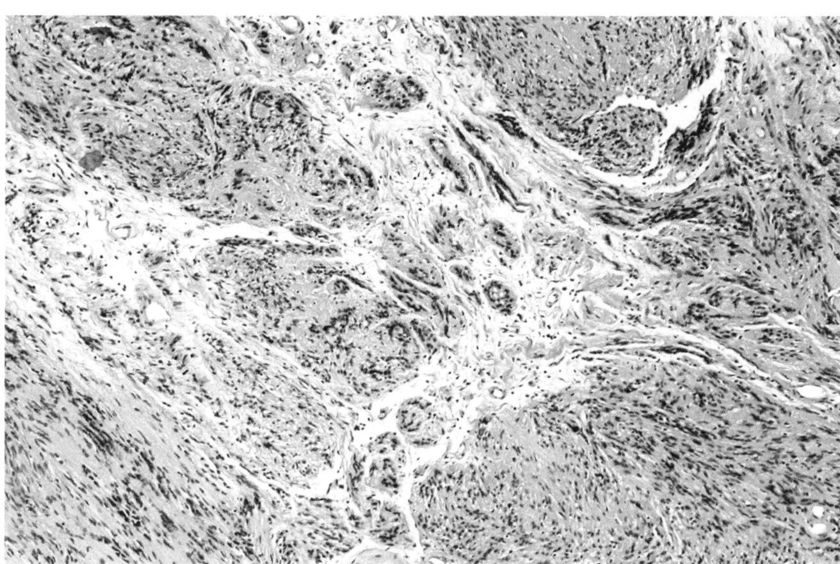

FIGURE 27-58. Schwannoma with alternating Antoni A and B areas.

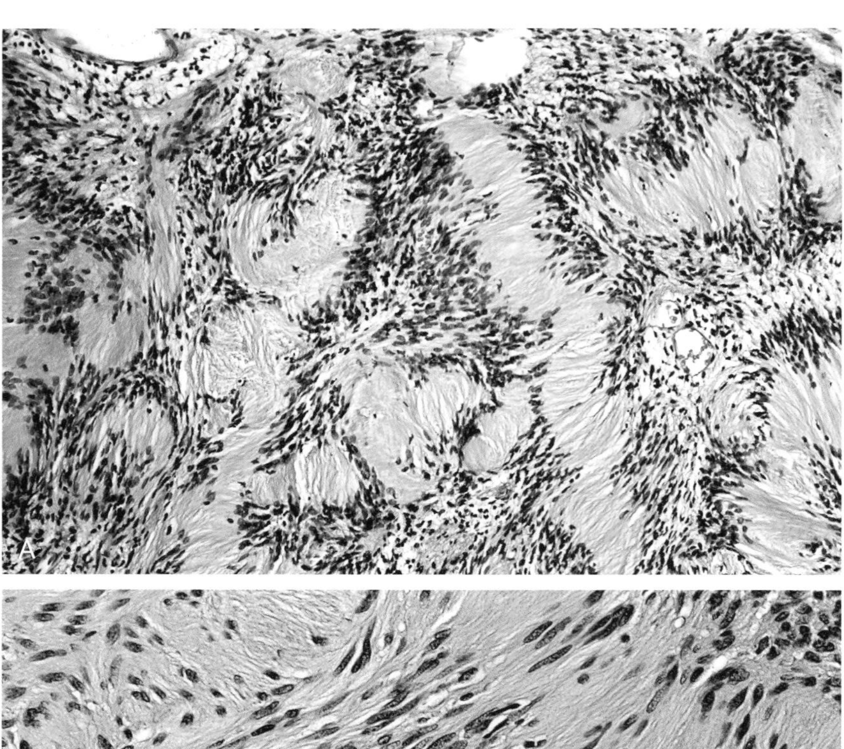

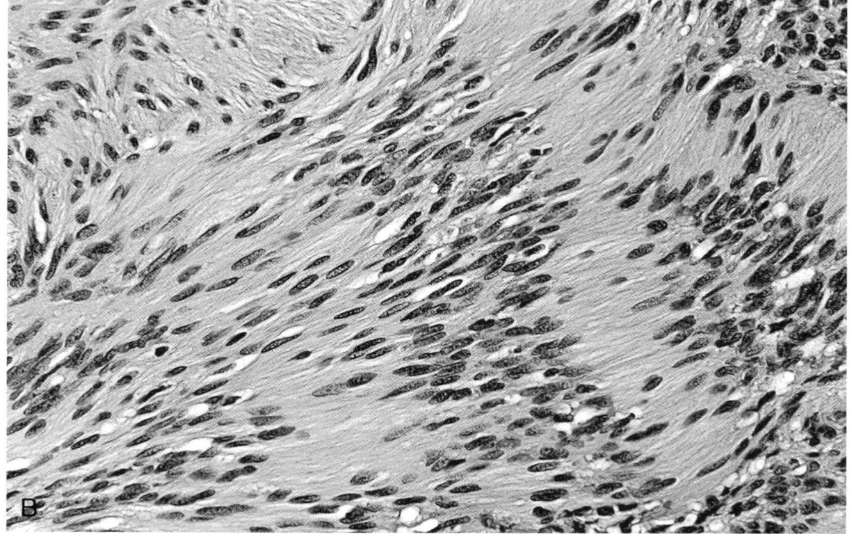

FIGURE 27-59. (A) Antoni A areas illustrating nuclear palisading with Verocay bodies. (B) High-power view shows nuclear palisading.

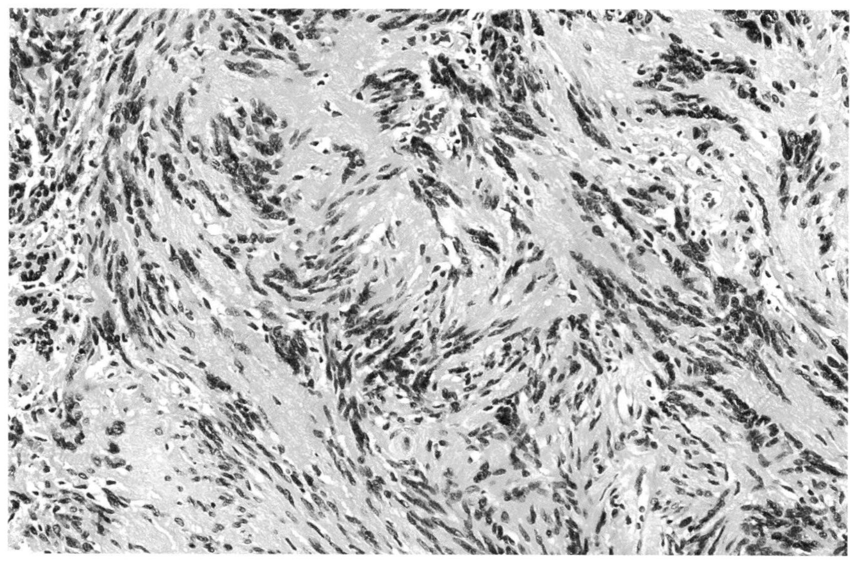

FIGURE 27-60. Antoni A areas with short fascicles and focal nuclear palisading.

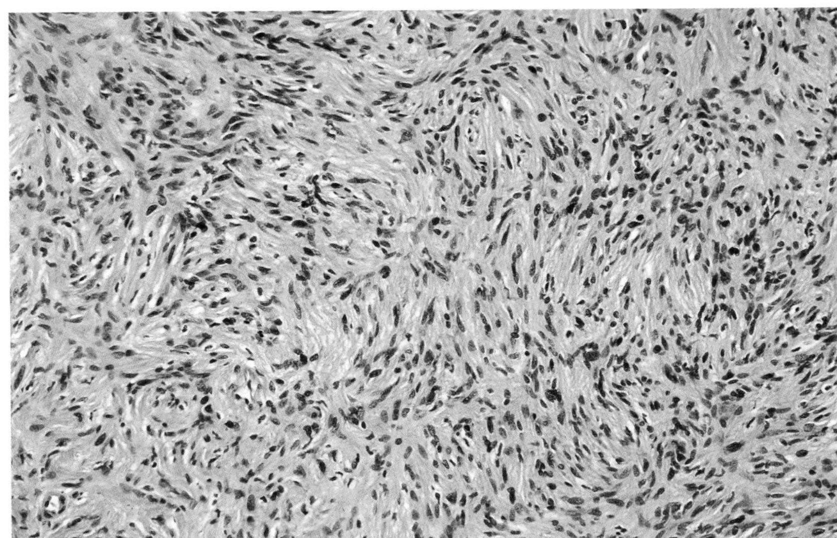

FIGURE 27-61. Antoni A areas with ill-defined fascicles without nuclear palisading.

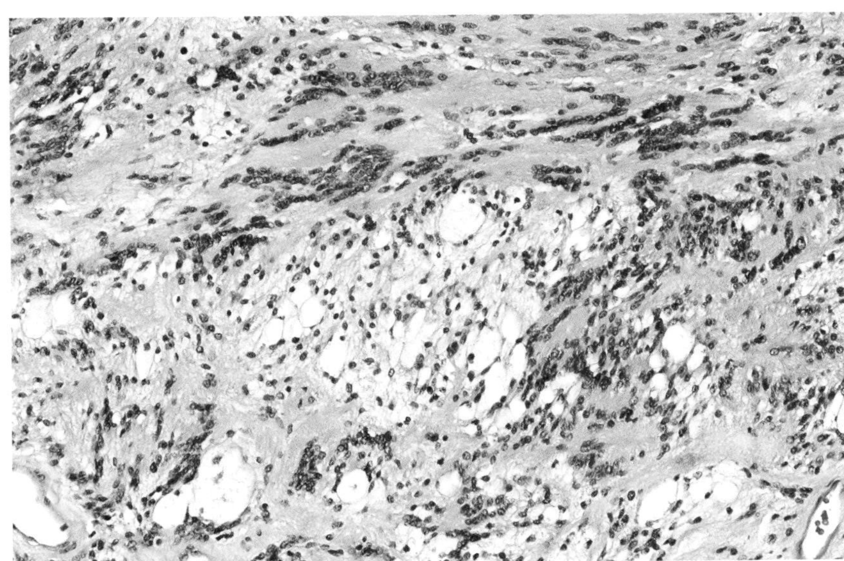

FIGURE 27-62. Transition between Antoni A areas and loosely textured Antoni B areas (center).

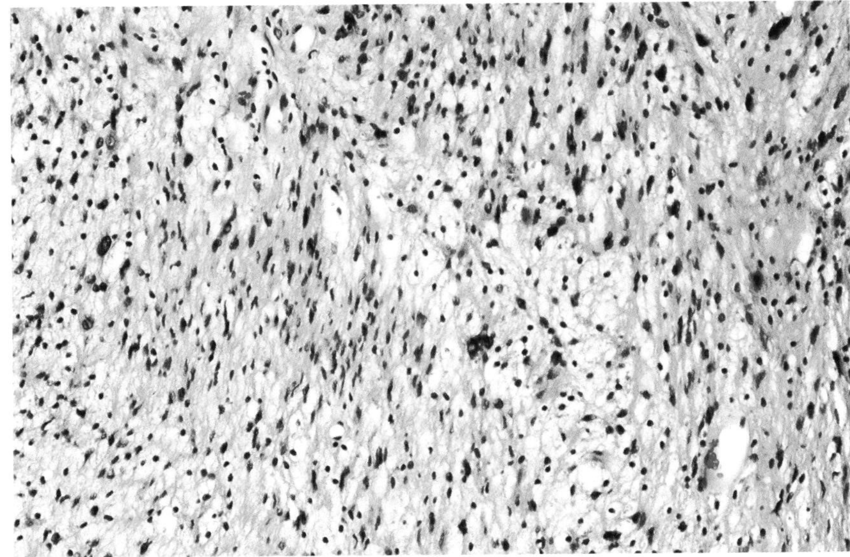

FIGURE 27-63. Antoni B areas in a schwannoma.

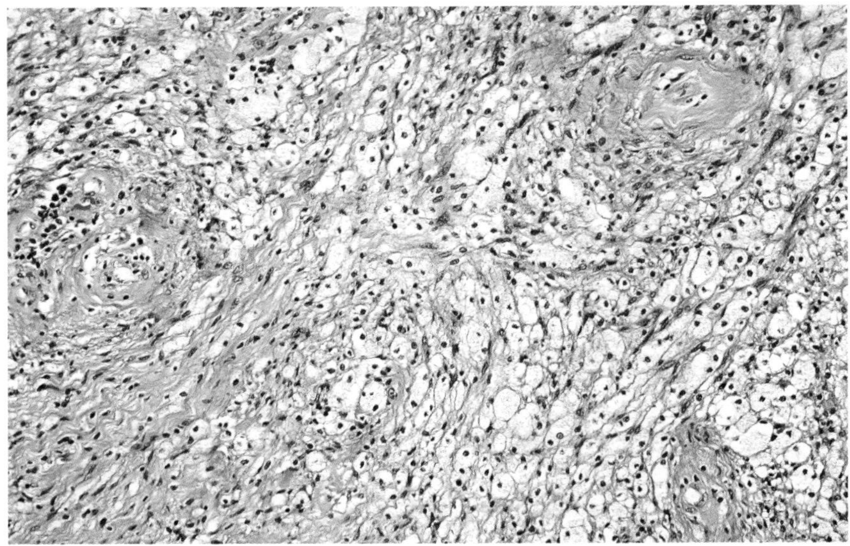

FIGURE 27-64. Antoni B areas with xanthomatous change.

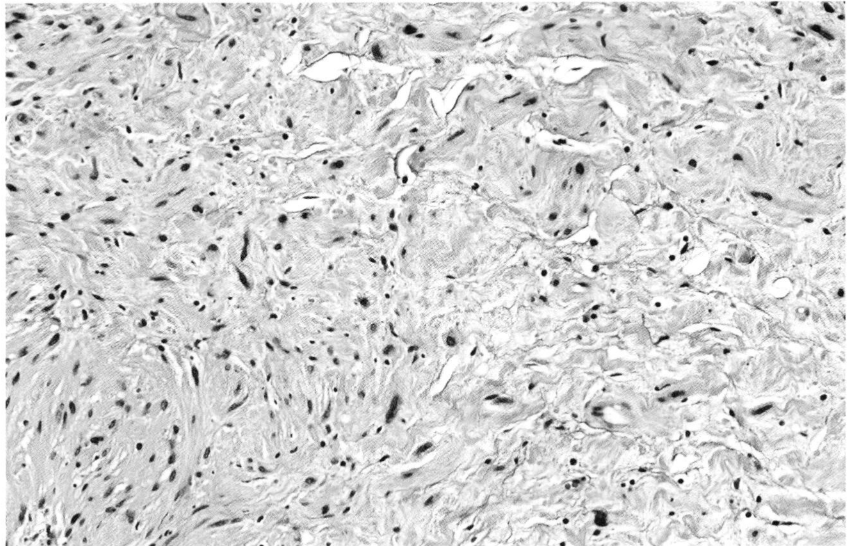

FIGURE 27-65. Antoni B areas with hyalinization.

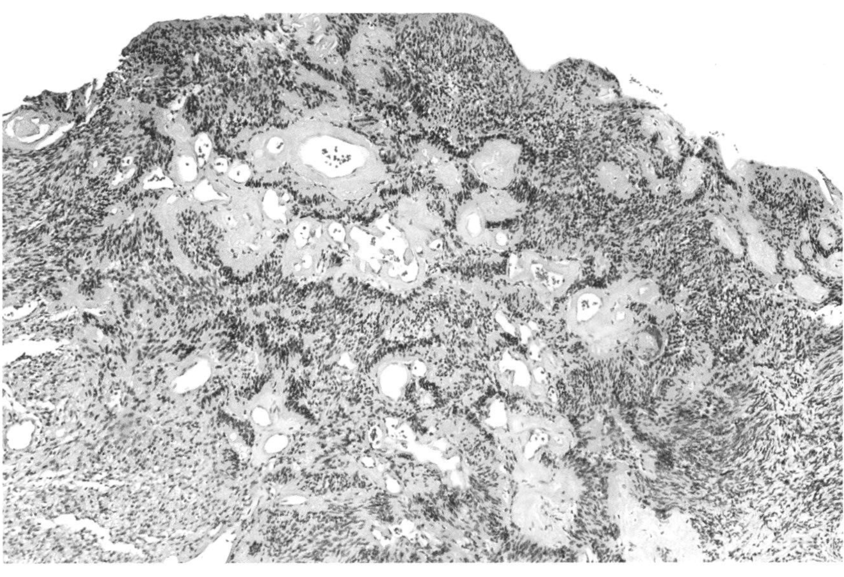

FIGURE 27-66. Ectatic irregularly shaped vessels with surrounding hyalinization are a common feature of schwannomas.

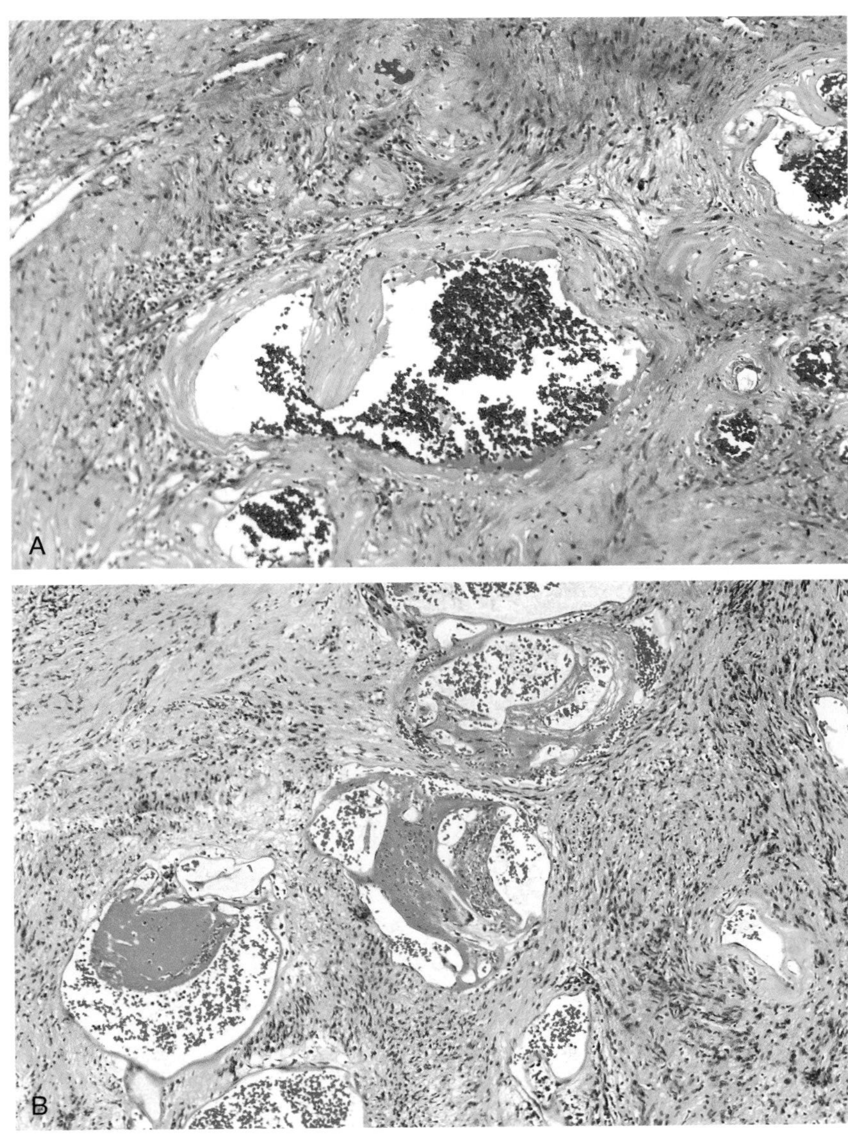

FIGURE 27-67. Hyalinized (A) and partially thrombosed (B) vessels in a schwannoma.

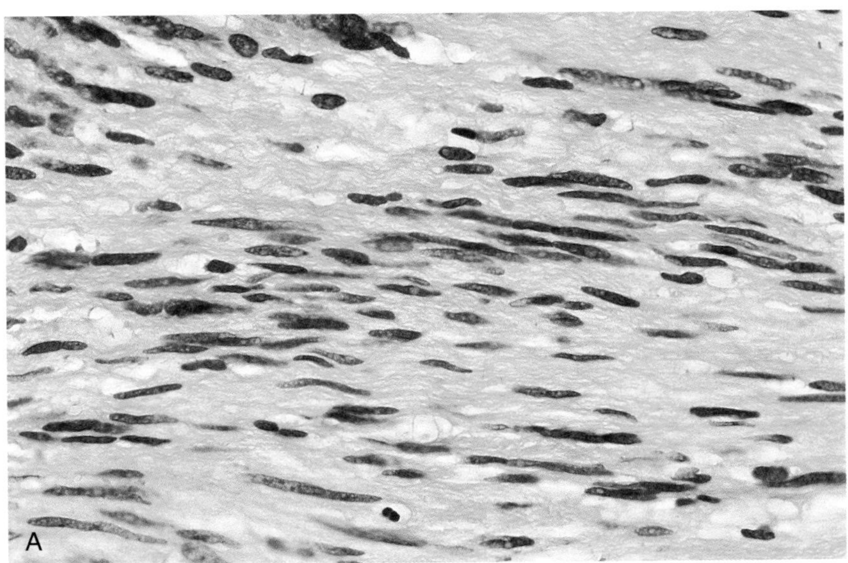

FIGURE 27-68. Differentiated Schwann cells (A) expressing S-100 protein (B) in a schwannoma.
Continued

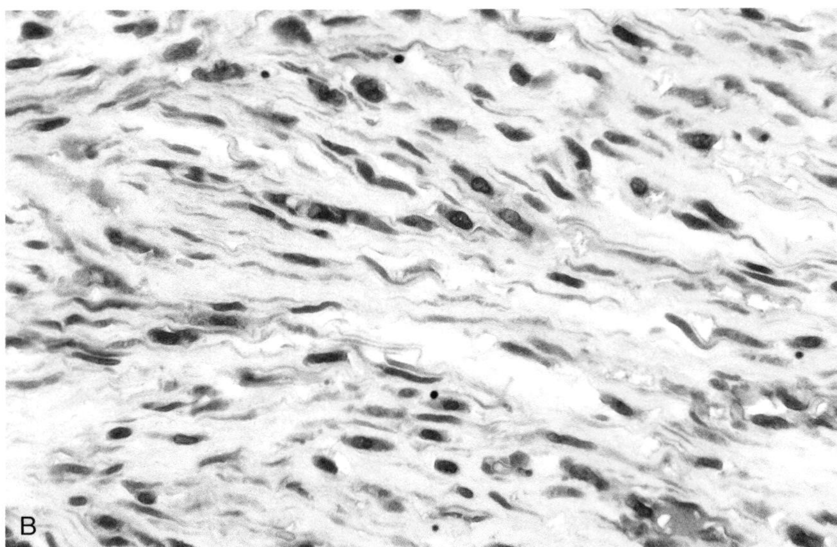

FIGURE 27-68, cont'd

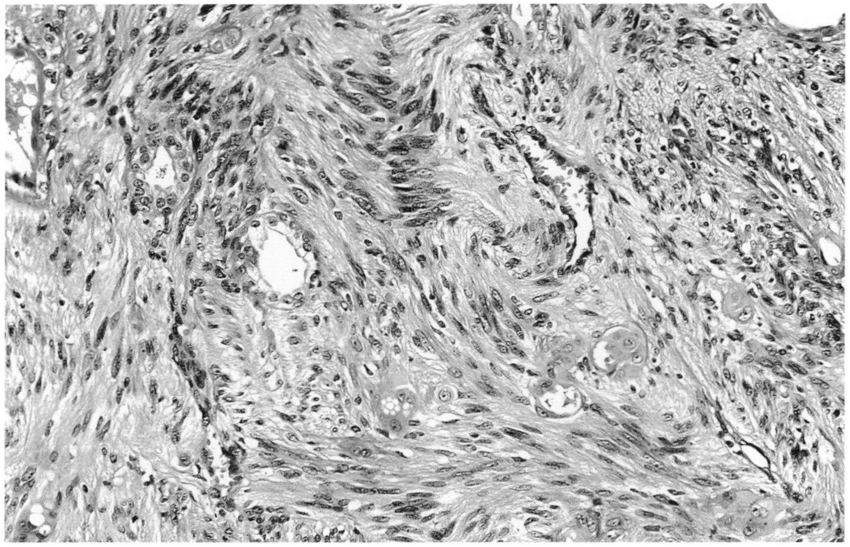

FIGURE 27-69. Schwannoma with benign glands and squamous islands.

hypocellular Antoni B areas (see Figs. 27-66 and 27-67). Their gaping, tortuous lumens are often filled with thrombus material in various stages of organization, and their walls are thickened by dense fibrosis. Glands and benign epithelial structures may occur in schwannoma (Fig. 27-69).[77,78] Judging from the number and type of glands, this seems to represent true epithelial differentiation in the tumor rather than entrapment or induced proliferation of normal structures. On occasion, schwannomas develop cystic spaces lined by Schwann cells that assume a round or epithelioid appearance. This change may be confused with true epithelial differentiation (Fig. 27-70). These tumors have been referred to as *pseudoglandular schwannomas*.[79] Rarely, schwannomas contain a significant population of small lymphocyte-like Schwann cells arranged around collagen nodules forming giant rosettes (Figs. 27-71 to 27-73) or around vessels forming perivascular rosettes.[80] These have been referred to as *neuroblastoma-like schwannoma*.

Ultrastructural and Immunohistochemical Findings

Electron microscopy has provided some of the best evidence in support of the separate nature of schwannomas and neurofibromas. In contrast to the neurofibroma, which contains a mixture of cell types, the schwannoma consists almost exclusively of Schwann cells.[81] These cells have attenuated cell processes that emanate from the cell body and lie in undulating layers adjacent to the cell body.[68-73,76-84] Basal lamina consisting of electron-dense material (measuring approximately 50 nm) coats the surface of the Schwann cell and lies in redundant

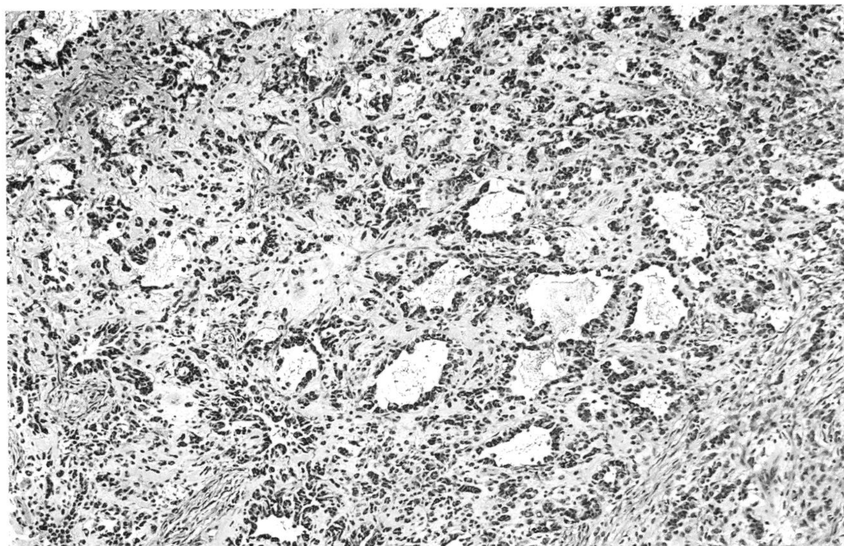

FIGURE 27-70. Schwannoma with cystic spaces resembling glands or dilated lymphatics (a so-called pseudoglandular schwannoma).

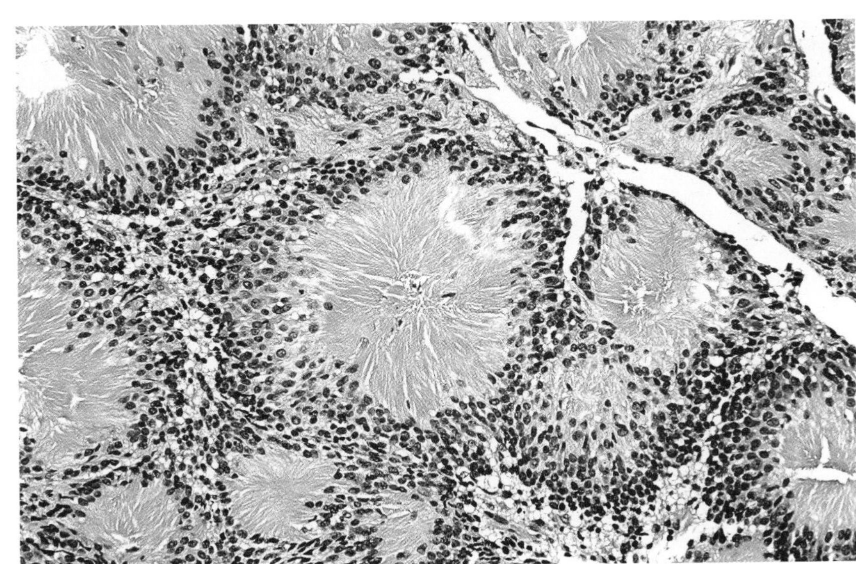

FIGURE 27-71. Neuroblastoma-like schwannoma composed of rounded Schwann cells forming rosettes.

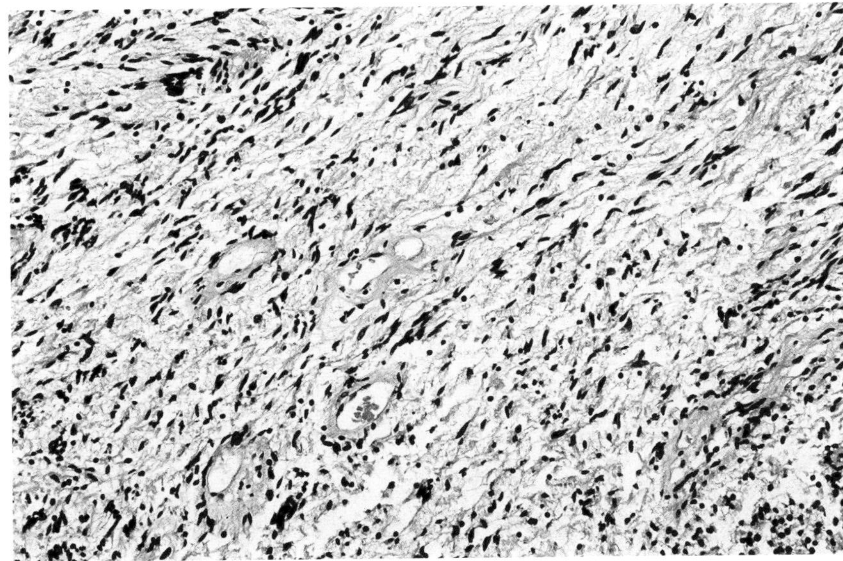

FIGURE 27-72. Neuroblastoma-like schwannoma showing more conventional feature.

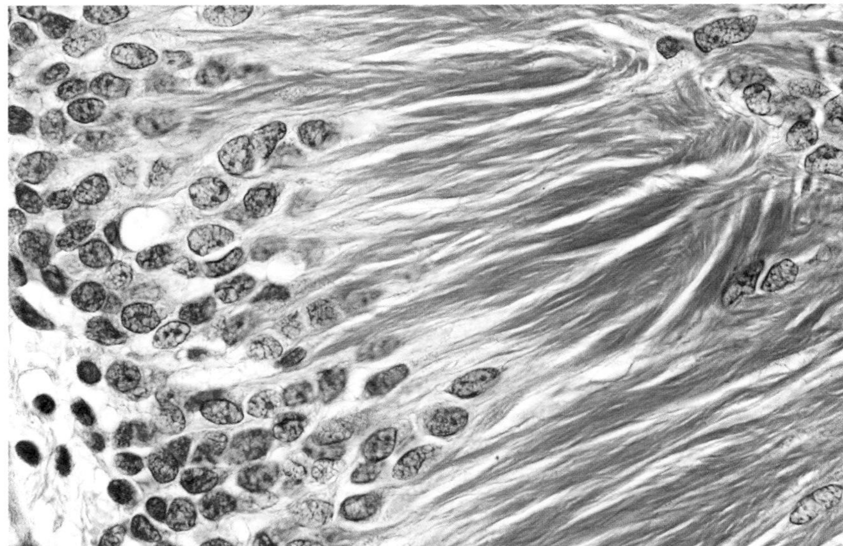

FIGURE 27-73. Giant rosette in a schwannoma formed by the radial arrangement of Schwann cells around a collagen core (Masson trichrome stain).

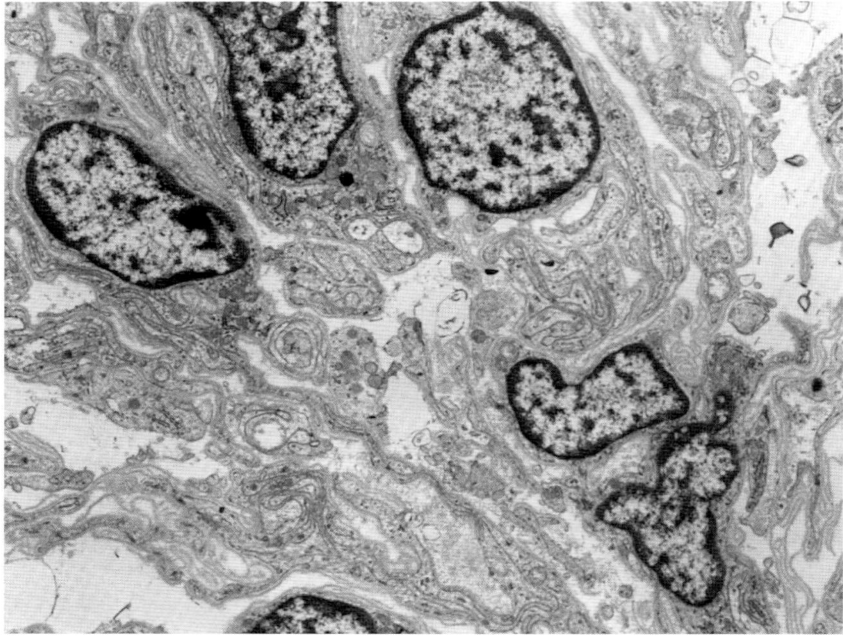

FIGURE 27-74. Electron micrograph of a schwannoma. Cells give off long cytoplasmic processes, which lie in layers adjacent to the cell body and are invested by well-formed continuous basal lamina. *(From Taxy JB, Battifora H. In: Trump B, Jones RT, editors. Diagnostic electron microscopy. New York: Wiley; 1980.)*

stacks between the cells along with typical and long-spacing collagen (Fig. 27-74). The cytoplasm of the Schwann cell contains a flattened, occasionally invaginated nucleus, microfibrils, occasional lysosomes, and scattered mitochondria. In Antoni B areas, the Schwann cells have increased numbers of lysosomes and myelin figures with only a fragmented basal lamina, suggesting that these are degenerated Antoni A areas.

In concert with ultrastructural observations, most cells in schwannomas have the antigenic phenotype of Schwann cells. S-100 protein is strongly expressed by most cells in a schwannoma (see Fig. 27-68), in contrast to the cells of neurofibroma, which variably express the antigen. Nuclear staining for SOX10, a recently characterized marker of neural crest differentiation, has proven to be an excellent marker for schwannomas and is also expressed in the schwann cell component of neurofibromas.[84a] Leu-7 and occasionally glial fibrillary acidic protein are present in these tumors. Although the expression of S-100 protein is usually diminished in the Antoni B areas, immunostaining for this protein is so consistent and of such intensity that it serves as an important diagnostic tool. It is most valuable for diagnosing a severely degenerated schwannoma in which the amount of myxoid change or fibrosis obscures the neoplastic nature of the lesion altogether. It usually also distinguishes deeply situated schwannomas from well-differentiated leiomyosarcomas. This important differential point is especially difficult in biopsy material from large intra-abdominal or retroperitoneal masses. The difficulty can be further compounded by the fact that schwannomas and leiomyosarcomas can display equivalent degrees of nuclear palisading. Whereas S-100 protein immunostaining is nearly always observed in schwannomas, it is seldom observed in leiomyosarcomas. SOX10 can also be used to the same purpose since it is essentially never expressed in leiomyosarcomas.[84a]

Discussion

Schwannomas are benign with only anecdotal cases of malignant transformation.[85-87] Among the well over 1000 schwannomas that have been seen, there has been only one instance of true malignant transformation. In that case, the original tumor had the features of a classic schwannoma, whereas the recurrent tumor, 8 years later, had areas of malignancy. The patient later succumbed to metastatic disease. Woodruff et al.[88] presented nine acceptable cases, including two of their own, in a comprehensive review of the literature. As a group, these tumors occur in adults without NF1 but with a long-standing mass. Unlike neurofibromas, in which supervening malignancy resembles a spindle cell sarcoma, malignancy in schwannomas often has an epithelioid appearance. Areas of a conventional schwannoma are identified alongside confluent expanses of large, round, atypical eosinophilic cells (Fig. 27-75CD).[89] McMenamin and Fletcher[90] reported several additional cases of malignant transformation. Noting microscopic collections of epithelioid cells in schwannomas, they suggested that they represent the early stage of malignant transformation. Additionally, they noted schwannomas with malignant transformation to epithelioid angiosarcoma (Fig. 27-75AB).

Schwannoma with Degenerative Change (Ancient Schwannoma)

Ancient schwannomas are those displaying marked nuclear atypia of a degenerative type. They are usually large tumors of long duration, and a significant number are located in deep structures such as the retroperitoneum. Degenerative changes include cyst formation, calcification, hemorrhage, and hyalinization (Figs. 27-76 to 27-81). The tumor itself is usually infiltrated by large numbers of siderophages and histiocytes. One of the most treacherous aspects of this tumor is the degree of nuclear atypia encountered. The Schwann cell nuclei are large, hyperchromatic, and often multilobed but lack mitotic figures (see Figs. 27-77 to 27-81). These tumors behave as ordinary

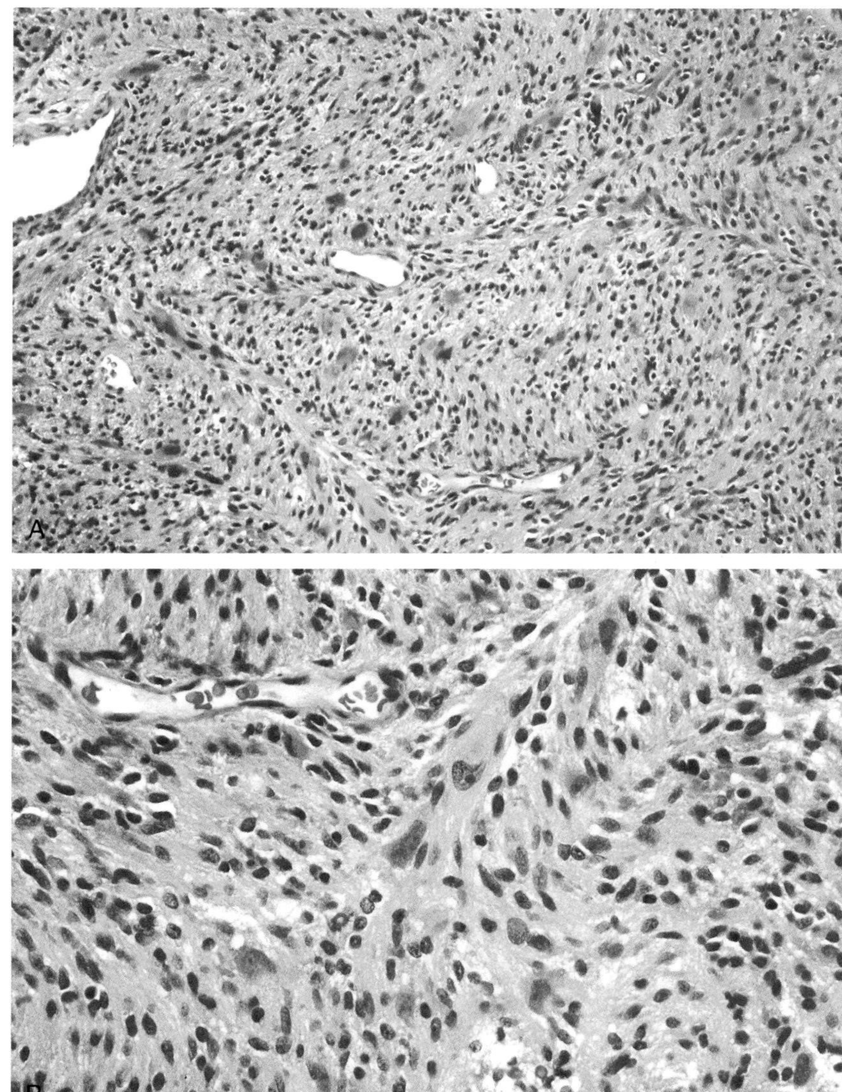

FIGURE 27-75. Schwannoma with scattered atypical (A, B) cells and frank malignant change (C, D). Scattered atypical cells within otherwise benign schwannoma (A, B) have been described as the precursor lesion to frank malignancy, which is diagnosed by confluent areas of obviously malignant cells (C, D). *Continued*

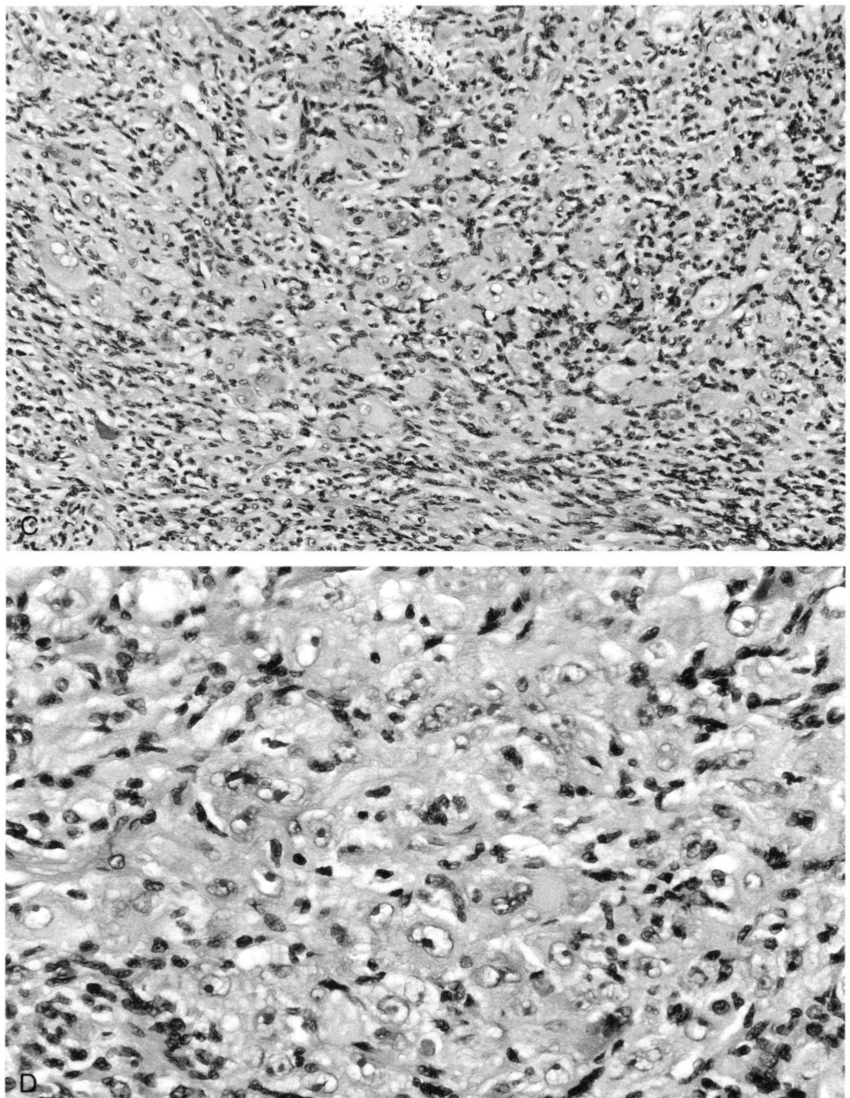

FIGURE 27-75, cont'd

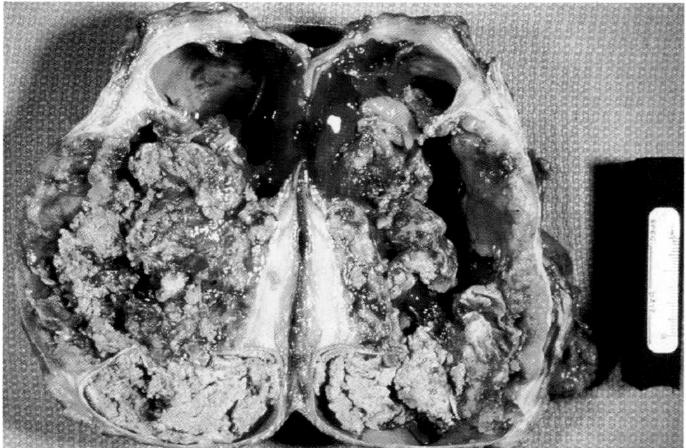

FIGURE 27-76. Gross specimen of a schwannoma of the retroperitoneum with extensive degenerative changes (ancient schwannoma). Tumors are characterized by areas of old and new hemorrhage, cyst formation, and calcification.

schwannomas; therefore, the nuclear atypia can be dismissed as a degenerative change.

Cellular Schwannoma

Cellular schwannoma is a well-recognized variant of schwannoma[91-95] that, because of its cellularity, mitotic activity, and occasional presence of bone destruction, is diagnosed as malignant in more than one-fourth of cases.[96] Lesions reported as plexiform MPNST of infancy and childhood[97] and congenital neural hamartoma (fascicular schwannoma)[98] are cellular schwannomas.[99] Defined as a schwannoma composed predominantly or exclusively of Antoni A areas that lack Verocay bodies, cellular schwannoma occurs in a similar age group as classic schwannoma but tends to develop more often in deep structures such as the posterior mediastinum and retroperitoneum. Only about one-fourth develop in the deep soft tissues of the extremities. It may present as a palpable

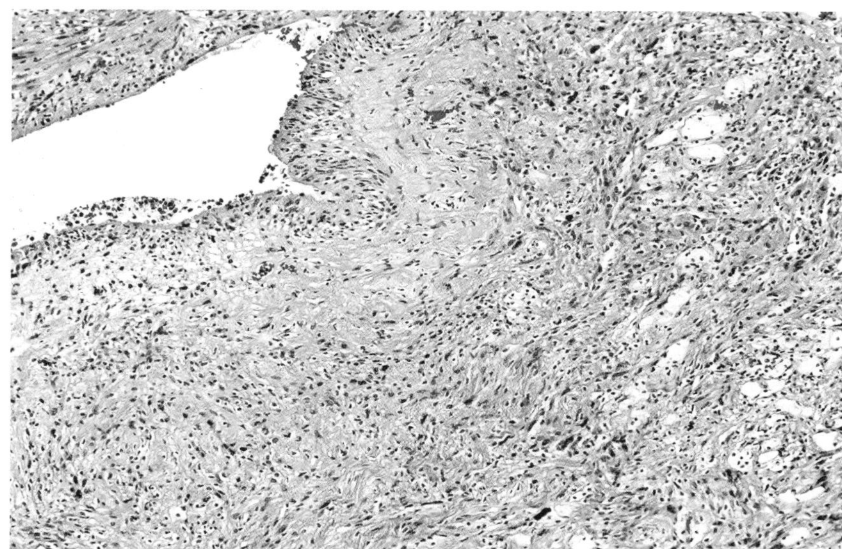

FIGURE 27-77. Ancient schwannoma with cyst formation and interstitial hyalinization.

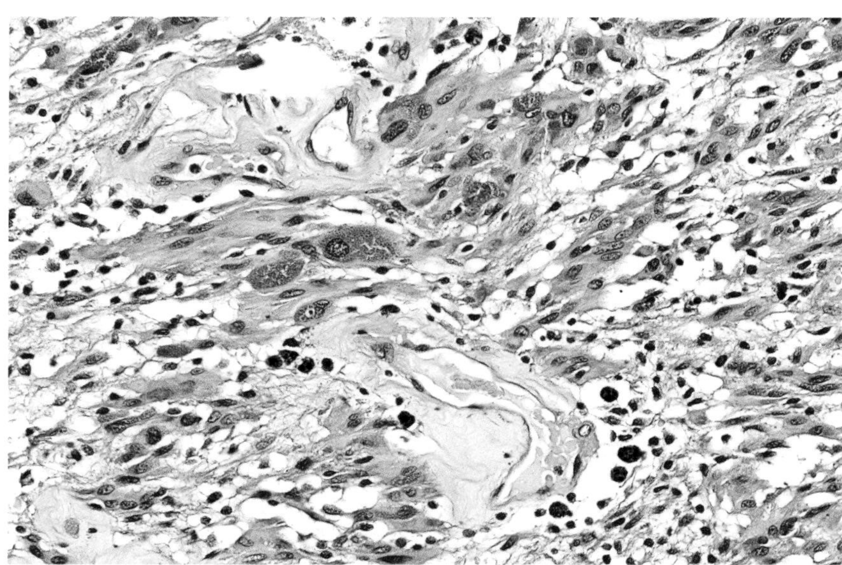

FIGURE 27-78. Ancient schwannoma with degenerative atypia and perivascular hyalinization. Note the lipofuscin-like pigment in the Schwann cells.

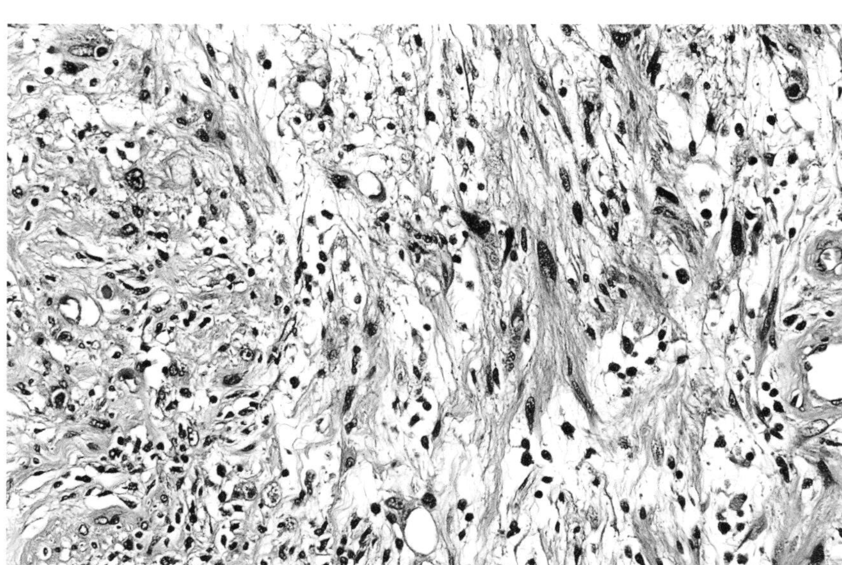

FIGURE 27-79. Ancient schwannoma.

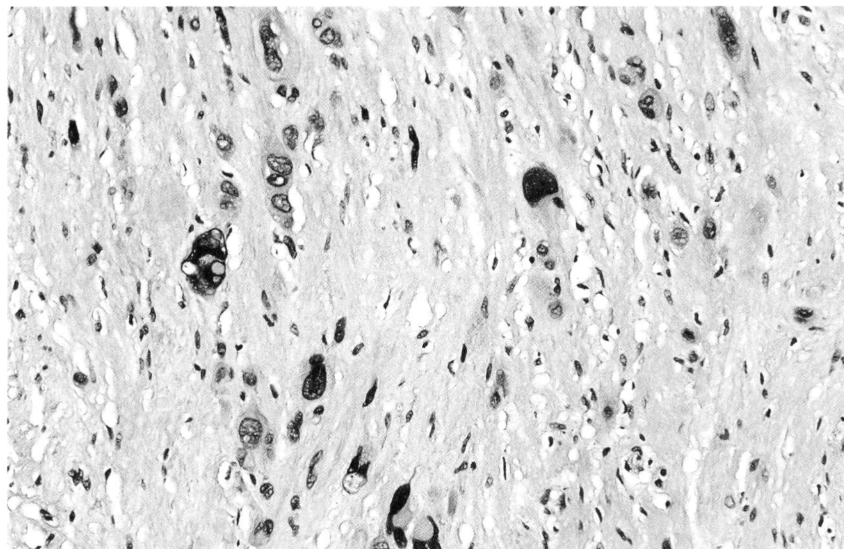

FIGURE 27-80. Ancient schwannoma with extensive hyalinization.

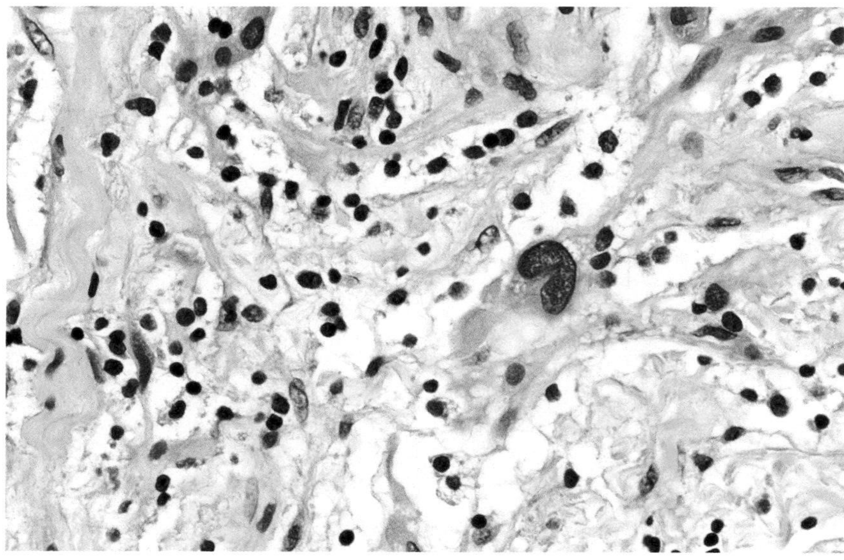

FIGURE 27-81. Degenerative atypia in an ancient schwannoma.

asymptomatic mass noted radiographically or as a mass producing neurologic symptoms. Like classic schwannomas, the lesions appear circumscribed, if not encapsulated, and occasionally are multinodular or plexiform. Usually homogeneously tan in color, they commonly have hemorrhage but seldom display cystic degeneration (Fig. 27-82).[57] Underneath their capsule, they may contain lymphoid aggregates. Antoni A areas dominate the histologic picture but small amounts of Antoni B may be present, usually not exceeding 10% of the lesion.[57] In addition to short, intersecting fascicles and whorls of Schwann cells, the Antoni A areas may display long, sweeping fascicles of Schwann cells sometimes arranged in a herringbone fashion (Figs. 27-83 and 27-84). The presence of this pattern often suggests the diagnosis of fibrosarcoma or leiomyosarcoma to those unfamiliar with cellular schwannomas.

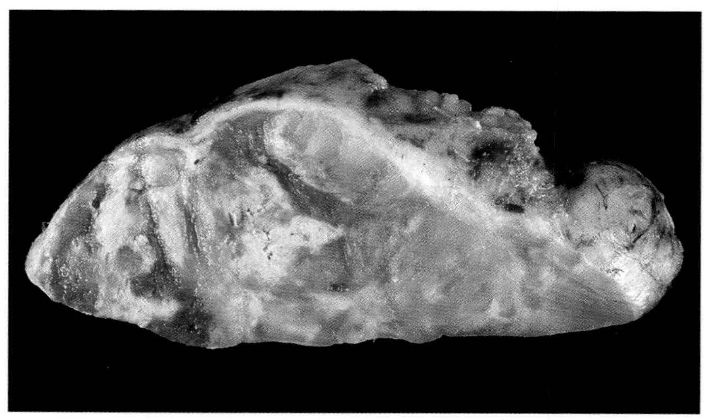

FIGURE 27-82. Cellular schwannoma with a characteristic tawny yellow color.

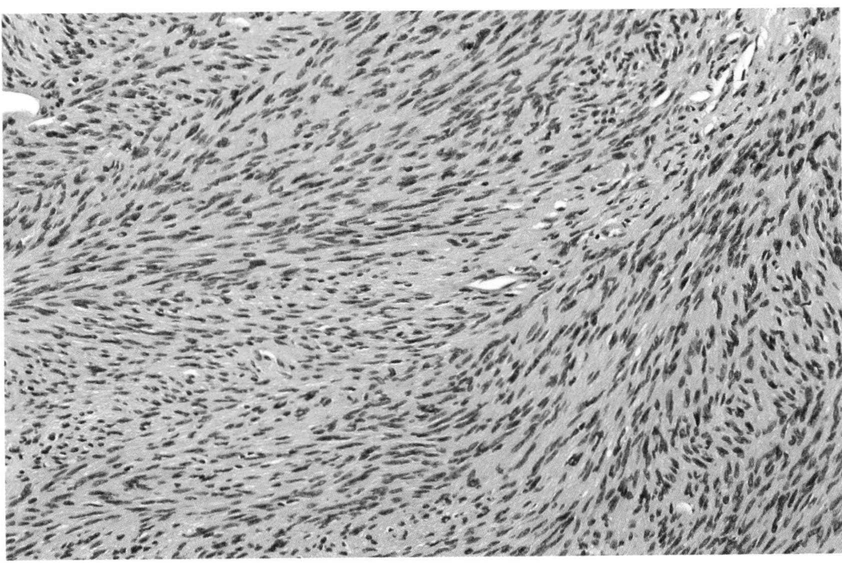

FIGURE 27-83. Cellular schwannoma with long fascicles of Schwann cells without Antoni B areas or Verocay bodies.

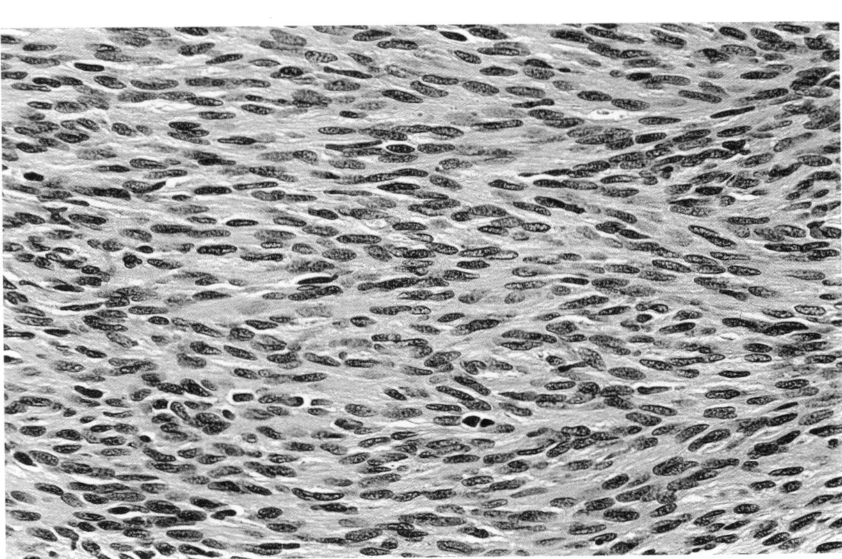

FIGURE 27-84. Cellular schwannoma consisting of differentiated Schwann cells without mitotic activity.

Mitotic activity may be observed but usually is low (less than 4 mitoses per 10 high-power fields [HPF]).[94] Focal areas of necrosis are seen in up to 10% of cases. The cells fringing the necrotic zones, however, are differentiated Schwann cells and lack the hyperchromatism and anaplasia so typical of those surrounding areas of zonal necrosis in MPNSTs. Like classic schwannomas, the cellular schwannoma displays diffuse, strong immunoreactivity for S-100 protein. Most cellular schwannomas are diploid with a low S-phase fraction (6% to 7%).[91]

Important factors that suggest a benign diagnosis include cellularity that is disproportionately high compared with the levels of mitotic activity and atypia, sharp circumscription if not encapsulation, perivascular hyalinization, occasionally focal Antoni B areas, and invariably strong, diffuse immunoreactivity for S-100 protein. Staining for S-100 protein is an invaluable adjunct for this diagnosis, particularly if one is dealing with material obtained by small-needle biopsies of large retroperitoneal or mediastinal masses. In fact, malignancy is rarely diagnosed based on needle biopsies of differentiated spindle cell tumors if staining for S-100 protein is strongly positive because of the possibility of a cellular schwannoma.

Although initial skepticism was expressed about the biologic behavior of cellular schwannomas, with some suggesting that they were in fact a low-grade MPNST, several large studies with extended follow-up information[91,93,94,100] have reaffirmed their benignancy. More than 100 cases have been reported, with nearly one-third having follow-up periods of more than 5 years. Fewer than 5% of patients have developed recurrences, and none has developed metastatic disease. In most of the cases reported by White et al.,[94] treatment was conservative and consisted of surgical excision only. That these truly represent variants of schwannoma is indicated not only by histologic but also by ultrastructural and cytogenetic similarities.[101]

Plexiform Schwannoma

About 5% of schwannomas grow in a plexiform or multinodular pattern,[102] which may or may not be apparent macroscopically (Figs. 27-85 to 27-87). Unlike plexiform neurofibromas, which are considered nearly pathognomonic of NF1, the association of plexiform schwannomas with NF1 or NF2 is considerably weaker.[102] Of the approximately 50 cases reported in the literature, there have been only a few cases associated with NF1[100,103,104] or NF2.[105-107] Plexiform schwannomas usually occur in the skin and infrequently in deep sites. Like classic schwannoma, they are encapsulated but, as a group, are more cellular and, therefore, qualify also as cellular schwannomas. It is important to be aware of this fact because there is a risk of misinterpreting a lesion as a sarcoma arising in a plexiform neurofibroma. Attention to the fact that the lesion does not have a level of atypia commensurate with the mitotic activity, lacks geographic necrosis, and displays strong S-100 protein staining provides good support for benignancy in these cases.

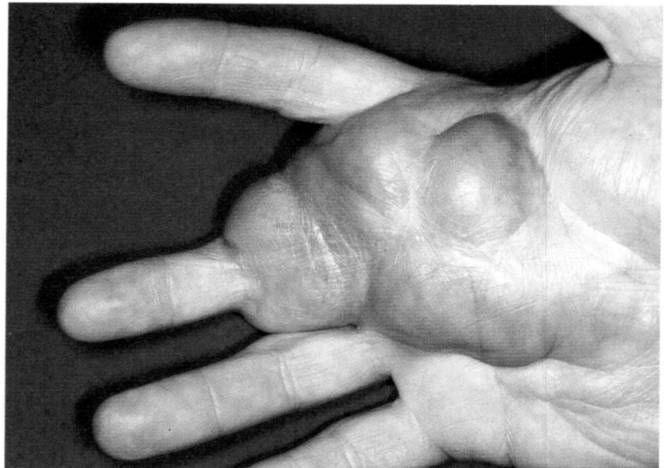

FIGURE 27-85. Plexiform schwannoma.

Epithelioid Schwannoma

Schwannomas consisting predominantly or exclusively of epithelioid Schwann cells have been termed *epithelioid schwannoma*.[108,109] Many of the cases reported as benign epithelioid peripheral nerve sheath tumor of soft tissues are examples of epithelioid schwannoma. Although most authors consider these lesions to be variants of schwannoma, others regard them as benign epithelioid nerve sheath tumors of indeterminate type.[110]

These tumors develop as small (1 to 2 cm) circumscribed or encapsulated masses in the skin and the superficial soft tissue, usually of the extremities. With only a rare exception, these lesions are not associated with NF1 or NF2.[110] The tumor is composed of small rounded Schwann cells arranged singly, in small aggregates, or in cords within a collagenous or partially myxoid stroma (Fig. 27-88). Areas of conventional

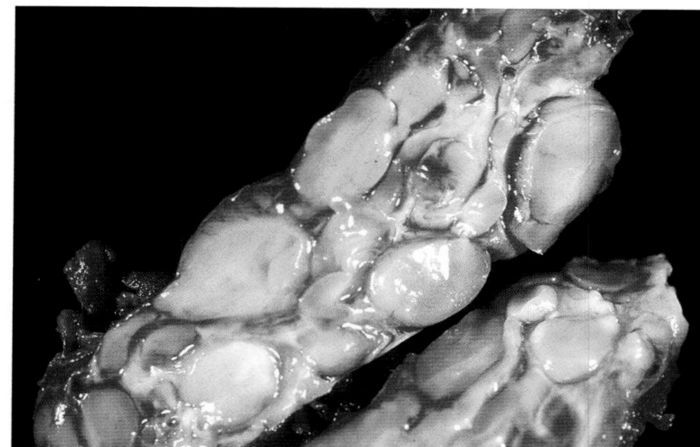

FIGURE 27-86. Gross specimen of a plexiform schwannoma illustrating a multinodular pattern of growth.

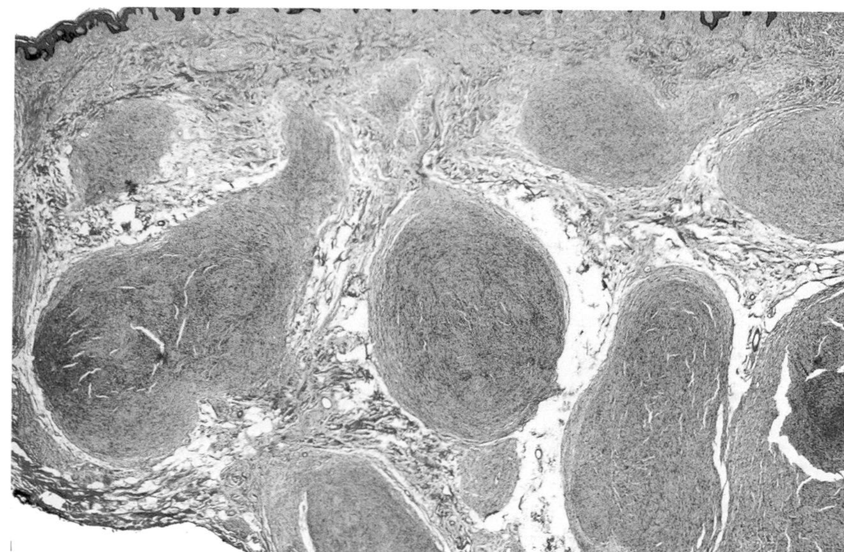

FIGURE 27-87. Plexiform schwannoma involving the dermis.

schwannoma may be seen in some tumors. The epithelioid Schwann cells are small and rounded with sharp cytoplasmic borders and occasionally intranuclear cytoplasmic (pseudo) inclusions. A small subset displays nuclear atypia with prominent nucleoli and low levels of mitotic activity.[108] The cells may be associated with dense collagen cores forming irregular collagen rosettes similar to those seen in the neuroblastoma-like schwannoma. Immunohistochemistry is helpful, if not essential, in establishing the diagnosis. The cells strongly express S100 protein and SOX10 and often additional Schwann cell markers such as glial fibrillary acidic protein (GFAP) and low affinity nerve growth factor receptor (Fig. 27-89A).[110] In addition, immunostains for type IV collagen or laminin outlines a latticework of basement membrane material around individual cells and groups of cells (Fig. 27-89B). The combination of these two stains is highly suggestive of the diagnosis because few tumors coexpress these two antigens to this degree. Electron microscopy shows that the cells resemble differentiated Schwann cells. The behavior of these lesions is benign. In fact, even those with some nuclear atypia and mitotic activity have behaved well. These lesions should be distinguished from epithelioid MPNST, lesions of high nuclear grade, which lack a capsule and a network of basal lamina encircling cells.

NEUROFIBROMATOSIS 2 (NF2; BILATERAL VESTIBULAR SCHWANNOMAS)

Neurofibromatosis 2 is an autosomal dominant disease with an incidence of 1 of 25,000 to 40,000 live births, which has as its hallmark bilateral vestibular schwannomas. It is the result of inactivating germline mutations of the tumor suppressor gene *NF2* located on chromosome 22. Approximately 50% of NF2 cases arise as *de novo* mutations, a subset of which 20% to 30% are patients with mild mosaic disease in which only a fraction of cells contain a mutated *NF2* gene. These cases may

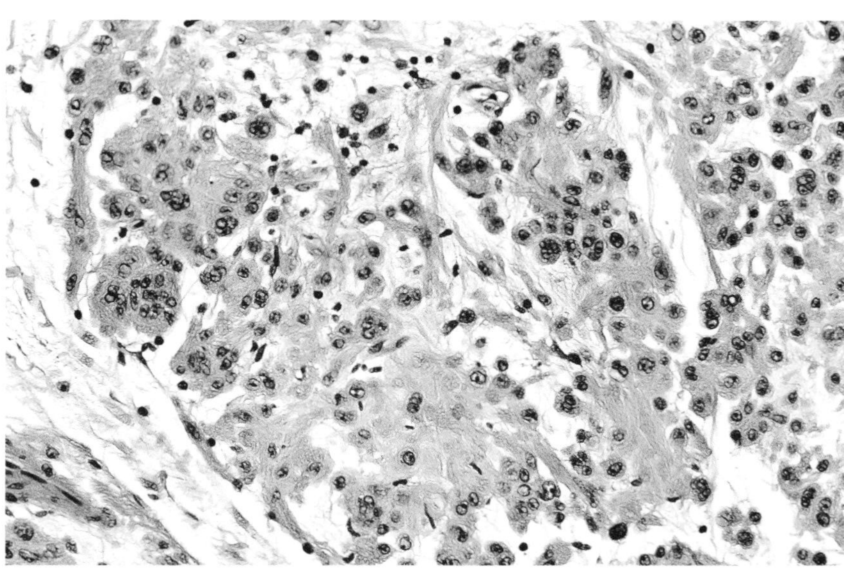

FIGURE 27-88. Epithelioid schwannoma. Note the cohesive nests of bland epithelioid cells.

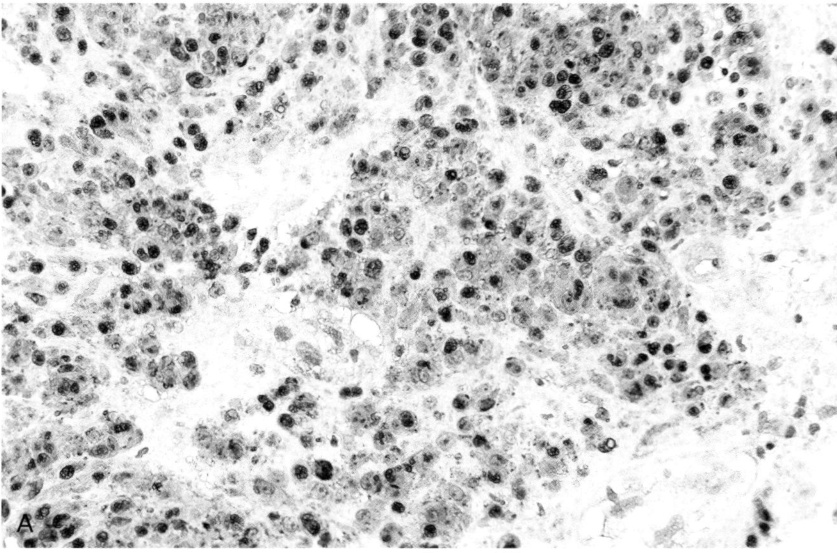

FIGURE 27-89. Epithelioid schwannoma with S-100 protein (A) and intricate pattern of type IV collagen immunoreactivity (B). The latter is reflective of basal lamina material surrounding the cells. *Continued*

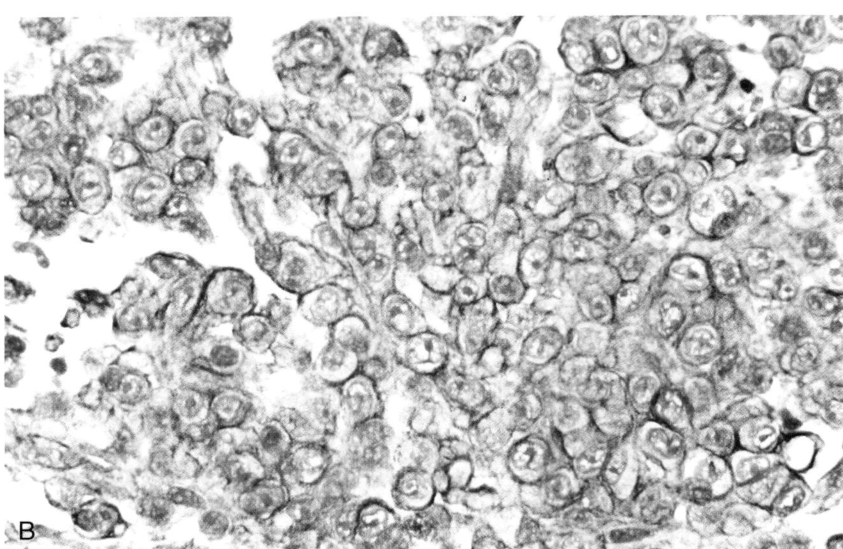

FIGURE 27-89, cont'd

be difficult to diagnose based on blood samples of peripheral lymphocytes alone and may require analysis of the multiple tumors.[111] *NF2* mutations are varied and encompass truncating mutations leading to nonfunctional product, missense mutations, and large deletions with no gene product. There appears to be some correlation between disease severity and mutational status. Patients with nonsense or frameshift mutations have severe disease, whereas those with missense mutations, in-frame deletions, and large deletions have a mild form.[112]

The *NF2* gene encodes the protein merlin or schwannomin, a 595 amino acid member of the moesin-ezrin-radixin cytoskeleton-associated proteins.[113] This protein is expressed in Schwann cells, meningeal cells, and the lens of the eye where it localizes to regions of the cell membrane engaged in cell contact and mobility. The mechanisms by which the loss of this protein results in tumorigenesis are not well understood. Merlin has several binding partners, including transmembrane and cytoskeletal proteins and signaling molecules/kinases. It is not clear whether merlin's association with one particular partner is responsible for tumor suppression or whether it is a collective association with several partners.[45] A number of studies indicate that merlin controls contact-dependent inhibition of proliferation in several cells types through interaction with its extracellular matrix CD44. Other lines of evidence have shown that merlin stabilizes large actin-cytoskeleton-associated membrane signaling complexes.

The onset of NF2 is usually during adolescence or early adult life, with the development of tinnitus or hearing loss due to the presence of bilateral vestibular schwannomas that usually affect the vestibular portion of the eighth cranial nerve. Café au lait spots and neurofibromas are rare or absent in this form of neurofibromatosis. In addition to vestibular schwannomas, other central nervous system tumors occur commonly, including schwannomas of other cranial nerves, meningioma, ependymoma, and glioma. Approximately one-half to two-thirds of patients with NF2 also develop cutaneous schwannomas, but schwannomas in the absence of bilateral vestibular schwannomas (schwannomatosis) is a different disease (see schwannomatosis). Because half of NF2 patients do not have a family history of NF2, and many present with meningiomas, spinal cord tumors, or peripheral schwannomas before the development of vestibular schwannomas, the NIH diagnostic criteria proposed in 1997 have recently been expanded under the less stringent Manchester system (Box 27-2).[113,114]

BOX 27-2 Manchester Criteria for Diagnosis of Neurofibromatosis 2

A. Bilateral vestibular schwannoma.
B. First-degree family relative with NF2 and unilateral vestibular schwannoma or any two* of the following: meningioma, schwannoma, glioma, neurofibroma, posterior subcapsular lenticular opacity.
C. Unilateral vestibular schwannoma and any two* of the following: meningioma, schwannoma, glioma, neurofibroma, posterior subcapsular lenticular opacity.
D. Multiple meningiomas (two or more) and unilateral vestibular schwannoma or any two* of the following: schwannoma, glioma, neurofibroma, cataract.

*Note any two means two individual tumors or cataracts.
From Evans DG, Huson SM, Donnai D, et al. A clinical study of type 2 neurofibromatosis. *Q J Med* 1992;84:603–618.

NF2-associated schwannomas are histologically similar to sporadic ones and do not undergo malignant transformation. Patients, nonetheless, experience significant morbidity and mortality. Prior to 1990, the life expectancy following diagnosis averaged 15 years. Although survival has improved, most patients eventually become completely deaf or disabled as a result of poor balance, visual problems, or muscle weakness caused by spinal cord tumors.[111] By far the strongest predictor of mortality is age at diagnosis. In addition, patients referred to specialty centers have a significantly lower mortality. Once a diagnosis of NF2 is established, screening of young family members is strongly recommended so that appropriate interventions can be planned.

SCHWANNOMATOSIS

Formerly considered by some as an attenuated form of NF2, multiple schwannomas or schwannomatosis[115] is currently considered a completely different disease. The majority of cases of schwannomatosis are sporadic, but there are well-documented familial cases that follow an autosomal dominant pattern of inheritance with reduced penetrance.[116] Men and women are equally affected. Patients present with multiple, often painful schwannomas involving skin or soft tissue. In some patients, the schwannomas have a striking segmental distribution affecting the length of a nerve. Although some patients develop cranial or spinal nerve schwannomas, they do not develop the variety of central nervous system tumors seen in NF2, such as astrocytoma, ependymoma, and meningioma. Based on a large international clinical database, revised diagnostic criteria for schwannomatosis have been proposed (Table 27-3).[116]

By molecular and linkage analysis of familial cases, the schwannomatosis locus has been identified on chromosome 22 proximal to *NF2*. Recently, a germline mutation of *INI1/SMARCB1*, which is located within a short distance of *NF2*, has been identified in one-third of families with schwannomatosis and 7% of individuals with sporadic schwannomatosis.[117] In patients with germline mutations, a second hit with loss of *INI1/SMARCB1* occurs. Bi-allelic inactivation of *NF2* is also found within a subset of patients with schwannomatosis, suggesting the concept of a four-hit theory of tumorigenesis.

Patients with schwannomatosis enjoy a normal life expectancy, although the quality of life can be compromised by symptomatic schwannomas. The very recent report of malignant transformation of a schwannoma in a patient with schwannomatosis and a germline mutation of *INI1/SMARCB1* suggests a cautionary note, however. That patient also had two offspring with an atypical teratoid/rhabdoid tumor,[118] a rare tumor also known to be associated with *INI1/SMARCB1* mutation.

TABLE 27-3 Revised Clinical Criteria for Diagnosis of Schwannomatosis

DEFINITE	POSSIBLE
Age >30 years AND two or more nonintradermal schwannomas, at least one with histologic confirmation AND no evidence of vestibular tumor on high quality MRI scan AND no known constitutional *NF2* mutation OR One pathologically confirmed nonvestibular schwannoma plus a first-degree relative who meets above criteria	Age <30 years AND two or more nonintradermal schwannomas, at least one with histologic confirmation AND no evidence of vestibular tumor on high quality MRI scan AND no known constitutional *NF2* mutation OR Age <45 years AND two or more nonintradermal schwannomas at least one with histologic confirmation AND no symptoms of 8th nerve dysfunction AND no known constitutional *NF2* mutation
Segmental schwannomatosis Meets criteria for either definite or possible schwannomatosis but limited to one limb or five or fewer contiguous segments of the spine	

From MacCollin M, Chiocca EA, Evans DG, et al. Diagnostic criteria for schwannomatosis. Neurology 2005;64:1838–1845.

PERINEURIOMA

Perineurioma is a soft tissue tumor composed of cells resembling normal perineurium.[119] Because neurofibromas contain a subpopulation of perineurial cells and rare nerve sheath tumors have hybrid features between neurofibroma and perineurioma,[120-122] the term *perineurioma* is traditionally used for tumors in which the vast majority of cells show perineurial differentiation. It was first described in 1978 by Lazarus and Trombetta[123] on the basis of ultrastructural findings. The tumor was slow to gain wide recognition because of the inability to diagnose the lesion by light microscopy alone. Greater familiarity with its features coupled with additional immunohistochemical markers to document perineurial differentiation has resulted in more frequent and consistent diagnosis. All perineuriomas, including the variants, express antigens that are identical to normal perineurium. Even with these enhanced diagnostic markers, they are still far less common than neurofibromas and schwannomas. There are several forms of perineurioma: intraneural, extraneural (soft tissue), sclerosing, and reticular.

Intraneural Perineurioma

Intraneural perineurioma, originally termed *localized hypertrophic neuropathy*, is a rare condition that has been shown to be an intraneural clonal proliferation of perineurial cells. The lesions usually develop in a nerve in the upper extremity of a young individual. Characteristic signs and symptoms include muscle weakness, denervation changes seen by electromyography, and, in extreme cases, muscle atrophy. The affected nerve displays a fusiform expansion extending several centimeters in length (Fig. 27-90). On a cross section, the entire nerve is expanded by the formation of tiny "onion bulbs" consisting of concentric layers of perineurial cells ensheathing a central axon and Schwann cell (Fig. 27-91). The perineurial cells occasionally spin off the sheath and communicate with adjacent ones. Because of the highly organized nature of these lesions, the usual impression is that of a reactive or reparative process. However, with immunostains for EMA and S-100 protein, the striking preponderance of perineurial cells becomes readily apparent. Immunostains for EMA highlight the ensheathing perineurial cells, leaving the central portion of the onion bulb devoid of staining. With S-100 protein or neurofilament protein immunostains, highlighting Schwann cells and axons respectively, a reverse staining pattern is noted (Fig. 27-92).

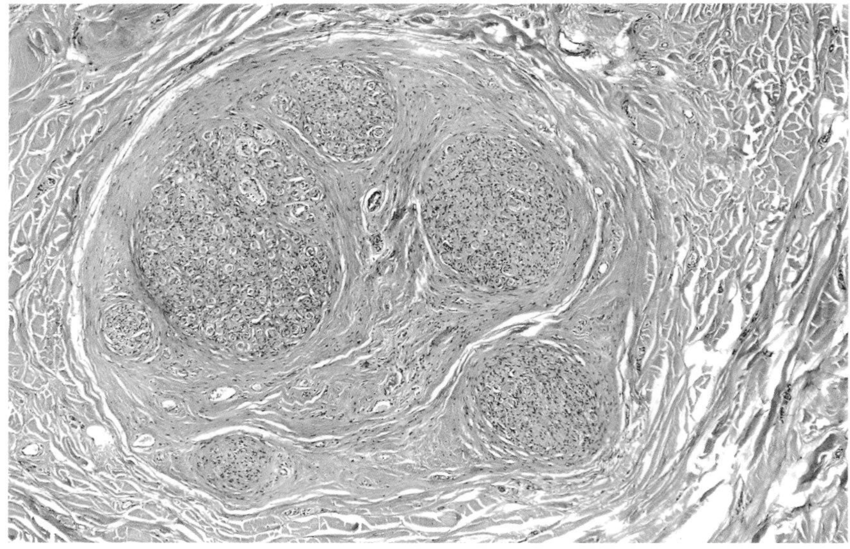

FIGURE 27-90. Intraneural perineurioma.

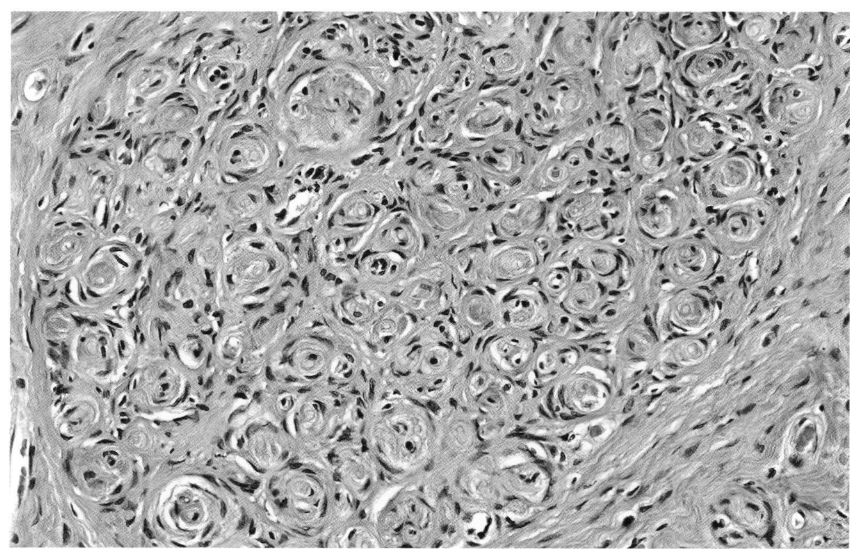

FIGURE 27-91. Intraneural perineurioma with onion-bulb expansion of the nerve sheath.

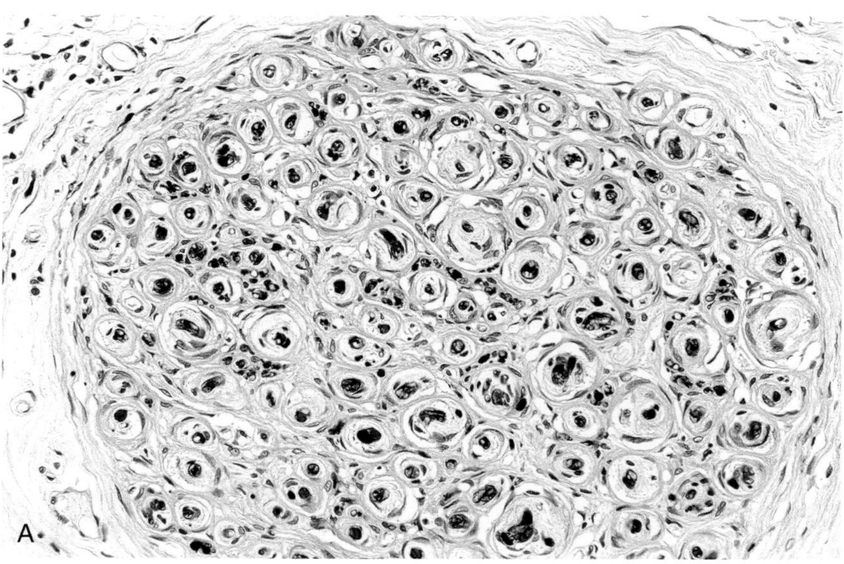

FIGURE 27-92. Intraneural perineurioma. S-100 protein immunostain decorates Schwann cells but not perineurial cells (A).

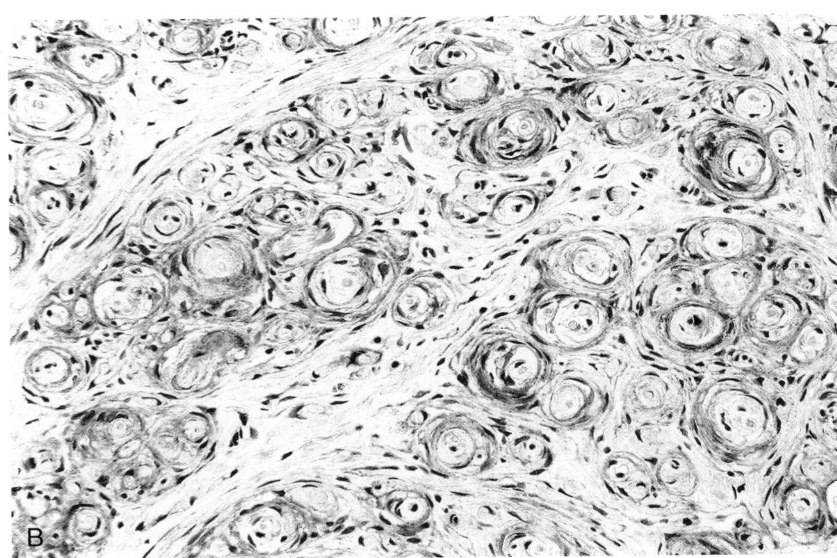

FIGURE 27-92, cont'd. Epithelial membrane antigen (EMA) immunostain shows reverse pattern with positively staining perineurial component and no staining of Schwann cells (B).

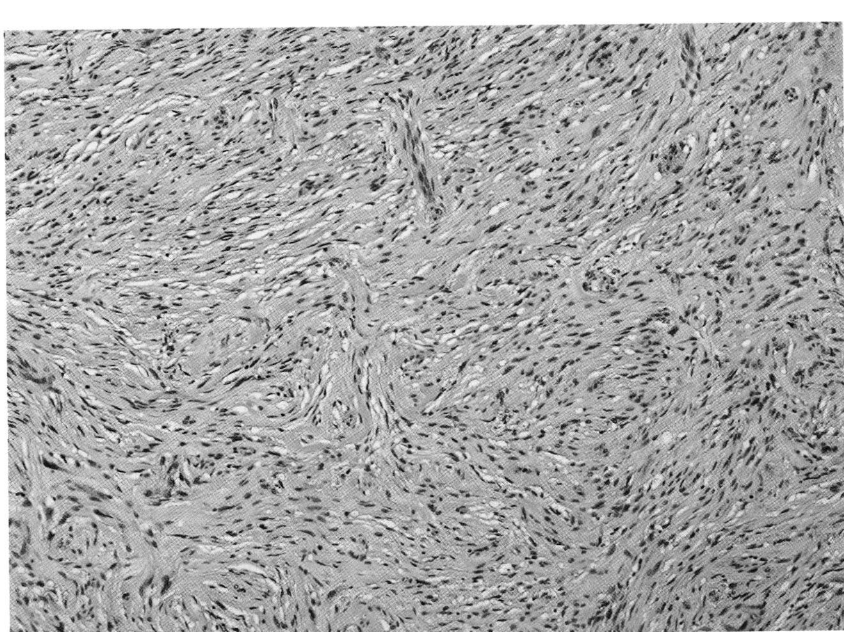

FIGURE 27-93. Extraneural (soft tissue) perineurioma with slender perineurial cells arranged in short fascicles.

The question of whether the intraneural perineurioma is a true neoplasm or an unusual reactive process has been debated and is reflected in the variety of terms used for this lesion. The best evidence to date suggests that they are indeed neoplastic. These lesions are associated with significant proliferative activity (as reflected by MIB-1 and proliferating cell nuclear antigen immunoreactivity) and clonal alterations of chromosome 22.[124]

The behavior of intraneural perineurioma has been uniformly benign, with neither recurrences nor metastases reported. Nonetheless, there are no standard guidelines for the treatment of this condition. MRI has been successful in determining the extent of nerve involvement,[125] but, because complete resection with nerve grafting does not completely restore function,[126] this option should be carefully weighed against the degree of nerve compromise.

Soft Tissue (Extraneural) Perineurioma

Soft tissue perineurioma, although more common than its intraneural counterpart, is still relatively uncommon.[127-131] It occurs equally in the sexes and affects primarily adults. Most involve the superficial soft tissues of the extremities and trunk, but approximately 30% develop in deep soft tissue and rarely in visceral locations.[128] They are not associated with *NF1* or *NF2*. Although alterations of chromosome 22 have been reported, they have not been identified in *NF2* locus per se.[127,132]

The lesions are circumscribed white masses ranging in size from 1 cm to nearly 20 cm with an average of about 4 cm.[128] The most common appearance of a soft tissue perineurioma is a spindle cell lesion composed of slender fibroblast-like cells with long streamer-like cell processes arranged in a storiform, whorled, pacinian, or short fascicular pattern (Figs. 27-93 to

27-97). The lesions vary in their cellularity, although most are hypocellular. Those with little stroma and a storiform pattern resemble dermatofibrosarcoma protuberans or benign fibrous histiocytoma, whereas those that are myxoid are often compared to myxoid neurofibromas. Highly collagenized perineuriomas provide a close mimicry to low-grade fibromyxoid sarcoma. Unfortunately, EMA, a characteristic marker of perineurioma, can also be seen in low-grade fibromyxoid sarcomas. On the other hand, MUC4, a relatively new marker, is a remarkably sensitive maker of low grade fibromyxoid sarcoma which can be employed diagnostically. The distinction between the two can also be facilitated by molecular analysis to determine the presence of the low-grade fibromyxoid sarcoma-associated translocation.

The diagnosis of perineurioma is suggested in some perineuriomas by widely separated slender processes that may appear to ramify within or dissect through the matrix (see Fig. 27-94). Ossification occurs rarely.[133] Approximately 20% of perineuriomas have atypical features that include scattered atypical cells, low levels of mitotic activity (less than 13/30 HPF), increased cellularity, and infiltration of muscle. So far, these lesions have not pursued a significantly different course from typical cases.[128]

Definitionally, all benign perineuriomas are EMA-positive and S-100 protein-negative (see Fig. 27-97), an immunophenotype that mirrors the normal perineurial cell. In addition, the majority of perineuriomas also express claudin-1,[134] a tight junction-associated protein, and GLUT1, human erythrocyte glucose transporter,[135] barrier function proteins present in normal perineurial cells.[136,137] Because EMA staining in perineuriomas is membranous, it may be difficult to appreciate if the cell processes are widely separated. Consequently, high-power examination of the tumor may be necessary. Claudin-1, on the other hand, is more diffusely and robustly expressed

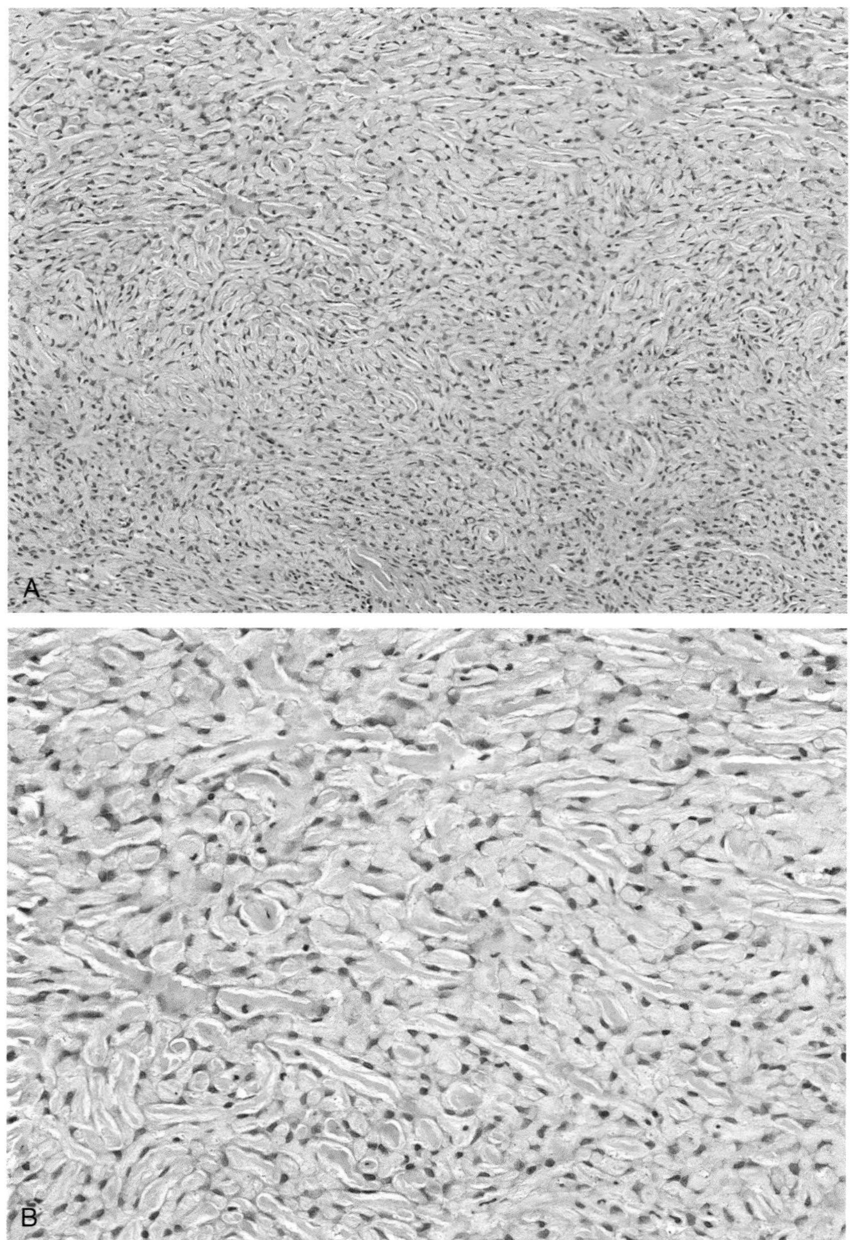

FIGURE 27-94. Soft tissue perineurioma showing anastomosing pattern of cells (A, B).

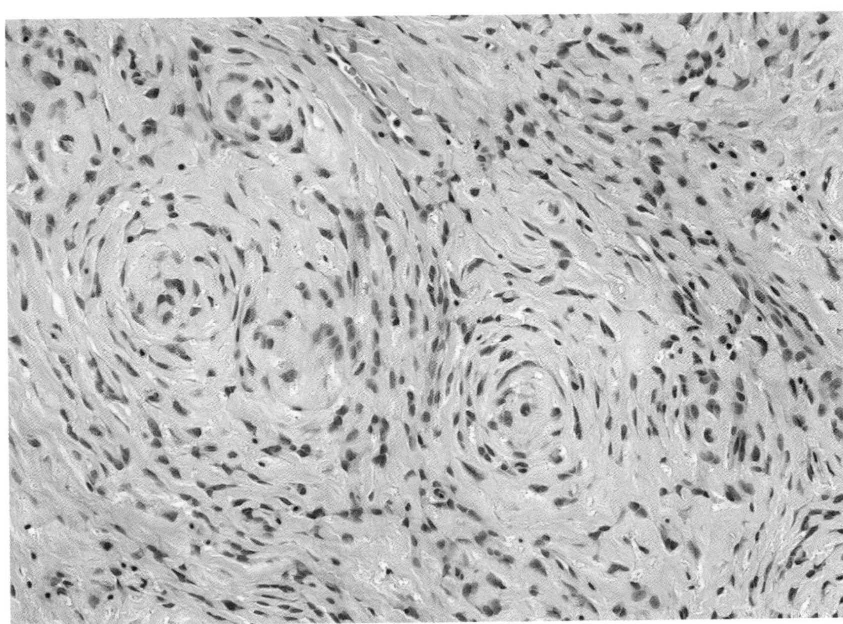

FIGURE 27-95. Whorled structures in a perineurioma.

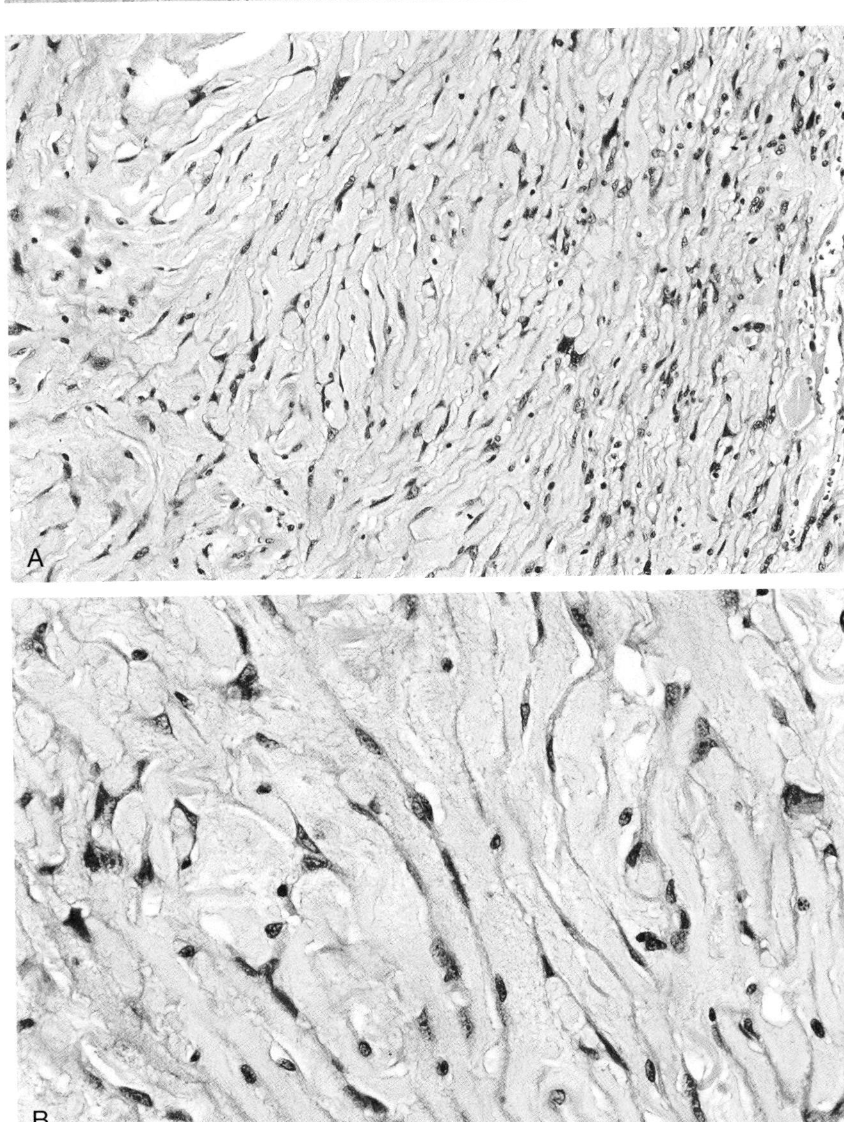

FIGURE 27-96. (A) Extraneural (soft tissue) perineurioma with cytologic atypia. (B) High-power view illustrating slender cell processes. The tumor behaved in an aggressive fashion.

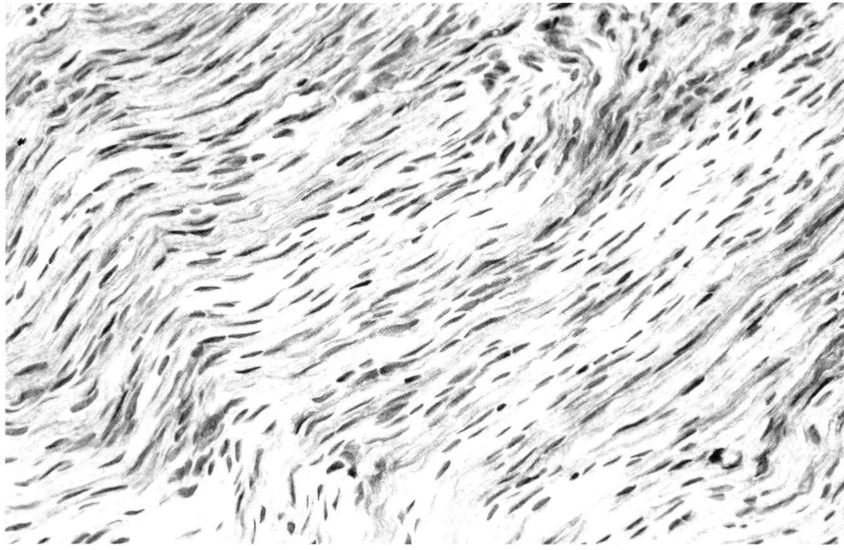

FIGURE 27-97. EMA immunostaining of a perineurioma.

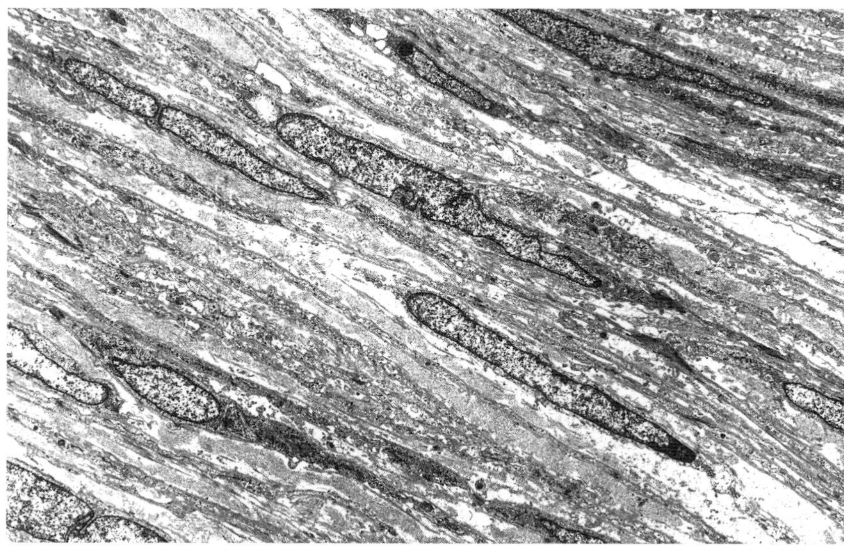

FIGURE 27-98. Electron micrograph of a perineurioma showing slender elongated cells invested with basal lamina.

and, therefore, is easier to interpret. Type IV collagen and laminin, two components of the basement membrane, also decorate the abundant basal lamina elaborated by the perineurial cell. This finding, however, is not specific for perineurial tumors and is seen in a variety of other soft tissue lesions, particularly conventional schwannomas. Between 20% and 60% of perineuriomas express CD34 and actin.[1] Electron microscopic identification may be used in lieu of immunohistochemistry, although the relative ease and low cost of immunohistochemistry has decreased its popularity. The attributes of perineurial cells include slender, nontapered processes containing large numbers of pinocytotic vesicles and partial investment with basal lamina (Figs. 27-98 and 27-99).

Most perineuriomas possess little or no atypia and no mitotic activity; however, in the experience of Hornick and Fletcher,[128] 14 of 81 cases of perineuriomas had one or more atypical features, including mitotic activity (as high as 13/30 HPF), occasional pleomorphic cells, hypercellular foci, or infiltration of skeletal muscle (1 case). Only 2 of 81 cases recurred and none metastasized within a mean follow-up period of 41 months, suggesting that none of these features per se predict malignancy.

Sclerosing Perineurioma

An unusual variant of soft tissue perineurioma has been described by Fetsch and Miettinen[138] as *sclerosing perineurioma*.[135,139] These lesions occur primarily in young men and affect the hand exclusively. Unlike the foregoing forms of perineurioma, the cells vary from spindled to distinctly rounded and are arranged in cords, trabeculae, and chains within a densely sclerotic stroma (Fig. 27-100). In addition to EMA and GLUT1 [135] positivity, nearly half of the lesions

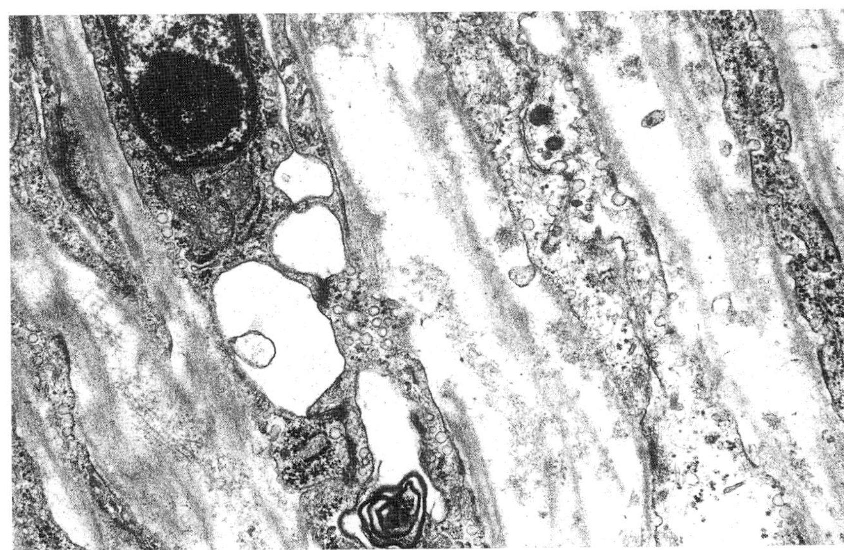

FIGURE 27-99. Electron micrograph of a perineurioma. A process of the perineurial cell is invested in basal lamina and has surface-oriented pinocytotic vesicles.

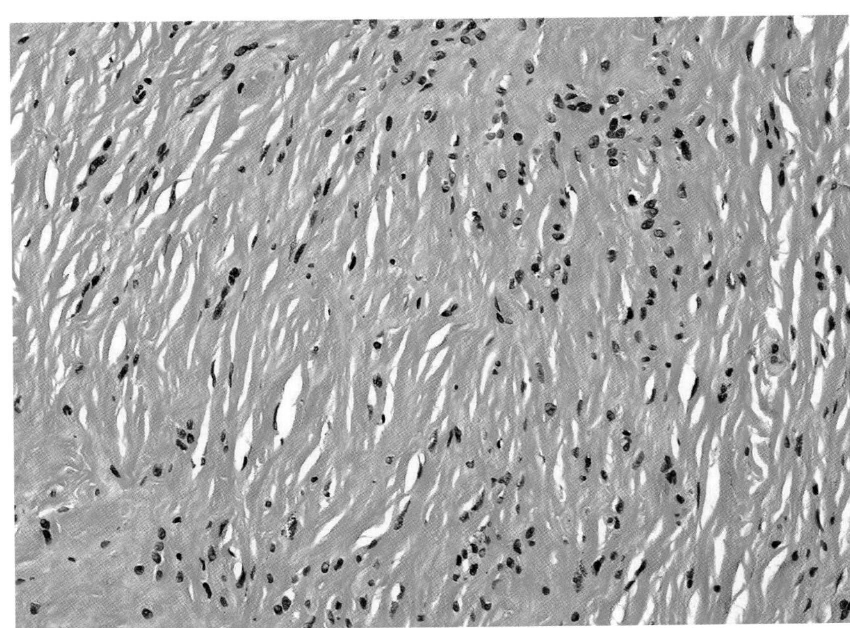

FIGURE 27-100. Sclerosing perineurioma.

also express smooth muscle or muscle-specific actin. The differential diagnosis includes a variety of epithelioid lesions (e.g., epithelioid hemangioendothelioma, adnexal tumors) and fibrosing lesions (fibroma of the tendon sheath, calcifying fibrous pseudotumor, fibrosing tenosynovial giant cell tumor). Because it is a recently recognized tumor, it is likely that many perineuriomas were previously diagnosed as fibrous histiocytoma, dermatofibrosarcoma protuberans, neurofibroma, or meningioma. Although it is occasionally possible to suspect the diagnosis of a perineurioma when distinct whorls are present in a tumor or when a presumed neurofibroma fails to stain for S-100 protein, the diagnosis must be confirmed with immunohistochemistry. Rearrangements/deletions of 10q[140] and deletions of *NF2* have been documented in this form of perineurioma.[140]

Reticular Perineurioma

Reticular perineurioma is a variant of perineurioma characterized by a lace-like arrangement of cells that results in the formation of microscopic cysts (Fig. 27-101).[141-144] Aside from the unusual histologic appearance, they appear to be similar to classic perineurioma.

Perineurial MPNST (Malignant Perineurioma)

By convention, the term *perineurioma* is used to refer to lesions with histologically benign or, at most, minimally atypical features, as described previously. However, tumors possessing the cytoarchitectural features of benign perineurioma, including

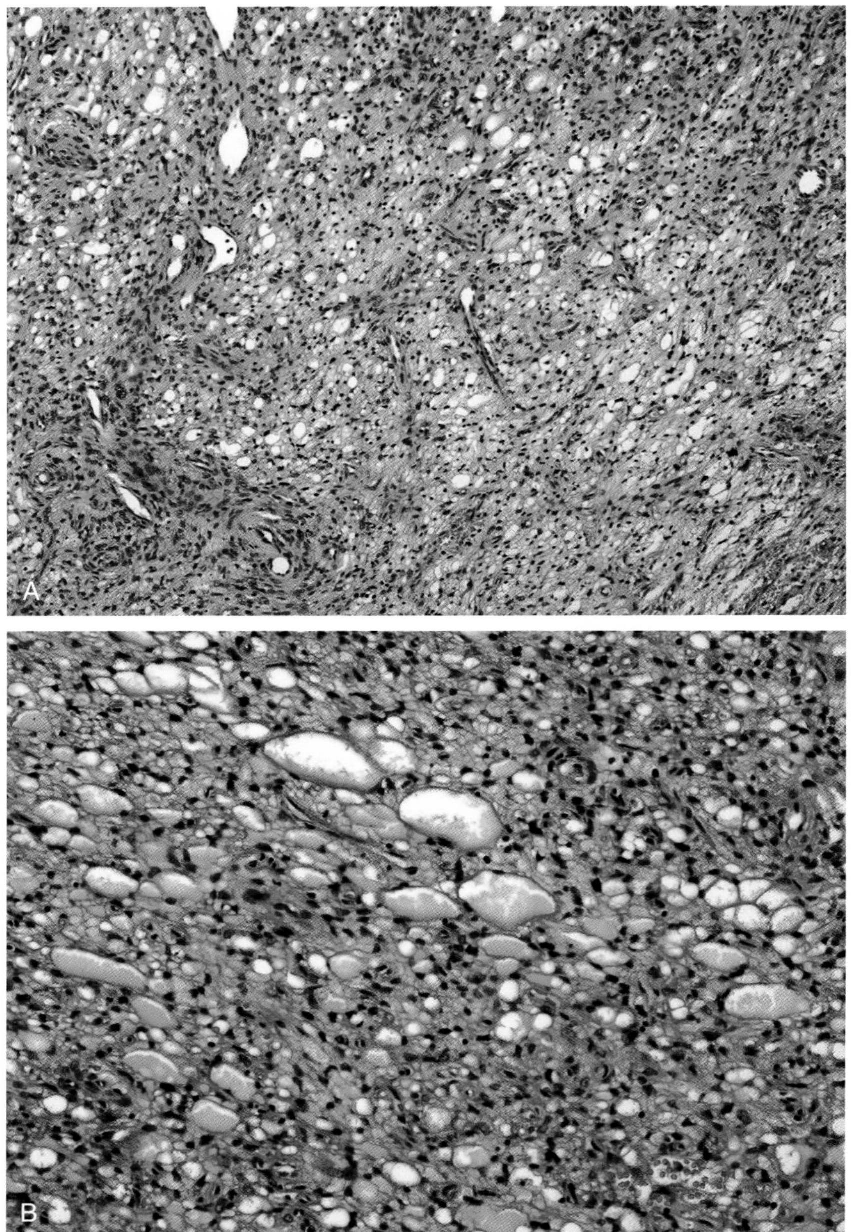

FIGURE 27-101. Reticular perineurioma (A) illustrating microscopic cysts (B).

cellular whorls and cells with thread-like cytoplasmic processes, and also significant atypia and mitotic activity that would qualify as overt malignancy, have been recognized and designated perineurial MPNST (Figs. 27-102 and 27-103).[145] Seven such cases were recognized among 121 MPNST from the Mayo Clinic. Clinically, these tumors had a similar presentation similar to other MPNST, although none was associated with a neurofibroma or occurred in a patient with NF1. Four of the tumors were high grade, and three were low grade. Four of the seven cases recurred, and two metastasized.

GRANULAR CELL TUMOR

The granular cell tumor is a benign neural tumor characterized by large granular-appearing eosinophilic cells. Reactive granular lesions consisting of collections of granular-appearing histiocytes at sites of trauma comprise a separate, unrelated entity (see Chapter 11).[146]

Granular cell tumors are small, painless nodules presenting typically in the dermis or subcutis, although deep soft tissues and organs are occasionally involved. The majority occur in adults, and women are affected twice as often as men (Fig. 27-104). About 10% to 15% of patients have multiple lesions that appear synchronously or metachronously over time. Multiple granular cell tumors have been reported in LEOPARD syndrome associated with mutations in *PTPN11*.[147]

Pathologic Findings

Granular cell tumors are poorly circumscribed nodules usually less than 3 cm in diameter with a pale yellow-tan appearance. About two-thirds of the nodules are located in the dermal or

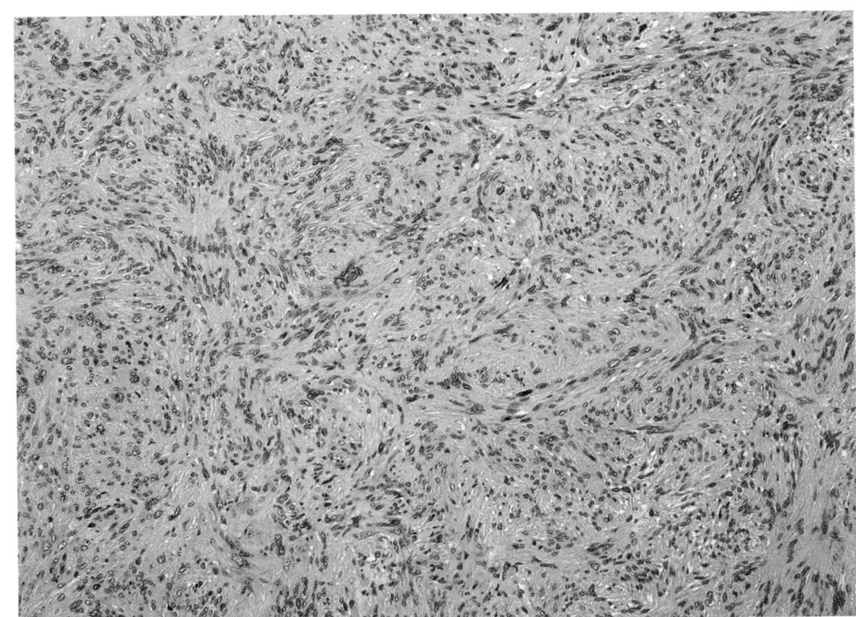

FIGURE 27-102. Perineurial malignant peripheral nerve sheath tumor illustrating generalized nuclear atypia.

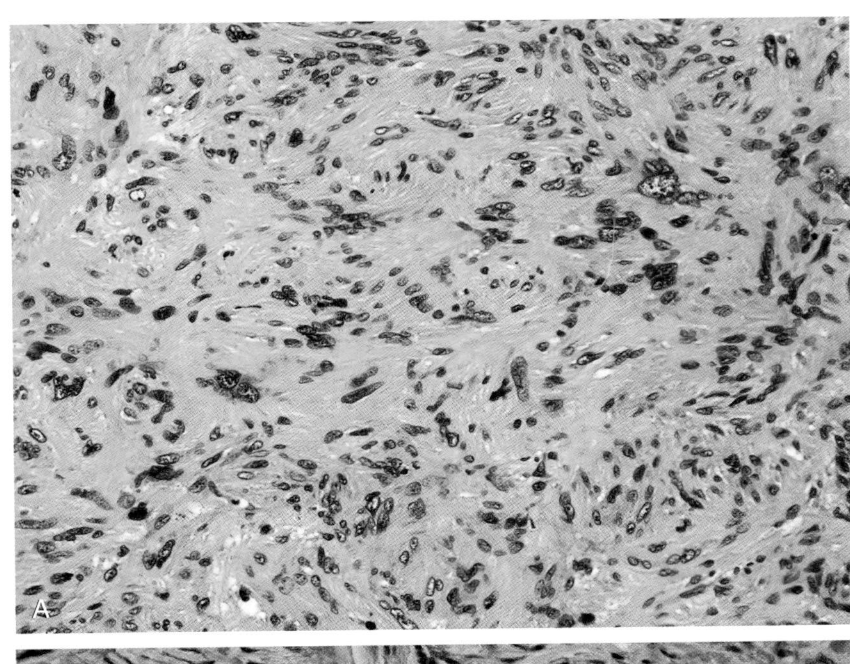

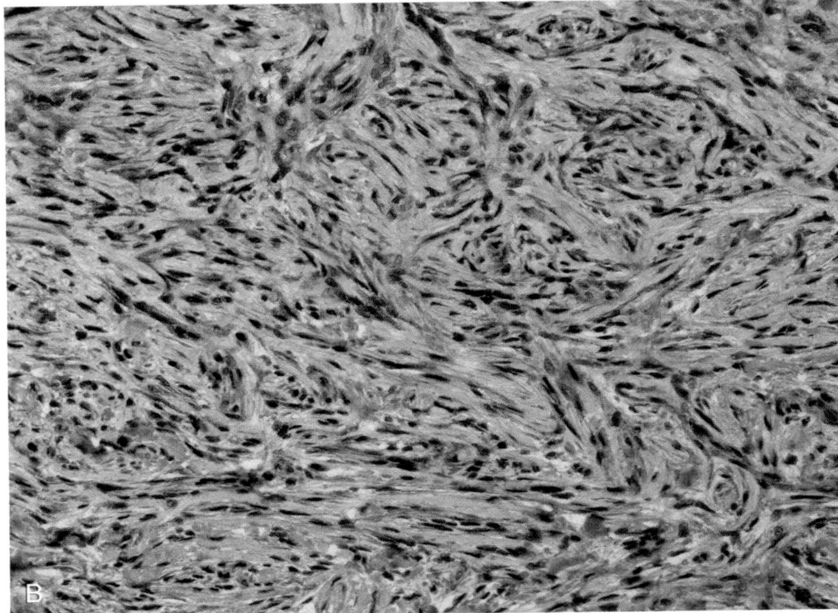

FIGURE 27-103. Perineurial malignant peripheral nerve sheath tumor (malignant perineurioma) (A). Tumor was strongly and diffusely claudin-1 positive (B).

subcutaneous tissues where they are associated with marked pseudoepitheliomatous hyperplasia of the skin, a feature that can result in a mistaken diagnosis of squamous cell carcinoma (Fig. 27-105). The cells are disposed in ribbons or nests divided by slender fibrous connective tissue septa or in large sheets with no particular cellular arrangement. Older lesions frequently exhibit marked desmoplasia, and some of these can be identified by the presence of only a few scattered nests of granular cells in a dense mass of collagen. Tumors tend to grow along muscle fibers and along nerve sheath (Fig. 27-106). Rarely, benign granular cell tumor may be identified in lymph nodes (Fig. 27-107).

The cells of granular cell tumor are rounded, polygonal, or slightly spindled in character, with nuclei ranging from small and dark to large with vesicular chromatin (Figs. 27-108 and 27-109). Mild to moderate amounts of nuclear atypia may be seen, but in and of itself is not indicative of malignancy

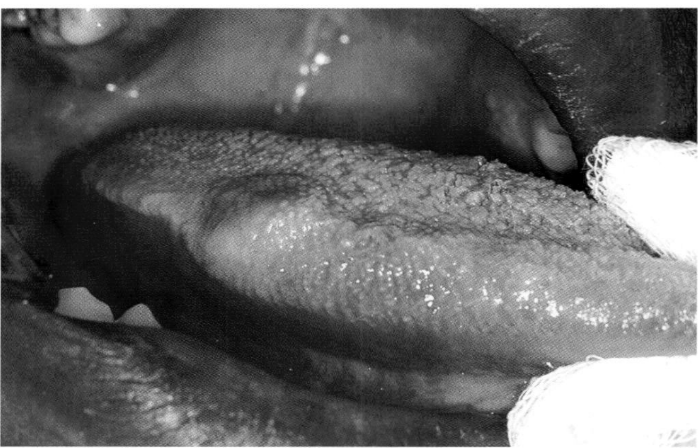

FIGURE 27-104. Granular cell tumor of the tongue.

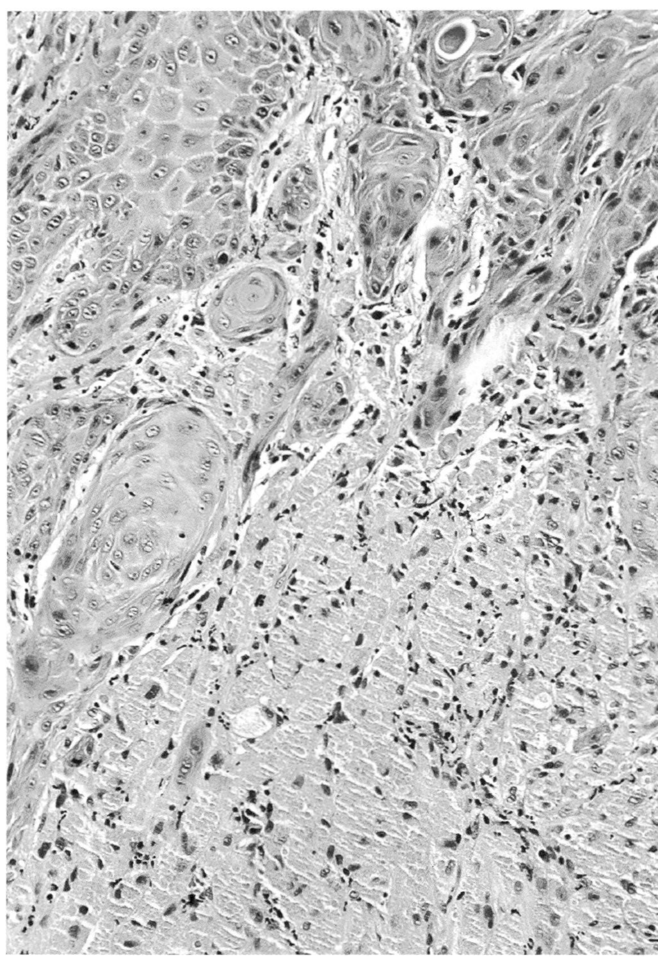

FIGURE 27-105. Granular cell tumor with pseudoepitheliomatous hyperplasia of the overlying skin.

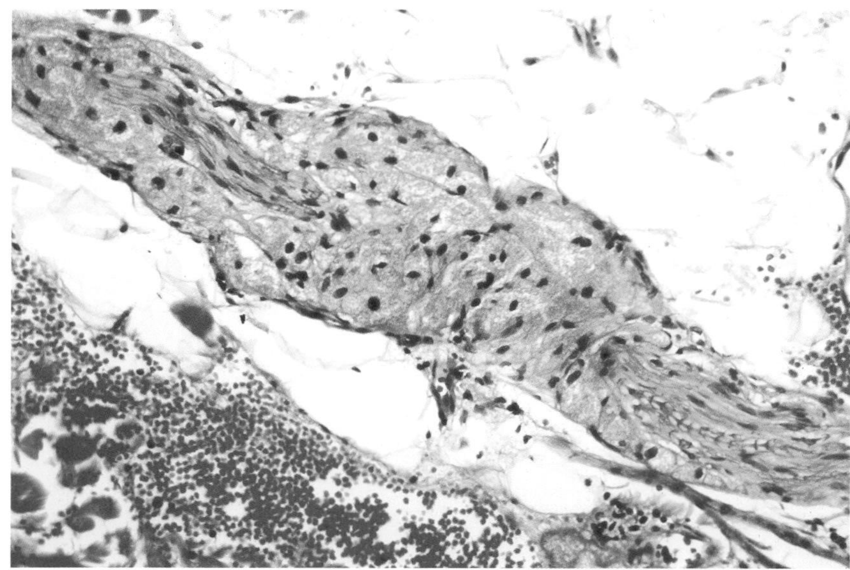

FIGURE 27-106. Granular cell tumor involving a small nerve.

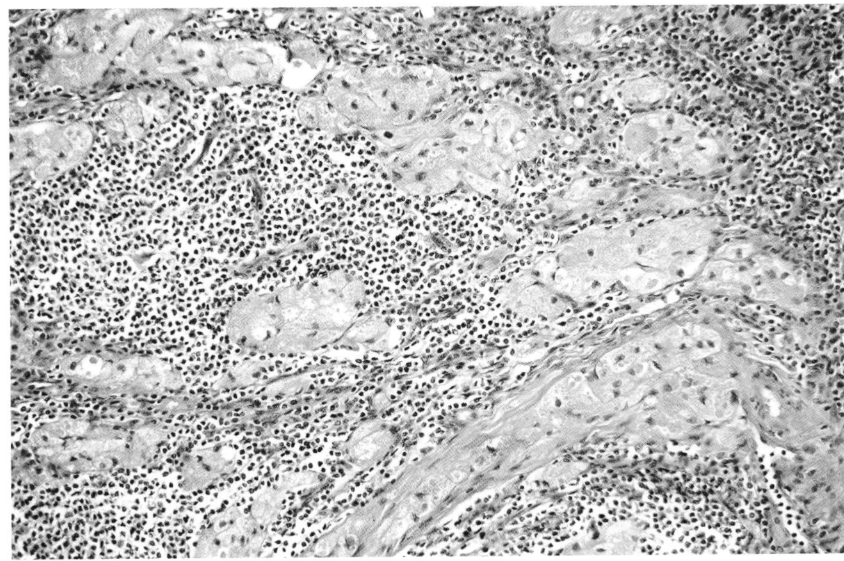

FIGURE 27-107. Granular cell tumor involving a lymph node.

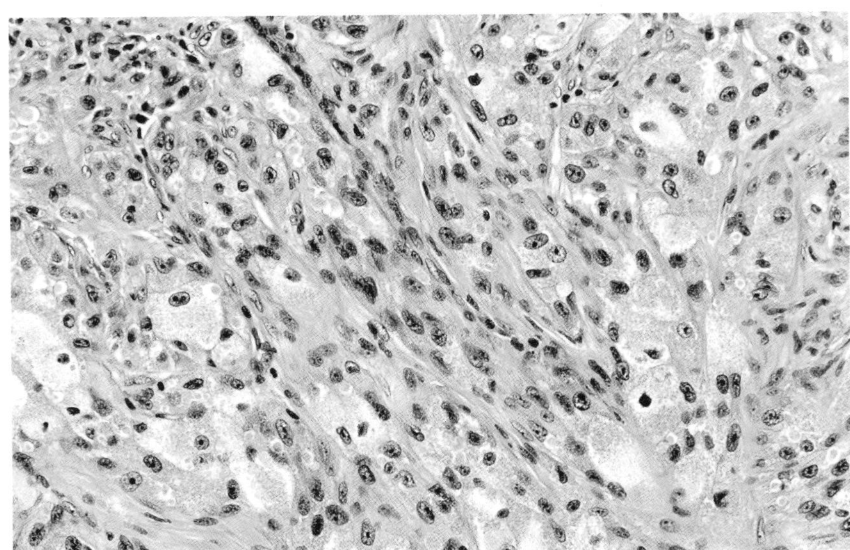

FIGURE 27-108. Granular cell tumor with spindled and rounded tumor cells.

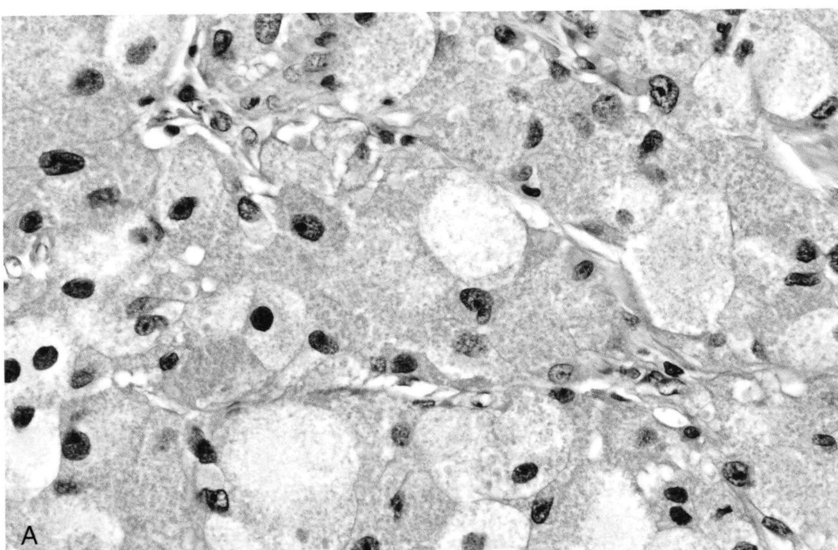

FIGURE 27-109. Granular cell tumor with a range of nuclear appearances. Some nuclei are small and dark (A), *Continued*

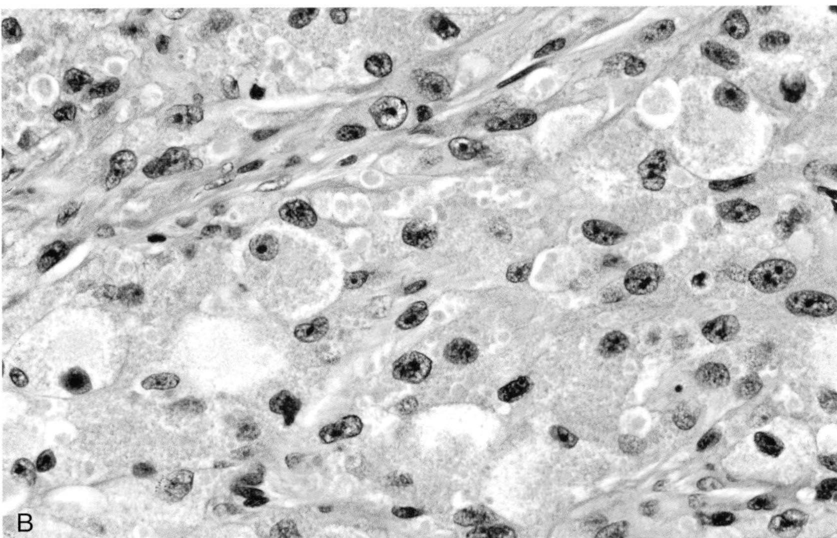

FIGURE 27-109, cont'd. and others are larger with a vesicular nuclear chromatin pattern (B).

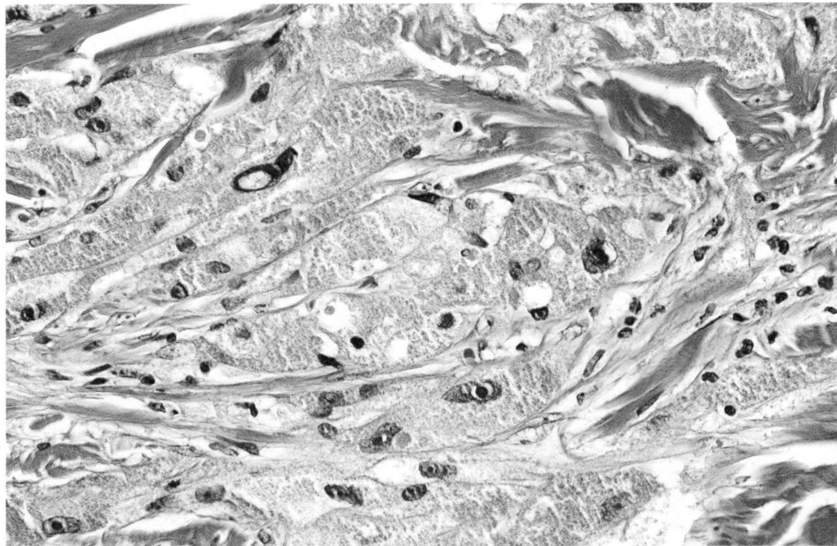

FIGURE 27-110. Benign granular cell tumor with atypical cells. This change does not per se indicate malignancy.

(Fig. 27-110). The eosinophilic cytoplasm is fine to coarsely granular. The granules, representing phagolysosomes, are strongly periodic acid-Schiff (PAS)-positive and diastase-resistant (Fig. 27-111). Smaller cells containing coarse particles that are strongly PAS-positive are interspersed between the granular cells (interstitial cells, angulate body cells).

The tumors express S-100 protein (Fig. 27-112), neuron-specific enolase, laminin, and various myelin proteins. Because the characteristic granules are lysosomal in nature, they are also strongly positive for CD68 (Kp1).[148,149] The cells do not react with antibodies for neurofilament proteins or GFAP.[146,150,151]

Ultrastructurally, the granular cell tumor contains intracellular granules consisting of membrane-bound, autophagic, vacuoles containing myelin figures and fragmented rough endoplasmic reticulum and mitochondria. According to some authors, myelinated and nonmyelinated axon-like structures are also present (Figs. 27-113 and 27-114). There are also small interstitial cells with angulated bodies containing packets of parallel microtubules (Fig. 27-115), microfilaments, and lipid material as well as cells with multiple cytoplasmic processes, partly surrounded by incomplete basal laminae.

Differential Diagnosis

A number of benign mesenchymal tumors have a granular appearance. The coarsely granular cytoplasm and the absence of cross-striations and glycogen distinguish the benign granular cell tumor from rhabdomyoma; the absence of lipid droplets distinguishes it from hibernoma and fibroxanthoma. Reactive histiocytic proliferations that occur in sites of injury or surgical trauma (e.g., scars of cesarean section) may simulate a benign granular cell tumor. The granular cells in these lesions are arranged in sheets or coarse nodules that circumscribe areas of necrotic debris (see Chapter 11).[146,152]

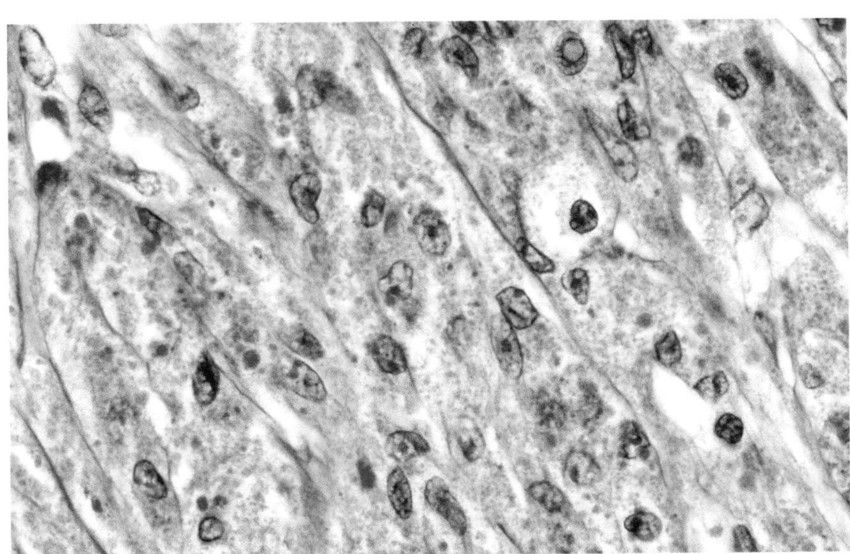

FIGURE 27-111. Periodic acid-Schiff (PAS)-positive diastase-resistant bodies in a granular cell tumor.

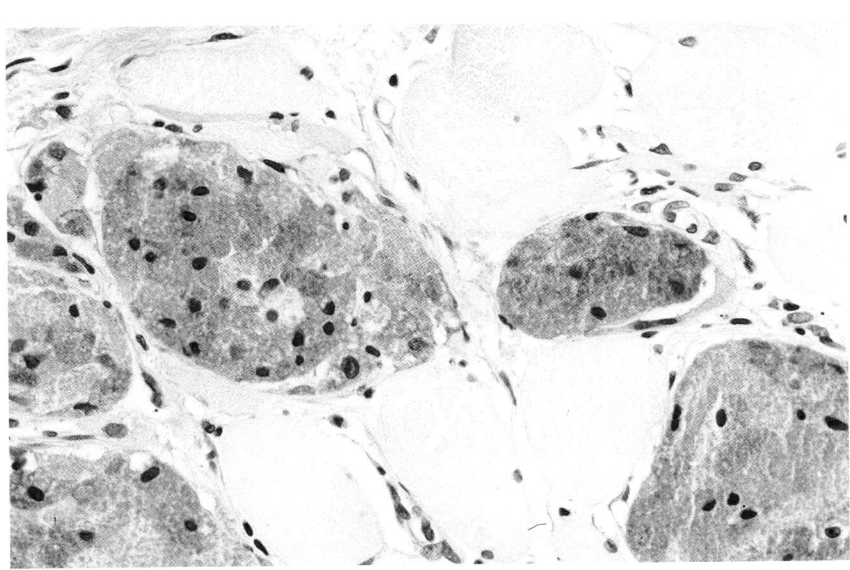

FIGURE 27-112. S-100 protein immunoreactivity in a granular cell tumor.

Discussion

Although originally considered to be a muscle tumor, the expression of S-100 protein, myelin proteins (P0 and P2), and myelin-associated glycoprotein has secured this lesion a position among benign nerve sheath tumors.[150,153] Despite their often infiltrative growth that evokes a striking desmoplasia, the lesions are benign. Of 92 cases reported by Strong et al.,[154] six recurred, one of them after 10 years. Therefore, local surgical excision is curative in nearly all cases.

Malignant Granular Cell Tumor

Malignant granular tumors are extremely rare, as evidenced from Fanburg-Smith et al.[155] having culled only 46 cases from the archives of the Armed Forces Institute of Pathology. In most respects, malignant tumors are similar to benign ones except they tend to be larger. Some patients give a history of recent growth in a long-standing lesion, suggesting malignant transformation of a preexisting benign lesion.

Although, in the earlier literature, a variety of malignant soft tissue tumors were labeled malignant granular cell tumors (e.g., granular cell leiomyosarcoma), this diagnosis should be restricted to neoplasms that are histologically similar to benign granular cell tumors but that have a constellation of histologic features that portend an increased risk for metastasis.[155] Such features include necrosis, spindling, vesicular nuclei with prominent nucleoli, increased mitotic activity (greater than 2 mitoses/10 HPF), high nucleocytoplasmic ratio, and pleomorphism. Tumors with three or more of these features are considered malignant and have an approximately 40% risk of causing death (Figs. 27-116 and 27-117). Tumors with fewer than three features (termed *atypical granular cell tumor*) have an excellent outcome with no metastases. This system provides a systematic approach to identifying lesions with a significant

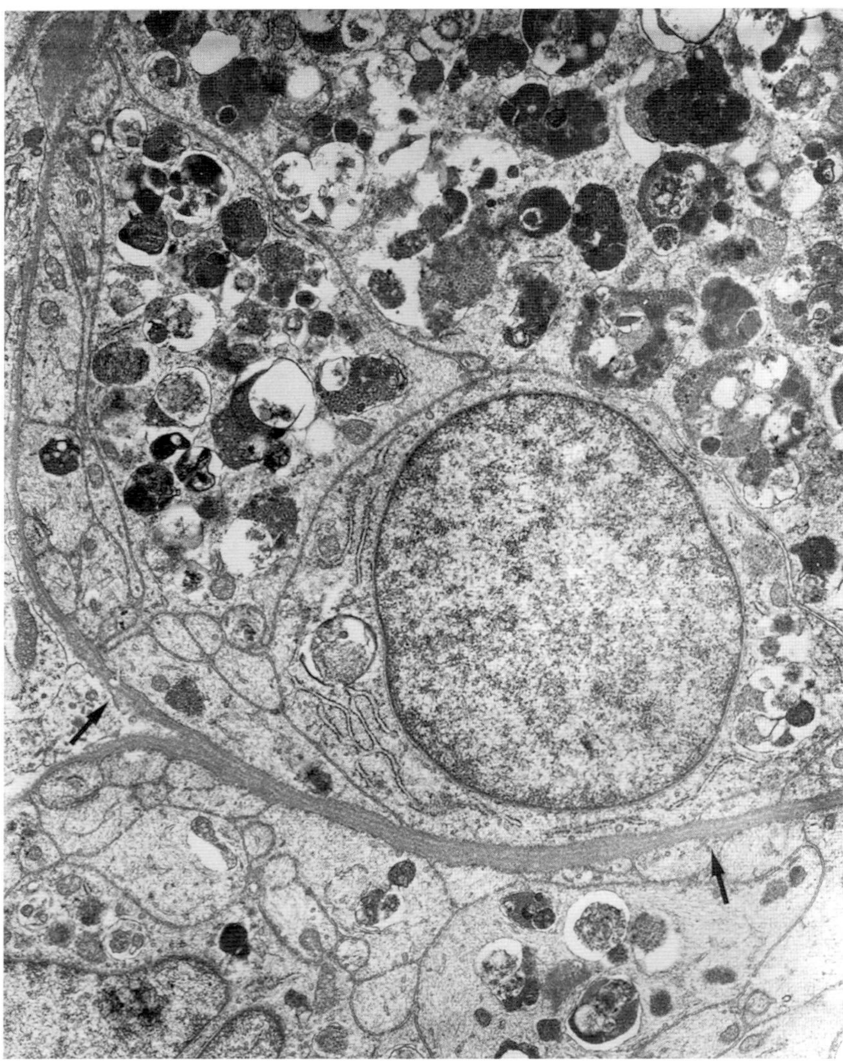

FIGURE 27-113. Ultrastructure of granular cell tumor. Large autophagic granules in the cytoplasm of the tumor cell are surrounded by a distinct basal lamina (arrows). *(Courtesy of Dr. Zelma Molnar, Veterans Administration Hospital, Hines, IL.)*

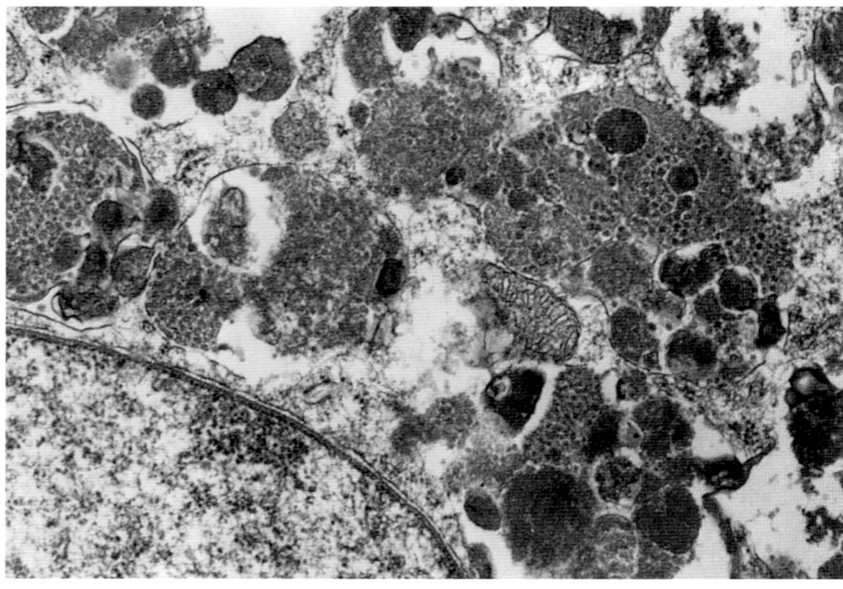

FIGURE 27-114. Large vacuoles containing finely granular structures and small masses of electron-dense material.

risk of metastasis. When using this system, it is usually required that features, such as spindling and atypia, be prominent in the tumor and not simply a focal change.

Malignant granular cell tumors usually recur before they metastasize, and the interval between diagnosis and metastasis is characteristically several years. Common metastatic sites are lymph node, lung, liver, and bone.

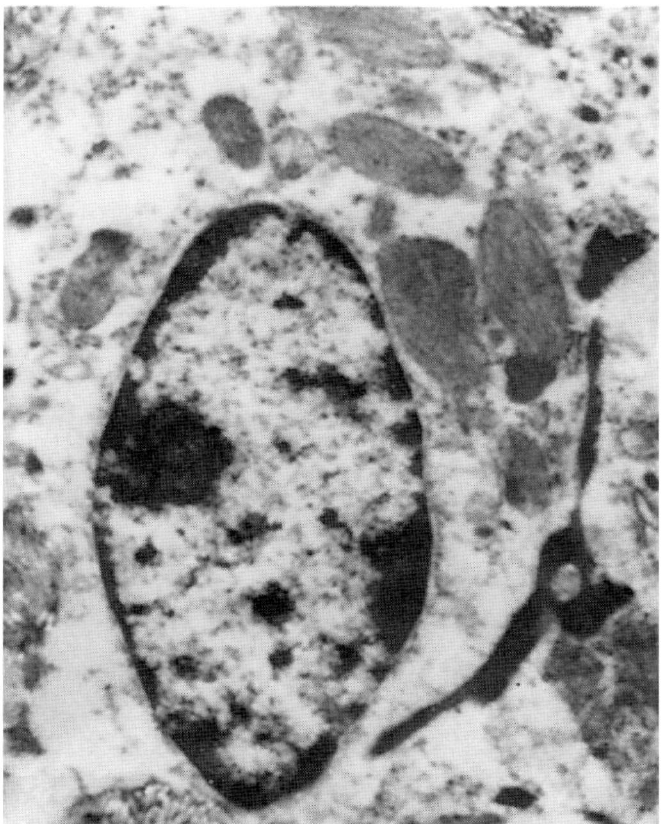

FIGURE 27-115. Angulated bodies in interstitial cell of a granular cell tumor (x7800).

CONGENITAL (GINGIVAL) GRANULAR CELL TUMOR

Congenital (gingival) granular cell tumor and its synonym, congenital epulis, refer to a gingival tumor of infants having granular features. Although superficially resembling an adult granular cell tumor, it is considered a totally different tumor with characteristic hallmarks that include location on labial aspect of the dental ridge with a predilection for the upper jaw, prominent vascularity with scattered lymphocytes and remnants of odontogenic epithelium, and no expression of S-100 protein (Fig. 27-118).[156]

A typical lesion is a small (1 cm), round or ovoid, protruding nodule covered by a smooth mucosal surface and firmly attached to the gum by a broad base or pedicle. Ulceration of the mucosa is uncommon, and there is no pseudoepitheliomatous hyperplasia of the mucosa.[157] Congenital granular cell tumors stabilize in their growth after birth, and some regress spontaneously. Lack et al.[156] reported that lesions treated later in the neonatal period were smaller and exhibited some evidence of involution.

NERVE SHEATH MYXOMA

Nerve sheath myxoma is a superficial myxoid tumor first described in 1969 by Harkin and Reed. Since that report, there has been considerable debate as to its line of differentiation and its relationship to another cutaneous myxoid lesion, the neurothekeoma. Based on analysis of over 300 cases from the Armed Forces Institute of Pathology, Fetsch et al.[158] mounted a compelling argument that nerve sheath myxoma is a true nerve sheath tumor perhaps related to schwannoma and unrelated to the neurothekeoma. Differential gene expression profiling supports this view. Nerve sheath myxomas have molecular signatures very similar to dermal schwannomas, whereas all subtypes of neurothekeomas resemble the profile of fibrous histiocytomas.[159] Neurothekeomas, therefore, are discussed with benign fibrohistiocytic tumors in Chapter 11. The two lesions are compared in Table 27-4.

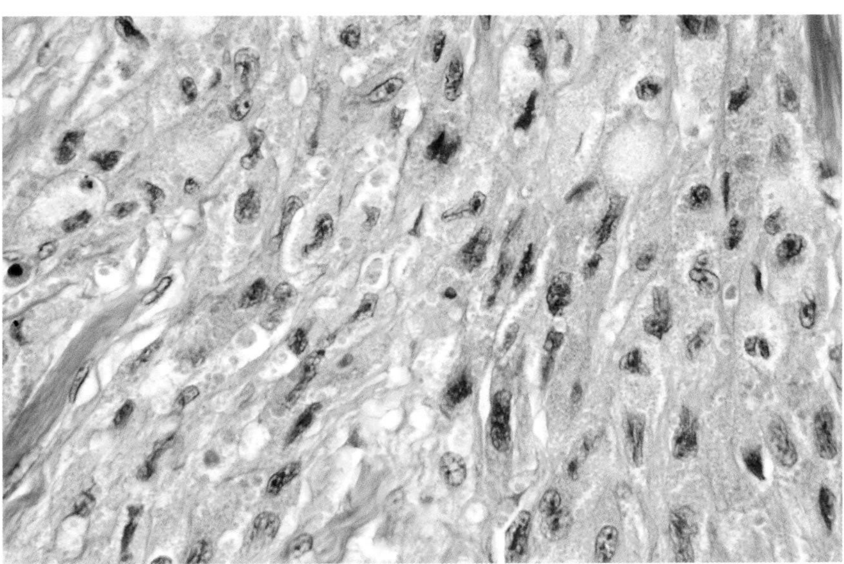

FIGURE 27-116. Malignant granular cell tumor with nuclear atypia, spindling, and prominent nucleoli.

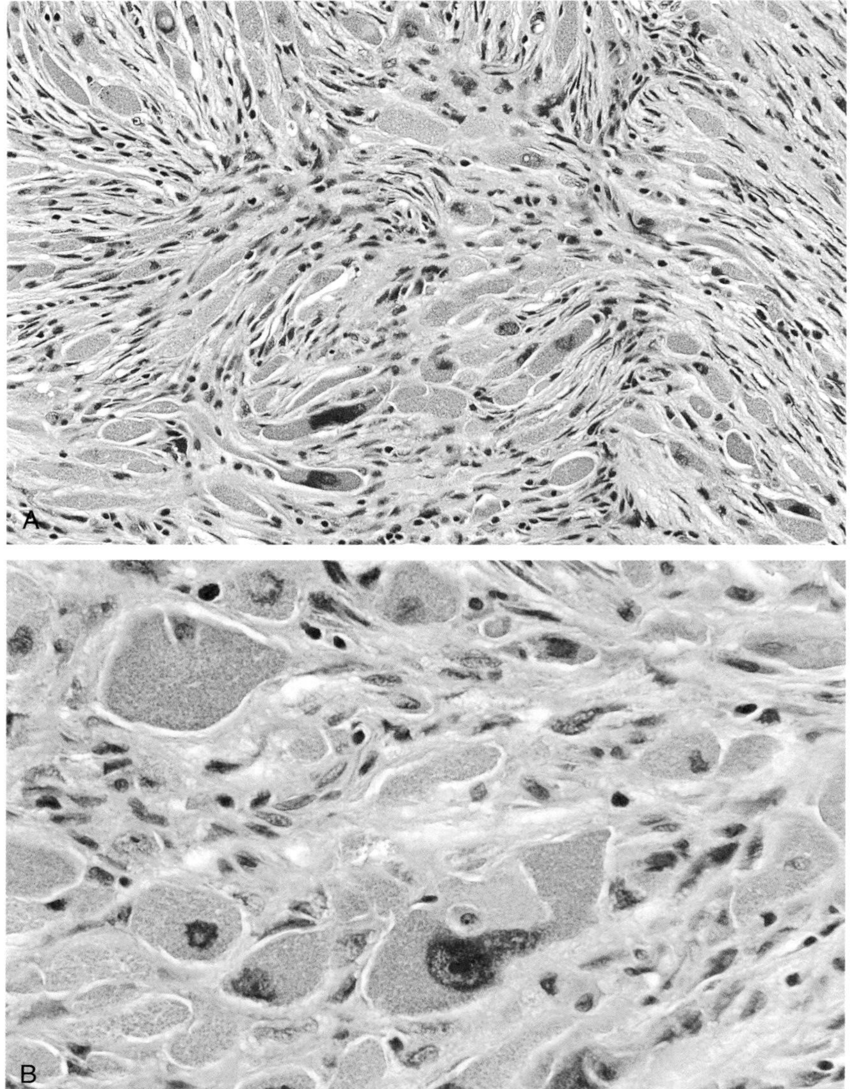

FIGURE 27-117. (A, B) Malignant granular cell tumor illustrating profound nuclear atypia, prominent nucleoli, and spindling. Mitotic figures were also identified.

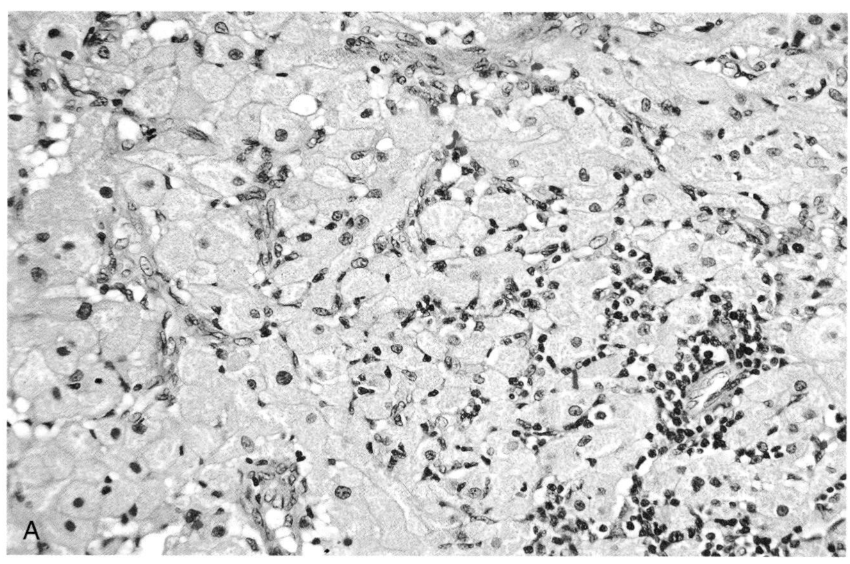

FIGURE 27-118. (A, B) Congenital granular cell tumor.

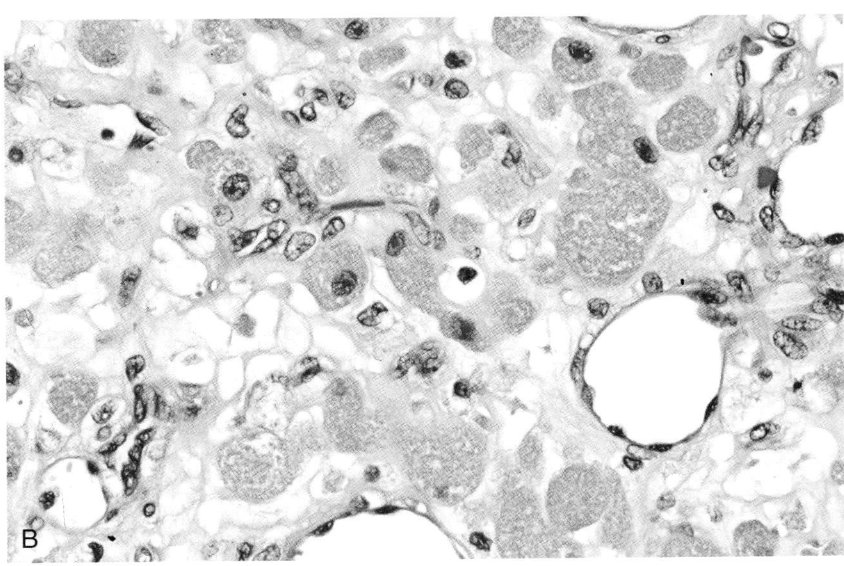

FIGURE 27-118, cont'd

TABLE 27-4 Comparison of Nerve Sheath Myxoma and Neurothekeoma

	NERVE SHEATH MYXOMA	NEUROTHEKEOMA
Age	All Ages	Children—Young Adults
Location	Dermis/subcutis of extremities	Dermis/subcutis of upper body
Histologic features	Coarse myxoid nodules composed of cords, clusters, syncytia of rounded or multipolar Schwann cells	Smaller variably myxoid and cellular nodules composed of small rounded cells and occasional giant cells
S-100 protein	Virtually all	–
GFAP	Virtually all	–
NKI/C3	–	Virtually all
MiTF	–	+

From Rios JJ, Diaz-Cano SJ, Rivera-Hueto F, et al. Cutaneous ganglion cell choristoma. Report of a case. J Cutan Pathol 1991;18(6):469–473.

GFAP, glial fibrillary acidic protein.

Nerve sheath myxomas are far rarer than neurothekeomas. They occur at all ages and affect the genders equally. Nearly 90% of cases develop on the extremity, particularly the fingers and knee. These slowly growing tumors of the dermis and/or subcutis are composed of irregularly shaped nodules bordered by fibrous bands and contain an abundant myxoid matrix (Figs. 27-119 and 27-120). The cells vary from small epithelioid cells arranged in cords or syncytial aggregates to large multipolar ones, some containing large vacuoles of stromal mucin, creating a ring appearance. The cells strongly express S-100 protein (Fig. 27-121), GFAP, neuron-specific enolase, and CD57. CD34 perineurial cells are present but are not numerous.

Although benign, nearly 50% recur, in large part, because of incomplete excisions.

EXTRACRANIAL MENINGIOMA

Extracranial meningiomas are rare tumors that occur in the skin or soft tissue of the scalp or along the vertebral axis.[160,161] In extremely rare cases, they may even develop in areas where meningeal rests do not occur. By definition, an extracranial meningioma is not associated with an underlying meningioma of the neuraxis. Extracranial extension of an intracranial tumor should always be considered before accepting a meningioma in soft tissue or skin as a primary tumor. Although true extracranial meningiomas probably arise from ectopic arachnoid lining cells, their precise presentation and localization suggest at least two pathogenetic mechanisms.[160]

One form of extracranial meningioma, termed *type I* by Lopez et al.,[160] arises in the skin of the scalp, forehead, and paravertebral areas and, as a result, may be mistaken clinically for cutaneous lesions, including epidermal inclusion cyst, skin tag, and nevus. The pathogenesis is probably similar to that of meningocele and is believed to be the result of abnormalities of neural tube closure with relocation of meningeal tissue in the surrounding skin and subcutis (Fig. 27-122). This proposal explains the congenital nature of the type I tumor and its distribution, which coincides with that of meningocele. The similarity of this tumor to meningocele is heightened by its histologic appearance. Although some consist of solid, isolated nests of meningothelial cells in the skin, others may contain a rudimentary stalk or cystic cavity (Fig. 27-123). These lesions occupy an intermediate position in the spectrum between meningocele and extracranial meningioma and have been named *meningeal hamartomas*. The type I meningioma is benign, although persistence of a connection with the central nervous system can lead to postoperative meningitis or neurologic deficits.

The second form of extracranial meningioma (type II) (Fig. 27-124) may occur at any age, but adults are usually affected. These tumors are situated in the vicinity of the sensory organs (eye, ear, nose) or along the paths of the cranial and spinal nerves. Symptoms associated with the tumor are related to its size, location, and growth rate. Histologically, these lesions are indistinguishable from the ordinary intracranial meningioma. The solid nests of meningothelial cells are arranged in sheets or whorls and occasionally are punctuated by psammoma bodies (Fig. 27-125). In addition to surgical removal, appropriate studies to exclude an intracranial component are recommended for these more deeply situated tumors.

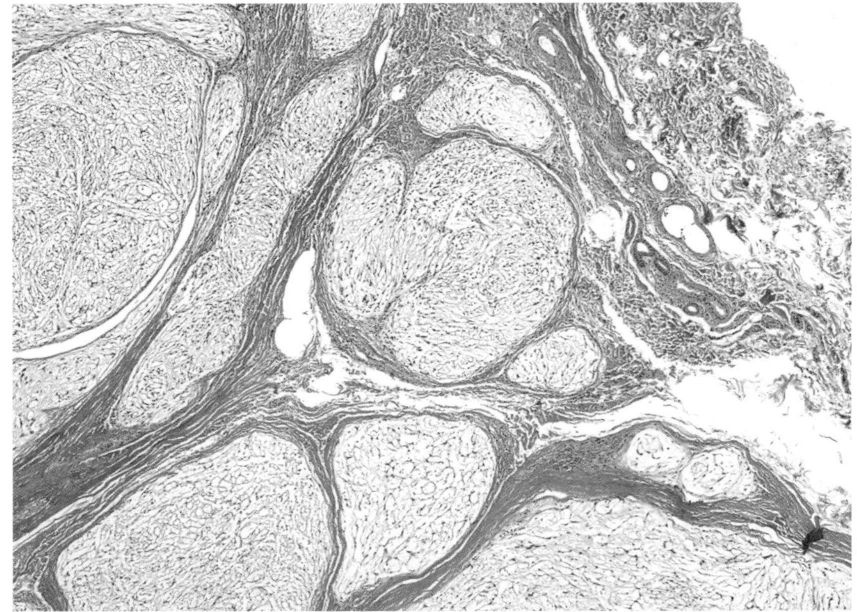

FIGURE 27-119. Nerve sheath myxoma illustrating large irregular myxoid nodules.

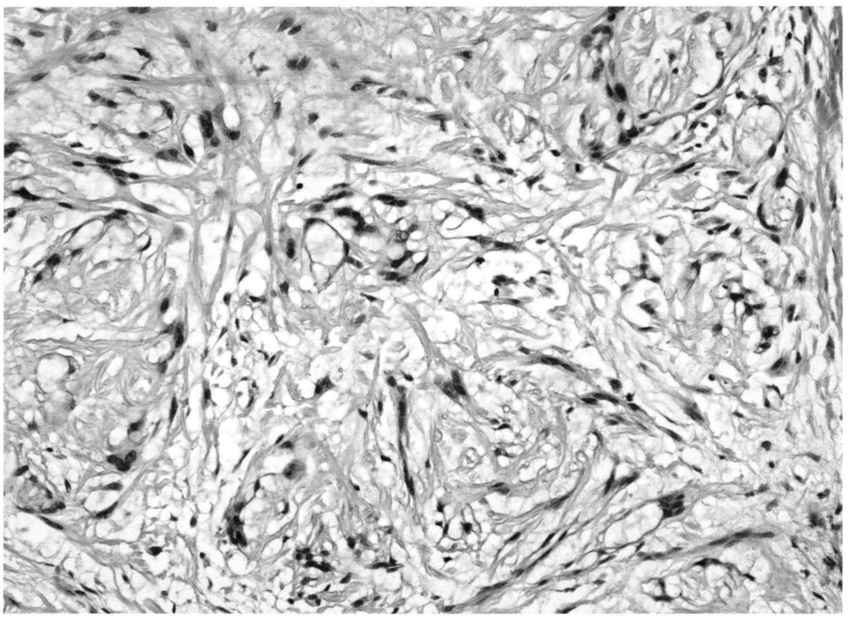

FIGURE 27-120. Nerve sheath myxoma illustrating spindled and multipolar Schwann cells.

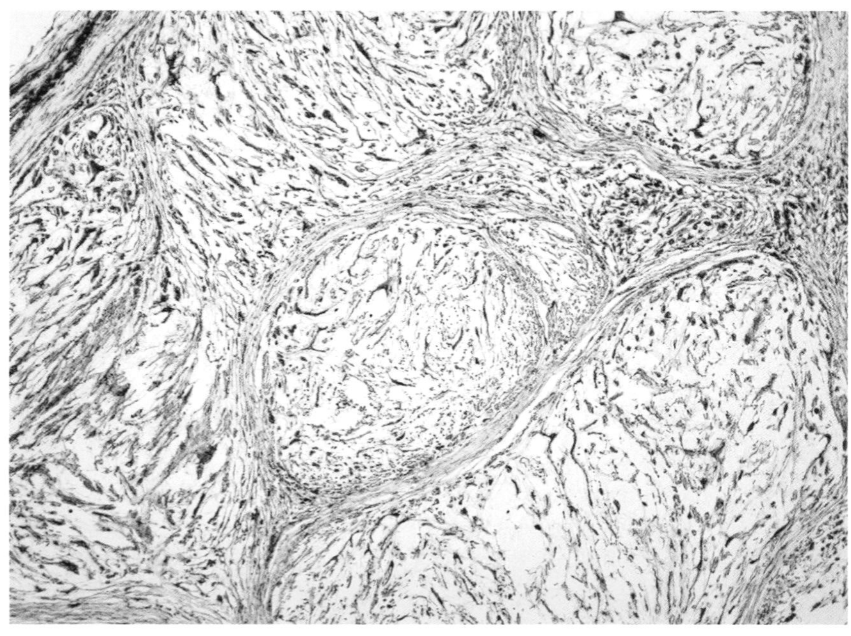

FIGURE 27-121. Nerve sheath myxoma showing strong S-100 protein expression.

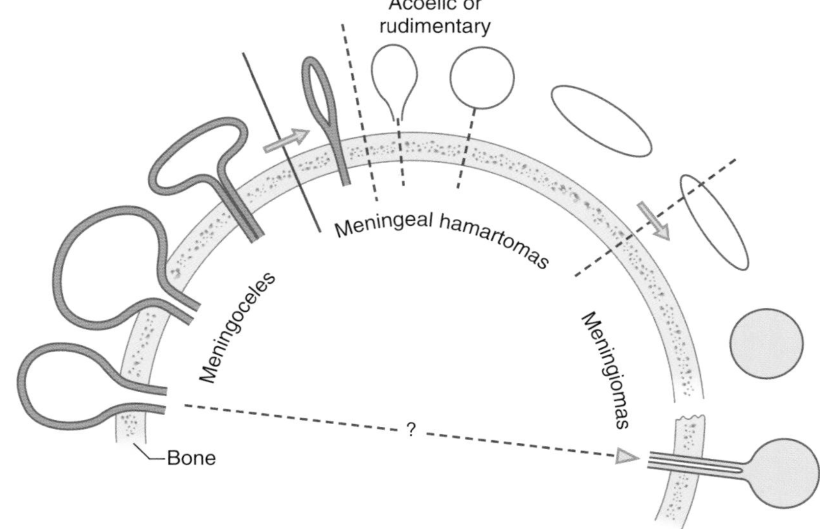

FIGURE 27-122. Histogenesis of cutaneous meningiomas. Note the possible relations between meningoceles, meningeal hamartomas, and type I extracranial meningiomas. The first retain their connections with the central nervous system and are predominantly cystic, whereas the last two lose the connections and are solid. *(From Lopez DA, Silvers DN, Helwig EB. Cutaneous meningiomas: a clinicopathologic study. Cancer 1974; 34:728.)*

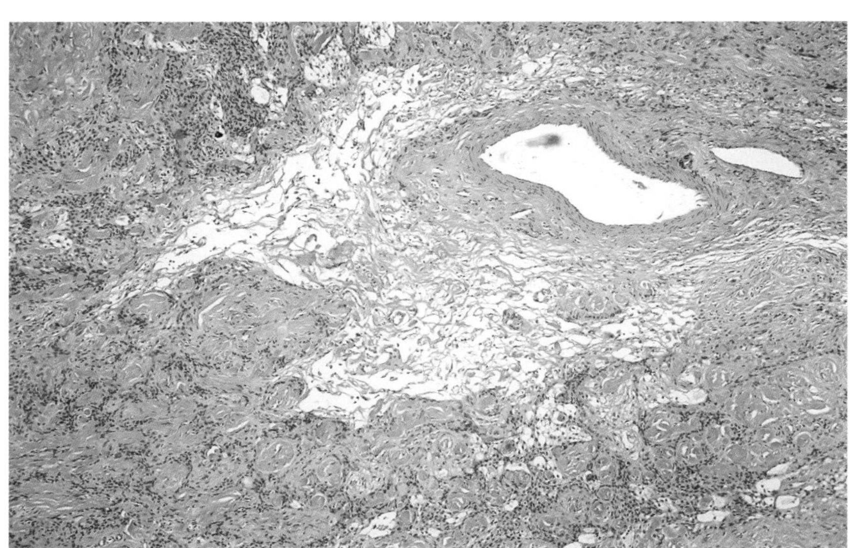

FIGURE 27-123. Type I ectopic meningioma from a child. Note the partially cystic central area.

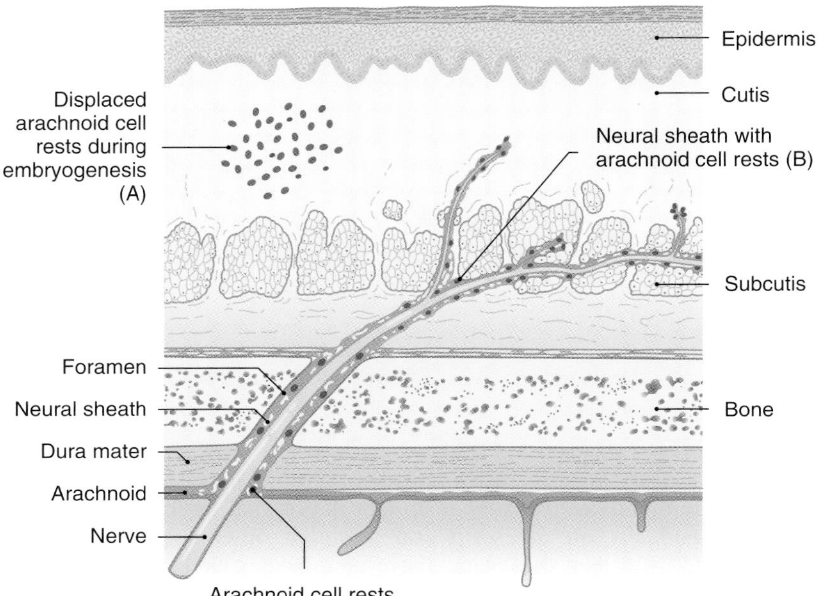

FIGURE 27-124. Primary cutaneous meningiomas. There are two possible origins of primary cutaneous meningiomas. (A) Type I may result from abnormalities of neural tube closure with resultant ectopic arachnoid cell rests. (B) Type II, which occurs in adults and follows the distribution of the sensory organs and nerves, probably is derived from arachnoid rests in nerve sheaths. *(From Lopez DA, Silvers DN, Helwig EB. Cutaneous meningiomas: a clinicopathologic study. Cancer 1974; 34:728.)*

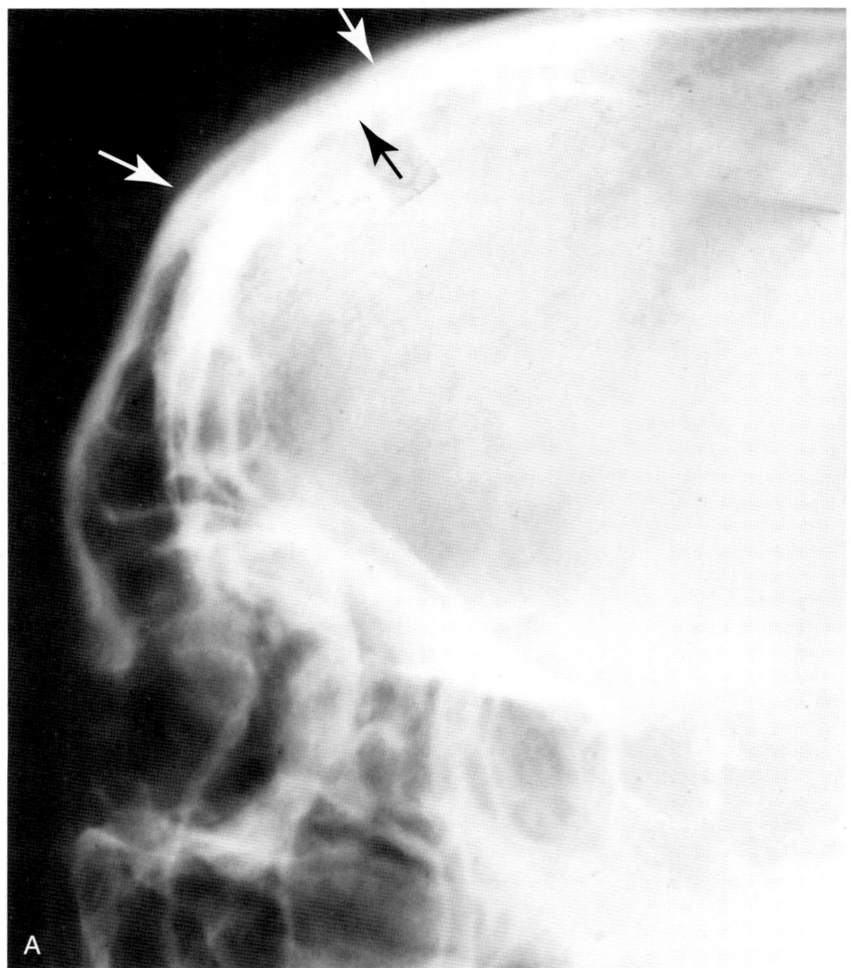

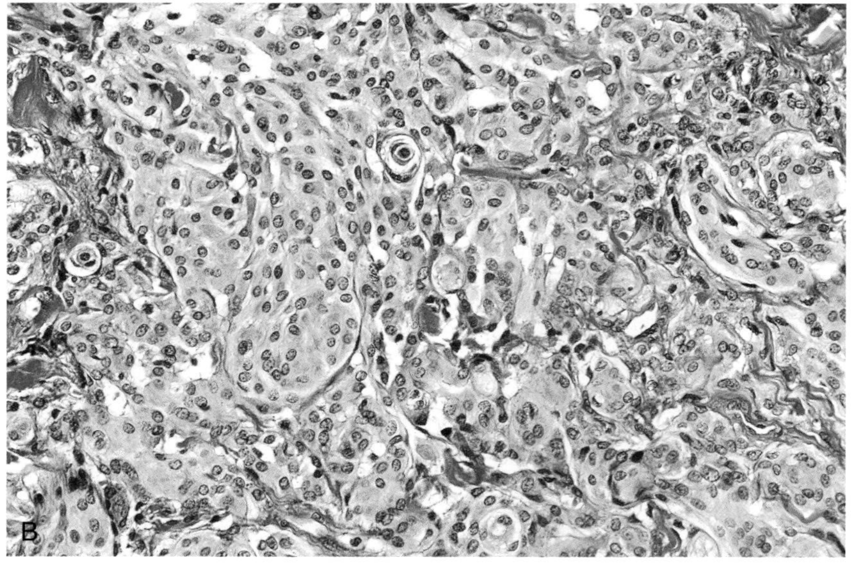

FIGURE 27-125. Primary cutaneous meningioma of the frontal area of the scalp. (A) Radiograph demonstrates extracranial location of frontal mass. The outer table of the skull is partly eroded (between the white arrows), whereas the inner table is intact (black arrow). (B) Tumor consists of whorls of plump epithelioid cells indistinguishable from cells of the intracranial form of meningioma.

GLIAL HETEROTOPIAS

Like ectopic meningeal rests, ectopic deposits of glial tissue occur occasionally on the scalp and rarely in other soft tissue sites.[162-164] Over the years, they have been called a variety of names, including *nasal glioma*, *glial hamartoma*, and *heterotopic glial tissue*.[165] The common presentation of a glial heterotopia is that of a small polypoid mass at the root of the nose or to one side of the bridge of the nose in an infant, which grows commensurately with the infant. In most cases, the lesions lack a communication with the brain; in the few that do communicate with the brain, the connection

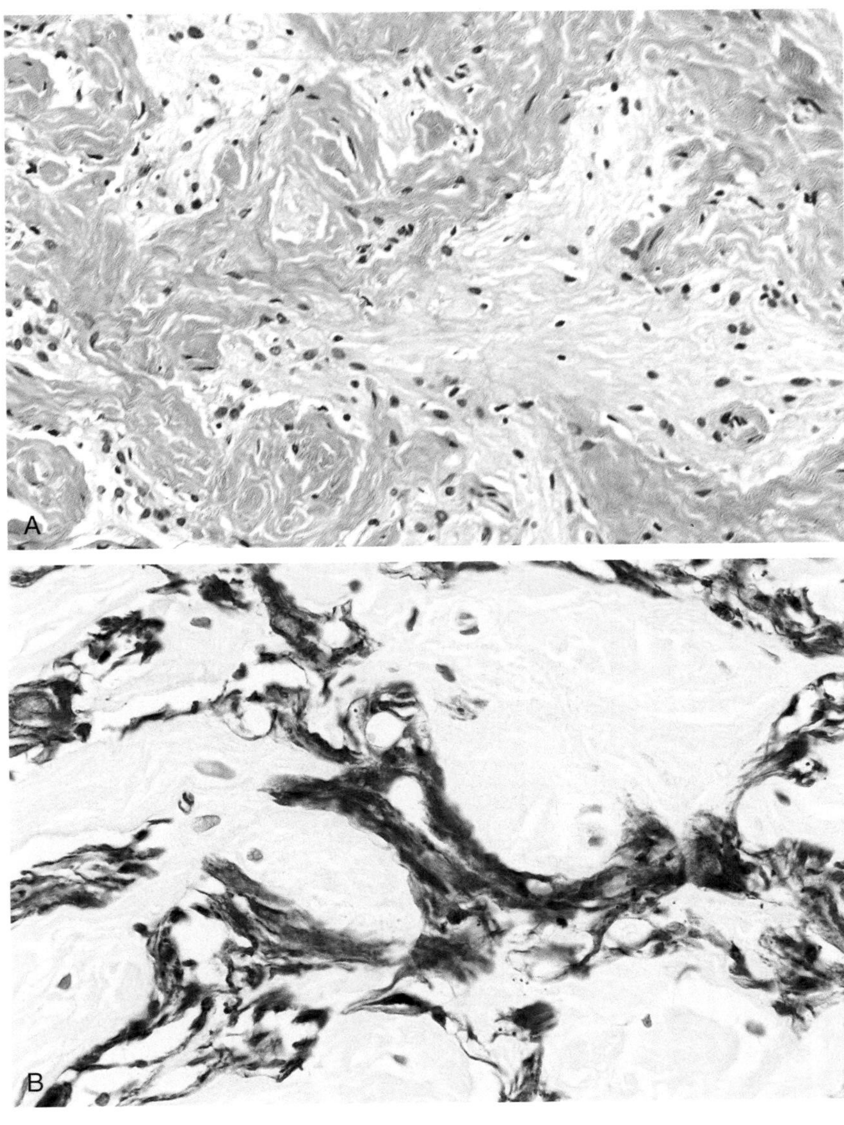

FIGURE 27-126. (A) Glial heterotopia with lightly staining glial tissue interspersed between collagen (dark areas). (B) Immunostaining for glial fibrillary acidic protein highlights glial tissue against the negatively staining backdrop of collagen.

occurs through the cribriform plate so that rhinorrhea may be an accompanying symptom. Histologically, the lesions consist of mats of mature glial tissue that, in addition to astrocytes, may contain neurons (Fig. 27-126). Gemistocytic change of the astrocytes and calcification is occasionally present.[166] Although most glial heterotopias may be viewed as variants of encephalocele, in which the communication with the brain is lost, glial heterotopias also occur in other somatic soft tissue of adults, suggesting other pathogenetic mechanisms as well.

References

1. Pina-Oviedo S, Ortiz-Hidalgo C. The normal and neoplastic perineurium: a review. Adv Anat Pathol 2008;15(3):147–64.
2. Shapiro L, Juhlin EA, Brownstein MH. "Rudimentary polydactyly": an amputation neuroma. Arch Dermatol 1973;108(2):223–5.
3. Raue F, Frank-Raue K. Update multiple endocrine neoplasia type 2. Fam Cancer 2010;9(3):449–57.
4. Carney JA, Hayles AB. Alimentary tract manifestations of multiple endocrine neoplasia, type 2b. Mayo Clin Proc 1977;52(9):543–8.
5. Dembinski AS, Jones JW. Intra-abdominal pacinian neuroma: a rare lesion in an unusual location. Histopathology 1991;19(1):89–90.
6. Fletcher CD, Theaker JM. Digital pacinian neuroma: a distinctive hyperplastic lesion. Histopathology 1989;15(3):249–56.
7. Fraitag S, Gherardi R, Wechsler J. Hyperplastic pacinian corpuscles: an uncommonly encountered lesion of the hand. J Cutan Pathol 1994; 21(5):457–60.
8. Hart WR, Thompson NW, Hildreth DH, et al. Hyperplastic pacinian corpuscles: a cause of digital pain. Surgery 1971;70(5):730–5.
9. Rhode CM, Jennings WD Jr. Pacinian corpuscle neuroma of digital nerves. South Med J 1975;68(1):86–9.
10. Albrecht S, Kahn HJ, From L. Palisaded encapsulated neuroma: an immunohistochemical study. Mod Pathol 1989;2(4):403–6.
11. Argenyi ZB, Cooper PH, Santa Cruz D. Plexiform and other unusual variants of palisaded encapsulated neuroma. J Cutan Pathol 1993;20(1) 34–9.
12. Dakin MC, Leppard B, Theaker JM. The palisaded, encapsulated neuroma (solitary circumscribed neuroma). Histopathology 1992;20(5): 405–10.
13. Fletcher CD. Solitary circumscribed neuroma of the skin (so-called palisaded, encapsulated neuroma). A clinicopathologic and immunohistochemical study. Am J Surg Pathol 1989;13(7):574–80.
14. Jokinen CH, Ragsdale BD, Argenyi ZB. Expanding the clinicopathologic spectrum of palisaded encapsulated neuroma. J Cutan Pathol 2010;37(1): 43–8.
15. Argenyi ZB, Santa Cruz D, Bromley C. Comparative light-microscopic and immunohistochemical study of traumatic and palisaded

encapsulated neuromas of the skin. Am J Dermatopathol 1992;14(6):504–10.
16. Adams 2nd WR. Morton's neuroma. Clin Podiatr Med Surg 2010;27(4):535–45.
17. Hassouna H, Singh D. Morton's metatarsalgia: pathogenesis, aetiology and current management. Acta Orthop Belg 2005;71(6):646–55.
18. Reed RJ, Bliss BO. Morton's neuroma. Regressive and productive intermetatarsal elastofibrositis. Arch Pathol 1973;95(2):123–9.
19. Robinson S, Cohen AR. Cowden disease and Lhermitte-Duclos disease: an update. Case report and review of the literature. Neurosurg Focus 2006;20(1):E6.
20. Devroede G, Lemieux B, Massé S, et al. Colonic hamartomas in tuberous sclerosis. Gastroenterology 1988;94(1):182–8.
21. Kanter AS, Hyman NH, Li SC. Ganglioneuromatous polyposis: a premalignant condition. Report of a case and review of the literature. Dis Colon Rectum 2001;44(4):591–3.
22. Mendelsohn G, Diamond MP. Familial ganglioneuromatous polyposis of the large bowel. Report of a family with associated juvenile polyposis. Am J Surg Pathol 1984;8(7):515–20.
23. Shekitka KM, Sobin LH. Ganglioneuromas of the gastrointestinal tract. Relation to Von Recklinghausen disease and other multiple tumor syndromes. Am J Surg Pathol 1994;18(3):250–7.
24. Haggitt RC, Reid BJ. Hereditary gastrointestinal polyposis syndromes. Am J Surg Pathol 1986;10(12):871–87.
25. Koch CA, Brouwers FM, Rosenblatt K, et al. Adrenal ganglioneuroma in a patient presenting with severe hypertension and diarrhea. Endocr Relat Cancer 2003;10(1):99–107.
26. Reindl T, Degenhardt P, Luck W, et al. [The VIP-secreting tumor as a differential diagnosis of protracted diarrhea in pediatrics]. Klin Padiatr 2004;216(5):264–9.
27. Duffy S, Jhaveri M, Scudierre J, et al. MR imaging of a posterior mediastinal ganglioneuroma: fat as a useful diagnostic sign. AJNR Am J Neuroradiol 2005;26(10):2658–62.
28. Dundr P, Dudorkinová D, Povysil C, et al. Pigmented composite paraganglioma-ganglioneuroma of the urinary bladder. Pathol Res Pract 2003;199(11):765–9.
29. Usuda H, Emura I. Composite paraganglioma-ganglioneuroma of the urinary bladder. Pathol Int 2005;55(9):596–601.
30. de Montpreville VT, Mussot S, Gharbi N, et al. Paraganglioma with ganglioneuromatous component located in the posterior mediastinum. Ann Diagn Pathol 2005;9(2):110–14.
31. Kimura N, Watanabe T, Fukase M, et al. Neurofibromin and NF1 gene analysis in composite pheochromocytoma and tumors associated with von Recklinghausen's disease. Mod Pathol 2002;15(3):183–8.
32. Matias-Guiu X, Garrastazu MT. Composite phaeochromocytoma-ganglioneuroblastoma in a patient with multiple endocrine neoplasia type IIA. Histopathology 1998;32(3):281–2.
33. Geoerger B, Hero B, Harms D, et al. Metabolic activity and clinical features of primary ganglioneuromas. Cancer, 2001;91(10):1905–13.
34. Drago G, Pasquier B, Pasquier D, et al. Malignant peripheral nerve sheath tumor arising in a "de novo" ganglioneuroma: a case report and review of the literature. Med Pediatr Oncol 1997;28(3):216–22.
35. de Chadarevian JP, MaePascasio J, Halligan GE, et al. Malignant peripheral nerve sheath tumor arising from an adrenal ganglioneuroma in a 6-year-old boy. Pediatr Dev Pathol 2004;7(3):277–84.
36. Barrett R, Cramer F. Tumors of the peripheral nerves and so-called "ganglia" of the peroneal nerve. Clin Orthop Relat Res 1963;27:135–46.
37. Cobb CA 3rd, Moiel RH. Ganglion of the peroneal nerve. Report of two cases. J Neurosurg 1974;41(2):255–9.
38. Gurdjian ES, Larsen RD, Lindner DW. Intraneural cyst of the peroneal and ulnar nerves. Report of two cases. J Neurosurg 1965;23(1):76–8.
39. Markel SF, Enzinger FM. Neuromuscular hamartoma—a benign 'triton tumor" composed of mature neural and striated muscle elements. Cancer Metastasis Rev 1982;49(1):140–4.
40. Maher CO, Spinner RJ, Giannini C, et al. Neuromuscular choristoma of the sciatic nerve. J Neurosurg 2002;96:1123–6.
41. Boyaci S, Moray M, Aksoy K, et al. Intraocular neuromuscular choristoma: a case report and literature review. Neurosurgery 2011;68(2):E551–5.
42. O'Connell JX, Rosenberg AE. Multiple cutaneous neuromuscular choristomas. Report of a case and a review of the literature. Am J Surg Pathol 1990;14(1):93–6.
43. Van Dorpe J, Sciot R, De Vos R, et al. Neuromuscular choristoma (hamartoma) with smooth and striated muscle component: case report with immunohistochemical and ultrastructural analysis. Am J Surg Pathol 1997;21(9):1090–5.
44. Brasfield RD, Das Gupta TK. Von Recklinghausen's disease: a clinicopathological study. Ann Surg 1972;175(1):86–104.
45. McClatchey AI. Neurofibromatosis. Annu Rev Pathol 2007;2:191–216.
46. Barker D, Wright E, Nguyen K, et al. Gene for von Recklinghausen neurofibromatosis is in the pericentromeric region of chromosome 17. Science (New York, N.Y.) 1987;236(4805):1100–2.
47. Theos A, Korf BR. Pathophysiology of neurofibromatosis type 1. Ann Intern Med 2006;144(11):842–9.
48. Weiss B, Bollag G, Shannon K. Hyperactive Ras as a therapeutic target in neurofibromatosis type 1. Am J Med Genet 1999;89(1):14–22.
49. Arun D, Gutmann DH. Recent advances in neurofibromatosis type 1. Curr Opin Neurol 2004;17(2):101–5.
50. Crowe FW, Schull WJ, Neel JV. A clinical, pathological, and genetic study of multiple neurofibromatosis. Springfield, IL: Charles C Thomas Publishers; 1956.
51. Riccardi VM. Von Recklinghausen neurofibromatosis. N Engl J Med 1981;305(27):1617–27.
52. Canale DJ, Bebin J. Von Recklinghausen disease of the nervous system, in Handbook of clinical neurology, B.G. In: Vinken PJ, editor. New York: Elsevier; 1972. p. 132.
53. Bird CC, Willis RA. The histogenesis of pigmented neurofibromas. J Pathol 1969;97(4):631–7.
54. Fetsch JF, Michal M, Miettinen M. Pigmented (melanotic) neurofibroma: a clinicopathologic and immunohistochemical analysis of 19 lesions from 17 patients. Am J Surg Pathol 2000;24(3):331–43.
55. Lin BT, Weiss LM, Medeiros LJ. Neurofibroma and cellular neurofibroma with atypia: a report of 14 tumors. Am J Surg Pathol 1997;21(12):1443–9.
56. Jokinen CH, Argenyi ZB. Atypical neurofibroma of the skin and subcutaneous tissue: clinicopathologic analysis of 11 cases. J Cutan Pathol 2010;37:35–42.
57. Scheithauer BW, Woodruff JM, Erlandson RA. Tumors of the peripheral nervous system. Washington, D.C.: Armed Forces Institute of Pathology; 1999.
58. Packer RJ, Gutmann DH, Rubenstein A, et al. Plexiform neurofibromas in NF1: toward biologic-based therapy. Neurology 2002;58(10):1461–70.
59. Gupta A, Cohen BH, Ruggieri P, et al. Phase I study of thalidomide for the treatment of plexiform neurofibroma in neurofibromatosis 1. Neurology 2003;60(1):130–2.
60. Hosoi K. Multiple neurofibromatosis (von Recklinghausen's disease) with special reference to malignant transformation. Arch Surg 1931;22:258.
61. Sorensen SA, Mulvihill JJ, Nielsen A. Long-term follow-up of von Recklinghausen neurofibromatosis. Survival and malignant neoplasms. N Engl J Med 1986;314(16):1010–15.
62. Evans DG, Baser ME, McGaughran J, et al. Malignant peripheral nerve sheath tumours in neurofibromatosis 1. J Med Genet 2002;39(5):311–14.
63. De Raedt T, Brems H, Wolkenstein P, et al. Elevated risk for MPNST in NF1 microdeletion patients. Am J Hum Genet 2003;72(5):1288–92.
64. Kluwe L, Friedrich RE, Peiper M, et al. Constitutional NF1 mutations in neurofibromatosis 1 patients with malignant peripheral nerve sheath tumors. Hum Mutat 2003;22(5):420.
65. Guccion JG, Enzinger FM. Malignant Schwannoma associated with von Recklinghausen's neurofibromatosis. Virchows Arch A Pathol Anat Histol 1979;383(1):43–57.
66. Dasgupta B, Gutmann DH. Neurofibromatosis 1: closing the GAP between mice and men. Curr Opin Genet Dev, 2003;13(1):20–7.
67. Zhu Y, Ghosh P, Charnay P, et al. Neurofibromas in NF1: Schwann cell origin and role of tumor environment. Science 2002;296(5569):920–2.
68. Yang FC, Ingram DA, Chen S, et al. Neurofibromin-deficient Schwann cells secrete a potent migratory stimulus for Nf1+/− mast cells. J Clin Invest 2003;112(12):1851–61.
69. Perry A, Kunz SN, Fuller CE, et al. Differential NF1, p16, and EGFR patterns by interphase cytogenetics (FISH) in malignant peripheral nerve sheath tumor (MPNST) and morphologically similar spindle cell neoplasms. J Neuropathol Exp Neurol 2002;61(8):702–9.
70. Kourea HP, Cordon-Cardo C, Dudas M, et al. Expression of p27(kip) and other cell cycle regulators in malignant peripheral nerve sheath tumors and neurofibromas: the emerging role of p27(kip) in malignant transformation of neurofibromas. Am J Pathol 1999;155(6):1885–91.
71. Kourea HP, Orlow I, Scheithauer BW, et al. Deletions of the INK4A gene occur in malignant peripheral nerve sheath tumors but not in neurofibromas. Am J Pathol 1999;155(6):1855–60.
72. Nielsen GP, Stemmer-Rachamimov AO, Ino Y, et al. Malignant transformation of neurofibromas in neurofibromatosis 1 is associated with CDKN2A/p16 inactivation. Am J Pathol 1999;155(6):1879–84.

73. Antinheimo J, Sankila R, Carpén O, et al. Population-based analysis of sporadic and type 2 neurofibromatosis-associated meningiomas and schwannomas. Neurology 2000;54(1):71–6.
74. Stemmer-Rachminov AO, Xu L, Gonzalez-Agosti C, et al. Universal absence of merlin, but not other ERM family members, in schwannomas. Am J Pathol 1997;151:1649–54.
75. Roche PH, Bouvier C, Chinot O, et al. Genesis and biology of vestibular schwannomas. Prog Neurol Surg 2008;21:24–31.
76. Stout AP. The peripheral manifestations of specific nerve sheath tumor (neurilemoma). Am J Cancer 1935;24:751.
77. Brooks JJ, Draffen RM. Benign glandular schwannoma. Arch Pathol Lab Med 1992;116(2):192–5.
78. Fletcher CD, Madziwa D, Heyderman E, et al. Benign dermal Schwannoma with glandular elements–true heterology or a local 'organizer' effect? Clin Exp Dermatol 1986;11(5):475–85.
79. Chan JK, Fok KO. Pseudoglandular schwannoma. Histopathology, 1996;29(5):481–3.
80. Goldblum JR, Beals TF, Weiss SW. Neuroblastoma-like neurilemoma. Am J Surg Pathol 1994;18(3):266–73.
81. Lassmann H, Jurecka W, Lassmann G, et al. Different types of benign nerve sheath tumors. Light microscopy, electron microscopy and autoradiography. Virchows Arch A Pathol Anat Histol 1977;375(3): 197–210.
82. Fisher ER, Vuzevski VD. Cytogenesis of schwannoma (neurilemoma), neurofibroma, dermatofibroma, and dermatofibrosarcoma as revealed by electron microscopy. Am J Clin Pathol 1968;49(2): 141–54.
83. Razzuk MA, Urschel HC Jr, Martin JA, et al. Electron microscopical observations on mediastinal neurolemmoma, neurofibroma, and ganglioneuroma. Ann Thorac Surg 1973;15(1):73–83.
84. Waggener JD. Ultrastructure of benign peripheral nerve sheath tumors. Cancer 1966;19(5):699–709.
84a. Karamchandani JR, Nielsen TO, van de Rijn M, et al. SOX10 and S100 in the diagnosis of soft-tissue neoplasms. Appl Immunhistochem Mol Morphol 2012;20:445–50.
85. Hanada M, Tanaka T, Kanayama S, et al. Malignant transformation of intrathoracic ancient neurilemoma in a patient without von Recklinghausen's disease. Acta Pathol Jpn 1982;32(3):527–36.
86. Nayler SJ, Leiman G, Omar T, et al. Malignant transformation in a schwannoma. Histopathology 1996;29(2):189–92.
87. Rasbridge SA, Browse NL, Tighe JR, et al. Malignant nerve sheath tumor arising in a benign ancient schwannoma. Histopathology 1989;14: 525–8.
88. Woodruff JM, Selig AM, Crowley K, et al. Schwannoma (neurilemoma) with malignant transformation. A rare, distinctive peripheral nerve tumor. Am J Surg Pathol 1994;18(9):882–95.
89. Carstens PH, Schrodt GR. Malignant transformation of a benign encapsulated neurilemoma. Am J Clin Pathol 1969;51(1):144–9.
90. McMenamin ME, Fletcher CDM. Expanding the spectrum of malignant change in schwannomas: epithelioid malignant change, epithelioid malignant peripheral nerve sheath tumor, and epithelioid angiosarcoma. Am J Surg Pathol 2001;25:13–25.
91. Casadei GP, Scheithauer BW, Hirose T, et al. Cellular schwannoma. A clinicopathologic, DNA flow cytometric, and proliferation marker study of 70 patients. Cancer 1995;75(5):1109–19.
92. Fletcher CD, Davies SE. McKee PH. Cellular schwannoma: a distinct pseudosarcomatous entity. Histopathology 1987;11(1):21–35.
93. Lodding P, Kindblom LG, Angervall L, et al. Cellular schwannoma. A clinicopathologic study of 29 cases. Virchows Arch A Pathol Anat Histopathol 1990;416(3):237–48.
94. White W, Shiu MH, Rosenblum MK, et al. Cellular schwannoma. A clinicopathologic study of 57 patients and 58 tumors. Cancer 1990; 66(6):1266–75.
95. Woodruff JM, Godwin TA, Erlandson RA, et al. Cellular schwannoma: a variety of schwannoma sometimes mistaken for a malignant tumor. Am J Surg Pathol 1981;5(8):733–44.
96. Trassard M, Le Doussal V, Bui BN, et al. Angiosarcoma arising in a solitary schwannoma (neurilemoma) of the sciatic nerve. Am J Surg Pathol 1996;20(11):1412–17.
97. Meis-Kindblom JM, Enzinger FM. Plexiform malignant peripheral nerve sheath tumor of infancy and childhood. Am J Surg Pathol 1994; 18(5):479–85.
98. Argenyi ZB, Goodenberger ME. Strauss JS. Congenital neural hamartoma ("fascicular schwannoma"). A light microscopic, immunohistochemical, and ultrastructural study. Am J Dermatopathol 1990;12(3): 283–93.
99. Woodruff JM, Scheithauer BW, Kurtkaya-Yapicier O, et al. Congenital and childhood plexiform (multinodular) cellular schwannoma: a troublesome mimic of malignant peripheral nerve sheath tumor. Am J Surg Pathol 2003;27(10):1321–9.
100. Fletcher CD, Davies SE. Benign plexiform (multinodular) schwannoma: a rare tumour unassociated with neurofibromatosis. Histopathology 1986;10(9):971–80.
101. Stenman G, Kindblom LG, Johansson M, et al. Clonal chromosome abnormalities and in vitro growth characteristics of classical and cellular schwannomas. Cancer Genet Cytogenet 1991;57(1):121–31.
102. Woodruff JM, Marshall ML, Godwin TA, et al. Plexiform (multinodular) schwannoma. A tumor simulating the plexiform neurofibroma. Am J Surg Pathol 1983;7(7):691–7.
103. Iwashita T, Enjoji M, Plexiform neurilemoma: a clinicopathologic and immunohistochemical analysis of 23 tumors from 20 patients. Virchows Arch [Pathol Anat] 1986;422:305–9.
104. Kao GF, Laskin WB, Olsen TG. Solitary cutaneous plexiform neurilemoma (schwannoma): a clinicopathologic, immunohistochemical, and ultrastructural study of 11 cases. Mod Pathol 1989;2:20–6.
105. Ishida T, Kuroda M, Motoi T, et al. Phenotypic diversity of neurofibromatosis 2: association with plexiform schwannoma. Histopathology 1998;32(3):264–70.
106. Reith JD, Goldblum JR. Multiple cutaneous plexiform schwannomas. Report of a case and review of the literature with particular reference to the association with types 1 and 2 neurofibromatosis and schwannomatosis. Arch Pathol Lab Med 1996;120(4):399–401.
107. Val-Bernal JF, Figols J. Vazquez-Barquero A. Cutaneous plexiform schwannoma associated with neurofibromatosis type 2. Cancer 1995; 76(7):1181–6.
108. Kindblom LG, Meis-Kindblom JM, Havel G, et al. Benign epithelioid schwannoma. Am J Surg Pathol 1998;22(6):762–70.
109. Smith K, Mezebish D, Williams JP, et al. Cutaneous epithelioid schwannomas: a rare variant of a benign peripheral nerve sheath tumor. J Cutan Pathol 1998;25(1):50–5.
110. Laskin WB, Fetsch JF, Lasota J, et al. Benign epithelioid peripheral nerve sheath tumors of the soft tissues: clinicopathologic spectrum of 33 cases. Am J Surg Pathol 2005;29(1):39–51.
111. Evans DG. Neurofibromatosis type 2 (NF2): a clinical and molecular review. Orphanet J Rare Dis 2009;4:16.
112. Evans DG, Baser ME, O'Reilly B, et al. Management of the patient and family with neurofibromatosis 2: a consensus conference statement. Br J Neurosurg 2005;19(1):5–12.
113. Baser ME, Evans RDG, Gutmann DH. Neurofibromatosis 2. Curr Opin Neurol 2003;16(1):27–33.
114. Evans DG, Huson SM, Donnai D, et al. A clinical study of type 2 neurofibromatosis. Q J Med 1992;84(304):603–18.
115. MacCollin M, Woodfin W, Kronn D, et al. Schwannomatosis: a clinical and pathologic study. Neurology 1996;46(4):1072–9.
116. MacCollin M, Chiocca EA, Evans DG, et al. Diagnostic criteria for schwannomatosis. Neurology 2005;64(11):1838–45.
117. Hadfield KD, Newman WG, Bowers NL, et al. Molecular characterization of SMARCB1 and NF2 in familial and sporadic schwannmatosis. J Med Genet 2012;45:332–9.
118. Carter JM, O'Hara C, Dundas G, et al. Epithelioid malignant peripheral nerve sheath tumor arising in a schwannoma, in a patient with "neuroblastoma-like" schwannomatosis and a novel germline SMARCB1 mutation. Am J Surg Pathol 2012;36(1):154–60.
119. Macarenco RS, Ellinger F, Oliveira AM. Perineurioma: a distinctive and underrecognized peripheral nerve sheath neoplasm. Arch Pathol Lab Med 2007;131(4):625–36.
120. Michal M, Kazakov DV, Belousova I, et al. A benign neoplasm with histopathological features of both schwannoma and retiform perineurioma (benign schwannoma-perineurioma): a report of six cases of a distinctive soft tissue tumor with a predilection for the fingers. Virchows Arch 2004;445(4):347–53.
121. Zamecnik M, Michal M. Perineurial cell differentiation in neurofibromas. Report of eight cases including a case with composite perineurioma-neurofibroma features. Pathol Res Pract 2001;197(8):537–44.
122. Hornick JL, Bundock EA. Fletcher CD. Hybrid schwannoma/ perineurioma: clinicopathologic analysis of 42 distinctive benign nerve sheath tumors. Am J Surg Pathol 2009;33(10):1554–61.
123. Lazarus SS, Trombetta LD. Ultrastructural identification of a benign perineurial cell tumor. Cancer 1978;41(5):1823–9.
124. Emory TS, Scheithauer BW, Hirose T, et al. Intraneural perineurioma. A clonal neoplasm associated with abnormalities of chromosome 22. Am J Clin Pathol 1995;103(6):696–704.

125. Simmons Z, Mahadeen ZI, Kothari MJ, et al. Localized hypertrophic neuropathy: magnetic resonance imaging findings and long-term follow-up. Muscle Nerve 1999;22(1):28–36.
126. Jazayeri MA, Robinson JH, Legolvan DP. Intraneural perineurioma involving the median nerve. Plast Reconstr Surg 2000;105(6):2089–91.
127. Giannini C, Scheithauer BW, Jenkins RB, et al. Soft-tissue perineurioma. Evidence for an abnormality of chromosome 22, criteria for diagnosis, and review of the literature. Am J Surg Pathol 1997;21(2):164–73.
128. Hornick JL, Fletcher CD. Soft tissue perineurioma: clinicopathologic analysis of 81 cases including those with atypical histologic features. Am J Surg Pathol 2005;29(7):845–58.
129. Sciot R, Dal Cin P, Hagemeijer A, et al. Cutaneous sclerosing perineurioma with cryptic NF2 gene deletion. Am J Surg Pathol 1999;23(7):849–53.
130. Smith K, Skelton H. Cutaneous fibrous perineurioma. J Cutan Pathol 1998;25(6):333–7.
131. Tsang WY, Chan JK, Chow LT, et al. Perineurioma: an uncommon soft tissue neoplasm distinct from localized hypertrophic neuropathy and neurofibroma. Am J Surg Pathol 1992;16(8):756–63.
132. Lasota J, Wozniak A, Debiec-Rychter M, Loss of chromosome 22q and lack of NF2 mutations in perineuriomas [abstract 46]. Mod Pathol 2000;13:11A.
133. Rank JP, Rostad SW. Perineurioma with ossification: a case report with immunohistochemical and ultrastructural studies. Arch Pathol Lab Med 1998;122(4):366–70.
134. Folpe AL, Billings SD, McKenney JK, et al. Expression of claudin-1, a recently described tight junction-associated protein, distinguishes soft tissue perineurioma from potential mimics. Am J Surg Pathol 2002; 26(12):1620–6.
135. Yamaguchi U., Hasegawa T, Hirose T, et al. Sclerosing perineurioma: a clinicopathological study of five cases and diagnostic utility of immunohistochemical staining for GLUT1. Virchows Arch 2003;443(2):159–63.
136. Weidenheim KM, Campbell Jr WG. Perineural cell tumor. Immunocytochemical and ultrastructural characterization. Relationship to other peripheral nerve tumors with a review of the literature. Virchows Arch A Pathol Anat Histopathol 1986;408(4):375–83.
137. Hirose T, Tani T, Shimada T, et al. Immunohistochemical demonstration of EMA/Glut1-positive perineurial cells and CD34-positive fibroblastic cells in peripheral nerve sheath tumors. Mod Pathol 2003;16(4):293–8.
138. Fetsch JF, Miettinen M. Sclerosing perineurioma: a clinicopathologic study of 19 cases of a distinctive soft tissue lesion with a predilection for the fingers and palms of young adults. Am J Surg Pathol 1997;21(12):1433–42.
139. Burgues O, Monteagudo C, Noguera R, et al. Cutaneous sclerosing Pacinian-like perineurioma. Histopathology 2001;39(5):498–502.
140. Brock JE, Perez-Atayde AR, Kozakewich HP, et al. Cytogenetic aberrations in perineurioma: variation with subtype. Am J Surg Pathol 2005;29(9):1164–9.
141. Graadt van Roggen JF, McMenamin ME, Belchis DA, et al. Reticular perineurioma: a distinctive variant of soft tissue perineurioma. Am J Surg Pathol 2001;25(4):485–93.
142. Ushigome S, Takakuwa T, Hyuga M, et al. Perineurial cell tumor and the significance of the perineurial cells in neurofibroma. Acta Pathol Jpn 1986;36(7):973–87.
143. Michal M, Extraneural retiform perineuriomas. A report of four cases. Pathol Res Pract 1999;195(11):759–63.
144. Mentzel T, Kutzner H. Reticular and plexiform perineurioma: clinicopathological and immunohistochemical analysis of two cases and review of perineurial neoplasms of skin and soft tissues. Virchows Arch 2005;447(4):677–82.
145. Rosenberg AS, Langee CL, Stevens GL, et al. Malignant peripheral nerve sheath tumor with perineurial differentiation: "malignant perineurioma". J Cutan Pathol 2002;29(6):362–7.
146. Sobel HJ, Avrin E, Marquet E, et al. Reactive granular cells in sites of trauma. A cytochemical and ultrastructural study. Am J Clin Pathol 1974;61(2):223–34.
147. Schrader KA, Nelson TN, De Luca A, et al. Multiple granular cell tumors are an associated feature of LEOPARD syndrome caused by mutation in PTPN11. Clinical Genetics 2009;75(2):185–9.
148. Filie AC, Lage JM, Azumi N. Immunoreactivity of S100 protein, alpha-1-antitrypsin, and CD68 in adult and congenital granular cell tumors. Mod Pathol 1996;9(9):888–92.
149. Kurtin PJ, Bonin DM. Immunohistochemical demonstration of the lysosome-associated glycoprotein CD68 (KP-1) in granular cell tumors and schwannomas. Hum Pathol 1994;25(11):1172–8.
150. Mukai M. Immunohistochemical localization of S-100 protein and peripheral nerve myelin proteins (P2 protein, P0 protein) in granular cell tumors. Am J Pathol 1983;112(2):139–46.
151. Nakazato Y, Ishizeki J, Takahashi K, et al. Immunohistochemical localization of S-100 protein in granular cell myoblastoma. Cancer 1982;49(8):1624–8.
152. Sobel HJ, Churg J. Granular cells and granular cell lesions. Arch Pathol 1964;77:132–41.
153. Smolle J, Konrad K, Kerl H. Granular cell tumors contain myelin-associated glycoprotein. An immunohistochemical study using Leu 7 monoclonal antibody. Virchows Arch A Pathol Anat Histopathol 1985;406(1):1–5.
154. Strong EW, McDivitt RW, Brasfield RD. Granular cell myoblastoma. Cancer 1970;25(2):415–22.
155. Fanburg-Smith JC, Meis-Kindblom JM, Fante R, et al. Malignant granular cell tumor of soft tissue: diagnostic criteria and clinicopathologic correlation. Am J Surg Pathol 1998;22(7):779–94.
156. Lack EE, Perez-Atayde AR, McGill TJ, et al. Gingival granular cell tumor of the newborn (congenital "epulis"): ultrastructural observations relating to histogenesis. Hum Pathol 1982;13(7):686–9.
157. Lack EE, Worsham GF, Callihan MD, et al. Gingival granula cell tumors of the newborn (congenital "epulis"): a clinical and pathologic study of 21 patients. Am J Surg Pathol 1981;5(1):37–46.
158. Fetsch JF, Laskin WB, Miettinen M. Nerve sheath myxoma: a clinicopathologic and immunohistochemical analysis of 57 morphologically distinctive, S100 protein and GFAP positive myxoid peripheral nerve sheath tumors with a predilection for the extremities and a high local recurrence rate. Amer J Surg Pathol 2005;29(12):1615–24.
159. Sheth S, Li X, Binder S, et al. Differential gene expression profiles of neurothekeomas and nerve sheath myxomas by microarray analysis. Mod Pathol 2011;24(3):343–54.
160. Lopez DA, Silvers DN, Helwig EB. Cutaneous meningiomas–a clinicopathologic study. Cancer 1974;34(3):728–44.
161. Theaker JM, Fleming KA. Meningioma of the scalp: a case report with immunohistological features. J Cutan Pathol 1987;14(1):49–53.
162. Rios JJ, Diaz-Cano SJ, Rivera-Hueto F, et al. Cutaneous ganglion cell choristoma. Report of a case. J Cutan Pathol 1991;18(6):469–73.
163. Shepherd NA, Coates PJ, Brown AA. Soft tissue gliomatosis–heterotopic glial tissue in the subcutis: a case report. Histopathology 1987;11(6):655–60.
164. Skelton HG, Smith KJ. Glial heterotopia in the subcutaneous tissue overlying T-12. J Cutan Pathol 1999;26(10):523–7.
165. Orkin M, Fisher I. Heterotopic brain tissue (heterotopic neural rest). Case report with review of related anomalies. Arch Dermatol 1966;94(6):699–708.
166. Penner CR, Thompson L. Nasal glial heterotopia: a clinicopathologic and immunophenotypic analysis of 10 cases with a review of the literature. Ann Diagn Pathol 2003;7(6):354–9.
167. *National Institutes of Health Consensus Development Conference Statement of Neurofibromatosis*. Bethesda, MD: US Department of Health and Human Services; July 13-5, 1987.

Malignant Peripheral Nerve Sheath Tumors

CHAPTER CONTENTS

MALIGNANT PERIPHERAL NERVE SHEATH TUMOR

Malignant tumors arising from or displaying differentiation along the lines of the various elements of the nerve sheath (e.g., Schwann cell, perineural cell, fibroblast) are collectively referred to as *malignant peripheral nerve sheath tumors (MPNSTs)*. Because MPNSTs recapitulate the appearance of various cells of the nerve sheath, they range in appearance from tumors that resemble a neurofibroma to those resembling a fibrosarcoma. Rarely, tumors arising from nerves or neurofibromas display aberrant lines of differentiation. For example, angiosarcomas may arise in nerves or in preexisting neurofibromas. By convention, these tumors are not considered MPNSTs but are classified according to their aberrant line of differentiation. Although primitive neuroectodermal tumors may also rarely arise from peripheral nerves, they are considered along with Ewing sarcoma (see Chapter 33).

The diagnosis of MPNST has traditionally been one of the most difficult and elusive among soft tissue tumors in the past because of a lack of standardized diagnostic criteria. Even today, there are no specific biomarkers that can be used to establish the diagnosis with certainty. Although there is a general agreement that a sarcoma can usually be considered an MPNST if it arises from a peripheral nerve or a neurofibroma, there has been less agreement about the diagnostic criteria for tumors occurring outside of these settings. As a result, the incidence of this sarcoma, as reported in the literature, has varied depending on the stringency of the diagnostic criteria.

A sarcoma is assumed to be an MPNST if one of three criteria can be met: (1) the tumor arises from a peripheral nerve and shows no aberrant or heterologous line of differentiation; (2) it arises from a preexisting benign nerve sheath tumor, usually a neurofibroma; or (3) the tumor displays a constellation of histologic features that are seen in tumors arising in the foregoing situations and are considered typical of malignant Schwann cell tumors. These features include the (1) dense and hypodense fascicles alternating in a marble-like pattern consisting of (2) asymmetrically tapered spindled cells with irregular buckled nuclei or (3) immunohistochemical or electron microscopic evidence of Schwann cell differentiation in the context of a fibrosarcomatous-appearing tumor. In addition, there are features that are less specific but frequently occur in Schwann cell tumors, including nuclear palisading, whorled structures that vaguely suggest large tactoid structures, peculiar hyperplastic perivascular change, and, occasionally, heterologous elements (e.g., cartilage, bone, skeletal muscle). Clearly, these criteria allow inclusion of only MPNSTs that are reasonably well differentiated or have not yet obscured their site of origin. Nonetheless, this approach offers an acceptable degree of diagnostic reproducibility and eliminates the potpourri of spindle cell tumors that have been diagnosed as MPNSTs in the past.

Clinical Findings

MPNSTs account for approximately 5% to 10% of all soft tissue sarcomas, and about one-fourth to one-half occur in the setting of neurofibromatosis 1 (NF1).[1-6] This range probably reflects differences in diagnostic criteria and patient referral patterns. In most large studies, the percentage of patients with MPNST with and without NF1 is roughly equal.[2,5] Although the lifetime risk of developing an MPNST in the setting of NF1 is about 10%,[7,8] the risk approaches 30% in patients with symptomatic plexiform neurofibromas. In addition, patients with large rearrangements of the *NF1* gene, so-called microdeletions, have a lifetime risk of MPNST of 16% to 26%.[9] This is postulated to be the result of inactivation of additional tumor suppressor genes, tentatively identified as ADAP2 and RNF135, adjacent to the microdeletion.[10]

Patients with NF1 develop sarcomas usually after a relatively long latency (10 to 20 years), and, in some cases, the MPNSTs are multiple. MPNSTs in childhood are recognized but infrequent.[11-13] The exact mechanism of malignant transformation or tumor progression in NF1 is not fully understood but involves a multistep process in which genes other than the *NF1* gene also participate (see later text). Aside from the foregoing genetic predilection to develop MPNST, little is known about the pathogenesis of sporadic tumors in humans.

About 10% to 20% of cases occur as a result of therapeutic or occupational irradiation after a latent period of more than 15 years.[1,3,14-16] These tumors do not differ significantly from other MPNSTs.

The MPNST is typically a disease of adult life because most tumors occur in patients 20 to 50 years of age with a median age of about 35.[1,5,17-22] Patients with NF1 usually present at a slightly earlier age and have larger tumors than those with sporadic lesions. Men predominate in studies that report a high percentage of patients with NF1 because of the slight bias for men in this disease.[1,3,17,20] In sporadic cases of MPNST, the gender ratio is roughly equal.

Like other sarcomas, these lesions present as enlarging masses that are usually noted several months before diagnosis. Pain is variable but is more prevalent in those patients with NF1. In fact, pain or a sudden enlargement of a preexisting mass in this setting should lead to immediate biopsy to exclude the possibility of malignant transformation of a neurofibroma. Fluorodeoxyglucose positron emission tomography, which allows visualization of glucose metabolism by cells, has been reasonably successful in identifying malignant change in plexiform neurofibromas[23] and may give some indication of the grade of the lesion.[24] MPNSTs that arise from major nerves typically give rise to a striking constellation of sensory and motor symptoms, including projected pain, paresthesias, and weakness. The symptoms rarely antedate the detection of a mass.

Most MPNSTs arise in association with major nerve trunks, including the sciatic nerve, brachial plexus, and sacral plexus. Consequently, the most common anatomic sites include the proximal portions of the upper and lower extremities and the trunk. Comparatively few arise in the head and neck, a feature that contrasts with the distribution of the schwannoma.

Gross Findings

In its classic form, an MPNST arises as a large fusiform or eccentric mass in a major nerve (Fig. 28-1). Thickening of the nerve proximally and distally to the main mass usually indicates spread of the neoplasm along the epineurium and perineurium. In NF1 patients, MPNST may develop in a preexisting neurofibroma (Fig. 28-2). Most of these lesions are deeply

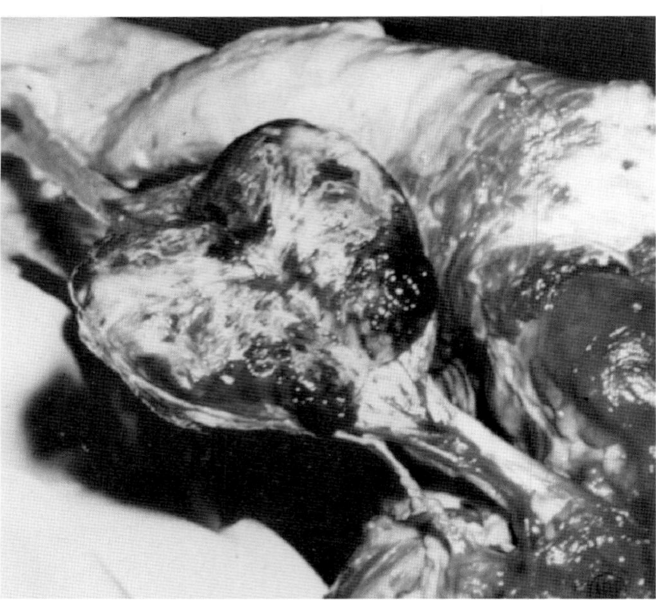

FIGURE 28-1. MPNST arising as a large fusiform mass from the sciatic nerve. Cut section of tumor shows prominent hemorrhage and necrosis.

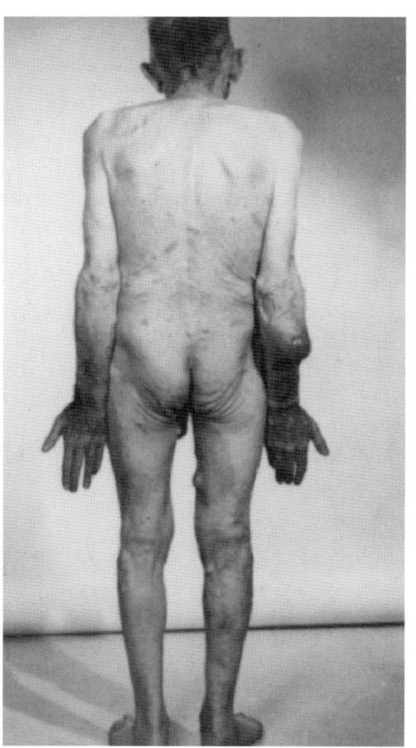

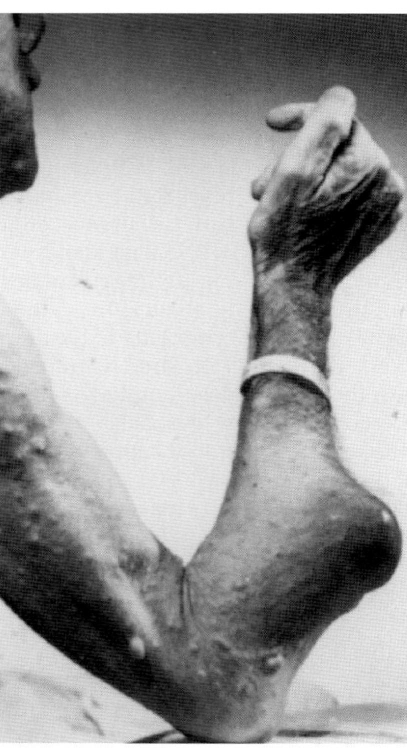

FIGURE 28-2. MPNST of the arm in a patient with long-standing neurofibromatosis.

situated; only rare ones arise from superficial neurofibromas. Regardless of the clinical setting, the gross appearance of the MPNST is essentially similar to that of other soft tissue sarcomas. It is usually large, averaging more than 5 cm in diameter and has a fleshy, opaque, white-tan surface marked by areas of secondary hemorrhage and necrosis. This appearance contrasts with the white mucoid appearance of the typical neurofibroma.

Microscopic Findings

Most MPNSTs resemble fibrosarcomas in their overall organization (Figs. 28-3 to 28-6) with certain modifications. Classically, the cells recapitulate the features of the normal Schwann cell. Unlike the symmetrically spindled cells of fibrosarcoma, they have irregular contours. In profile, the nuclei are wavy, buckled, or comma-shaped, whereas, when viewed en face, they are asymmetrically oval (Fig. 28-7). The cytoplasm is lightly stained and usually indistinct. The cells can range from spindled in shape to fusiform or even rounded so that the lesion can mimic a fibrosarcoma or even a round cell sarcoma (Fig. 28-8). The cells are arranged in sweeping fascicles, but there is greater variation in organization than in the fibrosarcoma. Densely cellular fascicles alternate with hypocellular, myxoid zones (see Fig. 28-6), which swirl and interdigitate with one another, creating a marble-like effect (see Fig. 28-3). Others display a peculiar nodular, curlicue, or whorled arrangement of spindled cells (Figs. 28-9 and 28-10), crudely suggesting tactoid differentiation. Nuclear palisading may be present, but, in the cases by the authors of this edition, it occurs in fewer than 10% of all MPNSTs and, when present, is usually of a focal nature (Fig. 28-11).

There are several other subtle features that are quite characteristic of MPNST. Because they are not completely specific, they must be evaluated in the context of the foregoing discussion before a given tumor is labeled MPNST. These features include hyaline bands (Fig. 28-12) and nodules, which, in a cross section, can be likened to giant rosettes (see Fig. 28-12B), extensive perineural and intraneural spread of tumor (Fig. 28-13), and a peculiar proliferation of tumor in

Text continued on p. 863

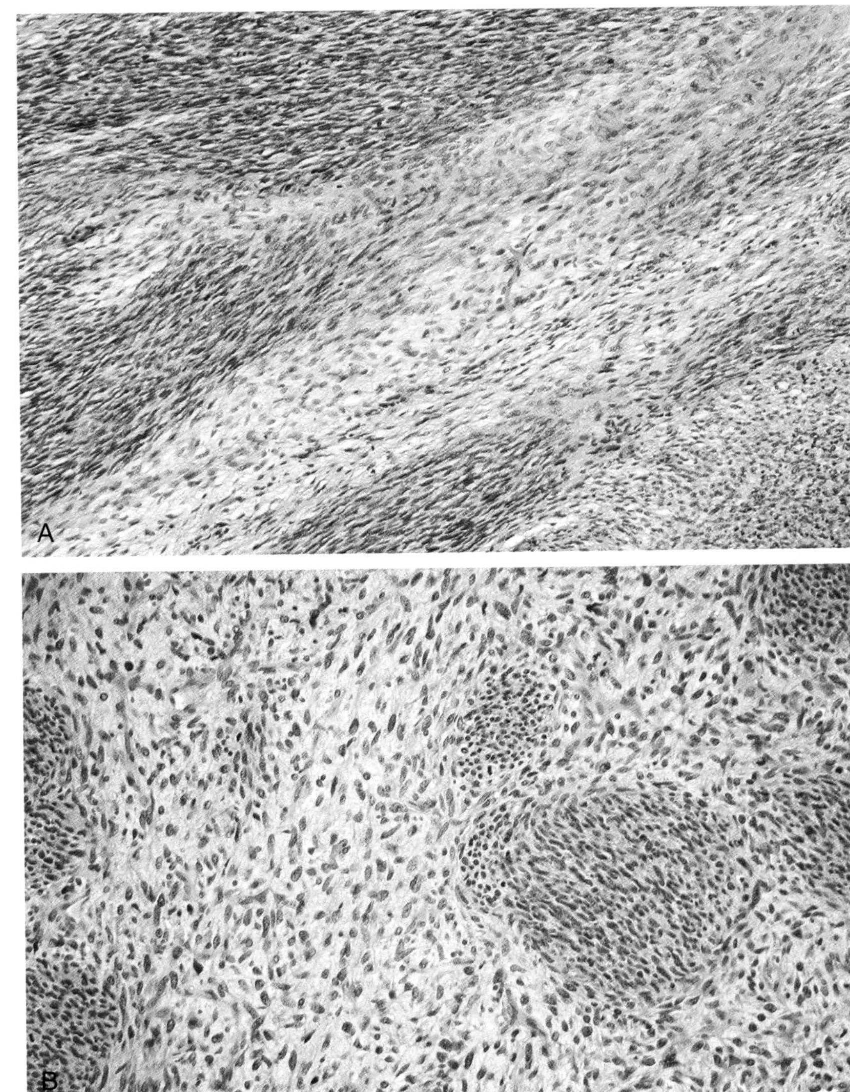

FIGURE 28-3. (A, B) Typical appearance of an MPNST with densely cellular areas alternating with less cellular ones, creating a marbleized appearance.

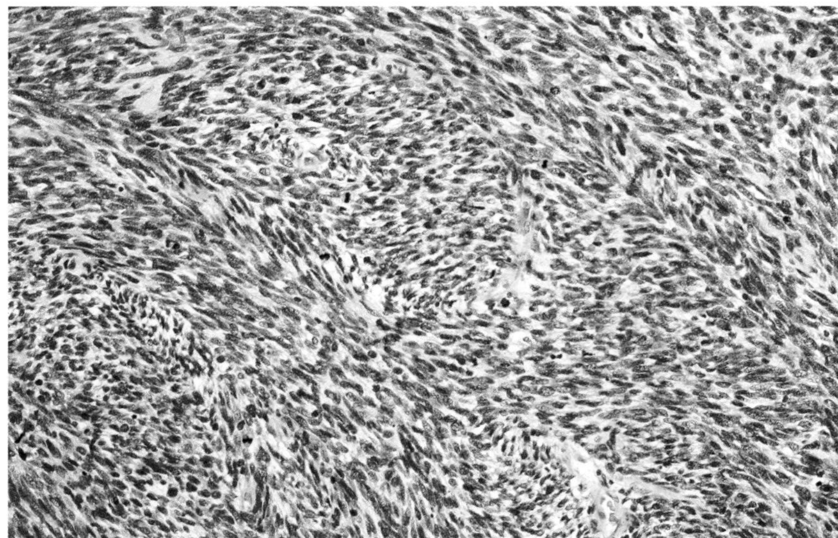

FIGURE 28-4. MPNST consisting exclusively of dense fascicles of spindled cells, similar to a fibrosarcoma.

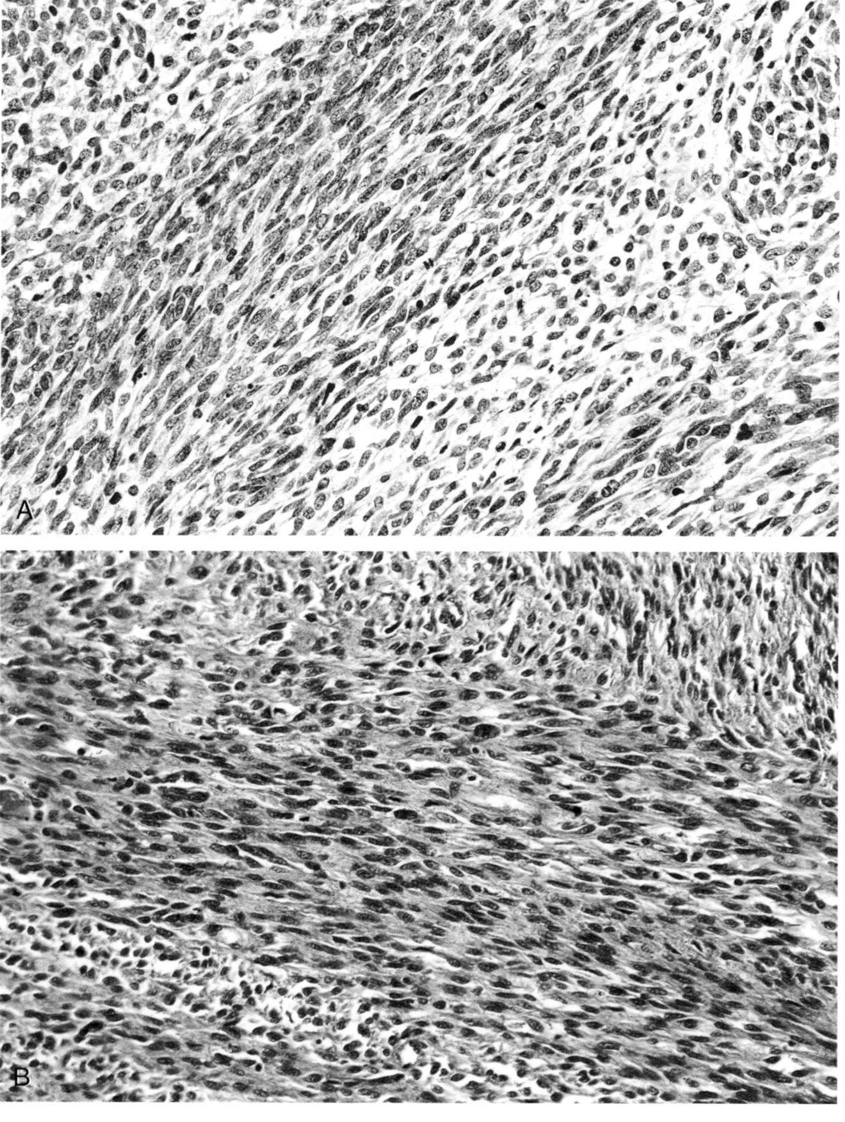

FIGURE 28-5. (A, B) Cellular fascicles of an MPNST.

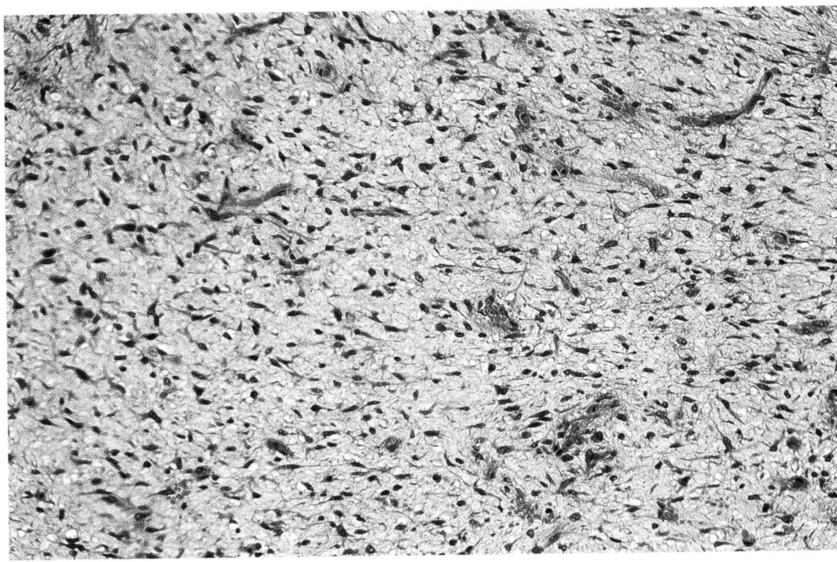

FIGURE 28-6. Myxoid area in an MPNST showing randomly arranged Schwann cells.

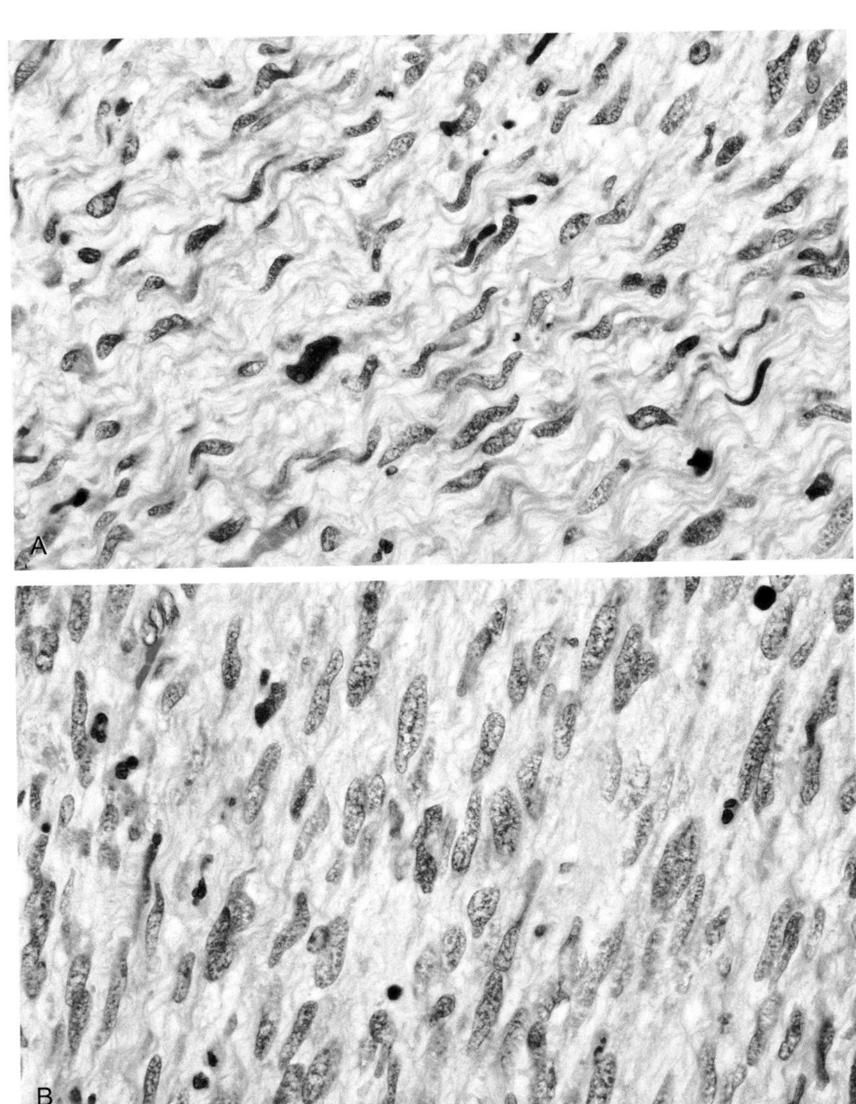

FIGURE 28-7. Cells in an MPNST with well-differentiated areas (A) in which cells have an irregular, buckled shape characteristic of Schwann cells to less differentiated areas (B). *Continued*

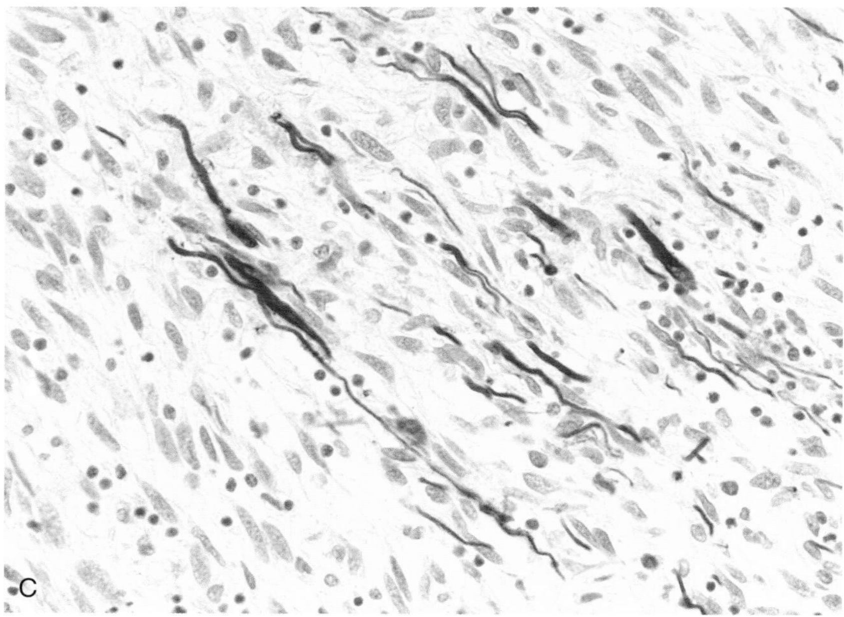

FIGURE 28-7, cont'd. (C) S-100 protein immunostain shows focal weak staining of cells in an MPNST.

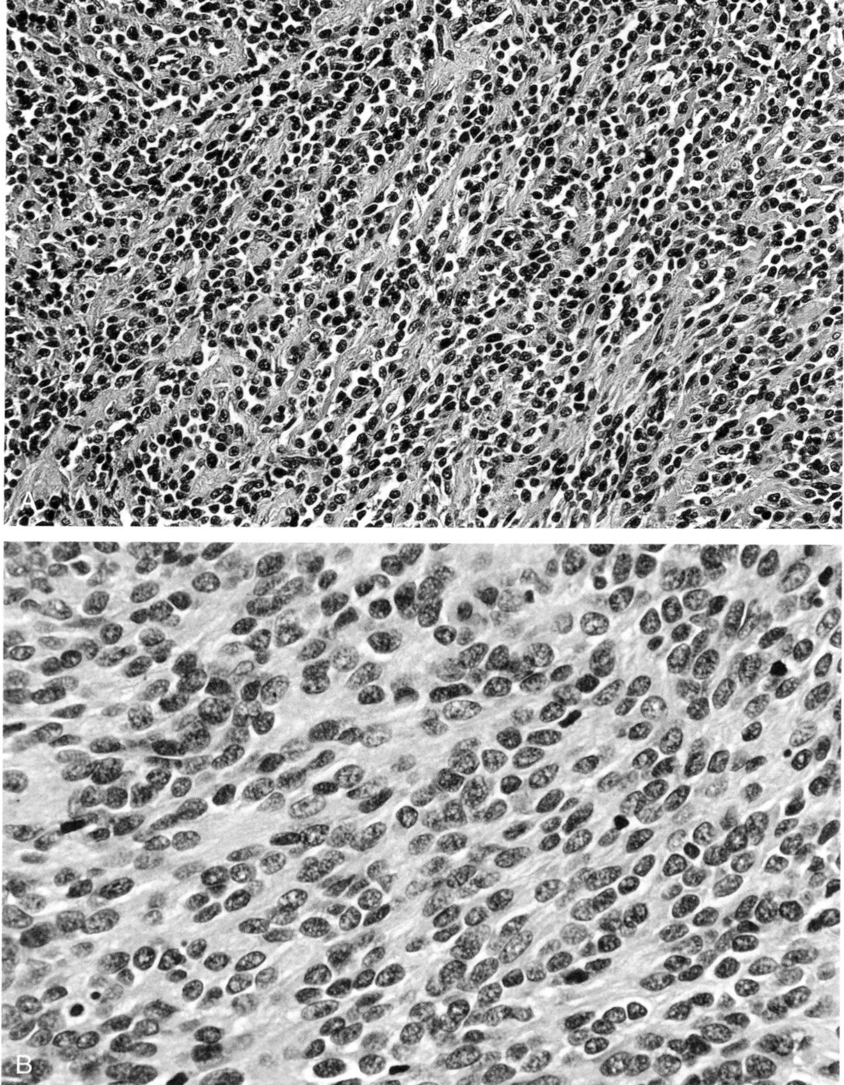

FIGURE 28-8. MPNST with areas composed of rounded (A) or short fusiform (B) cells. In *B* sample, vague palisading of nuclei can be seen.

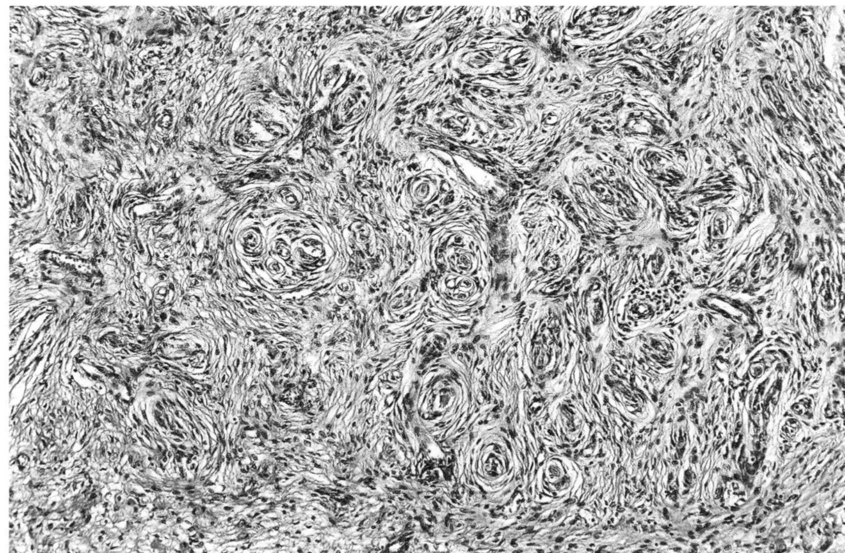

FIGURE 28-9. Low-grade MPNST with a curlicue arrangement of cells.

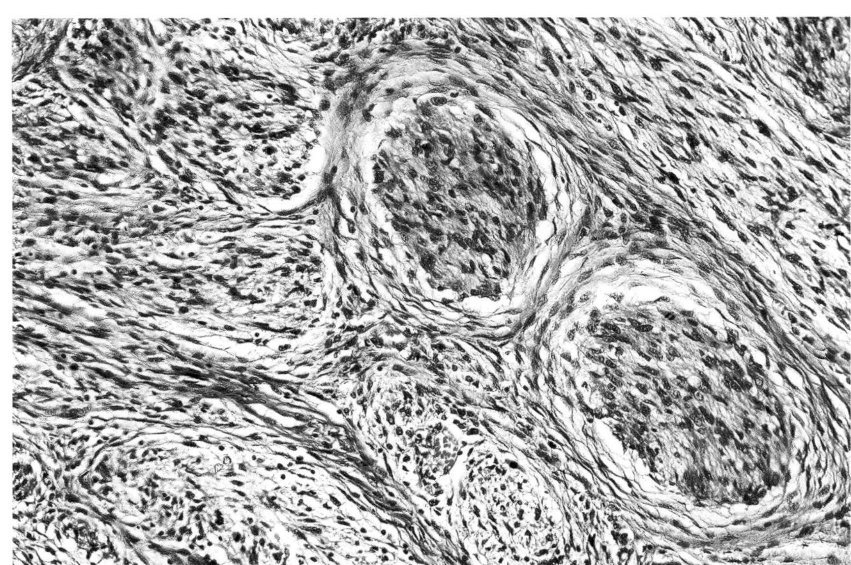

FIGURE 28-10. Whorled structures in an MPNST.

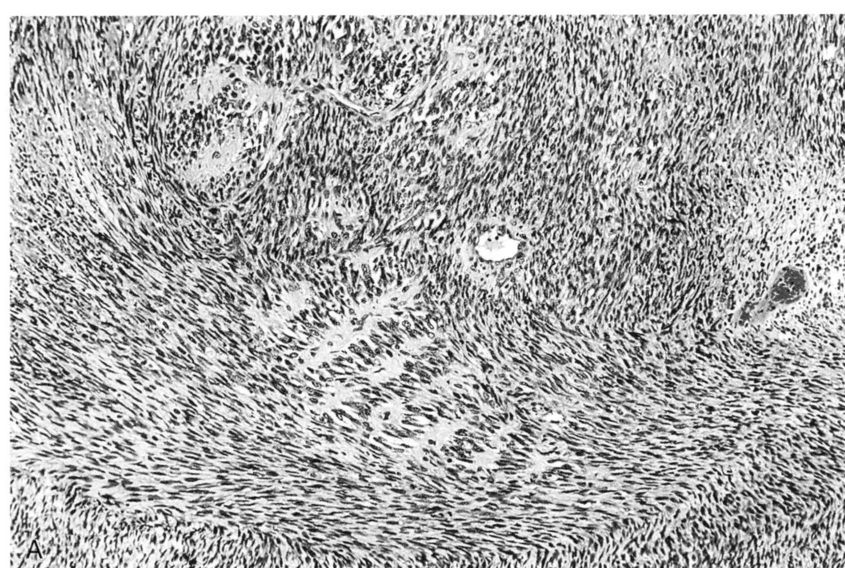

FIGURE 28-11. (A, B) Nuclear palisading is an uncommon feature in an MPNST. It may also be seen in schwannomas and some leiomyosarcomas. *Continued*

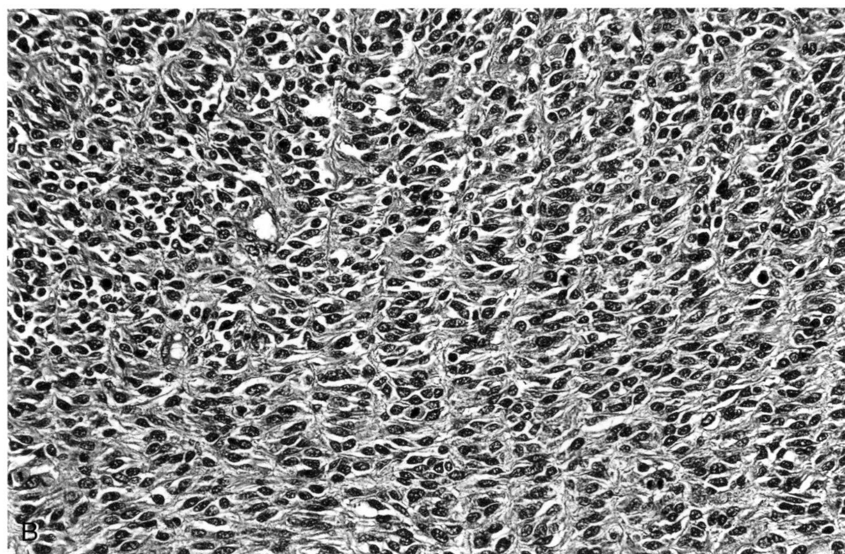

FIGURE 28-11, cont'd

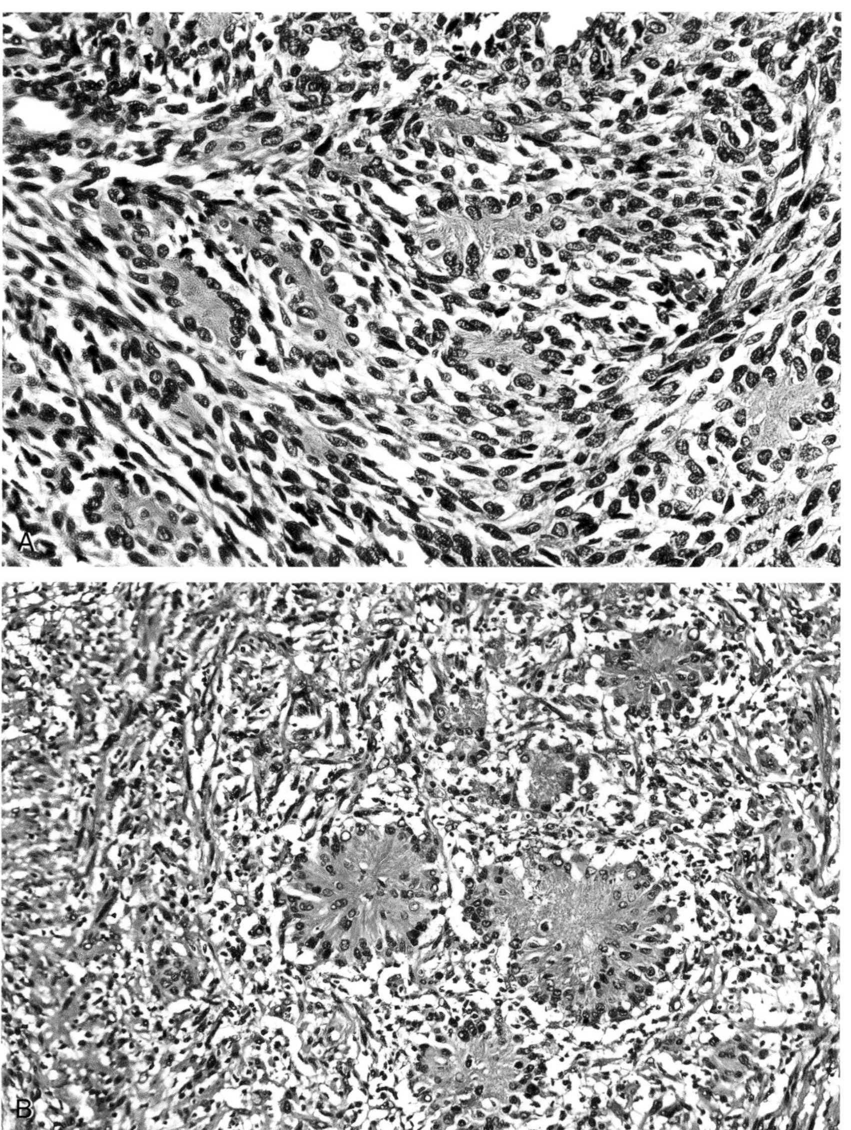

FIGURE 28-12. Hyalinized cords (A) and nodules (B) are uncommon but distinctive features of MPNSTs.

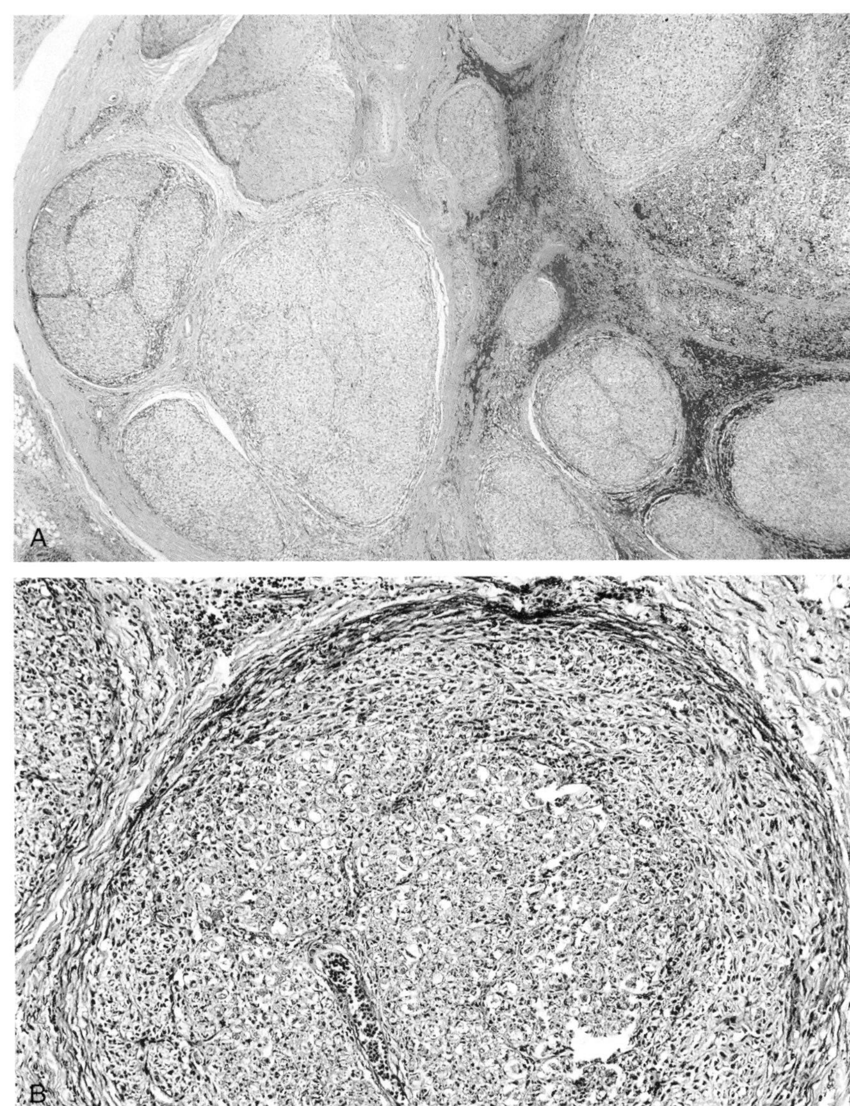

FIGURE 28-13. (A) Replacement of a peripheral nerve by an MPNST. (B) High-power view showing insinuation of a tumor between the nerve fascicles.

the subendothelial zones of vessels so that the neoplastic cells appear to herniate into the lumen (Fig. 28-14). Small vessels may also proliferate in the walls of or around large vessels (see Fig. 28-14B). Heterologous elements, present in about 10% to 15% of MPNST, seem to be more common in MPNSTs than in other sarcomas.[13,25] Mature islands of cartilage and bone are the most common elements (Fig. 28-15), whereas skeletal muscle, mucin-secreting glands, and squamous islands are rare.

Although most MPNSTs conform to this description, a small percentage appear quite different. Some of these tumors closely resemble neurofibromas, except they manifest a greater degree of cellularity, pleomorphism, and mitotic activity. These MPNSTs are typically found in the setting of von Recklinghausen disease and have sometimes been termed *malignant neurofibromas.* If the lesion fulfills the criteria of malignancy as detailed in Chapter 27, it is referred to as a *low-grade malignant peripheral nerve sheath tumor arising in a neurofibroma.* At the opposite end of the spectrum are anaplastic MPNSTs, which may be difficult to distinguish from other pleomorphic sarcomas (Fig. 28-16). They are composed of plump, spindled, and giant cells intermixed with hemorrhage and necrosis similar to that seen in glioblastoma multiforme. Although these pleomorphic tumors have been documented more often in the setting of von Recklinghausen disease, this may reflect the general reluctance to diagnose an anaplastic MPNST outside of the setting of NF1. Diagnosis of these tumors depends on identifying areas of typical MPNST. Infrequently, MPNSTs contain areas of primitive neuroepithelial differentiation consisting of cords or nests of small round cells[26] and, in extraordinary cases, even rosettes (Fig. 28-17). Primitive neuroepithelial differentiation appears to be a more common feature of MPNST in children.[27]

Immunohistochemical Findings

The application of immunohistochemistry to the diagnosis of MPNST has been of limited value. None of the conventional markers has proven to be sensitive and specific enough to

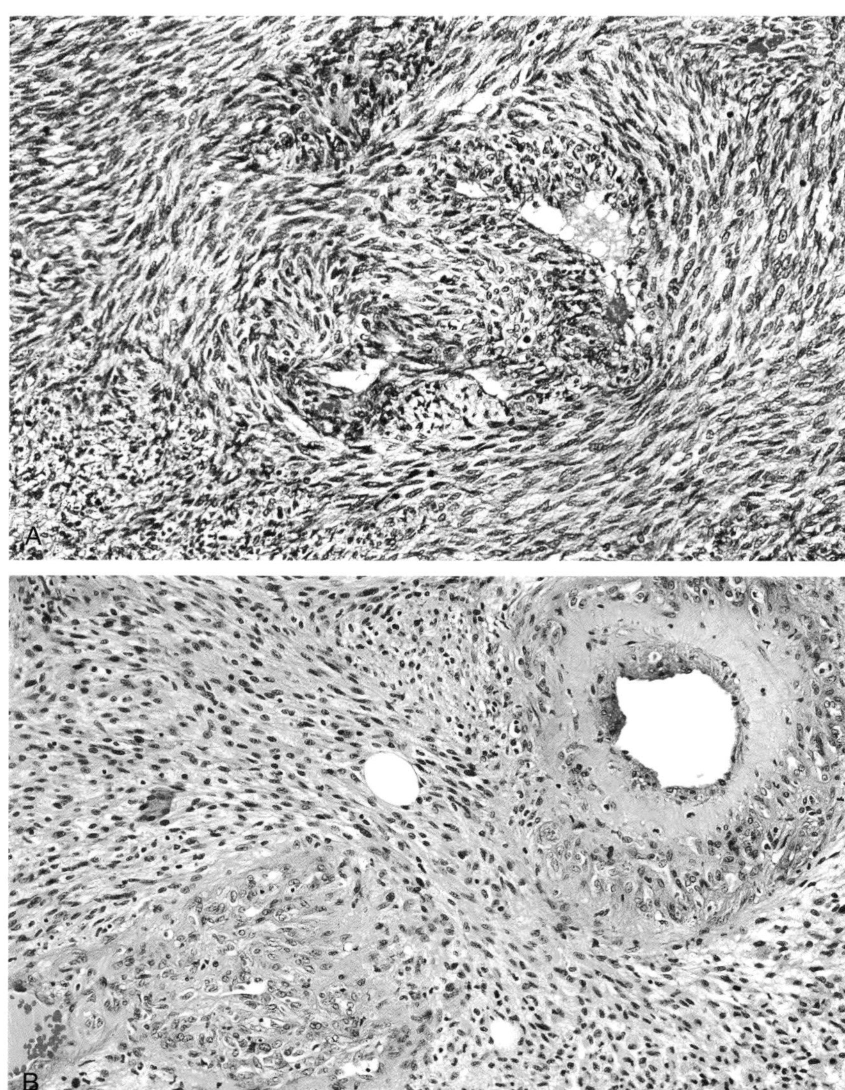

FIGURE 28-14. Peculiar changes around small vessels in MPNST. The tumor appears to herniate into lumens of vessels (A), whereas there is a small proliferation of small vessels in the walls of large vessels in the MPNST (B).

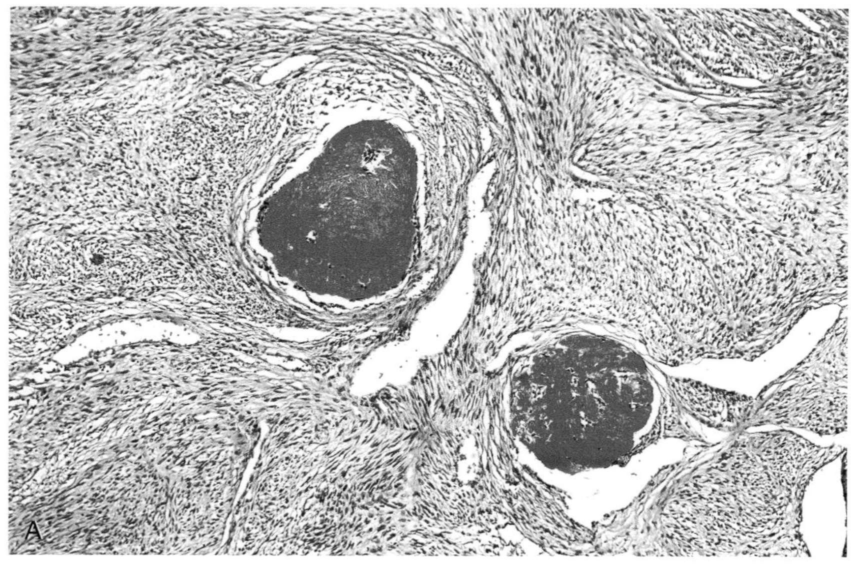

FIGURE 28-15. Heterologous elements in an MPNST are most often bone (A) and cartilage (B).

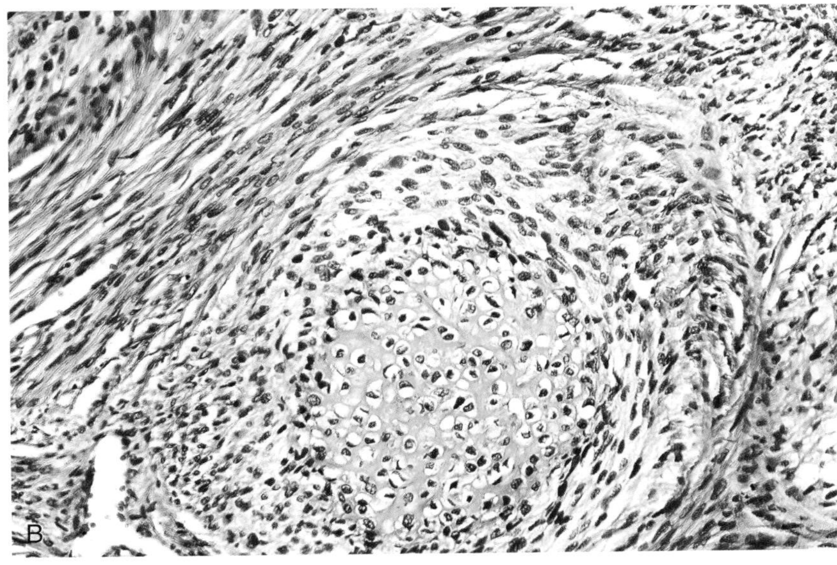

FIGURE 28-15, cont'd

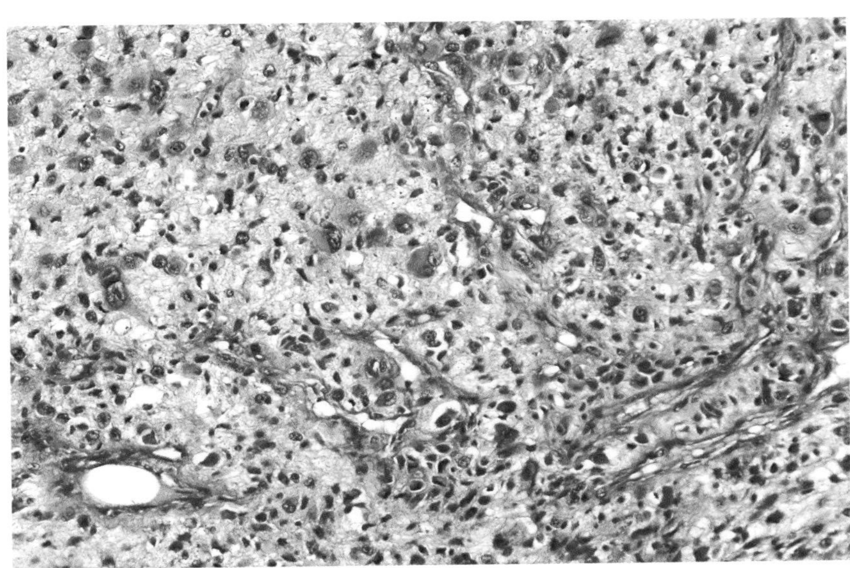

FIGURE 28-16. Pleomorphic areas in an MPNST.

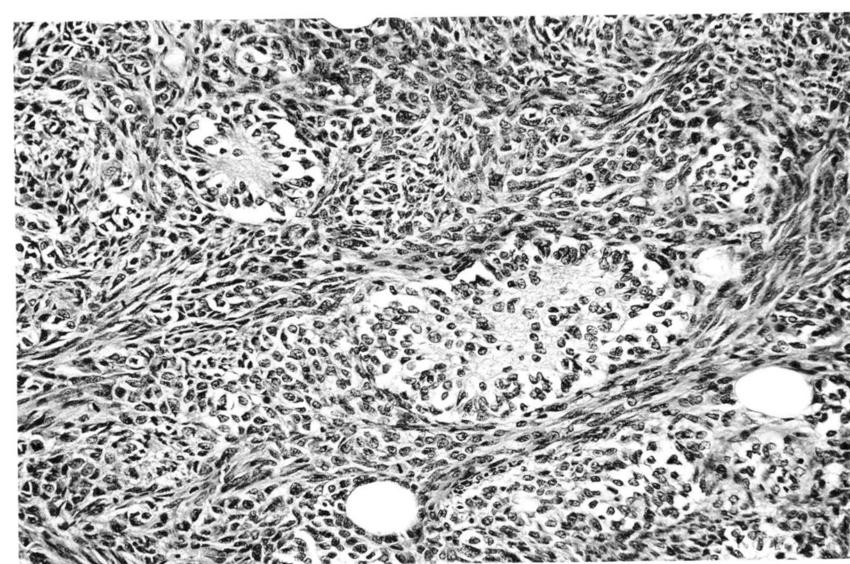

FIGURE 28-17. Primitive neuroectodermal differentiation in the form of a rosette in an MPNST.

establish the diagnosis of MPNST with certainty. Therefore, immunostains are best used in situations in which the differential diagnosis has been winnowed down and in which other tumors that resemble MPNST, such as synovial sarcoma, have been excluded by molecular studies.

S-100 protein has been the classic and most widely used antigen for documenting nerve sheath differentiation. Between 50% and 90% of MPNSTs express the antigen but usually focally only (see Fig. 28-7C).[5,28-31] Although its presence is often used to infer nerve sheath differentiation in a monomorphic-appearing spindle cell sarcoma, it is expressed in a significant percentage of synovial sarcomas (as well as other lesions such as cellular schwannoma and spindled melanoma that also enter the differential diagnosis). Therefore, interest in developing additional markers or panels that would assist in this distinction has been ongoing. Transducer-like enhancer of split 1, also known as TLE1, is strongly expressed in a nuclear pattern in 80% to 100% of genetically proven synovial sarcoma[32-35] and only weakly expressed in a minority (2% to 15%) of MPNSTs,[35,36] indicating its utility in this situation. A combination of S-100 protein and nestin expression reportedly has a high predictive value for the diagnosis of MPNST[37] as does HMGA2,[38] compared to synovial sarcoma.

SOX10, a neural crest transcription factor critical for development and maturation of Schwann cells from neural crest shows early promise for the diagnosis of MPNST. In a study by Nonaka et al.,[39] antibodies to SOX10 performed with better sensitivity and specificity for the diagnosis of MPNST than S-100 protein. Of 45 S-100 protein negative MPNSTs reported by Nonaka et al.,[39] approximately one-third expressed SOX10 to a variable degree. Moreover, there was an example of an MPNST positive for S-100 protein but negative for SOX10.[39]

CD34 is expressed in some MPNSTs and is likely a reflection of perineurial differentiation. A p53 immunoreactivity is also detected in more than half of MPNSTs, in contrast to its usual absence from neurofibromas.[40-42] Antibodies to CD57 (Leu 7 and HNK1), which react with myelin basic proteins, decorate about one-half of MPNSTs.[31]

Despite the limitations of immunohistochemistry for diagnostic purposes, some have advocated its use as a prognostic marker. Many, but not all, studies suggest that elevated Ki67 expression is associated with decreased survival in MPNST.[5,43] Nuclear expression of p53, which is present in about 80% of MPNSTs, is associated with a poor disease-specific survival, and lack of S-100 protein expression is associated with a five-fold increase risk of metastasis even in patients whose tumors were completely resected.[5] Although a combination of antigens (e.g., Ki-67, p53, VEGF, and pMEK) reliably discriminates neurofibromas from MPNST, this distinction rarely requires more than histologic sections.

Differential Diagnosis

Most MPNSTs are easily diagnosed as malignant tumors, and the major challenge resides in distinguishing them from other sarcomas such as fibrosarcoma, monophasic synovial sarcoma, and leiomyosarcoma. As implied previously, fibrosarcoma and synovial sarcoma have a more uniform fascicular pattern, contain symmetric fusiform cells resembling fibroblasts, and clearly lack features of neural differentiation. Monophasic synovial sarcoma often contains densely hyalinized or calcified areas (or both) in combination with areas, suggesting rudimentary epithelial differentiation in the form of clusters of round cells with clear cytoplasm. Immunostains, as detailed previously, and molecular studies are important diagnostic adjuncts.

Leiomyosarcoma can usually be distinguished from MPNST without undue difficulty. Its cells have deeply eosinophilic cytoplasm, centrally placed blunt-ended nuclei, and juxtanuclear vacuoles. In a Masson trichrome stain, its cytoplasm is fuchsinophilic with longitudinal striations. The cytoplasm of MPNST is usually less fuchsinophilic without longitudinal striations. An important diagnostic problem is the distinction of neurofibromas with one or more unusual features from an MPNST. This occurs typically with borderline neurofibromatous lesions of von Recklinghausen disease. A diagnosis of malignancy depends on the findings of enhanced cellularity, diffuse atypia, and usually at least a low level of mitotic activity. This problem is discussed in greater detail in Chapter 27. In rare instances, one encounters a typical neurofibroma in which small foci may appear malignant by virtue of the foregoing criteria. These lesions have been interpreted as *neurofibroma with focal malignant change*, and conservative excision is recommended if the focus constitutes a small portion of the entire neurofibroma and the focus appears totally removed by the excision. Preliminary follow-up in these cases supports this conservative approach to management.

The criterion of mitotic activity does not apply to schwannoma. Otherwise typical schwannomas displaying mitotic activity pursue a benign course, and only very rarely has this tumor been known to undergo malignant degeneration. When material from a small biopsy specimen is evaluated, it is hazardous to attempt to distinguish a cellular schwannoma from an MPNST solely on the basis of mitotic activity. In this situation, a larger sample of the mass is necessary to determine whether the tumor has an Antoni A and B pattern, perivascular hyalinization, Verocay bodies, or other typical features.

In the evaluation of MPNST, it is important to remember that desmoplastic melanomas, particularly those with neurotropic features, can be mistaken for MPNST. Desmoplastic melanoma present as fibrosing dermal lesions typically of the head and neck. In many instances, they are associated with a junctional component of atypical melanocytes and are composed of spindled cells with a decidedly Schwann cell appearance. The features that favor a desmoplastic melanoma over an MPNST are the dermal location, presence of junctional component, lymphoid response, and strong expression of S-100 protein.

Molecular and Cytogenetic Findings

The development of MPNST from neurofibroma appears to be a multistep process in which a number of genes participate, leading to a gain in function of some and a loss of function of others. Patients with NF1 have germline inactivation of NF1. Evidence, furthermore, supports the view that both alleles are inactivated in neurofibromas[44] and MPNST,[45] and that Schwann cells derived from NF1-deleted (neurofibromin-deficient) animals acquire increased proliferative capacity and angioinvasive properties (see Chapter 27).[46,47] The progression of a neurofibroma to an MPNST is associated with a number of additional chromosomal alterations.[48-51] The most common alterations are genomic gains involving 17q, 7p, 5p, 8q, and 12q. Less common alterations are genomic losses of 9p, 13q, and 1p. The 9p includes notably the *CDKN2* gene, a cyclin-dependent kinase inhibitor that is inactivated in more than 50% of MPNSTs but not in neurofibromas.[52,53] This gene produces two protein products, p16 and p19. The former negatively regulates cell cycling through the *Rb* pathway, whereas the latter negatively regulates cycling through the p53 pathway. Studies of sporadic and NF1-associated MPNSTs have demonstrated consistent absence of p16[54,55] in the face of normal expression of other cell cycle component proteins by Western blot analysis,[54] leading the authors to conclude that p16 inactivation is sufficient for abnormal stimulation of the cell cycle without involvement of other components.[54] However, others using immunohistochemical methods report diminished or absent expression of both p16 and p27,[56] but they point out that these alterations were not reliable in separating neurofibromas from low-grade peripheral nerve sheath tumors. That *p53* is ultimately affected in MPNST is suggested by positive immunostaining for p53 in a large number of MPNSTs, particularly high-grade ones, but not in neurofibromas.[40-42,56] Protein expression of the checkpoint with forkhead-associated domain and ring finger, another mitotic checkpoint gene, is also reduced in MPNST and has been correlated with high mitotic activity.[57]

With array-based methods, it has been possible to analyze a panoply of genes that are differentially expressed by MPNSTs compared to neurofibromas and normal Schwann cells. The major trend in malignant transformation is toward downregulation as opposed to upregulation of genes, the latter represented principally by genes involved in cell proliferation.[58] Schwann cell differentiation genes (*SOX10*, *CNP*, *PMP22*, and *NGFR*) are consistently downregulated, whereas neural crest stem cell genes (*SOX9* and *TWIST1*) are upregulated relative to normal Schwann cells. There is, however, great variability in the expression of cell cycle regulators attributable to the wide range in growth rates of these tumors.[59] Using comparative genomic hybridization, others have correlated specific regions of copy level gains to poor patient survival in the disease. The candidate genes in these locations include *SOX5* (12p12.1), *NOP2* and *MLF2* (12p13), *FOXM1* (12p13) and *FKBP1A* (20p13), and *CDK4* (12q13) and *TSPAN31* (12q13-q14). In multivariate analysis, gains in *CDK4* were the most significant predictor of poor survival.[60]

Clinical Behavior

Most MPNSTs are high-grade sarcomas, with a high probability of producing local recurrence and distant metastasis. Although the prognosis reported in the early literature for this disease was dismal, the survival reported from large cancer referral centers in which patients have undergone sophisticated radiologic imaging and extensive surgery often coupled with adjuvant radiation or chemotherapy has improved. Nevertheless, the challenges in treating this disease remain daunting. Unlike other sarcomas, they usually present as the American Joint Committee on Cancer (AJCC) stage III lesions and, as a group, are relatively chemoresistant. Therefore, the development of nomograms that account for such differences among sarcoma types has been an important advance.[61]

Based on three large referral studies,[4-6] local recurrences develop in about 40% of patients within a year of the original surgery on average. Factors that predict recurrence include anatomic site, tumor size, and adequacy of margins (Table 28-1). Lesions in the head and neck or retroperitoneum where adequate excisions are more difficult have a higher recurrence rate. Metastases develop in 40% to 60% of patients within 12 months of surgery on average. Increased risk of metastasis is noted in tumors that are large, are AJCC stage III, require chemotherapy, or lack S-100 protein immunostaining. Prognostic variables that predict survival vary from study to study. However, size seems to be a consistent determinant for outcome in most studies. Patients presenting with metastatic disease have a notably poor course and, in fact, are excluded from the statistical analysis in large studies. Clearly, such studies report better outcomes than if all patients were included. At one time, it was believed that MPNSTs associated with NF1 had a significantly worse outcome than sporadic ones. That has largely been disproven by numerous authors. Observed differences can be attributed to other factors, such as size or location, rather than intrinsic properties of the tumor.

Two-thirds of metastases develop in the lung, whereas the remainder develop in other sites, including the liver, brain, bone, and adrenal. Fewer than 10% of patients with metastasis developed regional node deposits, indicating that routine lymph node dissections do not play an important role in the

TABLE 28-1 MPNST-Specific Mortality in Patients With Complete Surgical Excision (85 Patients)

5-YR ACTUARIAL	DISEASE-SPECIFIC DEATH RATES	*p*
Univariable Prognostic Factors		
Presentation Status		
Recurrent	40.2%	0.83
Primary	54.3%	
NF1 Syndrome		
Present	58.2%	0.18
Absent	42.9%	
Site		
Head/neck	55.7%	0.75
Trunk	46.7%	0.17
Extremity	46.6%	
Tumor Size		
>= 10 cm	71.4%	0.003
<10 cm	33.3%	
Margin Status		
Positive	46.2%	0.92
Negative	54.3%	
S-100 Protein Immunostaining		
Positive	31.0%	0.002
Negative	77.9%	

Modified from Zou C, Smith KD, Liu J, et al. Clinical, pathological, and molecular variables predictive of malignant peripheral nerve sheath tumor outcome. Ann Surg 2009;249(6):1014–1022.

treatment of this disease. This also emphasizes that metastatic spindle cell lesions with Schwann cell-like features are apt to be metastatic desmoplastic or neurotropic melanomas or some other spindle cell tumor mimicking MPNST. However, lymph node metastasis may be seen in the presence of widely metastatic disease. One should also be aware of the propensity of this tumor to spread for considerable distances along the nerve sheath, and there are reports of tumors entering the subarachnoid space of the spinal cord through this route. Therefore, it is wise to obtain a frozen section of the nerve margins to assess the adequacy of the excision.

Although MPNST does not occur often in the pediatric age group, it appears to have a course roughly comparable to adults. Meis et al.,[27] in a retrospective review based on consultation material, noted metastasis in 50% of patients at 2 years. A report from two large centers, however, reported a 5-year survival of 51% and 10-year survival of 41%.[62] Multivariate analysis identified the absence of NF1, IRS groups I or II, and location on an extremity as independent favorable prognostic factors.[63] Others have related the prognosis closely to whether the patient underwent radical surgery. Survival at 10 years was 80% for patients who had undergone radical surgery compared to only 14% for those who did not.[62]

MALIGNANT PERIPHERAL NERVE SHEATH TUMOR WITH RHABDOMYOBLASTIC DIFFERENTIATION (MALIGNANT TRITON TUMOR)

In the broadest sense, a Triton tumor is any neoplasm with both neural and skeletal muscle differentiation; included are the neuromuscular hamartoma (benign Triton tumor), medulloblastoma with rhabdomyosarcoma, rhabdomyosarcoma with ganglion cells (ectomesenchymoma), and MPNST with rhabdomyosarcoma.[25,64-66] The term *malignant Triton tumor* is usually applied only to the MPNST with rhabdomyosarcoma because it is the most widely recognized of the foregoing entities.[65,67-69] This composite neoplasm was first described in 1938 by Masson and Martin who suggested that the neural elements in the tumor induced differentiation of skeletal muscle in much the same fashion as normal nerve was believed to induce the regeneration of skeletal muscle in the Triton salamander. As a result, these tumors were eventually accorded the name of the amphibian.

Malignant Triton tumors are rare variants of MPNST. Slightly more than half occur in patients with NF1,[64,70,71] and one has been reported in the setting of Li-Fraumeni syndrome.[72] Although no consistent cytogenetic abnormality has been reported in this tumor, most have displayed clonal abnormalities involving various breakpoints along chromosome 1.[73,74]

The tumor develops most commonly in the fourth decade and may affect any soft tissue sites and rarely internal organs. The hallmark of this tumor is the presence of rhabdomyoblasts scattered throughout a backdrop indistinguishable from an ordinary MPNST (Figs. 28-18 and 28-19). The number of rhabdomyoblasts varies greatly from tumor to tumor and even from area to area in the same tumor. They are usually relatively mature, and their abundant eosinophilic cytoplasm contrasts sharply with the pale-staining cytoplasm of the Schwann cells. Cross-striations can be identified but, as in rhabdomyosarcomas, are more readily identified in cells with elongated tapered cytoplasm. Both desmin and nuclear regulatory proteins (MyoD1 and myogenin) can be demonstrated in the rhabdomyoblasts (see Fig. 28-19B). Occasionally, other lines of divergent differentiation, such as cartilage, are present.

Malignant Triton tumors are aggressive tumors, which based on a retrospective literature review have a 5-year survival rate of 10%.[64]

MALIGNANT PERIPHERAL NERVE SHEATH TUMOR WITH GLANDS (GLANDULAR MALIGNANT SCHWANNOMA)

In 1892, Garre reported a patient with von Recklinghausen disease and an MPNST of the sciatic nerve. Scattered throughout the schwannian background of the tumor were numerous well-differentiated glands. Since that time, very few additional

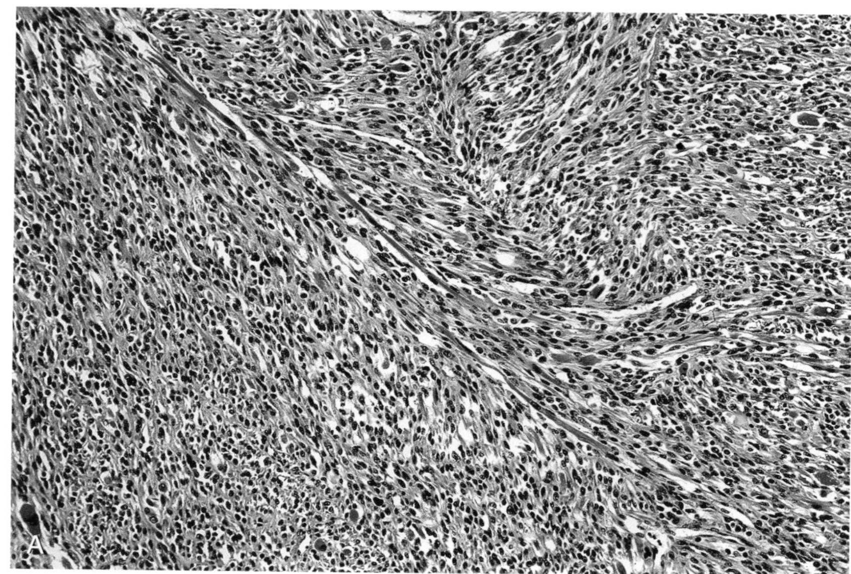

FIGURE 28-18. (A) MPNST with rhabdomyoblastic differentiation (malignant Triton tumor).

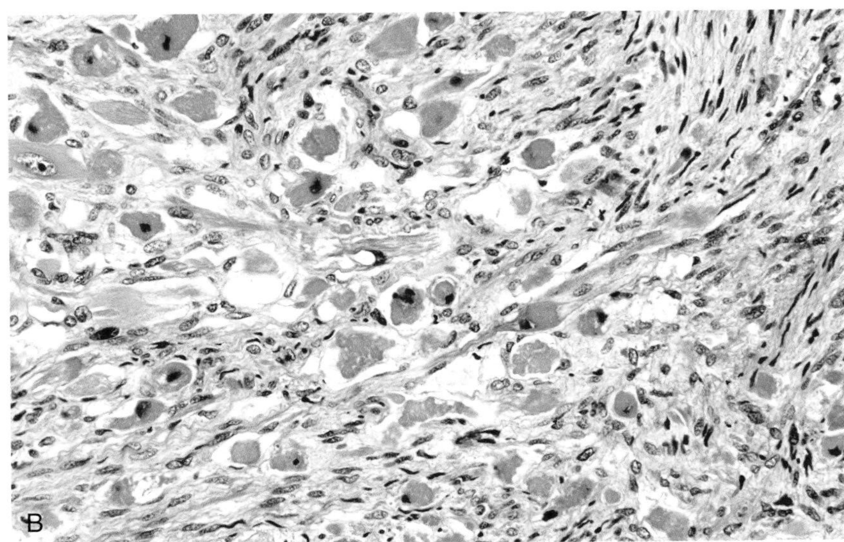

FIGURE 28-18, cont'd. (B) Rounded or elongated large rhabdomyoblasts are scattered throughout the tumor.

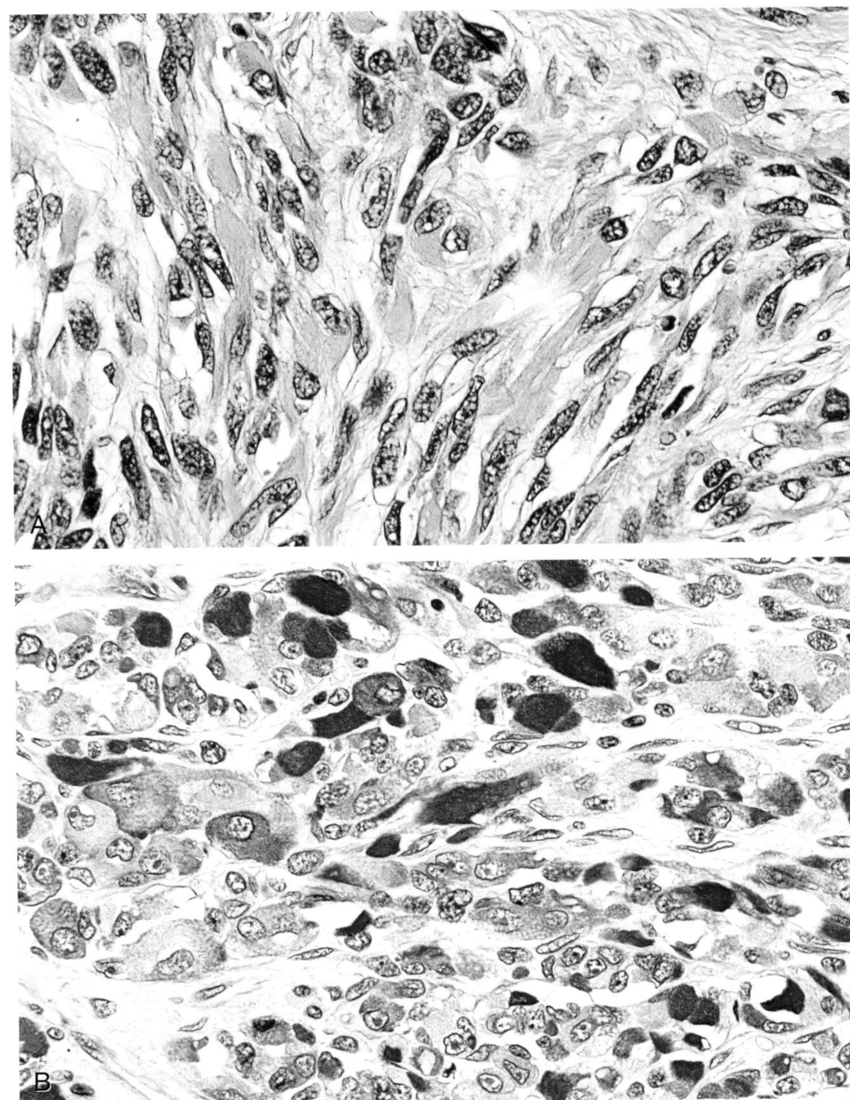

FIGURE 28-19. Rhabdomyoblasts in an MPNST (A) showing desmin immunoreactivity (B).

tumors have been reported, probably making it among the rarest of MPNST with divergent differentiation.[75-80] Almost all of these tumors have occurred in patients with NF1, a fact that surely accounts for the young median age (about 30 years)[69] of affected patients. The tumors usually arise from major nerves, including the sciatic, median, brachial plexus, and spinal nerves.

Characteristically, they have a spindle-cell background indistinguishable from ordinary MPNST and may contain other heterologous elements such as muscle, cartilage, and bone. The glands are usually few in number and are made up of well-differentiated, nonciliated cuboidal or columnar cells with clear cytoplasm and occasional goblet cells (Figs. 28-20 to 28-22). Rarely they appear malignant. Intracellular and extracellular mucin, histochemically identical to conventional epithelial mucins, can be demonstrated in the glands (see Fig. 28-21). Rarely squamous islands in addition to glands are encountered (see Fig. 28-22). Somatostatin immunoreactivity was noted in the glands of one glandular schwannoma.[81]

It may be difficult to distinguish these tumors from biphasic synovial sarcomas because the glandular elements may be virtually identical. It is principally the spindled element that distinguishes them, although obviously the presence of goblet cells or neuroendocrine differentiation favors the diagnosis of a glandular MPNST. In synovial sarcomas, the spindled element resembles a conventional fibrosarcoma and may be secondarily hyalinized or calcified. Subtle degrees of epithelial differentiation may also be evident in the spindled stroma of the synovial sarcoma. This feature is not present in glandular MPNST because the epithelial elements invariably arise rather abruptly from the stroma. The immunologic phenotypes of synovial sarcoma and glandular MPNST differ. The former often contains keratin-positive cells in the spindled zones (and, occasionally, S-100 protein-positive ones), whereas the latter displays only focal S-100 protein positivity. The addition of other neural antigens, such as NGFR, also known as *nerve growth factor receptor*, may improve the sensitivity and specificity of the diagnosis.[82]

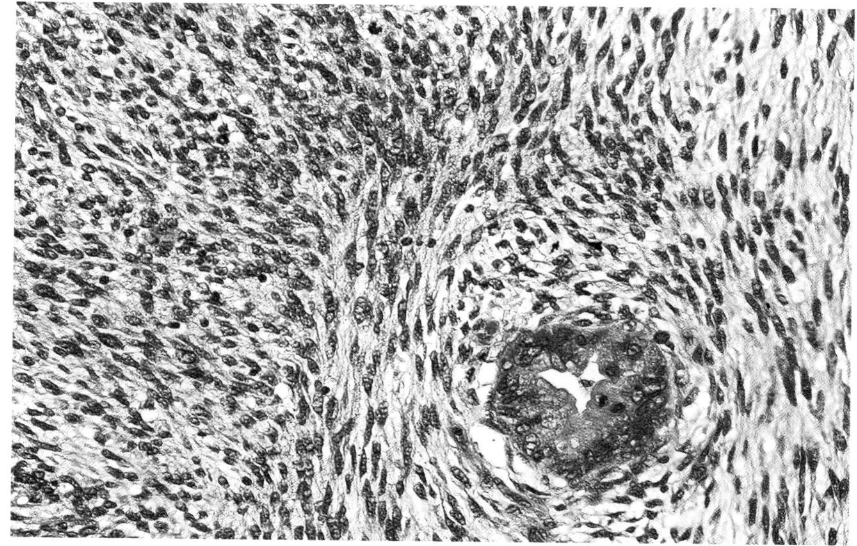

FIGURE 28-20. MPNST with glandular differentiation. Glands, in this case, appear malignant.

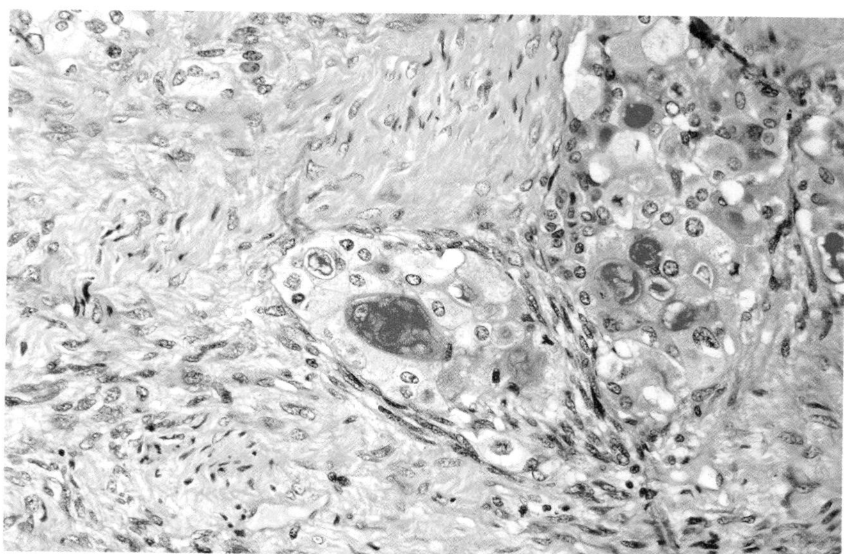

FIGURE 28-21. Glands in an MPNST containing carminophilic mucin.

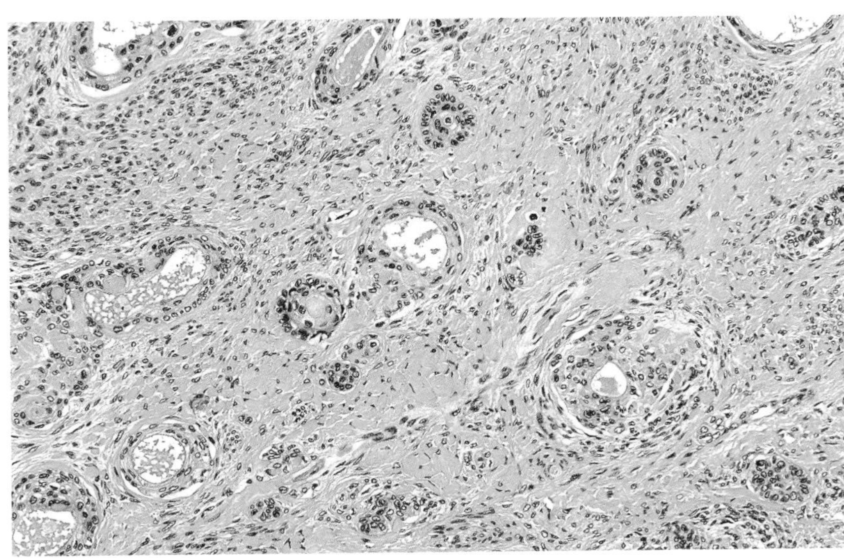

FIGURE 28-22. MPNST with glands and squamous islands.

Although the glandular elements set this tumor apart as a peculiar histologic variant, they serve essentially no role in grading the tumor or predicting its biologic behavior. Tumors with a highly malignant schwannian component may be expected to do poorly regardless of the degree of differentiation of the glands. Most tumors reported in the literature seem to fall into this category. On the other hand, tumors with a low-grade schwannian element may do extremely well, as illustrated by the fact that the two patients with tumors of this type reported by Woodruff and Christensen[83] are alive and well. It should be noted in passing, however, that certain rare (benign) schwannomas with glandular elements should be clearly distinguished from glandular MPNST. Usually, they are superficial lesions with glands that resemble adnexal structures, leading some to question whether they are entrapped elements.

MALIGNANT PERIPHERAL NERVE SHEATH TUMOR WITH ANGIOSARCOMA

Slightly more than 20 angiosarcomas arising in nerve sheath tumors have been reported, making these tumors largely curiosities.[84-89] Most have developed in patients with NF1 and not surprisingly, therefore, were associated with either plexiform neurofibroma, MPNST, or both. Anecdotal reports attest to the fact that angiosarcoma may also occur in benign schwannomas,[87] normal nerves,[88] and sporadic MPNST.[89] Because of the strong association with NF1, these tumors usually occur in young individuals. They are indistinguishable from MPNST and have conventional-appearing angiosarcomas that may be microscopic or macroscopic in size. The prognosis is poor, and most of the patients have succumbed to the disease.

EPITHELIOID MALIGNANT PERIPHERAL NERVE SHEATH TUMOR

Epithelioid MPNST, accounting for fewer than 5% of MPNST, closely resembles carcinoma or melanoma by virtue of the fact that the tumor is composed predominantly or exclusively of Schwann cells with a polygonal epithelioid appearance.[90-95]

Although often confused with melanomas, there is convincing evidence that these tumors represent nerve sheath tumors rather than melanomas or metastatic carcinomas. First, the tumors follow a distribution similar to that of the ordinary MPNST, with most occurring in patients 20 to 50 years of age. The median age is in the fourth decade, and males are affected slightly more often than females. Most of the tumors reported in the literature originated in major nerves, including the sciatic, tibial, peroneal, facial, antebrachial cutaneous, and digital nerves. In the experience by the authors of this edition, 8 of 10 deeply situated epithelioid MPNST originated from a major nerve, including the sciatic nerve (three cases) and the brachial plexus, femoral, radial, and median nerves (one case each). It is the cases in which origin from a nerve or neurofibroma cannot be documented that pose the most challenging and sometimes irresolvable problems in diagnosis. Although this form of MPNST may occur in NF1, it seems to occur less frequently than in ordinary MPNST. Lodding et al.[93] encountered 1 case in their series of 16, whereas none of 26 patients had the disease in the cases from the authors of this edition.[92] MPNST with epithelioid features is a recognized pattern of malignant transformation of schwannomas, including one that arose in a patient with schwannomatosis and germline *SMARCB1* mutation.[96]

Histologically, the tumor is variable. In cases from the authors of this edition, the most characteristic appearance is that of short cords of large epithelioid cells arranged in a vague nodular pattern (Figs. 28-23 to 28-27). The cells in these tumors usually have large, round nuclei with prominent melanoma-like nucleoli (see Fig. 28-25). The tumors may appear densely cellular or myxoid (see Fig. 28-25B), depending on the accumulation of acid mucin between the cords, and there is often subtle blending of the epithelioid areas with spindled areas resembling the conventional MPNST (Fig. 28-28) However, the term *epithelioid MPNST* should be reserved for tumors in which the predominant pattern is epithelioid. Although the combination of all of these features is usually sufficient to make the correct diagnosis, many tumors lack this distinctive appearance. In fact, most tumors reported

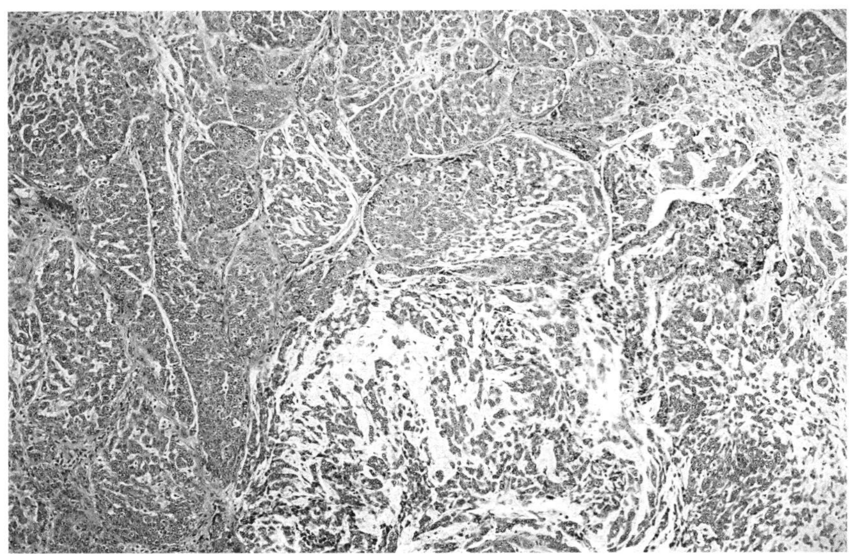

FIGURE 28-23. Epithelioid MPNST showing vague nodular growth. The tumor varies from slightly myxoid to cellular.

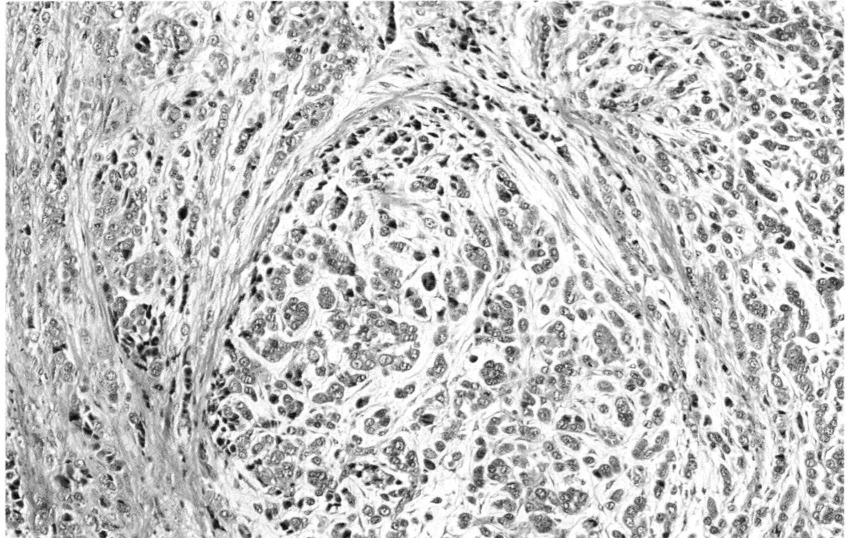

FIGURE 28-24. Epithelioid MPNST with cords of epithelioid cells.

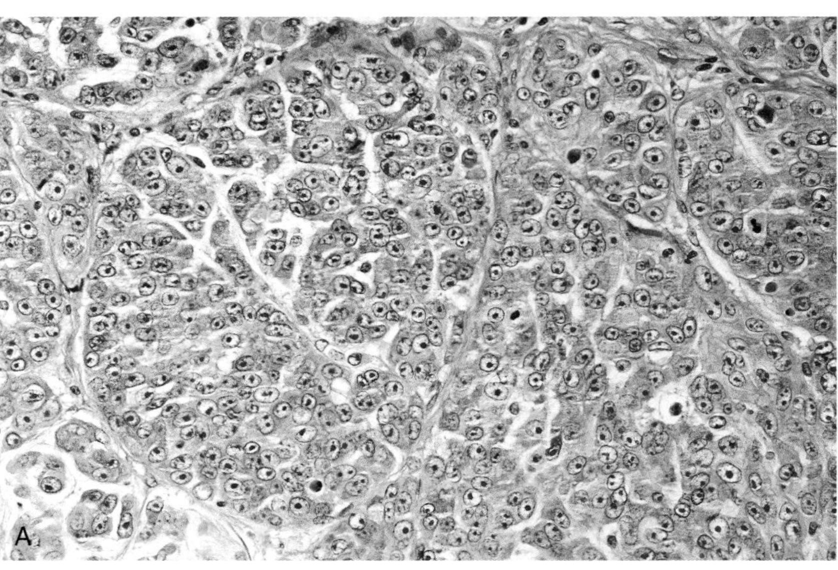

FIGURE 28-25. Epithelioid MPNST showing the polygonal shape of cells and prominent nucleoli (A).

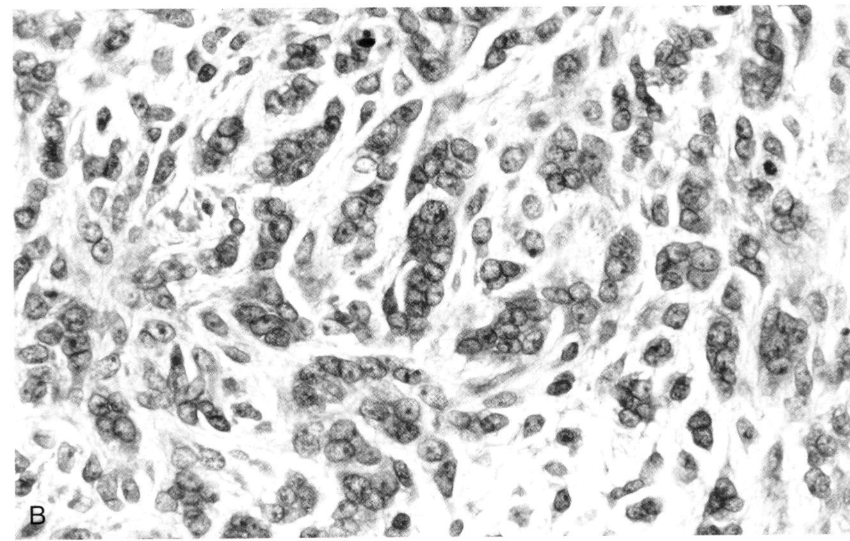

FIGURE 28-25, cont'd. In some areas, groups of cells are separated by myxoid stroma (B).

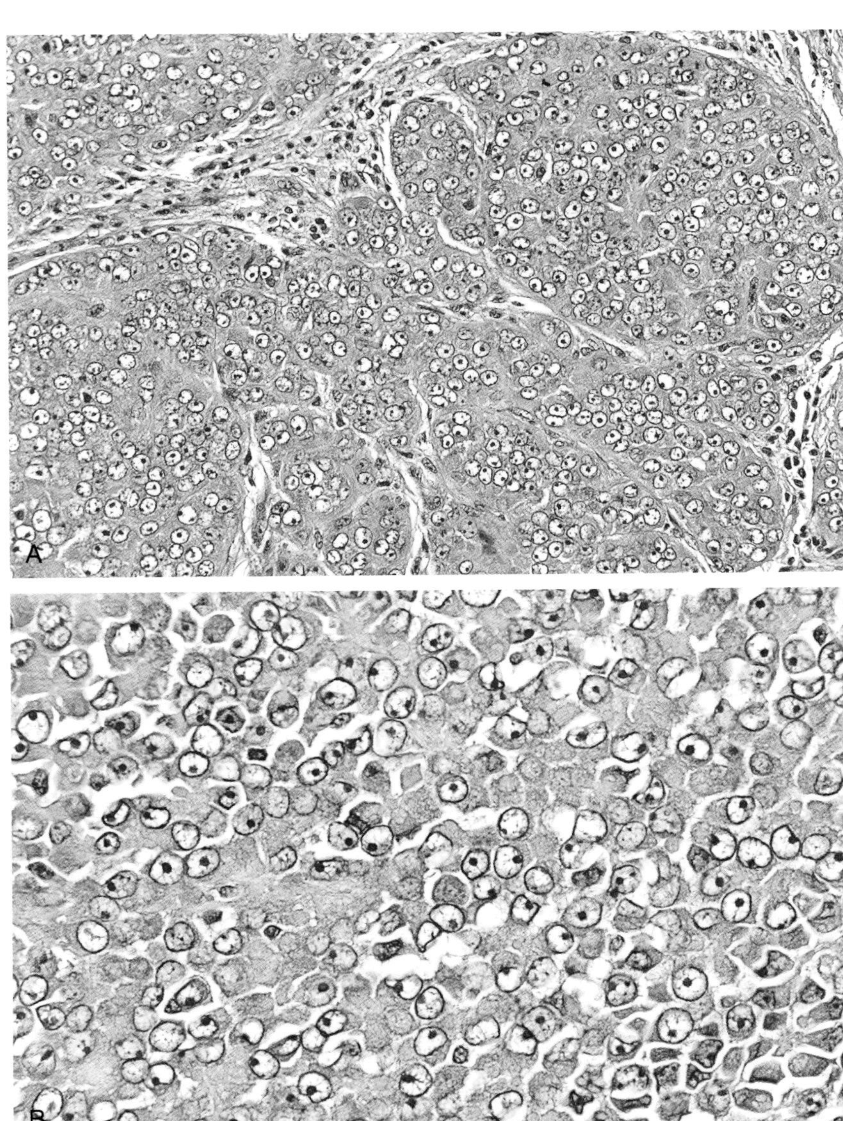

FIGURE 28-26. (A) Epithelioid MPNST with rhabdoid cells. (B) High-power view of rhabdoid cells shows a glassy perinuclear zone.

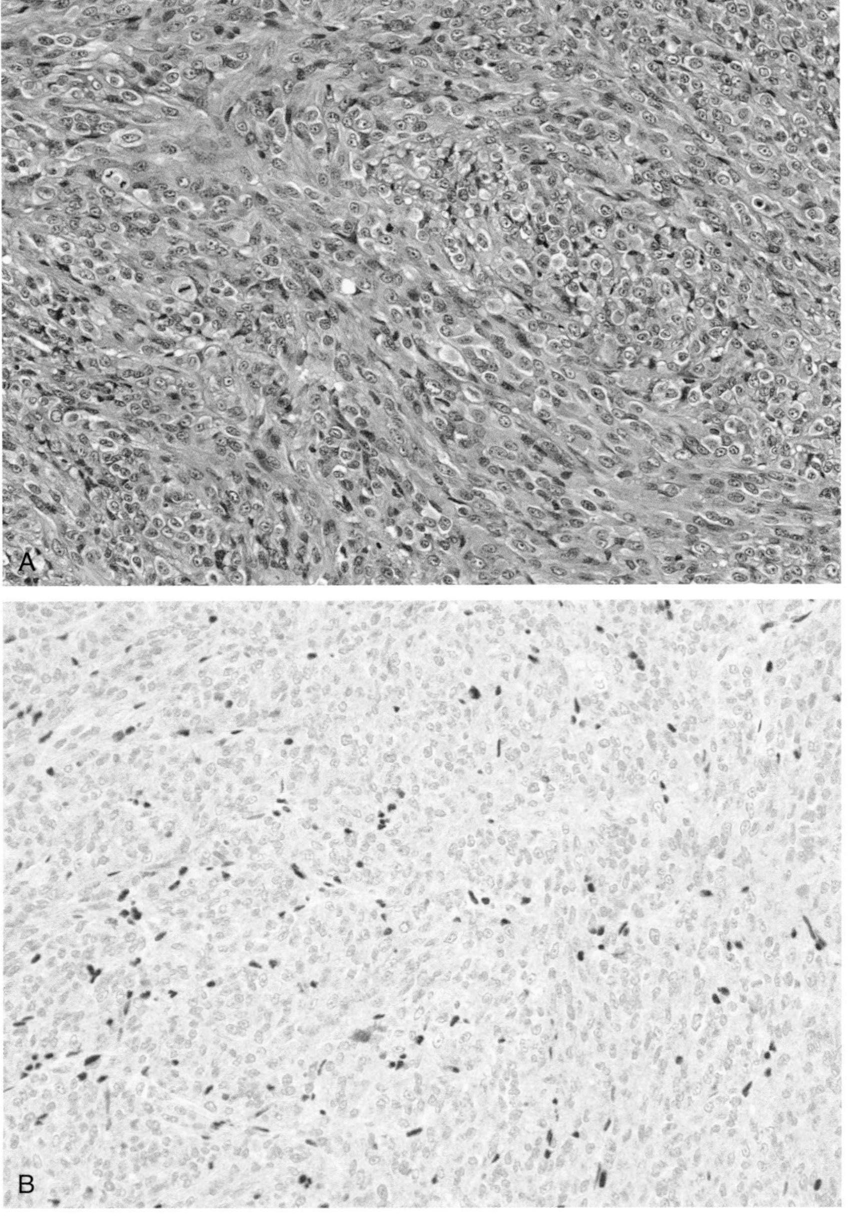

FIGURE 28-27. (A) Epithelioid MPNST showing (B) INI1 inactivation (loss of staining). Normal cells display nuclear staining.

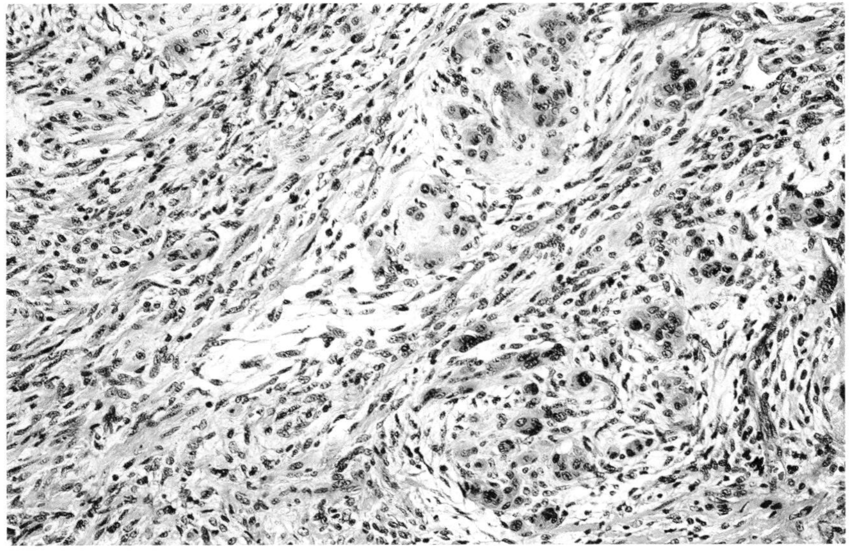

FIGURE 28-28. MPNST with focal epithelioid differentiation.

in the literature have resembled melanomas or carcinomas and have consisted simply of small nests of epithelioid cells admixed with a spindled component.

There are a number of rather unusual forms of epithelioid MPNST that deserve comment. Some contain a predominance of clear cells, and others are made up of rhabdoid cells with a prominent glassy eosinophilic perinuclear zone corresponding ultrastructurally to the presence of whorls of intermediate filaments (see Fig. 28-26). As an interesting correlate, some epithelioid MPNSTs show loss of SMARCB1 immunostaining (see later text) as is encountered in other tumors with a rhabdoid phenotype (see Fig. 28-27). Still other tumors consist of sheets of rounded pleomorphic cells suggestive of a pleomorphic carcinoma (Fig. 28-29).

Consequently, the diagnosis has largely depended on an established origin from a nerve. In the absence of this feature, the diagnosis is sometimes suspected by a delicate mesenchymal pattern of collagenization and a transition to spindled schwannian areas (see Fig. 28-28). Unlike many melanomas, neither melanin pigment nor glycogen can be demonstrated in the cytoplasm of these tumors. In one unique case that was reviewed, the diagnosis of malignant epithelioid schwannoma was established by virtue of the presence of true rosettes in a tumor that otherwise resembled melanoma (see Fig. 28-17). It should be emphasized that a clear-cut distinction from melanoma or carcinoma is not always possible on routine sections, a dilemma compounded by the fact that, occasionally, metastatic spindled melanomas are virtually indistinguishable from MPNST.

About 80% of these tumors are strongly and diffusely positive for S-100 protein, a pattern of immunoreactivity that contrasts with conventional MPNST (Fig. 28-30).[92] They do not express melanoma-associated antigens, and only rarely is keratin present. Therefore, the presence of either keratin or melanin-related antigens in a malignant epithelioid tumor argues against the diagnosis of epithelioid MPNST. About one-half also lack SMARCB1 immunostaining,[97] a finding that contrasts with malignant melanoma. Immunostaining for pericellular type IV collagen, a consistent feature of schwannoma, is of limited use in distinguishing epithelioid MPNST from melanoma because they share considerable overlap.[92]

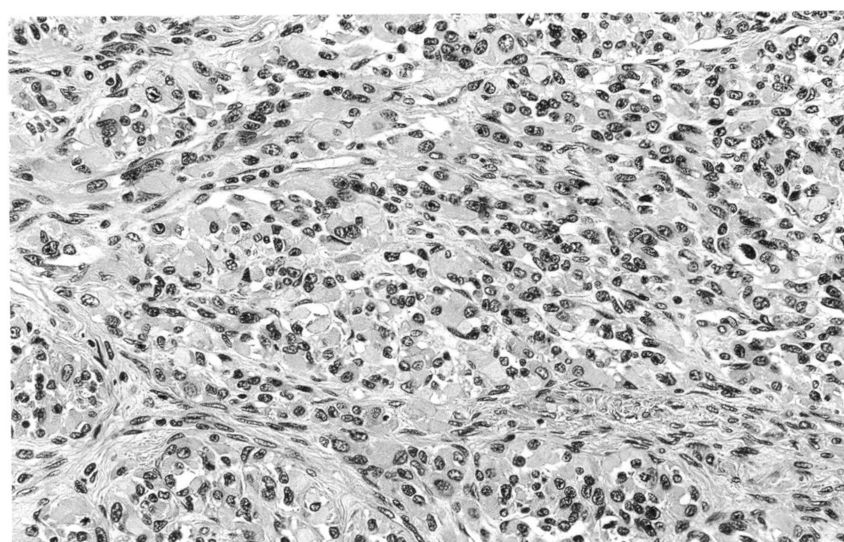

FIGURE 28-29. Epithelioid MPNST composed of pleomorphic epithelioid cells.

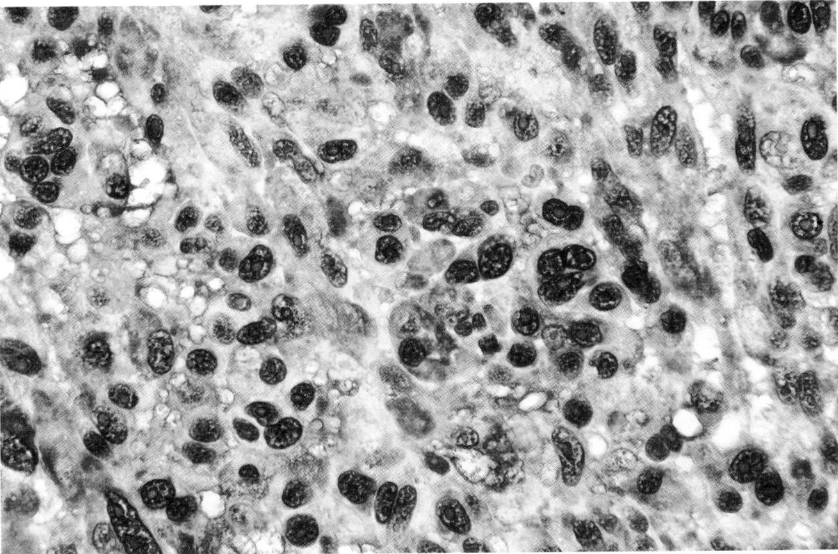

FIGURE 28-30. S-100 protein immunostaining in an epithelioid MPNST.

Epithelioid MPNSTs are aggressive lesions; at least half of the patients reported in the literature developed distant metastases, usually in the lung. In the experience of the authors of this edition, with 10 patients with tumors in deep soft tissue, 3 developed metastatic disease.[92] Because of the melanoma-like appearance of these tumors, the question has been raised as to whether they commonly spread to regional lymph nodes. Lodding et al.[93] noted lymph node metastasis in 3 of their 14 cases, but the authors of this edition had no instances of lymph node metastasis in 16 cases.[92]

EXTRASPINAL (SOFT TISSUE) EPENDYMOMA

Soft tissue ependymomas are rare tumors that occur in subcutaneous locations dorsal to the sacrum and coccyx or in deep soft tissue anterior to the sacrum and posterior to the rectum. Many that occur in the latter location represent ependymomas of the cauda equina that have extended through the sacral foramina to present as presacral masses.[98] Those situated dorsally to the sacrum represent the more significant group in terms of soft tissue tumors; consequently, this discussion is restricted to this group. Pathogenetically, the dorsal coccygeal ependymoma may arise from normal remnants of the neural tube (coccygeal medullary vestige) or from abnormal remnants resulting from embryologic malformations. The latter contention is supported by the fact that a significant proportion of patients with this tumor[99] have developmental abnormalities such as spina bifida.

Characteristically, these tumors present as long-standing masses that are often diagnosed preoperatively as pilonidal cysts, teratomas, or sweat gland tumors. Although a few have proved to be extensive at the time of initial surgery,[99] most are encapsulated and easily separated from the fascia overlying the sacrum and coccyx. Grossly, they are myxoid multilobulated masses with focal areas of hemorrhage and necrosis (Fig. 28-31). Most resemble the ependymomas arising from the cauda equina and are of the myxopapillary type. Cuboidal or columnar cells are arranged on fibrovascular stalks in a papillary configuration (Fig. 28-32). Secondary perivascular

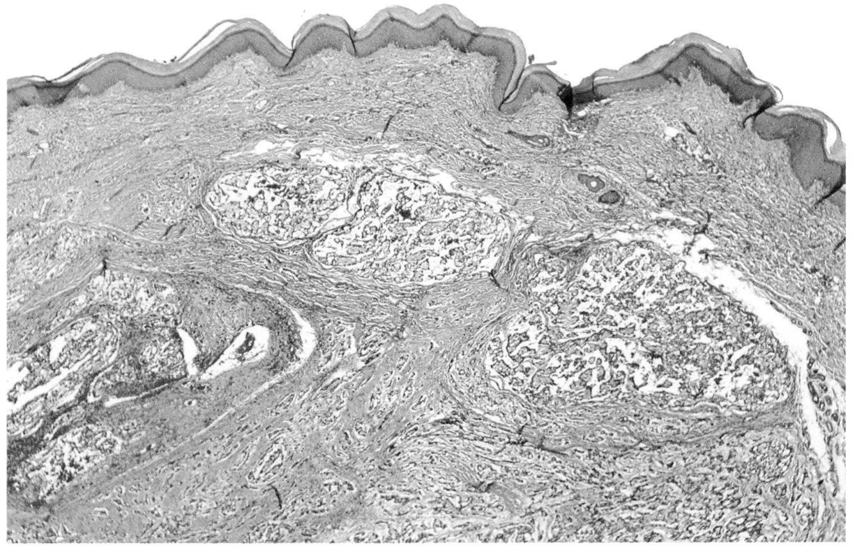

FIGURE 28-31. Extraspinal ependymoma presenting in a dorsococcygeal location.

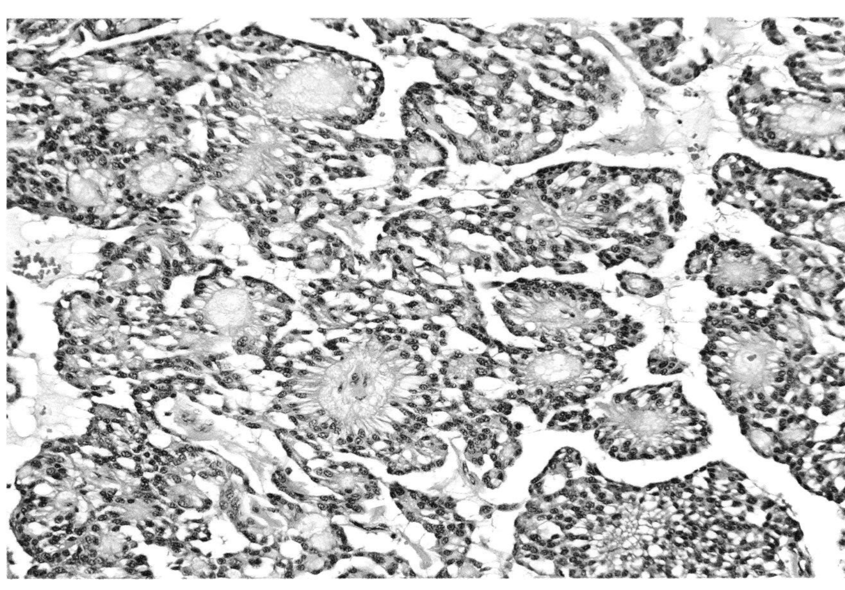

FIGURE 28-32. Extraspinal ependymoma. Tumor resembles a myxopapillary ependymoma of the cauda equina and contains perivascular pseudorosettes and papillary structures.

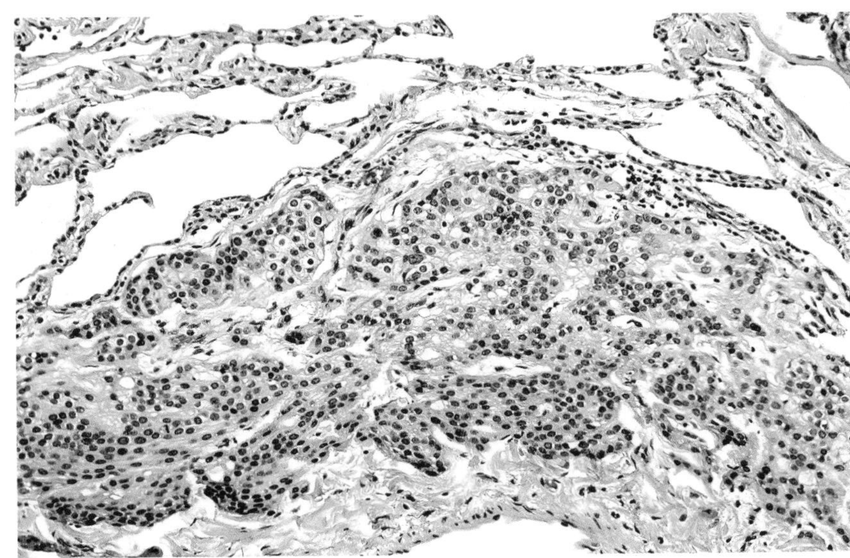

FIGURE 28-33. Extraspinal ependymoma metastatic to lung. Nests of tumor may mimic the pattern of carcinoma or carcinoid tumor.

degenerative changes result in the peculiar myxoid and hyalinized appearance that characterizes the myxopapillary ependymoma. In cases where the degeneration is not marked, the tumor may resemble the more cellular papillary ependymoma of the brain. The cells are usually well differentiated with apically polarized nuclei. Occasionally, blepharoplasts are demonstrated by means of special stains (phosphotungstic acid-hematoxylin stain). Carminophilic intracytoplasmic mucin is not present in these cells, despite its presence in the closely related choroid plexus papilloma.[98] Ultrastructurally, these cells have many of the features of normal ependymal cells. They contain microvilli and lateral desmosomes at their apical surfaces, whereas elaborate interdigitations of the plasma membrane and underlying basement membrane material characterize the basal surfaces. Parallel arrays of fine filaments and occasional microtubules are found in the cytoplasm.

Although ependymomas are, in general, low-grade neoplasms and usually pose problems in control of local disease only, dorsal coccygeal ependymomas have a greater propensity to metastasize than their intraspinal counterparts. This has been ascribed to their easier accessibility to lymphatic channels and to the longer survival time associated with these tumors. Of the few cases reported, local recurrence has developed in 25%, and death has ensued in one-half.[100] Three of 17 reported dorsal coccygeal ependymomas metastasized to regional (inguinal) nodes or the lung. Metastasis to the lung may be mistaken for a carcinoid tumor (Fig. 28-33). Distant metastasis is a late event, usually occurring 10 years or more after diagnosis of the primary tumor. Adequate treatment of these tumors consists of wide local excision with irradiation for residual or inoperable disease. The protracted course of this disease underscores the need for extended follow-up care and even resection of isolated metastases if and when they appear.

References

1. Ducatman BS, Scheithauer BW, Piepgras DG, et al. Malignant peripheral nerve sheath tumors. A clinicopathologic study of 120 cases. Cancer 1986;57(10):2006–21.
2. Hruban RH, Shiu MH, Senie RT, et al. Malignant peripheral nerve sheath tumors of the buttock and lower extremity. A study of 43 cases. Cancer 1990;66(6):1253–65.
3. Wong WW, Hirose T, Scheithauer BW, et al. Malignant peripheral nerve sheath tumor: analysis of treatment outcome. Int J Radiat Oncol Biol Phys 1998;42(2):351–60.
4. Okada K, Hasegawa T, Tajino T, et al. Clinical relevance of pathological grades of malignant peripheral nerve sheath tumor: a multi-institution TMTS study of 56 cases in Northern Japan. Ann Surg Oncol 2007; 14(2):597–604.
5. Zou C, Smith KD, Liu J, et al. Clinical, pathological, and molecular variables predictive of malignant peripheral nerve sheath tumor outcome. Ann Surg 2009;249(6):1014–22.
6. Anghileri M, Miceli R, Fiore M, et al. Malignant peripheral nerve sheath tumors: prognostic factors and survival in a series of patients treated at a single institution. Cancer 2006;107:1065–74.
7. Ferner RE, O'Doherty MJ. Neurofibroma and schwannoma. Curr Opin Neurol 2002;15(6):679–84.
8. Evans DG, Baser ME, McGaughran J. Malignant peripheral nerve sheath tumor in neurofibromatosis 1. J Med Genet 2002;39:311–14.
9. De Raedt T, Brems H, Wolkenstein P. Elevated rsik for MPNST in NF1 microdeletions patients. Amer J Hum Genet 2003;72:1288–92.
10. Pasmant E, Masliah-Planchon J, Lévy P, et al. Identification of genes potentially involved in the increased risk of malignancy in NF-1-microdeleted patients. Mol Med 2010;17:79–87.
11. Carli M, Morgan M, Bisogno G, et al. Malignant peripheral nerve sheath tumors in childhood (MPNST): a combined experience of the Italian and German co-operative studies: SIOP XXVII meeting. Med Pediatr Oncol 1995;25:243.
12. Coffin CM, Dehner LP. Peripheral neurogenic tumors of the soft tissues in children and adolescents: a clinicopathologic study of 139 cases. Pediatr Pathol 1989;9(4):387–407.
13. deCou JM, Rao BN, Parham DM, et al. Malignant peripheral nerve sheath tumors: the St. Jude Children's Research Hospital experience. Ann Surg Oncol 1995;2(6):524–9.
14. Ducatman BS, Scheithauer BW. Postirradiation neurofibrosarcoma. Cancer 1983;51(6):1028–33.
15. Foley KM, Woodruff JM, Ellis FT, et al. Radiation-induced malignant and atypical peripheral nerve sheath tumors. Ann Neurol 1980;7(4): 311–18.
16. Kourea HP, Bilsky MH, Leung DH, et al. Subdiaphragmatic and intrathoracic paraspinal malignant peripheral nerve sheath tumors: a clinicopathologic study of 25 patients and 26 tumors. Cancer 1998;82(11): 2191–203.
17. Guccion JG, Enzinger FM. Malignant Schwannoma associated with von Recklinghausen's neurofibromatosis. Virchows Arch A Pathol Anat Histol 1979;383(1):43–57.

18. Bojsen-Moller M, Myhre-Jensen O. A consecutive series of 30 malignant schwannomas. Survival in relation to clinico-pathological parameters and treatment. Acta Pathol Microbiol Immunol Scand A 1984;92(3):147–55.
19. D'Agostino AN, Soule EH, Miller RH. Primary malignant neoplasms of nerves (malignant neurilemomas) in patients without manifestations of multiple neurofibromatosis (von Recklinghausen's disease). Cancer 1963;16:1003–14.
20. D'Agostino AN, Soule EH, Miller RH. Sarcomas of the peripheral nerves and somatic soft tissues associated with multiple neurofibromatosis (von Recklinghausen's disease). Cancer 1963;16:1015–27.
21. Daimaru Y, Hashimoto H, Enjoji M. Malignant peripheral nerve-sheath tumors (malignant schwannomas). An immunohistochemical study of 29 cases. Am J Surg Pathol 1985;9(6):434–44.
22. Sorensen SA, Mulvihill JJ, Nielsen A. Long-term follow-up of von Recklinghausen neurofibromatosis. Survival and malignant neoplasms. N Engl J Med 1986;314(16):1010–15.
23. Ferner RE, Lucas JD, O'Doherty MJ, et al. Evaluation of (18)fluorodeoxyglucose positron emission tomography ((18)FDG PET) in the detection of malignant peripheral nerve sheath tumours arising from within plexiform neurofibromas in neurofibromatosis 1. J Neurol Neurosurg Psychiatry 2000;68(3):353–7.
24. Brenner W, Friedrich RE, Gawad KA, et al. Prognostic relevance of FDG PET in patients with neurofibromatosis type-1 and malignant peripheral nerve sheath tumours. Eur J Nucl Med Mol Imaging 2006; 33(4):428–32.
25. Daimaru Y, Hashimoto H, Enjoji M. Malignant "triton" tumors: a clinicopathologic and immunohistochemical study of nine cases. Hum Pathol 1984;15(8):768–78.
26. Abe S, Imamura T, Park P, et al. Small round-cell type of malignant peripheral nerve sheath tumor. Mod Pathol 1998;11(8):747–53.
27. Meis JM, Enzinger FM, Martz KL, et al. Malignant peripheral nerve sheath tumors (malignant schwannomas) in children. Am J Surg Pathol 1992;16(7):694–707.
28. Matsunou H, Shimoda T, Kakimoto S, et al. Histopathologic and immunohistochemical study of malignant tumors of peripheral nerve sheath (malignant schwannoma). Cancer 1985;56(9):2269–79.
29. Nakajima T, Watanabe S, Sato Y, et al. An immunoperoxidase study of S-100 protein distribution in normal and neoplastic tissues. Am J Surg Pathol 1982;6(8):715–27.
30. Weiss SW, Langloss JM, Enzinger FM. Value of S-100 protein in the diagnosis of soft tissue tumors with particular reference to benign and malignant Schwann cell tumors. Lab Invest 1983;49(3):299–308.
31. Wick MR, Swanson PE, Scheithauer BW, et al. Malignant peripheral nerve sheath tumor. An immunohistochemical study of 62 cases. Am J Clin Pathol 1987;87(4):425–33.
32. Knosel T, Heretsch S, Altendorf-Hoffmann A. TLE1 is a robust diagnostic biomarker for synovial sarcomas and correlates with t(X;18): analysis of 319 cases. Eur J Cancer 2010;46(6):1170–6.
33. Foo WC, Cruise MW, Wick MR, et al. Immunohistochemical staining for TLE1 distinguishes synovial sarcoma frm histologic mimics. Am J Clin Pathol 2011;135(6):839–44.
34. Jagdis A, Rubin BP, Tubbs RR, et al. Prospective evaluation of TLE1 as a diagnostic immunohistochemical marker in synovial sarcoma. Am J Surg Pathol 2009;33(12):1743–51.
35. Terry J, Saito T, Subramanian S, et al. TLE1 as a diagnostic immunohistochemical marker for synovial sarcoma emerging from gene expression profiling studies. Am J Surg Pathol 2007;31(2):240–6.
36. Kosemehmetoglu K, Vrana JA, Folpe AL. TLE1 expression is not specific for synovial sarcoma: a whole section study of 163 soft tissue and bone neoplasms. Mod Pathol 2009;22(7):872–8.
37. Olsen SH, Thomas DG, Lucas DR. Cluster analysis of immunohistochemical profiles in synovial sarcoma, malignant peripheral nerve sheath tumor, and Ewing sarcoma. Mod Pathol 2006;19(5):659–68.
38. Hui P, Li N, Johnson C, et al. HMGA proteins in malignant peripheral nerve sheath tumor and synovial sarcoma: preferential expression of HMGA2 in malignant peripheral nerve sheath tumor. Mod Pathol 2005; 18(11):1519–26.
39. Nonaka D, Chiriboga L, Rubin BP. Sox10: a pan-schwannian and melanocytic marker. Am J Surg Pathol 2008;32(9):1291–8.
40. Halling KC, Scheithauer BW, Halling AC, et al. p53 expression in neurofibroma and malignant peripheral nerve sheath tumor. An immunohistochemical study of sporadic and NF1-associated tumors. Am J Clin Pathol 1996;106(3):282–8.
41. Kindblom LG, Ahlden M, Meis-Kindblom JM, et al. Immunohistochemical and molecular analysis of p53, MDM2, proliferating cell nuclear antigen and Ki67 in benign and malignant peripheral nerve sheath tumours. Virchows Arch 1995;427(1):19–26.
42. McCarron KF, Goldblum JR. Plexiform neurofibroma with and without associated malignant peripheral nerve sheath tumor: a clinicopathologic and immunohistochemical analysis of 54 cases. Mod Pathol 1998;11(7): 612–17.
43. Liapis H, Marley EF, Lin Y, et al. p53 and Ki67 proliferating cell nuclear atnigen in benign and malignant peipheral nerve sheath tumors in children. Pediatr Dev Pathol 1999;2:377–84.
44. Sawada S, Florell S, Purandare SM, et al. Identification of NF1 mutations in both alleles of a dermal neurofibroma. Nat Genet 1996;14(1):110–12.
45. Menon AG, Anderson KM, Riccardi VM, et al. Chromosome 17p deletions and p53 gene mutations associated with the formation of malignant neurofibrosarcomas in von Recklinghausen neurofibromatosis. Proc Natl Acad Sci U S A 1990;87(14):5435–9.
46. Kim HA, Ling B, Ratner N. Nf1-deficient mouse Schwann cells are angiogenic and invasive and can be induced to hyperproliferate: reversion of some phenotypes by an inhibitor of farnesyl protein transferase. Mol Cell Biol 1997;17(2):862–72.
47. Kim HA, Rosenbaum T, Marchionni MA, et al. Schwann cells from neurofibromin deficient mice exhibit activation of p21ras, inhibition of cell proliferation and morphological changes. Oncogene 1995;11(2): 325–35.
48. Berner JM, Sorlie T, Mertens F, et al. Chromosome band 9p21 is frequently altered in malignant peripheral nerve sheath tumors: studies of CDKN2A and other genes of the pRB pathway. Genes Chromosomes Cancer 1999;26(2):151–60.
49. Mechtersheimer G, Otaño-Joos M, Ohl S, et al. Analysis of chromosomal imbalances in sporadic and NF1-associated peripheral nerve sheath tumors by comparative genomic hybridization. Genes Chromosomes Cancer 1999;25(4):362–9.
50. Mertens F, Rydholm A, Bauer HF, et al. Cytogenetic findings in malignant peripheral nerve sheath tumors. Int J Cancer 1995;61(6): 793–8.
51. Schmidt H, Würl P, Taubert H, et al. Genomic imbalances of 7p and 17q in malignant peripheral nerve sheath tumors are clinically relevant. Genes Chromosomes Cancer 1999;25(3):205–11.
52. Kourea HP, Cordon-Cardo C, Dudas M, et al. Expression of p27(kip) and other cell cycle regulators in malignant peripheral nerve sheath tumors and neurofibromas: the emerging role of p27(kip) in malignant transformation of neurofibromas. Am J Pathol 1999;155(6):1885–91.
53. Kourea HP, Orlow I, Scheithauer BW, et al. Deletions of the INK4A gene occur in malignant peripheral nerve sheath tumors but not in neurofibromas. Am J Pathol 1999;155(6):1855–60.
54. Agesen TH, Florenes VA, Molenaar WM, et al. Expression patterns of cell cycle components in sporadic and neurofibromatosis type 1-related malignant peripheral nerve sheath tumors. J Neuropathol Exp Neurol 2005;64(1):74–81.
55. Sabah M, Cummins R, Leader M, et al. Loss of p16 (INK4A) expression is associated with allelic imbalance/loss of heterozygosity of chromosome 9p21 in microdissected malignant peripheral nerve sheath tumors. Appl Immunohistochem Mol Morphol 2006;14(1):97–102.
56. Zhou H, Coffin CM, Perkins SL, et al. Malignant peripheral nerve sheath tumor: a comparison of grade, immunophenotype, and cell cycle/growth activation marker expression in sporadic and neurofibromatosis 1-related lesions. Am J Surg Pathol 2003;27(10):1337–45.
57. Kobayashi C, Oda Y, Takahira T, et al. Aberrant expression of CHFR in malignant peripheral nerve sheath tumors. Mod Pathol 2006;19(4): 524–32.
58. Subramanian S, Thayanithy V, West RB, et al. Genome-wide transcriptome analyses reveal p53 inactivation mediated loss of miR-34a expression in malignant peripheral nerve sheath tumours. J Pathol 2010; 220(1):58–70.
59. Miller SJ, Rangwala F, Williams J, et al. Large-scale molecular comparison of human schwann cells to malignant peripheral nerve sheath tumor cell lines and tissues. Cancer Res 2006;66(5):2584–91.
60. Yu J, Deshmukh H, Payton JE, et al. Array-based comparative genomic hybridization identifies CDK4 and FOXM1 alterations as independent predictors of survival in malignant peripheral nerve sheath tumor. Clin Cancer Res 2011;17(7):1924–34.
61. Eilber FC, Brennan MF, Eilber FR. Validation of the postoperative nomogram for 12 year sarcoma-specific mortality. Cancer Metastasis Rev 2004;101:2270–5.
62. Casanova M, Ferrari A, Spreafico F, et al. Malignant peripheral nerve sheath tumors in children: a single-institution twenty-year experience. J Pediatr Hematol Oncol 1999;21(6):509–13.

63. Carli M, Ferrari A, Mattke A, et al. Pediatric malignant peripheral nerve sheath tumor: the Italian and German soft tissue sarcoma cooperative group. J Clin Oncol 2005;23(33):8422–30.
64. Brooks JS, Freeman M, Enterline HT. Malignant "Triton" tumors. Natural history and immunohistochemistry of nine new cases with literature review. Cancer 1985;55(11):2543–9.
65. Ordonez NG, Tornos C. Malignant peripheral nerve sheath tumor of the pleura with epithelial and rhabdomyoblastic differentiation: report of a case clinically simulating mesothelioma. Am J Surg Pathol 1997;21(12):1515–21.
66. Woodruff JM, Chernik NL, Smith MC, et al. Peripheral nerve tumors with rhabdomyosarcomatous differentiation (malignant "Triton" tumors). Cancer 1973;32(2):426–39.
67. Heffner DK, Gnepp DR. Sinonasal fibrosarcomas, malignant schwannomas, and "Triton" tumors. A clinicopathologic study of 67 cases. Cancer 1992;70(5):1089–101.
68. Travis JA, Sandberg AA, Neff JR, et al. Cytogenetic findings in malignant triton tumor. Genes Chromosomes Cancer 1994;9(1):1–7.
69. Wong SY, Teh M, Tan YO, et al. Malignant glandular triton tumor. Cancer 1991;67(4):1076–83.
70. Ducatman BS, Scheithauer BW. Malignant peripheral nerve sheath tumors with divergent differentiation. Cancer 1984;54(6):1049–57.
71. Terzic A, Bode B, Gratz KW, et al. Prognostic factors for the malignant triton tumor of the the head and neck. Head and neck pathology 2009;31(5):679–88.
72. Chao MM, Levine JE, Ruiz RE, et al. Malignant triton tumor in a patient with Li-Fraumeni syndrome and a novel TP53 mutation. Pediatr Blood Cancer 2007;49(7):1000–4.
73. Velagaleti GV, Miettinen M, Gatalica Z. Malignant peripheral nerve sheath tumor with rhabdomyoblastic differentiation (malignant triton tumor) with balanced t(7;9)(q11.2;p24) and unbalanced translocation der(16)t(1;16)(q23;q13). Cancer Genet Cytogenet 2004;149(1):23–7.
74. Hennig Y, Loschke S, Katenkamp D, et al. A malignant triton tumor with an unbalanced translocation (1;13)(q10;q10) and an isochromosome (8)(q10) as the sole karyotypic abnormalities. Cancer Genet Cytogenet 2000;118(1):80–2.
75. Smith TA, Machen SK, Fisher C, et al. Usefulness of cytokeratin subsets for distinguishing monophasic synovial sarcoma from malignant peripheral nerve sheath tumor. Am J Clin Pathol 1999;112(5):641–8.
76. Christensen WN, Strong EW, Bains MS, et al. Neuroendocrine differentiation in the glandular peripheral nerve sheath tumor. Pathologic distinction from the biphasic synovial sarcoma with glands. Am J Surg Pathol 1988;12(6):417–26.
77. Cross PA, Clarke NW. Malignant nerve sheath tumour with epithelial elements. Histopathology 1988;12(5):547–9.
78. DeSchryver K, Santa Cruz DJ. So-called glandular schwannoma: ependymal differentiation in a case. Ultrastruct Pathol 1984;6(2–3):167–75.
79. Foraker AG. Glandlike elements in a peripheral neurosarcoma. Cancer 1948;1(2):286–93.
80. Michel SL. Epithelial elements in a malignant neurogenic tumor of the tibial nerve. Am J Surg 1967;113(3):404–8.
81. Warner TF, Louie R, Hafez GR, et al. Malignant nerve sheath tumor containing endocrine cells. Am J Surg Pathol 1983;7(6):583–90.
82. Woodruff JM. Peripheral nerve tumors showing glandular differentiation (glandular schwannomas). Cancer 1976;37(5):2399–413.
83. Woodruff JM, Christensen WN. Glandular peripheral nerve sheath tumors. Cancer 1993;72(12):3618–28.
84. Bricklin AS, Rushton HW. Angiosarcoma of venous origin arising in radial nerve. Cancer 1977;39(4):1556–8.
85. Brown RW, Tornos C, Evans HL. Angiosarcoma arising from malignant schwannoma in a patient with neurofibromatosis. Cancer 1992;70(5):1141–4.
86. Chaudhuri B, Ronan SG, Manaligod JR. Angiosarcoma arising in a plexiform neurofibroma: a case report. Cancer 1980;46(3):605–10.
87. Meis JM, Kindblom LG, Enzinger FM. Angiosarcoma arising in peripheral nerve sheath tumors: report of 5 additional cases. Lab Invest 1994;70:80A.
88. Mentzel T, Katenkamp D. Intraneural angiosarcoma and angiosarcoma arising in benign and malignant peripheral nerve sheath tumours: clinicopathological and immunohistochemical analysis of four cases. Histopathology 1999;35(2):114–20.
89. Morphopoulos GD, Banerjee SS, Ali HH, et al. Malignant peripheral nerve sheath tumour with vascular differentiation: a report of four cases. Histopathology 1996;28(5):401–10.
90. Alvira MM, Mandybur TK, Menefee MG. Light microscopic and ultrastructural observations of a metastasizing malignant epithelioid schwannoma. Cancer 1976;38(5):1977–82.
91. Cohn I. Epithelial neoplasms of peripheral and cranial nerves: report of three cases: review of the literature. Arch Surg 1928;17:117.
92. Laskin WB, Weiss SW, Bratthauer GL. Epithelioid variant of malignant peripheral nerve sheath tumor (malignant epithelioid schwannoma). Am J Surg Pathol 1991;15(12):1136–45.
93. Lodding P, Kindblom LG, Angervall L. Epithelioid malignant schwannoma. A study of 14 cases. Virchows Arch A Pathol Anat Histopathol 1986;409(4):433–51.
94. McCormack LJ, Hazard JB, Dickson JA. Malignant epithelioid neurilemoma (schwannoma). Cancer 1954;7(4):725–8.
95. Taxy JB, Battifora H. Epithelioid schwannoma: diagnosis by electron microscopy. Ultrastruct Pathol 1981;2(1):19–24.
96. Carter JM, O'Hara C, Dundas G, et al. Epithelioid malignant peripheral nerve sheath tumor arising in a schwannoma, in a patient with "neuroblastoma-like" schwannomatosis and a novel germline SMARCB1 mutation. Am J Surg Pathol 2012;36(1):154–60.
97. Hollmann TJ, Hornick JL. INI1-deficient tumors: diagnostic features and molecular genetics. Am J Surg Pathol 2011;35(10):e47–e363.
98. Wolff M, Santiago H, Duby MM. Delayed distant metastasis from a subcutaneous sacrococcygeal ependymoma. Case report, with tissue culture, ultrastructural observations, and review of the literature. Cancer 1972;30(4):1046–67.
99. Anderson MS. Myxopapillary ependymomas presenting in the soft tissue over the sacrococcygeal region. Cancer 1966;19(4):585–90.
100. Timmerman W, Bubrick MP. Presacral and postsacral extraspinal ependymoma: report of a case and review of the literature. Dis Colon Rectum 1984;27(2):114–19.

Soft Tissue Tumors Showing Melanocytic Differentiation

CHAPTER CONTENTS

(MALIGNANT) MELANOTIC SCHWANNOMA

A rare form of pigmented neural tumor commonly arising from the sympathetic nervous system was described in 1932 by Millar[1] as malignant melanotic tumor of ganglion cells, discussed under the term *melanocytic schwannoma* by Fu et al.,[2] and redesignated *psammomatous melanotic schwannoma* by Carney,[3] who noted its association with Carney syndrome. Melanotic schwannoma is a distinctive neoplasm of adult life that differs significantly from classic schwannoma, despite the similarity in the names.[1-11] The tumor arises commonly from the spinal or autonomic nerves near the midline. However, a number of cases have been reported in the stomach and in bone and soft tissues. Unusual sites include the heart, bronchus, liver, and skin.[3] In some series, more than 50% of patients with the tumor have evidence of Carney syndrome, which includes myxomas of the heart, skin, and breast, spotty pigmentation caused by lentigenes, blue nevus and the distinctive epithelioid blue nevus,[4] endocrine overactivity manifested by Cushing disease (pigmented nodular adrenal disease), acromegaly (pituitary adenoma), or sexual precocity (Sertoli cell tumor). However, other series of melanotic schwannoma have noted an association with Carney syndrome in 5% or less of affected patients.[11-14] The tumor typically develops at an earlier age (average 22.5 years) in patients with Carney syndrome than in those without the syndrome (average 33.2 years).[3] About 20% of patients with melanotic schwannomas have multiple tumors, and, in such patients, there is an even higher probability that other manifestations of Carney syndrome will be present.[3] The symptoms related specifically to the tumor depend on its location and rate of growth, but, most commonly, they are pain and neurologic symptoms in the affected part. Most striking is a case reported by Fu et al.,[2] in which the patient lost sympathetic nerve function in the ipsilateral lower extremity.

The tumors are usually circumscribed or encapsulated and vary from black-brown to gray-blue (Fig. 29-1). The neoplastic

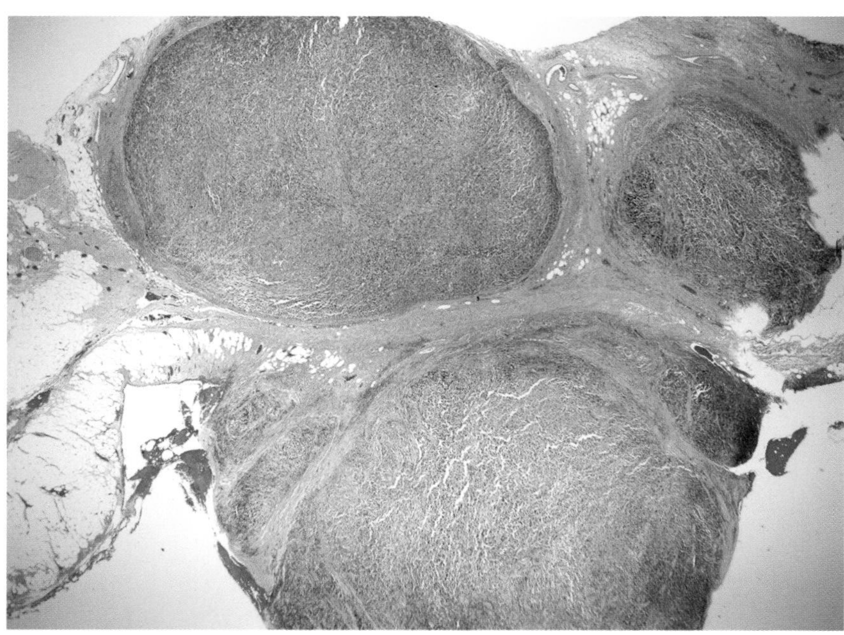

FIGURE 29-1. Melanotic schwannoma presenting as a multinodular, heavily-pigmented paraspinal mass.

cells grow in fascicles or sheets, vary in shape from polygonal to spindled, and blend gradually from one to another (Fig. 29-2). This feature, coupled with the ill-defined borders of the cytoplasm, often imparts a syncytial quality to the tumors that is somewhat reminiscent of a schwannoma. It is often difficult to make out cellular detail in these tumors because of the heavy pigment deposits (Fig. 29-3). Usually, there are at least focal areas with little or no pigment, so the character of the cells can be evaluated. Likewise, the nuclei may display clear intranuclear cytoplasmic (pseudo) inclusions characteristic of Schwann cells (Fig. 29-4). Nuclear hyperchromatism may be marked, and the nucleoli are often prominent (Fig. 29-5). Occasionally, there is vague palisading or formation of whorled structures so that the tumor resembles a schwannoma or neurofibroma. Psammoma bodies are present in most cases, although extensive sampling may be required to identify them (Fig. 29-6).[3]

The melanin pigment may be coarsely clumped or finely granular and varies from area to area. Tinctorially, it is similar to dermal melanin and stains positively with the Fontana stain and negatively for iron and periodic acid-Schiff (PAS). In this respect, it differs from the faint and focal pigment seen in conventional schwannomas, which is neural melanin. By immunohistochemistry, these tumors strongly express S-100 protein and various melanocytic markers, including HMB-45, Melan-A, and tyrosinase.[12] Ultrastructurally, there is a spectrum of maturation, including premelanosomes and melanosomes, strongly suggesting that the pigment is synthesized by

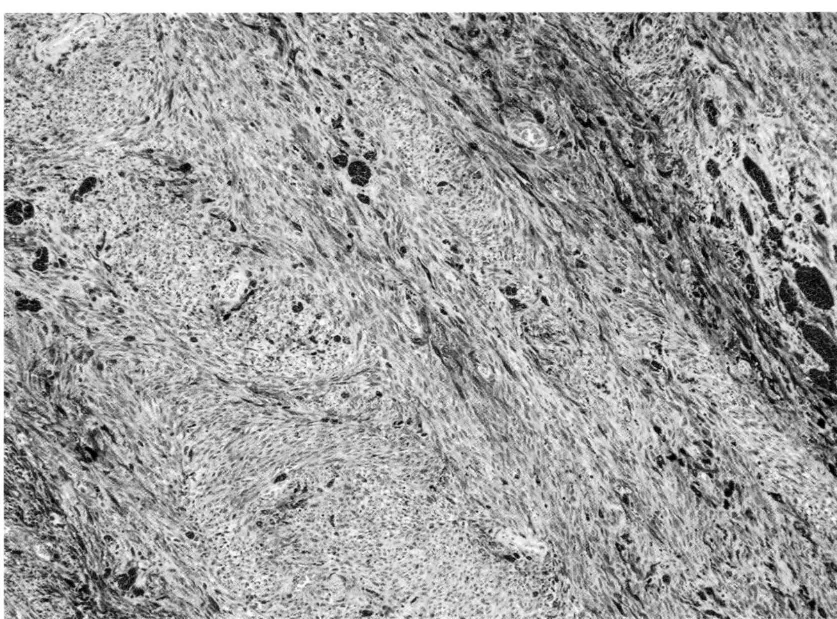

FIGURE 29-2. Melanotic schwannoma, consisting of a heavily-pigmented, fascicular proliferation of relatively uniform spindled cells.

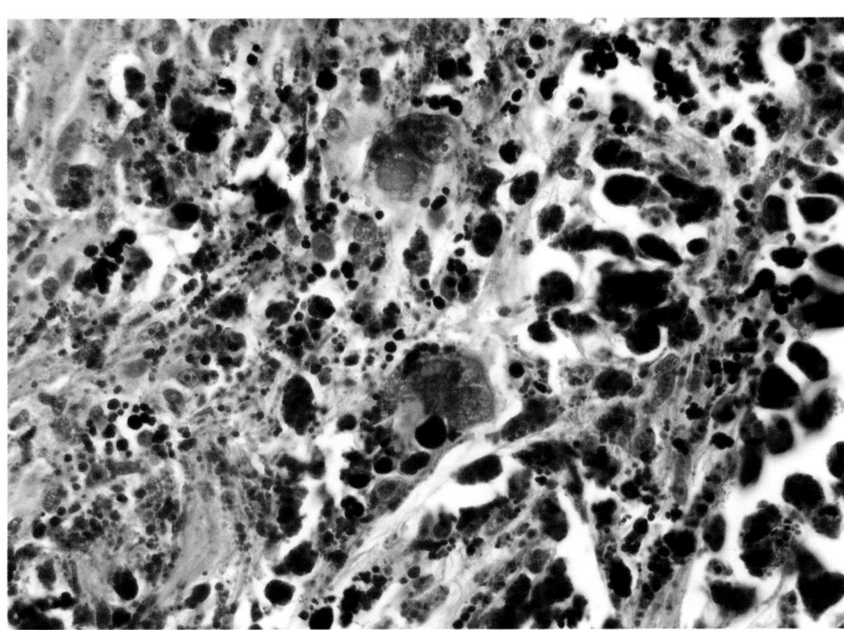

FIGURE 29-3. In some cases of melanotic schwannoma, the abundant intracytoplasmic melanin pigment may largely obscure the underlying cells. Note the striking nuclear pleomorphism and intranuclear pseudoinclusions.

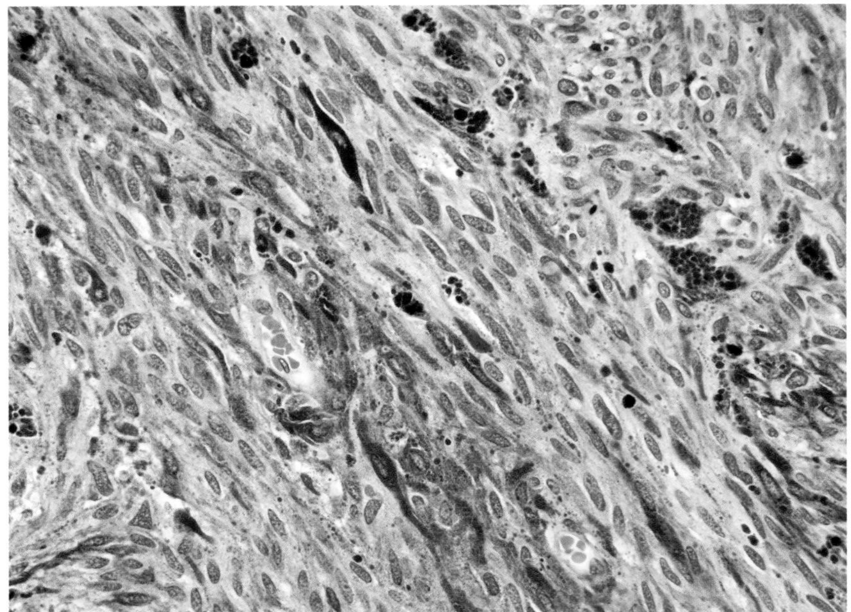

FIGURE 29-4. Higher power view of melanotic schwannoma, showing a fascicular proliferation of uniform, generally bland schwannian-appearing spindled cells with abundant melanin pigment and occasional intranuclear pseudoinclusions.

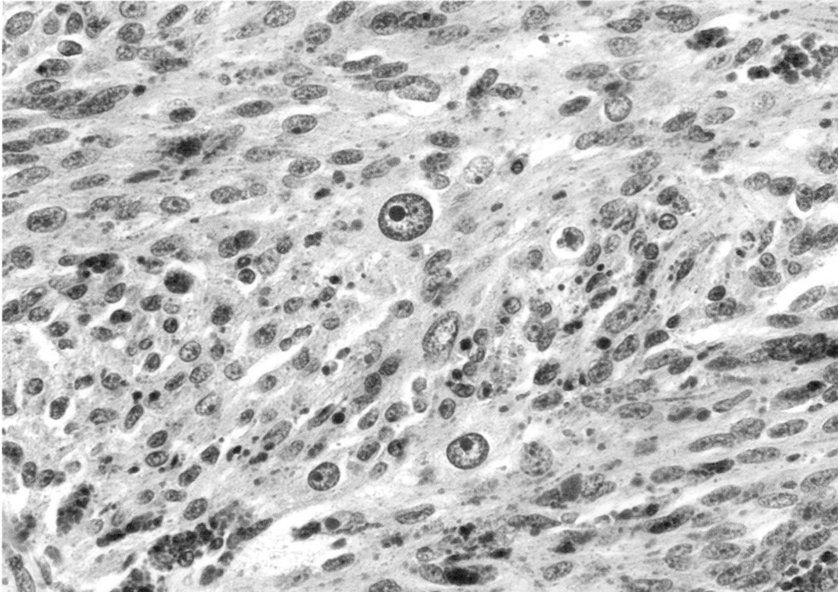

FIGURE 29-5. Some melanotic schwannomas show marked nucleomegaly and prominent melanoma-like nucleoli.

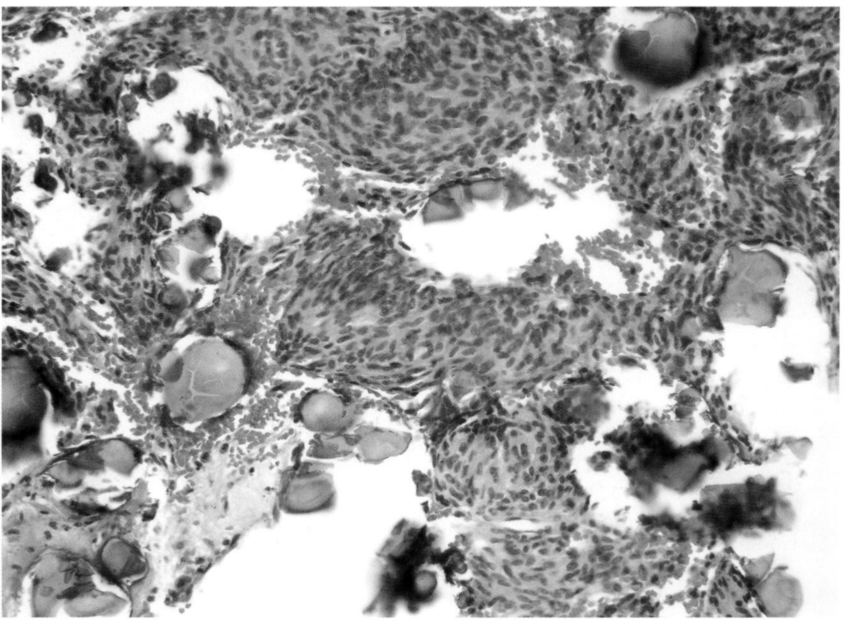

FIGURE 29-6. Psammoma bodies in melanotic schwannoma.

the tumor cell. Except for the presence of melanosomes, the cells resemble Schwann cells with elaborate cytoplasmic processes that interdigitate or spiral in the manner of mesaxons. Relatively little is known about the genetic events underlying melanotic schwannomas. Very recent gene expression profiling studies show these tumors to have a clearly different expression profile than do conventional schwannomas or melanomas, supporting their classification as a distinct entity.[12]

The biologic behavior of these tumors is difficult to predict, and metastases can occur in the absence of overt malignant features. Neither tumor size nor ploidy predicts malignant behavior. In the past, it was thought that most of these lesions had a benign, indolent course. Metastases, for example, were reported in only 13% of patients with melanotic schwannomas and Carney syndrome.[3] A review of approximately 60 cases in the literature has disclosed metastasis in 26%.[11] Furthermore, only 53% of patients followed for more than 5 years were disease-free, suggesting that long-term follow-up is required to fully judge metastatic risk. A recent study of 40 cases of melanotic schwannoma, presented in abstract form, found a local recurrence rate of 32% and a metastatic rate of 44%, with a greater risk for metastases seen in those tumors showing a mitotic rate of greater than 2/10 high-power fields (HPF)[12] (Fig. 29-7). Therefore, although all may be potentially malignant, those showing significant mitotic activity have a particularly high risk for aggressive clinical behavior. When metastases develop, they, too, abound with melanin pigment (Fig. 29-8).

The usual problem in differential diagnosis is distinguishing this tumor from a metastatic malignant melanoma. Primary melanotic schwannomas usually do not have the

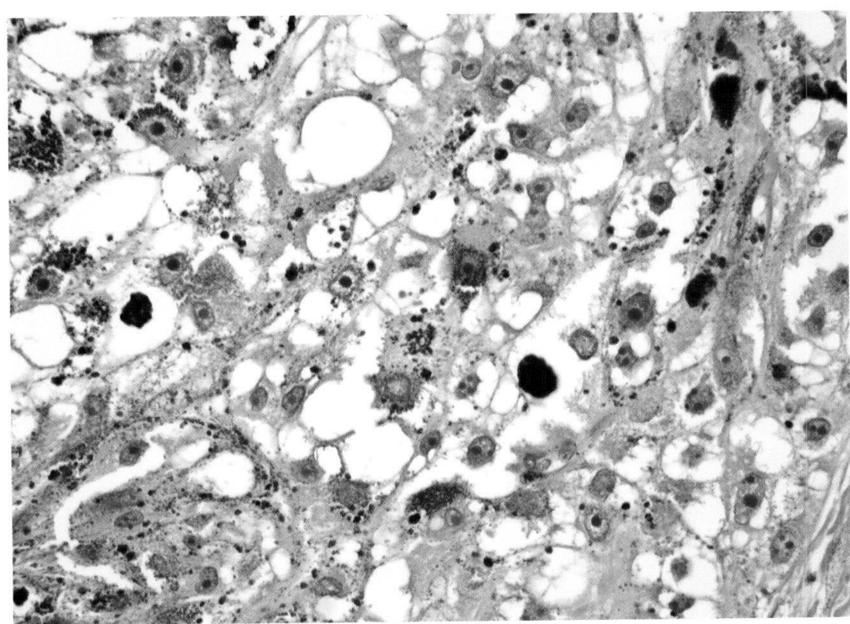

FIGURE 29-7. The presence of elevated mitotic activity (greater than 2 MF/10 HPF) has been associated with adverse outcome in patients with melanotic schwannoma.

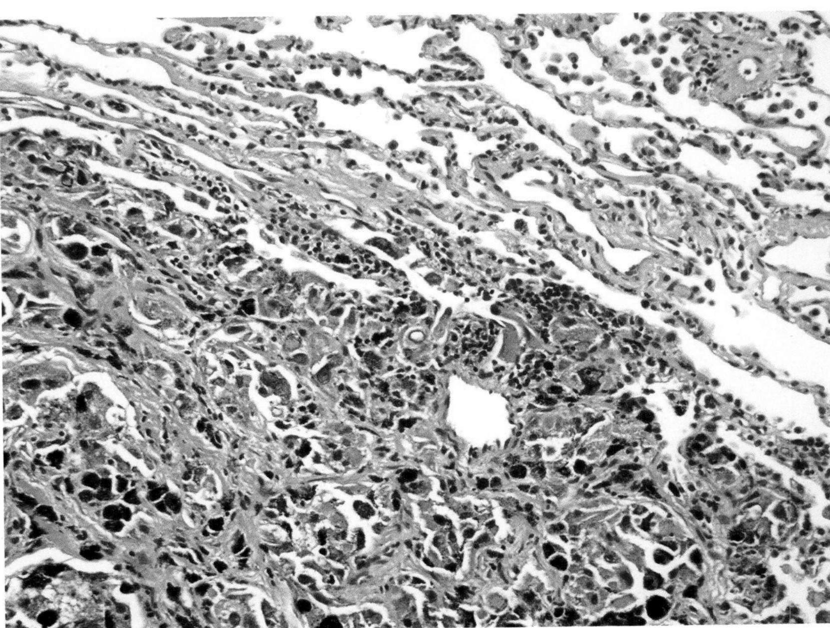

FIGURE 29-8. Lung metastasis in a patient with melanotic schwannoma. The overall risk of metastases is greater than 40% in some series, and all of these tumors should be considered potentially malignant.

degree of nuclear atypia or mitotic activity expected in a metastatic melanoma. The peculiar syncytial quality of the cells and, particularly, the psammomatous calcification are important features of melanotic schwannoma that metastatic melanomas lack.

MELANOTIC NEUROECTODERMAL TUMOR OF INFANCY (RETINAL ANLAGE TUMOR, MELANOTIC PROGONOMA)

First described in 1918 by Krompecher, melanotic neuroectodermal tumor of infancy, a rare tumor of disputed histogenesis, has been referred to as *congenital melanocarcinoma*, *melanotic adamantinoma*, *retinal anlage tumor*, *melanotic progonoma*, and *pigmented epulis of infancy*.[15-38] Although most current studies support a neural crest origin of this tumor, there is little evidence that the tumor specifically represents retinal anlage. Therefore, the preference is for the less fanciful term *melanotic neuroectodermal tumor of infancy*.

Clinical Findings

The tumor usually develops during the first year of life and presents as a protruding mass in the upper or lower jaw. The skin or mucosa is tightly stretched over the lesion, but it is rarely, if ever, ulcerated. Radiographically, the tumor is a cystic radiolucent lesion with a capacity for local destruction and displacement of the developing teeth (Fig. 29-9). Patients with this tumor in unusual sites, such as the anterior fontanelle, epididymis,[20,21,38] mediastinum,[31] and brain,[36] develop symptoms referable to those sites. The few cases reported in the uterus[31] and shoulder[29] and those in adults[30] should be disregarded because they represent different lesions altogether. One of these tumors has been encountered in the soft tissues of the extremity, and it has also been reported in long bone.[39]

Gross and Microscopic Findings

Grossly, the tumor ranges in color from slate gray to blue-black, depending on the amount of melanin pigment. It is composed of irregular alveolar spaces lined by cuboidal cells containing varying amounts of melanin pigment (Fig. 29-10). In addition, small, round, less well-differentiated cells resembling those of neuroblastoma lie in the alveolar space or as isolated nests in a fibrous stroma (Fig. 29-11). Neurofibrillary material resembling glial tissue may be seen in association with these cells in the alveolar spaces. In two exceptional cases, glial tissue was found outside of the epithelial islands. One case was a tumor arising in the brain in which the entire stroma was glial,[36] and the second was a tumor arising in a glial heterotopia of the oropharynx.[27]

The cuboidal cells have the electron microscopic features of epithelial and melanocytic cells.[18] They are bounded by basal laminae and elaborately interdigitate laterally with neighboring cells, forming desmosomes. Both mature and immature melanosomes similar to those of melanocytes and melanoma cells are present in the cytoplasm. Functionally, they share certain properties of the melanocyte in that melanization of these cells may be increased by agents that induce similar changes in melanocytes of animals.[18] Immunohistochemically, the cuboidal cells express cytokeratin and HMB-45. Neuron-specific enolase, CD57, and synaptophysin are variably present in the epithelial cells and the small neuroblastic element.

The round, less well-differentiated cells contain few organelles but are believed to be neuroblastic by virtue of their elongated cell processes, dense-core vesicles,[18] and intracytoplasmic neurofilamentous material.[18,22] Their association with glial-like areas and, in one case, with ganglioneuromatous areas[18] provides further support for this contention.

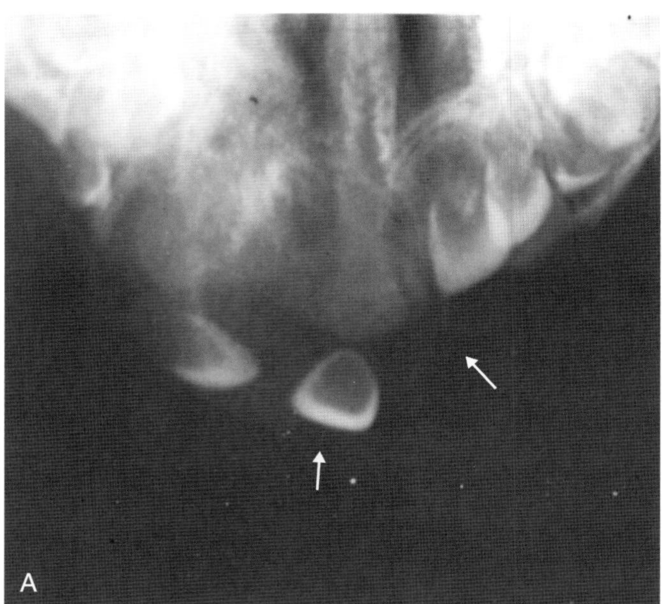

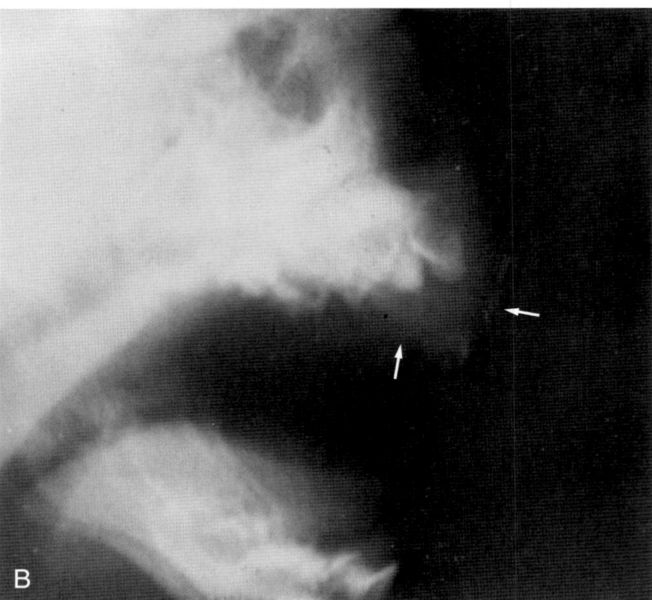

FIGURE 29-9. Radiograph of pigmented neuroectodermal tumor of infancy (retinal anlage tumor) in the maxilla. Tumor is a vaguely outlined soft tissue mass (*arrows*) with destruction of the maxilla (A) and displacement of teeth (B).

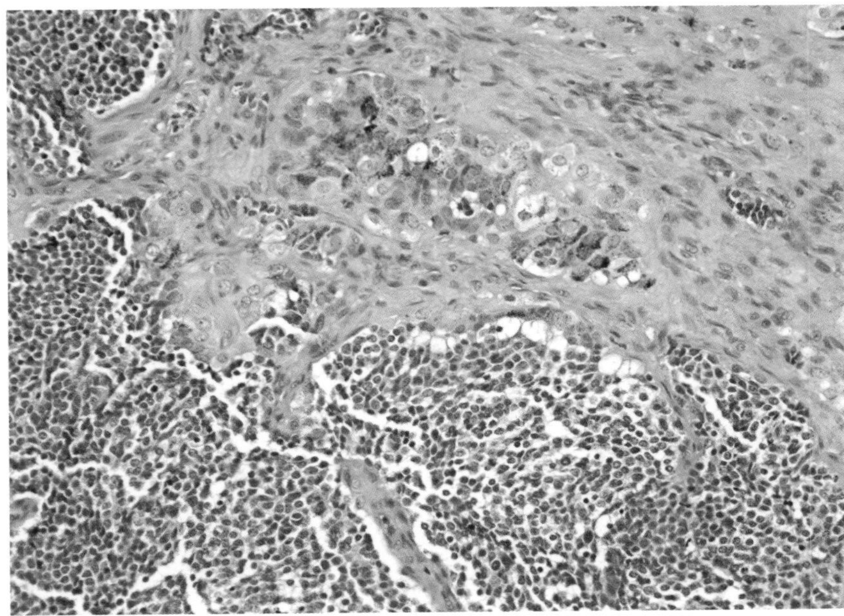

FIGURE 29-10. Melanotic neuroectodermal tumor of infancy, composed of irregular alveolar spaces lined by cuboidal cells containing varying amounts of melanin pigment.

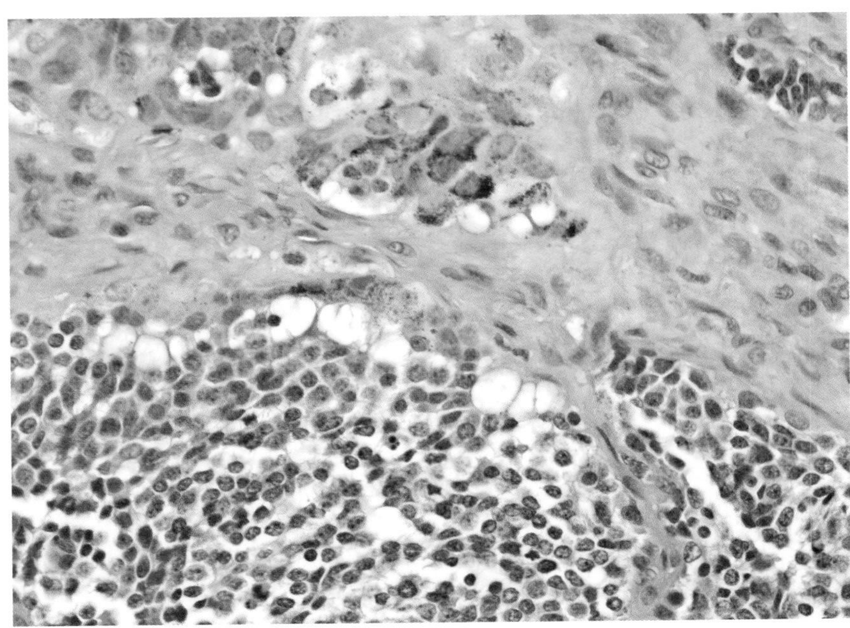

FIGURE 29-11. Neuroblastoma-like round cells adjacent to larger melanin-containing cells in melanotic neuroectodermal tumor of infancy.

Discussion

Traditionally, this tumor was considered benign, but, in a large series from the Armed Forces of Pathology (also recognized as the AFIP), nearly half of those with follow-up information recurred, and 5% to 10% of cases reported in the literature have produced metastasis.[18,24,28] One case, a stillborn, was noted to have multiple metastases at delivery.[28] A second case, a tumor of the epididymis, produced micrometastases in regional lymph nodes[24]; and two others metastasized as primitive neuroblastic tumors devoid of melanin.[18,24] Although metastasis is a relatively uncommon event, attempts to eradicate the tumor at the time of initial surgery are endorsed. Unfortunately, to date, it has not been possible to predict recurrence or metastasis in this disease.

The histogenesis of this tumor has been controversial. The concepts of a congenital melanoma and an odontogenic tumor are now obsolete for various reasons. The former does not account for the primitive neuroblastic component, and the latter does not take into consideration tumors at sites where there are no odontogenic rests. To date, the most appealing theory is that the tumor is derived from neural crest.[16,18] This concept allows latitude in the distribution of the lesions, accounts for the presence of pigmented and neuroblastic elements, and explains the rare tumor associated with increased levels of vanillylmandelic acid.[16,18] It does not seem necessary to compare this tumor specifically to the developing retina; in fact, the embryologic evidence against this possibility has been extensively summarized.[16] It seems more probable that this tumor merely reflects a primitive stage or degree of differentiation common to many types of pigmented neuroepithelium. No specific genetic aberration has been identified in these tumors.

CLEAR CELL SARCOMA OF TENDON AND APONEUROSIS

Described by Enzinger[40] in 1965, the clear cell sarcoma is a rare melanin-producing soft tissue sarcoma. Although, unfortunately, it is also referred to as *malignant melanoma of soft parts*, it is clinically, genetically, and biologically distinct from cutaneous melanoma, despite certain histologic similarities. In contrast to cutaneous melanoma, clear cell sarcomas invariably arise in the deep soft tissue of the distal extremities, and 70% possess a consistent balanced translocation t(12;22)(q13;q12)[41-47] that is not found in melanoma and is believed to be an early, if not primary, event in tumorigenesis. This translocation fuses *EWSR1* on chromosome 22 with *ATF1*,[48] a member of the CREB transcription factor family on chromosome 12. This results in four fusion transcripts that are differentially expressed among tumors.[49] The fusion protein mimics the action of melanocyte stimulating hormone by binding to and constitutively activating the promoter for MiTF, the melanocyte master transcription factor.[50] Recent evidence suggests that MiTF is a critical oncogenic target because it not only mediates melanin production in these tumors but also EWSR1-ATF1-induced tumor growth.[50,51]

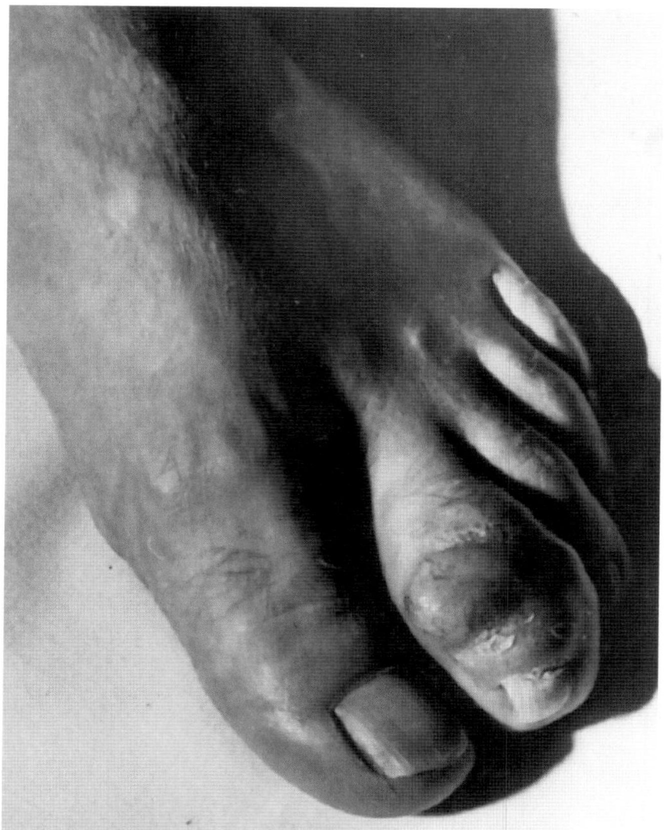

FIGURE 29-12. Clear cell sarcoma of the second toe.

Clinical Findings

Clear cell sarcoma mainly affects young adults between the ages of 20 and 40 years with a median age of about 30 years. Approximately 40% of cases occur on the foot and ankle (Fig. 29-12) with another 30% on the knee, thigh, and hand.[52-55] The head and neck region and the trunk are distinctly unusual sites (Table 29-1). Clear cell sarcomas present as a slowly enlarging, occasionally painful mass, which is usually present about 2 years at the time of diagnosis, although a significant percentage has been present for 5 years or longer. They arise in deep soft tissue, and, unless the lesion is extremely large or distal, the overlying skin and dermis are usually not involved.

TABLE 29-1 Anatomic Distribution of 141 Clear Cell Sarcomas

LOCATION	NO. OF PATIENTS	(%)
Head and neck	1	0.8
Trunk	3	2.1
Upper extremity	31	22.0
Lower extremity (foot 28; knee 21; heel 15; ankle 11)	106	75.1
Total	141	100.00

Data from Montgomery EA, Meis JM, Ramos AG, et al. Clear cell sarcoma of tendons and aponeurosis: a clinicopathologic study of 58 cases with analysis of prognostic factors. Int J Surg Pathol 1993;1:59.

Pathologic Findings

Macroscopically, the tumor consists of a lobulated or multinodular gray-white mass firmly attached to tendons or aponeuroses (Figs. 29-13 and 29-14), which averages between 2 and 6 cm. The cut surface may be marred by focal hemorrhage, necrosis, or cystic change. In a small proportion of cases, the melanin may be prominent enough to be visualized as foci of dark brown or black discoloration (see Fig. 29-14).

Histologically, tumors consist of compact nests or fascicles of predominantly fusiform or spindled cells with a clear cytoplasm bordered and defined by a delicate framework of fibrocollagenous tissue contiguous with adjacent tendons or aponeuroses (Figs. 29-15 to 29-22). The cells have highly distinctive features consisting of nuclei with a vesicular nuclear chromatin pattern and prominent basophilic nucleoli reminiscent of malignant melanoma. The cytoplasm varies from clear to weakly eosinophilic (Fig. 29-23A) and contains large amounts of intracellular glycogen. Clear cells and eosinophilic cells coexist in different portions of the same neoplasm with focal transitions between the two (see Fig. 29-21). A highly characteristic feature is the multinucleated tumor giant cells with 10 to 15 peripherally placed nuclei (see Fig. 29-19). In general, clear cell sarcomas are neither pleomorphic nor mitotically highly active, although this observation does not necessarily apply to recurrent or metastatic lesions.

Melanin is present in over 50% of clear cell sarcomas but is usually not abundant enough to be seen on hematoxylin-eosin stain. It can be detected with appropriate histochemical

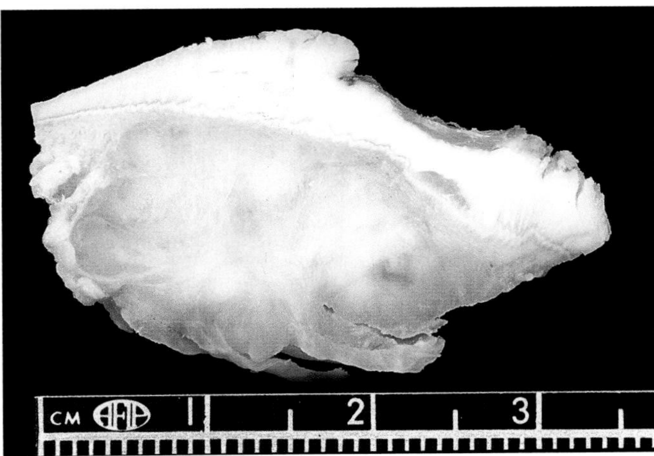

FIGURE 29-13. Clear cell sarcoma diffusely infiltrating a tendon (top) and skeletal muscle (bottom).

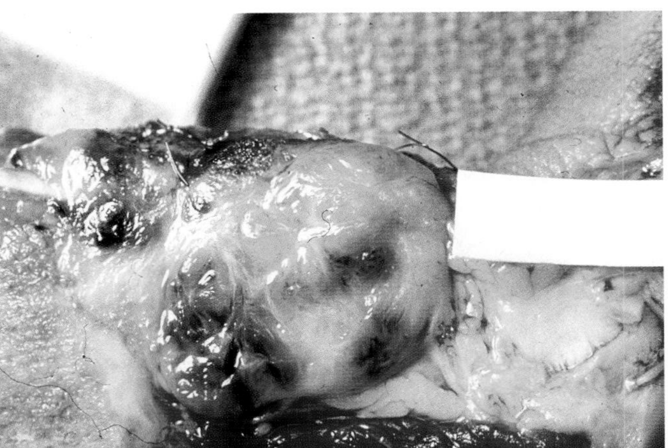

FIGURE 29-14. Clear cell sarcoma showing pigmented areas.

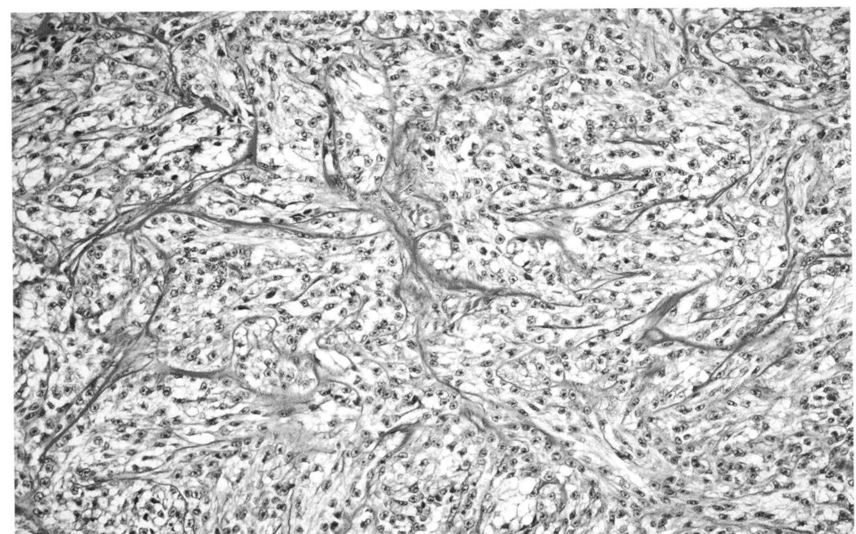

FIGURE 29-15. Clear cell sarcoma. Fibrous tissue septa divide the tumor into well-defined nests and groups of pale-staining tumor cells.

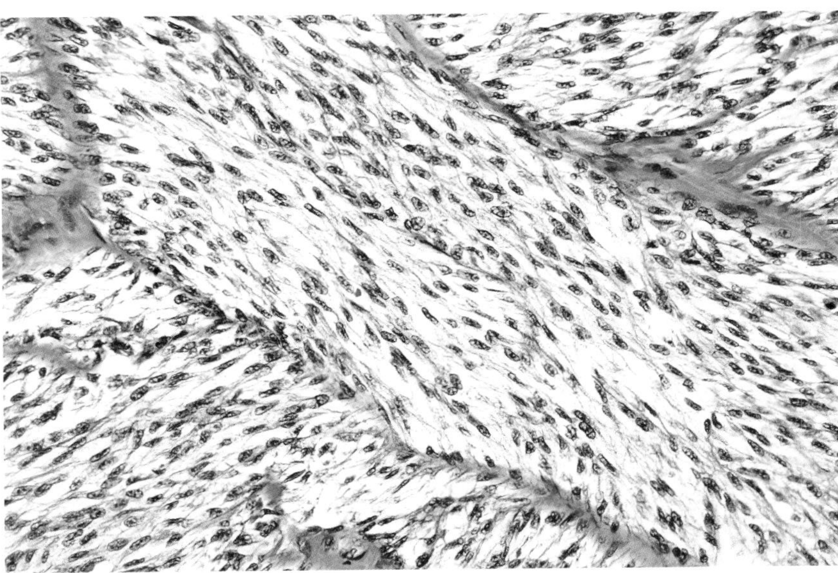

FIGURE 29-16. Clear cell sarcoma showing arrangement of the pale-staining tumor cells in short fascicles separated by dense fibrous septa.

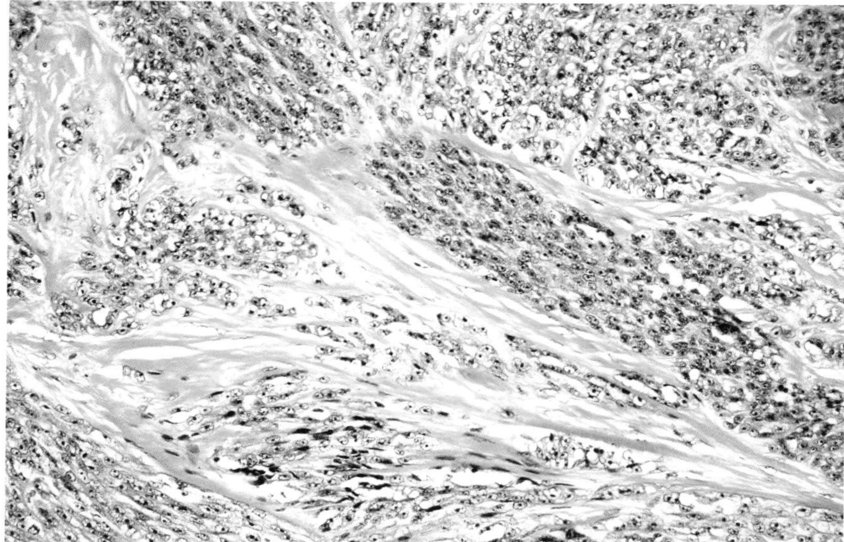

FIGURE 29-17. Clear cell sarcoma subdivided by dense fibrous bands.

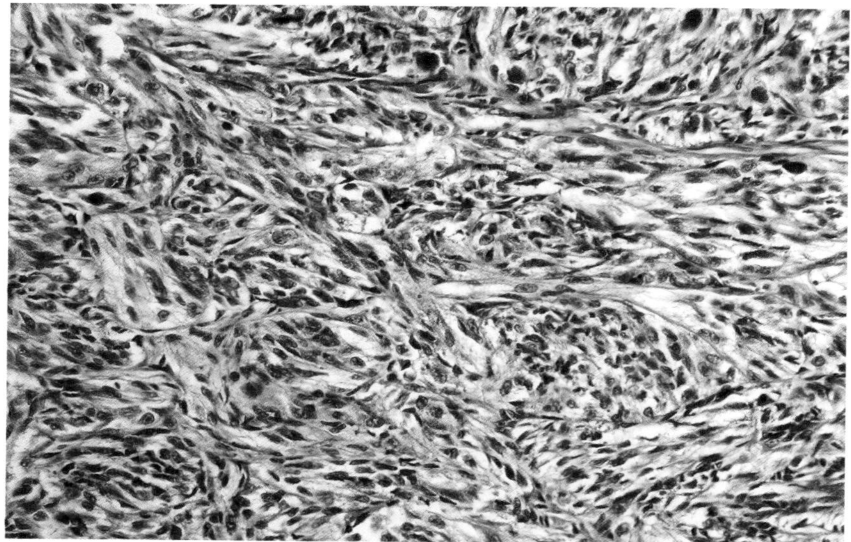

FIGURE 29-18. Clear cell sarcoma with cytoplasmic melanin pigment.

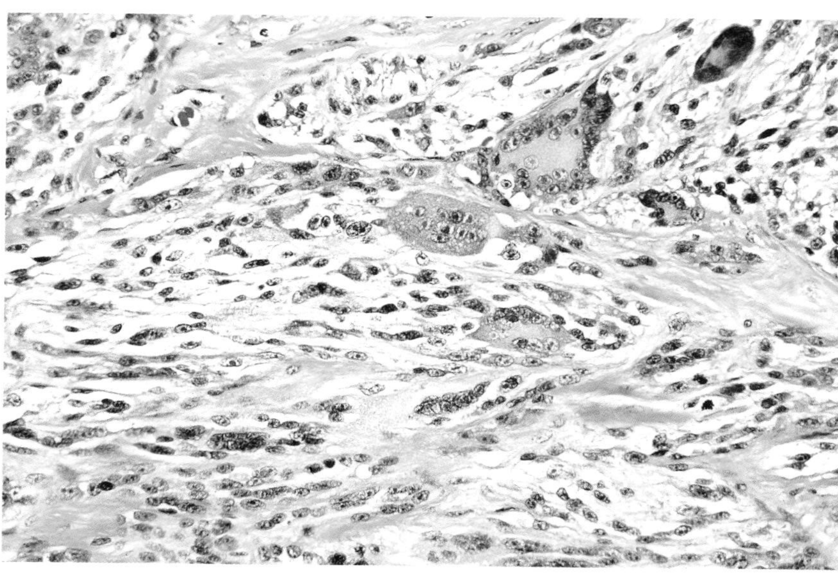

FIGURE 29-19. Clear cell sarcoma with scattered multinucleated giant cells. The giant cells have a wreath of peripherally placed nuclei of uniform size and shape.

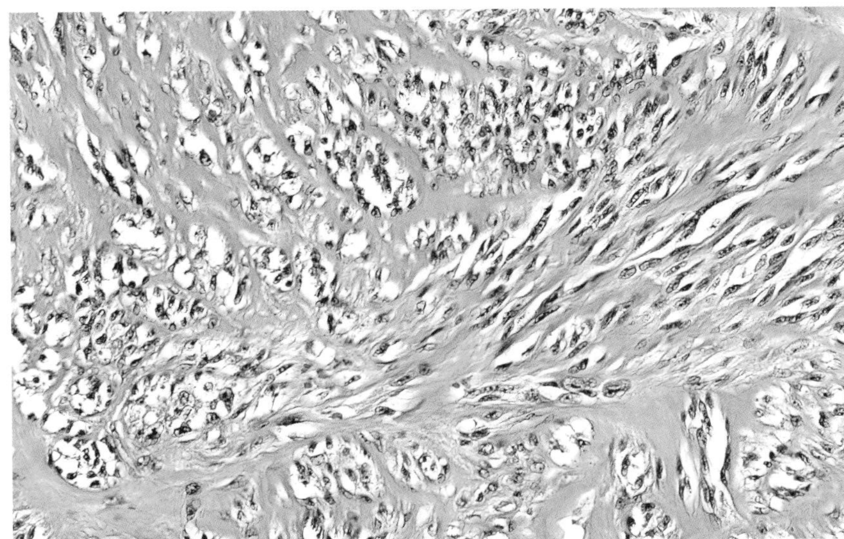

FIGURE 29-20. Clear cell sarcoma with areas of dense hyalinization.

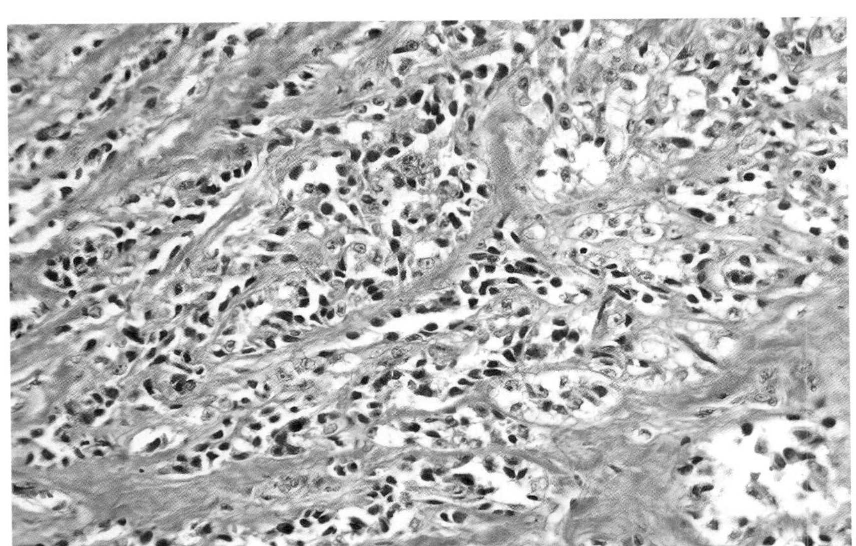

FIGURE 29-21. Clear cell sarcoma with degeneration. Cells can acquire a small cell appearance that is misleading.

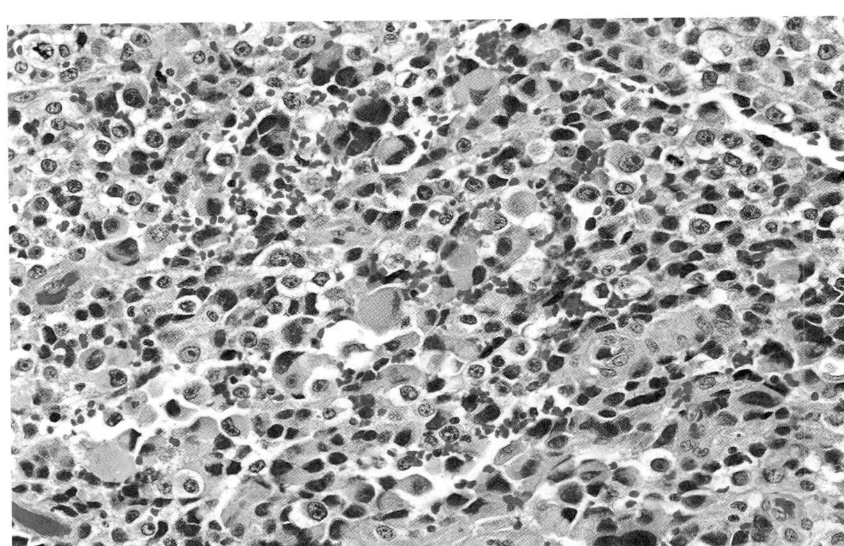

FIGURE 29-22. Metastatic clear cell sarcoma with marked pleomorphism and essentially no spindling. Metastatic deposits of this type resemble carcinoma or melanoma.

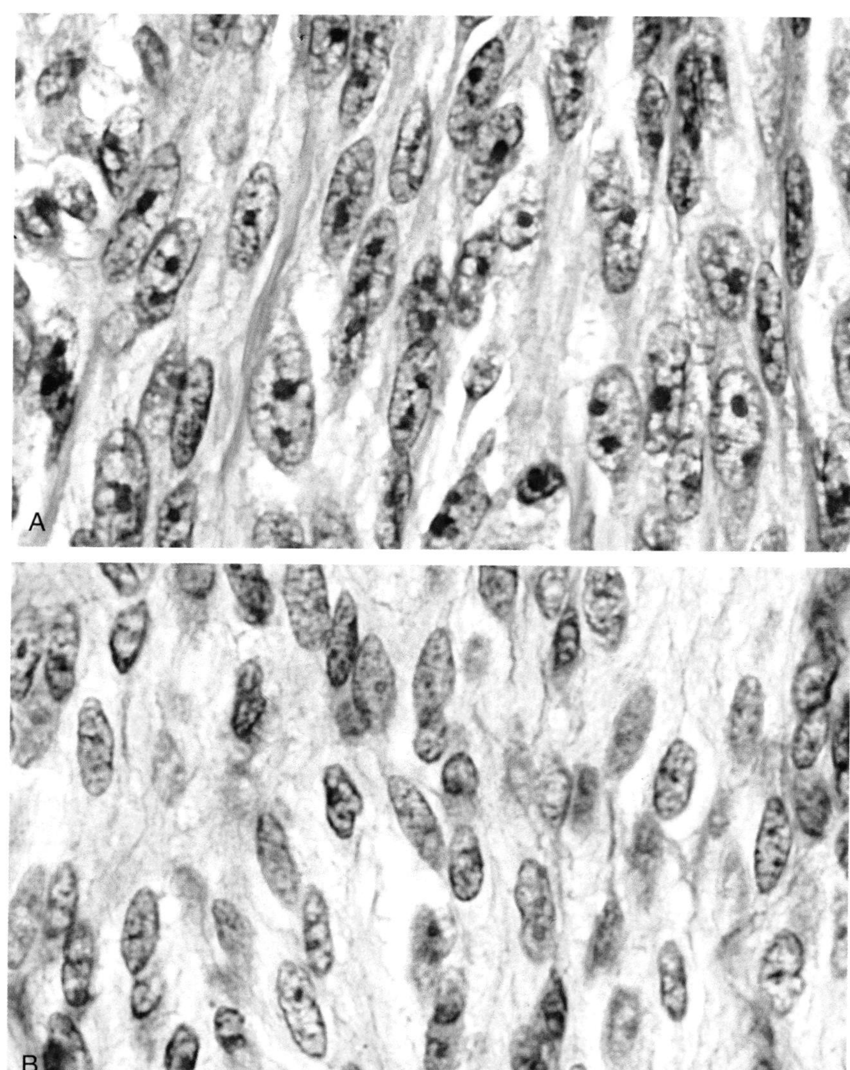

FIGURE 29-23. Comparison of cytologic features of clear cell sarcoma and a cellular blue nevus at the same magnification. (A) Clear cell sarcoma has prominent vesicular nuclei with a large single nucleolus. (B) Cellular blue nevus cells are smaller with a less vesicular nuclear chromatin pattern and small, pinpoint nucleoli.

(Fontana or Warthin-Starry) or immunohistochemical stains (Fig. 29-24). Virtually all clear cell sarcomas diffusely express S-100 protein (Fig. 29-25), and most also express antigens associated with melanin synthesis (HMB-45, Melan-A, Mel-CAM, MiTF).[56-58] Neuron-specific enolase, CD57, and LN3 have also been noted in these lesions.

Ultrastructurally, the tumor consists of oval or fusiform cells with rounded nuclei, evenly dispersed chromatin at the nuclear membrane, and a large, centrally placed, single nucleolus. The cytoplasm contains multiple, rounded and swollen mitochondria, membrane-bound vesicles, and ribosomes and polyribosomes in varying numbers. There are also aggregates of rough endoplasmic reticulum, scanty amounts of glycogen, and occasional lipid droplets. Mononuclear and multinuclear cells display similar ultrastructural characteristics. Melanosomes in varying stages of development are present, in most cases.[55,59] Some show dense pigmentation, and others exhibit the typical lamellar, striated, or barrel-stave internal structure of premelanosomes (Fig. 29-26). Basal laminae surround groups of closely apposed neoplastic cells. Collagen fibers are abundant in the extracellular spaces. Benson et al.[60] also described occasional cells with stubby or finger-like dendritic processes, a few of which contained longitudinally aligned filaments.

Differential Diagnosis

Because cytologic features are of paramount importance in the diagnosis of clear cell sarcoma, care must be exercised to evaluate optimally preserved areas only. Poorly preserved or degenerated clear cell sarcomas having shriveled cells that cling to the fibrous bands are easily misconstrued as a round cell sarcoma, particularly alveolar rhabdomyosarcoma. In well-preserved material, however, the differential diagnosis typically includes, on the one hand, sarcomas with a predominant fascicular growth pattern such as fibrosarcoma, synovial sarcoma, and malignant peripheral nerve sheath tumor, and, on the other hand, melanin-producing tumors such as cellular blue nevus and nodular malignant melanoma. The distinctive cytologic features of clear cell sarcoma, including prominent melanoma-like nucleoli, clear cytoplasm, and immunophenotypic profile, set this lesion apart from the spindle cell sarcomas noted previously.

The distinction of clear cell sarcoma from other melanin-producing lesions can be more problematic and may require correlation of the histologic, clinic, and molecular data. In general, clear cell sarcomas originate in deep structures, rarely involve the dermis, and have a predominantly and relatively uniform spindle-cell appearance that contrasts with the epithelioid appearance of nodular melanomas. However, in ambiguous situations, molecular genetic analysis is highly recommended because the t(12;22) that characterizes clear cell sarcoma has not been identified in malignant melanoma. Conversely, *BRAF* mutations, often found in conventional melanomas, are absent in clear cell sarcomas.[49] Cellular blue nevus can occur in a similar age and location and have certain common histologic features, including spindled cells and giant cells with clear cytoplasm. Cellular blue nevi typically are dermal-based lesions with a peripheral zone that resembles a neurofibroma by virtue of the interdigitation of slender pigmented dendritic cells with surrounding collagen. The cells lack atypia and have small, pinpoint nucleoli (see Fig. 29-23B). Recurrent cellular blue nevi, however, can acquire more atypical cytologic features so that a distinction from clear cell sarcoma is not always possible. In these situations, review of the original material and/or molecular genetic analysis is essential. The recently described paraganglioma-like dermal melanocytic tumor, while having cells with a clear to eosinophilic cytoplasm, comprises zellballen-like nests of cells of distinctly low nuclear grade (Fig. 29-27). These lesions, based in the dermis, rarely extend to deep structures. At this point, all have behaved in a benign fashion.[61] Dermal perivascular epithelioid cell neoplasms, later discussed in depth, typically show lesser degrees of nuclear atypia than do clear cell sarcoma, lack S-100 protein expression, and coexpress muscle and melanocytic markers.

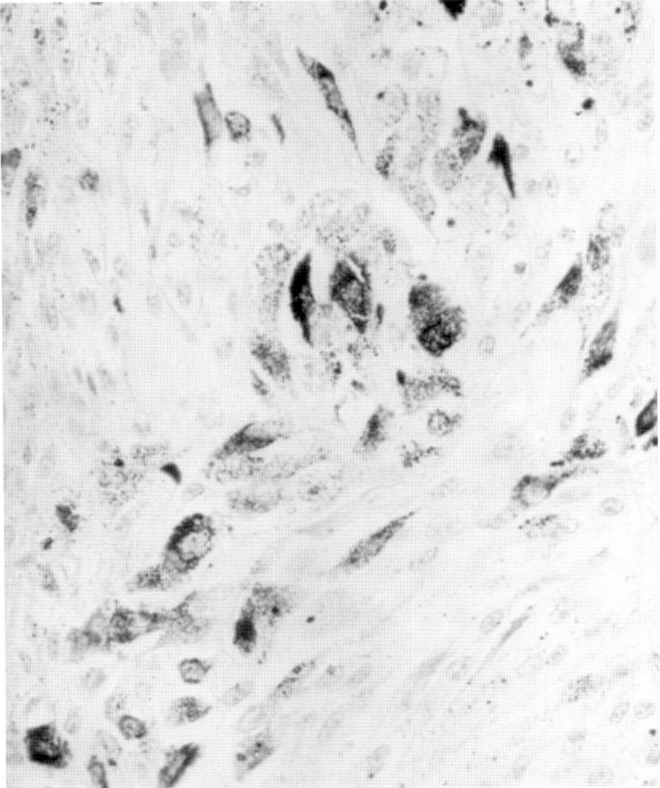

FIGURE 29-24. Clear cell sarcoma. Fontana stain reveals melanin pigment in some of the tumor cells.

Discussion

Clear cell sarcoma is an extremely rare tumor for which it has been difficult to amass outcome and therapeutic data in a large patient population. For example, only 28 pediatric patients were referred to the Italian and German Soft Tissue Sarcoma Cooperative Group over a 20-year period from 1980 to 2000.[54] Nevertheless, there is agreement based on the largest

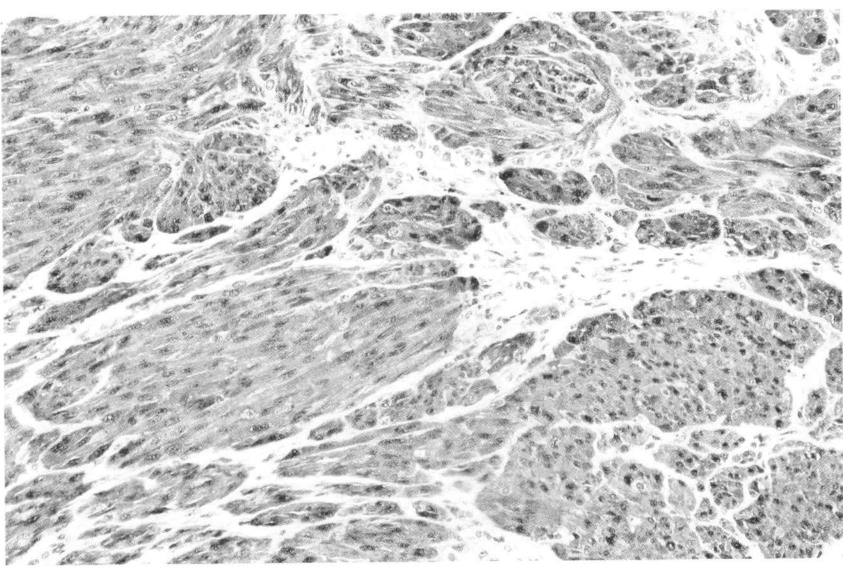

FIGURE 29-25. Strong S-100 protein immunostaining in a clear cell sarcoma.

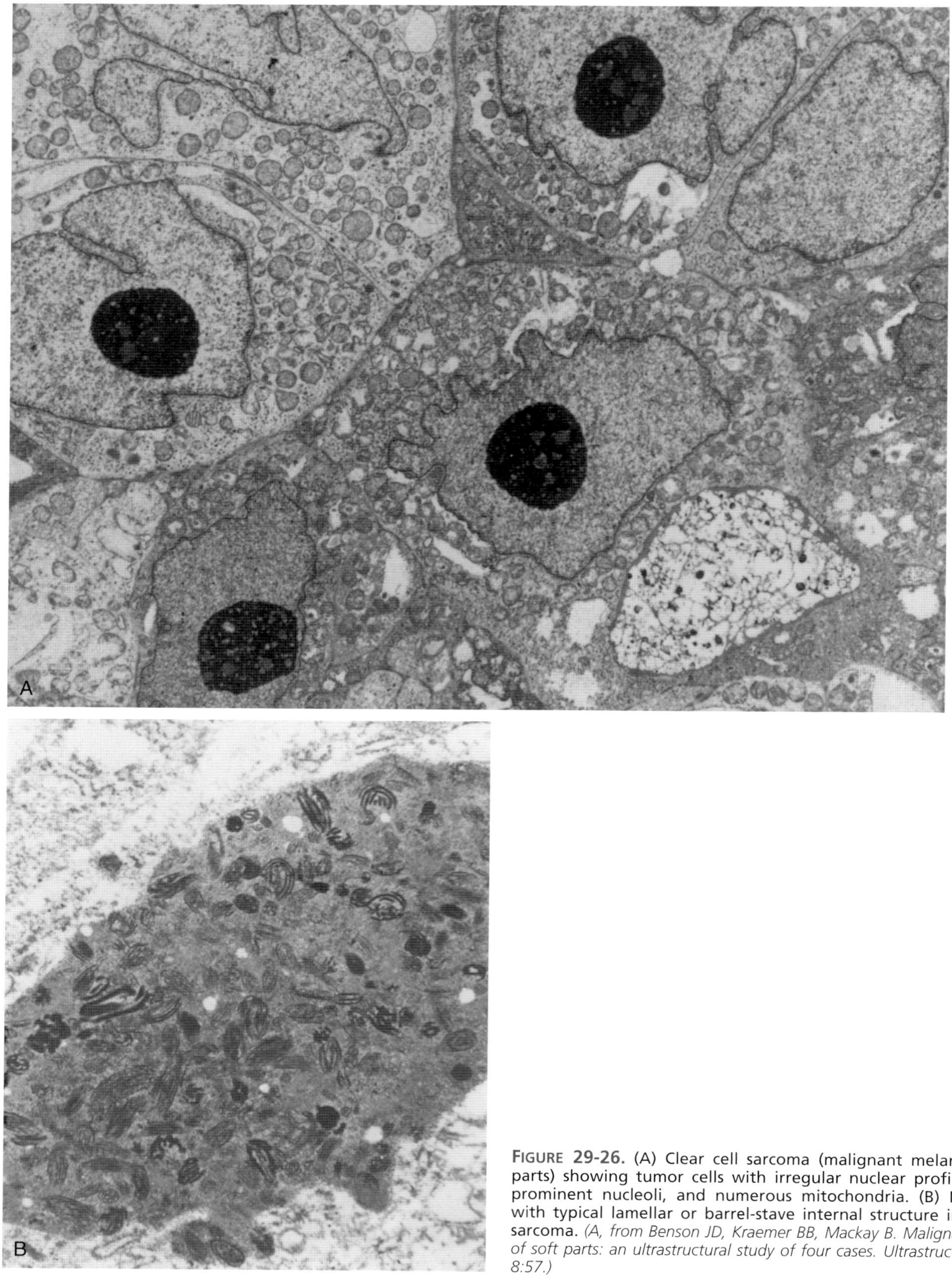

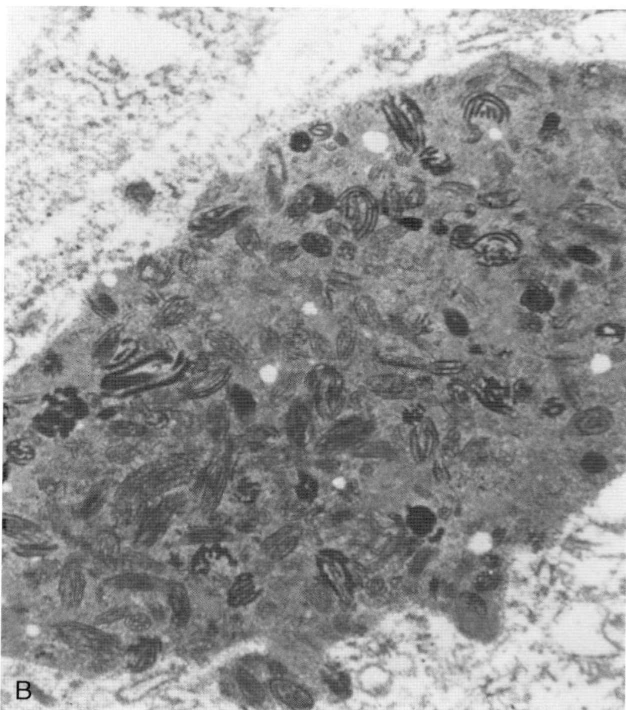

FIGURE 29-26. (A) Clear cell sarcoma (malignant melanoma of soft parts) showing tumor cells with irregular nuclear profiles, strikingly prominent nucleoli, and numerous mitochondria. (B) Melanosomes with typical lamellar or barrel-stave internal structure in a clear cell sarcoma. *(A, from Benson JD, Kraemer BB, Mackay B. Malignant melanoma of soft parts: an ultrastructural study of four cases. Ultrastruct Pathol 1985; 8:57.)*

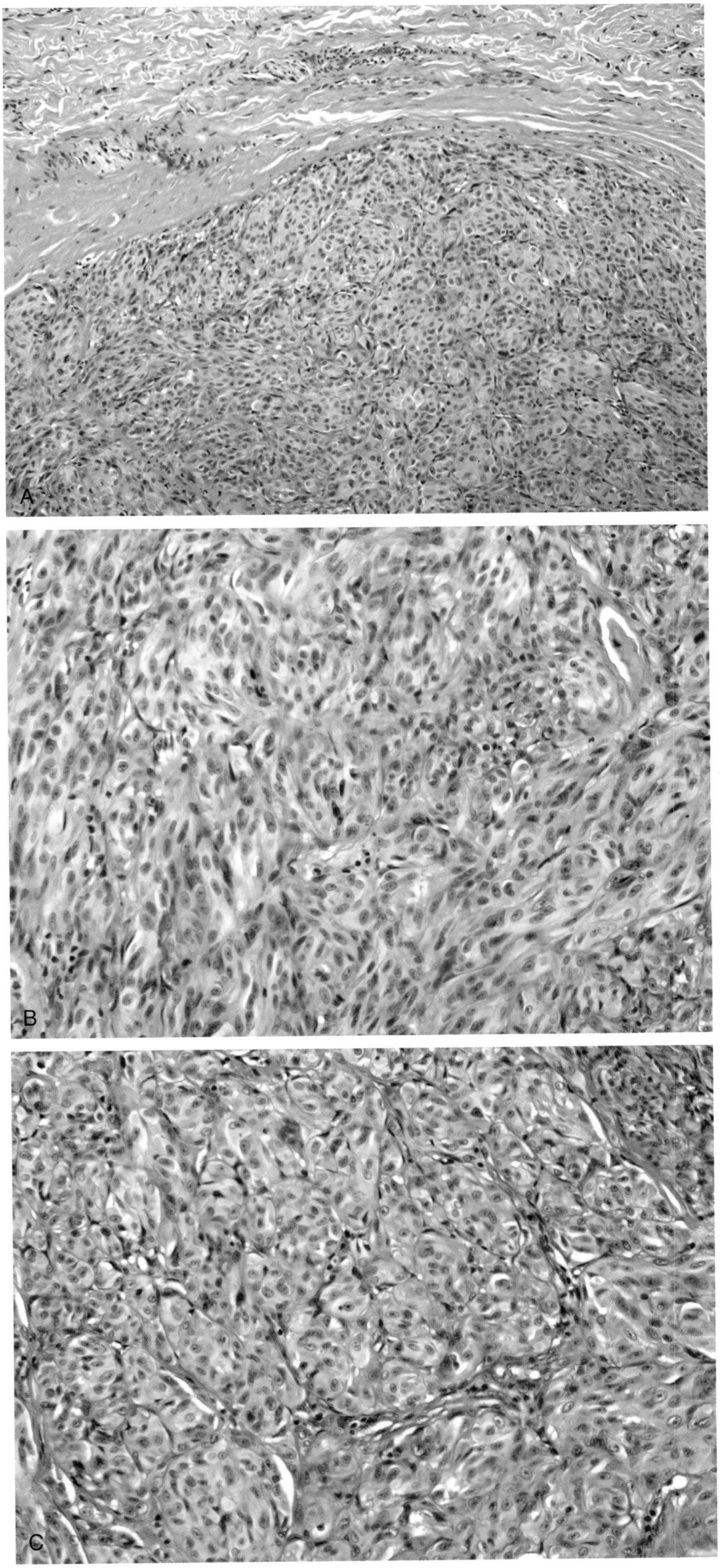

A

B

C

FIGURE 29-27. Paraganglioma-like dermal melanocytic tumor (A) showing zellballen-like nests of slightly spindled (B) to rounded cells (C).

studies that this is a high-grade sarcoma.[40,52-55,62] Recurrences, which reflect the adequacy of initial surgery, range from 14% to 39%, whereas metastases to lung or lymph node develop in approximately one-half of patients within an interval of 2 to 8 years. Late metastases after 10 to 20 years have been reported in patients with repeated local recurrences. Because patients who develop local recurrences or regional lymph node metastases eventually develop distant metastases, there is a clear need for controlling local disease and for long-term surveillance. Given the risk for regional lymph node metastases in this disease, there has been recent interest in performing a sentinel lymph node biopsy. A recent report describes the feasibility of identifying and excising sentinel nodes,[63] but there are insufficient data on which to base a therapeutic recommendation.

Clear cell sarcoma has traditionally been considered an upgradable sarcoma, and, for that reason, several studies have attempted to identify other prognostic factors. Size[52,53,55] and necrosis[52,53] have proved to be the most robust prognostic factors[52,53,55] with tumors greater than 5 cm having a significantly worse outcome than those that are smaller. Other factors, such as age, location, depth, or proliferation index, have been found to be independent prognostic factors. Radical surgery is the mainstay of therapy, and chemotherapy has proven to have little efficacy.[54]

CLEAR CELL SARCOMA-LIKE TUMOR OF GASTROINTESTINAL TRACT (MALIGNANT GASTROINTESTINAL NEUROECTODERMAL TUMOR)

Clear cell sarcoma-like tumor of the gastrointestinal tract (CCSLGT), originally described as osteoclast-rich tumor of the gastrointestinal tract with features resembling clear cell sarcoma of soft parts[64] is extremely rare, with fewer than 25 reported cases.[64-73] A case morphologically corresponding to this entity had been previously published by Alpers and Beckwith[74] as a malignant neuroendocrine tumor of the jejunum with osteoclast-like tumor giant cells. Since the description of this tumor by Zambrano et al.,[64] only 18 definite and 4 probable additional examples have been reported.[65,75] The largest and most recent series was published by Stockman et al.,[65] who coined the term *malignant gastrointestinal neuroectodermal tumor* to describe these rare lesions. Although this term has considerable merit, it remains to be seen whether it will be widely embraced.

Clinical Features

CCSLGT typically arises in young to middle aged adults and most often involves the small intestine, although any part of the gastrointestinal tract may be affected.[65,75] The tumor is typically centered within the wall of the bowel, with secondary involvement of the mucosa and serosa. CCSLGT is highly malignant with aggressive local recurrence, lymph node or visceral metastasis, or death from disease in 18 of 24 (75%) reported cases, generally in less than 36 months.[65,75] This behavior is in contrast to the more indolent behavior of classic clear cell sarcoma of soft tissue. There are no data on the possible role of adjuvant therapies in the treatment of CCSLGT.

Pathologic Features

The tumors grow in solid sheets, pseudopapillary formations and alveolar formations, generally without the well-formed nests that characterize soft tissue-type clear cell sarcoma (Fig. 29-28).[65,75] The neoplastic cells are usually round to oval with only infrequent spindling and contain a moderate amount of clear to lightly eosinophilic cytoplasm. The nuclei of CCSLGT are centrally located and round with irregularly dispersed chromatin and either inapparent or small nucleoli, in most instances (Fig. 29-29). Macronucleoli of the type seen in conventional melanoma and soft tissue-type clear cell sarcoma are only infrequently identified. Mitotic activity may be brisk, and necrosis is frequently present. Perhaps the most distinctive feature of CCSLGT is the presence of osteoclast-like multinucleated giant cells admixed with the neoplastic cells (Fig. 29-30).[64] The number of osteoclast-like giant cells varies greatly from field to field within a given CCSLGT with some areas containing large numbers of such cells and other areas lacking them entirely. Occasional cases of CCSLGT lack osteoclast-like giant cells, however.[65] Neoplastic giant cells of the type seen in soft tissue clear cell sarcoma are absent.

Ultrastructurally, the cells of CCSLGT are poorly differentiated with primitive cell junctions, scarce intracellular filaments, and variable amounts of glycogen. Melanosomes have not been identified in any case studied to date, although occasional dense core granules have been reported to be present.[64,73] Very recently, Stockman et al.[65] have shown features suggestive of neuroectodermal differentiation in CCSLGT, including dense-core secretory granules, secretory vesicles, and synapse-like structures.

By immunohistochemistry, all CCSLGT reported to date have shown an identical immunophenotype with expression of S-100 protein and absent expression of markers of melanocytic differentiation, such as HMB-45, Melan A, MiTF, and tyrosinase (Fig. 29-31).[65,75] SOX10, a transcription factor frequently expressed by nerve sheath and melanocytic tumors, is frequently positive. All cases studied to date have been CD117 (C-kit)-negative. Occasional cases may express synaptophysin, CD57, and/or neuron-specific enolase.

Cytogenetic and Molecular Genetic Features

Traditional karyotyping, reverse transcription polymerase chain reaction analysis, and/or fluorescence in situ hybridization (FISH) study have been performed on 19 CCSLGT. Of these, 6 cases have contained *EWSR1-CREB1* fusions, 8 cases have contained *EWSR1-ATF1* fusions, and 3 cases contained an *EWSR1* rearrangement by FISH, with an unknown partner. Two studied cases have not shown rearrangements in *EWSR1*, *ATF1*, or *CREB1*.[64,65,71,73]

Discussion

Although some investigators have regarded CCSLGT as simply a variant of clear cell sarcoma lacking melanocytic differentiation, the preponderance of evidence suggests that CCSLGT represents a distinct entity. From a clinical perspective, CCSLGT shows much more aggressive behavior than does soft tissue clear cell sarcoma, with metastatic disease in less than

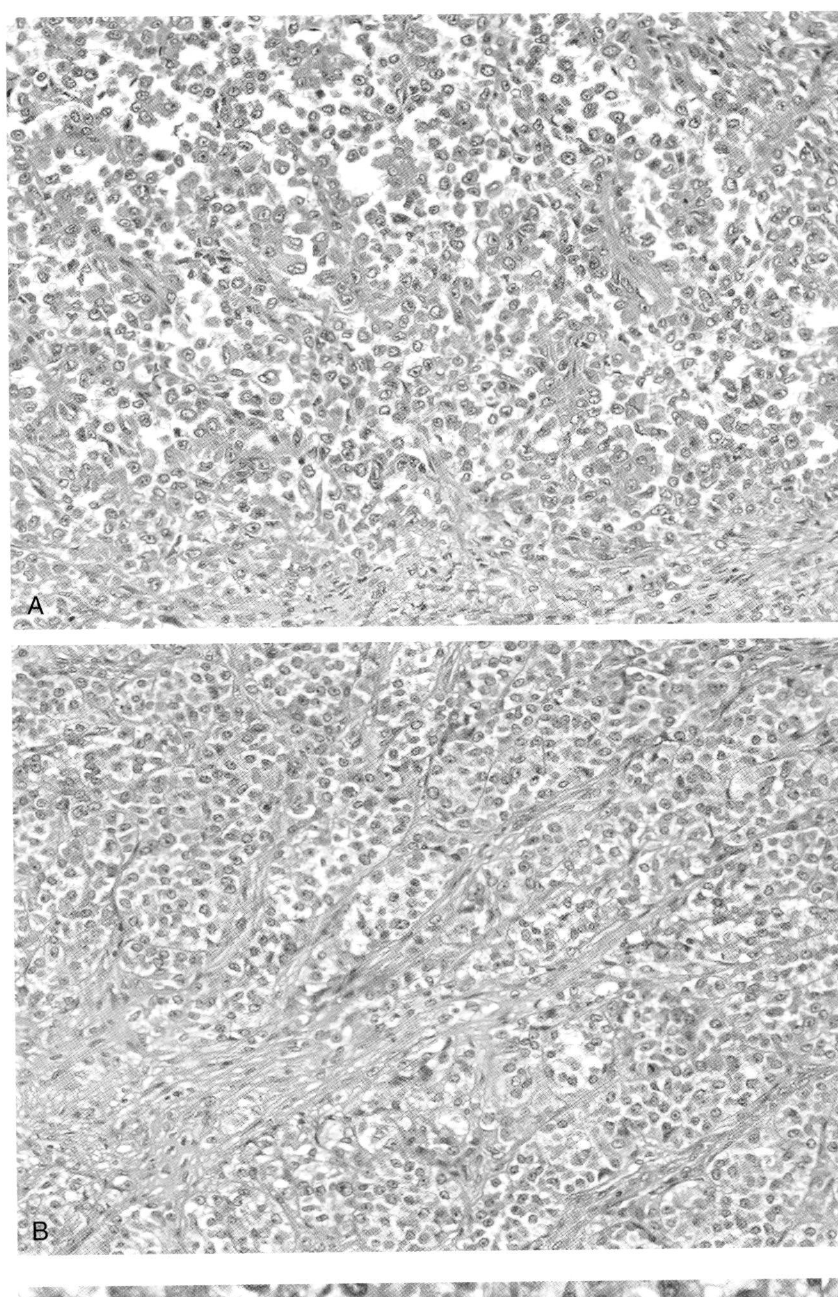

FIGURE 29-28. Pseudopapillary (A) and solid/nested (B) growth patterns in clear cell sarcoma-like gastrointestinal tumor.

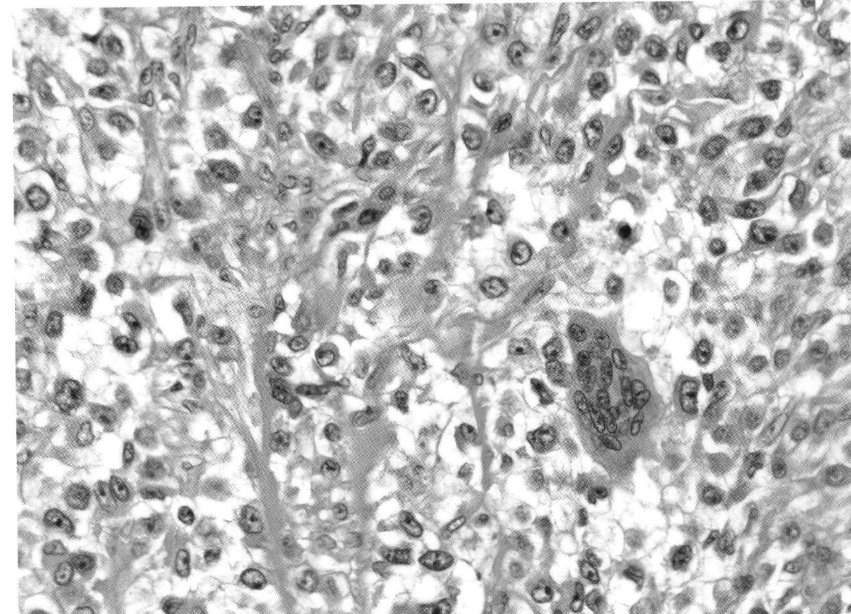

FIGURE 29-29. Higher power view of clear cell sarcoma-like gastrointestinal tumor, showing primitive cells with a moderate amount of clear to lightly eosinophilic cytoplasm, vesicular nuclei, and small nucleoli. Note the osteoclast-like giant cell.

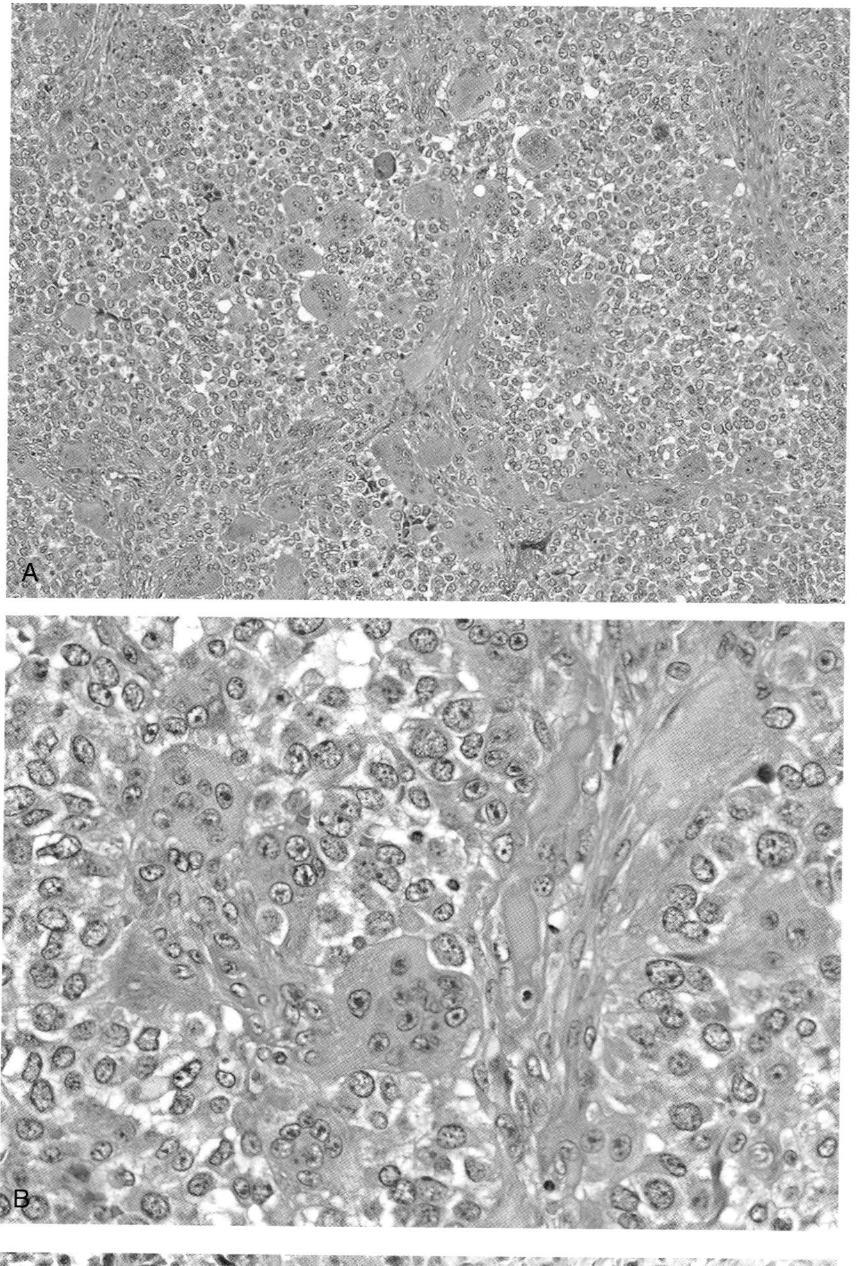

FIGURE 29-30. Numerous osteoclast-like giant cells in clear cell sarcoma-like gastrointestinal tumor (A). In contrast to clear cell sarcoma of soft parts, Touton-type neoplastic giant cells are absent (B).

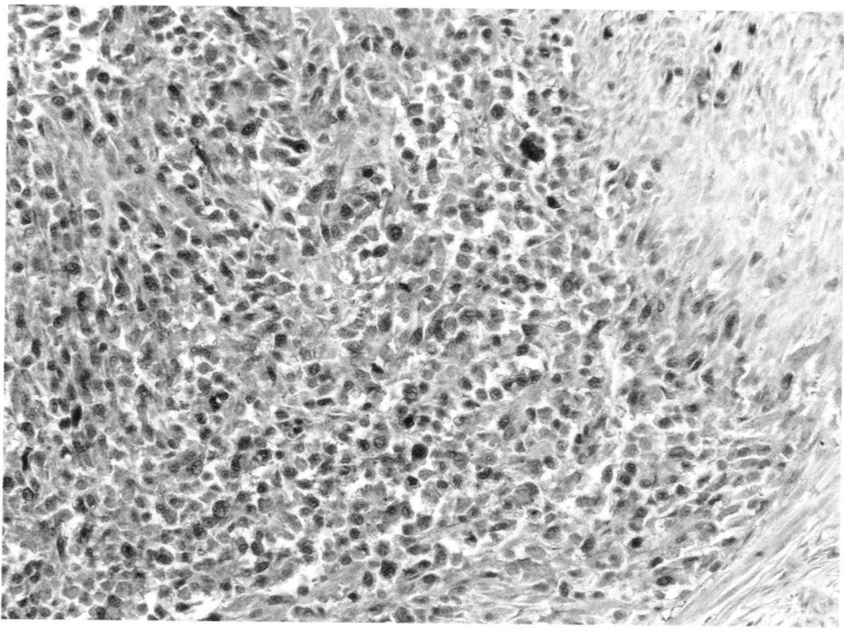

FIGURE 29-31. Although clear cell sarcoma-like gastrointestinal tumors typically show strong S-100 protein expression (shown), expression of more specific melanocytic markers (e.g., HMB-45, Melan-A) is not seen.

36 months in almost all reported cases, as compared with the much more protracted survival of patients with clear cell sarcoma. Morphologically, CCSLGT shares some features with clear cell sarcoma, such as clear to lightly eosinophilic cytoplasm and a tendency toward nested growth but more often shows dissimilar features, including sheet-like, pseudoalveolar and pseudopapillary growth, inapparent or small nucleoli, and perhaps, most notably, osteoclast-like giant cells, instead of Touton-type neoplastic giant cells. At the immunophenotypic level, CCSLGT and clear cell sarcoma share expression of S-100 protein but differ very significantly in terms of expression of specific melanocytic markers, the expression of which has never been documented in CCSLGT. Perhaps the most compelling evidence linking CCSLGT and clear cell sarcoma is the presence of EWSR1-ATF1 and EWS1-CREB1 fusions in both tumors, but even this may not be conclusive proof of a link. Indeed, it is now known that these same fusions may be seen in a wholly dissimilar soft tissue neoplasm, angiomatoid (malignant) fibrous histiocytoma,[76,77] and in a salivary gland tumor, hyalinizing clear cell carcinoma.[78]

Differential Diagnosis

CCSLGT may be distinguished from clear cell sarcoma involving the gastrointestinal tract[72] and metastatic melanoma by virtue of its distinctive morphologic features, including the presence of osteoclast-like giant cells and its absent expression of specific melanocytic markers. Gastrointestinal stromal tumors differ morphologically from CCSLGT and express CD117, protein kinase C-theta, and DOG1, markers not reported to be positive in CCSLGT.[79-81]

PERIVASCULAR EPITHELIOID CELL FAMILY OF TUMORS

The term *perivascular epithelioid cell tumor (PEComa)* has been applied to a growing family of tumors composed of histologically and immunohistochemically distinctive perivascular epithelioid cells. This family includes renal and extrarenal angiomyolipoma (AML), lymphangiomyomatosis (LAM), clear cell sugar tumor (CCST) of the lung, and a number of extrapulmonary spindled and epithelioid neoplasms that have been referred to by a variety of names, including *primary extrapulmonary sugar tumor (PEST)*,[82] clear cell myomelanocytic tumor,[83] and abdominopelvic sarcoma of perivascular epithelioid cells.[84]

The concept of a family of tumors composed of these distinctive perivascular epithelioid cells has evolved over the last century. Renal AML and its association with tuberous sclerosis complex (TSC) has been recognized for many years.[85] In the late 1960s and early 1970s, LAM and CCST were formally described.[86,87] Valensi[88] reported the association between LAM and TSC in 1973, and the next year, Monteforte and Kohnen[89] noted the association between AML and LAM. A breakthrough observation occurred in 1991, when Pea et al.[90] identified HMB-45 immunoreactivity and premelanosomes in renal AML. Identical observations were made in hepatic AML,[91] pulmonary CCST,[92] and LAM,[93] thereby solidifying the concept that AML, LAM, and CCST were related to one another morphologically, immunohistochemically, and through their association with TSC. The PEComa family of tumors subsequently grew quickly following the 1996 report by Zamboni et al.[94] of a pancreatic tumor that was morphologically identical to CCST. PEComa of both epithelioid and spindle-cell type have been reported in a wide variety of intra-abdominal, bone, soft tissue, and visceral sites, including the falciform ligament/ligamentum teres, mesentery, uterus, heart, thigh, and gastrointestinal tract. The following discussion will focus on AML, LAM, non-AML, and non-LAM PEComas.

Angiomyolipoma

The term *angiomyolipoma (AML)* should be reserved for a specific lesion arising most commonly in one or both kidneys as a solitary or multicentric mass; rarely, the mass is a pedunculated growth or presents as a satellite nodule outside of the renal capsule. Multiple and bilateral lesions are less common than solitary ones and are more often encountered in patients with tuberous sclerosis.[85]

Clinical Findings

AML occurs more commonly in women than in men, with a median age in the fifth decade of life. In about two-thirds of cases, it causes symptoms such as abdominal or flank pain, hematuria, or chills and fever. Less commonly, it is asymptomatic and is discovered as an incidental finding at operation for some unrelated cause or at autopsy. Rarely, sudden, severe flank pain and shock are caused by rupture of the tumor and massive perirenal or retroperitoneal hemorrhage.[95] Rare instances of associated hypertension have been recorded.[96] Most lesions occur in the kidney, although hepatic examples are well-recognized as well.[97,98] The precise classification of cases reported as angiomyolipoma in such locations as the nasal cavity,[99] oral cavity,[100] colon,[101] lung,[102] and skin[103] is debatable, and it is more likely that these represent vascular leiomyomas with adipocytic metaplasia.

Approximately one-third of patients present with manifestations of TSC, ranging from hyperpigmented spots, shagreen patches, periungual fibromas, and angiofibromas to renal cysts, cardiac rhabdomyoma, and gliosis and calcification of the cerebral cortex with mental deficiency.[104,105] There are also rare cases in which the tumor is associated with LAM[106,107] and renal cell carcinoma.[108] CT scans and MRI reveal a fatty mass with intermixed soft tissue densities, except in those cases in which the absence of fat or hemorrhage obscures the radiologic findings.[109]

Pathologic Findings

Grossly, the lesion presents as a yellow to gray mass, varying in size from a few centimeters to 20 cm or more (average 9 cm). Large lesions may become attached to the diaphragm or liver. Focal hemorrhage is present in about half of the cases. The tumor is usually well delineated from the surrounding renal parenchyma (Fig. 29-32). Some tumors extend into the inferior vena cava,[110] and others involve perirenal lymph nodes,[111] both of which may contribute to a presumed diagnosis of malignancy.

Microscopically, AML shows triphasic histology with tortuous, thick-walled blood vessels, irregularly arranged sheets and bundles of myoid-appearing perivascular epithelioid cells,

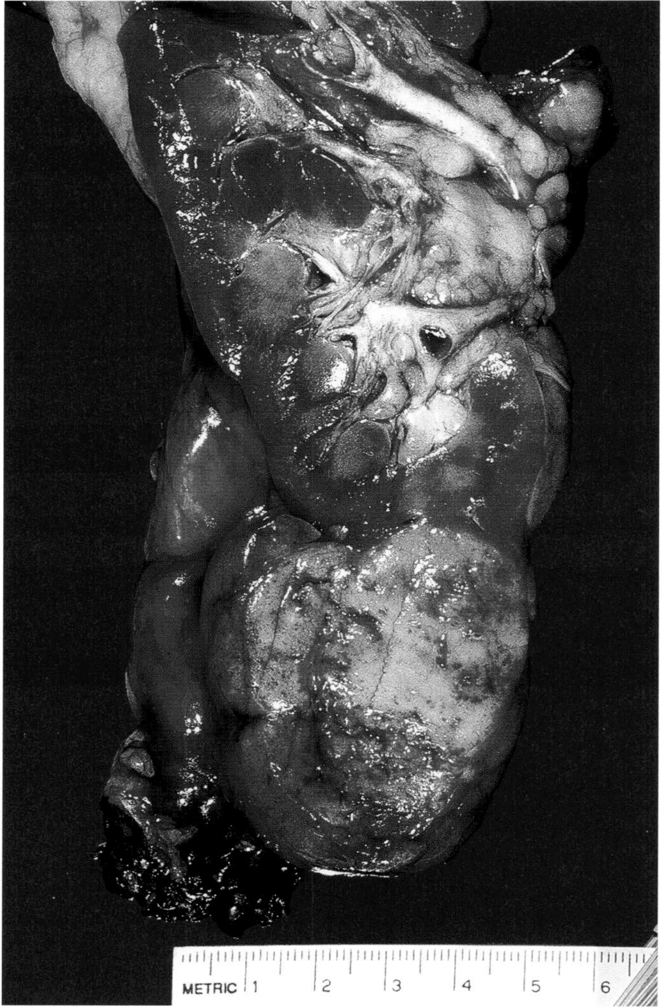

FIGURE 29-32. Angiomyolipoma of the kidney. The lesion, well circumscribed, is broadly attached to one pole of the kidney. Focal hemorrhage within the nodule is apparent.

and lipid-distended perivascular epithelioid cells (so-called *adipocytes*). Both abnormal, thick-walled vessels showing little elastica and hyalinization of the media and normal-appearing blood vessels are present in AML, the latter most likely representing in-growth of normal host blood vessels (Figs. 29-33 and 29-34).[112] In some cases, the myoid cells display a striking degree of cellular pleomorphism with hyperchromatic nuclei, occasional multinucleated giant cells, and necrotic foci (Fig. 29-35). Epithelioid cells containing spherical granules and dense PAS-positive, needle-shaped or rhomboid crystals similar to those in juxtaglomerular tumors may be present, although these cells do not stain for renin (Fig. 29-36).[113-115] Some cases of AML show profound cystic change, which may obscure the recognition of this tumor.[116]

Immunohistochemically, the myoid and lipid-distended cells of AML show a myomelanocytic immunophenotype with coexpression of smooth muscle actin and melanocytic markers (e.g., HMB-45, Melan-A, tyrosinase, MiTF) (Fig. 29-37).[90,117-119] Desmin expression is less common but may be present. A significant percentage of cases stain for progesterone receptors and, less commonly, estrogen receptors.[120-122] CD117 (*KIT*) is also expressed in the majority of tumors.[117]

Ultrastructurally, many of these myoid cells contain myofilaments, glycogen particles, and electron-dense granules. As previously mentioned, premelanosomes are often identified.[85]

Cytogenetic Findings

Although relatively few of these lesions have been studied by cytogenetics, some have been found to show trisomy 7 or 8,[123,124] and others reveal loss of heterozygosity of TSC genes on chromosomes 9q34 (*TSC1*) and 16p13 (*TSC2*).[120,125] Loss of hamartin and tuberin expression, the products of *TSC1* and *TSC2* genes, respectively, can be detected in AML with *TSC1* and *TSC2* mutations.[126] Loss of tuberin and hamartin expression results in loss of control of cell signaling related to the mTOR pathway, with a variety of downstream effects.[127]

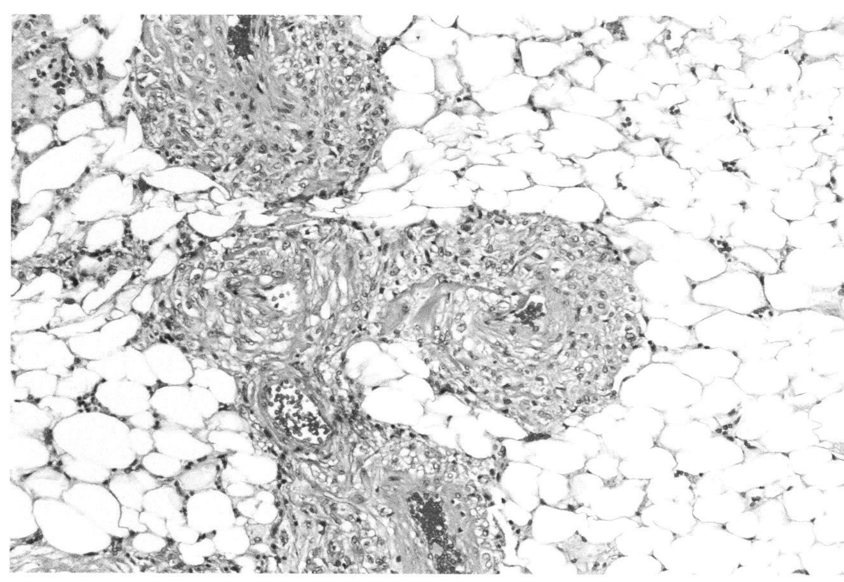

FIGURE 29-33. Angiomyolipoma with the basic components of the tumor: mature adipose tissue and smooth muscle surrounding thick-walled, medium-sized, vascular channels.

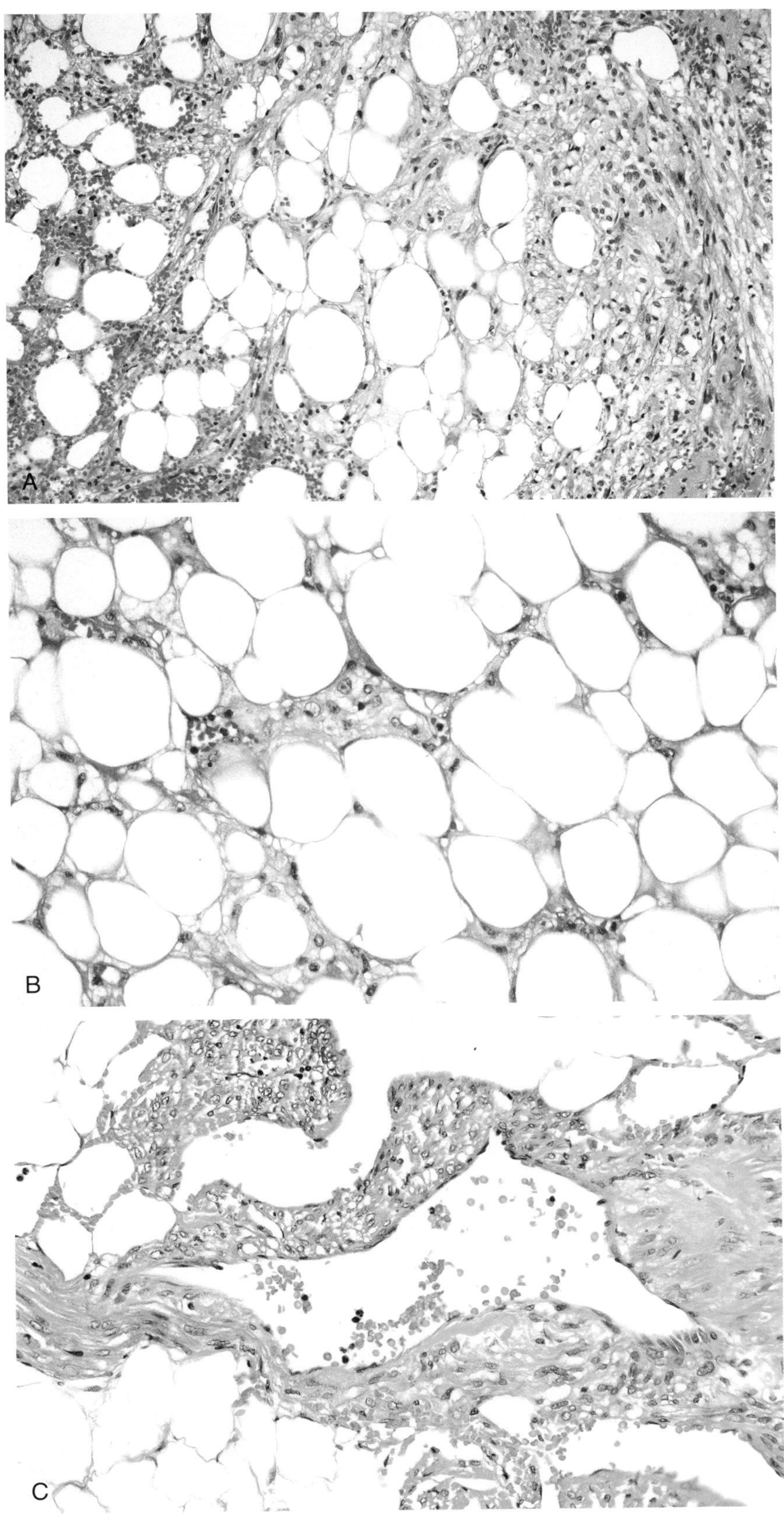

FIGURE 29-34. (A) Angiomyolipoma exhibiting an admixture of mature fat cells and vacuolated smooth muscle cells. (B) Isolated vacuolated smooth muscle cells in an angiomyolipoma. Areas such as this could be mistaken for liposarcoma, particularly when the cells show cytologic atypia. (C) Angiomyolipoma with collections of vacuolated smooth muscle cells arranged around dilated vascular spaces.

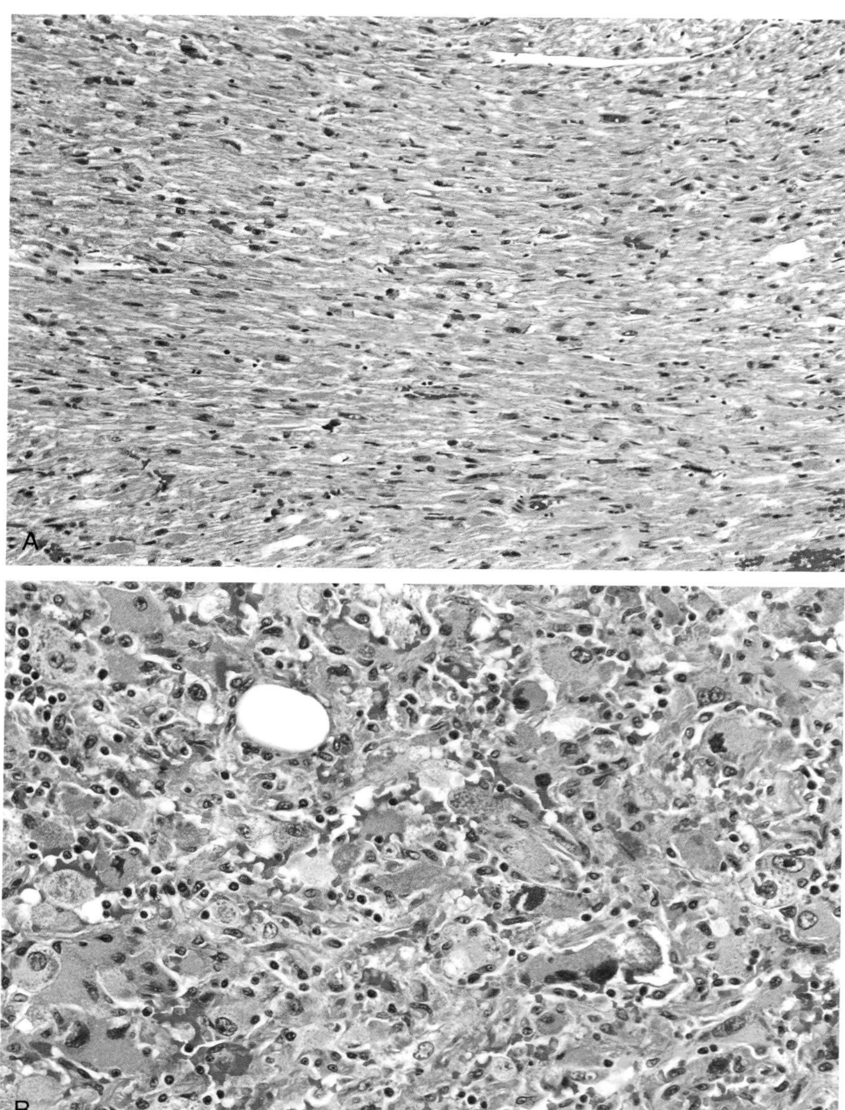

FIGURE 29-35. (A) Angiomyolipoma with an area composed of atypical spindle-shaped smooth muscle cells arranged in fascicles. These areas could be confused for leiomyosarcoma or dedifferentiated liposarcoma with divergent leiomyosarcomatous differentiation. (B) Angiomyolipoma exhibiting striking variation in the size and shape of smooth muscle elements, with rare cells showing marked cytologic atypia, a feature that has been mistaken for evidence of malignancy.

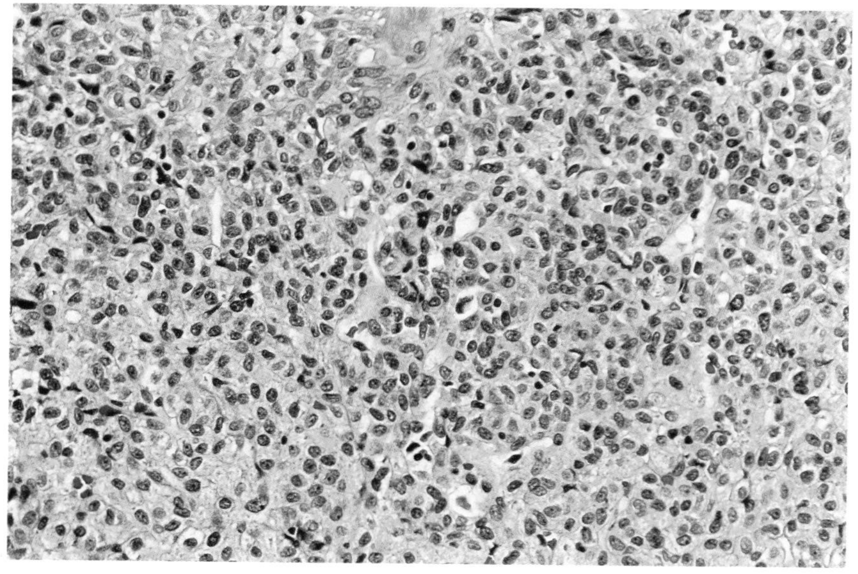

FIGURE 29-36. Angiomyolipoma composed of uniform small epithelioid smooth muscle cells, a feature that could be mistaken for renal cell carcinoma, particularly in patients with tuberous sclerosis.

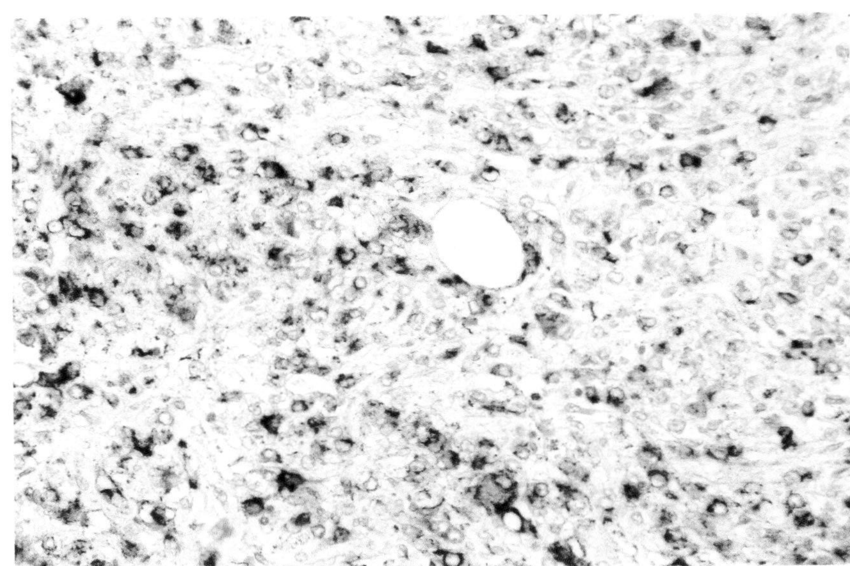

FIGURE 29-37. HMB-45 immunoreactivity in the myoid cells of an angiomyolipoma.

Differential Diagnosis

Although the histologic appearance of the tumor is characteristic and should not cause difficulty with the diagnosis, rare cases of AML are mistaken for sarcomas or carcinomas. Those tumors that have a prominent fatty component may be mistaken for liposarcoma, particularly when they present as large retroperitoneal masses. The presence of convoluted thick-walled blood vessels, small, inconspicuous clusters of perivascular epithelioid cells and immunoreactivity for HMB-45 allows for their distinction. AML with an inconspicuous fatty component may be confused with leiomyosarcoma, particularly those that are large, hypercellular, and pleomorphic. This distinction may be particularly challenging on a needle biopsy specimen. The myoid cells of AML tend to be plumper and paler than those found in leiomyosarcoma, and HMB-45 or Melan-A immunoreactivity can be extremely useful in this setting. Given that both renal cell carcinoma and AML are associated with TSC, some epithelioid AML are confused with renal cell carcinoma, and vice versa. Again, immunohistochemistry for melanocytic markers may be very helpful in this differential diagnosis. The possibility of epithelioid AML should also be considered whenever one has difficulty classifying epithelioid renal neoplasm, showing nuclear pleomorphism but little mitotic activity.

Discussion

Typical renal AML virtually always acts in a clinically benign fashion, even those with atypical features. There is no evidence that the presence of regional or systemic lymph node involvement, perirenal satellite tumors, or angiomyolipomatous growth in other organs reflects malignant potential.[85,128] There are, however, very rare examples of otherwise typical AML that have transformed to an overtly sarcomatous epithelioid or spindled neoplasm with subsequent malignant behavior.[129,130] On the other hand, epithelioid renal AML does harbor metastatic potential, especially those cases showing necrosis and/or marked nuclear atypia.[131-137] In their review of the literature, Hornick and Fletcher[131] approximated that one-third of reported epithelioid AML have resulted in metastases, occasionally resulting in patient death. Several of the cases reported by Pea et al.[132] of renal cell carcinoma, which they reclassified as monotypic epithelioid AML, were

TABLE 29-2 Proposed Risk Stratification System for Epithelioid Angiomyolipomas

EVALUATED PARAMETERS	RISK CATEGORY	RISK OF DISEASE PROGRESSION (%)
Tuberous sclerosis complex (TSC) and/or concurrent angiomyolipoma	Low (0-1 adverse parameters)	15
Tumor size greater than 7 cm	Intermediate (2-3 adverse parameters)	64
Carcinoma-like growth pattern	High (4-5 adverse parameters)	100
Extrarenal extension and/or involvement of the renal vein		
Necrosis		

Modified from Nese N, Martignoni G, Fletcher CD, et al. Pure epithelioid PEComas (so-called epithelioid angiomyolipoma) of the kidney: a clinicopathologic study of 41 cases: detailed assessment of morphology and risk stratification. Am J Surg Pathol 2011;35(2):161–176.

characterized by an aggressive clinical course. Similarly, L'Hostis et al.[138] reported a case of a monophasic epithelioid pleomorphic AML that metastasized to the liver and paravertebral region resulting in the patient's death 2 years after presentation. Nese et al.[139] have very recently proposed a risk stratification system for the evaluation of epithelioid renal AML (Table 29-2). For unclear reasons, hepatic AML, including epithelioid variants, usually act in a clinically benign fashion, with rare exception.[140]

AML typically grows slowly and is adequately treated by partial nephrectomy. Small, asymptomatic tumors may require careful follow-up only, although total nephrectomy may be necessary for large tumors. Cases have also been treated successfully by therapeutic embolization or cryotherapy.[141]

Lymphangiomyoma and Lymphangiomyomatosis

LAM is a rare disease characterized by a proliferation of perivascular epithelioid cells[142,143] around lymphatics and lymph nodes of the mediastinum, retroperitoneum, and the pulmonary interstitium.[144] Localized lesions are referred to as *lymphangiomyoma*, whereas extensive lesions involving large segments of the lymphatic chain with or without pulmonary involvement are designated *LAM*. LAM and tuberous sclerosis appear to be overlapping diseases. Patients with pulmonary LAM and tuberous sclerosis-associated renal AMLs share a common allelic loss of the *TSC2* gene.[145,146] In addition, 1% of patients with tuberous sclerosis have changes in the lung very similar to LAM. Conversely, 15% of patients with LAM have AMLs. However, pulmonary LAM, unlike tuberous sclerosis, affects essentially women only, with exceedingly rare cases reported in men. These rare cases are typically seen in men who have TSC.[147]

Clinical Findings

The disease occurs almost exclusively in women, usually during the reproductive years (mean age about 40 years). Progressive dyspnea, the most common symptom, can be related to the almost constant presence of chylous pleural effusion or to pulmonary involvement, which occurs in about half of the patients.[148-151] Other symptoms include pneumothorax, hemoptysis, and rarely abdominal pain, chylous ascites, and chyluria.

Radiographic studies can be helpful for diagnosing this condition. Lymphangiography indicates obstruction in the major lymphatic ducts (Fig. 29-38A), ectatic lymph vessels distal to the obstruction, occasionally lymphatic–venous connections, and general loss of lymph node architecture (Fig. 29-38B). Chest radiographs demonstrate changes highly characteristic of this condition (Fig. 29-39). In the fully developed case, there is a coarse reticular nodular infiltrate with bulla. Numerous thin-walled cysts are noted on high-resolution CT, and pulmonary function studies indicate severe diffusion impairment.

Pathologic Findings

At surgery, these lesions are red to gray spongy masses that preferentially replace the thoracic duct and mediastinal lymph nodes (Fig. 29-40). Less often, they involve the retroperitoneal lymph nodes only; in particularly dramatic cases, the entire lymphatic chain from neck to inguinal region is transformed into multiple confluent masses. Chylous effusion is encountered, in most cases, and, in some instances, the pleural surfaces are noted to weep fluid, suggesting the presence of numerous abnormal communications between the lymphatics and the pleural surface. When the process affects the lungs as well, the organ has a honeycomb appearance with formation of numerous blebs or bullae.

Histologically, the lymphangiomyoma has a remarkably uniform appearance. The perivascular epithelioid cells are arranged in short fascicles around a ramifying network of endothelium-lined spaces (Figs. 29-41 to 29-43) and have an abundant grainy eosinophilic cytoplasm and nuclei devoid of pleomorphism and mitotic activity (Fig. 29-44). Occasionally, foci of lymphocytes are scattered between the muscle cells; in many instances, they represent vestiges of preexisting lymph nodes. The vascular spaces are usually empty but are sometimes filled with eosinophilic material containing fat droplets and occasional lymphocytes.

In the lung, the pathologic changes are extensive and severe (Figs. 29-45 and 29-46). The primary lesion is a haphazard proliferation of perivascular epithelioid cells that surround arterioles, venules, and lymphatics (see Fig. 29-45A), and which diffusely thicken the alveolar septa. Secondary changes ensue, including bulla formation, as a result of air trapping by obstructed bronchioles, and hemorrhage and hemosiderin deposition as a result of venule destruction. Although the

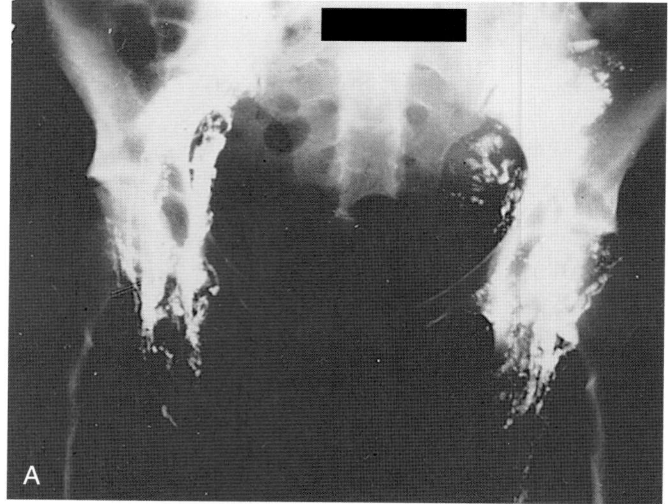

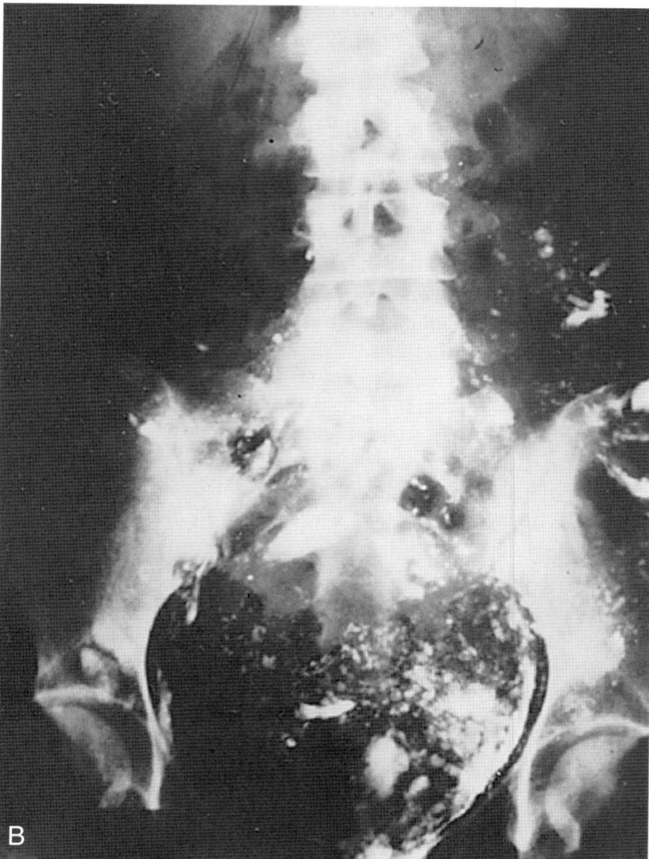

FIGURE 29-38. Lymphangiogram of a patient with lymphangiomyomatosis. (A) Initial film shows markedly dilated lymphatic vessels suggesting proximal obstruction. (B) Follow-up film (48 hours) shows amorphous collections of contrast material indicative of a loss of normal lymph node architecture. *(Courtesy of Dr. Van Vliet, Grand Rapids, MI.)*

macroscopic appearance of honeycombing may initially suggest the diagnosis of end-stage interstitial fibrosis, the two lesions are quite different histologically. LAM is characterized by an exclusive proliferation of perivascular epithelioid cells that can be identified after applying a trichrome stain by their cytoplasmic fuchsinophilia (see Fig. 29-45B). The muscle proliferation that accompanies end-stage interstitial fibrosis (muscular cirrhosis) is less striking and is always associated with areas of fibrosis.

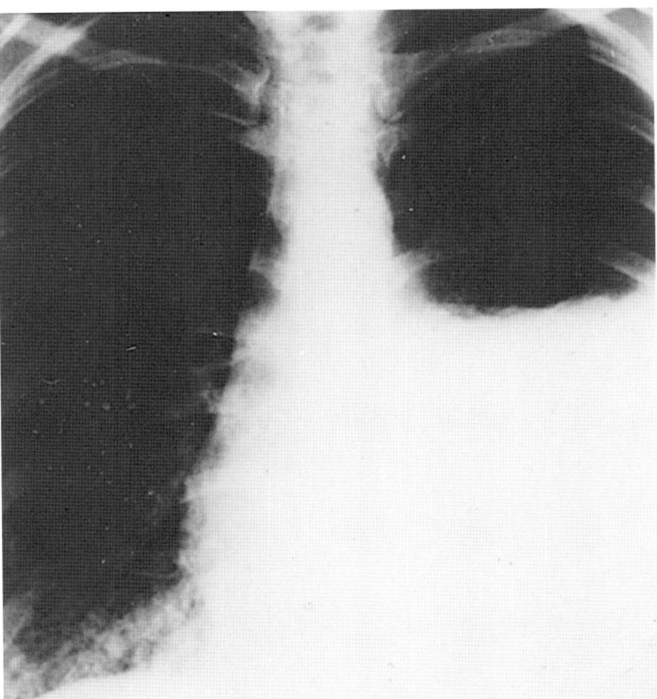

FIGURE 29-39. Chest radiograph in a patient with lymphangiomyomatosis. Lung volume is unaltered despite extensive interstitial disease. Massive (chylous) effusion is present on the left. *(Courtesy of Dr. Van Vliet, Grand Rapids, MI.)*

Differential Diagnosis

The full-blown case rarely presents diagnostic difficulty. Problems arise in limited forms of the disease when only one or two lymph nodes in the mediastinum or retroperitoneum are examined. Partial replacement of a lymph node might initially suggest the diagnosis of metastatic leiomyosarcoma (Fig. 29-47). The most helpful histologic feature is the consistent orientation of the perivascular epithelioid cells around endothelial spaces. Leiomyosarcomas show no predictable or consistent polarization toward vessels and, except in extremely well-differentiated cases, they usually have more pleomorphism and mitotic activity. The presence of lipid droplets in the fluid bathing the perivascular epithelioid cells in lymphangiomyomas is also suggestive of the diagnosis. Because the cells of LAM express melanocytic markers, these can be used to make this distinction as well.

Discussion

The clinical course of patients with this disease is variable. Those with localized lesions may survive for long periods following surgical excision, but patients with pulmonary involvement usually experience progressive pulmonary insufficiency. Approximately 30% to 70% of patients with pulmonary disease will die within 10 years of diagnosis. Estrogen and progesterone receptor proteins have been detected in pulmonary or abdominal tissue in this disease, and some patients have responded to progesterone or antiestrogen treatment.[152-156] Recently, heart-lung transplantation has been used as a definitive treatment, although recurrences of the disease have been noted in the transplanted lung.[157] Recent evidence strongly suggests that LAM represents an unusual form of estrogen-mediated benign metastasis of tuberin-null perivascular epithelioid cells, rather than a primary pulmonary process.[158,159]

PEComa (Excluding AML, LAM, and Pulmonary CCST)

Although AML, LAM, and pulmonary CCST are well described, relatively little is known about other members of

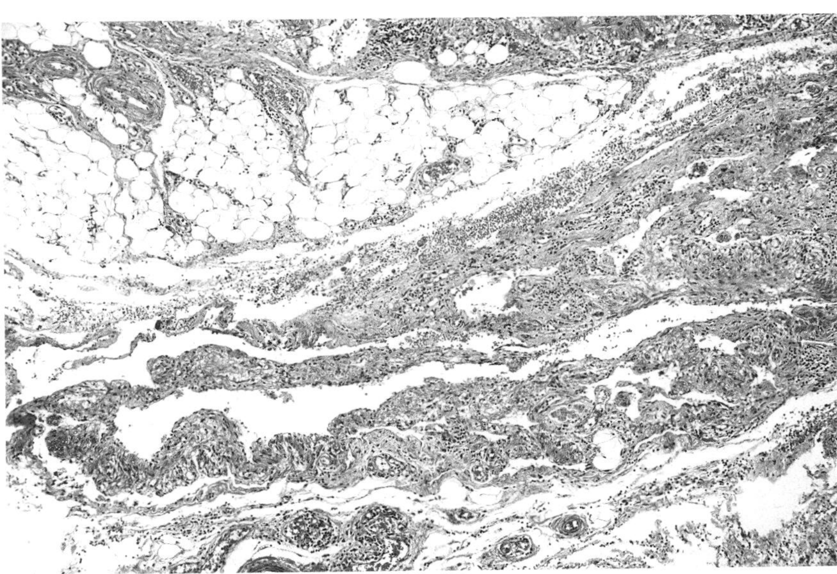

FIGURE 29-40. Lymphangiomyomatosis involving large lymphatic channels.

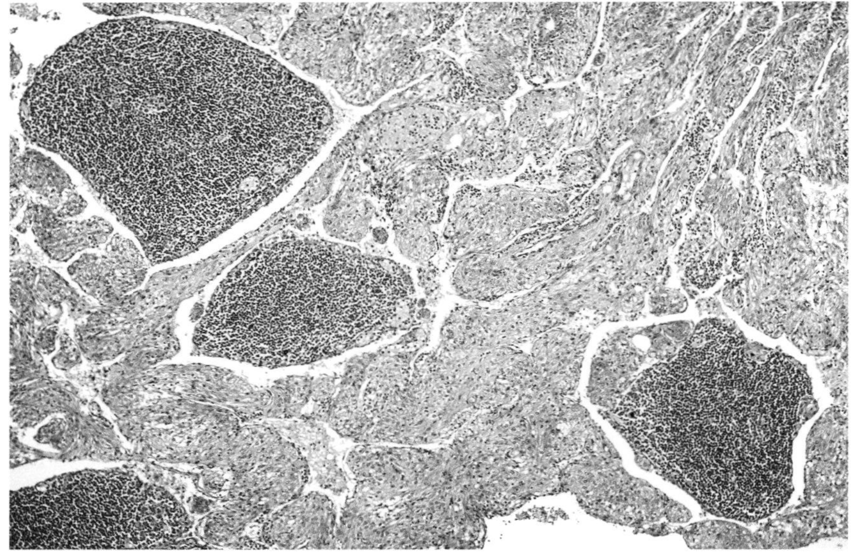

FIGURE 29-41. Lymphangiomyoma.

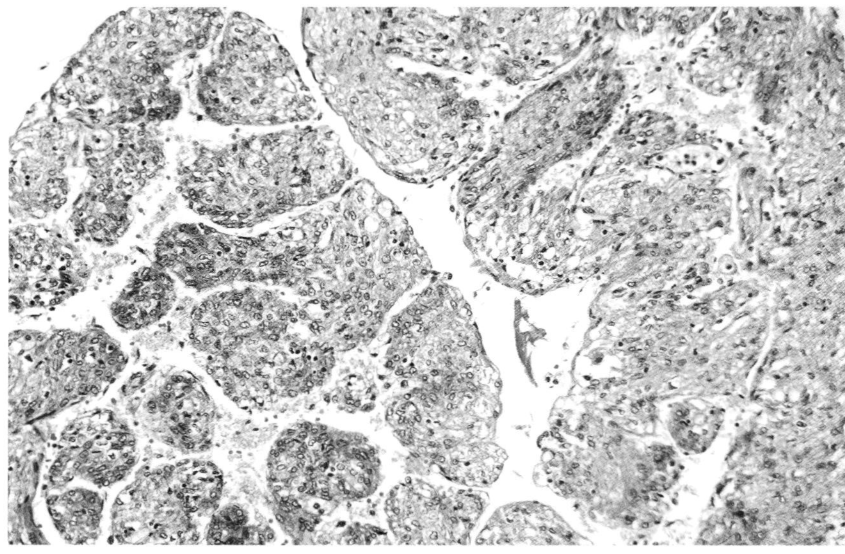

FIGURE 29-42. Lymphangiomyoma with the classic pericytoma pattern.

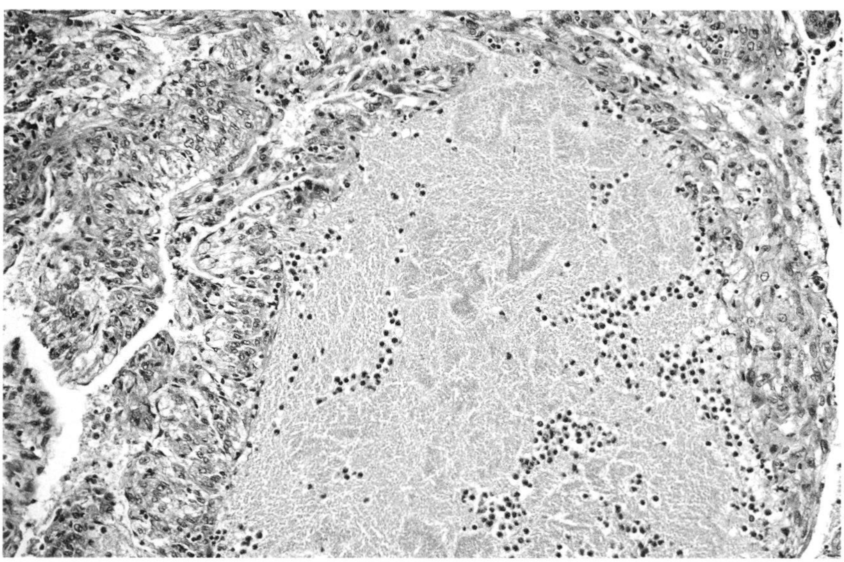

FIGURE 29-43. Lymphangiomyoma with lymph fluid in vascular spaces.

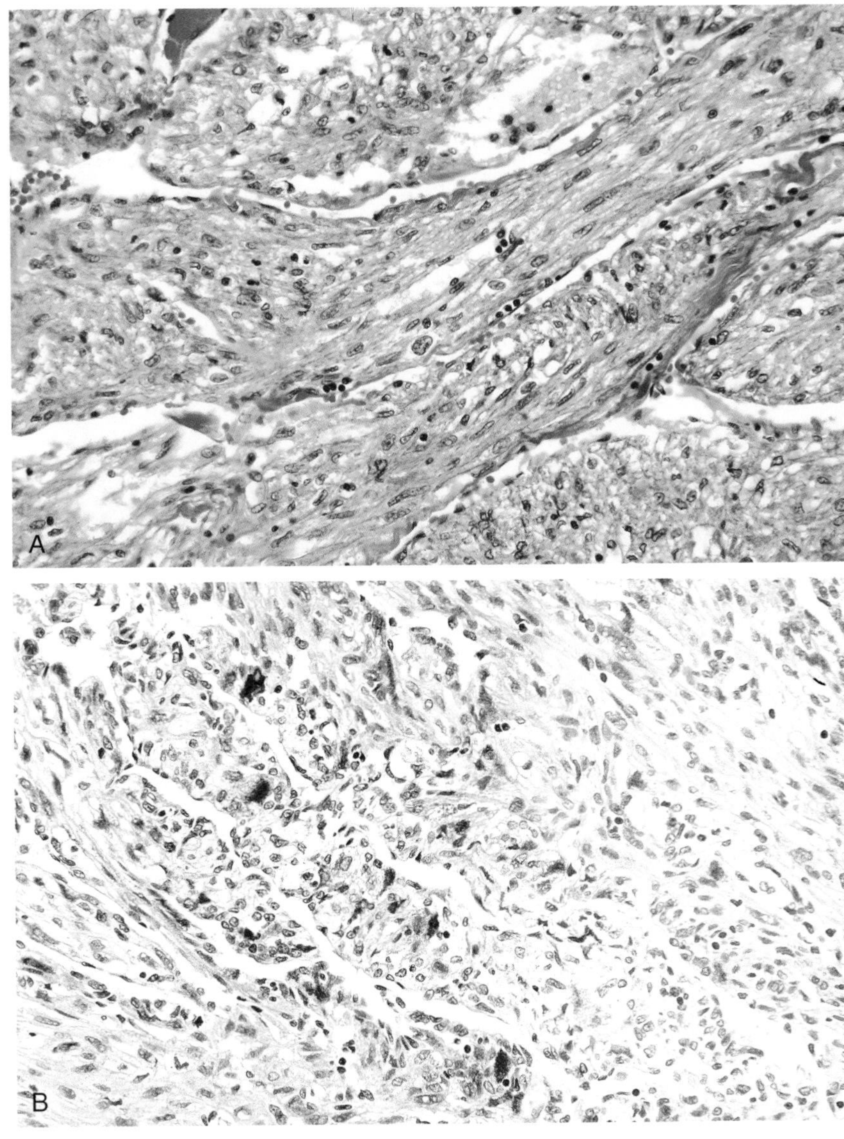

FIGURE 29-44. Lymphangiomyoma with distinctive partially vacuolated smooth muscle cells surrounding endothelium-lined spaces (A). These perivascular epithelioid clear cells coexpress smooth muscle and melanin markers. (B) This field shows focal positivity using HMB-45 antibody.

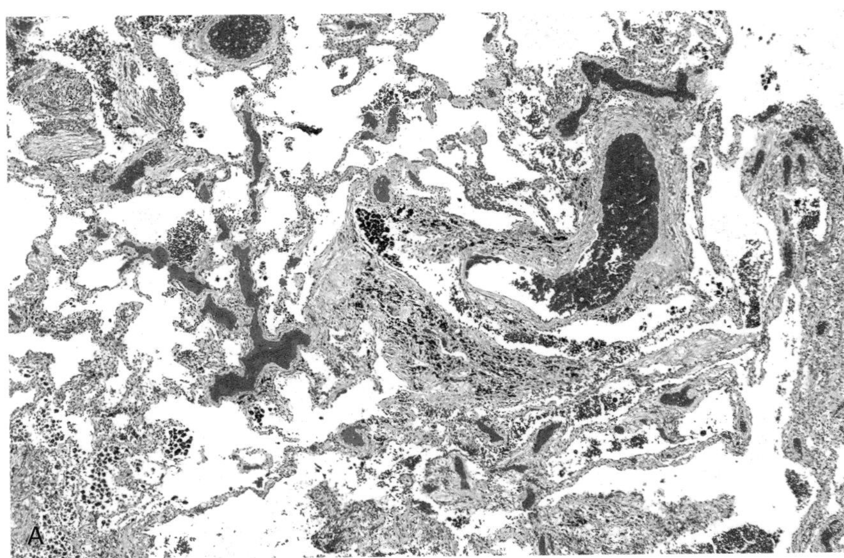

FIGURE 29-45. Lymphangiomyomatosis of the lung (A) with characteristic perivascular epithelioid cells (PEC) *Continued*

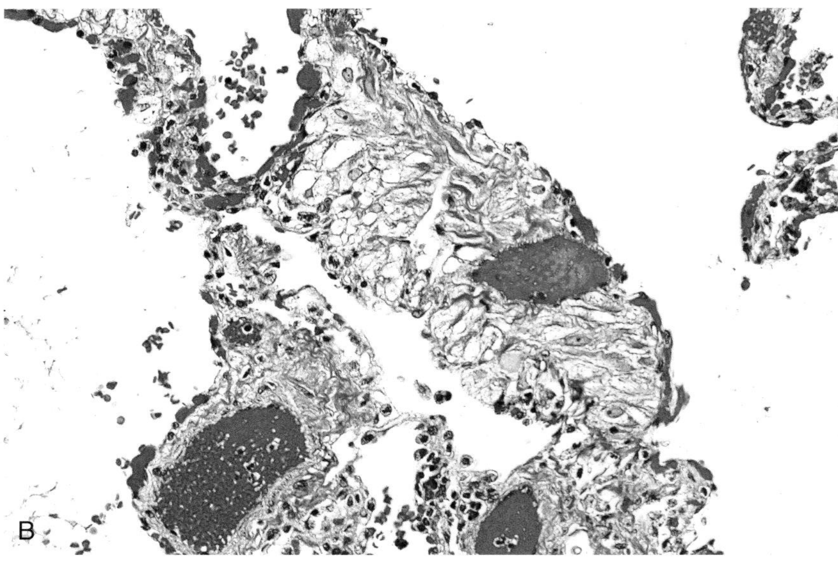

FIGURE 29-45, cont'd. (B) (Trichrome stain).

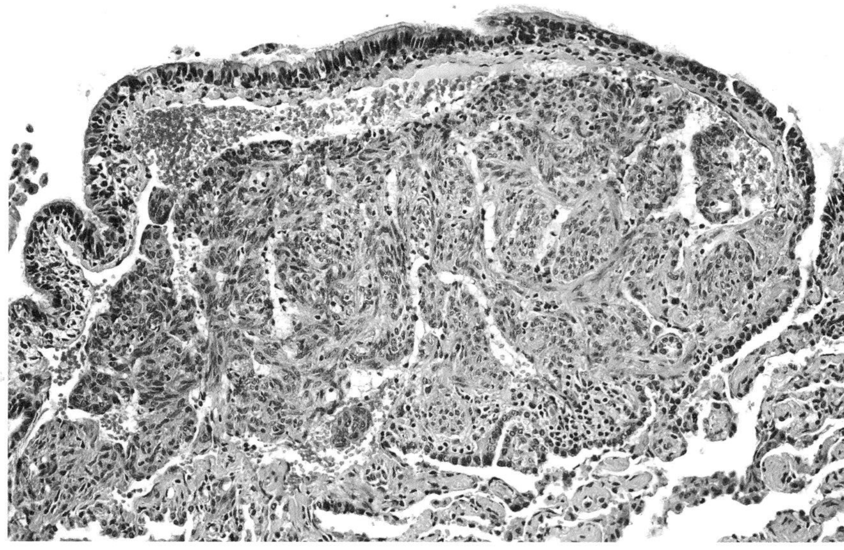

FIGURE 29-46. End-stage lung involved by lymphangiomyomatosis.

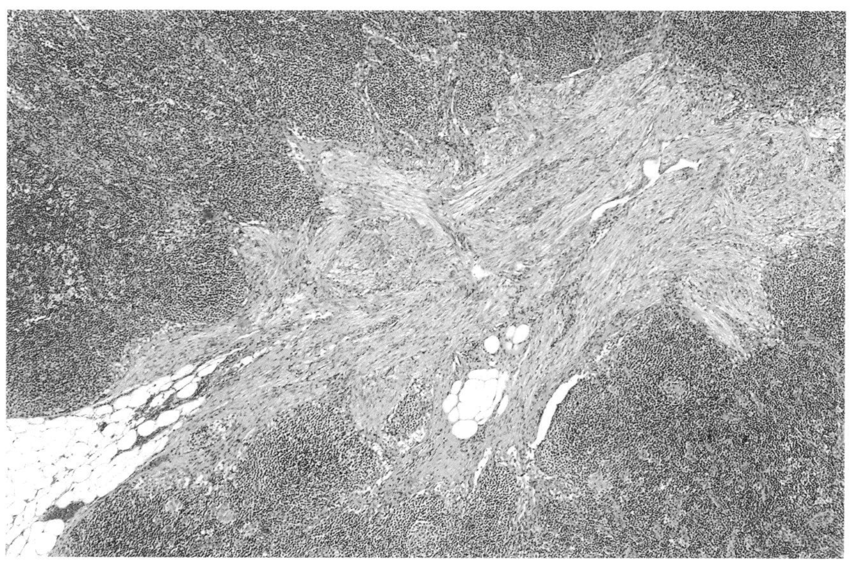

FIGURE 29-47. Lymph node partially involved by lymphangiomyomatosis.

the PEComa family, which includes lesions described under the rubrics of PEST, clear cell myomelanocytic tumor, abdominopelvic sarcoma of perivascular epithelioid cells, and PEComa arising in visceral sites, bone, and soft tissue. Since the initial report of a PEST arising in the pancreas, similar lesions have been described in virtually every anatomic site. In 2005, Folpe et al.[160] reported details of 26 PEComas of soft tissue and gynecologic origin and reviewed the literature on this topic.

Clinical Findings

These tumors can arise in patients of virtually any age, although the peak incidence is in the fourth decade of life.[160] There is a striking female predominance, even if one excludes those tumors that arise in gender-specific sites such as the uterus and prostate. Overall, the female-to-male ratio is approximately 7 to 1. Although a hormonal influence is possible, very few PEComas (aside from AML and LAM) have been evaluated for estrogen or progesterone receptor expression. Up to 40% of these tumors arise in gynecologic locations, most commonly the uterus.[161,162] An equivalent percentage of cases arise in the somatic soft tissues/skin[160,163,164]; viscera[165-167] and bone[168] PEComas are less common. Symptoms are related to the site of origin. Tumor size ranges widely, but most are between 4 and 6 cm at the time of excision. Very few patients with these tumors (less than 10%) show signs of TSC.[160]

Pathologic Findings

PEComas are generally grossly circumscribed, but some are histologically infiltrative into the surrounding soft tissue. The cut surface may be solid, firm, or even myxoid, and areas of hemorrhage or necrosis may be grossly appreciated (Fig. 29-48).

Histologically, PEComas are composed of clear to lightly eosinophilic cells that are arranged into nests, fascicles, and occasionally sheets, often with a radial arrangement around blood vessels (Figs. 29-49 to 29-53). Overall cellularity is usually low to moderate, but some cases are highly cellular. An admixture of epithelioid and spindled cells is common; some cases are predominantly spindled, identical to so-called *clear cell myomelanocytic tumor*,[160] and some are predominantly epithelioid, identical to CCST or monotypic epithelioid AML. Most tumors are composed of relatively uniform nuclei of low nuclear grade, but some have higher-grade nuclei and prominent nuclear pleomorphism that is identifiable at low magnification. Multinucleated giant cells are common, and, occasionally, one may encounter giant cells with a central eosinophilic zone surrounded by a peripheral clear zone, reminiscent of the spider cells seen in adult rhabdomyoma (Fig. 29-54). Prominent stromal sclerosis may be present.[169] Most tumors have few, if any, mitotic figures (MF), but some, especially those of higher nuclear grade, may have prominent mitotic activity (greater than 5 MF/50 HPF), including atypical MF (Fig. 29-55). Coagulative necrosis and angiolymphatic invasion are uncommonly identified.

Immunohistochemical and Ultrastructural Findings

PEComas typically show immunohistochemical evidence of both smooth muscle and melanocytic differentiation. In the study by Folpe et al.,[160] HMB-45 was the most sensitive melanocytic marker (96% of cases) (Fig. 29-56), followed by Melan-A (72%) and MiTF (50%) (Fig. 29-57). All of their cases expressed at least one melanocytic marker. Smooth muscle actin was found in 80% of cases and was typically stronger in epithelioid cells. Desmin was expressed in 36% of cases. Overall, 20 of 24 cases (83%) coexpressed smooth muscle actin and HMB-45 and/or Melan-A. Interestingly, this study found one-third of cases to stain for S-100 protein, a potential diagnostic pitfall in distinguishing this lesion from melanoma or clear cell sarcoma. However, all of the S-100 protein-positive tumors also stained for one or more muscle markers. Although uncommon, rare cells may also stain for pancytokeratins. CD117 (*KIT*) expression is similarly uncommon. Ultrastructural analysis reveals evidence of both smooth muscle and melanocytic differentiation in the form of premelanosomes (Fig. 29-58).[82]

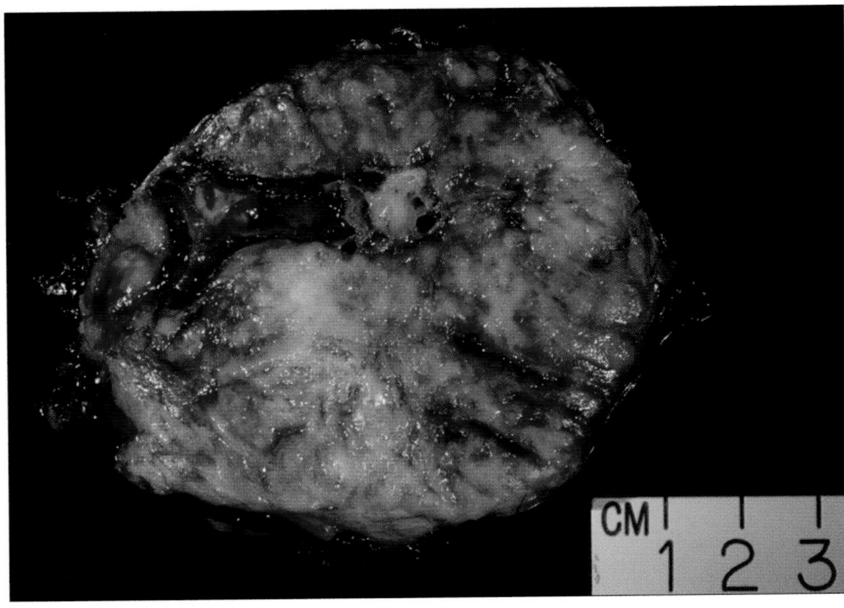

FIGURE 29-48. Gross appearance of a soft tissue PEComa. The cut surface has a variegated appearance, including focal areas of necrosis.

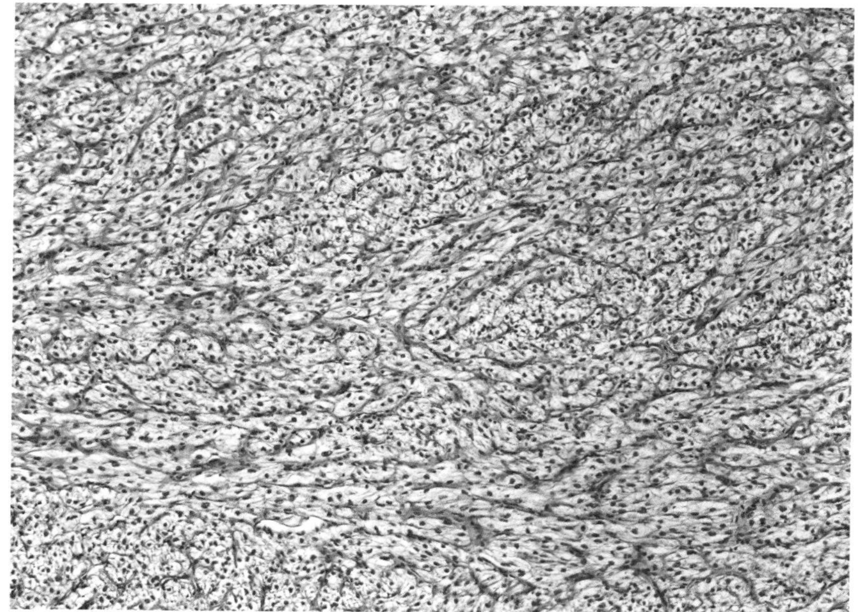

FIGURE 29-49. PEComa of soft tissue composed predominantly of nests of epithelioid cells with cleared-out cytoplasm.

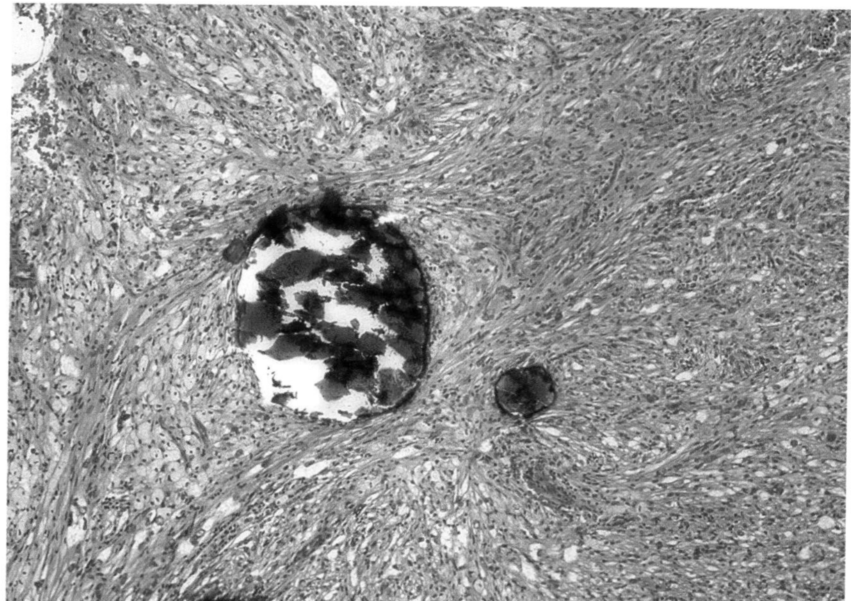

FIGURE 29-50. Higher-magnification view of nests of epithelioid cells in a PEComa of soft tissue.

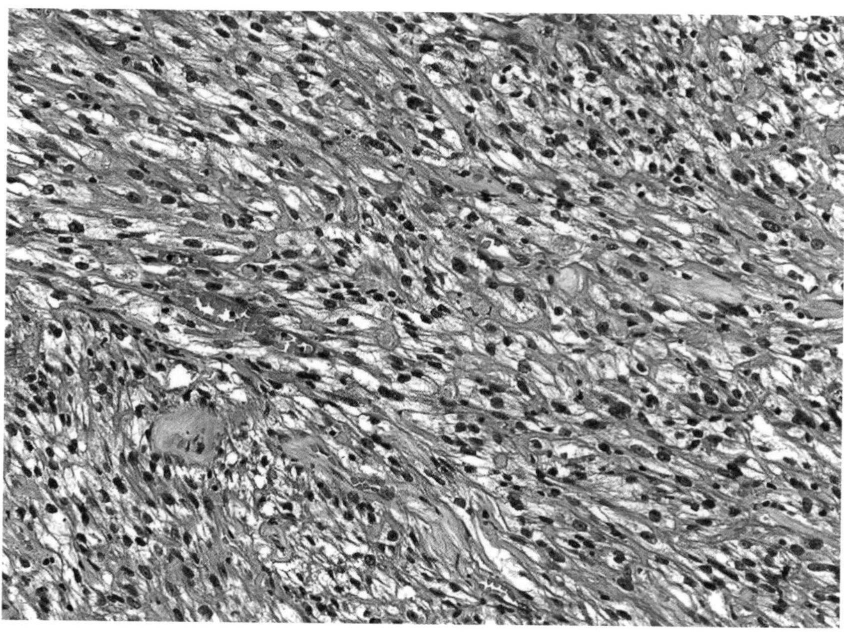

FIGURE 29-51. High-magnification view of cells with a spindled morphology in a soft tissue PEComa.

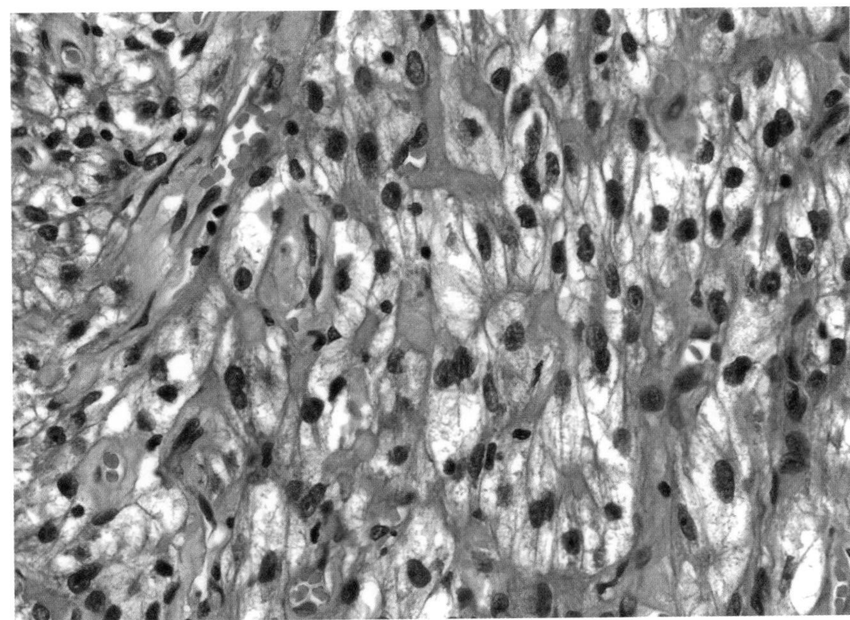

FIGURE 29-52. Soft tissue PEComa with uniform-appearing nuclei.

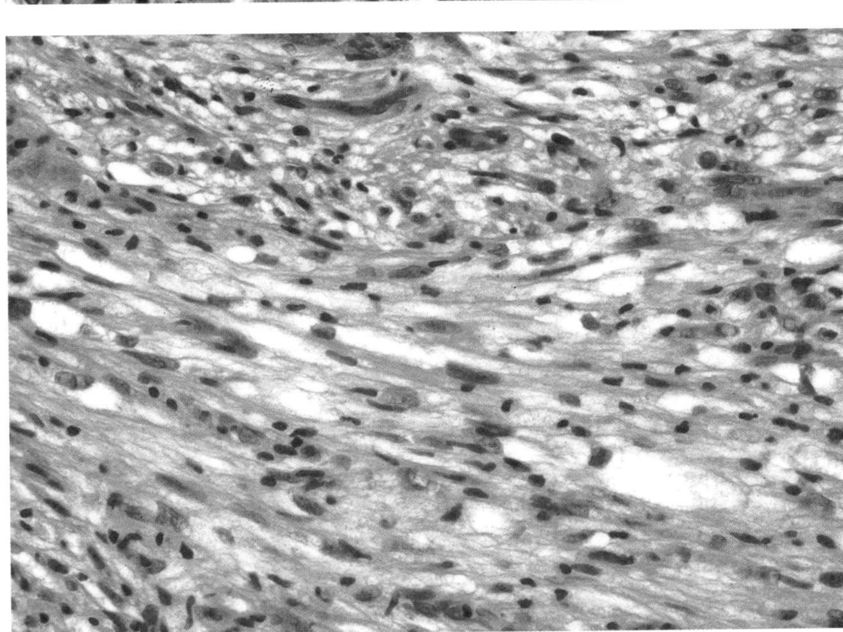

FIGURE 29-53. Bland-appearing spindled cells in soft tissue PEComa.

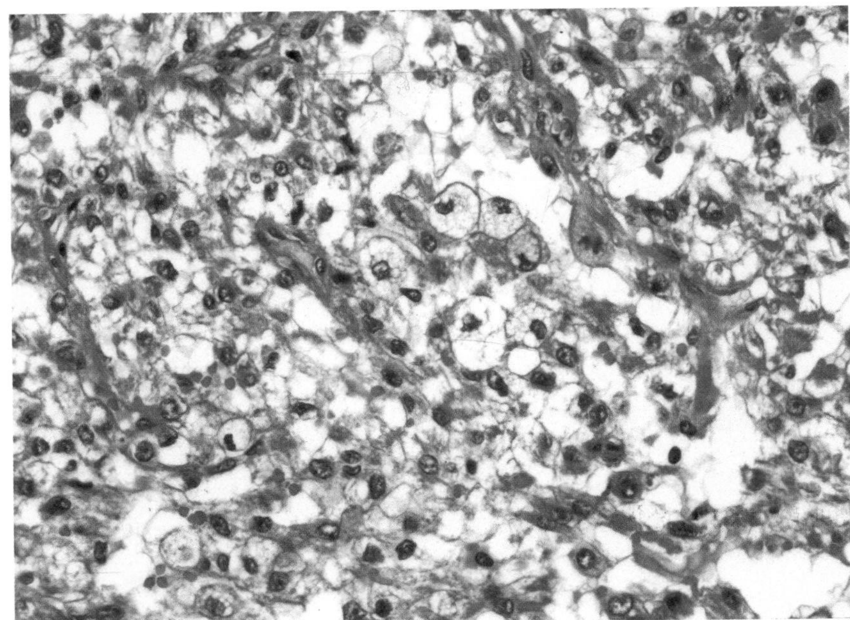

FIGURE 29-54. Cells reminiscent of spider cells seen in adult rhabdomyoma in a case of soft tissue PEComa.

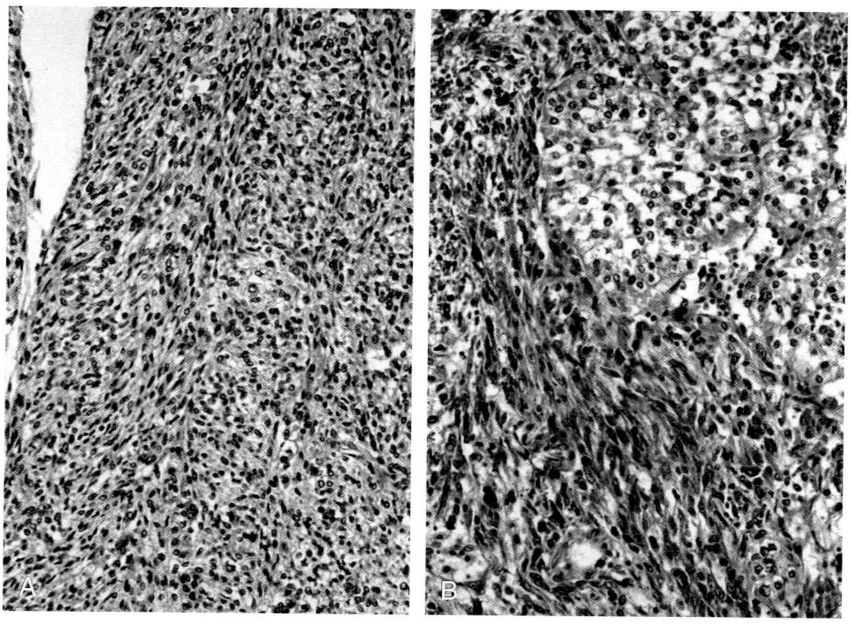

FIGURE 29-55. (A) Highly cellular focus in a malignant PEComa. (B) High-magnification view of highly cellular focus in a malignant PEComa.

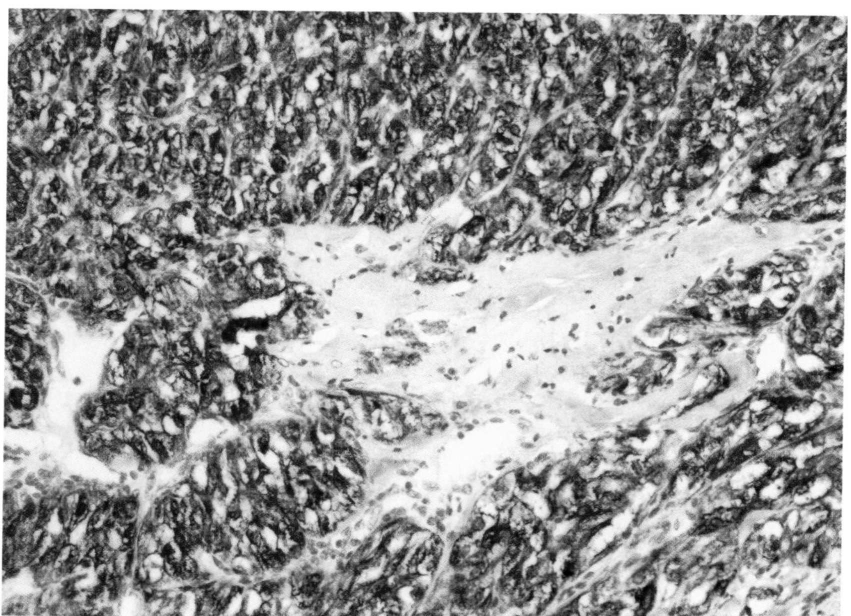

FIGURE 29-56. HMB-45 immunoreactivity in a soft tissue PEComa.

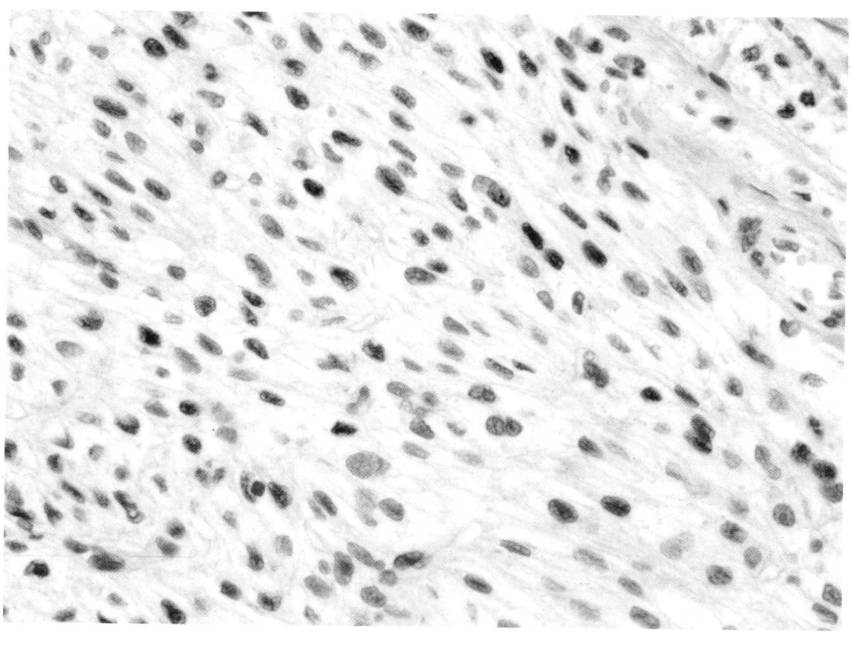

FIGURE 29-57. Nuclear immunoreactivity for MiTF in a soft tissue PEComa.

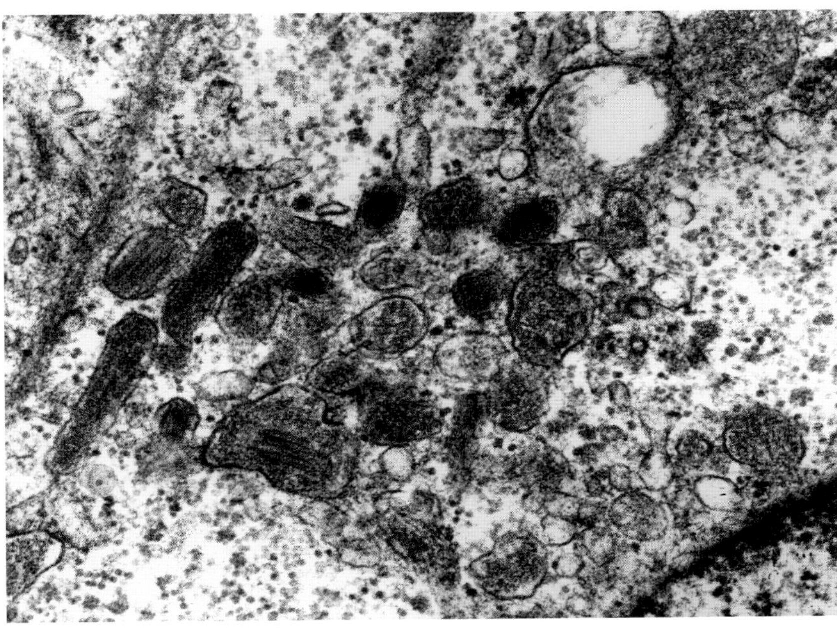

FIGURE 29-58. Ultrastructural appearance of a soft tissue PEComa characterized by the presence of premelanosomes.

Cytogenetic Findings

Relatively few cases of PEComa have been karyotyped, and a specific cytogenetic aberration has not been identified. The presence of a t(3;10) has been reported in one clear cell myomelanocytic tumor.[83] Pan et al.[170] performed comparative genomic hybridization on a number of PEComas and found frequent losses on chromosomes 19, 16p, 17p, 1p, and 18p and gains on chromosomes X, 12q, 3q, 5, and 2q. A small number of PEComas have been reported to show rearrangement of the *TFE3* gene and expression of TFE3 protein by immunohistochemistry.[160,171-174]

Differential Diagnosis

The differential diagnosis of PEComa is quite broad and dictated by the location of the tumor and predominant morphology (spindled versus epithelioid). Given the consistent expression of melanocytic markers, it is easy to understand how this lesion could be confused with either a melanoma or clear cell sarcoma. In addition, up to one-third of PEComas stain for S-100 protein, although strong, diffuse S-100 protein staining is typical of melanoma and clear cell sarcoma. Expression of muscle markers usually allows for this distinction, although not all PEComas express these antigens. As noted, one should be wary of diagnosing PEComa in an HMB-45-positive, S-100 protein-positive, actin-negative tumor.[160] Identification of the specific t(12;22) resulting in an *EWSR1/ATF-1* gene fusion can be invaluable in distinguishing clear cell sarcoma from PEComa.

Intra-abdominal PEComas can be confused with a gastrointestinal stromal tumor (GIST) because both may show an admixture of spindled and epithelioid cells. PEComas are typified by their characteristic clear to lightly eosinophilic cytoplasm and elaborate capillary vasculature. CD117 is expressed in some PEComas but is a far more consistent feature in GIST. CD34 is also expressed in the majority of GISTs but is not characteristic of PEComa. *DOG1* expression has not been reported in PEComa. Immunohistochemical demonstration of melanocytic differentiation is the most reliable way to distinguish PEComa from GIST.

Clear cell carcinomas (e.g., cervix, vagina, renal cell carcinoma) also enter the differential diagnosis, especially for PEComas with an epithelioid morphology. Clear cell carcinomas strongly express cytokeratins and do not express melanocytic markers.

PEComas can also be confused with true smooth muscle tumors, either spindled or epithelioid, especially when they arise in the abdomen or uterus. In the original report of clear cell myomelanocytic tumor by Folpe et al.,[83] a number of cases had been previously published as leiomyosarcomas of the ligamentum teres. Silva et al.[175] recently identified a subset of uterine smooth muscle tumors with mixed epithelioid and spindled features that harbored HMB-45-positive cells; these authors argued against designating these tumors as PEComas on the basis of simply identifying rare HMB-45-positive cells in an otherwise typical smooth muscle tumor. Morphologically, true smooth muscle tumors are composed of cells with diffuse cytoplasmic eosinophilia, perinuclear vacuoles, and cigar-shaped nuclei, and they usually lack the delicate capillary network seen in most PEComas. Multinucleated giant cells and spider-like cells are characteristic of PEComa. Unfortunately, there is significant overlap in immunophenotype because, as mentioned previously, morphologically typical uterine smooth muscle tumors occasionally express HMB-45, although they do not express Melan-A. Therefore, the coexpression of smooth muscle actin and Melan-A or MiTF would strongly favor a PEComa.

Discussion

Given the relative rarity of this group of tumors and that it was not delineated until the mid-1990s, it has not been possible to fully define criteria for malignancy in PEComas. In the study by Folpe et al.,[160] follow-up information in 26 patients (median follow-up period of 30 months) revealed local recurrence and metastases in 13% and 21% of patients, respectively. The most common sites of metastasis included the liver, lung, and bone. Similarly, in their review of the literature, 7% of patients were found to have local recurrence, and 20% developed metastatic disease. Overall, close to 80% of patients were alive with no evidence of disease as of their last follow-up. Tumor size greater than 8 cm, mitotic activity greater than 1 MF/50 HPF, and coagulative necrosis were found to be associated with aggressive clinical behavior. In their evaluation of previously published cases with sufficient morphologic detail, tumor size greater than 5 cm, infiltrative growth pattern, high nuclear grade, coagulative necrosis, and mitotic activity greater than 1 MF/50 HPF were associated with aggressive clinical behavior. So, Folpe et al.[160] proposed a provisional classification of PEComas into benign, uncertain malignant potential, and malignant categories (Tables 29-3 and 29-4). Benign tumors had no worrisome features (i.e., less than 5 cm, noninfiltrative, low to moderate nuclear grade and cellularity, mitotic activity less than 1 MF/50 HPF, no coagulative necrosis or vascular invasion). Tumors of uncertain malignant potential had either nuclear pleomorphism/multinucleated giant cells only or tumor size greater than 5 cm. Tumors with two or more worrisome features were classified as malignant. There have been a number of case reports and small series of malignant PEComas[84,176,177]; some of these patients have been treated with adjuvant therapy (including Gleevec),[178] but the efficacy of such therapy is not known. A role for inhibitors of the mTOR pathway in the treatment of unresectable AML and malignant PEComas has recently been demonstrated.[179,180]

TABLE 29-3 Proposed Classification of PEComas

CATEGORY	HISTOLOGIC CRITERIA
Benign	No worrisome features (greater than 5 cm, noninfiltrative, not high nuclear grade, not high cellularity, mitotic activity greater than 1 MF/50 HPF, no necrosis, no vascular invasion
Uncertain malignant potential	Nuclear pleomorphism/multinucleated giant cells only OR size greater than 5 cm
Malignant	Two or more worrisome features (greater than 5 cm, infiltrative, high nuclear grade, high cellularity, mitotic activity greater than 1 MF/50 HPF, necrosis, vascular invasion

Modified from Folpe AL, Mentzel T, Lehr HA, et al. Perivascular epithelioid cell neoplasms of soft tissue and gynecologic origin: a clinicopathologic study of 26 cases and review of the literature. Am J Surg Pathol 2005;29(12):1558–1575.

TABLE 29-4 Risk of Aggressive Clinical Behavior of PEComa Based Upon Histologic Classification

CATEGORY	AGGRESSIVE BEHAVIOR
Benign	0/22 (0%)
Uncertain malignant potential	2/23 (7%)
Malignant	12/17 (71%)

Modified from Folpe AL, Mentzel T, Lehr HA, et al. Perivascular epithelioid cell neoplasms of soft tissue and gynecologic origin: a clinicopathologic study of 26 cases and review of the literature. Am J Surg Pathol 2005;29(12):1558–1575.

References

1. Millar WG. A malignant melanotic tumor of ganglion cells arising from thoracic sympathetic ganglion. J Pathol Bacteriol 1932;35:351.
2. Fu YS, Kaye GI, Lattes R. Primary malignant melanocytic tumors of the sympathetic ganglia, with an ultrastructural study of one. Cancer [Case Reports Research Support, U.S. Gov't, P.H.S.] 1975;36(6):2029–41.
3. Carney JA. Psammomatous melanotic schwannoma. A distinctive, heritable tumor with special associations, including cardiac myxoma and the Cushing syndrome. Am J Surg Pathol 1990;14(3):206–22.
4. Carney JA, Ferreiro JA. The epithelioid blue nevus. A multicentric familial tumor with important associations, including cardiac myxoma and psammomatous melanotic schwannoma. Am J Surg Pathol 1996;20(3): 259–72.
5. Font RL, Truong LD. Melanotic schwannoma of soft tissues. Electron-microscopic observations and review of literature. Am J Surg Pathol [Case Reports Research Support, Non-U.S. Gov't] 1984;8(2):129–38.
6. Killeen RM, Davy CL, Bauserman SC. Melanocytic schwannoma. Cancer [Case Reports Review] 1988;62(1):174–83.
7. Krausz T, Azzopardi JG, Pearse E. Malignant melanoma of the sympathetic chain: with a consideration of pigmented nerve sheath tumours. Histopathology [Case Reports] 1984;8(5):881–94.
8. Leger F, Vital C, Rivel J, et al. Psammomatous melanotic schwannoma of a spinal nerve root. Relationship with the Carney complex. Pathol Res Pract [Case Reports] 1996;192(11):1142–6; discussion 7.
9. Lowman RM, Livolsi VA. Pigmented (melanotic) schwannomas of the spinal canal. Cancer [Case Reports] 1980;46(2):391–7.
10. Mennemeyer RP, Hallman KO, Hammar SP, et al. Melanotic schwannoma. Clinical and ultrastructural studies of three cases with evidence of intracellular melanin synthesis. Am J Surg Pathol 1979;3(1):3–10.
11. Vallat-Decouvelaere AV, Wassef M, Lot G, et al. Spinal melanotic schwannoma: a tumour with poor prognosis. Histopathology [Case Reports] 1999;35(6):558–66.
12. Torres-Mora J, Dry S, Li X, et al. Melanotic schwannoma: A clinicopathological study of 32 cases. Mod Pathol 2012;25(Suppl. 2):21A.
13. Zhang HY, Yang GH, Chen HJ, et al. Clinicopathological, immunohistochemical, and ultrastructural study of 13 cases of melanotic schwannoma. Chin Med J [Research Support, Non-U.S. Gov't] 2005; 118(17):1451–61.
14. Kindblom LG, Meis-Kindblom JM, Nelson JS, et al. Melanotic schwannoma. A study of 42 cases. Mod Pathol 1995;8(1):7.
15. Allen MS Jr, Harrison W, Jahrsdoerfer RA. "Retinal anlage" tumors. Melanotic progonoma, melanotic adamantinoma, pigmented epulis, melanotic neuroectodermal tumor of infancy, benign melanotic tumor of infancy. Am J Clin Pathol 1969;51(3):309–14.
16. Borello ED, Gorlin RJ. Melanotic neuroectodermal tumor of infancy–a neoplasm of neural crese origin. Report of a case associated with high urinary excretion of vanilmandelic acid. Cancer [Case Reports Review] 1966;19(2):196–206.
17. Cutler LS, Chaudhry AP, Topazian R. Melanotic neuroectodermal tumor of infancy: an ultrastructural study, literature review, and reevaluation. Cancer [Case Reports Review] 1981;48(2):257–70.
18. Dehner LP, Sibley RK, Sauk JJ Jr, et al. Malignant melanotic neuroectodermal tumor of infancy: a clinical, pathologic, ultrastructural and tissue culture study. Cancer [Case Reports Research Support, U.S. Gov't, P.H.S. Review] 1979;43(4):1389–410.
19. Dooling EC, Chi JG, Gilles FH. Melanotic neuroectodermal tumor of infancy: its histological similarities to fetal pineal gland. Cancer [Case Reports Comparative Study Research Support, U.S. Gov't, P.H.S.] 1977;39(4):1535–41.
20. Duckworth R, Seward GR. A melanotic ameloblastic odontoma. Oral Surg Oral Med Oral Pathol 1965;19:73–85.
21. Eaton WL, Ferguson JP. A retinoblastic teratoma of the epididymis; case report. Cancer [Case Reports] 1956;9(4):718–20.
22. Frank GL, Koten JW. Melanotic hamartoma ("retinal anlage tumour") of the epididymis. J Pathol Bacteriol 1967;93(2):549–54.
23. Hayward AF, Fickling BW, Lucas RB. An electron microscope study of a pigmented tumour of the jaw of infants. Br J Cancer 1969;23(4): 702–8.
24. Johnson RE, Scheithauer BW, Dahlin DC. Melanotic neuroectodermal tumor of infancy. A review of seven cases. Cancer 1983;52(4):661–6.
25. Kapadia SB, Frisman DM, Hitchcock CL, et al. Melanotic neuroectodermal tumor of infancy. Clinicopathological, immunohistochemical, and flow cytometric study. Am J Surg Pathol 1993;17(6):566–73.
26. Koudstaal J, Oldhoff J, Panders AK, et al. Melanotic neuroectodermal tumor of infancy. Cancer 1968;22(1):151–61.

27. Lee SC, Henry MM, Gonzalez-Crussi F. Simultaneous occurrence of melanotic neuroectodermal tumor and brain heterotopia in the oropharynx. Cancer [Case Reports] 1976;38(1):249–53.
28. Lindahl F. Malignant melanotic progonoma. One case. Acta Pathol Microbiol Scand A 1970;78(5):532–6.
29. Lurie HI, Isaacson C. A melanotic progonoma in the scapula region. Cancer [Case Reports] 1961;14:1088–9.
30. Lurie HI. Congenital melanocarcinoma, melanotic adamantinoma, retinal anlage tumor, progonoma, and pigmented epulis of infancy. Summary and review of the literature and report of the first case in an adult. Cancer 1961;14:1090–108.
31. Misugi K, Okajima H, Newton WA Jr, et al. Mediastinal origin of a melanotic progonoma or retinal anlage tumor: ultrastructural evidence for neural crest origin. Cancer 1965;18:477–84.
32. Navas Palacios JJ. Malignant melanotic neuroectodermal tumor: light and electron microscopic study. Cancer Chemother Rep 1980;46: 529.
33. Pettinato G, Manivel C, d'Amore ES, et al. Melanotic neuroectodermal tumor of infancy: an immunohistochemical study. Histopathology 1988;12:425.
34. Schulz DM. A malignant, melanotic neoplasm of the uterus, resembling the retinal anlage tumors; report of a case. Am J Clin Pathol [Case Reports] 1957;28(5):524–32.
35. Stirling RW, Powell G, Fletcher CD. Pigmented neuroectodermal tumour of infancy: an immunohistochemical study. Histopathology 1988;12(4):425–35.
36. Stowens D, Lin TH. Melanotic progonoma of the brain. Hum Pathol [Case Reports] 1974;5(1):105–13.
37. Williams AO. Melanotic ameloblastoma ("progonoma") of infancy showing osteogenesis. J Pathol Bacteriol [Case Reports] 1967;93(2): 545–8.
38. Zone RM. Retinal anlage tumor of the epididymis: a case report. J Urol [Case Reports] 1970;103(1):106–7.
39. Rekhi B, Suryavanshi P, Desai S, et al. Melanotic neuroectodermal tumor of infancy in thigh of an infant–a rare case report with diagnostic implications. Skeletal Radiol 2011;40(8):1079–84.
40. Enzinger FM. Clear-cell sarcoma of tendons and aponeuroses. An analysis of 21 cases. Cancer 1965;18:1163–74.
41. Bridge JA, Borek DA, Neff JR, et al. Chromosomal abnormalities in clear cell sarcoma. Implications for histogenesis. Am J Clin Pathol 1990;93(1): 26–31.
42. Bridge JA, Sreekantaiah C, Neff JR, et al. Cytogenetic findings in clear cell sarcoma of tendons and aponeuroses. Malignant melanoma of soft parts. Cancer Genet Cytogenet 1991;52(1):101–6.
43. Reeves BR, Fletcher CD, Gusterson BA. Translocation t(12;22)(q13;q13) is a nonrandom rearrangement in clear cell sarcoma. Cancer Genet Cytogenet 1992;64(2):101–3.
44. Rodriguez E, Sreekantaiah C, Reuter VE, et al. t(12;22)(q13;q13) and trisomy 8 are nonrandom aberrations in clear-cell sarcoma. Cancer Genet Cytogenet [Case Reports] 1992;64(2):107–10.
45. Stenman G, Kindblom LG, Angervall L. Reciprocal translocation t(12;22)(q13;q13) in clear-cell sarcoma of tendons and aponeuroses. Genes Chromosomes Cancer 1992;4(2):122–7.
46. Mrozek K, Karakousis CP, Perez-Mesa C, et al. Translocation t(12;22) (q13;q12.2-12.3) in a clear cell sarcoma of tendons and aponeuroses. Genes Chromosomes Cancer [Case Reports Research Support, U.S. Gov't, P.H.S. Review] 1993;6(4):249–52.
47. Travis JA, Bridge JA. Significance of both numerical and structural chromosomal abnormalities in clear cell sarcoma. Cancer Genet Cytogenet [Case Reports] 1992;64(2):104–6.
48. Zucman J, Delattre O, Desmaze C, et al. EWS and ATF-1 gene fusion induced by t(12;22) translocation in malignant melanoma of soft parts. Nat Genet [Research Support, Non-U.S. Gov't] 1993;4(4):341–5.
49. Panagopoulos I, Mertens F, Isaksson M, et al. Absence of mutations of the BRAF gene in malignant melanoma of soft parts (clear cell sarcoma of tendons and aponeuroses). Cancer Genet Cytogenet 2005;156(1): 74–6.
50. Davis IJ, Kim JJ, Ozsolak F, et al. Oncogenic MITF dysregulation in clear cell sarcoma: defining the MiT family of human cancers. Cancer Cell 2006;9(6):473–84.
51. Jishage M, Fujino T, Yamazaki Y, et al. Identification of target genes for EWS/ATF-1 chimeric transcription factor. Oncogene [Research Support, Non-U.S. Gov't] 2003;22(1):41–9.
52. Lucas DR, Nascimento AG, Sim FH. Clear cell sarcoma of soft tissues. Mayo Clinic experience with 35 cases. Am J Surg Pathol 1992;16(12): 1197–204.
53. Montgomery EA, Meis JM, Ramos AG, et al. Clear cell sarcoma of tendons and aponeurosis: a clinicopathologic study of 58 cases with analysis of prognostic factors. Int J Surg Pathol 1993;1:59.
54. Ferrari A, Casanova M, Bisogno G, et al. Clear cell sarcoma of tendons and aponeuroses in pediatric patients: a report from the Italian and German Soft Tissue Sarcoma Cooperative Group. Cancer 2002;94(12): 3269–76.
55. Sara AS, Evans HL, Benjamin RS. Malignant melanoma of soft parts (clear cell sarcoma). A study of 17 cases, with emphasis on prognostic factors. Cancer 1990;65(2):367–74.
56. Kindblom LG, Lodding P, Angervall L. Clear-cell sarcoma of tendons and aponeuroses. An immunohistochemical and electron microscopic analysis indicating neural crest origin. Virchows Arch A Pathol Anat Histopathol 1983;401(1):109–28.
57. Mechtersheimer G, Tilgen W, Klar E, et al. Clear cell sarcoma of tendons and aponeuroses: case presentation with special reference to immunohistochemical findings. Hum Pathol [Case Reports Research Support, Non-U.S. Gov't] 1989;20(9):914–17.
58. Swanson PE, Wick MR. Clear cell sarcoma. An immunohistochemical analysis of six cases and comparison with other epithelioid neoplasms of soft tissue. Arch Pathol Lab Med 1989;113(1):55–60.
59. Kubo T. Clear-cell sarcoma of patellar tendon studied by electron microscopy. Cancer 1969;24(5):948–53.
60. Benson JD, Kraemer BB, Mackay B. Malignant melanoma of soft parts: an ultrastructural study of four cases. Ultrastruct Pathol 1985;8(1): 57–70.
61. Deyrup AT, Althof P, Zhou M, et al. Paraganglioma-like dermal melanocytic tumor: a unique entity distinct from cellular blue nevus, clear cell sarcoma, and cutaneous melanoma. Am J Surg Pathol 2004;28(12): 1579–86.
62. Chung EB, Enzinger FM. Malignant melanoma of soft parts. A reassessment of clear cell sarcoma. Am J Surg Pathol 1983;7(5):405–13.
63. Picciotto F, Zaccagna A, Derosa G, et al. Clear cell sarcoma (malignant melanoma of soft parts) and sentinel lymph node biopsy. Eur J Dermatol [Case Reports] 2005;15(1):46–8.
64. Zambrano E, Reyes-Mugica M, Franchi A, et al. An osteoclast-rich tumor of the gastrointestinal tract with features resembling clear cell sarcoma of soft parts: reports of 6 cases of a GIST simulator. Int J Surg Pathol 2003;11(2):75–81.
65. Stockman DL, Miettinen M, Suster S, et al. Malignant gastrointestinal neuroectodermal tumor: clinicopathologic, immunohistochemical, ultrastructural, and molecular analysis of 16 cases with a reappraisal of clear cell sarcoma-like tumors of the gastrointestinal tract. Am J Surg Pathol 2012;36(6):857–68.
66. Ekfors TO, Kujari H, Isomaki M. Clear cell sarcoma of tendons and aponeuroses (malignant melanoma of soft parts) in the duodenum: the first visceral case. Histopathology 1993;22(3):255–9.
67. Donner LR, Trompler RA, Dobin S. Clear cell sarcoma of the ileum: the crucial role of cytogenetics for the diagnosis. Am J Surg Pathol 1998;22(1):121–4.
68. Pauwels P, Debiec-Rychter M, Sciot R, et al. Clear cell sarcoma of the stomach. Histopathology 2002;41(6):526–30.
69. Covinsky M, Gong S, Rajaram V, et al. EWS-ATF1 fusion transcripts in gastrointestinal tumors previously diagnosed as malignant melanoma. Hum Pathol 2005;36(1):74–81.
70. Fukuda T, Kakihara T, Baba K, et al. Clear cell sarcoma arising in the transverse colon. Pathol Int 2000;50(5):412–16.
71. Huang W, Zhang X, Li D, et al. Osteoclast-rich tumor of the gastrointestinal tract with features resembling those of clear cell sarcoma of soft parts. Virchows Arch 2006;448(2):200–3.
72. Abdulkader I, Cameselle-Teijeiro J, de Alava E, et al. Intestinal clear cell sarcoma with melanocytic differentiation and EWS [corrected] rearrangement: report of a case. Int J Surg Pathol 2008;16(2): 189–93.
73. Antonescu CR, Nafa K, Segal NH, et al. EWS-CREB1: a recurrent variant fusion in clear cell sarcoma–association with gastrointestinal location and absence of melanocytic differentiation. Clin Cancer Res 2006; 12(18):5356–62.
74. Alpers CE, Beckstead JH. Malignant neuroendocrine tumor of the jejunum with osteoclast-like giant cells. Enzyme histochemistry distinguishes tumor cells from giant cells. Am J Surg Pathol 1985;9(1): 57–64.
75. Kosemehmetoglu K, Folpe AL. Clear cell sarcoma of tendons and aponeuroses, and osteoclast-rich tumour of the gastrointestinal tract with features resembling clear cell sarcoma of soft parts: a review and update. J Clin Pathol 2010;63(5):416–23.

76. Antonescu CR, Dal Cin P, Nafa K, et al. EWSR1-CREB1 is the predominant gene fusion in angiomatoid fibrous histiocytoma. Genes Chromosomes Cancer 2007;46(12):1051–60.
77. Rossi S, Szuhai K, Ijszenga M, et al. EWSR1-CREB1 and EWSR1-ATF1 fusion genes in angiomatoid fibrous histiocytoma. Clin Cancer Res 2007;13(24):7322–8.
78. Antonescu CR, Katabi N, Zhang L, et al. EWSR1-ATF1 fusion is a novel and consistent finding in hyalinizing clear-cell carcinoma of salivary gland. Genes Chromosomes Cancer 2011;50(7):559–70.
79. Miettinen M, Wang ZF, Lasota J. DOG1 antibody in the differential diagnosis of gastrointestinal stromal tumors: a study of 1840 cases. Am J Surg Pathol 2009;33(9):1401–8.
80. Motegi A, Sakurai S, Nakayama H, et al. PKC theta, a novel immunohistochemical marker for gastrointestinal stromal tumors (GIST), especially useful for identifying KIT-negative tumors. Pathol Int 2005; 55(3):106–12.
81. Fletcher CD, Berman JJ, Corless C, et al. Diagnosis of gastrointestinal stromal tumors: a consensus approach. Hum Pathol 2002;33(5): 459–65.
82. Tazelaar HD, Batts KP, Srigley JR. Primary extrapulmonary sugar tumor (PEST): a report of four cases. Mod Pathol 2001;14(6):615–22.
83. Folpe AL, Goodman ZD, Ishak KG, et al. Clear cell myomelanocytic tumor of the falciform ligament/ligamentum teres: a novel member of the perivascular epithelioid clear cell family of tumors with a predilection for children and young adults. Am J Surg Pathol 2000;24(9): 1239–46.
84. Bonetti F, Martignoni G, Colato C, et al. Abdominopelvic sarcoma of perivascular epithelioid cells. Report of four cases in young women, one with tuberous sclerosis. Mod Pathol 2001;14(6):563–8.
85. Eble JN. Angiomyolipoma of kidney. Semin Diagn Pathol 1998;15(1): 21–40.
86. Frack MD, Simon L, Dawson BH. The lymphangiomyomatosis syndrome. Cancer 1968;22(2):428–37.
87. Liebow AA, Castleman B. Benign clear cell ("sugar") tumors of the lung. Yale J Biol Med 1971;43(4):213–22.
88. Valensi QJ. Pulmonary lymphangiomyoma, a probable forme frust of tuberous sclerosis. A case report and survey of the literature. Am Rev Respir Dis 1973;108(6):1411–15.
89. Monteforte WJ Jr, Kohnen PW. Angiomyolipomas in a case of lymphangiomyomatosis syndrome: relationships to tuberous sclerosis. Cancer 1974;34(2):317–21.
90. Pea M, Bonetti F, Zamboni G, et al. Melanocyte-marker-HMB-45 is regularly expressed in angiomyolipoma of the kidney. Pathology 1991;23(3):185–8.
91. Weeks DA, Malott RL, Arnesen M, et al. Hepatic angiomyolipoma with striated granules and positivity with melanoma–specific antibody (HMB-45): a report of two cases. Ultrastruct Pathol 1991;15(4-5): 563–71.
92. Gaffey MJ, Mills SE, Askin FB, et al. Clear cell tumor of the lung. A clinicopathologic, immunohistochemical, and ultrastructural study of eight cases. Am J Surg Pathol 1990;14(3):248–59.
93. Chan JK, Tsang WY, Pau MY, et al. Lymphangiomyomatosis and angiomyolipoma: closely related entities characterized by hamartomatous proliferation of HMB-45-positive smooth muscle [see comments]. Histopathology 1993;22(5):445–55.
94. Zamboni G, Pea M, Martignoni G, et al. Clear cell "sugar" tumor of the pancreas. A novel member of the family of lesions characterized by the presence of perivascular epithelioid cells. Am J Surg Pathol 1996;20(6): 722–30.
95. Unlu C, Lamme B, Nass P, et al. Retroperitoneal haemorrhage caused by a renal angiomyolipoma. Emerg Med J [Case Reports] 2006;23(6): 464–5.
96. Springer AM, Saxena AK, Willital GH. Angiomyolipoma with hypertension mimicking a malignant renal tumor. Pediatr Surg Int [Case Reports] 2002;18(5-6):526–8.
97. Majid S, White D, Sarkar S. An unusual cause for the incidental finding of multiple liver lesions. Diagnosis: multiple fatty vascular lesions of angiomyolipomas. Gut [Case Reports] 2006;55(7):983, 1029.
98. Xu AM, Zhang SH, Zheng JM, et al. Pathological and molecular analysis of sporadic hepatic angiomyolipoma. Hum Pathol [Comparative Study] 2006;37(6):735–41.
99. Erkilic S, Kocer NE, Mumbuc S, et al. Nasal angiomyolipoma. Acta Otolaryngol [Case Reports] 2005;125(4):446–8.
100. Piattelli A, Fioroni M, Rubini C, et al. Angiomyolipoma of the palate. Report of a case. Oral Oncol [Case Reports Research Support, Non-U.S. Gov't Review] 2001;37(3):323–5.
101. Sharara AI, Tawil A. Angiomyolipoma of the colon. Clinical gastroenterology and hepatology: the official clinical practice journal of the American Gastroenterological Association [Case Reports] 2005;3(9): A35.
102. Kasuno K, Ueda S, Tanaka A, et al. Pulmonary angiomyolipoma recurring 26 years after nephrectomy for angiomyolipoma: benign clinical course. Clin Nephrol [Case Reports] 2004;62(6):469–72.
103. Tsuruta D, Maekawa N, Ishii M. Cutaneous angiomyolipoma. Dermatology [Case Reports Letter] 2004;208(3):231–2.
104. Patel U, Simpson E, Kingswood JC, et al. Tuberose sclerosis complex: analysis of growth rates aids differentiation of renal cell carcinoma from atypical or minimal-fat-containing angiomyolipoma. Clin Radiol 2005;60(6):665–73; discussion 3–4.
105. Henske EP. Tuberous sclerosis and the kidney: from mesenchyme to epithelium, and beyond. Pediatr Nephrol [Research Support, N.I.H., Extramural Research Support, Non-U.S. Gov't Research Support, U.S. Gov't, P.H.S. Review] 2005;20(7):854–7.
106. De Pauw RA, Boelaert JR, Haenebalcke CW, et al. Renal angiomyolipoma in association with pulmonary lymphangioleiomyomatosis. Am J Kidney Dis [Case Reports Review] 2003;41(4):877–83.
107. Cohen MM, Pollock-BarZiv S, Johnson SR. Emerging clinical picture of lymphangioleiomyomatosis. Thorax [Research Support, Non-U.S. Gov't] 2005;60(10):875–9.
108. Jimenez RE, Eble JN, Reuter VE, et al. Concurrent angiomyolipoma and renal cell neoplasia: a study of 36 cases. Mod Pathol 2001;14(3): 157–63.
109. Israel GM, Hindman N, Hecht E, et al. The use of opposed-phase chemical shift MRI in the diagnosis of renal angiomyolipomas. AJR Am J Roentgenol 2005;184(6):1868–72.
110. Coumbaras M, Dahan H, Strauss C, et al. [Renal angiomyolipoma complicated by extension to the renal vein and inferior vena cava]. J Radiol [Case Reports Review] 2006;87(5):572–4.
111. Gogus C, Safak M, Erekul S, et al. Angiomyolipoma of the kidney with lymph node involvement in a 17-year old female mimicking renal cell carcinoma: a case report. Int Urol Nephrol [Case Reports] 2001;33(4):617–18.
112. Karbowniczek M, Yu J, Henske EP. Renal angiomyolipomas from patients with sporadic lymphangiomyomatosis contain both neoplastic and non-neoplastic vascular structures. Am J Pathol 2003;162(2): 491–500.
113. Eble JN, Amin MB, Young RH. Epithelioid angiomyolipoma of the kidney: a report of five cases with a prominent and diagnostically confusing epithelioid smooth muscle component. Am J Surg Pathol 1997;21(10):1123–30.
114. Belanger EC, Dhamanaskar PK, Mai KT. Epithelioid angiomyolipoma of the kidney mimicking renal sarcoma. Histopathology [Letter] 2005;47(4):433–5.
115. Mai KT, Perkins DG, Collins JP. Epithelioid cell variant of renal angiomyolipoma. Histopathology [Case Reports] 1996;28(3):277–80.
116. Davis CJ, Barton JH, Sesterhenn IA. Cystic angiomyolipoma of the kidney: a clinicopathologic description of 11 cases. Mod Pathol 2006;19(5):669–74.
117. Makhlouf HR, Ishak KG, Shekar R, et al. Melanoma markers in angiomyolipoma of the liver and kidney: a comparative study. Arch Pathol Lab Med [Comparative Study] 2002;126(1):49–55.
118. Jungbluth AA, King R, Fisher DE, et al. Immunohistochemical and reverse transcription-polymerase chain reaction expression analysis of tyrosinase and microphthalmia-associated transcription factor in angiomyolipomas. Appl Immunohistochem Mol Morphol 2001;9(1): 29–34.
119. Zavala-Pompa A, Folpe AL, Jimenez RE, et al. Immunohistochemical study of microphthalmia transcription factor and tyrosinase in angiomyolipoma of the kidney, renal cell carcinoma, and renal and retroperitoneal sarcomas: comparative evaluation with traditional diagnostic markers. Am J Surg Pathol 2001;25(1):65–70.
120. Henske EP, Ao X, Short MP, et al. Frequent progesterone receptor immunoreactivity in tuberous sclerosis-associated renal angiomyolipomas. Mod Pathol 1998;11(7):665–8.
121. Colombat M, Boccon-Gibod L, Carton S. An unusual renal angiomyolipoma with morphological lymphangioleiomyomatosis features and coexpression of oestrogen and progesterone receptors. Virchows Arch [Case Reports] 2002;440(1):102–4.
122. Logginidou H, Ao X, Russo I, et al. Frequent estrogen and progesterone receptor immunoreactivity in renal angiomyolipomas from women with pulmonary lymphangioleiomyomatosis. Chest 2000;117 (1):25–30.

123. Wullich B, Henn W, Siemer S, et al. Clonal chromosome aberrations in three of five sporadic angiomyolipomas of the kidney. Cancer Genet Cytogenet 1997;96(1):42–5.
124. Dal Cin P, Sciot R, Van Poppel H, et al. Chromosome analysis in angiomyolipoma. Cancer Genet Cytogenet 1997;99(2):132–4.
125. El-Hashemite N, Zhang H, Henske EP, et al. Mutation in TSC2 and activation of mammalian target of rapamycin signalling pathway in renal angiomyolipoma. Lancet [Research Support, Non-U.S. Gov't Research Support, U.S. Gov't, P.H.S.] 2003;361(9366):1348–9.
126. Plank TL, Logginidou H, Klein-Szanto A, et al. The expression of hamartin, the product of the TSC1 gene, in normal human tissues and in TSC1- and TSC2-linked angiomyolipomas. Mod Pathol 1999;12(5): 539–45.
127. Folpe AL, Kwiatkowski DJ. Perivascular epithelioid cell neoplasms: pathology and pathogenesis. Hum Pathol 2010;41(1):1–15.
128. Brecher ME, Gill WB, Straus FH 2nd. Angiomyolipoma with regional lymph node involvement and long-term follow-up study. Hum Pathol [Case Reports] 1986;17(9):962–3.
129. Ferry JA, Malt RA, Young RH. Renal angiomyolipoma with sarcomatous transformation and pulmonary metastases. Am J Surg Pathol 1991; 15(11):1083–8.
130. Cibas ES, Goss GA, Kulke MH, et al. Malignant epithelioid angiomyolipoma ('sarcoma ex angiomyolipoma') of the kidney: a case report and review of the literature. Am J Surg Pathol [Case Reports Review] 2001;25(1):121–6.
131. Hornick JL, Fletcher CD. PEComa: what do we know so far? Histopathology 2006;48(1):75–82.
132. Pea M, Bonetti F, Martignoni G, et al. Apparent renal cell carcinomas in tuberous sclerosis are heterogeneous: the identification of malignant epithelioid angiomyolipoma. Am J Surg Pathol 1998;22(2): 180–7.
133. Martignoni G, Pea M, Bonetti F, et al. Carcinomalike monotypic epithelioid angiomyolipoma in patients without evidence of tuberous sclerosis: a clinicopathologic and genetic study. Am J Surg Pathol 1998;22(6): 663–72.
134. Christiano AP, Yang X, Gerber GS. Malignant transformation of renal angiomyolipoma. J Urol [Case Reports] 1999;161(6):1900–1.
135. Lowe BA, Brewer J, Houghton DC, et al. Malignant transformation of angiomyolipoma. J Urol [Case Reports] 1992;147(5):1356–8.
136. Yamamoto T, Ito K, Suzuki K, et al. Rapidly progressive malignant epithelioid angiomyolipoma of the kidney. J Urol [Case Reports] 2002; 168(1):190–1.
137. Warakaulle DR, Phillips RR, Turner GD, et al. Malignant monotypic epithelioid angiomyolipoma of the kidney. Clin Radiol [Case Reports] 2004;59(9):849–52.
138. L'Hostis H, Deminiere C, Ferriere JM, et al. Renal angiomyolipoma: a clinicopathologic, immunohistochemical, and follow-up study of 46 cases. Am J Surg Pathol 1999;23(9):1011–20.
139. Nese N, Martignoni G, Fletcher CD, et al. Pure epithelioid PEComas (so-called epithelioid angiomyolipoma) of the kidney: a clinicopathologic study of 41 cases: detailed assessment of morphology and risk stratification. Am J Surg Pathol 2011;35(2):161–76.
140. Dalle I, Sciot R, de Vos R, et al. Malignant angiomyolipoma of the liver: a hitherto unreported variant. Histopathology [Case Reports] 2000;36(5):443–50.
141. Silverman SG, Tuncali K, vanSonnenberg E, et al. Renal tumors: MR imaging-guided percutaneous cryotherapy–initial experience in 23 patients. Radiology [Research Support, Non-U.S. Gov't] 2005;236(2): 716–24.
142. Bonetti F, Pea M, Martignoni G, et al. Clear cell ("sugar") tumor of the lung is a lesion strictly related to angiomyolipoma–the concept of a family of lesions characterized by the presence of the perivascular epithelioid cells (PEC). Pathology 1994;26(3):230–6.
143. Bonetti F, Pea M, Martignoni G, et al. Cellular heterogeneity in lymphangiomyomatosis of the lung. Hum Pathol 1992;22:727.
144. Taylor JR, Ryu J, Colby TV, et al. Lymphangioleiomyomatosis. Clinical course in 32 patients. N Engl J Med 1990;323(18):1254–60.
145. Carsillo T, Astrinidis A, Henske EP. Mutations in the tuberous sclerosis complex gene TSC2 are a cause of sporadic pulmonary lymphangioleiomyomatosis. Proc Natl Acad Sci U S A 2000;97(11):6085–90.
146. Strizheva GD, Carsillo T, Kruger WD, et al. The spectrum of mutations in TSC1 and TSC2 in women with tuberous sclerosis and lymphangiomyomatosis. Am J Respir Crit Care Med 2001;163(1):253–8.
147. Schiavina M, Di Scioscio V, Contini P, et al. Pulmonary lymphangioleiomyomatosis in a karyotypically normal man without tuberous sclerosis complex. Am J Respir Crit Care Med 2007;176(1):96–8.
148. Cornog JL Jr, Enterline HT. Lymphangiomyoma, a benign lesion of chyliferous lymphatics synonymous with lymphangiopericytoma. Cancer 1966;19(12):1909–30.
149. Corrin B, Liebow AA, Friedman PJ. Pulmonary lymphangiomyomatosis. A review. Am J Pathol 1975;79(2):348–82.
150. Enterline HT, Roberts B. Lymphangiopericytoma; case report of a previously undescribed tumor type. Cancer 1955;8(3):582–7.
151. Wolff M. Lymphangiomyoma: clinicopathologic study and ultrastructural confirmation of its histogenesis. Cancer 1973;31(4):988–1007.
152. Colley MH, Geppert E, Franklin WA. Immunohistochemical detection of steroid receptors in a case of pulmonary lymphangioleiomyomatosis. Am J Surg Pathol [Case Reports] 1989;13(9):803–7.
153. Brentani MM, Carvalho CR, Saldiva PH, et al. Steroid receptors in pulmonary lymphangiomyomatosis. Chest [Case Reports] 1984;85(1): 96–9.
154. McCarty KS Jr, Mossler JA, McLelland R, et al. Pulmonary lymphangiomyomatosis responsive to progesterone. N Engl J Med [Research Support, U.S. Gov't, P.H.S.] 1980;303(25):1461–5.
155. Tomasian A, Greenberg MS, Rumerman H. Tamoxifen for lymphangioleiomyomatosis. N Engl J Med [Case Reports Letter] 1982;306(12): 745–6.
156. Ohori NP, Yousem SA, Sonmez-Alpan E, et al. Estrogen and progesterone receptors in lymphangioleiomyomatosis, epithelioid hemangioendothelioma, and sclerosing hemangioma of the lung. Am J Clin Pathol [Research Support, Non-U.S. Gov't] 1991;96(4):529–35.
157. Bittmann I, Rolf B, Amann G, et al. Recurrence of lymphangioleiomyomatosis after single lung transplantation: new insights into pathogenesis. Hum Pathol [Case Reports] 2003;34(1):95–8.
158. Karbowniczek M, Astrinidis A, Balsara BR, et al. Recurrent lymphangiomyomatosis after transplantation: genetic analyses reveal a metastatic mechanism. Am J Respir Crit Care Med 2003;167(7):976–82.
159. Yu JJ, Robb VA, Morrison TA, et al. Estrogen promotes the survival and pulmonary metastasis of tuberin-null cells. Proc Natl Acad Sci U S A 2009;106(8):2635–40.
160. Folpe AL, Mentzel T, Lehr HA, et al. Perivascular epithelioid cell neoplasms of soft tissue and gynecologic origin: a clinicopathologic study of 26 cases and review of the literature. Am J Surg Pathol 2005; 29(12):1558–75.
161. Vang R, Kempson RL. Perivascular epithelioid cell tumor ('PEComa') of the uterus: a subset of HMB-45-positive epithelioid mesenchymal neoplasms with an uncertain relationship to pure smooth muscle tumors. Am J Surg Pathol 2002;26(1):1–13.
162. Bosincu L, Rocca PC, Martignoni G, et al. Perivascular epithelioid cell (PEC) tumors of the uterus: a clinicopathologic study of two cases with aggressive features. Mod Pathol [Case Reports Research Support, Non-U.S. Gov't] 2005;18(10):1336–42.
163. Mentzel T, Reibhauer S, Rutten A, et al. Cutaneous clear cell myomelanocytic tumor: a new member of the growing family of perivascular epithelioid cell tumors (PEComas). Clinicopathological and immunohistochemical analysis of seven cases. Histopathology 2005;46(5): 498–504.
164. de Saint Aubain Somerhausen N, Gomez Galdon M, Bouffioux B, et al. Clear cell 'sugar' tumor (PEComa) of the skin: a case report. J Cutan Pathol [Case Reports] 2005;32(6):441–4.
165. Pan CC, Yang AH, Chiang H. Malignant perivascular epithelioid cell tumor involving the prostate. Arch Pathol Lab Med 2003;127(2): E96–8.
166. Pan CC, Yu IT, Yang AH, et al. Clear cell myomelanocytic tumor of the urinary bladder. Am J Surg Pathol 2003;27(5):689–92.
167. Yamamoto H, Oda Y, Yao T, et al. Malignant perivascular epithelioid cell tumor of the colon: report of a case with molecular analysis. Pathol Int [Case Reports] 2006;56(1):46–50.
168. Insabato L, De Rosa G, Terracciano LM, et al. Primary monotypic epithelioid angiomyolipoma of bone. Histopathology 2002;40(3):286–90.
169. Hornick JL, Fletcher CD. Sclerosing PEComa: clinicopathologic analysis of a distinctive variant with a predilection for the retroperitoneum. Am J Surg Pathol 2008;32(4):493–501.
170. Pan CC, Jong YJ, Chai CY, et al. Comparative genomic hybridization study of perivascular epithelioid cell tumor: molecular genetic evidence of perivascular epithelioid cell tumor as a distinctive neoplasm. Hum Pathol 2006;37(5):606–12.
171. Tanaka M, Kato K, Gomi K, et al. Perivascular epithelioid cell tumor with SFPQ/PSF-TFE3 gene fusion in a patient with advanced neuroblastoma. Am J Surg Pathol 2009;33(9):1416–20.
172. Argani P, Aulmann S, Illei PB, et al. A distinctive subset of PEComas harbors TFE3 gene fusions. Am J Surg Pathol 2010;34(10):1395–406.

173. Dickson BC, Brooks JS, Pasha TL, et al. TFE3 expression in tumors of the microphthalmia-associated transcription factor (MiTF) family. Int J Surg Pathol 2011;19(1):26–30.
174. Kuroda N, Goda M, Kazakov DV, et al. Perivascular epithelioid cell tumor of the nasal cavity with TFE3 expression. Pathol Int 2009;59(10):769–70.
175. Silva EG, Deavers MT, Bodurka DC, et al. Uterine epithelioid leiomyosarcomas with clear cells: reactivity with HMB-45 and the concept of PEComa. Am J Surg Pathol 2004;28(2):244–9.
176. Dimmler A, Seitz G, Hohenberger W, et al. Late pulmonary metastasis in uterine PEComa. J Clin Pathol 2003;56(8):627–8.
177. Greene LA, Mount SL, Schned AR, et al. Recurrent perivascular epithelioid cell tumor of the uterus (PEComa): an immunohistochemical study and review of the literature. Gynecol Oncol 2003;90(3):677–81.
178. Rigby H, Yu W, Schmidt MH, et al. Lack of response of a metastatic renal perivascular epithelial cell tumor (PEComa) to successive courses of DTIC based-therapy and imatinib mesylate. Pediatr Blood Cancer [Case Reports] 2005;45(2):202–6.
179. Dabora SL, Franz DN, Ashwal S, et al. Multicenter phase 2 trial of sirolimus for tuberous sclerosis: kidney angiomyolipomas and other tumors regress and VEGF- D levels decrease. PLoS One 2011;6(9):e23379.
180. Shitara K, Yatabe Y, Mizota A, et al. Dramatic tumor response to everolimus for malignant epithelioid angiomyolipoma. Jpn J Clin Oncol 2011;41(6):814–16.

Cartilaginous and Osseous Soft Tissue Tumors

CHAPTER CONTENTS

Benign extraosseous cartilaginous lesions are uncommon and usually present as tumor-like masses. In the past, the term *soft part* or *extraskeletal chondroma* was used arbitrarily for small, well-defined solitary nodules of hyaline cartilage that are unattached to bone and occur primarily in the distal extremities, especially the fingers and hand. The same designation has been used for the rare chondroma-like lesions that occur in the gastrointestinal and respiratory tracts. These lesions, however, must be distinguished from the cartilaginous rests of branchial origin that are usually found in the soft tissues of the lateral neck in infants and small children and from the metaplastic cartilage encountered in some benign lipomatous (chondroid lipoma) and fibromatous (calcifying aponeurotic fibroma) neoplasms; they must also be distinguished from multiple cartilaginous nodules in the synovium (synovial chondromatosis) and from the cartilage in myositis ossificans and its variants.

Chondrosarcomas also occur as primary soft tissue neoplasms, but they are much less common than primary chondrosarcomas of bone and are of two types: *extraskeletal myxoid chondrosarcoma* and *mesenchymal chondrosarcoma*. Extraskeletal myxoid chondrosarcoma will not be discussed in this chapter because there is actually little evidence for true chondroid differentiation in this tumor. Rather, this entity will be fully discussed in Chapter 33 as one of the translocation-associated sarcomas.

Well-differentiated extraosseous chondrosarcomas resembling hyaline cartilage are rare. In fact, if this tumor is encountered in soft tissue, it is more likely an extension or metastasis of a bone tumor than a primary soft tissue neoplasm. Well-differentiated chondrosarcomas do arise from the synovium (sometimes secondary to synovial chondromatosis) and from the periosteum (periosteal chondrosarcoma). They also appear following radiation therapy or injection of radioactive material, usually after a latent period of many years. Rare examples of chondrosarcoma also occur in parenchymal organs. In some locations (e.g., bladder), they usually represent part of a carcinosarcoma.

This chapter will also address soft tissue lesions with osseous differentiation, including (1) myositis ossificans and related non-neoplastic, heterotopic ossifications; (2) fibrodysplasia (myositis) ossificans progressiva (FOP); and (3) extraskeletal osteosarcoma.

Myositis ossificans, by far the most common of the lesions, is a localized, self-limiting ossifying process that follows mechanical trauma, in most cases. Identical lesions also occur in persons with no apparent history of preceding injury, and, in some of these cases, an infectious process has been suggested as a possible cause or initiating factor. Although most of these lesions originate in muscle tissue, morphologically similar proliferations also arise in the subcutis, tendons, fasciae, and periosteum. Depending on their location, these heterotopic ossifications have been variously classified as *panniculitis ossificans*, *fasciitis ossificans*, *florid reactive periostitis*, and *fibro-osseous pseudotumor of digits*.

Not further discussed in the chapter are other rare heterotopic ossifications that occur after various kinds of soft tissue injury. These lesions have been described in surgical scars, particularly those of the abdomen,[1,2] in burns[3] and in association with dislocations of the elbow and other joints, and total hip arthroplasty,[4] among others. Repeated minor soft tissue trauma is also the cause of the drill bone or shooter bone in the deltoid and pectoralis muscles, the rider bone in the adductor muscles of the thigh, and the shoemaker's bone in the rectus muscle of the lower abdominal wall—all lesions that are rarely encountered today but have been repeatedly described in the earlier literature.

In addition to these more deeply seated lesions, localized bone formations in the dermis and subcutis are not particularly rare. They may be solitary or multiple, and they occur spontaneously or in connection with a variety of neoplastic (e.g., linear basal cell nevus, basal cell carcinoma, chondroid syringoma, calcifying epithelioma) and non-neoplastic (e.g., scars, acne, puncture wounds, injections, organizing hematomas, pseudohypoparathyroidism, dermatomyositis) processes. Many of these lesions have been reported as *osteoma cutis*, but they, too, seem to be products of metaplasia rather than neoplasia.[5]

Fibrodysplasia ossificans progressiva (myositis ossificans progressiva) is a heritable disorder in which massive crippling ossification occurs following diffuse fibroblastic proliferation in muscle and associated soft tissues, especially those of the back, shoulder, and neck. The process has its onset during early childhood and follows a relentless clinical course with total disability in its later stages. Microscopically, the early phase of the lesion may be confused with fibromatosis, but this process can be definitively identified radiographically in nearly all cases by the presence of microdactylia and other malformations of the hands and feet.

Extraskeletal osteosarcoma is a highly malignant tumor that afflicts a much older age group than osteosarcoma of bone. Occasionally, it occurs in radiation-damaged tissues. With vanishingly rare exceptions, there is no convincing evidence that it ever occurs as a malignant transformation of heterotopic ossification, including myositis ossificans.[6]

EXTRASKELETAL CHONDROMA (CHONDROMA OF SOFT PARTS)

Extraskeletal chondroma is a benign cartilaginous tumor that occurs predominantly in the hands and feet. Its variable histologic appearance not infrequently leads to a mistaken diagnosis of chondrosarcoma. There are two large series of this entity, including a report of 70 cases from the Mayo Clinic[7] and 104 cases from the files of the Armed Forces Institute of Pathology (commonly recognized as the AFIP).[8]

Clinical Findings

The tumor occurs primarily in the soft tissues of the hands and feet, usually with no connection to the underlying bone. The single most common site is the fingers, where more than 80% are found. Less frequent sites include the hands, toes, feet, and trunk; unusual cases have been described in the dura,[9] auricle,[10] parotid gland,[11] and fallopian tube.[12] Extraskeletal chondroma grows as a slowly enlarging nodule or mass that seldom causes pain or tenderness; the tumor mainly affects adults 30 to 60 years of age and is rare in children.[13] There is a slight male predominance. Nearly all are solitary. Dellon et al.[14] described an unusual and questionable case with bilateral chondromas in the right index and left ring fingers of a patient with renal failure because multiple chondroid lesions are more likely forms of synovial chondromatosis. The association of pulmonary chondroma, gastric epithelioid stromal tumor, and extra-adrenal paraganglioma is known as *Carney triad*.

Radiographically, the lesion is well demarcated and does not involve bone, although some tumors cause compression deformities or bone erosion. Discrete, irregular, ring-like or curvilinear calcifications are often demonstrable (Fig. 30-1).[15]

Pathologic Findings

Chondromas are firm, well-demarcated, oval-round masses. Occasionally, they are soft or friable with focal cystic change. Nearly all are small, seldom exceeding 3 cm in greatest diameter. They may be attached to the tendon or tendon sheath. Microscopically, they vary in appearance. About two-thirds consist of mature hyaline cartilage arranged in distinct lobules with sharp borders (Fig. 30-2). Some are altered by focal fibrosis (*fibrochondroma*) or ossification (*osteochondroma*)[16]; others show myxoid change (*myxochondroma*), sometimes together with focal hemorrhage. About one-third display focal or diffuse calcification, usually a late feature that may completely obscure the cartilaginous nature of the tumor and mimic tumoral calcinosis.[17] The calcified material is granular, floccular, or crystalline and often outlines the contours of the chondrocytes in a lace-like pattern (Figs. 30-3 to 30-5). Calcification tends to be more pronounced in the center than at the periphery of the lobule. It is often accompanied by cellular degeneration and necrosis, which accounts for the softened gross appearance of some of these tumors. Cells with periodic acid-Schiff-positive, diastase-resistant intracytoplasmic hyaline globules, possibly representing a glycoproteinaceous secretory product, may be occasionally encountered.[18]

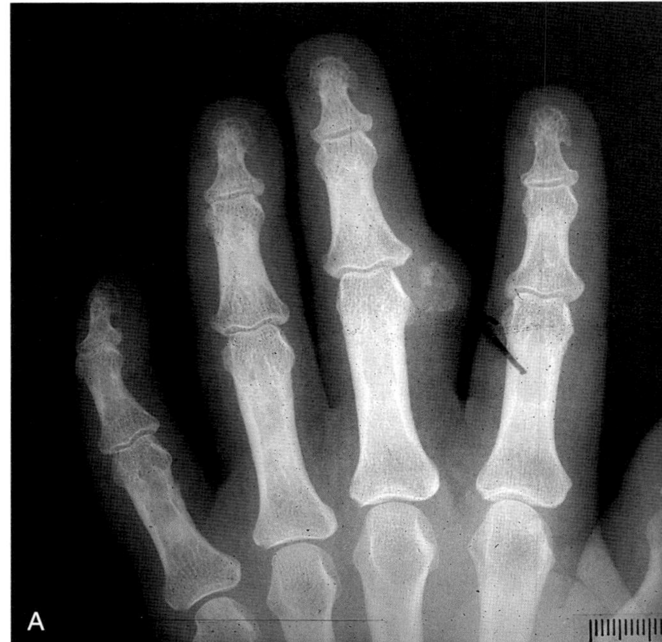

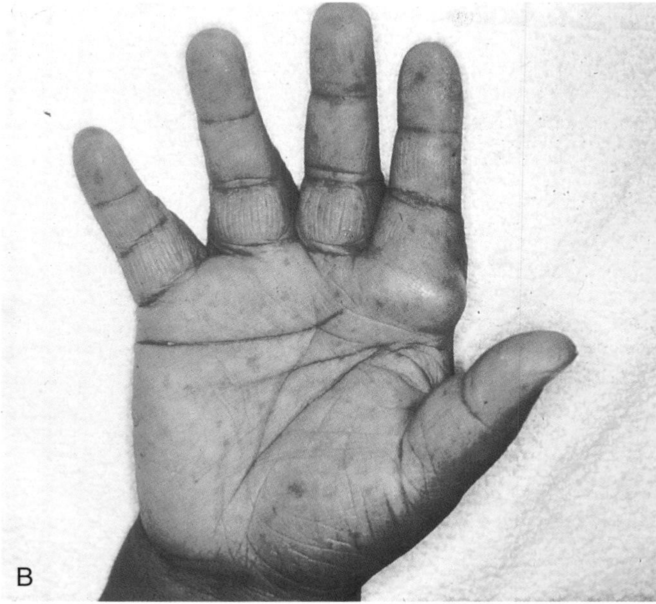

FIGURE 30-1. Chondroma of soft parts. (A) Radiograph of the left third finger showing a small soft tissue mass with foci of calcification. (B) Chondroma of soft parts at the base of the right second finger.

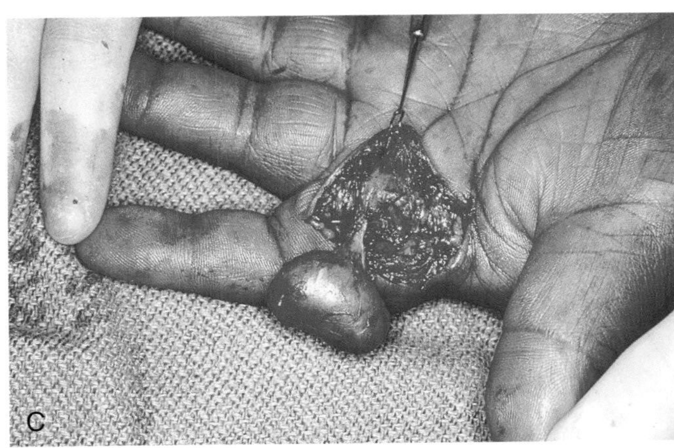

FIGURE 30-1, cont'd. (C) Intraoperative specimen of enucleated chondroma of soft parts.

A striking feature that occurs in about 15% of cases is a granuloma-like proliferation of epithelioid and multinucleated giant cells reminiscent of a fibroxanthoma or a giant cell tumor (Figs. 30-6 and 30-7).[19,20] This proliferation is most conspicuous at the tumor margin and along the interlobular vascular channels. There are also rare extraskeletal chondromas in which the presence of plump immature-appearing cells in a myxoid background simulates a chondrosarcoma. In general, however, these tumors can be recognized as chondromas by the presence of more mature, less cellular cartilaginous areas at the periphery. Other examples, such as the series of eight cases reported by Cates et al.,[21] exhibit features that closely simulate those of chondroblastoma.

Like normal chondrocytes, the cells of the extraskeletal chondroma are positive for S-100 protein. The matrix is rich in types I and III collagen, whereas there seems to be reduced amounts of types II and IV collagen.

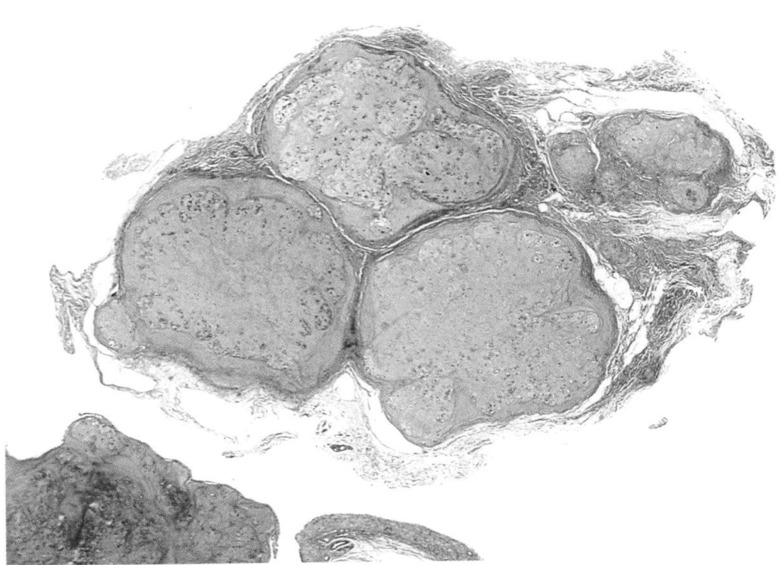

FIGURE 30-2. Cross-section of a chondroma of soft parts showing circumscription and a multinodular growth pattern.

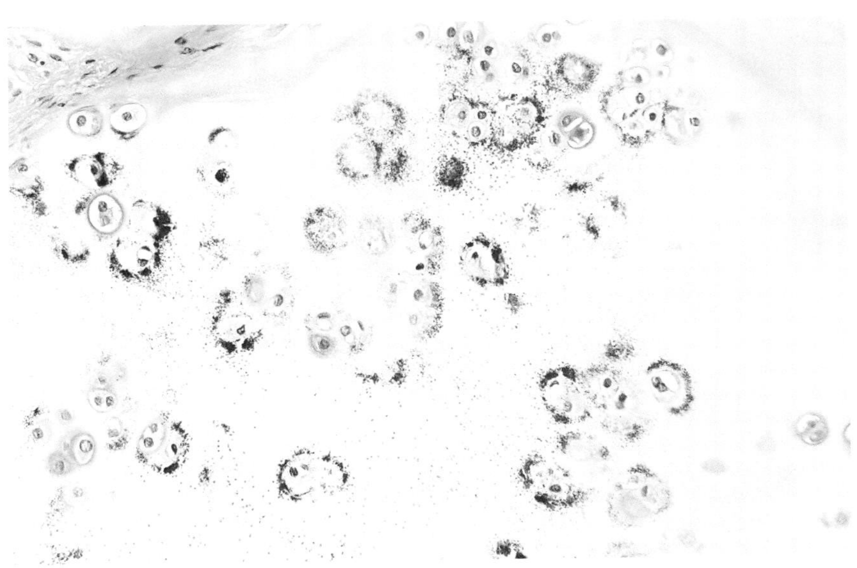

FIGURE 30-3. Chondroma of soft parts consisting of mature hyaline cartilage with nests of benign-appearing cells in lacunae.

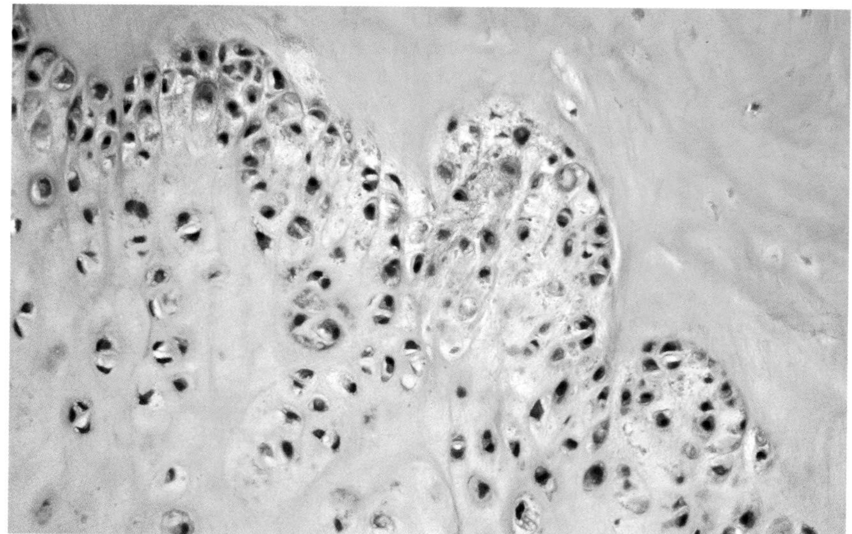

FIGURE 30-4. Chondroma of soft parts with a hypercellular zone at the periphery of a lobule.

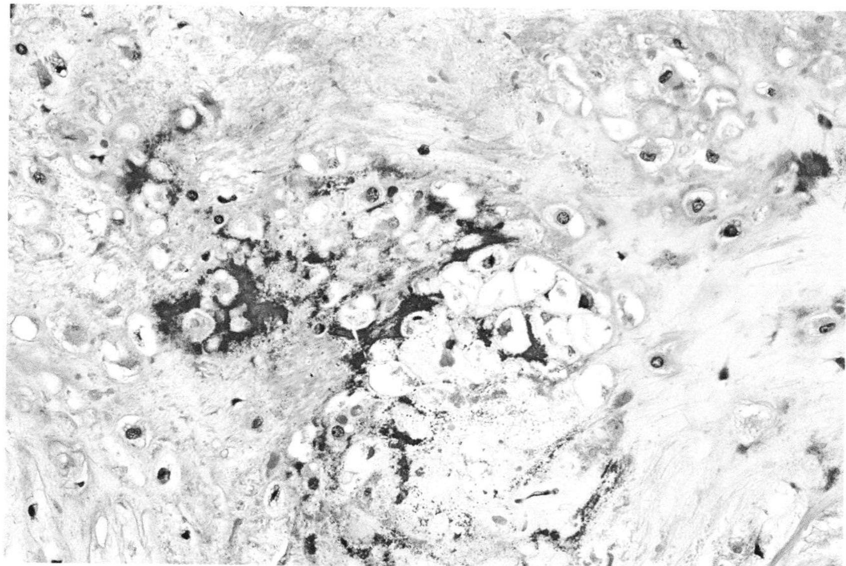

FIGURE 30-5. Calcified chondroma of soft parts. Calcium deposits surround and partly replace the cartilage cells.

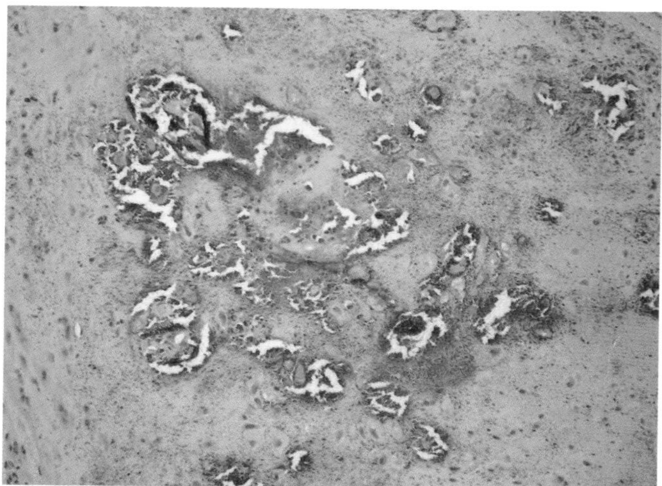

FIGURE 30-6. Calcified chondroma of soft parts. *(Photograph courtesy of Dr. John X. O'Connell.)*

Clonal chromosomal abnormalities have been identified in some extraskeletal chondromas, including monosomy 6, trisomy 5, and rearrangements of chromosome 11.[22-24] Sakai et al.[25] described a rare case of extraskeletal chondroma with three clones, including t(6;12)(q12;p11.2), t(3;7)(q13;p12), and der(2)t(2;18)(p11.2;q11.2).

Differential Diagnosis

Distinction from other benign lesions should not be difficult. *Calcifying aponeurotic fibroma* is characterized by short bar-like foci of cartilaginous metaplasia in a dense, poorly circumscribed fibromatous background. It occurs in the hand rather than in the distal portion of the digits and almost always affects patients younger than 25 years. *Tumoral calcinosis* may mimic a heavily calcified chondroma, but it lacks cartilage and usually shows a distinct histiocytic response to the calcified material. *Giant cell tumor of tendon sheath* has a more uniform

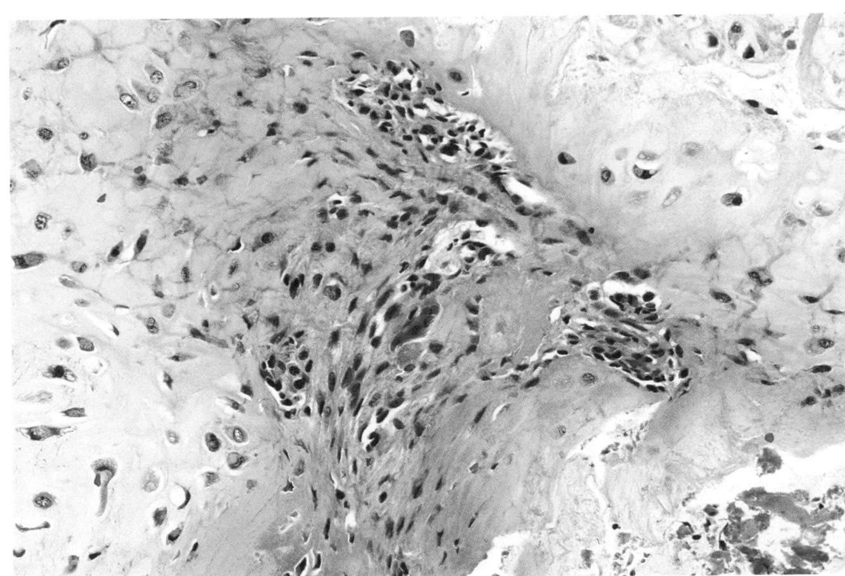

FIGURE 30-7. High-power view of interlobular septa in a chondroma of soft parts. Rare multinucleated giant cells are seen.

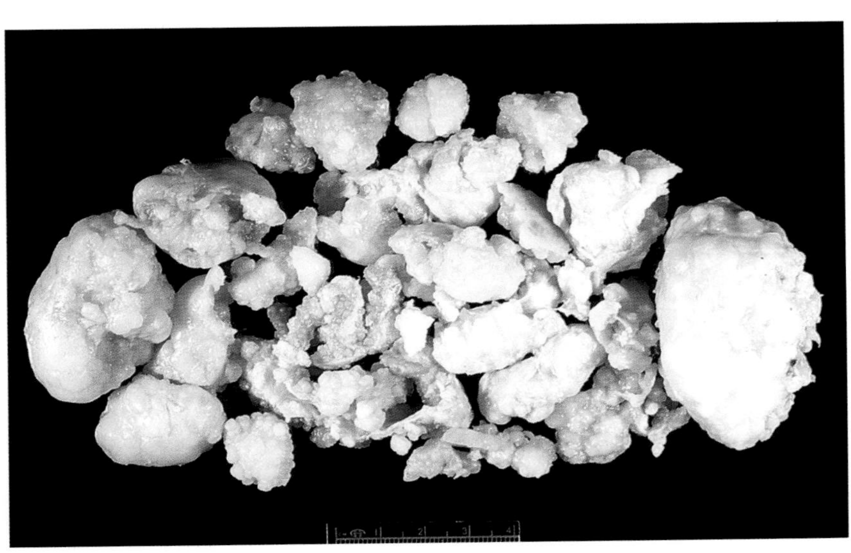

FIGURE 30-8. Conglomerate of variably sized nodules of synovial chondromatosis.

cellular pattern and rarely has metaplastic cartilage or bone. Radiography usually allows distinction from *periosteal* or *juxtacortical chondroma*, a small well-circumscribed tumor located underneath the periosteum that causes erosion of the underlying cortex with ledges or buttresses at the margin of the tumor and from *subungual osteochondroma*, a lesion that has cartilage overlying well-developed bone.

Synovial chondromatosis differs from extraskeletal chondroma by its occurrence in large joints, such as the knee, hip, elbow, or shoulder joint and the formation of numerous, small, metaplastic cartilaginous or osteocartilaginous nodules of varying size attached to the synovial membrane of the joint, tendon sheath, or lining of the adjacent extra-articular bursa (Figs. 30-8 to 30-10).[26] These synovial nodules often become detached and are found as loose bodies in the joint space. Some are hypercellular with clustering of tumor cells and increased mitotic activity. Most become calcified or ossified and can be readily demonstrated by routine radiography as multiple, small, discrete radiopaque bodies (loose bodies or joint mice). *Nonmineralized loose bodies* are demonstrable on arthrograms, CT scans, bone scans, or MRI as multiple filling defects outlined by contrast material.[27] As in extraskeletal chondromas, hypercellularity, binucleate cells, and nuclear atypia are compatible with a benign clinical course. However, rare instances of *chondrosarcoma* arising in synovial chondromatosis have been reported.[28]

Drawing a sharp line between *extraskeletal myxoid chondrosarcoma* and the *myxoid variant of chondroma* may be difficult, especially with those rare tumors that exhibit a moderate degree of cellular pleomorphism. Usually, however, the cartilage cells of chondromas are better differentiated, especially in the peripheral portion of the tumor; they tend to be less cellular and smaller; and, as a rule, they occur in the soft tissues of the hands and feet, unusual locations for extraskeletal myxoid chondrosarcoma. Finally, a significant subset of extraskeletal myxoid chondrosarcomas show evidence of a

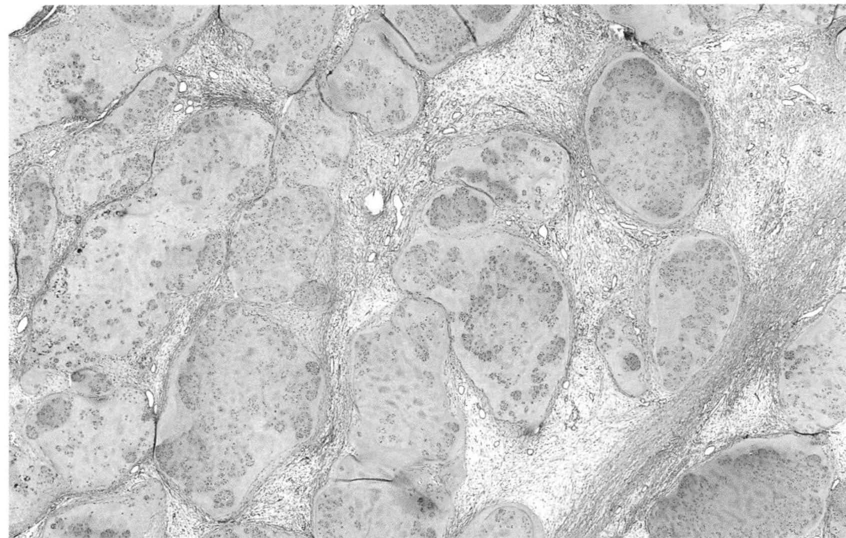

FIGURE 30-9. Synovial chondromatosis of the left knee.

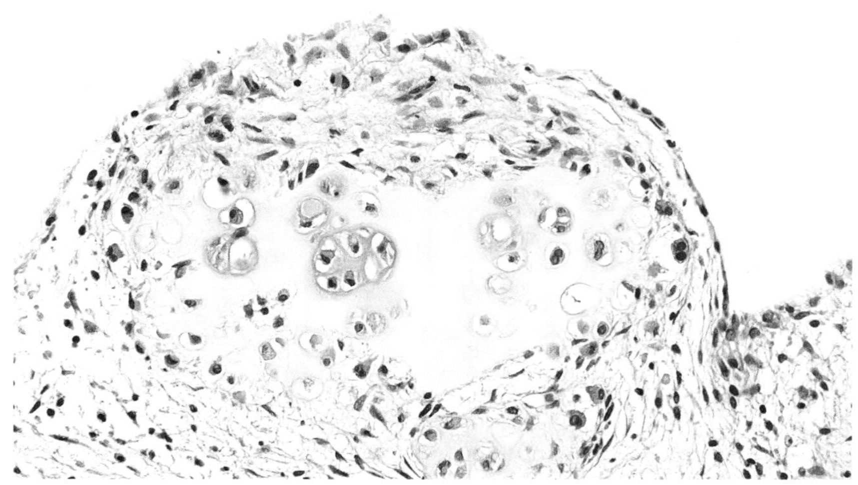

FIGURE 30-10. High-power view of synovial chondromatosis with a nodule of metaplastic cartilage underneath the synovium.

t(9;22), and analysis by fluorescence in situ hybridization (FISH) or reverse transcription polymerase chain reaction (RT-PCR) for evidence of an aberration of the *EWSR1* gene can be helpful in difficult cases.

Discussion

Although some of the chondroblastic or myxoid forms of extraskeletal chondroma cause concern because of their atypical cellular features, there is no evidence that these tumors behave differently from the well-differentiated forms composed of adult-type hyaline cartilage. A few tumors have been seen that recurred locally, but all were treated effectively by reexcising the tumor. Overall, up to 15% of cases recur locally.[7,8] It is noteworthy that transformation of extraskeletal chondroma to chondrosarcoma has never been encountered, although this is by no means rare with chondroid lesions of bone. Local excision is the preferred mode of therapy.

EXTRASKELETAL MESENCHYMAL CHONDROSARCOMA

Extraskeletal mesenchymal chondrosarcoma is a malignant cartilaginous tumor composed of two components: sheets of primitive mesenchymal cells and interspersed islands of well-differentiated hyaline cartilage. Because of the latter, extraskeletal mesenchymal chondrosarcoma has traditionally been considered a variant of chondrosarcoma. More recent data suggest that this is a translocation-associated sarcoma, as later discussed in greater detail. Because of its prominent vascular pattern, several cases reported in the earlier literature were initially interpreted as hemangiopericytoma with cartilaginous differentiation.[29] Mesenchymal chondrosarcoma is a rare tumor that is two to three times more common in bone than in soft tissue.[30-33] Unlike extraskeletal myxoid chondrosarcoma, it is a rapidly growing tumor with a high incidence of metastasis.

Clinical Findings

This neoplasm differs from other forms of chondrosarcoma by its preponderance in young adults 15 to 35 years of age and its slightly more frequent occurrence in females than in males. The tumor may also occur in young children[34] and has been described as a congenital lesion.[35] The principal anatomic sites of extraskeletal mesenchymal chondrosarcoma are the region of the head and neck, particularly the orbit, the cranial and spinal dura mater, and the occipital portion of the neck, followed by the lower extremities, especially the thigh (Table 30-1).[36] Rare examples of this tumor have been described in virtually every anatomic site, including the pancreas,[37] retroperitoneum,[38] and mediastinum.[39]

TABLE 30-1 Anatomic Distribution of 51 Extraskeletal Mesenchymal Chondrosarcomas

ANATOMIC LOCATION	NO. OF PATIENTS	PERCENTAGE (%)
Upper extremities	6	12
Lower extremities	18	35
Orbit	5	10
Trunk	8	16
Dura/meninges	11	21
Head and neck	3	6
Total	51	100

Data from Guccion JG, Font RL, Enzinger FM, et al. Extraskeletal mesenchymal chondrosarcoma. Arch Pathol 1973;95(5):336–340; Huvos AG, Rosen G, Dabska M, et al. Mesenchymal chondrosarcoma. A clinicopathologic analysis of 35 patients with emphasis on treatment. Cancer 1983;51(7):1230–1237; and Nakashima Y, Unni KK, Shives TC, et al. Mesenchymal chondrosarcoma of bone and soft tissue. A review of 111 cases. Cancer 1986;57(12):2444–2453.

Orbital lesions tend to produce exophthalmos, orbital pain, blurring of vision, and headaches; intracranial and intraspinal tumors are accompanied by vomiting, headaches, and various motor and sensory defects.[40] Tumors in the extremities usually manifest as a painless, slowly enlarging mass situated in the musculature. Cases have been reviewed in which a metastasis from a primary mesenchymal chondrosarcoma of bone mimicked a soft tissue tumor, and so a bone survey is essential, particularly when the tumor occurs in an unusual location. In most cases, radiography reveals a well-defined soft tissue mass, often with irregular radiopaque stipplings, arcs, flecks, or streaks as the result of focal calcification or bone formation in cartilaginous areas. CT scans, MRI, and angiography are helpful for outlining the tumor prior to surgical therapy.[41]

Pathologic Findings

Grossly, mesenchymal chondrosarcoma presents as a multilobulated circumscribed mass that shows considerable variation in size. Cut sections show a mixture of fleshy soft gray-white tissue with scattered foci of irregularly sized cartilage and bone. At times, there are also small areas of hemorrhage and necrosis, but hemorrhage is much less prominent than in extraskeletal myxoid chondrosarcoma.

Microscopically, mesenchymal chondrosarcoma exhibits a characteristic pattern composed of sheets of undifferentiated round, oval, or spindle-shaped cells with an abrupt transition with small well-defined nodules of well-differentiated, relatively low-grade-appearing hyaline cartilage, frequently with central calcification and ossification (Figs. 30-11 to 30-15). The undifferentiated cells have ovoid or elongated hyperchromatic nuclei and scanty, poorly outlined cytoplasm; they are arranged in small aggregates or in a hemangiopericytoma-like pattern around sinusoidal vascular channels lined by a single layer of endothelium. Solid cellular and richly vascular patterns may be present in different portions of the same neoplasm. The cartilaginous foci are usually well defined, but

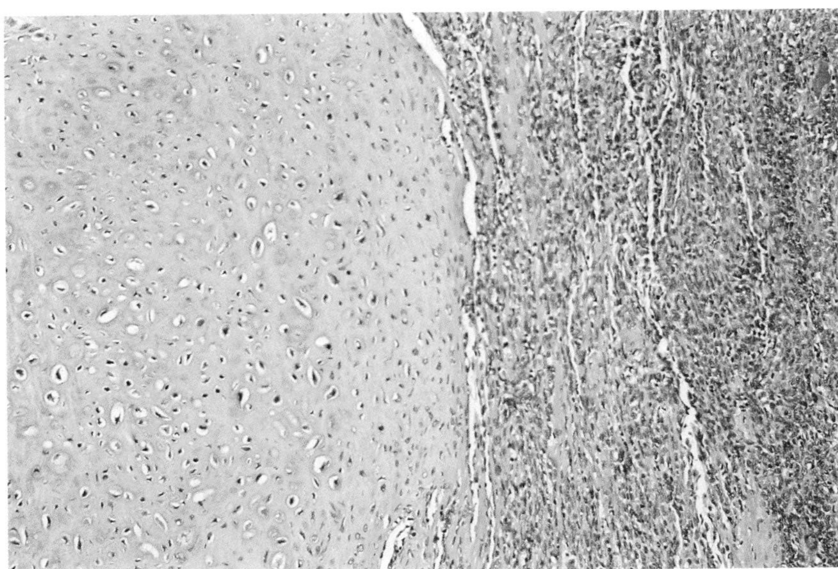

FIGURE 30-11. Low-power view of a mesenchymal chondrosarcoma with the characteristic bimorphic picture: islands of well-differentiated cartilage surrounded by sheets of small, undifferentiated tumor cells.

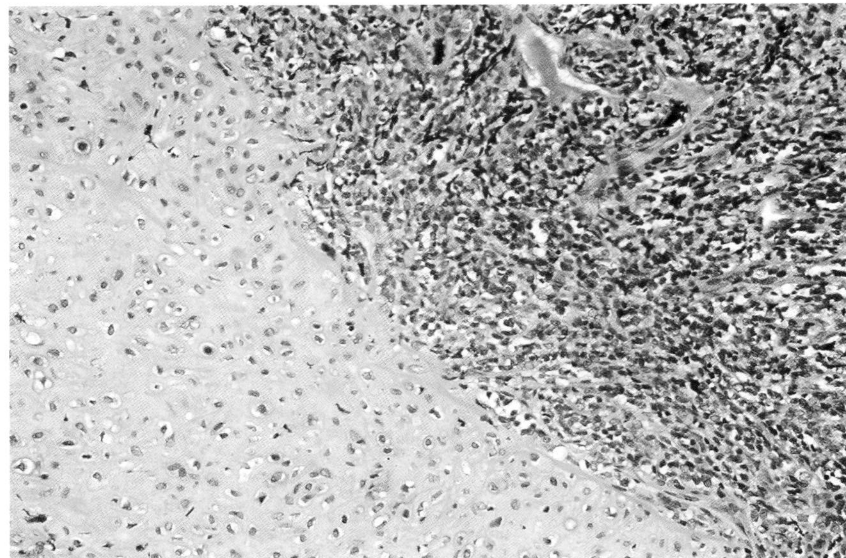

FIGURE 30-12. Sharp demarcation between small, undifferentiated tumor cells and well-differentiated cartilage in a mesenchymal chondrosarcoma.

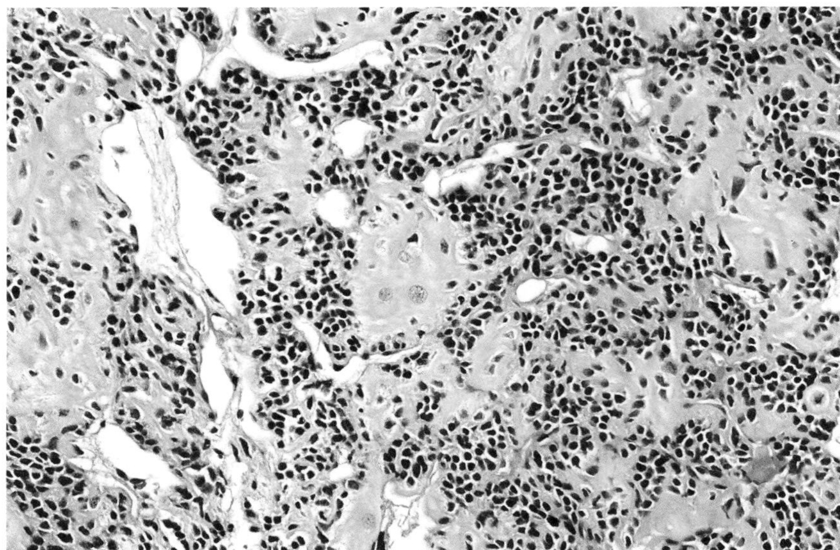

FIGURE 30-13. Extraskeletal mesenchymal chondrosarcoma with an intimate admixture of islands of cartilaginous tissue and small round cells.

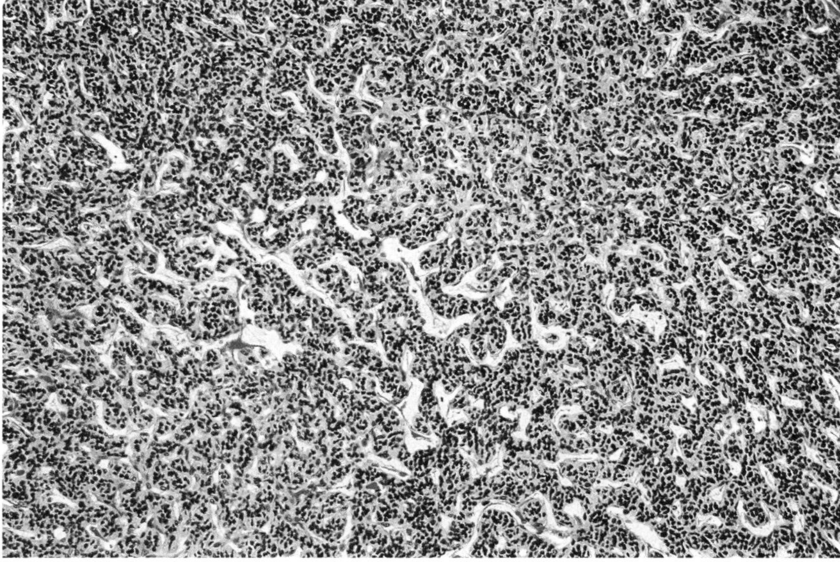

FIGURE 30-14. Small round cells surround a prominent hemangiopericytoma-like vasculature in an extraskeletal mesenchymal chondrosarcoma.

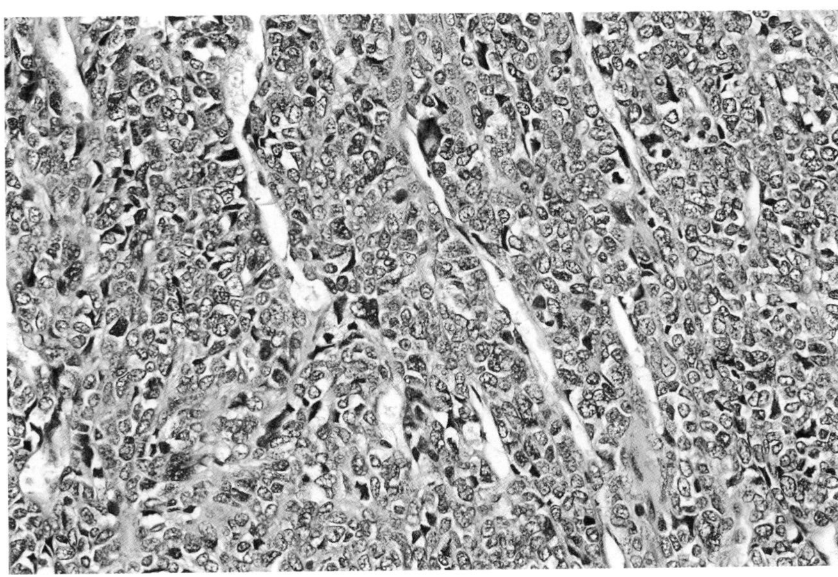

FIGURE 30-15. High-power view of small round cells surrounding hemangiopericytoma-like vessels in an extraskeletal mesenchymal chondrosarcoma.

there are also poorly circumscribed cartilaginous areas that gradually blend with the undifferentiated tumor cells. Spindle cell areas, with or without collagen formation, are present in some cases but are rarely a prominent feature.

Immunohistochemically, the cartilaginous portion of the tumor typically shows strong S-100 protein positivity, whereas only isolated cells in the undifferentiated areas stain for this antigen.[42,43] The round cells typically do not stain for broad-spectrum cytokeratins, but up to 35% show focal epithelial membrane antigen (EMA) staining.[44] Interestingly, up to 50% may also show focal desmin immunoreactivity, but stains for MyoD1 and myogenin are negative.[44]

In the absence of the cartilaginous foci, the undifferentiated areas may closely resemble other round cell sarcomas, particularly the Ewing family of tumors. Although early reports on the product of the *MIC2* gene (CD99) indicated that the undifferentiated areas of extraskeletal mesenchymal chondrosarcoma were negative for this antigen,[45] a subsequent report by Granter et al.[46] found that all 11 of their cases showed strong membranous immunoreactivity for CD99 in these undifferentiated areas. Similarly, Hoang et al.[47] found CD99 staining in 17 of 21 cases. These divergent results are likely a result of the use of different antibodies and different antigen retrieval techniques. Consistent CD99 membranous immunoreactivity has been found in mesenchymal chondrosarcoma and, therefore, it is believed that this marker does not allow distinction of extraskeletal mesenchymal chondrosarcoma from the Ewing family of tumors. FLI1, a marker found in many, but not all, cases of the Ewing family of tumors, is typically negative in mesenchymal chondrosarcoma.[48]

Wehrli et al.[49] reported on the utility of Sox9, a transcription factor thought to be a master regulator of chondrogenesis, in distinguishing mesenchymal chondrosarcoma from other small round blue cell tumors. In their study, 21 of 22 mesenchymal chondrosarcomas showed nuclear staining in both the primitive mesenchymal cells and the cartilaginous component. All other types of small round blue cell tumors were negative for this antigen. Similarly, several other studies also found consistent Sox9 staining in mesenchymal chondrosarcoma.[50,51]

Cytogenetic and Molecular Genetic Findings

Recently, Wang et al.[52] identified a novel, recurrent *HEY1-NCOA2* [(8;8)(q21;q13)] fusion in mesenchymal chondrosarcoma. In their study, all 9 cases of mesenchymal chondrosarcoma showed evidence of this fusion by either RT-PCR or FISH, but 15 samples of other types of chondrosarcoma lacked this fusion.

Differential Diagnosis

Although typical mesenchymal chondrosarcomas pose no particular diagnostic problem, recognition of this tumor may be difficult with small biopsy or needle-biopsy specimens that demonstrate only one of the two tissue elements. In particular, tumors without the cartilaginous element may be easily mistaken for a member of the Ewing family of tumors or *poorly differentiated synovial sarcoma* with a prominent hemangiopericytoma-like pattern. Metaplastic cartilage may occur in poorly differentiated synovial sarcoma, but it is much less common than foci of calcification or bone. Careful search for a biphasic pattern or epithelial differentiation with antibodies for cytokeratin or EMA is indicated in difficult cases. Because CD99 does not allow distinction of mesenchymal chondrosarcoma from the Ewing family of tumors or even poorly differentiated synovial sarcoma, molecular analysis for evidence of *EWSR1* or *SYT* aberrations can be extremely useful. Paraffin-embedded tissue is routinely used for FISH analysis using dual-color, break-apart *EWSR1* and *SYT* probes.

Distinction from differentiated forms of *extraskeletal chondrosarcoma* may also cause some diagnostic difficulty. These rare tumors, however, always display a more uniform pattern and lack the contrasting differentiated and undifferentiated areas.

Discussion

Mesenchymal chondrosarcoma is a fully malignant tumor that pursues an aggressive clinical course and metastasizes in a high percentage of cases.[31,36,53] Nakashima et al.[31] reported 5- and 10-year survival rates of 54.6% and 27.3%, respectively. The principal metastatic site is the lung. Lymph node metastasis is less common than with extraskeletal myxoid chondrosarcoma. Several patients have followed a protracted clinical course with late metastases, but there seems to be no reliable prognostic relation to the patient's age or degree of cellular differentiation. Combined radical surgery and chemotherapy or radiotherapy appears to be the treatment of choice.[51]

NON-NEOPLASTIC HETEROTOPIC OSSIFICATIONS

Myositis Ossificans

Myositis ossificans is a benign ossifying process that is generally solitary and well circumscribed. It is found most commonly in the musculature, but it may also occur in other tissues, including tendons and subcutaneous fat (sometimes referred to as *panniculitis ossificans*). Distinguishing between traumatic and nontraumatic forms of myositis ossificans serves little purpose because both forms are morphologically identical and are assuredly secondary to some kind of injury.

Histologically, the early stage of myositis ossificans has immature and highly cellular zones that are often confused with extraskeletal osteosarcoma. The late stage of myositis ossificans, on the other hand, consists almost entirely of mature lamellar bone and is sometimes misinterpreted as an osteoma. The term *myositis ossificans* is a misnomer because the lesion is not necessarily confined to the musculature, is devoid of bone in its early proliferative phase, and lacks a significant degree of inflammation.[54] If inflammation is present, it is usually minimal and is mostly evident in the tissues surrounding the lesion. For these reasons, myositis ossificans and related processes have also been designated as *pseudomalignant osseous tumors of soft tissues* and *extraosseous localized, non-neoplastic bone and cartilage formation*, both terms that more accurately define this process.[54] Nevertheless, these terms have not been widely applied in the literature and, for this reason, the conventional term *myositis ossificans* is retained for this chapter.

Clinical Findings

The initial complaint, noted within hours or days after injury, is pain or tenderness, followed by a diffuse, doughy soft tissue swelling. Later, usually during the second or third week after onset, the swelling becomes more circumscribed and indurated and gradually changes into a mass that is distinctly outlined and firm to stony on palpation.

The condition chiefly affects young, vigorous, athletically active adolescents and adults, predominantly males,[55,56] but it may also be found in older persons and females. Myositis ossificans is rare in small children.[57] In about 80% of cases, the lesion involves the limbs; the favored sites in the lower extremity are the quadriceps muscle and the gluteus muscle and in the upper extremity the flexor muscles, especially the brachialis muscle. Trauma-induced lesions have also been described in the head and neck, particularly in the masseter temporalis and sternocleidomastoid muscles.[58] Rare examples of a histologically identical lesion may also arise within nerves.[59] Deep-seated lesions may involve both muscle and underlying periosteum. Rarely, similar lesions arise in the mesentery, usually in middle-aged to elderly men (median age 49 years) following significant abdominal surgery or trauma.[60,61] These patients usually present with bowel obstruction.

Radiographically, at the initial stage, plain films show a slight increase in soft tissue density. Calcification is rarely seen before the end of the third week after injury and initially presents as rather faint, irregular, floccular radiopacities, sometimes described as the dotted veil pattern of myositis ossificans.[62] As the lesion progresses and becomes increasingly calcified, it presents as a well-outlined soft tissue mass that is most densely calcified at its periphery. Calcification becomes clearly apparent radiographically 4 to 6 weeks after the onset of the lesion; it proceeds from the periphery toward the center of the process, but even in late lesions the central core tends to remain uncalcified (Figs. 30-16 and 30-17). The appearance

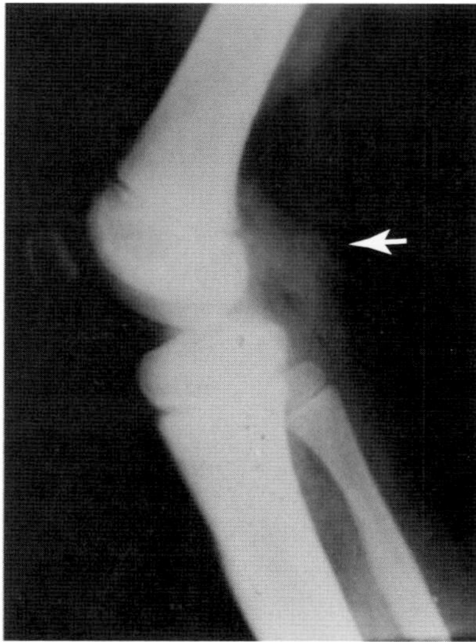

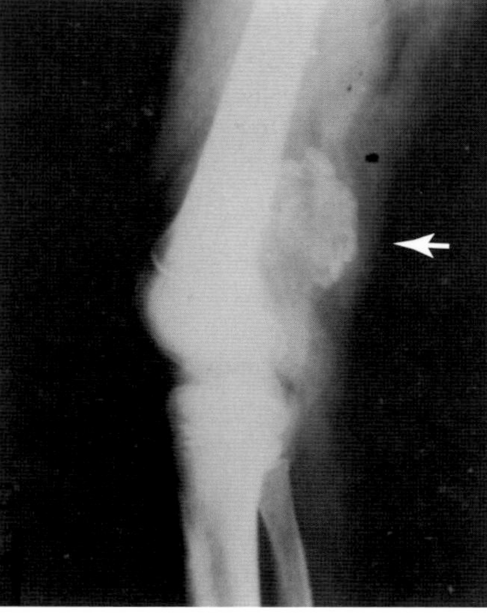

FIGURE 30-16. Myositis ossificans of the popliteal fossa showing evidence of progressive ossification within a 22-day period.

of myositis ossificans on CT and MRI is quite characteristic and often leads to the correct diagnosis.[63]

Pathologic Findings

Grossly, most of the lesions measure 3 to 6 cm in greatest diameter. They tend to be well circumscribed and cut with a gritty sensation; they are white, soft, and rather gelatinous (or hemorrhagic) in the center and yellow-gray with a rough granular surface at the periphery.

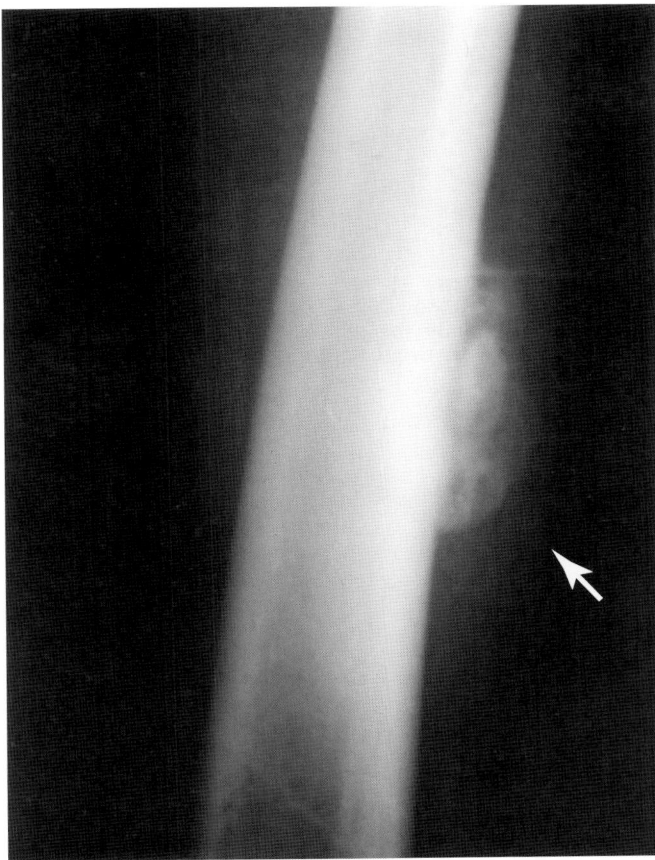

FIGURE 30-17. Radiograph of myositis ossificans (arrow) of the upper thigh. The lesion had been present for 5 weeks.

Histologically, myositis ossificans is characterized by the presence of a distinct zonal pattern that reflects different degrees of cellular maturation, a pattern that is most conspicuous in lesions of 3 weeks' or more duration. In these cases, the innermost portion of the lesion is composed of immature, loosely textured, often richly vascular fibroblastic tissue bearing a close resemblance to nodular fasciitis or granulation tissue (Fig. 30-18). The constituent fibroblasts and myofibroblasts display a mild degree of cellular pleomorphism and rather prominent mitotic activity. They are intermingled with a varying number of macrophages, chronic inflammatory cells, fibrinous material, and not infrequently multinucleated giant cells. In addition, there may be prominent endothelial proliferation, focal hemorrhage, fibrin, and entrapped atrophic or necrotic muscle fibers.[64]

Peripheral to these areas is an intermediate zone in which the cells become condensed into ill-defined trabeculae consisting of a mixture of fibroblasts, osteoblasts, and varying amounts of osteoid separated by thin-walled, ectatic vascular channels (Figs. 30-19 to 30-21). Farther toward the periphery, the osteoid increasingly undergoes calcification and evolves into mature lamellar bone (Fig. 30-22). Not infrequently, islets of immature or mature cartilage are present and precede bone formation. Characteristically, bone formation is most prominent at the margin of the lesion, often with rimming of the osteoid by a monolayer of osteoblasts showing little variation in size and shape. The bone is separated from the surrounding muscle tissue by a zone of loose, myxoid, or compressed fibrous tissue. The surrounding muscle often shows atrophic changes, sometimes together with a mild inflammatory infiltrate and focal sarcolemmal proliferation. In some lesions, particularly those arising in the subcutaneous fat, the zonal pattern is absent or inconspicuous. Older lesions consist of only mature lamellar bone together with interspersed fat cells, fibrous tissue, and thin-walled vascular spaces indistinguishable from osteoma.

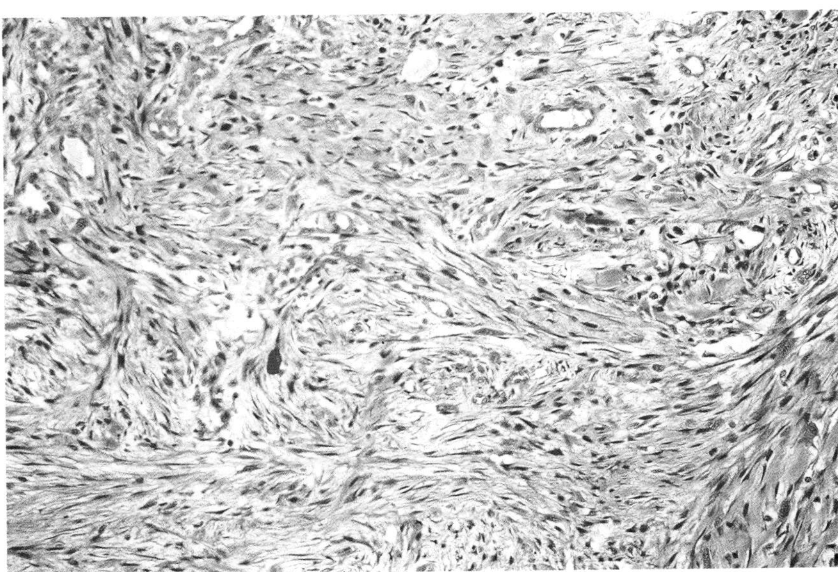

FIGURE 30-18. Central portion of myositis ossificans showing fibroblastic/myofibroblastic proliferation closely resembling nodular fasciitis.

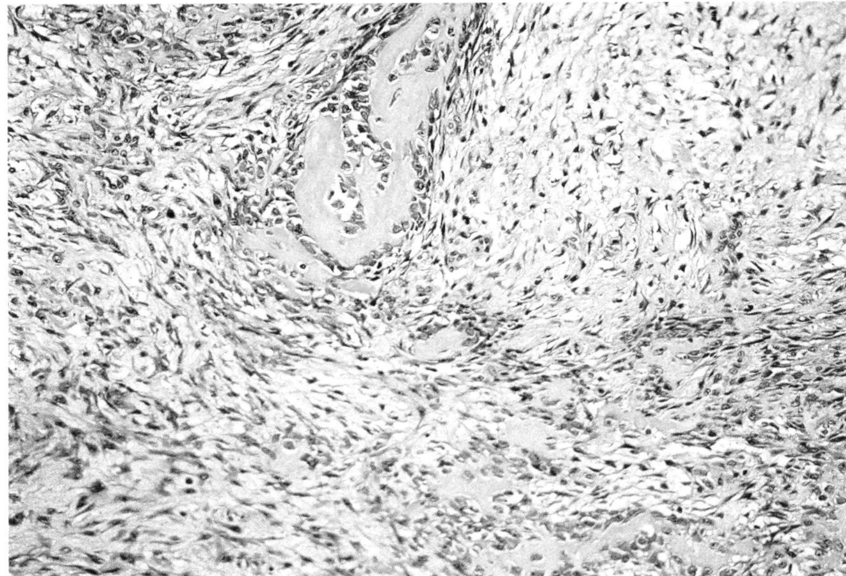

FIGURE 30-19. Intermediate portion of myositis ossificans with transition from proliferating spindle-shaped cells to trabeculae of osteoid lined by plump osteoblasts.

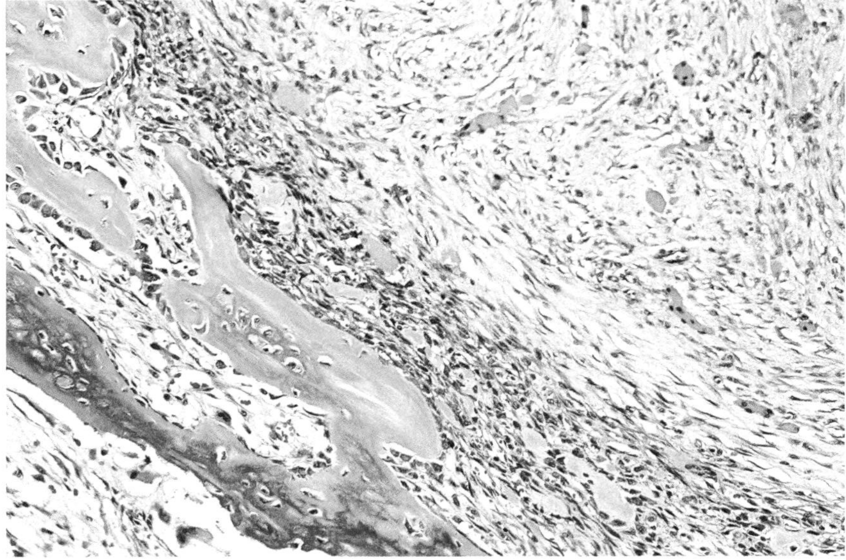

FIGURE 30-20. Osteoblast-lined osteoid adjacent to spindle cell proliferation resembling nodular fasciitis in a case of myositis ossificans.

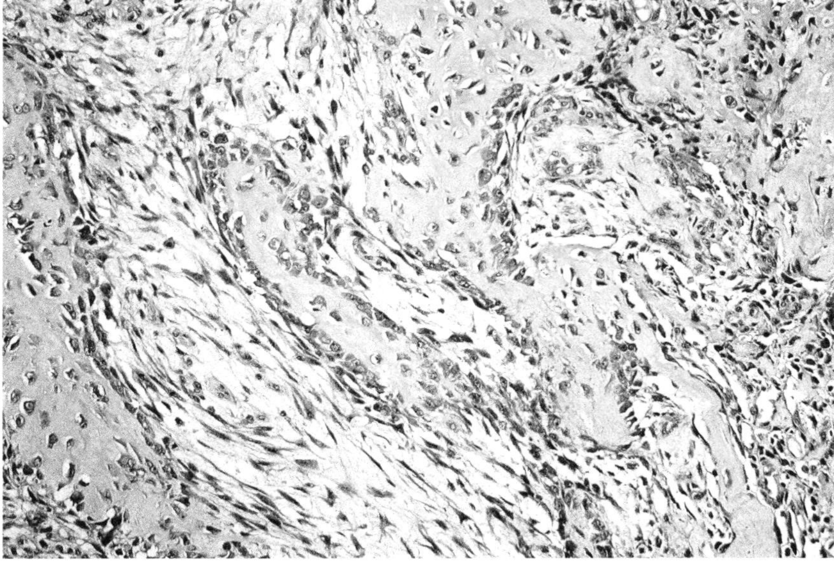

FIGURE 30-21. Myositis ossificans. Numerous osteoblasts are seen lining osteoid, surrounded by a cytologically bland proliferation of spindle-shaped cells.

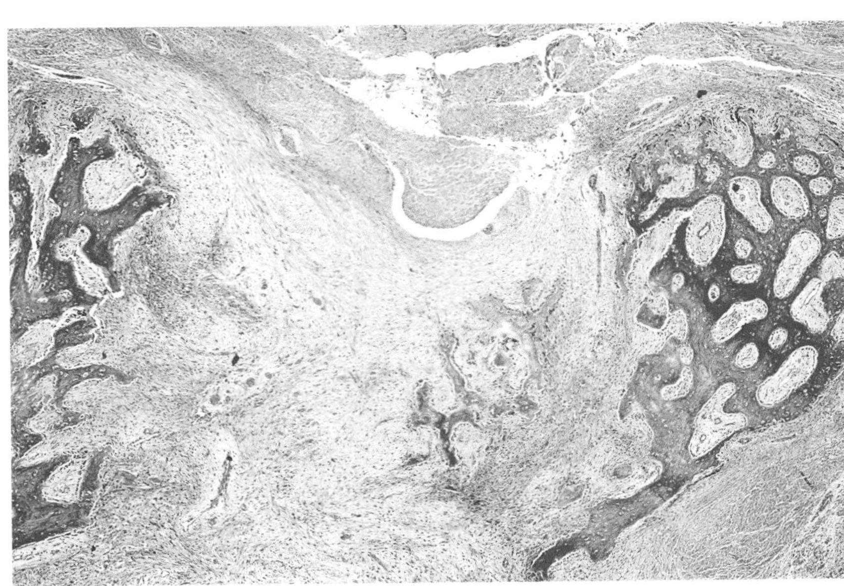

FIGURE 30-22. Low-magnification view of a peripheral portion of myositis ossificans displaying a zone of osteoid trabeculae rimmed by osteoblasts, underneath which is a proliferation of spindle-shaped cells.

TABLE 30-2 Differential Diagnostic Features of Myositis Ossificans, Fibro-Osseous Pseudotumor of the Digits, and Extraskeletal Osteosarcoma

LESION	PEAK AGE	SITE	ZONING	PLEOMORPHISM	ATYPICAL MITOSES
Myositis ossificans	Second to third decades	Muscles of lower or upper extremities	Immature central areas, mature lamellar bone at periphery	Absent to mild	Absent
Fibro-osseous pseudotumor	Second to third decades	Digits	Usually absent	Absent to mild	Absent
Extraskeletal osteosarcoma	Sixth to seventh decades	Muscles of lower or upper extremities	If present, has central osteoid or bone and atypical spindled cells at periphery	Moderate to severe	Present

Malignant Transformation of Myositis Ossificans

No convincing cases of malignant transformation of myositis ossificans have been seen, but there are several accounts in the literature in which transformation of myositis ossificans into extraskeletal osteosarcoma is claimed.[65,66] In most of these cases, the presence of myositis ossificans is poorly documented, and in only a few is the diagnosis based on biopsy. In some of the reported cases, long duration and dedifferentiation of a well-differentiated osteosarcoma may have simulated an origin in myositis ossificans. Regardless, for all practical purposes, myositis ossificans is a benign pseudosarcomatous lesion and should be treated as one.

Differential Diagnosis

It is of paramount importance to distinguish this lesion from *extraskeletal osteosarcoma* (Table 30-2). This is best accomplished on the basis of the characteristic zoning phenomenon of myositis ossificans, that is, the presence of immature cellular areas in the center and more mature, ossifying areas with osteoblastic rimming at the periphery. In sharp contrast, osteosarcoma displays a more disorderly growth of hyperchromatic and often pleomorphic cells with lace-like rather than trabecular osteoid formation and sometimes a reverse zoning effect (i.e., osteoid or bone formation in the interior and older portion of the lesion and immature spindle cell formation at its margin). Moreover, unlike myositis ossificans, extraskeletal osteosarcoma shows a greater degree of cellular atypia, no subsidence of growth at the periphery, and infiltration of neighboring tissues in a destructive manner. Mitotic figures are present in the immature portions of myositis ossificans and osteosarcoma, but several clearly atypical or tripolar forms point toward malignancy. Confusion of myositis ossificans with osteosarcoma is most likely with small biopsy specimens obtained during the initial proliferative phase or obtained from the cellular center of an early lesion.

The differential diagnosis may also be a problem in cases in which the lesion lacks the characteristic zoning phenomenon and grows in an irregular multifocal or multilobulated fashion, as in most cases of fibro-osseous pseudotumor involving the distal portions of the fingers or toes (discussed later). Because extraskeletal osteosarcomas occur rarely in young persons, consideration of the age of the patient may help reach a correct diagnosis.

Although exceedingly uncommon, a soft tissue metastasis of a silent osteoblastic carcinoma or melanoma can masquerade as myositis ossificans. Benign lesions also may be confused with myositis ossificans, including purely reactive lesions such as nodular fasciitis, proliferative myositis, posttraumatic periostitis, and exuberant fracture callus. Proliferative myositis may have minute foci of osteoid or bone, but, characteristically, this feature is associated with a diffuse proliferation of plump fibroblasts resembling ganglion cells. Posttraumatic periostitis manifests as an ossified mass that is attached to bone with a broad base. Exuberant callus is usually associated with a discernible fracture line on standard radiographs.

Discussion

The pathogenesis of myositis ossificans is still poorly understood. In cases with a definite history of traumatic injury, it can be assumed that the process commences with tissue necrosis or hemorrhage, or both, followed by exuberant reparative fibroblastic/myofibroblastic and vascular proliferation, eventually leading to progressive ossification. The exact environmental or humoral conditions that favor ossification as opposed to a nonossifying reactive myofibroblastic proliferation are not understood. Detachment and intramuscular implantation of periosteal cells are not necessary prerequisites for ossification because this process also takes place in the subcutis and at other sites that are a considerable distance from bone. Similarly, the occurrence of ectopic ossifications in patients with paraplegia and patients with tetanus may be explained by trauma resulting from passive exercise rather than disturbed neurotrophic factors.

A satisfactory explanation for nontraumatic cases of myositis ossificans is even more problematic. It is likely that minor injury such as a spontaneous muscle tear or a similar disruptive lesion associated with heavy manual labor, weight lifting, or some other strenuous exercise or activity has been overlooked or forgotten; yet it is difficult to exclude the possibility that some of these cases are caused or initiated by an infectious process. Lagier and Cox[67] reported a patient who had had an anti-influenza vaccination 15 days before the onset of the lesion. There are also examples of this lesion developing following trigger point injection.[68]

Because myositis ossificans is a benign, self-limiting process, the prognosis is excellent, and there is no need for further therapy once the diagnosis of myositis ossificans has been established. Although quite challenging, this lesion can occasionally be diagnosed by core biopsy or even fine-needle aspiration.[69] If the lesion is partly excised at an early phase of its growth, it may continue to grow for a limited period; in these cases, repeated radiographic examinations should be obtained during the follow-up period to document the maturation of the lesion and the absence of destructive growth. Spontaneous regression of myositis ossificans has also been observed.[70]

Fibro-Osseous Pseudotumor of the Digits

Fibro-osseous pseudotumor of the digits, a heterotopic ossification closely related to myositis ossificans, occurs in the subcutaneous tissue of the digits and has been described under various names, including *florid reactive periostitis of the tubular bones of hands and feet*,[71] *pseudomalignant osseous tumor of the soft tissues*,[72] and *parosteal fasciitis*.[73] This lesion appears to be closely related to bizarre parosteal osteochondromatous proliferation (Nora lesion) and acquired osteochondroma. Clinically, this process presents as a painful, localized, fusiform, often erythematous swelling in the soft tissues of the fingers, especially the region of the proximal phalanx[74-76] (Fig. 30-23) and, less commonly, the toes.[77] It predominantly

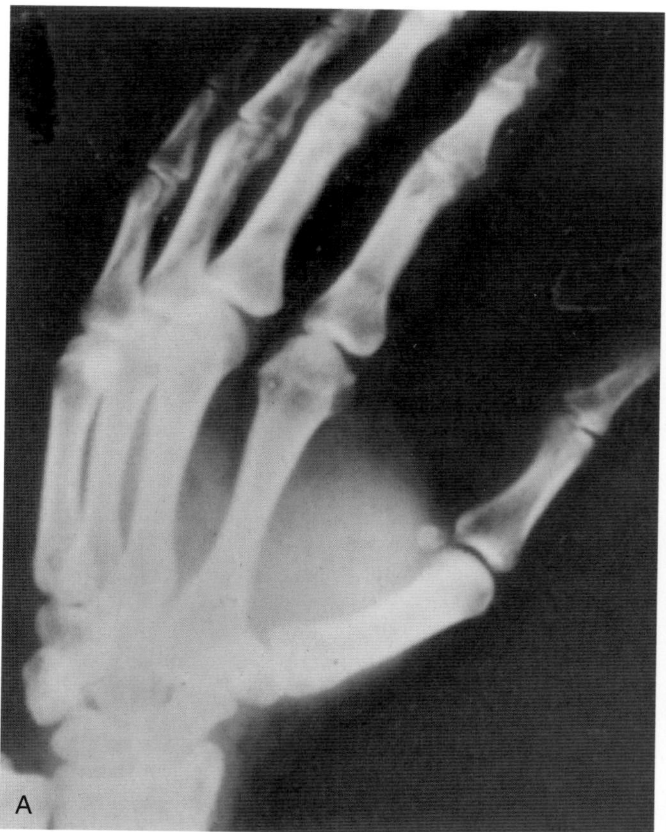

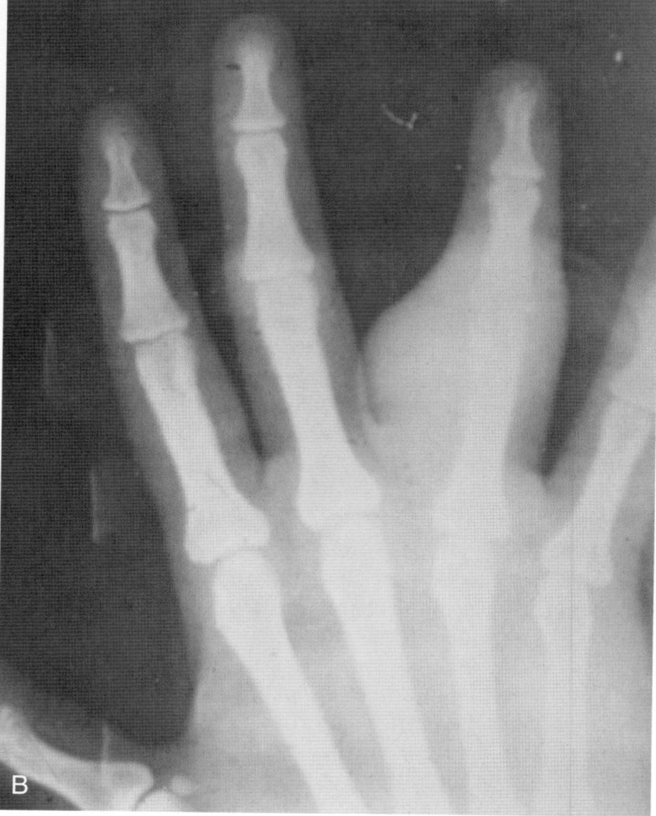

FIGURE 30-23. Radiographs of fibro-osseous pseudotumor of the thenar eminence (A) and the right ring finger (B).

affects young adults and, unlike myositis ossificans, is more common in women.

Radiographically, fibro-osseous pseudotumor of the digits is usually an ill-defined soft tissue mass with focal calcification that lacks the typical zoning pattern of myositis ossificans.[78] There may be thickening of the adjacent periosteum, and rare cases erode adjacent bone. Histologically, the lesion closely resembles myositis ossificans but lacks its orderly zonal pattern; it consists merely of an irregular, often nodular mixture of loosely arranged fibroblasts, a prominent myxoid matrix, and deposits of osteoid rimmed by uniform osteoblasts (Figs. 30-24 to 30-27). Multinucleated giant cells may be seen, and, in some cases, there is a mild lymphoplasmacytic infiltrate. Immunohistochemically, the spindle-shaped cells express smooth muscle actin and calponin, suggesting myofibroblastic differentiation.[76]

The major differential diagnosis is with *extraskeletal osteosarcoma*. The latter lesion typically occurs in older patients and rarely involves the digits. Furthermore, extraskeletal osteosarcoma is characterized by more pleomorphic hyperchromatic cells and atypical mitotic figures. *Bizarre parosteal osteochondromatous proliferation* (*Nora lesion*), similar to fibro-osseous pseudotumor, predominantly involves the short tubular bones of the hands and feet of young adults.[79] Given the overlapping clinical and histologic features, Nora lesion could represent an intermediate step between fibro-osseous pseudotumor of the digits and acquired osteochondroma (Turret exostosis). Nora lesion presents as a well-delineated mass attached to the bone surface. Histologically, a zonal architecture is apparent at low magnification with central or basally located new bone surrounded by a peripheral cap of cartilage. The cartilage often shows foci of hypercellularity with binucleated cells, which may result in a misinterpretation of malignancy if the entire clinical and radiographic picture is not considered.

As with the conventional form of myositis ossificans, the exact pathogenetic mechanism of this process is not clear. In the series by Dupree and Enzinger,[74] a history of trauma was

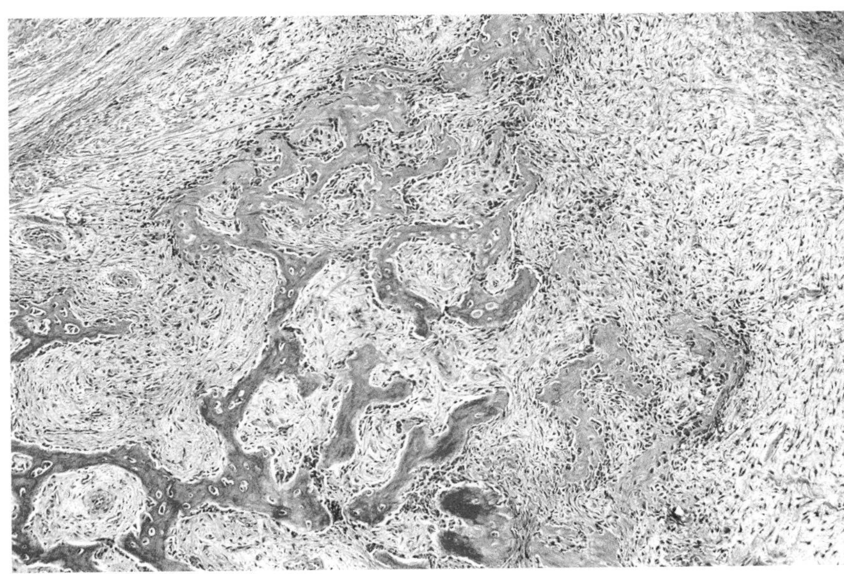

FIGURE 30-24. Fibro-osseous pseudotumor of the right index finger showing a peripheral zone of proliferating spindle cells and a central zone of osteoid.

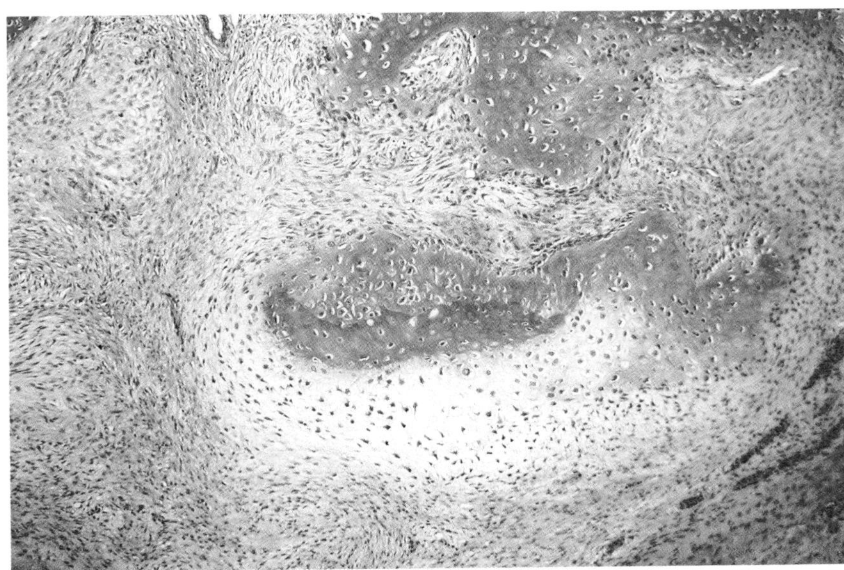

FIGURE 30-25. Fibro-osseous pseudotumor with osteoblast-rimmed osteoid material and a surrounding chondroid zone.

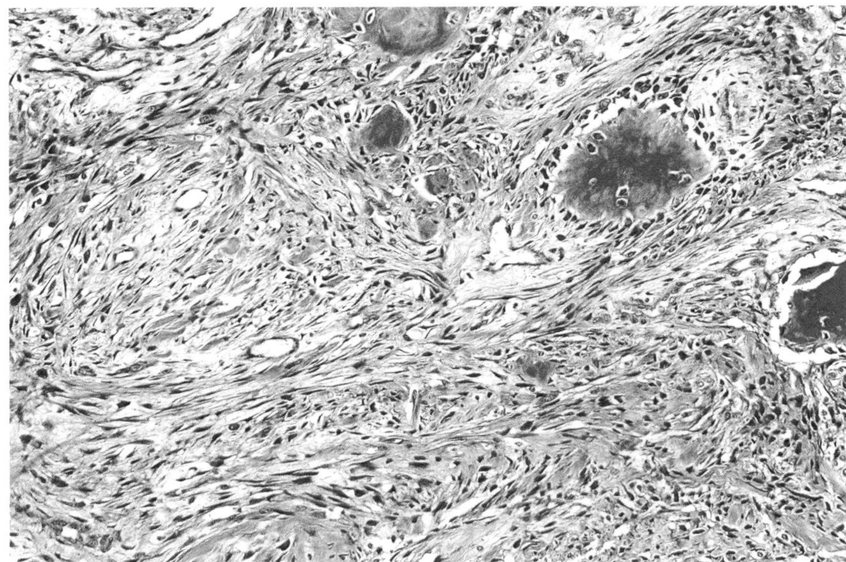

FIGURE 30-26. High-magnification view of fibro-osseous pseudotumor with proliferation of spindle-shaped cells adjacent to trabeculae of osteoid resembling myositis ossificans.

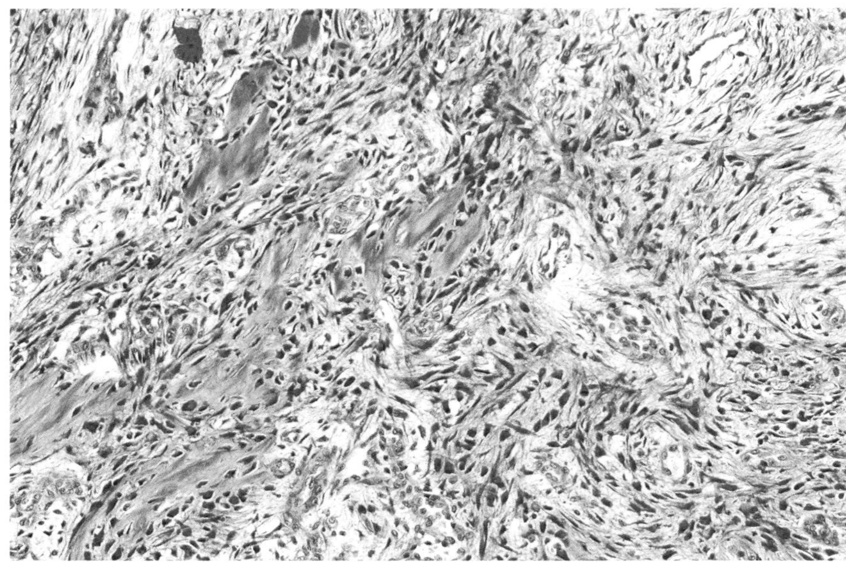

FIGURE 30-27. Fibro-osseous pseudotumor with an admixture of proliferating cytologically bland spindle-shaped cells and osteoid.

provided in only 9 of 21 patients. Most patients are cured by complete excision, but local recurrences do occur but are generally related to inadequate excision.[80]

FIBRODYSPLASIA (MYOSITIS) OSSIFICANS PROGRESSIVA

Fibrodysplasia (myositis) ossificans progressiva (FOP) is a rare, slowly progressive autosomal dominant disorder that principally affects children under the age of 10 years. It is characterized by progressive fibroblastic proliferation and subsequent calcification and ossification of subcutaneous fat, muscles, tendons, aponeuroses, and ligaments. The disorder is often associated with congenital symmetric malformations of the digits, especially microdactyly or adactyly of the thumbs and great toes, which precede onset of the fibroblastic proliferations and calcifications.[81-83] Its prevalence in children, diffuse or multinodular soft tissue involvement, progressive clinical course, and increased familial incidence distinguish it from localized myositis ossificans.

Clinical Findings

The disease typically has its onset between birth and 6 years of age, although in rare instances it arises in older children and even in young adults. Males and females are about equally affected, and there is no predilection for any particular race. As in localized myositis ossificans, FOP presents as a painful, doughy soft tissue swelling that most commonly begins in the upper paraspinal muscles and spreads from the axial to the appendicular skeleton, typically from cranial to caudal and from the proximal to the distal extremities (Fig. 30-28).[82] This

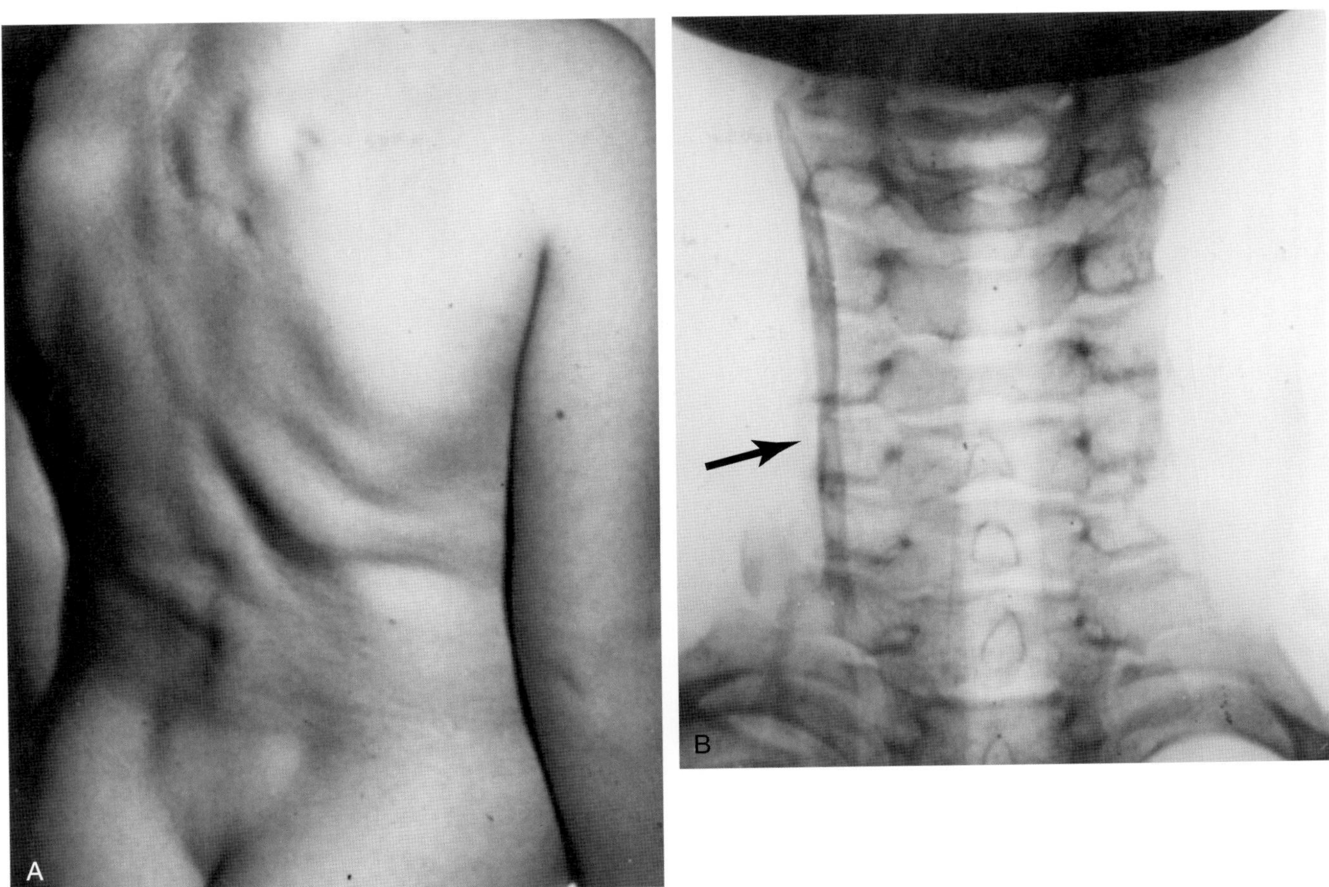

FIGURE 30-28. (A) Fibrodysplasia (myositis) ossificans progressiva involving the back of a child with ill-defined, indurated nodules caused by focal fibroblastic proliferation and ossification of the musculature. (B) Radiograph of linear ossification of paraspinal muscles (arrow). *(Courtesy of Prof. Dr. Günther Möbius, Schwerin.)*

typical progression may be modified by injury, immunization or surgery, because these would initiate a lesion at that particular site.[81] The preosseous lesion is a highly vascular fibroblastic proliferation that is histologically similar to that seen in the infantile forms of fibromatosis. During the later stages, the fibroblastic proliferation is replaced by endochondral ossification with mature lamellar bone having bone marrow elements that may involve an entire muscle from origin to insertion.[84] This causes progressive muscle stiffening, immobilization, and contraction deformities, leading to severe changes in posture and gait as well as increasing difficulties in respiration. In fact, patients with FOP are much more likely to suffer a catastrophic fall resulting in traumatic brain injury, intracranial hemorrhage, or death than are those without this disease.[85] Involvement of the masseter muscle may impair normal mastication and result in severe weight loss.[86] Many patients die during early adult life from respiratory failure or pneumonia, with a median age at death of 40 years.[87]

Malformation or the absence of one or more digits is an almost constant finding that helps distinguish this disease from infantile forms of fibromatosis and often allows for early diagnosis, thereby preventing the deleterious effects of a biopsy[88,89] (Box 30-1). The malformations are usually present at birth or appear soon thereafter; in the earliest stage, they are best identified radiographically (Fig. 30-29). They consist mainly of bilateral shortening of the fingers (microdactyly),

BOX 30-1 Digital Malformations Associated with Fibrodysplasia Ossificans Progressiva

- Malformation/absence of one or more digits
- Bilateral shortening of the fingers (microdactyly)
- Absence of both thumbs and great toes (adactyly)
- Digital deviations, particularly bilateral hallux valgus

absence of both thumbs and great toes (adactyly), or digital deviations, particularly valgus position of the great toe (bilateral hallux valgus). Sometimes the significance of these osseous malformations is not immediately recognized, and surgical correction is attempted, precipitating ectopic ossification. Additional radiographic changes, which appear at a later stage of the disease, consist of bony bridges in muscles and tendons; contractures and ankylosis of the shoulder, elbow, spine, and other joints[90]; and proximal tibial osteochondromas, a lesion found in up to 90% of patients[91] (Fig. 30-30). CT scans and MRI may help demonstrate early changes of the

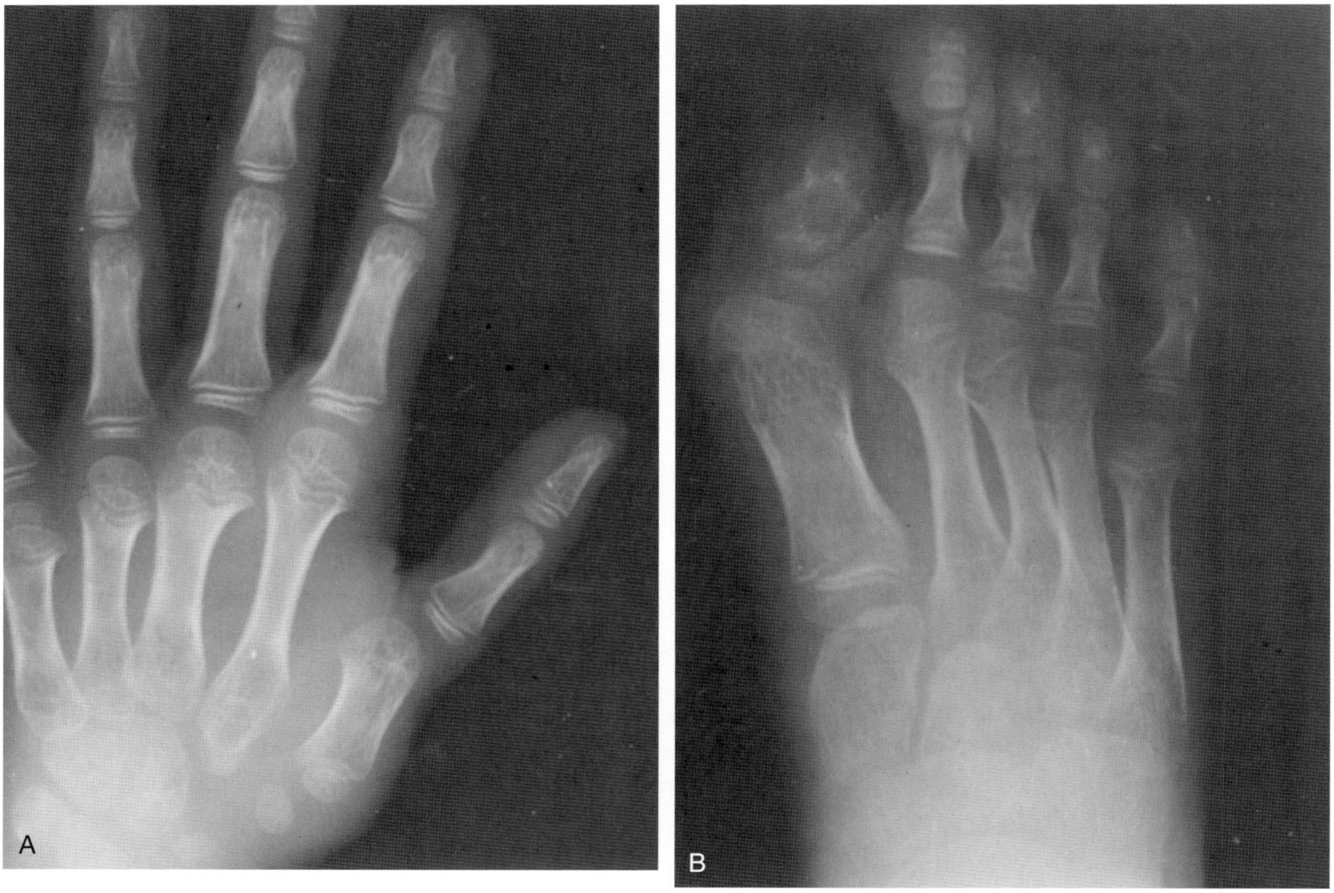

FIGURE 30-29. Fibrodysplasia (myositis) ossificans progressiva. (A) Radiograph shows shortening and deviation of the thumb. (B) Radiograph shows malformation of the great toe, a relatively common radiographic finding in this disease.

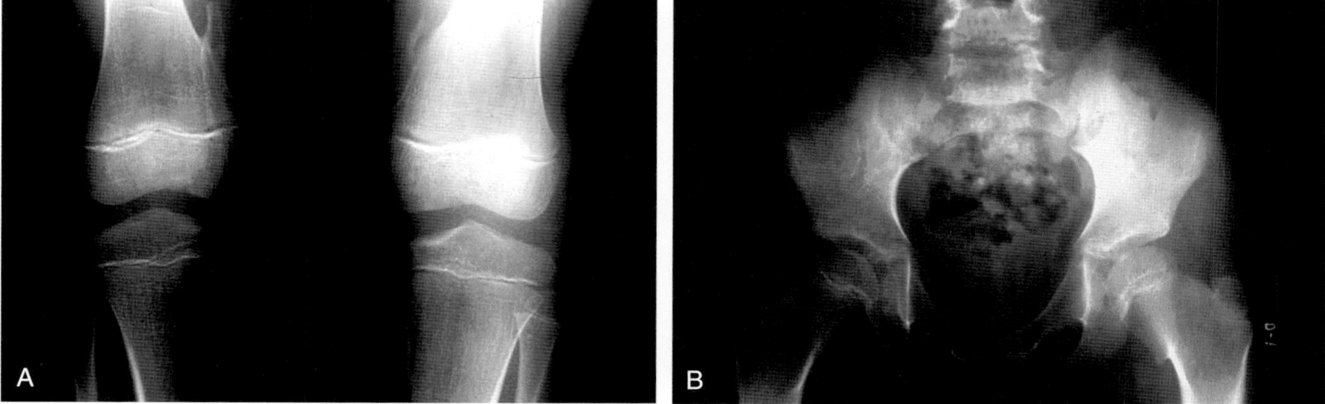

FIGURE 30-30. (A) Radiograph of both knees of a 7-year-old boy with fibrodysplasia (myositis) ossificans progressiva. Ossification is demonstrated along the medial femoral condyles bilaterally as well as the medial left tibial metaphysis along sites of ligamentous insertions producing pseudoexostoses. (B) Radiograph of the pelvis of the same patient showing bilateral broad, short femoral necks and small pseudoexostoses along the medial femoral metaphyses.

disease (Fig. 30-31).[92] Laboratory findings are generally unremarkable, except for elevated alkaline phosphatase levels. Basic fibroblast growth factor, a potent stimulator of angiogenesis, has been found to be significantly elevated in the urine in patients with acute flare-ups of FOP but not during disease quiescence.[93]

Pathologic Findings

There are essentially two stages of the disease. The first consists of nodular swelling of muscle and subcutis caused by interstitial edema, perivascular lymphocytic inflammation, and a loose proliferation of fibroblasts, usually in the endomysium and perimysium (Fig. 30-32).[94] During the second stage, collagen is laid down between the fibroblasts, followed by variable muscular atrophy, calcification, ossification of the collagenized fibrous tissue, and formation of mature bone and cartilage. Unlike localized myositis ossificans, the ossification occurs in the center of the nodules. The nodules often interconnect, leading eventually to the formation of bony bridges that replace muscles, tendons, and ligaments. Gannon et al.[95] found that the cells in the early preosseous fibroblastic stage are immunoreactive for bone morphogenetic protein 2/4 (BMP4, discussed later), whereas the cells of infantile fibromatosis do not stain for this antigen.

Genetic Aspects of Fibrodysplasia Ossificans Progressiva

FOP is a rare disease inherited in an autosomal dominant pattern.[96] Most cases are a result of new mutations, probably related to the low reproductive fitness of affected individuals.[97] There is also phenotypic variability because some patients have a milder form of this disorder.[98] Janoff et al.[99] reported a fascinating case in which this disease occurred in two half-sisters with the same unaffected mother and different unaffected fathers, suggesting that the mother had a mutant gene in numerous ova but that the mutant gene was present in few or no somatic cells (gonadal mosaicism).

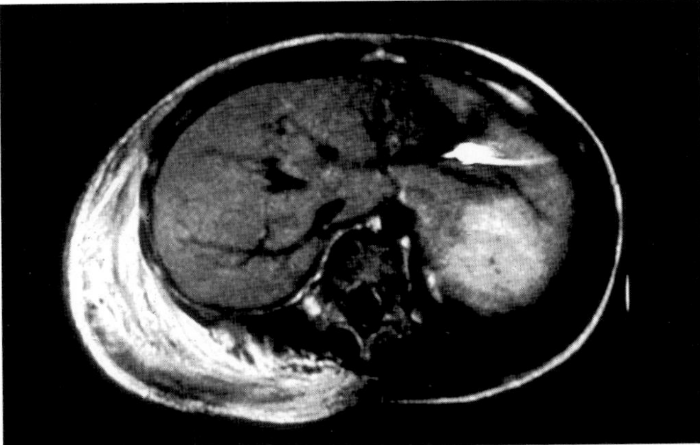

FIGURE 30-31. Fibrodysplasia (myositis) ossificans progressiva. MRI of the same patient depicted in Figure 30-30 reveals a large soft tissue mass that extends along the deep and superficial muscles of the back from the lower neck to the lower thoracic spine.

Over the past few years, the underlying genetic defect in FOP has been elucidated. Most cases are related to a point mutation of the BMP type 1 receptor *ACVR1* gene, resulting in its constitutive activation.[100,101] Mutations in this gene (also known as *ALK2*) result in downstream upregulation of *Smad1* and *Smad2* that induce osteoblastic differentiation and skeletal metamorphosis.[100,102,103] A number of mutation variants have also been described, resulting in atypical or milder forms of the disease, with apparent genotypic-phenotypic correlations.[98,104-106]

Discussion

The outlook for patients with FOP is poor, and the disease usually proves fatal within a period of 10 to 15 years, frequently as the result of severe respiratory insufficiency caused by progressive immobilization of the thorax (thoracic insufficiency syndrome). Biopsy and trauma may lead to the development of new lesions and should be avoided. Unfortunately, this is a fairly common problem. In a study of 138 patients with well-documented FOP, Kitterman et al.[107] reported an incorrect initial diagnosis in 87% of patients. The mean duration between onset of symptoms and an established diagnosis was 4.1 years. Sixty-seven percent of patients had unnecessary diagnostic (biopsy) procedures, and 68% received inappropriate therapy. Most important, 49% of patients developed permanent loss of mobility secondary to invasive interventions resulting in posttraumatic ossification. Therefore, a high index of clinical suspicion is necessary to initiate confirmatory

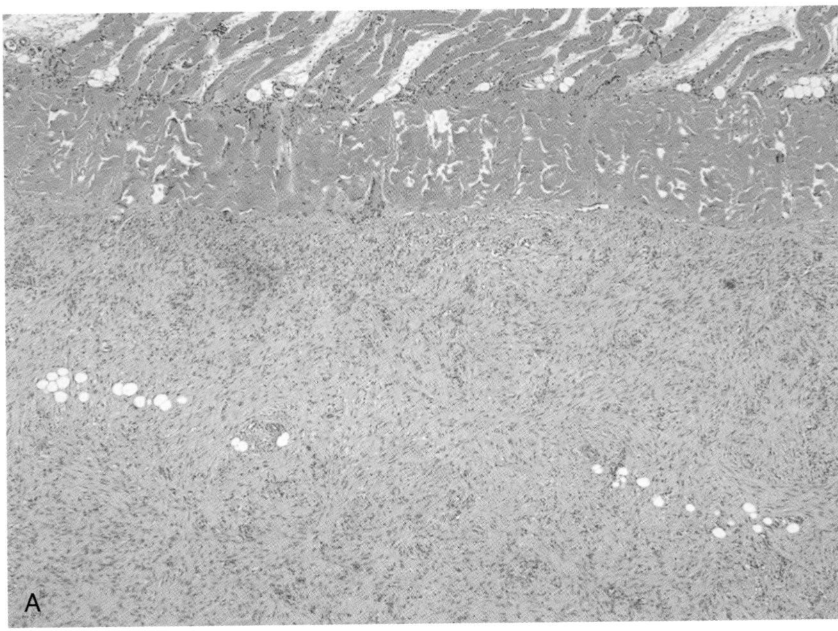

FIGURE 30-32. (A) Low-magnification view of fibrodysplasia (myositis) ossificans progressiva. A loosely textured fibroblastic proliferation superficially resembling nodular fasciitis is apparent.
Continued

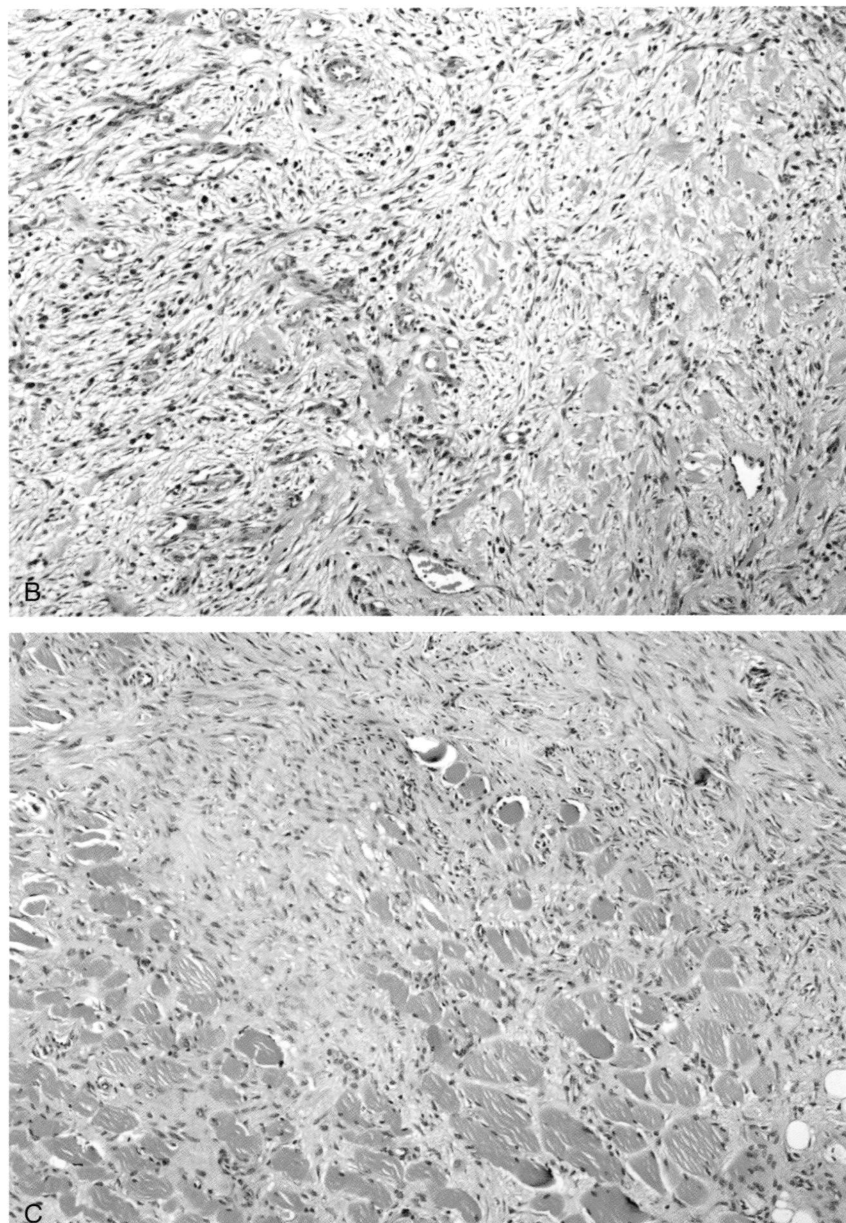

FIGURE 30-32, cont'd. (B) Spindled to stellate-shaped cells are deposited in a myxoid matrix and associated with dense collagen. (C) The proliferation is seen interdigitating between skeletal muscle fibers.

diagnostic genetic testing as well as to avoid harmful diagnostic and therapeutic procedures.

A variety of therapeutic modalities have been used with minimal success. Dietary measures, steroids, and agents binding minerals or blocking calcification (ethylenediaminetetraacetic acid; 1-hydroxyethylidene-1, 1-diphosphonic acid) have been tried with disappointing results.[108] High doses of intravenous disodium etidronate may be helpful for decreasing pain, swelling, and acute flare-ups of this disease, but excessive use can result in rickets-like osseous abnormalities.[109] Recently, studies have found nuclear retinoic acid receptor-γ agonists to potently inhibit heterotopic ossification in mice.[110] Small doses of fractionated radiation therapy may also be effective.[111]

The differential diagnosis includes the battered child syndrome, ectopic bone formation with multiple congenital anomalies, pseudohypoparathyroidism, and dermatomyositis with multiple calcifications. As mentioned earlier, the initial noncalcified fibrous proliferation of FOP may be mistaken for an infantile form of fibromatosis. Clinical suspicion resulting in diagnostic genetic testing is the best way to make a definitive diagnosis.

EXTRASKELETAL OSTEOSARCOMA

Extraskeletal osteosarcoma is a malignant mesenchymal neoplasm that produces osteoid, bone, or chondroid material, and is located in the soft tissues without attachment to the skeleton. Compared to osteosarcoma of bone, extraskeletal osteosarcoma is quite rare, accounting for only 1% to 2% of all soft tissue sarcomas.[112] Although there are some similarities with skeletal osteosarcomas, extraskeletal osteosarcomas are distinctive, particularly with respect to their morphologic appearance.

Excluded from the chapter are osteosarcomas arising in the breast, urinary bladder, prostate, and other visceral organs because, in many of these tumors, there is a participating epithelial component suggesting carcinosarcoma. Also excluded are malignant mesenchymomas, a rather nebulous entity that exhibits, by definition, two or more well-defined malignant mesenchymal components.

There are few reliable data in the literature as to the incidence of extraskeletal osteosarcoma. Allan and Soule[113] encountered 26 cases among 2100 soft tissue sarcomas, an incidence of 1.24%. In a study of the Swedish Cancer Registry, only four extraskeletal osteosarcomas among 242 osteosarcomas of bone were identified.[114] They calculated an annual incidence of two to three cases per million of population.

Clinical Findings

Although osteosarcomas of bone occur chiefly during the first two decades of life, extraskeletal osteosarcomas are rarely encountered in patients under 40 years of age.[115] In a series of 40 extraskeletal osteosarcomas reported from the Mayo Clinic, the mean age was 50.7 years (range 23 to 81 years),[116] and in a series of 25 cases from Denmark, patients ranged in age from 35 to 82 years, with a mean age of 67 years.[117] The data as to the gender incidence vary, and both male and female predominance has been reported.

There are no specific signs or symptoms. Generally, the tumor presents as a progressively enlarging soft tissue mass that is painful in about one-third of patients. Large tumors may ulcerate through the skin but usually only after biopsy or some other surgical procedure. The duration of symptoms varies from a few weeks to many years, although most present within 6 to 8 months following the initiation of symptoms.[118]

Among the various anatomic sites, the muscles of the thigh are most commonly affected; the large muscles of the pelvic and shoulder girdles are other relatively common sites.[119] Most tumors are deep-seated and fixed to the underlying tissues, but occasional lesions are freely movable and are confined to the subcutis or even the dermis.[120] There are also reports of extraskeletal osteosarcomas arising in unusual locations, including the mesentery,[121] mediastinum,[122] omentum,[123] and esophagus.[124] The laboratory findings show no specific abnormalities. Alkaline phosphatase is usually normal with localized disease, but it is often elevated in the presence of metastases. With conventional radiographs, CT scan, and MRI, extraskeletal osteosarcoma manifests as a soft tissue mass with spotty to massive calcifications and no evidence of bone involvement (Figs. 30-33 to 30-35).[125]

Pathogenesis

Mechanical injury has been hypothesized to be a causative agent, but the etiologic significance of trauma is difficult to assess. Preceding trauma has been reported in up to one-quarter of patients.[116] There are anecdotal reports of osteosarcoma arising at the sites of a previous injection or fracture. Unlike osteosarcoma of bone, the tumor has not been reported in siblings.

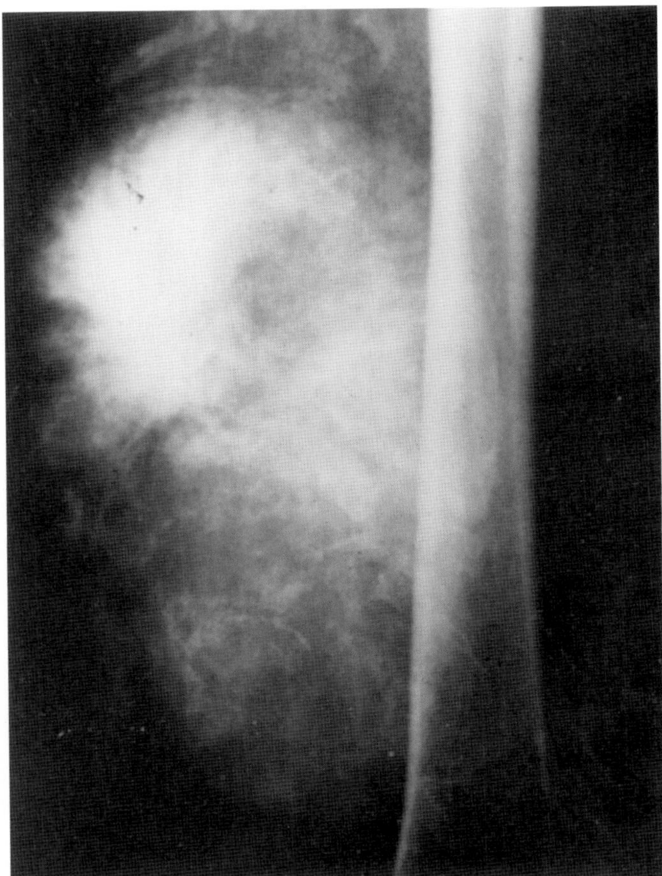

FIGURE 30-33. Radiograph of extraskeletal osteosarcoma of the mid-thigh demonstrating a soft tissue mass with extensive ossification. *(From Chung EB, Enzinger FM. Extraskeletal osteosarcoma. Cancer 1987;60:1132.)*

Radiation-Induced Extraskeletal Osteosarcoma

Since Martland described the postradiation development of osteosarcoma in patients engaged in the manufacture of luminous watch dials, numerous cases of both skeletal and extraskeletal postradiation osteosarcomas have been reported in the literature.[126,127] Most extraskeletal osteosarcomas occurred in patients who underwent radiation therapy for a malignant neoplasm, most commonly breast carcinoma.[128,129] In most instances, the tumor becomes apparent 4 years or more after radiotherapy. Assessment of these cases is facilitated by the presence of chronic radiodermatitis in the skin overlying the tumor or radiation change in the surrounding muscle tissue. There are also sporadic cases that developed following diagnostic procedures with radioactive thorium dioxide (Thorotrast). One of these, an extraskeletal osteosarcoma of the mandibular region in a 51-year-old man,

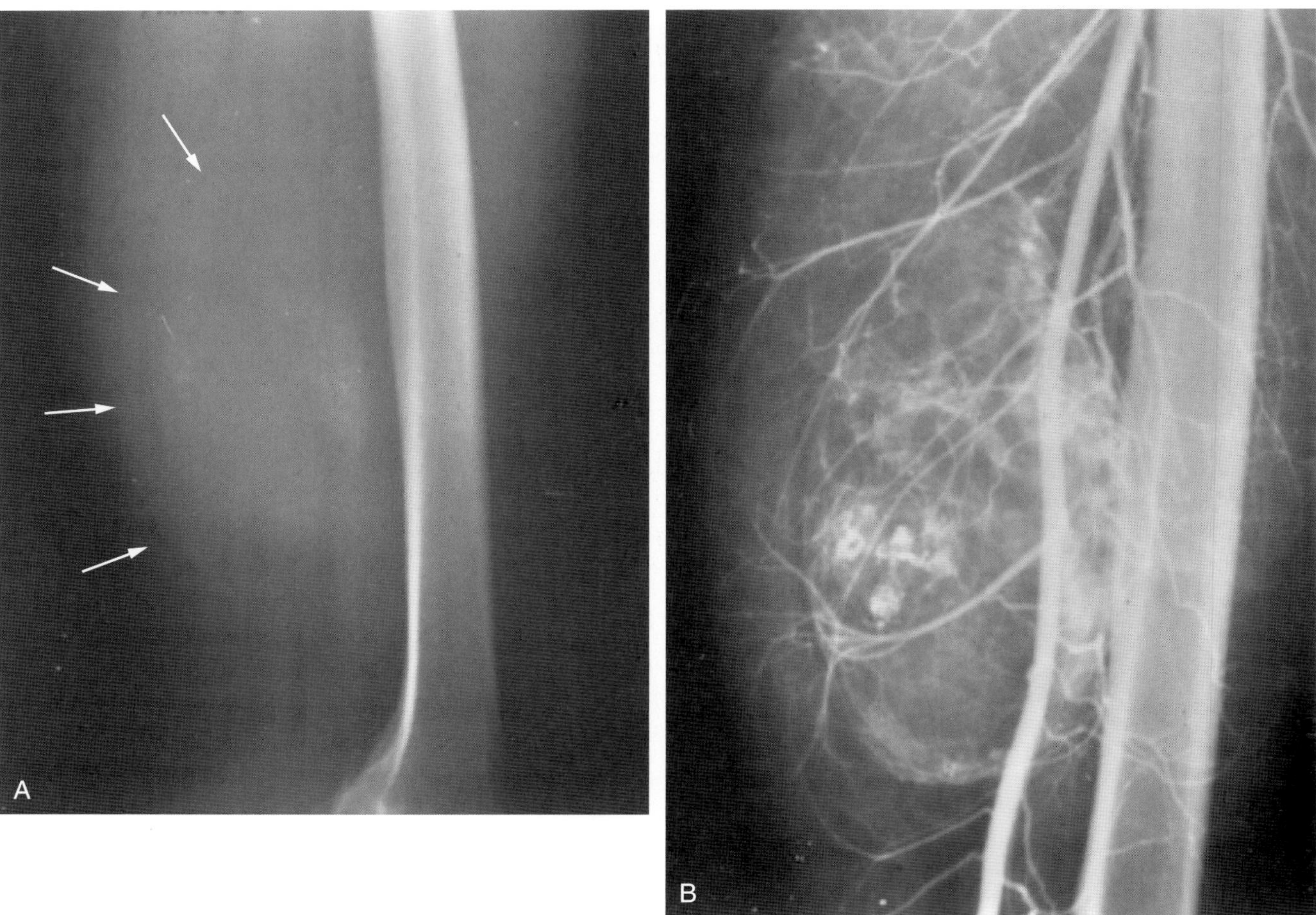

FIGURE 30-34. (A) Radiograph of extraskeletal osteosarcoma shows a soft tissue mass with areas of ossification (arrows). (B) There is a moderate degree of vascularization in the angiogram with focal neovascularity and stretching and displacement of arteries.

appeared 30 years after a Thorotrast angiogram of the carotid artery.[130]

Pathologic Findings

The tumor varies in its gross appearance from a well-circumscribed mass with a distinct pseudocapsule to an infiltrating tumor without discernible borders. Frequently, it is firm to stony on palpation. Less often, it presents as a soft or multicystic mass. On section, it usually displays a granular white surface with yellow flecks and multiple foci of necrosis and hemorrhage. Most tumors measure 5 to 10 cm when excised.

Microscopically, extraskeletal osteosarcomas have in common the presence of neoplastic osteoid and bone, occasionally with neoplastic cartilage. There is a striking variation in the relative prominence of this material and the associated osteoblastic and fibroblastic elements. Extraskeletal osteosarcomas, like osteosarcomas of bone, range from tumors that resemble fibrosarcoma or a high-grade pleomorphic sarcoma (*fibroblastic osteosarcoma*) to extremely cellular tumors with an irregular round or spindle cell pattern with considerable pleomorphism and mitotic activity (*osteoblastic osteosarcoma*) (Fig. 30-36A). The vast majority of extraskeletal osteosarcomas closely resemble an undifferentiated pleomorphic sarcoma (malignant fibrous histiocytoma [MFH]-like) except for the presence of osteoid deposition (Fig. 30-36B). Usually, the osteoid is deposited in a fine, ramifying, lace-like or coarsely trabecular pattern, occasionally showing transitions toward sheaths of osteoid or mature-appearing bone (Figs. 30-37 to 30-39). Unlike myositis ossificans in which the most mature portion is located at the periphery, there is often a reverse zoning phenomenon (i.e., central deposition of osteoid material and atypical spindle cell proliferation at the periphery). Atypical cartilage of variable cellularity, with or without myxoid areas or focal bone formation (Fig. 30-40), is present in many cases but rarely predominates (*chondroblastic osteosarcoma*).[131] There are also a varying number of benign and malignant multinucleated giant cells of the osteoclastic type that are often associated with hemorrhage (*osteoclastic* or *giant cell osteosarcoma*) (Fig. 30-41). The vascular pattern varies substantially. Very rarely, lesions with markedly dilated vascular spaces resembling a vascular tumor (*telangiectatic osteosarcoma*) occur (Fig. 30-42), although this variant is extremely uncommon in extraskeletal osteosarcomas.[132] Well-differentiated forms resembling parosteal osteosarcoma[133] and, even more rarely, tumors with a small cell pattern (*small cell*

Text continued on p. 943

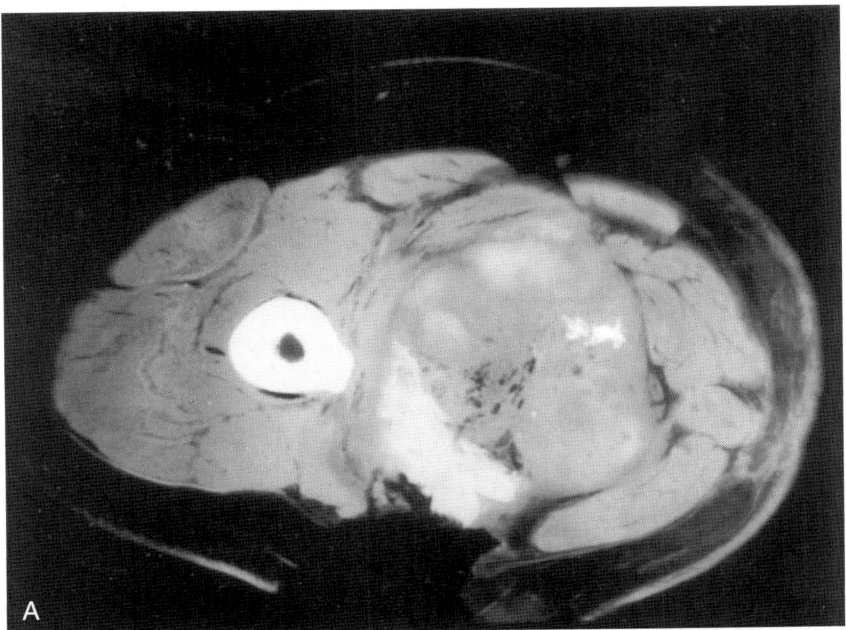

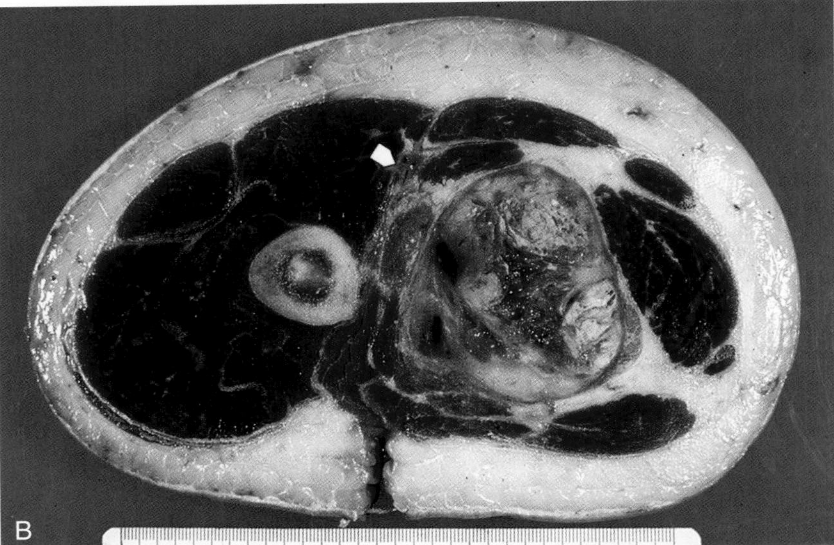

FIGURE 30-35. Computed tomography scan (A) and cross-section of extraskeletal osteosarcoma of the thigh (B). Note the circumscription of the tumor, areas of hemorrhage, and the absence of bone involvement.

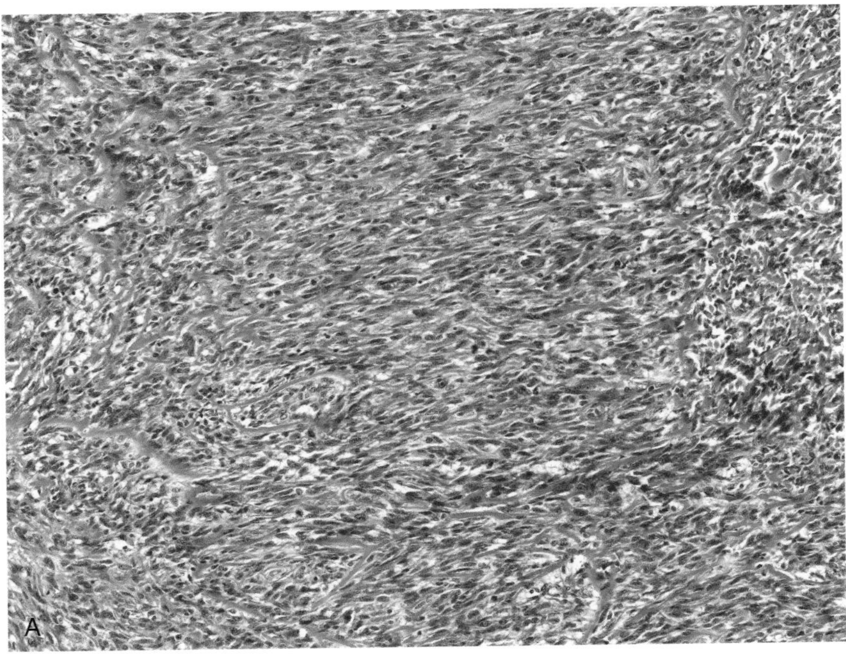

FIGURE 30-36. (A) Fibrosarcoma-like area of an extraskeletal osteosarcoma. *Continued*

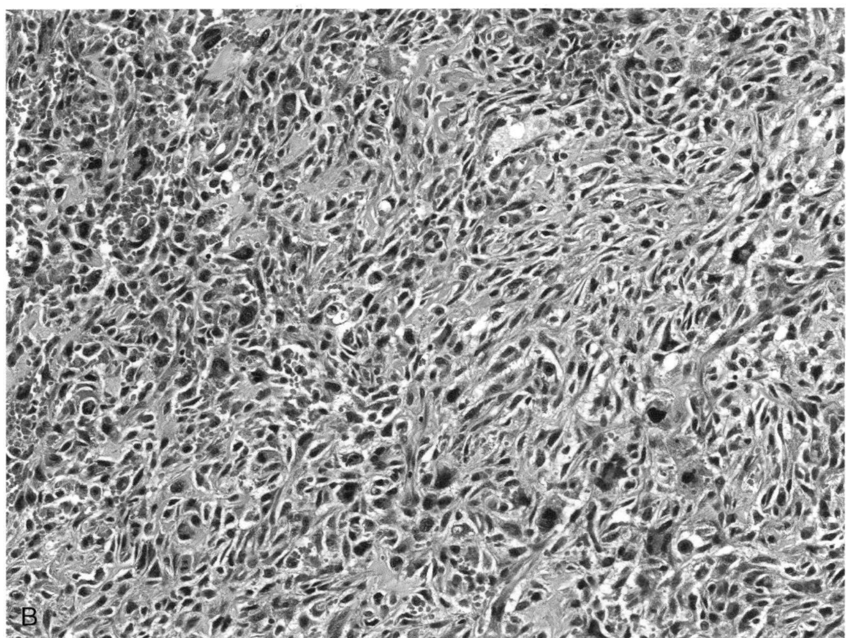

FIGURE 30-36, cont'd. (B) Malignant fibrous histiocytoma-like area of an extraskeletal osteosarcoma.

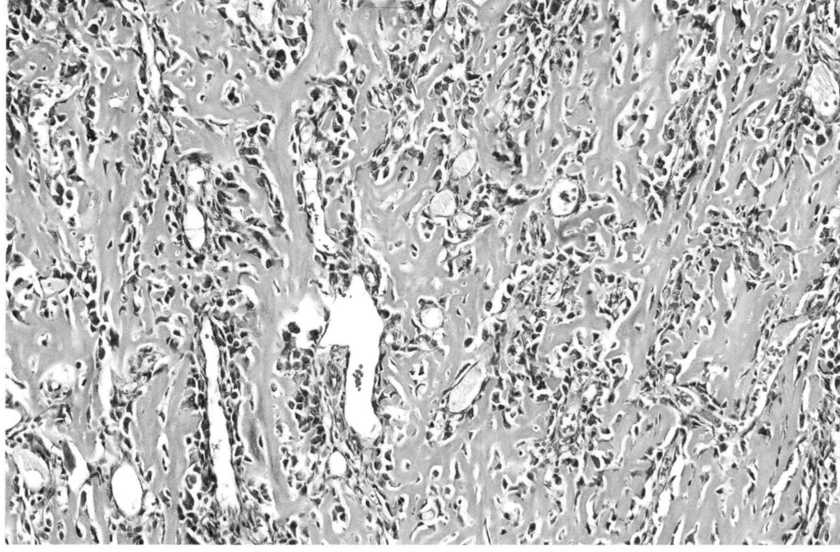

FIGURE 30-37. Extraskeletal osteosarcoma with large hyperchromatic cells separated by hyalinized collagen and osteoid.

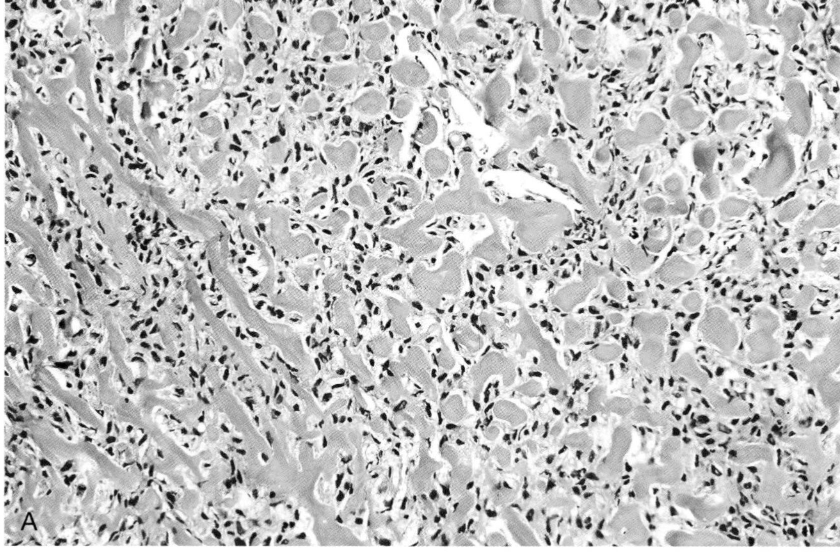

FIGURE 30-38. Extraskeletal osteosarcoma of the retroperitoneum. (A) Malignant cells are compressed by osteoid material.

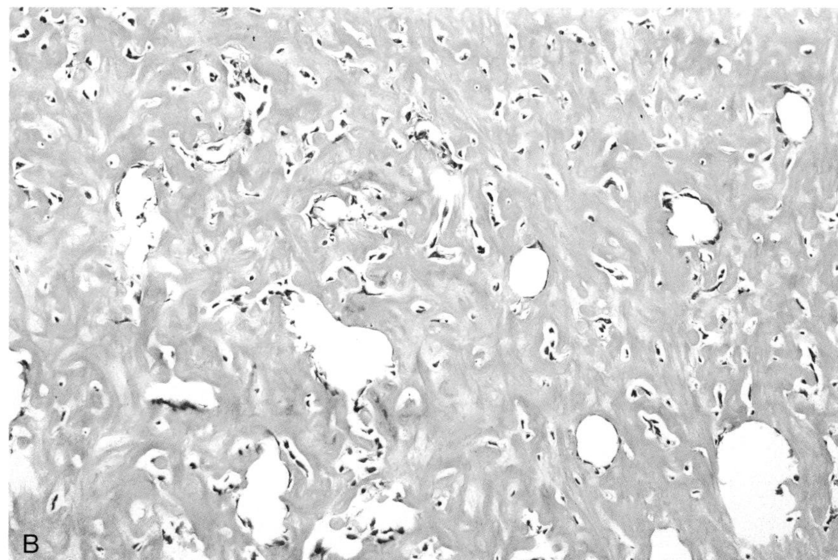

FIGURE 30-38, cont'd. (B) In this portion of the tumor, there is a broad expanse of osteoid with relatively few malignant cells.

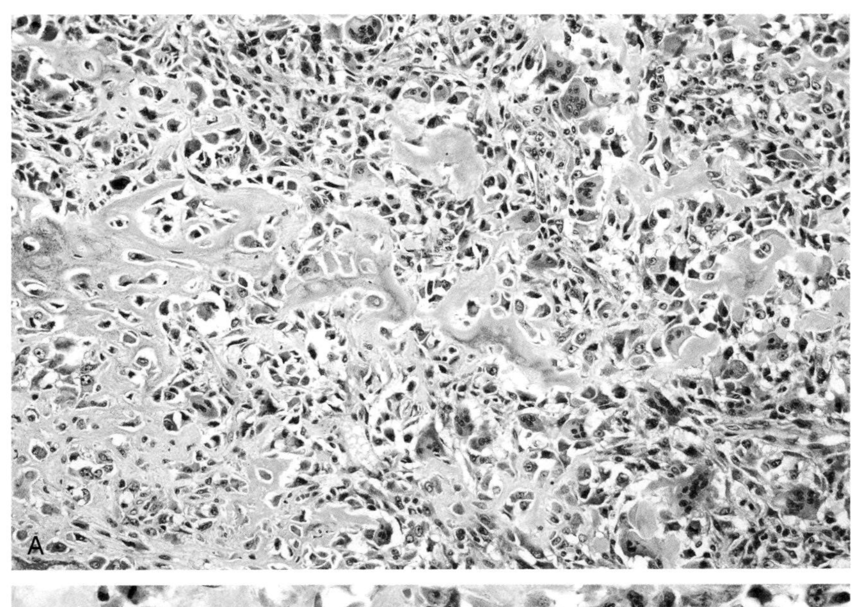

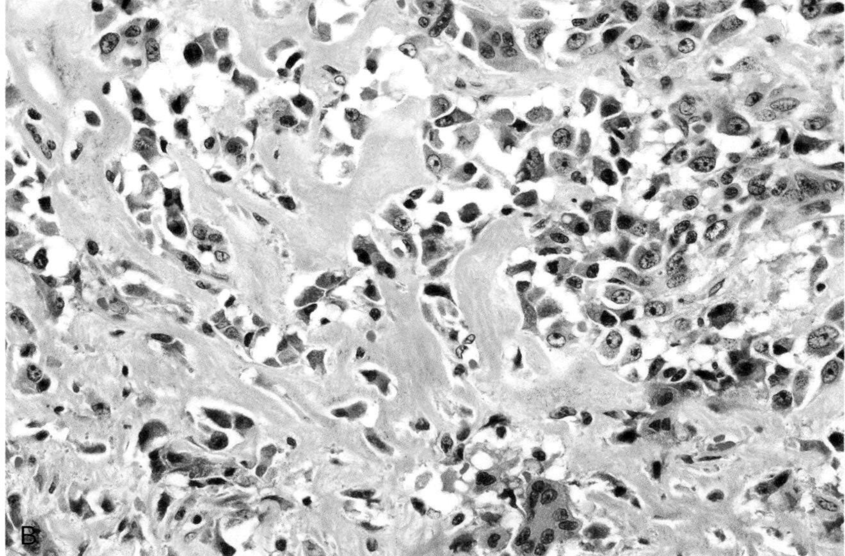

FIGURE 30-39. (A) Extraskeletal osteosarcoma of the thigh. Bands of osteoid material are seen between pleomorphic spindle-shaped and epithelioid cells. (B) High-magnification view of malignant cells depositing osteoid in an extraskeletal osteosarcoma.

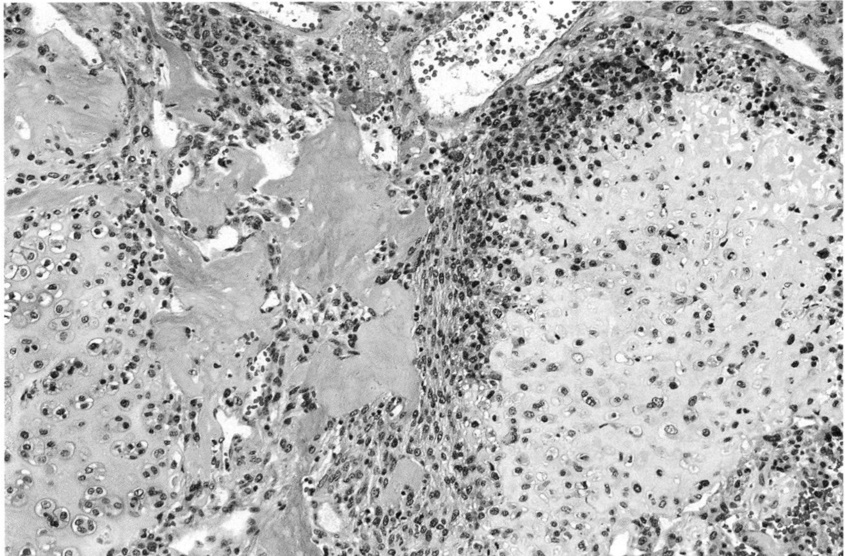

FIGURE 30-40. Osteoblastic osteosarcoma with chondroblastic and osteoblastic areas adjacent to one another.

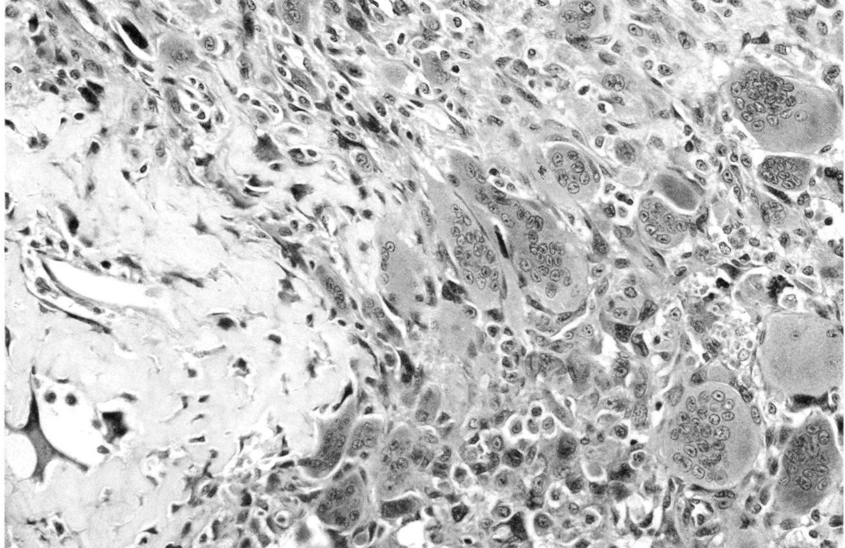

FIGURE 30-41. Osteoclast-like giant cells in an extraskeletal osteosarcoma.

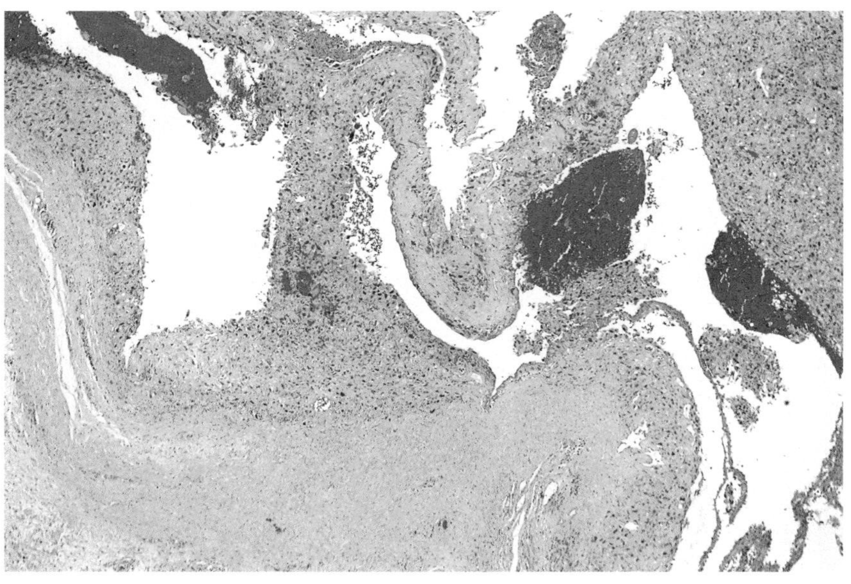

FIGURE 30-42. Telangiectatic extraskeletal osteosarcoma with markedly dilated blood-filled spaces lined by pleomorphic tumor cells.

osteosarcoma) have also been described (Fig. 30-43).[134] Metastatic lesions closely resemble their primary neoplasms.

Immunohistochemical Findings

In recent years, monoclonal antibodies to osteocalcin and osteonectin have been used in an attempt to recognize skeletal and extraskeletal osteosarcoma.[135] Fanburg-Smith et al.[135] found that an antibody to osteocalcin was 82% sensitive for extraskeletal osteosarcoma neoplastic cells, with immunostaining of neoplastic cells away from bone in 91% of cases and in 75% for bony tumor matrix. They reported 100% specificity for osteoblasts because this antigen was nonreactive in all non-bone cells. However, an antibody to osteonectin was not specific for osteoblasts. These markers have not been found to be particularly helpful in solidifying this diagnosis.

Differential Diagnosis

It can be quite challenging to distinguish extraskeletal osteosarcoma from other benign and malignant bone- and cartilage-forming soft tissue lesions. The differentiation from *myositis ossificans* and other reactive reparative processes has already been discussed in the chapter (see Table 30-2). Among malignant tumors, metaplastic bone may be found in synovial sarcoma, epithelioid sarcoma, malignant melanoma, and a number of other mesenchymal or epithelial neoplasms. In most of these neoplasms, osteoid or bone is confined to a small portion of the tumor and is relatively well differentiated without the disorderly pattern and cellular pleomorphism of osteosarcoma. For some of them, however, it is exceedingly difficult to reach a definitive diagnosis and to exclude osteosarcoma. In fact, at times, the only distinguishing feature between extraskeletal osteosarcoma and other high-grade pleomorphic (MFH-like) tumors with metaplastic bone is the relatively small amounts of neoplastic osteoid and bone in the latter tumor. The presence of the osseous and chondroid elements in the fibrous septa and pseudocapsule favors a pleomorphic sarcoma.[136] Bane et al.,[137] on the other hand, propose that the production of any neoplastic osteoid or bone in a pleomorphic sarcoma, no matter how focal, warrants a diagnosis of osteosarcoma. Therefore, the distinction between extraskeletal osteosarcoma and a high-grade pleomorphic sarcoma with bone is sometimes arbitrary, residing with the definitional criteria of the author.

Parosteal osteosarcoma may also make its appearance as a bulky lobulated, densely ossified soft tissue mass focally indistinguishable from an extraskeletal osteosarcoma. In most cases, this relatively low-grade tumor can be identified by its greater overall differentiation, its broad attachment to a thickened cortical bone, and its tendency to encircle the shaft of the bone and cause cortical erosion.[138] Differential diagnostic considerations must also include *periosteal osteosarcoma*,[139] a more aggressive and less-well-differentiated osteoblastic tumor that is often marked by a prominent chondroblastic component, and the rare *high-grade surface osteosarcoma*.[140]

Discussion

The outlook for patients with extraskeletal osteosarcoma is grave, and most patients with this tumor succumb to metastatic disease within 2 to 3 years after the initial diagnosis. In the series by Bane et al.,[137] 13 of 26 (50%) tumors recurred locally and 16 (61.5%) metastasized; five patients had distant metastases at presentation. Similarly, Lee et al.[116] reported local recurrences and distant metastases in 45% and 65% of patients, respectively, with 33 of 40 (83%) patients dying of tumor during the follow-up period. The lungs constitute the most common metastatic site, followed by the liver, bones, regional lymph nodes, and soft tissue. Despite the dismal prognosis, combination therapy with radical surgery (possibly limb-sparing segmental resection as an alternative to amputation), radiotherapy, and sequential preoperative or postoperative multiagent chemotherapy should be carried out in the hope of improving survival. In a multi-institutional study of 20 patients from the Japanese Musculoskeletal Oncology

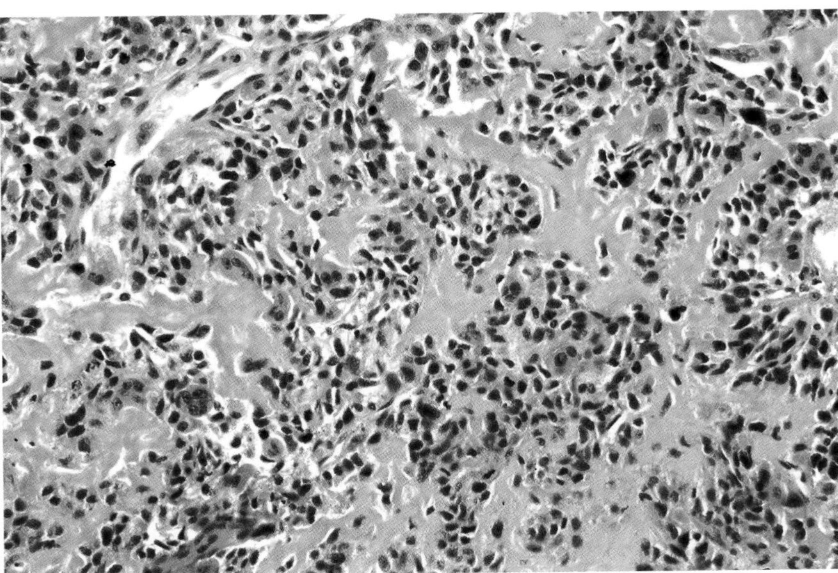

FIGURE 30-43. Extraskeletal osteosarcoma composed predominantly of small round cells adjacent to bands of osteoid.

Group, a response rate of 45% was reported in patients treated with multiagent chemotherapy.[141]

Tumor size, histologic subtype, and proliferation index have been proposed as prognostic variables. Bane et al.[137] found that a tumor size of 5 cm or more was an unfavorable prognostic indicator, although tumor size was not found to be of prognostic significance in other series.[116] Chung and Enzinger[119] found that patients with the fibroblastic type of extraskeletal osteosarcoma had a slightly better prognosis than those with other histologic subtypes, whereas Lee et al.[116] reported that patients with the chondroblastic type fared slightly better.

References

1. Patel RM, Weiss SW, Folpe AL. Heterotopic mesenteric ossification: a distinctive pseudosarcoma commonly associated with intestinal obstruction. Am J Surg Pathol 2006;30(1):119–22.
2. Wilson JD, Montague CJ, Salcuni P, et al. Heterotopic mesenteric ossification ("intraabdominal myositis ossificans"): report of five cases. Am J Surg Pathol 1999;23(12):1464–70.
3. Maender C, Sahajpal D, Wright TW. Treatment of heterotopic ossification of the elbow following burn injury: recommendations for surgical excision and perioperative prophylaxis using radiation therapy. J Shoulder Elbow Surg 2010;19(8):1269–75.
4. Vanden Bossche L, Vanderstraeten G. Heterotopic ossification: a review. J Rehabil Med 2005;37(3):129–36.
5. Myllylä RM, Haapasaari KM, Palatsi R, et al. Multiple miliary osteoma cutis is a distinct disease entity: four case reports and review of the literature. Br J Dermatol 2011;164(3):544–52.
6. Konishi E, Kusuzaki K, Murata H, et al. Extraskeletal osteosarcoma arising in myositis ossificans. Skeletal Radiol 2001;30(1):39–43.
7. Dahlin C, Salvador H. Cartilaginous tumors of the soft tissues of the hands and feet. Mayo Clin Proc 1974;49:721.
8. Chung EB, Enzinger FM. Chondroma of soft parts. Cancer 1978;41(4):1414–24.
9. Bergmann M, Pinz W, Blasius S, et al. Chondroid tumors arising from the meninges–report of 2 cases and review of the literature. Clin Neuropathol 2004;23(4):149–53.
10. Kwon H, Kim HY, Jung SN, et al. Extraskeletal chondroma in the auricle. J Craniofac Surg 2010;21(6):1990–1.
11. Aslam MB, Haqqani MT. Extraskeletal chondroma of parotid gland. Histopathology 2006;48(4):465–7.
12. Varras M, Akrivis C, Tsoukalos G, et al. Tubal ectopic pregnancy associated with an extraskeletal chondroma of the fallopian tube: case report. Clin Exp Obstet Gynecol 2008;35(1):83–5.
13. Smida M, Abdenaji W, Douira-Khomsi W, et al. Childhood soft tissue chondroma. Two cases report. Tunis Med 2011;89(4):379–82.
14. Dellon AL, Weiss SW, Mitch WE. Bilateral extraosseous chondromas of the hand in a patient with chronic renal failure. J Hand Surg Am 1978;3(2):139–41.
15. Bansal M, Goldman AB, DiCarlo EF, et al. Soft tissue chondromas: diagnosis and differential diagnosis. Skeletal Radiol 1993;22(5):309–15.
16. Singh VK, Shah G, Singh PK, et al. Extraskeletal ossifying chondroma in Hoffa's fat pad: an unusual cause of anterior knee pain. Singapore Med J 2009;50(5):e189–92.
17. Le Corroller T, Bouvier-Labit C, Champsaur P. Diffuse mineralization of forearm extraskeletal chondroma. Joint Bone Spine 2008;75(4):479–81.
18. del Rosario AD, Bui HX, Singh J, et al. Intracytoplasmic eosinophilic hyaline globules in cartilaginous neoplasms: a surgical, pathological, ultrastructural, and electron probe x-ray microanalytic study. Hum Pathol 1994;25(12):1283–9.
19. Yamada T, Irisa T, Nakano S, et al. Extraskeletal chondroma with chondroblastic and granuloma-like elements. Clin Orthop Relat Res 1995;(315):257–61.
20. Isayama T, Iwasaki H, Kikuchi M. Chondroblastoma-like extraskeletal chondroma. Clin Orthop Relat Res 1991;(268):214–17.
21. Cates JM, Rosenberg AE, O'Connell JX, et al. Chondroblastoma-like chondroma of soft tissue: an underrecognized variant and its differential diagnosis. Am J Surg Pathol 2001;25(5):661–6.
22. Bridge JA, Bhatia PS, Anderson JR, et al. Biologic and clinical significance of cytogenetic and molecular cytogenetic abnormalities in benign and malignant cartilaginous lesions. Cancer Genet Cytogenet 1993;69(2):79–90.
23. Tallini G, Dorfman H, Brys P, et al. Correlation between clinicopathological features and karyotype in 100 cartilaginous and chordoid tumours. A report from the Chromosomes and Morphology (CHAMP) Collaborative Study Group. J Pathol 2002;196(2):194–203.
24. Buddingh EP, Naumann S, Nelson M, et al. Cytogenetic findings in benign cartilaginous neoplasms. Cancer Genet Cytogenet 2003;141(2):164–8.
25. Sakai Junior N, Abe KT, Formigli LM, et al. Cytogenetic findings in 14 benign cartilaginous neoplasms. Cancer Genet 2011;204(4):180–6.
26. McKenzie G, Raby N, Ritchie D. A pictorial review of primary synovial osteochondromatosis. Eur Radiol 2008;18(11):2662–9.
27. Walker EA, Murphey MD, Fetsch JF. Imaging characteristics of tenosynovial and bursal chondromatosis. Skeletal Radiol 2011;40(3):317–25.
28. Sah AP, Geller DS, Mankin HJ, et al. Malignant transformation of synovial chondromatosis of the shoulder to chondrosarcoma. A case report. J Bone Joint Surg Am 2007;89(6):1321–8.
29. Reeh MJ. Hemangiopericytoma with cartilaginous differentiation involving orbit. Arch Ophthalmol 1966;75(1):82–3.
30. Huvos AG, Rosen G, Dabska M, et al. Mesenchymal chondrosarcoma. A clinicopathologic analysis of 35 patients with emphasis on treatment. Cancer 1983;51(7):1230–7.
31. Nakashima Y, Unni KK, Shives TC, et al. Mesenchymal chondrosarcoma of bone and soft tissue. A review of 111 cases. Cancer 1986;57(12):2444–53.
32. Cesari M, Bertoni F, Bacchini P, et al. Mesenchymal chondrosarcoma. An analysis of patients treated at a single institution. Tumori 2007;93(5):423–7.
33. Bertoni F, Picci P, Bacchini P, et al. Mesenchymal chondrosarcoma of bone and soft tissues. Cancer 1983;52(3):533–41.
34. De Cecio R, Migliaccio I, Falleti J, et al. Congenital intracranial mesenchymal chondrosarcoma: case report and review of the literature in pediatric patients. Pediatr Dev Pathol 2008;11(4):309–13.
35. Tuncer S, Kebudi R, Peksayar G, et al. Congenital mesenchymal chondrosarcoma of the orbit: case report and review of the literature. Ophthalmology 2004;111(5):1016–22.
36. Guccion JG, Font RL, Enzinger FM, et al. Extraskeletal mesenchymal chondrosarcoma. Arch Pathol 1973;95(5):336–40.
37. Bu X, Dai X. Primary mesenchymal chondrosarcoma of the pancreas. Ann R Coll Surg Engl 2010;92(3):W10–12.
38. Taori K, Patil P, Attarde V, et al. Primary retroperitoneal extraskeletal mesenchymal chondrosarcoma: a computed tomography diagnosis. Br J Radiol 2007;80(959):e268–70.
39. Suster S, Moran CA. Malignant cartilaginous tumors of the mediastinum: clinicopathological study of six cases presenting as extraskeletal soft tissue masses. Hum Pathol 1997;28(5):588–94.
40. Misra V, Singh PA. Cytodiagnosis of extraosseous mesenchymal chondrosarcoma of meninges: a case report. Acta Cytol 2008;52(3):366–8.
41. Gelderblom H, Hogendoorn PC, Dijkstra SD, et al. The clinical approach towards chondrosarcoma. Oncologist 2008;13(3):320–9.
42. Devoe K, Weidner N. Immunohistochemistry of small round-cell tumors. Semin Diagn Pathol 2000;17(3):216–24.
43. Swanson PE, Lillemoe TJ, Manivel JC, et al. Mesenchymal chondrosarcoma. An immunohistochemical study. Arch Pathol Lab Med 1990;114(9):943–8.
44. Fanburg-Smith JC, Auerbach A, Marwaha JS, et al. Immunoprofile of mesenchymal chondrosarcoma: aberrant desmin and EMA expression, retention of INI1, and negative estrogen receptor in 22 female-predominant central nervous system and musculoskeletal cases. Ann Diagn Pathol 2010;14(1):8–14.
45. Devaney K, Abbondanzo SL, Shekitka KM, et al. MIC2 detection in tumors of bone and adjacent soft tissues. Clin Orthop Relat Res 1995;(310):176–87.
46. Granter SR, Renshaw AA, Fletcher CD, et al. CD99 reactivity in mesenchymal chondrosarcoma. Hum Pathol 1996;27(12):1273–6.
47. Hoang MP, Suarez PA, Donner LR, et al. Mesenchymal chondrosarcoma: a small cell neoplasm with polyphenotypic differentiation. Int J Surg Pathol 2000;8(4):291–301.
48. Lee AF, Hayes MM, Lebrun D, et al. FLI-1 distinguishes Ewing sarcoma from small cell osteosarcoma and mesenchymal chondrosarcoma. Appl Immunohistochem Mol Morphol 2011;19(3):233–8.
49. Wehrli BM, Huang W, De Crombrugghe B, et al. Sox9, a master regulator of chondrogenesis, distinguishes mesenchymal chondrosarcoma from other small blue round cell tumors. Hum Pathol 2003;34(3):263–9.

50. Fanburg-Smith JC, Auerbach A, Marwaha JS, et al. Reappraisal of mesenchymal chondrosarcoma: novel morphologic observations of the hyaline cartilage and endochondral ossification and beta-catenin, Sox9, and osteocalcin immunostaining of 22 cases. Hum Pathol 2010;41(5):653–62.
51. Shakked RJ, Geller DS, Gorlick R, et al. Mesenchymal chondrosarcoma: clinicopathologic study of 20 cases. Arch Pathol Lab Med 2012;136(1):61–75.
52. Wang L, Motoi T, Khanin R, et al. Identification of a novel, recurrent HEY1-NCOA2 fusion in mesenchymal chondrosarcoma based on a genome-wide screen of exon-level expression data. Genes Chromosomes Cancer 2012;51(2):127–39.
53. Dantonello TM, Int-Veen C, Leuschner I, et al. Mesenchymal chondrosarcoma of soft tissues and bone in children, adolescents, and young adults: experiences of the CWS and COSS study groups. Cancer 2008;112(11):2424–31.
54. Ackerman LV. Extra-osseous localized non-neoplastic bone and cartilage formation (so-called myositis ossificans): clinical and pathological confusion with malignant neoplasms. J Bone Joint Surg Am 1958;40-A(2):279–98.
55. Beiner JM, Jokl P. Muscle contusion injury and myositis ossificans traumatica. Clin Orthop Relat Res 2002;(Suppl. 403):S110–19.
56. Muir B. Myositis ossificans traumatica of the deltoid ligament in a 34 year old recreational ice hockey player with a 15 year post-trauma follow-up: a case report and review of the literature. J Can Chiropr Assoc 2010;54(4):229–42.
57. Lasry F, Touki A, Abkari A, et al. A rare cause of painful cervical swelling: myositis ossificans progressiva in childhood. Report of a case. Joint Bone Spine 2005;72(4):335–7.
58. Conner GA, Duffy M. Myositis ossificans: a case report of multiple recurrences following third molar extractions and review of the literature. J Oral Maxillofac Surg 2009;67(4):920–6.
59. Katz LD, Lindskog D, Eisen R. Neuritis ossificans of the tibial, common peroneal and lateral sural cutaneous nerves. J Bone Joint Surg Br 2011;93(7):992–4.
60. Patel S, Richards A, Trehan R, et al. Post-traumatic myositis ossificans of the sternocleidomastoid following fracture of the clavicle: a case report. Cases J 2008;1(1):413.
61. Hashash JG, Zakhary L, Aoun EG, et al. Heterotopic mesenteric ossification. Colorectal Dis 2012;14(1):e29–30.
62. Martin DA, Senanayake S. Images in clinical medicine. Myositis ossificans. N Engl J Med 2011;364(8):758.
63. Tyler P, Saifuddin A. The imaging of myositis ossificans. Semin Musculoskelet Radiol 2010;14(2):201–16.
64. de Silva MV, Reid R. Myositis ossificans and fibroosseous pseudotumor of digits: a clinicopathological review of 64 cases with emphasis on diagnostic pitfalls. Int J Surg Pathol 2003;11(3):187–95.
65. Konishi E, Kusuzaki K, Murata H, et al. Extraskeletal osteosarcoma arising in myositis ossificans. Skeletal Radiol 2001;30(1):39–43.
66. Järvi OH, Kvist HT, Vainio PV. Extraskeletal retroperitoneal osteosarcoma probably arising from myositis ossificans. Acta Pathol Microbiol Scand 1968;74(1):11–25.
67. Lagier R, Cox JN. Pseudomalignant myositis ossificans. A pathological study of eight cases. Hum Pathol 1975;6(6):653–65.
68. Shin SJ, Kang SS. Myositis ossificans of the elbow after a trigger point injection. Clin Orthop Surg 2011;3(1):81–5.
69. Barwad A, Banik T, Gorsi U, et al. Fine needle aspiration cytology of myositis ossificans. Diagn Cytopathol 2011;39(6):432–4.
70. Nisolle JF, Delaunois L, Trigaux JP. Myositis ossificans of the chest wall. Eur Respir J 1996;9(1):178–9.
71. Mathew SE, Madhuri V, Alexander M, et al. Florid reactive periostitis of the forearm bones in a child. J Bone Joint Surg Br 2011;93(3):418–20.
72. Patel MR, Desai SS. Pseudomalignant osseous tumor of soft tissue: a case report and review of the literature. J Hand Surg Am 1986;11(1):66–70.
73. Park C, Park J, Lee KY. Parosteal (nodular) fasciitis of the hand. Clin Radiol 2004;59(4):376–8.
74. Dupree WB, Enzinger FM. Fibro-osseous pseudotumor of the digits. Cancer 1986;58(9):2103–9.
75. Spjut HJ, Dorfman HD. Florid reactive periostitis of the tubular bones of the hands and feet. A benign lesion which may simulate osteosarcoma. Am J Surg Pathol 1981;5(5):423–33.
76. Chaudhry IH, Kazakov DV, Michal M, et al. Fibro-osseous pseudotumor of the digit: a clinicopathological study of 17 cases. J Cutan Pathol 2010;37(3):323–9.
77. Tan KB, Tan SH, Aw DC, et al. Fibro-osseous pseudotumor of the digit: presentation as an enlarging erythematous cutaneous nodule. Dermatol Online J 2010;16(12):7.
78. Sundaram M, Wang L, Rotman M, et al. Florid reactive periostitis and bizarre parosteal osteochondromatous proliferation: pre-biopsy imaging evolution, treatment and outcome. Skeletal Radiol 2001;30(4):192–8.
79. Berber O, Dawson-Bowling S, Jalgaonkar A, et al. Bizarre parosteal osteochondromatous proliferation of bone: clinical management of a series of 22 cases. J Bone Joint Surg Br 2011;93(8):1118–21.
80. Craver RD, Correa-Gracian H, Heinrich S. Florid reactive periostitis. Hum Pathol 1997;28(6):745–7.
81. Trigui M, Ayadi K, Zribi M, et al. Fibrodysplasia ossificans progressiva: diagnosis and surgical management. Acta Orthop Belg 2011;77(2):139–44.
82. Tran L, Stein N, Miller S. Fibrodysplasia ossificans progressiva: early diagnosis is critical yet challenging. J Pediatr 2010;157(5):860.e1.
83. Kaplan FS, Le Merrer M, Glaser DL, et al. Fibrodysplasia ossificans progressiva. Best Pract Res Clin Rheumatol 2008;22(1):191–205.
84. Kaplan FS, Tabas JA, Gannon FH, et al. The histopathology of fibrodysplasia ossificans progressiva. An endochondral process. J Bone Joint Surg Am 1993;75(2):220–30.
85. Glaser DL, Rocke DM, Kaplan FS. Catastrophic falls in patients who have fibrodysplasia ossificans progressiva. Clin Orthop Relat Res 1998;(346):110–16.
86. Herford AS, Boyne PJ. Ankylosis of the jaw in a patient with fibrodysplasia ossificans progressiva. Oral Surg Oral Med Oral Pathol Oral Radiol Endod 2003;96(6):680–4.
87. Kaplan FS, Zasloff MA, Kitterman JA, et al. Early mortality and cardiorespiratory failure in patients with fibrodysplasia ossificans progressiva. J Bone Joint Surg Am 2010;92(3):686–91.
88. Nakashima Y, Haga N, Kitoh H, et al. Deformity of the great toe in fibrodysplasia ossificans progressiva. J Orthop Sci 2010;15(6):804–9.
89. Kartal-Kaess M, Shore EM, Xu M, et al. Fibrodysplasia ossificans progressiva (FOP): watch the great toes! Eur J Pediatr 2010;169(11):1417–21.
90. Baysal T, Elmali N, Kutlu R, et al. The stone man: myositis (fibrodysplasia) ossificans progressiva. Eur Radiol 1998;8(3):479–81.
91. Deirmengian GK, Hebela NM, O'Connell M, et al. Proximal tibial osteochondromas in patients with fibrodysplasia ossificans progressiva. J Bone Joint Surg Am 2008;90(2):366–74.
92. Shiva Kumar R, Keerthiraj B, Kesavadas C. Teaching NeuroImages: MRI in fibrodysplasia ossificans progressiva. Neurology 2010;74(6):e20.
93. Kaplan F, Sawyer J, Connors S, et al. Urinary basic fibroblast growth factor. A biochemical marker for preosseous fibroproliferative lesions in patients with fibrodysplasia ossificans progressiva. Clin Orthop Relat Res 1998;(346):59–65.
94. Gannon FH, Valentine BA, Shore EM, et al. Acute lymphocytic infiltration in an extremely early lesion of fibrodysplasia ossificans progressiva. Clin Orthop Relat Res 1998;(346):19–25.
95. Gannon FH, Kaplan FS, Olmsted E, et al. Bone morphogenetic protein 2/4 in early fibromatous lesions of fibrodysplasia ossificans progressiva. Hum Pathol 1997;28(3):339–43.
96. Shore EM, Kaplan FS. Inherited human diseases of heterotopic bone formation. Nat Rev Rheumatol 2010;6(9):518–27.
97. Kaplan FS, McCluskey W, Hahn G, et al. Genetic transmission of fibrodysplasia ossificans progressiva. Report of a family. J Bone Joint Surg Am 1993;75(8):1214–20.
98. Kaplan FS, Xu M, Seemann P, et al. Classic and atypical fibrodysplasia ossificans progressiva (FOP) phenotypes are caused by mutations in the bone morphogenetic protein (BMP) type I receptor ACVR1. Hum Mutat 2009;30(3):379–90.
99. Janoff HB, Muenke M, Johnson LO, et al. Fibrodysplasia ossificans progressiva in two half-sisters: evidence for maternal mosaicism. Am J Med Genet 1996;61(4):320–4.
100. Fukuda T, Kohda M, Kanomata K, et al. Constitutively activated ALK2 and increased SMAD1/5 cooperatively induce bone morphogenetic protein signaling in fibrodysplasia ossificans progressiva. J Biol Chem 2009;284(11):7149–56.
101. Kaplan FS, Pignolo RJ, Shore EM. The FOP metamorphogene encodes a novel type I receptor that dysregulates BMP signaling. Cytokine Growth Factor Rev 2009;20(5-6):399–407.
102. Kaplan FS, Shen Q, Lounev V, et al. Skeletal metamorphosis in fibrodysplasia ossificans progressiva (FOP). J Bone Miner Metab 2008;26(6):521–30.
103. van Dinther M, Visser N, de Gorter DJ, et al. ALK2 R206H mutation linked to fibrodysplasia ossificans progressiva confers constitutive

activity to the BMP type I receptor and sensitizes mesenchymal cells to BMP-induced osteoblast differentiation and bone formation. J Bone Miner Res 2010;25(6):1208–15.

104. Ohte S, Shin M, Sasanuma H, et al. A novel mutation of ALK2, L196P, found in the most benign case of fibrodysplasia ossificans progressiva activates BMP-specific intracellular signaling equivalent to a typical mutation, R206H. Biochem Biophys Res Commun 2011;407(1): 213–18.
105. Gregson CL, Hollingworth P, Williams M, et al. A novel ACVR1 mutation in the glycine/serine-rich domain found in the most benign case of a fibrodysplasia ossificans progressiva variant reported to date. Bone 2011;48(3):654–8.
106. Song GA, Kim HJ, Woo KM, et al. Molecular consequences of the ACVR1(R206H) mutation of fibrodysplasia ossificans progressiva. J Biol Chem 2010;285(29):22542–53.
107. Kitterman JA, Kantanie S, Rocke DM, et al. Iatrogenic harm caused by diagnostic errors in fibrodysplasia ossificans progressiva. Pediatrics 2005;116(5):e654–61.
108. Francis MD, Valent DJ. Historical perspectives on the clinical development of bisphosphonates in the treatment of bone diseases. J Musculoskelet Neuronal Interact 2007;7(1):2–8.
109. Dua T, Kabra M, Kalra V. Familial fibrodysplasia ossificans progressiva: trial with etidronate disodium. Indian Pediatr 2001;38(11): 1305–9.
110. Shimono K, Tung WE, Macolino C, et al. Potent inhibition of heterotopic ossification by nuclear retinoic acid receptor-γ agonists. Nat Med 2011;17(4):454–60.
111. Soldić Z, Murgić J, Radić J, et al. Radiation therapy in treatment of fibrodysplasia ossificans progressiva: a case report and review of the literature. Coll Antropol 2011;35(2):611–14.
112. Klein MJ, Siegal GP. Osteosarcoma: anatomic and histologic variants. Am J Clin Pathol 2006;125(4):555–81.
113. Allan CJ, Soule EH. Osteogenic sarcoma of the somatic soft tissues. Clinicopathologic study of 26 cases and review of literature. Cancer 1971;27(5):1121–33.
114. Lorentzon R, Larsson SE, Boquist L. Extra-osseous osteosarcoma: a clinical and histopathological study of four cases. J Bone Joint Surg Br 1979;61-B(2):205–8.
115. Siraj F, Jain D, Chopra P. Extraskeletal osteosarcoma of abdominal wall in a child. Ann Diagn Pathol 2011;15(2):131–4.
116. Lee JS, Fetsch JF, Wasdhal DA, et al. A review of 40 patients with extraskeletal osteosarcoma. Cancer 1995;76(11):2253–9.
117. Lidang Jensen M, Schumacher B, Myhre Jensen O, et al. Extraskeletal osteosarcomas: a clinicopathologic study of 25 cases. Am J Surg Pathol 1998;22(5):588–94.
118. Goldstein-Jackson SY, Gosheger G, Delling G, et al. Extraskeletal osteosarcoma has a favourable prognosis when treated like conventional osteosarcoma. J Cancer Res Clin Oncol 2005;131(8):520–6.
119. Chung EB, Enzinger FM. Extraskeletal osteosarcoma. Cancer 1987; 60(5):1132–42.
120. Papachristou DJ, Goodman M, Cieply K, et al. Extraskeletal osteosarcoma of subcutaneous soft tissue with lymph node and skin metastasis: a case report with fluorescence in situ hybridization analysis. Pathol Oncol Res 2012;18(1):107–10.
121. Heukamp LC, Knoblich A, Rausch E, et al. Extraosseous osteosarcoma arising from the small intestinal mesentery. Pathol Res Pract 2007; 203(6):473–7.
122. Hishida T, Yoshida J, Nishimura M, et al. Extraskeletal osteosarcoma arising in anterior mediastinum: brief report with a review of the literature. J Thorac Oncol 2009;4(7):927–9.
123. Tao SX, Tian GQ, Ge MH, et al. Primary extraskeletal osteosarcoma of omentum majus. World J Surg Oncol 2011;9(1):25.
124. Erra S, Costamagna D, Durando R. A rare case of extraskeletal osteosarcoma of the esophagus: an example of difficult diagnosis. G Chir 2010;31(1-2):24–7.
125. Murphey MD, Robbin MR, McRae GA, et al. The many faces of osteosarcoma. Radiographics 1997;17(5):1205–31.
126. Orta L, Suprun U, Goldfarb A, et al. Radiation-associated extraskeletal osteosarcoma of the chest wall. Arch Pathol Lab Med 2006;130(2): 198–200.
127. Laskin WB, Silverman TA, Enzinger FM. Postradiation soft tissue sarcomas. An analysis of 53 cases. Cancer 1988;62(11):2330–40.
128. Silver SA, Tavassoli FA. Primary osteogenic sarcoma of the breast: a clinicopathologic analysis of 50 cases. Am J Surg Pathol 1998;22(8): 925–33.
129. Ottaviani G, Jaffe N. The etiology of osteosarcoma. Cancer Treat Res 2009;152:15–32.
130. Hasson J, Hartman KS, Milikow E, et al. Thorotrast-induced extraskeletal osteosarcoma of the cervical region. Report of a case. Cancer 1975;36(5):1827–33.
131. Salamanca J, Dhimes P, Pinedo F, et al. Extraskeletal cutaneous chondroblastic osteosarcoma: a case report. J Cutan Pathol 2008;35(2): 231–5.
132. Lee KH, Joo JK, Kim DY, et al. Mesenteric extraskeletal osteosarcoma with telangiectatic features: a case report. BMC Cancer 2007;7:82.
133. Fukunaga M. Extraskeletal osteosarcoma histologically mimicking parosteal osteosarcoma. Pathol Int 2002;52(7):492–6.
134. Yang JY, Kim JM. Small cell extraskeletal osteosarcoma. Orthopedics 2009;32(3):217.
135. Fanburg-Smith JC, Bratthauer GL, Miettinen M. Osteocalcin and osteonectin immunoreactivity in extraskeletal osteosarcoma: a study of 28 cases. Hum Pathol 1999;30(1):32–8.
136. Bhagavan BS, Dorfman HD. The significance of bone and cartilage formation in malignant fibrous histiocytoma of soft tissue. Cancer 1982;49(3):480–8.
137. Bane BL, Evans HL, Ro JY, et al. Extraskeletal osteosarcoma. A clinicopathologic review of 26 cases. Cancer 1990;65(12):2762–70.
138. Funovics PT, Bucher F, Toma CD, et al. Treatment and outcome of parosteal osteosarcoma: biological versus endoprosthetic reconstruction. J Surg Oncol 2011;103(8):782–9.
139. Cesari M, Alberghini M, Vanel D, et al. Periosteal osteosarcoma: a single-institution experience. Cancer 2011;117(8):1731–5.
140. Staals EL, Bacchini P, Bertoni F. High-grade surface osteosarcoma: a review of 25 cases from the Rizzoli Institute. Cancer 2008;112(7): 1592–9.
141. Torigoe T, Yazawa Y, Takagi T, et al. Extraskeletal osteosarcoma in Japan: multiinstitutional study of 20 patients from the Japanese Musculoskeletal Oncology Group. J Orthop Sci 2007;12(5):424–9.

Miscellaneous Benign Soft Tissue Tumors and Pseudotumors

CHAPTER CONTENTS

This chapter discusses a heterogeneous group of benign tumors or pseudotumors, many of which are characterized by abundant myxoid stroma (intramuscular myxoma, juxta-articular myxoma, cutaneous myxoma, and ganglion, among others); there is evidence that the cells in these lesions are fibroblastic or have some features of myofibroblasts.

TUMORAL CALCINOSIS

Tumoral calcinosis is a distinct clinical and histologic entity that is characterized by tumor-like periarticular deposits of calcium that are found foremost in the regions of the hip, shoulder, and elbow. The disorder occurs predominantly in otherwise healthy children, adolescents, and young adults, is more often multiple than solitary, and not infrequently affects two or more siblings of the same family. Unlike similar calcifications associated with renal insufficiency, hypervitaminosis D, and milk-alkali syndrome, there are no demonstrable abnormalities in calcium metabolism.

Tumoral calcinosis encompasses a heterogeneous group of disorders that are characterized by tumor-like periarticular deposits of calcium hydroxyapatite. The term *tumoral calcinosis* was coined by Inclan[1] in 1943, but this condition was recognized as an entity much earlier. In 1899, Duret[2] observed this process in siblings: a 17-year-old girl and her younger brother who had multiple calcifications in the vicinity of the hip and elbow joint. Later, in 1935, Teutschlaender[3] gave a detailed account of another typical case, an 11-year-old girl with multiple lesions in the shoulder and elbow regions that had their onset at age 2 years. He thought that this process was secondary to fat necrosis and used the term *lipid calcinosis*. Since these descriptions, numerous other acceptable examples of this growth have been reported under various names, including *calcifying bursitis*,[4] *calcareous tendinitis*,[5] and *Kikuyu bursa*.[6] In New Guinea, the natives aptly refer to it as *hip stones*.[7]

Clinical Findings

There are essentially three forms of tumoral calcinosis (Fig. 31-1). The most common form is sporadic (nonfamilial) and idiopathic. This form has its onset during the first and second decades of life and is rare in patients older than 50 years. It affects Caucasian and African-Americans roughly equally, and there is a slight female preponderance. Most patients present with a solitary large, firm, subcutaneous calcified mass that is slowly growing and usually asymptomatic; it is typically located in the vicinity of a large joint, especially the trochanteric and gluteal regions of the hip and the lateral portion of the shoulder and the posterior elbow (Table 31-1). It is less commonly seen in the hands, feet, and knees,[8,9] and rare cases have been described in the scalp,[10] neck region,[11] and paraspinal region.[12] The lesion is firmly attached to the underlying fascia, muscle, or tendon and may even infiltrate these structures, but it is unrelated to bone, and the underlying joints are unaffected. Most of these patients are in otherwise good health.

There is also a familial form of tumoral calcinosis that comes in two varieties: hyperphosphatemic or normophosphatemic familial tumoral calcinosis, both of which are inherited in an autosomal recessive manner but are characterized by distinct genetic mutations. The hyperphosphatemic form, which appears to lie on a spectrum with the so-called *hyperostosis-hyperphosphatemic syndrome*, is characterized by mutations in *GALNT3*,[13-16] *FGF23*,[17-19] or the *KL* gene.[20] Biallelic mutations in *GALNT3* prevent degradation of the phosphaturic hormone fibroblast growth factor 23 (FGF23),[21] but defective function of any of these three genes results in hyperphosphatemia and ectopic calcifications.[22] In contrast, the normophosphatemic variant is associated with absence of functional *SAMD9*, a putative tumor suppressor gene.[22-24]

Both hereditary forms of this disease have a predilection for young males, especially African-Americans. These patients characteristically have elevation of serum phosphate and vitamin D, unless they have the normophosphatemic variant. The lesions are often multifocal and may be associated with a number of other bony abnormalities, including calcifications in the shaft of long bones and cranium as well as ocular and dental abnormalities.[25]

Finally, there is also a secondary form of tumoral calcinosis resulting from conditions that promote ectopic calcifications.[26] This is a wide range of conditions, which includes chronic

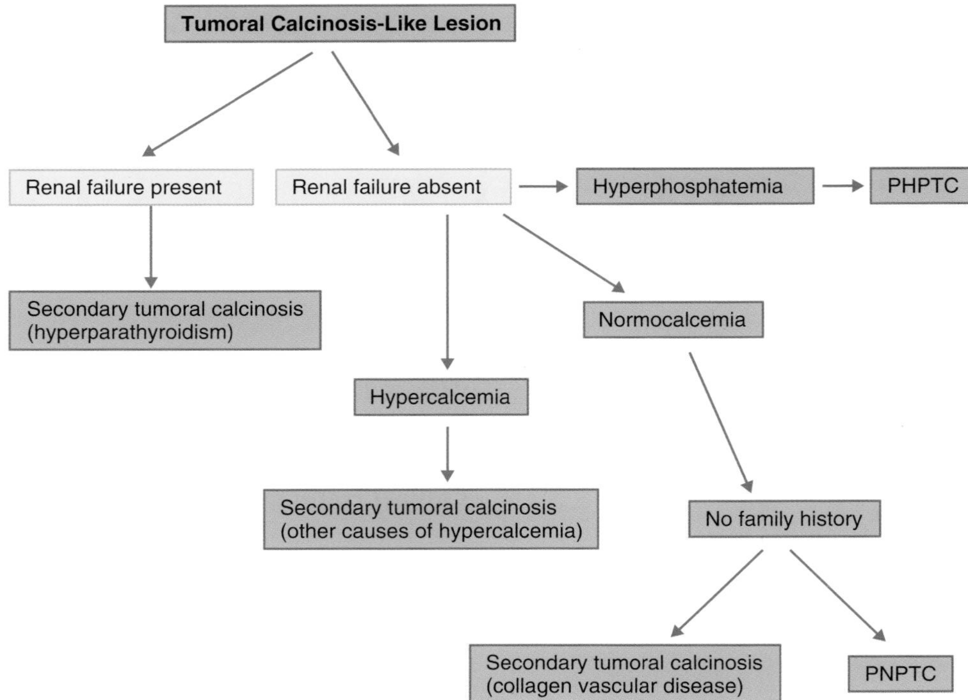

FIGURE 31-1. An algorithmic approach to tumoral calcinosis-like lesions. PHPTC, primary hyperphosphatemic tumoral calcinosis; PNPTC, primary normophosphatemic tumoral calcinosis. *Modified from Laskin WB, Miettinen M, Fetsch JF. Calcareous lesions of the distal extremities resembling tumoral calcinosis (tumoral calcinosis-like lesions): clinicopathologic study of 43 cases emphasizing a pathogenesis-based approach to classification. Am J Surg Pathol 2007;31(1):15–25.*

TABLE 31-1 Anatomic Locations of 105 Cases of Tumoral Calcinosis

SITE	NO. OF CASES	PERCENTAGE (%)
Hips	33	31
Buttocks	27	26
Upper extremities	16	15
Lower extremities	12	11
Spine/sacrum	7	7
Miscellaneous	10	10
Total	105	100

Modified from Pakasa NM, Kalengayi RM. Tumoral calcinosis: a clinicopathological study of 111 cases with emphasis on the earliest changes. Histopathology 1997;31(1):18–24.

renal failure, typically associated with secondary hyperparathyroidism,[27] systemic sclerosis,[28] sarcoidosis,[29] and primary hyperparathyroidism,[30] among many others. Treatment of the calcific lesions is best done by treating the underlying disorder.

Examination with radiography, CT, and MRI reveals a subcutaneous conglomerate of multiple, rounded opacities separated by radiolucent lines (fibrous septa) imparting a chicken-wire pattern of lucencies with distinct fluid levels in some of the nodules (Figs. 31-2 and 31-3).[31] Despite the large amounts of calcium in the lesion in patients with idiopathic tumoral calcinosis, there is no evidence of osteoporosis in the skeleton as in patients with renal insufficiency and secondary hyperparathyroidism.

Pathologic Findings

Study of the gross specimen discloses a firm, rubbery mass that is unencapsulated, extends into the adjacent muscles and tendons, and is usually 5 to 15 cm in greatest diameter. On sectioning, the mass consists of a framework of dense fibrous tissue containing spaces filled with yellow-gray, pasty, calcareous material or chalky, milky liquid that is easily washed out, resulting in irregular cystic cavities.

Microscopically, active and inactive phases of the disease can be distinguished, often together in the same lesion (Figs. 31-4 and 31-5). Slavin et al.[32] proposed a three-stage classification scheme to describe these lesions, spanning from cellular lesions devoid of calcification to cellular cystic lesions with calcification, and, finally, hypocellular calcified lesions. In the active (cellular) phase, a central mass of amorphous or granular calcified material is bordered by a florid proliferation of mononucleated or multinucleated macrophages, osteoclast-like giant cells, fibroblasts, and chronic inflammatory elements.[33] Fibrohistiocytic nodules may be seen during the early proliferative phase and are characterized by fibroblast-like cells, foamy histiocytes, occasional multinucleated macrophages, and hemosiderin-laden macrophages. During the inactive phase, there is merely calcified material surrounded by dense fibrous material extending into the adjacent tissues or a cystic space surrounded by calcium deposits. Sometimes the calcified material forms small psammoma body-like masses with concentric layering of calcium (calcospherites) that bear a superficial resemblance to ova of parasites.

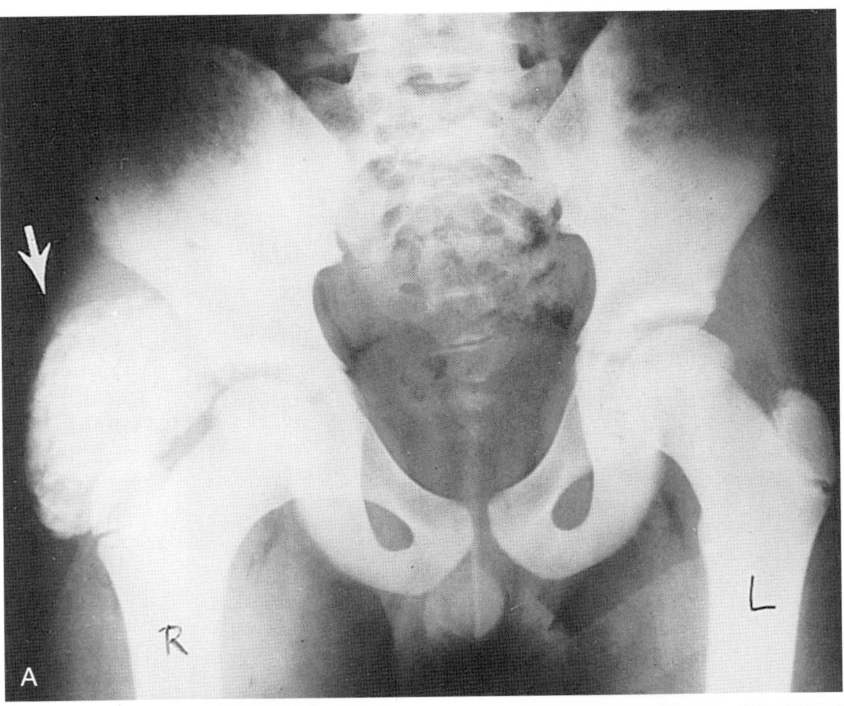

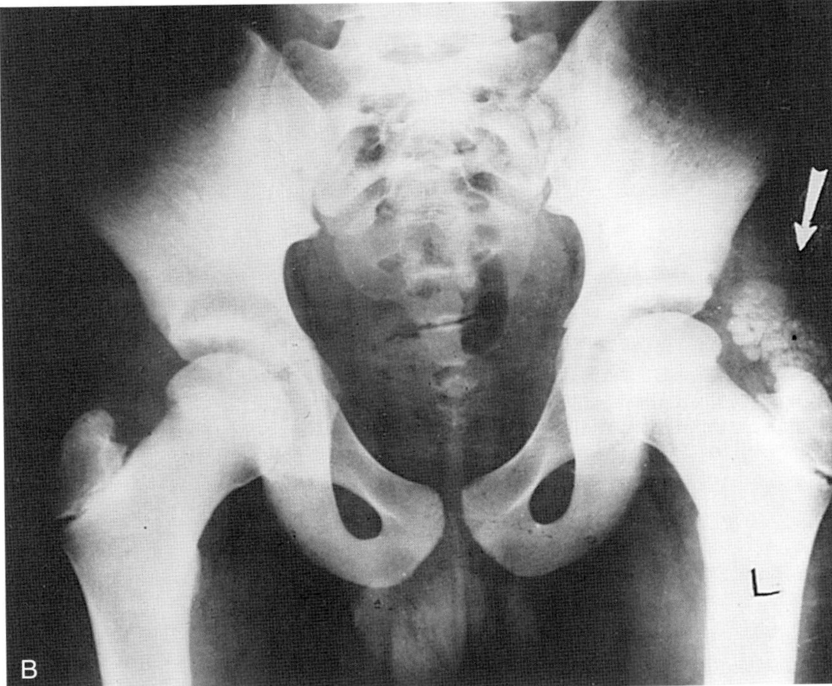

FIGURE 31-2. Radiograph of tumoral calcinosis involving the soft tissues of both hips *(arrows)*. Nine months after the calcified mass in the right hip (A) was removed, a second mass developed in the left hip (B).

Differential Diagnosis

Morphologically, the lesions of tumoral calcinosis are identical regardless of whether they are idiopathic, familial, or secondary. Patients with chronic renal disease and secondary hyperparathyroidism are usually older than those with idiopathic tumoral calcinosis, have additional calcifications in visceral organs such as the kidney, lung, heart, and stomach, and have abnormally low calcium levels.[34] There are also tumoral calcinosis-like lesions and vascular calcifications associated with hyperphosphatemia in patients with end-stage renal disease undergoing hemodialysis.[27] Similar calcifying soft tissue lesions, but associated with hypercalcemia, occur in patients with primary hyperparathyroidism[30] and milk-alkali syndrome (Burnett syndrome),[35] a rare condition associated with prolonged antacid therapy for peptic ulcer. Patients with excessive osteolysis and mobilization of calcium in destructive neoplastic and infectious lesions of bone may also develop lesions that can resemble tumoral calcinosis. More recently, Laskin et al.[9] described a group of tumoral calcinosis-like

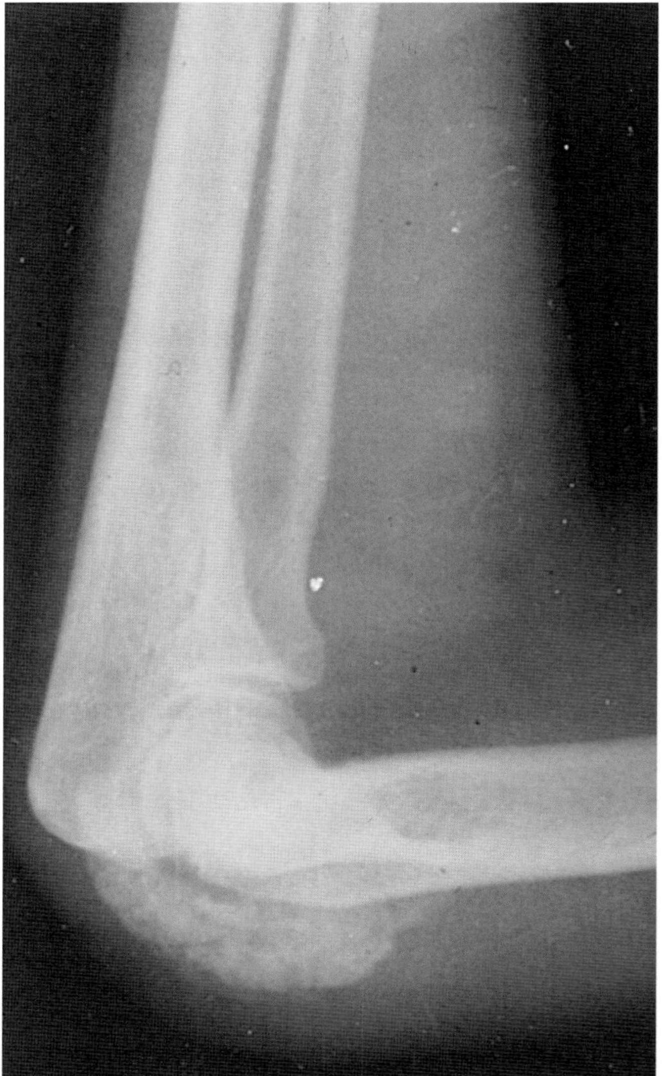

FIGURE 31-3. Tumoral calcinosis in the right elbow region of an 18-year-old man. The radiograph shows a calcified mass in the elbow region.

lesions that arise in an acral location and are smaller in size and seem to be pathogenetically distinct from tumoral calcinosis. In all of these lesions, a detailed clinical history and laboratory data aid in reaching a reliable diagnosis (see Table 31-1).

Calcinosis universalis and *calcinosis circumscripta* likewise are located in the skin and subcutis and are associated with normal serum calcium and phosphorus levels. Calcinosis universalis forms multiple nodules or plaques that occur mainly in children and are associated in about half of the cases with manifestations of scleroderma, systemic lupus erythematosus, or dermatomyositis.[36] It may ultimately lead to limited mobility, contractures, and ankylosis. Calcinosis circumscripta, on the other hand, chiefly affects middle-aged women and most commonly involves the hand and wrist, including tendon sheaths. It is associated in a large percentage of cases with Raynaud's disease or scleroderma, sclerodactyly, or polymyositis.[37] The CREST syndrome is a related condition involving *c*alcinosis cutis, *R*aynaud phenomenon, *e*sophageal hypomotility, *s*clerodactyly, and *t*elangiectasis.

There are also dystrophic calcifications, as in calcareous tendinitis or tenosynovitis, that show a similar microscopic picture but are smaller and develop in damaged tissue secondary to minor injury, ischemic necrosis, or a necrotizing infectious process.[38] Calcifications of tendons and ligaments have also been reported in patients undergoing long-term therapy with etretinate, a synthetic vitamin A derivative prescribed for acne, psoriasis, and various keratinization disorders.[39] Other forms of calcification, such as those of the scrotal skin, are not uncommon, but the exact cause is still not clear.[40]

Discussion

Although there are different familial and nonfamilial causes of tumoral calcinosis, the constellation of histologic features is fairly consistent. The largest study in the literature by Pakasa and Kalengayi[33] is composed of patients with familial, idiopathic, and secondary tumoral calcinosis, and, therefore, the observations made in that large series are not restricted to a single entity. Minor repeated trauma and tissue injury seem to

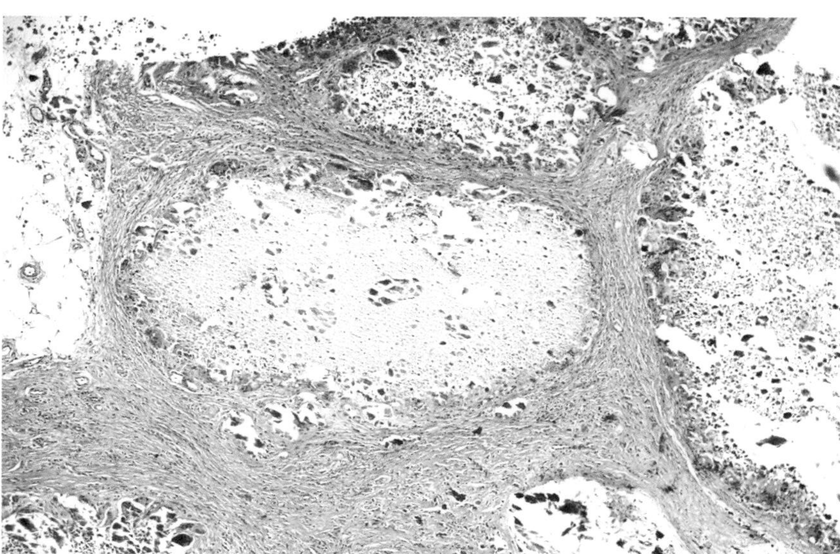

FIGURE 31-4. Tumoral calcinosis. Amorphous calcified material bordered by a florid proliferation of macrophages and multinucleated, osteoclast-like giant cells. The nodules are separated by bands of dense fibrous tissue.

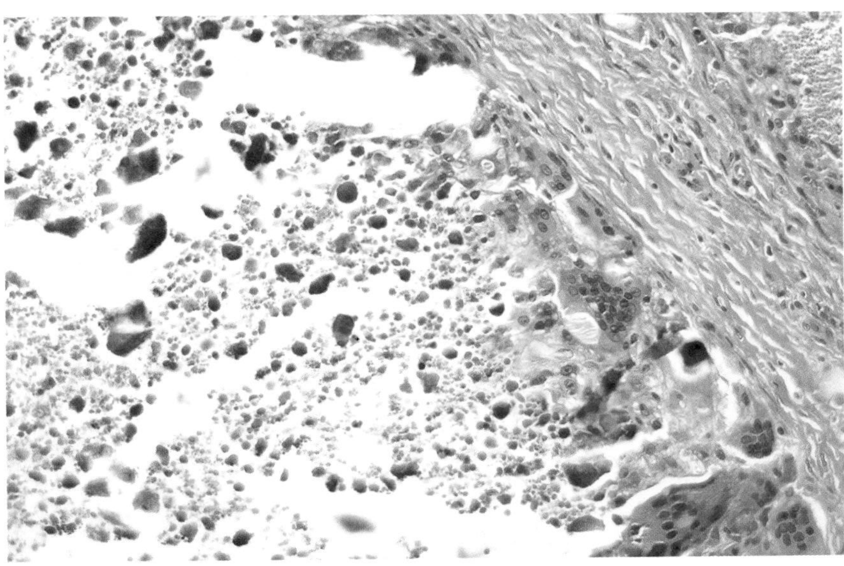

FIGURE 31-5. Tumoral calcinosis with a characteristic mixture of calcified material, histiocytes, and multinucleated giant cells.

play a role in the calcifying process in some cases, serving as a trigger mechanism in genetically susceptible individuals, leading to a chain of events that begins with hemorrhage, fat necrosis, fibrosis and collagenization, and ends with collagenolysis and, ultimately, calcification.

For familial and idiopathic lesions, surgical excision is the treatment of choice.[30] Although the majority of patients with idiopathic lesions are cured, familial lesions have a propensity to locally recur. A number of medical therapies have been attempted, with limited success. Treatment of the underlying systemic cause in patients with secondary tumoral calcinosis is critical for effective management.

INTRAMUSCULAR MYXOMA

There is a dizzying array of benign mesenchymal lesions characterized by abundant myxoid matrix, a small number of inconspicuous stellate- or spindle-shaped cells, and a poorly developed vascular pattern. Most are composed of modified fibroblasts that produce excessive amounts of glycosaminoglycans rich in hyaluronic acid and little collagen. Chief among them is the intramuscular myxoma, a benign mesenchymal lesion that is of particular importance because it is almost always cured by local excision yet is easily mistaken for a low-grade myxoid sarcoma.

Clinical Findings

Intramuscular myxoma is a tumor of adult life that occurs primarily in patients 40 to 70 years of age.[41-43] It is rare in young adults and virtually nonexistent in children and adolescents.[44] About two-thirds of the patients are women.[45,46] There is no evidence of increased familial incidence.

The clinical manifestations are nonspecific, and it is difficult to diagnose this tumor before biopsy and microscopic examination. In most patients, the sole presenting sign is a painless, palpable mass that is slightly movable and often fluctuant. Pain or tenderness is present in fewer than one-fourth

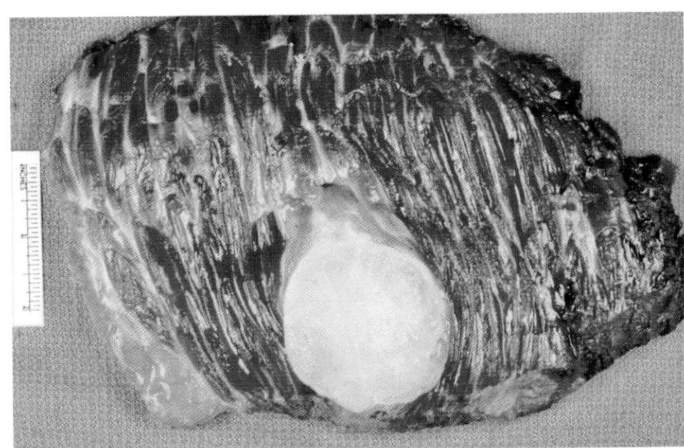

FIGURE 31-6. Intramuscular myxoma showing a uniform yellowish-white cut surface. The tumor characteristically appears well circumscribed.

of patients.[41] As one would expect, pain and occasional numbness, paresthesia, and muscle weakness distal to the lesion are mostly associated with tumors of large size. Because of the relative lack of symptoms, most are present for several months or even years before they are excised. The rate of growth varies, but there is no close relation between size and clinical duration. A history of trauma is rarely given, and the tumor is not etiologically related to thyroid dysfunction, as in myxedema.

By far, the most frequent sites of the tumor are the large muscles of the thigh, shoulder, buttocks, and upper arm (Fig. 31-6). Unusual examples have been reported in the muscles of the head and neck,[47] the forearm,[48] and even the small muscles of the hand.[49] The exact location in the musculature varies: some tumors are completely surrounded by muscle tissue, and others are firmly attached on one side to muscle fascia. There are also myxomas of identical appearance that arise from the periosteum, subchondral epiphysis, and joint capsule, discussed later. Angiographic examination reveals a poorly vascularized soft tissue mass surrounded by well-vascularized muscle tissue.[50] MRI reveals a well-defined, usually homogeneous tumor exhibiting low signal intensity relative to skeletal muscle on T1-weighted images and a hyperintense appearance relative to muscle on T2-weighted images.[51]

Multiple Intramuscular Myxomas and Fibrous Dysplasia

Although most intramuscular myxomas are solitary, there are occasional patients in whom two or more myxomas are present, usually in the same region of the body. Microscopically, these tumors are in no way different from the solitary intramuscular myxomas. Nearly all are associated with monostotic or polyostotic fibrous dysplasia of bone, generally in the same anatomic region where the myxomas are located (Fig. 31-7) (Mazabraud syndrome).[52,53] In this setting, females are affected more commonly than males, even more so than in solitary cases. Often there is a long interval between the appearances of the two processes. In most cases, the fibrous dysplasia is noted during the growth period, whereas the multiple myxomas, like their solitary forms, become apparent many years later during adult life. On occasion, multiple intramuscular myxomas are detected before the osseous lesions. If specifically sought, radiologically evident bone abnormalities are seen in many patients with intramuscular myxomas.[46] In the case reported by Mazabraud et al.,[54] an osteosarcoma developed in a patient with fibrous dysplasia and multiple myxomas, a phenomenon that has been noted by others. Activating missense mutations in the Arg201 codon of the gene encoding the alpha subunit of G_S (*GNAS1*), the G protein that stimulates cAMP formation, have been recognized in fibrous dysplasia of bone and McCune-Albright syndrome, a syndrome consisting of polyostotic fibrous dysplasia, sexual precocity, and café-au-lait spots.[55,56] Subsequently, these same mutations have been identified in intramuscular myxomas with and without fibrous dysplasia.[57] In a recent study by Delaney et al.,[58] 8 of 28 (29%) sporadic intramuscular myxomas were found to have *GNAS1* mutations using a conventional polymerase chain reaction (PCR) technique. However, using a more sensitive COLD (*co*amplification at *l*ower *d*enaturation temperature) PCR technique, 17 of 28 (61%) sporadic lesions harbored this mutation, which was not detected in any of the low-grade myxofibrosarcomas.

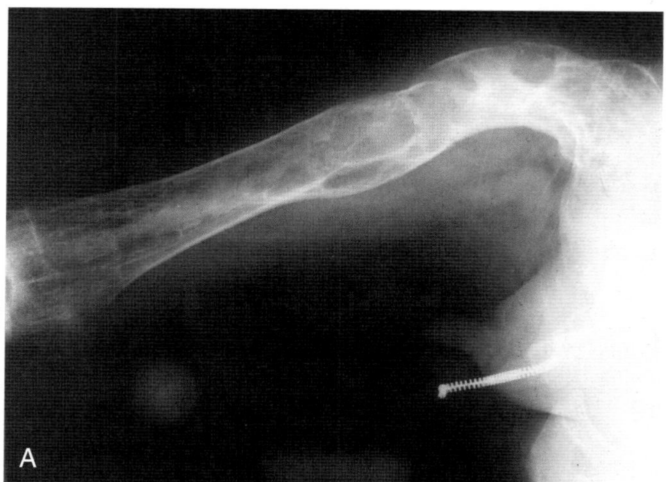

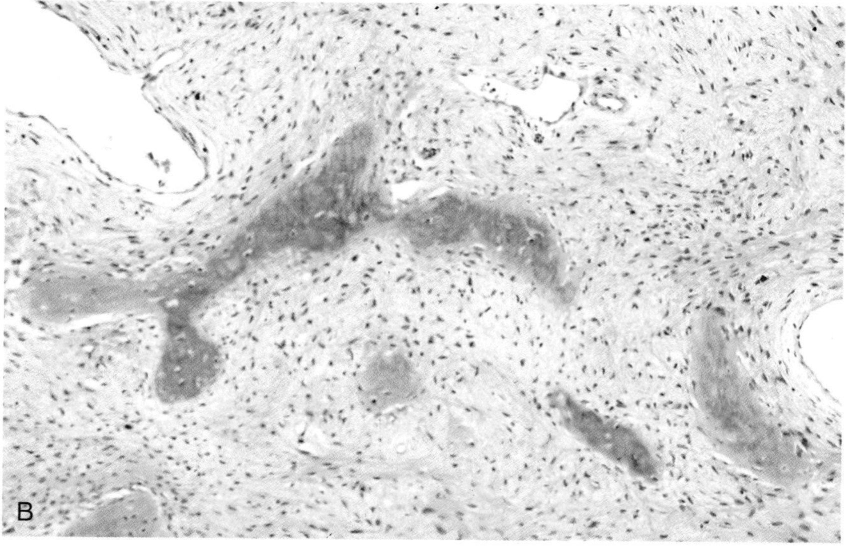

FIGURE 31-7. Patient with multiple intramuscular myxomas and fibrous dysplasia. (A) Characteristic radiographic features of fibrous dysplasia involving the humerus show a shepherd's crook deformity. (B) Histologic appearance of fibrous dysplasia. An intramuscular myxoma was found in the soft tissues adjacent to the humerus.

Pathologic Findings

The gross appearance is characteristic and varies little from case to case. Most tumors are ovoid or globular and have a glistening gray-white or white appearance, depending on the relative amounts of collagen and myxoid material (Fig. 31-8). They consist of a mass of stringy, gelatinous material with occasional small fluid-filled, cyst-like spaces, and they are covered by bundles of skeletal muscle or fascial tissue (Fig. 31-9). Although on gross examination most of the tumors appear to be well circumscribed, many infiltrate the adjacent musculature or are surrounded by edematous muscle tissue, which may serve as a natural cleavage plane for the surgeon. The size varies greatly; the majority measure 5 to 10 cm in greatest diameter, but some lesions are 20 cm or larger.

On histologic examination, the tumor varies little in its appearance and is composed of relatively small numbers of inconspicuous cells, abundant mucoid material, and a loose meshwork of reticulin fibers (Figs. 31-10 to 31-14). Characteristically, mature collagen fibers and vascular structures are sparse. Fluid-filled cystic spaces are seen occasionally (Fig. 31-15), but they are rarely a prominent feature. The constituent cells have small, hyperchromatic, pyknotic-appearing nuclei and scanty cytoplasm that sometimes extends along the reticulin fibers with multiple processes, giving the cell a stellate appearance (Figs. 31-16 and 31-17). There is little cellular pleomorphism, and there are no multinucleated giant cells. In some cases, there are also scattered macrophages with small intracellular droplets of lipid material (Fig. 31-18). The small size of these droplets and the absence of nuclear deformation or scalloping afford their distinction from lipoblasts. At the periphery, where the tumor merges with the surrounding muscle, fat cells and atrophic muscle fibers are occasionally scattered in the mucoid substance. These residual muscle fibers can be misinterpreted as evidence of rhabdomyoblastic differentiation, resulting in a misdiagnosis of rhabdomyosarcoma.

Some intramuscular myxomas show focal areas of hypercellularity and hypervascularity, which may cause further confusion with a low-grade myxoid sarcoma (so-called *cellular myxoma*) (Fig. 31-19).[59,60] In the study by Nielsen et al.,[59] 38 of 51 (76%) cases of intramuscular myxoma had hypercellular zones that comprised 10% to 80% of the tumor. However, even in these hypercellular zones, the cells lack nuclear atypia, and there is a paucity of mitotic figures and an absence of necrosis. Areas of more typical hypocellular intramuscular myxoma allow their definitive recognition.

Immunohistochemically, the cells may stain for actins, suggesting focal myofibroblastic differentiation. The macrophages containing lipid droplets are negative for S100 protein, unlike true lipoblasts. The cells are suspended in large amounts of mucoid material that stains positively with Alcian blue and colloidal iron stains and is depolymerized by prior treatment of the sections with hyaluronidase.[43] Ultrastructurally, the cells show evidence of fibroblastic differentiation.[50]

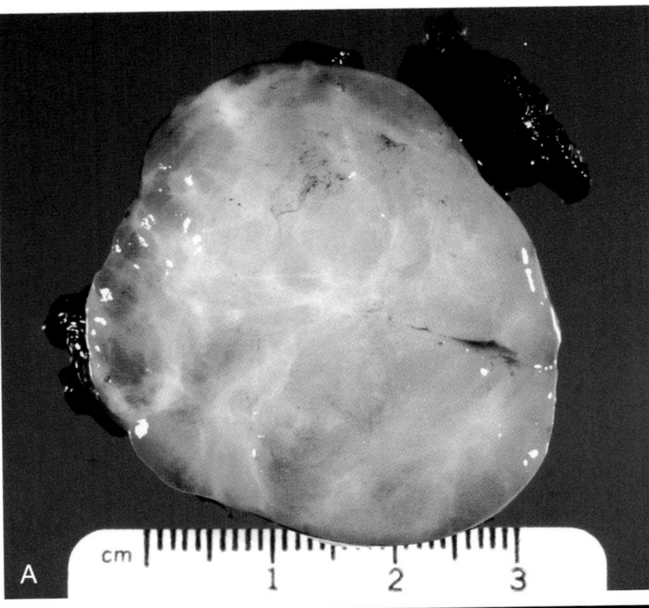

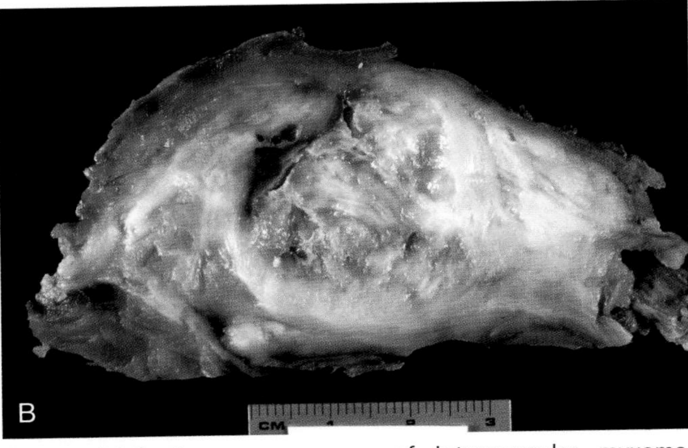

FIGURE 31-8. Gross appearances of intramuscular myxoma. (A) The tumor has a mucoid, gelatinous cut surface with thin fibrous septa. (B) Fibrous-appearing intramuscular myxoma.

Differential Diagnosis

Numerous benign and low-grade malignant myxoid neoplasms are apt to be confused with intramuscular myxoma (Table 31-2). At times, the tumor is difficult to distinguish from myxolipoma, myxoid neurofibroma, nerve sheath myxoma, chondroma with myxoid change and nodular fasciitis, conditions discussed in previous chapters. More important, intramuscular myxoma may be confused with low-grade myxoid sarcomas of various types. *Low-grade myxofibrosarcoma*, similar to intramuscular myxoma, predominantly affects adults and most often arises as an irregular infiltrating subcutaneous mass, although it can arise in deeper soft tissues. At the low end of the histologic spectrum, myxofibrosarcoma is a hypocellular neoplasm composed of spindle-shaped cells deposited in an abundant myxoid stroma. However, the cells always demonstrate a greater degree of nuclear hyperchromasia and cytologic atypia than those of intramuscular myxoma. Many of these neoplasms also have prominent curvilinear blood vessels, often with perivascular tumoral condensation. *Myxoid liposarcoma* is characterized by a regular plexiform vasculature with spindle-shaped or stellate cells with mild cytologic atypia deposited in a myxoid stroma. In addition, the identification of cells with adipocytic differentiation, including well-formed lipoblasts, is useful for this distinction. *Extraskeletal myxoid chondrosarcoma* is a multinodular tumor

Text continued on p. 958

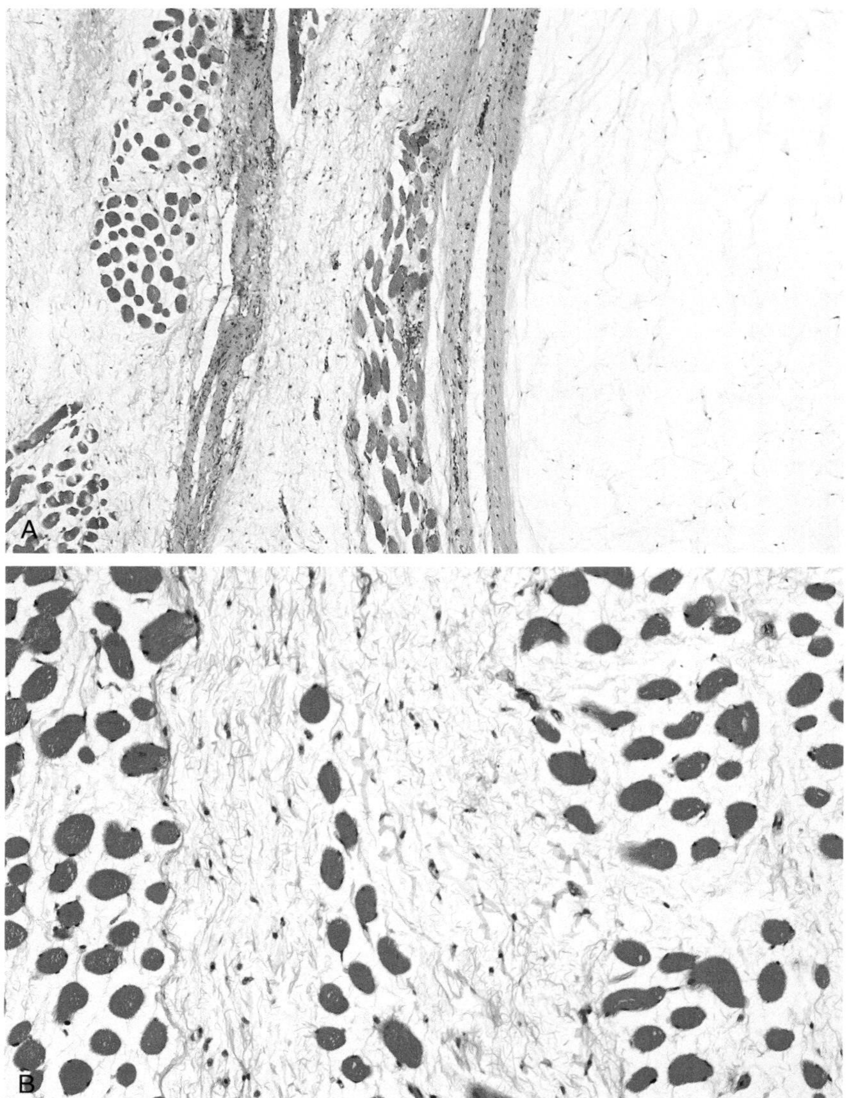

FIGURE 31-9. Intramuscular myxoma. Although grossly well circumscribed, the tumor infiltrates the surrounding skeletal muscle (A). Higher-magnification appearance of the peripheral portion of an intramuscular myxoma with atrophy of the surrounding skeletal muscle (B).

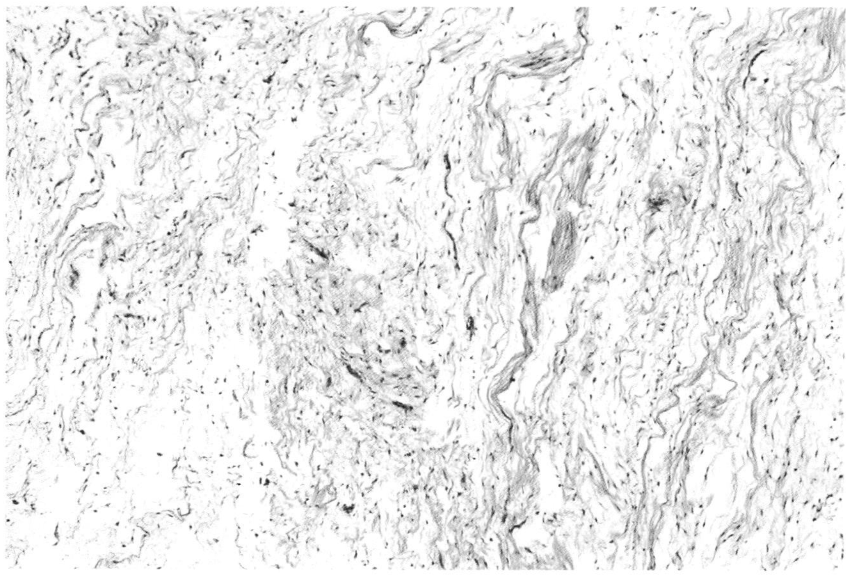

FIGURE 31-10. Low-magnification appearance of intramuscular myxoma characterized by a paucity of cells, abundance of mucoid material, and almost complete absence of vascular structures.

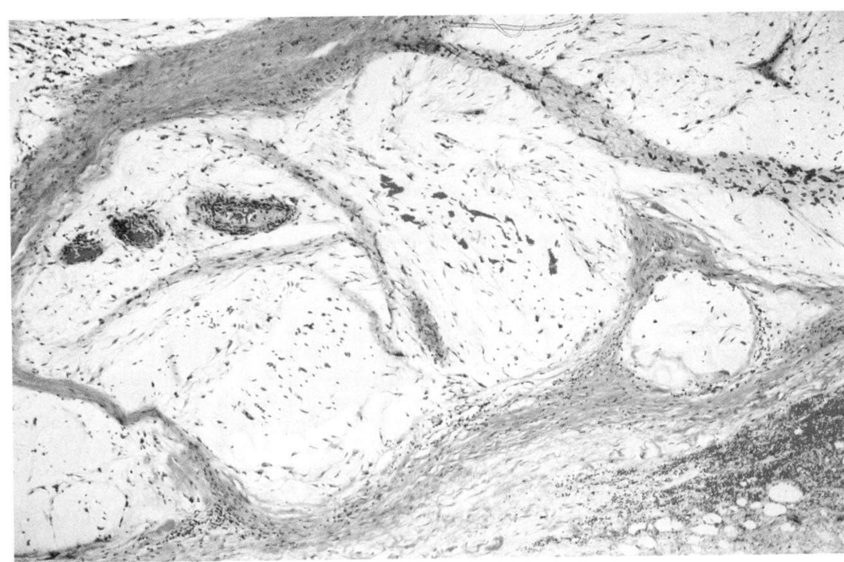

FIGURE 31-11. Intramuscular myxoma. Intersecting fibrous septa give the tumor a multilobular appearance.

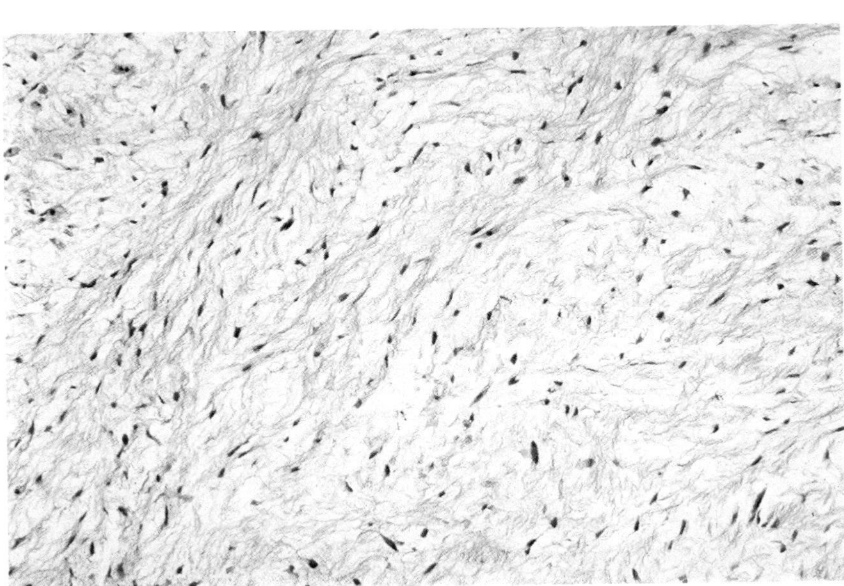

FIGURE 31-12. Intramuscular myxoma. The tumor cells are widely separated by abundant mucoid material and generally do not touch one another.

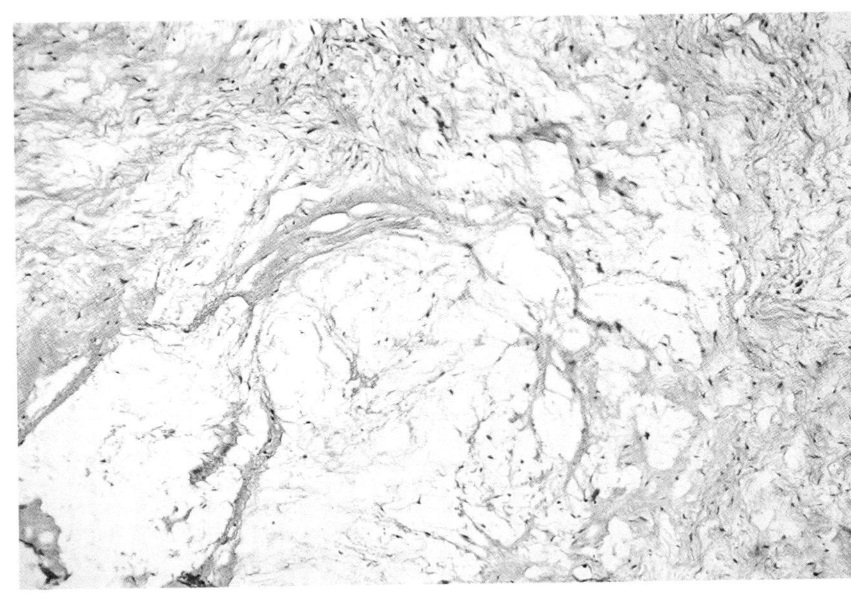

FIGURE 31-13. Intramuscular myxoma with prominent fluid-filled cystic spaces.

FIGURE 31-14. Hemorrhagic zone in an otherwise typical intramuscular myxoma.

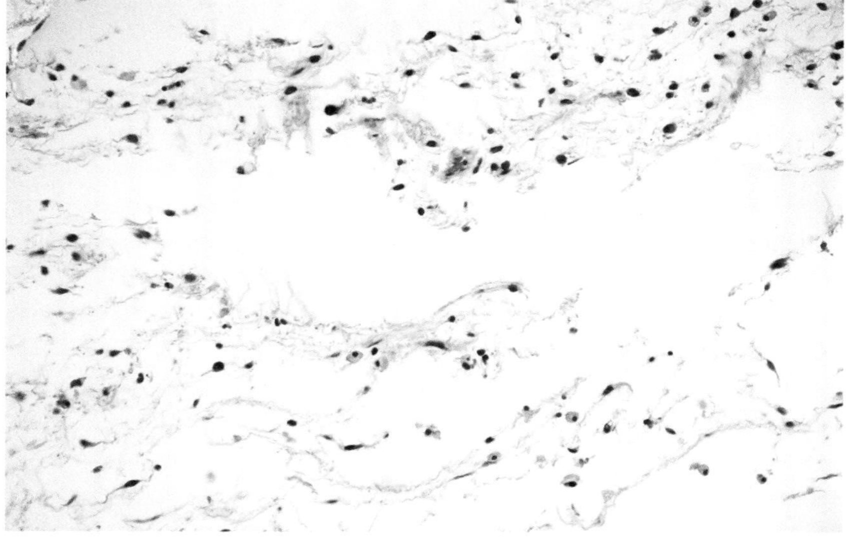

FIGURE 31-15. Cystic area in an intramuscular myxoma.

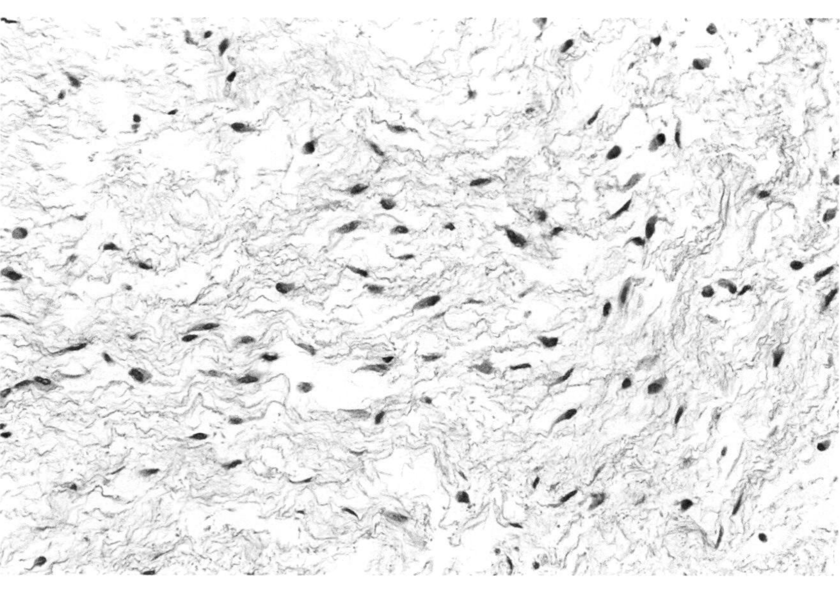

FIGURE 31-16. Intramuscular myxoma. The tumor is composed of cytologically bland spindled and stellate-shaped cells that are widely separated by myxoid stroma.

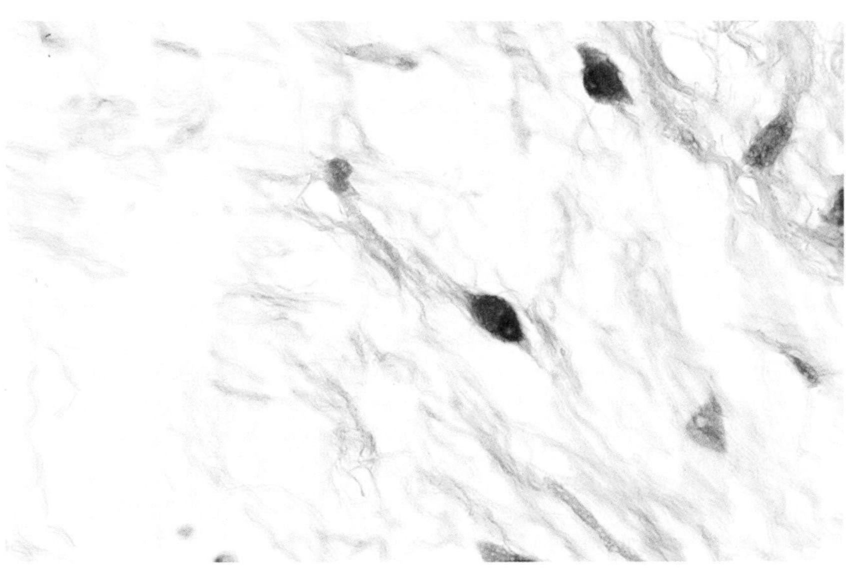

FIGURE 31-17. High-magnification appearance of pyknotic cells with tapered cytoplasm in an intramuscular myxoma.

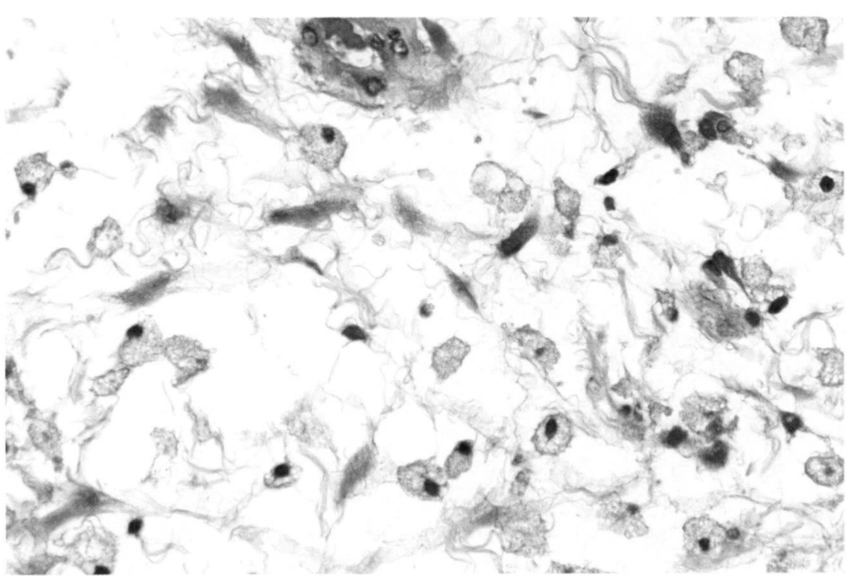

FIGURE 31-18. Intramuscular myxoma with collection of macrophages with small intracellular droplets of lipid material.

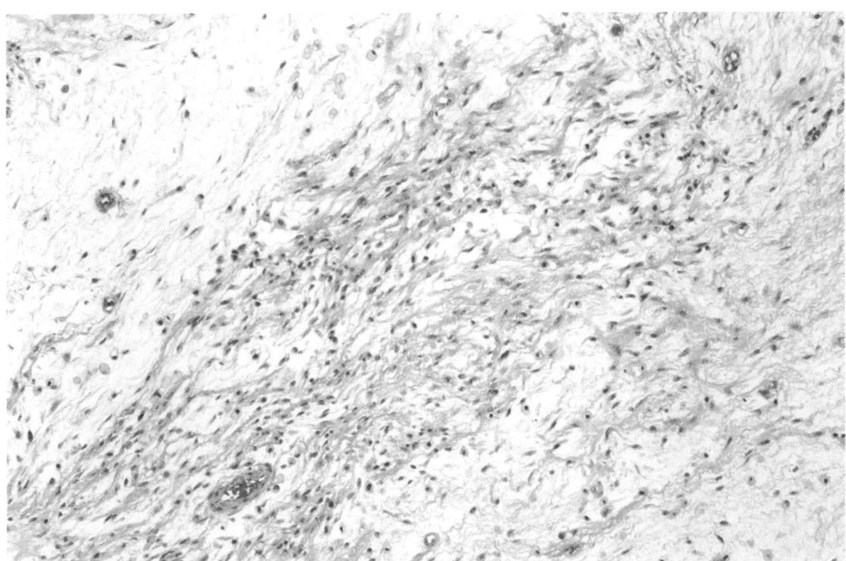

FIGURE 31-19. Hypercellular focus in an otherwise typical intramuscular myxoma.

TABLE 31-2 Differential Diagnosis of Intramuscular Myxoma

TUMOR TYPE	PLEOMORPHISM	VASCULARITY	MATRIX
Intramuscular myxoma	–	Inconspicuous	Hyaluronic acid
Myxoid liposarcoma	+	Fine, plexiform	Hyaluronic acid
Myxoid chondrosarcoma	+	Irregular	Chondroitin sulfate
Myxofibrosarcoma	+++	Coarse, curvilinear	Hyaluronic acid

composed of nests and cords of cells with densely eosinophilic cytoplasm deposited in a chondroitin sulfate-rich stroma. Although blood vessels are often not conspicuous, these lesions frequently show areas of hemorrhage and hemosiderin deposition at the periphery of the nodules. Immunostaining for S-100 protein, when positive, is useful for recognizing this entity, although fewer than one-half of all cases stain for this antigen. Perhaps the most difficult distinction is from a *low-grade fibromyxoid sarcoma (Evans tumor)*, especially when dealing with a cellular intramuscular myxoma. Low-grade fibromyxoid sarcoma arises in the deep soft tissues of young adults. Histologically, this tumor is composed of cytologically uniform spindle-shaped cells deposited in a variably collagenous and myxoid matrix, often with a swirling arrangement of tumor cells around thin-walled capillaries. The transition between fibrous and myxoid zones is often abrupt. In difficult cases, evaluation for evidence of a t(7;16) or MUC4 expression by immunohistochemistry characteristic of this tumor can be extremely helpful. Paraffin-embedded tissue can be used for evaluation by fluorescence in situ hybridization using a probe to the *FUS* gene, which is characteristically rearranged in the Evans tumor.

Discussion

Despite their frequently large size and prominent myxoid appearance, intramuscular myxomas are benign and rarely recur locally, even when incompletely excised. In the series by Nielsen et al.,[59] none of the 32 patients for whom follow-up information was available developed a local recurrence, including those with hypercellular lesions. In the rare examples that do recur, reexcision is typically curative.

JUXTA-ARTICULAR MYXOMA

Juxta-articular myxoma is an uncommon lesion marked by the accumulation of mucinous material in the vicinity of the large joints, most commonly the knee (almost 90% of cases) but occasionally near the shoulder, elbow, hip, or ankle (Table 31-3).[45,61-64] It almost always arises in adults, particularly men, with a predilection for the third through fifth decades of life. In the largest series to date, the patients ranged in age from 16 to 83 years, with a median age of 43 years.[61] The growth typically presents as a swelling or mass that is sometimes rapidly enlarging and is not infrequently associated with pain or tenderness.[62] These lesions may be associated with antecedent trauma and can arise adjacent to a joint with osteoarthritis. Some lesions are discovered incidentally during total knee or hip arthroplasty.[61] When in the region of the knee, they are frequently referred to as *parameniscal cyst*, *cystic myxomatous tumor*, or *periarticular myxoma*. The radiologic features are similar to those found with intramuscular myxoma.[65]

TABLE 31-3 Anatomic Location of 65 Juxta-Articular Myxomas

SITE	NO. OF CASES	PERCENTAGE (%)
Knee	57	88.0
Shoulder	3	4.5
Elbow	3	4.5
Hip	1	1.5
Ankle	1	1.5
Total	65	100.0

Modified from Meis JM, Enzinger FM. Juxta-articular myxoma: a clinical and pathologic study of 65 cases. Hum Pathol 1992;23(6):639–646.

Grossly, most lesions are 2 to 6 cm, but some are as large as 12 cm at the time of excision. They typically have a mucoid, cystic, or multicystic appearance on a cut section. Histologically, juxta-articular myxoma closely resembles intramuscular myxoma and is composed of scattered small, spindled, or stellate-shaped fibroblast-like cells deposited in a richly myxoid matrix that often contains variously sized thin- or thick-walled cystic spaces (Fig. 31-20). Occasionally, there are hypercellular areas with slight cellular pleomorphism, features that may arouse suspicion of a low-grade myxoid sarcoma. The process involves not only the periarticular soft tissues and the overlying cutaneous fat, but also the joint capsule, tendons, and rarely skeletal muscle. Some lesions have areas of hemorrhage and hemosiderin deposition with scattered chronic inflammation and reactive fibroblastic proliferation. This lesion has the same immunohistochemical and ultrastructural features as its intramuscular counterpart.

Juxta-articular myxoma is benign but is apt to recur after incomplete excision. In the series by Meis and Enzinger,[61] recurrences appeared in 10 of the 29 patients for whom follow-up information was available, including one lesion that recurred four times.

The pathogenesis of this condition is not clear, but it may represent an exuberant reactive fibroblastic proliferation with overproduction of mucin. On the other hand, Sciot et al.[66] described a case with clonal chromosomal changes, including trisomy 7 and a translocation between chromosomes 8 and 22. Unlike intramuscular myxoma, this lesion does not have mutations in the *GNAS1* gene.[67]

CUTANEOUS MYXOMA (SUPERFICIAL ANGIOMYXOMA)

Cutaneous myxoma, also known as *superficial angiomyxoma*, was first described by Carney et al.[68,69] in their 1986 study of the superficial myxoid tumors, which occurred in the setting of Carney complex, which had been described one year earlier. This lesion was later more fully characterized by Allen et al.[70] in 1988 and Calonje et al.[71] in 1999. Cutaneous myxoma should be distinguished from the other cutaneous myxoid lesions with which it may be confused because it has a propensity for local recurrence.

Cutaneous myxoma arises slightly more commonly in males, predominantly middle-aged adults with a peak incidence between 20 and 40 years of age.[71,72] These lesions can arise essentially anywhere in the superficial tissues but there is a predilection for the trunk, lower extremities, and head and neck; some arise in the genital region (vulva, mons pubis, scrotum/inguinal) of both males and females.[73-75] Histologically, identical lesions may arise in the setting of Carney complex, particularly those that are multiple and arise in the eyelids and external ear.[76] Clinically, most appear as slowly growing polypoid or papulonodular cutaneous lesions that may be confused with a cyst, skin tag, or neurofibroma.

Pathologic Findings

Grossly, cutaneous myxomas are usually well circumscribed, but some are poorly demarcated. The majority are between 1 and 5 cm and have a gray to white, glistening, gelatinous cut surface. Thin fibrous septa traverse the neoplasm, resulting in a vaguely multinodular tumor. Cysts that are sometimes filled with keratinous debris may be identified grossly.

As seen by light microscopy, this lesion has a lobular or multinodular appearance at low magnification (Figs. 31-21 and 31-22); most are histologically poorly circumscribed with extension into the underlying subcutaneous tissue and

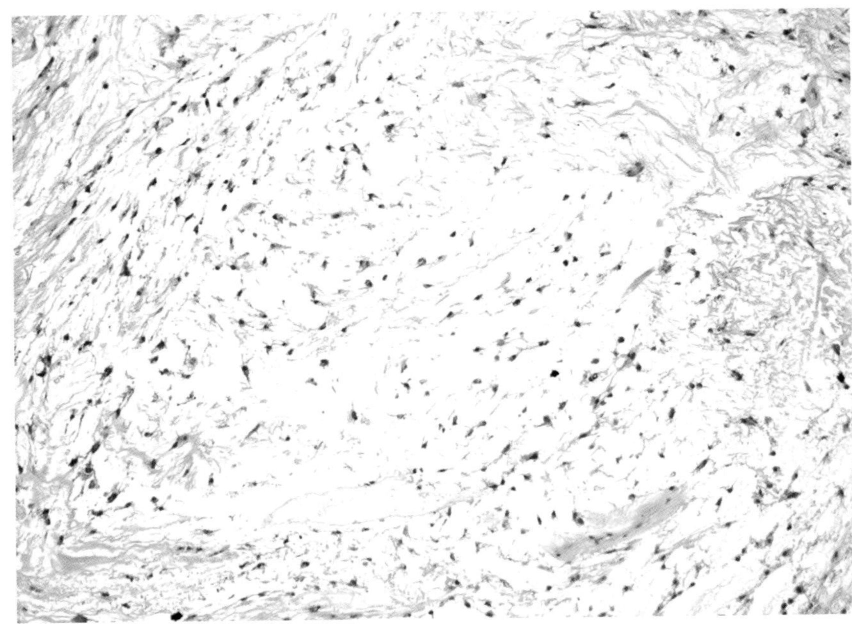

FIGURE 31-20. Juxta-articular myxoma composed of a hypocellular proliferation of bland spindled cells evenly deposited in a myxoid stroma. The histology is essentially identical to that seen in intramuscular myxoma.

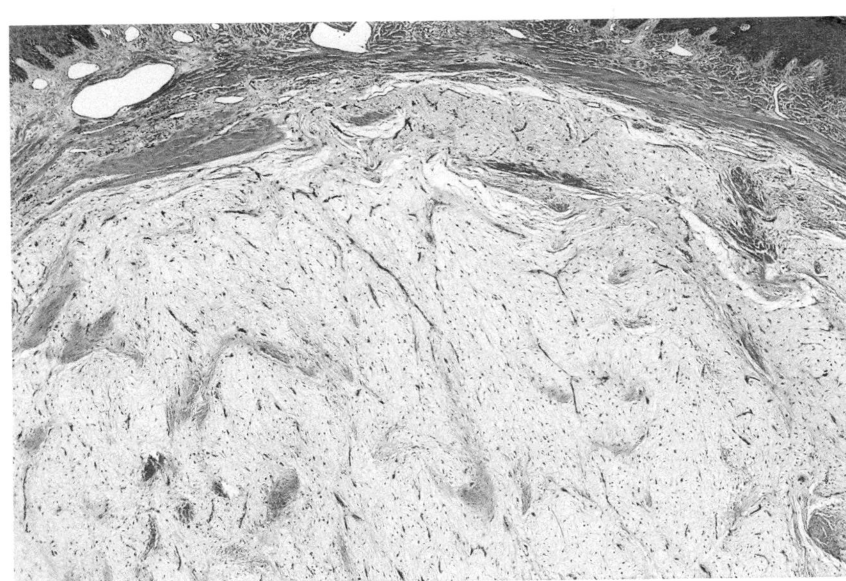

FIGURE 31-21. Cutaneous myxoma (superficial angiomyxoma). At low magnification, the tumor is hypocellular with prominent myxoid stroma; it appears fairly well circumscribed at its superficial aspect.

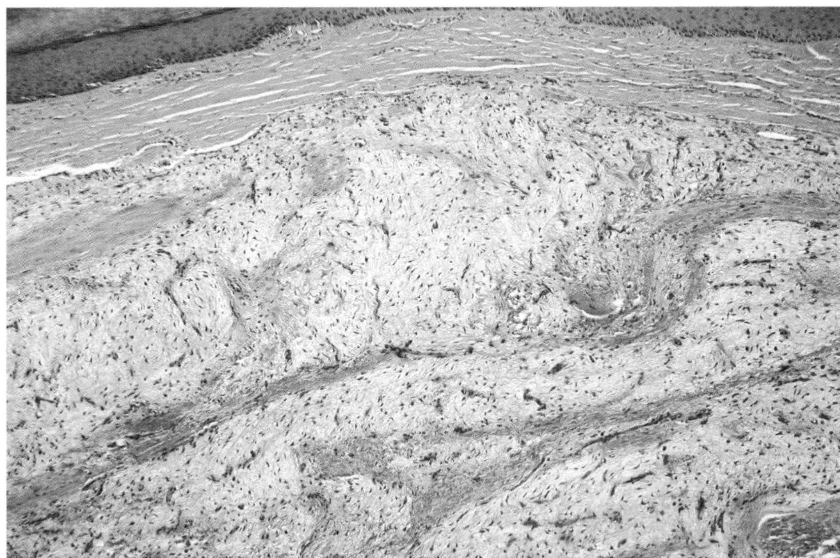

FIGURE 31-22. Multilobular appearance of a cutaneous myxoma.

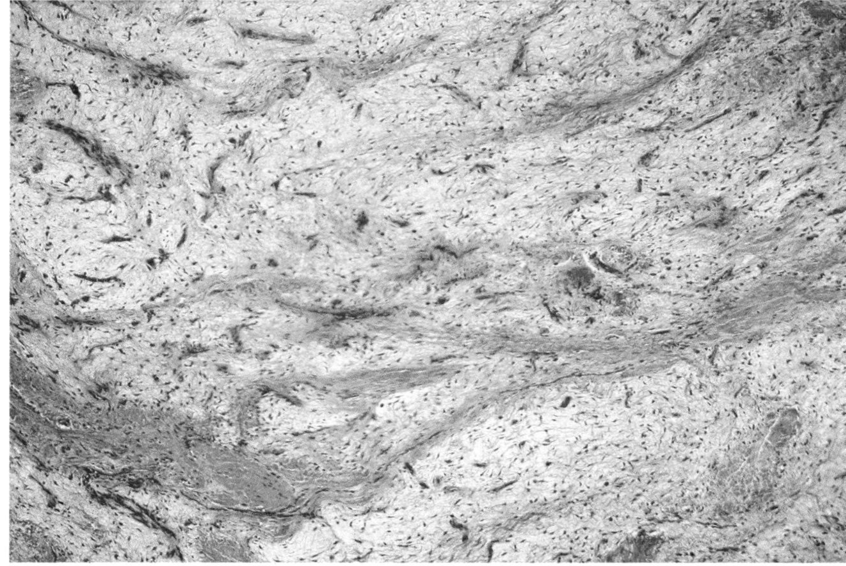

FIGURE 31-23. Cutaneous myxoma. Fibrous septa subdivide the tumor into ill-defined lobules.

rarely skeletal muscle. A sparse proliferation of spindled to stellate-shaped cells is deposited in an extensive myxoid stroma, sometimes forming cysts or irregular clefts, that is sensitive to hyaluronidase digestion (Fig. 31-23). The cells have indistinct cell borders and oval nuclei with inconspicuous nucleoli; mitotic figures are rare. Binucleated or multinucleated cells may be seen, as are scattered cells with intranuclear cytoplasmic pseudoinclusions. There is often a prominent vasculature that is focally arborizing, reminiscent of that seen in myxoid liposarcoma (Fig. 31-24). Other vascular alterations, including perivascular hyalinization, perivascular lymphocytes, and fibrin thrombi may be seen. A mixed inflammatory infiltrate is common, particularly stromal neutrophils, a feature unique to this tumor when compared to other cutaneous myxoid lesions.[71] Up to one-quarter of these tumors have epithelial structures consisting of basaloid buds, epithelial strands, or epidermoid (keratin-filled) cysts, possibly as a result of entrapment of adnexal structures by the neoplasm (Figs. 31-25 to 31-27).[70,71,77]

Immunohistochemically, the tumor cells consistently express CD34 but rarely stain for cytokeratins or S-100 protein.[71] Some cells stain for smooth muscle actin, muscle-specific actin, or desmin, suggesting focal myofibroblastic differentiation.[78]

Differential Diagnosis

The differential diagnosis of cutaneous myxoma is extensive and includes many benign and low-grade malignant myxoid lesions, including aggressive angiomyxoma, focal cutaneous mucinosis, digital mucous cyst, dermal nerve sheath myxoma (myxoid neurothekeoma), myxoid neurofibroma, superficial acral fibromyxoma, myxoid liposarcoma, and myxofibrosarcoma.

Some cutaneous myxomas arise in the genital region and so may be confused with *aggressive angiomyxoma*. The latter lesion, however, tends to be much larger, involves deeper

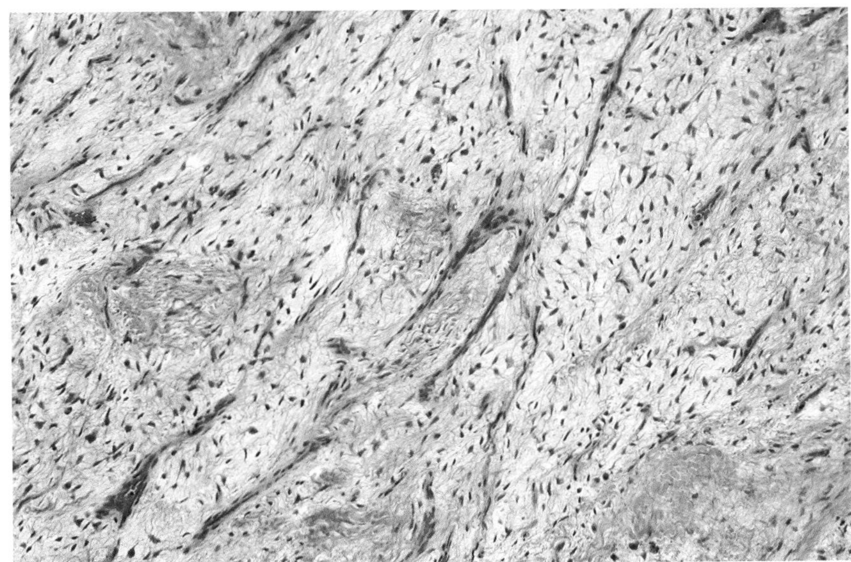

FIGURE 31-24. Cutaneous myxoma. A prominent arborizing vasculature is present, mimicking that found in myxoid liposarcoma.

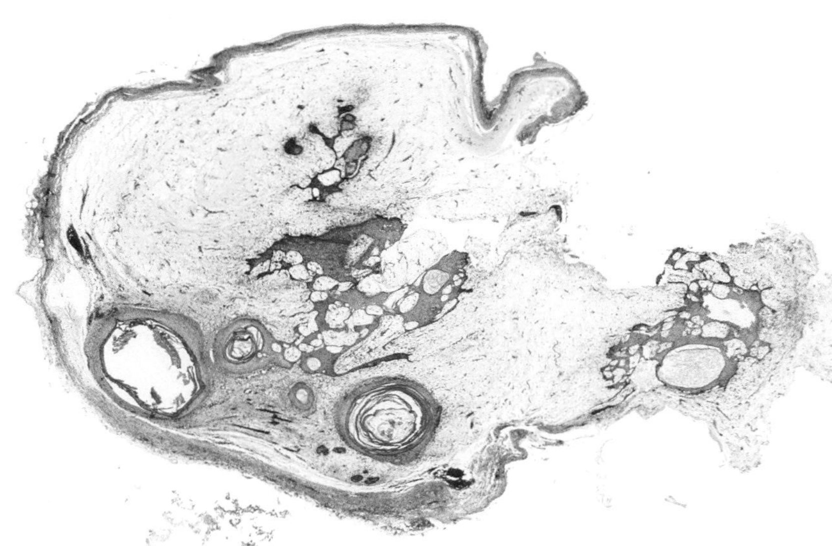

FIGURE 31-25. Cutaneous myxoma in a patient with Carney complex. Note the adnexal structures surrounded by myxoid matrix.

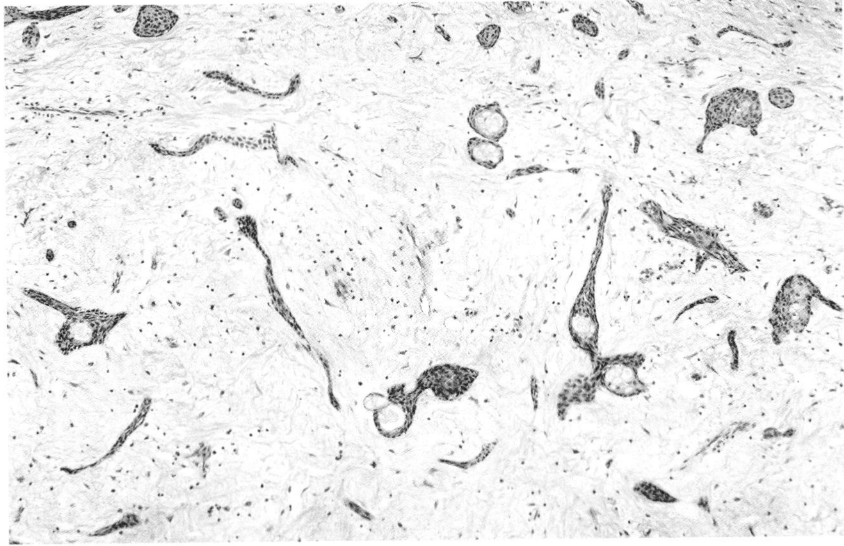

FIGURE 31-26. Cutaneous myxoma in a patient with Carney complex. Numerous epithelial strands are found in the substance of the neoplasm.

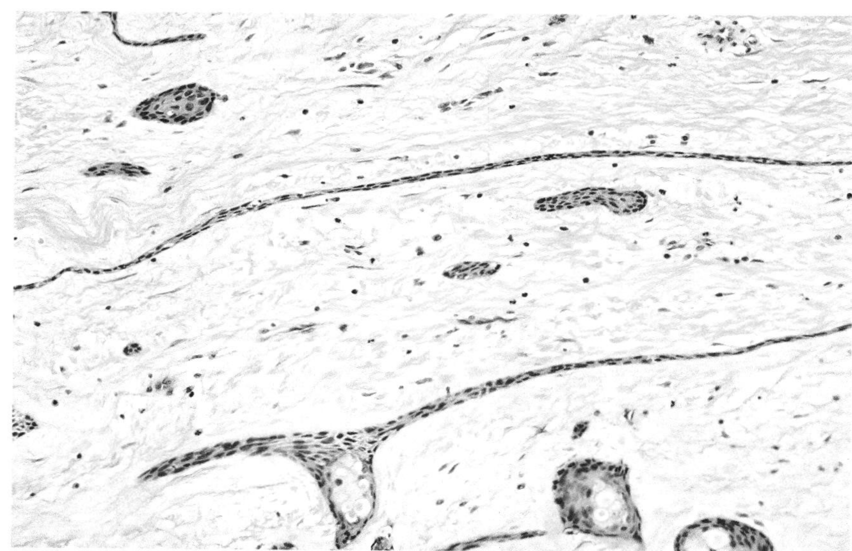

FIGURE 31-27. High-magnification view of elongated epithelial strands that appear to be compressed by the surrounding neoplasm in a cutaneous myxoma in a patient with Carney complex.

structures, usually in the female pelvic region, and has a vascular pattern that differs from that of cutaneous myxoma. *Focal cutaneous mucinosis* lacks the lobular architecture, stromal neutrophils, and epithelial structures found in cutaneous myxoma. *Digital mucous cyst* is easily distinguished given its almost exclusive location on the fingers. Similarly, *superficial acral fibromyxoma* arises almost exclusively on the fingers and toes of middle-aged adults.[79] *Nerve sheath myxoma* has a more pronounced lobular growth pattern and is characterized by plumper cells that are usually positive for S-100 protein. *Myxoid neurofibroma* is composed of cells with wavy or buckled nuclei that are also S-100 protein-positive.

Myxoid liposarcoma is usually more deeply located and larger than cutaneous myxoma and is characterized by a chicken-wire plexiform vasculature with scattered lipoblasts. *Myxofibrosarcoma* has a greater degree of nuclear atypia and hyperchromasia as well as curvilinear vessels often lined by hyperchromatic tumor cells.

Discussion

Cutaneous myxoma has a propensity for local recurrence if incompletely excised. In the series by Allen et al.,[70] 8 of 20 (40%) tumors recurred, including 5 of 8 (63%) tumors with epithelial components. Calonje et al.[71] reported a recurrence rate of 30%, including one case that recurred three times. In the latter series, recurrences developed a median of 12 months following initial excision. No cutaneous myxoma has been reported to metastasize. Although Allen et al.[70] noted that recurrences were more common in tumors with epithelial elements, the smaller series of cases arising in the genital region reported by Fetsch et al.[73] did not confirm this association.

CARNEY COMPLEX

The triad of cutaneous and cardiac myxomas, spotty pigmentation, and endocrine overactivity was first described by Carney et al.[68] in 1985. The disorder is familial and is transmitted as an autosomal dominant trait and principally affects young adults.[69] Most individuals with the complex harbor a mutation of the *PRKAR1A* gene (located at 17q22-24), which encodes for the regulatory R1 alpha subunit of protein kinase A.[80,81]

The cutaneous myxomas arising in this complex have a predilection for the eyelids and range from small sessile papules to large pedunculated, finger-like masses; they are multiple, in most cases, and are characterized by an appearance during early adulthood (mean age 18 years).[69] The lesions are found in the dermis or subcutaneous tissue, are usually sharply circumscribed, and are characterized by cytologically bland spindled and stellate-shaped cells deposited in an abundant myxoid stroma with a prominent capillary vasculature, identical to sporadic cutaneous myxomas discussed in the previous section. They are often associated with a basaloid proliferation of the surface epithelium, which may cause misclassification of some of these lesions as basal cell carcinoma or trichofolliculoma. In 1994, Ferreiro and Carney[76] reported the association of myxomas of the external ear with Carney complex. Of the 152 patients with this complex known to these authors at that time, 22 (14%) had myxomas of the external ear. Furthermore, 22 of 26 (85%) patients with external ear myxomas were found to have Carney complex. Multifocal myxoid fibroadenomas and myxomatosis of the breast are also occasional components of this complex.[82]

The most serious components of the syndrome are psammomatous melanotic schwannoma and cardiac myxoma. Cardiac myxomas, regardless of their association with this syndrome, may be associated with peripheral tumor emboli, and up to 24% of all patients with cardiac myxomas die of its complications (Fig. 31-28).[83]

The spotty skin pigmentation includes lentigines that predominantly affect the face, particularly the vermilion border of the lips, and blue nevi, including epithelioid blue nevi.[84-86] Endocrine overactivity may be caused by the presence of primary pigmented nodular adrenocortical disease resulting in the Cushing syndrome,[87,88] pituitary adenoma resulting in acromegaly,[89] or sexual precocity associated with testicular

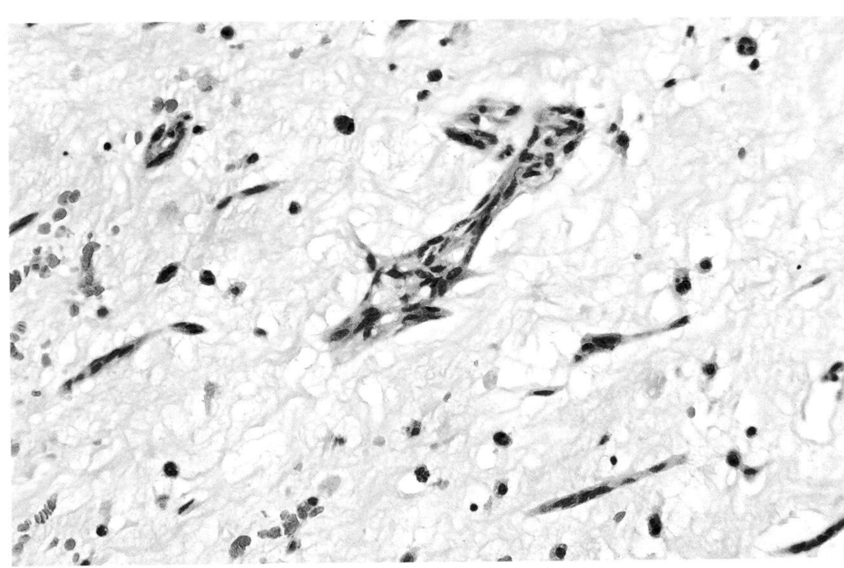

FIGURE 31-28. Cardiac myxoma in a patient with Carney complex.

lesions, particularly large-cell calcifying Sertoli cell tumor.[90] Thyroid gland abnormalities ranging from follicular hyperplasia to cystic carcinoma have been associated with Carney complex.[91,92] Recently, patients with Carney complex were also found to have an increased risk of pancreatic ductal and acinar neoplasms.[93]

GANGLION (GANGLION CYST)

Ganglion is by far the most common and best known of the more superficially located myxoid lesions. It occurs as a unilocular or multilocular cystic or myxoid mass on the dorsal surface of the wrist in young persons, especially women, generally 25 to 45 years of age. Less often, it is found on the volar surface of the wrist or fingers and the dorsum of the foot and toes.[94,95] It is, in fact, the most common lesion of the hand and wrist, accounting for 50% to 70% of all masses in this location. In about half of the cases, the condition is associated with tenderness or mild pain and causes interference of function. A history of trauma is given in about 50% of cases.

Ganglia usually measure 1 to 3 cm in diameter. They are frequently attached to the joint capsule and tendon sheaths and probably are the result of excessive mucin production by fibroblasts rather than disintegration of preformed fibrous structures. There is no communication between the ganglion and the joint space. Some of these lesions are easily confused with myxomas, especially during the initial myxoid stage of development. Most, however, are readily recognized by their location and the presence of multiple thick-walled cystic spaces of variable size in association with myxoid areas. Focal myxoid change is noted in the earliest stage. Subsequently, microscopic cysts develop and coalesce into larger ones until, finally, the lesion assumes its typical form of a dominant cyst (Figs. 31-29 to 31-31). Most of these lesions can be treated nonoperatively, but a select group is surgically excised with a low rate of recurrence. Ganglion-like lesions may also arise in the subperiosteal region or bone.[96]

AMYLOID TUMOR (AMYLOIDOMA)

Although systemic amyloid deposition is much more common, localized deposits of amyloid may result in a mass (amyloidoma), and these deposits have been reported in virtually every anatomic site. Amyloidomas may arise in association with immunocytic dyscrasias, including multiple myeloma and plasmacytoid lymphoma, but they may occur in patients on long-term hemodialysis, as well as those with chronic infectious or inflammatory diseases (tuberculosis, osteomyelitis, rheumatoid arthritis).[97,98] Some occur in patients with no clinical evidence of immunocytic dyscrasia or any other coexisting or preexisting disease; these lesions are rare and are found mainly in the soft tissues[99,100] or as solitary or multiple nodules in the respiratory,[101] urinary,[102] or gastrointestinal tracts.[103] There are also reports of localized amyloid tumors in the region of the head and neck,[104] bone,[105] and nervous system.[106] Amyloid tumors have rarely been reported at the site of insulin injections.

Grossly, amyloidomas consist of a lobulated nodule or mass with a white-yellow or pink-yellow waxy surface. Microscopic examination discloses amorphous faintly eosinophilic material that is periodic-acid-Schiff-positive and metachromatic with the crystal violet stain. The deposits are typically surrounded by histiocytes and multinucleated giant cells associated with a variable lymphoplasmacytic infiltrate.[107] The plasma cells usually show no evidence of immaturity or cellular atypia (Figs. 31-32 and 31-33). In most cases, the interspersed vessel walls are diffusely thickened by amyloid deposits. Elastic stains help distinguish the tumor from elastofibroma, and the absence of a fibroblastic proliferation distinguishes it from tumoral calcinosis. Definitionally, amyloid stains positively with a Congo red stain and displays an apple-green color birefringence under polarized light (Fig. 31-34), a reflection of its beta pleated sheet configuration. The subtypes of amyloid can be differentiated by immunohistochemical demonstration of the kappa and lambda light chains in AL (primary) amyloid, amyloid A protein in AA (secondary) amyloid, and β_2-microglobulin in hemodialysis-associated

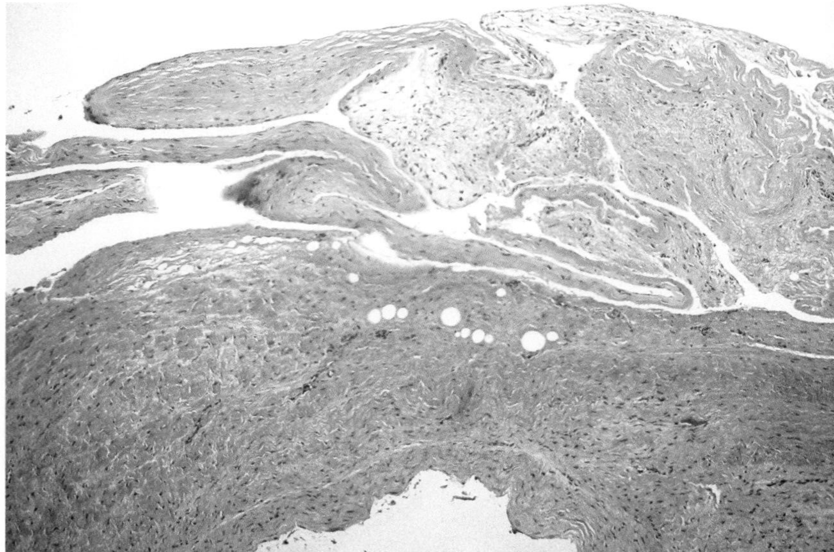

FIGURE 31-29. Low-magnification view of a ganglion cyst with multiple irregular thick-walled cystic spaces and focal myxoid change in the surrounding matrix.

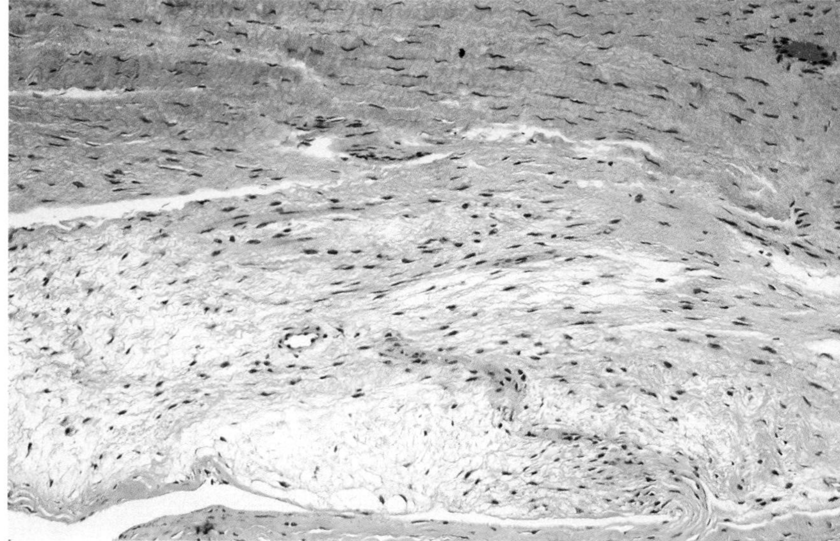

FIGURE 31-30. High-magnification view of focal myxoid change with bland spindle-shaped cells in a ganglion cyst.

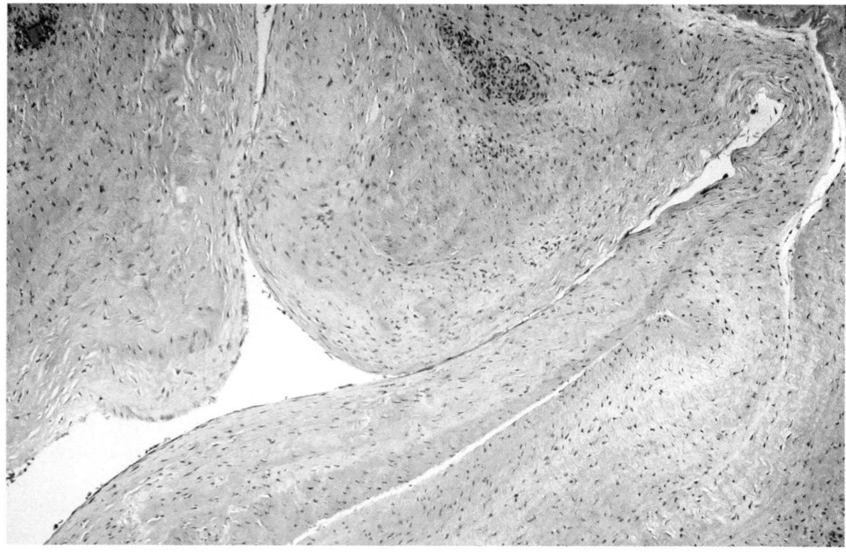

FIGURE 31-31. Ganglion. Dominant cyst with prominent myxoid change in the surrounding soft tissue.

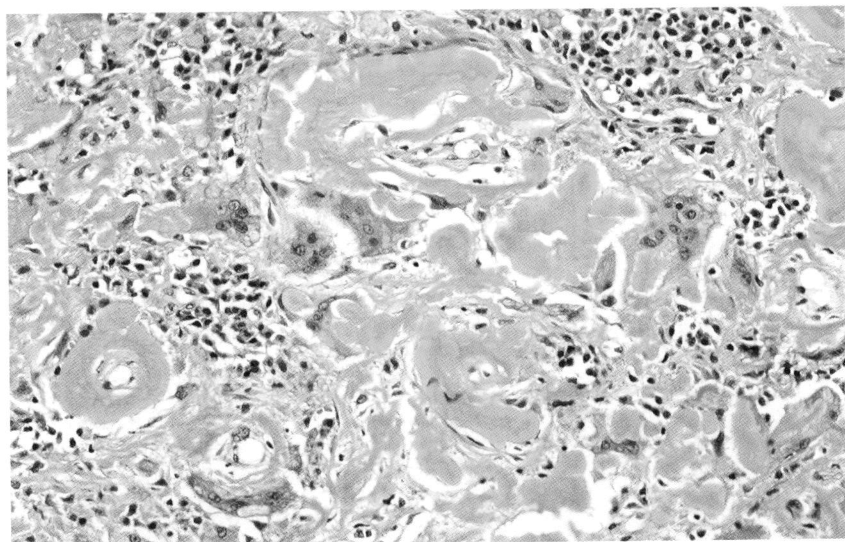

FIGURE 31-32. Amyloid tumor with amorphous deposits of amyloid associated with foreign body-type giant cells and plasma cells.

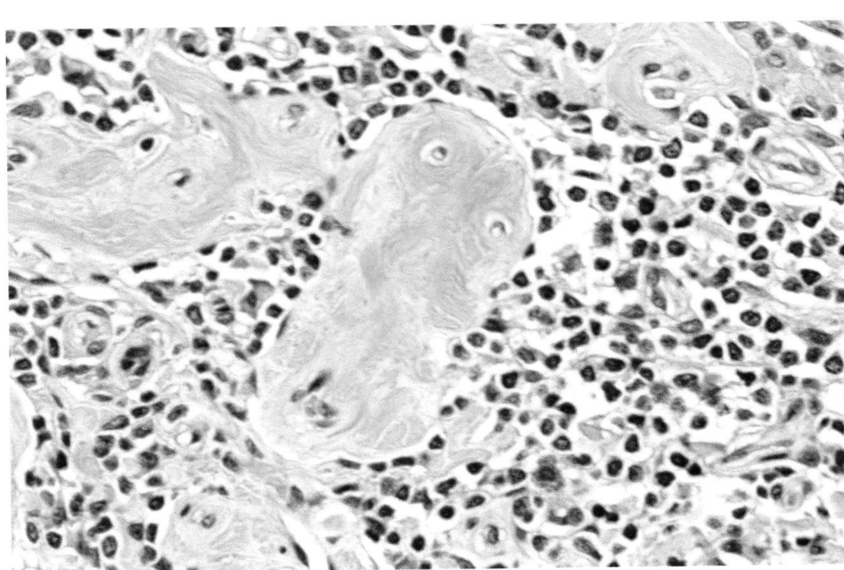

FIGURE 31-33. High magnification of amyloid tumor with prominent plasma cell infiltrates surrounding deposits of amyloid.

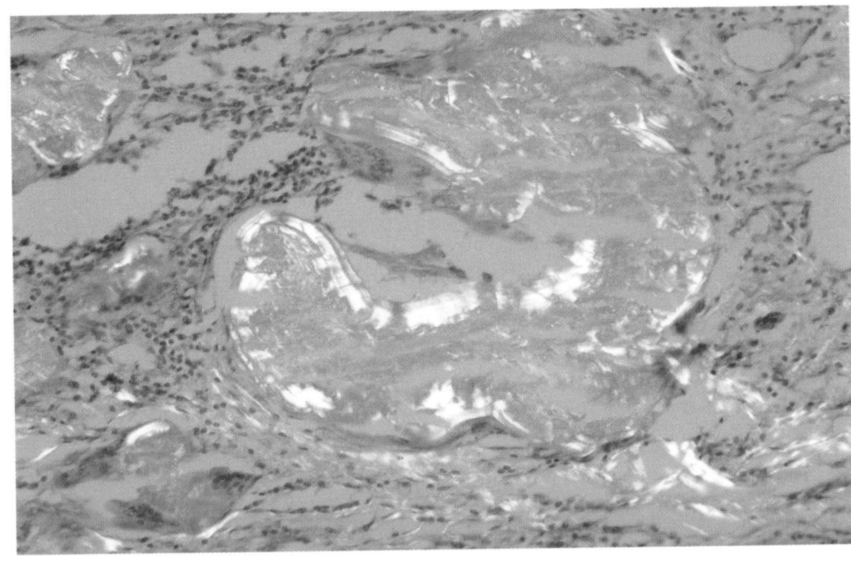

FIGURE 31-34. Apple-green color birefringence under polarized light in an amyloid tumor.

amyloid.[108] Electron microscopy shows that the amyloid consists of fine, straight, nonbranching fibrils that measure 70 to 100 nm in diameter.

Early reports often provided no information as to the type of amyloid comprising the tumor-like mass. More recent reports have described deposits of both the AA[109] and AL[110] types with few reports of β_2-microglobulin amyloid.[111] Laeng et al.[112] detected monoclonal rearrangements of the heavy-chain immunoglobulin gene in amyloidomas of the nervous system, providing strong support for the concept that at least some of these lesions are composed of AL-producing B-cell clones capable of terminal differentiation. Of the 14 soft tissue amyloidomas reported by Krishnan et al.,[113] 10 were associated with plasmacytoid lymphoma (nine cases) or myeloma (one case). In their review of the literature of amyloidoma of bone, Pambuccian et al.[114] found all lesions to be composed of AL amyloid, with many patients progressing to generalized disease.

References

1. Inclan A. Tumoral calcinosis. JAMA 1943;121:490.
2. Duret MH. Tumeurs multiples et singulieres des bourses sereuses (endotheliomes peut etre d'origine parasitaire). Bull Mem Soc Anat (Paris) 1899;74:725.
3. Teutschlaender O. Zur kenntnis der progressiven lipocalcinogranulomatose der muskulatur. Virchows Arch 1935;295:424.
4. Mens J, van der Korst JK. Calcifying supracoracoid bursitis as a cause of chronic shoulder pain. Ann Rheum Dis 1984;43(5):758–9.
5. Jakobeit C, Winiarski B, Jakobeit S, et al. Ultrasound-guided, high-energy extracorporeal - shock-wave treatment of symptomatic calcareous tendinopathy of the shoulder. ANZ J Surg 2002;72(7):496–500.
6. Lobo M. Radiography of "Kikuyu Bursa." Radiography 1974;40(477): 207–9.
7. Murthy DP. Tumoral calcinosis: a study of cases from Papua New Guinea. J Trop Med Hyg 1990;93(6):403–7.
8. Hutt N, Baghla DP, Gulati V, et al. Acral post-traumatic tumoral calcinosis in pregnancy: a case report. J Med Case Reports 2011;5:89.
9. Laskin WB, Miettinen M, Fetsch JF. Calcareous lesions of the distal extremities resembling tumoral calcinosis (tumoral calcinosislike lesions): clinicopathologic study of 43 cases emphasizing a pathogenesis-based approach to classification. Am J Surg Pathol 2007;31(1):15–25.
10. Jacob JJ, Thomas N, Seshadri MS. Tumoral calcinosis of the scalp: An unusual site for a rare tumor. Laryngoscope 2007;117(1):179–80.
11. Emlakcioğlu E, Kara M, Ozcan HN, et al. Thoracic outlet syndrome with involvement of the cervical sympathetics because of idiopathic tumoral calcinosis. Am J Phys Med Rehabil 2011;90(9):765–7.
12. Dray N, Rao AG, Silver RM. Paraspinal tumoral calcinosis in a child with systemic sclerosis/myositis overlap. Pediatr Radiol 2011;41(9): 1216–18.
13. Yancovitch A, Hershkovitz D, Indelman M, et al. Novel mutations in GALNT3 causing hyperphosphatemic familial tumoral calcinosis. J Bone Miner Metab 2011;29(5):621–5.
14. Barbieri AM, Filopanti M, Bua G, et al. Two novel nonsense mutations in GALNT3 gene are responsible for familial tumoral calcinosis. J Hum Genet 2007;52(5):464–8.
15. Joseph L, Hing SN, Presneau N, et al. Familial tumoral calcinosis and hyperostosis-hyperphosphataemia syndrome are different manifestations of the same disease: novel missense mutations in GALNT3. Skeletal Radiol 2010;39(1):63–8.
16. Topaz O, Shurman DL, Bergman R, et al. Mutations in GALNT3, encoding a protein involved in O-linked glycosylation, cause familial tumoral calcinosis. Nat Genet 2004;36(6):579–81.
17. Bergwitz C, Banerjee S, Abu-Zahra H, et al. Defective O-glycosylation due to a novel homozygous S129P mutation is associated with lack of fibroblast growth factor 23 secretion and tumoral calcinosis. J Clin Endocrinol Metab 2009;94(11):4267–74.
18. Garringer HJ, Malekpour M, Esteghamat F, et al. Molecular genetic and biochemical analyses of FGF23 mutations in familial tumoral calcinosis. Am J Physiol Endocrinol Metab 2008;295(4):E929–37.
19. Larsson T, Yu X, Davis SI, et al. A novel recessive mutation in fibroblast growth factor-23 causes familial tumoral calcinosis. J Clin Endocrinol Metab 2005;90(4):2424–7.
20. Ichikawa S, Imel EA, Kreiter ML, et al. A homozygous missense mutation in human KLOTHO causes severe tumoral calcinosis. J Clin Invest 2007;117(9):2684–91.
21. Ichikawa S, Baujat G, Seyahi A, et al. Clinical variability of familial tumoral calcinosis caused by novel GALNT3 mutations. Am J Med Genet A 2010;152A(4):896–903.
22. Sprecher E. Familial tumoral calcinosis: from characterization of a rare phenotype to the pathogenesis of ectopic calcification. J Invest Dermatol 2010;130(3):652–60.
23. Chefetz I, Ben Amitai D, Browning S, et al. Normophosphatemic familial tumoral calcinosis is caused by deleterious mutations in SAMD9, encoding a TNF-alpha responsive protein. J Invest Dermatol 2008;128(6): 1423–9.
24. Topaz O, Indelman M, Chefetz I, et al. A deleterious mutation in SAMD9 causes normophosphatemic familial tumoral calcinosis. Am J Hum Genet 2006;79(4):759–64.
25. Martinez S, Vogler JB 3rd, Harrelson JM, et al. Imaging of tumoral calcinosis: new observations. Radiology 1990;174(1):215–22.
26. McGregor DH, Mowry M, Cherian R, et al. Nonfamilial tumoral calcinosis associated with chronic renal failure and secondary hyperparathyroidism: report of two cases with clinicopathological, immunohistochemical, and electron microscopic findings. Hum Pathol 1995;26(6):607–13.
27. Chu HY, Chu P, Lin YF, et al. Uremic tumoral calcinosis in patients on peritoneal dialysis: clinical, radiologic, and laboratory features. Perit Dial Int 2011;31(4):430–9.
28. Primetis E, Dalakidis A, Papacharalampous X, et al. Extensive tumoral calcinosis in a patient with systemic sclerosis. Am J Orthop 2010; 39(10):E108–10.
29. Carter JD, Warner E. Clinical images: tumoral calcinosis associated with sarcoidosis. Arthritis Rheum 2003;48(6):1770.
30. Möckel G, Buttgereit F, Labs K, et al. Tumoral calcinosis revisited: pathophysiology and treatment. Rheumatol Int 2005;25(1):55–9.
31. Martinez S. Tumoral calcinosis: 12 years later. Semin Musculoskelet Radiol 2002;6(4):331–9.
32. Slavin RE, Wen J, Kumar D, et al. Familial tumoral calcinosis. A clinical, histopathologic, and ultrastructural study with an analysis of its calcifying process and pathogenesis. Am J Surg Pathol 1993;17(8):788–802.
33. Pakasa NM, Kalengayi RM. Tumoral calcinosis: a clinicopathological study of 111 cases with emphasis on the earliest changes. Histopathology 1997;31(1):18–24.
34. Tong MK, Siu YP. Tumoral calcinosis in end stage renal disease. Postgrad Med J 2004;80(948):601.
35. Wiggins HE, Karian BK, Smith BM. A sublingual-submandibular calcific mass associated with tumoral calcinosis in a patient with suspected milk-alkali syndrome. Oral Surg Oral Med Oral Pathol 1975;40(1): 8–18.
36. Dönmez O, Durmaz O. Calcinosis cutis universalis with pediatric systemic lupus erythematosus. Pediatr Nephrol 2010;25(7):1375–6.
37. Ardolino AM, Milne BW, Patel PA, et al. Digital calcinosis circumscripta: case series and review of the literature. Journal of Pediatric Orthopaedics Part B/European Paediatric Orthopaedic Society, Pediatric Orthopaedic Society of North America. 2011. Available at: http://www.ncbi.nlm.nih.gov/pubmed/21654339. Accessed September 19, 2011.
38. Shon W, Folpe AL. Tenosynovitis with psammomatous calcification: a poorly recognized pseudotumor related to repetitive tendinous injury. Am J Surg Pathol 2010;34(6):892–5.
39. Gollnick HP. Oral retinoids–efficacy and toxicity in psoriasis. Br J Dermatol 1996;135(Suppl. 49):6–17.
40. Dubey S, Sharma R, Maheshwari V. Scrotal calcinosis: idiopathic or dystrophic? Dermatol Online J 2010;16(2):5.
41. Enzinger FM. Intramuscular myxoma: a review and follow-up study of 34 cases. Am J Clin Pathol 1965;43:104–13.
42. Ireland DC, Soule EH, Ivins JC. Myxoma of somatic soft tissues. A report of 58 patients, 3 with multiple tumors and fibrous dysplasia of bone. Mayo Clin Proc 1973;48(6):401–10.
43. Kindblom LG, Stener B, Angervall L. Intramuscular myxoma. Cancer 1974;34(5):1737–44.
44. Ishoo E. Intramuscular myxoma presenting as a rare posterior neck mass in a young child: case report and literature review. Arch Otolaryngol Head Neck Surg 2007;133(4):398–401.

45. Allen PW. Myxoma is not a single entity: a review of the concept of myxoma. Ann Diagn Pathol 2000;4(2):99–123.
46. Miettinen M, Höckerstedt K, Reitamo J, et al. Intramuscular myxoma–a clinicopathological study of twenty-three cases. Am J Clin Pathol 1985;84(3):265–72.
47. Papadogeorgakis N, Petsinis V, Nikitakis N, et al. Intramuscular myxoma of the masseter muscle. A case report. Oral Maxillofac Surg 2009; 13(1):37–40.
48. Ly JQ, Bau JL, Beall DP. Forearm intramuscular myxoma. AJR Am J Roentgenol 2003;181(4):960.
49. Abu Hassan FO, Shomaf M. Intramuscular myxoma of the hypothenar muscles. Strategies Trauma Limb Reconstr 2009;4(2):103–6.
50. Hashimoto H, Tsuneyoshi M, Daimaru Y, et al. Intramuscular myxoma. A clinicopathologic, immunohistochemical, and electron microscopic study. Cancer 1986;58(3):740–7.
51. Yao MS, Chen CY, Chin-Wei Chien J, et al. Magnetic resonance imaging of gluteal intramuscular myxoma. Clin Imaging 2007;31(3):214–16.
52. Case DB, Chapman CN Jr, Freeman JK, et al. Best cases from the AFIP: atypical presentation of polyostotic fibrous dysplasia with myxoma (Mazabraud syndrome). Radiographics 2010;30(3):827–32.
53. Zoccali C, Teori G, Prencipe U, et al. Mazabraud's syndrome: a new case and review of the literature. Int Orthop 2009;33(3):605–10.
54. Mazabraud A, Semat P, Roze R. [Apropos of the association of fibromyxomas of the soft tissues with fibrous dysplasia of the bones]. Presse Med 1967;75(44):2223–8.
55. Lietman SA, Ding C, Levine MA. A highly sensitive polymerase chain reaction method detects activating mutations of the GNAS gene in peripheral blood cells in McCune-Albright syndrome or isolated fibrous dysplasia. J Bone Joint Surg Am 2005;87(11):2489–94.
56. Lumbroso S, Paris F, Sultan C. Activating Gs(alpha) mutations: analysis of 113 patients with signs of McCune-Albright syndrome–a European Collaborative Study. J Clin Endocrinol Metab 2004;89(5):2107–13.
57. Okamoto S, Hisaoka M, Ushijima M, et al. Activating Gs(alpha) mutation in intramuscular myxomas with and without fibrous dysplasia of bone. Virchows Arch 2000;437(2):133–7.
58. Delaney D, Diss TC, Presneau N, et al. GNAS1 mutations occur more commonly than previously thought in intramuscular myxoma. Mod Pathol 2009;22(5):718–24.
59. Nielsen GP, O'Connell JX, Rosenberg AE. Intramuscular myxoma: a clinicopathologic study of 51 cases with emphasis on hypercellular and hypervascular variants. Am J Surg Pathol 1998;22(10):1222–7.
60. van Roggen JF, McMenamin ME, Fletcher CD. Cellular myxoma of soft tissue: a clinicopathological study of 38 cases confirming indolent clinical behaviour. Histopathology 2001;39(3):287–97.
61. Meis JM, Enzinger FM. Juxta-articular myxoma: a clinical and pathologic study of 65 cases. Hum Pathol 1992;23(6):639–46.
62. Minkoff J, Stecker S, Irizarry J, et al. Juxta-articular myxoma: a rare cause of painful restricted motion of the knee. Arthroscopy 2003;19(10): E6–13.
63. Echols PG, Omer GE Jr, Crawford MK. Juxta-articular myxoma of the shoulder presenting as a cyst of the acromioclavicular joint: a case report. J Shoulder Elbow Surg 2000;9(2):157–9.
64. Körver RJ, Theunissen PH, van de Kreeke WT, et al. Juxta-articular myxoma of the knee in a 5-year-old boy: a case report and review of the literature (2009: 12b). Eur Radiol 2010;20(3):764–8.
65. King DG, Saifuddin A, Preston HV, et al. Magnetic resonance imaging of juxta-articular myxoma. Skeletal Radiol 1995;24(2):145–7.
66. Sciot R, Dal Cin P, Samson I, et al. Clonal chromosomal changes in juxta-articular myxoma. Virchows Arch 1999;434(2):177–80.
67. Okamoto S, Hisaoka M, Meis-Kindblom JM, et al. Juxta-articular myxoma and intramuscular myxoma are two distinct entities. Activating Gs alpha mutation at Arg 201 codon does not occur in juxta-articular myxoma. Virchows Arch 2002;440(1):12–15.
68. Carney JA, Gordon H, Carpenter PC, et al. The complex of myxomas, spotty pigmentation, and endocrine overactivity. Medicine (Baltimore) 1985;64(4):270–83.
69. Carney JA, Headington JT, Su WP. Cutaneous myxomas. A major component of the complex of myxomas, spotty pigmentation, and endocrine overactivity. Arch Dermatol 1986;122(7):790–8.
70. Allen PW, Dymock RB, MacCormac LB. Superficial angiomyxomas with and without epithelial components. Report of 30 tumors in 28 patients. Am J Surg Pathol 1988;12(7):519–30.
71. Calonje E, Guerin D, McCormick D, et al. Superficial angiomyxoma: clinicopathologic analysis of a series of distinctive but poorly recognized cutaneous tumors with tendency for recurrence. Am J Surg Pathol 1999;23(8):910–17.
72. Clarke LE. Fibrous and fibrohistiocytic neoplasms: an update. Dermatol Clin 2012;30(4):643–56.
73. Fetsch JF, Laskin WB, Tavassoli FA. Superficial angiomyxoma (cutaneous myxoma): a clinicopathologic study of 17 cases arising in the genital region. Int J Gynecol Pathol 1997;16(4):325–34.
74. Basak S, Rogers S, Solomonsz AF. Superficial angiomyxoma of the vulva: a case report of a rare cutaneous tumour. J Obstet Gynaecol 2011;31(4):360–1.
75. Kim HS, Kim GY, Lim SJ, et al. Giant superficial angiomyxoma of the vulva: a case report and review of the literature. J Cutan Pathol 2010;37(6):672–7.
76. Ferreiro JA, Carney JA. Myxomas of the external ear and their significance. Am J Surg Pathol 1994;18(3):274–80.
77. Toth A, Nemeth T, Szucs A, et al. Retropharyngeal superficial angiomyxoma. J Laryngol Otol 2010;124(9):1017–20.
78. Meer S, Beavon I. Intraoral superficial angiomyxoma. Oral Surg Oral Med Oral Pathol Oral Radiol Endod 2008;106(5):e20–3.
79. Fetsch JF, Laskin WB, Miettinen M. Superficial acral fibromyxoma: a clinicopathologic and immunohistochemical analysis of 37 cases of a distinctive soft tissue tumor with a predilection for the fingers and toes. Hum Pathol 2001;32(7):704–14.
80. Wilkes D, McDermott DA, Basson CT. Clinical phenotypes and molecular genetic mechanisms of Carney complex. Lancet Oncol 2005;6(7): 501–8.
81. Veugelers M, Wilkes D, Burton K, et al. Comparative PRKAR1A genotype-phenotype analyses in humans with Carney complex and prkar1a haploinsufficient mice. Proc Natl Acad Sci USA 2004;101(39): 14222–7.
82. Carney JA, Toorkey BC. Myxoid fibroadenoma and allied conditions (myxomatosis) of the breast. A heritable disorder with special associations including cardiac and cutaneous myxomas. Am J Surg Pathol 1991;15(8):713–21.
83. Amano J, Kono T, Wada Y, et al. Cardiac myxoma: its origin and tumor characteristics. Ann Thorac Cardiovasc Surg 2003;9(4):215–21.
84. Horvath A, Stratakis CA. Carney complex and lentiginosis. Pigment Cell Melanoma Res 2009;22(5):580–7.
85. Carney JA, Ferreiro JA. The epithelioid blue nevus. A multicentric familial tumor with important associations, including cardiac myxoma and psammomatous melanotic schwannoma. Am J Surg Pathol 1996;20(3): 259–72.
86. Carney JA, Stratakis CA. Epithelioid blue nevus and psammomatous melanotic schwannoma: the unusual pigmented skin tumors of the Carney complex. Semin Diagn Pathol 1998;15(3):216–24.
87. Kirschner LS, Taymans SE, Stratakis CA. Characterization of the adrenal gland pathology of Carney complex, and molecular genetics of the disease. Endocr Res 1998;24(3-4):863–4.
88. Groussin L, Horvath A, Jullian E, et al. A PRKAR1A mutation associated with primary pigmented nodular adrenocortical disease in 12 kindreds. J Clin Endocrinol Metab 2006;91(5):1943–9.
89. Zhang Y, Nosé V. Endocrine tumors as part of inherited tumor syndromes. Adv Anat Pathol 2011;18(3):206–18.
90. Petersson F, Bulimbasic S, Sima R, et al. Large cell calcifying Sertoli cell tumor: a clinicopathologic study of 1 malignant and 3 benign tumors using histomorphology, immunohistochemistry, ultrastructure, comparative genomic hybridization, and polymerase chain reaction analysis of the PRKAR1A gene. Hum Pathol 2010;41(4):552–9.
91. Nosé V. Thyroid cancer of follicular cell origin in inherited tumor syndromes. Adv Anat Pathol 2010;17(6):428–36.
92. Tran T, Gianoukakis AG. Familial thyroid neoplasia: impact of technological advances on detection and monitoring. Curr Opin Endocrinol Diabetes Obes 2010;17(5):425–31.
93. Gaujoux S, Tissier F, Ragazzon B, et al. Pancreatic ductal and acinar cell neoplasms in Carney complex: a possible new association. J Clin Endocrinol Metab 2011;9(11):E1888–95.
94. Talawadekar GD, Damodaran P, Jain SA. Hourglass ganglion cyst of the foot: a case report. J Foot Ankle Surg 2010;49(5):489.e11–12.
95. Casal D, Bilhim T, Pais D, et al. Paresthesia and hypesthesia in the dorsum of the foot as the presenting complaints of a ganglion cyst of the foot. Clin Anat 2010;23(5):606–10.
96. Kural C, Sungur I, Cetinus E. Bilateral lunate intraosseous ganglia. Orthopedics 2010;33(7):514.
97. Glenner GG. Amyloid deposits and amyloidosis. The beta-fibrilloses (first of two parts). N Engl J Med 1980;302(23):1283–92.
98. Glenner GG. Amyloid deposits and amyloidosis: the beta-fibrilloses (second of two parts). N Engl J Med 1980;302(24):1333–43.

99. Maheshwari AV, Muro-Cacho CA, Kransdorf MJ, et al. Soft-tissue amyloidoma of the extremities: a case report and review of literature. Skeletal Radiol 2009;38(3):287–92.
100. Pasternak S, Wright BA, Walsh N. Soft tissue amyloidoma of the extremities: report of a case and review of the literature. Am J Dermatopathol 2007;29(2):152–5.
101. Yang MC, Blutreich A, Das K. Nodular pulmonary amyloidosis with an unusual protein composition diagnosed by fine-needle aspiration biopsy: a case report. Diagn Cytopathol 2009;37(4):286–9.
102. Kato H, Toei H, Furuse M, et al. Primary localized amyloidosis of the urinary bladder. Eur Radiol 2003;13(Suppl. 6):L109–12.
103. Koczka CP, Goodman AJ. Gastric amyloidoma in patient after remission of Non-Hodgkin's Lymphoma. World J Gastrointest Oncol 2009;1(1): 93–6.
104. Parmar H, Rath T, Castillo M, et al. Imaging of focal amyloid depositions in the head, neck, and spine: amyloidoma. AJNR Am J Neuroradiol 2010;31(7):1165–70.
105. Factor RE, Layfield LJ, Grossmann AH, et al. Fine-needle aspiration diagnosis of an intraosseous amyloidoma. Diagn Cytopathol 2011. Available at: http://www.ncbi.nlm.nih.gov/pubmed/21548115. Accessed July 21, 2011.
106. Jährig A, Spaar FW, Lindermeyer J, et al. A historical cerebral amyloidoma (SPA) classified retrospectively as ALλ-type. A case report. Amyloid 2011;18(Suppl. 1):109–11.
107. Mukhopadhyay S, Damron TA, Valente AL. Recurrent amyloidoma of soft tissue with exuberant giant cell reaction. Arch Pathol Lab Med 2003;127(12):1609–11.
108. Feiner HD. Pathology of dysproteinemia: light chain amyloidosis, non-amyloid immunoglobulin deposition disease, cryoglobulinemia syndromes, and macroglobulinemia of Waldenström. Hum Pathol 1988; 19(11):1255–72.
109. Gouvêa AF, Ribeiro AC, León JE, et al. Head and neck amyloidosis: clinicopathological features and immunohistochemical analysis of 14 cases. J Oral Pathol Med 2012;41(2):178–85.
110. Coriu D, Badelita S, Talmaci R, et al. Bortezomib in systemic AL amyloidosis: a single center experience. Amyloid 2011;18(Suppl. 1):143–5.
111. Okuda I, Ubara Y, Takaichi K, et al. Genital beta2-microglobulin amyloidoma in a long-term dialysis patient. Am J Kidney Dis 2006; 48(3):e35–9.
112. Laeng RH, Altermatt HJ, Scheithauer BW, et al. Amyloidomas of the nervous system: a monoclonal B-cell disorder with monotypic amyloid light chain lambda amyloid production. Cancer 1998;82(2):362–74.
113. Krishnan J, Chu WS, Elrod JP, et al. Tumoral presentation of amyloidosis (amyloidomas) in soft tissues. A report of 14 cases. Am J Clin Pathol 1993;100(2):135–44.
114. Pambuccian SE, Horyd ID, Cawte T, et al. Amyloidoma of bone, a plasma cell/plasmacytoid neoplasm. Report of three cases and review of the literature. Am J Surg Pathol 1997;21(2):179–86.

Soft Tissue Tumors of Intermediate Malignancy of Uncertain Type

CHAPTER CONTENTS

In previous editions of this textbook, several entities of uncertain type were placed into either benign or malignant categories. Although these entities still remain an enigma with regard to line of cellular differentiation, larger clinicopathologic studies of each of these entities have revealed a better understanding of their clinical behavior. Although some of these entities were initially placed into the benign category (e.g., ossifying fibromyxoid tumor and pleomorphic hyalinizing angiectatic tumor [PHAT] of soft parts), it is clear that these lesions have a significant risk for local recurrence and can even metastasize on occasion. Similarly, other entities of uncertain type were originally categorized among the malignant tumors (myxoinflammatory fibroblastic sarcoma) but, given the lower risk for metastasis, especially with adequate therapy, behave less aggressively than the other lesions in this category. So, there is ample justification to categorize these tumors with those of intermediate malignancy, albeit of uncertain lineage.

OSSIFYING FIBROMYXOID TUMOR OF SOFT TISSUE

Ossifying fibromyxoid tumor of soft tissue, first described in a series of 59 cases from the Armed Forces Institute of Pathology (AFIP) in 1989,[1] is a rare tumor of uncertain differentiation that most commonly arises in the extremities. Close to 200 cases have been reported in the literature, in three large series,[1-3] as well as numerous case reports or small series. Although the original description of this tumor by Enzinger et al.[1] emphasized the bland morphologic appearance and typically benign clinical behavior, even in this series there was an indication that exceptional examples act in a clinically aggressive fashion. Several subsequent reports described tumors with typical features that unexpectedly metastasized, or tumors that had atypical or overtly malignant histologic features, some of which behaved aggressively.[4-7] Although some have suggested that malignant ossifying fibromyxoid tumors represent instead other tumor types,[8] two very recent studies have clearly confirmed the existence of atypical and malignant forms of this tumor.[3,9] So, it seems reasonable to consider ossifying fibromyxoid tumor a neoplasm of uncertain differentiation, spanning a morphologic and clinical spectrum from benign-appearing lesions that almost always behave in a benign fashion to histologically malignant lesions with a high risk for aggressive behavior.

Clinical Findings

Ossifying fibromyxoid tumor almost exclusively affects adults (mean age near 50 years), with only rare examples documented in children.[10,11] Men are affected more commonly than women. Most patients present with a small, painless, well-defined, often lobulated subcutaneous mass that involves the extremities in approximately 70% of cases (Table 32-1). Less commonly involved sites include the trunk, head and neck, mediastinum, and retroperitoneum.[12-16] Radiographic studies usually reveal a well-circumscribed mass with an incomplete ring of peripheral calcification and scattered calcifications in the substance of the neoplasm (Fig. 32-1).[17] Erosion of underlying bone and periosteal reaction is rarely seen.[1]

Pathologic Findings

Grossly, ossifying fibromyxoid tumor is usually well circumscribed, spherical, lobulated or multinodular, and typically covered by a thick fibrous pseudocapsule (Fig. 32-2). Most measure 3 to 5 cm, but occasional lesions are 15 cm or larger.[3] On a cut section, the tumor is tan-white and often has a gritty texture, as one would expect in a tumor that frequently has calcifications.

Microscopically, the majority are located in the subcutaneous tissue, but some are attached to tendons, fascia, or involve the underlying skeletal muscle. A typical ossifying fibromyxoid tumor is composed of uniform round, ovoid, or spindle-shaped cells arranged in nests and cords and deposited in a variably myxoid and collagenous stroma (Figs. 32-3 to 32-7). In approximately 70% of cases, there is an incomplete shell of lamellar bone found at the periphery of the nodules, either within or immediately beneath a dense fibrous pseudocapsule and sometimes extending into the substance of the tumor (Fig. 32-8). Bone is found in approximately 75% of histologically

TABLE 32-1 Anatomic Location of 59 Cases of Ossifying Fibromyxoid Tumor

SITE	NO. OF CASES
Upper extremity	20 (34%)
Shoulder/upper arm	10
Elbow/forearm	4
Hands/fingers	6
Lower extremity	20 (34%)
Buttock/thigh	11
Knee/lower leg	4
Foot	5
Trunk	11 (19%)
Chest wall	9
Abdomen	1
Flank	1
Head and neck	8 (13%)
Total	59 (100%)

Modified from Enzinger FM, Weiss SW, Liang CY. Ossifying fibromyxoid tumor of soft parts: a clinicopathological analysis of 59 cases. Am J Surg Pathol 1989;13:817–827.

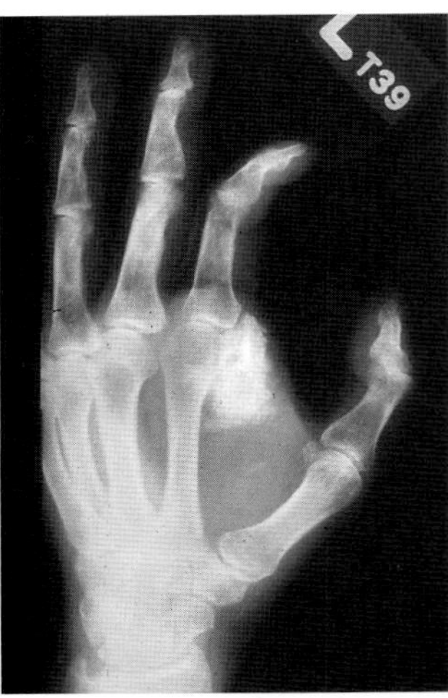

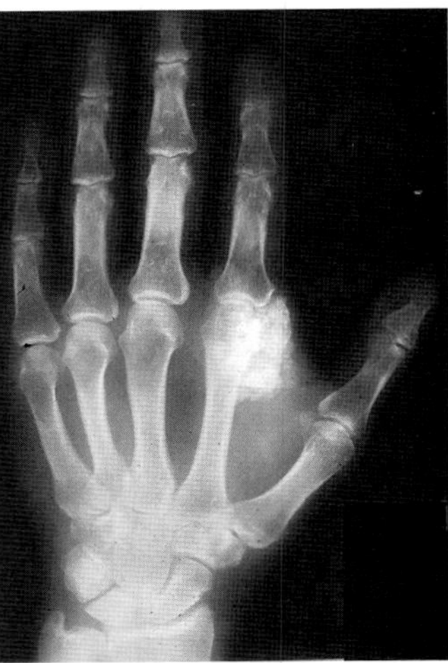

FIGURE 32-1. Typical radiographic appearance of ossifying fibromyxoid tumor of soft tissue. The tumor is well circumscribed and has extensive calcification.

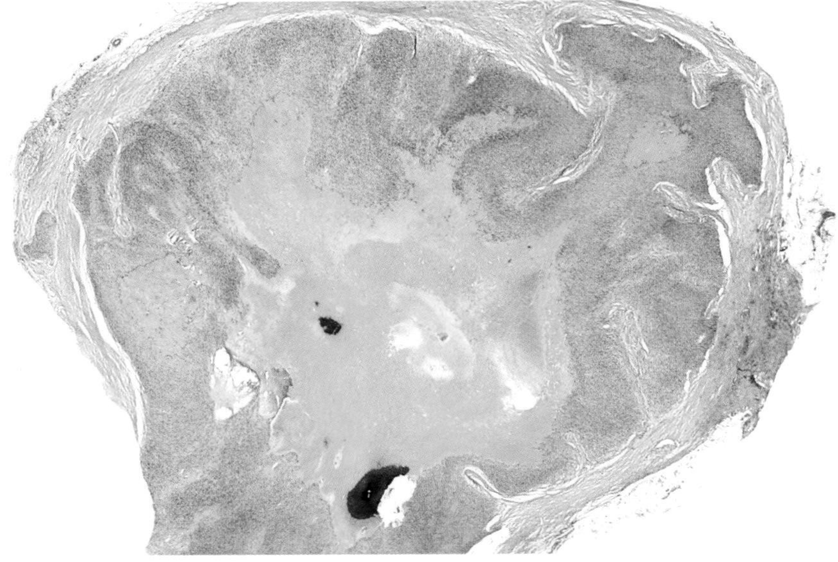

FIGURE 32-2. Ossifying fibromyxoid tumor of soft tissue. A pseudocapsule almost completely surrounds the neoplasm.

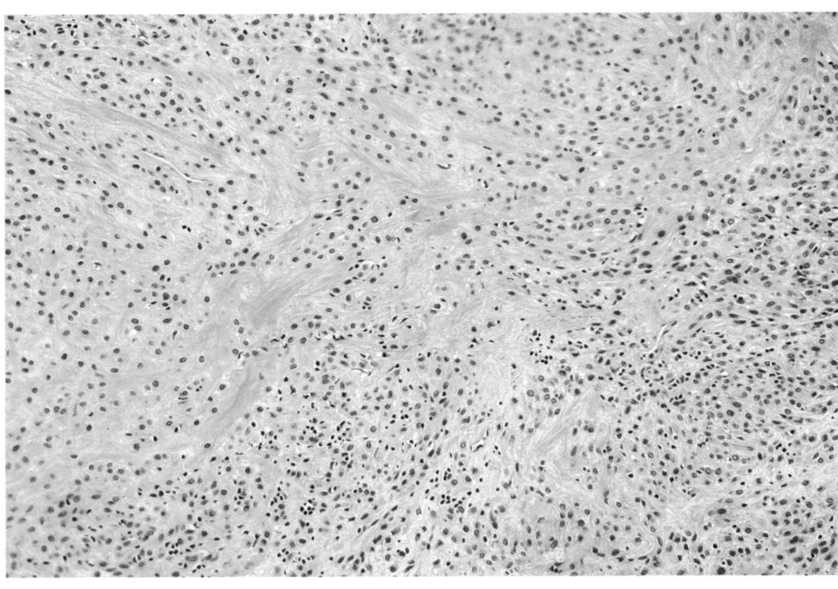

FIGURE 32-3. Low-magnification appearance of an ossifying fibromyxoid tumor. The cells are arranged in a variety of patterns and deposited in a variably hyalinized and myxoid matrix.

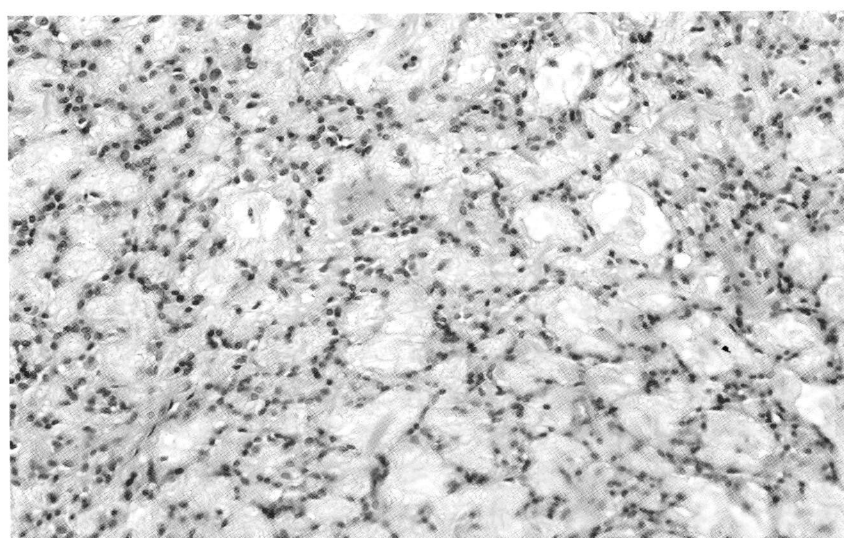

FIGURE 32-4. Ossifying fibromyxoid tumor. Cords of small tumor cells are suspended in a myxoid matrix.

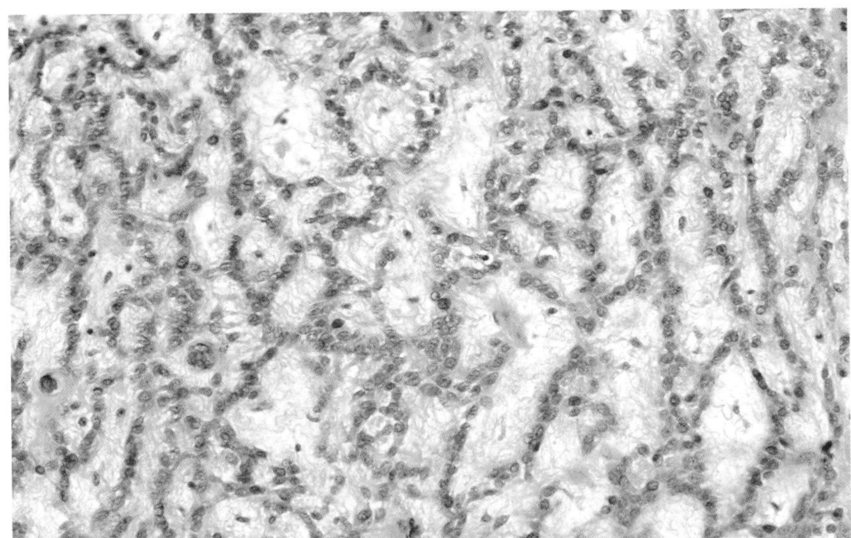

FIGURE 32-5. Thin cords of epithelioid tumor cells in an ossifying fibromyxoid tumor.

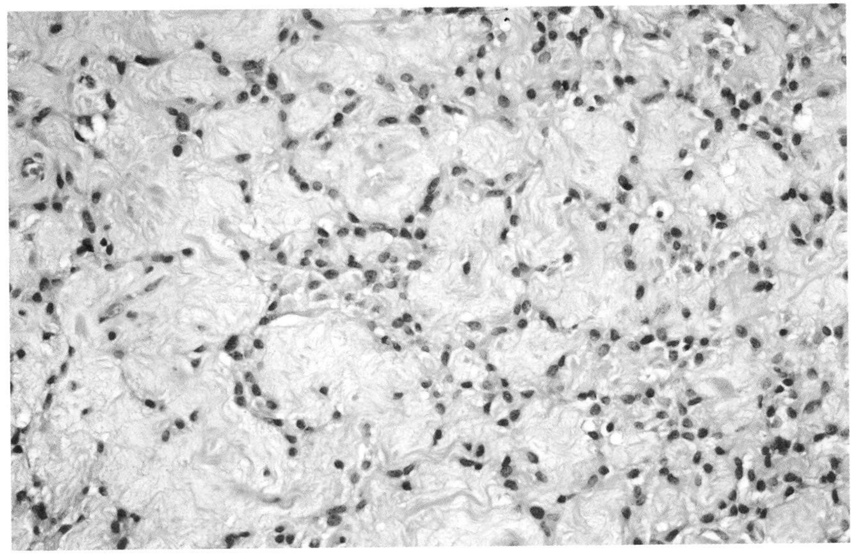

FIGURE 32-6. Less-cellular zone in an ossifying fibromyxoid tumor.

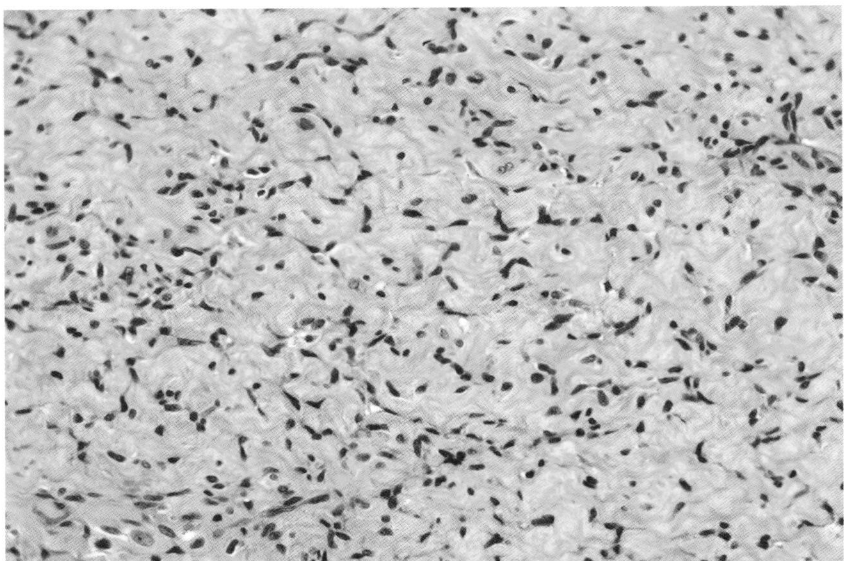

FIGURE 32-7. Fibrous zone in an ossifying fibromyxoid tumor, with compression of cords of tumor cells.

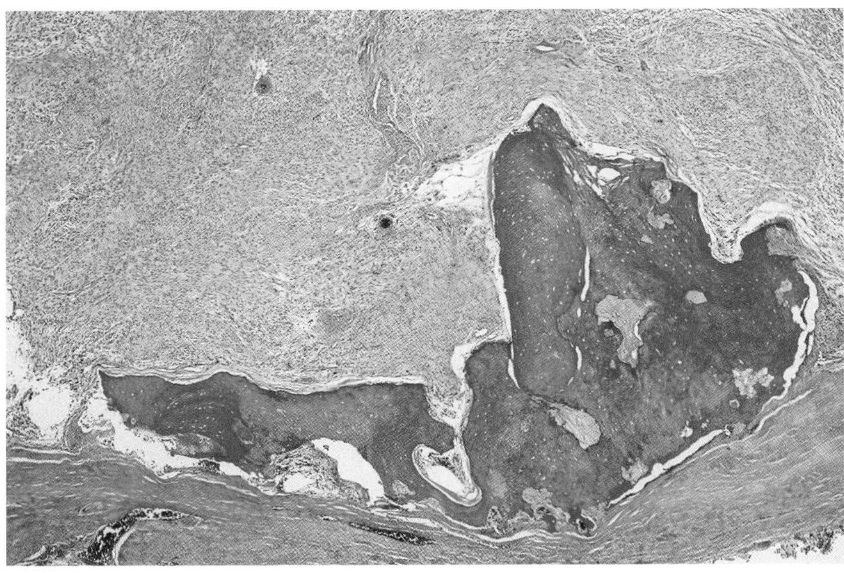

FIGURE 32-8. Ossifying fibromyxoid tumor with an incomplete rim of lamellar bone.

typical tumors, as compared with approximately 50% of those showing atypical histologic features.[2,3]

The constituent cells, which vary little in size and shape, are characterized by pale-staining vesicular nuclei with minute nucleoli and small amounts of eosinophilic cytoplasm (Fig. 32-9). The cells may be deposited in a variety of patterns, including cords, nests, or sheets; or they may be randomly distributed in a fibromyxoid matrix. Small pseudorosette-like structures are commonly present. Some lesions are predominantly myxoid with an abundant stroma of Alcian blue-positive, hyaluronidase-sensitive acid mucopolysaccharides, occasionally forming microcysts.[2,6] Other tumors are predominantly collagenous. Small foci of calcification and very rarely metaplastic cartilage may also be seen in the tumor nodules. Most have a rich vasculature, with many vessels exhibiting perivascular hyalinization and others subintimal fibrin deposition or thrombosis.

As thoroughly described by Folpe and Weiss,[2] Graham et al.[3] and others,[4] subsets of ossifying fibromyxoid tumors have atypical or overtly malignant features, usually consisting of some combination of high nuclear grade, high cellularity, or increased mitotic activity (greater than 2 mitotic figures [MF]/50 high-power fields [HPF]). It should be emphasized that these cases maintain the overall cytoarchitectural features of typical ossifying fibromyxoid tumor and may be conceptualized as representing a phenomenon akin to myxoid and round cell liposarcoma, rather than dedifferentiation. Some malignant ossifying fibromyxoid tumors show areas resembling sclerosing epithelioid fibrosarcoma, with densely hyalinized collagen and epithelioid cells.[2] Osteoid and/or woven bone may be present within the center of malignant-appearing tumors, and their presence is not indicative of osteosarcoma in a tumor otherwise showing morphologic features of ossifying fibromyxoid tumor. In general, confident diagnosis of

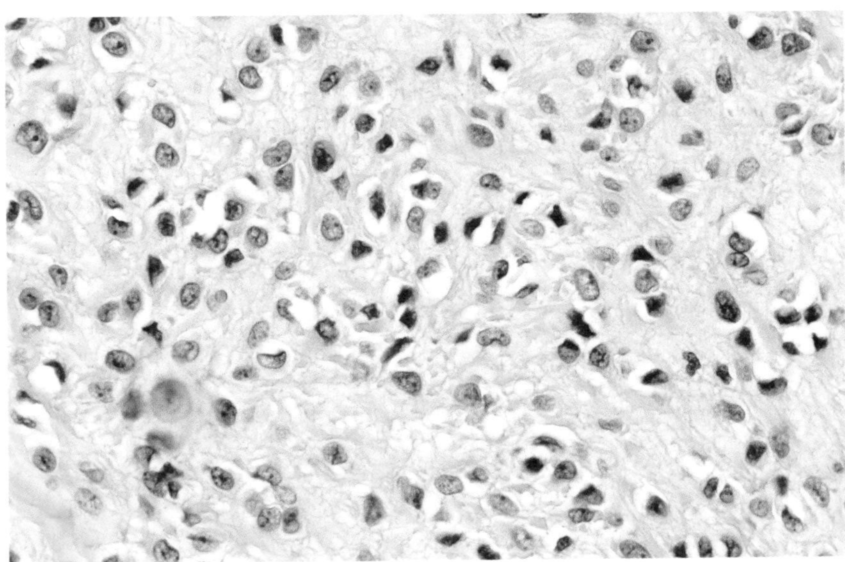

FIGURE 32-9. High-magnification view of bland epithelioid cells with vacuolated or eosinophilic cytoplasm in an ossifying fibromyxoid tumor.

malignant ossifying fibromyxoid tumor requires identification of areas of typical ossifying fibromyxoid tumor, either adjacent to malignant zones or present in an earlier manifestation of a recurrent lesion (Figs. 32-10 to 32-12).[3] Exceptionally, the tumor is composed exclusively of malignant-appearing areas. The clinical significance of these areas will be discussed later in detail.

Immunohistochemical and Ultrastructural Findings

Immunohistochemically, the cells are positive for vimentin and express S-100 protein in about 70% of cases (see Fig. 32-12), but immunoreactivity for the latter tends to be less intense and uniform than in schwannoma.[18,19] It is not uncommon for entirely typical ossifying fibromyxoid tumors to show only patchy S-100 protein expression. Atypical or malignant areas express S-100 protein less often than typical areas.[2,3] Scattered cells are positive for desmin and/or neurofilament protein in about 40% and 80% of tumors, respectively (Fig. 32-13). The cells may also occasionally express CD56, CD57, neuron-specific enolase, glial fibrillary acidic protein, smooth muscle actin, or cytokeratins.[2,3] Loss of expression of the SMARCB1/INI1 tumor suppressor gene product in a distinctive mosaic pattern has been reported by Graham et al.[3] in approximately 70% of tested cases, reflecting hemizygous loss of the *SMARCB1* locus and other regions of 22q, as determined by fluorescence in situ hybridization (FISH).[3,9]

In their original series, Enzinger et al.[1] noted ultrastructural features suggesting both cartilaginous and schwannian differentiation. The cells have irregular cell borders with short processes and intracellular microfilaments. In addition, well-developed and occasionally reduplicated external lamina may be present (Fig. 32-14).[1,20] However, ossifying fibromyxoid tumor lacks certain characteristic ultrastructural features of both cartilaginous and Schwann cell tumors. Other features that have been noted include ribosome-lamellar complexes.[2] It has also been suggested that the cells have some ultrastructural features of myoepithelial cells[21] or might possibly be derived from osteoprogenitor cells.

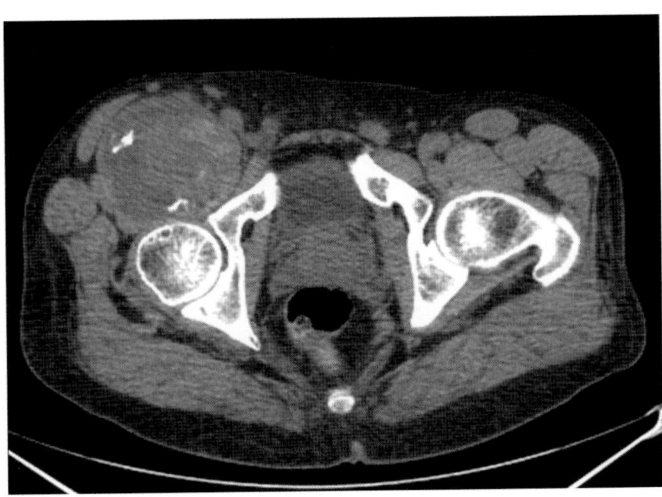

FIGURE 32-10. CT of a *de novo* malignant ossifying fibromyxoid tumor, showing a large soft tissue mass in the inguinal region, with a partial shell of bone. This patient presented with simultaneous lung and pleura metastases.

Cytogenetic and Molecular Genetic Findings

Very few cases of ossifying fibromyxoid tumor have been studied by cytogenetics, and, until very recently, no consistent aberration was identified. Nishio et al.[22] reported a histologically and clinically malignant tumor that showed a complex karyotype demonstrating t(3;11)(p21;p15), t(5;13)(q13;q34), and deletions of 12q13, 9p22, and 8p21, among others. Sovani et al.[23] reported an ossifying fibromyxoid tumor with loss of chromosome 6, extra material of unknown origin attached to the long arm of chromosome 12, and an unbalanced translocation involving chromosomes 6 and 14. Kawashima et al.[24] reported a case showing 46,XY,-Y, add(1)(q42), add(6)(p21),

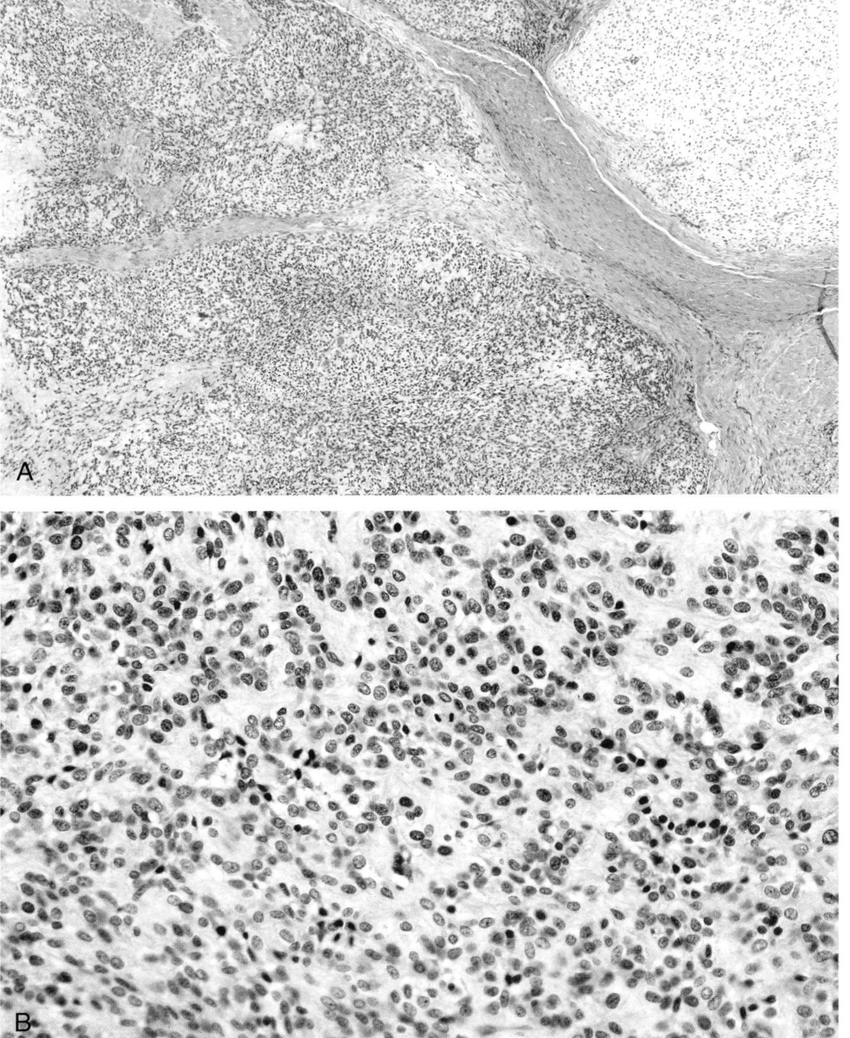

FIGURE 32-11. (A) Low-magnification view of a malignant ossifying fibromyxoid tumor showing the characteristic multilobular appearance. Some of the lobules are strikingly cellular. (B) High-magnification view of a cellular focus in a malignant ossifying fibromyxoid tumor.

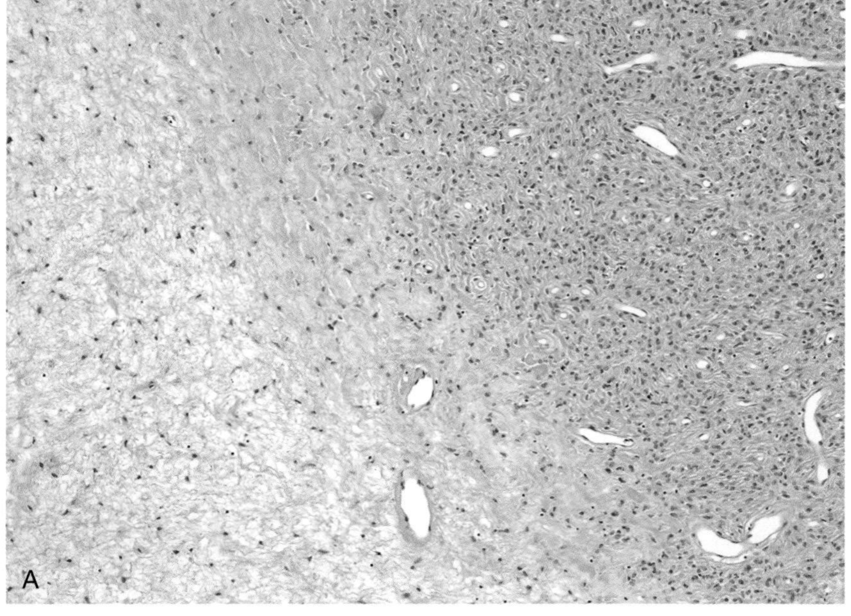

FIGURE 32-12. Primary ossifying fibromyxoid tumor showing typical histologic features (A).

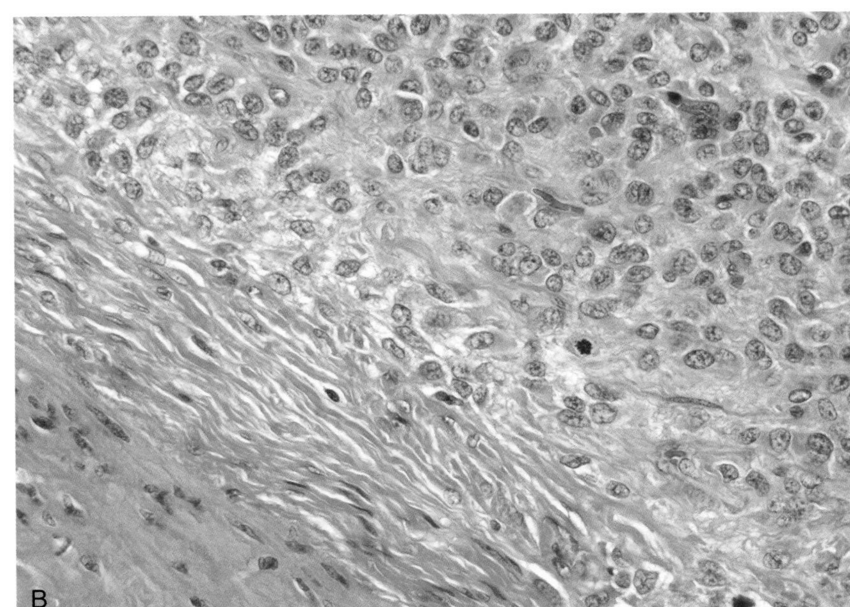

FIGURE 32-12, cont'd. In contrast, this patient's recurrent tumor, 3 years after initial resection, showed histologic features of malignancy, including high nuclear grade, high cellularity, and elevated mitotic activity (B).

FIGURE 32-13. Expression of S-100 protein (A), desmin (B), and neurofilament protein (C) in ossifying fibromyxoid tumor. *Continued*

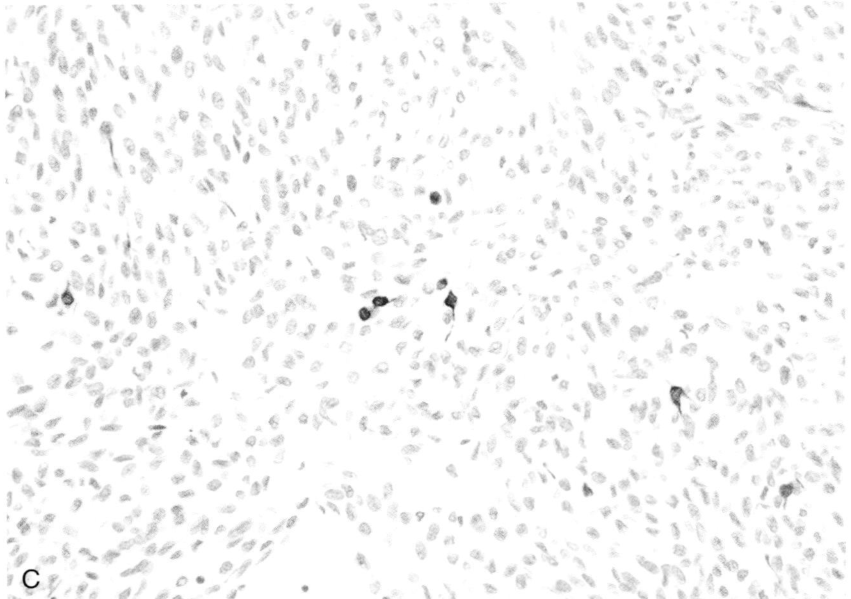

FIGURE 32-13, cont'd

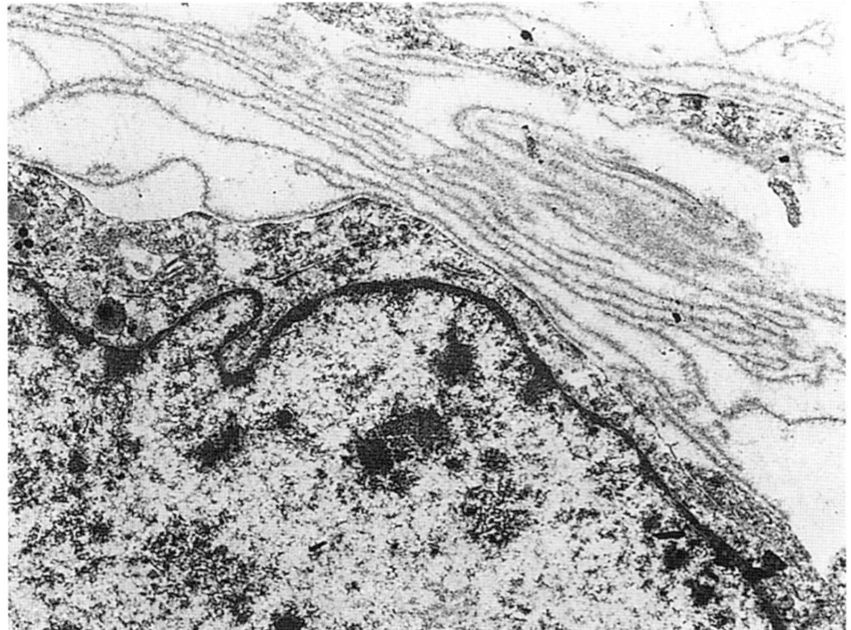

FIGURE 32-14. Electron micrograph of an ossifying fibromyxoid tumor with reduplication and scroll formation of external laminae, suggesting a tumor with neural differentiation. *(From Enzinger FM, Weiss SW, Liang CY. Ossifying fibromyxoid tumor of soft parts: a clinicopathological analysis of 59 cases. Am J Surg Pathol 1989;13:817.)*

t(10;18)(q26;q11), der(11)t(11;15)(q23;q15), add(12)(q13), ins(14;?)(q13;?),-15,+mar. One of the cases reported by Folpe and Weiss[2] showed a complex karyotype, including a t(11;19)(q11;q13) and abnormalities of chromosomes 1 and 3.

Very recently, however, Gebre-Medhin et al.[9] have shown three ossifying fibromyxoid tumors, including one typical, one atypical, and one malignant case, to have complex karyotypes, including different structural rearrangements of chromosome band 6p21. Mapping of this breakpoint by FISH demonstrated rearrangements of the *PHF1* gene, a transcriptional repressor previously shown to be consistently rearranged in endometrial stromal sarcomas.[25,26] This finding was further confirmed by interphase FISH, showing *PHF1* rearrangements in four of four typical, two of three atypical, and one of six malignant ossifying fibromyxoid tumors tested (Fig. 32-15).[9] Confirmatory reverse transcription polymerase chain reaction (RT-PCR) analysis of one case demonstrated an *EP400/PHF1* fusion transcript. *PHF1* is known to interact with polycomb group proteins, regulators of homeotic (*Hox*) genes, including *PRC2*, and dysregulation of *PRC2* target genes may underlie the pathogenesis of ossifying fibromyxoid tumors.[9]

FISH analyses of ossifying fibromyxoid tumors by Graham et al.[3] and Gebre-Medhin[9] have also consistently noted hemizygous loss of chromosome 22 or 22q, including, but not limited to, the *SMARCB1* locus (Fig. 32-16). It is currently unclear what role this plays in the pathogenesis of ossifying fibromyxoid tumors.

Differential Diagnosis

The differential diagnosis includes benign and malignant epithelioid nerve sheath tumors (epithelioid neurofibroma, epithelioid schwannoma, epithelioid malignant peripheral nerve sheath tumor), chondroid syringoma (cutaneous mixed tumor), myxoid chondrosarcoma, and epithelioid smooth muscle tumors.

Ossifying fibromyxoid tumor has many features in common with nerve sheath tumors. However, ossifying fibromyxoid tumor has not been documented to arise from a peripheral nerve, and the architectural and cytologic features are not typical of either epithelioid neurofibroma or epithelioid schwannoma. The cells lack the cytologic atypia characteristic of epithelioid malignant peripheral nerve sheath tumors.

The general absence of epithelial markers in ossifying fibromyxoid tumor helps exclude chondroid syringoma as a diagnostic consideration. The lobulated architecture and arrangement of the neoplastic cells into cord-like structures bear some resemblance to extraskeletal myxoid chondrosarcoma, but the stroma of ossifying fibromyxoid tumor varies between myxoid and collagenous, and the neoplastic cells have less eosinophilic cytoplasm than those of myxoid chondrosarcoma. Histochemically, periodic acid-Schiff (PAS) staining usually reveals abundant intracytoplasmic glycogen in the cells of myxoid chondrosarcoma, a feature lacking in ossifying fibromyxoid tumors. The ultrastructural characteristics of the two tumors are also quite distinctive. Epithelioid smooth muscle tumors usually express myoid antigens and lack S-100 protein, and they exhibit ultrastructural evidence of myoid differentiation.

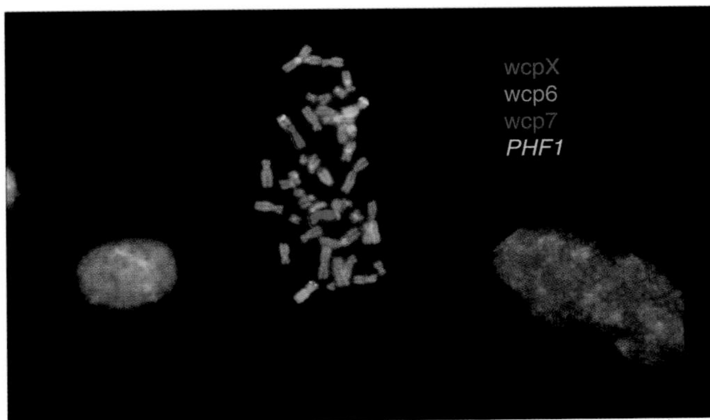

FIGURE 32-15. Break-apart FISH in a case of malignant ossifying fibromyxoid tumor, demonstrating *PHF1* rearrangement.

Discussion

The behavior of ossifying fibromyxoid tumor is highly variable. The vast majority of these tumors are histologically benign and have the characteristic features described in the original series from the AFIP (typical ossifying fibromyxoid tumor). Not unexpectedly, most of these pursue a benign clinical course. However, it has been noted that on rare occasion even histologically typical tumors may locally recur and metastasize. For example, Yoshida et al.[5] described a case lacking malignant features but which locally recurred, metastasized, and ultimately killed the patient. In the original report of typical ossifying fibromyxoid tumors by Enzinger et al.,[1] 11 of 41 (27%) patients for whom follow-up information was available experienced one or more recurrences. In addition, one patient with three recurrences developed a similar tumor in the contralateral thigh that was presumed to be a metastasis. The patient committed suicide shortly after discovery of the contralateral lesion. One additional patient developed a recurrence that showed histologic progression with increased bone production, originally interpreted as representing well-differentiated osteosarcoma. Combining the results of their study with those of the three largest previously published series,[1,6,19] Folpe and Weiss[2] estimated the overall recurrence and metastatic rates of typical ossifying fibromyxoid tumor to be 17% and 5%, respectively, suggesting that this tumor be

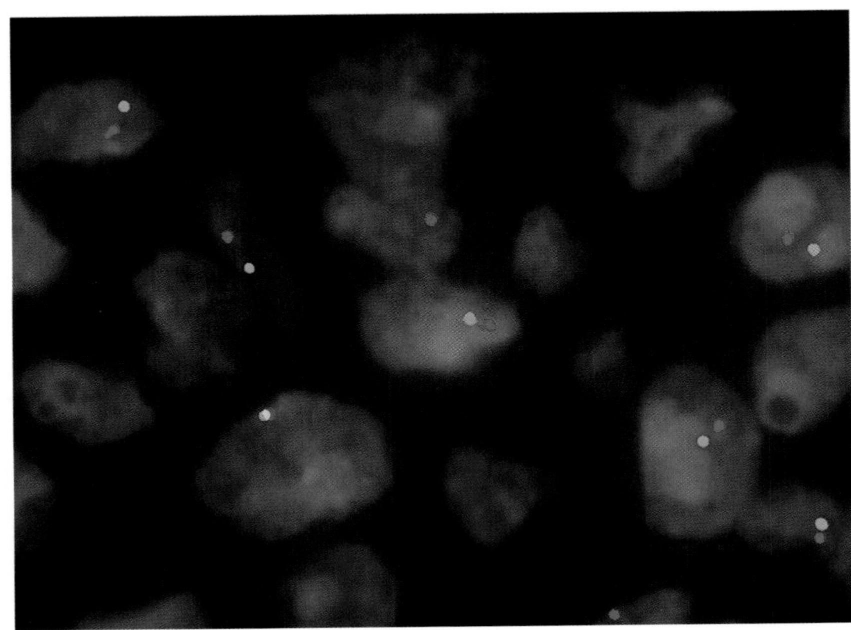

FIGURE 32-16. FISH in a case of ossifying fibromyxoid tumor, showing only one signal for SMARCB1 (green signal) and for PANX2 (control, red signal), consistent with monosomy 22 or loss of one 22q. Abnormalities in 22q are common in ossifying fibromyxoid tumors. *(Courtesy of Dr. Armita Bahrami, St. Jude Children's Research Hospital, Memphis, TN)*

TABLE 32-2 Proposed Classification of Ossifying Fibromyxoid Tumors

	DIAGNOSTIC CRITERIA
Typical OFMT	Low nuclear grade and low cellularity with mitotic activity <2 MF/50 HPF
Atypical OFMT	Tumors deviating from typical OFMT but not meeting criteria for malignant OFMT
Malignant OFMT	High nuclear grade or high cellularity and mitotic activity >2 MF/50 HPF

Modified from Folpe AL, Weiss SW. Ossifying fibromyxoid tumor of soft parts: a clinicopathologic study of 70 cases with emphasis on atypical and malignant variants. Am J Surg Pathol 2003;27:421–431.

OFMT, ossifying fibromyxoid tumor; MF, mitotic figure; HPF, high-power field.

TABLE 32-3 Risk of Local Recurrence and Metastasis in 45 Cases of Ossifying Fibromyxoid Tumor with Follow-Up

	NO. CASES WITH FOLLOW-UP	LOCAL RECURRENCES (%)	METASTASES (%)
Typical OFMT	25	3 (12)	1 (4)
Atypical OFMT	16	2 (13)	1 (6)
Malignant OFMT	10	6 (60)	6 (60)

Modified from Folpe AL, Weiss SW. Ossifying fibromyxoid tumor of soft parts: a clinicopathologic study of 70 cases with emphasis on atypical and malignant variants. Am J Surg Pathol 2003;27:421–431.

OFMT, ossifying fibromyxoid tumor.

considered a lesion with a low risk of distant metastasis (intermediate or borderline malignancy). It is, however, likely that the true metastatic rate for a typical ossifying fibromyxoid tumor is less than 5% because a recent very large series of typical lesions documented no metastases.[8]

As mentioned previously, some of these tumors have atypical histologic features, including high nuclear grade, increased cellularity, and increased mitotic activity. Williams et al.[7] described a series of nine head and neck tumors, one of which was histologically malignant (high cellularity, high nuclear grade, and a mitotic rate of 5 MF/10 HPF) and locally recurred within the 2-year follow-up period. In 1995, Kilpatrick et al.[4] reported six atypical and malignant ossifying fibromyxoid tumors. All of the tumors in this report had histologic features of malignancy, including areas of increased cellularity, increased mitotic activity, or deposition of centrally placed osteoid. Although meaningful follow-up was not available in four of these cases, one patient, a 68-year-old man with a 9-cm deep soft tissue mass adjacent to the greater trochanter, developed a local recurrence and histologically proven pulmonary metastases.

More recently, Folpe and Weiss[2] described 70 cases of ossifying fibromyxoid tumor with an emphasis on atypical and malignant variants. Twenty cases (29%) were histologically typical and showed low cellularity, low nuclear grade, and fewer than 2 MF/50 HPF. Most of the cases in this series (45 cases; 64%) showed a mixture of typical and atypical areas, and five cases (7%) showed essentially no areas of typical ossifying fibromyxoid tumor. By univariate analysis, high cellularity, high nuclear grade, and mitotic activity of greater than 2 MF/50 HPF were significantly associated with both local recurrence and metastasis. An infiltrative growth pattern was associated with local recurrence but not metastasis. None of the other features evaluated showed any correlation with an adverse clinical outcome. Therefore, the authors suggested that tumors with high nuclear grade or those with high cellularity and mitotic activity of greater than 2 MF/50 HPF should be regarded as sarcomas with significant potential for metastasis. Of the 10 cases in this category with clinical follow-up, 6 developed metastatic disease. Cases deviating from typical ossifying fibromyxoid tumors, but falling short of malignant ossifying fibromyxoid tumors, have a metastatic rate (6%) roughly similar to typical tumors (4%) and are classified as atypical ossifying fibromyxoid tumors (Tables 32-2 and 32-3).[2] The validity of this classification system has recently been confirmed by Graham et al.,[3] who documented adverse events in 33% of patients with malignant ossifying fibromyxoid tumors with follow-up (all showing some typical areas), including two patients with local recurrences, three patients with distant metastases, and three deaths from disease. No adverse events were seen in patients with typical tumors.

Line of Differentiation

The line of differentiation of ossifying fibromyxoid tumor has been the subject of considerable debate over the years, with investigators favoring cartilaginous, osteogenous, or myoepithelial differentiation. Until recently, however, the most widely accepted theory was that ossifying fibromyxoid tumor represented an unusual peripheral nerve sheath tumor, on the basis of its encapsulation, expression of nerve sheath-related markers such as S-100, CD57 and GFAP, and some ultrastructural features.[27]

More recent data have shed considerable new light on this subject. A very recent gene expression profiling and proteomic study of ossifying fibromyxoid tumor have suggested limited neural differentiation, with upregulation of neuron-related genes such as *EAAT4* and *HuC*, and downregulation of Schwann cell-associated genes such as peripheral myelin protein 22 (*PMP22*) and myelin expression factor 2 (*MYEF2*).[3] Additionally, cluster and principal component analyses show ossifying fibromyxoid tumor to clearly segregate from true nerve sheath tumors, such as schwannoma and nerve sheath myxoma (Fig. 32-17).[3] Proteomic data show expression of proteins related to neuronal, schwannian, and cartilaginous differentiation.[3] These findings and, more important, the very recent finding by Gebre-Medhin et al.[9] of *PHF1* rearrangements in these tumors strongly suggest that ossifying fibromyxoid tumors are translocation-associated neoplasms showing a scrambled phenotype, as originally hypothesized by Folpe and Weiss[2] in 2003.

MYXOINFLAMMATORY FIBROBLASTIC SARCOMA (INFLAMMATORY MYXOHYALINE TUMOR OF THE DISTAL EXTREMITIES WITH VIROCYTE OR REED-STERNBERG-LIKE CELLS, ACRAL MYXOINFLAMMATORY FIBROBLASTIC SARCOMA)

In 1998, Montgomery et al.[28] reported 49 cases of a previously undescribed tumor of the distal extremities with unusual

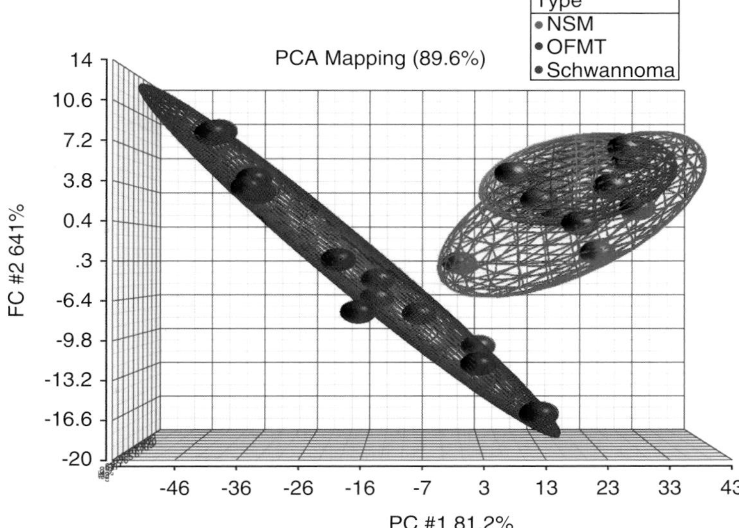

FIGURE 32-17. Principal component analysis mapping of gene expression profiling data from ossifying fibromyxoid tumors, as compared with true nerve sheath tumors. Histologically benign and malignant ossifying fibromyxoid tumors cluster together (*blue*), and apart from nerve sheath myxomas (*red*) and schwannomas (*green*).

histologic features often prompting a misdiagnosis of an inflammatory or infectious process. Because of the presence of scattered bizarre cells with vesicular nuclei and macronucleoli and a prominent inflammatory background, the authors coined the term *inflammatory myxohyaline tumor of distal extremities with virocyte or Reed-Sternberg-like cells.* In this initial report, local recurrences occurred in almost one-fourth of the patients, although none developed metastatic disease. Shortly thereafter, Meis-Kindblom and Kindblom[29] reported a series describing the identical tumor, including one patient with biopsy-proven metastasis and used the term *acral myxoinflammatory fibroblastic sarcoma* to emphasize the occasionally aggressive clinical course. Similar cases were also reported by Michal et al.[30] as inflammatory myxoid tumor of the soft parts with bizarre giant cells. Because it has become clear that these lesions may involve nonacral locations, the World Health Organization (commonly recognized as WHO) has recommended use of the term *myxoinflammatory fibroblastic sarcoma* for this lesion.[31]

Clinical Findings

Although the age range is broad, most patients with this tumor are in the fourth and fifth decades of life.[28-30] Males and females are affected equally, and most patients present with a slowly growing, painless, ill-defined mass of the distal extremities. The upper extremities are affected more commonly than the lower extremities, with the single most common site being the soft tissues of the fingers and hand, although some lesions arise in the lower arm and wrist. On the lower extremities, these tumors may arise in the toes, feet, ankles, and lower legs (Table 32-4). There are few cases reported in the literature that have arisen in extra-acral sites.[32,33] Some patients report mild pain and decreased mobility of the affected site, and occasionally there is a history of antecedent trauma, which serves to bring the tumor to clinical attention. Given its location, the lesion is often thought to represent a ganglion cyst or some form of tenosynovitis. Magnetic resonance imaging findings are not diagnostic but typically reveal a poorly circumscribed mass with involvement of the underlying tendon sheath.[34]

TABLE 32-4 Anatomic Distribution of 95 Myxoinflammatory Fibroblastic Sarcomas (Inflammatory Myxohyaline Tumors) of the Distal Extremities[22, 23]

ANATOMIC SITE	NO. OF CASES
Upper extremities	65 (68%)
Fingers/hands	53
Wrist/lower arm	10
Miscellaneous	2
Lower extremities	30 (32%)
Toes/feet	16
Ankles/lower leg	13
Miscellaneous	1

Pathologic Findings

Grossly, the tumor is multinodular and poorly circumscribed, and it is often removed piecemeal by the surgeon (Fig. 32-18). Gelatinous-appearing areas are conspicuous in the lesions with extensive myxoid change. The tumors range in size from 1 to 8 cm (mean 3 to 4 cm).

At low magnification, the tumor is multinodular and poorly circumscribed and frequently involves surrounding tendon sheaths and the synovium of adjacent joints (Fig. 32-19). Most arise in the subcutaneous tissue, but some involve the dermis and others focally infiltrate skeletal muscle. Destruction or invasion of underlying bony structures has not been reported.

The most striking feature at low magnification is that of a dense inflammatory infiltrate merging with myxoid or hyaline zones (Figs. 32-20 and 32-21). In most cases, leukocytes and plasma cells predominate, although neutrophils and eosinophils are conspicuous in some tumors (Fig. 32-22).[35] Germinal centers are occasionally encountered. The amount of myxoid and hyalinized stroma varies from case to case. Some tumors are composed predominantly of hypocellular myxoid zones

(Fig. 32-23), whereas other tumors may have only focal myxoid change. Hyaline zones contain a sparse mixture of inflammatory and neoplastic cells and often resemble the hyalinized zones of inflammatory myofibroblastic tumor (Fig. 32-24). Hemosiderin deposition may be conspicuous.

Examination of more cellular zones reveals bizarre atypical cells deposited in a hyalinized or myxoid stroma and allows for recognition of this lesion as a neoplastic process. These atypical cells range in shape from plump spindled cells to histiocytoid or epithelioid cells (Fig. 32-25). The spindled cells have a moderate degree of nuclear atypia, whereas the larger epithelioid cells often have large vesicular nuclei with macronucleoli and prominent eosinophilic cytoplasm, imparting a close similarity to virocytes or Reed-Sternberg cells (Figs. 32-26 and 32-27). Despite the marked degree of nuclear atypia, there is a paucity of mitotic figures, typically with fewer than 2 MF/50 HPF. Ganglion-like cells resembling those seen in proliferative fasciitis may be widely scattered throughout the neoplasm or form small nodular collections. Some bizarre cells have multivacuolated cytoplasm simulating lipoblasts (Fig. 32-28), and others appear to engulf inflammatory cells.[36] Multinucleated giant cells, including Touton-type giant cells, are occasionally encountered (Fig. 32-29). In addition, there is often an intermingling of round mononuclear cells with bland nuclear features and small amounts of amphophilic cytoplasm. Necrosis is rarely present. In rare cases, areas of typical myxoinflammatory fibroblastic sarcoma are juxtaposed to a low-grade, hemosiderin-rich spindle cell proliferation, identical to that seen in so-called *hemosiderotic fibrolipomatous tumor* or *early* PHAT (see later text).[37,38]

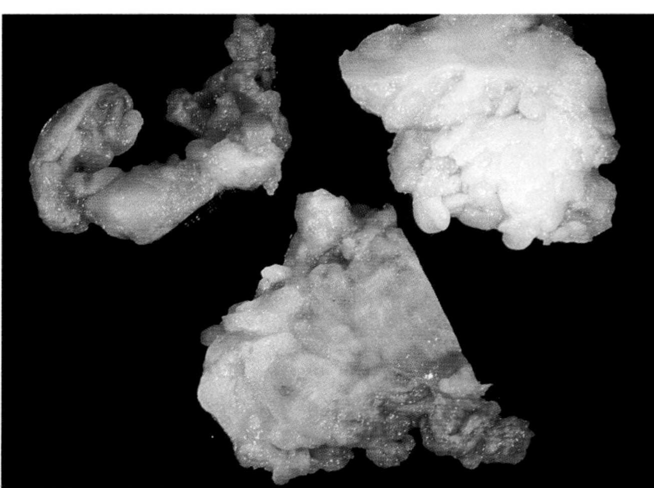

FIGURE 32-18. Gross specimen of a myxoinflammatory fibroblastic sarcoma showing multinodular focally gelatinous mass. *(From Montgomery EA, Devaney KO, Giordano TJ, et al. Inflammatory myxohyaline tumor of distal extremities with virocyte or Reed-Sternberg-like cells: a distinctive lesion with features simulating inflammatory conditions, Hodgkin's disease, and various sarcomas. Mod Pathol 1998;11:384.)*

Immunohistochemical and Ultrastructural Findings

The mononuclear and larger bizarre cells consistently stain for vimentin, with variable immunoreactivity for CD68, CD34, and smooth muscle actin (Table 32-5).[28,29] Immunostains for S-100 protein, HMB-45, desmin, epithelial membrane antigen (EMA), CD45, CD15, and CD30 are typically negative. Focal immunoreactivity for cytokeratins is sometimes found. The lymphocytic infiltrate is predominantly composed of T cells with a smaller component of B cells.

Ultrastructurally, the bizarre neoplastic cells characteristically have a single, often clefted nucleus with one or more large nucleoli and occasional intranuclear cytoplasmic inclusions.[29] There are abundant rough endoplasmic reticulum and mitochondria, as well as densely packed perinuclear whorls of intermediate filaments, although actin-type and thin filaments are not seen. Small lipid droplets, glycogen, and scattered lysosomes may also be seen in the cytoplasm. Overall, the ultrastructural features are most consistent with a tumor showing fibroblastic differentiation.[32]

Text continued on p. 985

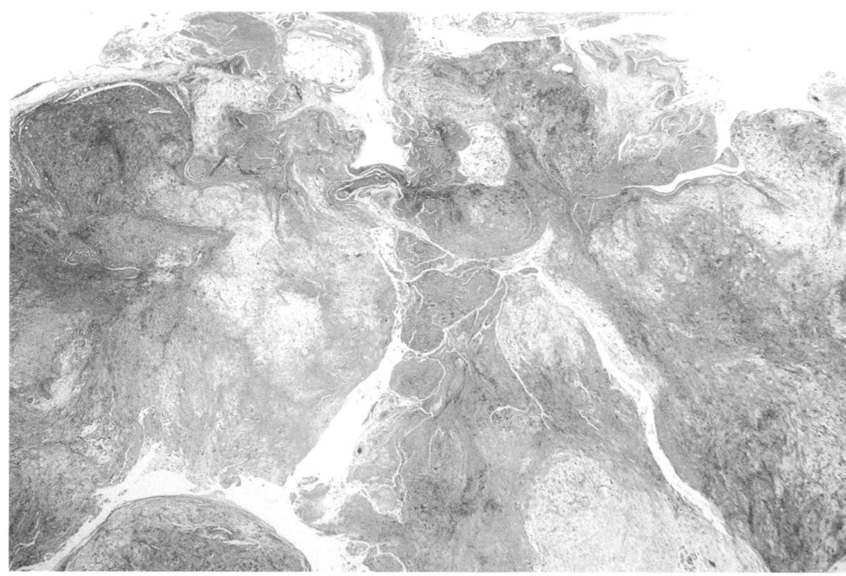

FIGURE 32-19. Low-power view of myxoinflammatory fibroblastic sarcoma illustrating a mixture of myxoid, hyaline, and inflammatory zones.

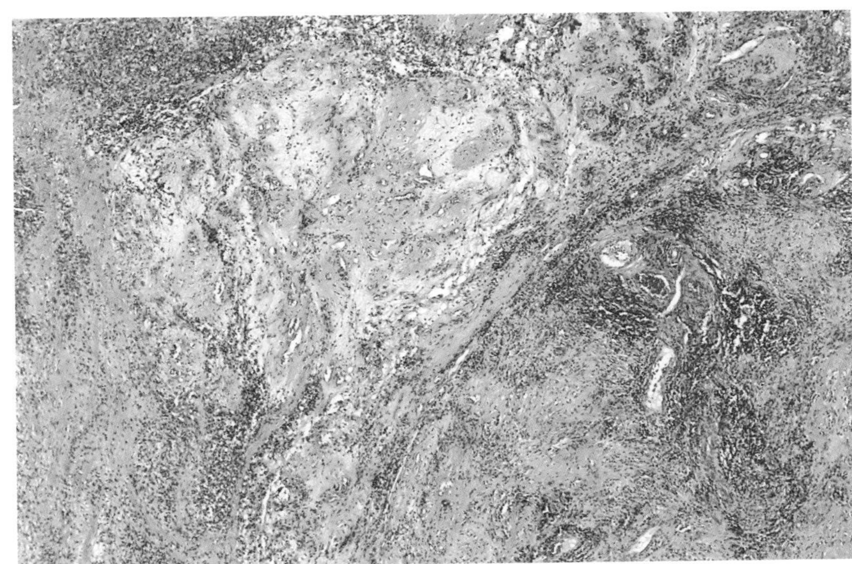

FIGURE 32-20. Admixture of myxoid, hyaline, and inflammatory zones in a myxoinflammatory fibroblastic sarcoma.

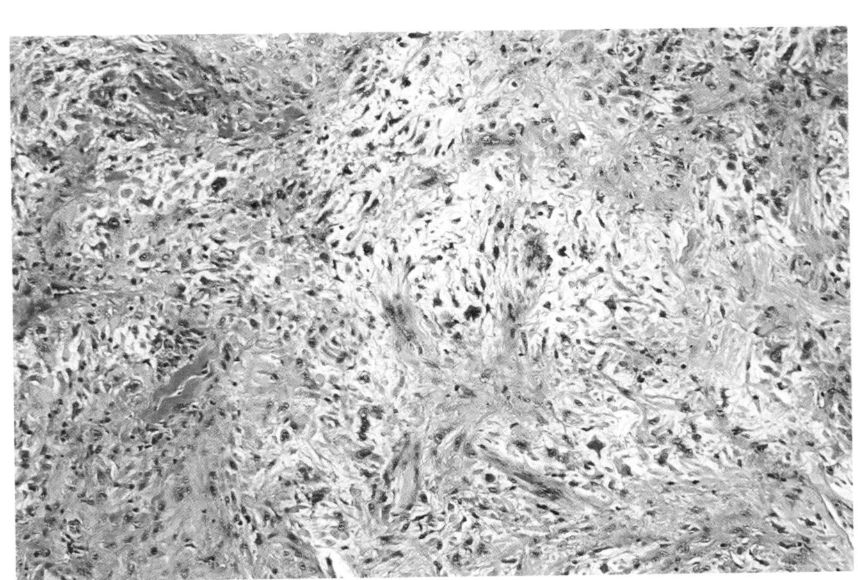

FIGURE 32-21. Myxoinflammatory fibroblastic sarcoma. Note the transition between myxoid and hyaline zones.

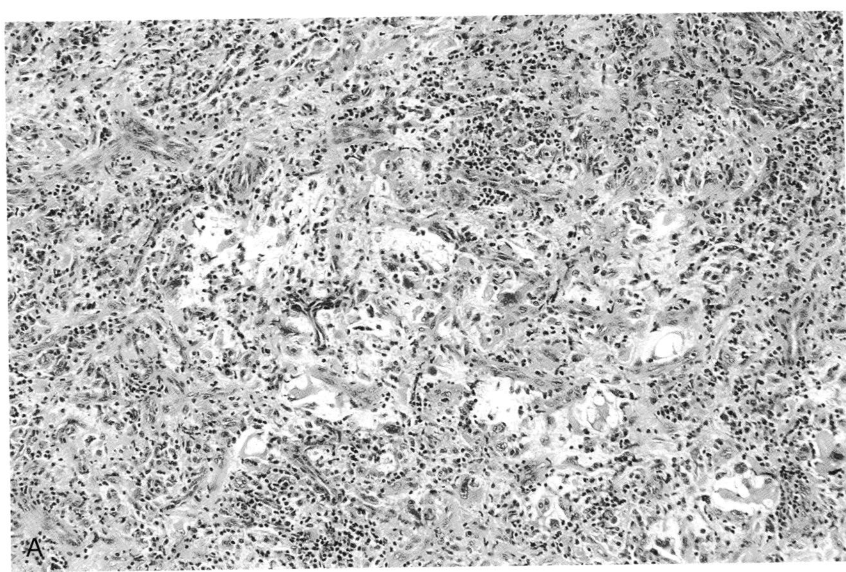

FIGURE 32-22. (A, B) Myxoinflammatory fibroblastic sarcoma with prominent inflammatory zones.

Continued

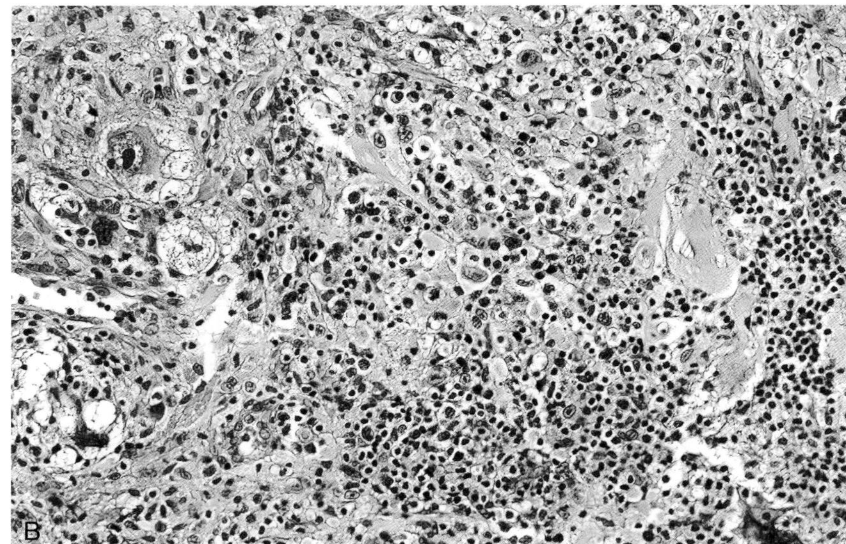

FIGURE 32-22, cont'd

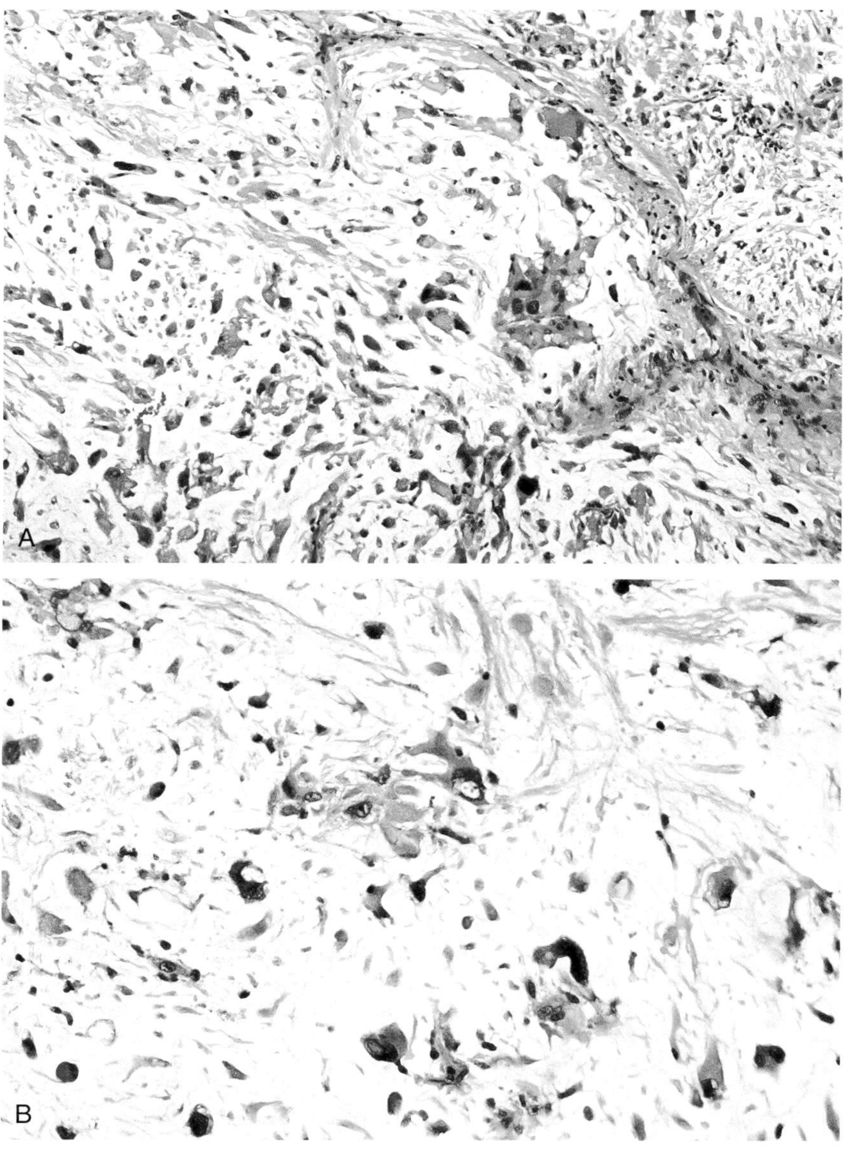

FIGURE 32-23. (A) Low-magnification view of a myxoid zone in a myxoinflammatory fibroblastic sarcoma. (B) Higher-magnification view of cells with smudgy nuclei in a myxoid zone of a myxoinflammatory fibroblastic sarcoma.

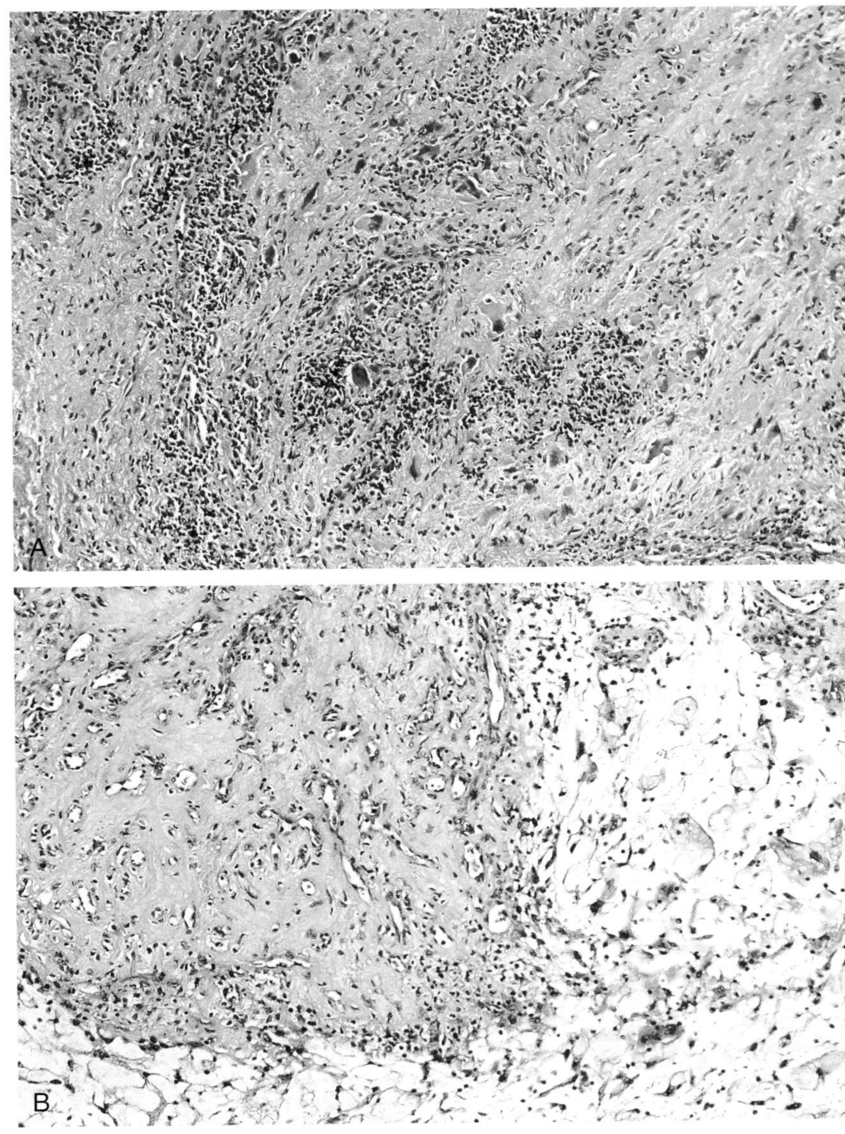

FIGURE 32-24. Myxoinflammatory fibroblastic sarcoma. (A) Hyaline area with prominent inflammatory component. (B) Sharp transition between myxoid and hyaline zones.

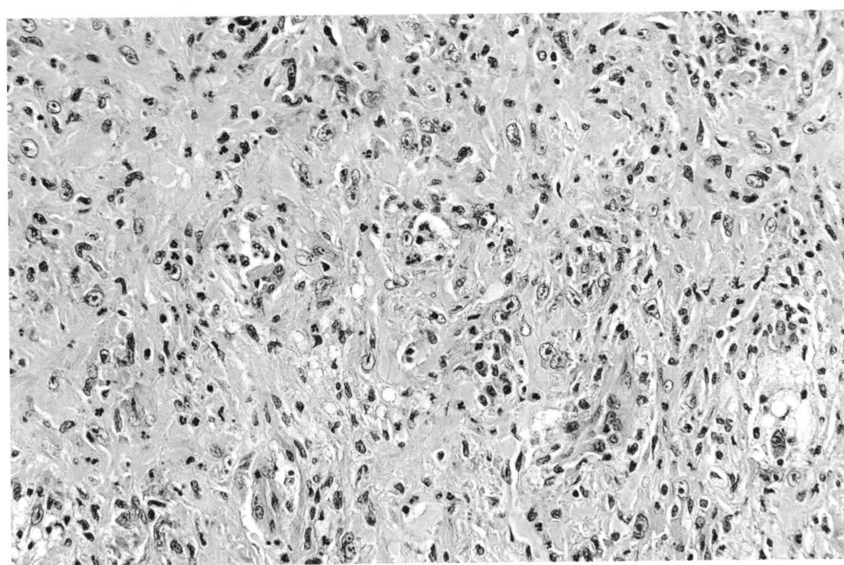

FIGURE 32-25. Myxoinflammatory fibroblastic sarcoma. Neoplastic cells range from spindled to epithelioid.

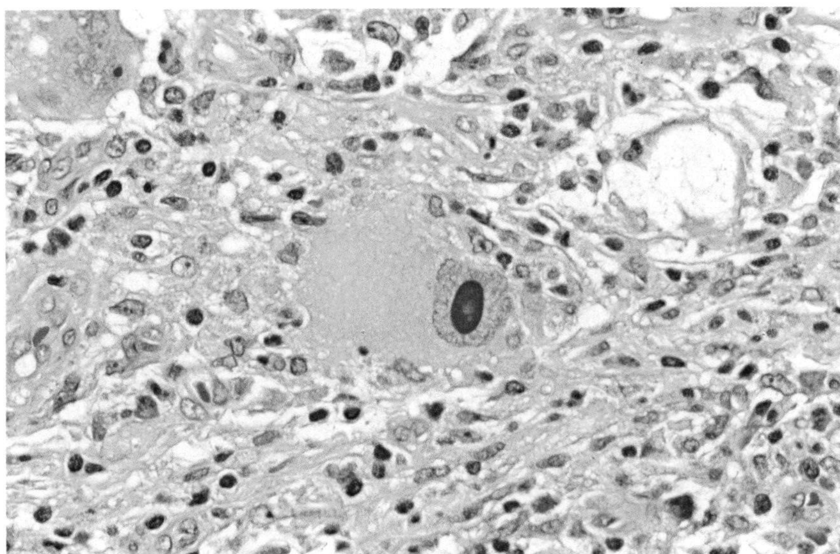

FIGURE 32-26. Enlarged tumor cell with a large eosinophilic nucleolus resembling a virocyte in a myxoinflammatory fibroblastic sarcoma.

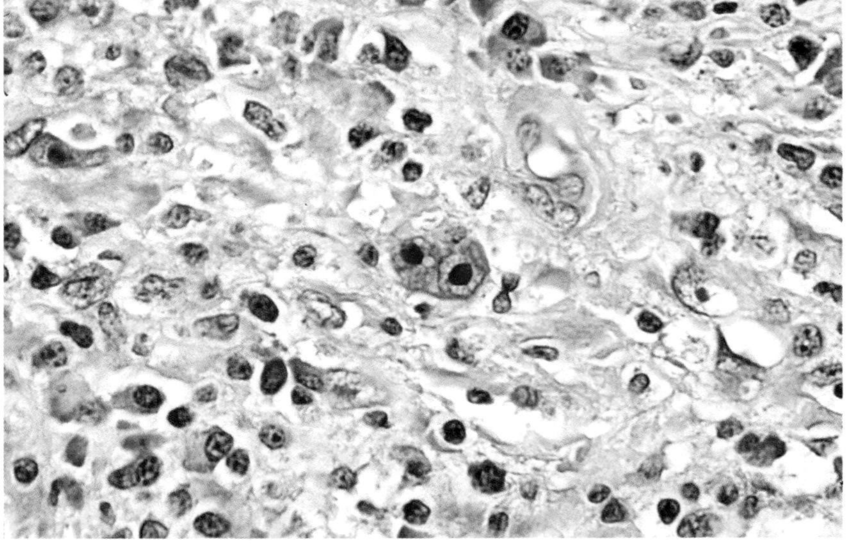

FIGURE 32-27. Myxoinflammatory fibroblastic sarcoma with cells resembling Reed-Sternberg cells.

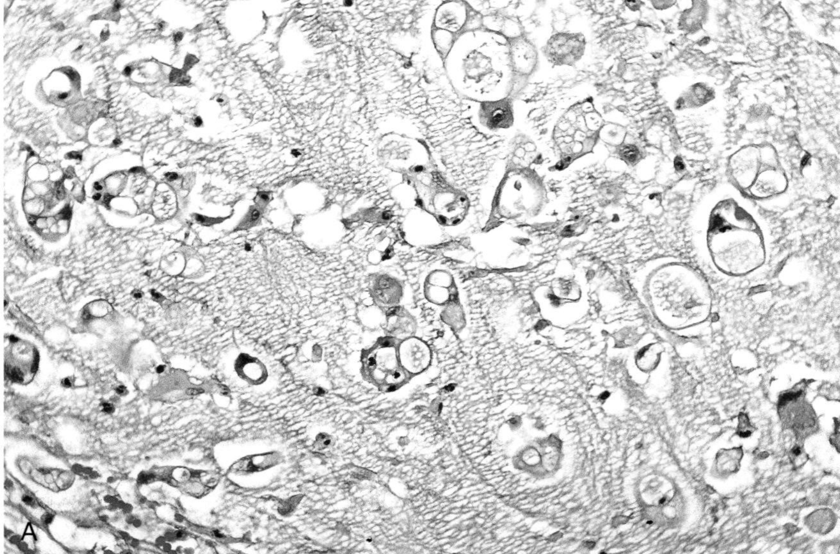

FIGURE 32-28. Myxoid zones in a myxoinflammatory fibroblastic sarcoma. (A) Bizarre cells are distended with stromal mucin.

FIGURE 32-28, cont'd. (B) Pseudolipoblasts are prominent in this tumor.

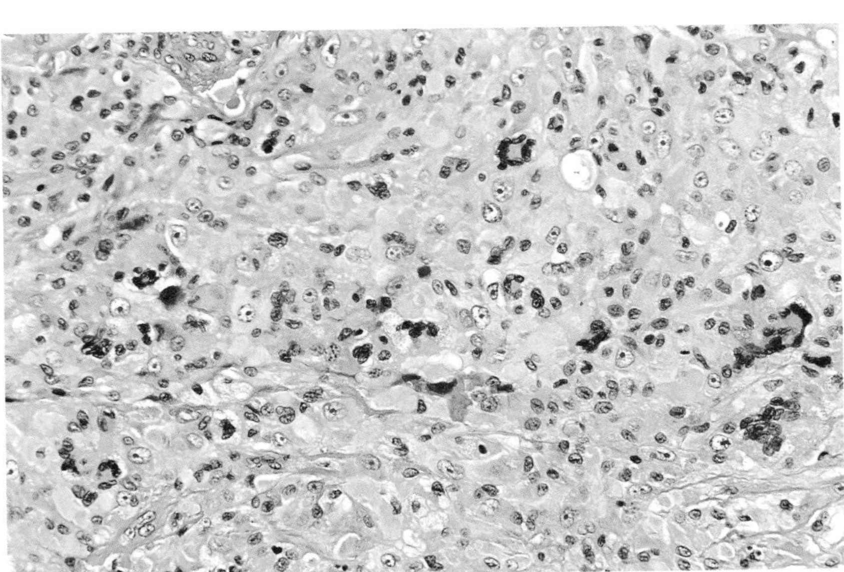

FIGURE 32-29. Scattered multinucleated giant cells in a cellular zone of myxoinflammatory fibroblastic sarcoma.

TABLE 32-5 Immunohistochemical Data on Myxoinflammatory Fibroblastic Sarcomas (Inflammatory Myxohyaline Tumors) of the Distal Extremities[22, 23]

MARKER	NO. OF CASES STAINED
Vimentin	35/35 (100%)
CD68	23/35 (66%)
CD34	7/25 (28%)
Cytokeratin	4/38 (11%)
Smooth muscle actin	2/33 (6%)
CD15	0/5
CD30	0/12
EMA	0/28
S-100 protein	0/44
Desmin	0/6

EMA, epithelial membrane antigen.

Genetic Findings

In 2001, Lambert et al.[39] reported a single case of myxoinflammatory fibroblastic sarcoma with a t(1;10)(p22;q24) and loss of chromosomes 3 and 13. This finding was confirmed by Hallor et al.,[40] in 2009, who identified this same translocation or der (10)(t1;10) as well as aberrations in chromosome 3 in four of five studied cases. Using a variety of molecular methods, Hallor et al.[40] were able to show this translocation to contain a unique fusion gene, *TGFBR3-MGEA5*, resulting in transcriptional upregulation of *NPM3* and *FGF8*, two genes located downstream to *MGEA5*. Additional support for a critical role of this gene fusion in myxoinflammatory fibroblastic sarcoma has recently been provided by Antonescu et al.,[37] who identified it by FISH in 5 of 7 tested cases, as well as in 12 of 14 hemosiderotic fibrolipomatous tumors and 3 of 3 cases showing mixed histologic features of these two tumors. As will be discussed later, an identical t(1;10)(p22;q24) has also been reported in hemosiderotic fibrolipomatous tumor[40,41] and in tumors showing hybrid features of hemosiderotic fibrolipomatous tumor and myxoinflammatory fibroblastic sarcoma.[38]

Differential Diagnosis

Because of the wide array of appearances of this tumor, the differential diagnosis, in part, depends on the cellularity of the lesion and the relative amount of myxoid and hyaline stroma. An infectious or inflammatory process is often considered, given the prominent inflammatory background, cells with virocyte-like nuclei, and necrosis. Special stains for microbial organisms are invariably negative as are immunohistochemical stains for cytomegalovirus. Montgomery et al.[28] analyzed 10 cases by PCR for the presence of Epstein-Barr virus (EBV); 4 patients were found to harbor EBV, but the level of amplification was compatible with latent, rather than active, viral infection.

Giant cell tumor of the tendon sheath is often a diagnostic consideration given the location of the tumor, the prominent inflammatory component, and the presence of Touton-like giant cells and hemosiderin. Recognition of the large bizarre cells, which are widely scattered in some cases, is critical for distinguishing these lesions. This tumor also has histologic features that overlap with those found in inflammatory myofibroblastic tumor, although the cells of myxoinflammatory fibroblastic sarcoma are more bizarre than those seen in the latter and lack the well-developed immunohistochemical and ultrastructural features of myofibroblasts. Moreover, the acral location of most myxoinflammatory fibroblastic sarcomas is not characteristic of inflammatory myofibroblastic tumor. Finally, ALK-1 protein positivity is frequently found in inflammatory myofibroblastic tumor, particularly those arising in the abdomen.

For those tumors with prominent myxoid stroma, there are a number of benign and malignant myxoid lesions that could be considered. The large bizarre cells characteristic of myxoinflammatory fibroblastic sarcoma would not be found in any benign myxoid soft tissue neoplasm. Distinction from myxofibrosarcoma/myxoid undifferentiated pleomorphic sarcoma is the most difficult aspect of the differential diagnosis; both tumors have enough distinguishing characteristics to support the contention that they are distinct entities. Focal areas of high-grade pleomorphic sarcoma may be seen in myxofibrosarcoma, whereas high-grade areas would not be found in myxoinflammatory fibroblastic sarcoma. Additional differences include the alternating myxoid and hyalinized zones, a more striking inflammatory infiltrate, the presence of virocyte-like cells, and the acral location typical of myxoinflammatory fibroblastic sarcoma.

The presence of Reed-Sternberg-like cells also raises the possibility of Hodgkin lymphoma in some cases. Immunohistochemically, the large atypical cells lack expression of CD15 and CD30, as one would expect to find in the Reed-Sternberg cells of Hodgkin lymphoma.

Discussion

In the series of 51 cases reported by Montgomery et al.,[28] follow-up information was obtained in 27 patients with a median follow-up period of 53 months. Of these 27 patients, 6 (22%) developed at least one local recurrence 15 months to 10 years after the initial excision, but none developed metastatic disease. In the subsequent study of 44 cases by Meis-Kindblom and Kindblom,[29] follow-up information obtained in 32 patients revealed a local recurrence rate of 67%, including 8 patients who had two local recurrences and 5 who had at least three local recurrences. The rather striking difference in recurrence rates between these studies probably reflects a difference in the referral base. The cases reported from the AFIP were largely ascertained retrospectively,[29] and many were not originally diagnosed as sarcoma, whereas those reported by Montgomery et al.[28] were ascertained prospectively and all were diagnosed as low-grade sarcomas and treated more aggressively. One patient reported by Meis-Kindblom and Kindblom[29] developed a histologically documented inguinal lymph node metastasis 1.5 years after the initial excision. A second patient developed suspected pulmonary metastases 2 years after the first local recurrence and 5 years after the initial presentation, although the metastases were not documented histologically (Table 32-6). Sakaki et al.[42] reported an acral tumor that metastasized only 3 months after initial excision. Exceptional cases have been reviewed that progressed to a high-grade pleomorphic (malignant fibrous histiocytoma-like) sarcoma. Wide local excision without adjuvant therapy appears to be adequate treatment for this tumor.

PLEOMORPHIC HYALINIZING ANGIECTATIC TUMOR OF SOFT PARTS

Initially described in 1996 in a series of 14 cases by Smith et al.,[43] pleomorphic hyalinizing angiectatic tumor (PHAT) of soft parts is a rare yet distinctive tumor with locally aggressive behavior. Since its initial description, fewer than 100 additional cases of PHAT have been reported in the literature,[44-51] and it is likely that this neoplasm continues to be mistaken for other entities, in particular, undifferentiated pleomorphic sarcoma and schwannoma. Accurate recognition

TABLE 32-6 Clinical Behavior of Myxoinflammatory Fibroblastic Sarcomas (Inflammatory Myxohyaline Tumors) of the Distal Extremities

STUDY	NO. OF CASES WITH FOLLOW-UP	FOLLOW-UP INTERVAL (MEDIAN)	LOCAL RECURRENCE	METASTASIS
Meis-Kindblom et al.[29]	36	6 months to 45 years (5 years)	24/36 (67%)	2/36 (6%)
Montgomery et al.[28]	27	6 months to 10 years (53 months)	6/27 (22%)	0/27 (0%)

of this neoplasm is of clinical importance given its propensity for local recurrence.

Clinical Findings

PHAT of soft parts characteristically arises in adults as a slowly enlarging mass that is often present for several years before coming to clinical attention. In the series of 41 cases reported by Folpe and Weiss,[44] patients ranged in age from 10 to 79 years, with a median age of 51 years. In most cases, the clinical impression is that of a hematoma, a benign neoplasm, or even Kaposi sarcoma. There may be a slight female predilection. The single most common site of the tumor is the subcutaneous tissue of the lower extremities. In the original series of 14 cases described by Smith et al.,[43] 11 tumors arose in the subcutaneous tissue, including 8 in the lower extremities and 1 each in the buttock, chest wall, and arm. However, three tumors arose in skeletal muscle, one each in the shoulder, thigh, and chest wall. In the more recent and larger series by Folpe and Weiss,[44] the most common site was the lower extremity (ankle/foot in 15 cases and lower leg in 10 cases), followed by the thigh, perineum, buttock, and arm (Table 32-7). Single cases arose in the axilla, back, and hand. The tumor ranges in size from less than 1 cm to up to 20 cm in greatest dimension, but most are in the range of 5 to 7 cm. Many patients have noted the presence of tumor for a significant period of time prior to seeking treatment.

Pathologic Findings

Grossly, most tumors have a lobulated appearance with a cut surface that varies in color from white-tan to maroon (Fig. 32-30). Rare examples have a prominent cystic component, and others show conspicuous myxoid change. The tumors are not encapsulated; although some have fairly well-demarcated borders, most show diffusely infiltrative margins with trapping of normal tissues at the tumor periphery.

Microscopically, the most striking feature at low magnification is the presence of clusters of thin-walled ectatic blood vessels scattered throughout the lesion. The vessels range in size from small to macroscopic, and they tend to be distributed in small clusters (Figs. 32-31 and 32-32). Typically, the ectatic vessels are lined by endothelium with a thick subjacent rim of amorphous eosinophilic material that is often surrounded by lamellated collagen. Some vessels contain organizing intraluminal thrombi with papillary endothelial hyperplasia. Hyaline material emanates from the vessels and extends into the stroma of the neoplasm, trapping neoplastic cells. The constituent cells are plump, spindled, and rounded with pleomorphic nuclei arranged in sheets or occasionally in fascicles reminiscent of fibrosarcoma (Fig. 32-33). In general, the cells have hyperchromatic, pleomorphic nuclei, and lack discernible cytoplasmic differentiation. Not uncommonly, intranuclear cytoplasmic inclusions are prominent (Fig. 32-34). Despite the striking degree of nuclear pleomorphism, mitotic figures are scarce (usually less than 1 MF/50 HPF). Occasional tumor cells, particularly those adjacent to ectatic vessels, contain intracytoplasmic hemosiderin. The tumors have a variable inflammatory infiltrate, most prominently mast cells, although in some lesions lymphocytes, plasma cells, and eosinophils are conspicuous. Foci of psammomatous calcification are occasionally present.

In the series reported by Folpe and Weiss,[44] the authors emphasized the identification of a pattern at the periphery of some tumors, which they termed *early PHAT*. These areas are characterized by low to, at most, moderate cellularity composed of bland, hemosiderin-laden spindled cells with wavy nuclei arranged in fascicles (Fig. 32-35). The cells infiltrate the surrounding adipocytes in a manner reminiscent of dermatofibrosarcoma protuberans. Sometimes, these peripheral zones have clusters of abnormally arranged ectatic blood vessels with fibrin deposition, although the vascular changes are far less impressive than those found more centrally (Fig. 32-36). Abundant, finely granular intracytoplasmic hemosiderin pigment is a conspicuous feature. Other features characteristic of PHAT, including pleomorphic cells with intranuclear pseudoinclusions and a mixed inflammatory infiltrate, may be found in early PHAT with careful searching. As will be

TABLE 32-7 Anatomic Location of 41 Cases of Pleomorphic Hyalinizing Angiectatic Tumor

ANATOMIC LOCATION	NO. OF CASES
Ankle/foot	15
Lower leg	10
Thigh	6
Perineum	3
Buttock	2
Arm	2
Axilla	1
Back	1
Hand	1
Total	41

Data from Imlay SP, Argenyi ZB, Stone MS, et al. Cutaneous parachordoma. A light microscopic and immunohistochemical report of two cases and review of the literature. J Cutan Pathol [Case Reports Review] 1998; 25(5):279–284.

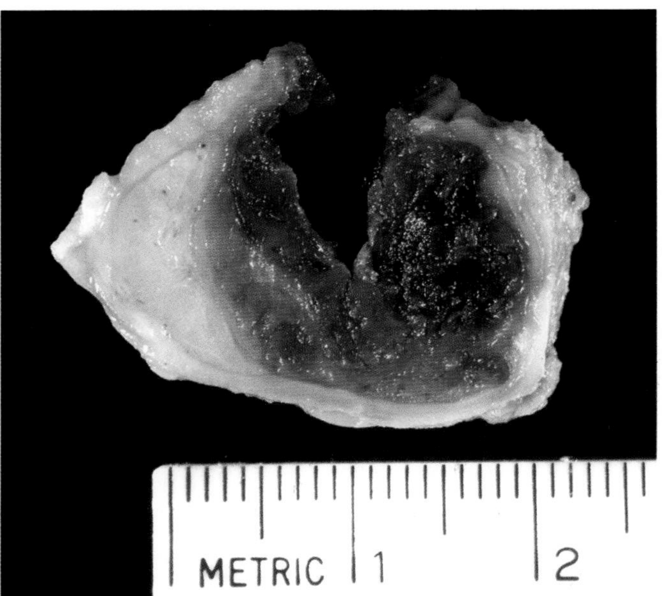

FIGURE 32-30. Pleomorphic hyalinizing angiectatic tumor. Gross specimen with a hemorrhagic appearance.

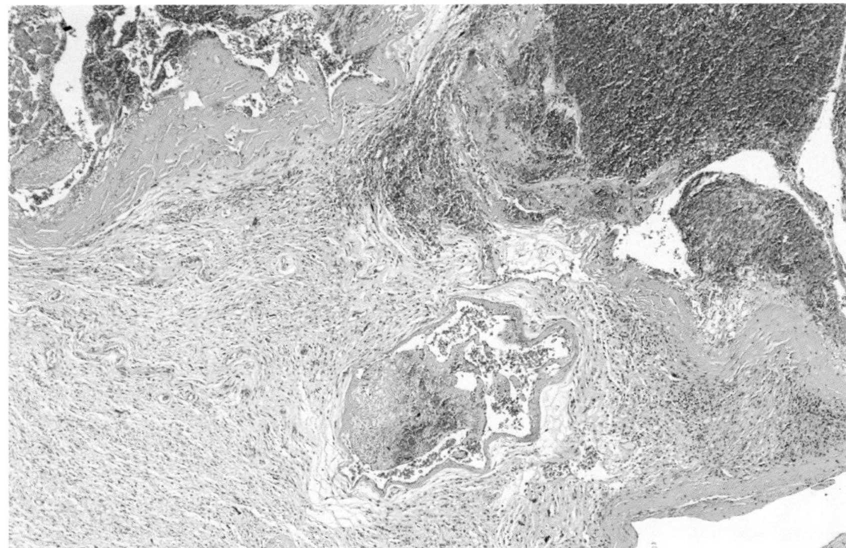

FIGURE 32-31. Pleomorphic hyalinizing angiectatic tumor with clusters of thin-walled ectatic vessels, a characteristic feature of this tumor.

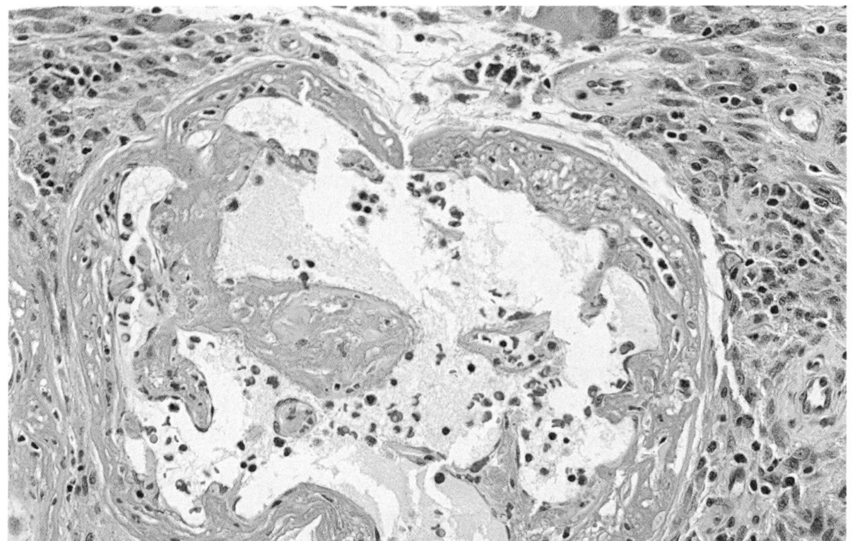

FIGURE 32-32. Characteristic high-power view of a vessel in a pleomorphic hyalinizing angiectatic tumor.

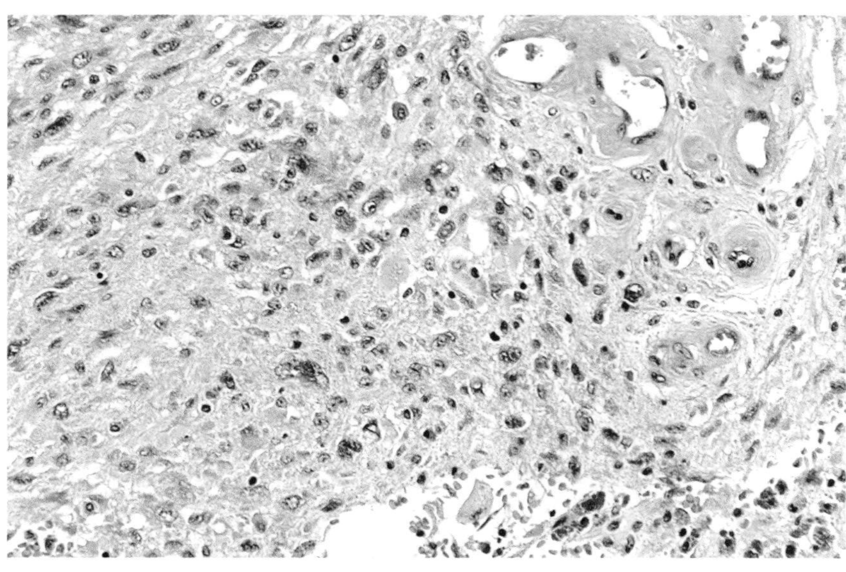

FIGURE 32-33. Pleomorphic nuclei in a pleomorphic hyalinizing angiectatic tumor. Despite the marked nuclear pleomorphism, mitotic figures are scarce.

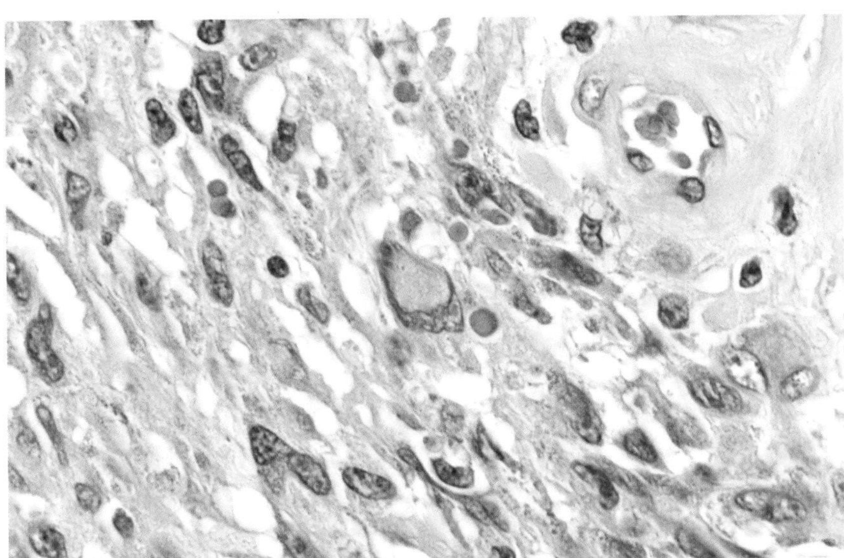

FIGURE 32-34. Pleomorphic hyalinizing angiectatic tumor with prominent intranuclear cytoplasmic inclusions.

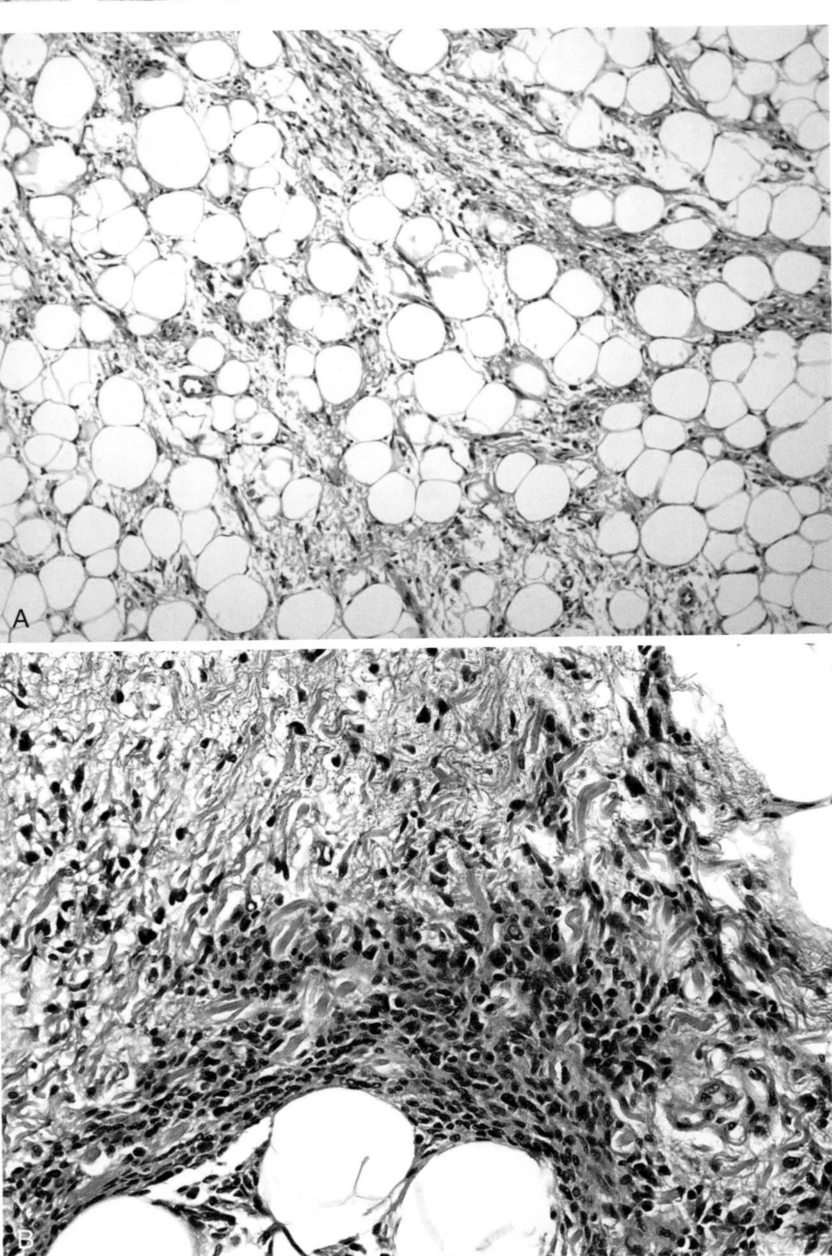

FIGURE 32-35. (A) Early PHAT characterized by a proliferation of bland spindled cells infiltrating mature adipose tissue. (B) Higher-magnification view of a more-cellular zone of early PHAT. Focal hemosiderin deposition and occasional nuclear pseudoinclusions are apparent.

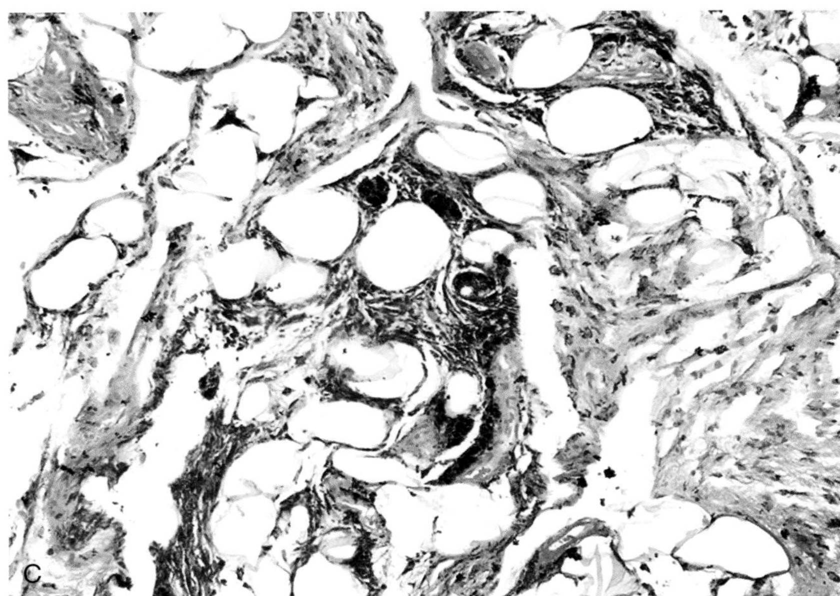

FIGURE 32-35, cont'd. (C) Prussian Blue stain for iron in early PHAT.

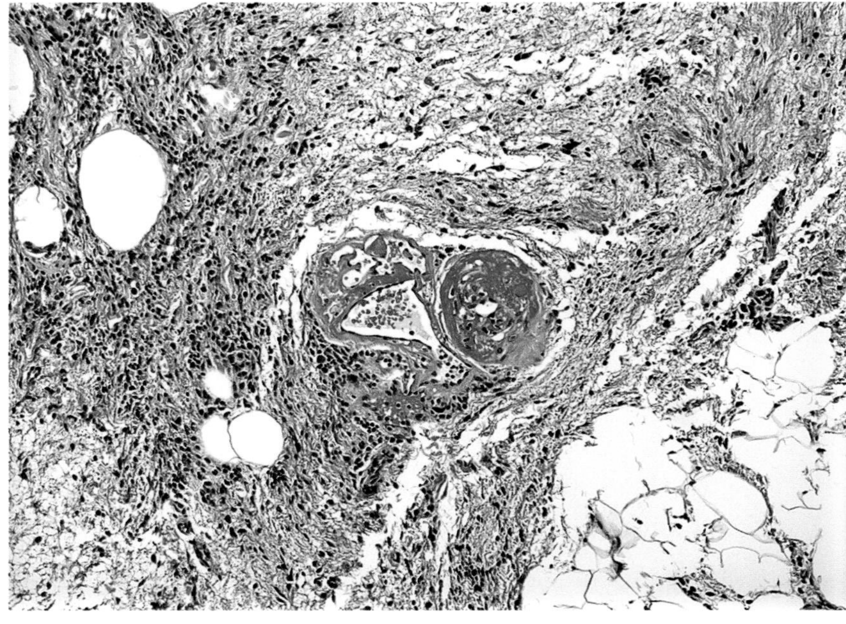

FIGURE 32-36. Damaged blood vessel in early PHAT.

discussed later, the morphologic features of early PHAT are identical to those of hemosiderotic fibrolipomatous tumor.

Immunohistochemical and Ultrastructural Findings

By immunohistochemistry, the lesional cells express CD34 and vimentin but are negative for actins, desmin, cytokeratin, EMA, von Willebrand factor, and CD31. Groisman et al.[48] reported immunoreactivity for vascular endothelial growth factor (VEGF), a secreted protein implicated in tumor-associated angiogenesis, in both tumoral and endothelial cells. The spindled cells of early PHAT are also CD34-positive.[44]

Few PHATs have been evaluated by electron microscopy.[47] The neoplastic cells lack specific evidence of differentiation and generally contain large numbers of cytoplasmic filaments that have been confirmed to represent vimentin filaments by immunoelectron microscopy.[43] Overall, the cells have features suggesting fibroblastic differentiation.[47]

Genetic Findings

There is awareness of only a single PHAT that has been analyzed by cytogenetic methods. Wei et al.[52] have very recently reported a case showing mixed features of classical and early PHAT, and showing two unbalanced translocations involving chromosomes 1 and 3 and chromosomes 1 and 10, with a karyotype of 45,XX,der(1)t(1;3)(p31;q12),-3,der(10)t(1;10)(p31;q25)[11]/46,XX[4]. These unbalanced translocations are quite similar, although not identical, to those seen in myxoinflammatory fibroblastic sarcoma, hemosiderotic fibrolipomatous tumor, and hybrid lesions. Three PHAT of the distal extremities have also been seen, both containing classical and early PHAT, which showed rearrangements of *TGFRB3* and *MGEA5* by FISH (Fig. 32-37) (Folpe AL and Antonescu CR, unpublished observations, 2012).

Differential Diagnosis

PHAT of soft parts bears a striking resemblance to schwannoma, although several light microscopic and immunohistochemical features allow their distinction. Unlike schwannoma, PHAT is not encapsulated, usually grows in an infiltrative manner, lacks distinct Antoni A and B zones, and does not express S-100 protein.

The tumor also resembles psammomatous melanotic schwannoma, by virtue of the occasional presence of psammoma bodies in PHAT. Furthermore, intranuclear inclusions are commonly seen in both tumors. Unlike psammomatous melanotic schwannoma, which coexpresses S-100 protein and HMB-45, PHAT lacks these antigens.

The pronounced nuclear pleomorphism in the absence of specific features of differentiation often suggests the diagnosis of undifferentiated pleomorphic sarcoma. Despite the striking cellularity of many PHATs, this tumor lacks significant mitotic activity, displays intranuclear cytoplasmic inclusions, and expresses CD34, a constellation of findings not characteristic of undifferentiated pleomorphic sarcomas. Conversely, ectatic, fibrin-filled blood vessels may be seen in some undifferentiated pleomorphic sarcomas, and one should be very hesitant to diagnosis PHAT in lesions occurring in atypical locations, showing appreciable mitotic activity and lacking other typical features of PHAT, including early PHAT. Cases of high-grade myxofibrosarcoma closely mimicking PHAT have been reported.[53,54]

Discussion

The clinical behavior of PHAT is characterized by local recurrence in up to 50% of cases, but metastases have not been documented. In the original study by Smith et al.,[43] follow-up information available for eight patients revealed that four (50%) developed local recurrence, including one patient with an aggressive recurrence necessitating amputation and another who suffered multiple recurrences over a 25-year period. In the larger and more recent study by Folpe and Weiss,[44] 6 of 18 (33%) patients with follow-up information developed local recurrences. In addition, one case in their study showed histologic progression to a myxoid pleomorphic sarcoma in a recurrence. A small number of other cases of PHAT showing progression to myxoid sarcoma have also been reported.[55,56] Wide local excision is recommended as the best therapeutic approach whenever possible.

Because of the paucity of reports, its lineage has yet to be elucidated. The absence of S-100 protein immunoreactivity essentially negates the possibility of an unusual neural neoplasm. Some have suggested that PHAT is related to solitary fibrous tumor (SFT) and giant cell angiofibroma given the overlapping histologic and immunohistochemical features,[45,46] but the expression of CD34 in PHAT seems to be a less consistent finding than in other neoplasms.

The most striking histologic feature of PHAT is the hyalinizing angiectatic vasculature. This may reflect, in part, the slow growth of the tumor, as suggested by the low Ki-67 index and S-phase fraction.[43,45] It has also been suggested that deposition of hyaline material leads to progressive vascular obliteration and tumoral hypoxia, which, in turn, promotes VEGF production by the neoplastic cells, resulting in active angiogenesis.[48]

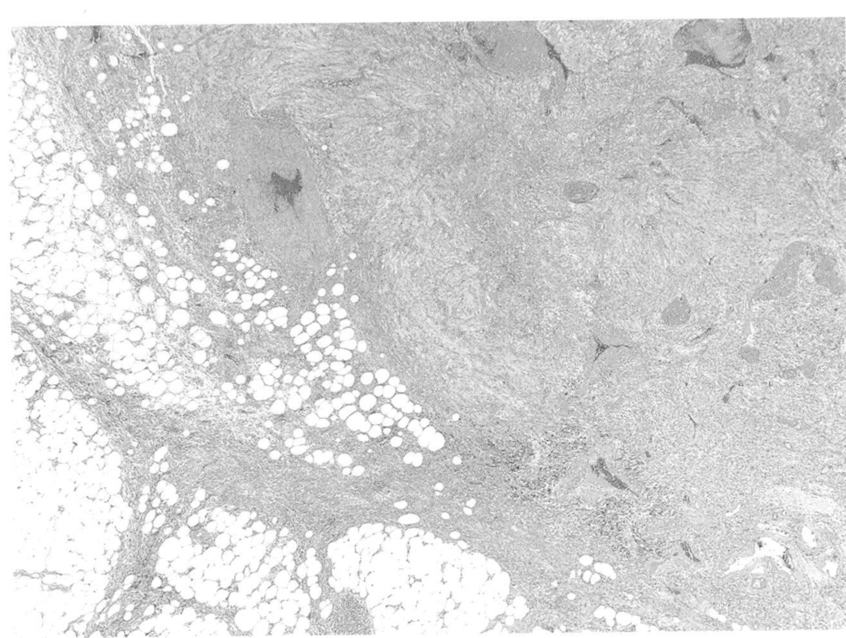

FIGURE 32-37. PHAT, arising in the foot of a 39-year-old woman, showing features of both classical and early PHAT. This tumor was positive for *TGFBR3-MGEA5* rearrangement by FISH.

Myxoinflammatory Fibroblastic Sarcoma, Hemosiderotic Fibrolipomatous Tumor and Pleomorphic Hyalinizing Angiectatic Tumor: A Family of Related Neoplasms?

Hemosiderotic fibrolipomatous tumor, originally described as *hemosiderotic fibrohistiocytic lipomatous lesion* by Marshall-Taylor and Fanburg-Smith,[57] typically occurs in the foot/ankle region of middle-aged patients and consists of an admixture of fat, moderately cellular fascicles of spindled cells with intracytoplasmic hemosiderin, macrophages, chronic inflammatory cells, and a focally myxoid stroma, identical to early PHAT. This lesion also shows vascular hyalinization, small aggregates of damaged capillary-sized vessels, and scattered pleomorphic cells. Although initially considered to be reactive in nature, hemosiderotic fibrolipomatous tumor is now considered neoplastic, based on its high rate of local recurrence (50%) and the presence of the recurrent unbalanced t(1;10)(p22;q24) (*TGRBR3-MGEA5*).[37]

As noted previously, this same translocation has also been identified in myxoinflammatory fibroblastic sarcoma and in tumors showing hybrid features of myxoinflammatory fibroblastic sarcoma and hemosiderotic fibrolipomatous tumor (Fig. 32-38). Although it is curious that areas resembling hemosiderotic fibrolipomatous tumor are unusual in typical myxoinflammatory fibroblastic sarcoma, both in this textbook authors' experience and in the published literature, there seems little doubt that these are closely related lesions, likely representing different morphologic manifestations of the same underlying genetic event. Furthermore, as noted by Folpe and Weiss,[44] the morphologic features of hemosiderotic lipomatous tumor are essentially identical to those of the low-grade

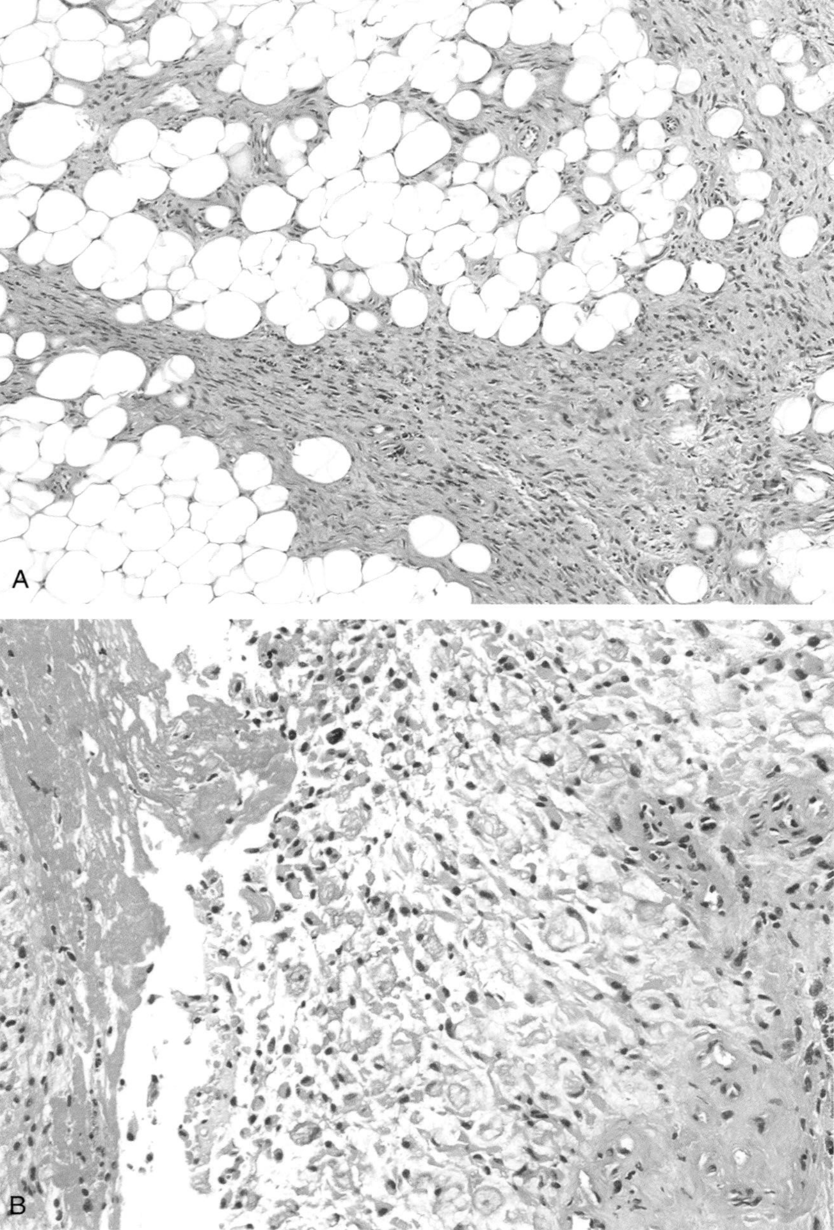

FIGURE 32-38. Hybrid hemosiderotic fibrolipomatous tumor (A) and myxoinflammatory fibroblastic sarcoma (B). This tumor was positive for *TGFBR3-MGEA5* rearrangement by FISH.

spindle cell proliferation frequently found at the periphery of classical PHAT, so-called early PHAT. Although Antonescu et al.[37] were not able to demonstrate *TGRBR3-MGEA5* rearrangements in three tested PHATs (including one with an early component), three cases of combined PHAT were positive for this gene fusion by FISH, as noted previously. Additionally, similar (but not identical) aberrations involving chromosomes 1 and 10 have been reported by Wei et al.[52] Therefore, it is likely that myxoinflammatory fibroblastic sarcoma, PHAT, and hemosiderotic fibrolipomatous tumor represent different morphologic manifestations of a single genetic entity, characterized clinically by distal extremity location, locally aggressive growth, and very low metastatic potential.

MYOEPITHELIOMA/MIXED TUMOR OF SOFT TISSUE (PARACHORDOMA)

The previous edition of this textbook viewed parachordoma and myoepithelioma of soft tissue as related, if not necessarily entirely identical, entities. Over the past several years, it has become increasingly clear that the clinicopathologic similarities between these two entities greatly outweigh any minor morphologic differences and that both tumors show rearrangements of the *EWSR1* gene in many instances.[58-61] WHO currently regards myoepithelioma and parachordoma as synonyms, with the former as the preferred term.

Parachordoma was first described by Laskowski[62] in 1951 as *chordoma periphericum* but was more fully described in a series of 10 cases by Dabska[63] in 1977. Although the authors believed at the time that they were describing chordomas arising in a paramidline or peripheral location, over time it became apparent their lesions were histologically distinct from true chordomas. Since that time, fewer than 60 cases have been described in the literature, mostly in the form of case reports or small series.[64-72] This small number of reported cases reflects both the rarity of this tumor as well as the increasing tendency of pathologists to label these lesions as *myoepithelioma*.

The term *myoepithelioma/mixed tumor of soft tissue* was first introduced by Kilpatrick and Fletcher[73] in 1997, in a series of 19 cases. Subsequently, more than 200 soft tissue myoepithelial tumors have been published, in four large series[61,74-76] and a large number of case reports.

Clinical Findings

Myoepitheliomas arise in patients of all ages, but there is a peak incidence in the second through fourth decades of life.[64,74] However, a significant number of myoepitheliomas arise in pediatric patients, often showing malignant histologic features and an aggressive clinical course (myoepithelial carcinoma).[75] There is no significant gender predilection, and most patients present with a slowly enlarging, painless mass in the deep soft tissue of the extremities, usually in the muscles of the thigh, groin, calf, upper arm, or forearm (Table 32-8). The head and neck are also relatively common locations for these tumors. The tumor may be situated primarily in the subcutis or deep to the fascia; less often, the lesion may be centered in or secondarily involve the dermis.[58-60,76-78]

Pathologic Findings

Grossly, myoepitheliomas form a nodular mass ranging in size from 1 to 12 cm in greatest dimension, but most are 3 to 7 cm (Fig. 32-39). In the series from Brigham and Women's Hospital, tumor size ranged from slightly less than 1 cm to up to 20 cm (mean 4.7), although histologically benign tumors were significantly smaller than histologically malignant tumors (3.8 cm and 5.9 cm, respectively).[74] Most are grossly well circumscribed and have a yellow-white to tan cut surface that is glistening, myxoid, or gelatinous. Necrosis is rarely a prominent feature.

The histologic appearance of mixed tumor/myoepithelioma spans a morphologic spectrum similar to that observed in their counterparts in the salivary gland (Figs. 32-40 and 32-41). Myoepitheliomas show a predominantly reticular growth pattern with cords of epithelioid, ovoid, or spindled cells deposited in a variably collagenous or chondromyxoid stroma. Although grossly well circumscribed, there are frequently small nests of cells that are separated from the main tumor and trail off into the surrounding soft tissue structures, sometimes evoking a desmoplastic stromal response (Fig. 32-42). In some cases, the cells are arranged in nests or large sheets, but mixed architectural patterns are common.[74] Tumors classically described as *parachordoma* consist of small nests of pale-staining cells, somewhat resembling the cells of the notochord. Most of the cells are round, eosinophilic cells arranged in cords, chains, or pseudoacini reminiscent of

TABLE 32-8 Anatomic Distribution of 101 Soft Tissue Myoepithelial Tumors

ANATOMIC LOCATION	NO. OF CASES
Lower limb/limb girdle	41
Upper limb/limb girdle	35
Head and neck	15
Trunk	10
Total	101

Modified from Hornick JL, Fletcher CD. Myoepithelial tumors of soft tissue: a clinicopathologic and immunohistochemical study of 101 cases with evaluation of prognostic parameters. Am J Surg Pathol 2003; 27:1183–1196.

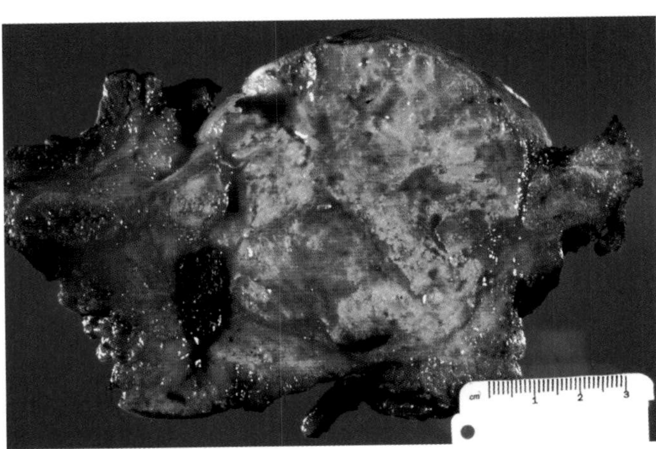

FIGURE 32-39. Gross appearance of a myoepithelioma arising in the chest wall of a 55-year-old man.

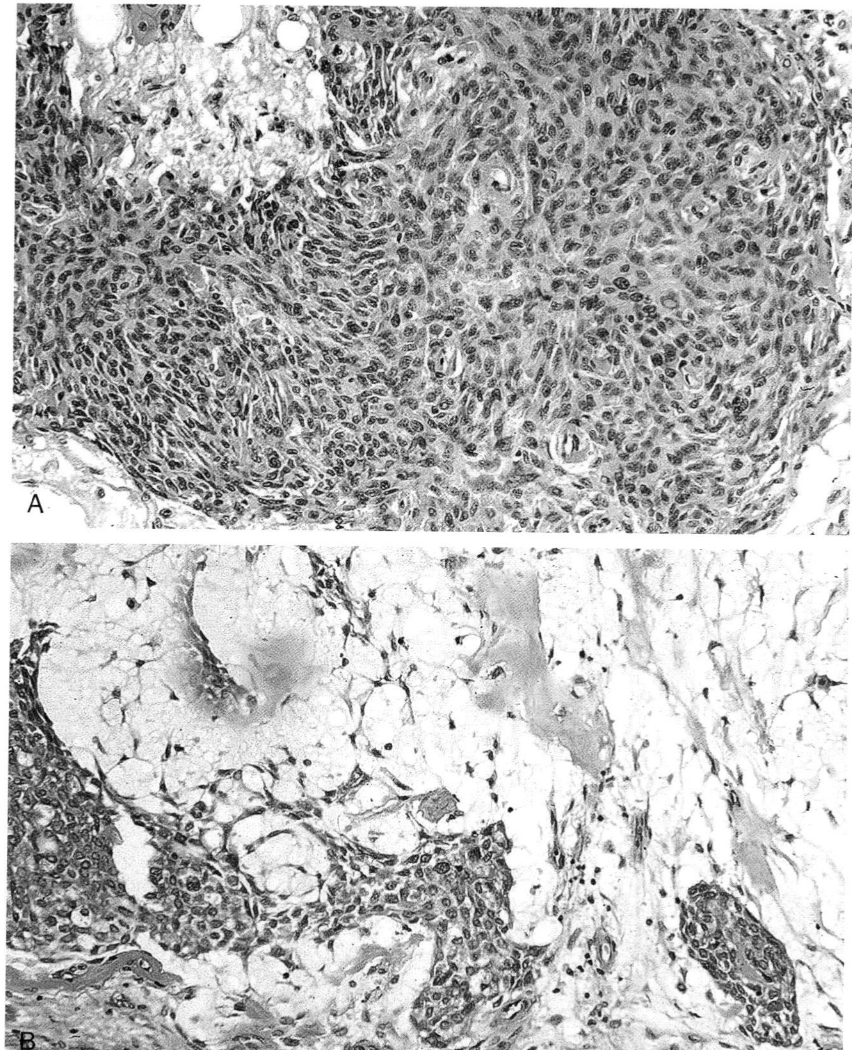

FIGURE 32-40. (A) Soft tissue myoepithelioma with a solidly cellular proliferation of spindled cells merging with epithelioid cells. (B) Nests of spindled cells deposited in an abundant myxoid stroma in a soft tissue myoepithelioma. *(Case courtesy of Dr. Christopher Fletcher, Brigham and Women's Hospital, Boston, MA.)*

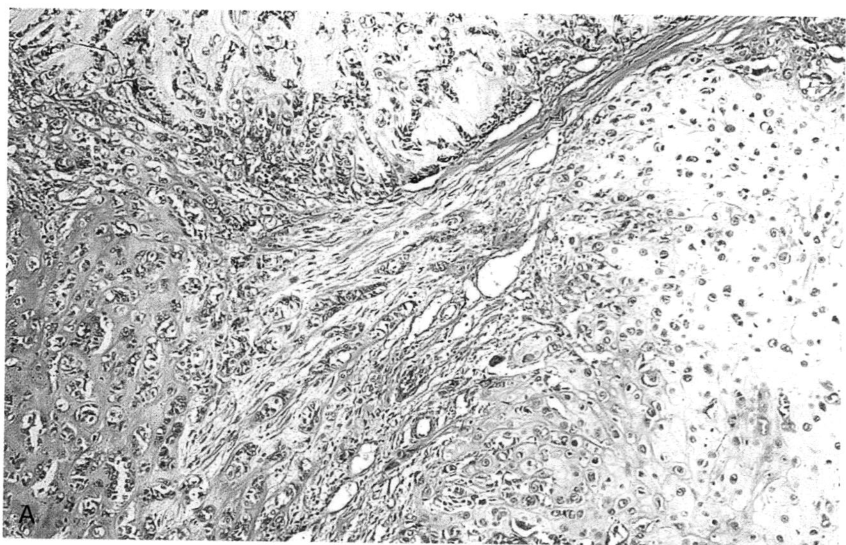

FIGURE 32-41. (A) Low-magnification view of a soft tissue mixed tumor showing an admixture of cords of epithelioid cells and metaplastic cartilage.

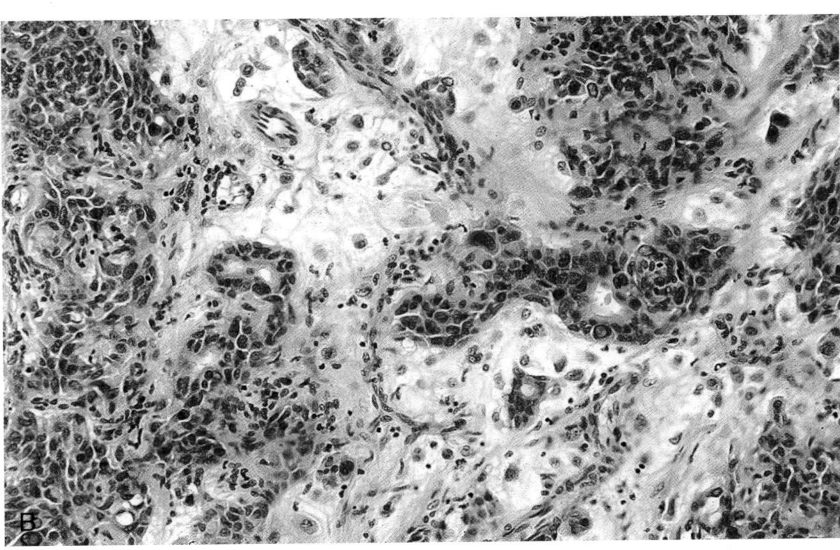

FIGURE 32-41, cont'd. (B) Ductal differentiation in a soft tissue mixed tumor. *(Case courtesy of Dr. Christopher Fletcher, Brigham and Women's Hospital, Boston, MA.)*

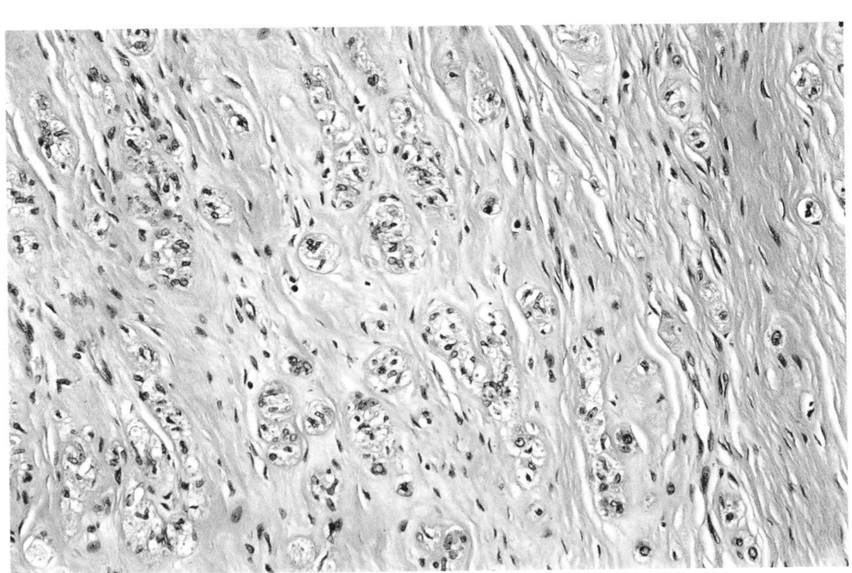

FIGURE 32-42. Periphery of a myoepithelioma with infiltrating small nests and single cells in a desmoplastic background.

myxoid chondrosarcoma (Figs. 32-43 to 32-50). Not uncommonly, the cells show a transition to spindle-shaped cells (see Fig. 32-47) or small, round glomoid cells (see Fig. 32-48).[64] All lesions have a population of cells with vacuolated cytoplasm resembling physaliferous cells found in chordomas (see Figs. 32-49 and 32-50). Parachordoma-like areas may be seen in a minority of otherwise typical myoepitheliomas, emphasizing the unity of these tumors. The stroma varies in character from case to case and in different areas of the same tumor (Fig. 32-51). Metaplastic cartilage, bone, or both can be seen in a small percentage of cases.

Most myoepitheliomas show only a mild degree of nuclear atypia, and mitotic figures are inconspicuous, usually with less than 1 MF/20 HPF.[64,73,74,76] However, some have cytologically malignant features and are composed of larger cells with vesicular or coarse chromatin and prominent nucleoli (Fig. 32-52).[74,75] In the series by Hornick and Fletcher,[74] 61 of 101 tumors were classified as histologically benign, whereas 40 tumors were felt to be histologically malignant based upon the cytologic features (malignant myoepithelioma, malignant mixed tumor, or myoepithelial carcinoma). Some histologically malignant tumors show small foci of classical benign-appearing areas; others have foci of heterologous chondrosarcomatous or osteosarcomatous differentiation.[74] A greater percentage of pediatric myoepithelial tumors appear to show atypical features.[75]

Immunohistochemical and Ultrastructural Findings

The cells of myoepithelioma consistently coexpress epithelial markers (cytokeratins and/or EMA) and S-100 protein (Fig. 32-53).[64,74,76,79] Myoepitheliomas are more often positive with antibodies directed against broad spectrum (e.g., AE1/AE3) and low-molecular weight cytokeratins (e.g., Cam 5.2), and less often for high molecular weight cytokeratins (e.g.,

Text continued on p. 1000

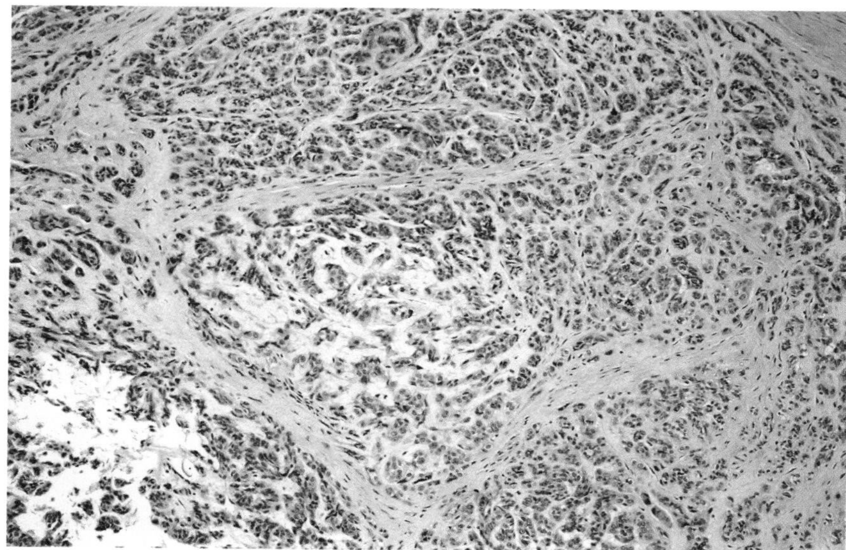

FIGURE 32-43. Myoepithelioma showing multinodular masses of epithelioid to spindle cells, with a variably myxochondroid matrix.

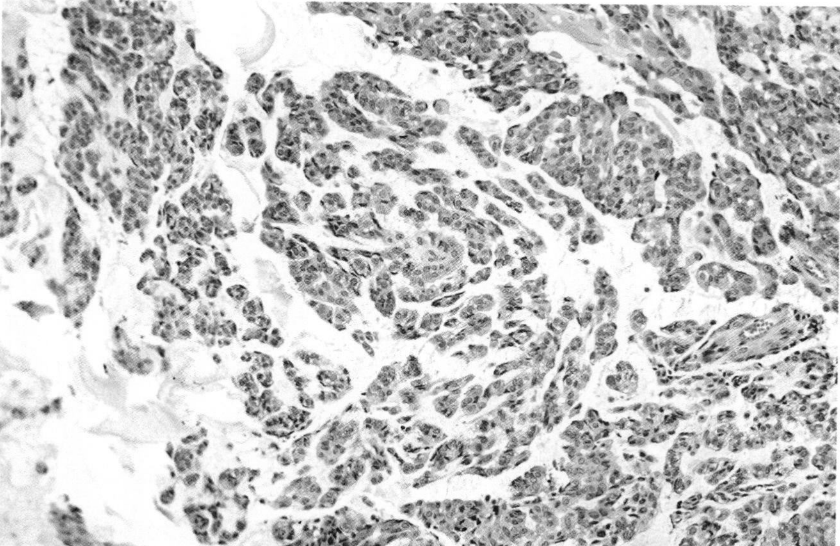

FIGURE 32-44. Myoepithelioma. Nests of epithelioid cells are suspended in a myxoid matrix.

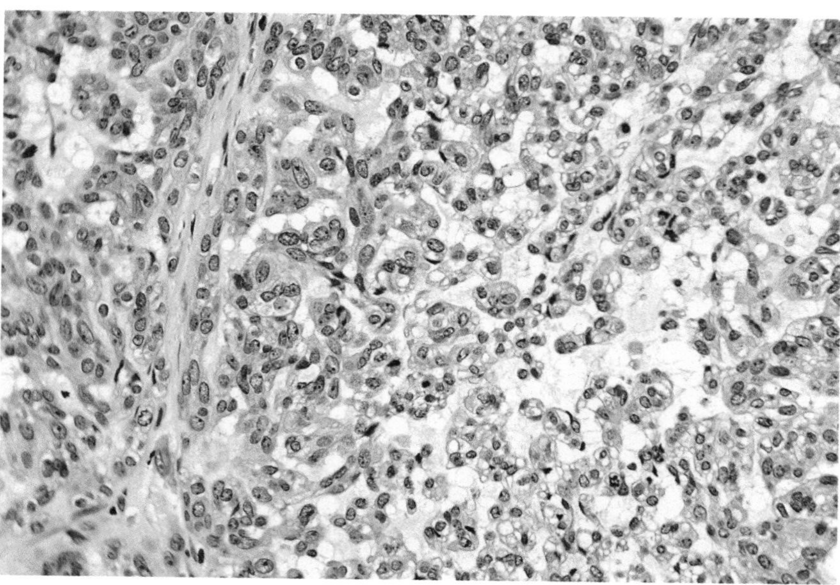

FIGURE 32-45. Myoepithelioma. Nests and cords of epithelioid to spindle-shaped cells are deposited in a myxochondroid matrix.

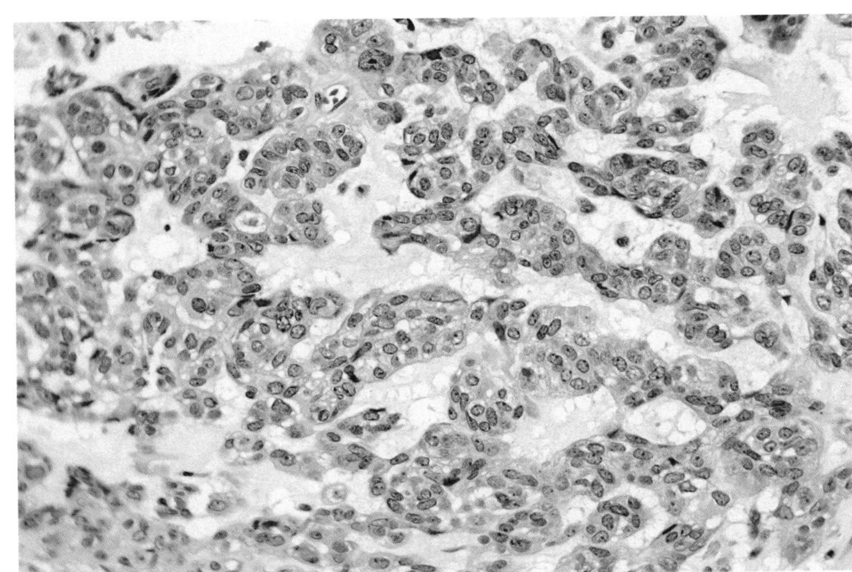

FIGURE 32-46. Nests of uniform-appearing epithelioid cells suspended in a myxochondroid matrix in a myoepithelioma.

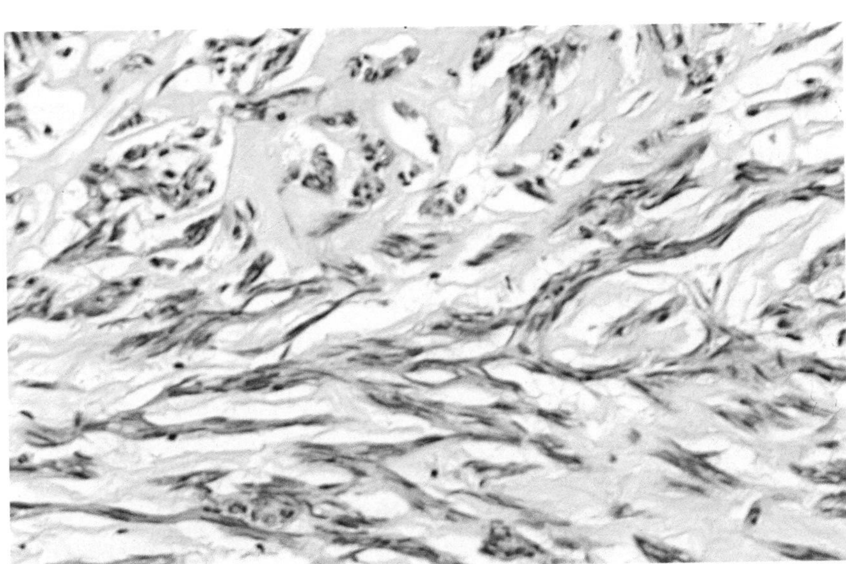

FIGURE 32-47. Focus of spindle cells in myoepithelioma.

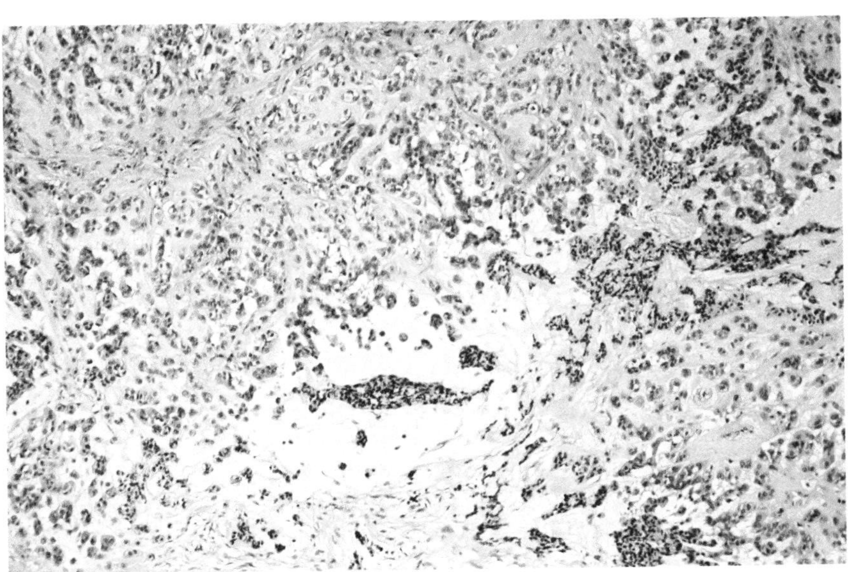

FIGURE 32-48. Transition from large epithelioid cells to small glomoid cells in a myoepithelioma.

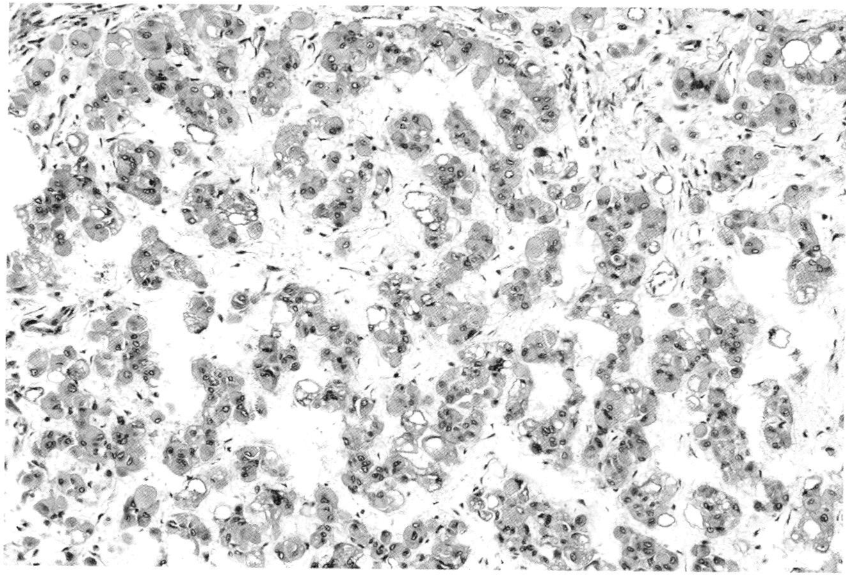

FIGURE 32-49. Chordoma-like area in a myoepithelioma. Nests of large cells with abundant eosinophilic and vacuolated cytoplasm are suspended in a myxochondroid matrix.

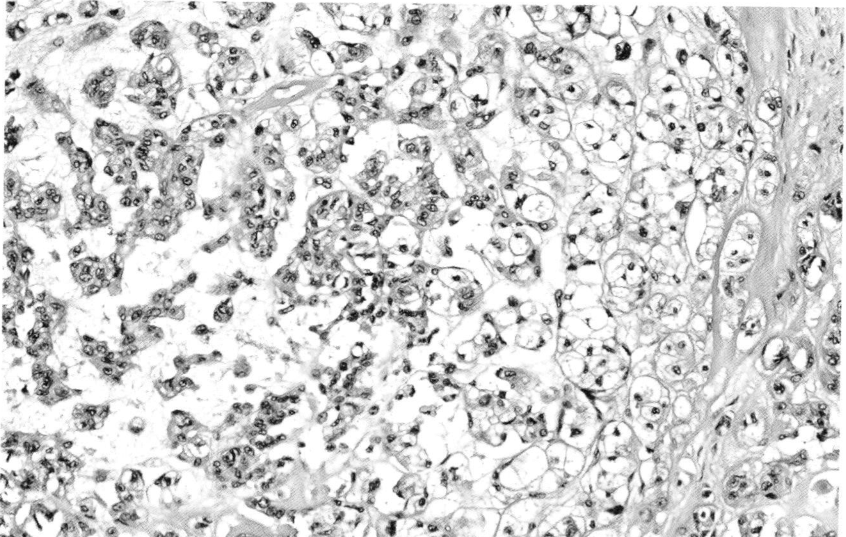

FIGURE 32-50. Myoepithelioma. Transition from eosinophilic cells to cells with clear, vacuolated cytoplasm.

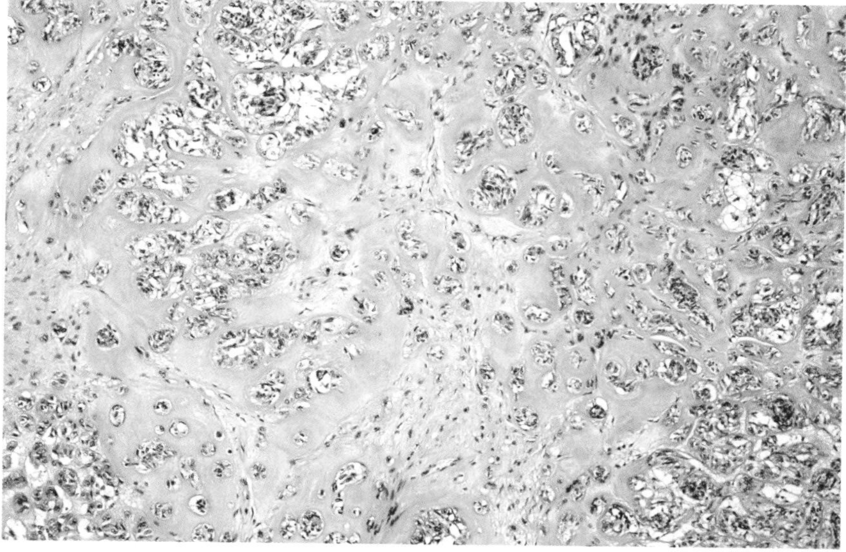

FIGURE 32-51. Myoepithelioma with a densely hyalinized matrix.

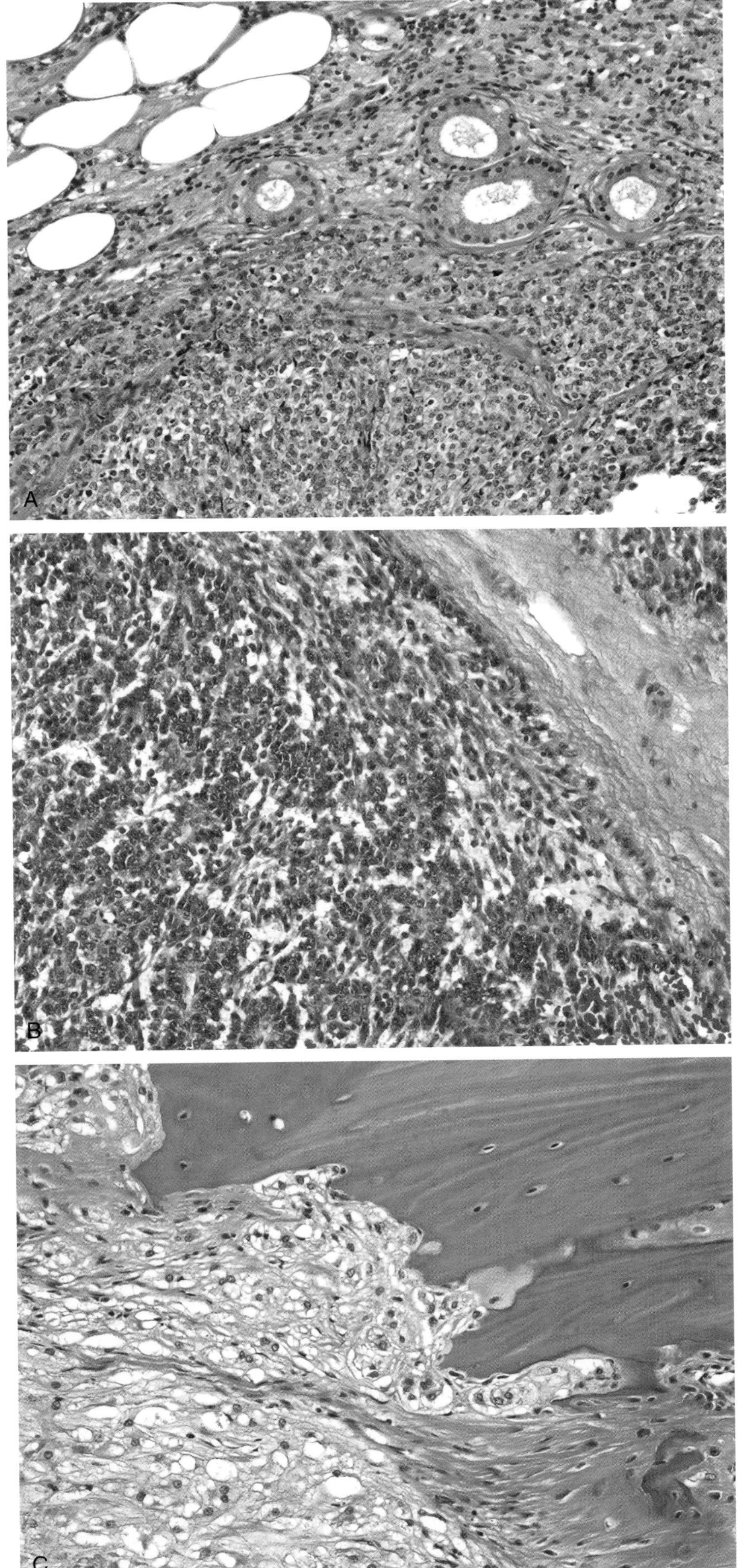

FIGURE 32-52. Small cell pattern in a superficially located malignant myoepithelioma (A). Malignant myoepithelioma with spindled and plasmacytoid features (B). Malignant myoepithelioma of soft tissue, invading subjacent bone (C).

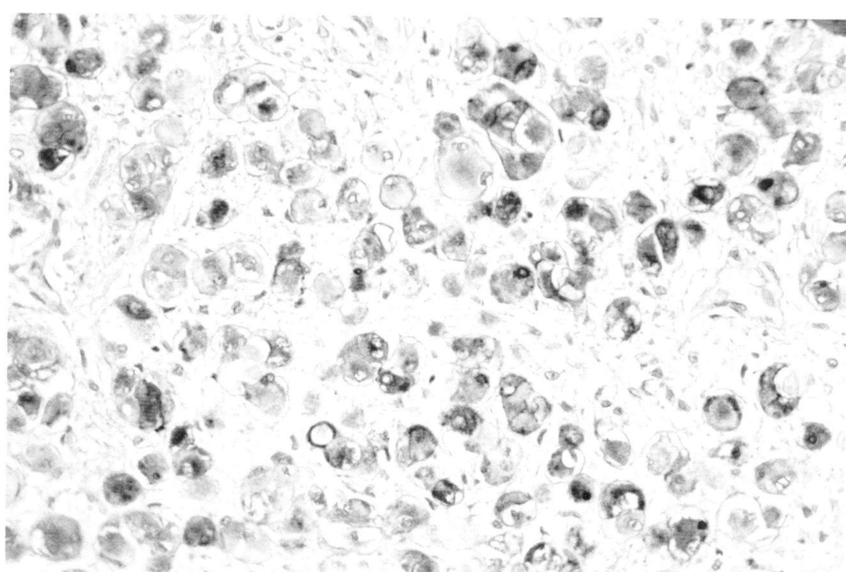

FIGURE 32-53. Myoepithelioma with strong immunoreactivity for high-molecular-weight cytokeratin.

34βE12 and CK14), EMA, CK7, and CK20.[64,74,80] Cytokeratin expression in myoepithelial tumors may, however, be very limited in extent. Expression of other myoepithelial markers, including muscle actins, GFAP, calponin, and p63, is seen in 15% to 50% of cases.[64,74]

By electron microscopy, myoepithelioma is most often composed of cells showing incomplete epithelial differentiation, with primitive cell junctions, fragmented basal lamina, and microvillous projections.[81-86] Some show better developed epithelial features, with tumor cells surrounded by basal lamina and containing cytoplasmic filaments and intercellular junctions.[87-89]

Cytogenetic and Molecular Genetic Findings

Soft tissue myoepitheliomas are characterized most often by the presence of *EWSR1* gene rearrangements, with a variety of different fusion partners. In 2008, Brandal et al.[90] described a soft tissue myoepithelioma showing a t(1;22)(q23;q12) resulting in a *EWSR1-PBX1* fusion, and, in 2009, these same authors described a second case showing a t(19;22)(q13;q12) resulting in an *EWSR1-ZNF444* fusion.[91] Shortly thereafter, Gleason and Fletcher[75] reported *EWSR1* rearrangement by FISH in two pediatric malignant myoepithelial tumors. These preliminary results were confirmed in a much larger series of 66 myoepithelial tumors studied by Antonescu et al.[61] Antonescu et al.[61] found *EWSR1* rearrangements by FISH in 30 (45%) cases (chiefly those in deep soft tissue). RT-PCR studies performed on these 30 cases showed *EWSR1-POU5F1* (5 cases), *EWSR1-PBX1* (5 cases), and *EWSR1-ZNF444* (1 case) fusions, with 19 cases lacking an identifiable fusion partner.[61] One case was found to have a fusion involving *FUS*, rather than *EWSR1*. Interestingly, all tumors with ductal differentiation and all salivary gland myoepithelial tumors were *EWSR1*-negative. Antonescu et al.[61] suggested a possible association between fusion type and morphology in soft tissue myoepithelial tumors: *EWSR1-POU5F1* tumors often occur in younger patients and have a clear cell appearance, and *EWSR1-PBX1* tumors have a bland sclerotic appearance or clear cell morphology. However, too few cases were evaluated to allow definite conclusions. *EWSR1* rearrangements have subsequently been shown by Flucke et al.[59,60] to occur in significant subsets of myoepithelial tumors of the skin as well, including one case with a proven *EWSR1-ATF1* fusion.[58] In contrast, true mixed tumors of the skin and soft tissue have been shown to harbor *PLAG1* rearrangements, similar to their salivary gland counterparts, rather than *EWSR1* rearrangements.[92] Other cytogenetic abnormalities that have been reported in myoepithelioma (parachordoma) include trisomy 15 and monosomies of chromosomes 1, 16, and 17,[64] der2(2)5(2;4),del (3q) and loss of chromosomes 9, 19, 20, and 22,[93] loss of chromosomes 1, 2, and 6 and a small der(5)t(1p;5q),[94] and der(17)t(15;17)(q11;p12).[95]

Differential Diagnosis

Given the morphologic heterogeneity of this group of tumors, the differential diagnosis is quite broad and depends, in large part, upon the predominant cell type and stromal component. If ducts are present, the diagnosis of mixed tumor is straightforward. Most commonly, considerations include extraskeletal myxoid chondrosarcoma, ossifying fibromyxoid tumor, and chordoma.

Distinction from extraskeletal myxoid chondrosarcoma may be particularly challenging. This tumor typically shows a multinodular pattern with cords of eosinophilic spindled to ovoid cells deposited in a myxoid matrix. There is such a significant degree of morphologic overlap with parachordoma/mixed tumor/myoepithelioma that immunohistochemistry and/or molecular diagnostic testing is often required. However, the presence of dense sclerosis, hemorrhage, hemosiderin, and hematoidin pigment surrounding nodules of tumor, characteristic of extraskeletal myxoid chondrosarcoma but not myoepithelioma, may be quite helpful in this distinction. Myoepitheliomas typically coexpress cytokeratin (or EMA) and S-100 protein, whereas extraskeletal myxoid chondrosarcoma expresses S-100 protein in a minority of cases and does not typically express cytokeratins. It is important to keep in mind that both extraskeletal myxoid chondrosarcoma and myoepithelioma commonly show rearrangements involving the *EWSR1* locus. FISH for the *NR4A3* gene, rearranged in extraskeletal myxoid chondrosarcoma but not to date in myoepithelioma, may be helpful in resolving this differential diagnosis.[60]

Ossifying fibromyxoid tumor also enters the differential diagnosis. This tumor is a lobulated neoplasm composed of cords or nests of uniform, pale-staining, ovoid cells deposited in a variably myxoid or hyalinized stroma with a rim of metaplastic bone at the periphery in 70% of cases. Most ossifying fibromyxoid tumors express S-100 protein and about 50% desmin. Focal cytokeratin positivity is very uncommon. *EWSR1* rearrangements have not been shown in ossifying fibromyxoid tumor.[61]

Chordoma, particularly extra-axial chordoma, is also a consideration, especially for tumors with a focal or predominant parachordoma-like pattern. Myoepithelial tumors and chordomas show significant immunohistochemical overlap with respects to cytokeratin and S-100 protein expression, although chordomas are more likely to express high molecular weight cytokeratins.[64,70,80,81] Immunohistochemistry for the specific notochordal marker brachyury, expressed by virtually all chordomas but no myoepithelial tumors, may be very helpful (Fig. 32-54).[96]

Myoepithelial carcinoma (malignant myoepithelioma) may be confused with metastatic carcinoma, metastatic melanoma, and even epithelioid sarcoma, especially the proximal type.

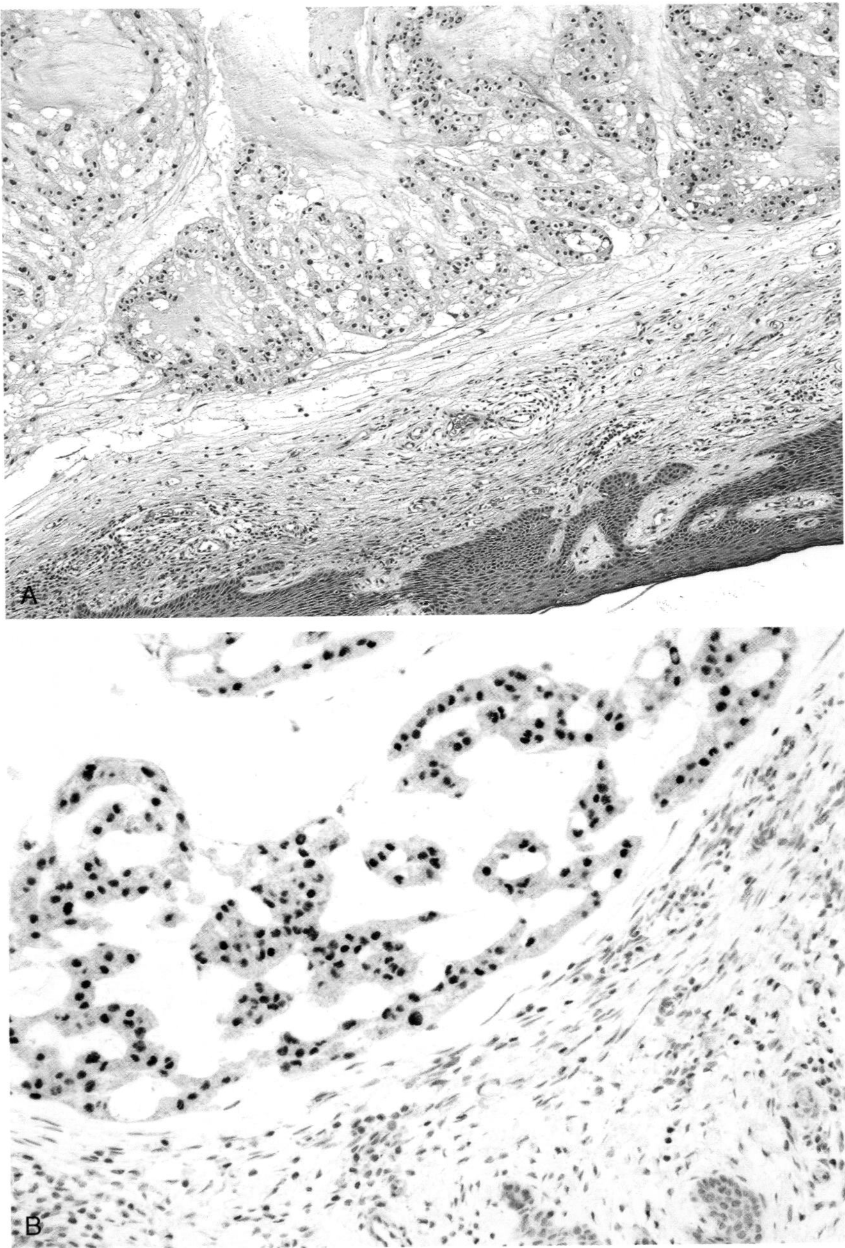

FIGURE 32-54. Extra-axial chordoma (chordoma periphericum) arising in the subcutaneous soft tissue of the groin (A). Brachyury expression confirms true notochordal differentiation, distinguishing this tumor from myoepithelioma (B).

Clearly, knowledge of a history of a primary carcinoma or a melanoma elsewhere is of paramount importance. In the absence of such a history, immunohistochemistry can be extremely helpful in distinguishing among these lesions. Immunoreactivity for muscle markers (e.g., calponin, desmin), S-100 protein, and GFAP support a diagnosis of myoepithelial carcinoma over metastatic carcinoma. Melanomas typically coexpress S-100 protein and melanocytic antigens such as HMB-45 or Melan A, and they rarely express cytokeratins, GFAP, or muscle markers. Epithelioid sarcoma frequently expresses cytokeratin and EMA but not S-100 protein, GFAP, or myogenic markers. Loss of expression of *SMARCB1* is seen in approximately 90% of epithelioid sarcomas but may also be seen in malignant myoepitheliomas.[97]

Discussion

Although most mixed tumor/myoepitheliomas of soft tissue are histologically and clinically benign, some cases locally recur, and others are either histologically malignant, clinically malignant, or both. In the series of 12 cutaneous and soft tissue myoepitheliomas by Michal and Miettinen,[87] one patient developed metastatic disease and died as a direct result of the tumor. Similarly, of the 10 patients with clinical follow-up information in the series by Kilpatrick et al.,[98] 2 patients developed local recurrence, and 2 additional patients developed lung and lymph node metastases and died of their tumor. In the much larger subsequent series reported by Hornick and Fletcher,[74] of the 33 histologically benign cases with follow-up, 6 (18%) locally recurred, but none metastasized (mean follow-up of 36 months). Of the 31 histologically malignant cases with follow-up, 13 (42%) recurred and 10 (32%) metastasized (mean follow-up of 50 months). Four patients died of metastatic tumor with metastatic sites, including lung, mediastinum, spine, orbit, bone, brain, and other unusual soft tissue sites (Table 32-9). There was no apparent correlation between margin status and risk of local recurrence, but local recurrence and metastasis were significantly more likely in patients with histologically malignant tumors. These authors suggested that the presence of at least moderate cytologic atypia (prominent nucleoli, vesicular or coarse chromatin, nuclear pleomorphism) warrants classification as a malignant myoepithelioma/myoepithelial carcinoma.[74] Most

TABLE 32-9 Risk of Local Recurrence and Metastasis in 64 Cases of Soft Tissue Myoepithelioma with Follow-Up

HISTOLOGIC CATEGORY	NO. OF CASES	LOCAL RECURRENCE (%)	METASTASES (%)
Benign myoepithelial tumors	33	6 (18)	0 (0)
Malignant myoepithelial tumors	31	13 (42)	10 (32)

Modified from Hornick JL, Fletcher CD. Myoepithelial tumors of soft tissue: a clinicopathologic and immunohistochemical study of 101 cases with evaluation of prognostic parameters. Am J Surg Pathol 2003; 27:1183–1196.

cases previously reported as parachordoma have behaved in an indolent fashion, chiefly with locally recurring potential.[64] Two cases of parachordoma have been reported with metastatic disease.[99,100]

SOLITARY FIBROUS TUMOR (HEMANGIOPERICYTOMA)

The term *hemangiopericytoma* was first coined by Stout and Murray for tumors thought to originate from the pericytes, a modified dendritic-like smooth muscle cell encircling blood vessels (see Chapter 26). Unfortunately, the original descriptions by Stout[101-103] were vague, and it is clear that he included a number of lesions, such as myofibroma, under this rubric. It was not until the 1976 paper by Enzinger and Smith[104] that a more useful architectural and cytologic description of hemangiopericytoma was set forth. Their classical description emphasized the staghorn, partially hyalinized vessels surrounded by small rounded and fusiform cells that displayed no obvious light microscopic features of differentiation. Just as important, these authors made clear the importance of distinguishing hemangiopericytomas from other lesions that could have a pericytic vascular pattern, notably high-grade synovial sarcomas. In addition, they defined features that were associated with malignancy. The importance of this paper seemed forgotten over the years as the term *hemangiopericytoma* grew increasingly unpopular because pericytic differentiation could be confirmed in only a minority of cases ultrastructurally,[105-108] and actin, a marker of pericytes, was infrequently present in these lesions.[109-112] Moreover, as a diagnosis of exclusion, diagnostic reproducibility among pathologists was often poor.[113]

The waning popularity of the diagnosis of hemangiopericytoma also coincided with the increasing popularity of the diagnosis of SFT, a pleural-based lesion first described by Klemperer and Rabin.[114] The observation that similar lesions occurred outside of the pleura and had overlapping features with classical hemangiopericytoma, including CD34 immunoreactivity, paved the way for the popular belief that all hemangiopericytomas were (or should become) SFTs. This was not based on any quantum leap in the understanding of either tumor but rather observed histologic similarities between the two and a preference of one term over the other. Which term is better is debatable, and what lineage these lesions recapitulate is uncertain. Nevertheless, the acknowledgment that the two are similar, if not identical, is useful and has been endorsed by WHO.[115] This classification now considers lesions previously classified as *hemangiopericytoma* as *cellular phase* of SFT. The term *solitary fibrous tumor* will be used for tumors previously labeled *hemangiopericytoma-solitary fibrous tumor* in the previous edition of this book.

Clinical Features

SFT is primarily a tumor of adult life that affects the sexes equally. It is located almost exclusively in deep soft tissue, particularly the thigh, pelvic fossa, retroperitoneum, and serosal surfaces.[116] Tumors in these locations often chiefly show cellular features, and, as noted previously, were previously labeled *hemangiopericytoma*. Although formerly believed to be restricted to the pleura, tumors showing features of classical SFT have been increasingly recognized in extrapulmonary sites.[117-120] Specific symptoms relate to the location of the tumor. Those in somatic soft tissue present as painless enlarging masses, whereas those within the abdominal cavity produce symptoms referable to impingement on specific organs. Serosal lesions are preferentially located on the pleura where they are usually discovered as incidental findings during workup for another abnormality. Most are rounded, sharply outlined, homogeneous densities or masses on a pedicle that shifts with positional changes (Fig. 32-55). Less commonly, they grow endophytically into the lung[121] or as a plaque-like mass over the fissures.

Hypoglycemia has been reported in about 5% of SFT, most often those located in the pelvis and retroperitoneum, and may lead to symptoms of sweating, headache, disorientation, convulsions, and even coma. It is mediated through the production of insulin-like growth factors by the tumor.[122-124] Insulin-like growth factors and insulin-like growth factor receptor mRNA can be identified in tumor cells even in the absence of clinical hypoglycemia.[125,126] Hypoglycemic symptoms abate with tumor removal. In addition, the insulin-like growth factors stimulate proliferation of tumor cells through an autocrine loop that can be abolished when the receptors are inactivated.

FIGURE 32-55. Radiograph of a solitary fibrous tumor of the pleura. Note the circumscribed mass in the left chest.

Pathologic Findings

SFTs grow in deep soft tissue as a circumscribed mass (Fig. 32-56) or as exophytic lesions from the serosal surfaces (Fig. 32-57). Most measure 5 to 10 cm in diameter and have a gray-white to red-brown color on a cut section. Hemorrhage and cystic degeneration may be seen.

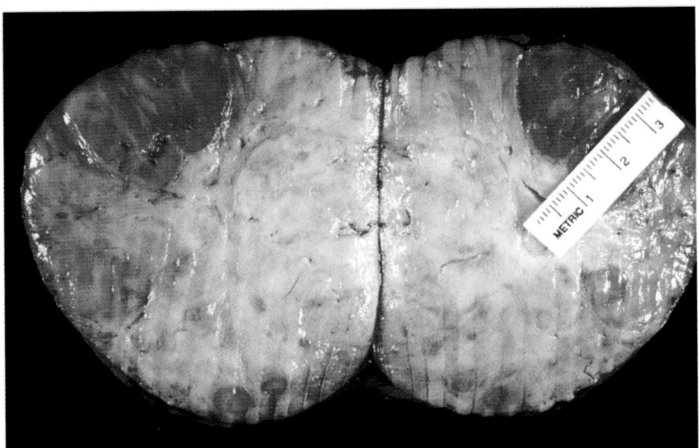

FIGURE 32-56. Gross specimen of a cellular solitary fibrous tumor (hemangiopericytoma).

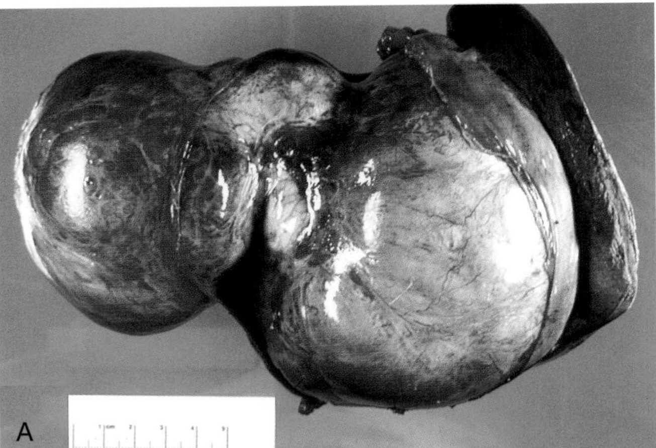

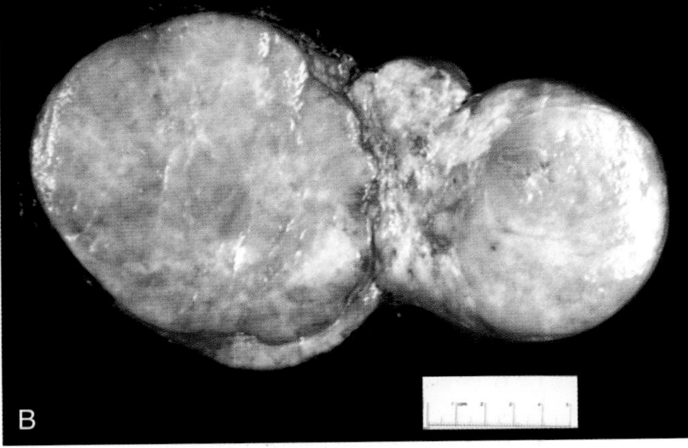

FIGURE 32-57. Solitary fibrous tumor growing as an exophytic mass from the surface of the liver (A). Cut section shows a dense white interior (B).

SFTs are highly variable in appearance, depending on the relative proportion of cells and fibrous stroma. The cellular end of this spectrum corresponds to classical hemangiopericytoma (Figs. 32-58 to 32-65) and the hyalinized end to classical solitary fibrous tumor. However, it should be emphasized that many cases have hybrid features (Fig. 32-66). The cellular phase of SFT consists of tightly packed round to fusiform cells with indistinct cytoplasmic borders that are arranged around an elaborate vasculature. The vessels form a continuous, ramifying vascular network that exhibits striking variation in caliber. As a rule, the dilated, branching vessels divide and communicate with small or minute vessels that may be partly compressed and obscured by the surrounding cellular proliferation. Typically, the dividing sinusoidal vessels have a staghorn or antler-like configuration (see Fig. 32-58). Commonly, the vessels, particularly large ones, are invested with a thick coat of collagen that extends into the interstitium (see Fig. 32-60). Myxoid change is common (see Fig. 32-62) and, when extreme, may produce an appearance similar to a myxoid liposarcoma. However, the presence of coarse-walled vessels, interstitial hyalinization, and the absence of lipoblasts are important features that distinguish these hemangiopericytomas from myxoid liposarcomas. Similar changes have been observed in classical SFT.[127]

Lesions having features of classical SFT consist principally of spindle cells (Figs. 32-67 to 32-71). The arrangement of the cells varies from area to area in the same tumor. In some zones, the cells are arranged in short, ill-defined fascicles, whereas in others they are arranged randomly in what has been described as a patternless pattern. A characteristic feature of the lesion, which usually suggests the diagnosis even at low power, is the striking hyalinization. In these areas, the cells are usually arranged singly or in small parallel clusters next to dense collagen. Artifactual cracks develop between the cells and collagen or between groups of collagen fibers (see Fig. 32-69). Gaping staghorn vessels, although occasionally present, are not as striking as in classical hemangiopericytoma (see Fig. 32-71).

Text continued on p. 1010

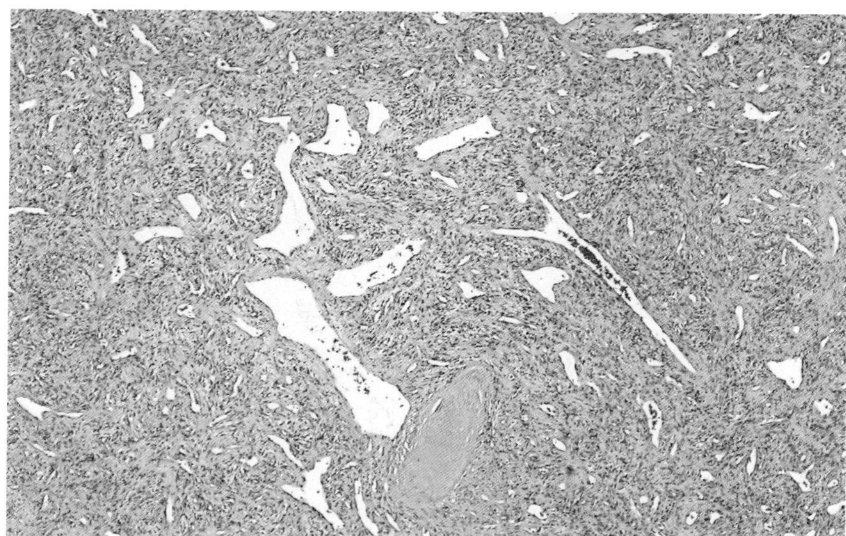

FIGURE 32-58. Cellular solitary fibrous tumor with a richly vascular pattern consisting of large and small vessels lined by a single layer of flattened endothelial cells.

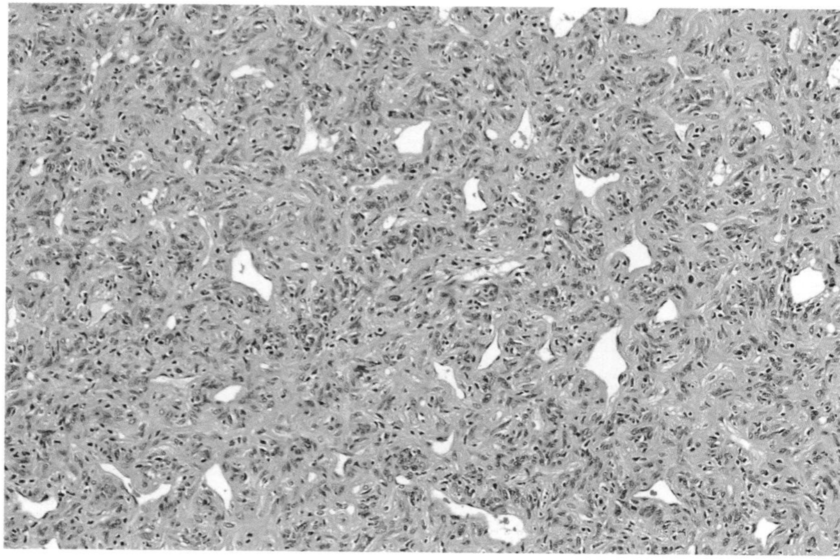

FIGURE 32-59. Cellular solitary fibrous tumor with predominantly small vessels.

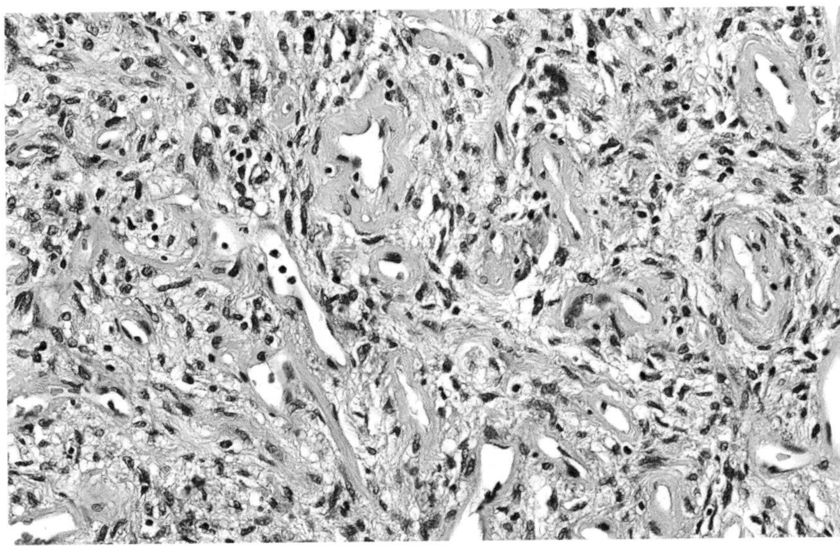

FIGURE 32-60. Cellular solitary fibrous tumor with perivascular hyalinization.

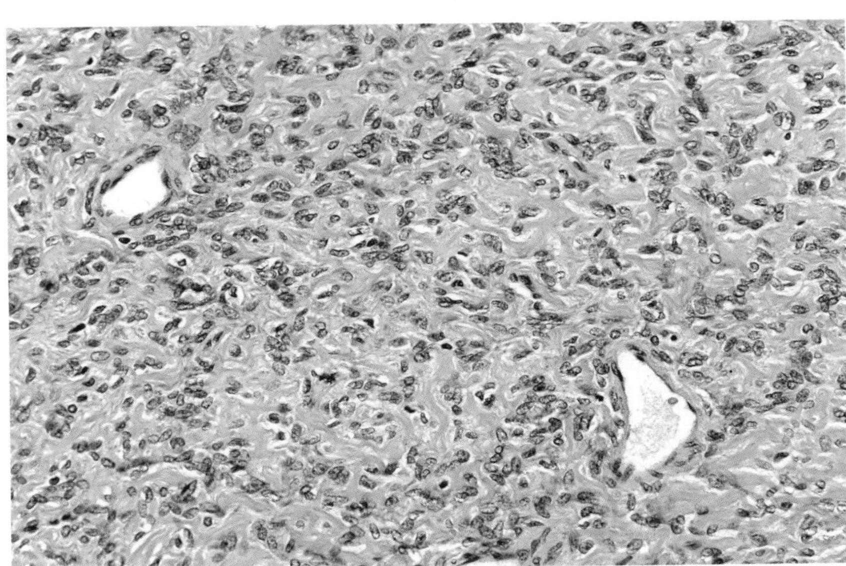

FIGURE 32-61. Cellular solitary fibrous tumor with interstitial hyalinization.

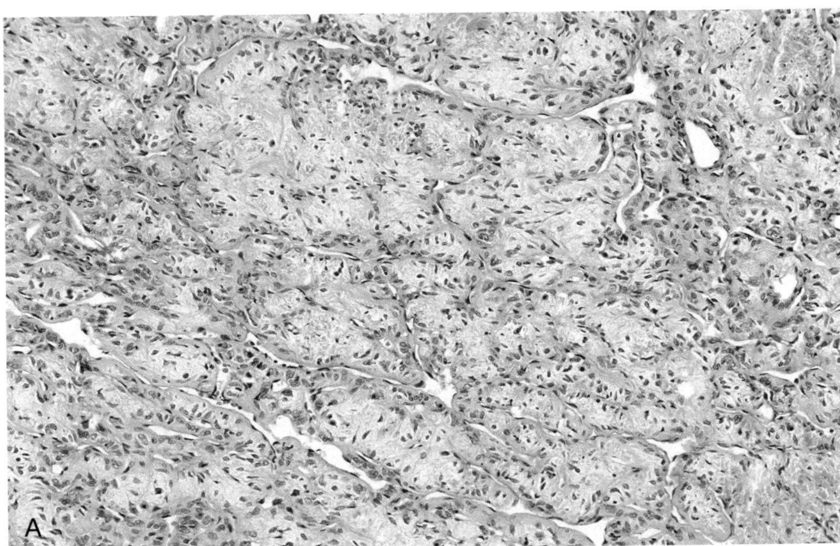

FIGURE 32-62. (A) Myxoid change in a solitary fibrous tumor. *Continued*

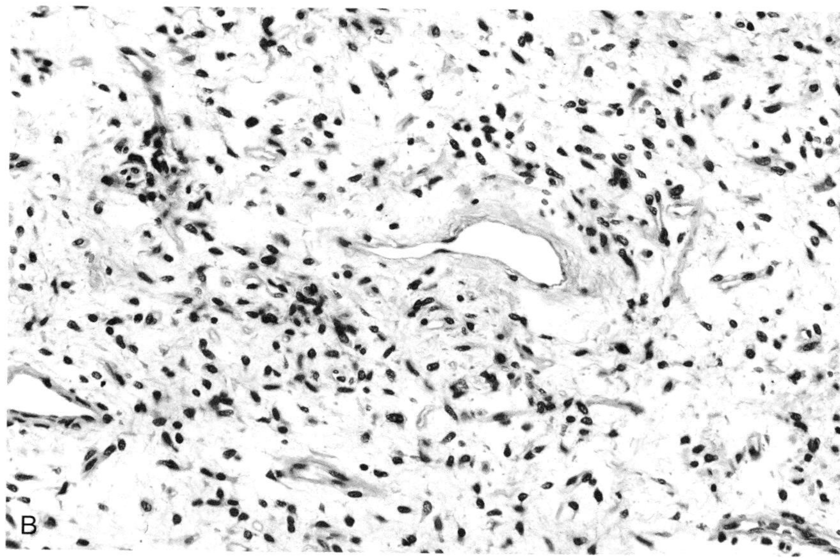

FIGURE 32-62, cont'd. (B) At high power, vessels are seen to be thicker and less elaborate than those in a myxoid liposarcoma.

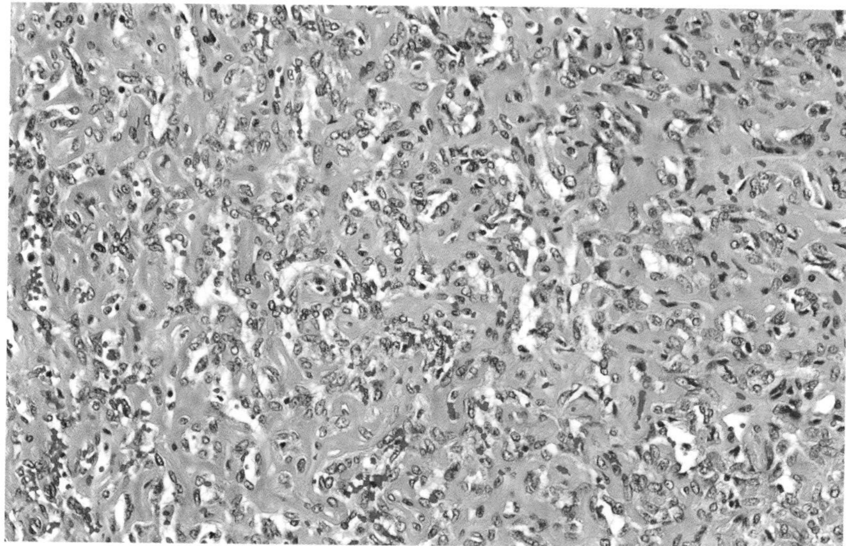

FIGURE 32-63. Pseudovascular pattern as a result of loss of cellular cohesion in a myxoid solitary fibrous tumor.

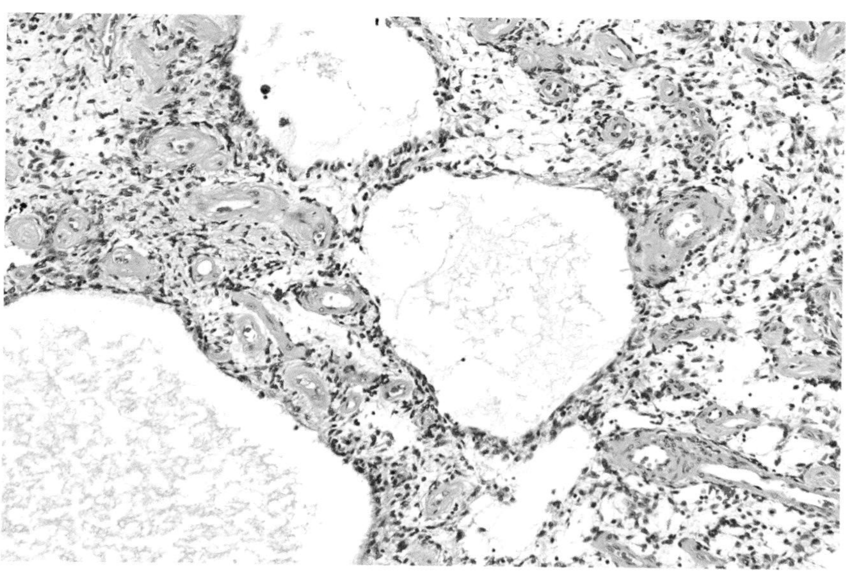

FIGURE 32-64. Cystic change in a myxoid solitary fibrous tumor.

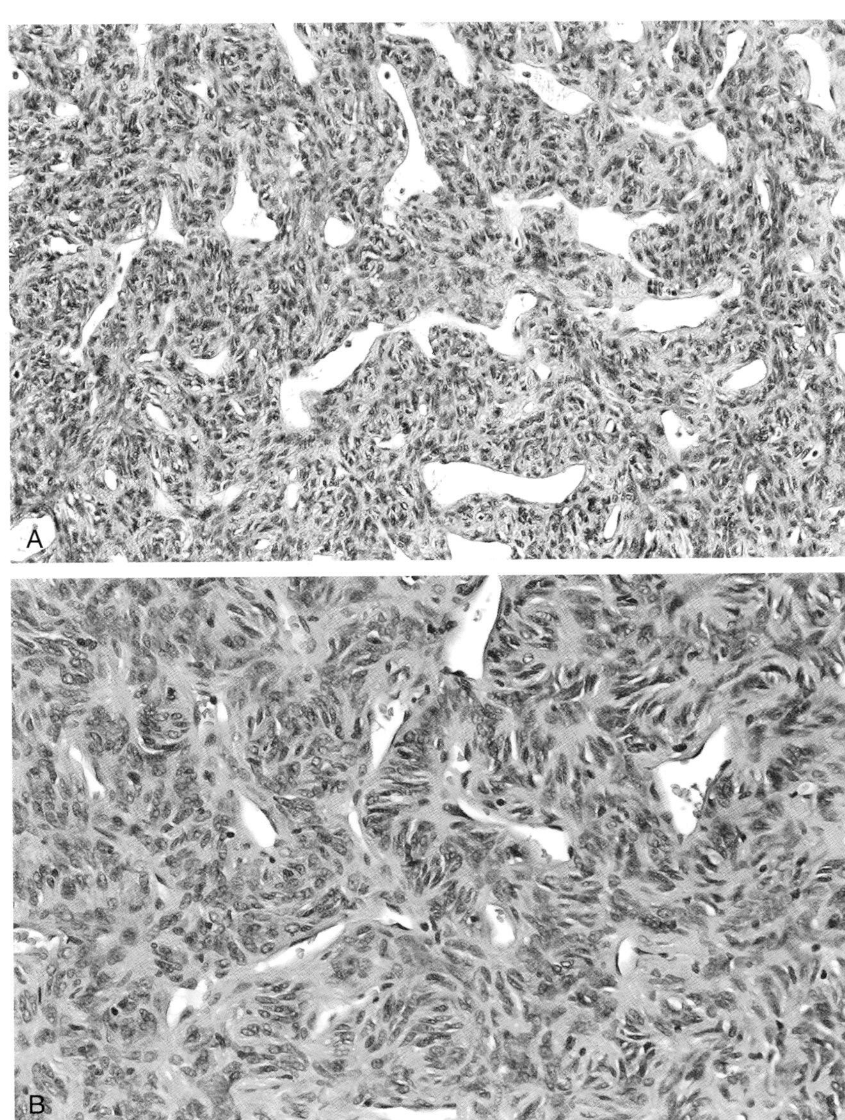

FIGURE 32-65. (A, B) The cells in cellular solitary fibrous tumor range from round/ovoid to slightly spindled.

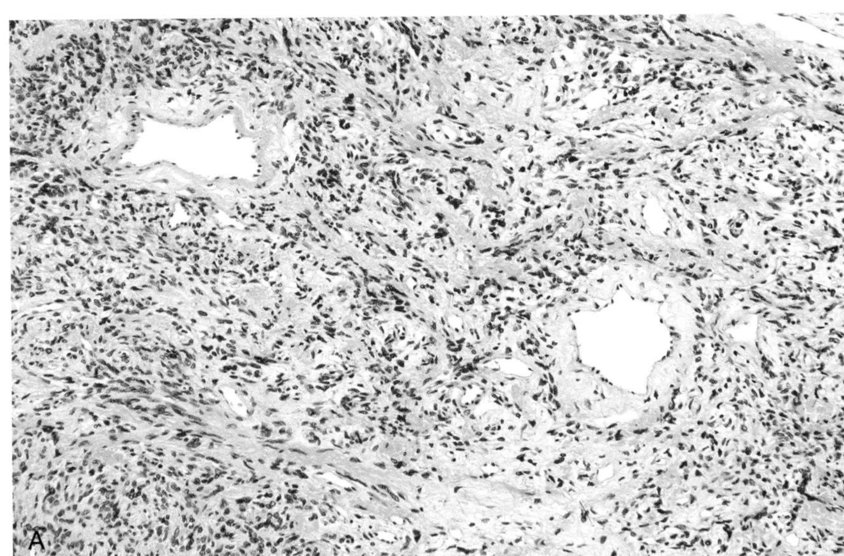

FIGURE 32-66. Tumor with features intermediate between a classical hemangiopericytoma and a classical solitary fibrous tumor. Tumor has a pericytic vascular pattern (A) but shows areas of interstitial hyalinization (B), and more spindling of the tumor cells (C). *Continued*

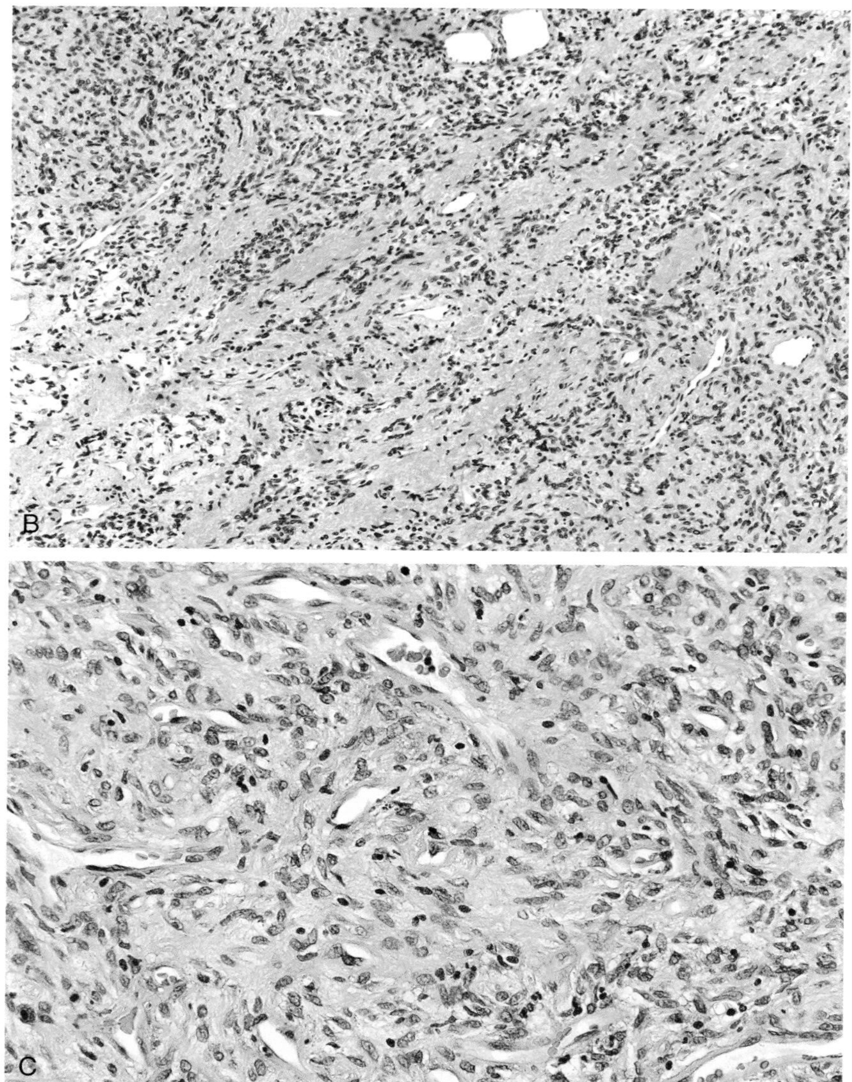

FIGURE 32-66, cont'd

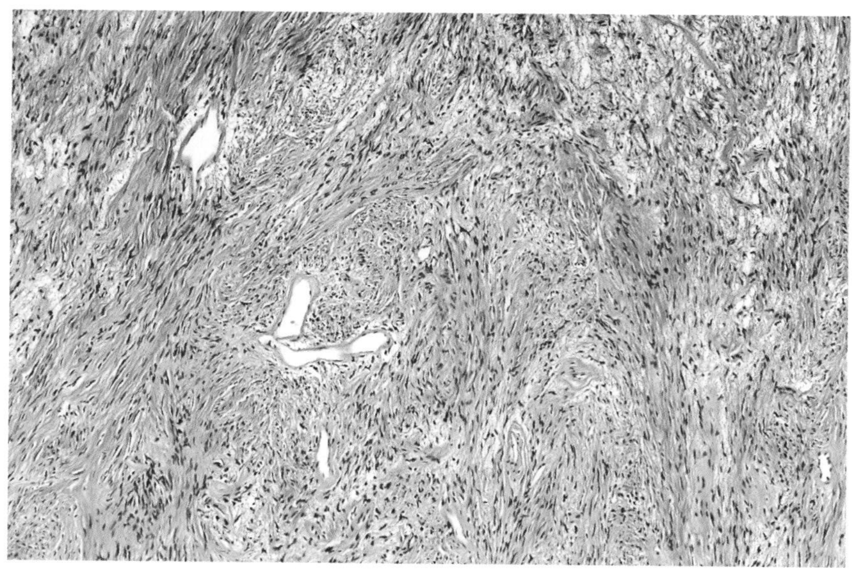

FIGURE 32-67. Solitary fibrous tumor with a heavily hyalinized area and focally prominent staghorn vessels.

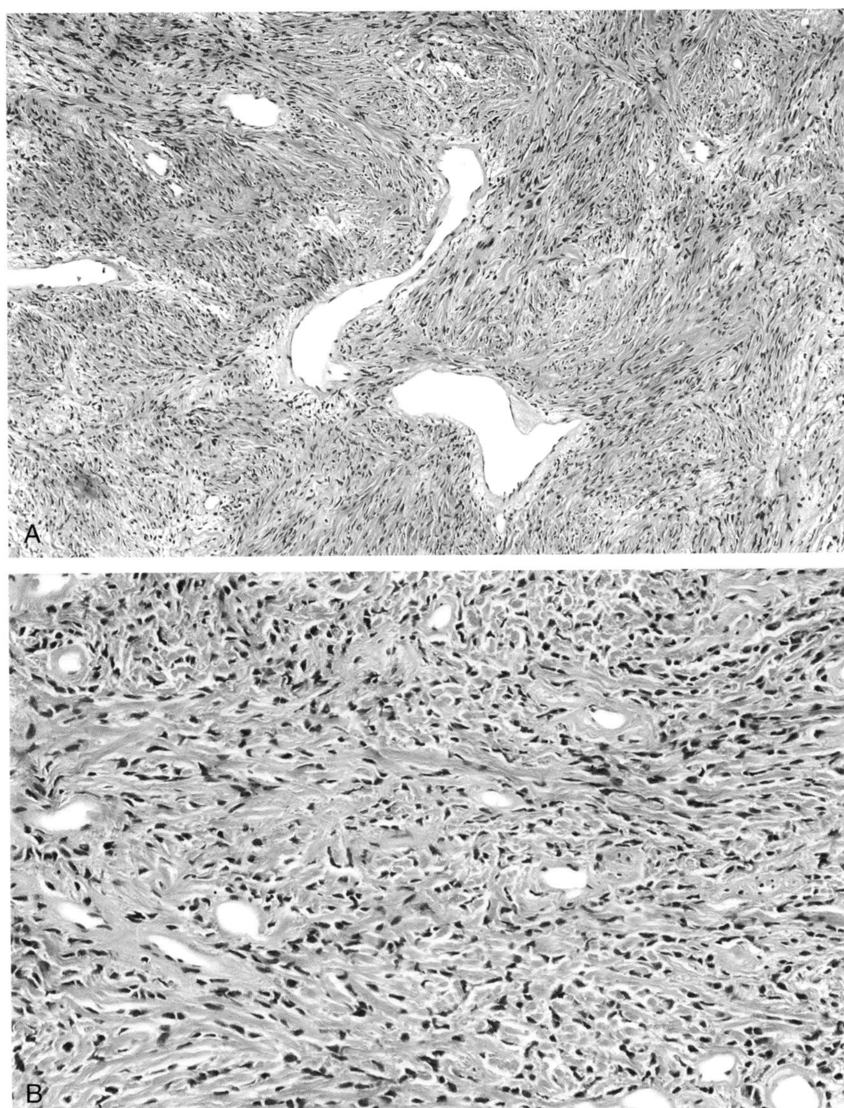

FIGURE 32-68. Solitary fibrous tumor showing a pericytic pattern (A) and patternless pattern (B) consisting of small fusiform cells randomly arranged between collagen bundles.

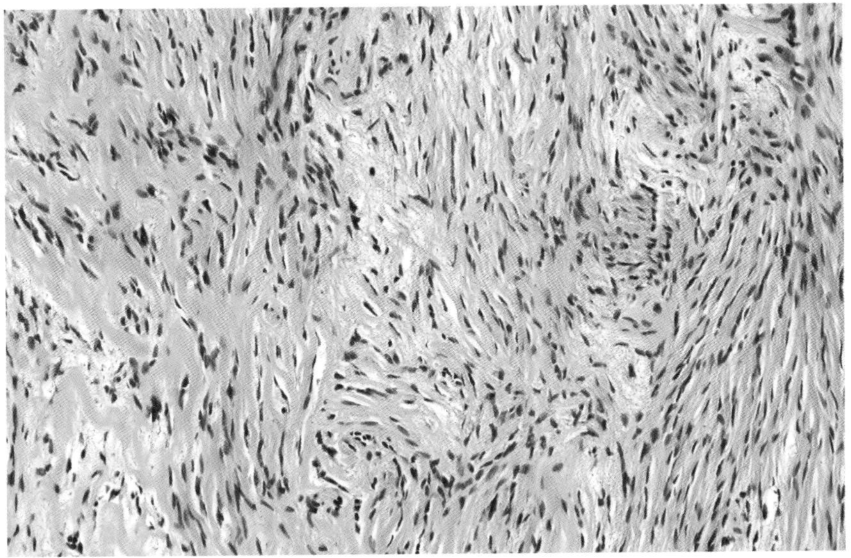

FIGURE 32-69. Solitary fibrous tumor with a characteristic cracking artifact between the cells and collagen.

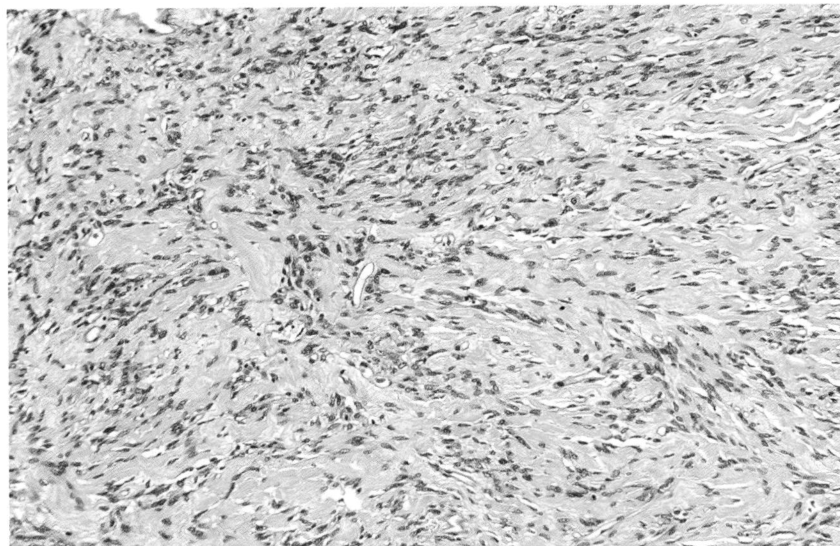

FIGURE 32-70. Solitary fibrous tumor with a staggered or grouped arrangement of cells in the collagen.

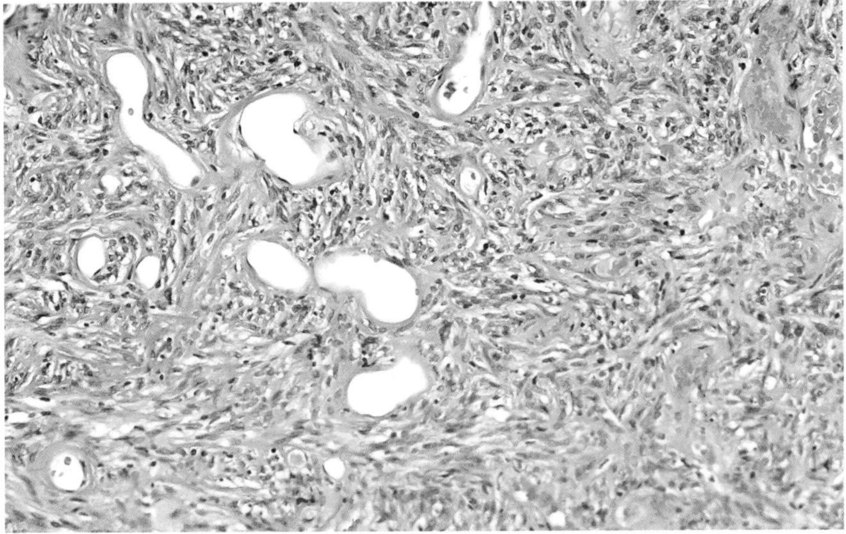

FIGURE 32-71. Solitary fibrous tumor with a hemangiopericytoma-like area.

A small subset of SFT contains a variable amount of fat as an integral part of the tumor[128-130] and may be mistaken for well-differentiated or dedifferentiated liposarcomas (see later text). Unusual features that can confuse the histologic picture of SFT are the presence of pseudovascular spaces created by the loss of cellular cohesion (see Fig. 32-68), cystic change (see Fig. 32-64), and giant cells (see later text).

Immunohistochemical and Ultrastructural Findings

Cellular SFTs express CD34 but usually in a smaller percentage of cases and to a lesser degree than do more classical, hyalinized tumors (Fig. 32-72). SFTs of pleural and extrapleural origin typically express CD34 (80% to 90%), CD99 (70%), bcl2 (30%),[108,131-136] EMA (30%), and actin (20%). Desmin, cytokeratin, and S-100 protein are usually absent.[108] The high sensitivity of CD34 for SFTs has resulted in a more accurate and consistent diagnosis of the entity, undoubtedly accounting for the increasing number of SFTs now diagnosed at extrathoracic sites (Fig. 32-73). Anomalous cytokeratin expression may be seen, particularly in histologically malignant tumors.

Most early ultrastructural studies attempted to draw parallels between the cells of classical hemangiopericytoma and normal pericytes.[105,137] However, fewer than 30% of reported cases provided convincing evidence of pericytic differentiation.[108] Neoplastic cells are described as having rounded nuclei, an organelle-poor cytoplasm containing occasional arrays of microfilaments, cell processes, and poorly developed junctions. It has been pointed out that the cells comprising these tumors are fundamentally undifferentiated,[106] and it is only because of their topographic relation to blood vessels and their close association with periendothelial basement membrane that a relation to normal pericytes is inferred.[106] Moreover, mesenchymal cells that reside farther from the capillary may not display a close association with basement membrane.[105] SFTs seem to display considerable cellular heterogeneity. They contain fibroblasts, pericytes, undifferentiated perivascular cells, and endothelial cells, leading some

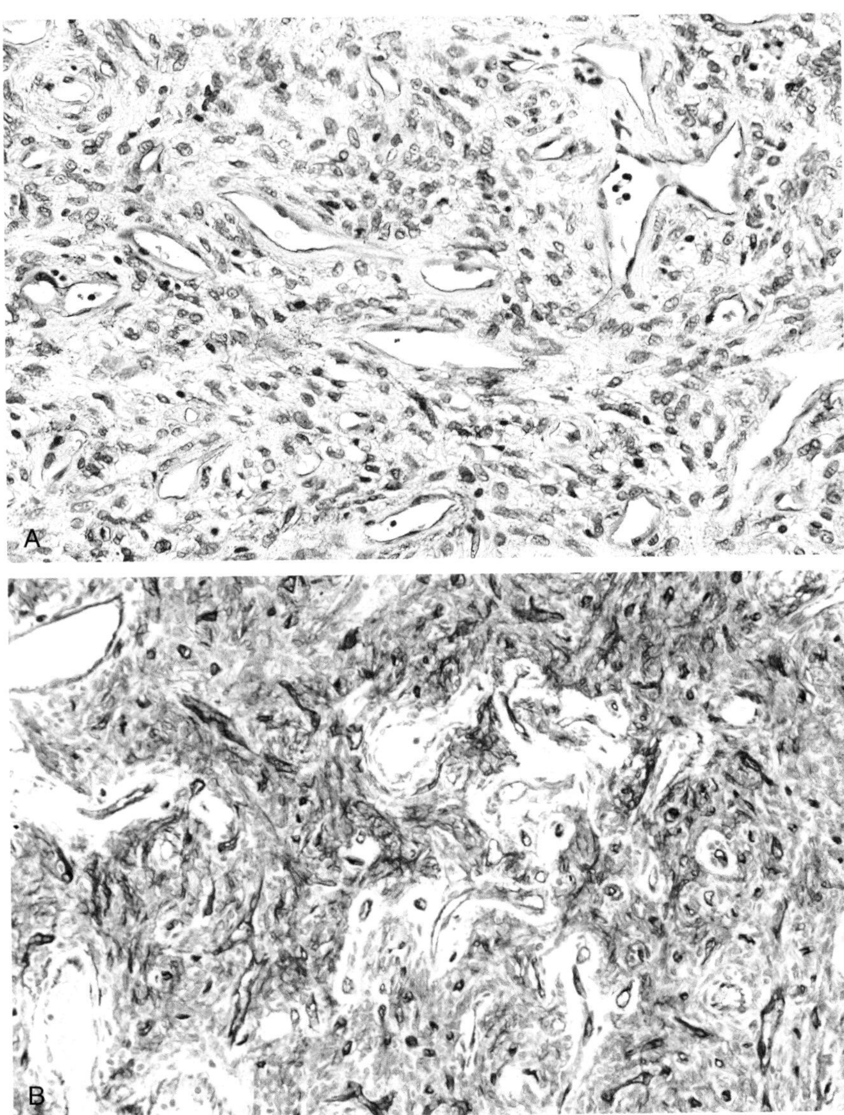

FIGURE 32-72. CD34 immunostain in cellular solitary fibrous tumor. Most tumors are positive, but staining may be relatively focal (A) or occasionally diffuse (B).

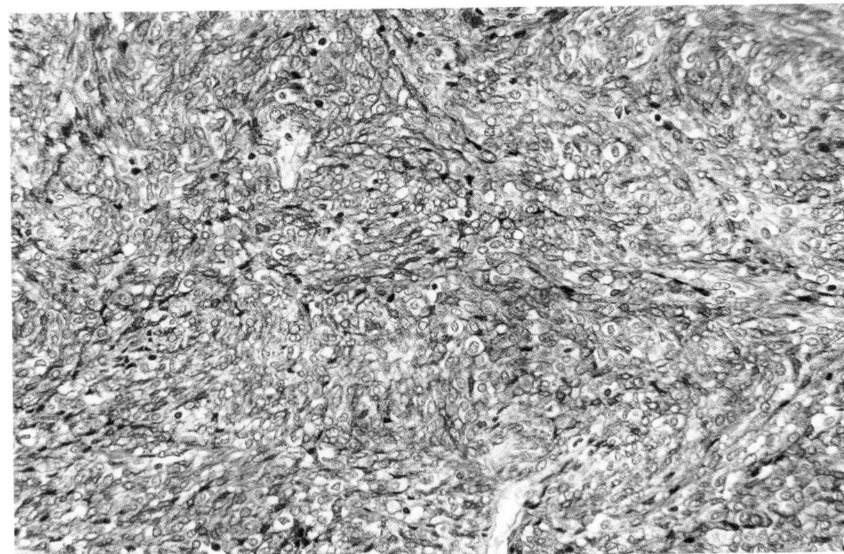

FIGURE 32-73. CD34 immunostain in a solitary fibrous tumor showing diffuse staining.

to conclude that they arise from pluripotential perivascular cells.[138,139]

Differential Diagnosis

The differential diagnosis of SFT is lengthy and includes both benign and malignant lesions having a prominent pericytic vascular pattern.

Fibrous histiocytoma, particularly its deep subcutaneous form, usually displays a more prominent, more uniform spindle-cell pattern than hemangiopericytoma, often with a distinct storiform arrangement of the tumor cells. There are, however, occasional examples of this tumor in which distinction may be exceedingly difficult, and many of these lesions seem to occur in the orbit.

Synovial sarcoma, in about 10% to 20% of cases, exhibits a distinctive but focal hemangiopericytoma-like pattern. This pattern usually occurs in high-grade round cell areas of the synovial sarcoma. The caliber of the vascular channels does not have a broad range as is seen in hemangiopericytomas. Synovial sarcomas are almost always associated with distinct spindle cells, hyalinized-calcified areas, glands, and expression of cytokeratin. CD34 expression is not seen in synovial sarcoma, a useful negative finding in cases where the differential diagnosis includes SFT with anomalous cytokeratin expression.

Mesenchymal chondrosarcoma frequently shows a hemangiopericytoma-like vascular pattern in the closely packed small-cell areas but is readily recognizable by the presence of islands of well-differentiated cartilage or, much less frequently, bone. Ill-defined foci of immature cartilage may also be present in the small-cell component (see Chapter 30).

Juxtaglomerular tumors that secrete renin and cause hypertension may also be misinterpreted as hemangiopericytomas,[140-143] especially those rare lesions that occur in extrarenal locations such as the retroperitoneum. In most of these neoplasms, large epithelioid cells and thick-walled vessels are present, and some contain PAS-positive renin crystals.

In the past, many phosphaturic mesenchymal tumors (PMTs) were erroneously labeled as hemangiopericytomas. Recognition of the distinctive matrix produced by PMTs and clinical investigation for associated osteomalacia should allow for the ready distinction of these two entities.

Cytogenetic Findings

Several balanced translocations have been observed in cellular SFT, including t(12;19),[144,145] t(13;22),[146] and t(3;12).[147] The single most common abnormality is rearrangements of the long arm of chromosome 12, a site similar to those affected in lipomas and leiomyomas. A variety of chromosomal abnormalities have been reported in SFT, including malignant variants, but until extremely recently no consistent aberration has been identified.[148-159] However, in 2013 Mohajeri and colleagues identified a pathognomonic NAB2/STAT6 gene fusion in solitary fibrous tumors, strongly suggesting that solitary fibrous tumors are translocation-associated neoplasms.[159a]

Discussion

The clinical behavior of SFT (including cases reported as hemangiopericytoma) has traditionally been a problematic area, largely because of inclusional criteria. Studies often do not make clear whether cellular SFT, classical SFT, or both were analyzed. Frequently, the proportion of lesions with overtly malignant versus conventional features is not clear. Therefore, there is pressing need to analyze the entire spectrum of lesions in a standard fashion to determine whether there are inherent differences between the two ends of this spectrum.

The majority of SFT are histologically benign. However, a small percentage of cases possess atypical features (Figs. 32-74 and 32-75). The criteria for malignancy in tumors previously classified as hemangiopericytoma vary from study to study. The criteria proposed by Enzinger and Smith[104] for malignancy in classical hemangiopericytoma (cellular SFT) identify overtly malignant or high-grade lesions but fail to address low-grade lesions. In their study, large size (greater than 5 cm), increased mitotic rate (greater than 4 MF/10 HPF), high cellularity, presence of immature and pleomorphic tumor cells, and foci of hemorrhage and necrosis predicted a highly

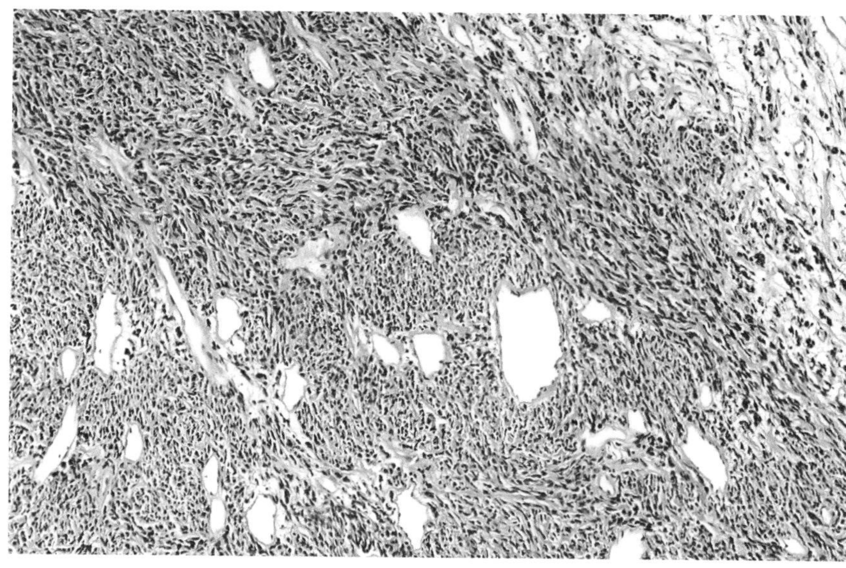

FIGURE 32-74. Malignant solitary fibrous tumor with heightened cellularity. Tumor also contained areas of histologically benign solitary fibrous tumor.

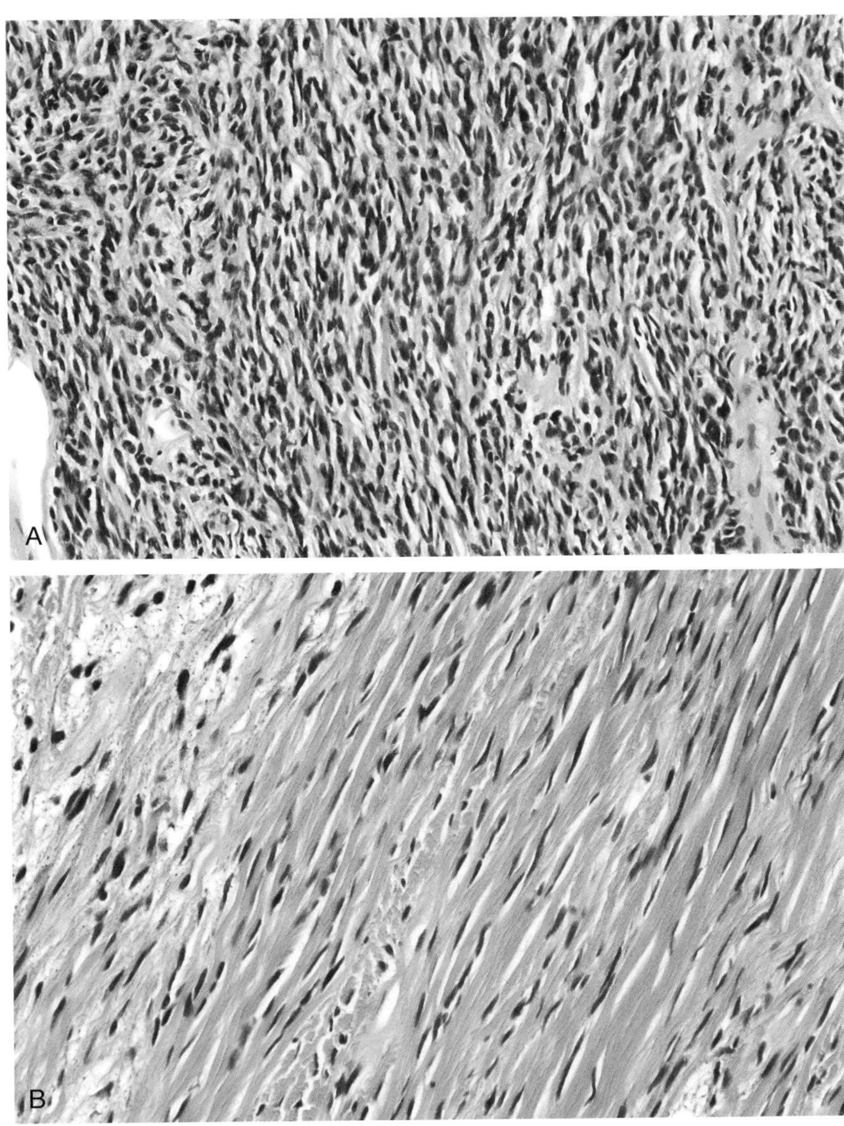

FIGURE 32-75. (A) Malignant area of a malignant solitary fibrous tumor. (B) High-power view of benign areas for comparison. Same case as in Figure 32-72.

malignant course (Fig. 32-76). McMaster et al.,[116] in a review of 60 cases from the Mayo Clinic, used similar but less stringent criteria for malignant behavior: either a slight degree of anaplasia and 1 MF/10 HPF or a moderate degree of cellular anaplasia and 1 MF/20 HPF. Middleton et al.[111] associated recurrence or metastasis with a trabecular pattern, necrosis, mitoses, vascular invasion, and cellular atypia. Lesions with the features reported by Enzinger and Smith[104] are identified as malignant, although the term *low malignant potential* is used for lesions with lower levels of mitotic activity (1 to 3 MF/10 HPF), especially if they have any degree of atypia and cellularity. The term *malignant hemangiopericytoma* is archaic and should be avoided, particularly for round cell sarcomas that simply have a pericytic vascular pattern, as most prove to be sarcomas of other types (e.g., synovial sarcoma). Malignancy in classical SFT has been assessed on very similar parameters and is defined by high cellularity, greater than 4 MF/10 HPF, and hemorrhage/necrosis.[131,160,161] A subset of SFT shows an abrupt transition from typical areas to high-grade pleomorphic sarcoma; the term *dedifferentiated solitary fibrous tumor* has been proposed for these lesions but is not widely accepted.[162,163]

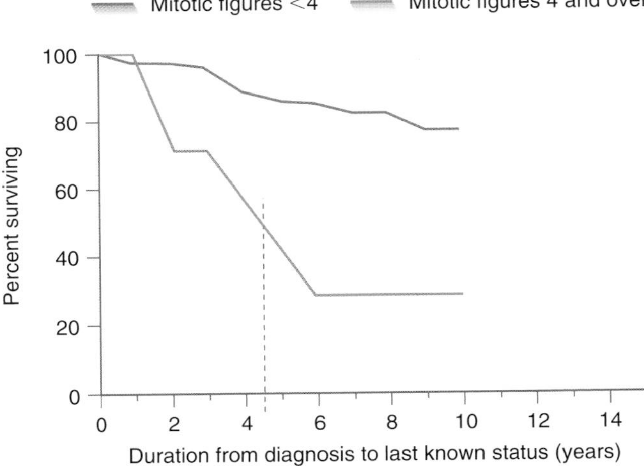

FIGURE 32-76. Actuarial survival rate of patients with hemangiopericytoma and relative survival, based on the number of mitotic figures. Mitotic figures and necrosis are the two most important criteria when distinguishing benign from malignant hemangiopericytomas. *(From Enzinger FM, Smith BH. Hemangiopericytoma: an analysis of 106 cases. Hum Pathol 1976; 7:61.)*

Overall, thoracic and extrathoracic SFTs are quite similar clinically and biologically.[160] The majority have rather banal or benign histologic features and pursue a favorable course. Those that have malignant areas, generally defined as areas of high cellularity, greater than 4 MF/10 HPF, and hemorrhage/necrosis,[160,161] are at risk for metastasis. This principle is well illustrated by the following studies. In the most extensive series of thoracic SFTs reported from a single institution, two-thirds were judged benign on the basis of a number of histologic parameters.[164] All but two of the patients in this group were free of disease following simple excision or wedge resection of the lung. Malignant tumors had a more variable outcome. Approximately one-half of the patients were cured of their tumors following excision, whereas the remainder developed recurrences, metastases, or both (Table 32-10). Overall, the metastatic rate of SFTs was 9% (16 of 169 with follow-up information). In addition to the criteria mentioned previously, nonpedunculated growth and an atypical location (e.g., parietal pleura, interlobar fissure, mediastinum, or endophytic growth into lung) were also correlated with more aggressive behavior (Table 32-11). Two other studies reaffirmed these observations. Vallat-Decouvelaere et al.[131] reported their experience from a large consultation service and indicated that approximately 10% of extrathoracic SFTs have atypical features (cellularity, atypia, greater than 4 MF/10 HPF, necrosis) or a history of local recurrence. Eight of 10 patients in this category developed local recurrences, and 5 died of distant metastasis. A more recent study of 79 cases of both thoracic and extrathoracic lesions also found that large size (greater than 10 cm) and presence of malignant areas predicted metastasis.[160] However, size and malignant areas were not independent variables.

A recent series of SFTs from Memorial Sloan-Kettering Cancer Center (New York, NY) found 2- and 5-year survival rates of 93% and 80%, respectively, although it is unclear whether this series included histologically malignant tumors.[165] Most recently, the authors of a study of 110 cases of SFT, treated at the MD Anderson Cancer Center (Houston, TX), have proposed a risk stratification system for patients with this disease (Table 32-12). This system appears to accurately stratify patients with this disease, with a much greater risk for metastasis and death from disease seen in patients with moderate or high-risk tumors, as compared with low-risk tumors.[166]

TABLE 32-10 Clinical Behavior of Intrathoracic Solitary Fibrous Tumors

HISTOLOGIC DIAGNOSIS*	RECURRENCE (%)	METASTASES (%)
Benign	2	0
Malignant†	39	22

Data from England DM, Hochholzer L, McCarthy MJ. Localized benign and malignant fibrous tumors of the pleura: a clinicopathologic review of 223 cases. Am J Surg Pathol 1989; 13:640–658.

* There were 98 benign tumors with follow-up ranging from 1 to 317 months (median 57 months) and 71 malignant tumors with follow-up ranging from 2 to 372 months (median 31 months).

† Tumors were classified as malignant, based on one or more of the following features in any portion of tumor: high cellularity with crowded overlapping nuclei, greater than 4 MF/10 HPF, nuclear atypia, pleomorphic giant cells, and atypical mitoses.

TABLE 32-11 Features Associated with Malignancy in Solitary Fibrous Tumors

THORACIC[164]	SOFT TISSUE[118]
Histologic features	
Increased cellularity	Increased cellularity
Pleomorphism	Pleomorphism
Mitoses (>4 MF/10 HPF)	Mitoses (>4 MF/10 HPF)
Clinical/gross features	
Nonpedunculated	
Atypical location (parietal pleura, parenchyma)	
Size >10 cm	
Necrosis/hemorrhage	

Variants of Solitary Fibrous Tumor

Lipomatous Solitary Fibrous Tumor

Lipomatous SFT is a rare variant that contains a variable amount of mature fat as an integral part of the tumor (Figs. 32-77 and 32-78).[128-130] Microscopically, they consist of areas of histologically benign SFT admixed with microscopic or macroscopic areas of mature fat. In the typical case, about one-fourth to three-fourths of the tumor is mature fat. In some areas, spindling of the pericytic areas creates a resemblance to a spindle cell lipoma. To date, all of the lesions with follow-up information have behaved in a benign fashion, although a few have recurred. The principal significance of this variant is that it is easily mistaken for a well-differentiated liposarcoma, particularly when only a small biopsy specimen is available. In these situations, it is helpful to be apprised of the clinical features that suggest a relatively circumscribed, rather than infiltrative, mass.

Meningeal (Cranial and Intraspinal) Hemangiopericytoma-Solitary Fibrous Tumor

Meningeal hemangiopericytomas are indistinguishable from hemangiopericytoma-SFTs at other sites and are no longer considered variants of meningioma.[112,167,168] Unlike conventional meningiomas, meningeal hemangiopericytoma-SFTs lack EMA, and they do not display mutations in the NF2 locus on chromosome 22.[169,170] They express vimentin as the sole intermediate filament. They occur at a younger age than meningiomas, grow more often along the sinuses, bleed profusely at operation, have a tendency to recur, and may metastasize to extracranial sites. Guthrie et al.,[171] in a review of 44 meningeal hemangiopericytoma-SFTs, reported 5- and 15-year survival rates of 67% and 23%, respectively. Mena et al.,[172] in another large series, noted a recurrence rate of 60.6% and a metastatic rate of 23.4%.

Solitary Fibrous Tumor with Giant Cells (Giant Cell Angiofibroma)

A giant-cell-rich form of SFT was described by Dei Tos et al.[173] as giant cell angiofibroma. Although originally identified in the orbital region, this tumor may occur in diverse locations.[174] It displays all of the features of a classical SFT but is identified by pseudovascular spaces (resulting from a loss of cellular-stromal cohesion) lined by multinucleated stromal giant cells (Figs. 32-79 to 32-82).

TABLE 32-12 Risk Stratification Model for Solitary Fibrous Tumor

RISK FACTOR	SCORE	METASTASIS-FREE RATE (5 YEARS; 10 YEARS)	DISEASE-SPECIFIC SURVIVAL (5 YEARS; 10 YEARS)
Age			
<55 years	0		
≥55 years	1		
Tumor size (cm)			
<5	0		
5 to <10	1		
10 to <15	2		
≥15	3		
Mitotic figures/10 HPF			
0	0		
1-3	1		
≥4	2		
Risk	Score		
Low	0-2	100%	100%
Moderate	3-4	77%; 64%	93%; 93%
High	5-6	15%; 0%	60%; 0%

Adapted from Demicco EG, Park MS, Araujo DM, et al. Solitary fibrous tumor: a clinicopathological study of 110 cases and proposed risk assessment model. Mod Pathol 2012;25(9):1298–1306.

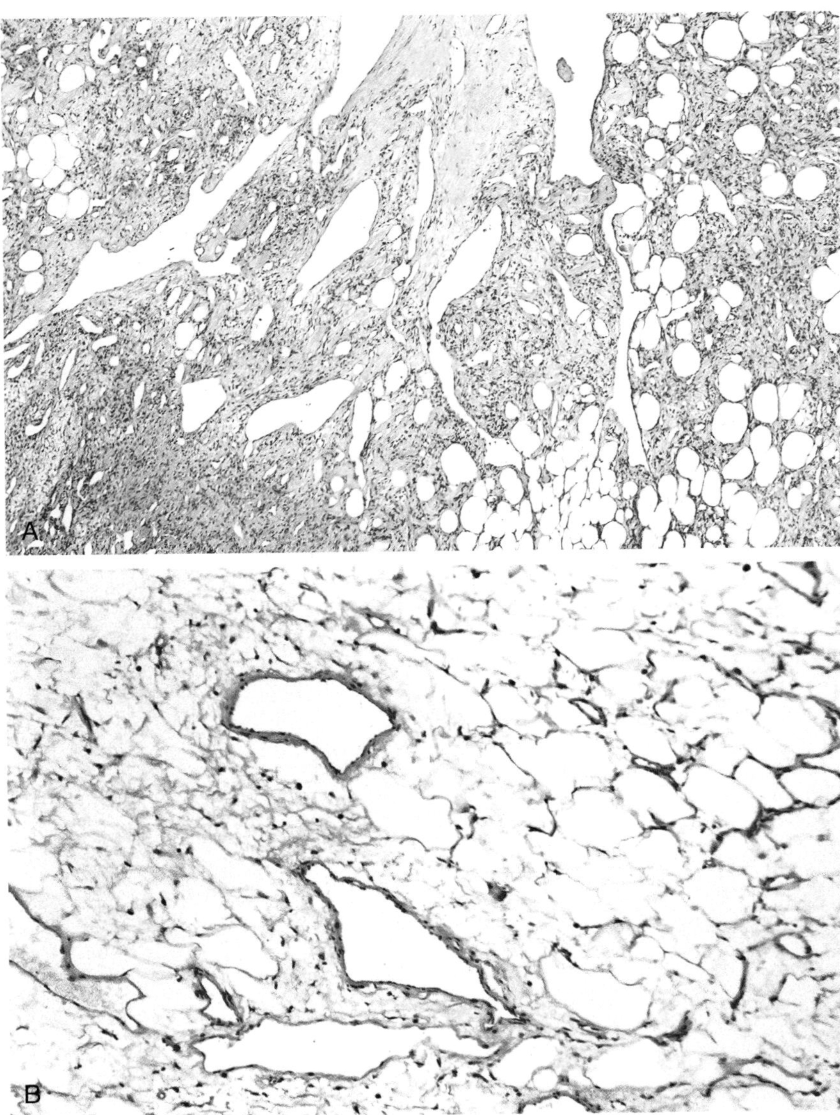

FIGURE 32-77. Lipomatous solitary fibrous tumor, showing a range of appearances, from areas having focal fat only (A) to those that are predominantly fatty (B).

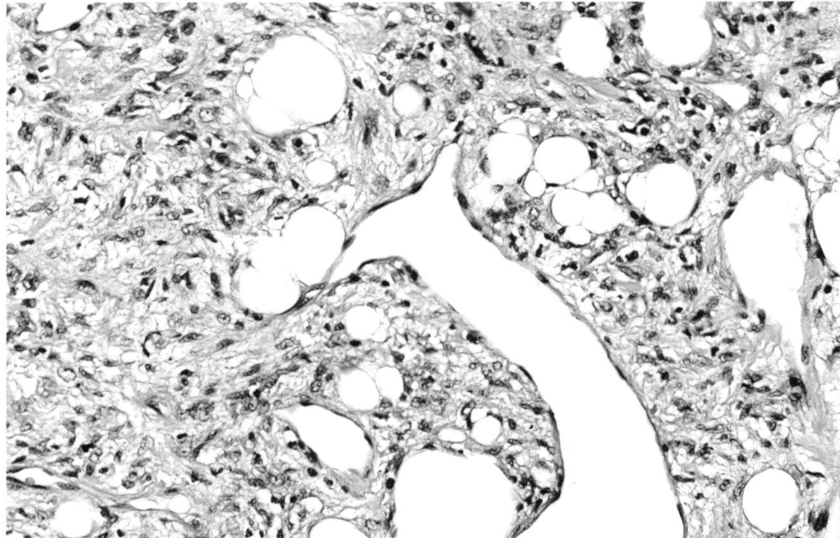

FIGURE 32-78. Lipomatous solitary fibrous tumor.

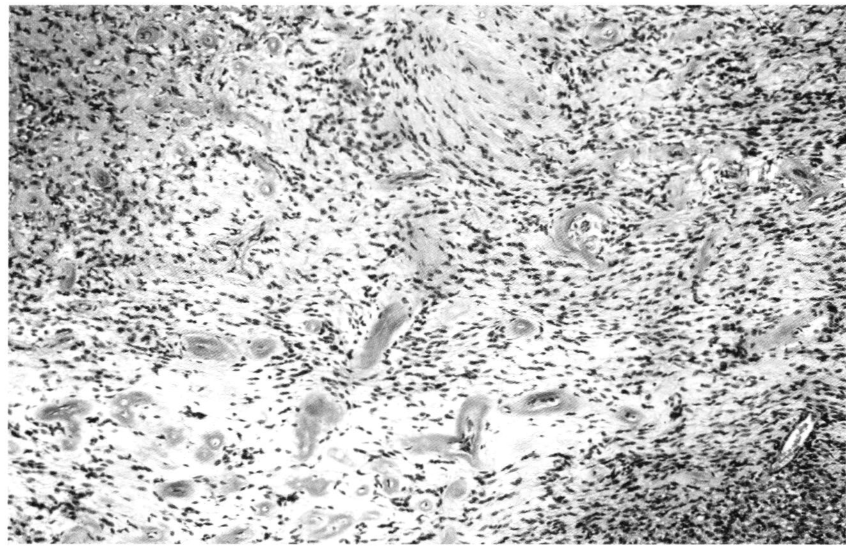

FIGURE 32-79. Giant cell angiofibroma with cellular proliferation of spindle-shaped cells between small blood vessels with marked perivascular hyalinization.

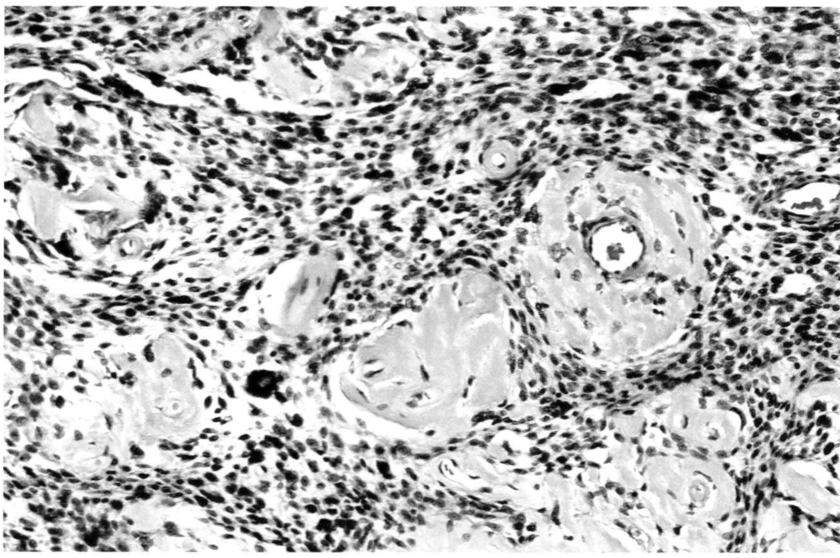

FIGURE 32-80. High-power view of a giant cell angiofibroma with cellular spindle cell proliferation between hyalinized blood vessels and scattered multinucleated floret-like giant cells.

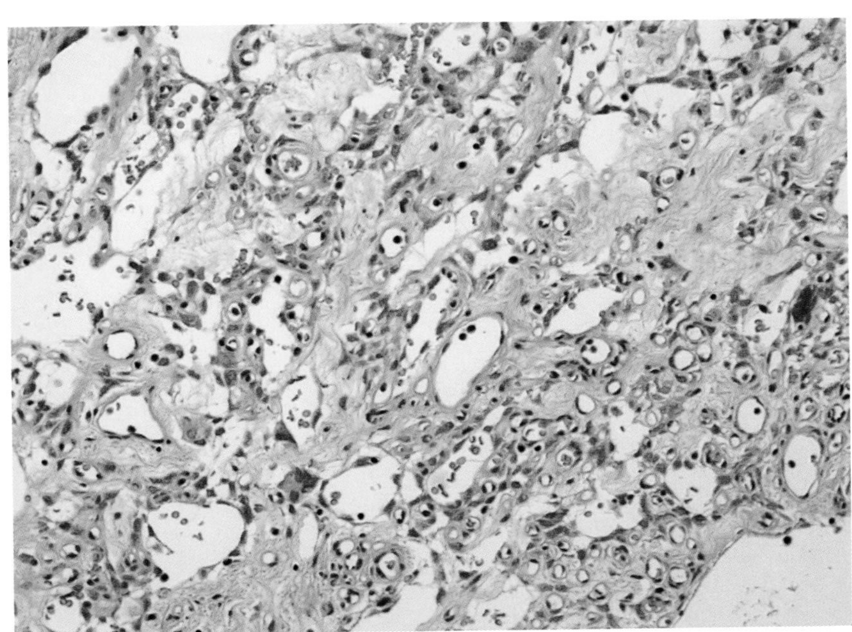

FIGURE 32-81. Scattered multinucleated giant cells in a giant cell angiofibroma.

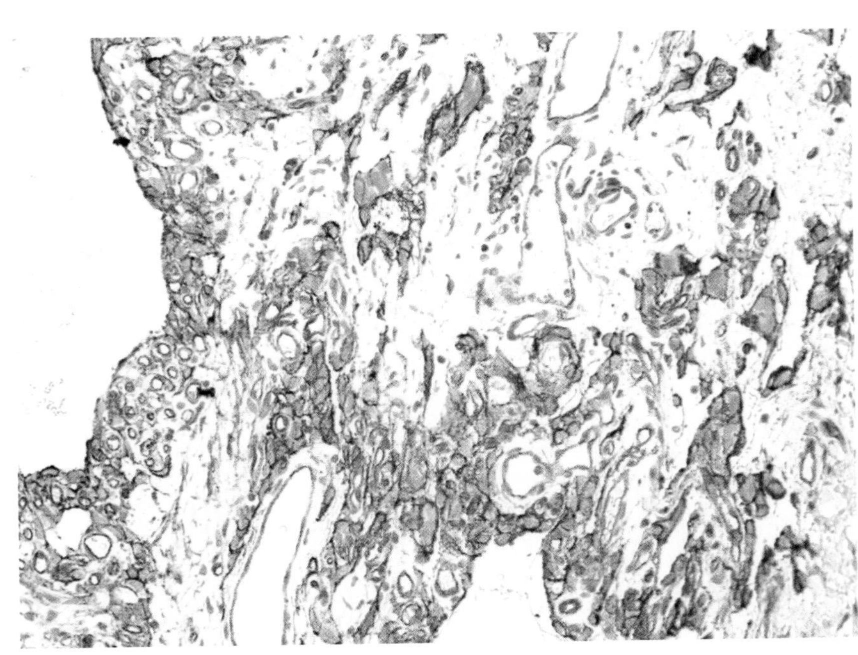

FIGURE 32-82. CD34 immunoreactivity in a giant cell angiofibroma.

INFANTILE HEMANGIOPERICYTOMA

Infantile hemangiopericytoma deserves separate consideration because of its different histologic picture and clinical behavior from adult cellular SFT. It is unclear at the present time whether these lesions are related to SFT, a myofibroma, or are a distinct entity altogether.

These lesions mostly occur in infants during the first year of life and, like juvenile hemangiomas, are usually located in the subcutis and oral cavity.[175,176] Tumors in older children and deep-seated tumors in the muscle, mediastinum, and abdomen have also been described.[177,178] Alpers et al.[175] reported an infantile hemangiopericytoma of the tongue and sublingual region that was discovered at birth, grew in an infiltrative manner, and recurred rapidly after local excision. After 30 months, the child was well with no evidence of further recurrence or metastasis. All lesions in this textbook authors' cases have been solitary, but there are rare accounts of patients with multiple tumors.[179] One was associated with Kasabach-Merritt syndrome.[179]

Microscopically, infantile hemangiopericytoma bears a close resemblance to the adult type, but many lesions, especially superficial ones, are multilobulated, often with distinct intravascular and perivascular satellite nodules outside of the main tumor mass (Fig. 32-83A) and frequent endovascular growth (Fig. 32-83B). There is often increased mitotic activity and focal necrosis, features that indicate a poor prognosis for adult-type hemangiopericytomas but generally do not with

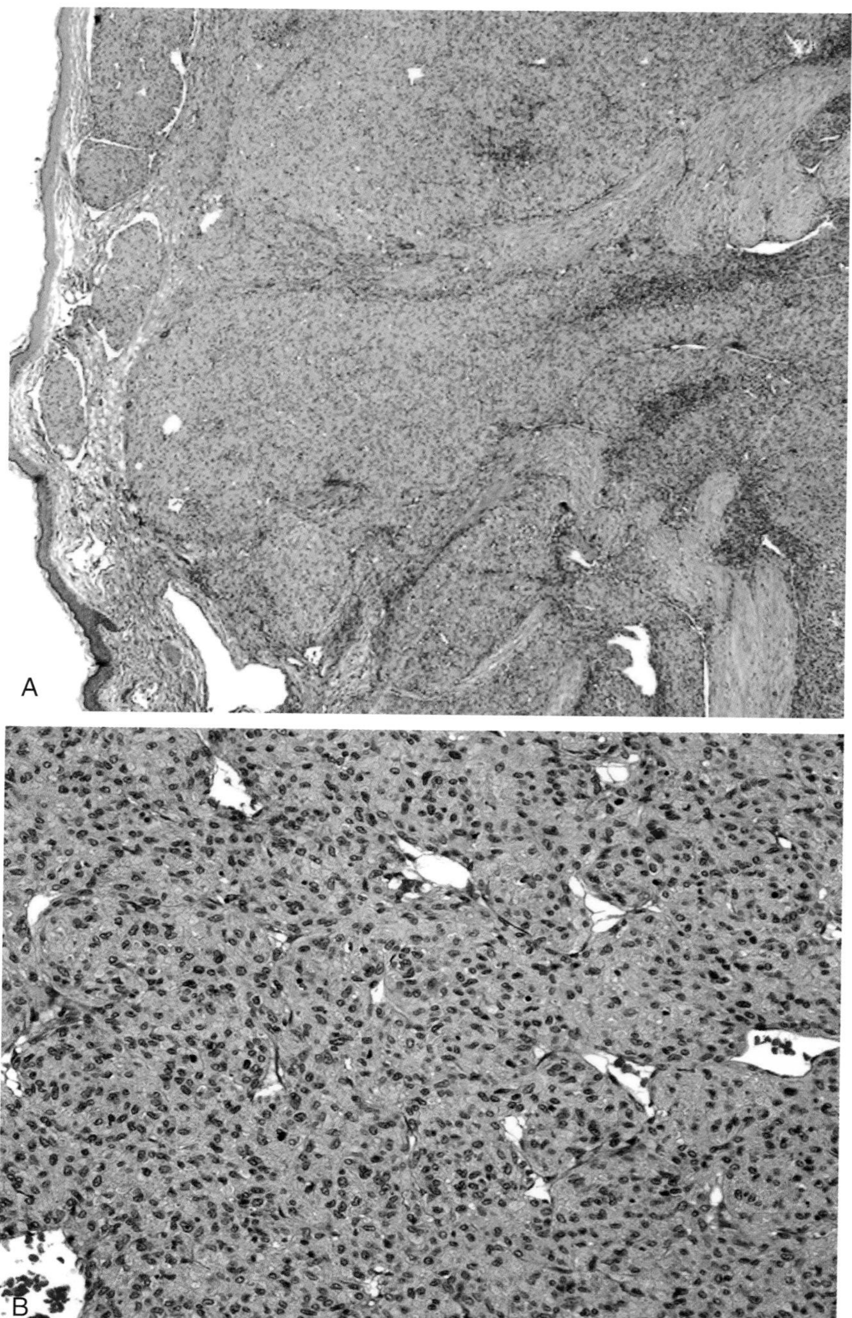

FIGURE 32-83. (A) Low-magnification view of infantile hemangiopericytoma with the typical multilobular arrangement of tumor cells. (B) Higher-magnification view of infantile hemangiopericytoma.

the infantile form. Judging from this textbook authors' cases and the literature, most of these tumors tend to follow a benign clinical course; they are curable by local excision or may regress spontaneously.[179,180] In rare instances, however, there may be local infiltrative growth or recurrence and even metastasis.[181] Deep-seated lesions and those occurring in older children seem to pursue a more aggressive clinical course than superficial ones that appear during the first years of life.

The hemangiopericytoma-like pattern found in the lobular or tufted hemangioma (a variant of lobular capillary hemangioma marked by dermal or subcutaneous capillary or vascular lobules), infantile myofibromatosis, and infantile fibrosarcoma must be distinguished from that of infantile hemangiopericytoma (see Chapters 9 and 21). Other benign and malignant neoplasms that may cause diagnostic difficulty include the juvenile hemangioma, glomus tumor, angiosarcoma, vascular forms of leiomyoma and leiomyosarcoma, endometrial stromal sarcoma, malignant peripheral nerve sheath tumor, mesothelioma, and liposarcoma.

PHOSPHATURIC MESENCHYMAL TUMOR

The term *phosphaturic mesenchymal tumor, mixed connective tissue variant* was first introduced by Weidner and Santa Cruz[182] in 1987, as a unifying concept for what had previously been considered a heterogeneous group of bone and soft tissue tumors associated with phosphate wasting and osteomalacia (tumor-induced osteomalacia [TIO]). The existence of this tumor as a discrete entity was first further validated by Folpe et al.[183] and subsequently by Bahrami et al,[184] clearly showing that greater than 90% of TIO-associated mesenchymal tumors correspond morphologically to PMT. Although Weidner and Santa Cruz[182] originally described four types of PMT (mixed connective tissue type, osteoblastoma-like, ossifying fibroma-like, and nonossifying fibroma-like), these are now believed to represent minor morphologic variants in soft tissue and bone locations, rather than discrete entities.

Clinical Features

PMTs most often occur in middle-aged adults in soft tissue, bone, and sinonasal locations.[183,184] Extremely rare examples have been reported in infants.[185] Most PMT/mixed connective tissue present as small, inapparent lesions that may require very careful clinical examination and radionuclide scans (e.g., octreotide scans, fluorodeoxyglucose positron emission tomography) for localization in some cases. A long history of osteomalacia is usually present but is not required for diagnosis (Fig. 32-84). The great majority of putative nonphosphaturic PMT represent superficial soft tissue tumors identified prior to becoming symptomatic, although instances have also been seen in which patients were diagnosed with osteomalacia following identification of their tumor.[184] The overwhelming majority of PMT are histologically and clinically benign, with complete excision resulting in the resolution of phosphate wasting and osteomalacia.

TIO, in most instances, is the result of excess production of FGF-23, a phosphaturic hormone that acts to inhibit renal proximal tubule phosphate reuptake.[186-190] Elevated serum FGF-23 can be demonstrated in patients with PMT-associated TIO, and FGF-23 expression can be demonstrated by RT-PCR in routinely processed tissues, both in PMT presenting with TIO and those without this history.[184] However, low-level expression of FGF-23 can also be identified in occasional cases of fibrous dysplasia,[191] aneurysmal bone cyst, and chondromyxoid fibroma of bone,[192] presumably reflecting normal low-level expression of this gene in bone. Therefore, there is only a limited role for FGF-23 RT-PCR in the diagnosis of PMT. It is hoped that quantitative RT-PCR assays may be more valuable in this respect. Rare PMTs with known TIO are FGF-23 negative, presumably reflecting production of other phosphaturic hormones, such as frizzled-4 and MEPE.[193]

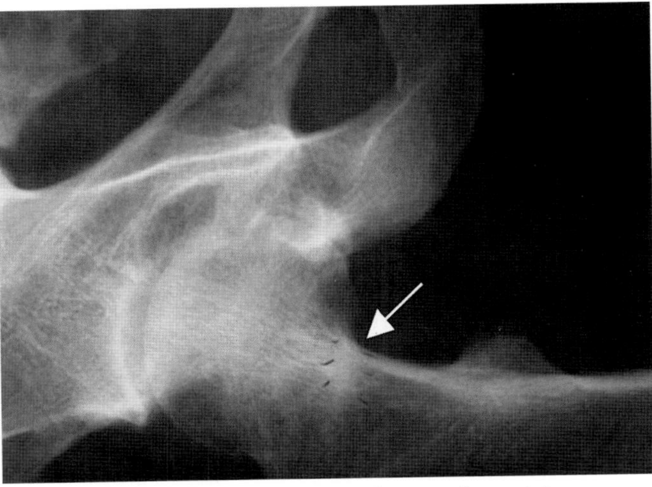

FIGURE 32-84. Femoral neck stress fracture (arrow) in a young adult male with long-standing tumor-induced osteomalacia, secondary to an occult phosphaturic mesenchymal tumor *(Courtesy of Dr. Jack Lawson, Yale-New Haven Hospital, New Haven, CT.)*

Histologically, benign PMTs behave in a clinically benign fashion, although they frequently recur locally if incompletely excised. Histologically, malignant PMTs have significant potential for aggressive local recurrence, distant metastasis, and adverse patient outcome.[183]

Pathologic Findings

Most PMTs present as nonspecific soft tissue or bone masses, often with a component of fat. Some tumors may be highly calcified. Microscopically, PMTs are characterized by a hypocellular to moderately cellular proliferation of bland, spindled to stellate cells, which produce an unusual smudgy basophilic matrix (Fig. 32-85). The tumor vasculature is usually very well-developed and may be hemangiopericytoma-like, capillary sized, or rarely consist of dilated thick-walled vessels. The tumor matrix calcifies in a distinctive grungy or flocculent fashion to form flower-like crystals and areas resembling primitive cartilage or osteoid.[182-184] In turn, this calcified matrix serves as a stimulus for the recruitment of osteoclasts and bland fibrohistiocytic spindled cells, producing areas resembling giant cell tumor of bone or fibrous histiocytoma. Rarely, these lesions may undergo aneurysmal bone cyst-like changes, including formation of woven bone within the center and at the periphery of the tumor. A variable component of mature adipose tissue is also frequently present, particularly in the sinuses. For unknown reasons, craniofacial sinus PMTs less often contain calcified matrix,[183] although typical PMT may occur in these locations.[194] Dermal PMT may grow in an infiltrative fashion, reminiscent of dermatofibrosarcoma protuberans (Fig. 32-86). A small number of histologically malignant PMTs have been reported; these cases show frankly sarcomatous features, including high nuclear grade, high cellularity, necrosis and elevated mitotic activity, resembling undifferentiated pleomorphic sarcoma (Fig. 32-87).[183] A preexisting component of benign-appearing PMT can typically be identified in these cases, either in the primary tumor or in an earlier presentation.

Immunohistochemical and Ultrastructural Features

PMT typically expresses vimentin only.[183] Rare cases have shown limited expression of CD34, smooth muscle actin, PGP9.5, S-100 protein, synaptophysin, and dentin matrix protein-1.[195-198] These findings are nonspecific and do not point toward any particular cell lineage. The blood vessels within PMT have a lymphatic phenotype with expression of lymphatic endothelium-associated markers such as LYVE-1.[199] Expression of FGF-23 protein has been documented in some cases, although commercially available antibodies to

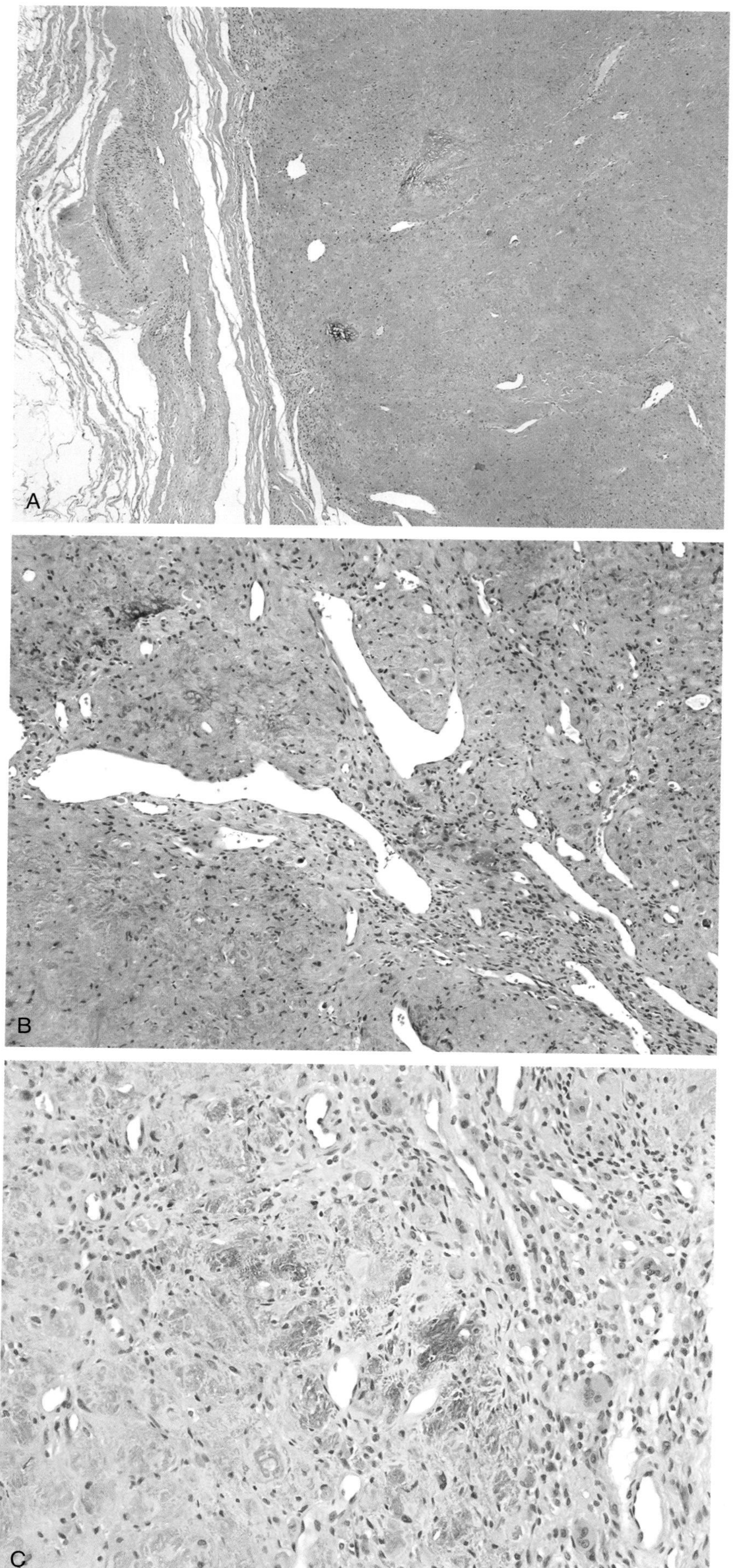

FIGURE 32-85. Phosphaturic mesenchymal tumor, presenting as a generally well-circumscribed, hypocellular soft tissue mass with abundant basophilic matrix (A). A hemangiopericytoma-like vascular pattern is often present (B). Amorphous calcifying matrix in PMT (C).

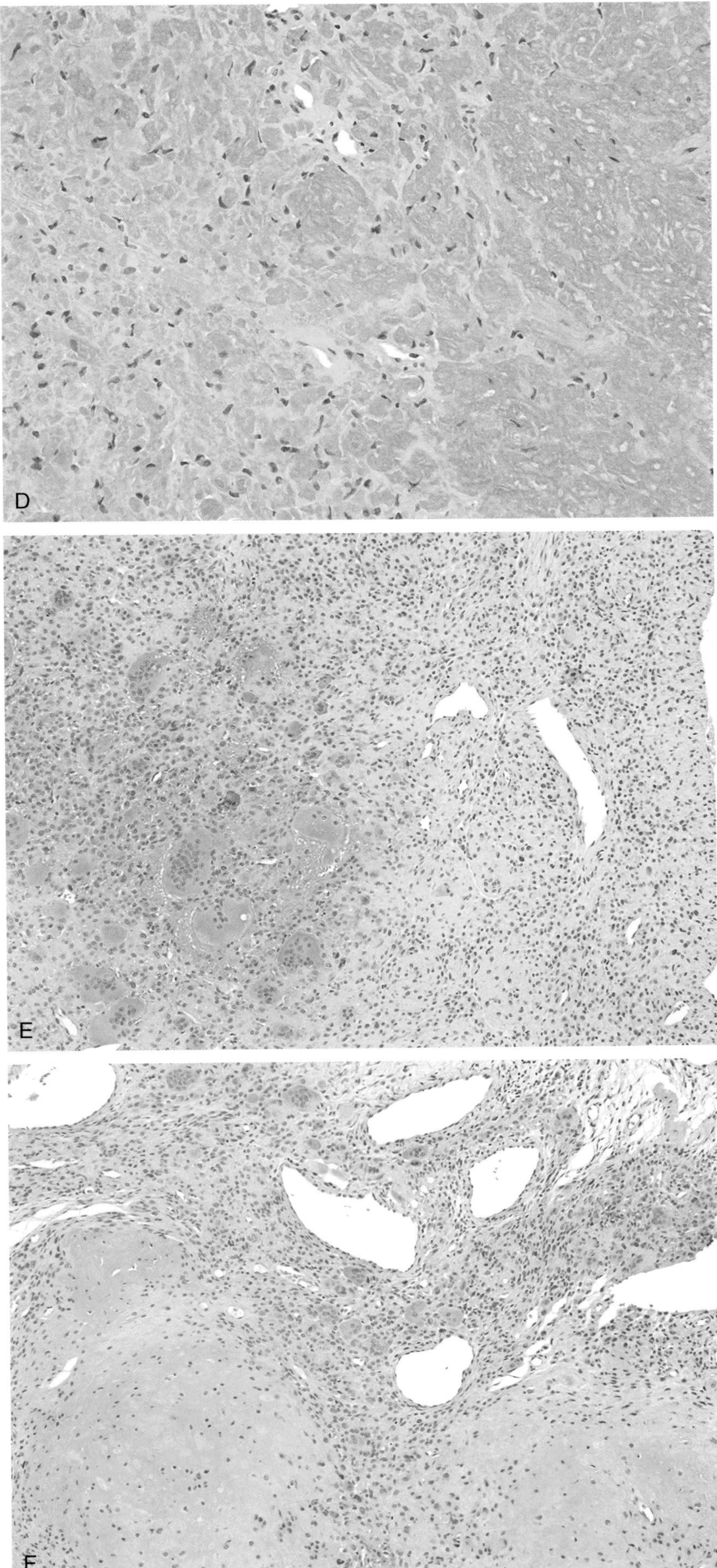

FIGURE 32-85, cont'd. Very bland spindled cells and abundant calcifying matrix in PMT (D). The calcified matrix of PMT serves to recruit osteoclast-like giant cells, which may be many in number, mimicking various giant cell rich tumors (E). At times, the matrix in PMT may resemble osteoid or chondroid (F).

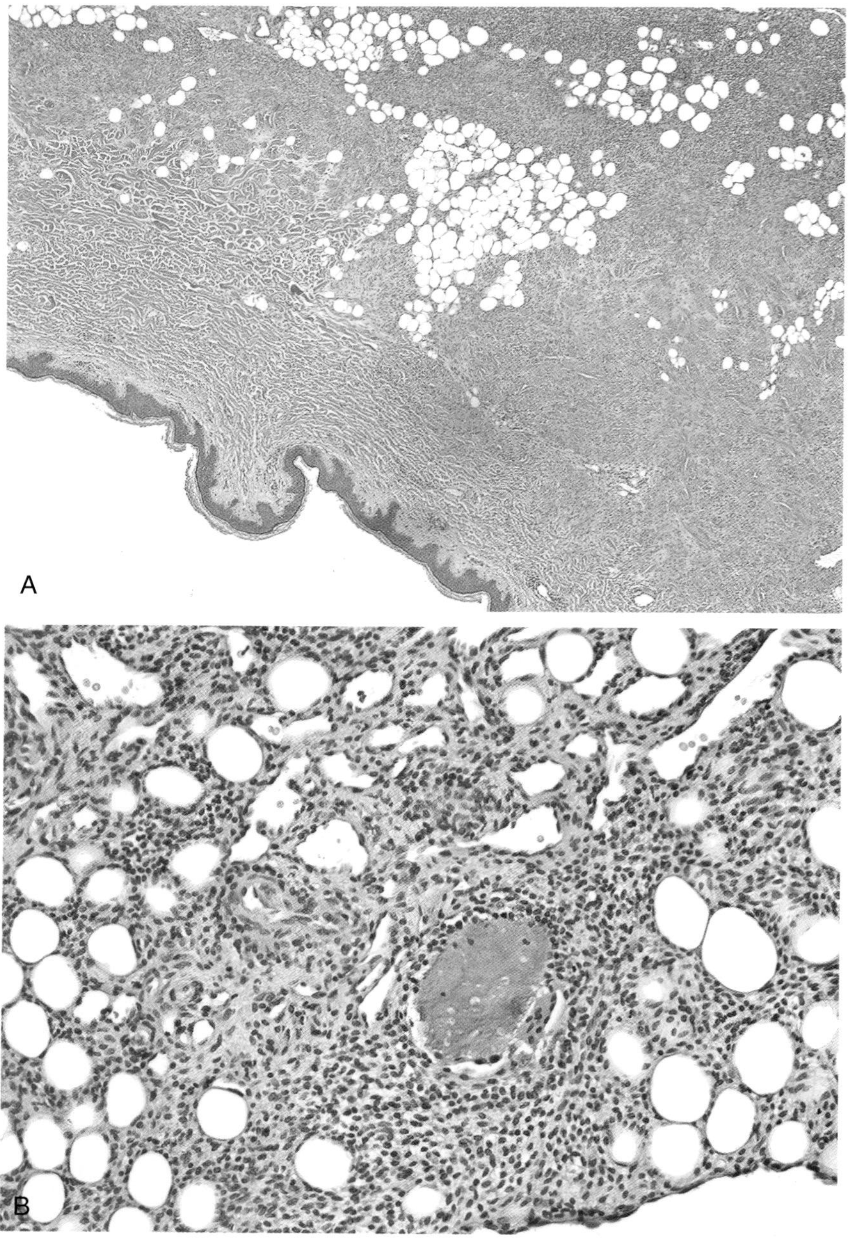

FIGURE 32-86. Dermal phosphaturic mesenchymal tumor, growing in an infiltrative, dermatofibrosarcoma-like pattern into the subcutaneous fat (A). Bland spindled cells, numerous small vessels, and a focus of calcified matrix in a dermal PMT (B).

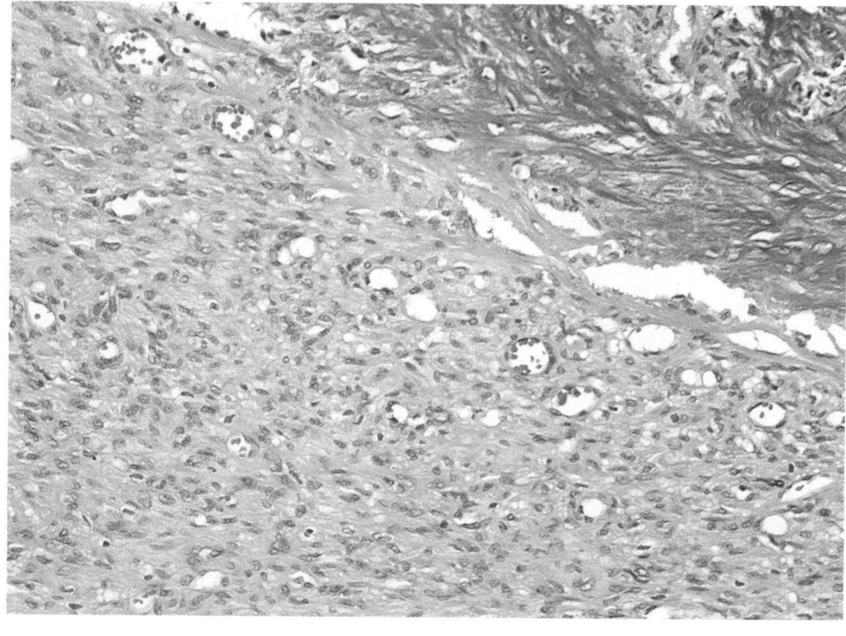

FIGURE 32-87. Malignant phosphaturic mesenchymal tumor, with areas resembling undifferentiated pleomorphic sarcoma.

FGF-23 have questionable specificity and are not widely available.[183]

Very few cases of PMT have been studied ultrastructurally.[182,196] The neoplastic cells are oval to polygonal with indented nuclei, a moderate number of cytoplasmic organelles, variable amounts of intermediate filaments, and interdigitating cell processes or filopodia. The intercellular matrix contains collagen fibers and matrix granules, sometimes forming crystals.

Genetic Findings

To date, a specific genetic event has not been identified in PMT. Only two cases of PMT have been karyotyped, showing 46,Y,t(X;3;14)(q13;p25;q21)[15]/46XY[5] and 46,XY,add(2)(q31),add(4)(q31.1) [2]/ 92,slx2 [3]/ 46,sl,der(2)t(2;4)(q14.2;p14), der(4)t(2;4)(q14.2;p14),add(4)(q31.1)[10]/46,sdl,add(13)(q34)[4]/92,sdl2x2[1].[200]

Differential Diagnosis

In most cases, PMT will have been resected expressly for treatment of known TIO, and the diagnosis is straightforward. Unsuspected PMT may be confused with SFT, hemangiomas, giant cell tumors, spindle cell lipomas, and various cartilaginous tumors, among others. Recognition of the unique constellation of histologic features shown by PMT, in particular the distinctive calcified matrix, is the key to distinguishing it from other tumors. Typical SFT shows a uniformly distributed, thick-walled branching vasculature, expresses CD34, and lacks calcified matrix. Chondromas of soft parts may show a pattern of calcification that mimics PMT and often contain osteoclast-like giant cells but lack the bland spindle cells, myxoid change, and fat of PMT. Giant cell tumors of bone and soft tissue lack the distinctive spindle cells and matrix of PMT. Mesenchymal chondrosarcoma is clearly a malignant-appearing lesion showing an admixture of round cells, hemangiopericytoma-like spindled areas, and relatively mature cartilage. The distinction of malignant PMT from matrix-producing sarcomas, such as osteosarcoma and chondrosarcoma, requires identification of areas of more typical PMT.

References

1. Enzinger FM, Weiss SW, Liang CY. Ossifying fibromyxoid tumor of soft parts. A clinicopathological analysis of 59 cases. Am J Surg Pathol 1989;13(10):817–27.
2. Folpe AL, Weiss SW. Ossifying fibromyxoid tumor of soft parts: a clinicopathologic study of 70 cases with emphasis on atypical and malignant variants. Am J Surg Pathol [Review] 2003;(4):421–31.
3. Graham RP, Dry S, Li X, et al. Ossifying fibromyxoid tumor of soft parts: a clinicopathologic, proteomic, and genomic study. Am J Surg Pathol 2011;35(11):1615–25.
4. Kilpatrick SE, Ward WG, Mozes M, et al. Atypical and malignant variants of ossifying fibromyxoid tumor. Clinicopathologic analysis of six cases. Am J Surg Pathol [Case Reports] 1995;19(9):1039–46.
5. Yoshida H, Minamizaki T, Yumoto T, et al. Ossifying fibromyxoid tumor of soft parts. Acta Pathol Jpn [Case Reports] 1991;41(6):480–6.
6. Zamecnik M, Michal M, Simpson RH, et al. Ossifying fibromyxoid tumor of soft parts: a report of 17 cases with emphasis on unusual histological features. Ann Diagn Pathol 1997;1(2):73–81.
7. Williams SB, Ellis GL, Meis JM, et al. Ossifying fibromyxoid tumour (of soft parts) of the head and neck: a clinicopathological and immunohistochemical study of nine cases. J Laryngol Otol 1993;107(1):75–80.
8. Miettinen M, Finnell V, Fetsch JF. Ossifying fibromyxoid tumor of soft parts–a clinicopathologic and immunohistochemical study of 104 cases with long-term follow-up and a critical review of the literature. Am J Surg Pathol 2008;32(7):996–1005.
9. Gebre-Medhin S, Nord KH, Moller E, et al. Recurrent rearrangement of the PHF1 gene in ossifying fibromyxoid tumors. Am J Pathol 2012; 181(3):1069–77.
10. Aminudin CA, Sharaf I, Hamzaini AH, et al. Ossifying fibromyxoid tumour in a child. Med J Malaysia [Case Reports] 2004;59(Suppl F): 49–51.
11. Al-Mazrou KA, Mansoor A, Payne M, et al. Ossifying fibromyxoid tumor of the ethmoid sinus in a newborn: report of a case and literature review. Int J Pediatr Otorhinolaryngol [Case Reports Review] 2004; 68(2):225–30.
12. Williams RW, Case CP, Irvine GH. Ossifying fibromyxoid tumour of soft parts–a new tumour of the parotid/zygomatic arch region. Br J Oral Maxillofac Surg 1994;32(3):174–7.
13. Ijiri R, Tanaka Y, Misugi K, et al. Ossifying fibromyxoid tumor of soft parts in a child: a case report. J Pediatr Surg 1999;34(8): 1294–6.
14. Ekfors TO, Kulju T, Aaltonen M, et al. Ossifying fibromyxoid tumour of soft parts: report of four cases including one mediastinal and one infantile. APMIS 1998;106(12):1124–30.
15. Nakayama F, Kuwahara T. Ossifying fibromyxoid tumor of soft parts of the back. J Cutan Pathol 1996;23(4):385–8.
16. Thompson J, Castillo M, Reddick RL, et al. Nasopharyngeal nonossifying variant of ossifying fibromyxoid tumor: CT and MR findings. AJNR Am J Neuroradiol 1995;16(5):1132–4.
17. Schaffler G, Raith J, Ranner G, et al. Radiographic appearance of an ossifying fibromyxoid tumor of soft parts. Skeletal Radiol [Case Reports] 1997;26(10):615–18.
18. Miettinen M. Ossifying fibromyxoid tumor of soft parts. Additional observations of a distinctive soft tissue tumor. Am J Clin Pathol [Case Reports Research Support, Non-U.S. Gov't] 1991;95(2): 142–9.
19. Schofield JB, Krausz T, Stamp GW, et al. Ossifying fibromyxoid tumour of soft parts: immunohistochemical and ultrastructural analysis. Histopathology 1993;22(2):101–12.
20. Donner LR. Ossifying fibromyxoid tumor of soft parts: evidence supporting Schwann cell origin. Hum Pathol [Case Reports] 1992;23(2): 200–2.
21. Min KW, Seo IS, Pitha J. Ossifying fibromyxoid tumor: modified myoepithelial cell tumor? Report of three cases with immunohistochemical and electron microscopic studies. Ultrastruct Pathol [Case Reports] 2005;29(6):535–48.
22. Nishio J, Iwasaki H, Ohjimi Y, et al. Ossifying fibromyxoid tumor of soft parts. Cytogenetic findings. Cancer genetics and cytogenetics [Case Reports] 2002;133(2):124–8.
23. Sovani V, Velagaleti GV, Filipowicz E, et al. Ossifying fibromyxoid tumor of soft parts: report of a case with novel cytogenetic findings. Cancer Genet Cytogenet 2001;127(1):1–6.
24. Kawashima H, Ogose A, Umezu H, et al. Ossifying fibromyxoid tumor of soft parts with clonal chromosomal aberrations. Cancer Genet Cytogenet 2007;176(2):156–60.
25. Chiang S, Ali R, Melnyk N, et al. Frequency of known gene rearrangements in endometrial stromal tumors. Am J Surg Pathol 2011;35(9): 1364–72.
26. Micci F, Panagopoulos I, Bjerkehagen B, et al. Consistent rearrangement of chromosomal band 6p21 with generation of fusion genes JAZF1/PHF1 and EPC1/PHF1 in endometrial stromal sarcoma. Cancer Res 2006;66(1):107–12.
27. Fisher C, Hedges M, Weiss SW. Ossifying fibromyxoid tumor of soft parts with stromal cyst formation and ribosome-lamella complexes. Ultrastruct Pathol [Case Reports] 1994;18(6):593–600.
28. Montgomery EA, Devaney KO, Giordano TJ, et al. Inflammatory myxohyaline tumor of distal extremities with virocyte or Reed-Sternberg-like cells: a distinctive lesion with features simulating inflammatory conditions, Hodgkin's disease, and various sarcomas. Mod Pathol 1998;11(4): 384–91.
29. Meis-Kindblom JM, Kindblom LG. Acral myxoinflammatory fibroblastic sarcoma: a low-grade tumor of the hands and feet. Am J Surg Pathol 1998;22(8):911–24.
30. Michal M. Inflammatory myxoid tumor of the soft parts with bizarre giant cells. Pathol Res Pract 1998;194(8):529–33.
31. Fletcher CD, Unni KK, Mertens F. Pathology and genetics of tumors of soft tissue and bone. Lyon, France: IARC Press; 2002.

32. Jurcic V, Zidar A, Montiel MD, et al. Myxoinflammatory fibroblastic sarcoma: a tumor not restricted to acral sites. Ann Diagn Pathol 2002;6(5):272–80.
33. McFarlane R, Meyers AD, Golitz L. Myxoinflammatory fibroblastic sarcoma of the neck. J Cutan Pathol [Case Reports] 2005;32(5):375–8.
34. Tateishi U, Hasegawa T, Onaya H, et al. Myxoinflammatory fibroblastic sarcoma: MR appearance and pathologic correlation. AJR Am J Roentgenol [Research Support, Non-U.S. Gov't] 2005;184(6):1749–53.
35. Alkuwari E, Gravel DH. A 30-year-old man with a soft tissue mass on the right elbow. Inflammatory myxohyaline tumor of the distal extremities with prominent eosinophilic infiltrate. Arch Pathol Lab Med [Case Reports] 2006;130(3):e35–6.
36. Kinkor Z, Mukensnabl P, Michal M. Inflammatory myxohyaline tumor with massive emperipolesis. Pathol Res Pract [Case Reports] 2002; 198(9):639–42.
37. Antonescu CR, Zhang L, Nielsen GP, et al. Consistent t(1;10) with rearrangements of TGFBR3 and MGEA5 in both myxoinflammatory fibroblastic sarcoma and hemosiderotic fibrolipomatous tumor. Genes Chromosomes Cancer 2011;50(10):757–64.
38. Elco CP, Marino-Enriquez A, Abraham JA, et al. Hybrid myxoinflammatory fibroblastic sarcoma/hemosiderotic fibrolipomatous tumor: report of a case providing further evidence for a pathogenetic link. Am J Surg Pathol 2010;34(11):1723–7.
39. Lambert I, Debiec-Rychter M, Guelinckx P, et al. Acral myxoinflammatory fibroblastic sarcoma with unique clonal chromosomal changes. Virchows Arch [Case Reports] 2001;438(5):509–12.
40. Hallor KH, Sciot R, Staaf J, et al. Two genetic pathways, t(1;10) and amplification of 3p11-12, in myxoinflammatory fibroblastic sarcoma, haemosiderotic fibrolipomatous tumour, and morphologically similar lesions. J Pathol 2009;217(5):716–27.
41. Wettach GR, Boyd LJ, Lawce HJ, et al. Cytogenetic analysis of a hemosiderotic fibrolipomatous tumor. Cancer Genet Cytogenet 2008;182(2): 140–3.
42. Sakaki M, Hirokawa M, Wakatsuki S, et al. Acral myxoinflammatory fibroblastic sarcoma: a report of five cases and review of the literature. Virchows Arch 2003;442(1):25–30.
43. Smith ME, Fisher C, Weiss SW. Pleomorphic hyalinizing angiectatic tumor of soft parts. A low-grade neoplasm resembling neurilemoma. Am J Surg Pathol 1996;20(1):21–9.
44. Folpe AL, Weiss SW. Pleomorphic hyalinizing angiectatic tumor: analysis of 41 cases supporting evolution from a distinctive precursor lesion. Am J Surg Pathol 2004;28(11):1417–25.
45. Fukunaga M, Ushigome S. Pleomorphic hyalinizing angiectatic tumor of soft parts. Pathol Int 1997;47(11):784–8.
46. Gallo C, Murer B, Roncaroli F. [Pleomorphic hyalinizing angiectasic soft-tissue tumor. Description of a case]. Pathologica 1997;89(5): 531–5.
47. Capovilla M, Birembaut P, Cucherousset J, et al. Pleomorphic hyalinizing angiectatic tumor of soft parts: ultrastructural analysis of a case with original features. Ultrastruct Pathol [Case Reports] 2006;30(1):59–64.
48. Groisman GM, Bejar J, Amar M, et al. Pleomorphic hyalinizing angiectatic tumor of soft parts: immunohistochemical study including the expression of vascular endothelial growth factor. Arch Pathol Lab Med 2000;124(3):423–6.
49. Husek K, Vesely K. Pleomorphic hyalinizing angiectatic tumor. Cesk Patol 2001;37(4):177–81.
50. Fujiwara M, Yuba Y, Wada A, et al. Pleomorphic hyalinizing angiectatic tumor of soft parts: report of a case and review of the literature. J Dermatol [Case Reports Review] 2004;31(5):419–23.
51. Lee JC, Jiang XY, Karpinski RH, et al. Pleomorphic hyalinizing angiectatic tumor of soft parts. Surgery [Case Reports] 2005;137(1):119–21.
52. Wei S, Pan Z, Siegal GP, et al. Complex analysis of a recurrent pleomorphic hyalinizing angiectatic tumor of soft parts. Hum Pathol 2012; 43(1):121–6.
53. Capovilla M, Birembaut P. Primary cutaneous myxofibrosarcoma mimicking pleomorphic hyalinizing angiectatic tumor (PHAT): a potential diagnostic pitfall. Am J Dermatopathol 2006;28(3):276–7; author reply 7–8.
54. Mitsuhashi T, Barr RJ, Machtinger LA, et al. Primary cutaneous myxofibrosarcoma mimicking pleomorphic hyalinizing angiectatic tumor (PHAT): a potential diagnostic pitfall. Am J Dermatopathol 2005; 27(4):322–6.
55. Illueca C, Machado I, Cruz J, et al. Pleomorphic hyalinizing angiectatic tumor: a report of 3 new cases, 1 with sarcomatous myxofibrosarcoma component and another with unreported soft tissue palpebral location. Appl Immunohistochem Mol Morphol 2012;20(1):96–101.
56. Kazakov DV, Pavlovsky M, Mukensnabl P, et al. Pleomorphic hyalinizing angiectatic tumor with a sarcomatous component recurring as high-grade myxofibrosarcoma. Pathol Int 2007;57(5):281–4.
57. Marshall-Taylor C, Fanburg-Smith JC. Hemosiderotic fibrohistiocytic lipomatous lesion: ten cases of a previously undescribed fatty lesion of the foot/ankle. Mod Pathol 2000;13(11):1192–9.
58. Flucke U, Mentzel T, Verdijk MA, et al. EWSR1-ATF1 chimeric transcript in a myoepithelial tumor of soft tissue: a case report. Hum Pathol 2012;43(5):764–8.
59. Flucke U, Palmedo G, Blankenhorn N, et al. EWSR1 gene rearrangement occurs in a subset of cutaneous myoepithelial tumors: a study of 18 cases. Mod Pathol 2011;24(11):1444–50.
60. Flucke U, Tops BB, Verdijk MA, et al. NR4A3 rearrangement reliably distinguishes between the clinicopathologically overlapping entities myoepithelial carcinoma of soft tissue and cellular extraskeletal myxoid chondrosarcoma. Virchows Arch 2012;460(6):621–8.
61. Antonescu CR, Zhang L, Chang NE, et al. EWSR1-POU5F1 fusion in soft tissue myoepithelial tumors. A molecular analysis of sixty-six cases, including soft tissue, bone, and visceral lesions, showing common involvement of the EWSR1 gene. Genes Chromosomes Cancer 2010; 49(12):1114–24.
62. Laskowski J. Zarys onkologii. Pathology of tumors. Warsaw: PZWL; 1995. p. 91.
63. Dabska M. Parachordoma: a new clinicopathologic entity. Cancer 1977;40(4):1586–92.
64. Folpe AL, Agoff SN, Willis J, et al. Parachordoma is immunohistochemically and cytogenetically distinct from axial chordoma and extraskeletal myxoid chondrosarcoma. Am J Surg Pathol 1999;23(9):1059–67.
65. Gimferrer JM, Baldo X, Montero CA, et al. Chest wall parachordoma. Eur J Cardiothorac Surg [Case Reports] 1999;16(5):573–5.
66. Hemalatha AL, Srinivasa MR, Parshwanath HA. Parachordoma of tibia–a case report. Indian J Pathol Microbiol [Case Reports] 2003;46(3):454–5.
67. Hirokawa M, Manabe T, Sugihara K. Parachordoma of the buttock: an immunohistochemical case study and review. Jpn J Clin Oncol [Case Reports Review] 1994;24(6):336–9.
68. Karabela-Bouropoulou V, Skourtas C, Liapi-Avgeri G, et al. Parachordoma. A case report of a very rare soft tissue tumor. Pathol Res Pract [Case Reports] 1996;192(9):972–8; discussion 9–81.
69. Ishida T, Oda H, Oka T, et al. Parachordoma: an ultrastructural and immunohistochemical study. Virchows Arch A Pathol Anat Histopathol [Case Reports Research Support, Non-U.S. Gov't] 1993;422(3):239–45.
70. Imlay SP, Argenyi ZB, Stone MS, et al. Cutaneous parachordoma. A light microscopic and immunohistochemical report of two cases and review of the literature. J Cutan Pathol [Case Reports Review] 1998;25(5): 279–84.
71. Koh JS, Chung JH, Lee SY, et al. Parachordoma of the tibia: report of a rare case. Pathol Res Pract [Case Reports] 2000;196(4):269–73.
72. Sangueza OP, White CR Jr. Parachordoma. Am J Dermatopathol [Case Reports] 1994;16(2):185–8.
73. Kilpatrick SE, Hitchcock MG, Kraus MD, et al. Mixed tumors and myoepitheliomas of soft tissue: a clinicopathologic study of 19 cases with a unifying concept [see comments]. Am J Surg Pathol 1997;21(1): 13–22.
74. Hornick JL, Fletcher CD. Myoepithelial tumors of soft tissue: a clinicopathologic and immunohistochemical study of 101 cases with evaluation of prognostic parameters. Am J Surg Pathol 2003;27(9):1183–96.
75. Gleason BC, Fletcher CD. Myoepithelial carcinoma of soft tissue in children: an aggressive neoplasm analyzed in a series of 29 cases. Am J Surg Pathol 2007;31(12):1813–24.
76. Michal M, Miettinen M. Myoepitheliomas of the skin and soft tissues. Report of 12 cases. Virchows Arch 1999;434(5):393–400.
77. Kutzner H, Mentzel T, Kaddu S, et al. Cutaneous myoepithelioma: an under-recognized cutaneous neoplasm composed of myoepithelial cells. Am J Surg Pathol 2001;25(3):348–55.
78. Hornick JL, Fletcher CD. Cutaneous myoepithelioma: a clinicopathologic and immunohistochemical study of 14 cases. Hum Pathol 2004; 35(1):14–24.
79. Mentzel T. [Myoepithelial neoplasms of skin and soft tissues]. Pathologe [Review] 2005;26(5):322–30.
80. Scolyer RA, Bonar SF, Palmer AA, et al. Parachordoma is not distinguishable from axial chordoma using immunohistochemistry. Pathol Int [Case Reports Comparative Study] 2004;54(5):364–70.
81. Fisher C, Miettinen M. Parachordoma: a clinicopathologic and immunohistochemical study of four cases of an unusual soft tissue neoplasm. Ann Diagn Pathol 1997;1(1):3–10.

82. Niezabitowski A, Limon J, Wasilewska A, et al. Parachordoma–a clinicopathologic, immunohistochemical, electron microscopic, flow cytometric, and cytogenetic study. Gen Diagn Pathol 1995;141(1):49–55.
83. Fisher C. Parachordoma exists–but what is it? Adv Anat Pathol 2000;7(3):141–8.
84. Carstens PH. Chordoid tumor: a light, electron microscopic, and immunohistochemical study. Ultrastruct Pathol [Case Reports Review] 1995; 19(4):291–5.
85. Shin HJ, Mackay B, Ichinose H, et al. Parachordoma. Ultrastruct Pathol [Case Reports] 1994;18(1-2):249–56.
86. Povysil C, Matejovsky Z. A comparative ultrastructural study of chondrosarcoma, chordoid sarcoma, chordoma and chordoma periphericum. Pathol Res Pract [Comparative Study] 1985;179(4-5):546–59.
87. Kuhnen C, Herter P, Kasprzynski A, et al. [Myoepithelioma of soft tissue—case report with clinicopathologic, ultrastructural, and cytogenetic findings]. Pathologe [Case Reports] 2005;26(5):331–7.
88. Colombat M, Lesourd A, Moughabghab M, et al. [Soft tissue myoepithelioma, a rare tumor. A case report]. Ann Pathol [Case Reports] 2003;23(1):55–8.
89. Bisceglia M, Cardone M, Fantasia L, et al. Mixed tumors, myoepitheliomas, and oncocytomas of the soft tissues are likely members of the same family: a clinicopathologic and ultrastructural study. Ultrastruct Pathol [Case Reports] 2001;25(5):399–418.
90. Brandal P, Panagopoulos I, Bjerkehagen B, et al. Detection of a t(1;22)(q23;q12) translocation leading to an EWSR1-PBX1 fusion gene in a myoepithelioma. Genes Chromosomes Cancer 2008;47(7):558–64.
91. Brandal P, Panagopoulos I, Bjerkehagen B, et al. t(19;22)(q13;q12) Translocation leading to the novel fusion gene EWSR1-ZNF444 in soft tissue myoepithelial carcinoma. Genes Chromosomes Cancer 2009; 48(12):1051–6.
92. Bahrami A, Dalton JD, Krane JF, et al. A subset of cutaneous and soft tissue mixed tumors are genetically linked to their salivary gland counterpart. Genes Chromosomes Cancer 2012;51(2):140–8.
93. Tihy F, Scott P, Russo P, et al. Cytogenetic analysis of a parachordoma. Cancer Genet Cytogenet [Case Reports] 1998;105(1):14–19.
94. Tong G, Perle MA, Desai P, et al. Parachordoma or chordoma periphericum? Case report of a tumor of the thoracic wall. Diagn Cytopathol [Case Reports] 2003;29(1):18–23.
95. Pauwels P, Dal Cin P, Roumen R, et al. Intramuscular mixed tumour with clonal chromosomal changes. Virchows Arch [Case Reports] 1999;434(2):167–71.
96. Tirabosco R, Mangham DC, Rosenberg AE, et al. Brachyury expression in extra-axial skeletal and soft tissue chordomas: a marker that distinguishes chordoma from mixed tumor/myoepithelioma/parachordoma in soft tissue. Am J Surg Pathol 2008;32(4):572–80.
97. Hollmann TJ, Hornick JL. INI1-deficient tumors: diagnostic features and molecular genetics. Am J Surg Pathol 2011;35(10):e47–63.
98. Kilpatrick SE, Hitchcock MG, Kraus MD, et al. Mixed tumors and myoepitheliomas of soft tissue: a clinicopathologic study of 19 cases with a unifying concept. Am J Surg Pathol 1997;21(1):13–22.
99. Miettinen M, Karaharju E, Jarvinen H. Chordoma with a massive spindle-cell sarcomatous transformation. A light- and electron-microscopic and immunohistological study. Am J Surg Pathol [Case Reports Research Support, Non-U.S. Gov't] 1987;11(7):563–70.
100. Abe S, Imamura T, Harasawa A, et al. Parachordoma with multiple metastases. J Comput Assist Tomogr [Case Reports] 2003;27(4):634–8.
101. Stout AP. Hemangiopericytoma; a study of 25 cases. Cancer 1949;2(6): 1027–54, illust.
102. Stout AP, Murray MR. Hemangiopericytoma: a vascular tumor featuring Zimmermann's pericytes. Ann Surg 1942;116(1):26–33.
103. Stout AP. Tumors featuring pericytes; glomus tumor and hemangiopericytoma. Lab Invest 1956;5(2):217–23.
104. Enzinger FM, Smith BH. Hemangiopericytoma. An analysis of 106 cases. Hum Pathol 1976;7(1):61–82.
105. Battifora H. Hemangiopericytoma: ultrastructural study of five cases. Cancer 1973;31(6):1418–32.
106. Erlandson RA, Woodruff JM. Role of electron microscopy in the evaluation of soft tissue neoplasms, with emphasis on spindle cell and pleomorphic tumors. Hum Pathol [Review] 1998;29(12):1372–81.
107. Dardick I, Hammar SP, Scheithauer BW. Ultrastructural spectrum of hemangiopericytoma: a comparative study of fetal, adult, and neoplastic pericytes. Ultrastruct Pathol [Comparative Study Research Support, Non-U.S. Gov't] 1989;13(2-3):111–54.
108. Gengler C, Guillou L. Solitary fibrous tumour and haemangiopericytoma: evolution of a concept. Histopathology [Review] 2006;48(1): 63–74.
109. Schurch W, Skalli O, Lagace R, et al. Intermediate filament proteins and actin isoforms as markers for soft-tissue tumor differentiation and origin. III. Hemangiopericytomas and glomus tumors. Am J Pathol 1990;136(4):771–86.
110. Nemes Z. Differentiation markers in hemangiopericytoma. Cancer 1992;69(1):133–40.
111. Middleton LP, Duray PH, Merino MJ. The histological spectrum of hemangiopericytoma: application of immunohistochemical analysis including proliferative markers to facilitate diagnosis and predict prognosis. Hum Pathol 1998;29(6):636–40.
112. D'Amore ES, Manivel JC, Sung JH. Soft-tissue and meningeal hemangiopericytomas: an immunohistochemical and ultrastructural study. Hum Pathol 1990;21(4):414–23.
113. Fletcher CD. Haemangiopericytoma—a dying breed? Reappraisal of an 'entity' and its variants: a hypothesis. Curr Diagn Pathol 1994;1(1): 19–23.
114. Klemperer P, Rabin CB. Primary neoplasms of the pleura: a report of five cases. Arch Pathol 1931;11:385.
115. Guillou L, Fletcher JA, Fletcher CD, et al. Extrapleural solitary fibrous tumor and hemangiopericytoma. In: Fletcher CD, Unni KK, Mertens F, editors. World Health Organization classification of tumours: pathology and genetics of tumours of soft tissue and bone. Pathology ed. Lyon: IARC Press; 2002. p. 86–90.
116. McMaster MJ, Soule EH, Ivins JC. Hemangiopericytoma. A clinicopathologic study and long-term followup of 60 patients. Cancer 1975;36(6):2232–44.
117. Brunnemann RB, Ro JY, Ordonez NG, et al. Extrapleural solitary fibrous tumor: a clinicopathologic study of 24 cases. Mod Pathol 1999;12(11): 1034–42.
118. Fukunaga M, Naganuma H, Nikaido T, et al. Extrapleural solitary fibrous tumor: a report of seven cases. Mod Pathol 1997;10(5):443–50.
119. Hasegawa T, Matsuno Y, Shimoda T, et al. Extrathoracic solitary fibrous tumors: their histological variability and potentially aggressive behavior. Hum Pathol 1999;30(12):1464–73.
120. Young RH, Clement PB, McCaughey WT. Solitary fibrous tumors ("fibrous mesotheliomas") and potentially aggressive behavior. Hum Pathol 1999;114:493.
121. Yousem SA, Flynn SD. Intrapulmonary localized fibrous tumor. Intraparenchymal so-called localized fibrous mesothelioma. Am J Clin Pathol [Case Reports] 1988;89(3):365–9.
122. Fukasawa Y, Takada A, Tateno M, et al. Solitary fibrous tumor of the pleura causing recurrent hypoglycemia by secretion of insulin-like growth factor II. Pathol Int [Case Reports] 1998;48(1):47–52.
123. Masson EA, MacFarlane IA, Graham D, et al. Spontaneous hypoglycaemia due to a pleural fibroma: role of insulin like growth factors. Thorax [Case Reports] 1991;46(12):930–1.
124. Benn JJ, Firth RG, Sonksen PH. Metabolic effects of an insulin-like factor causing hypoglycaemia in a patient with a haemangiopericytoma. Clin Endocrinol (Oxf) [Case Reports] 1990;32(6):769–80.
125. Hoog A, Sandberg Nordqvist AC, Hulting AL, et al. High-molecular weight IGF-2 expression in a haemangiopericytoma associated with hypoglycaemia. APMIS [Case Reports Research Support, Non-U.S. Gov't Review] 1997;105(6):469–82.
126. Pavelic K, Spaventi S, Gluncic V, et al. The expression and role of insulin-like growth factor II in malignant hemangiopericytomas. J Mol Med (Berl) [Research Support, Non-U.S. Gov't] 1999;77(12):865–9.
127. de Saint Aubain Somerhausen N, Rubin BP, Fletcher CD. Myxoid solitary fibrous tumor: a study of seven cases with emphasis on differential diagnosis. Mod Pathol 1999;12(5):463–71.
128. Ceballos KM, Munk PL, Masri BA, et al. Lipomatous hemangiopericytoma: a morphologically distinct soft tissue tumor. Arch Pathol Lab Med 1999;123(10):941–5.
129. Folpe AL, Devaney K, Weiss SW. Lipomatous hemangiopericytoma: a rare variant of hemangiopericytoma that may be confused with liposarcoma. Am J Surg Pathol 1999;23(10):1201–7.
130. Guillou L, Gebhard S, Coindre JM. Lipomatous hemangiopericytoma: a fat-containing variant of solitary fibrous tumor? Clinicopathologic, immunohistochemical, and ultrastructural analysis of a series in favor of a unifying concept. Hum Pathol 2000;31(9):1108–15.
131. Vallat-Decouvelaere AV, Dry SM, Fletcher CD. Atypical and malignant solitary fibrous tumors in extrathoracic locations: evidence of their comparability to intra-thoracic tumors. Am J Surg Pathol 1998;22(12): 1501–11.
132. Suster S, Nascimento AG, Miettinen M, et al. Solitary fibrous tumors of soft tissue. A clinicopathologic and immunohistochemical study of 12 cases. Am J Surg Pathol 1995;19(11):1257–66.

133. van de Rijn M, Lombard CM, Rouse RV. Expression of CD34 by solitary fibrous tumors of the pleura, mediastinum, and lung. Am J Surg Pathol [Research Support, U.S. Gov't, Non-P.H.S.] 1994;18(8):814–20.
134. Chilosi M, Facchettti F, Dei Tos AP, et al. bcl-2 expression in pleural and extrapleural solitary fibrous tumours. J Pathol 1997;181(4): 362–7.
135. Hanau CA, Miettinen M. Solitary fibrous tumor: histological and immunohistochemical spectrum of benign and malignant variants presenting at different sites. Hum Pathol 1995;26(4):440–9.
136. Hasegawa T, Hirose T, Seki K, et al. Solitary fibrous tumor of the soft tissue. An immunohistochemical and ultrastructural study. Am J Clin Pathol [Case Reports] 1996;106(3):325–31.
137. Nunnery EW, Kahn LB, Reddick RL, et al. Hemangiopericytoma: a light microscopic and ultrastructural study. Cancer [Case Reports] 1981; 47(5):906–14.
138. Ide F, Obara K, Mishima K, et al. Ultrastructural spectrum of solitary fibrous tumor: a unique perivascular tumor with alternative lines of differentiation. Virchows Arch 2005;446(6):646–52.
139. Briselli M, Mark EJ, Dickersin GR. Solitary fibrous tumors of the pleura: eight new cases and review of 360 cases in the literature. Cancer 1981;47(11):2678–89.
140. Gherardi GJ, Arya S, Hickler RB. Juxtaglomerular body tumor: a rare occult but curable cause of lethal hypertension. Hum Pathol [Case Reports] 1974;5(2):236–40.
141. Robertson PW, Klidjian A, Harding LK, et al. Hypertension due to a renin-secreting renal tumour. Am J Med 1967;43(6):963–76.
142. Warshaw BL, Anand SK, Olson DL, et al. Hypertension secondary to a renin-producing juxtaglomerular cell tumor. J Pediatr 1979;94(2): 247–50.
143. Ohmori H, Motoi M, Sato H, et al. Extrarenal renin-secreting tumor associated with hypertension. Acta Pathol Jpn [Case Reports] 1977; 27(4):567–86.
144. Henn W, Wullich B, Thoennes M, et al. Recurrent t(12;19)(q13;q13.3) in intracranial and extracranial hemangiopericytoma. Cancer Genet Cytogenet 1993;71:3009.
145. Sreekantaiah C, Bridge JA, Rao UN, et al. Clonal chromosomal abnormalities in hemangiopericytoma. Cancer Genet Cytogenet [Research Support, Non-U.S. Gov't Research Support, U.S. Gov't, P.H.S.] 1991; 54(2):173–81.
146. Limon J, Rao U, Dal Cin P, et al. Translocation (13;22) in a hemangiopericytoma. Cancer Genet Cytogenet [Case Reports] 1986;21(4): 309–18.
147. Mandahl N, Orndal C, Heim S, et al. Aberrations of chromosome segment 12q13-15 characterize a subgroup of hemangiopericytomas. Cancer [Case Reports Research Support, Non-U.S. Gov't] 1993;71(10): 3009–13.
148. Cerda-Nicolas M, Lopez-Gines C, Gil-Benso R, et al. Solitary fibrous tumor of the orbit: morphological, cytogenetic and molecular features. Neuropathology 2006;26(6):557–63.
149. de Leval L, Defraigne JO, Hermans G, et al. Malignant solitary fibrous tumor of the pleura: report of a case with cytogenetic analysis. Virchows Arch 2003;442(4):388–92.
150. Debiec-Rychter M, de Wever I, Hagemeijer A, et al. Is 4q13 a recurring breakpoint in solitary fibrous tumors? Cancer Genet Cytogenet 2001;131(1):69–73.
151. Hoshino M, Ogose A, Kawashima H, et al. Malignant solitary fibrous tumor of the soft tissue: a cytogenetic study. Cancer Genet Cytogenet 2007;177(1):55–8.
152. Martin AJ, Summersgill BM, Fisher C, et al. Chromosomal imbalances in meningeal solitary fibrous tumors. Cancer Genet Cytogenet 2002;135(2):160–4.
153. Qian YW, Malliah R, Lee HJ, et al. A t(12;17) in an extraorbital giant cell angiofibroma. Cancer Genet Cytogenet 2006;165(2):157–60.
154. Rakheja D, Wilson KS, Meehan JJ, et al. Extrapleural benign solitary fibrous tumor in the shoulder of a 9-year-old girl: case report and review of the literature. Pediatr Dev Pathol 2004;7(6):653–60.
155. Swelam WM, Cheng J, Ida-Yonemochi H, et al. Oral solitary fibrous tumor: a cytogenetic analysis of tumor cells in culture with literature review. Cancer Genet Cytogenet 2009;194(2):75–81.
156. Torabi A, Lele SM, DiMaio D, et al. Lack of a common or characteristic cytogenetic anomaly in solitary fibrous tumor. Cancer Genet Cytogenet 2008;181(1):60–4.
157. Torres-Olivera FJ, Vargas MT, Torres-Gomez FJ, et al. Cytogenetic, fluorescence in situ hybridization, and immunohistochemistry studies in a malignant pleural solitary fibrous tumor. Cancer Genet Cytogenet 2009;189(2):122–6.
158. Yamazaki K, Eyden BP. Pulmonary lipomatous hemangiopericytoma: report of a rare tumor and comparison with solitary fibrous tumor. Ultrastruct Pathol 2007;31(1):51–61.
159. Dal Cin P, Sciot R, Fletcher CD, et al. Trisomy 21 in solitary fibrous tumor. Cancer Genet Cytogenet 1996;86(1):58–60.
159a. Mohajeri A, Tayebwa J, Collin A, et al. Comprehensive genetic analysis identifies a pathognomonic NAB2/STAT6 fusion gene, nonrandom secondary genomic imbalances, and a characteristic gene expression profile in solitary fibrous tumor. Genes Chromosomes Cancer 2013; doi: 10.1002/gcc.22083 [Epub ahead of print].
160. Gold JS, Antonescu CR, Hajdu C, et al. Clinicopathologic correlates of solitary fibrous tumors. Cancer 2002;94(4):1057–68.
161. Nielsen GP, O'Connell JX, Dickersin GR, et al. Solitary fibrous tumor of soft tissue: a report of 15 cases, including 5 malignant examples with light microscopic, immunohistochemical, and ultrastructural data. Mod Pathol 1997;10(10):1028–37.
162. Collini P, Negri T, Barisella M, et al. High-grade sarcomatous overgrowth in solitary fibrous tumors: a clinicopathologic study of 10 cases. Am J Surg Pathol 2012;36(8):1202–15.
163. Mosquera JM, Fletcher CD. Expanding the spectrum of malignant progression in solitary fibrous tumors: a study of 8 cases with a discrete anaplastic component–is this dedifferentiated SFT? Am J Surg Pathol 2009;33(9):1314–21.
164. England DM, Hochholzer L, McCarthy MJ. Localized benign and malignant fibrous tumors of the pleura. A clinicopathologic review of 223 cases. Am J Surg Pathol 1989;13(8):640–58.
165. Espat NJ, Lewis JJ, Leung D, et al. Conventional hemangiopericytoma: modern analysis of outcome. Cancer 2002;95(8):1746–51.
166. Demicco EG, Park MS, Araujo DM, et al. Solitary fibrous tumor: a clinicopathological study of 110 cases and proposed risk assessment model. Mod Pathol 2012;25(9):1298–306.
167. Carneiro SS, Scheithauer BW, Nascimento AG, et al. Solitary fibrous tumor of the meninges: a lesion distinct from fibrous meningioma. A clinicopathologic and immunohistochemical study. Am J Clin Pathol 1996;106(2):217–24.
168. Iwaki T, Fukui M, Takeshita I, et al. Hemangiopericytoma of the meninges: a clinicopathologic and immunohistochemical study. Clin Neuropathol 1988;7(3):93–9.
169. Joseph JT, Lisle DK, Jacoby LB, et al. NF2 gene analysis distinguishes hemangiopericytoma from meningioma. Am J Pathol [Research Support, Non-U.S. Gov't Research Support, U.S. Gov't, Non-P.H.S. Research Support, U.S. Gov't, P.H.S.] 1995;147(5):1450–5.
170. Perry A, Scheithauer BW, Nascimento AG. The immunophenotypic spectrum of meningeal hemangiopericytoma: a comparison with fibrous meningioma and solitary fibrous tumor of meninges. Am J Surg Pathol 1997;21(11):1354–60.
171. Guthrie BL, Ebersold MJ, Scheithauer BW, et al. Meningeal hemangiopericytoma: histopathological features, treatment, and long-term follow-up of 44 cases. Neurosurgery 1989;25(4):514–22.
172. Mena H, Ribas JL, Pezeshkpour GH, et al. Hemangiopericytoma of the central nervous system: a review of 94 cases. Hum Pathol [Case Reports] 1991;22(1):84–91.
173. Dei Tos AP, Seregard S, Calonje E, et al. Giant cell angiofibroma. A distinctive orbital tumor in adults. Am J Surg Pathol 1995;19(11): 1286–93.
174. Guillou L, Gebhard S, Coindre JM. Orbital and extraorbital giant cell angiofibroma: a giant cell-rich variant of solitary fibrous tumor? Clinicopathologic and immunohistochemical analysis of a series in favor of a unifying concept. Am J Surg Pathol 2000;24(7):971–9.
175. Alpers CE, Rosenau W, Finkbeiner WE, et al. Congenital (infantile) hemangiopericytoma of the tongue and sublingual region. Am J Clin Pathol [Case Reports] 1984;81(3):377–82.
176. Baker DL, Oda D, Myall RW. Intraoral infantile hemangiopericytoma: literature review and addition of a case. Oral Surg Oral Med Oral Pathol [Case Reports Review] 1992;73(5):596–602.
177. Eimoto T. Ultrastructure of an infantile hemangiopericytoma. Cancer [Case Reports] 1977;40(5):2161–70.
178. Kauffman SL, Stout AP. Hemangiopericytoma in children. Cancer 1960;13:695–710.
179. Chung KC, Weiss SW, Kuzon WM Jr. Multifocal congenital hemangiopericytomas associated with Kasabach-Merritt syndrome. Br J Plast Surg 1995;48(4):240–2.
180. Chen KT, Kassel SH, Medrano VA. Congenital hemangiopericytoma. J Surg Oncol [Case Reports] 1986;31(2):127–9.
181. Jakobiec FA, Howard GM, Jones IS, et al. Hemangiopericytoma of the orbit. Am J Ophthalmol 1974;78(5):816–34.

182. Weidner N, Santa Cruz D. Phosphaturic mesenchymal tumors. A polymorphous group causing osteomalacia or rickets. Cancer 1987;59(8):1442–54.
183. Folpe AL, Fanburg-Smith JC, Billings SD, et al. Most osteomalacia-associated mesenchymal tumors are a single histopathologic entity: an analysis of 32 cases and a comprehensive review of the literature. Am J Surg Pathol 2004;28(1):1–30.
184. Bahrami A, Weiss SW, Montgomery E, et al. RT-PCR analysis for FGF23 using paraffin sections in the diagnosis of phosphaturic mesenchymal tumors with and without known tumor induced osteomalacia. Am J Surg Pathol 2009;33(9):1348–54.
185. Jung GH, Kim JD, Cho Y, et al. A 9-month-old phosphaturic mesenchymal tumor mimicking the intractable rickets. J Pediatr Orthop B 2010;19(1):127–32.
186. Shimada T, Mizutani S, Muto T, et al. Cloning and characterization of FGF23 as a causative factor of tumor-induced osteomalacia. Proceedings of the National Academy of Sciences of the United States of America [Research Support, Non-U.S. Gov't] 2001;98(11):6500–5.
187. Shimada T, Urakawa I, Yamazaki Y, et al. FGF-23 transgenic mice demonstrate hypophosphatemic rickets with reduced expression of sodium phosphate cotransporter type IIa. Biochemical and biophysical research communications 2004;314(2):409–14.
188. Bowe AE, Finnegan R, Jan de Beur SM, et al. FGF-23 inhibits renal tubular phosphate transport and is a PHEX substrate. Biochem Biophys Res Commun 2001;284(4):977–81.
189. Kumar R. Phosphatonin–a new phosphaturetic hormone? (lessons from tumour- induced osteomalacia and X-linked hypophosphataemia). Nephrol Dial Transplant 1997;12(1):11–13.
190. Kumar R. New insights into phosphate homeostasis: fibroblast growth factor 23 and frizzled-related protein-4 are phosphaturic factors derived from tumors associated with osteomalacia. Curr Opin Nephrol Hypertens 2002;11(5):547–53.
191. Riminucci M, Collins MT, Fedarko NS, et al. FGF-23 in fibrous dysplasia of bone and its relationship to renal phosphate wasting. J Clin Invest 2003;112(5):683–92.
192. Krishnamurthy S, Inwards CY, Oliveira AM, et al. Frequent expression of fibroblast growth factor-23 (FGF-23) mRNA in aneurysmal bone cyst (ABC). Mod Pathol 2011;24(Supplement 1):17A.
193. Berndt T, Craig TA, Bowe AE, et al. Secreted frizzled-related protein 4 is a potent tumor-derived phosphaturic agent. J Clin Invest 2003; 112(5):785–94.
194. Shelekhova KV, Kazakov DV, Michal M. Sinonasal phosphaturic mesenchymal tumor (mixed connective tissue variant): report of 2 cases. Am J Surg Pathol 2010;34(4):596–7.
195. Shelekhova KV, Kazakov DV, Hes O, et al. Phosphaturic mesenchymal tumor (mixed connective tissue variant): a case report with spectral analysis. Virchows Arch 2006;448(2):232–5.
196. Cheung FM, Ma L, Wu WC, et al. Oncogenic osteomalacia associated with an occult phosphaturic mesenchymal tumour: clinico-radiologico-pathological correlation and ultrastructural studies. Hong Kong Med J 2006;12(4):319–21.
197. Stone MD, Quincey C, Hosking DJ. A neuroendocrine cause of oncogenic osteomalacia. J Pathol 1992;167(2):181–5.
198. Toyosawa S, Tomita Y, Kishino M, et al. Expression of dentin matrix protein 1 in tumors causing oncogenic osteomalacia. Mod Pathol 2004; 17(5):573–8.
199. Williams K, Flanagan A, Folpe A, et al. Lymphatic vessels are present in phosphaturic mesenchymal tumours. Virchows Arch 2007;451(5):871–5.
200. Graham RP, Folpe AL, Oliveira AM, et al. A cytogenetic analysis of 2 cases of phosphaturic mesenchymal tumor mixed connective tissue type. Hum Pathol 2012;43(8):1334–8.

Malignant Soft Tissue Tumors of Uncertain Type

CHAPTER CONTENTS

The neoplasms described in this comprehensive chapter are a heterogeneous group of tumors of uncertain histogenesis because they have no known normal tissue counterpart. Each is characterized by its own distinctive clinical and pathologic features. This heterogeneous group of tumors can be further subdivided into those that are translocation-associated (Ewing family of tumors, extraskeletal myxoid chondrosarcoma, synovial sarcoma, alveolar soft part sarcoma, desmoplastic small round cell tumor) and those that are not (epithelioid sarcoma, malignant extrarenal rhabdoid tumor [MERT]).

Chromosomal aberrations have been found in virtually all tumor types, some of which are primary and clearly central to the pathogenesis of a given tumor, and others are secondary, probably occurring later in tumor development and progression.[1] Approximately 20% of soft tissue sarcomas are characterized by a specific balanced translocation resulting in the creation of a fusion gene. The ability to detect these translocations (fluorescence in situ hybridization [FISH] or reverse transcription polymerase chain reaction [RT-PCR]) has diagnostic, prognostic, and therapeutic implications. Although all of these elements will be addressed in the chapter, a detailed discussion related to primary molecular events in various sarcomas and their downstream signaling pathways is thoroughly discussed in Chapter 4.

EWING FAMILY OF TUMORS (EXTRASKELETAL EWING SARCOMA/PERIPHERAL PRIMITIVE NEUROECTODERMAL TUMOR)

There has been a remarkable evolution in the concepts regarding the histogenesis and relation of skeletal and extraskeletal Ewing sarcoma (ES) and peripheral neuroepithelioma (also sometimes referred to as *primitive neuroectodermal tumor*). In 1918, Stout[2] reported the case of a 42-year-old man with an ulnar nerve tumor composed of undifferentiated round cells that formed rosettes. Three years later, Ewing[3] reported a round cell neoplasm in the radius of a 14-year-old girl, calling it a *diffuse endothelioma of bone* and proposed an endothelial derivation. Over the next decades, there was much debate regarding the histogenesis of this neoplasm. It was not until 1975 that Angervall and Enzinger[4] described the first ES arising in soft tissue (extraskeletal ES). Subsequent reports confirmed the clinical and pathologic features of this tumor.

At about the same time, Seemayer et al.[5] described peripheral neuroectodermal tumors (PNET) arising in the soft tissues that were unrelated to structures of the peripheral or sympathetic nervous system; subsequently, Jaffe et al.[6] reported identical tumors in bone. In 1979, Askin et al.[7] described the malignant small cell tumor of the thoracopulmonary region (Askin tumor) as having histologic features similar to those of PNET but with a unique clinicopathologic profile. With the advent of immunohistochemical, cytogenetic, and molecular genetic techniques, it is now clear that these tumors represent ends of a morphologic spectrum known as the Ewing family of tumors (EFT).[8,9]

Identification of a common cytogenetic abnormality, t(11;22)(q24;q12), in ES[10] and PNET[11] clearly supports the contention that these neoplasms are histogenetically related. Since these early reports, numerous additional studies have found this translocation or variants involving 22q12, the site of the ES (*EWSR1*) gene, in almost all EFT.[12] The following discussion elaborates on this spectrum of tumors arising in extraskeletal locations.

Clinical Features

Most patients with EFT are adolescents or young adults, the majority of whom are less than 30 years of age.[13] In those studies that attempt to distinguish ES from PNET, there tends to be a broader age range in PNET, with a significant number of patients over the age of 40 years, although the mean ages are similar.[14-18] There is a slight male predilection, and the disease is very uncommon in non-Caucasians.[19] There is no evidence of familial predisposition or an association with environmental factors. Although some patients treated for EFT develop secondary neoplasms (such as radiation-induced osteosarcoma or therapy-related acute myeloid leukemia), EFT rarely occurs as a second neoplasm after therapy for another tumor.[20]

EFT may arise virtually anywhere but is most common in the deep soft tissues of the extremities. The most common anatomic sites are the upper thigh and buttock followed by the upper arm and shoulder. Tumors that are intimately attached to a major nerve may give rise to signs and symptoms related to diminished neurologic function. Less common, the tumor arises in the paravertebral soft tissues or chest wall generally in close association with the vertebrae or the ribs (Fig. 33-1). Well-characterized examples of EFT, often with molecular confirmation, have been reported in virtually every anatomic site.

In general, the tumor presents as a rapidly growing, deeply located mass measuring 5 to 10 cm in greatest diameter. Superficially located cases do occur but are uncommon.[21,22] The tumor is painful in about one-third of cases. If peripheral nerves or the spinal cord are involved, there may be progressive sensory or motor disturbances. As with other round cell sarcomas, the preoperative duration of symptoms is usually less than 1 year. Unlike neuroblastoma, catecholamine levels are within normal limits. CT, MRI, and PET scans are a routine part of the evaluation to determine anatomic relationships, presence of distant disease, and to evaluate the extent of therapeutic response to adjuvant therapy.[23]

Pathologic Findings

The gross appearance of the tumor varies. In general, it is multilobulated, soft, and friable; it rarely exceeds 10 cm in greatest diameter. The cut surface has a gray-yellow or gray-tan appearance, often with large areas of necrosis, cyst formation, or hemorrhage. Despite the extensive necrosis, calcification is rare.

There is a spectrum of histologic change in this family of tumors; in the older literature, criteria distinguishing ES, so-called *atypical ES* (large cell variant), and PNET were varied, as discussed later (Table 33-1). In a large clinicopathologic study of EFT, based on morphologic criteria alone, Llombart-Bosch et al.[24] classified 280 cases as conventional ES, 53 as PNET, and 80 as atypical ES. Because these lesions comprise a spectrum of histogenetically related tumors, the precise criteria for designating a tumor as an extraskeletal ES, atypical ES, or PNET are less critical, so, therefore, cases across the spectrum can be classified as EFT. The morphologic spectrum of this family of tumors continues to expand to include adamantinoma-like cases,[25-27] cytokeratin-positive tumors,[28-30] and rare desmin-positive cases.[31,32] The morphologic and immunophenotypic diversity was the focus of a study of 66 genetically confirmed EFT cases by Folpe et al.[27] As later discussed, cases with classical morphologic features can be accurately diagnosed using light microscopy with ancillary immunohistochemistry. However, given the wide morphologic spectrum, genetic confirmation is essential for the diagnosis of unusual morphologic variants of EFT.

The histologic features of typical ES include a solidly packed, lobular pattern of strikingly uniform round cells (Figs. 33-2 and 33-3). The individual cells have a round or ovoid nucleus with a distinct nuclear membrane, fine powdery chromatin, and one or two inapparent or small nucleoli. There are no multinucleated giant cells. The cytoplasm is ill-defined, scanty, and pale staining; and, in many cases, it is irregularly vacuolated as a result of intracellular deposits of glycogen (Figs. 33-4 and 33-5). Intracellular glycogen is present in most cases, but the amount varies from tumor to tumor and sometimes in different portions of the same neoplasm. In addition, glycogen droplets may compress and indent the nucleus (Fig. 33-6). The number of mitotic figures varies, and, in many cases, the paucity of mitotic figures contrasts with the immature appearance of the neoplastic cells.

Although the tumor is richly vascular, the thin-walled vessels are compressed and obscured by the closely packed tumor cells; the rich vascularity is often discernible in areas of degeneration and necrosis only (Fig. 33-7). In fact, the association of distinct vascular structures with degenerated or necrotic ghost cells is a common, striking feature (filigree pattern) (Fig. 33-8). Aside from the prominent vascularity, there is occasionally a pseudovascular or pseudoalveolar pattern caused by small fluid-filled pools or blood lakes amid the solidly arranged tumor cells (Fig. 33-9), a feature occasionally misinterpreted as angiosarcoma or alveolar rhabdomyosarcoma by those unfamiliar with this secondary change. In the study by Folpe et al.,[27] 74% of cases had features of typical ES.

In some cases, the cells show moderate nuclear enlargement, irregular nuclear contours, and frequent prominent nucleoli, corresponding to atypical or large cell ES (Fig. 33-10).[24]

Text continued on p. 1034

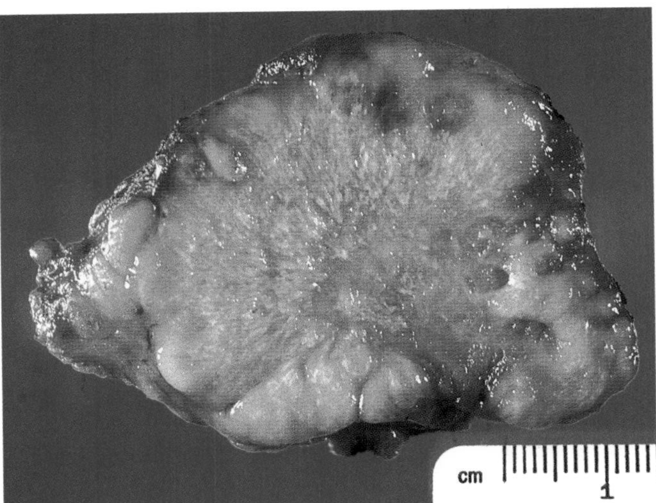

FIGURE 33-1. Gross photograph of EFT from the chest wall of a 10-year-old boy. Foci of necrosis are apparent.

TABLE 33-1 Spectrum of Light Microscopic Features Across the Ewing Family of Tumors

FEATURE	CLASSICAL EWING SARCOMA	ATYPICAL EWING SARCOMA	PNET
Cell shape	Uniform, round	Irregular	Irregular
Chromatin	Fine	Coarse	Coarse
Nucleoli	Pinpoint	More prominent	Prominent
Glycogen	Abundant	Moderate	Scant
Rosettes	Absent	Absent	Present

Modified from Navarro S, Cavazanna AO, Llombart-Bosch A, et al. Comparison of Ewing's sarcoma of bone and peripheral neuroepithelioma: an immunocytochemical and ultrastructural analysis of two primitive neuroectodermal neoplasms. Arch Pathol Lab Med 1994;118:608–615.

PNET, peripheral neuroectodermal tumor.

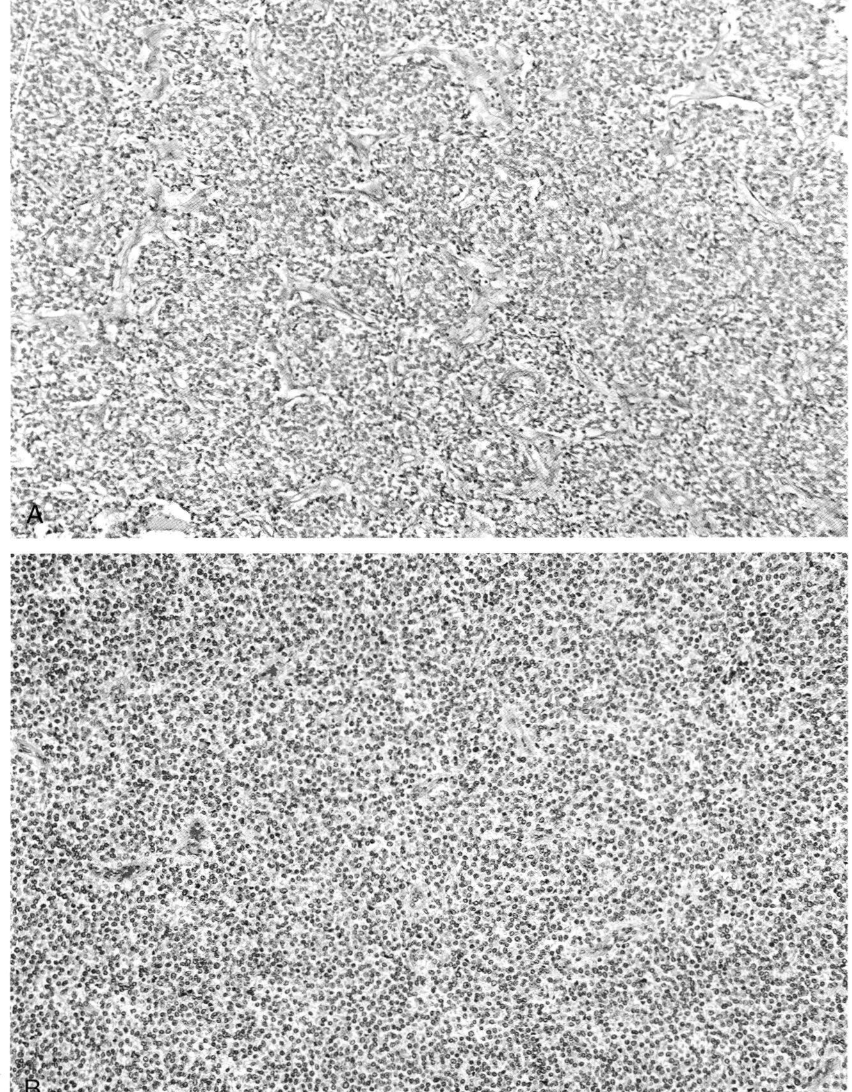

FIGURE 33-2. (A) Low-power view of extraskeletal EFT characterized by a lobular round cell pattern of striking uniformity. (B) Typical low-power view of the monotonous appearance of this tumor.

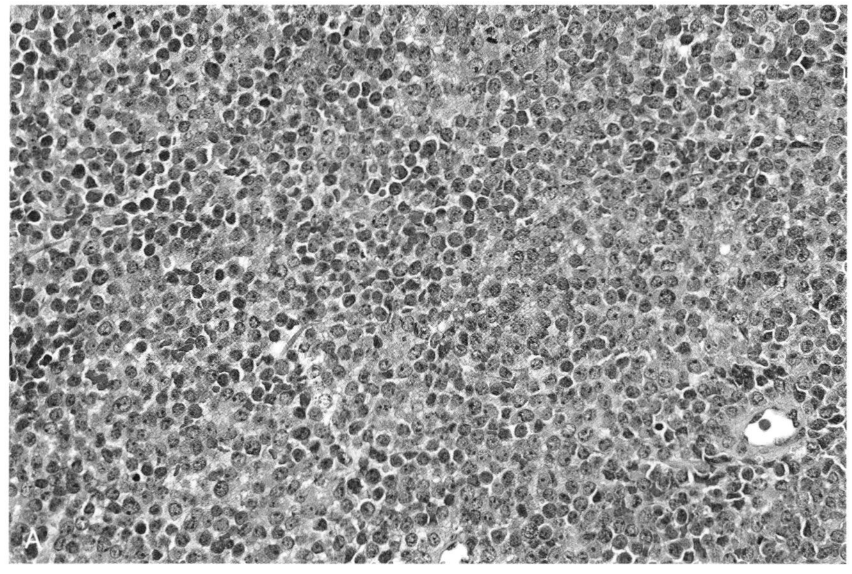

FIGURE 33-3. (A) Extraskeletal EFT composed of a monotonous proliferation of round cells. Homer Wright rosettes are not seen.

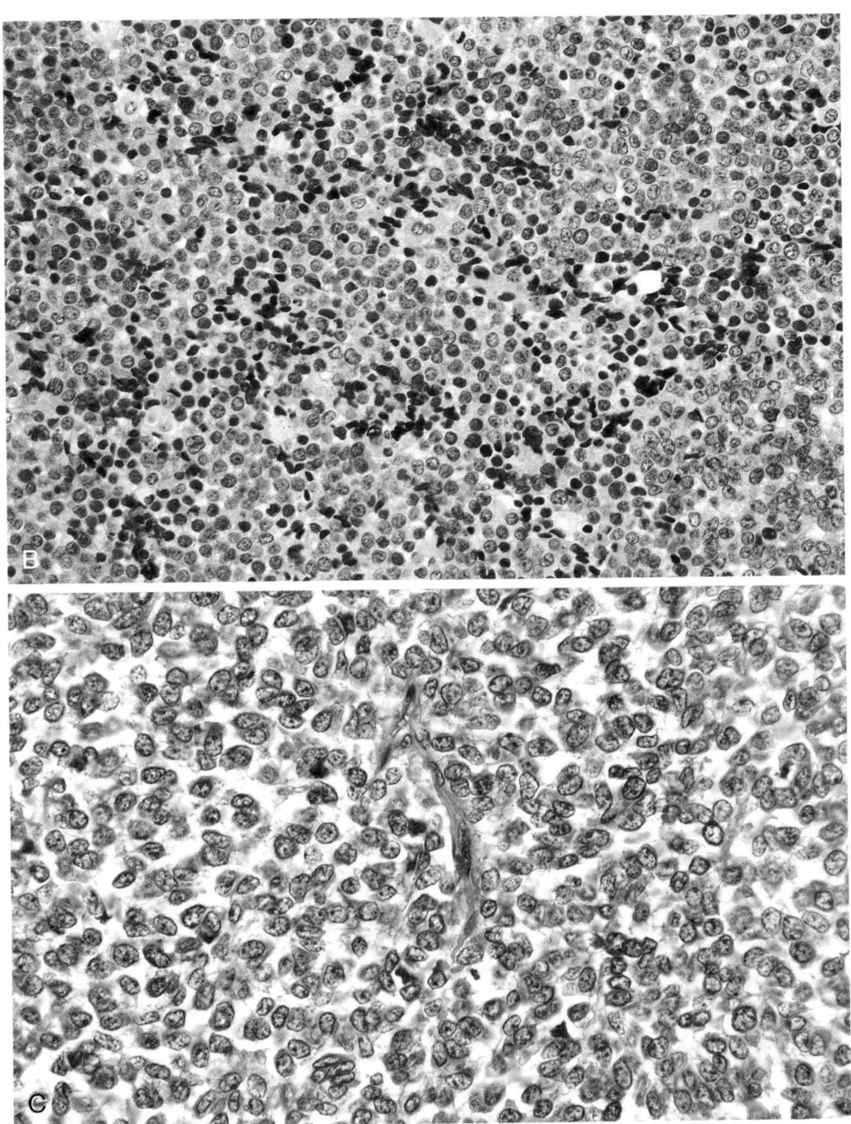

FIGURE 33-3, cont'd. (B) Admixture of small round cells with crushed darker-staining cells. (C) High-power view of round cell proliferation in extraskeletal EFT.

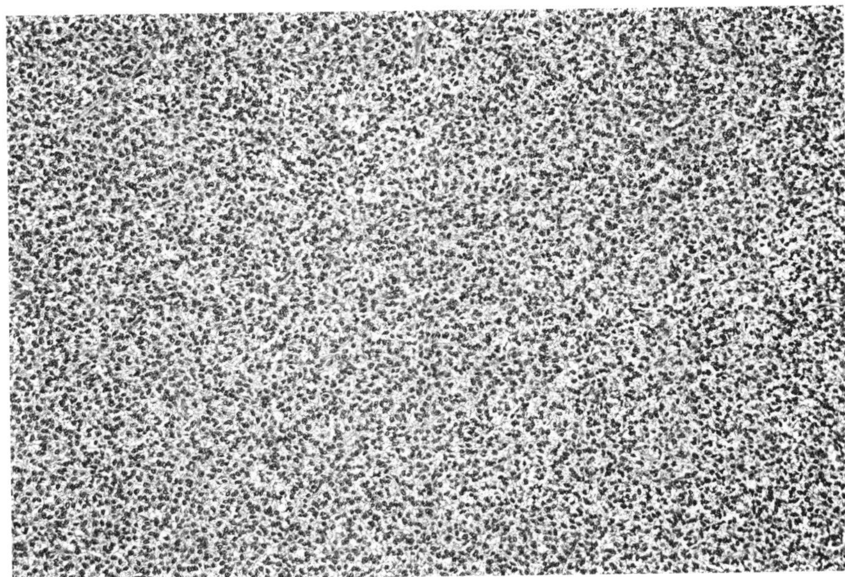

FIGURE 33-4. Low-power view of extraskeletal EFT composed of cells with abundant cleared-out cytoplasm secondary to glycogen deposition.

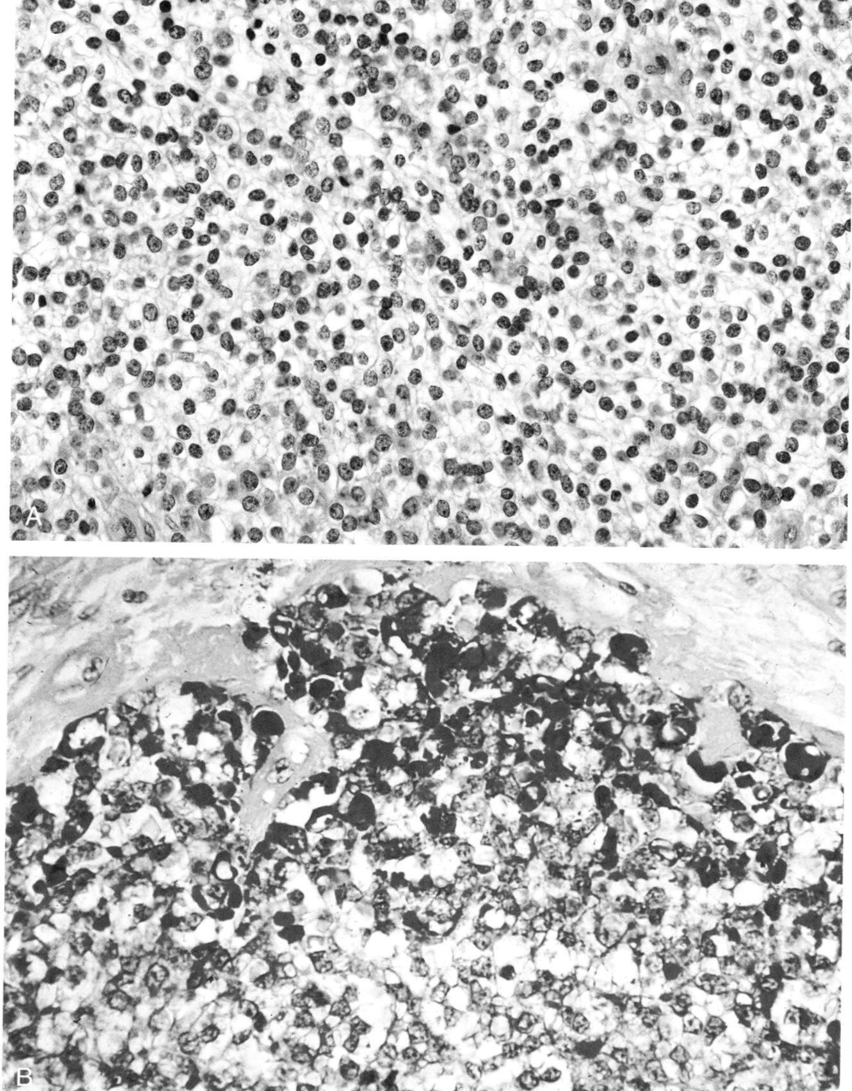

FIGURE 33-5. (A) Cells with abundant cleared-out cytoplasm and clearly defined cell borders in extraskeletal EFT. (B) PAS preparation reveals intracellular glycogen, especially in the peripheral portion of the tumor.

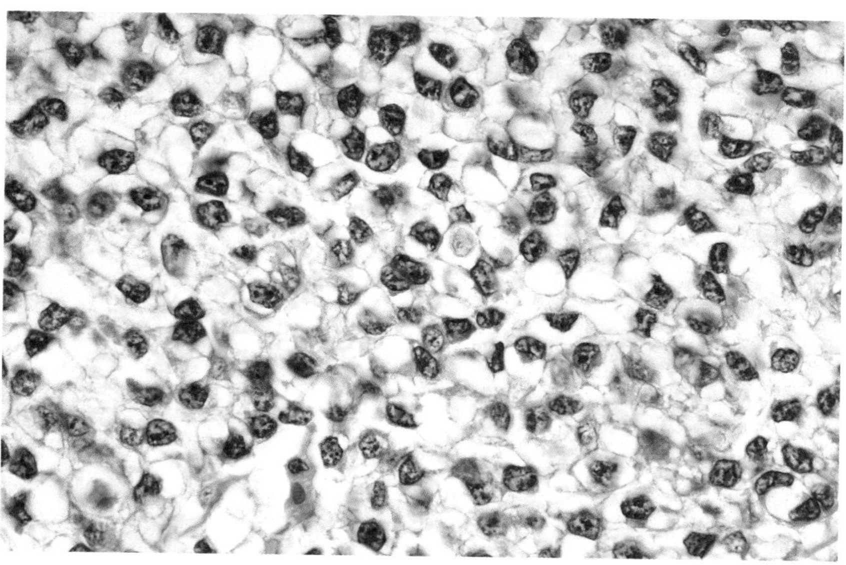

FIGURE 33-6. Extraskeletal EFT. Cytoplasmic vacuoles secondary to the deposition of intracellular glycogen often indent the nuclei.

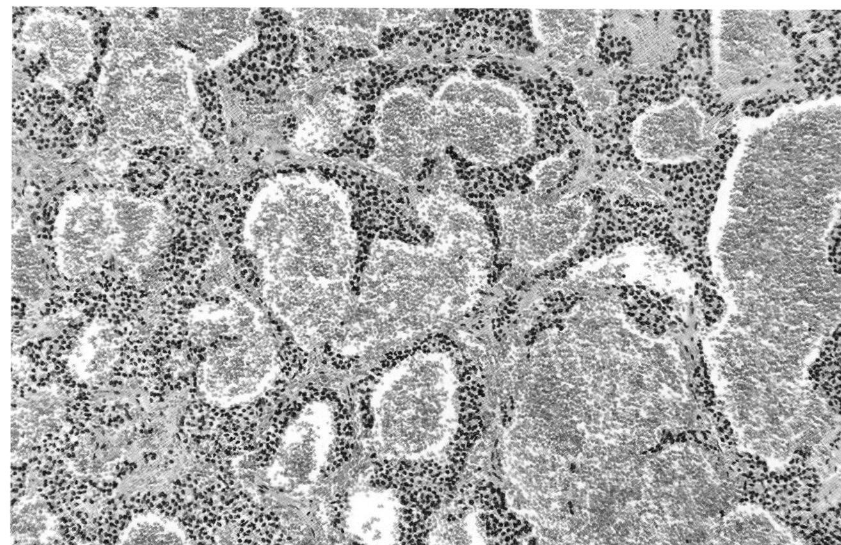

FIGURE 33-7. Hemorrhagic zone in extraskeletal EFT resembling a vascular neoplasm.

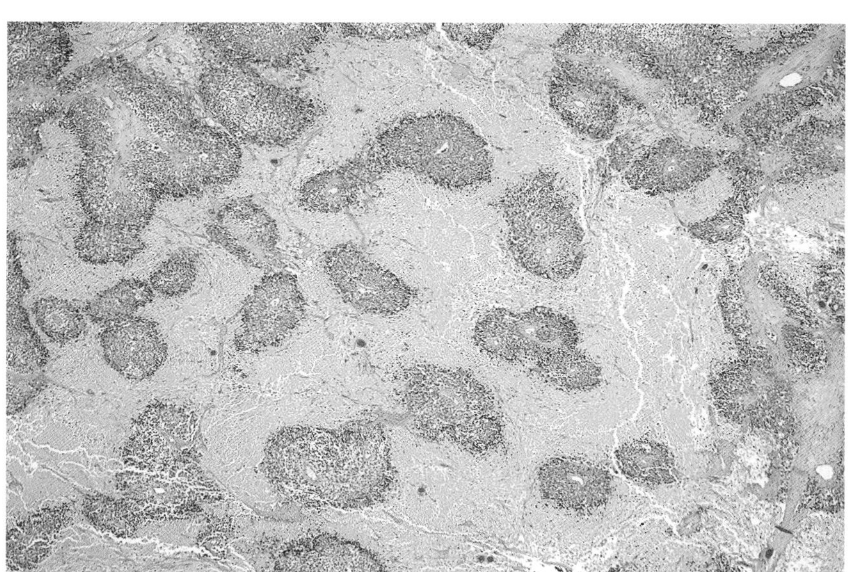

FIGURE 33-8. Extensive zones of necrosis in extraskeletal EFT. There is maintenance of the tumor cells around blood vessels.

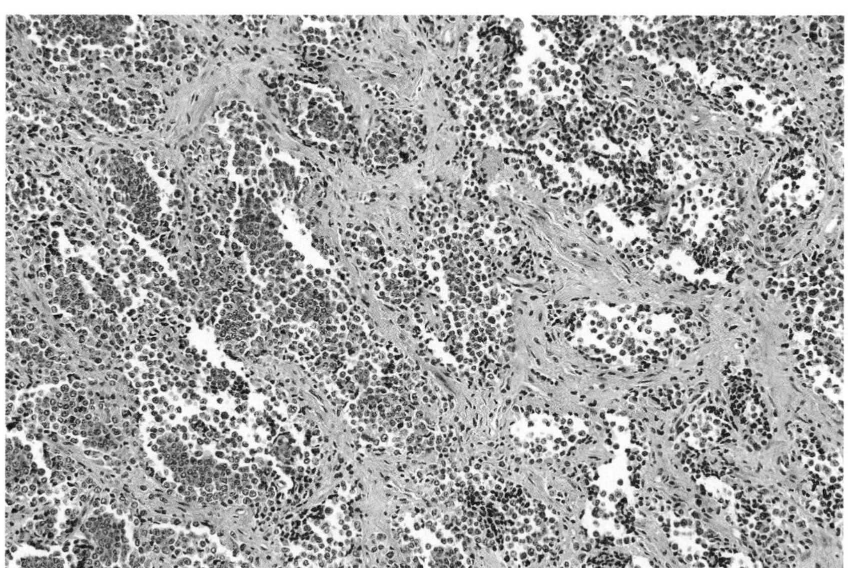

FIGURE 33-9. Pseudoalveolar pattern in an extraskeletal EFT superficially resembling an alveolar rhabdomyosarcoma.

EFT with a prominent spindle-cell pattern can also be seen, albeit rare. In these cases, an elaborate hemangiopericytoma-like vascular pattern may be present, thereby closely simulating a poorly differentiated synovial sarcoma.[24,27] Rarely, the stroma can be extensively hyalinized and densely eosinophilic, reminiscent of sclerosing epithelioid fibrosarcoma or sclerosing rhabdomyosarcoma, but typical areas of EFT are usually present and assist in accurate classification.

One of the most difficult and least well-characterized variants of EFT is the so-called *adamantinoma-like* variant, which accounted for 5% of the cases reported by Folpe et al.[27] These tumors show a distinctly nested, epithelioid growth pattern with striking stromal desmoplasia (Fig. 33-11). The nests of tumor cells may display prominent peripheral nuclear palisading and contain large polygonal cells with irregularly contoured, hyperchromatic nuclei, prominent nucleoli, and moderate amounts of cytoplasm.[24,26,27] Rarely, squamous pearls may be seen.[33] As later discussed, the immunophenotype of this variant is quite unusual because they typically show strong, uniform expression of pancytokeratins and focal staining for high-molecular-weight cytokeratins.[27]

The typical PNET comprising about 15% of cases is composed of sheets or lobules of small round cells containing darkly staining, round, or oval nuclei (Fig. 33-12). The cytoplasm is indistinct except in areas where the cells are more mature and the elongated hair-like cytoplasmic extensions coalesce to form rosettes (Figs. 33-13 and 33-14). Most of the rosettes are similar to those seen in neuroblastomas and contain a central solid core of neurofibrillary material (Homer Wright rosette). Rarely, the rosettes resemble those of retinoblastoma and contain a central lumen or

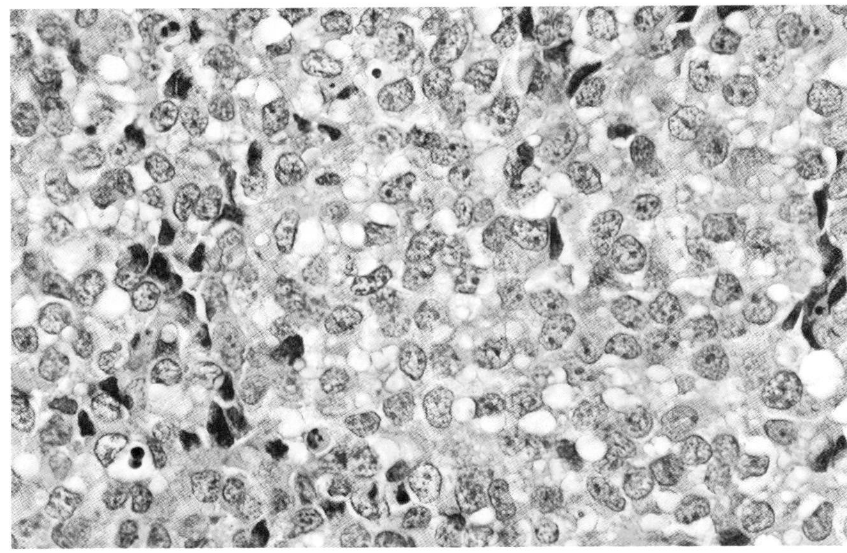

FIGURE 33-10. High-power view of large cells in extraskeletal EFT. The cells have vesicular chromatin and prominent nucleoli. Such tumors have been described as atypical or large-cell variants of EFT.

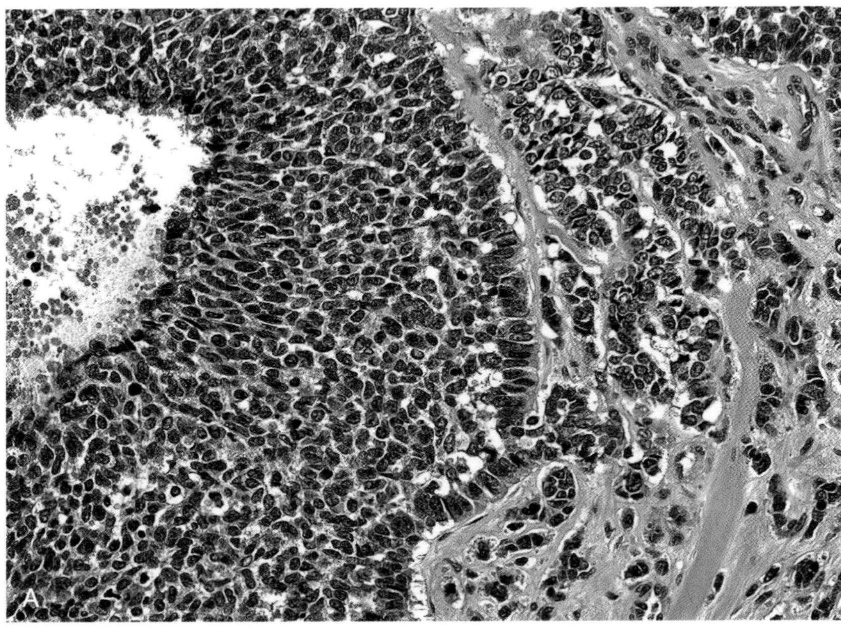

FIGURE 33-11. (A) Unusual case of an adamantinoma-like EFT.

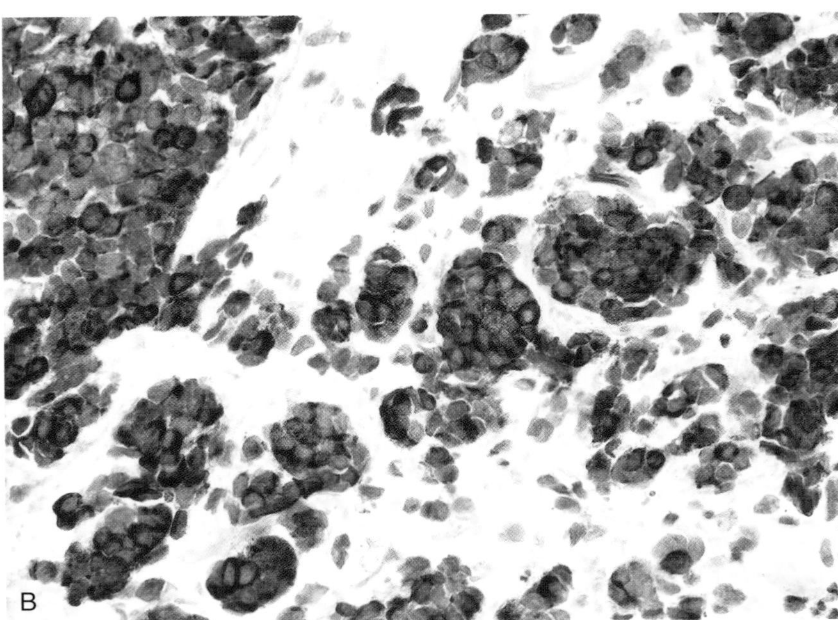

FIGURE 33-11, cont'd. (B) Strong cytokeratin immunoreactivity in an adamantinoma-like EFT.

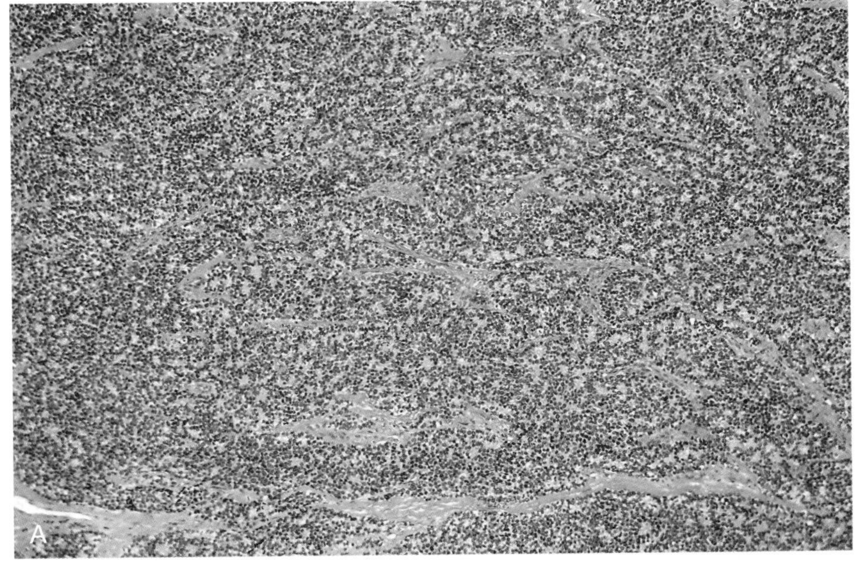

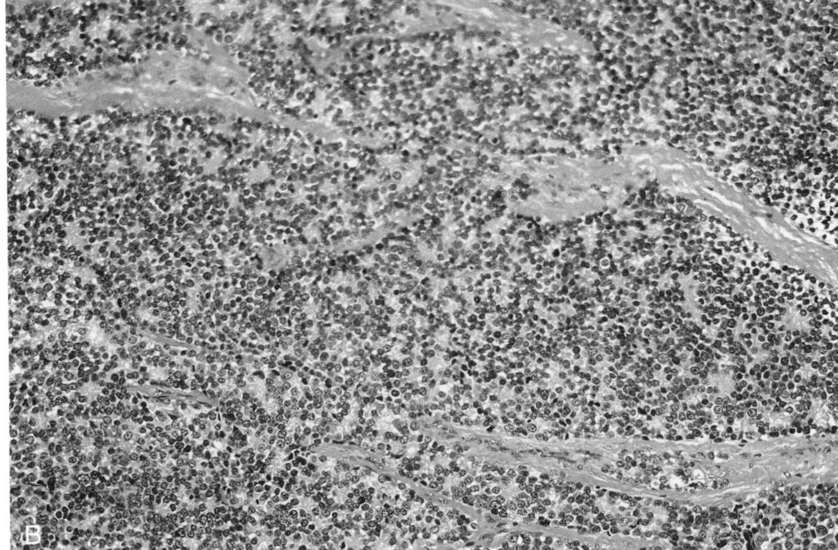

FIGURE 33-12. (A, B) Primitive neuroectodermal tumor (peripheral neuroepithelioma) with distinctive lobular architecture and numerous Homer Wright rosettes apparent at low magnification.

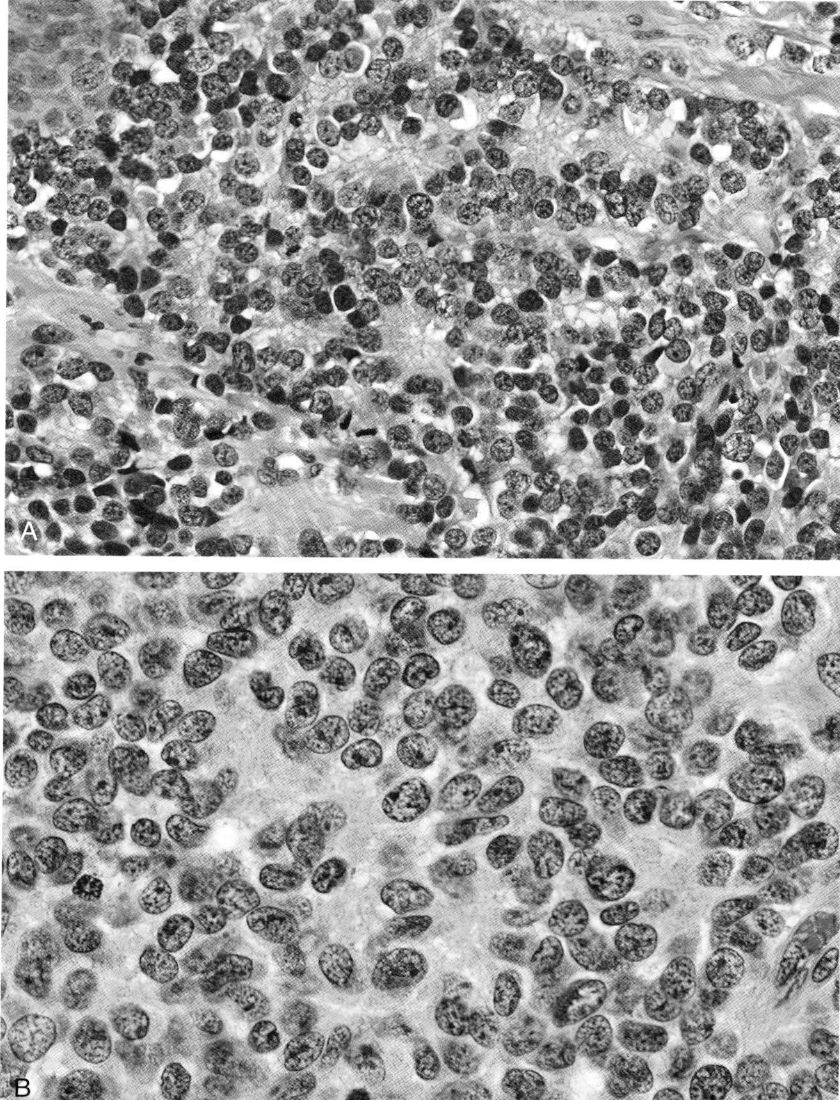

FIGURE 33-13. (A, B) Primitive neuroectodermal tumor (peripheral neuroepithelioma). Large cells with vesicular nuclei and prominent nucleoli surround a central fibrillary core (Homer Wright rosettes).

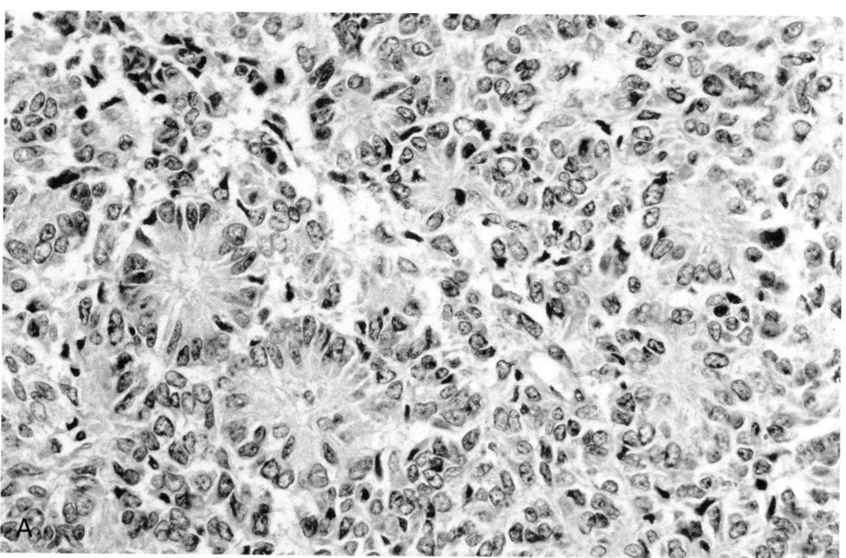

FIGURE 33-14. Primitive neuroectodermal tumor (peripheral neuroepithelioma) with round cell areas containing rosettes (A) and spindled areas

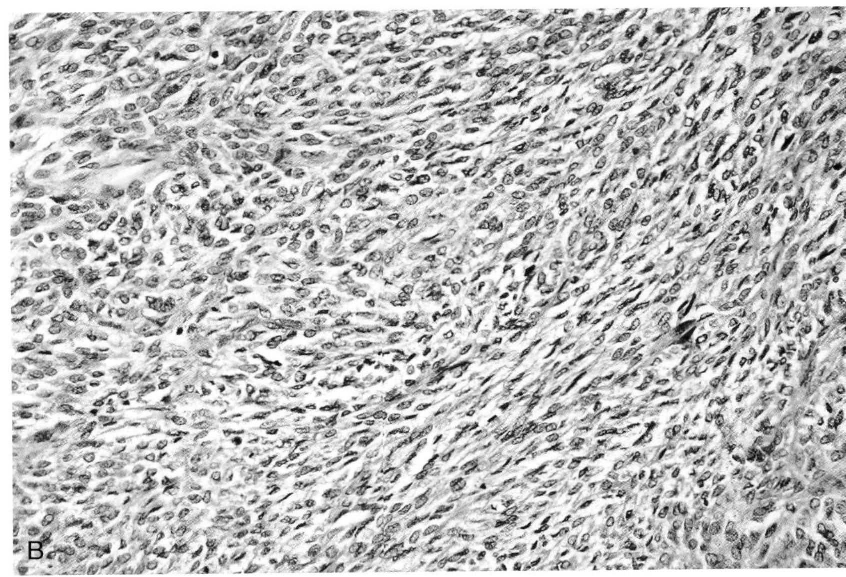

FIGURE 33-14, cont'd. (B) coexisting in the same tumor.

TABLE 33-2 Spectrum of Ultrastructural Features Across the Ewing Family of Tumors

FEATURE	CLASSICAL EWING SARCOMA	ATYPICAL EWING SARCOMA	PNET
Organelles	Scarce	Moderate	Abundant
Dense-core granules	Absent	Rare	Abundant
Neurotubules	Absent	Rare	Abundant
Neuritic processes	Absent	Rare	Abundant

Modified from Navarro S, Cavazanna AO, Llombart-Bosch A, et al. Comparison of Ewing's sarcoma of bone and peripheral neuroepithelioma: an immunocytochemical and ultrastructural analysis of two primitive neuroectodermal neoplasms. Arch Pathol Lab Med 1994; 118:608–615.

PNET, peripheral neuroectodermal tumor.

vesicle (Flexner-Wintersteiner rosette). Some tumors are composed of cords or trabeculae of small round cells. These areas bear a resemblance to a carcinoid tumor or a small cell undifferentiated carcinoma, although, histogenetically, they are properly compared to primitive neuroepithelium. Rarely, EFT may show evidence of cartilaginous or osseous differentiation.[34]

Ultrastructural Features

Similar to the spectrum of histologic findings, there is also an ultrastructural spectrum of neural differentiation in the EFT family (Table 33-2). Extraskeletal ES has primitive undifferentiated cells with uniform round or ovoid nuclei, a smooth nuclear envelope, and finely granular chromatin with one or two small nucleoli (Fig. 33-15).[35,36] Characteristically, the cytoplasm contains few organelles.

On the other end of the spectrum, PNET is characterized by the presence of elongated cell processes that interdigitate with each other and contain small dense-core granules (neurosecretory granules) that measure 50 to 100 nm and occasionally contain microtubules.[35,37] The processes are most highly developed in the center of the rosette and in the neurofibrillary areas, where they form a tangled mass. They are also noted in areas that display little neurofibrillary differentiation by light microscopy.

Immunohistochemical Findings

For many years, a diagnosis of EFT was essentially an immunohistochemical diagnosis of exclusion. However, beginning in the early 1990s, numerous studies confirmed the utility of the product of the *MIC2* gene (HBA71 antigen, glycoprotein p30/32, or CD99) in recognizing this group of tumors, confirming the high sensitivity of this marker for EFT (Fig. 33-16).[27,38] The *MIC2* gene is a pseudoautosomal gene located on the short arms of the sex chromosomes; its product is a membranous glycoprotein (CD99) that can be detected immunohistochemically using a variety of antibodies, including 12E7 and O13. Although initially believed to be highly specific for EFT, it is apparent that virtually all other round cell tumors in the differential diagnosis, on occasion, show membranous immunoreactivity for CD99 (Table 33-3), including lymphomas, particularly T-lymphoblastic lymphoma[39] and precursor B-lymphoblastic lymphoma,[40] Merkel cell carcinoma,[41] small cell carcinoma,[42] rhabdomyosarcoma,[43] small cell osteosarcoma,[44] desmoplastic small round cell tumor,[45] and mesenchymal chondrosarcoma.[46] Notably, childhood neuroblastomas do not stain for this antigen. Therefore, although CD99 is highly sensitive for recognizing EFT, this marker should always be used as part of a panel of immunostains because it lacks specificity. Given the rarity of CD99 negativity in EFT, suspected cases should be confirmed by molecular techniques prior to rendering a definitive diagnosis.

Many EFT also stain for neural markers, including neuron-specific enolase, CD57, S-100 protein, synaptophysin, and PGP9.5.[47] Although PNET tend to express one or more of these neural markers with greater frequency than typical ES, there is significant overlap. However, it should be kept in mind

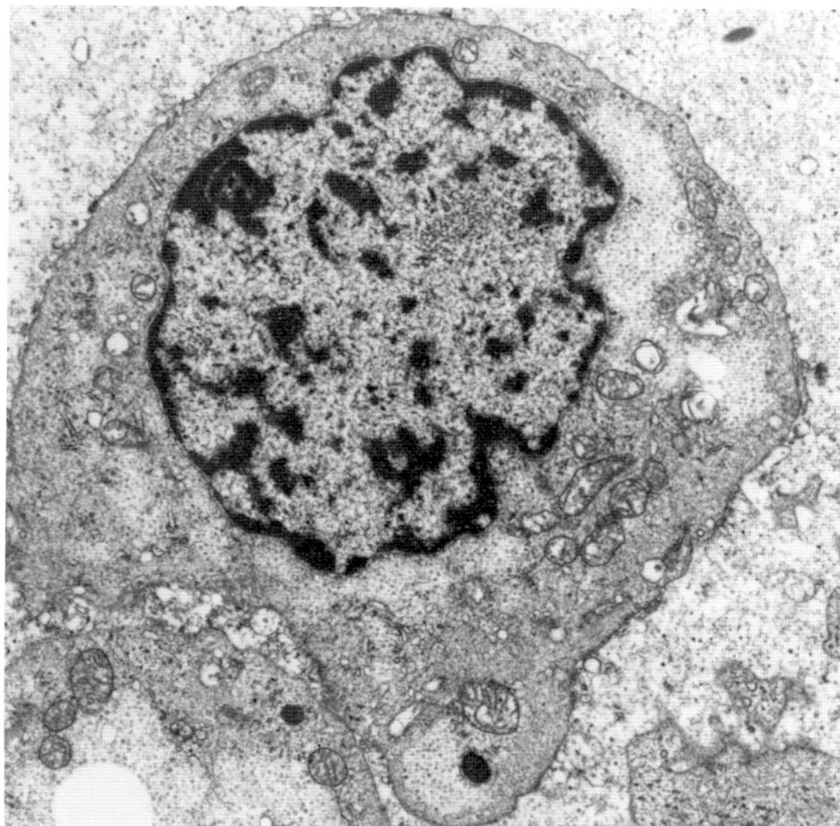

FIGURE 33-15. Electron microscopic view of EFT. This cell has a prominent nucleus with marginated chromatin, few organelles, and abundant glycogen.

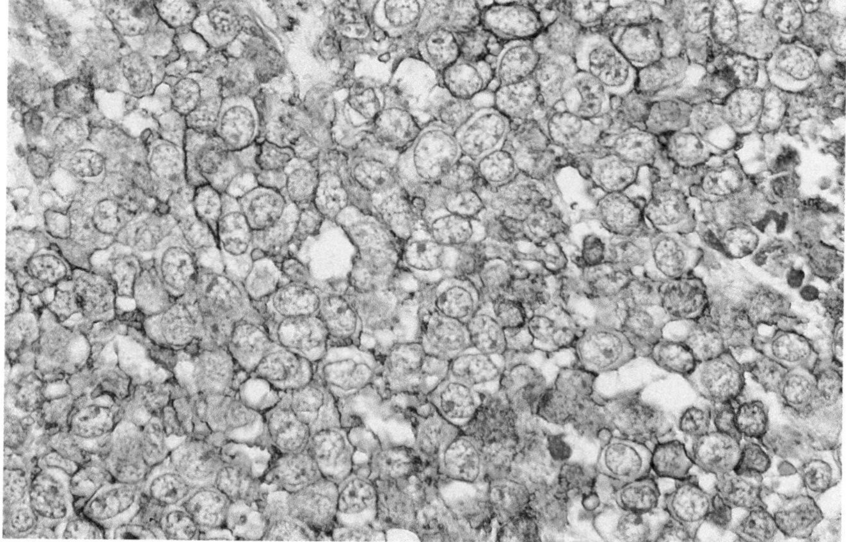

FIGURE 33-16. Strong membranous CD99 immunoreactivity in an extraskeletal EFT.

that in many of these studies the immunohistochemical expression of neural markers is used as one of the criteria to differentiate cases of typical ES from PNET, leading to the previous circular conclusion. Shanfeld et al.[48] found that the degree of immunohistochemical expression of neural markers in tumors that lack light microscopic evidence of neural differentiation was not predictive of clinical behavior. In addition, the extent of immunoexpression of these neural antigens has not been found to be related to the specific *EWSR1* gene fusion type.[49]

The recognition that EFT may express epithelial markers has become increasingly acknowledged and is a recognized diagnostic pitfall. Folpe et al.[27] found close to 25% of typical ES to be positive with the broad spectrum AE1/AE3 antibody, but these tumors did not express high-molecular-weight cytokeratins. These findings are similar to those of Gu et al.[29] and Collini et al.,[28] who found cytokeratin staining in 20% (either AE1/AE3 or CAM5.2) and 32% (antibody not stated) of cases, respectively. This cytokeratin immunoreactivity is usually focal and often dot-like, but it may be strong and diffuse on

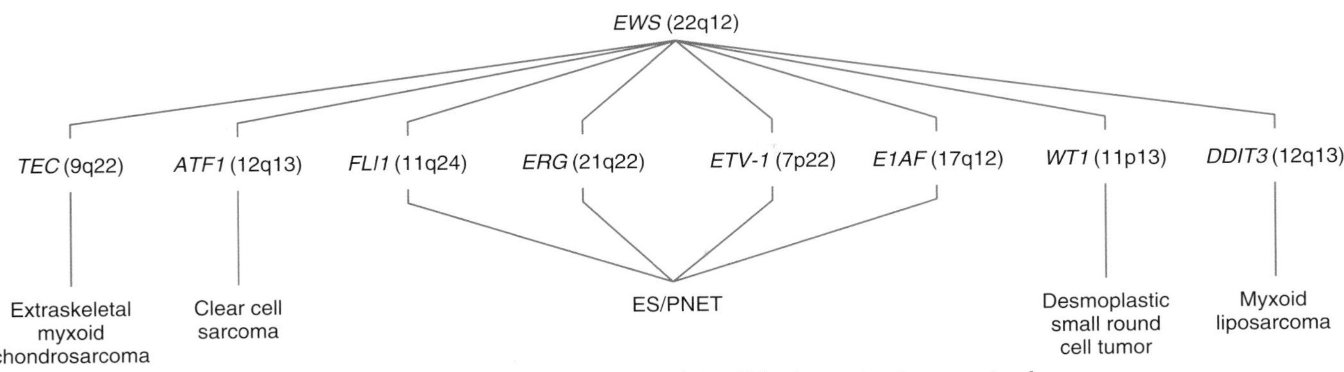

FIGURE 33-17. Critical role of the *EWSR1* gene (22q12) in the molecular genesis of sarcomas.

TABLE 33-3 Frequency of CD99 Immunoreactivity in Ewing Family of Tumors and Other Small Round Cell Tumors

DIAGNOSIS	POSITIVE (%)
EFT	95
T-lymphoblastic lymphoma	92
Poorly differentiated synovial sarcoma	50
Small cell osteosarcoma	23
Rhabdomyosarcoma	21
Desmoplastic small round cell tumor	16
Small cell carcinoma	9
Merkel cell carcinoma	9
Neuroblastoma	0

EFT, Ewing family of tumors.

occasion. The adamantinoma-like tumors typically strongly express AE1/AE3 and may even stain with antibodies to high-molecular-weight cytokeratins,[27] probably reflecting the complex epithelial differentiation in this variant.

The expression of desmin is quite rare, being found in only 1 of 56 (2%) cases in the study by Folpe et al.[27] Parham et al.[31] also reported two cases of desmin positivity in EFT, genetically confirmed. Neither MyoD1 nor myogenin are expressed in EFT, thereby minimizing any potential confusion with alveolar rhabdomyosarcoma.

As later described in detail, *FLI1*, a member of the E-twenty six (ETS) family of DNA-binding transcription factors, is involved in the t(11;22) translocation frequently observed in EFT. Polyclonal antibodies to the FLI1 protein have been developed, and FLI1 nuclear positivity has been reported in 71% to 84% of ES/PNET cases.[24,43] Rossi et al.,[50] using a monoclonal antibody, found all 15 cases of EFT stained for this antigen. Folpe et al.[27] found FLI1 positivity in 94% of EFT with known *EWSR1-FLI1* fusions, as well as one case with an *EWSR1-ERG* fusion. In the latter case, it was suggested that the polyclonal FLI1 antisera cross-reacted with a similar epitope found in the ERG protein because *ERG* and *FLI1* show considerable homology.[51] Despite the sensitivity of this marker, FLI1 is also frequently positive in lymphoblastic and other non-Hodgkin lymphomas, and rare examples of melanoma, Merkel cell carcinoma, and neuroblastoma.[24,43,50] Antibodies to ERG are also now available and are specific for these tumors with *ERG* rearrangement, showing only rare positivity in cases with *FLI1* rearrangements.[52]

Given the therapeutic success of imatinib mesylate (Gleevec) in the treatment of gastrointestinal stromal tumors, there has been considerable interest in evaluating the expression of CD117 in other tumors, including EFT. The frequency of CD117 expression in EFT reported in the literature varies considerably, ranging from 20% to 71%.[53-55] Folpe et al.[27] found CD117 staining in 24% of genetically confirmed cases. There are few cases that have been evaluated for mutations in the *KIT* gene; therefore, the clinical and potentially therapeutic significance of CD117 staining in EFT is not currently known.

Cytogenetic and Molecular Genetic Findings

The defining feature of the EFT family is the presence of nonrandom translocations leading to the fusion of the *EWSR1* gene on 22q12 with one of several members of the *ETS* family of transcription factors (Fig. 33-17).[56,57] The most frequent of these translocations is t(11;22)(q24;q12), detected in approximately 90% of cases,[58] resulting in fusion of the 3' end of the *FLI* gene on 11q24 with the 5' end of the *EWSR1* gene on 22q12. The fusion gene encodes an oncoprotein domain on *FLI1* generating aberrantly active transcription factors capable of DNA binding and malignant transformation.[51] The second most common translocation is t(21;22)(q22;q12), leading to the fusion of *EWSR1* to *ERG* at 21q22.[59] Less common alterations (fewer than 5% of cases) result in the fusion of *EWSR1* to *ETV1* at 7p22,[60] *ETV4* (also known as *E1AF*) at 17q12,[61] *FEV* at 2q33,[62] and *ZSG*, resulting in an inv(22).[63] The translocation breakpoints are restricted to introns 7 to 10 of the *EWSR1* gene and introns 3 to 9 of the *ETS*-related genes.[64] Fusion of *EWSR1* exon 7 to *FLI1* exon 6 (type 1 fusion) and *EWSR1* exon 7 to *FLI1* exon 5 (type 2) account for about 85% of *EWSR1-FLI1* fusions.[65,66] The ability to detect these fusions by molecular genetic techniques (FISH or RT-PCR) using fixed, paraffin-embedded tissues has greatly facilitated the diagnosis of these tumors.[67] For example, in the study by Bridge et al.,[67] FISH (using fixed, paraffin-embedded tissue) showed a sensitivity and specificity of 91% and 100%, respectively. RT-PCR using fixed tissues showed sensitivity and specificity of only 59% and 85%, respectively. However, RT-PCR can provide additional information regarding fusion type so that both techniques are complementary to one another. Interestingly, rare cases of EFT harbor translocations of *FUS* rather than *EWSR1*, including a t(16;21)(p11;q22) resulting in a *FUS-ERG* fusion[68] and a t(2;16)(q35;p11) resulting in a *FUS-FEV* fusion.[69] At present, according to the 2012 WHO classification, Ewing-like sarcomas that harbor alternate translocations are treated in a manner similar to conventional Ewing sarcoma.

Secondary cytogenetic abnormalities that occur in this group of tumors have been described, including trisomy 8,[70,71] trisomy 12,[72] and an unbalanced t(1;16) leading to gain of 1q and loss of 16q.[73] These cytogenetic abnormalities lack sufficient sensitivity and specificity for diagnostic purposes, but some have suggested a prognostic role.[74,75] In addition, alterations in *TP53* and *p16/p14ARF* are detected in up to 25% of EFT; these alterations are detected in a subset of patients who pursue an aggressive clinical course and are refractory to chemotherapy.[1]

Differential Diagnosis

Although a histogenetic relation between ES and PNET has been clearly established, the issue as to whether there is any clinical significance in differentiating between these lesions has been historically contentious. Part of the difficulty lies in the variability of criteria for classifying lesions as either ES or PNET. Whereas some studies require histologic evidence of rosette formation for a diagnosis of PNET, others require immunohistochemical evidence of neural differentiation, with or without rosettes. For example, in the study by Schmidt et al.,[18] a tumor was designated a PNET if it had Homer Wright rosettes on light microscopy or coexpressed two or more neural markers by immunohistochemistry. Using such criteria, the authors found that patients with PNET had a more aggressive clinical course than those with extraskeletal ES. Using identical criteria, however, others were unable to distinguish significant clinical differences between these tumors.[76,77] In the past, PNET was diagnosed if the tumor showed well-defined rosettes of the Homer Wright or Flexner-Wintersteiner type, if there were two or more positive neural markers, or if there was ultrastructural evidence of neural differentiation. Such arbitrary designations seem to be obsolete since recent studies (including those in which patients were uniformly treated) have failed to reveal significant clinical differences between these entities. Currently, all of these tumors are classified as members of the EFT, regardless of the presence or absence of light microscopic or immunohistochemical evidence of neural differentiation.

Neuroblastoma enters the differential diagnosis because of the young age of some patients with EFT, the frequent paravertebral location of the tumor, and the occasional presence of Homer Wright rosettes. Neuroblastoma develops at a relatively younger patient age than either EFT or alveolar rhabdomyosarcoma. In fact, about 25% of neuroblastomas are congenital, 50% are diagnosed by age 2, and 90% by age 5;[78] very few cases are diagnosed during adolescence or adult life.[79] These tumors arise in the distribution of sympathetic ganglia, in a paramidline position at any point between the base of the skull and the pelvis, in addition to the adrenal medulla and organs of Zuckerkandl. Up to 90% of patients have elevated urinary catecholamine metabolites.[80] Histologically, neuroblastoma is composed of sheets of small round cells that are divided into small lobules by delicate fibrovascular stroma (Figs. 33-18 to 33-24). The cells have round deeply staining nuclei and are almost devoid of cytoplasm. With progressive differentiation, the neuroblasts acquire attenuated cytoplasmic processes (neurites) that are polarized toward a central point to form Homer Wright rosettes. In addition, the stroma contains mats of neuropil, which are tangled networks of cell processes. In the most differentiated tumors, some cells show partial or complete ganglionic differentiation.

By immunohistochemistry, neuroblastomas express a number of neural antigens (NSE, PGP9.5, neurofilament protein) that may also be found in EFT. However, unlike EFT, neuroblastomas do not express CD99. Although NB-84 is a sensitive marker of neuroblastoma,[81] it lacks specificity and is expressed in up to 20% of EFT. Cytogenetically, neuroblastomas lack evidence of *EWSR1* aberrations (Table 33-4). Rather, they are characterized by deletions at 1p36 and 11q23, as well as gains of 17q.[82-84] These aberrations, along with *MYCN* amplification and TrkA expression, are important prognostic parameters in neuroblastoma.[85-87] However, this topic is beyond the scope of this discussion.

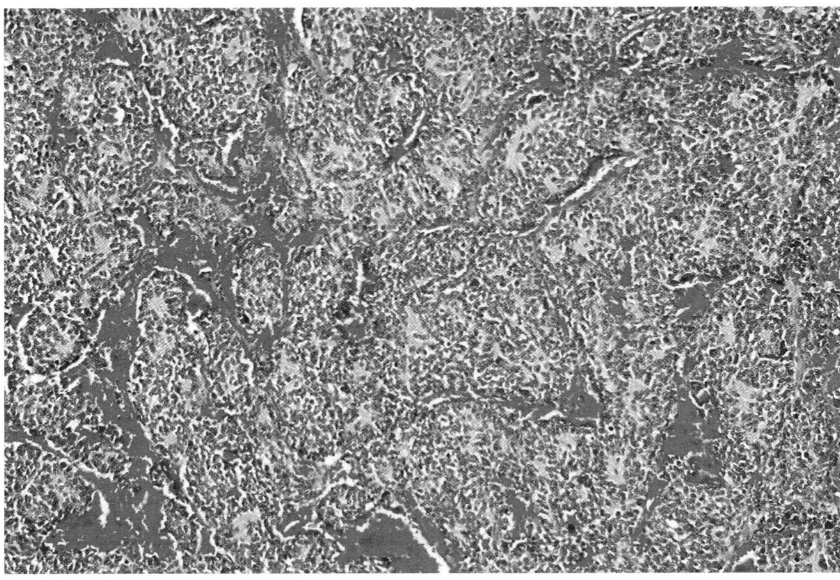

FIGURE 33-18. Poorly differentiated neuroblastoma with hemorrhagic fibrovascular septa that divide the tumor into small lobules.

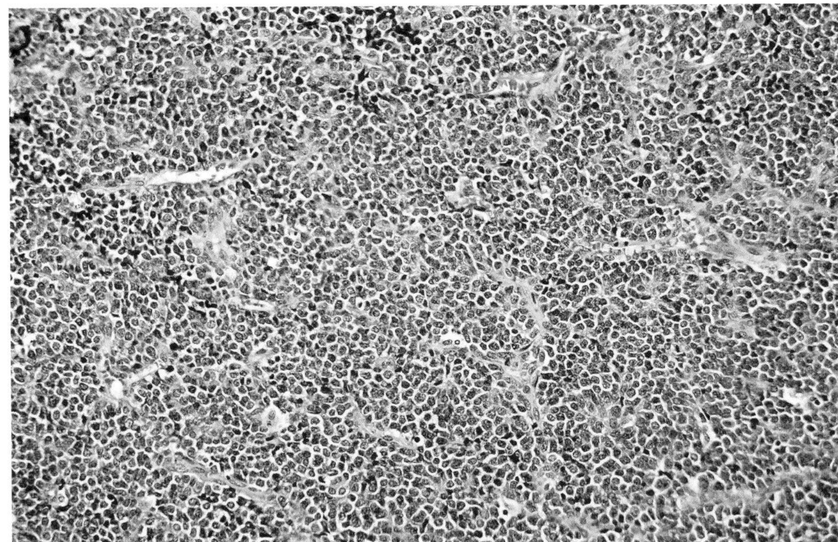

FIGURE 33-19. Poorly differentiated neuroblastoma composed of monotonous sheets of cells with little cytoplasm divided by fibrovascular septa.

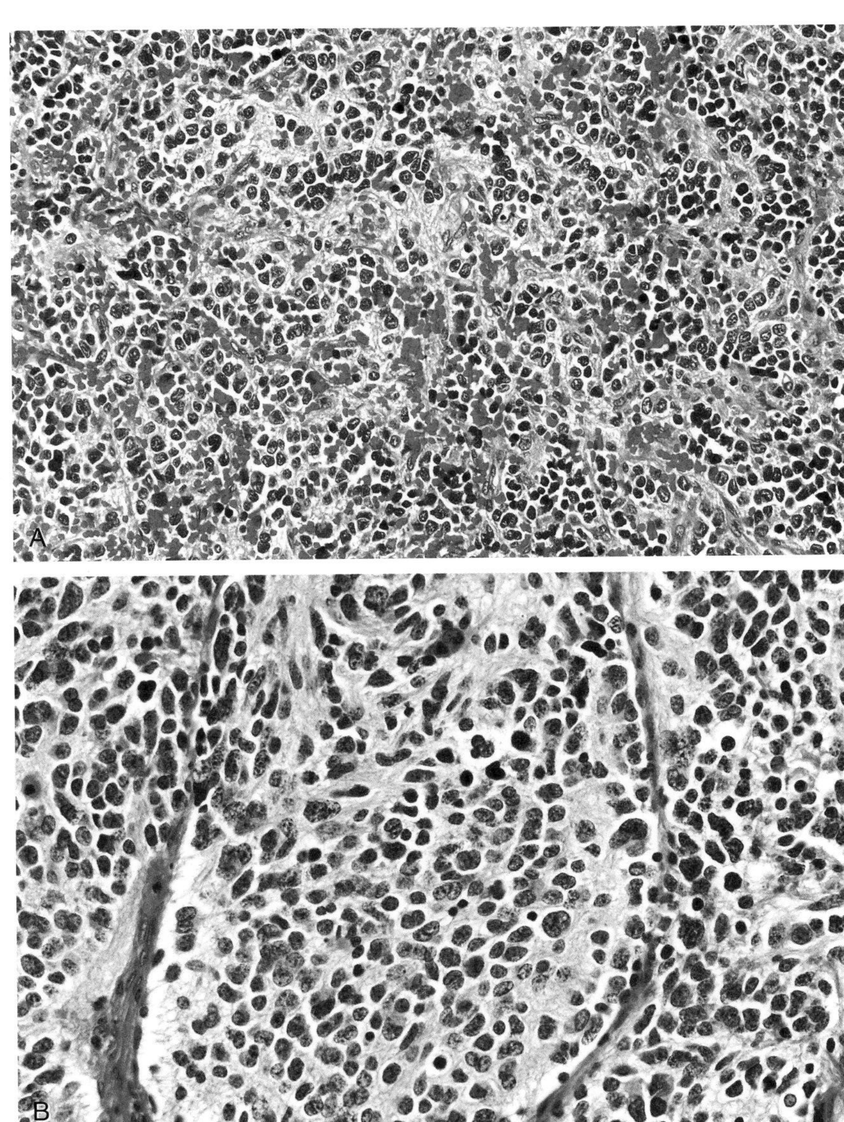

FIGURE 33-20. Low-power (A) and high-power (B) views of a poorly differentiated neuroblastoma composed of a sheet-like proliferation of monotonous small round cells with little cytoplasm.

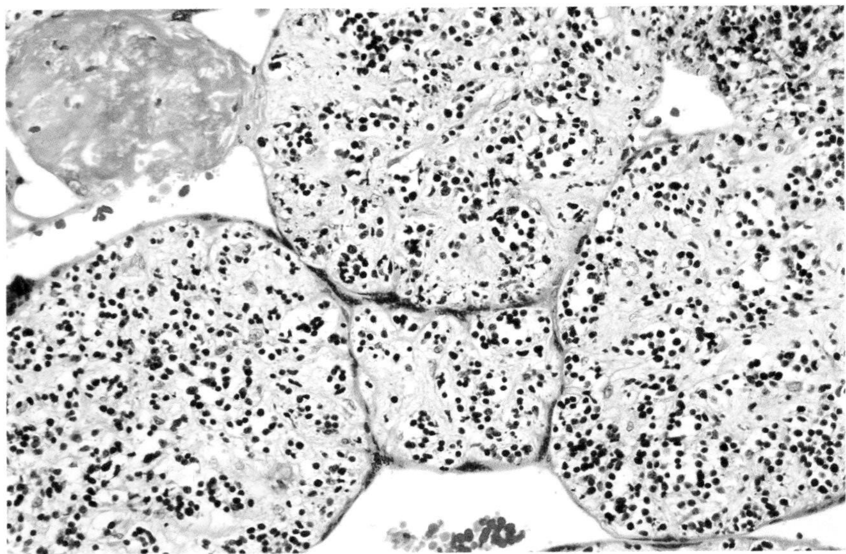

FIGURE 33-21. Congenital neuroblastoma involving the placenta. Tumor cells resemble nucleated erythrocytes and may be misinterpreted as evidence of erythroblastosis fetalis.

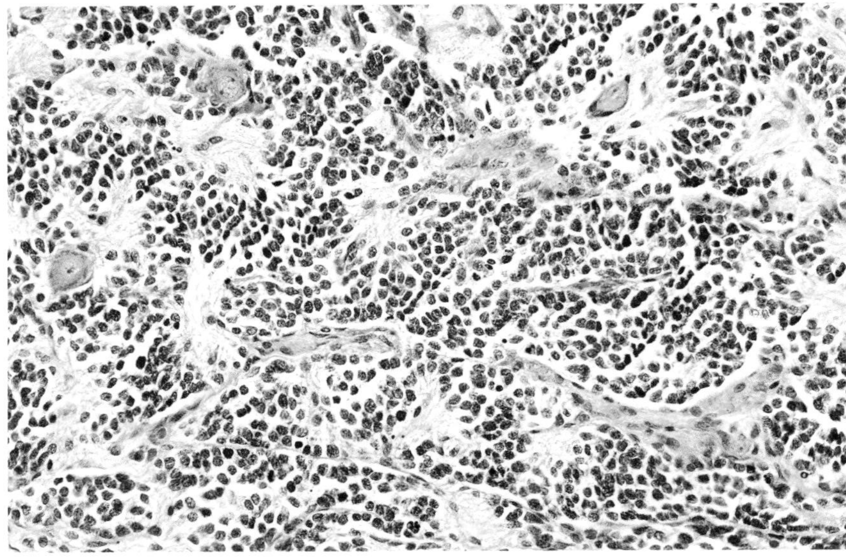

FIGURE 33-22. Poorly differentiated neuroblastoma. In this area of the tumor, the neuroblasts have attenuated cytoplasmic processes that are polarized toward a central point to form Homer Wright rosettes.

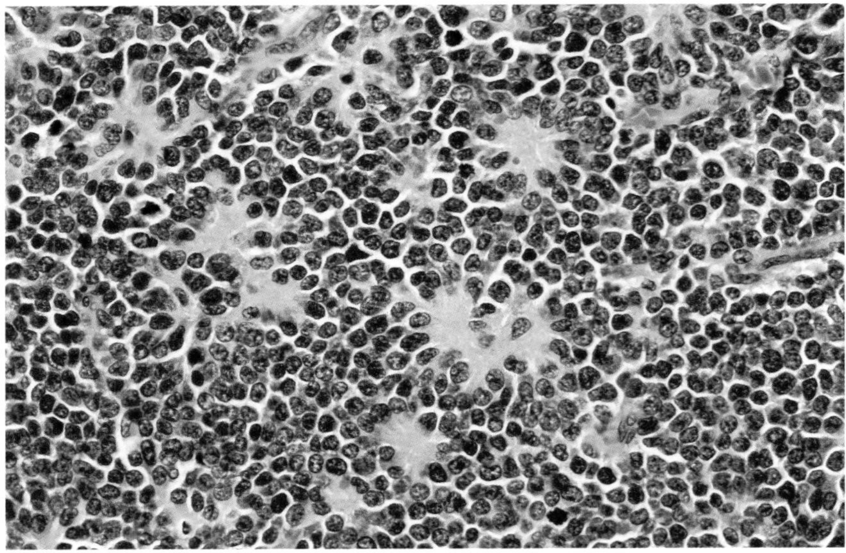

FIGURE 33-23. Homer Wright rosettes in a poorly differentiated neuroblastoma.

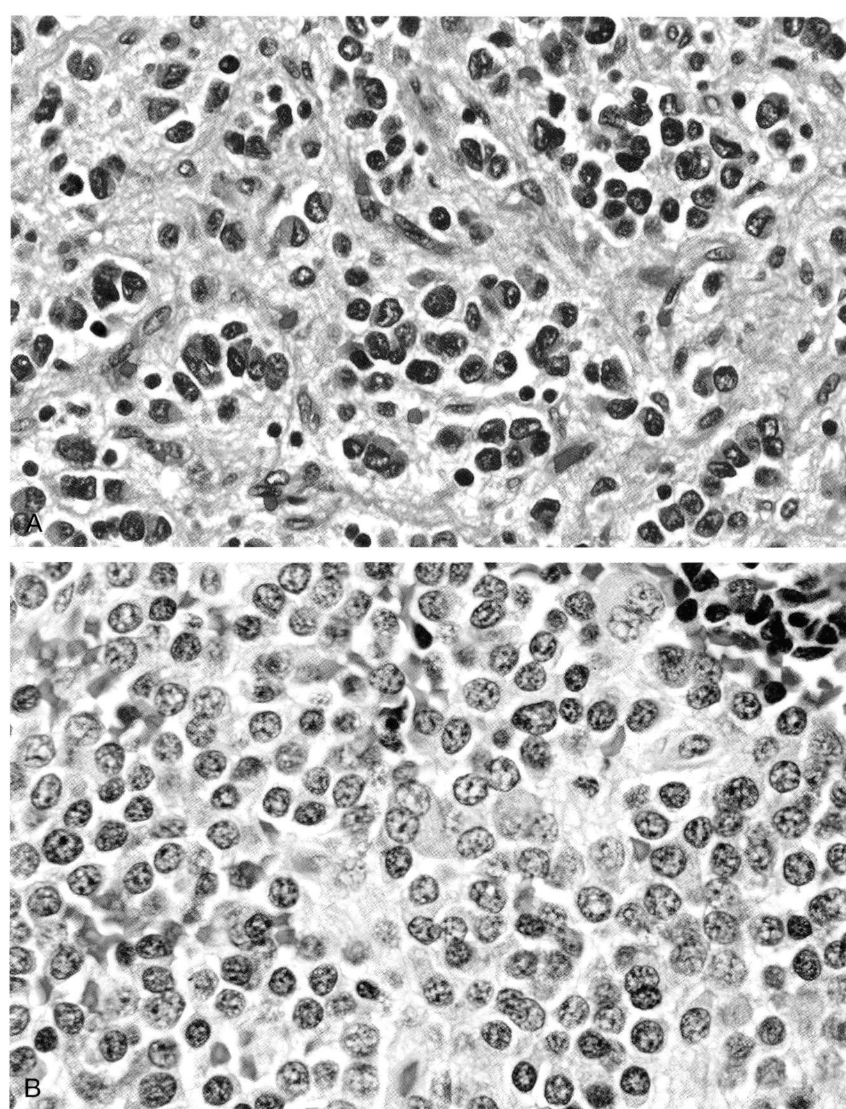

FIGURE 33-24. (A) Neuroblastoma composed predominantly of small round cells with little cytoplasm. Rare cells have a discernible rim of eosinophilic cytoplasm suggesting incipient ganglionic differentiation. (B) Neuroblastoma with focal ganglionic differentiation. A binucleated cell is apparent in the center of this photomicrograph.

TABLE 33-4 Cytogenetic Findings in Round Cell Tumors

TUMOR	CYTOGENETICS	GENES
Ewing family of tumors	t(11;22)(q24;q12)	*FLI1/EWSR1*
	t(21;22)(q22; q12)	*ERG/EWSR1*
	t(7;22)(p22;q12)	*ETV1/EWSR1*
	t(17;22)(q12;q12)	*E1AF/EWSR1*
	t(2;22)(q33;q12)	*FEV/EWSR1*
Alveolar rhabdomyosarcoma	t(2;13)(q35;q14)	*PAX3/FOXO1A*
	t(1;13)(p36;q14)	*PAX7/FOXO1A*
Neuroblastoma	$1p^-$	
Desmoplastic small round cell tumor	t(11;22)(p13;q12)	*WT1/EWSR1*
Round cell liposarcoma	t(12;16)(q13;p11)	*DDIT3/FUS*
	t(12;22)(q13;q12)	*DDIT3/EWSR1*
Poorly differentiated synovial sarcoma	t(X;18)(p11;q11)	*SS18/SSX-1 or SS18/SSX-2*

Alveolar rhabdomyosarcoma may display densely packed cellular areas, especially at its periphery, but, in general, its nuclei contain more chromatin and tend to be more irregular in outline. When multiple sections are examined, the solid round cell areas are nearly always associated with areas showing loss of cellular cohesion and a distinct alveolar pattern, multinucleated giant cells with marginally placed nuclei, and, in about 20% to 30% of cases, eosinophilic cells characteristic of rhabdomyoblasts with or without cross-striations. Furthermore, most rhabdomyosarcomas show positive immunostaining for myogenic markers, including myogenin and MyoD1. It must also be kept in mind that some

TABLE 33-5 Immunohistochemical Analysis of Round Cell Tumors

	CD99	TDT	MYOGENIN	CAM 5.2	DESMIN	WT1
EFT	+	–	–	20%	–	–
A-RMS	15%	–	+	50%	+	–
Lymphoma	>90%	+	–	–	–	–
DSRCT	20%	–	–	+	+	+

EFT, Ewing family of tumors; A-RMS, alveolar rhabdomyosarcoma; DSRCT, desmoplastic small round cell tumor.

alveolar rhabdomyosarcomas exhibit membranous staining for CD99 (Table 33-5). Detection of either t(1;13) or t(2;13) characteristic of alveolar rhabdomyosarcoma by cytogenetic or molecular genetic techniques is exceedingly useful for distinguishing alveolar rhabdomyosarcoma from EFT. The FISH method is preferred, using paraffin-embedded tissue and a probe for *FOXO1A* on a routine basis.

Malignant (non-Hodgkin) lymphoma is often suspected because of the undifferentiated appearance of the tumor cells. This diagnosis can be ruled out, in most cases, if attention is paid to the lobular arrangement and monotonous uniformity of the nuclei in EFT. The presence or absence of lymph node involvement may be significant because lymph node metastasis of EFT is rare. Furthermore, malignant lymphomas almost always express leukocyte common antigen. Because CD99 is found in most T-cell lymphoblastic lymphomas and some lymphoblastic lymphomas do not express leukocyte common antigen, a panel of antibodies that include T- and B-cell markers (e.g., CD20, CD79a, and TdT) to avoid an erroneous diagnosis is used routinely.

The *desmoplastic small round cell tumor* (DSRCT) typically presents in young adults, usually men, as a large intra-abdominal mass with multiple peritoneal implants. Rare examples of this tumor have also been described in the pleura, central nervous system, and peripheral soft tissues. Histologically, it is composed of sharply outlined islands of tumor cells separated by a desmoplastic stroma containing myofibroblasts and prominent vascularity. The tumor nests often show peripheral palisading and central necrosis. The individual tumor cells are relatively uniform, small, and round to oval with hyperchromatic nuclei, inconspicuous nucleoli, and scanty cytoplasm. Immunohistochemically, these lesions have a polyphenotypic profile, with coexpression of cytokeratin, vimentin, desmin, and neuron-specific enolase. The pattern of desmin immunoreactivity is unique, with a characteristic perinuclear pattern of staining. The majority of cases are also positive with antibodies directed against the carboxy-terminus of the WT1 protein. Up to 20% of these tumors can show membranous CD99 immunoreactivity. This tumor also has a unique cytogenetic abnormality: t(11;22)(p13;q22). The breakpoint on chromosome 22 is the same as that seen in EFT, but the locus on chromosome 11 involves the Wilms tumor gene (*WT1*), and therefore detection of an *EWSR1-WT1* fusion by RT-PCR is quite helpful. In the case of FISH, using dual-color, break-apart probes for *EWSR1*, one must correlate the FISH results with the clinical, morphologic, and immunohistochemical features because *EWSR1* aberrations do not distinguish DSRCT from EFT.

Metastatic pulmonary small cell carcinoma and *cutaneous neuroendocrine carcinoma* (*Merkel cell carcinoma*) must be considered in the differential diagnosis, particularly when the tumor occurs in patients older than 45 years and is located superficially. In general, metastatic pulmonary small cell carcinoma can be ruled out if a thorough clinical history and radiographic studies fail to reveal pulmonary involvement. Immunohistochemically, most pulmonary small cell carcinomas express TTF1, a marker that is absent in EFT.[88] The cells of Merkel cell carcinoma have large, closely packed nuclei and little cytoplasm, and they are frequently arranged in a trabecular pattern. This tumor is chiefly located in the dermis or subcutis, and two-thirds occur in patients over 60 years of age. Although cutaneous EFTs exist, they generally occur in much younger patients, with a peak incidence during the second decade of life. Immunohistochemically, virtually all Merkel cell carcinomas have a characteristic globular or punctate pattern of staining with antibodies to low-molecular-weight cytokeratins, and almost all of these tumors express cytokeratin 20, a marker generally absent in metastatic small cell carcinomas and EFT. Finally, most (but not all) pulmonary small cell carcinomas and Merkel cell carcinomas are negative for CD99.

Mesenchymal chondrosarcoma is a rare neoplasm that typically occurs in young adults, with an extraosseous location in approximately 20% of cases. Histologically, the neoplasm is characterized by a biphasic appearance of small nests or nodules of well-differentiated cartilage intimately admixed with undifferentiated round cells, often arranged around a hemangiopericytoma-like vascular pattern. Although the biphasic appearance is characteristic, it may not be seen on a small biopsy specimen, making distinction from EFT difficult. Immunohistochemically, mesenchymal chondrosarcoma usually expresses neural markers such as neuron-specific enolase and S-100 protein. The majority of mesenchymal chondrosarcomas show strong membranous CD99 immunoreactivity, adding to the difficulty in distinguishing this tumor from EFT, but these tumors lack *EWSR1* aberrations.

Small cell osteosarcoma, a rare variant of osteosarcoma, typically occurs in young patients and is composed of cells similar to those seen in EFT. The diagnosis can be made if osteoid is identified only, but osteoid may be only focally present in the tumor and is often not identified in small biopsy specimens. Most tumors express neural markers, including neuron-specific enolase and CD57, and some express cytokeratins, actins, and rarely CD99, but these lesions lack *EWSR1* aberrations.

Poorly differentiated synovial sarcoma is composed of small round cells often arranged around a hemangiopericytoma-like vasculature. However, unless one sees other areas of biphasic or monophasic synovial sarcoma, this lesion may be difficult to distinguish from EFT. Because only approximately 50% of poorly differentiated synovial sarcomas express cytokeratins and many show membranous CD99 immunoreactivity, the immunohistochemical distinction of poorly differentiated synovial sarcoma from EFT can be difficult. Cytokeratin subsets have been found to be useful in this regard because 60% to 70% of poorly differentiated synovial sarcomas stain for cytokeratins 7 and 19, whereas EFT rarely, if ever, express these antigens.[89] Furthermore, almost all cases of synovial sarcoma, including poorly differentiated tumors, show strong nuclear expression of TLE1, a marker that is not found in EFT. Finally, detection of t(X;18) by conventional cytogenetics or the resultant *SSX1-SS18* or *SSX2-SS18* fusion by molecular techniques serves as an important diagnostic aid in these cases as well.

Clinical Behavior and Therapy

Until the introduction of modern therapy, the outlook for patients with EFT was bleak, and only a small percentage of patients with this tumor survived. For instance, in the series of extraskeletal ES reported by Angervall and Enzinger[4] in 1975, 22 of the 35 patients with follow-up information died of metastatic disease, most commonly to the lung and skeleton. Similarly, many of the larger studies of PNET suggested that these tumors are highly aggressive neoplasms that rapidly give rise to metastatic disease and death. Jurgens et al.[90] cited a survival rate of approximately 50% at 3 years, whereas Kushner et al.[16] found that only 25% of patients with tumors larger than 5 cm were alive at 24 months. Although several older studies suggested that patients with PNET had a worse prognosis than those with extraskeletal ES, others have not found this to be the case. The data on this subject are difficult to interpret given the differences in diagnostic criteria for classifying tumors as extraskeletal ES or PNET, as previously discussed.

Parham et al.[76] studied 63 EFT from patients who were treated uniformly to determine the prognostic significance of neuroectodermal differentiation. Tumors were classified as PNET if they showed rosettes or immunohistochemical expression of at least two neural markers (or both). Using another classification scheme, tumors were classified as PNET if they showed rosettes or immunohistochemical expression of at least four neural markers (or both). Finally, using a third classification scheme, tumors that showed ultrastructural evidence of neural differentiation were classified as PNET. Using any of the previous classification schemes, the authors were unable to show any significant difference in clinical outcome for patients with or without neuroectodermal differentiation.

The prognosis for patients with EFT has steadily improved. About 75% of patients present with localized disease and the combination of surgery and/or radiotherapy and systemic chemotherapy result in a cure rate near 75% in this group.[91,92] However, little progress has been made for those patients who present with metastatic disease. The role of megatherapy (myeloablative high-dose chemotherapy, with or without total body irradiation following by stem cell infusion) in the treatment of metastatic disease remains unclear.[93,94] A number of ongoing clinical trials through the Children's Oncology Group and European Cooperative Groups continue to assess new potentially more efficacious protocols. With increased understanding of the molecular pathways, opportunities for targeted therapy have emerged. Potential targets can be broadly classified into those related to the *EWSR1-ETS* gene fusion (e.g., STAT3,[95] laminin β3[96]), receptor tyrosine kinases and associated signaling pathways (e.g., IGFR,[97] PDGF[98]), the p53 and retinoblastoma pathways,[99] angiogenesis,[100] and apoptosis.[101] Minimal residual disease can be detected in peripheral blood or bone marrow by RT-PCR, and detection of fusion transcript-positive cells in the blood seems to predict disease progression.[102]

Key prognostic factors that adversely influence the outcome of the disease are the presence of metastatic disease at the time of initial diagnosis, large tumor size, extensive necrosis (filigree pattern), central axis tumors, and poor response to initial chemotherapy.[91,103,104] Several studies have found that the type of *EWSR1-FLI1* fusion may be prognostically relevant because patients with type 1 fusions have been reported to have longer disease-free survival than those with other fusion types. De Alava et al.[64] found that patients with type 1 fusions have tumors with lower proliferative rates and generally respond better to chemotherapy. However, Ginsberg et al.[105] found no significant clinical differences between those with *EWSR1-FLI1* or *EWSR1-ERG* fusions. Several recent gene expression profile studies have identified expression profiles that are associated with the presence of metastases, prognosis, and response to therapy.[106-108]

EXTRASKELETAL MYXOID CHONDROSARCOMA

Extraskeletal myxoid chondrosarcoma is a morphologically distinctive neoplasm characterized by a multinodular architecture and cords or clusters of chondroblast-like cells deposited in an abundant myxoid matrix. It is categorized by the World Health Organization (WHO) as a tumor of uncertain differentiation because there is a paucity of convincing evidence of cartilaginous differentiation.

Extraskeletal myxoid chondrosarcoma has also been reported as *chordoid sarcoma*[109] and by Hajdu et al.[110] as *tendosynovial sarcoma*, a term coined for a group of neoplasms that have a close association with tendosynovial structures, including synovial sarcoma, epithelioid sarcoma, clear cell sarcoma, and extraskeletal myxoid chondrosarcoma. Myxoid chondrosarcoma occurs primarily in the deep tissues of the extremities, especially the musculature. Because a morphologically similar tumor also occurs in bone, radiographic examination, CT, or MRI is necessary to establish its soft tissue origin. It is a relatively slow-growing tumor but has a propensity for local recurrence and eventually pulmonary metastasis, sometimes many years after the initial diagnosis.

Clinical Findings

This tumor is quite uncommon and accounts for less than 3% of all soft tissue sarcomas.[111] It most commonly arises in patients older than 35 years, and only a few cases have been encountered in children and adolescents.[112] Most series have found a peak incidence during the fifth or sixth decades of life.[113-115] Men are affected about twice as often as women. The clinical signs and symptoms are nonspecific. Most patients present with a slowly growing, deep-seated mass that causes pain and tenderness in approximately one-third of cases. Complications such as ulceration and intratumoral hemorrhage may be encountered with large tumors. The duration of symptoms varies considerably, ranging from a few weeks to several years. Some patients have a history of trauma prior to discovery of the tumor, but as with other sarcomas the significance of this finding remains uncertain and is, in all likelihood, coincidental.

More than two-thirds of the tumors occur in the proximal extremities and limb girdles, especially the thigh and popliteal fossa, similar to myxoid liposarcoma.[113,116,117] Most are deep-seated, although occasional tumors are confined to the subcutis; the latter may be difficult to distinguish from myxoid forms of chondroma. Rare examples have been described in unusual locations, including the mediastinum,[118] vulva,[119] central nervous system,[120] and heart.[121] Radiography, CT, and MRI show a soft tissue mass with no distinctive radiologic features that would set the tumor apart from other types of soft tissue sarcoma.[122]

Pathologic Findings

Macroscopically, the neoplasm is a soft to firm, ovoid, lobulated to nodular, circumscribed mass surrounded by a dense fibrous pseudocapsule. On section, it has a gelatinous, gray to tan-brown surface, its color largely dependent on the extent of hemorrhage, a frequent feature of the tumor (Fig. 33-25). Occasionally, hemorrhage is so prominent that the tumor is mistaken for a hematoma. Highly cellular higher-grade tumors often have a fleshy consistency.

The size of the tumor varies from a few centimeters to 15 cm or more; most, however, are 4 to 7 cm in greatest diameter at the time of excision. Meis-Kindblom et al.[113] reported a size range from 1.1 to 25.0 cm and a median tumor size of 7 cm.

Microscopically, a characteristic multinodular pattern is clearly evident at low magnification (Fig. 33-26). The individual tumor nodules consist of round or slightly elongated cells of uniform shape and size separated by variable amounts of mucoid material (Figs. 33-27 to 33-31). The individual cells have small hyperchromatic nuclei and a narrow rim of deeply eosinophilic cytoplasm reminiscent of chondroblasts (Fig. 33-32). Occasional cells show cytoplasmic vacuolization. Unlike chondrosarcoma of bone, differentiated cartilage cells with distinct lacunae are rare. Mitotic figures are rare in typical cases but may be numerous in less well differentiated and more cellular forms of the tumor.[123,124]

Characteristically, the individual cells are arranged in short anastomosing cords, strands, or pseudoacini, often creating a lace-like appearance. Less frequently, the cellular elements are disposed in small loosely textured whorls or aggregates, reminiscent of an epithelial neoplasm. Rarely, cellular foci composed of fibroblastic/myofibroblastic spindle-shaped cells are present.[125] Indeed, if these features prevail throughout the tumor, a definitive diagnosis of chondrosarcoma may not be possible. Although most extraskeletal myxoid chondrosarcomas are highly myxoid tumors, a distinct subset is hypercellular with less myxoid stroma between the neoplastic cells; they are composed of sheets of large cells with vesicular nuclei and prominent nucleoli and are referred to as the *cellular variant of extraskeletal myxoid chondrosarcoma* (Fig. 33-33).[113,123] These tumors are best diagnosed by identifying typical less-cellular areas of extraskeletal myxoid chondrosarcoma or by cytogenetics/molecular genetics (discussed later). Some tumors are composed of a cellular proliferation of relatively small round cells closely resembling EFT (Fig. 33-34). Even more rarely, typical extraskeletal myxoid chondrosarcomas are associated with or progress to a high-grade pleomorphic sarcoma (dedifferentiated extraskeletal myxoid chondrosarcoma),[126] and still others may have rhabdoid features characterized by cells with large paranuclear hyaline inclusions.[127-130] Kohashi et al.[128] found loss of expression of SMARCB1 in 3 of 4 cases with rhabdoid features. Secondary changes such as fibrosis and hemorrhage are common, but calcification or bone formation is rare.

In the more typical tumors, the extracellular mucinous material is abundant and consists largely of chondroitin 4-sulfate, chondroitin 6-sulfate, and keratan sulfate.[131] It stains deeply with the colloidal iron stain and the Alcian blue

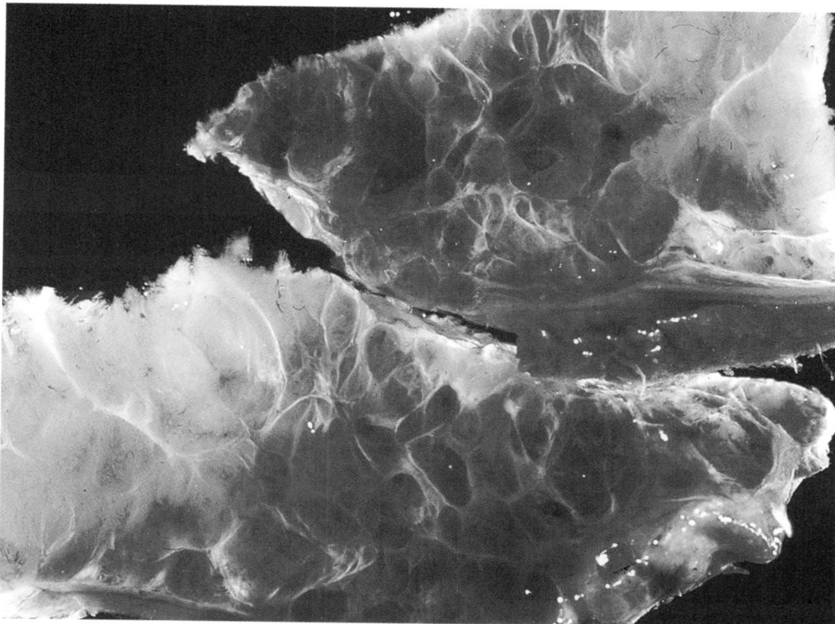

FIGURE 33-25. Gross appearance of an extraskeletal myxoid chondrosarcoma with a characteristic gelatinous appearance and a multinodular growth pattern. The dark appearance of some of the nodules is the result of hemorrhage.

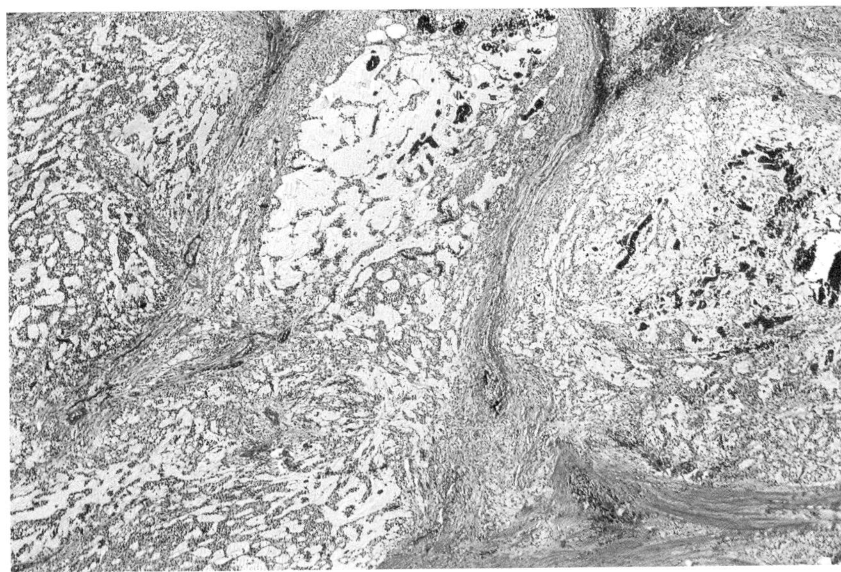

FIGURE 33-26. Low-power view of an extraskeletal myxoid chondrosarcoma with a characteristic nodular arrangement.

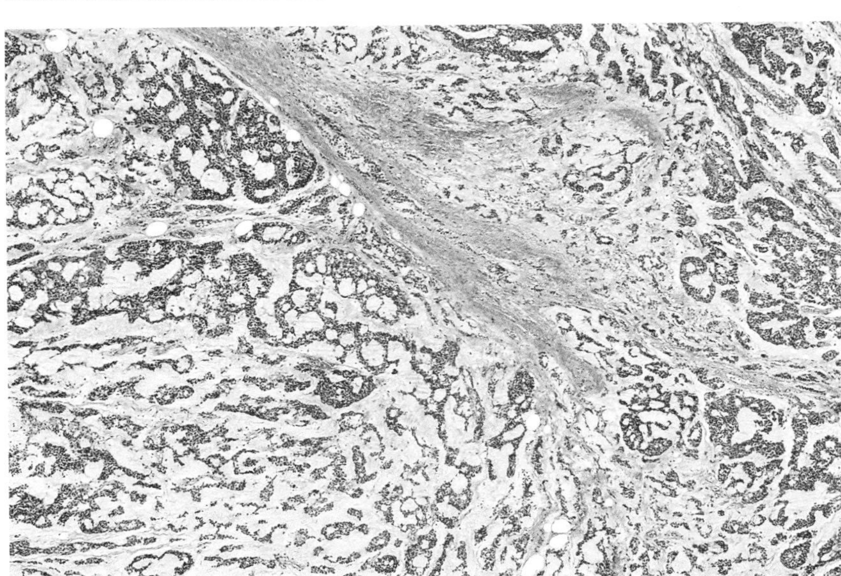

FIGURE 33-27. Extraskeletal myxoid chondrosarcoma. Cords of eosinophilic cells are deposited in an abundant myxoid stroma.

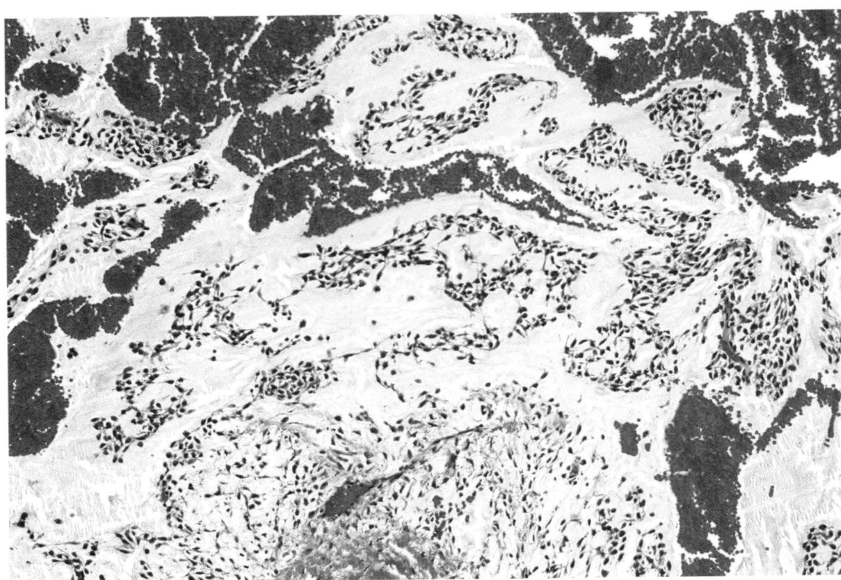

FIGURE 33-28. Characteristic alignment of tumor cells in strands and cords separated by large amounts of mucoid material in an extraskeletal myxoid chondrosarcoma. Note the areas of hemorrhage, a characteristic feature of this tumor.

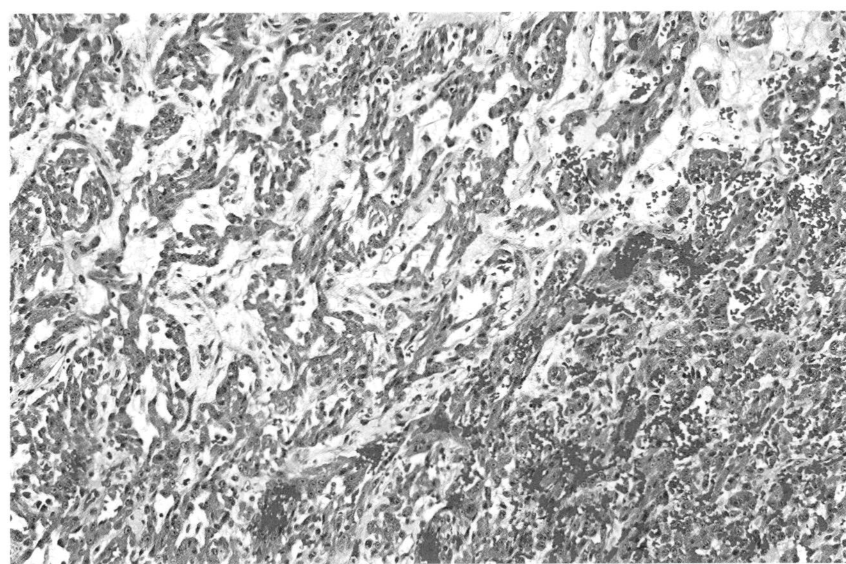

FIGURE 33-29. Extraskeletal myxoid chondrosarcoma. Cords of spindle-shaped cells with deeply eosinophilic cytoplasm are separated by mucoid material.

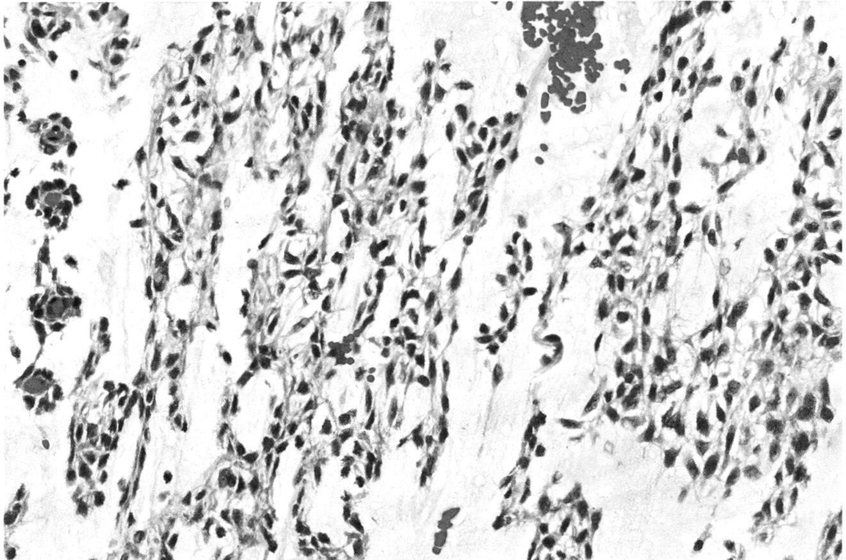

FIGURE 33-30. Extraskeletal myxoid chondrosarcoma with strands of small eosinophilic cells widely separated by mucoid material.

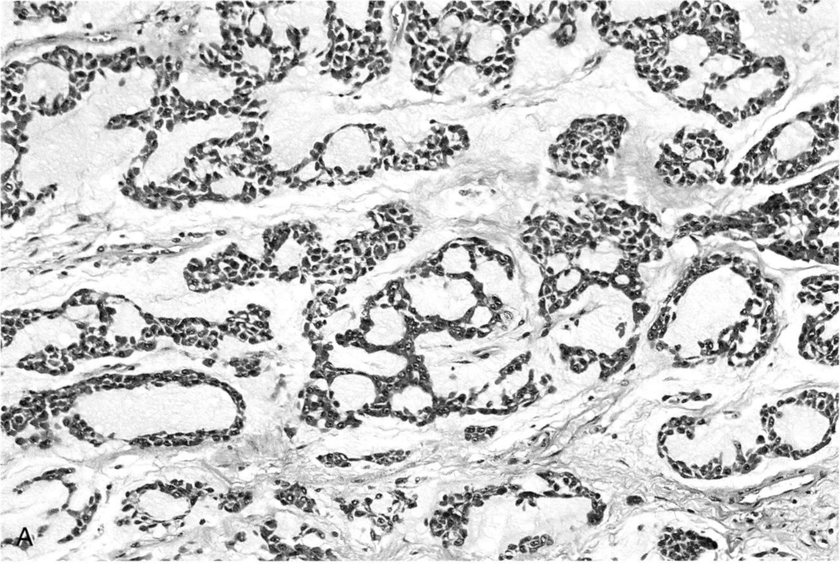

FIGURE 33-31. (A) Extraskeletal myxoid chondrosarcoma composed of cells arranged in a pseudoacinar pattern.

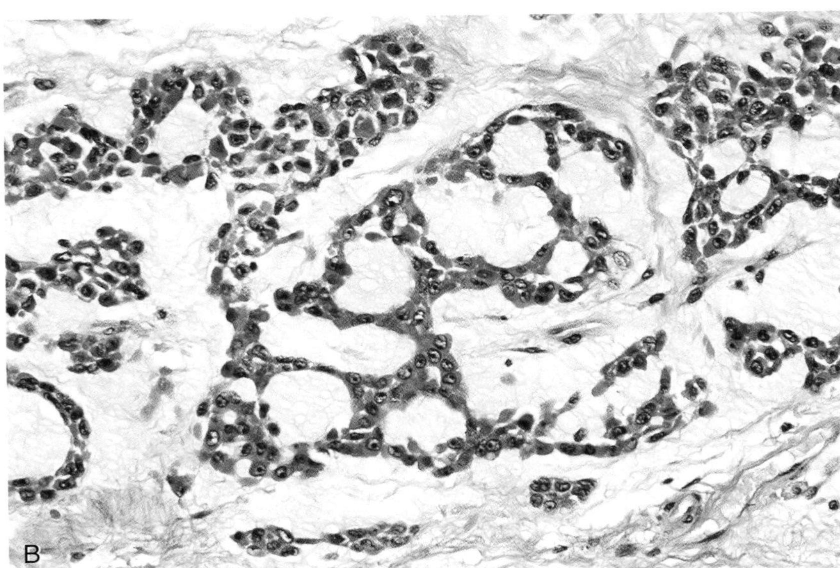

FIGURE 33-31, cont'd. (B) High-power view of densely eosinophilic epithelioid cells arranged in pseudoacini.

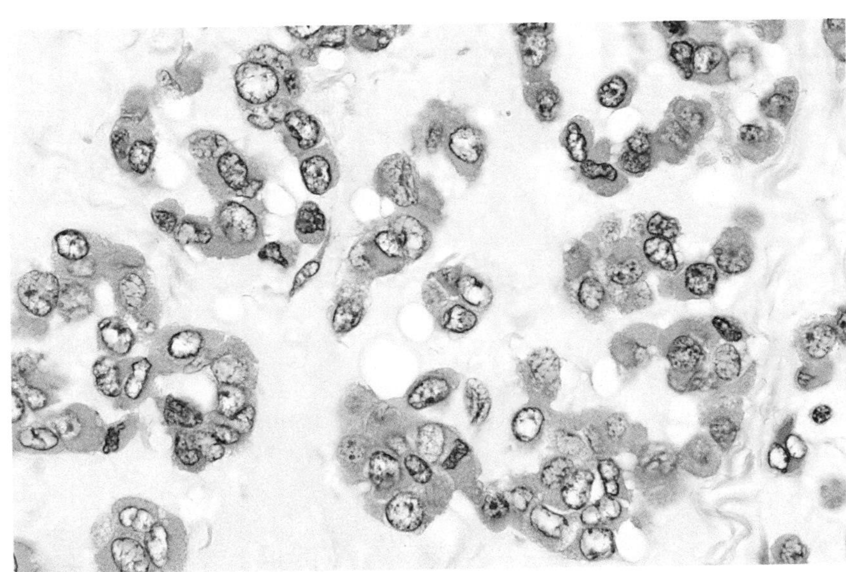

FIGURE 33-32. High-power view of neoplastic cells in an extraskeletal myxoid chondrosarcoma. The cells are surrounded by a rim of deeply eosinophilic cytoplasm.

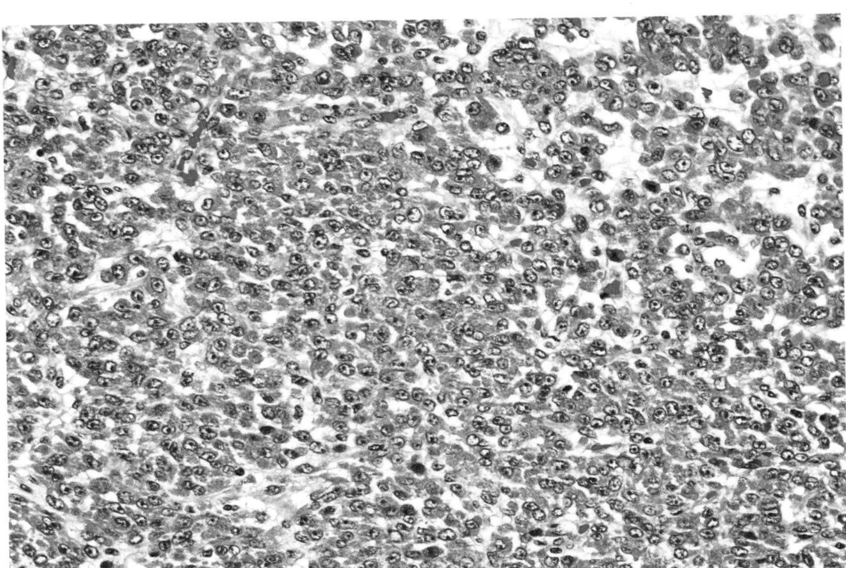

FIGURE 33-33. Cellular variant of an extraskeletal myxoid chondrosarcoma composed of large cells with vesicular nuclei and deeply eosinophilic cytoplasm. Other areas of typical myxoid chondrosarcoma were present in this tumor.

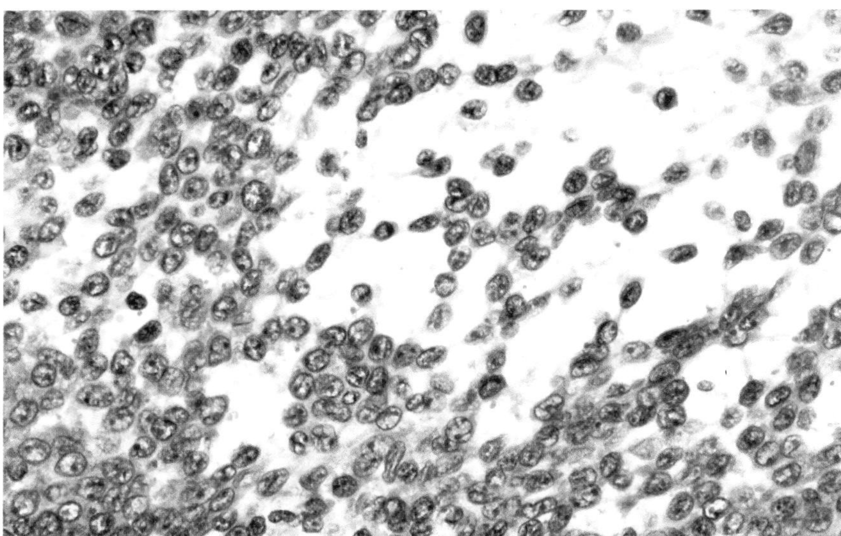

FIGURE 33-34. Cellular variant of extraskeletal myxoid chondrosarcoma composed of small round cells mimicking an extraskeletal EFT.

preparation; unlike other richly mucinous soft tissue tumors (with the exception of myxochondroma and chordoma), the staining reaction is not inhibited by pretreating the sections with hyaluronidase.

Immunohistochemical Findings

The cells of myxoid chondrosarcoma stain strongly for vimentin, but this is the only marker that is consistently positive. In contrast to true chondroid neoplasms, the majority of these tumors show an absence or only focal staining for S-100 protein.[132] As with many other types of sarcoma, rare cases show focal immunoreactivity for cytokeratins.[113] In addition, almost 30% of cases show scattered cells that are epithelial membrane antigen (EMA)-positive.[116] Some authors have found evidence of neuroendocrine differentiation, as evidenced by staining for neuron-specific enolase, chromogranin, or synaptophysin and/or identification of dense-core granules on ultrastructural examination.[133-135] Interestingly, the presence of neuroendocrine features has been associated with the relatively uncommon t(9;17)(q22;q11).[135,136] Others have found these cells to express microtubule-associated proteins-2 and class III β-tubulin, which are components of microtubules and are specifically localized in neurons and their derivatives.[137,138] This has been taken as further evidence of neural/neuroendocrine differentiation in at least some examples of extraskeletal myxoid chondrosarcoma. Some cases also express CD117.[139]

Cytogenetic and Molecular Genetic Findings

Extraskeletal myxoid chondrosarcoma is characterized most commonly by a balanced t(9;22)(q22;q12), which fuses *EWSR1* with *NR4A3* (also known as *NOR1*, *CHN*, or *TEC*).[140] Approximately 70% to 75% of cases harbor this translocation, but variant translocations include t(9;17)(q22;q11) that results in a *TAF15* (also known as *RBP56* or *TAF2N*) fusion with *NR4A3*,[136,141] a t(9;15)(q22;q21) resulting in a *NR4A3-TCF12*,[141] or even a t(3;9)(q12;q22) resulting in an *NR4A3-TFG* fusion.[142] Brody et al.[143] did not detect the *NR4A3-EWSR1* fusion in four cases of skeletal myxoid chondrosarcoma, suggesting that this lesion is pathogenetically distinct from its extraskeletal counterpart. Molecular assays using paraffin-embedded tissues (RT-PCR or FISH) can be extremely helpful in confirming this diagnosis.[136,144-146] In a study by Wang et al.,[146] 14 of 15 (93%) cases showed *EWSR1* aberrations by FISH.

The molecular consequences of these translocations are now being unraveled. Expression profiling studies have identified potential downstream targets, including *DKK1*, *NMB*, *DNER*, *CLCN3*, and *DEF6*.[147] Several studies, including an expression profiling study of genetically confirmed cases, have found high levels of expression of peroxisome proliferator-activated receptors-gamma (*PPARG*), a potential therapeutic target.[148,149]

Differential Diagnosis

Extraskeletal myxoid chondrosarcoma may be difficult to distinguish from a number of benign or malignant chondroid-like or myxoid lesions, including the *myxoid variant of extraskeletal (soft part) chondroma*. Extraskeletal chondromas usually occur in the soft tissues of the hands or feet—unusual locations for extraskeletal myxoid chondrosarcoma. They tend to be smaller, less cellular lesions without evidence of *EWSR1* aberrations. *Chondromyxoid fibroma* rarely occurs as a periosteal tumor or in soft tissue as secondary tissue implantations. It can be recognized by its greater degree of cellular pleomorphism and condensation of the tumor cells underneath a narrow, richly vascularized fibrous band that borders the individual tumor nodules. In addition, there may be multinucleated giant cells and foci of calcification or ossification, features rarely seen in myxoid chondrosarcomas.

Juxtacortical (parosteal) chondrosarcoma lacks the myxoid component and shows a broad attachment to the perichondrium or periosteum of the involved bone, sometimes with invasion of the underlying cortex and cortical irregularities on radiographs. *Chordoma*, especially its myxoid form, enters the differential diagnosis, but this diagnosis is unlikely if the tumor occurs outside of its usual location in the sacrococcygeal region, the base of the skull, or the cervical spine. Extraskeletal myxoid chondrosarcoma shows no radiographic evidence of bone involvement and lacks multivacuolated, physaliphorous tumor cells. Immunohistochemically, chordoma coexpresses S-100 protein, brachyury, and markers of epithelial differentiation (EMA and cytokeratins, particularly cytokeratins 8 and 19).

Myxoma and myxoid liposarcoma must also be considered in the differential diagnosis (Table 33-6). *Myxoma* displays a similar paucity of vascular structures, but it is less cellular because the cytologically bland cells are separated by abundant myxoid stroma. *Myxoid liposarcoma*, on the other hand, displays a striking plexiform vascular pattern and contains typical lipoblasts, especially at the margin of the tumor lobules. S-100 protein is found in approximately 40% of myxoid liposarcomas and does not help distinguish this tumor from extraskeletal myxoid chondrosarcoma. In difficult cases, molecular genetic analysis (RT-PCR or FISH) evaluating for aberrations of *EWSR1*, *FUS*, and *DDIT3* can be quite helpful (Table 33-7).

Still another problem is the distinction of extraskeletal myxoid chondrosarcoma from benign and malignant *mixed tumor/myoepithelioma*. These tumors display a curious modulation between epithelioid and spindled areas. Although the immunophenotype of deeply situated myoepithelial lesions is incompletely defined, this diagnosis is reserved for lesions that clearly express epithelial and myoepithelial markers, including cytokeratin, S-100 protein, calponin, and sometimes p63 and GFAP (Table 33-8). Recently, it has become clear that up to 50% of these tumors harbor *EWSR1* aberrations that can add further confusion in its distinction from extraskeletal myxoid chondrosarcoma.[150]

Myxopapillary ependymoma can be distinguished by its characteristic location in the sacrum, perivascular growth, positivity for GFAP, and the presence of glial-type microfilaments.

Discussion

Generally, extraskeletal myxoid chondrosarcoma is a relatively slow-growing tumor that recurs and eventually metastasizes in many cases. Of the 31 patients in the series by Enzinger and Shiraki,[114] 20 were alive at last follow-up, but 6 of these patients developed recurrence, and 4 died of metastatic disease. In the much larger study by Meis-Kindblom et al.,[113] local recurrences and metastasis developed in 48% and 16% of patients, respectively. Estimated 5-, 10-, and 15-year survival rates were 90%, 70%, and 60%, respectively. Ten-year survival rates ranging from 78% to 88% have been reported in more recent studies, but 10-year disease-free survival rates are much lower, ranging from 14% to 36%.[116,117,151]

Late recurrence and metastasis are common. In the series from the Armed Forces Institute of Pathology (AFIP), one patient developed a recurrence 18 years after the initial excision; in another case, pulmonary metastasis became evident 10 years after surgical removal of the tumor and 4 years after

TABLE 33-6 Light Microscopic Features of Extraskeletal Myxoid Chondrosarcoma and Differential Diagnostic Considerations

DIAGNOSIS	CELLULARITY	VASCULARITY	PLEOMORPHISM	MATRIX
Myxoma	1+	1+	0	HA
Myxoid liposarcoma	1+	3+ (fine)	1+	HA
Myxofibrosarcoma	1+ to 2+	3+ (coarse)	2+ to 3+	HA
Myxoid chondrosarcoma	1+ (cords)	1+	1+	CS

HA, hyaluronic acid; CS, chondroitin sulfate.

TABLE 33-7 Molecular Genetic Alterations in Extraskeletal Myxoid Chondrosarcoma and Other Myxoid Sarcomas in the Differential Diagnosis

DIAGNOSIS	TRANSLOCATIONS	GENES
Myxoid chondrosarcoma	t(9;22)(q22;q12)	*NR4A3; EWSR1*
	t(9;17)(q22;q11)	*NR4A3; RBP56*
Myxoid liposarcoma	t(12;16)(q13;p11)	*DDIT3; FUS*
	t(12;22)(q13;q12)	*DDIT3; EWSR1*
Myxofibrosarcoma	None characteristic	
Low-grade fibromyxoid sarcoma	t(7;16)(q34;p11)	*CREB3L2; FUS*
	t(11;16)(p11;p11)	*CREB3L1; FUS*

TABLE 33-8 Immunohistochemical Features of Extraskeletal Myxoid Chondrosarcoma and Differential Diagnostic Considerations

TUMOR	CAM5.2	CK7	CK19	EMA	S-100	CEA	ACTIN
Myxoid chondrosarcoma	–	–	–	–	±	–	–
Chordoma	+	±	+	+	+	+	–
Myxoid liposarcoma	–	–	–	–	±	–	–
Mixed tumor/myoepithelioma	+	–	–	+	+	–	±

removal of a regional lymph node metastasis.[114] The most frequent metastatic sites are the lungs, soft tissues, and lymph nodes.

Radical local excision with or without adjuvant radiotherapy seems to be the treatment of choice. Good results with high-dose irradiation have been reported,[109,117] but chemotherapy has not been found to be efficacious.[115] In a recent study of 87 patients with extraskeletal myxoid chondrosarcoma, Drilon et al.[115] found that 13% of patients presented with metastases, but for those that did not, 37% developed local recurrences a median of 3.2 years following excision and 26% developed distal recurrences. The 5-, 10-, and 15-year overall survival rates were 82%, 65%, and 58%, respectively. Twenty-one patients received chemotherapy, but no significant radiologic or clinical responses were found. Therefore, the best chance at cure is with early wide local excision (with or without radiation) for localized disease.[115,151]

Although there are some cases in which aggressive clinical behavior could be suggested by histologic features, such as high cellularity associated with high nuclear grade,[123] the largest study published to date by Meis-Kindblom et al.[113] found no association between cellularity and clinical outcome. In the study by Oliveira et al.,[116] tumor size of 10 cm or greater, high cellularity, mitotic activity greater than 2 mitotic figures/10 high-power fields (HPF), MIB-1 index greater than 10%, and anaplasia or the presence of rhabdoid cells were associated with more aggressive behavior. Meis-Kindblom et al.[113] found increasing patient age, large tumor size, and proximal tumor location to be predictive of an adverse outcome.

SYNOVIAL SARCOMA

Synovial sarcoma is a clinically and morphologically well-defined entity that, despite its name, is extremely uncommon in joint cavities and is encountered in areas with no apparent relation to synovial structures. It occurs primarily in the para-articular regions of the extremities, usually in close association with tendon sheaths, bursae, and joint capsules.

Its microscopic resemblance to developing synovium was suggested early in the literature, but there is no evidence that this tumor arises from or differentiates toward synovium. Indeed, there are such significant immunophenotypic and ultrastructural differences between synovial sarcoma and normal synovium that most regard the label *synovial sarcoma* a fanciful designation that has its roots in the descriptive works of the earlier literature. It should be noted in passing that the term *tendosynovial sarcoma*, coined by Hajdu et al.,[110] is not restricted to synovial sarcoma but embraces a collection of sarcomas, including epithelioid sarcoma, clear cell sarcoma, and extraskeletal myxoid chondrosarcoma and so has no diagnostic purposes. The reported data on the frequency of this tumor vary, but synovial sarcoma accounts for 5% to 10% of all soft tissue sarcomas.[152-154] In a review of over 6000 patients with soft tissue sarcomas seen at MD Anderson Cancer Center (Houston, TX), approximately 6% were synovial sarcomas.[153]

Histologically, there are two major categories of synovial sarcoma: biphasic and monophasic types. *Biphasic synovial sarcoma* has distinct epithelial and spindle cell components, in varying proportions. Of the *monophasic synovial sarcomas*, the vast majority is of the *monophasic fibrous type*, which itself is the most common subtype of synovial sarcoma. There is also a *monophasic epithelial type*, but this tumor is not reliably recognized and distinguished from adenocarcinoma without cytogenetic or molecular genetic studies. In practice, predominantly epithelial forms of synovial sarcoma are diagnosed by recognizing small spindle cell sarcoma areas, having cytogenetic/molecular genetic data, or both. Synovial sarcoma may also present as a poorly differentiated round cell sarcoma often arranged in a pericytomatous pattern (*poorly differentiated synovial sarcoma*), but this is not really a distinct subtype of synovial sarcoma; rather, it represents a form of tumor progression that can occur in either monophasic or biphasic tumors.

Clinical Findings

Age and Gender Incidence

Synovial sarcoma is most prevalent in adolescents and young adults 15 to 40 years of age. In a large series published by Ladanyi et al.,[155] the patients ranged in age from 6 to 82 years, with a mean age of 34 years. Forty-four percent of patients were under age 30 at diagnosis. The tumor may arise in children 10 years of age or younger, and there are several reports in the literature of this tumor arising in newborns.[156] Males are affected more often than females, with a male-to-female ratio of 1.2 to 1.0. There does not appear to be a predilection for any particular race.

Clinical Complaints

The most common presentation is that of a palpable, deep-seated swelling or mass associated with pain or tenderness in slightly more than half of the cases. Less frequently, pain or tenderness is the only manifestation of the disease. There may be minor limitation of motion, but severe functional disturbance is seldom encountered; when it does occur, it is nearly always associated with poorly differentiated, large tumors of long duration. Other clinical complaints are related to the location of the tumor. Primary or secondary involvement of nerves may cause projected pain, numbness, and paresthesia.

The preoperative duration of symptoms varies considerably. Generally, the tumor grows slowly and insidiously. In most cases, the preoperative duration is 2 to 4 years, but there are also cases in which a slow-growing mass or pain at the tumor site has been noted for as long as 20 years prior to surgery. Not infrequently, these cases are incorrectly diagnosed initially as arthritis, synovitis, or bursitis.

Trauma

Although most patients with synovial sarcoma fail to give a definitive history of antecedent trauma, there are patients with such a history in the textbook authors' cases and in the literature; most had sustained a minor or major injury during athletic or recreational activities. The interval between the episode of trauma and onset of the tumor varies considerably, ranging from a few weeks to as long as 40 years. It is likely that trauma is coincidental because synovial sarcoma predominates in parts of the body (extremities) that are most prone to injury. There are rare reports of synovial sarcoma arising in the field of previous therapeutic irradiation[157-159] and one case associated with a metal implant used for hip replacement surgery.[160]

TABLE 33-9 Synovial Sarcoma: AFIP, 345 Cases

ANATOMIC LOCATION	NO. OF CASES
Head-Neck	31 (9.0%)
Neck	12
Pharynx	7
Larynx	7
Other	5
Trunk	28 (8.1%)
Chest	10
Abdominal wall	9
Other	9
Upper Extremities	80 (23.2%)
Forearm-wrist	24
Shoulder	22
Elbow-upper arm	20
Hand	14
Lower Extremities	206 (59.7%)
Thigh-knee	102
Foot	45
Lower leg-ankle	33
Hip-groin	22
Other	4
Total	345 (100.0%)

AFIP, Armed Forces Institute of Pathology.

Anatomic Location

Synovial sarcomas occur predominantly in the extremities, where they tend to arise in the vicinity of large joints, especially the knee region (Table 33-9). They are intimately related to tendons, tendon sheaths, and bursal structures, usually just beyond the confines of the joint capsule; less frequently, they are attached to fascial structures, ligaments, aponeuroses, and interosseous membranes. They are rare in joint cavities; according to material by Namba et al.[161] and Bui-Mansfield et al.[162] and most reviews, intra-articular synovial sarcomas account for fewer than 5% of all cases.

In most series, 85% to 95% of all synovial sarcomas arise in the extremities, with a predilection for the lower extremities. In the lower extremities, most occur in the vicinity of the knee, with fewer arising in the foot, lower leg-ankle region, and hip-groin. Tumors arising in the upper extremities, which account for approximately 10% to 15% of all cases, are fairly evenly distributed among the forearm-wrist region, shoulder, elbow-upper arm region, and hand. Occasionally, one encounters minute (less than 1 cm) synovial sarcomas arising in the hands and feet; these tumors seem to follow a clinically favorable course.[163]

Following the extremities, the head and neck region is the second most common site of synovial sarcoma, accounting for up to 5% to 10% of all cases.[157] Most of these tumors seem to originate in the paravertebral connective tissue spaces and manifest as solitary retropharyngeal or parapharyngeal masses near the carotid bifurcation. Additional cases in this general area have been reported in the paranasal sinuses, mandible, parotid gland, and tonsil, among many others.[164] Because of the unusual location, synovial sarcomas in this region are often misdiagnosed.

About 5% of synovial sarcomas arise in the trunk, including the chest wall and abdominal wall.[165,166] Like synovial sarcomas at other sites, these neoplasms are usually deep-seated. Fetsch and Meis,[165] who reviewed 27 cases culled from the AFIP material, noted a large number of cystic tumors among their cases. The age and gender incidence of these tumors and their behavior correspond to those of synovial sarcomas at other sites.

Synovial sarcoma has been described at virtually every anatomic site, including the heart,[167] pleuropulmonary region,[168] kidney,[169] prostate,[170] retroperitoneum,[171] gastrointestinal tract,[172] and peripheral nerve,[173] among others. With tumors arising in these unusual sites, definitive recognition becomes more difficult and often requires confirmation by molecular genetic techniques.

Radiographic Findings

Radiographic studies may be extremely helpful for suggesting a preoperative diagnosis of synovial sarcoma, largely because of the presence of calcification.[174] Most synovial sarcomas present on routine films as round or oval, more or less lobulated swellings or masses of moderate density, usually located in close proximity to a large joint. The underlying bone tends to be uninvolved, but in about 15% to 20% of the cases, there is a periosteal reaction, superficial bone erosion, or invasion. Massive bone destruction, which is rare, is mostly caused by poorly differentiated synovial sarcomas of long duration and large size.

The most striking radiologic characteristic, found in 15% to 20% of synovial sarcomas, is the presence of multiple small, spotty radiopacities caused by focal calcification and, less frequently, bone formation.[175] In most instances, these changes consist merely of fine stippling, but, in some cases, large portions of the tumor are marked or even outlined by radiopaque masses (Figs. 33-35 to 33-37). Confusion with other tumors is possible, but radiopacities are not observed in most other forms of sarcoma, with the exception of extraskeletal osteosarcoma, a tumor that tends to occur in an older group of individuals.

CT and MRI are valuable tools for determining the site of origin and extent of the lesion. Like conventional radiographs, they show a para-articular heterogeneous septated mass, often with associated calcification or bone erosion.[176]

Gross Findings

The gross appearance varies, depending on the rate of growth and the location of the tumor. Slowly growing lesions tend to be sharply circumscribed, round, or multilobular; as a result of compression of adjacent tissues by the expansively growing tumor, they are completely or partially invested by a smooth, glistening pseudocapsule (Fig. 33-38). Cyst formation may be prominent, and occasional lesions present as multicystic masses (Fig. 33-39).[165,177] Most are firmly attached to surrounding tendons, tendon sheaths, or the exterior wall of the joint capsule; not infrequently, portions of these structures adhere to the gross specimen. On section, they are yellow to gray-white. They may attain a size of 15 cm or more, but most are between 3 and 6 cm at the time of excision. Calcification is common but rarely a discernible macroscopic feature. Less well-differentiated and more rapidly growing tumors tend to

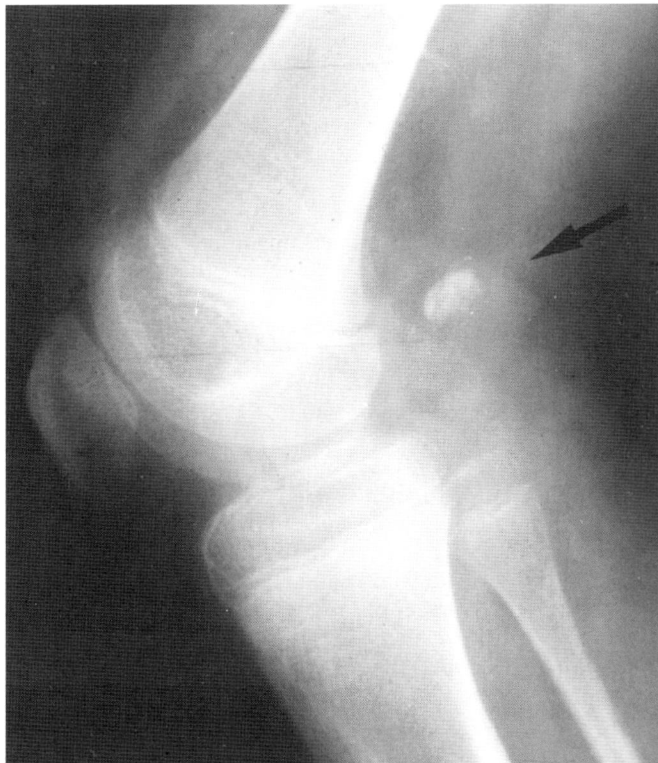

FIGURE 33-35. Radiograph of a synovial sarcoma originating in the popliteal fossa. Note the focal calcification in the tumor (*arrow*), a feature that is present in about 20% of these cases.

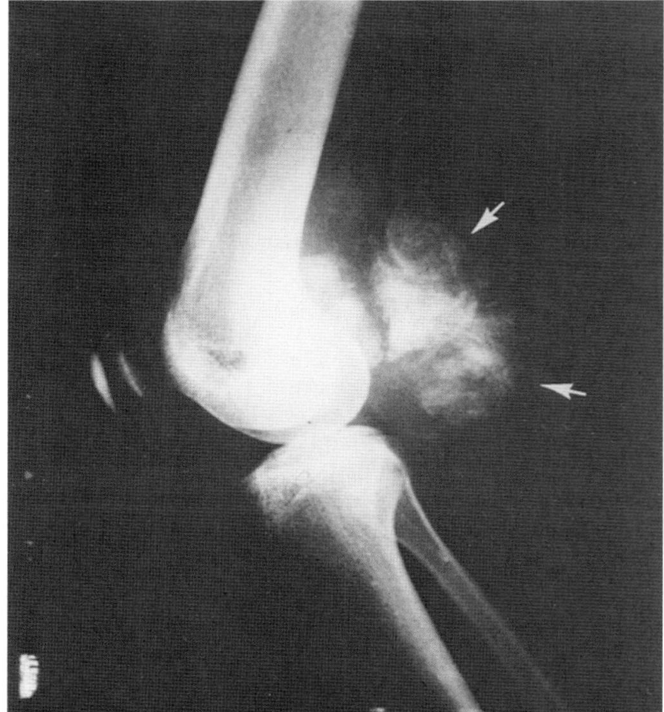

FIGURE 33-36. Massive calcification and ossification in a synovial sarcoma of the popliteal fossa (*arrows*). In general, tumors with extensive calcification carry a better prognosis than those without.

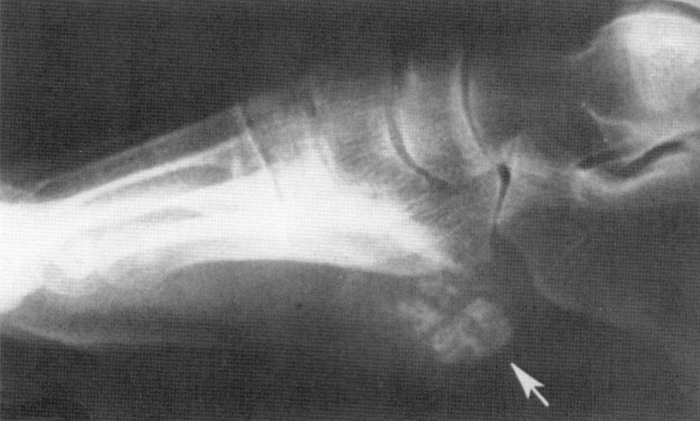

FIGURE 33-37. Radiograph of a synovial sarcoma of the planta pedis showing extensive calcification of the tumor (*arrow*).

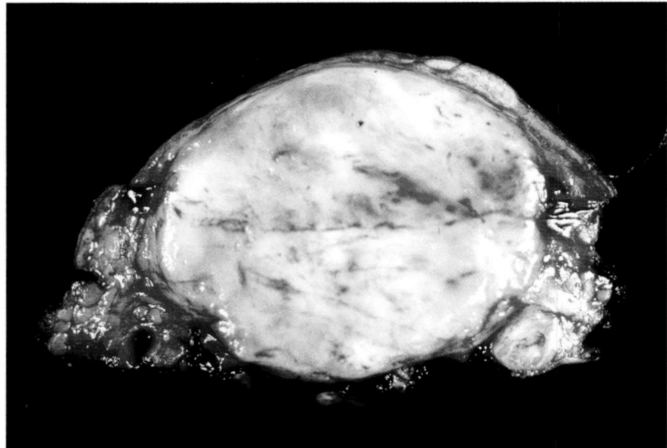

FIGURE 33-38. Photomicrograph of a high-grade monophasic fibrous synovial sarcoma. The tumor has a fleshy gray-tan appearance with focal hemorrhage.

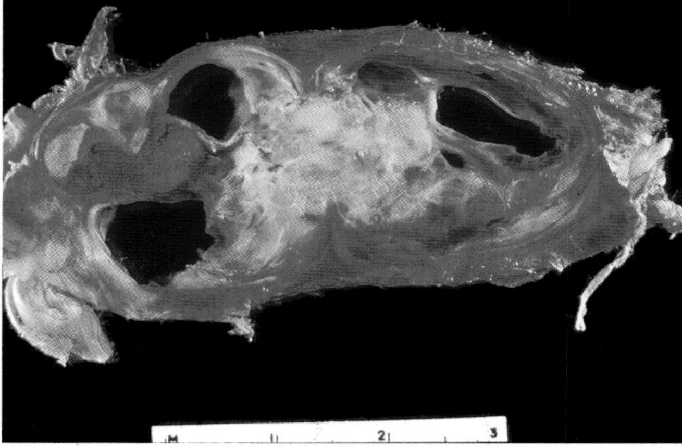

FIGURE 33-39. Multicystic synovial sarcoma of the knee region.

be poorly circumscribed and commonly exhibit a variegated and often friable or shaggy appearance, frequently with multiple areas of hemorrhage, necrosis, and cyst formation. Markedly hemorrhagic tumors may be confused with angiosarcomas or even organizing hematomas.

Microscopic Findings

Unlike most other types of sarcoma, the tumor is composed of two morphologically different types of cells: *epithelial cells*, resembling those of carcinoma, and fibrosarcoma-like *spindle cells*. Transitional forms between epithelial and spindle cells suggest a close relation, which is also supported by tissue culture, ultrastructural, immunohistochemical, and molecular genetic findings. Depending on the relative prominence of the two cellular elements and the degree of differentiation, synovial sarcomas form a continuous morphologic spectrum and can be broadly classified into the (1) *biphasic type*, with distinct epithelial and spindle cell components in varying proportions; (2) *monophasic fibrous type*; (3) rare *monophasic epithelial type* (or probably more appropriately epithelial predominant); and (4) *poorly differentiated* (*round cell*) *type*.

Biphasic Synovial Sarcoma

The classical synovial sarcoma—the biphasic type—is generally readily recognizable by the coexistence of morphologically different but histogenetically related epithelial cells and fibroblast-like spindle cells (Figs. 33-40 to 33-42). The epithelial cells are characterized by large, round or oval, vesicular nuclei and abundant pale-staining cytoplasm with distinctly outlined cellular borders. The cells are cuboidal to tall and columnar; they are arranged in solid cords, nests, or glandular structures that contain granular or homogeneous eosinophilic secretions (Figs. 33-43 and 33-44). The glandular spaces lined by epithelial cells must be distinguished from cleft-like artifacts that are the result of tissue shrinkage. Not infrequently, cuboidal or flattened epithelial cells also cover small villous or papillary structures often with spindle cells rather than connective tissue in the papillary core. A diagnosis of squamous cell carcinoma may also be suggested by focal squamous

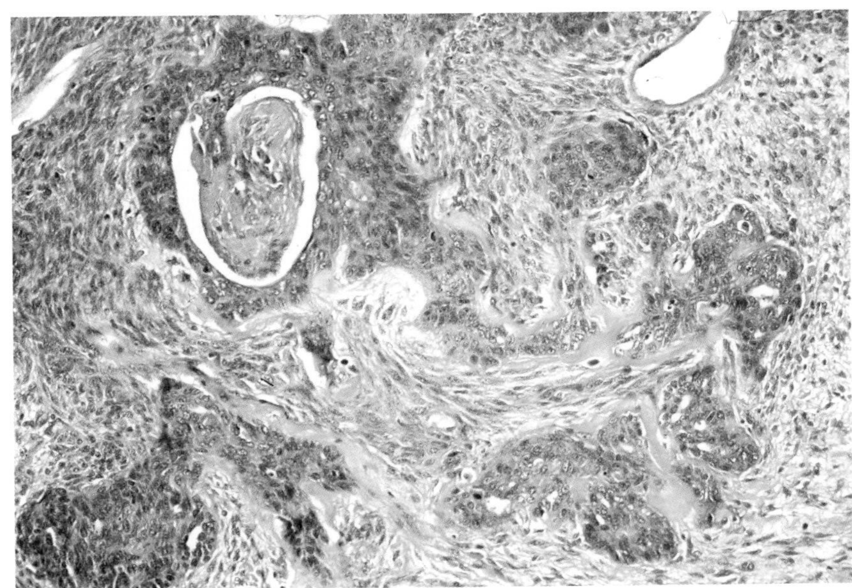

FIGURE 33-40. Biphasic synovial sarcoma showing close apposition of epithelial structures with malignant spindle cells.

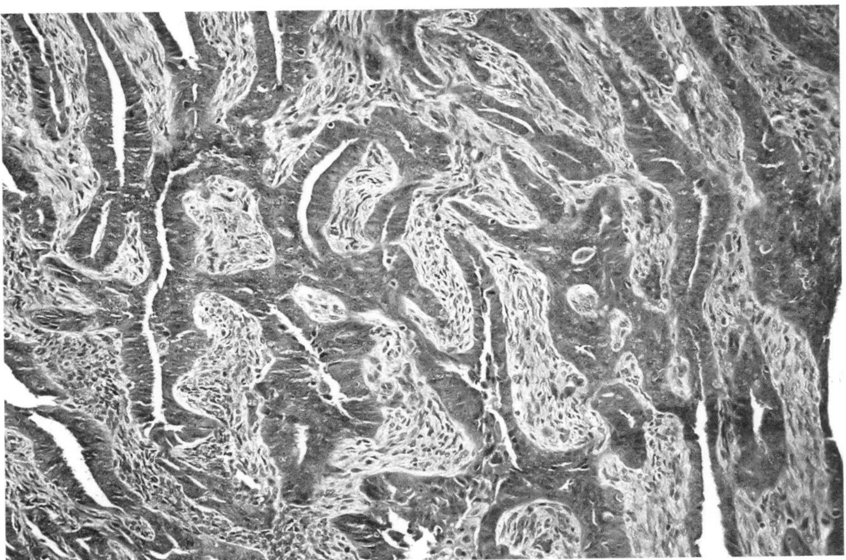

FIGURE 33-41. Typical biphasic synovial sarcoma with columnar epithelial cells surrounded by spindle cell elements.

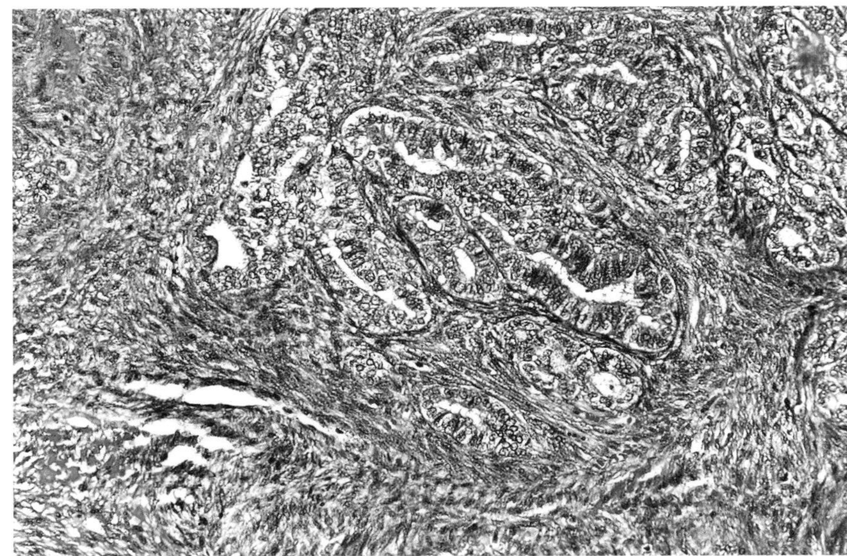

FIGURE 33-42. Biphasic synovial sarcoma with glandular epithelial structures adjacent to a malignant spindle cell component.

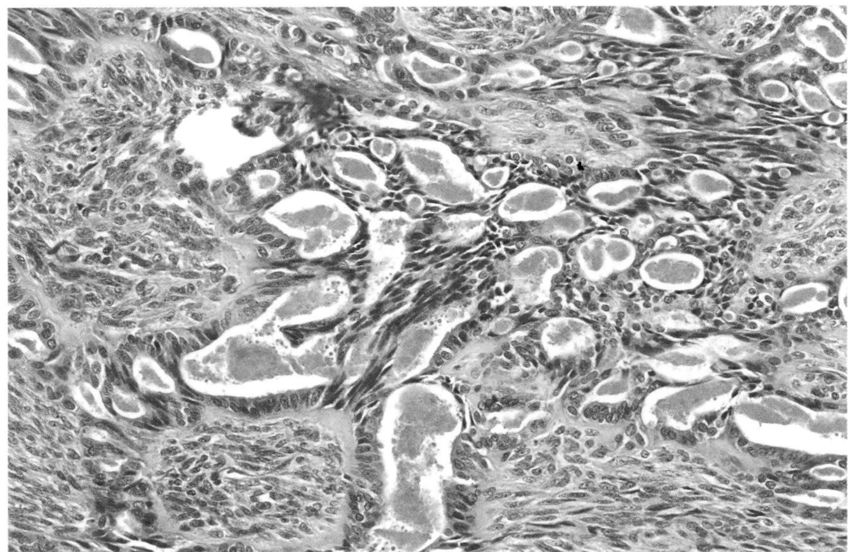

FIGURE 33-43. Biphasic synovial sarcoma. The epithelial structures have intraluminal eosinophilic secretions.

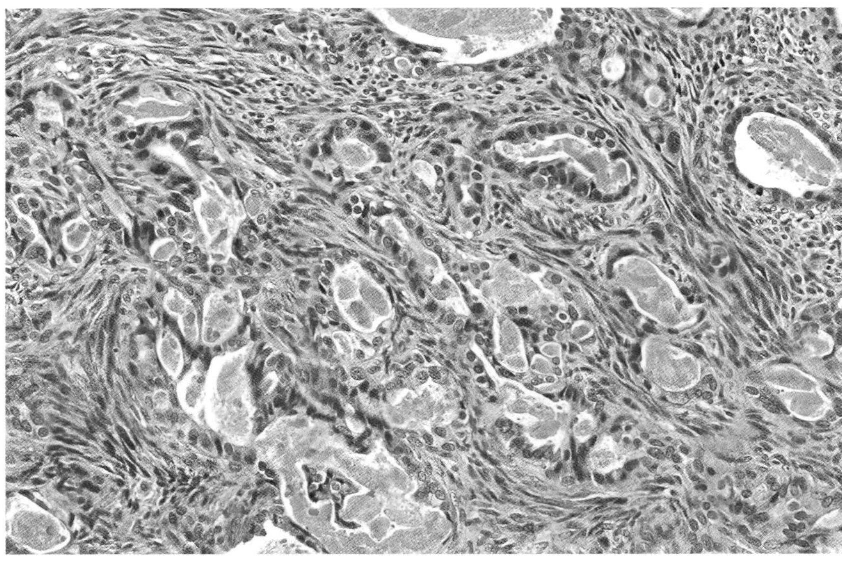

FIGURE 33-44. Biphasic synovial sarcoma with prominent intraluminal eosinophilic secretions in epithelial elements.

metaplasia, including the occasional formation of squamous pearls and keratohyaline granules.

The surrounding spindle cell component consists mostly of well-oriented, rather plump, spindle-shaped cells of uniform appearance with small amounts of indistinct cytoplasm and oval dark-staining nuclei. Generally, the cells form solid, compact sheets that are similar in many respects to fibrosarcoma (Figs. 33-45 and 33-46), except for the absence of long, sweeping fascicles or a herringbone pattern and a more irregular nodular arrangement. Mitotic figures in synovial sarcoma occur in both epithelial and spindle-shaped cells, but, as a rule, only the poorly differentiated forms of the tumor exhibit very high mitotic counts. Occasionally, there is nuclear palisading (Fig. 33-47), but in contrast to leiomyosarcomas and malignant peripheral nerve sheath tumors (MPNST), this feature is confined to a small portion of the tumor.

Commonly, the cellular portions of synovial sarcoma alternate with less cellular areas displaying hyalinization, myxoid change, or calcification. The collagen in the hyalinized zones may be diffusely distributed or form narrow bands or plaque-like masses sometimes associated with a markedly thickened basement membrane separating epithelial and spindle-cell elements (Fig. 33-48). The myxoid areas are generally less conspicuous and tend to occupy only a small, ill-defined portion of the tumor, although some cases are predominantly myxoid (Fig. 33-49).[178]

Calcification with or without ossification is another diagnostically important and characteristic feature that is present to a varying degree in about 20% of synovial sarcomas. It may be inconspicuous and consist merely of a few small irregularly distributed spherical concretions, or it may be extensive and occupy a large portion of the neoplasm (Fig. 33-50).[175,179] In general, calcification is preceded by hyalinization and is more pronounced at the periphery of the tumor than at its center. Rarely, chondroid changes are present and nearly always together with focal calcification and ossification.

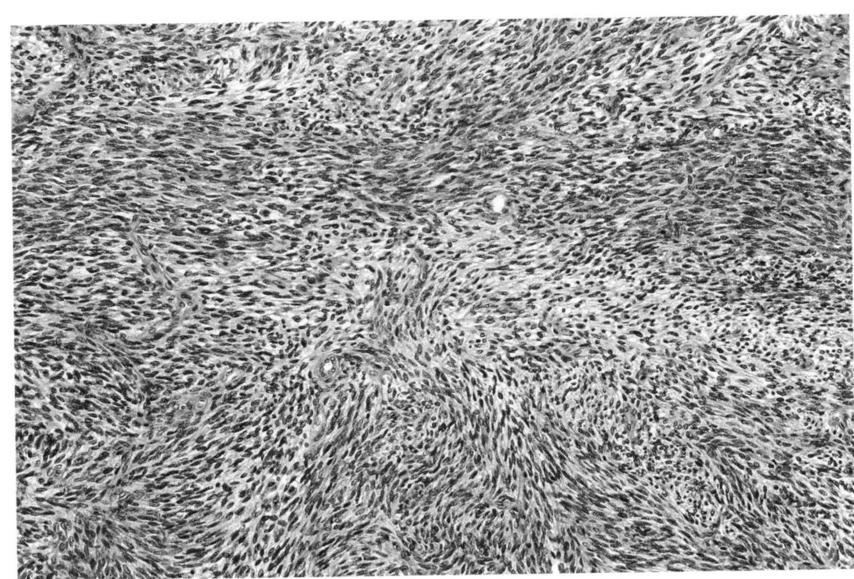

FIGURE 33-45. Fibrosarcoma-like area in a synovial sarcoma. Note the alternating darkly staining and lightly staining regions, imparting a marbled appearance.

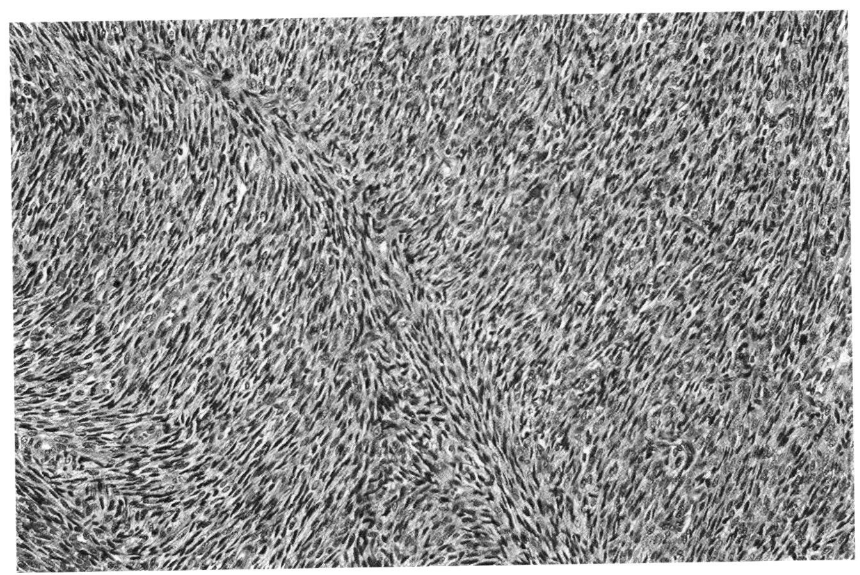

FIGURE 33-46. Fibrosarcoma-like area in a synovial sarcoma. The spindle cells are arranged in distinct fascicles.

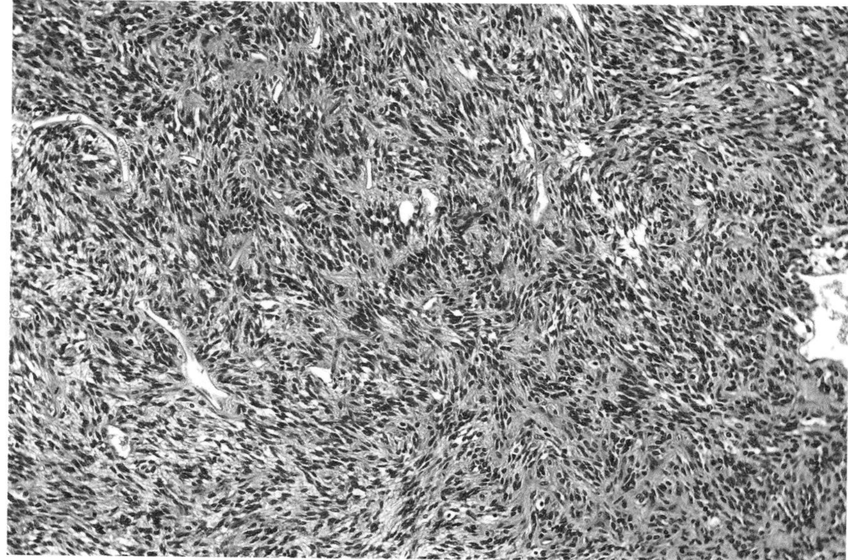

FIGURE 33-47. Synovial sarcoma with focal nuclear palisading reminiscent of a neural tumor.

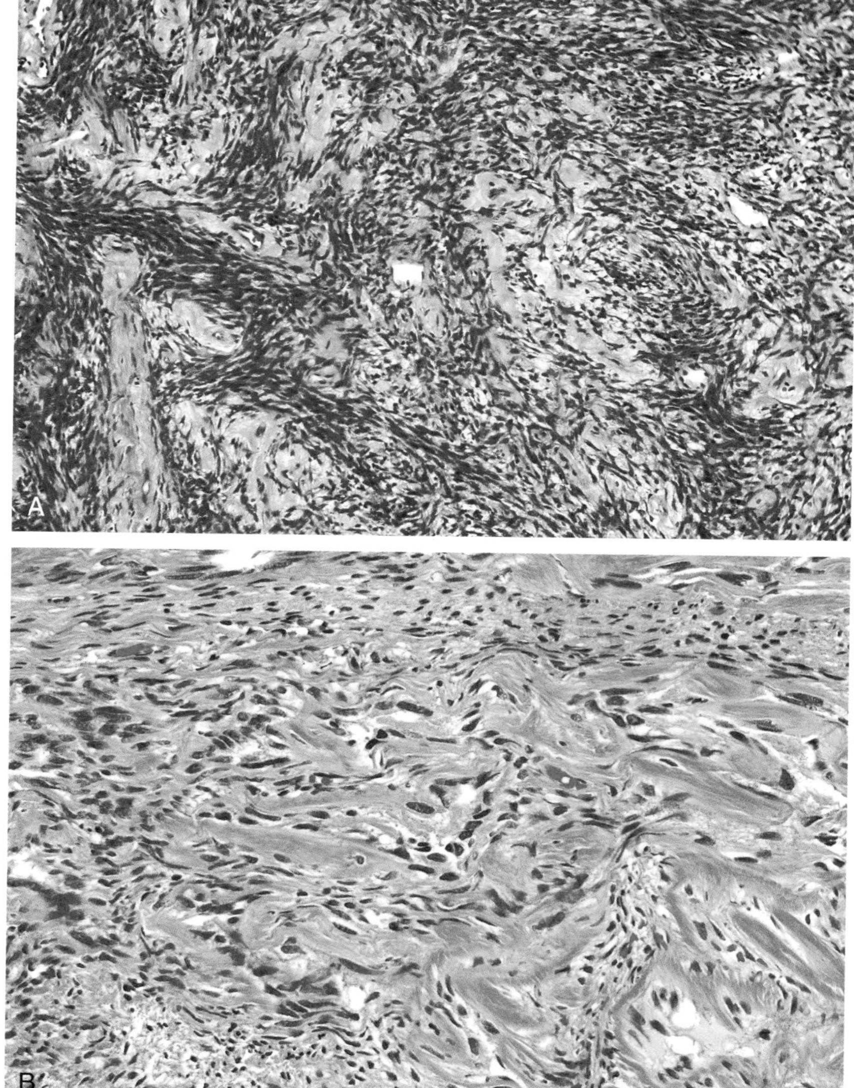

FIGURE 33-48. (A) Monophasic synovial sarcoma with prominent perivascular hyalinization. (B) Thick collagen bands separate malignant spindle cells in a monophasic synovial sarcoma. This pattern of hyalinization is characteristic of this tumor.

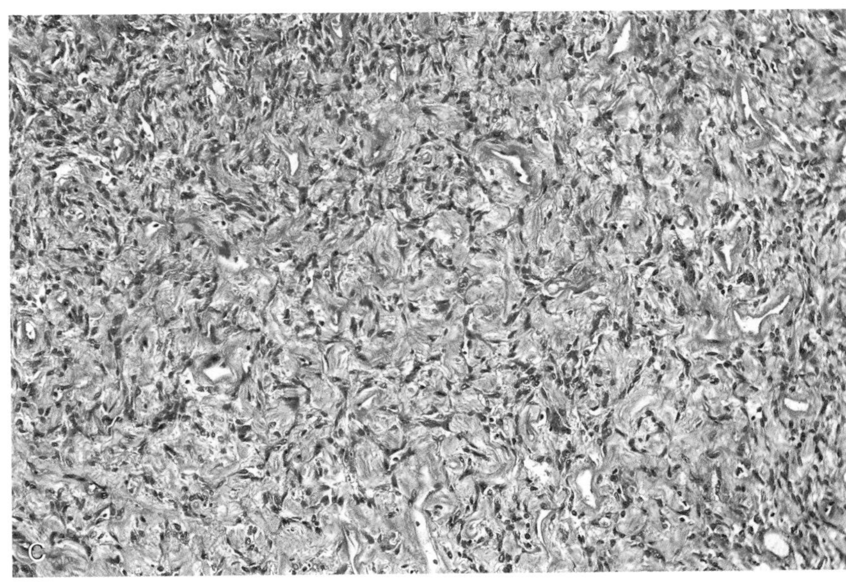

FIGURE 33-48, cont'd. (C) Extensive hyalinization in a synovial sarcoma with compression of neoplastic cells.

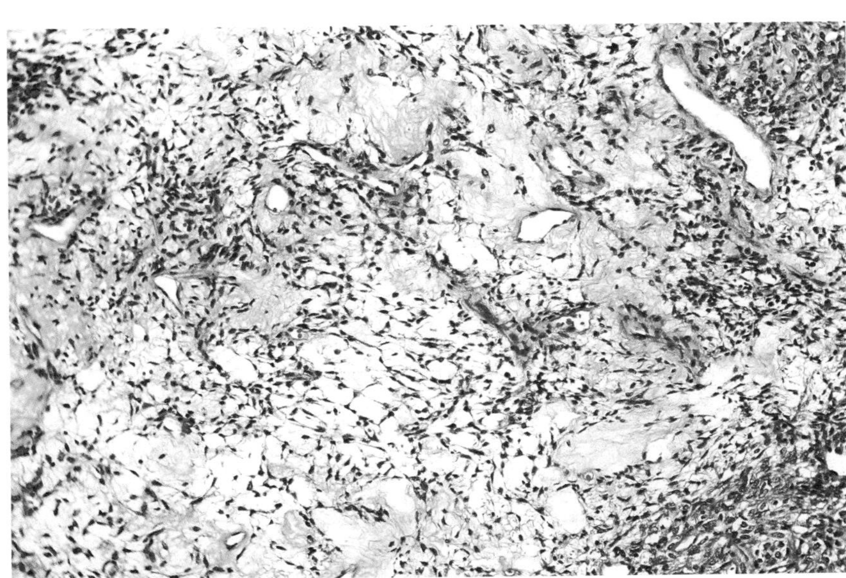

FIGURE 33-49. Prominent myxoid change in synovial sarcoma.

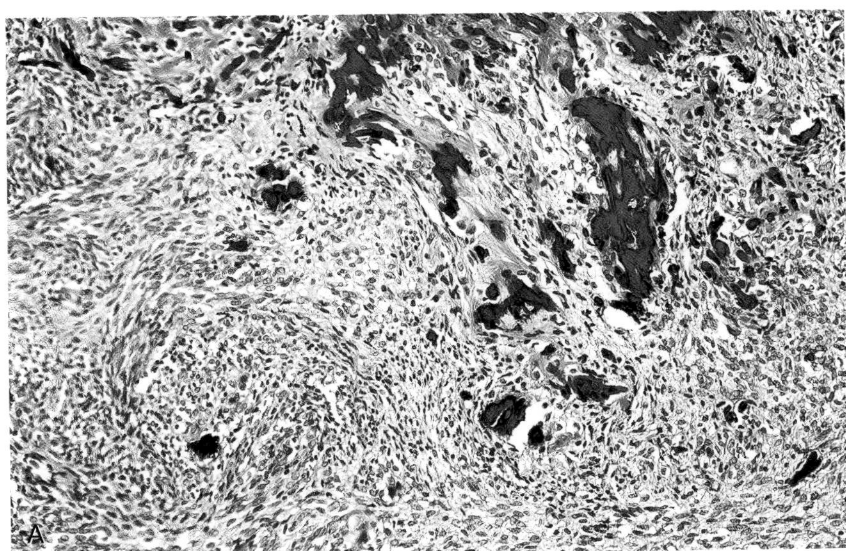

FIGURE 33-50. (A) Calcification in a synovial sarcoma, a common feature of this neoplasm.

Continued

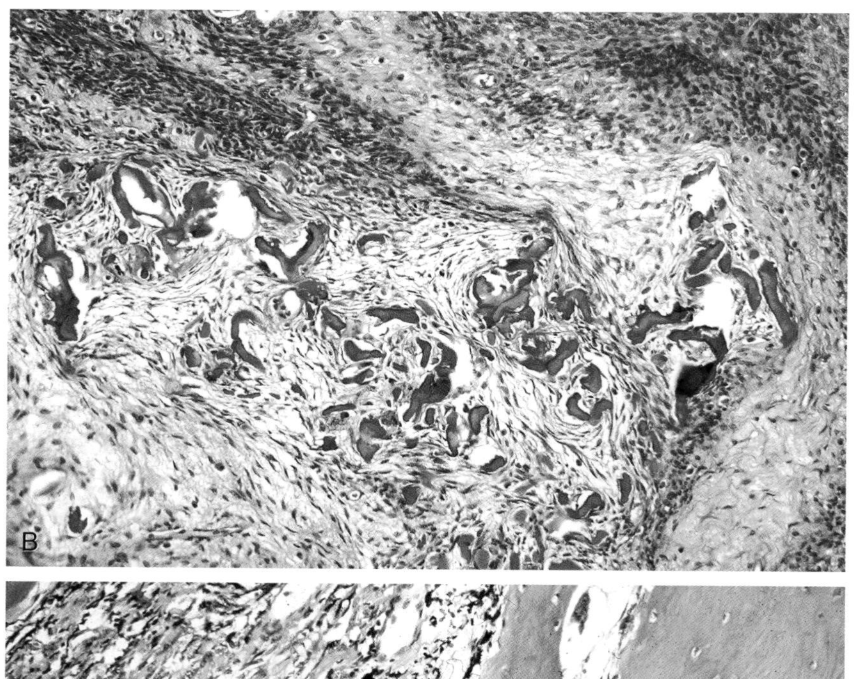

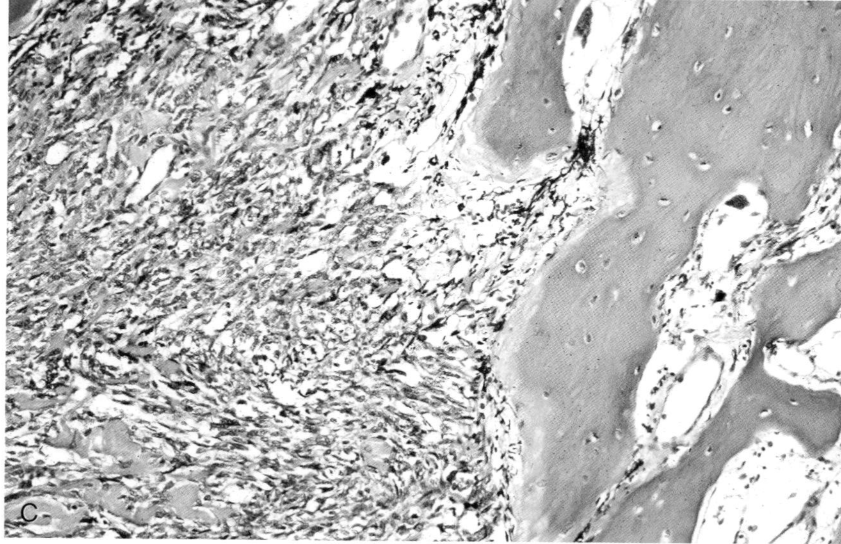

FIGURE 33-50, cont'd. (B) Note the focus of calcification in this small monophasic fibrous synovial sarcoma of the foot. (C) Monophasic fibrous type of synovial sarcoma with osseous metaplasia.

Mast cells are yet another conspicuous feature of synovial sarcoma; they show no particular distribution but are more numerous in the spindle cell than in the epithelial portions of the neoplasm. Inflammatory elements and multinucleated giant cells are rare.

The degree of vascularity varies. In some cases, it is a dominant feature with numerous dilated vascular spaces resembling hemangiopericytoma (Fig. 33-51); in others, there are merely a few scattered vascular structures. Some cases show prominent cystic changes (Fig. 33-52). Secondary changes such as hemorrhage are most prominent in poorly differentiated tumors. Scattered lipid macrophages, siderophages, multinucleated giant cells, and deposits of cholesterol may be present but are much less conspicuous in synovial sarcomas than in synovitis.

Monophasic Fibrous Synovial Sarcoma

The monophasic fibrous synovial sarcoma is a relatively common neoplasm and is far more common than the biphasic form. Because this type is closely related to the biphasic type and merely represents one extreme of its morphologic spectrum, the previously mentioned morphologic features of the spindle-cell portion of the biphasic type, such as cellular appearance, hyalinization, myxoid change, mast cell infiltrate, hemangiopericytomatous vasculature, and focal calcification, apply equally to the monophasic fibrous type.

In some cases, an obvious epithelial component can be identified by extensive sampling, in which case the tumor is more appropriately designated as a biphasic synovial sarcoma. Even in those cases without obvious epithelial differentiation, however, many monophasic fibrous synovial sarcomas have foci in which the cells have a more epithelioid morphology and appear to be more cohesive than the surrounding spindle-shaped cells. The cells in these foci have more eosinophilic cytoplasm but otherwise have the same nuclear features as the surrounding spindle-shaped cells. Such areas often show immunohistochemical evidence of epithelial differentiation (Fig. 33-53).

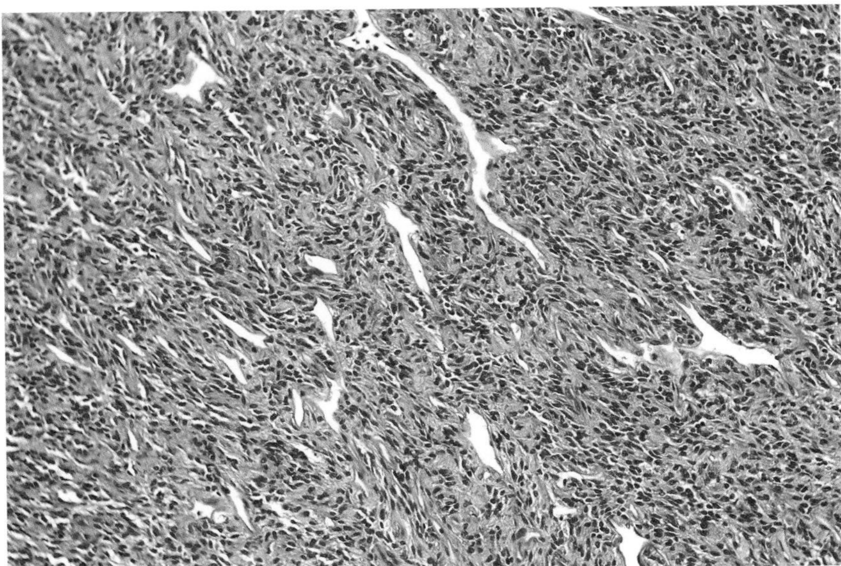

FIGURE 33-51. Prominent hemangiopericytomatous vasculature in a synovial sarcoma.

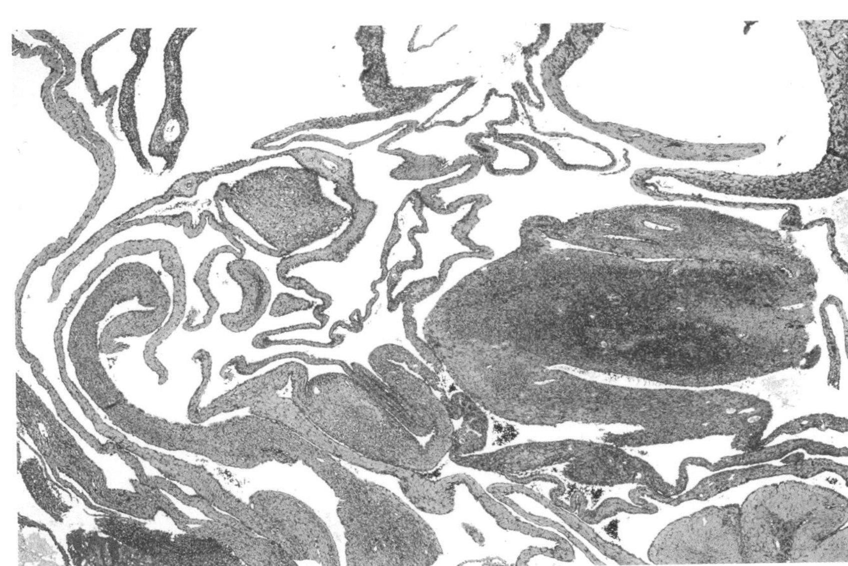

FIGURE 33-52. Cystic synovial sarcoma. Malignant spindle cells are seen in the thickened fibrous septa.

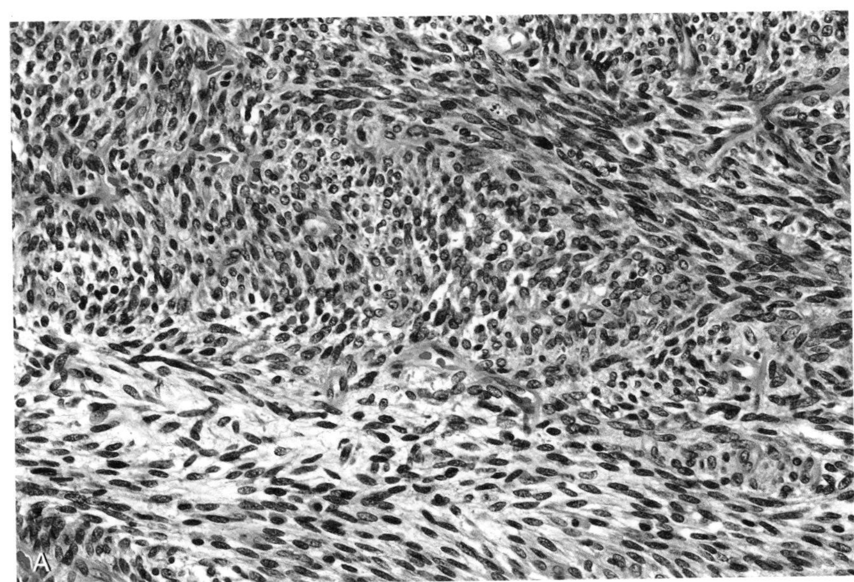

FIGURE 33-53. (A) High-magnification view of a monophasic fibrous synovial sarcoma. The malignant spindle cells are relatively uniform with respect to one another. *Continued*

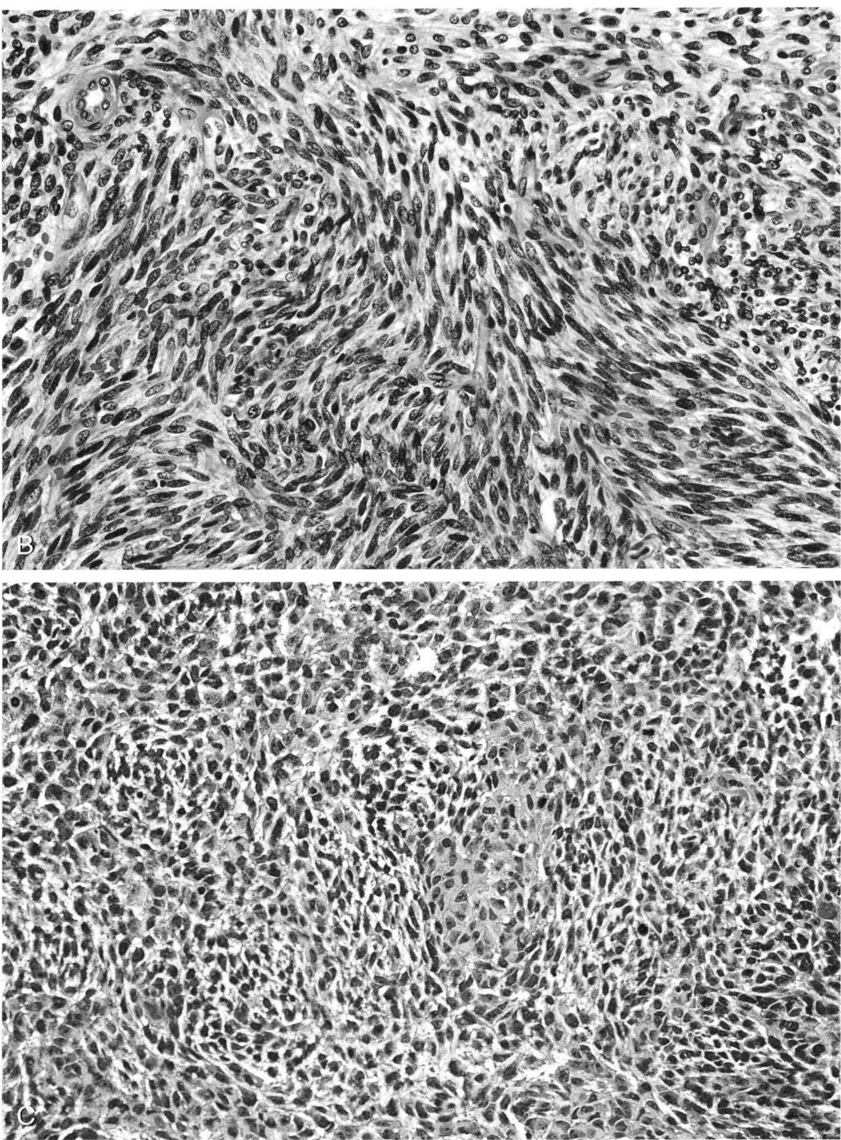

FIGURE 33-53, cont'd. (B) Uniform spindle cells in a monophasic fibrous synovial sarcoma. (C) Epithelioid area in a monophasic fibrous synovial sarcoma. A small group of cells have increased amounts of eosinophilic cytoplasm and appear more cohesive.

Monophasic Epithelial Synovial Sarcoma (Epithelial-Predominant Synovial Sarcoma)

What has been previously described about the diagnosis of the monophasic fibrous type of synovial sarcoma applies also to the monophasic epithelial synovial sarcoma, a rarely recognized neoplasm. It is often difficult or impossible to render this diagnosis with any degree of certainty without corroborating cytogenetic or molecular genetic data. In fact, it might be argued that this variant exists only conceptually as a means of validating the entire (epithelial) biphasic spectrum of synovial sarcoma. However, with the ability to analyze tumors for the characteristic translocation, it is now feasible to diagnose monophasic epithelial synovial sarcoma in tumors that otherwise would be misdiagnosed as other benign or malignant epithelial neoplasms. The most important differential considerations are metastatic carcinoma, melanoma, and adnexal tumors. However, other epithelioid mesenchymal tumors should also be considered, including epithelioid sarcoma and epithelioid MPNST. Several tumors of this type have been encountered, but all had minute foci of spindle-cell differentiation and, strictly speaking, were biphasic synovial sarcomas with an exceptionally prominent epithelial pattern (Figs. 33-54 to 33-56).

Poorly Differentiated Synovial Sarcoma

Poorly differentiated synovial sarcoma can be thought of as a form of tumor progression that can be superimposed on any of the other synovial sarcoma subtypes. Recognition of this subtype of synovial sarcoma is of practical importance not only because it poses a special problem in diagnosis, but also because it behaves more aggressively and metastasizes in a significantly higher percentage of cases.[180-182] The incidence of the poorly differentiated type among synovial sarcomas is difficult to estimate, but in the study by Machen et al.,[183] 21 of 34

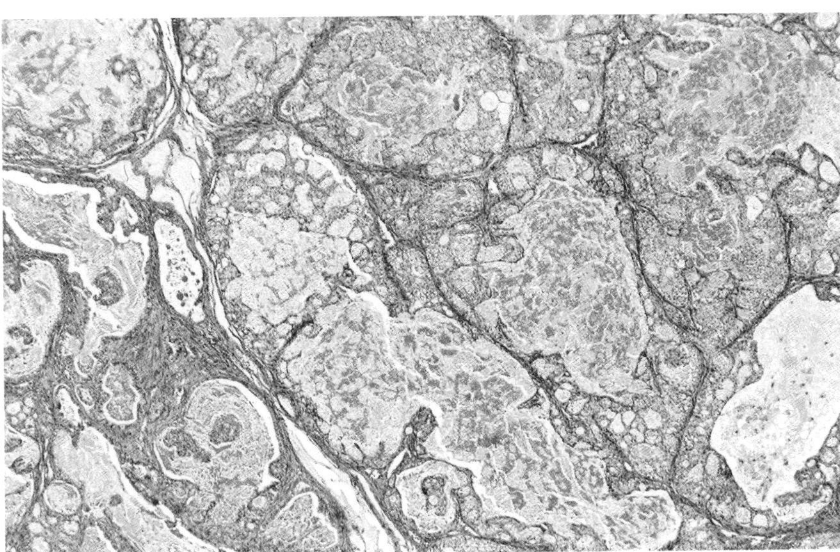

FIGURE 33-54. Predominantly epithelial-type synovial sarcoma. A cribriform glandular pattern was prominent throughout this neoplasm.

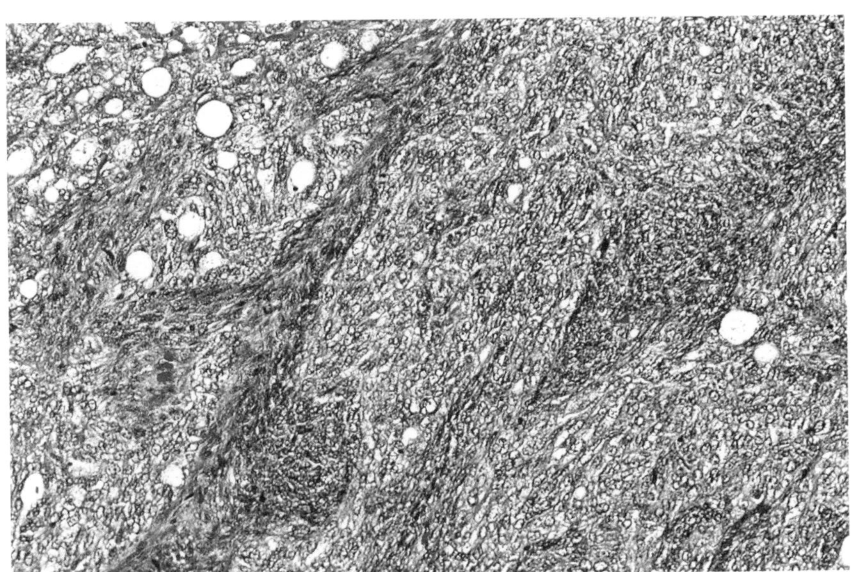

FIGURE 33-55. Predominantly epithelial-type synovial sarcoma. Small areas with a well-developed spindle cell pattern are present.

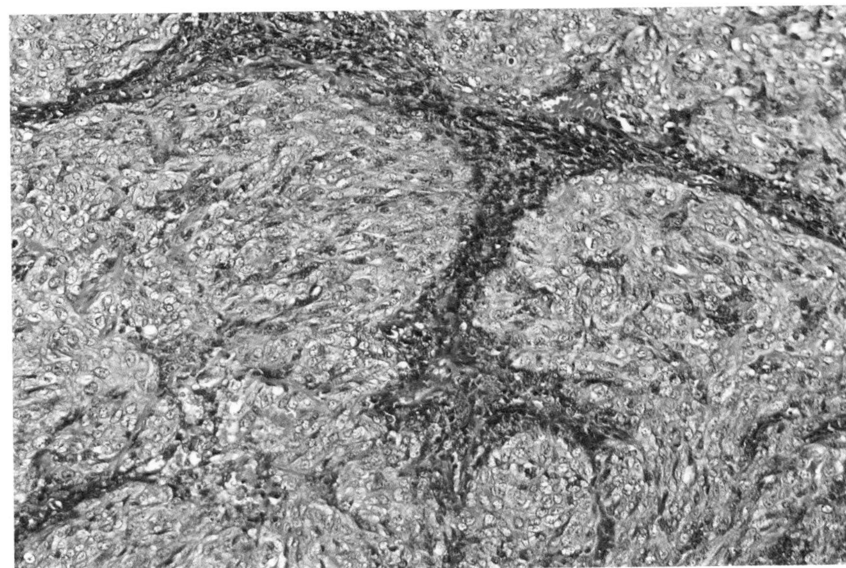

FIGURE 33-56. Predominantly epithelial-type synovial sarcoma. Most of this tumor was composed of sheets of cohesive epithelioid cells with only small foci of spindle-cell differentiation.

(62%) synovial sarcomas had poorly differentiated foci, in some cases accounting for up to 90% of the neoplasm. However, this pattern predominates in fewer than 20% of all cases of synovial sarcoma.

Histologically, poorly differentiated synovial sarcoma may have three patterns: (1) a large-cell or epithelioid pattern composed of variably sized rounded nuclei with prominent nucleoli (Fig. 33-57), (2) a small-cell pattern with nuclear features similar to other small round cell tumors, and (3) a high-grade spindle-cell pattern composed of spindle-shaped cells with high-grade nuclear features and a high mitotic rate (Fig. 33-58) often accompanied by necrosis.[184] These tumors often have a richly vascular pattern with dilated thin-walled vascular spaces resembling those of hemangiopericytoma. In fact, it appears that a high percentage of sarcomas interpreted as malignant hemangiopericytomas are in fact examples of poorly differentiated synovial sarcoma. Occasionally, cells with intracytoplasmic hyaline inclusions imparting a rhabdoid morphology may be found in poorly differentiated areas.[185]

Special Staining Procedures

Two distinctive types of mucinous material are present in synovial sarcomas. Secretions in the epithelial cells, intracellular clefts, and pseudoglandular spaces stain positively with the periodic acid-Schiff (PAS), colloidal iron, Alcian blue, and mucicarmine stains. The staining characteristics of the mucinous secretions remain unaltered after treatment of the secretions with diastase and hyaluronidase, but in general and in distinction to adenocarcinomas, the mucinous material is more conspicuous in the intracellular clefts and pseudoglandular spaces than in the secreting epithelial cells. In contrast to mesothelioma, granular intracellular glycogen that stains positively for PAS is never a striking feature of synovial sarcoma.

The second type of mucinous material, stromal, or mesenchymal mucin, which is elaborated by the spindle cells, also stains positively for colloidal iron and Alcian blue stains, but it is weakly carminophilic and stains negatively with the PAS preparation. It is present in the interstices of the spindle-cell

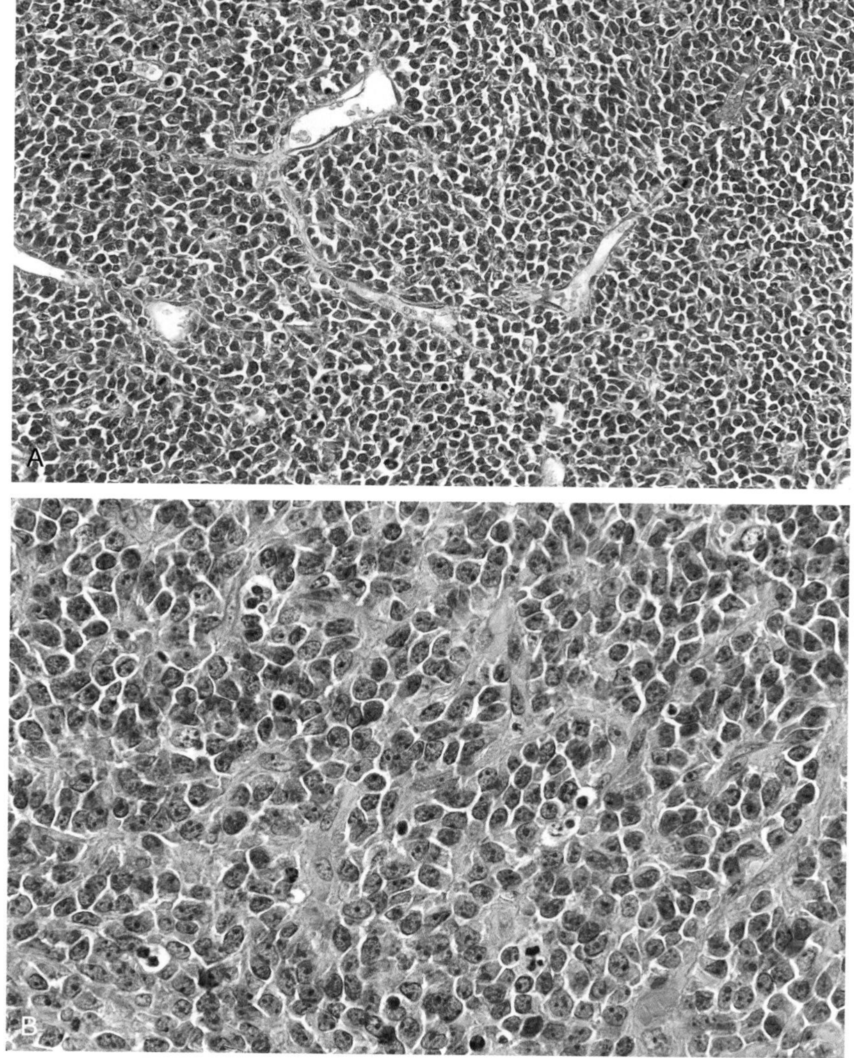

FIGURE 33-57. Poorly differentiated area of a synovial sarcoma. (A) Low-magnification view with a prominent hemangiopericytomatous vasculature. (B) Note the cytologic features of round cells in poorly differentiated synovial sarcoma.

areas and the loosely textured myxoid portions of the tumor. This material is rich in hyaluronic acid and, like other mesenchymal mucins, is completely removed by prior treatment with hyaluronidase.

Immunohistochemical Findings

Most synovial sarcomas display immunoreactivity for cytokeratins and EMA (Fig. 33-59). In an immunohistochemical study of 100 synovial sarcomas by Guillou et al.,[186] focal positivity for EMA and cytokeratin was found in 97% and 69% of cases, respectively. In this study, only 1 of 100 cases was negative for both of these epithelial markers. Approximately 90% of all synovial sarcomas are cytokeratin-positive. In general, the intensity of staining is more pronounced in the epithelial component than in the spindled component. In some lesions of the monophasic fibrous type, only a few isolated cells express these antigens, making it necessary to stain and examine multiple sections from different portions of the tumor (Fig. 33-60).[187] Poorly differentiated variants usually, but not always, express these epithelial markers. In the study by Folpe et al.,[181] all nine poorly differentiated synovial sarcomas stained for EMA, whereas only 30% and 50% stained for low- and high-molecular-weight cytokeratins, respectively. Similarly, van de Rijn et al.[180] found staining for EMA and cytokeratin in 95% and 42% of poorly differentiated synovial sarcomas, respectively. In contrast to other spindle cell sarcomas, the cells of synovial sarcoma specifically express cytokeratins 7 and 19.[187,188] In fact, these markers often decorate a much larger proportion of cells than either EMA or AE1/AE3. Miettinen et al.[187] evaluated 110 synovial sarcomas of all subtypes and found fairly consistent expression of CK7, CK19, CK8/18, and CK14 in the epithelial cells of biphasic tumors. However, the cells of monophasic synovial sarcoma had a more limited cytokeratin repertory, with focal expression of

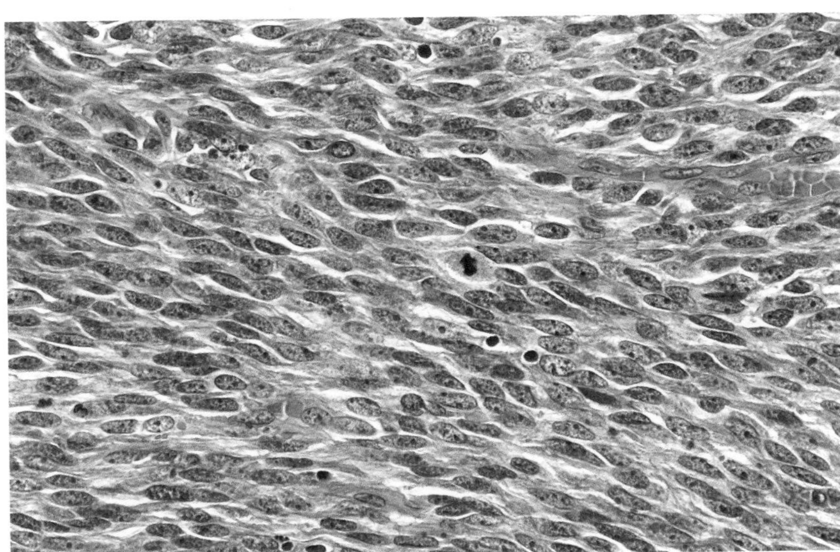

FIGURE 33-58. Poorly differentiated synovial sarcoma composed of spindle cells with high-grade nuclear features.

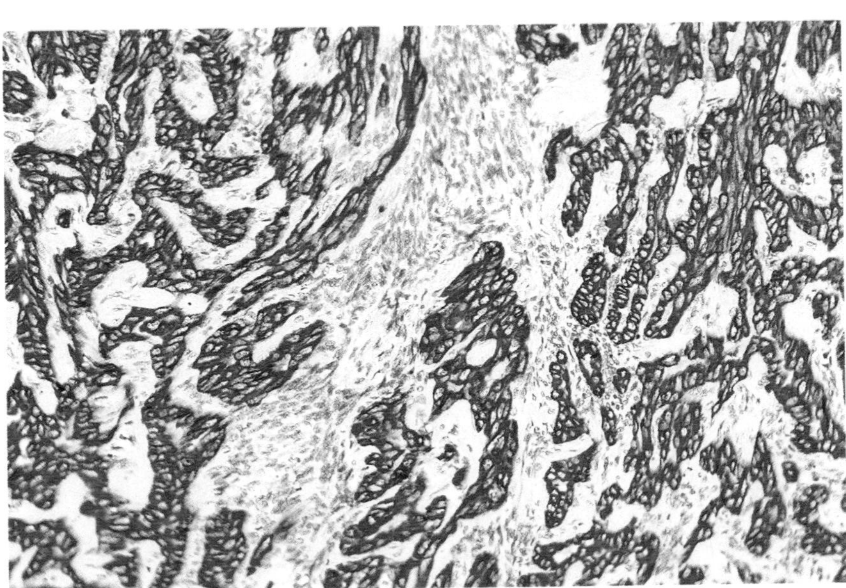

FIGURE 33-59. High-molecular-weight cytokeratin immunoreactivity highlights the epithelial elements in this biphasic synovial sarcoma.

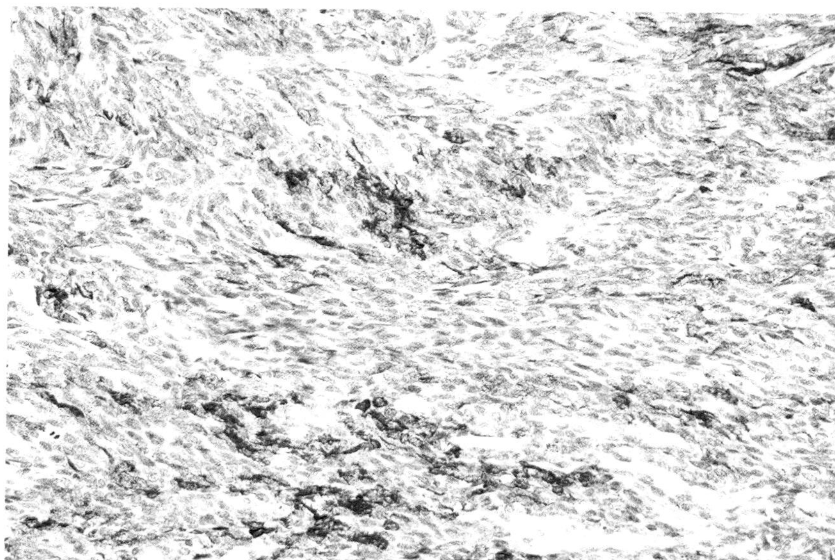

FIGURE 33-60. Focal immunoreactivity for cytokeratin 7 in a monophasic fibrous synovial sarcoma.

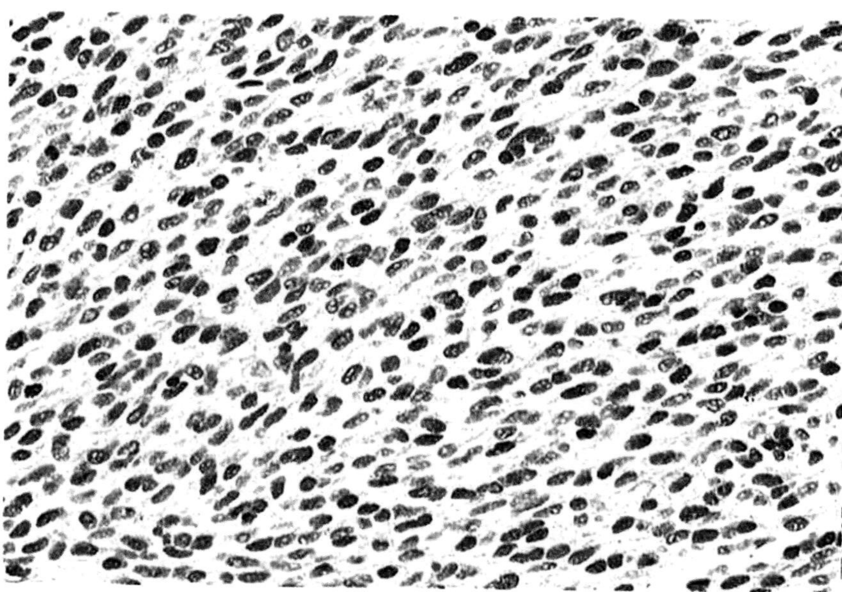

FIGURE 33-61. Strong nuclear TLE1 immunoreactivity in a monophasic fibrous synovial sarcoma.

CK7 (79%), CK19 (60%), and CK8/18 (45%). Poorly differentiated cells showed even more limited expression of CK7 (50%) and CK19 (61%). In a study of 60 t(X;18) *SS18-SSX*-positive cases, Pelmus et al.[189] found EMA to be the most sensitive epithelial marker.

Although not often emphasized, up to 30% of synovial sarcomas show focal immunoreactivity for S-100 protein.[188,189] Most of these S-100 protein-positive synovial sarcomas coexpress epithelial markers, but the occasional synovial sarcoma expresses S-100 protein in the absence of EMA or AE1/AE3, thereby causing confusion with an MPNST. In these cases, the detection of CK7 and/or CK19, TLE1 (discussed later) and/or molecular genetic studies may be useful for recognizing monophasic fibrous synovial sarcoma.

CD99, the product of the *MIC2* gene, can be immunohistochemically detected in the cytoplasm or cell membrane in 60% to 70% of synovial sarcomas.[189,190] BCL2 protein is diffusely expressed in virtually all synovial sarcomas, especially in the spindled cells, but is of limited diagnostic value because many other tumors express this antigen.[191,192] Unlike many other spindle cell tumors, synovial sarcoma is virtually always negative for CD34, although there are very rare exceptions. Calponin has also been found to be frequently expressed in synovial sarcoma, which may be useful in recognizing poorly differentiated variants because other round cell tumors are negative for this antigen.[193]

TLE1 has emerged as an extremely useful marker of synovial sarcoma, particularly in cytokeratin-negative cases[194-196] (Fig. 33-61). Gene expression profiling studies have consistently identified *TLE1* as an excellent discriminator of synovial sarcoma from other sarcomas. Terry et al.[196] found the TLE protein to be expressed in 91 of 94 molecularly confirmed synovial sarcomas, although it was very rarely expressed in other mesenchymal neoplasms. Similarly, all 35 molecularly confirmed synovial sarcomas tested by Jagdis et al.[195] showed strong and diffuse TLE1 immunoreactivity, whereas only 1 of 43 MPNSTs showed focal staining; the positive and negative predictive values in this study were 92% and 100%, respectively. However, not all studies have found this marker to be as useful. For example, Kosemehmetoglu et al.[197] found TLE1 staining in 53 of 143 (37%) nonsynovial sarcomas.

Other markers of interest include an immunohistochemical marker of SYT protein, which was found to be expressed in 41 of 47 cases of synovial sarcoma (typically strong diffuse nuclear staining), but up to 19% of nonsynovial sarcomas are also marked by this antibody.[198] As previously mentioned, rare synovial sarcomas have areas with rhabdoid morphology; however, Kohashi et al.[199] found decreased SMARCB1 expression in 69% of synovial sarcomas, regardless of the identification of rhabdoid features, suggesting post-transcriptional modification.

Ultrastructural Findings

The biphasic tumors are composed of epithelial and spindle cells with transitional forms showing features of both cell types. Frequently, the epithelial cells are disposed in clusters or gland-like structures, with microvilli or villous filopodia on the surfaces facing the intercellular or pseudoglandular spaces. In contrast to the cells of normal synovium, the epithelial cells are interconnected by junctional complexes, zonulae adherens, or desmosome-like structures, a finding supported by the consistent expression of tight junction-related proteins, including ZO-1, claudin, and occludin.[200] The ultrastructural features of the monophasic fibrous type are indistinguishable from those of the spindle-cell areas of the biphasic type. There are, however, identifying features of early epithelial differentiation, such as intercellular or cleft-like spaces of varying size bordered by multiple microvilli, as well as poorly developed junctions or desmosome-like structures.

Cytogenetic and Molecular Genetic Findings

A consistent, specific translocation, most commonly a balanced reciprocal translocation, t(X;18)(p11;q11), is found in virtually all synovial sarcomas, regardless of subtype.[201] This translocation involves the fusion of the *SS18* (also known as *SYT*) gene on chromosome 18 and either the *SSX1* or *SSX2* gene on the *X* chromosome (both at Xp11) or, rarely, with *SSX4* (also at Xp11).[155,202] The function of the SS18-SSX fusion protein has yet to be fully defined but fuses transcriptional activation (SYT) and repression (SSX) domains resulting in the dysregulation of gene expression.[203] DNA microarray expression profiling studies have shown upregulation of a number of genes, including *IGFBP2*, *IGF2*, and *ELF3*. A consistent finding has been the upregulation of genes involved with the Wnt signaling pathway, including *TLE1*.[204,205] *SS18-SSX1* and *SYT-SSX2* appear to be mutually exclusive gene fusions, and there is concordance of fusion type between primary tumors and their metastases.[206] Overall, approximately two-thirds of synovial sarcomas harbor an *SS18-SSX1* fusion and one-third reveal an *SS18-SSX2* fusion. Interestingly, several studies have found an association between fusion type and histology. The vast majority of tumors with *SS18-SSX2* are monophasic fibrous tumors, whereas almost all biphasic synovial sarcomas have an *SS18-SSX1* fusion.[207,208] The *SS18-SSX* fusion can be reliably detected by either RT-PCR or FISH.[209-211] These techniques are particularly useful for monophasic fibrous and poorly differentiated synovial sarcomas, which may be difficult to distinguish from other spindle cell and round cell sarcomas, respectively. It is also invaluable in distinguishing the rare monophasic epithelial (epithelial-predominant) type of synovial sarcoma from adenocarcinoma. Amary et al.[211] found RT-PCR and FISH to be complementary techniques, with sensitivities and specificities of 96% and 100%, respectively, when used in tandem. The authors of this textbook prefer to use paraffin-embedded tissue for analysis by FISH using a dual-color, break-apart *SS18* probe. In general, although it is not believed that molecular testing is required in every case, if the diagnosis of synovial sarcoma is in question for any reason, ancillary molecular diagnostic testing is used, provided that there is adequate tissue.

Differential Diagnosis

Distinguishing synovial sarcoma from other neoplasms may be difficult, and, in many instances, a reliable diagnosis is not possible without ancillary diagnostic techniques. The differential diagnosis depends on the subtype of synovial sarcoma.

Differential Diagnosis of Biphasic Synovial Sarcoma

In general, biphasic synovial sarcoma causes few diagnostic problems, especially if the tumor is located in the extremities near a large joint and occurs in a young adult. However, when the tumor arises in an unusual site, *carcinosarcoma*, *glandular MPNST*, and *malignant mesothelioma* enter the differential diagnosis. In carcinosarcomas of any site, the glandular element usually shows a significantly greater degree of nuclear pleomorphism than the epithelial component seen in biphasic synovial sarcoma. Similarly, the spindle-cell component of carcinosarcomas is usually more cytologically atypical. Glandular MPNST, a rare neoplasm, usually can be recognized by the presence of intestinal-type epithelium with goblet cells, the occasional association with rhabdomyosarcomatous elements, and the occurrence in patients with manifestations of neurofibromatosis type 1.[212]

Synovial sarcoma may arise in the pleuropulmonary region or peritoneum and, therefore, may cause confusion with malignant mesothelioma. However, the latter tumor typically presents in older patients, often male, usually with a history of significant asbestos exposure. Furthermore, malignant mesotheliomas involve the pleura or peritoneum diffusely and only rarely present as a localized mass. Histologically, malignant mesotheliomas with spindled and epithelial areas usually show a gradual transition between these two areas. Synovial sarcomas, on the other hand, have a sharp abutment of gland with stroma. There is some immunohistochemical overlap because synovial sarcomas express calretinin in over 50% of cases.[213] However, synovial sarcomas frequently express Ber-Ep4 and are negative for WT1. Finally, identification of a t(X;18) or *SS18-SSX* fusion would confirm a diagnosis of synovial sarcoma in difficult cases.

Differential Diagnosis of Monophasic Fibrous Synovial Sarcoma

The monophasic fibrous synovial sarcoma may resemble a number of other spindle cell neoplasms, including fibrosarcoma, leiomyosarcoma, MPNST, solitary fibrous tumor/hemangiopericytoma, and spindle cell carcinoma. Often, an immunohistochemical panel is necessary to make this distinction, and, in difficult cases, cytogenetic or molecular genetic techniques can confirm the diagnosis. This tumor can be distinguished from *fibrosarcoma* by its frequent location near large joints, its irregular and often multilobular growth pattern, the plump appearance of the nuclei, and the focal whorled arrangement of the spindle cells. In general, mitotic figures are less common than in fibrosarcomas. Additional factors that suggest a synovial sarcoma are the presence of mast cells, foci of calcification, the presence of a focal hemangiopericytoma-like vasculature, and the immunohistochemical demonstration of cytokeratin, EMA, and TLE1 in the neoplastic cells. It is clear that many so-called *fibrosarcomas* reported in the older literature are actually monophasic fibrous synovial sarcomas. In their reassessment of lesions diagnosed as fibrosarcoma at the Mayo Clinic over a 48-year period, Bahrami and Folpe[214] found that 13% were more properly classified as monophasic synovial sarcoma.

Some monophasic fibrous synovial sarcomas contain spindle cells with more eosinophilic cytoplasm, reminiscent of *leiomyosarcoma*. However, leiomyosarcomas typically have cells arranged in better-defined fascicles that intersect at right angles to each other. The nuclei are blunt-ended, often with a paranuclear vacuole, and the cytoplasm is more densely eosinophilic. Although some leiomyosarcomas express cytokeratins, particularly CK8/18, virtually all of these tumors stain strongly for smooth muscle actin, and many others express muscle-specific actin, h-caldesmon, or desmin.

MPNST may bear a close resemblance to monophasic fibrous synovial sarcoma (Table 33-10). Given the chemosensitivity of synovial sarcoma, this distinction is of more than academic interest. Obvious origin from a nerve suggests a diagnosis of MPNST, although rare examples of synovial sarcoma arise in peripheral nerves.[173] Synovial sarcomas do not arise from preexisting neurofibromas or in patients with neurofibromatosis type 1. Both MPNST and monophasic synovial sarcoma may have alternating areas of hypercellularity and hypocellularity, imparting a marbled appearance at low magnification. Neuroid-type whorls and perivascular or subintimal involvement of blood vessels by the neoplastic cells suggest a diagnosis of MPNST, although these findings are not entirely specific.

Cytologically, the cells of MPNST are often wavy or buckled and appear to have been pinched at one end, with bulbous protrusion of the opposite end of the nucleus. Immunohistochemically, approximately two-thirds of MPNST stain focally for S-100 protein. Because S-100 protein is found in up to 30% of synovial sarcomas, this marker alone cannot distinguish between these two neoplasms. Similarly, although up to 90% of synovial sarcomas express EMA or AE1/AE3, some examples of MPNST express these antigens as well. In this context, CK7 and CK19 may be useful in that virtually all synovial sarcomas express CK7, CK19, or both, whereas both of these antigens are rarely expressed in MPNST.[188] HMGA2 has been found to be consistently expressed in MPNST and only rarely in synovial sarcoma, suggesting that this marker may be a useful addition to the immunohistochemical panel.[215]

Finally, detection of an *SS18-SSX* fusion allows for a definitive diagnosis of synovial sarcoma. Although one study suggested that up to 75% of MPNST had a t(X;18),[216] subsequent studies by several groups have found the t(X;18) to be exclusive of synovial sarcoma.[217-219] Technical issues likely account for the false-positive cases in the study by O'Sullivan et al.[216,220] Coindre et al.[217] confirmed that MPNST are t(X;18)-negative sarcomas by analyzing 25 cases occurring in NF1 patients.

Many synovial sarcomas exhibit a prominent hemangiopericytoma-like vascular pattern, which can result in an erroneous diagnosis of *solitary fibrous tumor/hemangiopericytoma*. Typically, this vascular pattern is present as a focal phenomenon in synovial sarcoma. Immunohistochemical analysis should easily distinguish these lesions because synovial sarcomas typically express epithelial markers, TLE1, and lack CD34 expression, whereas solitary fibrous tumor/hemangiopericytoma has the opposite immunophenotype.

TABLE 33-10 Immunohistochemical and Molecular Genetic Features of Monophasic Fibrous Synovial Sarcoma Compared to Malignant Peripheral Nerve Sheath Tumor

	MSS (%)	MPNST (%)
AE1/AE3	90	30
CK7	85	Very rare
CK19	85	Very rare
S-100 protein	30	60
CD99	60-70	Rare
TLE1	95	Very rare
SYT aberration	++	–

MSS, monophasic synovial sarcoma; MPNST, malignant peripheral nerve sheath tumor.

Differential Diagnosis of Monophasic Epithelial (Epithelial-Predominant) Synovial Sarcoma

Distinction of purely epithelial forms of synovial sarcoma from *adnexal* or *metastatic carcinoma* is virtually impossible in the absence of a focal biphasic pattern. Fortunately, virtually all of these tumors, when carefully sampled, have focal spindle-cell areas that are sufficiently characteristic to allow a specific diagnosis. As previously mentioned, molecular diagnostic techniques should be used in suspected cases.

Differential Diagnosis of Poorly Differentiated Synovial Sarcoma

In most instances, poorly differentiated synovial sarcoma resembles a number of other small round cell neoplasms, including EFT, neuroblastoma, rhabdomyosarcoma, mesenchymal chondrosarcoma, and lymphoma, among others. A diagnosis of poorly differentiated synovial sarcoma is made simpler if one can identify a lower-grade component typical of either monophasic or biphasic synovial sarcoma. In the absence of such a component, or if only a small amount of tissue composed entirely of round cells is available, distinction from the aforementioned entities invariably requires ancillary diagnostic techniques.

Although CD99 is a highly sensitive marker of EFT, this antigen is found in up to 70% of synovial sarcomas, including poorly differentiated variants (Table 33-11). Furthermore, epithelial markers may be absent in poorly differentiated synovial

TABLE 33-11 Immunohistochemical and Molecular Genetic Features of Poorly Differentiated Synovial Sarcoma Compared to Ewing Family of Tumors

	PDSS (%)	EFT (%)
CD99	60-70	+
AE1/AE3	50-60	Rare
CAM5.2	50-60	30
CK7	70	Very rare
CK19	70	Very rare
SYT(SS18) aberration	+	–
EWSR1 aberration	–	+

PDSS, poorly differentiated synovial sarcoma; EFT, Ewing family of tumors.

sarcoma, and, although not well recognized, many EFTs express cytokeratins, especially low-molecular-weight isoforms.[28,29,43] CK7 and CK19 stains may be useful for this distinction because most poorly differentiated synovial sarcomas, including those that are negative with AE1/AE3 and EMA, express CK7, CK19, or both, whereas these antigens are typically absent in EFT.[89] Identification of the *EWSR1-FLI1* or *SS18-SSX* fusions are useful for confirming diagnoses of EFT and poorly differentiated synovial sarcoma, respectively.

Neuroblastoma arises from structures of the sympathetic nervous system during early childhood, characteristically has Homer Wright rosettes, and lacks expression of both CD99 and epithelial markers. *Rhabdomyosarcoma* can be excluded by the absence of desmin, myogenin, or MyoD1; appropriate T- and B-cell markers help exclude *lymphoma*.

Some poorly differentiated synovial sarcomas are composed of large epithelioid cells, sometimes accompanied by cells with rhabdoid features. These tumors may be difficult to distinguish from *metastatic carcinoma*, *epithelioid sarcoma*, and *MERT*. Recognition of a lower-grade area more typical of synovial sarcoma is the most useful way to distinguish these neoplasms. In the absence of such foci, a broad immunohistochemical panel coupled with molecular genetic studies can usually resolve this dilemma.

Discussion

Recurrence and Metastasis

Although traditionally considered to be a uniformly high-grade malignancy, advancements in therapy have lowered the incidence of recurrence and metastasis, with improved long-term survival. As one would expect, the prognosis is poorest in cases treated merely by local excision with inadequate margins and without any adjunctive therapy. In these cases, recurrence rates as high as 80% are reported.[221] With adequate surgical excision or with adjunctive radiotherapy, the recurrence rate has been reported to be significantly lower (less than 40%).[222] In most cases, the recurrent growth manifests within the first 2 years after initial therapy.

Metastatic lesions develop in about half of cases, most commonly to the lung, followed by the lymph nodes and the bone marrow. In a series by Machen et al.,[183] all patients who developed metastatic disease had involvement of one or both lungs; similarly, in the series of Ryan et al.,[223] the lung was affected in 94% of cases and the lymph nodes in 10%.

BOX 33-1 Favorable and Unfavorable Prognostic Factors by Multivariate Analysis for Synovial Sarcoma

Low Risk for Metastasis
- Patient age less than 25 years
- Tumor size less than 5 cm
- Absence of poorly differentiated areas

High Risk for Metastasis
- Patient age greater than 40 years
- Tumor size greater than or exactly 5 cm
- Poorly differentiated areas

Modified from Bergh P, Meis-Kindblom JM, Gherlinzoni F, et al. Synovial sarcoma: identification of low and high risk groups. *Cancer* 1999;85:2596.

There are numerous accounts of late metastasis and long periods of survival after metastasis. On the other hand, there are instances in which pulmonary metastasis is already present at the time of or prior to the initial diagnosis. Microscopically, the metastatic lesions are usually similar to the primary neoplasm, but metastases of biphasic tumors often exhibit a more prominent spindle-cell pattern than the primary lesion, a lesser degree of cellular differentiation, and increased mitotic activity. Care should be exercised when interpreting pulmonary metastasis of any spindle cell sarcoma to avoid interpreting entrapped alveolar spaces as evidence of biphasic differentiation.

Prognosis

Reported 5-year overall survival rates for synovial sarcoma range from 64% to 76%[224,225]; however, the numbers are far more dismal for those who present with metastases at the time of diagnosis. Numerous clinical and microscopic factors have been reported to influence survival (Box 33-1). Major clinical factors associated with a more favorable clinical outcome include age of the patient (15 years or younger),[225-228] tumor size smaller than 5 cm,[155,224,225,229-231] distal extremity location,[232] and low tumor stage.[224,232,233]

A wide array of histologic features has been reported to be of prognostic significance, but there is often disagreement among studies. There is still no agreement as to the prognostic significance of the microscopic subtype. Whereas some have found biphasic synovial sarcomas to behave in a more indolent fashion than monophasic tumors,[234] others have not found this to be so.[235] It is difficult to compare the results of these studies, however, because of great differences in the criteria used to distinguish the synovial sarcoma subtypes. In the study by Machen et al.,[183] the proportion of each tumor composed of spindled and epithelial areas was evaluated semiquantitatively and was not found to be of prognostic significance.

Two histologic patterns of synovial sarcoma have special clinical significance. Extensively calcified synovial sarcomas appear to have a better long-term prognosis. In a series of extensively calcified synovial sarcomas by Varela-Duran and Enzinger,[236] local recurrence and pulmonary metastases were detected in 32% and 29% of patients, respectively. In the study of extremity synovial sarcomas by Machen et al.,[183] 24% of cases had areas of calcification ranging from 5% to 20% of the tumors, but the presence or extent of calcification was not found to have an impact on clinical behavior. On the other hand, it is clear that tumors with poorly differentiated areas generally behave more aggressively and metastasize in a higher percentage of cases than those without these areas.[182,227,237,238] Thorough sampling of these tumors is required to determine the presence and extent of poorly differentiated areas. Other histologic features reported to have an adverse prognostic impact include the presence of rhabdoid cells,[239] extensive tumor necrosis,[240] high mitotic index (greater than 10 MF/10 HPF),[183,232,241] and high nuclear grade.[183] Potential biomarkers of poor prognosis include aberrant p53 expression,[242] aberrant beta-catenin expression,[238,243] expression of dysadherin,[244] expression of insulin-like growth factor 1 receptor[245] or insulin-like growth factor 2 (IGF2),[246] coexpression of hepatocyte growth factor and its receptor (c-MET),[242] and deletion of *PTEN*.[247]

Although there is some disagreement, some have found *SS18-SSX* fusion subtype to be an independent prognostic indicator. In the study by Kawai et al.,[208] a longer metastasis-free survival period in those patients with localized tumors and *SS18-SSX2* was observed. This contention was strongly supported by the much larger study by Ladanyi et al.[155] of 243 patients with synovial sarcoma. In this study, the median overall survival for the *SS18-SSX2* group was about twice that of the *SS18-SSX1* group (13.7 versus 6.1 years), and the 5-year survival rates were 73% and 53%, respectively. However, the impact of fusion type on survival was not significant when stratified for disease status at presentation. Among patients with localized disease at diagnosis, median overall survival for the *SS18-SSX2* group was about 50% longer than those in the *SS18-SSX1* group (13.7 years versus 9.2 years). By multivariate analysis, fusion type was the only independent factor to significantly impact overall survival. Nevertheless, a number of more recent studies have not found fusion type to have a prognostic impact.[211,237,248,249]

Therapy

Local control of synovial sarcoma is clearly related to the adequacy of initial surgical excision. Simple local excision without ancillary therapy is incapable of checking the growth and spread of the tumor, and most reviewers recommend extensive surgery as the therapy of choice, including radical local excision, often with removal of an entire muscle or muscle group, and amputation, depending mainly on the size of the tumor and its location. Because radical local excision is often impossible with tumors situated near a large joint—the favored location of synovial sarcoma—adjunctive radiotherapy in addition to local excision of the tumor is favored over amputation.[222,241,250,251]

Synovial sarcoma is a chemosensitive sarcoma. In particular, regimens that include ifosfamide and doxorubicin or epirubicin are efficacious, resulting in a partial or complete response in about 50% of patients.[233,252-254] There is also strong interest in potential targeted therapies for synovial sarcoma. For example, BCL2 is overexpressed in the vast majority of synovial sarcomas. The increased expression of this anti-apoptotic protein is not a result of gene amplification or rearrangement but rather is likely secondary to increased protein stability or transcriptional activation.[255] In vivo studies on synovial sarcoma cell lines have shown effective BCL2 blockade by G3139, an oligonucleotide that decreases BCL2 expression and induces apoptosis.[256] Several studies have shown overexpression of EGFR in up to 55% of synovial sarcomas,[247,257] and so the EGFR inhibitor gefitinib has been attempted in patients with locally advanced or metastatic synovial sarcomas that overexpress EGFR,[258,259] with variable success.

Line of Differentiation

There is still considerable debate as to the exact line of differentiation of this neoplasm. This uncertainty is also reflected in the 2012 WHO Soft Tissue Classification in which synovial sarcoma is placed among the tumors of uncertain differentiation. In the past, most discussion centered on whether synovial sarcomas arose from preformed synovium. The largely outdated concept that sarcomas arise from mature, preformed tissue has given way to a discussion as to whether these tumors have cellular features that resemble normal synovium. As previously mentioned, synovial sarcomas rarely arise in joint cavities, and these tumors may arise in locations in which normal synovial structures are rare or nonexistent, including the lung, heart, and abdominal wall. Furthermore, there are significant immunohistochemical and ultrastructural differences between the cells of synovial sarcoma and those of the synovial lining. Some reviewers believe that the term *synovial sarcoma* should be abandoned, but it is so well established in the literature that there seems little reason to alter it, at present, until there is a consensus as to the appropriate choice of alternate terms.

ALVEOLAR SOFT PART SARCOMA

Alveolar soft part sarcoma is a clinically and morphologically distinct soft tissue sarcoma first defined and named by Christopherson et al.[260] in 1952. Before this report, typical cases had been described under various designations, including malignant myoblastoma, angioendothelioma, and even liposarcoma. Since 1952, numerous examples have been reported and studied immunohistochemically and electron microscopically, but there is still uncertainty as to its exact nature. However, recent advances have been made in understanding the molecular pathogenesis and even the nature of the characteristic PAS-positive crystals. Alveolar soft part sarcomas are uniformly malignant; there is no benign counterpart of the tumor.

Alveolar soft part sarcoma is an uncommon neoplasm; its frequency among this textbook's authors' cases is estimated at 0.5% to 1.0% of all soft tissue sarcomas. It is even less common in other series. Ekfors et al.,[261] for example, found only one alveolar soft part sarcoma among 246 malignant soft tissue tumors in Finland, an incidence of 0.4%.

Clinical Findings

This tumor occurs principally in adolescents and young adults and is most frequently encountered in patients 15 to 35 years of age.[262-268] Female patients outnumber males, especially among patients under 25 years of age.[269] Infants and children are affected less frequently. There are two main locations of the tumor. When it occurs in adults, it is seen predominantly in the lower extremities, especially the anterior portion of the thigh. In a study of 102 alveolar soft part sarcomas by

Lieberman et al.,[262] 39.5% involved the soft tissues of the buttock or thigh. The tumor has also been described in a variety of unusual locations, including the female genital tract,[270] breast,[271] urinary bladder,[272] and bone,[273] among many other sites. When the tumor affects infants and children, it is often located in the region of the head and neck, especially the orbit and tongue; tumors in the head and neck tend to be smaller, probably because of earlier detection (Table 33-12).[274]

Alveolar soft part sarcoma usually presents as a slowly growing, painless mass that almost never causes functional impairment. Because of the relative lack of symptoms, it is easily overlooked; in a number of cases, metastasis to the lung or brain is the first manifestation of the disease.[267] Headache, nausea, and visual changes are often associated with cerebral metastasis. As a rule, the tumor is richly vascular, causing pulsation or a distinctly audible bruit, in some instances; massive hemorrhage may be encountered during surgical removal. Hypervascularity with prominent draining veins and prolonged capillary staining are usually demonstrable with angiography and CT scans. On MRI, the tumor typically demonstrates high signal intensity on both T2- and T1-weighted images.[275,276]

TABLE 33-12 Anatomic Distribution of 102 Alveolar Soft Part Sarcomas

LOCATION	NO. OF PATIENTS	PERCENTAGE (%)
Buttock/thigh	40	39.5
Leg/popliteal	17	16.6
Chest wall/trunk	13	12.9
Forearm	10	9.7
Arm	8	8.5
Back/neck	6	6.4
Tongue	4	3.2
Retroperitoneum	4	3.2
Total	102	100.0

Modified from Lieberman PH, Brennan MF, Kimmel M, et al. Alveolar soft-part sarcoma: a clinicopathologic study of half a century. Cancer 1989;63:1–13.

Pathologic Findings

The gross specimen tends to be poorly circumscribed, soft, and friable; on sectioning, it consists of yellow-white to gray-red tissue, often with large areas of necrosis and hemorrhage. Frequently, the tumor is surrounded by numerous tortuous vessels of large caliber.

The microscopic picture varies little from tumor to tumor, and the uniformity of the microscopic picture is one of its characteristic features. Dense fibrous trabeculae of varying thickness divide the tumor into compact groups or compartments of irregular size that, in turn, are subdivided into sharply defined nests or aggregates of tumor cells (Figs. 33-62 and 33-63). These cellular aggregates are separated from one another by thin-walled, sinusoidal vascular channels lined by a single layer of flattened endothelial cells. In most instances, the cellular aggregates exhibit central degeneration, necrosis, and loss of cohesion resulting in a pseudoalveolar pattern (Fig. 33-64). This pattern should not be confused with the more irregular alveolar pattern of alveolar rhabdomyosarcoma. Less frequently, the nest-like pattern is inconspicuous or absent entirely, and the tumor is merely composed of uniform sheets of large granular cells with few or no discernible vascular channels (Fig. 33-65). This more solid or compact type of alveolar soft part sarcoma occurs mainly in infants and children.

The individual cells are large, rounded, or more often polygonal and display little variation in size and shape. They have distinct cell borders and one or more vesicular nuclei with small nucleoli and abundant granular, eosinophilic, and sometimes vacuolated cytoplasm. Mitotic figures are scarce. Rare pleomorphic tumors have been reported in the literature (Fig. 33-66).[277]

At the margin of the tumor, there are usually numerous dilated veins, probably the result of multiple arteriovenous shunts in the neoplasm. Vascular invasion is a constant, striking finding that explains the tendency of the tumor to develop metastasis at an early stage of the disease (Fig. 33-67).

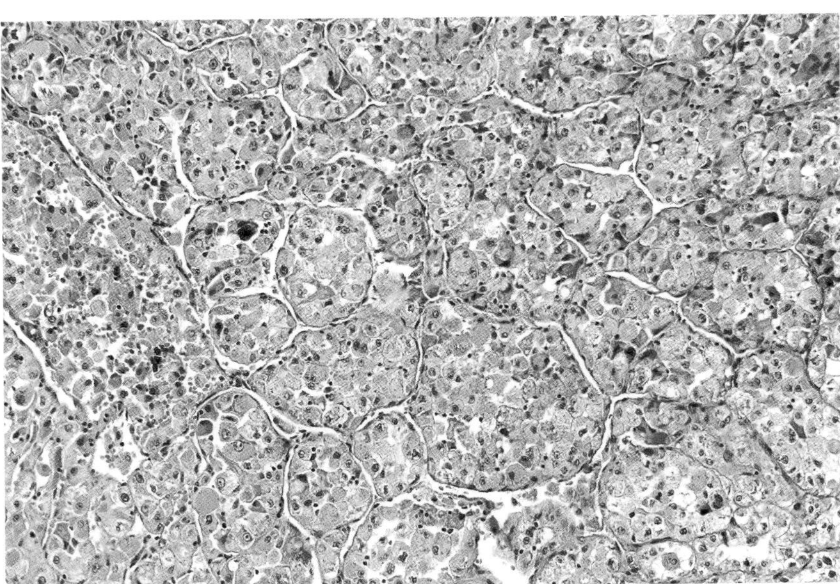

FIGURE 33-62. Alveolar soft part sarcoma with a typical organoid arrangement of tumor cells.

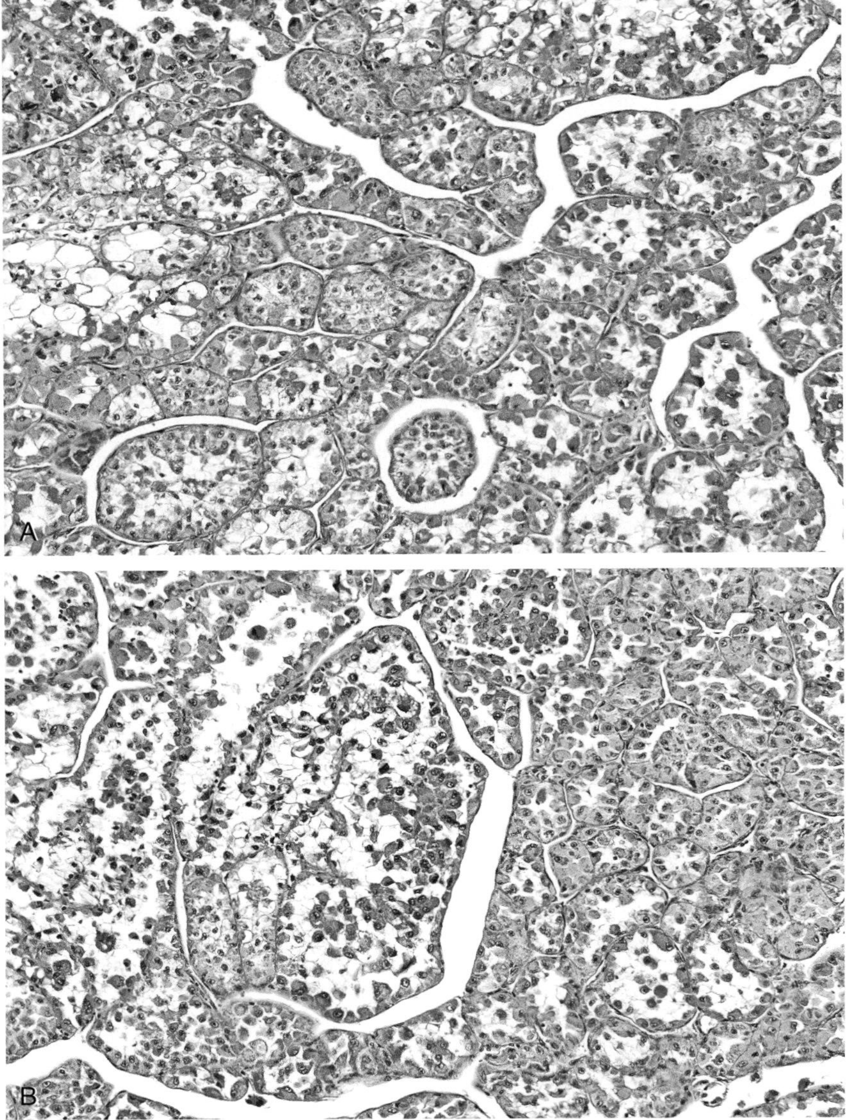

FIGURE 33-63. (A) Low-magnification view of alveolar soft part sarcoma composed of nests of large tumor cells with central loss of cellular cohesion resulting in a pseudoalveolar pattern. (B) Higher-power view revealing cell nests that are separated by thin-walled, sinusoidal vascular spaces.

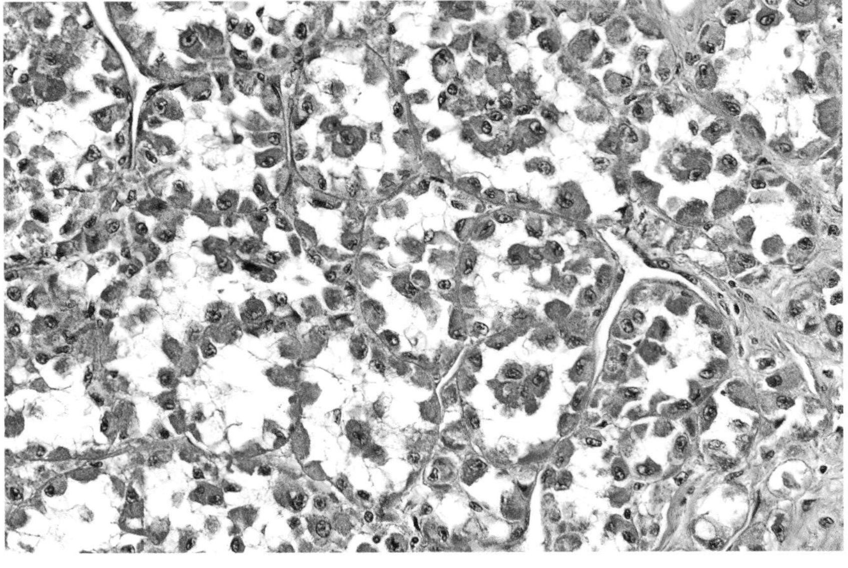

FIGURE 33-64. Prominent pseudoalveolar growth pattern in an alveolar soft part sarcoma.

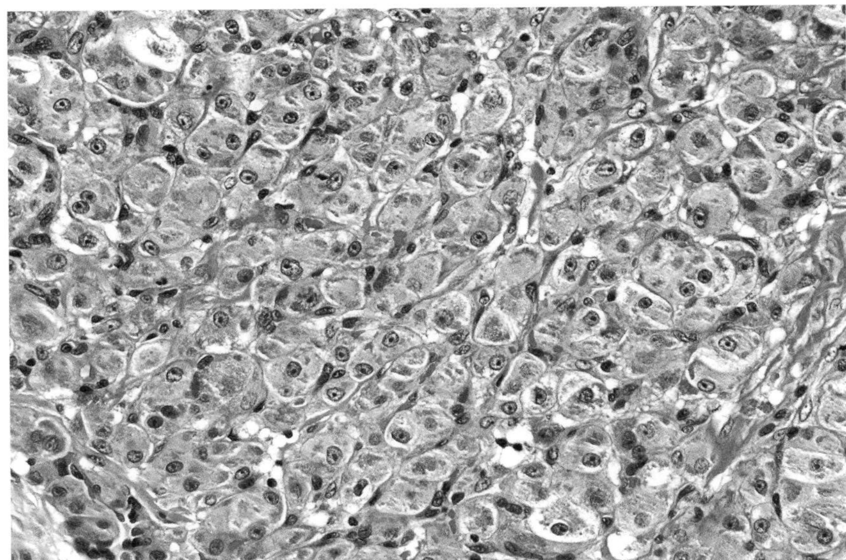

FIGURE 33-65. Alveolar soft part sarcoma arising in a child showing clustering and small nests of tumor cells.

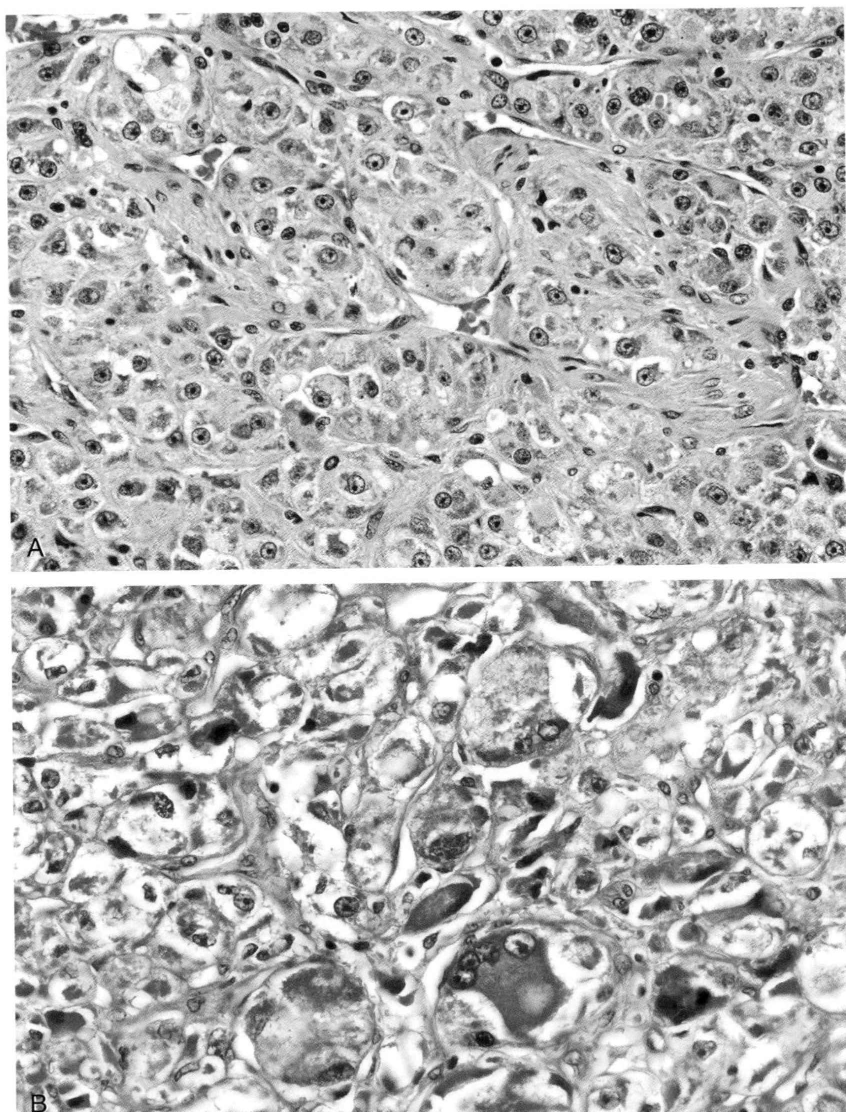

FIGURE 33-66. Range of cytologic atypia in alveolar soft part sarcomas. (A) This is the typical cytologic appearance of alveolar soft part sarcoma, with relatively uniform nuclei and prominent nucleoli. (B) Scattered atypical cells in an alveolar soft part sarcoma. *Continued*

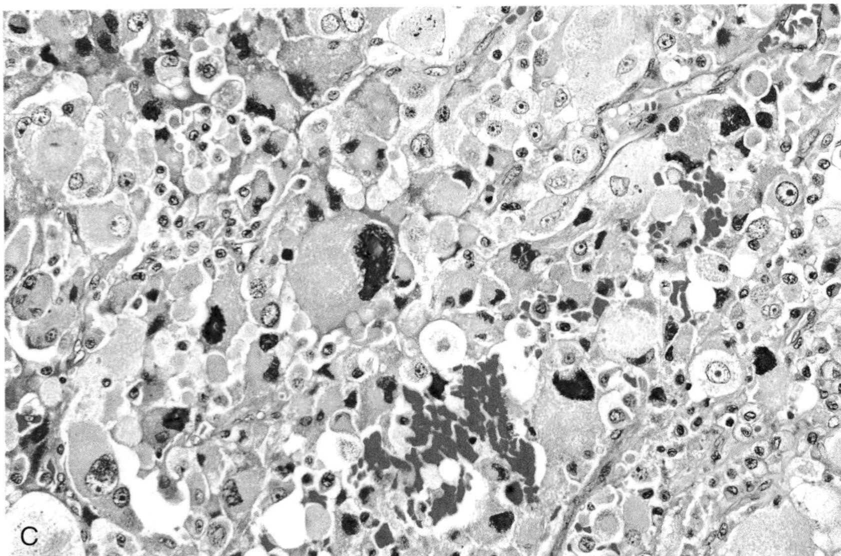

FIGURE 33-66, cont'd. (C) Marked cytologic atypia in an alveolar soft part sarcoma.

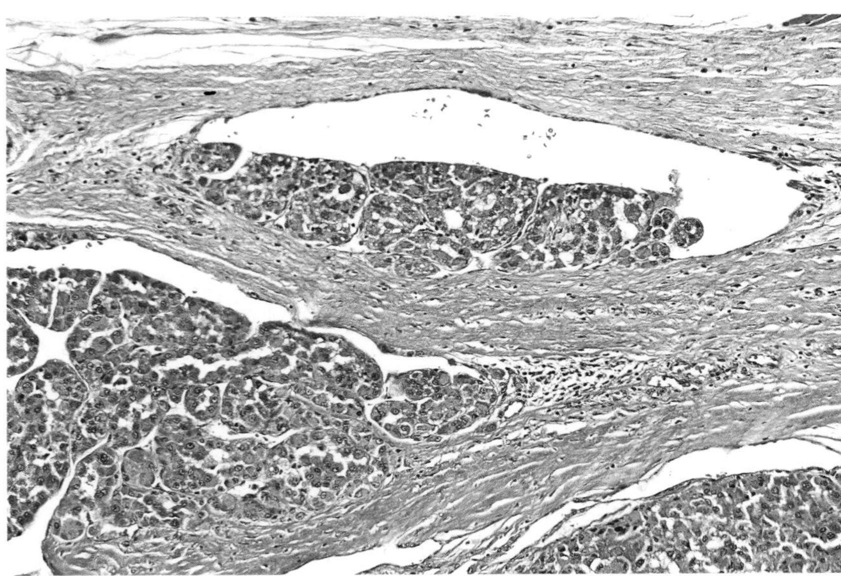

FIGURE 33-67. Dilated peripheral vein with tumor invasion.

Histochemical stains are useful for establishing the diagnosis in that PAS preparation reveals varying amounts of intracellular glycogen and characteristically PAS-positive, diastase-resistant rhomboid or rod-shaped crystals (Fig. 33-68). These crystals vary greatly in number from case to case. In some cases, they can be identified in almost every cell, whereas, in others, they are difficult to find or absent. In this textbook's authors' experience, the typical crystalline material is present in at least 80% of the tumors; in the remainder, there are merely PAS-positive granules, probably precursors of the crystals.

The nature of these crystals has been elucidated, although serendipitously. In the course of characterizing a monoclonal antibody to the monocarboxylate transporter 1 (MCT1) in a variety of tissues and tumors, Ladanyi et al.[278] noted expression on the surface and in the cytoplasm of the cells in examples of alveolar soft part sarcoma. MCT1 is one of a family of transporter proteins that catalyzes the rapid transport of monocarboxylates across plasma membranes. The protein is normally associated with the rough endoplasmic reticulin and is transported to the plasma membrane in association with its chaperone, CD147. Ladanyi et al.[278] found an abundance of MCT1 and CD147 on the surface of the cells of alveolar soft part sarcoma, as well as within the cytoplasm in the region of the characteristic crystals. Western blot analysis confirmed the nature of the protein and ultrastructural immunohistochemistry localized MCT1 and CD147 to the cytoplasmic crystals and their precursor granules.

Immunohistochemical Findings

Numerous immunohistochemical studies have attempted to elucidate the histogenesis of this unusual tumor, often

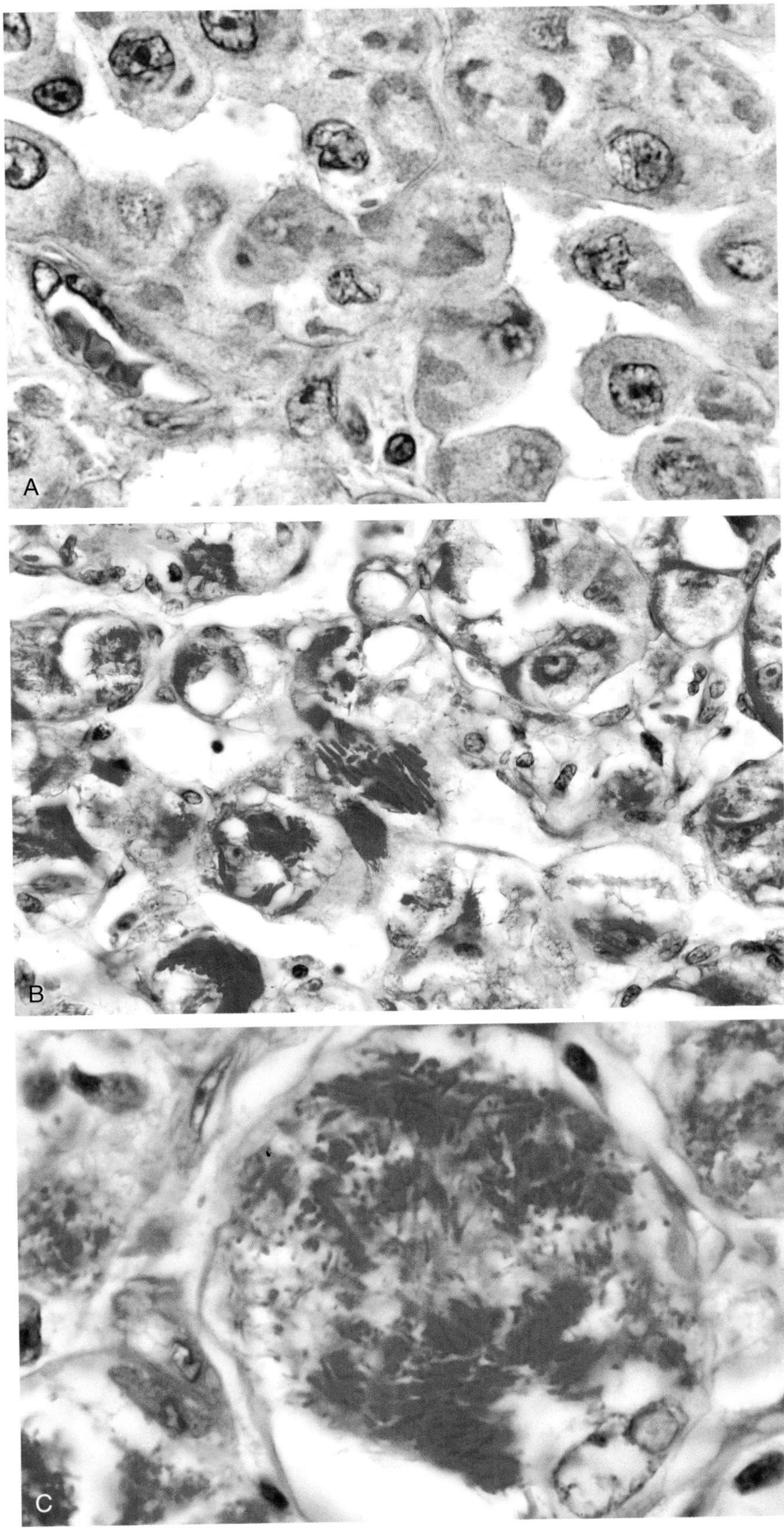

FIGURE 33-68. (A) High-magnification view of an alveolar soft part sarcoma. There is focal condensation of eosinophilic cytoplasm. (B) Periodic acid-Schiff (PAS) staining with diastase reveals varying amounts of intracellular crystalline material. (C) High-magnification view of crystalline material, diagnostic of alveolar soft part sarcoma.

resulting in contradictory results. The cells generally do not stain with antibodies against cytokeratin, EMA, neurofilaments, GFAP, serotonin, or synaptophysin; they occasionally express S-100 protein and neuron-specific enolase, but these markers are of no diagnostic value. The reports in regard to staining for muscle markers differ somewhat, but most have demonstrated muscle markers in less than 50% of tumors.[269,279]

In 1991, Rosai et al.[280] detected the myogenic nuclear regulatory protein MyoD1 by immunohistochemistry (confirmed by Western blot analysis) and suggested this as confirmatory evidence of its skeletal muscle nature. In contrast, Cullinane et al.[281] were unable to detect MyoD1 by Northern blot analysis. Using paraffin-embedded samples, Wang et al.[282] were unable to detect nuclear expression of MyoD1 in 12 alveolar soft part sarcomas, although there was considerable granular cytoplasmic immunoreactivity. Subsequent studies have failed to detect either MyoD1 or myogenin in alveolar soft part sarcoma,[283,284] effectively excluding classical skeletal muscle differentiation.

As discussed later, this tumor is characterized by aberrations of the *TFE3* gene on Xp11.2. As such, a number of studies have demonstrated nuclear immunoreactivity for this protein in most (but not all) alveolar soft part sarcomas.[285-288] For example, Tsuji et al.[288] found TFE3 staining in 22 of 24 (92%) cases, but 2 of 5 granular cell tumors also stained for this antigen. Similarly, Williams et al.[287] found TFE3 positivity in all 18 alveolar soft part sarcomas tested, but they also found staining in 4 granular cell tumors and 1 adrenal cortical carcinoma. CD147 (mentioned previously) is also frequently expressed in alveolar soft part sarcoma but appears to lack specificity.[288]

Ultrastructural Findings

Electron microscopy shows the cells to contain numerous mitochondria, prominent smooth endoplasmic reticulum, glycogen, and a well-developed Golgi apparatus. Characteristically, there are rhomboid, rod-shaped, or spicular crystals with a regular lattice pattern and sparse electron-dense secretory granules (Fig. 33-69). Both the crystals and dense granules are membrane-bound and consist of crystallized and uncrystallized filaments that are 4 to 6 nm in diameter, suggesting transitions between the two structures. The filaments are arranged in a parallel fashion with a periodicity of 10 nm.[289,290]

Cytogenetic and Molecular Genetic Findings

Cytogenetic studies of this tumor have identified a specific alteration, der(17)t(X;17)(p11.2q25).[291] This unbalanced translocation results in the fusion of the *TFE3* gene on Xp11.2 (a member of the basic-helix-loop-helix family of transcription factors) to *ASPSCR1* (also known as *ASPL* or *RCC17)* on 17q25. The resulting fusion gene encodes for a fusion protein that localizes to the nucleus and functions as an aberrant transcription factor.[291,292] Interestingly, this same gene fusion has been found in an unusual variant of pediatric renal cell carcinoma characterized by nested and pseudopapillary architecture, psammomatous calcifications, and epithelioid cells with abundant clear cytoplasm and well-defined cell borders.[293]

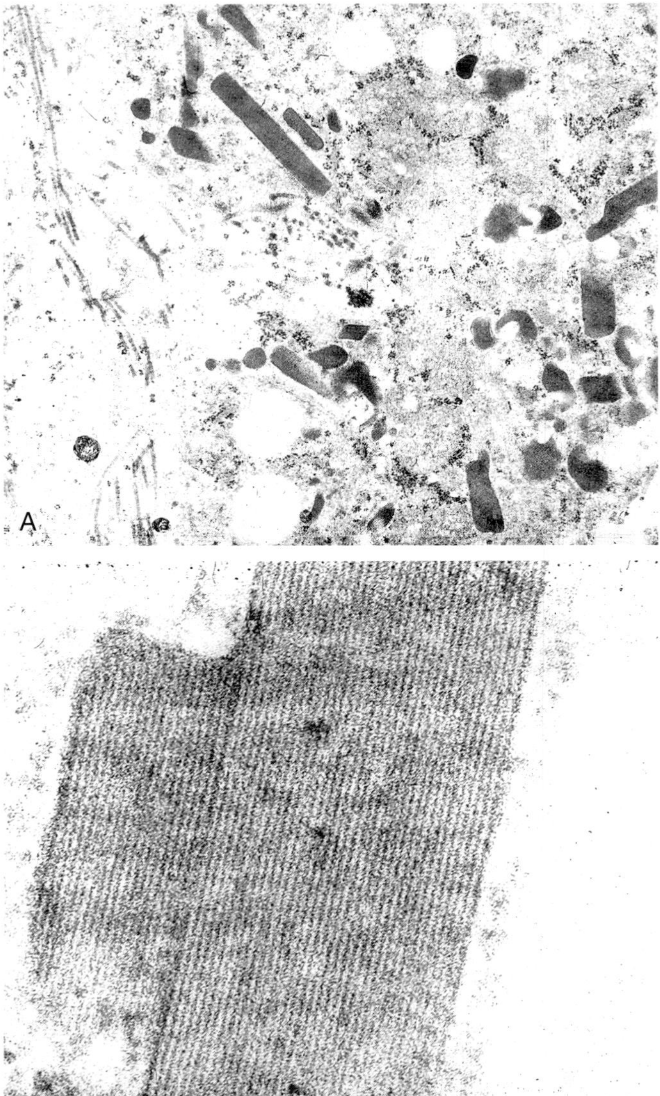

FIGURE 33-69. (A, B) Electron micrographs depicting intracellular crystalline structures in an alveolar soft part sarcoma.

However, among soft tissue sarcomas, the *ASPSCR1-TFE3* fusion appears to be both sensitive and specific. In the study by Tsuji et al.,[288] using fixed, paraffin-embedded tissues, the authors found evidence of this fusion (by RT-PCR) in 24 of 24 cases tested but in none of the 13 control tumors. Similar results were reported by others,[287,294] with documentation of this fusion in almost all cases of alveolar soft part sarcoma. Zhong et al.[295] developed a dual color, break-apart FISH probe that should also prove useful in diagnostically challenging cases.

Exactly how or whether the *ASPSCR1-TFE3* fusion is related to the accumulation of crystalline deposits of MCT1 and CD147 is not known. Saito et al.[296] suggested a role for DNA mismatch repair because inactivation of *hMSH2* and *hMLH1* was detected in some *ASPSCR1-TFE3*-positive alveolar soft part sarcomas.

Several expression profiling studies have found consistent upregulation of genes involved in angiogenesis, which is not entirely surprising given the obvious vascularity of this neoplasm.[297-299] Therefore, there is interest in anti-angiogenic targeted therapy.[300-302]

Differential Diagnosis

The differential diagnosis chiefly includes metastatic *renal cell carcinoma*, *paraganglioma*, and *granular cell tumor* (Table 33-13). Alveolar rhabdomyosarcoma is sometimes confused with alveolar soft part sarcoma more because of the similarity in name than the microscopic picture.

Renal cell carcinoma, primary or metastatic, often bears a striking resemblance to alveolar soft part sarcoma (Fig. 33-70), but, in most cases, it can be distinguished by the absence of the characteristic PAS-positive crystalline material. The pale-staining cytoplasm of its cells and the fat content of renal cell carcinoma are less reliable features because each may be encountered in degenerated forms of alveolar soft part sarcoma (Fig. 33-71). Immunoreactivity for EMA is useful for confirming a diagnosis of renal cell carcinoma because this antigen is absent in alveolar soft part sarcoma. Staining for TFE3 can be helpful, although it must be kept in mind that some pediatric renal cell carcinomas and granular cell tumors also express this antigen. Glycogen is present in both alveolar soft part sarcoma and renal cell carcinoma, but it is absent in *granular cell tumor* and *paraganglioma*. It is also noteworthy that the cells of granular cell tumor are less well defined, have a distinctly granular cytoplasm, and show strong S-100 protein staining.

The clinical features are also of value in the differential diagnosis. Primary renal cell carcinomas are usually demonstrable radiographically in the retroperitoneum. Renal cell carcinoma, paraganglioma, and malignant granular cell tumor chiefly affect patients over 40 years of age; they are rare in patients younger than 25 years. Moreover, there is no record that a bona fide paraganglioma has ever occurred in the extremities.

Clinical Behavior and Therapy

The ultimate prognosis is poor despite the relatively slow growth of the tumor. Of the 91 patients with follow-up information in the study from Memorial Sloan-Kettering Cancer Center (New York, NY), only 15% of patients were alive after 20 years.[262] Portera et al.[265] reported their experience in treating 74 patients with alveolar soft part sarcoma at MD Anderson Cancer Center. Thirty-five percent of patients presented with American Joint Committee on Cancer stage III or IV, but 65% of patients presented with stage IV disease. Five-year local recurrence free, distant recurrence free, disease free, and overall survival for 22 patients with localized disease at presentation were 88%, 84%, 71%, and 87%, respectively. In contrast, the median survival for patients with metastases was 40 months with a 5-year overall survival of 20%. All patients who had brain metastases had evidence of metastatic disease at other sites. Metastases tend to occur early in the course of the disease, and there are many reports of patients who present with pulmonary or brain metastasis. On the other hand,

TABLE 33-13 Differential Diagnostic Features of Alveolar Soft Part Sarcoma

LESION	GLYCOGEN	CRYSTALS	IMMUNOHISTOCHEMISTRY
Alveolar soft part sarcoma	+	+	Variable muscle markers; TFE3
Renal cell carcinoma	+	–	Epithelial membrane antigen
Paraganglioma	–	–	Neuroendocrine markers (synaptophysin, chromogranin); S-100 protein in sustentacular cells
Granular cell tumor	–	–	S-100 protein

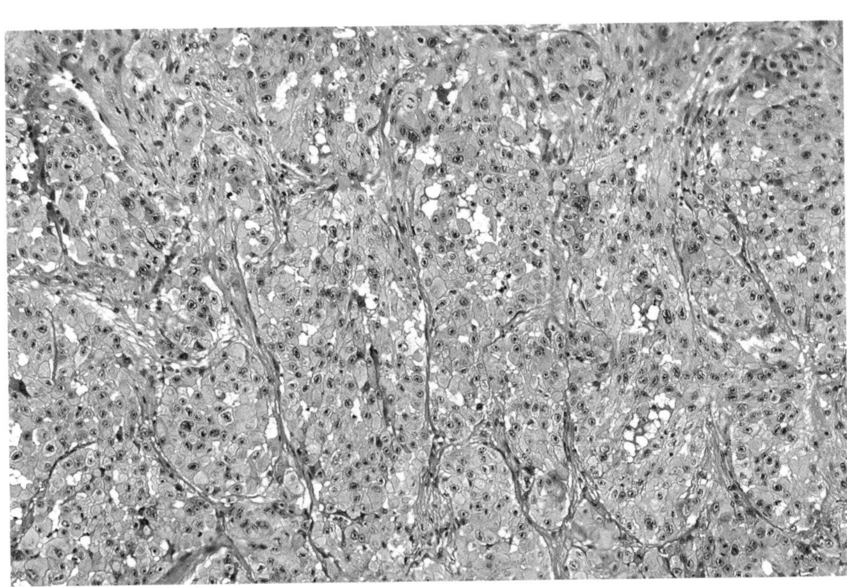

FIGURE 33-70. Metastatic renal cell carcinoma simulating an alveolar soft part sarcoma.

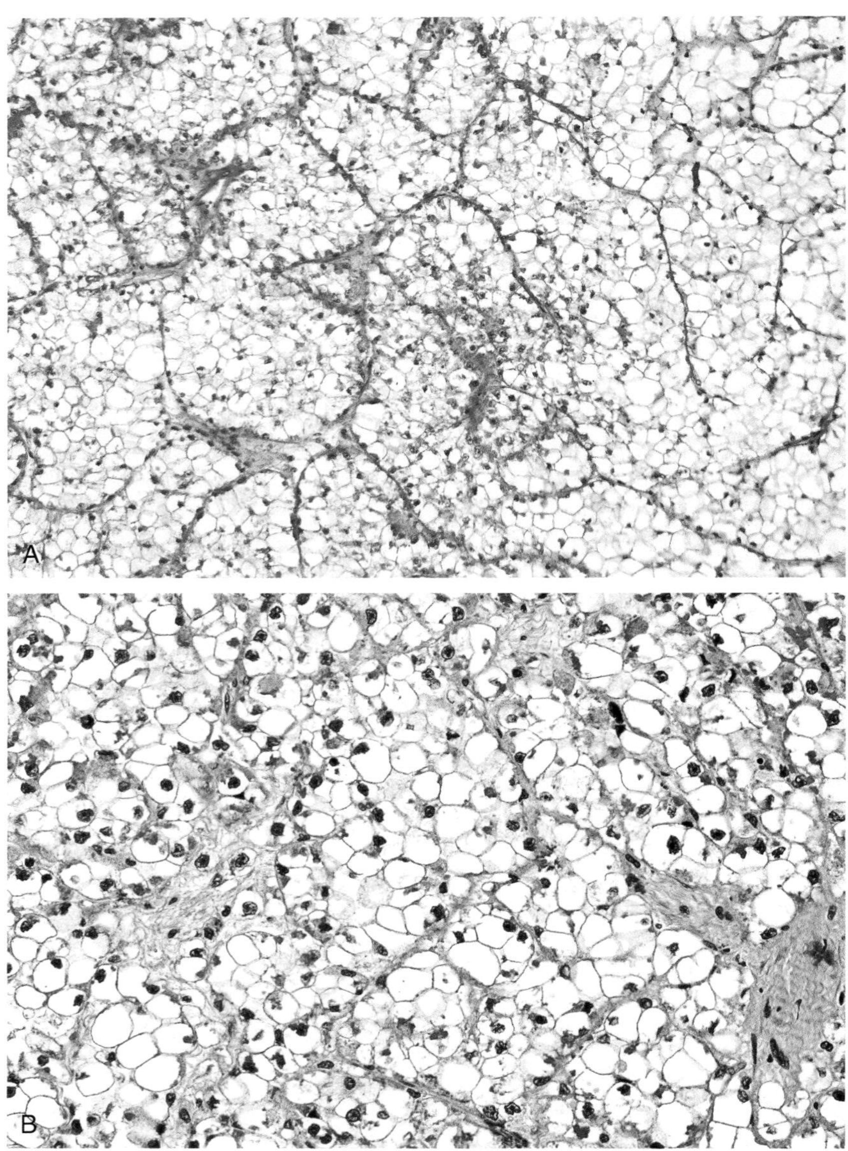

FIGURE 33-71. (A) Low-magnification view of alveolar soft part sarcoma simulating a renal cell carcinoma of clear cell type. The cytoplasmic clearing likely represents a degenerative feature of this tumor. (B) Higher-magnification view showing close simulation of a renal cell carcinoma by this alveolar soft part sarcoma.

metastasis may also be delayed for many years; Lillehei et al.[303] reported a patient who developed brain metastases 33 years after the initial presentation, emphasizing the need for long-term follow-up.

The most important prognostic parameters appear to be age at diagnosis, tumor size, and the presence of metastasis at presentation.[262,267] In the study by Lieberman et al.,[262] there was an increased risk of metastasis at presentation with increasing age because only 17% of patients who presented during the first decade of life had metastatic disease compared to 32% in patients older than 30 years of age. Improved prognosis in children may in part be related to the location of the tumor, early clinical detection, small size, and better resectability.[266,274] In addition, patients who present with metastatic disease tend to have primary tumors that are larger than those in patients who do not have metastasis at presentation.[262,266] Although the development of metastatic disease clearly portends a grave prognosis, resection of solitary brain metastases may be of prognostic benefit.[304] The principal metastatic sites are the lungs, followed by the brain and skeleton. Metastases to lymph nodes are infrequent.

Treatment is not particularly promising, and the relatively slow growth of the tumor must be considered when one is assessing the effect of therapy. Most reviewers recommend radical surgical excision of primary and metastatic lesions combined with radiotherapy or chemotherapy (or both), although most report limited success with systemic therapies.[268,305] There has been some initial success with the tyrosine kinase inhibitor sunitinib.[301,302,306]

Discussion

Despite numerous immunohistochemical and electron microscopic studies, the line of cellular differentiation of alveolar soft part sarcoma remains obscure. Over the years, several concepts concerning the nature of this tumor have been entertained.

Skeletal muscle differentiation has been suggested by many over the years, but a number of studies have also detracted from this concept. Fisher and Reidbord[307] first suggested the possibility of skeletal muscle differentiation on the basis of the resemblance of the membrane-bound crystals to those in nemaline myopathy and rhabdomyoma. This concept was strengthened by immunohistochemical studies that demonstrated the potential of the tumor cells to express desmin and muscle-specific actin. Although the initial detection of MyoD1 in a case of alveolar soft part sarcoma reported by Rosai et al.[280] seemed to lend support to the concept of skeletal muscle differentiation, others have been unable to duplicate this finding, and, therefore, there is no convincing evidence that alveolar soft part sarcomas exhibit skeletal muscle differentiation.

Still another histogenetic theory was offered by DeSchryver-Kecskemeti et al.,[308] who contended that the cytoplasmic granules of alveolar soft part sarcomas are similar to the renin granules of juxtaglomerular tumors and proposed the name *angioreninoma*. There is, however, no sign of hyperreninism (e.g., hypertension, hypokalemia, aldosteronism) in patients with alveolar soft part sarcoma; according to Mukai et al.,[309] immunostaining for renin is negative and plasma renin levels are normal.

DESMOPLASTIC SMALL ROUND CELL TUMOR

DSRCT is a relatively uncommon entity that typically involves the abdominal or pelvic peritoneum (or both) of young males and pursues an aggressive clinical course. The lesion is characterized by a proliferation of small round cells deposited in an abundant desmoplastic stroma and multiphenotypic differentiation by immunohistochemistry. This lesion has had a variety of names, including *desmoplastic small cell tumor with divergent differentiation*,[310] *intra-abdominal desmoplastic small round cell tumor*,[311] *malignant small cell epithelial tumor of the peritoneum* coexpressing mesenchymal-type intermediate filaments,[312] *intra-abdominal neuroectodermal tumor of childhood with divergent differentiation*,[313] and *desmoplastic small cell tumor with multiphenotypic differentiation*.[314] Given that this lesion clearly can occur in extra-abdominal locations as well as in adults, *desmoplastic small round cell tumor* is now the accepted name for this neoplasm.

Clinical Findings

Most patients with this tumor are 15 to 35 years of age, although patients as young as 5 years[315] and as old as the seventh and eighth decades of life have been reported.[316] In a study of 109 patients with this tumor by Gerald et al.,[317] the patients ranged in age from 6 to 49 years (mean 22 years). Males far outnumber females at a ratio of approximately 4 to 1.[317-319]

Most present with a large abdominal and/or pelvic mass with extensive peritoneal involvement, usually without an identifiable visceral site of origin (Table 33-14). The most common complaint is abdominal distension, often associated with pain and constipation. Other signs and symptoms include intestinal or ureteral obstruction, ascites, difficulty with urination, and impotence. Although most tumors arise in the abdomen/pelvis, this tumor has also been described in the paratesticular region,[320] ovary,[321] pleura,[322] central nervous system,[323] major salivary glands,[324,325] bone,[326] lung,[327] kidney,[328,329] and pancreas.[330]

Pathologic Findings

Grossly, the tumor forms a solid, large multilobulated mass that is white or gray-white on cross-section, sometimes distorted by cystic change and areas of necrosis. Microscopically, most tumors are composed of sharply demarcated nests of varying size with small round or oval cells embedded in a hypervascular desmoplastic stroma (Figs. 33-72 to 33-74). Large tumor cell nests often have central necrosis (Fig. 33-75). The neoplastic cells appear undifferentiated and have small hyperchromatic nuclei with inconspicuous nucleoli and scant amounts of eosinophilic cytoplasm (Fig. 33-76). In most cases, the nuclei are relatively uniform, but some tumors show foci with increased nuclear atypia, and rare tumors are composed predominantly of markedly atypical cells.[319] The cells may be arranged in a variety of patterns, including large nests with central necrosis, tubular-like structures, trabeculae separated by fibrovascular septa reminiscent of a zellballen pattern, and cords of single cells similar to lobular carcinoma of the breast (Fig. 33-77).[331] Typically, the cellular aggregates are surrounded and separated by abundant fibrous connective tissue with only a scattering of spindle-shaped fibroblasts and myofibroblasts. Occasionally, the tumor cells have more abundant cleared-out or vacuolated cytoplasm or even a signet ring-like appearance. A relatively common finding is the presence of rhabdoid-like foci in which the tumor cells have paranuclear intracytoplasmic hyaline inclusions composed of aggregates of intermediate filaments (Fig. 33-78). Other unusual features include Homer Wright-like rosettes, papillary areas, zones that resemble transitional cell carcinoma, and areas composed predominantly of cells with a spindled morphology.[319]

Immunohistochemical Findings

The tumor is characterized by a polyphenotypic profile with expression of epithelial, mesenchymal, and neural markers (Table 33-15). Virtually all tumors stain for epithelial markers, including cytokeratins and EMA. In the comprehensive study by Gerald et al.,[317] cytokeratins and EMA were expressed in 86% and 93% of cases, respectively. Occasionally, immunostains for cytokeratin reveal a dot-like pattern of

TABLE 33-14 Anatomic Distribution of 109 Cases of Desmoplastic Small Round Cell Tumor

LOCATION	NO. OF PATIENTS	PERCENTAGE (%)
Abdominal cavity	103	94
Thoracic region	4	4
Posterior cranial fossa	1	1
Hand	1	1
Total	109	100

From Gerald WL, Ladanyi M, de Alava E, et al. Clinical, pathologic, and molecular spectrum of tumors associated with t(11;22)(p13;q12): desmoplastic small round-cell tumor and its variants. J Clin Oncol 1998; 16:3028–3036.

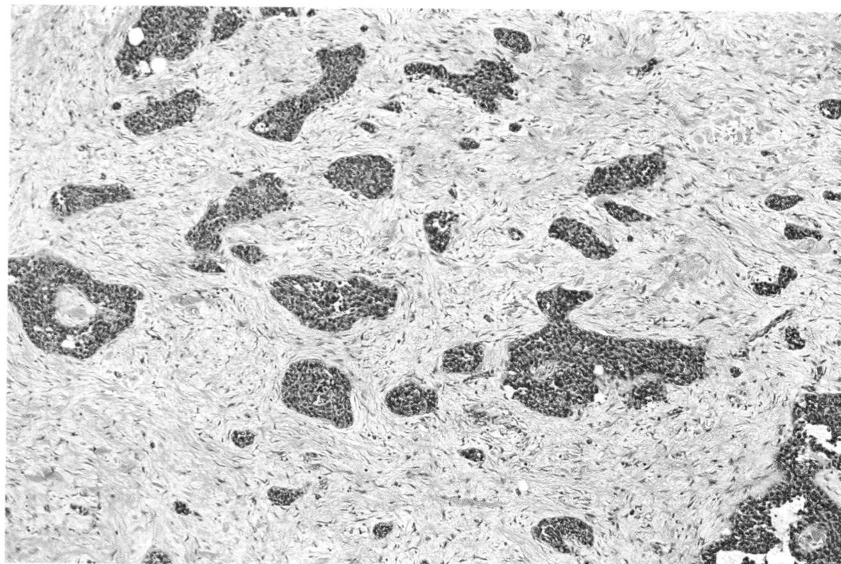

FIGURE 33-72. Desmoplastic small round cell tumor. Nests of undifferentiated tumor cells are surrounded by abundant fibrous stroma.

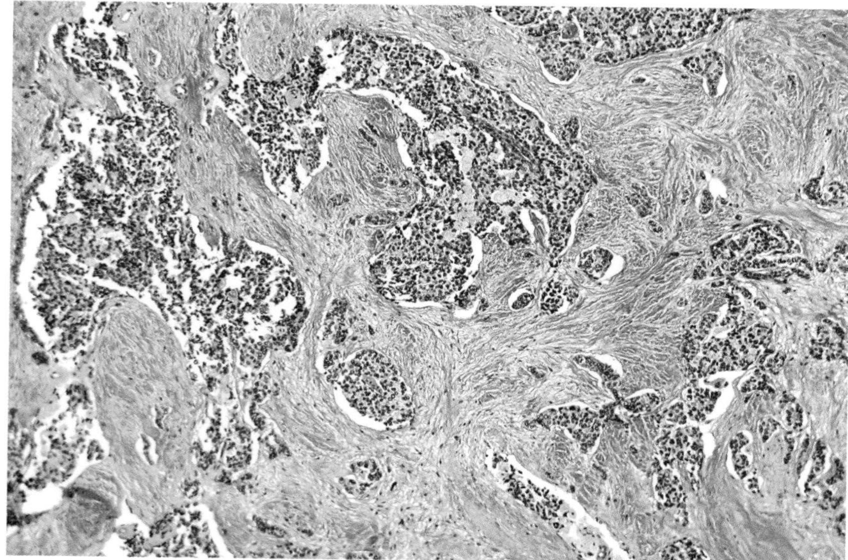

FIGURE 33-73. Nests of undifferentiated tumor cells are separated by a dense fibrous stroma in this desmoplastic small round cell tumor.

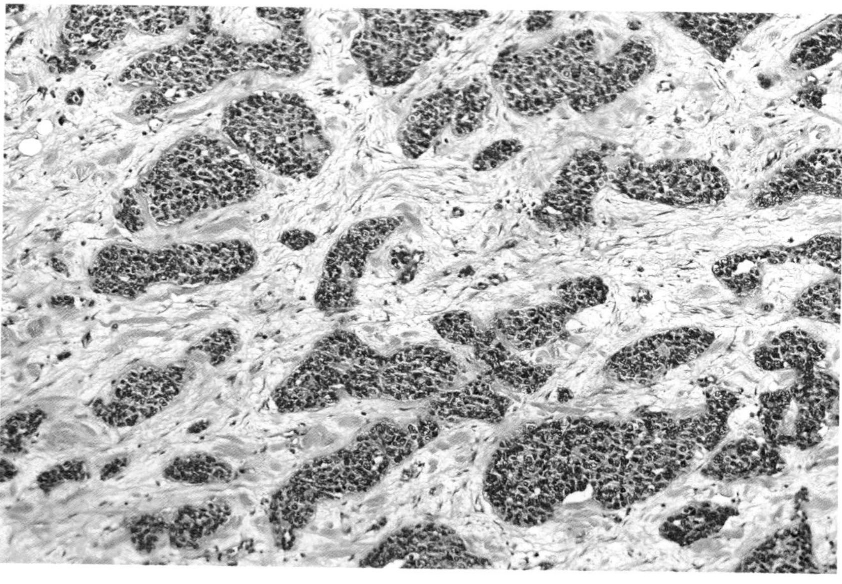

FIGURE 33-74. Prominent desmoplastic stroma surrounds varying-sized nests of tumor cells in a desmoplastic small round cell tumor.

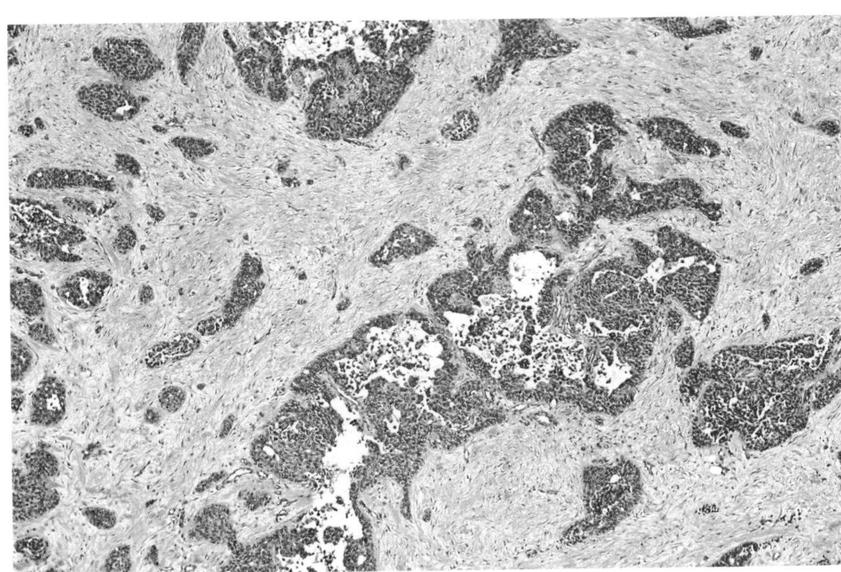

FIGURE 33-75. Desmoplastic small round cell tumor. Larger tumor nests show central necrosis.

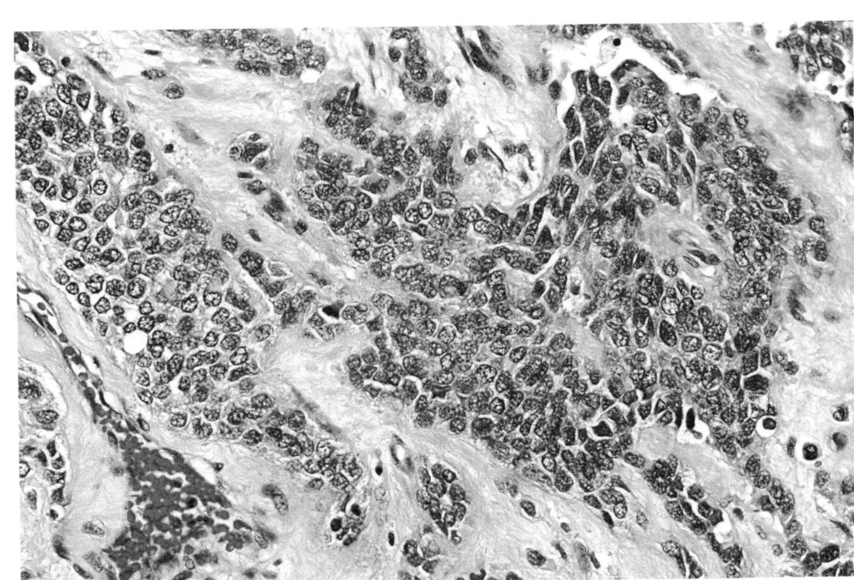

FIGURE 33-76. Desmoplastic small round cell tumor. The tumor cells appear undifferentiated and have small hyperchromatic nuclei with inconspicuous nucleoli.

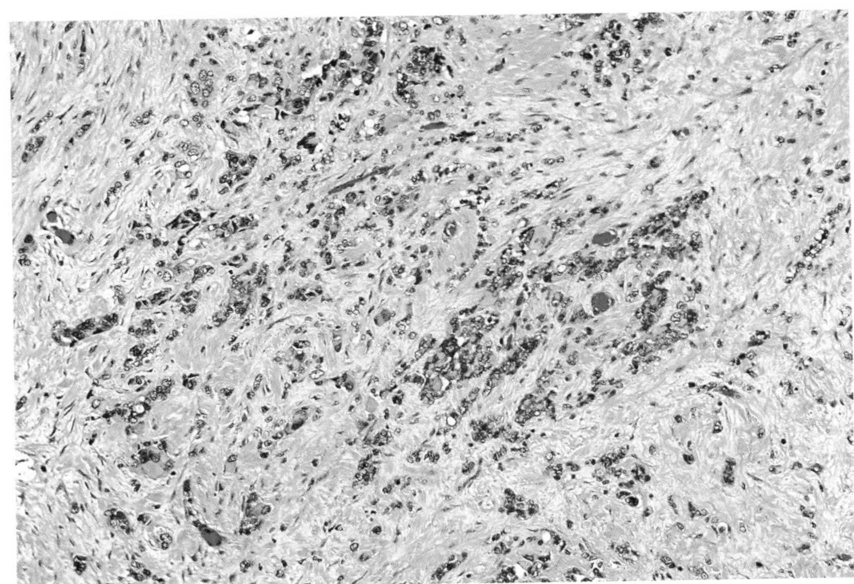

FIGURE 33-77. Desmoplastic small round cell tumor. Cords of cells are surrounded by a dense fibrous stroma mimicking lobular carcinoma of the breast.

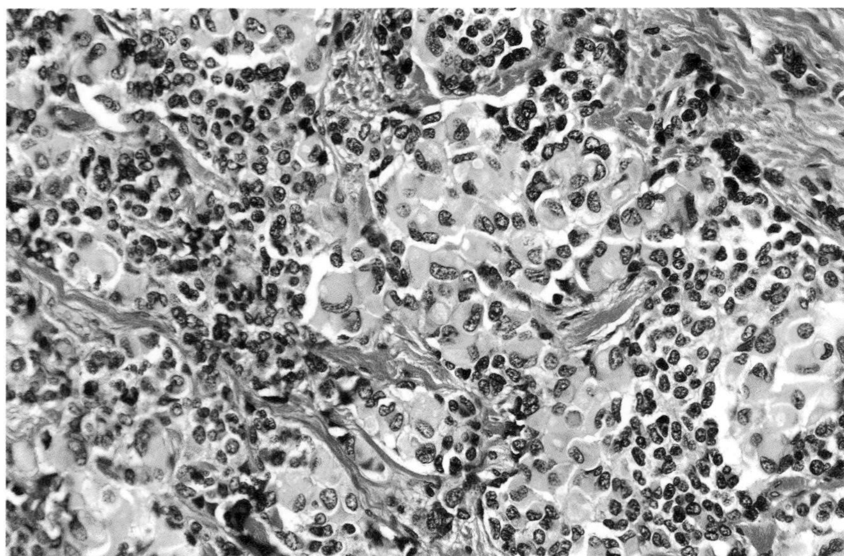

FIGURE 33-78. Focus of cells with a rhabdoid appearance in a desmoplastic small round cell tumor.

TABLE 33-15 Summary of Immunohistochemical Data on Desmoplastic Small Round Cell Tumors Reported in the Literature

MARKER	NO. POSITIVE	CASES (%)
Cytokeratin	97/107	91
Desmin	107/117	91
EMA	64/73	88
Vimentin	87/103	84
NSE	88/107	82
Synaptophysin	11/43	26
S-100 protein	13/74	18
Neurofilament protein	6/50	12
CD99	4/33	12
Chromogranin	7/64	11

Modified from Ordóñez NG. Desmoplastic small round cell tumor. II. An ultrastructural and immunohistochemical study with emphasis on new immunohistochemical markers. Am J Surg Pathol 1998;22:1314–1327.

cytoplasmic immunoreactivity. Stains for CK20 (positive in Merkel cell carcinoma) and CK5/6 (positive in malignant mesothelioma) are typically negative in DSRCT,[332] although epithelial markers, including MOC-31 and Ber-Ep4, are commonly expressed.

Virtually all DSRCT stain for vimentin, but perhaps the most useful diagnostic marker is desmin. Up to 90% of cases stain for this antigen, typically with a perinuclear dot-like or globular pattern, a unique pattern of desmin immunoreactivity peculiar to DSRCT (Fig. 33-79). Although often taken as evidence of myogenic differentiation, immunostains for nuclear myogenic regulatory proteins, including MyoD1 and myogenin, are negative; rare lesions express muscle-specific or smooth muscle actin.[332]

A variety of neural antigens have been detected in DSRCT, most commonly neuron-specific enolase and CD57, having been reported in 82% and 49% of cases, respectively.[332] However, immunoreactivity for more specific markers of neuroendocrine differentiation, including synaptophysin and chromogranin, are uncommon.

CD99 and NB-84 are markers that have been used in the differential diagnosis of small round cell neoplasms. Although CD99 is a highly sensitive marker for EFT, it is far from specific and has been detected in many other round cell neoplasms, including up to one-third of DSRCT.[332,333] Similarly, although NB-84 is a sensitive marker of neuroblastoma, it has been reported in other tumors, including up to 50% of DSRCT.[334]

As discussed later, the Wilms tumor gene (*WT1*) on 11p13 is central to the pathogenesis of DSRCT. Nuclear expression of WT1 (using antibodies to the carboxy terminus) is a consistent feature of this tumor.[335-338] In the study by Hill et al.,[337] all 11 DSRCT tested showed strong and diffuse nuclear staining, whereas all 11 EFT were negative for this antigen. Similar results were reported by Barnoud et al.[336]

A high-molecular-weight glycoprotein, CA-125 is often present in mucinous carcinomas of the ovary and adenocarcinomas of the uterine cervix and endometrium but has also been found to be expressed by the tumor cells in DSRCT.[332] Interestingly, some patients with DSRCT have elevated serum levels of CA-125, which may return to normal levels following aggressive treatment, thereby suggesting use to monitor disease status.[339]

The most striking ultrastructural feature of this tumor is the intracellular whorls and packets of microfilaments that are usually located near the nucleus, often compressing the nucleus or pushing it toward the periphery.[340]

Cytogenetic and Molecular Genetic Findings

The identification of a unique cytogenetic abnormality t(11;22)(p13;q12) in this tumor helped establish DSRCT as a distinct clinicopathologic entity.[341,342] The breakpoints involve the *EWSR1* gene on 22q12 and the Wilms tumor gene (*WT1*) on 11p13.[343] *WT1* is a tumor suppressor gene that encodes a zinc-finger-type transcription factor that normally represses promoters that control expression of growth factors such as platelet-derived growth factor-alpha (PDGFA).[344] The fusion protein appears to induce expression of PDGFA, a potent mitogen and chemoattractant for fibroblasts and endothelial cells, therefore serving as a potential link between the

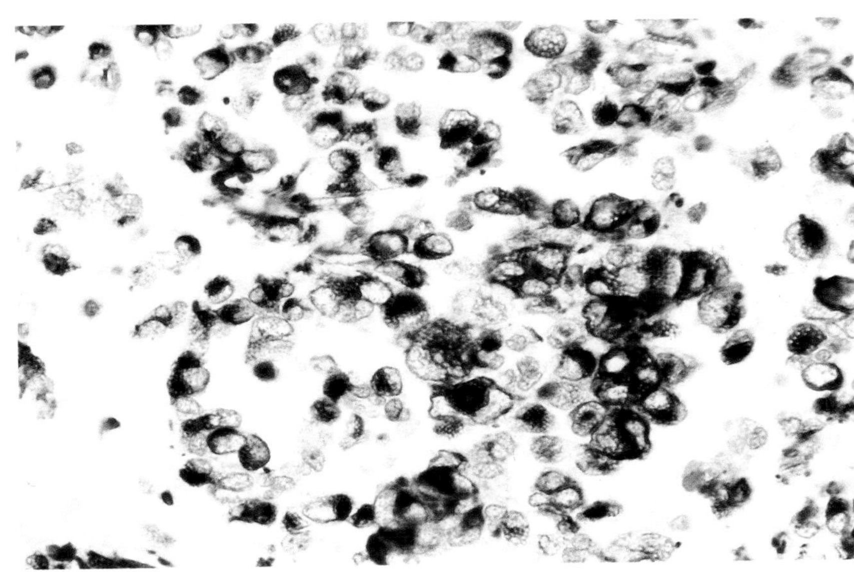

FIGURE 33-79. Typical perinuclear globular pattern of desmin immunoreactivity peculiar to desmoplastic small round cell tumors.

TABLE 33-16 Sensitivity and Specificity of the *EWSR1-WT1* Fusion for Desmoplastic Small Round Cell Tumor (DSRCT)

DIAGNOSIS	*EWSR1*-WT1-POSITIVE	%
DSRCT	11/12	92
Ewing family of tumors	0/8	0
Wilms tumor	0/17	0
Alveolar rhabdomyosarcoma	0/13	0
Nonalveolar rhabdomyosarcoma	0/9	0

Modified from de Alava E, Ladanyi M, Rosai J, et al. Detection of chimeric transcripts in desmoplastic small round cell tumor and related developmental tumors by reverse transcriptase polymerase chain reaction. A specific diagnostic assay. Am J Pathol 1995;147:1584–1591.

unique translocation and histologic characteristics of this tumor.[345]

The fusion can be detected by RT-PCR or FISH using frozen or fixed tissue.[346,347] Most commonly, this fusion involves exon 7 of *EWSR1* and exon 8 of *WT1*; rare variant fusions have been described.[348] Although the *EWSR1-WT1* fusion has been described in DSRCT only (Table 33-16), rare examples of DSRCT have been reported to have fusions characteristically identified in EFT, including *EWSR1-ERG*[349] and *EWSR1-FLI1*.[350] It is unclear whether these tumors might instead be better considered to represent variants of EFT.

Differential Diagnosis

DSRCT must be differentiated from other small round cell tumors, including EFT, alveolar rhabdomyosarcoma, neuroblastoma, lymphoma, poorly differentiated carcinoma, small cell carcinoma, Merkel cell carcinoma, and malignant mesothelioma. When arising in the typical clinicopathologic setting, DSRCT can be easily distinguished from these other entities, although ancillary techniques, including immunohistochemistry and molecular assays, are invariably required. The immunohistochemical expression of epithelial, mesenchymal, and neural antigens, particularly the perinuclear dot-like or globular pattern of desmin staining, is useful for arriving at a diagnosis. Given that the immunophenotypic features overlap with many of the aforementioned tumors, a panel of immunostains is generally required. In questionable cases, RT-PCR or FISH analysis for evidence of an *EWSR1-WT1* fusion is indicated.

The differential diagnosis of DSRCT continues to broaden as its pathologic profile expands; neoplasms, including sarcomatoid carcinoma, spindle cell sarcomas of various types, metastatic adenocarcinoma, and MERT, may occasionally be entertained as diagnostic considerations. As mentioned previously, a combination of immunohistochemical and molecular assays should allow for this distinction.

Discussion

DSRCT is a highly aggressive neoplasm with an extremely poor prognosis. In the series reported by Ordóñez et al.[351] in 1993, 16 of 22 patients died of disease within 8 to 50 months after the initial therapy. In a follow-up study published in 1998,[319] 25 of 35 patients for whom follow-up information was available died of widespread metastasis, and the remainder were alive with disease.[319] In a study from Memorial Sloan-Kettering Cancer Center, 13 of 32 patients treated with an extensive debulking procedure (greater than 90% of tumor removed) followed by systemic chemotherapy remained progression-free, although three of these patients died from toxicity related to treatment.[352] Although the prognosis remains dismal, improved survival is correlated with a complete or good response to multimodality therapy, including extensive surgical debulking.[353-355] Complete excision is often impossible because of the irregular outline of the tumor and the presence of multiple tiny implants in the peritoneum. A number of studies have found some patients to respond well to hyperthermic intraperitoneal chemotherapy.[356-358] Liver metastases may respond to yttrium microspheres,[359] and some can be effectively palliated through a combination of surgical debulking, chemotherapy, radiotherapy, and autologous bone marrow transplantation.[360]

The exact nature of this tumor is still uncertain. Some have speculated that DSRCT is derived from mesothelial or submesothelial cells, given the predominant location of this tumor in mesothelial-lined cavities and the immunohistochemical expression of both epithelial and mesenchymal antigens. The cells of DSRCT invariably express desmin, as do normal mesothelial cells, submesothelial mesenchymal cells, and some malignant mesotheliomas. However, there are a number of immunohistochemical differences between DSRCT and mesothelioma such as the expression of MOC-31, Ber-Ep4, and CD15 in DSRCT (usually absent in malignant mesotheliomas) and the absence of CK5/6 and thrombomodulin (usually present in malignant mesotheliomas). Furthermore, there is no ultrastructural evidence of mesothelial differentiation in DSRCT; as previously noted, some tumors arise in locations not lined by mesothelial cells.

CIC-REARRANGED FAMILY OF TUMORS

A subset of small round blue cell tumors closely resembling EFT but lacking aberrations of *EWSR1* has been recently identified, all of which show rearrangement of the *CIC* gene on 19q13.[361-366] Some of these tumors have a t(4;19)(q35;q13.1) involving the *DUX4* and *CIC* genes on chromosomes 4 and 19, respectively, whereas others show a t(10;19) involving a gene on chromosome 10q26 which is highly homologous to the *DUX4* gene on 4q35.[362]

Clinical Findings

These tumors generally arise in young patients, with a median age of 24 years, although the patients have ranged in age from 6 to 62 years.[361-366] The combined reports suggest a male predilection, and the most common location is in the deep soft tissues of the extremities. Rare cases have also been described in the pelvis, trunk, and head and neck. Patients typically present with a slowly enlarging painless soft tissue mass.

Pathologic Findings

This family of tumors closely resembles EFT and generally comprises small round cells with vesicular nuclei with fairly prominent nucleoli and amphophilic to slightly eosinophilic cytoplasm. The cells are often arranged into distinct lobules (Fig. 33-80), and extensive areas of geographic necrosis are typical (Fig. 33-81). Mitotic figures, including atypical mitotic figures, are easily identified. The cells tend to show more nuclear pleomorphism than is seen in classical ES (Fig. 33-82). Unusual features, including cytoplasmic clearing and tumor cells within myxoid stromal, have been described.

The tumor has no specific immunohistochemical phenotype, and they variably express CD99, with some cases showing diffuse membranous immunoreactivity reminiscent of EFT; others show only focal or patchy staining for this antigen (Fig. 33-83). They are generally negative for lymphoid, epithelial, myogenic, melanocytic, and neuroendocrine markers, but some cases show occasional positive cells for S-100 protein, desmin, or cytokeratins.

Cytogenetic and Molecular Genetic Findings

Obviously, the feature that defines this family of tumors is the presence of a *CIC* rearrangement, either with 4q35 or 10q26.3. Additional complex cytogenetic aberrations have

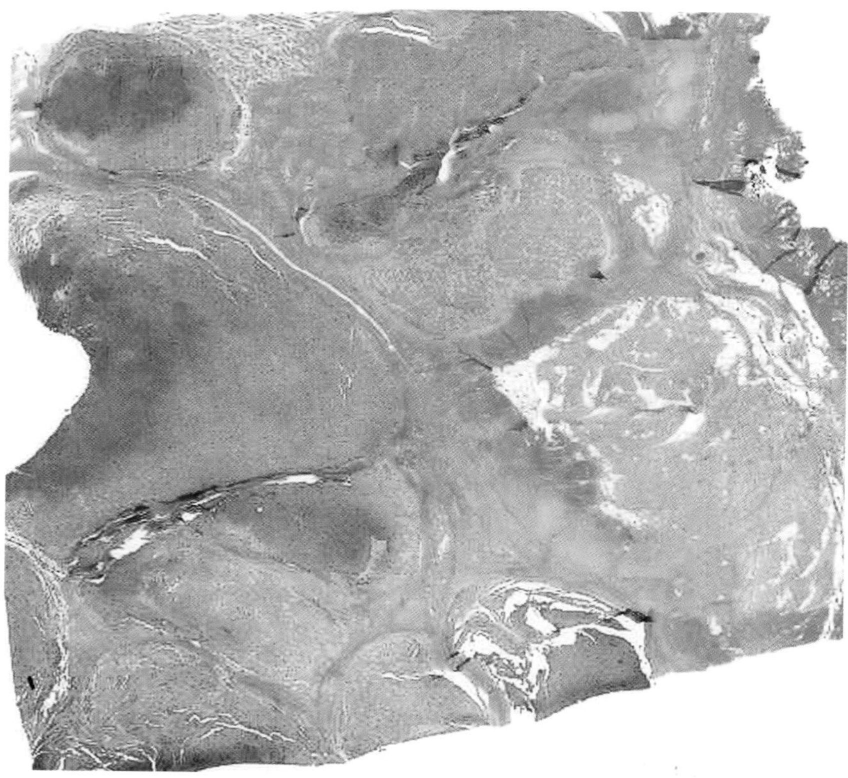

FIGURE 33-80. Low-magnification view of a CIC-DUX4 translocated sarcoma arising in the thigh of a 33-year old woman. Note the lobular growth pattern with fibrous septa. *(Photomicrograph courtesy of Dr. Darya Buehler, University of Wisconsin, Madison, WI.)*

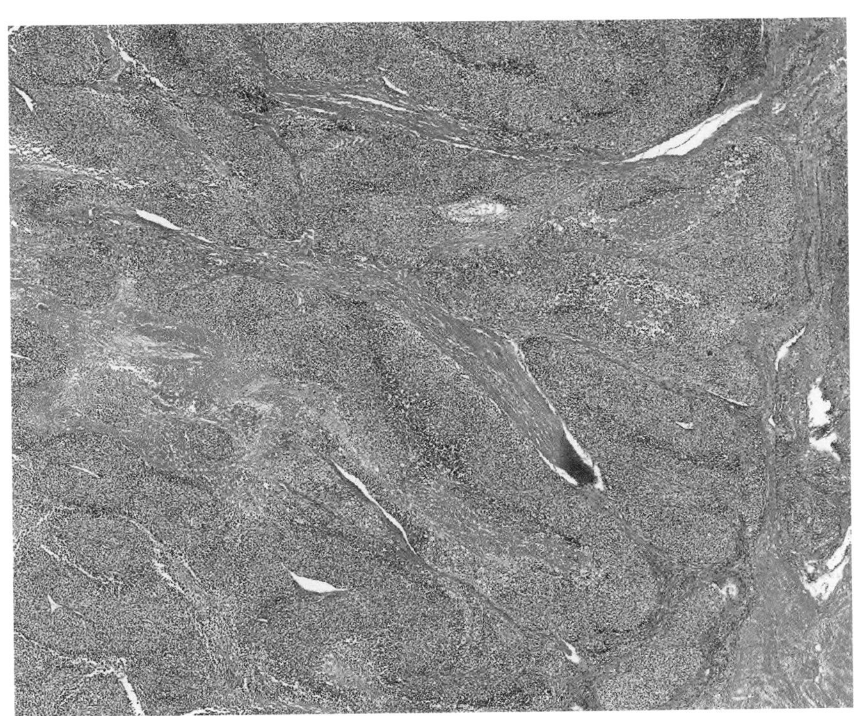

FIGURE 33-81. CIC-DUX4 translocated sarcoma with central area of necrosis surrounded by malignant round cells. *(Case provided by Dr. David Lucas, University of Michigan, Ann Arbor, MI.)*

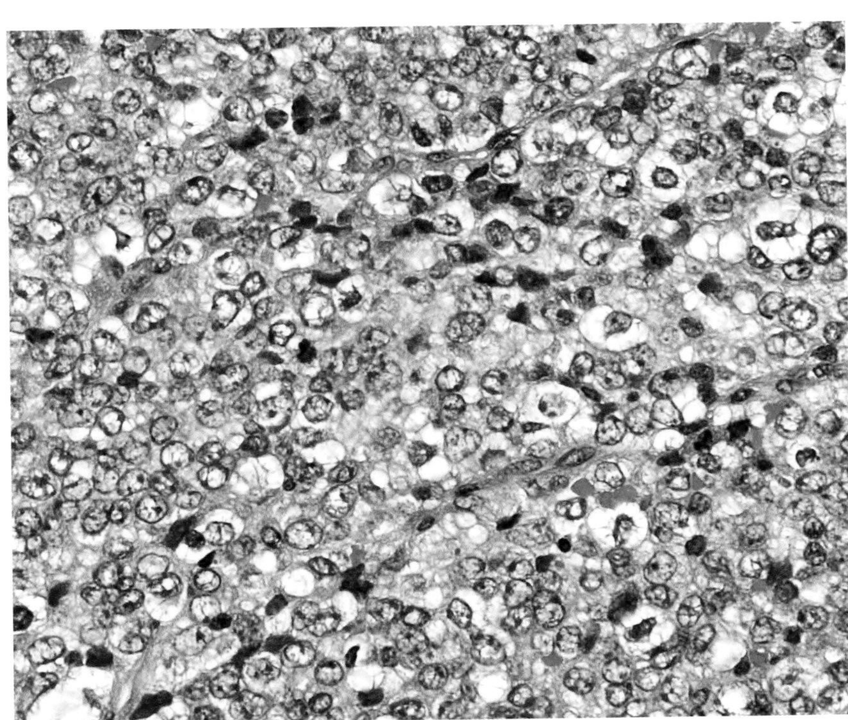

FIGURE 33-82. High-magnification view of the malignant cytology of the constituent cells in this CIC-DUX4 translocated sarcoma. *(Case provided by Dr. David Lucas, University of Michigan, Ann Arbor, MI.)*

been reported in occasional cases. The *CIC-DUX4* can be detected by either RT-PCR or FISH, using either frozen or paraffin-embedded tissues.[361,362]

Discussion

This appears to be a rare sarcoma and generally has been identified only after a comprehensive molecular genetic assessment of cases resembling EFT but lacking *EWSR1* aberrations. For example, Italiano et al.[362] studied 22 small round blue cell tumors that were negative for *EWSR1* gene rearrangements as well as for other pediatric sarcoma rearrangements. Of these, 15 cases showed *CIC* rearrangements, including 6 cases with a t(4;19) and 6 with a t(10;19), and 3 cases had an unknown fusion partner with *CIC*. Similarly, Graham et al.[361] identified 3 cases from a group of 19 undifferentiated soft tissue sarcomas. Exactly how or whether these tumors are related to EFT is not clear, but there is some evidence to suggest that this translocation results in upregulation of the *PEA* family of

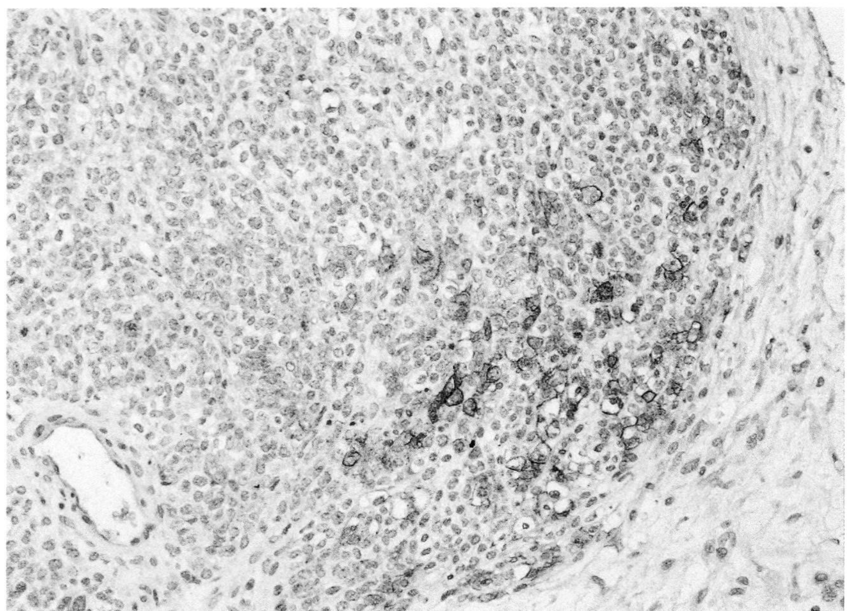

FIGURE 33-83. Focal membranous CD99 immunoreactivity in a CIC-DUX4 translocated sarcoma. (Photomicrograph courtesy of Dr. David Lucas, University of Michigan, Ann Arbor, MI.)

genes, a molecular alteration that is equivalent to the *EWSR1-ETS* fusion characteristic of EFT.[362,363]

Not unexpectedly, these tumors pursue a highly aggressive clinical course, with at least half of the patients developing metastatic disease, most commonly to the lungs. At this time, the role of adjuvant therapy is unclear in the treatment of these patients.

EPITHELIOID SARCOMA

The term *epithelioid sarcoma* has been applied to a morphologically distinctive neoplasm that is likely to be confused with a variety of benign and malignant conditions, especially a granulomatous process, a synovial sarcoma, or an ulcerating squamous cell carcinoma. The tumor mainly afflicts young adults; its principal sites are the fingers, hands, and forearms. In fact, epithelioid sarcoma is the most common soft tissue sarcoma in the hand and wrist.

Clinical Findings

Epithelioid sarcoma is most prevalent in adolescents and young adults 10 to 35 years of age (median age 26 years).[367-371] It is uncommon in children and older persons, but no age group is exempt. Male patients outnumber females by about 2 to 1,[367-371] and there is no predilection for any particular race. The tumor most commonly arises on the flexor surfaces of the fingers, hands and forearm, followed by the knee and lower leg, especially the pretibial region, the buttocks and thigh, the shoulder and arm, and the ankle, foot, and toe (Table 33-17). It is rare in the trunk and head and neck region, with the exception of the scalp. There are a number of reports in which epithelioid sarcoma arose on the penis and clinically mimicked Peyronie disease.[372] Other uncommon sites include the vulva,[373] esophagus,[374] oral cavity,[375] parotid gland,[376] and bone.[377]

TABLE 33-17 Anatomic Distribution of 215 Epithelioid Sarcomas

LOCATION	NO. OF PATIENTS	PERCENTAGE (%)
Hand/fingers	65	30
Forearm/wrist	37	17
Knee/lower leg	31	15
Buttock/thigh	22	10
Shoulder/arm	20	9
Ankle/foot/toes	19	9
Trunk	12	6
Head and neck	9	4
Total	215	100

From Chase DR, Enzinger FM. Epithelioid sarcoma: diagnosis, prognostic indicators, and treatment. Am J Surg Pathol 1985;9:241–263.

The tumor occurs in both the superficial and deep soft tissues. When located superficially, it usually presents as a firm nodule that may be solitary or multiple, has a callus-like consistency, and is often described as a woody hard knot or firm lump that is slowly growing and painless. Nodules situated in the dermis are often elevated above the skin surface and frequently become ulcerated weeks or months after they are first noted. Such lesions may be erroneously diagnosed as an indurated ulcer, draining abscess, or infected wart that fails to heal despite intensive therapy (Figs. 33-84 and 33-85). Deep-seated lesions are usually firmly attached to tendons, tendon sheaths, or fascial structures; they tend to be larger and less well defined and manifest as areas of induration or as multinodular lumpy masses, sometimes moving slightly with motion of the extremity (Fig. 33-86). Pain or tenderness is rarely a prominent symptom, with the exception of the tumors that encroach on large nerves. The size of the tumor varies substantially and ranges from a few millimeters to 15 cm or more, but most are 3 to 6 cm at the time of excision. Because many lesions are multinodular, determination of their exact size is often impossible.

Radiographic examination typically reveals a soft tissue mass with an occasional speckled pattern of calcification. Cortical thinning and erosion of underlying bone may be present, but invasion and destruction of adjacent bone are rare. MRI is useful for revealing the anatomic extent of the tumor and planning appropriate surgery.[378]

Pathologic Findings

Gross inspection usually reveals the presence of one or more nodules measuring 0.5 to 5.0 cm in greatest diameter. Deep-seated tumors, attached to tendons or fascia, tend to be larger and present as firm, multinodular masses with irregular outlines. The cut surface has a glistening gray-white or gray-tan mottled surface with focal yellow or brown areas caused by focal necrosis or hemorrhage.

There are two principal types of epithelioid sarcoma: the conventional (classical or distal) type and the proximal-type.

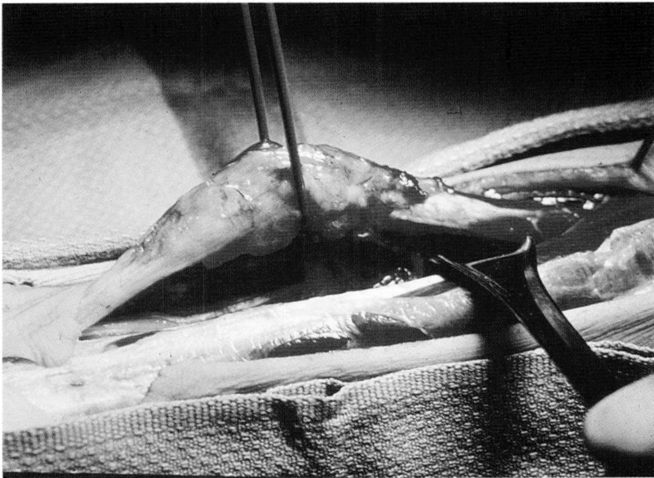

FIGURE 33-84. Recurrent ulcerating epithelioid sarcoma of the anterior tibial region in a 21-year-old man.

This discussion will focus on the former because the latter has distinctive features and will be discussed separately.

Histologically, the conventional type of epithelioid sarcoma has a distinct nodular arrangement of the tumor cells, a tendency to undergo central degeneration and necrosis, and an epithelioid appearance with cytoplasmic eosinophilia. The nodular pattern, probably the most conspicuous single feature of epithelioid sarcoma, varies somewhat. In some tumors, the nodules are well circumscribed; in others, they are less well defined and are often compacted into irregular multinodular masses (Figs. 33-87 and 33-88). Multiple nodules are less common in tissue obtained at the initial operation than in recurrent tumors. In rare cases, the presence of multiple small superficial satellite nodules near the operative site may mimic a dermatologic disease.[379] Necrosis of the tumor nodules is a common finding (Fig. 33-89); it is most prominent in the center of the nodules and, at times, is associated with hemorrhage and cystic change. Fusion of several necrotizing nodules results in a geographic lesion with scalloped margins (Fig. 33-90). When the tumor spreads within a fascia or aponeurosis, it forms festoon-like or garland-like bands punctuated by areas of necrosis. Not infrequently, the tumor grows along the neurovascular bundle and invests large vessels or nerves. Vascular invasion may be present, but it is rarely a prominent feature.

Lesions located or extending into the dermis often ulcerate through the skin and may simulate an ulcerating squamous cell carcinoma, especially because of the pronounced epithelioid appearance and eosinophilia of the tumor cells. This process occurs mainly in areas with small amounts of subcutaneous fat such as the fingers and the prepatellar and pretibial regions.

The constituent cellular elements range from large ovoid or polygonal cells with deeply eosinophilic cytoplasm to plump spindle-shaped cells (Figs. 33-91 to 33-93). In some cases, the spindle-cell pattern predominates (fibroma-like variant) and obscures the characteristic epithelioid features and nodularity (Figs. 33-94 and 33-95).[380,381] In general, cellular pleomorphism is minimal. Usually, epithelioid and spindle-shaped cells merge imperceptibly, and there is never the distinct

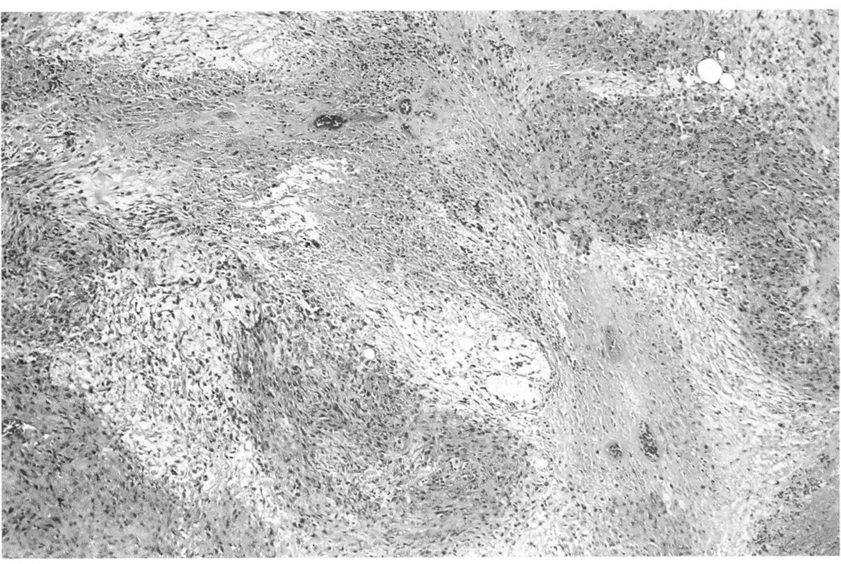

FIGURE 33-85. Ulcerating epithelioid sarcoma of the hand with indurated margins.

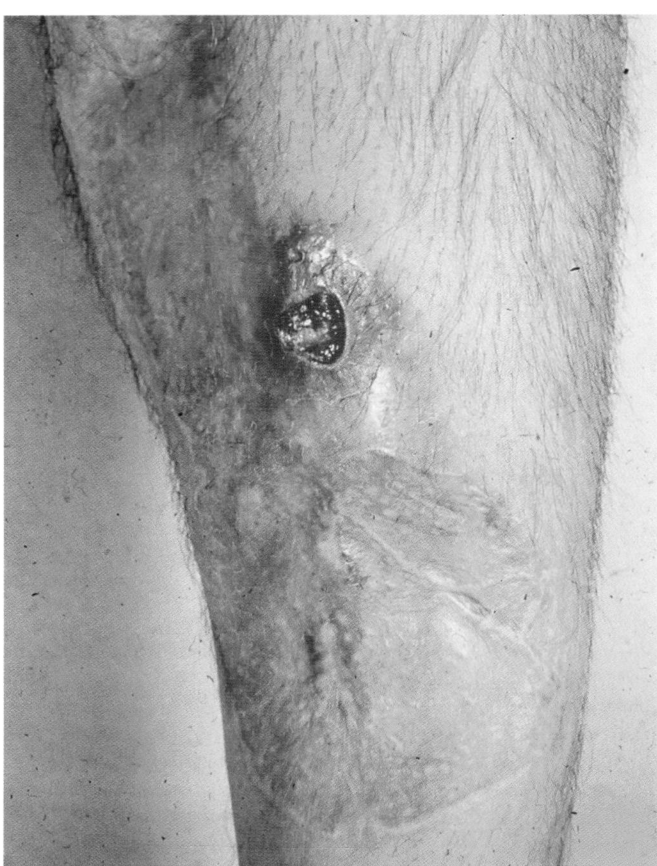

FIGURE 33-86. Epithelioid sarcoma of the wrist infiltrating the tendon of the flexor carpi ulnaris in a 28-year-old man. *(From Enzinger FM. Epithelioid sarcoma: a sarcoma simulating a granuloma or a carcinoma. Cancer 1970;26:1029.)*

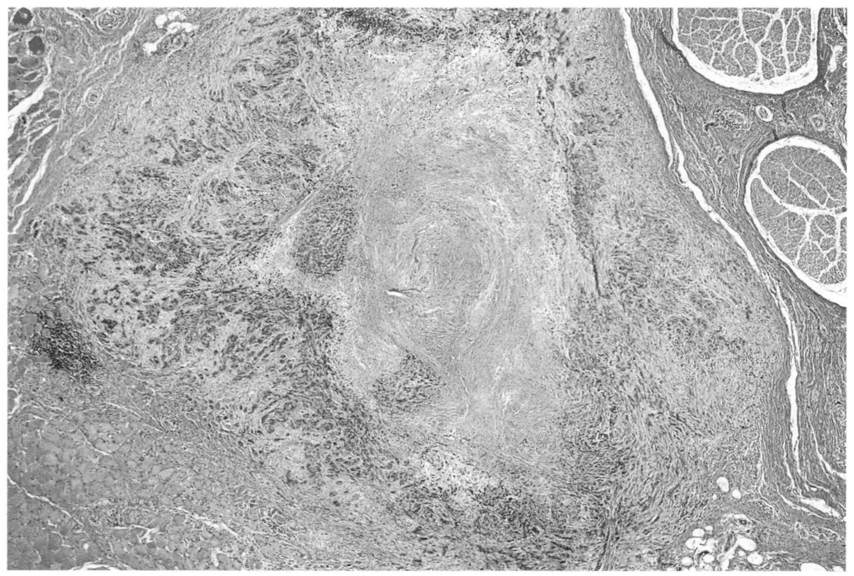

FIGURE 33-87. Typical low-magnification appearance of an epithelioid sarcoma with a pseudogranulomatous pattern.

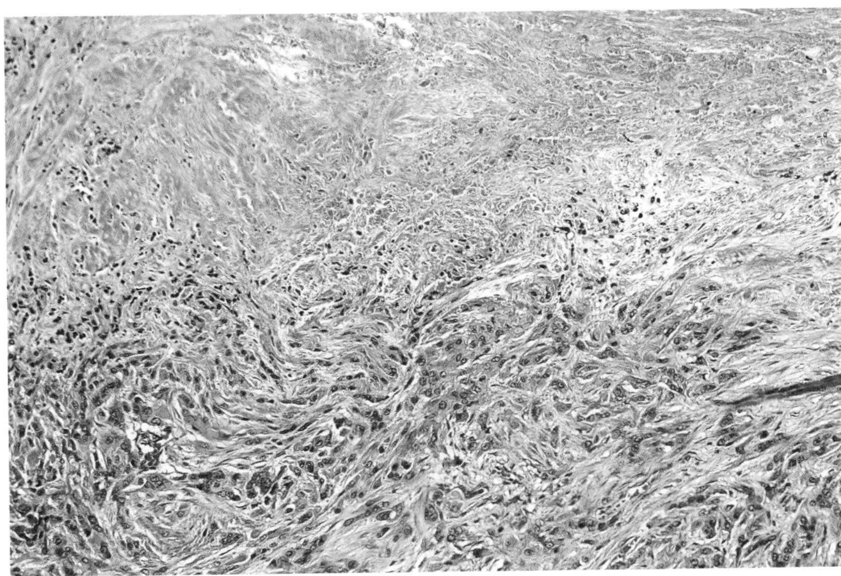

FIGURE 33-88. Epithelioid sarcoma. Note the nodules with central necrosis mimicking a necrotizing granulomatous process.

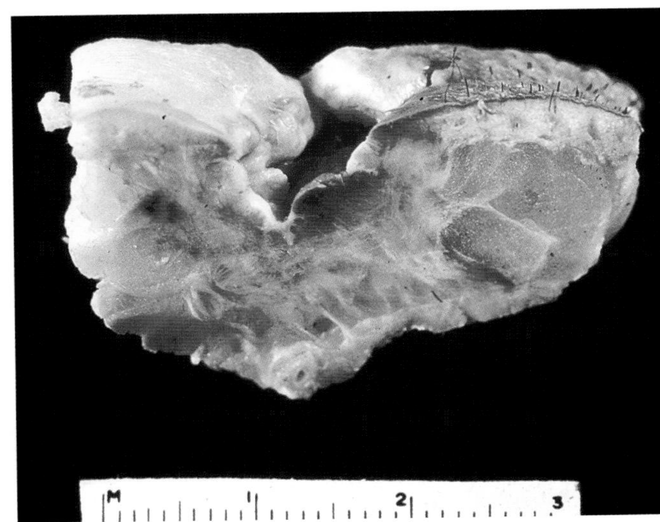

FIGURE 33-89. Epithelioid sarcoma with central necrosis of the tumor nodule.

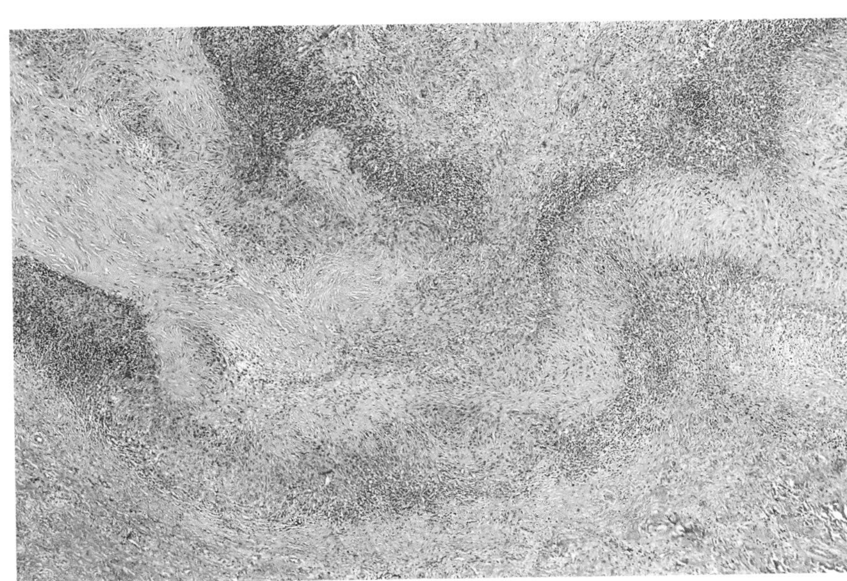

FIGURE 33-90. Epithelioid sarcoma. Fusion of several necrotizing nodules results in areas of geographic necrosis with scalloped margins.

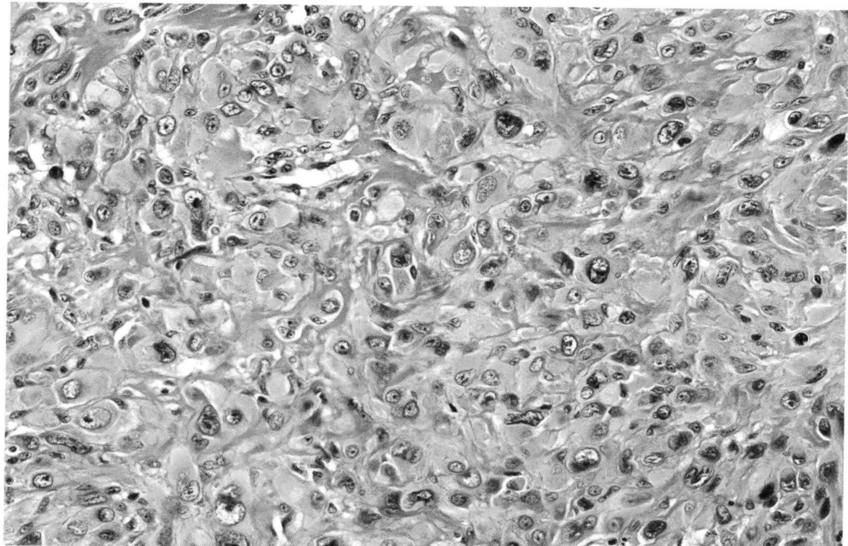

FIGURE 33-91. Cytologic features of malignant epithelioid cells in an epithelioid sarcoma.

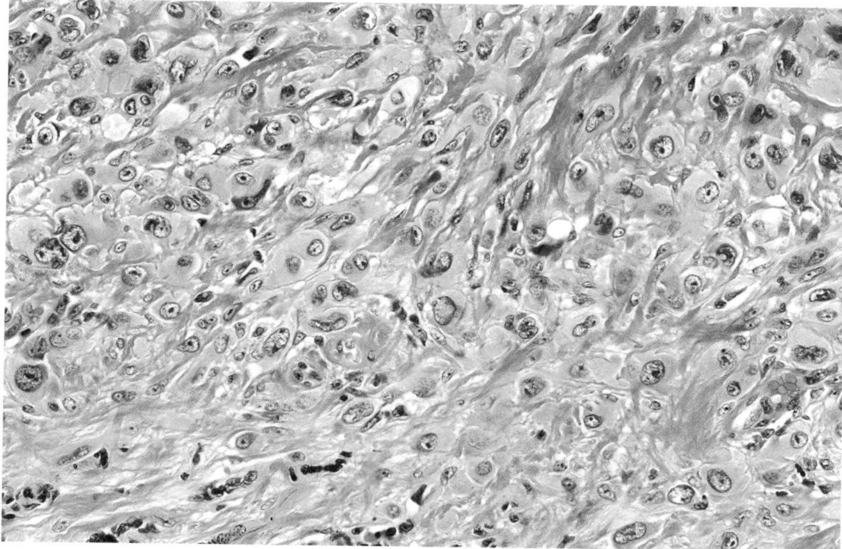

FIGURE 33-92. Close interplay between collagen and malignant epithelioid cells with densely eosinophilic cytoplasm in an epithelioid sarcoma.

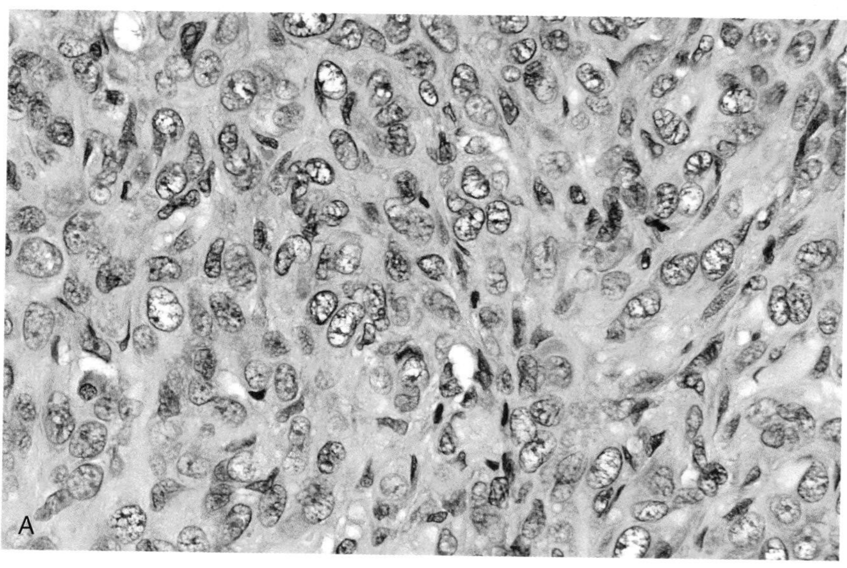

FIGURE 33-93. (A, B) Cytologic appearance of malignant epithelioid cells in epithelioid sarcoma. Most of the tumor cells have abundant deeply eosinophilic cytoplasm.

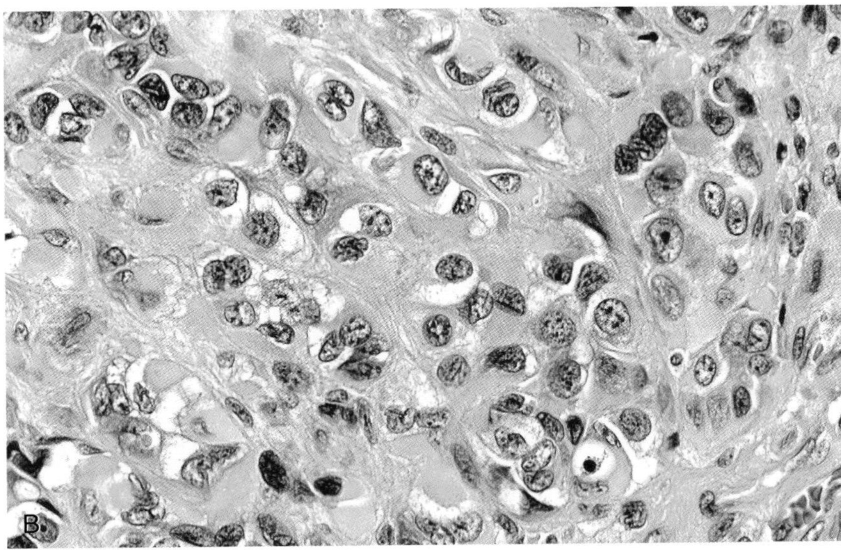

FIGURE 33-93, cont'd

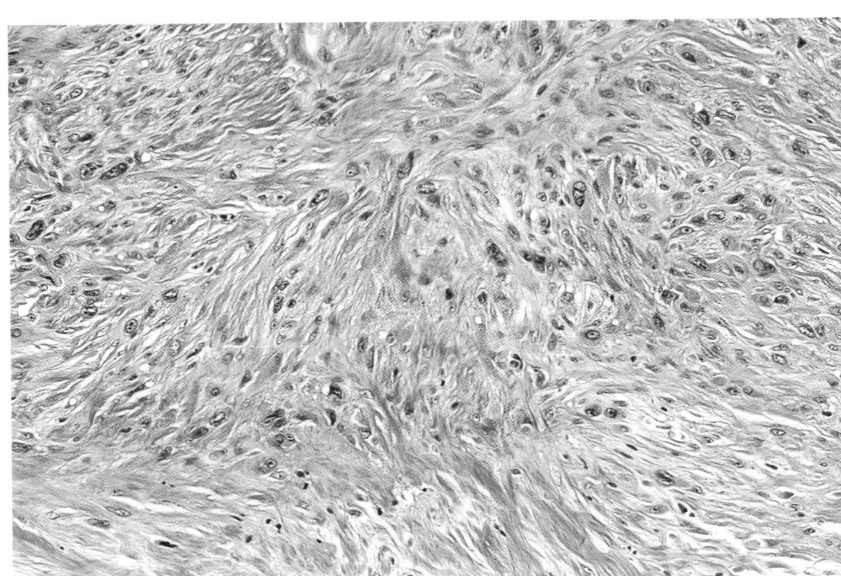

FIGURE 33-94. Epithelioid sarcoma with a predominantly spindle-cell pattern.

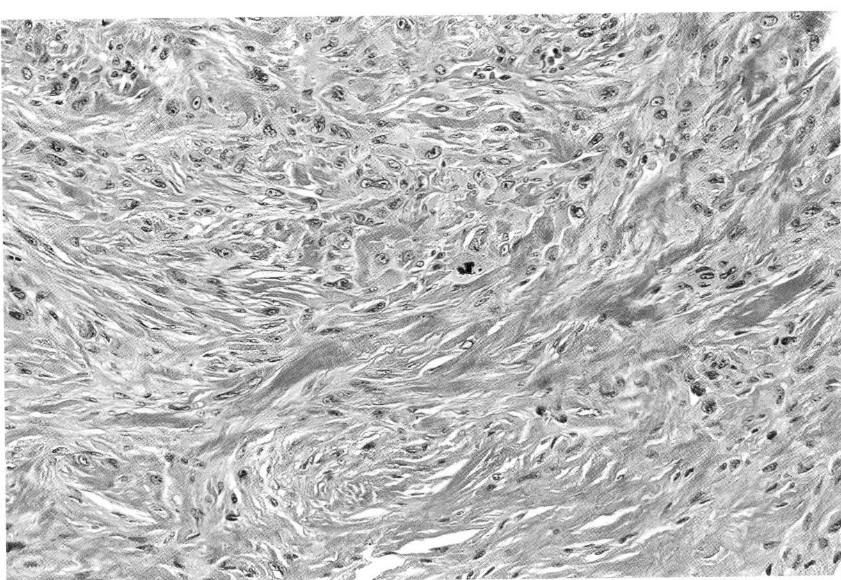

FIGURE 33-95. Interplay between dense collagen bundles and malignant spindle cells in an epithelioid sarcoma.

biphasic or pseudoglandular pattern that one encounters in biphasic synovial sarcoma (Fig. 33-96). In some tumors, the loss of cellular cohesion and secondary hemorrhage may closely simulate an angiosarcoma. Rare examples have prominent blood-filled spaces imparting an angiomatoid appearance.[382] Occasionally, the underlying nature of this tumor is even further obscured by myxoid change.[383,384] The presence of intracellular lipid droplets suggests the incipient lumen formation of endothelial cells seen in epithelioid hemangioendotheliomas. Intercellular deposition of dense hyalinized collagen is common and, together with the eosinophilic cytoplasm, contributes to the deeply eosinophilic appearance of the tumor. Calcification and bone formation are found in 10% to 20% of cases, but cartilaginous metaplasia is rare (Fig. 33-97).[385,386] Aggregates of chronic inflammatory cells along the peripheral margin of the tumor nodules are present in most cases and may mimic a chronic inflammatory process (Fig. 33-98).

Differential Diagnosis

The frequency with which epithelioid sarcoma is mistaken for a benign process is chiefly a result of its deceptively bland appearance during the initial stage of the disease. Small superficially located tumors with a nodular or multinodular pattern are likely to be mistaken for an inflammatory process, particularly a *necrotizing infectious granuloma, necrobiosis lipoidica, granuloma annulare,* or *rheumatoid nodule*. In contrast to the latter processes, the individual cells in epithelioid sarcoma tend to be more sharply defined, are larger and more eosinophilic, and stain positively for cytokeratins and EMA. The epithelioid features, nodularity, and immunostaining for cytokeratin also aid in differentiating epithelioid sarcoma from nodular fasciitis, fibrous histiocytoma, and fibromatosis.

Epithelioid sarcoma may also be mistaken for a wide array of epithelioid-appearing malignant soft tissue neoplasms. The cytologic features of the constituent cells are reminiscent of

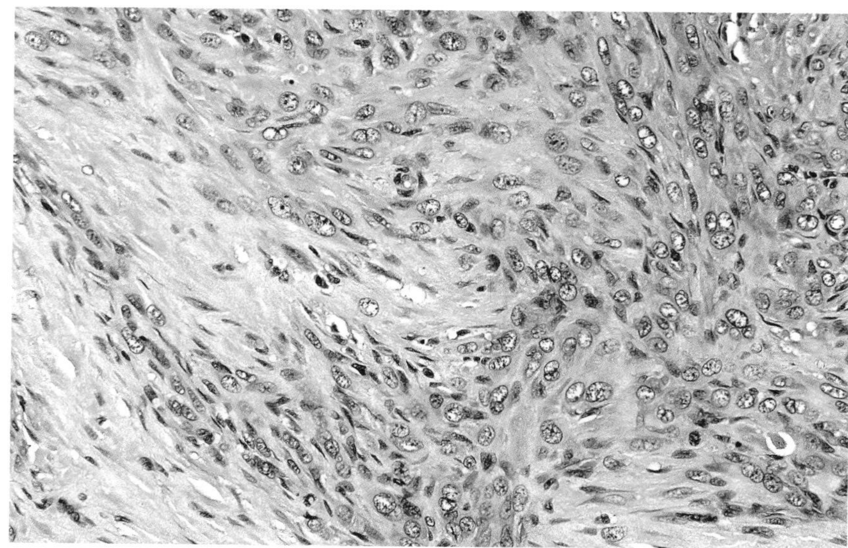

FIGURE 33-96. Transition from epithelioid to spindle cells and interdigitating collagen bundles in an epithelioid sarcoma.

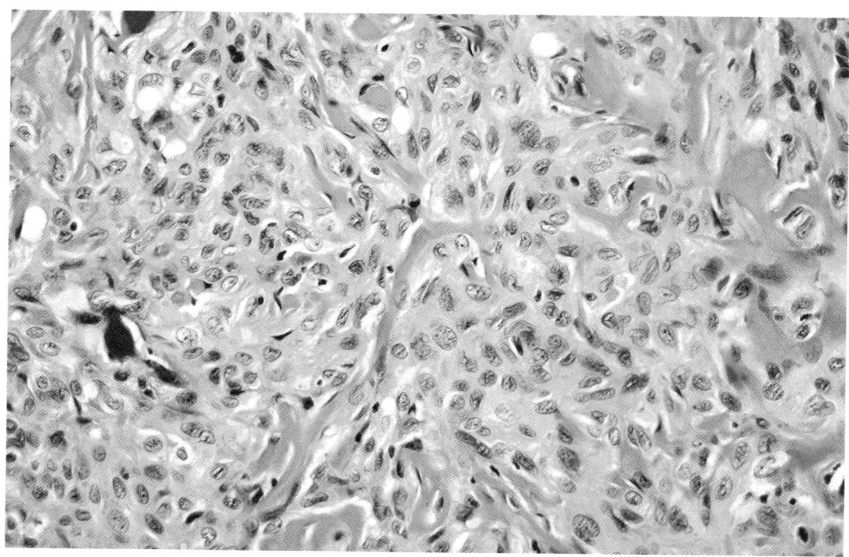

FIGURE 33-97. Focal calcifications in an epithelioid sarcoma, an unusual feature of this neoplasm.

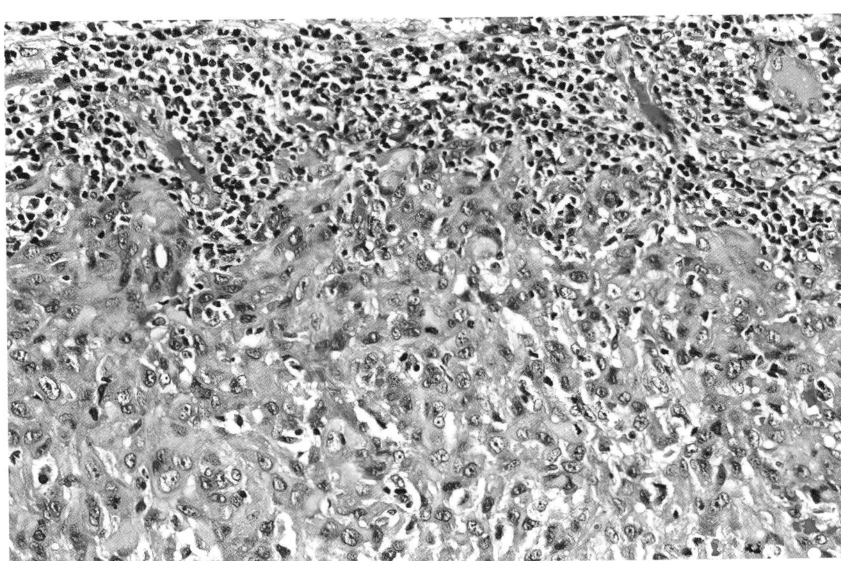

FIGURE 33-98. Aggregates of chronic inflammatory cells along the peripheral margin of a tumor nodule in an epithelioid sarcoma.

those seen in both *epithelioid MPNST* and *melanoma*. Unlike epithelioid sarcoma, epithelioid MPNST stains strongly for S-100 protein and virtually never expresses cytokeratins, although EMA may be rarely detected. A potential pitfall is the loss of SMARCB1 expression in up to 50% of epithelioid MPNST.[387] Similarly, malignant melanoma virtually always expresses S-100 protein, and many lesions also stain for HMB-45, Melan A, or other specific melanocytic antigens. Unlike epithelioid MPNST, melanoma consistently retains SMARCB1 expression.

Epithelioid sarcoma also has overlapping features with *epithelioid angiosarcoma*. Histologically, both are composed of large epithelioid cells with cytoplasmic vacuoles. Furthermore, epithelioid sarcoma may have a hemorrhagic pseudoangiosarcomatous pattern.[382,388] Confusion between these two entities is compounded by the fact that epithelioid angiosarcomas occasionally express cytokeratins and, contrarily, epithelioid sarcomas often express CD34. The absence of specific endothelial markers such as CD31 and ERG in epithelioid sarcoma allows their distinction. Furthermore, as shown by Hornick et al.,[387] epithelioid angiosarcoma consistently retains SMARCB1 positivity.

A variant of hemangioendothelioma has been reported, which shows histologic features strikingly similar to those seen in epithelioid sarcoma (*epithelioid sarcoma-like hemangioendothelioma*).[389-391] This tumor arises in the superficial or deep soft tissues, often in the extremities, of young to middle-aged adults. Histologically, it is characterized by solid sheets and nests of epithelioid to slightly spindled cells with cytoplasmic eosinophilia and only subtle evidence of vascular differentiation in the form of focal intracytoplasmic vacuolization. Like epithelioid sarcoma, the neoplastic cells consistently stain for cytokeratins and vimentin, but in addition they show clear-cut evidence of vascular endothelial differentiation by virtue of consistent expression of CD31 and FLI-1 (see Chapter 22).

Some epithelioid sarcomas are difficult to distinguish from ulcerating *squamous cell carcinoma*. However, epithelioid sarcoma lacks keratin pearls and dyskeratosis in the adjacent epithelium. Immunohistochemically, most epithelioid sarcomas stain for cyclin D1 (nuclear) and are negative for CK5/6, whereas squamous cell carcinomas typically have the opposite immunophenotype.[392,393]

Proximal-Type Epithelioid Sarcoma

In 1997, Guillou et al.[388] described a proximal-type epithelioid sarcoma characterized by its propensity to arise in axial locations (pelvis, perineum, genital tract), by its more aggressive behavior, and by its predominance of large epithelioid cells with marked cytologic atypia, frequently with intracytoplasmic hyaline inclusions, imparting a rhabdoid appearance to the tumor cells (Figs. 33-99 to 33-101). As described, these tumors have many features overlapping those of MERT, discussed elsewhere in the chapter. Although Guillou et al.[388] argued that a number of tumors reported as MERT arising in proximal locations represent this unusual form of epithelioid sarcoma, there is reasonable evidence to support the contention that proximal epithelioid sarcoma and MERT are distinct entities.[394,395]

Clinically, patients with this variant of epithelioid sarcoma tend to be older than those with the conventional/distal type. The mean age in the study of 18 cases by Guillou et al.[388] was 36 years, with most patients being between 20 and 40 years. Most tumors arise in central or axial locations, including the pelvis and perineal region, pubic region, vulva and buttocks, although rare examples have been reported in virtually every anatomic site, including the distal extremities.

Microscopically, proximal-type epithelioid sarcoma has a multinodular pattern of growth and is composed of large epithelioid cells with marked cytologic atypia, large vesicular nuclei, and prominent nucleoli. Paranuclear hyaline inclusions imparting a rhabdoid appearance are characteristic.[388,396-398] Although necrosis is common, the pseudogranulomatous pattern observed in classical epithelioid sarcoma is not present. The immunohistochemical and ultrastructural features are reportedly similar to those of classical epithelioid sarcoma.[394,395]

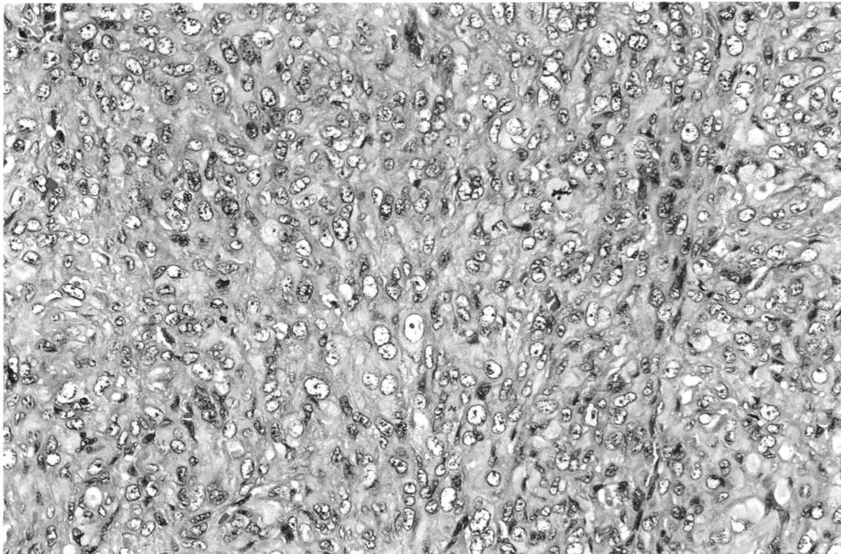

FIGURE 33-99. Proximal-type epithelioid sarcoma composed of sheets of large epithelioid cells with marked cytologic atypia.

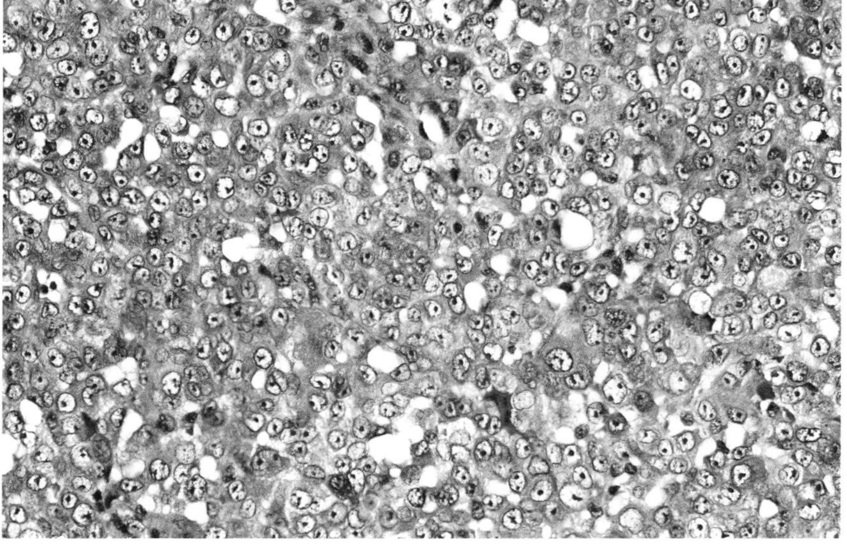

FIGURE 33-100. Sheets of large epithelioid cells with macronucleoli in a proximal-type epithelioid sarcoma.

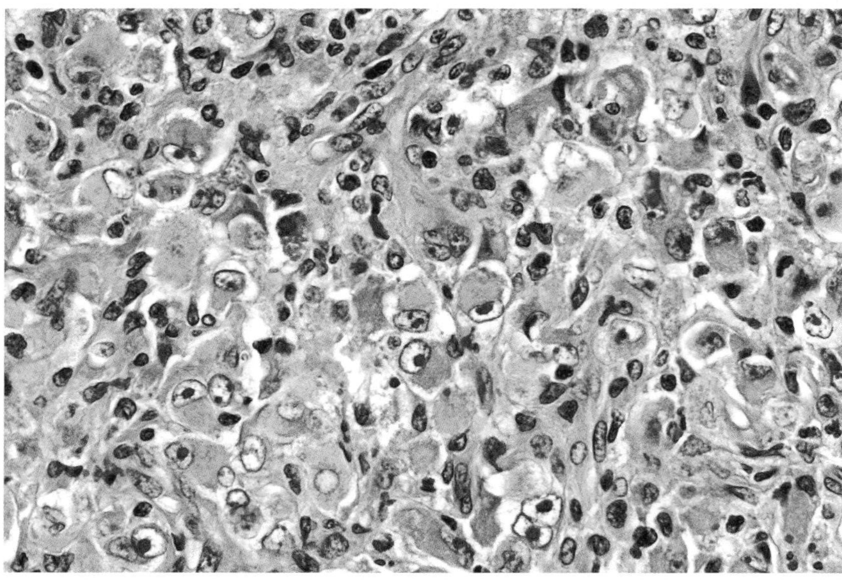

FIGURE 33-101. Proximal-type epithelioid sarcoma composed of large epithelioid cells with marked cytologic atypia and intracytoplasmic hyaline inclusions, imparting a rhabdoid appearance.

Immunohistochemical Findings

Most epithelioid sarcomas stain for both low- and high-molecular-weight cytokeratins (Fig. 33-102), EMA, and vimentin.[394,399,400] The degree of immunoreactivity, however, varies considerably from tumor to tumor and in different portions of the same neoplasm. In the large immunohistochemical study by Miettinen et al.,[395] the tumors stained for vimentin, EMA, CK8, and CK19 in 100%, 96%, 94%, and 72% of cases, respectively. Some cases also showed focal staining for CK7 and 34betaH12. Usually, the presence of cytokeratin is more pronounced in epithelioid areas than in spindled areas. Up to 60% of cases stain for CD34 (Fig. 33-103).[395,401] Some have found consistent strong CA-125 staining in this tumor, and some patients have elevated serum CA-125, raising the possibility that this could be used as a serum marker to monitor disease.[402-404] Antibodies directed against S-100 protein, neurofilament protein, carcinoembryonic antigen, von Willebrand factor, and CD31 are typically negative.

In recent years, a number of studies have focused on the immunohistochemical expression of SMARCB1 protein, the product of the *SMARCB1* gene (also known as *hSNF5*, *BAF47*, and *INI1*), a tumor suppressor gene located on the long arm of chromosome 22 (22a11.2).[405] Homozygous deletions or mutations of this gene are characteristic of malignant rhabdoid tumor of infancy and their central nervous system counterpart, atypical teratoid/rhabdoid tumor.[406-408] Because all normal cells show nuclear staining for this protein, loss of *SMARCB1* function results in a loss of immunoreactivity for this gene product, and virtually all malignant rhabdoid tumors and atypical teratoid/rhabdoid tumors show loss of SMARCB1 expression.[409-412] Numerous studies have demonstrated loss of SMARCB1 expression in both conventional (distal) and proximal-type epithelioid sarcomas, as well as those tumors that show hybrid features (Fig. 33-104).[387,411,413,414] For example, Hornick et al.[387] found complete loss of SMARCB1 expression in 127 of 136 (93%) epithelioid sarcomas, including 58 of 64 (91%) conventional types, 61 of 64 (95%) proximal types, and

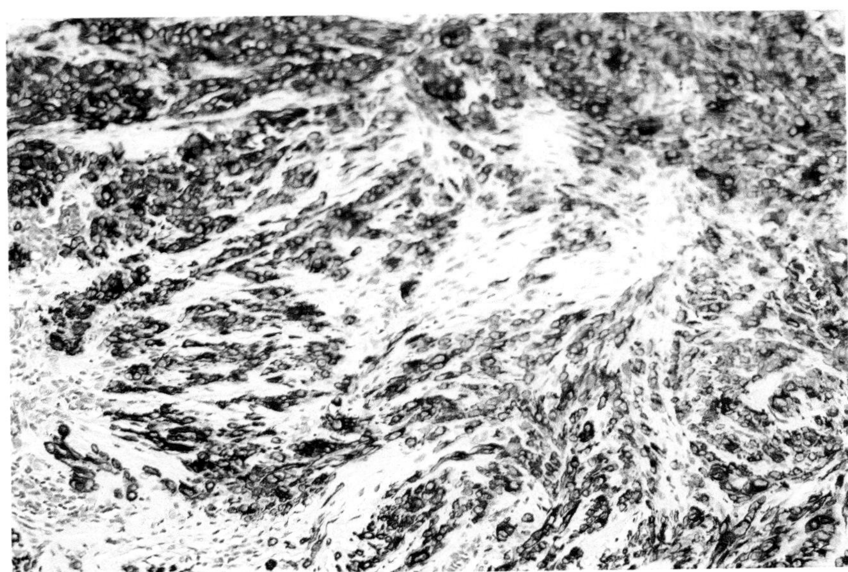

FIGURE 33-102. Strong cytokeratin immunoreactivity typical of epithelioid sarcoma.

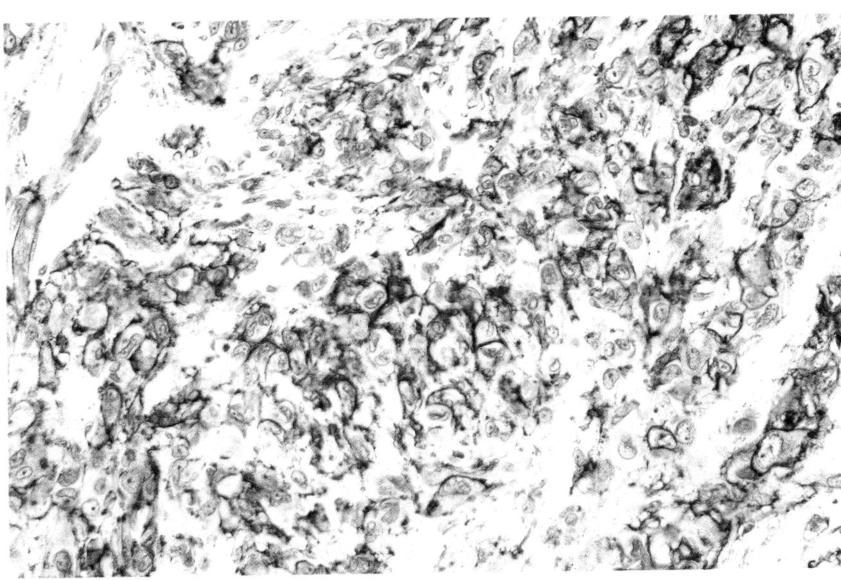

FIGURE 33-103. Membranous immunoreactivity for CD34 in an epithelioid sarcoma. This antigen is found in up to 70% of cases.

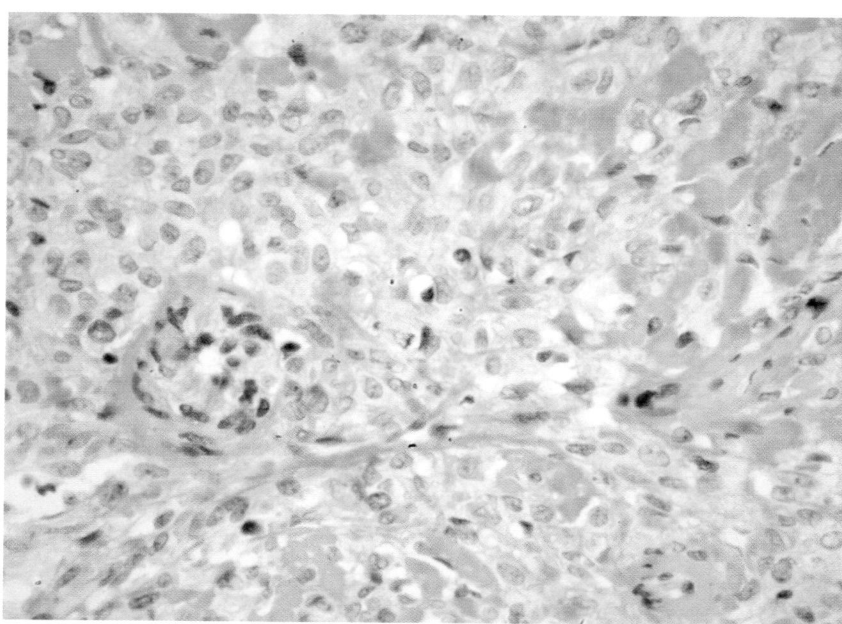

FIGURE 33-104. Epithelioid sarcoma showing loss of SMARCB1 staining in the neoplastic cells. Non-neoplastic cells entrapped within the tumor retain staining for this antigen.

in all 8 hybrid tumors tested. In addition, all 10 malignant rhabdoid tumors of infancy showed complete loss of this protein. Although 12 of 24 (50%) epithelioid MPNST and 2 of 22 (9%) myoepithelial carcinomas also showed loss of SMARCB1 staining, all other malignant epithelioid neoplasms tested, including metastatic carcinomas (54), metastatic testicular embryonal carcinomas (12), metastatic melanomas (20), epithelioid mesotheliomas (20), epithelioid angiosarcomas (20), epithelioid hemangioendotheliomas (10), anaplastic large cell lymphomas (7) and histiocytic sarcomas (5), showed retention of SMARCB1 staining. Similarly, Kohashi et al.[414] found loss of SMARCB1 protein in 27 of 29 (93%) conventional-type epithelioid sarcomas and 19 of 25 (76%) proximal-type tumors, although only 4 of 39 (10.3%) cases with loss of SMARCB1 staining analyzed at the DNA level showed homozygous deletions of the *SMARCB1* gene, all 4 of which were proximal-type epithelioid sarcomas. Therefore, the literature and this textbook's authors' experience suggest that loss of SMARCB1 staining is found in the vast majority (approximately 90%) of epithelioid sarcomas, regardless of type, and this finding can be extremely helpful in distinguishing this tumor from a variety of malignant epithelioid neoplasms. A superb review of SMARCB1 expression has been recently provided by Hollman and Hornick.[415]

Cytogenetic and Molecular Genetic Findings

A number of case reports and small series have found aberrations of the long arm of chromosome 22 (22q11) in both conventional and proximal-type epithelioid sarcomas,[416-419] including translocations. Quezado et al.[420] found loss of heterozygosity of chromosome 22q in 6 of 10 conventional-type lesions, and similar findings were reported by Lualdi et al.[421] Considering that the *SMARCB1* gene is located on 22q and the previously mentioned frequent loss of SMARCB1 protein in all types of epithelioid sarcoma, it is reasonable to suggest that *SMARCB1* gene deletions or mutations are central in the pathogenesis of epithelioid sarcoma, thereby linking it to malignant rhabdoid tumor of infancy and atypical teratoid/rhabdoid tumor because deletions of *SMARCB1* are clearly central to the pathogenesis of those tumors. However, alterations of this gene have been reported in varying frequencies in epithelioid sarcoma. Modena et al.[413] reported deletions of *SMARCB1* by FISH in 5 of 6 cases of proximal-type epithelioid sarcoma, but Kohashi et al.[414] found this alteration in only 4 of 39 (10.3%) epithelioid sarcomas, all of which were proximal-type lesions.

Clinical Course and Therapy

Epithelioid sarcoma has a high risk for local recurrence and metastasis and requires long-term follow-up, given that recurrence or metastasis may occur many years after the initial diagnosis. For the conventional type of epithelioid sarcoma, overall 5-year survival rates range from 50% to up to 85%,[368,422,423] and 10-year survival rates range from 42% to 55%.[423,424] In the large study from the AFIP, follow-up data, available in 202 patients, showed recurrence and metastatic rates of 77% and 45%, respectively; 32% of patients died as a direct result of their tumor.[368] The most common sites of metastasis were the lung (51%) and regional lymph nodes (34%) and less frequently the skin, central nervous system, and soft tissue (Table 33-18). The scalp was the site of metastasis in 22% of the cases. Similar findings were reported in the study of 106 patients by the French Sarcoma Group.[370] Of the 106 cases, 70 were conventional type, and 36 were proximal type. In the 80 patients with follow-up information, 54% presented with or developed metastatic disease, and 31% died of disease.

Multiple recurrences, often as the result of marginal resection, are a characteristic feature of the tumor. One of the patients reported by Chase and Enzinger[368] was treated for recurrent tumor growth in the left pretibial region on 11 occasions during a 16-year period. Another patient had 20 surgical procedures for recurrent growth within a period of 10 years. Recurrent tumors may form confluent nodules in the dermis

TABLE 33-18 Site of Metastatic Disease in 83 Metastasizing Epithelioid Sarcomas

LOCATION	NO. OF CASES	PERCENTAGE (%)
Lung	42	51
Lymph nodes	28	34
Scalp	18	22
Bone	11	13
Brain	11	13
Liver	10	12
Pleura	9	11

Modified from Chase DR, Enzinger FM. Epithelioid sarcoma: diagnosis, prognostic indicators, and treatment. Am J Surg Pathol 1985;9: 241–263.

BOX 33-2 Reported Adverse Prognostic Features for Epithelioid Sarcoma

Male gender
Nondistal extremity tumors
Large tumor size (greater than or exactly 5 cm)
Increased tumor depth
High mitotic index
Hemorrhage
Necrosis
Vascular invasion
Inadequate initial excision

or along tendons and fascial structures at or near the original tumor site. There are also cases where the skin adjacent and proximal to the tumor is studded with small, crater-like ulcerated nodules or plaques, a striking picture unlike that of any other recurrent soft tissue sarcoma.[379] In fact, the tendency for this tumor to track along an extremity some distance from the original scar suggests local metastasis, rather than local recurrence in the strict sense of the word. Recurrence generally develops within the first year after diagnosis, but recurrence may be late; in one of the cases reported by Chase and Enzinger,[368] it became apparent 25 years after the primary tumor was removed by local excision.

Intravascular growth and lymph node involvement are ominous features.[371,425] Metastasis may occur early in the course of disease (even before detection of the primary tumor), or it may occur many years following the initial diagnosis. Therefore, prognosis should be rendered with considerable caution, even if the patient appears to be well and free of a tumor 5 years after the initial diagnosis.

Prognosis depends on various factors, including the gender of the patient, the site, size and depth of the tumor, the number of mitotic figures, histologic subtype (proximal type being more aggressive), the presence or absence of hemorrhage, necrosis, vascular invasion, and the adequacy of the initial excision (Box 33-2).[368,370,371,388,426] In the series by Chase and Enzinger,[368] the survival rate for females was 78% compared to 64% for males. The improved outcome in females was even more pronounced in the series of Bos et al.,[424] who reported a 5-year survival rate of 80% in females compared to 40% in males.

Tumor site also appears to be prognostically important in that tumors arising in the distal extremities have a more favorable prognosis than those in the trunk and proximal portion of the limbs.[368,370,427] Tumor size greater than 5 cm is also associated with a more aggressive clinical course.[370,428,429] The expression of dysadherin, a membranous glycoprotein that downregulates E-cadherin and promotes metastasis, has been found to be a significant poor prognostic factor.[430] Several studies have found frequent overexpression of EGFR (with activation of components of the mTOR pathway), but gene amplification and kinase domain mutations are rare and have not been found to be prognostically significant.[431,432]

Accurate assessment and comparison of the efficacy of treatment is difficult, especially if the cases are derived from multiple sources, as in the AFIP material. It is clearly evident, however, that inadequate therapy (marginal resection) is associated with a more aggressive clinical course.[371,429] Adequate treatment requires early radical local excision or amputation if the primary tumor is situated in the fingers or toes. Amputation should also be considered as treatment for recurrent growth but does not seem to offer any benefit to patients with distant metastasis.[433] Regional lymph node dissection should be included among the therapeutic modalities because lymph node metastasis is a fairly common occurrence in epithelioid sarcoma. Some have suggested that a sentinel lymph node biopsy may be helpful in determining the need for a full dissection.[434] In all cases, surgical treatment should be combined with radiotherapy and multiagent chemotherapy over a prolonged period, similar to the chemotherapy given for other adult-type sarcomas. However, the true benefit of adjuvant therapy has yet to be fully shown.[435]

Discussion

There is still no consensus as to the line of cellular differentiation of epithelioid sarcoma. Not surprisingly, the relationship between epithelioid sarcoma and synovial sarcoma has been postulated in view of the intimate association of the tumor with tendons and aponeuroses, the mixture of epithelioid and spindled cellular elements, and the immunoreactivity for epithelial markers. There are, however, a number of contrasting features: the predominant location of epithelioid sarcoma in the hand, the consistent absence of pseudoglandular structures and intracellular mucin droplets, the lack of basal laminae ultrastructurally, and the absence of the t(X;18) characteristic of synovial sarcoma. Over the past years, it has also been suggested that epithelioid sarcoma is a tumor of primitive mesenchymal cells with fibroblastic and histiocytic differentiation,[436] a primitive mesenchymal tumor with differentiation along histiocytic and synovial lines,[437] a variant of fibrosarcoma,[438] a tumor of myofibroblasts altered by massive production of intermediate filaments,[439] a malignant giant cell tumor of the tendon sheath,[440] and a tumor related to nodular tenosynovitis and arising from synovioblastic mesenchyme.[441]

Finally, a brief discussion of the potential relationship between the proximal-type epithelioid sarcoma and MERT is warranted. Certainly, these tumors do share morphologic overlap, including the presence of cells with rhabdoid morphology. In addition, as previously mentioned, similar to MERT, the vast majority of epithelioid sarcomas, including the proximal-type, are characterized by inactivation of *SMARCB1* and loss of SMARCB1 protein expression. Clinically, both tumors are aggressive, although MERT is typically more rapidly fatal and there are some long-term survivors with proximal-type epithelioid sarcoma. Interestingly, patients with constitutional mutations in *SMARCB1* are predisposed to a variety of tumors, including MERT and atypical teratoid/rhabdoid tumor but they do not seem to develop epithelioid sarcoma.[442] Although proximal-type epithelioid sarcoma loses SMARCB1 immunoexpression, actual mutations of this gene seem to be rare and far less common than is found in MERT.[414] Finally, both tumors show immunohistochemical overlap with coexpression of epithelial markers and vimentin, and loss of SMARCB1 staining, but up to 60% of epithelioid sarcomas express CD34, a marker typically absent in MERT. Izumi et al.[430] found frequent expression of dysadherin in proximal-type epithelioid sarcoma but not in MERT.

MALIGNANT EXTRARENAL RHABDOID TUMOR

Malignant rhabdoid tumor of the kidney, initially described in 1978 and thought to be a rhabdomyosarcomatoid variant of Wilms tumor, has subsequently been defined as a distinct clinicopathologic entity different from Wilms tumor.[443,444] Most tumors arising in the kidney occur in children less than 1 year of age and have an aggressive clinical course. The majority of patients die of widespread metastatic disease within a short time from the initial diagnosis.

Subsequently, tumors with a histologic appearance similar to those arising in the kidney have been described in virtually every extrarenal anatomic site, most prominently the central nervous system, where they are referred to as *atypical teratoid/rhabdoid tumors*.[445] Lesions arising in the soft tissues most frequently occur in deep axial locations, including the paraspinal region and neck.[446] It is often difficult to determine from the descriptions of these tumors whether they represent pure extrarenal rhabdoid tumors composed exclusively of cells with a rhabdoid morphology (MERT) or whether they represent focal rhabdoid areas within a parent neoplasm of recognizable phenotype (composite extrarenal rhabdoid tumor [CERT]).[447] The term *MERT* as it pertains to soft tissue should be used for tumors with a predominant rhabdoid morphology in which no other clear line of differentiation can be documented. In this regard, it should be noted that carcinomas of various types may have rhabdoid features, most commonly renal cell carcinoma.[448] In addition, cells with rhabdoid features may be found in many types of sarcoma (e.g., epithelioid sarcoma,[449] DSRCT,[317] leiomyosarcoma,[450] synovial sarcoma,[451] rhabdomyosarcoma,[452] myxoid chondrosarcoma,[453] malignant mesothelioma,[454] meningioma,[455] and melanoma.[456] Clinically, MERTs occur over a much broader age range than those found in the kidney, although these lesions are still far more common in children. Like their renal counterparts, MERTs are generally characterized by aggressive clinical behavior because fewer than 50% of patients survive more than 5 years regardless of the type of therapy used.[447] As later described in greater detail, the histogenetic relationship between renal and extrarenal rhabdoid tumors (including those arising in the central nervous system) has been confirmed by the finding that they possess the same cytogenetic and molecular alterations.

Pathologic Findings

Grossly, MERT is usually less than 5 cm in greatest dimension, although size varies considerably. The cut surface is usually soft, fleshy, and gray to tan in color, frequently with foci of hemorrhage and necrosis.

The histologic hallmark of MERT is the presence of rhabdoid cells—large polygonal cells with eccentric vesicular nuclei, prominent nucleoli, and abundant cytoplasm containing juxtanuclear eosinophilic, PAS-positive hyaline inclusions or globules (Figs. 33-105 to 33-107). These inclusions correlate ultrastructurally to a paranuclear intracellular aggregate composed of compact bundles or whorls of intermediate filaments 10 nm in length (Figs. 33-108 to 33-110).[457] Some benign tumors, including pleomorphic adenomas and myoepitheliomas of the salivary glands, have intracytoplasmic hyaline inclusions, but these tumors lack the nuclear cytologic atypia to designate them as having a rhabdoid morphology. Evaluation of multiple sections may be required to determine whether

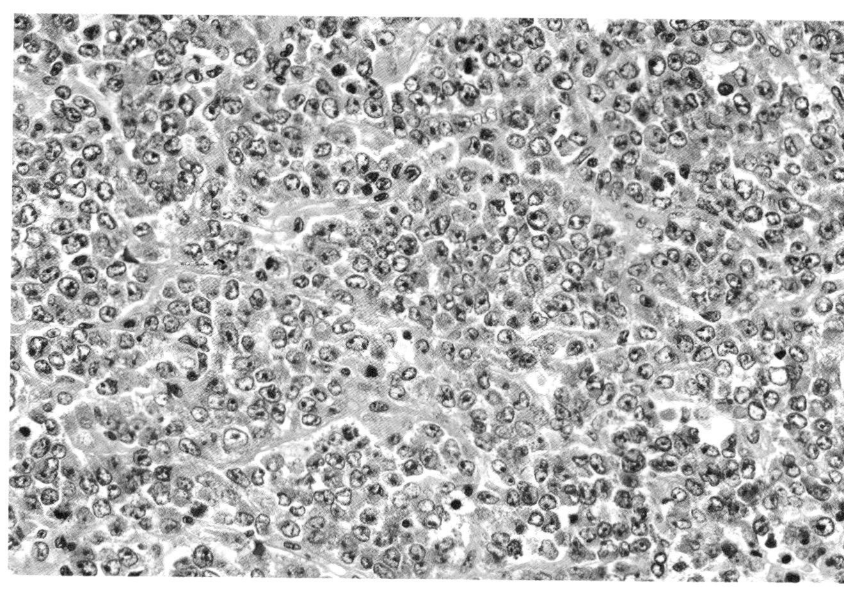

FIGURE 33-105. Malignant extrarenal rhabdoid tumor composed of nests of large epithelioid cells.

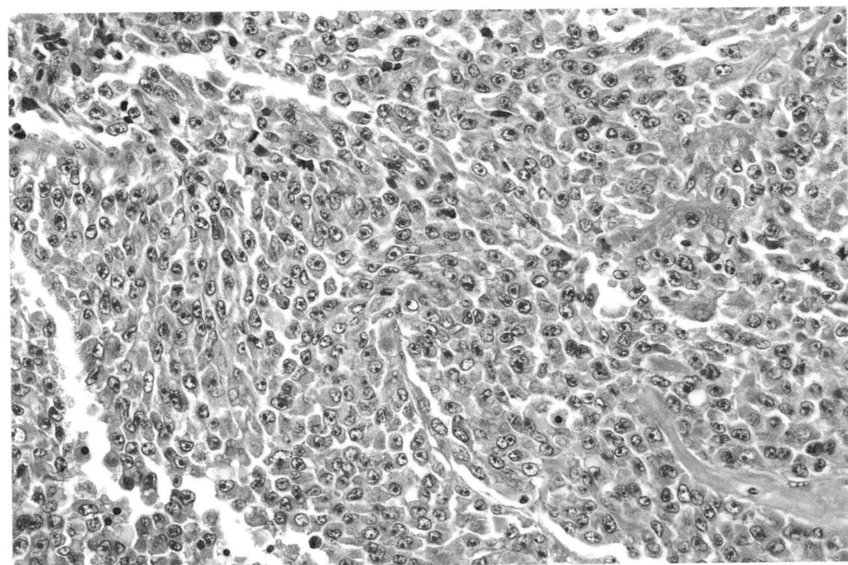

FIGURE 33-106. Sheets of large epithelioid cells with abundant eosinophilic cytoplasm in a malignant extrarenal rhabdoid tumor.

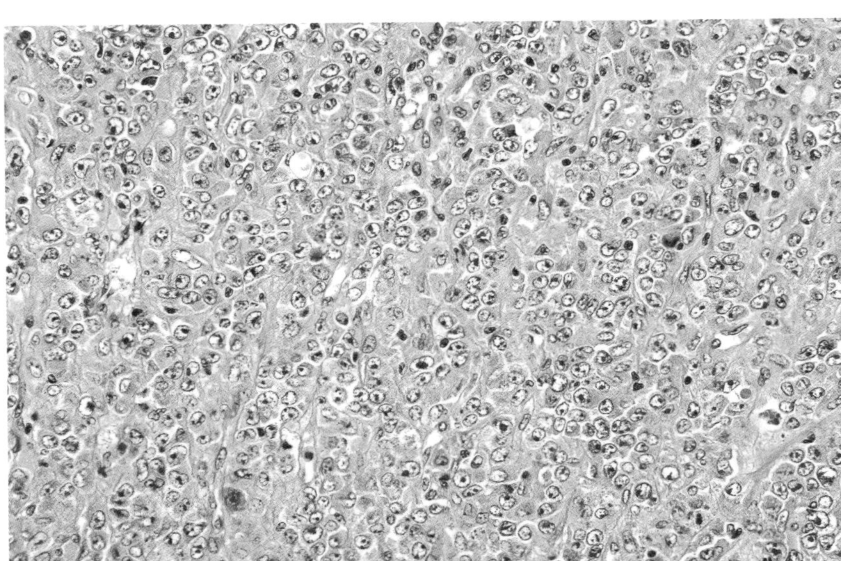

FIGURE 33-107. Malignant extrarenal rhabdoid tumor with a sheet of uniform large epithelioid cells having macronucleoli and abundant eosinophilic cytoplasm.

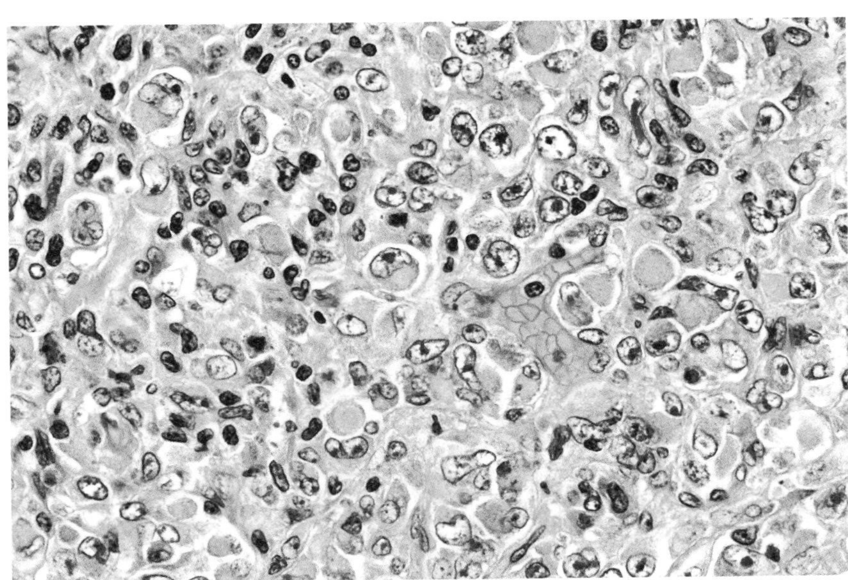

FIGURE 33-108. Malignant extrarenal rhabdoid tumor. The tumor cells have eccentric nuclei with macronucleoli.

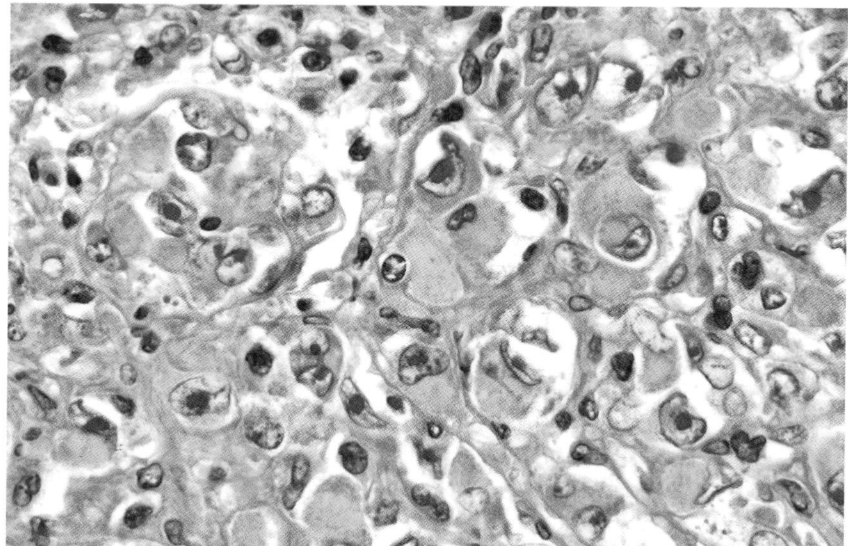

FIGURE 33-109. High-magnification view of paranuclear intracytoplasmic hyaline inclusions in a malignant extrarenal rhabdoid tumor.

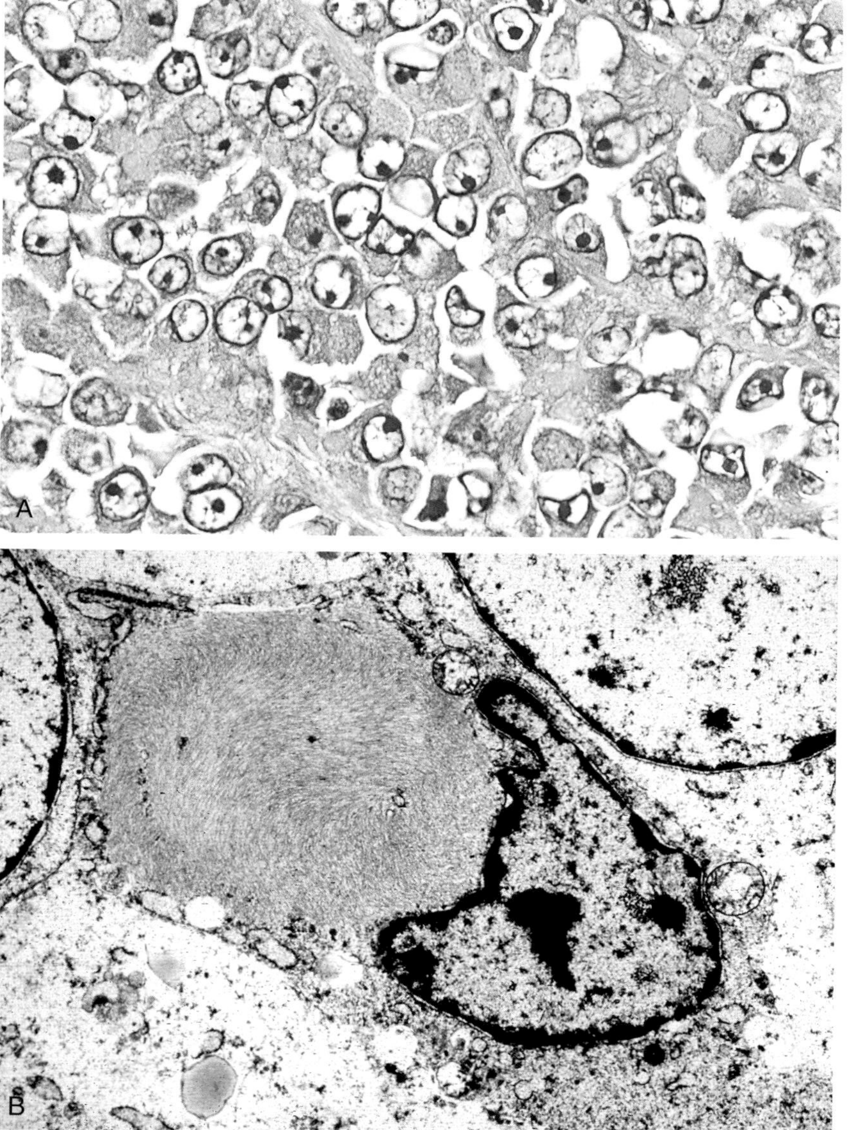

FIGURE 33-110. Malignant extrarenal rhabdoid tumor. (A) Cells with rhabdoid morphology. (B) Ultrastructural correlate, with a paranuclear whorl of intermediate filaments.

the rhabdoid cells are a component of CERT with a recognizable neoplastic phenotype (Fig. 33-111). In addition, ancillary techniques such as immunohistochemistry and molecular genetic analysis are usually necessary to recognize such a parent neoplasm, particularly if the rhabdoid cells comprise a substantial portion of the tumor, as well as to confirm the diagnosis of MERT.

Immunohistochemical and Ultrastructural Findings

A variety of antigens may be detected in the cells of MERT, including epithelial (Fig. 33-112), mesenchymal, and neural antigens.[446,458] Vimentin is the most consistently expressed marker, followed by EMA and cytokeratin. Less commonly, the cells express muscle specific actin, smooth muscle actin, CD99, CD57, synaptophysin, and S-100 protein. Numerous studies have reported consistent loss of expression of the SMARCB1 protein as a result of homozygous deletion or mutation of the *SMARCB1* gene.[410,459-461]

Judkins et al.[410] first reported the sensitivity and specificity of this marker in recognizing atypical teratoid/rhabdoid tumors of the central nervous system. Hoot et al.[459] evaluated this marker in a large number of renal and extrarenal rhabdoid tumors as well as an array of other pediatric soft tissue tumors (Table 33-19). In all 27 cases of renal or extrarenal rhabdoid tumor, including 21 tumors with either a chromosome 22 deletion or an *SMARCB1* mutation, there was no detectable expression of the SMARCB1 protein in any of the tumor cells. In contrast, nuclear expression of SMARCB1 protein was retained in all other tumors evaluated, including EFT (13 cases), Wilms tumor (6 cases), DSRCT (5 cases), and alveolar rhabdomyosarcoma (3 cases). Sigauke et al.[462] found

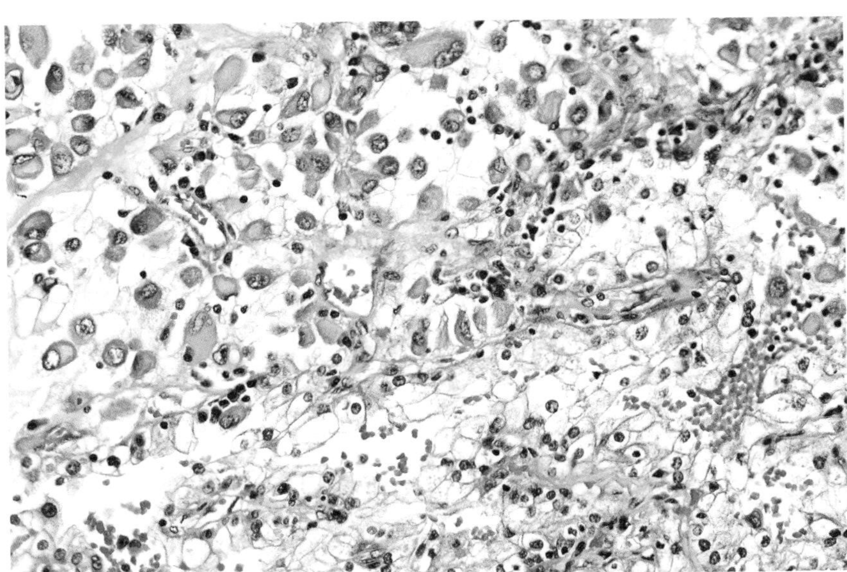

FIGURE 33-111. Composite extrarenal rhabdoid tumor with a typical clear cell renal cell carcinoma appearance at the bottom and cells with rhabdoid features near the top.

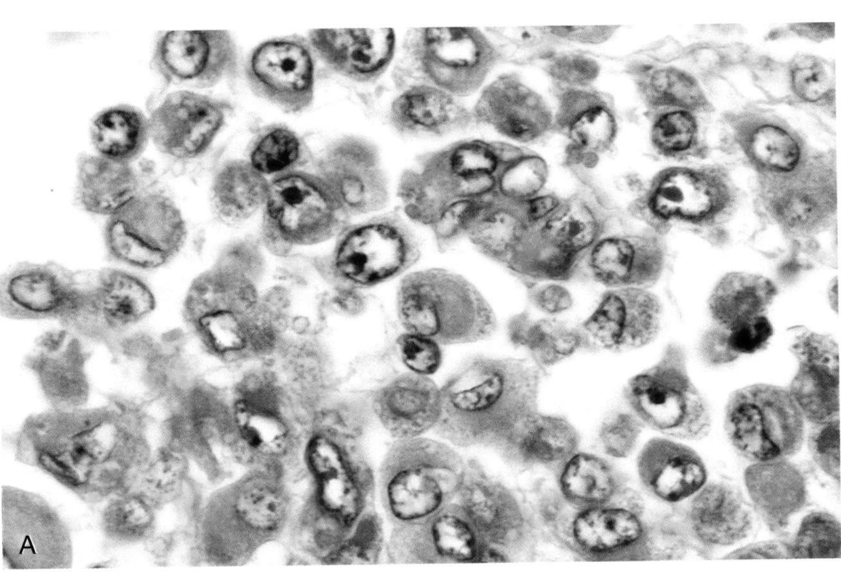

FIGURE 33-112. Malignant extrarenal rhabdoid tumor. (A) High-magnification view of rhabdoid cells.

Continued

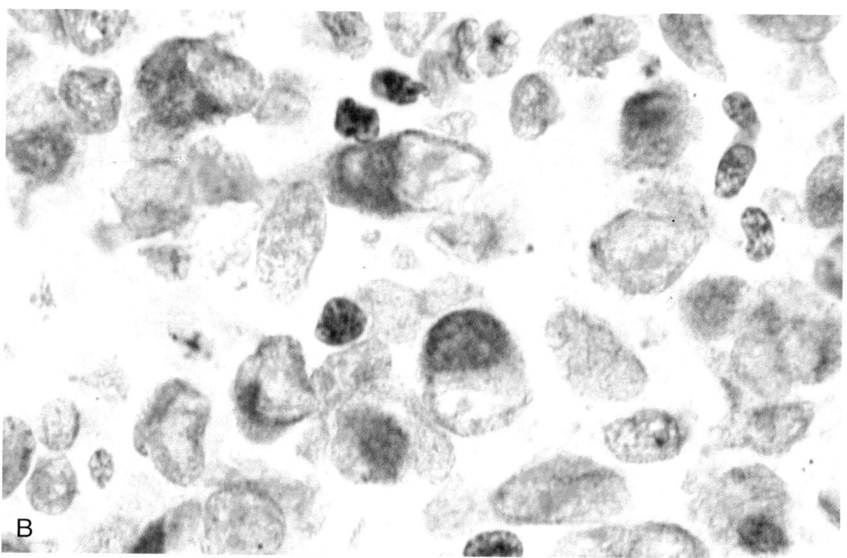

FIGURE 33-112, cont'd. (B) Paranuclear immunoreactivity for CAM5.2 in rhabdoid cells.

TABLE 33-19 Utility of Immunohistochemical Analysis of SMARCB1 in Distinguishing Renal and Extrarenal Malignant Rhabdoid Tumors from Other Pediatric Soft Tissue Tumors

TUMOR	SMARCB1 STAINING
Renal rhabdoid tumor	0/19
Extrarenal rhabdoid tumor	0/8
EFT	13/13
ARMS	3/3
ERMS	2/2
DSRCT	5/5
Clear cell sarcoma	4/4
Wilms tumor	6/6

Modified from Hoot A, Russo P, Judkins A, et al. Immunohistochemical analysis of hSNF5/INI1 distinguishes renal and extrarenal malignant rhabdoid tumors from other pediatric soft tissue tumors. Am J Surg Pathol 2004;22:1485–1491.

EFT, Ewing family of tumors; ARMS, alveolar rhabdomyosarcoma; ERMS, embryonal rhabdomyosarcoma; DSRCT, desmoplastic small round cell tumor.

an absence of expression of SMARCB1 protein in a large number of malignant rhabdoid tumors of the central nervous system, kidney, and soft tissue.

Ultrastructurally, rhabdoid cells are characterized by paranuclear aggregates or whorls of intermediate filaments 10 nm in size, predominantly composed of cytokeratin.[463]

Cytogenetic and Molecular Findings

The molecular alterations of renal and extrarenal rhabdoid tumors (including those arising in the central nervous system) have been elucidated over the past decade. Earlier cytogenetic studies consistently found 22q aberrations, including monosomy of chromosome 22, with or without partial deletion of the remaining chromosome 22.[464-466] Schofield et al.[467] reported loss of heterozygosity on 22q in 80% of renal rhabdoid tumors, suggesting the presence of a tumor suppressor gene at this locus. Subsequent studies consistently found deletions or mutations of the *SMARCB1* gene (also known as *hSNF5/INI1/BAF47*) in the vast majority of renal and extrarenal rhabdoid tumors, and atypical teratoid/rhabdoid tumors of the central nervous system.[406,407,468,469] *SMARCB1* is a member of the SWI/SNF chromatin-remodeling complex and is thought to have a direct role in activation and suppression of gene expression.[469] Germline mutations of the *SMARCB1* gene have been found in patients with multiple rhabdoid tumors (rhabdoid predisposition syndrome).[405,470] In a study of 50 patients with atypical teratoid/rhabdoid tumor and malignant rhabdoid tumors (renal and extrarenal), germline *SMARCB1* mutations were detected in 10 of 41 patients with central nervous system disease,[471] but germline mutations were not detected in 9 patients without central nervous system disease. Patients with germline mutations were younger at the time of diagnosis than those without germline mutations (5.5 versus 13 months, respectively) and had a far worse prognosis (0% 2-year survival versus 48%, respectively). Overall, up to 20% of rhabdoid tumors of all sites show no evidence of *SMARCB1* gene alterations. Genetic analysis of CERT by FISH has shown an absence of deletions of 22q11, indicating retained *SMARCB1* function,[472] and these tumors retain nuclear expression of SMARCB1 protein.[473] Alterations of the *SMARCB1* gene affect multiple pathways that may be central to the pathogenesis of this tumor, including the p16/INK4A, p14/ARF, and p21 (CIP1/WAF1) pathways.[474-476]

Discussion

Because of the definitional issues regarding MERT, it is difficult to cite meaningful studies from the literature. Sultan et al.[477] reported the clinicopathologic features of 229 tumors in the Surveillance, Epidemiology, and End Results (also recognized as SEER) database. Primary tumors were located in the central nervous system (35%), kidneys (20%), and extrarenal, non-central nervous system sites (45%). Although the vast majority of patients with central nervous system and renal tumors were younger than 18 years of age, 61% of patients with MERTs were older than 18 years. Age at diagnosis (2 to 18 years of age), localized tumor stage, and use of radiotherapy were significantly associated with improved survival.

It has been proposed that the rhabdoid phenotype represents a final common pathway for the evolution of many tumors to a higher-grade, more clinically aggressive neoplasm[469,478] analogous to the tumor progression seen with dedifferentiated sarcomas. There is ample evidence to support the existence of MERT as a clinicopathologic entity, rather than simply a pattern of tumor progression, a contention firmly based in the recognition of mutations of the *SMARCB1* gene, which are characteristic of this tumor.

The nature of this tumor remains an enigma, but recent evidence suggests a relationship to stem cell precursors. Vennetti et al.[479] found tumors of the central nervous system, kidney, and soft tissue express a number of stem cell-associated transcription factors, including glycipan-3, Sall4, T-cell leukemia/lymphoma1, and undifferentiated embryonic cell transcription factor 1. Their data also implicated EZH2 and the Id family of proteins, factors known to play a role in stem cell proliferation and differentiation.

References

1. Mertens F, Antonescu CR, Hohenberger P, et al. Translocation-related sarcomas. Semin Oncol 2009;36(4):312–23.
2. Stout A. Tumor of the ulnar nerve. Proc NY Pathol Soc 1918;18: 2–12.
3. Ewing J. Diffuse endothelioma of bone. Proc NY Pathol Soc 1921; 21:17–24.
4. Angervall L, Enzinger FM. Extraskeletal neoplasm resembling Ewing's sarcoma. Cancer 1975;36(1):240–51.
5. Seemayer TA, Thelmo WL, Bolande RP, et al. Peripheral neuroectodermal tumors. Perspect Pediatr Pathol 1975;2:151–72.
6. Jaffe R, Santamaria M, Yunis EJ, et al. The neuroectodermal tumor of bone. Am J Surg Pathol 1984;8(12):885–98.
7. Askin FB, Rosai J, Sibley RK, et al. Malignant small cell tumor of the thoracopulmonary region in childhood: a distinctive clinicopathologic entity of uncertain histogenesis. Cancer 1979;43(6):2438–51.
8. Dehner LP. Primitive neuroectodermal tumor and Ewing's sarcoma. Am J Surg Pathol 1993;17(1):1–13.
9. Dehner LP. The evolution of the diagnosis and understanding of primitive and embryonic neoplasms in children: living through an epoch. Mod Pathol 1998;11(7):669–85.
10. Aurias A, Rimbaut C, Buffe D, et al. Translocation involving chromosome 22 in Ewing's sarcoma. A cytogenetic study of four fresh tumors. Cancer Genet Cytogenet 1984;12(1):21–5.
11. Whang-Peng J, Triche TJ, Knutsen T, et al. Chromosome translocation in peripheral neuroepithelioma. N Engl J Med 1984;311(9): 584–5.
12. De Alava E, Pardo J. Ewing tumor: tumor biology and clinical applications. Int J Surg Pathol 2001;9(1):7–17.
13. Khoury JD. Ewing sarcoma family of tumors. Adv Anat Pathol 2005; 12(4):212–20.
14. Cavazzana AO, Ninfo V, Roberts J, et al. Peripheral neuroepithelioma: a light microscopic, immunocytochemical, and ultrastructural study. Mod Pathol 1992;5(1):71–8.
15. Hartman KR, Triche TJ, Kinsella TJ, et al. Prognostic value of histopathology in Ewing's sarcoma. Long-term follow-up of distal extremity primary tumors. Cancer 1991;67(1):163–71.
16. Kushner BH, Hajdu SI, Gulati SC, et al. Extracranial primitive neuroectodermal tumors. The Memorial Sloan-Kettering Cancer Center experience. Cancer 1991;67(7):1825–9.
17. Marina NM, Etcubanas E, Parham DM, et al. Peripheral primitive neuroectodermal tumor (peripheral neuroepithelioma) in children. A review of the St. Jude experience and controversies in diagnosis and management. Cancer 1989;64(9):1952–60.
18. Schmidt D, Herrmann C, Jürgens H, et al. Malignant peripheral neuroectodermal tumor and its necessary distinction from Ewing's sarcoma. A report from the Kiel Pediatric Tumor Registry. Cancer 1991;68(10): 2251–9.
19. Herzog CE. Overview of sarcomas in the adolescent and young adult population. J Pediatr Hematol Oncol 2005;27(4):215–18.
20. Tahasildar N, Goni V, Bhagwat K, et al. Ewing's sarcoma as second malignancy following a short latency in unilateral retinoblastoma. J Orthop Traumatol 2011;12(3):167–71.
21. Machado I, Llombart B, Calabuig-Fariñas S, et al. Superficial Ewing's sarcoma family of tumors: a clinicopathological study with differential diagnoses. J Cutan Pathol 2011;38(8):636–43.
22. Hasegawa SL, Davison JM, Rutten A, et al. Primary cutaneous Ewing's sarcoma: immunophenotypic and molecular cytogenetic evaluation of five cases. Am J Surg Pathol 1998;22(3):310–18.
23. Mar WA, Taljanovic MS, Bagatell R, et al. Update on imaging and treatment of Ewing sarcoma family tumors: what the radiologist needs to know. J Comput Assist Tomogr 2008;32(1):108–18.
24. Llombart-Bosch A, Machado I, Navarro S, et al. Histological heterogeneity of Ewing's sarcoma/PNET: an immunohistochemical analysis of 415 genetically confirmed cases with clinical support. Virchows Arch 2009;455(5):397–411.
25. Fujii H, Honoki K, Enomoto Y, et al. Adamantinoma-like Ewing's sarcoma with EWS-FLI1 fusion gene: a case report. Virchows Arch 2006;449(5):579–84.
26. Bridge JA, Fidler ME, Neff JR, et al. Adamantinoma-like Ewing's sarcoma: genomic confirmation, phenotypic drift. Am J Surg Pathol 1999;23(2):159–65.
27. Folpe AL, Goldblum JR, Rubin BP, et al. Morphologic and immunophenotypic diversity in Ewing family tumors: a study of 66 genetically confirmed cases. Am J Surg Pathol 2005;29(8):1025–33.
28. Collini P, Sampietro G, Bertulli R, et al. Cytokeratin immunoreactivity in 41 cases of ES/PNET confirmed by molecular diagnostic studies. Am J Surg Pathol 2001;25(2):273–4.
29. Gu M, Antonescu CR, Guiter G, et al. Cytokeratin immunoreactivity in Ewing's sarcoma: prevalence in 50 cases confirmed by molecular diagnostic studies. Am J Surg Pathol 2000;24(3):410–16.
30. Machado I, Navarro S, López-Guerrero JA, et al. Epithelial marker expression does not rule out a diagnosis of Ewing's sarcoma family of tumours. Virchows Archiv: An International Journal of Pathology 2011. Available at: http://www.ncbi.nlm.nih.gov/pubmed/21887539. Accessed September 21, 2011.
31. Parham DM, Dias P, Kelly DR, et al. Desmin positivity in primitive neuroectodermal tumors of childhood. Am J Surg Pathol 1992;16(5): 483–92.
32. Barisella M, Collini P, Orsenigo M, et al. Unusual myogenic and melanocytic differentiation of soft tissue pPNETs: an immunohistochemical and molecular study of 3 cases. Am J Surg Pathol 2010;34(7): 1002–6.
33. Fukunaga M, Ushigome S. Periosteal Ewing-like adamantinoma. Virchows Arch 1998;433(4):385–9.
34. Oda Y, Kinoshita Y, Tamiya S, et al. Extraskeletal primitive neuroectodermal tumour with massive osteo-cartilaginous metaplasia. Histopathology 2000;36(2):188–91.
35. Suh C-H, Ordóñez NG, Hicks J, et al. Ultrastructure of the Ewing's sarcoma family of tumors. Ultrastruct Pathol 2002;26(2):67–76.
36. Navarro S, Cavazzana AO, Llombart-Bosch A, et al. Comparison of Ewing's sarcoma of bone and peripheral neuroepithelioma. An immunocytochemical and ultrastructural analysis of two primitive neuroectodermal neoplasms. Arch Pathol Lab Med 1994;118(6):608–15.
37. Franchi A, Pasquinelli G, Cenacchi G, et al. Immunohistochemical and ultrastructural investigation of neural differentiation in Ewing sarcoma/PNET of bone and soft tissues. Ultrastruct Pathol 2001;25(3): 219–25.
38. Ambros IM, Ambros PF, Strehl S, et al. MIC2 is a specific marker for Ewing's sarcoma and peripheral primitive neuroectodermal tumors. Evidence for a common histogenesis of Ewing's sarcoma and peripheral primitive neuroectodermal tumors from MIC2 expression and specific chromosome aberration. Cancer 1991;67(7):1886–93.
39. Ozdemirli M, Fanburg-Smith JC, Hartmann DP, et al. Differentiating lymphoblastic lymphoma and Ewing's sarcoma: lymphocyte markers and gene rearrangement. Mod Pathol 2001;14(11):1175–82.
40. Ozdemirli M, Fanburg-Smith JC, Hartmann DP, et al. Precursor B-Lymphoblastic lymphoma presenting as a solitary bone tumor and mimicking Ewing's sarcoma: a report of four cases and review of the literature. Am J Surg Pathol 1998;22(7):795–804.
41. Perlman EJ, Lumadue JA, Hawkins AL, et al. Primary cutaneous neuroendocrine tumors. Diagnostic use of cytogenetic and MIC2 analysis. Cancer Genet Cytogenet 1995;82(1):30–4.
42. Lumadue JA, Askin FB, Perlman EJ. MIC2 analysis of small cell carcinoma. Am J Clin Pathol 1994;102(5):692–4.
43. Folpe AL, Hill CE, Parham DM, et al. Immunohistochemical detection of FLI-1 protein expression: a study of 132 round cell tumors with emphasis on CD99-positive mimics of Ewing's sarcoma/primitive neuroectodermal tumor. Am J Surg Pathol 2000;24(12):1657–62.

44. Devaney K, Abbondanzo SL, Shekitka KM, et al. MIC2 detection in tumors of bone and adjacent soft tissues. Clin Orthop Relat Res 1995;(310):176–87.
45. Gerald WL, Ladanyi M, De Alava E, et al. Clinical, pathologic, and molecular spectrum of tumors associated with t(11;22)(p13;q12): desmoplastic small round-cell tumor and its variants. J Clin Oncol 1998;16(9):3028–36.
46. Granter SR, Renshaw AA, Fletcher CD, et al. CD99 reactivity in mesenchymal chondrosarcoma. Hum Pathol 1996;27(12):1273–6.
47. Carter RL, al-Sams SZ, Corbett RP, et al. A comparative study of immunohistochemical staining for neuron-specific enolase, protein gene product 9.5 and S-100 protein in neuroblastoma, Ewing's sarcoma and other round cell tumours in children. Histopathology 1990;16(5):461–7.
48. Shanfeld R, Goldblum J. Immunohistochemical analysis of neural markers in peripheral primitive neuroectodermal tumors without light microscopic or ultrastructural evidence of neural differentiation. Appl Immunohistochem 1997;5:78–86.
49. Amann G, Zoubek A, Salzer-Kuntschik M, et al. Relation of neurological marker expression and EWS gene fusion types in MIC2/CD99-positive tumors of the Ewing family. Hum Pathol 1999;30(9):1058–64.
50. Rossi S, Orvieto E, Furlanetto A, et al. Utility of the immunohistochemical detection of FLI-1 expression in round cell and vascular neoplasm using a monoclonal antibody. Mod Pathol 2004;17(5):547–52.
51. Janknecht R. EWS-ETS oncoproteins: the linchpins of Ewing tumors. Gene 2005;363:1–14.
52. Wang WL, Patel NR, Caragea M, et al. Expression of ERG, an Ets family transcription factor, identifies ERG-rearranged Ewing sarcoma. Mod Pathol 2012;25(10):1378–83.
53. Ahmed A, Gilbert-Barness E, Lacson A. Expression of c-kit in Ewing family of tumors: a comparison of different immunohistochemical protocols. Pediatr Dev Pathol 2004;7(4):342–7.
54. Do I, Araujo ES, Kalil RK, et al. Protein expression of KIT and gene mutation of c-kit and PDGFRs in Ewing sarcomas. Pathol Res Pract 2007;203(3):127–34.
55. Scotlandi K, Manara MC, Strammiello R, et al. C-kit receptor expression in Ewing's sarcoma: lack of prognostic value but therapeutic targeting opportunities in appropriate conditions. J Clin Oncol 2003;21(10):1952–60.
56. Ladanyi M. EWS-FLI1 and Ewing's sarcoma: recent molecular data and new insights. Cancer Biol Ther 2002;1(4):330–6.
57. Delattre O, Zucman J, Melot T, et al. The Ewing family of tumors–a subgroup of small-round-cell tumors defined by specific chimeric transcripts. N Engl J Med 1994;331(5):294–9.
58. Delattre O, Zucman J, Plougastel B, et al. Gene fusion with an ETS DNA-binding domain caused by chromosome translocation in human tumours. Nature 1992;359(6391):162–5.
59. Im YH, Kim HT, Lee C, et al. EWS-FLI1, EWS-ERG, and EWS-ETV1 oncoproteins of Ewing tumor family all suppress transcription of transforming growth factor beta type II receptor gene. Cancer Res 2000;60(6):1536–40.
60. Jeon IS, Davis JN, Braun BS, et al. A variant Ewing's sarcoma translocation (7;22) fuses the EWS gene to the ETS gene ETV1. Oncogene 1995;10(6):1229–34.
61. Kaneko Y, Kobayashi H, Handa M, et al. EWS-ERG fusion transcript produced by chromosomal insertion in a Ewing sarcoma. Genes Chromosomes Cancer 1997;18(3):228–31.
62. Peter M, Mugneret F, Aurias A, et al. An EWS/ERG fusion with a truncated N-terminal domain of EWS in a Ewing's tumor. Int J Cancer 1996;67(3):339–42.
63. Mastrangelo T, Modena P, Tornielli S, et al. A novel zinc finger gene is fused to EWS in small round cell tumor. Oncogene 2000;19(33):3799–804.
64. De Alava E, Kawai A, Healey JH, et al. EWS-FLI1 fusion transcript structure is an independent determinant of prognosis in Ewing's sarcoma. J Clin Oncol 1998;16(4):1248–55.
65. Zoubek A, Pfleiderer C, Salzer-Kuntschik M, et al. Variability of EWS chimaeric transcripts in Ewing tumours: a comparison of clinical and molecular data. Br J Cancer 1994;70(5):908–13.
66. Zucman J, Melot T, Desmaze C, et al. Combinatorial generation of variable fusion proteins in the Ewing family of tumours. EMBO J 1993;12(12):4481–7.
67. Bridge RS, Rajaram V, Dehner LP, et al. Molecular diagnosis of Ewing sarcoma/primitive neuroectodermal tumor in routinely processed tissue: a comparison of two FISH strategies and RT-PCR in malignant round cell tumors. Mod Pathol 2006;19(1):1–8.
68. Shing DC, McMullan DJ, Roberts P, et al. FUS/ERG gene fusions in Ewing's tumors. Cancer Res 2003;63(15):4568–76.
69. Ng TL, O'Sullivan MJ, Pallen CJ, et al. Ewing sarcoma with novel translocation t(2;16) producing an in-frame fusion of FUS and FEV. J Mol Diagn 2007;9(4):459–63.
70. Sandberg AA, Bridge JA. Updates on cytogenetics and molecular genetics of bone and soft tissue tumors: Ewing sarcoma and peripheral primitive neuroectodermal tumors. Cancer Genet Cytogenet 2000;123(1):1–26.
71. Mugneret F, Lizard S, Aurias A, et al. Chromosomes in Ewing's sarcoma. II. Nonrandom additional changes, trisomy 8 and der(16)t(1;16). Cancer Genet Cytogenet 1988;32(2):239–45.
72. Maurici D, Perez-Atayde A, Grier HE, et al. Frequency and implications of chromosome 8 and 12 gains in Ewing sarcoma. Cancer Genet Cytogenet 1998;100(2):106–10.
73. Stark B, Mor C, Jeison M, et al. Additional chromosome 1q aberrations and der(16)t(1;16), correlation to the phenotypic expression and clinical behavior of the Ewing family of tumors. J Neurooncol 1997;31(1-2):3–8.
74. Ozaki T, Paulussen M, Poremba C, et al. Genetic imbalances revealed by comparative genomic hybridization in Ewing tumors. Genes Chromosomes Cancer 2001;32(2):164–71.
75. Hattinger CM, Pötschger U, Tarkkanen M, et al. Prognostic impact of chromosomal aberrations in Ewing tumours. Br J Cancer 2002;86(11):1763–9.
76. Parham DM, Hijazi Y, Steinberg SM, et al. Neuroectodermal differentiation in Ewing's sarcoma family of tumors does not predict tumor behavior. Hum Pathol 1999;30(8):911–18.
77. Siebenrock KA, Nascimento AG, Rock MG. Comparison of soft tissue Ewing's sarcoma and peripheral neuroectodermal tumor. Clin Orthop Relat Res 1996;(329):288–99.
78. Kim S, Chung DH. Pediatric solid malignancies: neuroblastoma and Wilms' tumor. Surg Clin North Am 2006;86(2):469–87, xi.
79. Esiashvili N, Goodman M, Ward K, et al. Neuroblastoma in adults: incidence and survival analysis based on SEER data. Pediatr Blood Cancer 2007;49(1):41–6.
80. Castleberry RP. Neuroblastoma. Eur J Cancer 1997;33(9):1430–7; discussion 1437–8.
81. Miettinen M, Chatten J, Paetau A, et al. Monoclonal antibody NB84 in the differential diagnosis of neuroblastoma and other small round cell tumors. Am J Surg Pathol 1998;22(3):327–32.
82. Maris JM, Guo C, Blake D, et al. Comprehensive analysis of chromosome 1p deletions in neuroblastoma. Med Pediatr Oncol 2001;36(1):32–6.
83. Guo C, White PS, Hogarty MD, et al. Deletion of 11q23 is a frequent event in the evolution of MYCN single-copy high-risk neuroblastomas. Med Pediatr Oncol 2000;35(6):544–6.
84. Łastowska M, Cotterill S, Bown N, et al. Breakpoint position on 17q identifies the most aggressive neuroblastoma tumors. Genes Chromosomes Cancer 2002;34(4):428–36.
85. Brodeur GM, Seeger RC, Schwab M, et al. Amplification of N-myc in untreated human neuroblastomas correlates with advanced disease stage. Science 1984;224(4653):1121–4.
86. Goto S, Umehara S, Gerbing RB, et al. Histopathology (International Neuroblastoma Pathology Classification) and MYCN status in patients with peripheral neuroblastic tumors: a report from the Children's Cancer Group. Cancer 2001;92(10):2699–708.
87. Brodeur GM. TRK-a expression in neuroblastomas: a new prognostic marker with biological and clinical significance. J Natl Cancer Inst 1993;85(5):344–5.
88. Matoso A, Singh K, Jacob R, et al. Comparison of thyroid transcription factor-1 expression by 2 monoclonal antibodies in pulmonary and non-pulmonary primary tumors. Appl Immunohistochem Mol Morphol 2010;18(2):142–9.
89. Machen SK, Fisher C, Gautam RS, et al. Utility of cytokeratin subsets for distinguishing poorly differentiated synovial sarcoma from peripheral primitive neuroectodermal tumour. Histopathology 1998;33(6):501–7.
90. Jürgens H, Bier V, Harms D, et al. Malignant peripheral neuroectodermal tumors. A retrospective analysis of 42 patients. Cancer 1988;61(2):349–57.
91. Balamuth NJ, Womer RB. Ewing's sarcoma. Lancet Oncol 2010;11(2):184–92.
92. Krasin MJ, Davidoff AM, Rodriguez-Galindo C, et al. Definitive surgery and multiagent systemic therapy for patients with localized Ewing

sarcoma family of tumors: local outcome and prognostic factors. Cancer 2005;104(2):367–73.
93. Burdach S, Van Kaick B, Laws HJ, et al. Allogeneic and autologous stem-cell transplantation in advanced Ewing tumors. An update after long-term follow-up from two centers of the European Intergroup study EICESS. Stem-Cell Transplant Programs at Düsseldorf University Medical Center, Germany and St. Anna Kinderspital, Vienna, Austria. Ann Oncol 2000;11(11):1451–62.
94. Drabko K, Zawitkowska-Klaczynska J, Wojcik B, et al. Megachemotherapy followed by autologous stem cell transplantation in children with Ewing's sarcoma. Pediatr Transplant 2005;9(5):618–21.
95. Lai R, Navid F, Rodriguez-Galindo C, et al. STAT3 is activated in a subset of the Ewing sarcoma family of tumours. J Pathol 2006;208(5):624–32.
96. Irifune H, Nishimori H, Watanabe G, et al. Aberrant laminin beta3 isoforms downstream of EWS-ETS fusion genes in Ewing family tumors. Cancer Biol Ther 2005;4(4):449–55.
97. Olmos D, Postel-Vinay S, Molife LR, et al. Safety, pharmacokinetics, and preliminary activity of the anti-IGF-1R antibody figitumumab (CP-751,871) in patients with sarcoma and Ewing's sarcoma: a phase 1 expansion cohort study. Lancet Oncol 2010;11(2):129–35.
98. Zwerner JP, May WA. PDGF-C is an EWS/FLI induced transforming growth factor in Ewing family tumors. Oncogene 2001;20(5):626–33.
99. Huang HY, Illei PB, Zhao Z, et al. Ewing sarcomas with p53 mutation or p16/p14ARF homozygous deletion: a highly lethal subset associated with poor chemoresponse. J Clin Oncol 2005;23(3):548–58.
100. Dalal S, Berry AM, Cullinane CJ, et al. Vascular endothelial growth factor: a therapeutic target for tumors of the Ewing's sarcoma family. Clin Cancer Res 2005;11(6):2364–78.
101. Fuchs B, Inwards CY, Janknecht R. Vascular endothelial growth factor expression is up-regulated by EWS-ETS oncoproteins and Sp1 and may represent an independent predictor of survival in Ewing's sarcoma. Clin Cancer Res 2004;10(4):1344–53.
102. Schleiermacher G, Peter M, Oberlin O, et al. Increased risk of systemic relapses associated with bone marrow micrometastasis and circulating tumor cells in localized ewing tumor. J Clin Oncol 2003;21(1):85–91.
103. Ahn HK, Uhm JE, Lee J, et al. Analysis of prognostic factors of pediatric-type sarcomas in adult patients. Oncology 2011;80(1-2):21–8.
104. Baldini EH, Demetri GD, Fletcher CD, et al. Adults with Ewing's sarcoma/primitive neuroectodermal tumor: adverse effect of older age and primary extraosseous disease on outcome. Ann Surg 1999;230(1):79–86.
105. Ginsberg JP, De Alava E, Ladanyi M, et al. EWS-FLI1 and EWS-ERG gene fusions are associated with similar clinical phenotypes in Ewing's sarcoma. J Clin Oncol 1999;17(6):1809–14.
106. Scotlandi K, Manara MC, Serra M, et al. Expression of insulin-like growth factor system components in Ewing's sarcoma and their association with survival. Eur J Cancer 2011;47(8):1258–66.
107. Ohali A, Avigad S, Cohen IJ, et al. High frequency of genomic instability in Ewing family of tumors. Cancer Genet Cytogenet 2004;150(1):50–6.
108. Schaefer KL, Eisenacher M, Braun Y, et al. Microarray analysis of Ewing's sarcoma family of tumours reveals characteristic gene expression signatures associated with metastasis and resistance to chemotherapy. Eur J Cancer 2008;44(5):699–709.
109. Hitchon H, Nobler MP, Wohl M, et al. The radiotherapeutic management of chordoid sarcoma. Am J Clin Oncol 1990;13(3):208–13.
110. Hajdu SI, Shiu MH, Fortner JG. Tendosynovial sarcoma: a clinicopathological study of 136 cases. Cancer 1977;39(3):1201–17.
111. Tsuneyoshi M, Enjoji M, Iwasaki H, et al. Extraskeletal myxoid chondrosarcoma–a clinicopathologic and electron microscopic study. Acta Pathol Jpn 1981;31(3):439–47.
112. Hachitanda Y, Tsuneyoshi M, Daimaru Y, et al. Extraskeletal myxoid chondrosarcoma in young children. Cancer 1988;61(12):2521–6.
113. Meis-Kindblom JM, Bergh P, Gunterberg B, et al. Extraskeletal myxoid chondrosarcoma: a reappraisal of its morphologic spectrum and prognostic factors based on 117 cases. Am J Surg Pathol 1999;23(6):636–50.
114. Enzinger FM, Shiraki M. Extraskeletal myxoid chondrosarcoma. An analysis of 34 cases. Hum Pathol 1972;3(3):421–35.
115. Drilon AD, Popat S, Bhuchar G, et al. Extraskeletal myxoid chondrosarcoma: a retrospective review from 2 referral centers emphasizing long-term outcomes with surgery and chemotherapy. Cancer 2008;113(12):3364–71.
116. Oliveira AM, Sebo TJ, McGrory JE, et al. Extraskeletal myxoid chondrosarcoma: a clinicopathologic, immunohistochemical, and ploidy analysis of 23 cases. Mod Pathol 2000;13(8):900–8.
117. McGrory JE, Rock MG, Nascimento AG, et al. Extraskeletal myxoid chondrosarcoma. Clin Orthop Relat Res 2001;(382):185–90.
118. Eguchi T, Yoshida K, Saito G, et al. Intrathoracic rupture of an extraskeletal myxoid chondrosarcoma. Gen Thorac Cardiovasc Surg 2011;59(5):367–70.
119. Sawada M, Tochigi N, Sasajima Y, et al. Primary extraskeletal myxoid chondrosarcoma of the vulva. J Obstet Gynaecol Res 2011;37(11):1706–10.
120. O'Brien J, Thornton J, Cawley D, et al. Extraskeletal myxoid chondrosarcoma of the cerebellopontine angle presenting during pregnancy. Br J Neurosurg 2008;22(3):429–32.
121. Geyer HL, Karlin N. Extraskeletal myxoid chondrosarcoma of the heart and review of current literature. Curr Oncol 2010;17(5):58–62.
122. Tateishi U, Hasegawa T, Nojima T, et al. MRI features of extraskeletal myxoid chondrosarcoma. Skeletal Radiol 2006;35(1):27–33.
123. Lucas DR, Fletcher CD, Adsay NV, et al. High-grade extraskeletal myxoid chondrosarcoma: a high-grade epithelioid malignancy. Histopathology 1999;35(3):201–8.
124. Reid R, De Silva MV, Paterson L. Poorly differentiated extraskeletal myxoid chondrosarcoma with t(9;22)(q22;q11) translocation presenting initially as a solid variant devoid of myxoid areas. Int J Surg Pathol 2003;11(2):137–41.
125. Abramovici LC, Steiner GC, Bonar F. Myxoid chondrosarcoma of soft tissue and bone: a retrospective study of 11 cases. Hum Pathol 1995;26(11):1215–20.
126. Tarkkanen M, Wiklund T, Virolainen M, et al. Dedifferentiated chondrosarcoma with t(9;22)(q34;q11-12). Genes Chromosomes Cancer 1994;9(2):136–40.
127. Kumar R, Rekhi B, Shirazi N, et al. Spectrum of cytomorphological features, including literature review, of an extraskeletal myxoid chondrosarcoma with t(9;22)(q22;q12) (TEC/EWS) results in one case. Diagn Cytopathol 2008;36(12):868–75.
128. Kohashi K, Oda Y, Yamamoto H, et al. SMARCB1/INI1 protein expression in round cell soft tissue sarcomas associated with chromosomal translocations involving EWS: a special reference to SMARCB1/INI1 negative variant extraskeletal myxoid chondrosarcoma. Am J Surg Pathol 2008;32(8):1168–74.
129. Oshiro Y, Shiratsuchi H, Tamiya S, et al. Extraskeletal Myxoid Chondrosarcoma with Rhabdoid Features, with Special Reference to Its Aggressive Behavior. Int J Surg Pathol 2000;8(2):145–52.
130. Sigauke E, Rakheja D, Maddox DL, et al. Absence of expression of SMARCB1/INI1 in malignant rhabdoid tumors of the central nervous system, kidneys and soft tissue: an immunohistochemical study with implications for diagnosis. Mod Pathol 2006;19(5):717–25.
131. Fletcher CD, Powell G, McKee PH. Extraskeletal myxoid chondrosarcoma: a histochemical and immunohistochemical study. Histopathology 1986;10(5):489–99.
132. Hisaoka M, Hashimoto H. Extraskeletal myxoid chondrosarcoma: updated clinicopathological and molecular genetic characteristics. Pathol Int 2005;55(8):453–63.
133. Goh YW, Spagnolo DV, Platten M, et al. Extraskeletal myxoid chondrosarcoma: a light microscopic, immunohistochemical, ultrastructural and immuno-ultrastructural study indicating neuroendocrine differentiation. Histopathology 2001;39(5):514–24.
134. Domanski HA, Carlén B, Mertens F, et al. Extraskeletal myxoid chondrosarcoma with neuroendocrine differentiation: a case report with fine-needle aspiration biopsy, histopathology, electron microscopy, and cytogenetics. Ultrastruct Pathol 2003;27(5):363–8.
135. Harris M, Coyne J, Tariq M, et al. Extraskeletal myxoid chondrosarcoma with neuroendocrine differentiation: a pathologic, cytogenetic, and molecular study of a case with a novel translocation t(9;17)(q22;q11.2). Am J Surg Pathol 2000;24(7):1020–6.
136. Panagopoulos I, Mertens F, Isaksson M, et al. Molecular genetic characterization of the EWS/CHN and RBP56/CHN fusion genes in extraskeletal myxoid chondrosarcoma. Genes Chromosomes Cancer 2002;35(4):340–52.
137. Hisaoka M, Okamoto S, Koyama S, et al. Microtubule-associated protein-2 and class III beta-tubulin are expressed in extraskeletal myxoid chondrosarcoma. Mod Pathol 2003;16(5):453–9.
138. Hu B, McPhaul L, Cornford M, et al. Expression of tau proteins and tubulin in extraskeletal myxoid chondrosarcoma, chordoma, and other chondroid tumors. Am J Clin Pathol 1999;112(2):189–93.
139. Hornick JL, Fletcher CD. Immunohistochemical staining for KIT (CD117) in soft tissue sarcomas is very limited in distribution. Am J Clin Pathol 2002;117(2):188–93.

140. Stenman G, Andersson H, Mandahl N, et al. Translocation t(9;22)(q22;q12) is a primary cytogenetic abnormality in extraskeletal myxoid chondrosarcoma. Int J Cancer 1995;62(4):398–402.
141. Sjögren H, Meis-Kindblom J, Kindblom LG, et al. Fusion of the EWS-related gene TAF2N to TEC in extraskeletal myxoid chondrosarcoma. Cancer Res 1999;59(20):5064–7.
142. Hisaoka M, Ishida T, Imamura T, et al. TFG is a novel fusion partner of NOR1 in extraskeletal myxoid chondrosarcoma. Genes Chromosomes Cancer 2004;40(4):325–8.
143. Brody RI, Ueda T, Hamelin A, et al. Molecular analysis of the fusion of EWS to an orphan nuclear receptor gene in extraskeletal myxoid chondrosarcoma. Am J Pathol 1997;150(3):1049–58.
144. Okamoto S, Hisaoka M, Ishida T, et al. Extraskeletal myxoid chondrosarcoma: a clinicopathologic, immunohistochemical, and molecular analysis of 18 cases. Hum Pathol 2001;32(10):1116–24.
145. Downs-Kelly E, Goldblum JR, Patel RM, et al. The utility of fluorescence in situ hybridization (FISH) in the diagnosis of myxoid soft tissue neoplasms. Am J Surg Pathol 2008;32(1):8–13.
146. Wang WL, Mayordomo E, Czerniak BA, et al. Fluorescence in situ hybridization is a useful ancillary diagnostic tool for extraskeletal myxoid chondrosarcoma. Mod Pathol 2008;21(11):1303–10.
147. Subramanian S, West RB, Marinelli RJ, et al. The gene expression profile of extraskeletal myxoid chondrosarcoma. J Pathol 2005;206(4):433–44.
148. Filion C, Motoi T, Olshen AB, et al. The EWSR1/NR4A3 fusion protein of extraskeletal myxoid chondrosarcoma activates the PPARG nuclear receptor gene. J Pathol 2009;217(1):83–93.
149. Koyama H, Boueres JK, Han W, et al. 5-Aryl thiazolidine-2,4-diones as selective PPARgamma agonists. Bioorg Med Chem Lett 2003;13(10):1801–4.
150. Antonescu CR, Zhang L, Chang NE, et al. EWSR1-POU5F1 fusion in soft tissue myoepithelial tumors. A molecular analysis of sixty-six cases, including soft tissue, bone, and visceral lesions, showing common involvement of the EWSR1 gene. Genes Chromosomes Cancer 2010;49(12):1114–24.
151. Kawaguchi S, Wada T, Nagoya S, et al. Extraskeletal myxoid chondrosarcoma: a multi-institutional study of 42 cases in Japan. Cancer 2003;97(5):1285–92.
152. Shi W, Indelicato DJ, Morris CG, et al. Long-term treatment outcomes for patients with synovial sarcoma: a 40-year experience at the University of Florida. Am J Clin Oncol 2013;36(1):83–8.
153. Herzog CE. Overview of sarcomas in the adolescent and young adult population. J Pediatr Hematol Oncol 2005;27(4):215–18.
154. Sultan I, Rodriguez-Galindo C, Saab R, et al. Comparing children and adults with synovial sarcoma in the Surveillance, Epidemiology, and End Results program, 1983 to 2005: an analysis of 1268 patients. Cancer 2009;115(15):3537–47.
155. Ladanyi M, Antonescu CR, Leung DH, et al. Impact of SYT-SSX fusion type on the clinical behavior of synovial sarcoma: a multi-institutional retrospective study of 243 patients. Cancer Res 2002;62(1):135–40.
156. Duband S, Morrison AL, Pasquier D, et al. First case report of a fetal synovial sarcoma confirmed by molecular detection of SYT-SSX fusion gene transcripts. Am J Perinatol 2008;25(8):517–20.
157. Al-Daraji W, Lasota J, Foss R, et al. Synovial sarcoma involving the head: analysis of 36 cases with predilection to the parotid and temporal regions. Am J Surg Pathol 2009;33(10):1494–503.
158. Deraedt K, Debiec-Rychter M, Sciot R. Radiation-associated synovial sarcoma of the lung following radiotherapy for pulmonary metastasis of Wilms' tumour. Histopathology 2006;48(4):473–5.
159. Egger JF, Coindre JM, Benhattar J, et al. Radiation-associated synovial sarcoma: clinicopathologic and molecular analysis of two cases. Mod Pathol 2002;15(9):998–1004.
160. Lamovec J, Zidar A, Cucek-Plenicar M. Synovial sarcoma associated with total hip replacement. A case report. J Bone Joint Surg Am 1988;70(10):1558–60.
161. Namba Y, Kawai A, Naito N, et al. Intraarticular synovial sarcoma confirmed by SYT-SSX fusion transcript. Clin Orthop Relat Res 2002;(395):221–6.
162. Bui-Mansfield LT, O'Brien SD. Magnetic resonance appearance of intraarticular synovial sarcoma: case reports and review of the literature. J Comput Assist Tomogr 2008;32(4):640–4.
163. Michal M, Fanburg-Smith JC, Lasota J, et al. Minute synovial sarcomas of the hands and feet: a clinicopathologic study of 21 tumors less than 1 cm. Am J Surg Pathol 2006;30(6):721–6.
164. Kusuma S, Skarupa DJ, Ely KA, et al. Synovial sarcoma of the head and neck: a review of its diagnosis and management and a report of a rare case of orbital involvement. Ear Nose Throat J 2010;89(6):280–3.
165. Fetsch JF, Meis JM. Synovial sarcoma of the abdominal wall. Cancer 1993;72(2):469–77.
166. Vera J, García MD, Marigil M, et al. Biphasic synovial sarcoma of the abdominal wall. Virchows Arch 2006;449(3):367–72.
167. Sakai M, Takami H, Joyama S, et al. Cardiac synovial sarcoma swinging through the aortic valve. Ann Thorac Surg 2011;92(3):1129.
168. Hartel PH, Fanburg-Smith JC, Frazier AA, et al. Primary pulmonary and mediastinal synovial sarcoma: a clinicopathologic study of 60 cases and comparison with five prior series. Mod Pathol 2007;20(7):760–9.
169. Karafin M, Parwani AV, Netto GJ, et al. Diffuse expression of PAX2 and PAX8 in the cystic epithelium of mixed epithelial stromal tumor, angiomyolipoma with epithelial cysts, and primary renal synovial sarcoma: evidence supporting renal tubular differentiation. Am J Surg Pathol 2011;35(9):1264–73.
170. Jun L, Ke S, Zhaoming W, et al. Primary synovial sarcoma of the prostate: report of 2 cases and literature review. Int J Surg Pathol 2008;16(3):329–34.
171. Alhazzani AR, El-Sharkawy MS, Hassan H. Primary retroperitoneal synovial sarcoma in CT and MRI. Urol Ann 2010;2(1):39–41.
172. Makhlouf HR, Ahrens W, Agarwal B, et al. Synovial sarcoma of the stomach: a clinicopathologic, immunohistochemical, and molecular genetic study of 10 cases. Am J Surg Pathol 2008;32(2):275–81.
173. Scheithauer BW, Amrami KK, Folpe AL, et al. Synovial sarcoma of nerve. Hum Pathol 2011;42(4):568–77.
174. Bixby SD, Hettmer S, Taylor GA, et al. Synovial sarcoma in children: imaging features and common benign mimics. AJR Am J Roentgenol 2010;195(4):1026–32.
175. Hisaoka M, Matsuyama A, Shimajiri S, et al. Ossifying synovial sarcoma. Pathol Res Pract 2009;205(3):195–8.
176. Kind M, Stock N, Coindre JM. Histology and imaging of soft tissue sarcomas. Eur J Radiol 2009;72(1):6–15.
177. Cummings NM, Desai S, Thway K, et al. Cystic primary pulmonary synovial sarcoma presenting as recurrent pneumothorax: report of 4 cases. Am J Surg Pathol 2010;34(8):1176–9.
178. Krane JF, Bertoni F, Fletcher CD. Myxoid synovial sarcoma: an underappreciated morphologic subset. Mod Pathol 1999;12(5):456–62.
179. Milchgrub S, Ghandur-Mnaymneh L, Dorfman HD, et al. Synovial sarcoma with extensive osteoid and bone formation. Am J Surg Pathol 1993;17(4):357–63.
180. Van de Rijn M, Barr FG, Xiong QB, et al. Poorly differentiated synovial sarcoma: an analysis of clinical, pathologic, and molecular genetic features. Am J Surg Pathol 1999;23(1):106–12.
181. Folpe AL, Schmidt RA, Chapman D, et al. Poorly differentiated synovial sarcoma: immunohistochemical distinction from primitive neuroectodermal tumors and high-grade malignant peripheral nerve sheath tumors. Am J Surg Pathol 1998;22(6):673–82.
182. De Silva MV, McMahon AD, Paterson L, et al. Identification of poorly differentiated synovial sarcoma: a comparison of clinicopathological and cytogenetic features with those of typical synovial sarcoma. Histopathology 2003;43(3):220–30.
183. Machen SK, Easley KA, Goldblum JR. Synovial sarcoma of the extremities: a clinicopathologic study of 34 cases, including semi-quantitative analysis of spindled, epithelial, and poorly differentiated areas. Am J Surg Pathol 1999;23(3):268–75.
184. Meis-Kindblom JM, Stenman G, Kindblom LG. Differential diagnosis of small round cell tumors. Semin Diagn Pathol 1996;13(3):213–41.
185. Paláu LMA, Thu Pham T, Barnard N, et al. Primary synovial sarcoma of the kidney with rhabdoid features. Int J Surg Pathol 2007;15(4):421–8.
186. Guillou L, Wadden C, Coindre JM, et al. "Proximal-type" epithelioid sarcoma, a distinctive aggressive neoplasm showing rhabdoid features. Clinicopathologic, immunohistochemical, and ultrastructural study of a series. Am J Surg Pathol 1997;21(2):130–46.
187. Miettinen M, Limon J, Niezabitowski A, et al. Patterns of keratin polypeptides in 110 biphasic, monophasic, and poorly differentiated synovial sarcomas. Virchows Arch 2000;437(3):275–83.
188. Smith TA, Machen SK, Fisher C, et al. Usefulness of cytokeratin subsets for distinguishing monophasic synovial sarcoma from malignant peripheral nerve sheath tumor. Am J Clin Pathol 1999;112(5):641–8.
189. Pelmus M, Guillou L, Hostein I, et al. Monophasic fibrous and poorly differentiated synovial sarcoma: immunohistochemical reassessment of 60 t(X;18)(SYT-SSX)-positive cases. Am J Surg Pathol 2002;26(11):1434–40.
190. Olsen SH, Thomas DG, Lucas DR. Cluster analysis of immunohistochemical profiles in synovial sarcoma, malignant peripheral nerve sheath tumor, and Ewing sarcoma. Mod Pathol 2006;19(5):659–68.

191. Suster S, Fisher C, Moran CA. Expression of bcl-2 oncoprotein in benign and malignant spindle cell tumors of soft tissue, skin, serosal surfaces, and gastrointestinal tract. Am J Surg Pathol 1998;22(7):863–72.
192. Krsková L, Kalinová M, Brízová H, et al. Molecular and immunohistochemical analyses of BCL2, KI-67, and cyclin D1 expression in synovial sarcoma. Cancer Genet Cytogenet 2009;193(1):1–8.
193. Fisher C, Montgomery E, Healy V. Calponin and h-caldesmon expression in synovial sarcoma; the use of calponin in diagnosis. Histopathology 2003;42(6):588–93.
194. Foo WC, Cruise MW, Wick MR, et al. Immunohistochemical staining for TLE1 distinguishes synovial sarcoma from histologic mimics. Am J Clin Pathol 2011;135(6):839–44.
195. Jagdis A, Rubin BP, Tubbs RR, et al. Prospective evaluation of TLE1 as a diagnostic immunohistochemical marker in synovial sarcoma. Am J Surg Pathol 2009;33(12):1743–51.
196. Terry J, Saito T, Subramanian S, et al. TLE1 as a diagnostic immunohistochemical marker for synovial sarcoma emerging from gene expression profiling studies. Am J Surg Pathol 2007;31(2):240–6.
197. Kosemehmetoglu K, Vrana JA, Folpe AL. TLE1 expression is not specific for synovial sarcoma: a whole section study of 163 soft tissue and bone neoplasms. Mod Pathol 2009;22(7):872–8.
198. He R, Patel RM, Alkan S, et al. Immunostaining for SYT protein discriminates synovial sarcoma from other soft tissue tumors: analysis of 146 cases. Mod Pathol 2007;20(5):522–8.
199. Kohashi K, Oda Y, Yamamoto H, et al. Reduced expression of SMARCB1/INI1 protein in synovial sarcoma. Mod Pathol 2010;23(7): 981–90.
200. Billings SD, Walsh SV, Fisher C, et al. Aberrant expression of tight junction-related proteins ZO-1, claudin-1 and occludin in synovial sarcoma: an immunohistochemical study with ultrastructural correlation. Mod Pathol 2004;17(2):141–9.
201. Sandberg AA, Bridge JA. Updates on the cytogenetics and molecular genetics of bone and soft tissue tumors. Synovial sarcoma. Cancer Genet Cytogenet 2002;133(1):1–23.
202. Brodin B, Haslam K, Yang K, et al. Cloning and characterization of spliced fusion transcript variants of synovial sarcoma: SYT/SSX4, SYT/SSX4v, and SYT/SSX2v. Possible regulatory role of the fusion gene product in wild type SYT expression. Gene 2001;268(1-2):173–82.
203. Dos Santos NR, De Bruijn DR, Van Kessel AG. Molecular mechanisms underlying human synovial sarcoma development. Genes Chromosomes Cancer 2001;30(1):1–14.
204. Nagayama S, Katagiri T, Tsunoda T, et al. Genome-wide analysis of gene expression in synovial sarcomas using a cDNA microarray. Cancer Res 2002;62(20):5859–66.
205. Nielsen TO, West RB, Linn SC, et al. Molecular characterisation of soft tissue tumours: a gene expression study. Lancet 2002;359(9314): 1301–7.
206. Panagopoulos I, Mertens F, Isaksson M, et al. Clinical impact of molecular and cytogenetic findings in synovial sarcoma. Genes Chromosomes Cancer 2001;31(4):362–72.
207. Antonescu CR, Kawai A, Leung DH, et al. Strong association of SYT-SSX fusion type and morphologic epithelial differentiation in synovial sarcoma. Diagn Mol Pathol 2000;9(1):1–8.
208. Kawai A, Woodruff J, Healey JH, et al. SYT-SSX gene fusion as a determinant of morphology and prognosis in synovial sarcoma. N Engl J Med 1998;338(3):153–60.
209. Guillou L, Coindre J, Gallagher G, et al. Detection of the synovial sarcoma translocation t(X;18) (SYT;SSX) in paraffin-embedded tissues using reverse transcriptase-polymerase chain reaction: a reliable and powerful diagnostic tool for pathologists. A molecular analysis of 221 mesenchymal tumors fixed in different fixatives. Hum Pathol 2001;32(1): 105–12.
210. Jin L, Majerus J, Oliveira A, et al. Detection of fusion gene transcripts in fresh-frozen and formalin-fixed paraffin-embedded tissue sections of soft-tissue sarcomas after laser capture microdissection and rt-PCR. Diagn Mol Pathol 2003;12(4):224–30.
211. Amary MF, Berisha F, Bernardi FD, et al. Detection of SS18-SSX fusion transcripts in formalin-fixed paraffin-embedded neoplasms: analysis of conventional RT-PCR, qRT-PCR and dual color FISH as diagnostic tools for synovial sarcoma. Mod Pathol 2007;20(4):482–96.
212. Huang L, Espinoza C, Welsh R. Malignant peripheral nerve sheath tumor with divergent differentiation. Arch Pathol Lab Med 2003;127(3): e147–50.
213. Miettinen M, Limon J, Niezabitowski A, et al. Calretinin and other mesothelioma markers in synovial sarcoma: analysis of antigenic similarities and differences with malignant mesothelioma. Am J Surg Pathol 2001;25(5):610–17.
214. Bahrami A, Folpe AL. Adult-type fibrosarcoma: a reevaluation of 163 putative cases diagnosed at a single institution over a 48-year period. Am J Surg Pathol 2010;34(10):1504–13.
215. Hui P, Li N, Johnson C, et al. HMGA proteins in malignant peripheral nerve sheath tumor and synovial sarcoma: preferential expression of HMGA2 in malignant peripheral nerve sheath tumor. Mod Pathol 2005;18(11):1519–26.
216. O'Sullivan MJ, Kyriakos M, Zhu X, et al. Malignant peripheral nerve sheath tumors with t(X;18). A pathologic and molecular genetic study. Mod Pathol 2000;13(11):1253–63.
217. Coindre JM, Hostein I, Benhattar J, et al. Malignant peripheral nerve sheath tumors are t(X;18)-negative sarcomas. Molecular analysis of 25 cases occurring in neurofibromatosis type 1 patients, using two different RT-PCR-based methods of detection. Mod Pathol 2002;15(6): 589–92.
218. Tamborini E, Agus V, Perrone F, et al. Lack of SYT-SSX fusion transcripts in malignant peripheral nerve sheath tumors on RT-PCR analysis of 34 archival cases. Lab Invest 2002;82(5):609–18.
219. Van de Rijn M, Barr FG, Collins MH, et al. Absence of SYT-SSX fusion products in soft tissue tumors other than synovial sarcoma. Am J Clin Pathol 1999;112(1):43–9.
220. Ladanyi M, Woodruff JM, Scheithauer BW, et al. Re: O'Sullivan MJ, Kyriakos M, Zhu X, Wick MR, Swanson PE, Dehner LP, Humphrey PA, Pfeifer JD: malignant peripheral nerve sheath tumors with t(X;18). A pathologic and molecular genetic study. Mod Pathol 2000;13:1336–46. *Mod Pathol* 2001;14(7):733–7.
221. Menendez LR, Brien E, Brien WW. Synovial sarcoma. A clinicopathologic study. Orthop Rev 1992;21(4):465–71.
222. Guadagnolo BA, Zagars GK, Ballo MT, et al. Long-term outcomes for synovial sarcoma treated with conservation surgery and radiotherapy. Int J Radiat Oncol Biol Phys 2007;69(4):1173–80.
223. Ryan JR, Baker LH, Benjamin RS. The natural history of metastatic synovial sarcoma: experience of the Southwest Oncology group. Clin Orthop Relat Res 1982;164:257–60.
224. Brennan B, Stevens M, Kelsey A, et al. Synovial sarcoma in childhood and adolescence: a retrospective series of 77 patients registered by the Children's Cancer and Leukaemia Group between 1991 and 2006. Pediatr Blood Cancer 2010;55(1):85–90.
225. Palmerini E, Staals EL, Alberghini M, et al. Synovial sarcoma: retrospective analysis of 250 patients treated at a single institution. Cancer 2009;115(13):2988–98.
226. Spillane AJ, A'Hern R, Judson IR, et al. Synovial sarcoma: a clinicopathologic, staging, and prognostic assessment. J Clin Oncol 2000;18(22): 3794–803.
227. Bergh P, Meis-Kindblom JM, Gherlinzoni F, et al. Synovial sarcoma: identification of low and high risk groups. Cancer 1999;85(12): 2596–607.
228. Italiano A, Penel N, Robin YM, et al. Neo/adjuvant chemotherapy does not improve outcome in resected primary synovial sarcoma: a study of the French Sarcoma Group. Ann Oncol 2009;20(3):425–30.
229. Deshmukh R, Mankin HJ, Singer S. Synovial sarcoma: the importance of size and location for survival. Clin Orthop Relat Res 2004;419: 155–61.
230. Brecht IB, Ferrari A, Int-Veen C, et al. Grossly-resected synovial sarcoma treated by the German and Italian Pediatric Soft Tissue Sarcoma Cooperative Groups: discussion on the role of adjuvant therapies. Pediatr Blood Cancer 2006;46(1):11–17.
231. Canter RJ, Qin LX, Maki RG, et al. A synovial sarcoma-specific preoperative nomogram supports a survival benefit to ifosfamide-based chemotherapy and improves risk stratification for patients. Clin Cancer Res 2008;14(24):8191–7.
232. Trassard M, Le Doussal V, Hacène K, et al. Prognostic factors in localized primary synovial sarcoma: a multicenter study of 128 adult patients. J Clin Oncol 2001;19(2):525–34.
233. Spurrell EL, Fisher C, Thomas JM, et al. Prognostic factors in advanced synovial sarcoma: an analysis of 104 patients treated at the Royal Marsden Hospital. Ann Oncol 2005;16(3):437–44.
234. Cagle LA, Mirra JM, Storm FK, et al. Histologic features relating to prognosis in synovial sarcoma. Cancer 1987;59(10):1810–14.
235. el-Naggar AK, Ayala AG, Abdul-Karim FW, et al. Synovial sarcoma. A DNA flow cytometric study. Cancer 1990;65(10):2295–300.
236. Varela-Duran J, Enzinger FM. Calcifying synovial sarcoma. Cancer 1982;50(2):345–52.
237. Guillou L, Benhattar J, Bonichon F, et al. Histologic grade, but not SYT-SSX fusion type, is an important prognostic factor in patients with synovial sarcoma: a multicenter, retrospective analysis. J Clin Oncol 2004;22(20):4040–50.

238. Hasegawa T, Yokoyama R, Matsuno Y, et al. Prognostic significance of histologic grade and nuclear expression of beta-catenin in synovial sarcoma. Hum Pathol 2001;32(3):257–63.
239. Oda Y, Hashimoto H, Tsuneyoshi M, et al. Survival in synovial sarcoma. A multivariate study of prognostic factors with special emphasis on the comparison between early death and long-term survival. Am J Surg Pathol 1993;17(1):35–44.
240. Golouh R, Vuzevski V, Bracko M, et al. Synovial sarcoma: a clinicopathological study of 36 cases. J Surg Oncol 1990;45(1):20–8.
241. Singer S, Baldini EH, Demetri GD, et al. Synovial sarcoma: prognostic significance of tumor size, margin of resection, and mitotic activity for survival. J Clin Oncol 1996;14(4):1201–8.
242. Oda Y, Sakamoto A, Satio T, et al. Molecular abnormalities of p53, MDM2, and H-ras in synovial sarcoma. Mod Pathol 2000;13(9): 994–1004.
243. Saito T, Oda Y, Sakamoto A, et al. Prognostic value of the preserved expression of the E-cadherin and catenin families of adhesion molecules and of beta-catenin mutations in synovial sarcoma. J Pathol 2000;192(3): 342–50.
244. Izumi T, Oda Y, Hasegawa T, et al. Dysadherin expression as a significant prognostic factor and as a determinant of histologic features in synovial sarcoma: special reference to its inverse relationship with E-cadherin expression. Am J Surg Pathol 2007;31(1):85–94.
245. Xie Y, Törnkvist M, Aalto Y, et al. Gene expression profile by blocking the SYT-SSX fusion gene in synovial sarcoma cells. Identification of XRCC4 as a putative SYT-SSX target gene. Oncogene 2003;22(48): 7628–31.
246. Sun Y, Gao D, Liu Y, et al. IGF2 is critical for tumorigenesis by synovial sarcoma oncoprotein SYT-SSX1. Oncogene 2006;25(7):1042–52.
247. Teng HW, Wang HW, Chen WM, et al. Prevalence and prognostic influence of genomic changes of EGFR pathway markers in synovial sarcoma. J Surg Oncol 2011;103(8):773–81.
248. Takenaka S, Ueda T, Naka N, et al. Prognostic implication of SYT-SSX fusion type in synovial sarcoma: a multi-institutional retrospective analysis in Japan. Oncol Rep 2008;19(2):467–76.
249. Ten Heuvel SE, Hoekstra HJ, Bastiaannet E, et al. The classic prognostic factors tumor stage, tumor size, and tumor grade are the strongest predictors of outcome in synovial sarcoma: no role for SSX fusion type or ezrin expression. Appl Immunohistochem Mol Morphol 2009;17(3): 189–95.
250. Randall RL, Schabel KL, Hitchcock Y, et al. Diagnosis and management of synovial sarcoma. Curr Treat Options Oncol 2005;6(6):449–59.
251. Al-Hussaini H, Hogg D, Blackstein ME, et al. Clinical features, treatment, and outcome in 102 adult and pediatric patients with localized high-grade synovial sarcoma. Sarcoma 2011;2011:231789.
252. Eilber FC, Brennan MF, Eilber FR, et al. Chemotherapy is associated with improved survival in adult patients with primary extremity synovial sarcoma. Ann Surg 2007;246(1):105–13.
253. Eilber FC, Dry SM. Diagnosis and management of synovial sarcoma. J Surg Oncol 2008;97(4):314–20.
254. Ferrari A, Gronchi A, Casanova M, et al. Synovial sarcoma: a retrospective analysis of 271 patients of all ages treated at a single institution. Cancer 2004;101(3):627–34.
255. Mancuso T, Mezzelani A, Riva C, et al. Analysis of SYT-SSX fusion transcripts and bcl-2 expression and phosphorylation status in synovial sarcoma. Lab Invest 2000;80(6):805–13.
256. Joyner DE, Albritton KH, Bastar JD, et al. G3139 antisense oligonucleotide directed against antiapoptotic Bcl-2 enhances doxorubicin cytotoxicity in the FU-SY-1 synovial sarcoma cell line. J Orthop Res 2006;24(3):474–80.
257. Bode B, Frigerio S, Behnke S, et al. Mutations in the tyrosine kinase domain of the EGFR gene are rare in synovial sarcoma. Mod Pathol 2006;19(4):541–7.
258. Blay JY, Ray-Coquard I, Alberti L, et al. Targeting other abnormal signaling pathways in sarcoma: EGFR in synovial sarcomas, PPAR-gamma in liposarcomas. Cancer Treat Res 2004;120:151–67.
259. Ray-Coquard I, Le Cesne A, Whelan JS, et al. A phase II study of gefitinib for patients with advanced HER-1 expressing synovial sarcoma refractory to doxorubicin-containing regimens. Oncologist 2008;13(4): 467–73.
260. Christopherson WM, Foote FW Jr, Stewart FW. Alveolar soft-part sarcomas; structurally characteristic tumors of uncertain histogenesis. Cancer 1952;5(1):100–11.
261. Ekfors TO, Kalimo H, Rantakokko V, et al. Alveolar soft part sarcoma: a report of two cases with some histochemical and ultrastructural observations. Cancer 1979;43(5):1672–7.
262. Lieberman PH, Brennan MF, Kimmel M, et al. Alveolar soft-part sarcoma. A clinico-pathologic study of half a century. Cancer 1989; 63(1):1–13.
263. Lieberman PH, Foote FW Jr, Stewart FW, et al. Alveolar soft-part sarcoma. JAMA 1966;198(10):1047–51.
264. Anderson ME, Hornicek FJ, Gebhardt MC, et al. Alveolar soft part sarcoma: a rare and enigmatic entity. Clin Orthop Relat Res 2005; 438:144–8.
265. Portera CA Jr, Ho V, Patel SR, et al. Alveolar soft part sarcoma: clinical course and patterns of metastasis in 70 patients treated at a single institution. Cancer 2001;91(3):585–91.
266. Casanova M, Ferrari A, Bisogno G, et al. Alveolar soft part sarcoma in children and adolescents: a report from the Soft-Tissue Sarcoma Italian Cooperative Group. Ann Oncol 2000;11(11):1445–9.
267. Ogose A, Yazawa Y, Ueda T, et al. Alveolar soft part sarcoma in Japan: multi-institutional study of 57 patients from the Japanese Musculoskeletal Oncology Group. Oncology 2003;65(1):7–13.
268. Pennacchioli E, Fiore M, Collini P, et al. Alveolar soft part sarcoma: clinical presentation, treatment, and outcome in a series of 33 patients at a single institution. Ann Surg Oncol 2010;17(12):3229–33.
269. Ordóñez NG. Alveolar soft part sarcoma: a review and update. Adv Anat Pathol 1999;6(3):125–39.
270. Hasegawa K, Ichikawa R, Ishii R, et al. A case of primary alveolar soft part sarcoma of the uterine cervix and a review of the literature. Int J Clin Oncol 2011. Available at: http://www.ncbi.nlm.nih.gov/pubmed/ 21519815. Accessed July 22, 2011.
271. Van Buren R, Stewart J 3rd. Alveolar soft part sarcoma presenting as a breast mass in a 13-year-old female. Diagn Cytopathol 2009;37(2): 122–4.
272. Amin MB, Patel RM, Oliveira P, et al. Alveolar soft-part sarcoma of the urinary bladder with urethral recurrence: a unique case with emphasis on differential diagnoses and diagnostic utility of an immunohistochemical panel including TFE3. Am J Surg Pathol 2006;30(10):1322–5.
273. Zhu FP, Lu GM, Zhang LJ, et al. Primary alveolar soft part sarcoma of vertebra: a case report and literature review. Skeletal Radiol 2009;38(8): 825–9.
274. Fanburg-Smith JC, Miettinen M, Folpe AL, et al. Lingual alveolar soft part sarcoma; 14 cases: novel clinical and morphological observations. Histopathology 2004;45(5):526–37.
275. Chen YD, Hsieh MS, Yao MS, et al. MRI of alveolar soft-part sarcoma. Comput Med Imaging Graph 2006;30(8):479–82.
276. Suh JS, Cho J, Lee SH, et al. Alveolar soft part sarcoma: MR and angiographic findings. Skeletal Radiol 2000;29(12):680–9.
277. Evans HL. Alveolar soft-part sarcoma. A study of 13 typical examples and one with a histologically atypical component. Cancer 1985;55(4): 912–17.
278. Ladanyi M, Antonescu CR, Drobnjak M, et al. The precrystalline cytoplasmic granules of alveolar soft part sarcoma contain monocarboxylate transporter 1 and CD147. Am J Pathol 2002;160(4):1215–21.
279. Miettinen M, Ekfors T. Alveolar soft part sarcoma. Immunohistochemical evidence for muscle cell differentiation. Am J Clin Pathol 1990;93(1): 32–8.
280. Rosai J, Dias P, Parham DM, et al. MyoD1 protein expression in alveolar soft part sarcoma as confirmatory evidence of its skeletal muscle nature. Am J Surg Pathol 1991;15(10):974–81.
281. Cullinane C, Thorner PS, Greenberg ML, et al. Molecular genetic, cytogenetic, and immunohistochemical characterization of alveolar soft-part sarcoma. Implications for cell of origin. Cancer 1992; 70(10):2444–50.
282. Wang NP, Bacchi CE, Jiang JJ, et al. Does alveolar soft-part sarcoma exhibit skeletal muscle differentiation? An immunocytochemical and biochemical study of myogenic regulatory protein expression. Mod Pathol 1996;9(5):496–506.
283. Gómez JA, Amin MB, Ro JY, et al. Immunohistochemical profile of myogenin and MyoD1 does not support skeletal muscle lineage in alveolar soft part sarcoma. Arch Pathol Lab Med 1999;123(6):503–7.
284. Cessna MH, Zhou H, Perkins SL, et al. Are myogenin and myoD1 expression specific for rhabdomyosarcoma? A study of 150 cases, with emphasis on spindle cell mimics. Am J Surg Pathol 2001;25(9):1150–7.
285. Argani P, Lal P, Hutchinson B, et al. Aberrant nuclear immunoreactivity for TFE3 in neoplasms with TFE3 gene fusions: a sensitive and specific immunohistochemical assay. Am J Surg Pathol 2003;27(6):750–61.
286. Pang LJ, Chang B, Zou H, et al. Alveolar soft part sarcoma: a bimarker diagnostic strategy using TFE3 immunoassay and ASPL-TFE3 fusion transcripts in paraffin-embedded tumor tissues. Diagn Mol Pathol 2008;17(4):245–52.

287. Williams A, Bartle G, Sumathi VP, et al. Detection of ASPL/TFE3 fusion transcripts and the TFE3 antigen in formalin-fixed, paraffin-embedded tissue in a series of 18 cases of alveolar soft part sarcoma: useful diagnostic tools in cases with unusual histological features. Virchows Arch 2011;458(3):291–300.
288. Tsuji K, Ishikawa Y, Imamura T. Technique for differentiating alveolar soft part sarcoma from other tumors in paraffin-embedded tissue: comparison of immunohistochemistry for TFE3 and CD147 and of reverse transcription polymerase chain reaction for ASPSCR1-TFE3 fusion transcript. Hum Pathol 2012;43(3):356–63.
289. Ordóñez NG, Mackay B. Alveolar soft-part sarcoma: a review of the pathology and histogenesis. Ultrastruct Pathol 1998;22(4):275–92.
290. Khanna P, Paidas CN, Gilbert-Barness E. Alveolar soft part sarcoma: clinical, histopathological, molecular, and ultrastructural aspects. Fetal Pediatr Pathol 2008;27(1):31–40.
291. Ladanyi M, Lui MY, Antonescu CR, et al. The der(17)t(X;17)(p11;q25) of human alveolar soft part sarcoma fuses the TFE3 transcription factor gene to ASPL, a novel gene at 17q25. Oncogene 2001;20(1):48–57.
292. Sandberg A, Bridge J. Updates on the cytogenetics and molecular genetics of bone and soft tissue tumors: alveolar soft part sarcoma. Cancer Genet Cytogenet 2002;136(1):1–9.
293. Argani P, Antonescu CR, Illei PB, et al. Primary renal neoplasms with the ASPL-TFE3 gene fusion of alveolar soft part sarcoma: a distinctive tumor entity previously included among renal cell carcinomas of children and adolescents. Am J Pathol 2001;159(1):179–92.
294. Pang LJ, Li F, Chang B, et al. [Detection of ASPL-TFE3 fusion gene by reverse transcriptase polymerase chain reaction in paraffin-embedded tumor tissues of alveolar soft part sarcoma]. Zhonghua Bing Li Xue Za Zhi 2004;33(6):508–12.
295. Zhong M, De Angelo P, Osborne L, et al. Dual-color, break-apart FISH assay on paraffin-embedded tissues as an adjunct to diagnosis of Xp11 translocation renal cell carcinoma and alveolar soft part sarcoma. Am J Surg Pathol 2010;34(6):757–66.
296. Saito T, Oda Y, Kawaguchi KI, et al. Possible association between tumor-suppressor gene mutations and hMSH2/hMLH1 inactivation in alveolar soft part sarcoma. Hum Pathol 2003;34(9):841–9.
297. Stockwin LH, Vistica DT, Kenney S, et al. Gene expression profiling of alveolar soft-part sarcoma (ASPS). BMC Cancer 2009;9:22.
298. Lazar AJ, Lahat G, Myers SE, et al. Validation of potential therapeutic targets in alveolar soft part sarcoma: an immunohistochemical study utilizing tissue microarray. Histopathology 2009;55(6):750–5.
299. Lazar AJ, Das P, Tuvin D, et al. Angiogenesis-promoting gene patterns in alveolar soft part sarcoma. Clin Cancer Res 2007;13(24):7314–21.
300. Conde N, Cruz O, Albert A, et al. Antiangiogenic treatment as a pre-operative management of alveolar soft-part sarcoma. Pediatr Blood Cancer 2011;57(6):1071–3.
301. Stacchiotti S, Negri T, Zaffaroni N, et al. Sunitinib in advanced alveolar soft part sarcoma: evidence of a direct antitumor effect. Ann Oncol 2011;22(7):1682–90.
302. Stacchiotti S, Tamborini E, Marrari A, et al. Response to sunitinib malate in advanced alveolar soft part sarcoma. Clin Cancer Res 2009;15(3):1096–104.
303. Lillehei KO, Kleinschmidt-DeMasters B, Mitchell DH, et al. Alveolar soft part sarcoma: an unusually long interval between presentation and brain metastasis. Hum Pathol 1993;24(9):1030–4.
304. Wang CH, Lee N, Lee LS. Successful treatment for solitary brain metastasis from alveolar soft part sarcoma. J Neurooncol 1995;25(2):161–6.
305. Reichardt P, Lindner T, Pink D, et al. Chemotherapy in alveolar soft part sarcomas. What do we know? Eur J Cancer 2003;39(11):1511–16.
306. Ghose A, Tariq Z, Veltri S. Treatment of multidrug resistant advanced alveolar soft part sarcoma with sunitinib. Am J Ther 2010. Available at: http://www.ncbi.nlm.nih.gov/pubmed/20634674. Accessed July 22, 2011.
307. Fisher ER, Reidbord H. Electron microscopic evidence suggesting the myogenous derivation of the so-called alveolar soft part sarcoma. Cancer 1971;27(1):150–9.
308. DeSchryver-Kecskemeti K, Kraus FT, Engleman W, et al. Alveolar soft-part sarcoma–A malignant angioreninoma: histochemical, immunocytochemical, and electron-microscopic study of four cases. Am J Surg Pathol 1982;6(1):5–18.
309. Mukai M, Torikata C, Iri H. Alveolar soft part sarcoma: an electron microscopic study especially of uncrystallized granules using a tannic acid-containing fixative. Ultrastruct Pathol 1990;14(1):41–50.
310. Gerald WL, Rosai J. Case 2. Desmoplastic small cell tumor with divergent differentiation. Pediatr Pathol 1989;9(2):177–83.
311. Gerald WL, Miller HK, Battifora H, et al. Intra-abdominal desmoplastic small round-cell tumor. Report of 19 cases of a distinctive type of high-grade polyphenotypic malignancy affecting young individuals. Am J Surg Pathol 1991;15(6):499–513.
312. Ordóñez NG, Zirkin R, Bloom RE. Malignant small-cell epithelial tumor of the peritoneum coexpressing mesenchymal-type intermediate filaments. Am J Surg Pathol 1989;13(5):413–21.
313. Variend S, Gerrard M, Norris PD, et al. Intra-abdominal neuroectodermal tumour of childhood with divergent differentiation. Histopathology 1991;18(1):45–51.
314. Gerald WL, Rosai J. Desmoplastic small cell tumor with multi-phenotypic differentiation. Zentralbl Pathol 1993;139(2):141–51.
315. Basade MM, Vege DS, Nair CN, et al. Intra-abdominal desmoplastic small round cell tumor in children: a clinicopathologic study. Pediatr Hematol Oncol 1996;13(1):95–9.
316. Reich O, Justus J, Tamussino KF. Intra-abdominal desmoplastic small round cell tumor in a 68-year-old female. Eur J Gynaecol Oncol 2000;21(2):126–7.
317. Gerald WL, Ladanyi M, De Alava E, et al. Clinical, pathologic, and molecular spectrum of tumors associated with t(11;22)(p13;q12): desmoplastic small round-cell tumor and its variants. J Clin Oncol 1998;16(9):3028–36.
318. Lae ME, Roche PC, Jin L, et al. Desmoplastic small round cell tumor: a clinicopathologic, immunohistochemical, and molecular study of 32 tumors. Am J Surg Pathol 2002;26(7):823–35.
319. Ordóñez NG. Desmoplastic small round cell tumor: I: a histopathologic study of 39 cases with emphasis on unusual histological patterns. Am J Surg Pathol 1998;22(11):1303–13.
320. García-González J, Villanueva C, Fernández-Aceñero MJ, et al. Paratesticular desmoplastic small round cell tumor: case report. Urol Oncol 2005;23(2):132–4.
321. Ota S, Ushijima K, Fujiyoshi N, et al. Desmoplastic small round cell tumor in the ovary: report of two cases and literature review. J Obstet Gynaecol Res 2010;36(2):430–4.
322. Parkash V, Gerald WL, Parma A, et al. Desmoplastic small round cell tumor of the pleura. Am J Surg Pathol 1995;19(6):659–65.
323. Neder L, Scheithauer BW, Turel KE, et al. Desmoplastic small round cell tumor of the central nervous system: report of two cases and review of the literature. Virchows Arch 2009;454(4):431–9.
324. Pang B, Leong CC, Salto-Tellez M, et al. Desmoplastic small round cell tumor of major salivary glands: report of 1 case and a review of the literature. Appl Immunohistochem Mol Morphol 2011;19(1):70–5.
325. Yin WH, Guo SP, Yang HY, et al. Desmoplastic small round cell tumor of the submandibular gland–a rare but distinctive primary salivary gland neoplasm. Hum Pathol 2010;41(3):438–42.
326. Yoshida A, Edgar MA, Garcia J, et al. Primary desmoplastic small round cell tumor of the femur. Skeletal Radiol 2008;37(9):857–62.
327. Muramatsu T, Shimamura M, Furuichi M, et al. Desmoplastic small round cell tumor of the lung. Ann Thorac Surg 2010;90(6):e86–7.
328. Wang LL, Perlman EJ, Vujanic GM, et al. Desmoplastic small round cell tumor of the kidney in childhood. Am J Surg Pathol 2007;31(4):576–84.
329. Da Silva RC, Medeiros Filho P, Chioato L, et al. Desmoplastic small round cell tumor of the kidney mimicking Wilms tumor: a case report and review of the literature. Appl Immunohistochem Mol Morphol 2009;17(6):557–62.
330. Qureshi SS, Shrikhande S, Ramadwar M, et al. Desmoplastic small round cell tumor of the pancreas: an unusual primary site for an uncommon tumor. J Indian Assoc Pediatr Surg 2011;16(2):66–8.
331. Dorsey BV, Benjamin LE, Rauscher F 3rd, et al. Intra-abdominal desmoplastic small round-cell tumor: expansion of the pathologic profile. Mod Pathol 1996;9(6):703–9.
332. Ordóñez NG. Desmoplastic small round cell tumor: II: an ultrastructural and immunohistochemical study with emphasis on new immunohistochemical markers. Am J Surg Pathol 1998;22(11):1314–27.
333. Zhang PJ, Goldblum JR, Pawel BR, et al. Immunophenotype of desmoplastic small round cell tumors as detected in cases with EWS-WT1 gene fusion product. Mod Pathol 2003;16(3):229–35.
334. Miettinen M, Chatten J, Paetau A, et al. Monoclonal antibody NB84 in the differential diagnosis of neuroblastoma and other small round cell tumors. Am J Surg Pathol 1998;22(3):327–32.
335. Barnoud R, Delattre O, Péoc'h M, et al. Desmoplastic small round cell tumor: RT-PCR analysis and immunohistochemical detection of the Wilms' tumor gene WT1. Pathol Res Pract 1998;194(10):693–700.
336. Barnoud R, Sabourin JC, Pasquier D, et al. Immunohistochemical expression of WT1 by desmoplastic small round cell tumor: a

comparative study with other small round cell tumors. Am J Surg Pathol 2000;24(6):830–6.
337. Hill DA, Pfeifer JD, Marley EF, et al. WT1 staining reliably differentiates desmoplastic small round cell tumor from Ewing sarcoma/primitive neuroectodermal tumor. An immunohistochemical and molecular diagnostic study. Am J Clin Pathol 2000;114(3):345–53.
338. Murphy AJ, Bishop K, Pereira C, et al. A new molecular variant of desmoplastic small round cell tumor: significance of WT1 immunostaining in this entity. Hum Pathol 2008;39(12):1763–70.
339. Khalbuss WE, Bui M, Loya A. A 19-year-old woman with a cervicovaginal mass and elevated serum CA 125. Desmoplastic small round cell tumor. Arch Pathol Lab Med 2006;130(4):e59–61.
340. Wills EJ. Peritoneal desmoplastic small round cell tumors with divergent differentiation: a review. Ultrastruct Pathol 1993;17(3-4):295–306.
341. Biegel JA, Conard K, Brooks JJ. Translocation (11;22)(p13;q12): primary change in intra-abdominal desmoplastic small round cell tumor. Genes Chromosomes Cancer 1993;7(2):119–21.
342. Sawyer JR, Tryka AF, Lewis JM. A novel reciprocal chromosome translocation t(11;22)(p13;q12) in an intraabdominal desmoplastic small round-cell tumor. Am J Surg Pathol 1992;16(4):411–16.
343. Ladanyi M, Gerald W. Fusion of the EWS and WT1 genes in the desmoplastic small round cell tumor. Cancer Res 1994;54(11):2837–40.
344. Lee SB, Haber DA. Wilms tumor and the WT1 gene. Exp Cell Res 2001;264(1):74–99.
345. Zhang PJ, Goldblum JR, Pawel BR, et al. PDGF-A, PDGF-Rbeta, TGFbeta3 and bone morphogenic protein-4 in desmoplastic small round cell tumors with EWS-WT1 gene fusion product and their role in stromal desmoplasia: an immunohistochemical study. Mod Pathol 2005;18(3):382–7.
346. Hill DA, O'Sullivan MJ, Zhu X, et al. Practical application of molecular genetic testing as an aid to the surgical pathologic diagnosis of sarcomas: a prospective study. Am J Surg Pathol 2002;26(8):965–77.
347. De Alava E, Ladanyi M, Rosai J, et al. Detection of chimeric transcripts in desmoplastic small round cell tumor and related developmental tumors by reverse transcriptase polymerase chain reaction. A specific diagnostic assay. Am J Pathol 1995;147(6):1584–91.
348. Antonescu CR, Gerald WL, Magid MS, et al. Molecular variants of the EWS-WT1 gene fusion in desmoplastic small round cell tumor. Diagn Mol Pathol 1998;7(1):24–8.
349. Ordi J, De Alava E, Torné A, et al. Intraabdominal desmoplastic small round cell tumor with EWS/ERG fusion transcript. Am J Surg Pathol 1998;22(8):1026–32.
350. Katz RL, Quezado M, Senderowicz AM, et al. An intra-abdominal small round cell neoplasm with features of primitive neuroectodermal and desmoplastic round cell tumor and a EWS/FLI-1 fusion transcript. Hum Pathol 1997;28(4):502–9.
351. Ordóñez NG, el-Naggar AK, Ro JY, et al. Intra-abdominal desmoplastic small cell tumor: a light microscopic, immunocytochemical, ultrastructural, and flow cytometric study. Hum Pathol 1993;24(8):850–65.
352. Schwarz RE, Gerald WL, Kushner BH, et al. Desmoplastic small round cell tumors: prognostic indicators and results of surgical management. Ann Surg Oncol 1998;5(5):416–22.
353. Kushner BH, Cheung NK, Kramer K, et al. Topotecan combined with myeloablative doses of thiotepa and carboplatin for neuroblastoma, brain tumors, and other poor-risk solid tumors in children and young adults. Bone Marrow Transplant 2001;28(6):551–6.
354. Hayes-Jordan A, Anderson PM. The diagnosis and management of desmoplastic small round cell tumor: a review. Curr Opin Oncol 2011;23(4):385–9.
355. Cao L, Ni J, Que R, et al. Desmoplastic small round cell tumor: a clinical, pathological, and immunohistochemical study of 18 Chinese cases. Int J Surg Pathol 2008;16(3):257–62.
356. Hayes-Jordan A, Anderson P, Curley S, et al. Continuous hyperthermic peritoneal perfusion for desmoplastic small round cell tumor. J Pediatr Surg 2007;42(8):E29–32.
357. Hayes-Jordan A, Green H, Fitzgerald N, et al. Novel treatment for desmoplastic small round cell tumor: hyperthermic intraperitoneal perfusion. J Pediatr Surg 2010;45(5):1000–6.
358. Msika S, Gruden E, Sarnacki S, et al. Cytoreductive surgery associated to hyperthermic intraperitoneal chemoperfusion for desmoplastic round small cell tumor with peritoneal carcinomatosis in young patients. J Pediatr Surg 2010;45(8):1617–21.
359. Subbiah V, Murthy R, Anderson PM. [90Y]yttrium microspheres radioembolotherapy in desmoplastic small round cell tumor hepatic metastases. J Clin Oncol 2011;29(11):e292–4.
360. Al Balushi Z, Bulduc S, Mulleur C, et al. Desmoplastic small round cell tumor in children: a new therapeutic approach. J Pediatr Surg 2009;44(5):949–52.
361. Graham C, Chilton-MacNeill S, Zielenska M, et al. The CIC-DUX4 fusion transcript is present in a subgroup of pediatric primitive round cell sarcomas. Hum Pathol 2012;43(2):180–9.
362. Italiano A, Sung YS, Zhang L, et al. High prevalence of CIC fusion with double-homeobox (DUX4) transcription factors in EWSR1-negative undifferentiated small blue round cell sarcomas. Genes Chromosomes Cancer 2012;51(3):207–18.
363. Kawamura-Saito M, Yamazaki Y, Kaneko K, et al. Fusion between CIC and DUX4 up-regulates PEA3 family genes in Ewing-like sarcomas with t(4;19)(q35;q13) translocation. Hum Mol Genet 2006;15(13):2125–37.
364. Rakheja D, Goldman S, Wilson KS, et al. Translocation (4;19)(q35;q13.1)-associated primitive round cell sarcoma: report of a case and review of the literature. Pediatr Dev Pathol 2008;11(3):239–44.
365. Richkind KE, Romansky SG, Finklestein JZ. t(4;19)(q35;q13.1): a recurrent change in primitive mesenchymal tumors? Cancer Genet Cytogenet 1996;87(1):71–4.
366. Yoshimoto M, Graham C, Chilton-MacNeill S, et al. Detailed cytogenetic and array analysis of pediatric primitive sarcomas reveals a recurrent CIC-DUX4 fusion gene event. Cancer Genet Cytogenet 2009;195(1):1–11.
367. Enzinger FM. Epitheloid sarcoma. A sarcoma simulating a granuloma or a carcinoma. Cancer 1970;26(5):1029–41.
368. Chase DR, Enzinger FM. Epithelioid sarcoma. Diagnosis, prognostic indicators, and treatment. Am J Surg Pathol 1985;9(4):241–63.
369. Prat J, Woodruff JM, Marcove RC. Epithelioid sarcoma: an analysis of 22 cases indicating the prognostic significance of vascular invasion and regional lymph node metastasis. Cancer 1978;41(4):1472–87.
370. Chbani L, Guillou L, Terrier P, et al. Epithelioid sarcoma: a clinicopathologic and immunohistochemical analysis of 106 cases from the French sarcoma group. Am J Clin Pathol 2009;131(2):222–7.
371. Jawad MU, Extein J, Min ES, et al. Prognostic factors for survival in patients with epithelioid sarcoma: 441 cases from the SEER database. Clin Orthop Relat Res 2009;467(11):2939–48.
372. Ormsby AH, Liou LS, Oriba HA, et al. Epithelioid sarcoma of the penis: report of an unusual case and review of the literature. Ann Diagn Pathol 2000;4(2):88–94.
373. Chiyoda T, Ishikawa M, Nakamura M, et al. Successfully treated case of epithelioid sarcoma of the vulva. The Journal of Obstetrics and Gynaecology Research 2011. Available at: http://www.ncbi.nlm.nih.gov/pubmed/21917072. Accessed October 1, 2011.
374. Maggiani F, Debiec-Rychter M, Ectors N, et al. Primary epithelioid sarcoma of the oesophagus. Virchows Arch 2007;451(4):835–8.
375. Hagström J, Mesimäki K, Apajalahti S, et al. A rare case of oral epithelioid sarcoma of the gingiva. Oral Surg Oral Med Oral Pathol Oral Radiol Endod 2011;111(4):e25–8.
376. Keelawat S, Shuangshoti S, Kittikowit W, et al. Epithelioid sarcoma of the parotid gland of a child. Pediatr Dev Pathol 2009;12(4):301–6.
377. Raoux D, Péoc'h M, Pedeutour F, et al. Primary epithelioid sarcoma of bone: report of a unique case, with immunohistochemical and fluorescent in situ hybridization confirmation of INI1 deletion. Am J Surg Pathol 2009;33(6):954–8.
378. Chao KC, Chen C, Hsieh SC, et al. MRI of epithelioid sarcoma of the thigh. Clin Imaging 2005;29(1):60–3.
379. Heenan PJ, Quirk CJ, Papadimitriou JM. Epithelioid sarcoma. A diagnostic problem. Am J Dermatopathol 1986;8(2):95–104.
380. Mirra JM, Kessler S, Bhuta S, et al. The fibroma-like variant of epithelioid sarcoma. A fibrohistiocytic/myoid cell lesion often confused with benign and malignant spindle cell tumors. Cancer 1992;69(6):1382–95.
381. Tan SH, Ong BH. Spindle cell variant of epithelioid sarcoma: an easily misdiagnosed tumour. Australas J Dermatol 2001;42(2):139–41.
382. Kaddu S, Wolf I, Horn M, et al. Epithelioid sarcoma with angiomatoid features: report of an unusual case arising in an elderly patient within a burn scar. J Cutan Pathol 2008;35(3):324–8.
383. Flucke U, Hulsebos TJ, Van Krieken JH, et al. Myxoid epithelioid sarcoma: a diagnostic challenge. A report on six cases. Histopathology 2010;57(5):753–9.
384. Fadare O. Myxoid epithelioid sarcoma: clinicopathologic analysis of 2 cases. Int J Surg Pathol 2009;17(2):147–52.
385. Chetty R, Slavin JL. Epithelioid sarcoma with extensive chondroid differentiation. Histopathology 1994;24(4):400–1.
386. Koplin SA, Nielsen GP, Hornicek FJ, et al. Epithelioid sarcoma with heterotopic bone: a morphologic review of 4 cases. Int J Surg Pathol 2010;18(3):207–12.

387. Hornick JL, Dal Cin P, Fletcher CD. Loss of INI1 expression is characteristic of both conventional and proximal-type epithelioid sarcoma. Am J Surg Pathol 2009;33(4):542–50.
388. Guillou L, Wadden C, Coindre JM, et al. "Proximal-type" epithelioid sarcoma, a distinctive aggressive neoplasm showing rhabdoid features. Clinicopathologic, immunohistochemical, and ultrastructural study of a series. Am J Surg Pathol 1997;21(2):130–46.
389. Billings SD, Folpe AL, Weiss SW. Epithelioid sarcoma-like hemangioendothelioma. Am J Surg Pathol 2003;27(1):48–57.
390. Hornick JL, Fletcher CD. Pseudomyogenic hemangioendothelioma: a distinctive, often multicentric tumor with indolent behavior. Am J Surg Pathol 2011;35(2):190–201.
391. Cai J, Peng F, Li L, et al. [Epithelioid sarcoma-like hemangioendothelioma: a clinicopathologic and immunohistochemical study of 3 cases]. Zhonghua Bing Li Xue Za Zhi 2011;40(1):27–31.
392. Lin L, Hicks D, Xu B, et al. Expression profile and molecular genetic regulation of cyclin D1 expression in epithelioid sarcoma. Mod Pathol 2005;18(5):705–9.
393. Lin L, Skacel M, Sigel JE, et al. Epithelioid sarcoma: an immunohistochemical analysis evaluating the utility of cytokeratin 5/6 in distinguishing superficial epithelioid sarcoma from spindled squamous cell carcinoma. J Cutan Pathol 2003;30(2):114–17.
394. Laskin WB, Miettinen M. Epithelioid sarcoma: new insights based on an extended immunohistochemical analysis. Arch Pathol Lab Med 2003;127(9):1161–8.
395. Miettinen M, Fanburg-Smith JC, Virolainen M, et al. Epithelioid sarcoma: an immunohistochemical analysis of 112 classical and variant cases and a discussion of the differential diagnosis. Hum Pathol 1999;30(8):934–42.
396. Kim HJ, Kim MH, Kwon J, et al. Proximal-type epithelioid sarcoma of the vulva with INI1 diagnostic utility. Ann Diagn Pathol 2011. Available at: http://www.ncbi.nlm.nih.gov/pubmed/21724432. Accessed July 21, 2011.
397. Hasegawa T, Matsuno Y, Shimoda T, et al. Proximal-type epithelioid sarcoma: a clinicopathologic study of 20 cases. Mod Pathol 2001; 14(7):655–63.
398. Tholpady A, Lonergan CL, Wick MR. Proximal-type epithelioid sarcoma of the vulva: relationship to malignant extrarenal rhabdoid tumor. Int J Gynecol Pathol 2010;29(6):600–4.
399. Miettinen M, Virtanen I, Damjanov H. Coexpression of keratin and vimentin in epithelioid sarcoma. Am J Surg Pathol 1985;9(6):460–3.
400. Armah HB, Parwani AV. Epithelioid sarcoma. Arch Pathol Lab Med 2009;133(5):814–19.
401. Fisher C. Epithelioid sarcoma of Enzinger. Adv Anat Pathol 2006; 13(3):114–21.
402. Hoshino M, Kawashima H, Ogose A, et al. Serum CA 125 expression as a tumor marker for diagnosis and monitoring the clinical course of epithelioid sarcoma. J Cancer Res Clin Oncol 2010;136(3):457–64.
403. Kato H, Hatori M, Kokubun S, et al. CA125 expression in epithelioid sarcoma. Jpn J Clin Oncol 2004;34(3):149–54.
404. Kato H, Hatori M, Watanabe M, et al. Epithelioid sarcomas with elevated serum CA125: report of two cases. Jpn J Clin Oncol 2003;33(3):141–4.
405. Roberts CW. Genetic causes of familial risk in rhabdoid tumors. Pediatr Blood Cancer 2006;47(3):235–7.
406. Rousseau-Merck MF, Versteege I, Legrand I, et al. hSNF5/INI1 inactivation is mainly associated with homozygous deletions and mitotic recombinations in rhabdoid tumors. Cancer Res 1999;59(13):3152–6.
407. Versteege I, Sévenet N, Lange J, et al. Truncating mutations of hSNF5/INI1 in aggressive paediatric cancer. Nature 1998;394(6689):203–6.
408. Bourdeaut F, Fréneaux P, Thuille B, et al. hSNF5/INI1-deficient tumours and rhabdoid tumours are convergent but not fully overlapping entities. J Pathol 2007;211(3):323–30.
409. Hoot AC, Russo P, Judkins AR, et al. Immunohistochemical analysis of hSNF5/INI1 distinguishes renal and extra-renal malignant rhabdoid tumors from other pediatric soft tissue tumors. Am J Surg Pathol 2004;28(11):1485–91.
410. Judkins AR. Immunohistochemistry of INI1 expression: a new tool for old challenges in CNS and soft tissue pathology. Adv Anat Pathol 2007;14(5):335–9.
411. Sigauke E, Rakheja D, Maddox DL, et al. Absence of expression of SMARCB1/INI1 in malignant rhabdoid tumors of the central nervous system, kidneys and soft tissue: an immunohistochemical study with implications for diagnosis. Mod Pathol 2006;19(5):717–25.
412. Haberler C, Laggner U, Slavc I, et al. Immunohistochemical analysis of INI1 protein in malignant pediatric CNS tumors: lack of INI1 in atypical teratoid/rhabdoid tumors and in a fraction of primitive neuroectodermal tumors without rhabdoid phenotype. Am J Surg Pathol 2006;30(11):1462–8.
413. Modena P, Lualdi E, Facchinetti F, et al. SMARCB1/INI1 tumor suppressor gene is frequently inactivated in epithelioid sarcomas. Cancer Res 2005;65(10):4012–19.
414. Kohashi K, Izumi T, Oda Y, et al. Infrequent SMARCB1/INI1 gene alteration in epithelioid sarcoma: a useful tool in distinguishing epithelioid sarcoma from malignant rhabdoid tumor. Hum Pathol 2009; 40(3):349–55.
415. Hollmann TJ, Hornick JL. INI1-deficient tumors: diagnostic features and molecular genetics. Am J Surg Pathol 2011;35(10):e47–63.
416. Cordoba JC, Parham DM, Meyer WH, et al. A new cytogenetic finding in an epithelioid sarcoma, t(8;22)(q22;q11). Cancer Genet Cytogenet 1994;72(2):151–4.
417. Debiec-Rychter M, Sciot R, Hagemeijer A. Common chromosome aberrations in the proximal type of epithelioid sarcoma. Cancer Genet Cytogenet 2000;123(2):133–6.
418. Feely MG, Fidler ME, Nelson M, et al. Cytogenetic findings in a case of epithelioid sarcoma and a review of the literature. Cancer Genet Cytogenet 2000;119(2):155–7.
419. Sonobe H, Ohtsuki Y, Sugimoto T, et al. Involvement of 8q, 22q, and monosomy 21 in an epithelioid sarcoma. Cancer Genet Cytogenet 1997;96(2):178–80.
420. Quezado MM, Abati AD, Albuquerque AV, et al. Morphologic diversity in malignant melanoma: the potential use of microdissection and the polymerase chain reaction for diagnosis. Mod Pathol 1998;11(10): 1010–15.
421. Lualdi E, Modena P, Debiec-Rychter M, et al. Molecular cytogenetic characterization of proximal-type epithelioid sarcoma. Genes Chromosomes Cancer 2004;41(3):283–90.
422. Baratti D, Pennacchioli E, Casali PG, et al. Epithelioid sarcoma: prognostic factors and survival in a series of patients treated at a single institution. Ann Surg Oncol 2007;14(12):3542–51.
423. Spillane AJ, Thomas JM, Fisher C. Epithelioid sarcoma: the clinicopathological complexities of this rare soft tissue sarcoma. Ann Surg Oncol 2000;7(3):218–25.
424. Bos GD, Pritchard DJ, Reiman HM, et al. Epithelioid sarcoma. An analysis of fifty-one cases. J Bone Joint Surg Am 1988;70(6):862–70.
425. Behranwala KA, A'Hern R, Omar AM, et al. Prognosis of lymph node metastasis in soft tissue sarcoma. Ann Surg Oncol 2004;11(7):714–19.
426. Gasparini P, Facchinetti F, Boeri M, et al. Prognostic determinants in epithelioid sarcoma. Eur J Cancer 2011;47(2):287–95.
427. Casanova M, Ferrari A, Collini P, et al. Epithelioid sarcoma in children and adolescents: a report from the Italian Soft Tissue Sarcoma Committee. Cancer 2006;106(3):708–17.
428. Evans HL, Baer SC. Epithelioid sarcoma: a clinicopathologic and prognostic study of 26 cases. Semin Diagn Pathol 1993;10(4):286–91.
429. Halling AC, Wollan PC, Pritchard DJ, et al. Epithelioid sarcoma: a clinicopathologic review of 55 cases. Mayo Clin Proc 1996;71(7): 636–42.
430. Izumi T, Oda Y, Hasegawa T, et al. Prognostic significance of dysadherin expression in epithelioid sarcoma and its diagnostic utility in distinguishing epithelioid sarcoma from malignant rhabdoid tumor. Mod Pathol 2006;19(6):820–31.
431. Xie X, Ghadimi MP, Young ED, et al. Combining EGFR and mTOR blockade for the treatment of epithelioid sarcoma. Clin Cancer Res 2011;17(18):5901–12.
432. Cascio MJ, O'Donnell RJ, Horvai AE. Epithelioid sarcoma expresses epidermal growth factor receptor but gene amplification and kinase domain mutations are rare. Mod Pathol 2010;23(4):574–80.
433. Whitworth PW, Pollock RE, Mansfield PF, et al. Extremity epithelioid sarcoma. Amputation vs local resection. Arch Surg 1991;126(12): 1485–9.
434. Blazer DG 3rd, Sabel MS, Sondak VK. Is there a role for sentinel lymph node biopsy in the management of sarcoma? Surg Oncol 2003; 12(3):201–6.
435. Jones RL, Constantinidou A, Olmos D, et al. Role of palliative chemotherapy in advanced epithelioid sarcoma. Am J Clin Oncol 2011. Available at: http://www.ncbi.nlm.nih.gov/pubmed/21422990. Accessed July 21, 2011.
436. Soule EH, Enriquez P. Atypical fibrous histiocytoma, malignant fibrous histiocytoma, malignant histiocytoma, and epithelioid sarcoma. A comparative study of 65 tumors. Cancer 1972;30(1):128–43.
437. Bloustein PA, Silverberg SG, Waddell WR. Epithelioid sarcoma: case report with ultrastructural review, histogenetic discussion, and chemotherapeutic data. Cancer 1976;38(6):2390–400.

438. Fisher ER, Horvat B. The fibrocytic deprivation of the so-called epithelioid sarcoma. Cancer 1972;30(4):1074–81.
439. Pisa R, Novelli P, Bonetti F. Epithelioid sarcoma: a tumor of myofibroblasts, or not? Histopathology 1984;8(2):353.
440. Fisher C. Epithelioid sarcoma: the spectrum of ultrastructural differentiation in seven immunohistochemically defined cases. Hum Pathol 1988;19(3):265–75.
441. Miettinen M, Lehto VP, Vartio T, et al. Epithelioid sarcoma. Ultrastructural and immunohistologic features suggesting a synovial origin. Arch Pathol Lab Med 1982;106(12):620–3.
442. Sévenet N, Sheridan E, Amram D, et al. Constitutional mutations of the hSNF5/INI1 gene predispose to a variety of cancers. Am J Hum Genet 1999;65(5):1342–8.
443. Beckwith JB, Palmer NF. Histopathology and prognosis of Wilms tumors: results from the First National Wilms' Tumor Study. Cancer 1978;41(5):1937–48.
444. Weeks DA, Beckwith JB, Mierau GW, et al. Rhabdoid tumor of kidney. A report of 111 cases from the National Wilms' Tumor Study Pathology Center. Am J Surg Pathol 1989;13(6):439–58.
445. Burger PC, Yu IT, Tihan T, et al. Atypical teratoid/rhabdoid tumor of the central nervous system: a highly malignant tumor of infancy and childhood frequently mistaken for medulloblastoma: a Pediatric Oncology Group study. Am J Surg Pathol 1998;22(9):1083–92.
446. Fanburg-Smith JC, Hengge M, Hengge UR, et al. Extrarenal rhabdoid tumors of soft tissue: a clinicopathologic and immunohistochemical study of 18 cases. Ann Diagn Pathol 1998;2(6):351–62.
447. Wick MR, Ritter JH, Dehner LP. Malignant rhabdoid tumors: a clinicopathologic review and conceptual discussion. Semin Diagn Pathol 1995;12(3):233–48.
448. Humphrey PA. Renal cell carcinoma with rhabdoid features. J Urol 2011;186(2):675–6.
449. Kim HJ, Kim MH, Kwon J, et al. Proximal-type epithelioid sarcoma of the vulva with INI1 diagnostic utility. Annals of Diagnostic Pathology 2011. Available at: http://www.ncbi.nlm.nih.gov/pubmed/21724432. Accessed October 1, 2011.
450. Clarke BA, Rahimi K, Chetty R. Leiomyosarcoma of the broad ligament with osteoclast-like giant cells and rhabdoid cells. Int J Gynecol Pathol 2010;29(5):432–7.
451. Jun SY, Choi J, Kang GH, et al. Synovial sarcoma of the kidney with rhabdoid features: report of three cases. Am J Surg Pathol 2004; 28(5):634–7.
452. Suárez-Vilela D, Izquierdo-Garcia FM, Alonso-Orcajo N. Epithelioid and rhabdoid rhabdomyosarcoma in an adult patient: a diagnostic pitfall. Virchows Arch 2004;445(3):323–5.
453. Oshiro Y, Shiratsuchi H, Tamiya S, et al. Extraskeletal myxoid chondrosarcoma with rhabdoid features, with special reference to its aggressive behavior. Int J Surg Pathol 2000;8(2):145–52.
454. Ordóñez NG. Mesothelioma with rhabdoid features: an ultrastructural and immunohistochemical study of 10 cases. Mod Pathol 2006; 19(3):373–83.
455. Wu YT, Ho JT, Lin YJ, et al. Rhabdoid papillary meningioma: a clinicopathologic case series study. Neuropathology: Official Journal of the Japanese Society of Neuropathology 2011. Available at: http://www.ncbi.nlm.nih.gov/pubmed/21382093. Accessed October 1, 2011.
456. Tallon B, Bhawan J. Primary rhabdoid melanoma with clonal recurrence. Am J Dermatopathol 2009;31(2):200–4.
457. Haas JE, Palmer NF, Weinberg AG, et al. Ultrastructure of malignant rhabdoid tumor of the kidney. A distinctive renal tumor of children. Hum Pathol 1981;12(7):646–57.
458. Perlman EJ. Pediatric renal tumors: practical updates for the pathologist. Pediatr Dev Pathol 2005;8(3):320–38.
459. Hoot AC, Russo P, Judkins AR, et al. Immunohistochemical analysis of hSNF5/INI1 distinguishes renal and extra-renal malignant rhabdoid tumors from other pediatric soft tissue tumors. Am J Surg Pathol 2004;28(11):1485–91.
460. Jackson EM, Shaikh TH, Gururangan S, et al. High-density single nucleotide polymorphism array analysis in patients with germline deletions of 22q11.2 and malignant rhabdoid tumor. Hum Genet 2007;122(2): 117–27.
461. Kohashi K, Oda Y, Yamamoto H, et al. Highly aggressive behavior of malignant rhabdoid tumor: a special reference to SMARCB1/INI1 gene alterations using molecular genetic analysis including quantitative real-time PCR. J Cancer Res Clin Oncol 2007;133(11):817–24.
462. Sigauke E, Rakheja D, Maddox DL, et al. Absence of expression of SMARCB1/INI1 in malignant rhabdoid tumors of the central nervous system, kidneys and soft tissue: an immunohistochemical study with implications for diagnosis. Mod Pathol 2006;19(5):717–25.
463. Itakura E, Tamiya S, Morita K, et al. Subcellular distribution of cytokeratin and vimentin in malignant rhabdoid tumor: three-dimensional imaging with confocal laser scanning microscopy and double immunofluorescence. Mod Pathol 2001;14(9):854–61.
464. Biegel JA. Genetics of pediatric central nervous system tumors. J Pediatr Hematol Oncol 1997;19(6):492–501.
465. Biegel JA, Allen CS, Kawasaki K, et al. Narrowing the critical region for a rhabdoid tumor locus in 22q11. Genes Chromosomes Cancer 1996;16(2):94–105.
466. Biegel JA, Rorke LB, Emanuel BS. Monosomy 22 in rhabdoid or atypical teratoid tumors of the brain. N Engl J Med 1989;321(13):906.
467. Schofield DE, Beckwith JB, Sklar J. Loss of heterozygosity at chromosome regions 22q11-12 and 11p15.5 in renal rhabdoid tumors. Genes Chromosomes Cancer 1996;15(1):10–17.
468. Biegel JA, Kalpana G, Knudsen ES, et al. The role of INI1 and the SWI/SNF complex in the development of rhabdoid tumors: meeting summary from the workshop on childhood atypical teratoid/rhabdoid tumors. Cancer Res 2002;62(1):323–8.
469. Biegel JA, Tan L, Zhang F, et al. Alterations of the hSNF5/INI1 gene in central nervous system atypical teratoid/rhabdoid tumors and renal and extrarenal rhabdoid tumors. Clin Cancer Res 2002;8(11):3461–7.
470. Janson K, Nedzi LA, David O, et al. Predisposition to atypical teratoid/rhabdoid tumor due to an inherited INI1 mutation. Pediatr Blood Cancer 2006;47(3):279–84.
471. Kordes U, Gesk S, Frühwald MC, et al. Clinical and molecular features in patients with atypical teratoid rhabdoid tumor or malignant rhabdoid tumor. Genes Chromosomes Cancer 2010;49(2):176–81.
472. Fuller CE, Pfeifer J, Humphrey P, et al. Chromosome 22q dosage in composite extrarenal rhabdoid tumors: clonal evolution or a phenotypic mimic? Hum Pathol 2001;32(10):1102–8.
473. Perry A, Fuller CE, Judkins AR, et al. INI1 expression is retained in composite rhabdoid tumors, including rhabdoid meningiomas. Mod Pathol 2005;18(7):951–8.
474. Katsumi Y, Iehara T, Miyachi M, et al. Sensitivity of malignant rhabdoid tumor cell lines to PD 0332991 is inversely correlated with p16 expression. Biochem Biophys Res Commun 2011;413(1):62–8.
475. Kuwahara Y, Charboneau A, Knudsen ES, et al. Reexpression of hSNF5 in malignant rhabdoid tumor cell lines causes cell cycle arrest through a p21(CIP1/WAF1)-dependent mechanism. Cancer Res 2010;70(5): 1854–65.
476. Venneti S, Le P, Martinez D, et al. p16INK4A and p14ARF tumor suppressor pathways are deregulated in malignant rhabdoid tumors. J Neuropathol Exp Neurol 2011;70(7):596–609.
477. Sultan I, Qaddoumi I, Rodríguez-Galindo C, et al. Age, stage, and radiotherapy, but not primary tumor site, affects the outcome of patients with malignant rhabdoid tumors. Pediatr Blood Cancer 2010;54(1):35–40.
478. Parham DM, Weeks DA, Beckwith JB. The clinicopathologic spectrum of putative extrarenal rhabdoid tumors. An analysis of 42 cases studied with immunohistochemistry or electron microscopy. Am J Surg Pathol 1994;18(10):1010–29.
479. Venneti S, Le P, Martinez D, et al. Malignant rhabdoid tumors express stem cell factors, which relate to the expression of EZH2 and Id proteins. Am J Surg Pathol 2011;35(10):1463–72.

Index

Page numbers followed by b, f, and t indicate boxes, figures, and tables, respectively.

D

E

F

G

N

O

W

X